Fibroblast Growth Factors

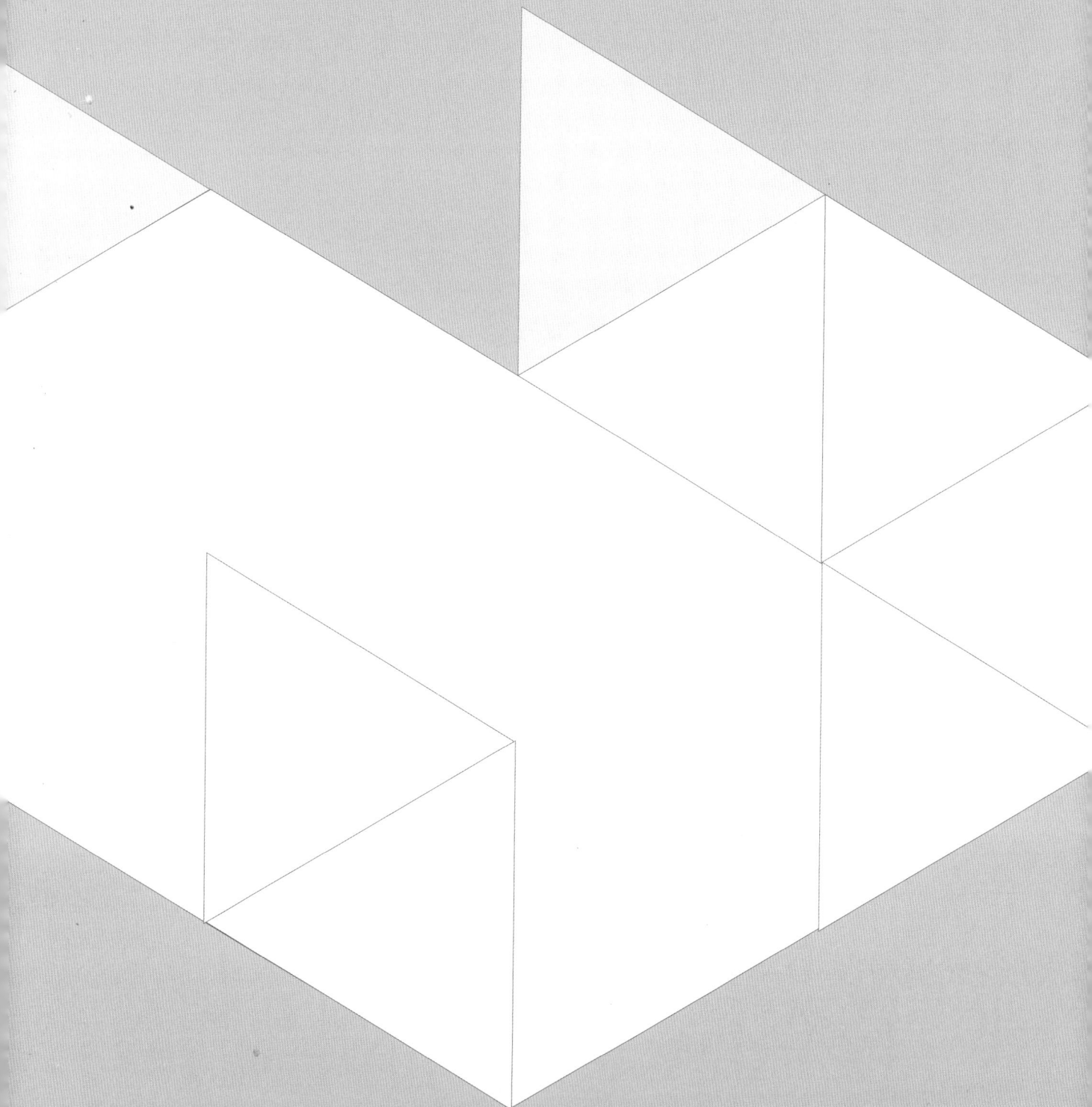

Fibroblast Growth Factors

Second edition

Xiaokun Li

高等教育出版社·北京

Preface

Professor Xiaokun Li invited me to write a preface for his new book titled Fibroblast Growth Factors (the second edition 2013-2018). It reminded me of what happened more than 27 years ago. At that time, Xiaokun Li and I were all young scientists. We were working together on rbFGF (recombinant basic Fibroblast Growth Factor), a new wound repair biopharmaceutic. That was the beginning of the age of biomedicine development for trauma in China. We have encountered many difficulties and frustrations, but we succeeded in this field. The rbFGF became one of the earliest approved new drugs for wound repair in China.

Fibroblast growth factors (FGFs) are one kind of growth factors. They act in a paracrine or endocrine fashion to carry out their functions in development, tissue homeostasis and metabolism. The bFGF is the second member in the FGF family of 23 members. In China, EGF (Epidermal Growth Factor) and bFGF have been approved for use in acute skin wounds and chronic ulcers. Up to now, the data show that topical application of a single growth factor is effective in accelerating acute or chronic wound healing. The average wound healing time in acute skin wounds can be shortened by 2 to 4 days when locally treated with growth factors. Also, those wounds such as "hard-to-heal" diabetic foot ulcers or pressure sores show significant improvement in the healing rate and the time compared with cohort controls. Importantly, besides its treatment efficacy, clinical evaluation and follow up on the healing of chronic cutaneous wounds confirmed its safety in that no adverse side-effects related to bFGF were observed. The results further established both the effectiveness and safety of using rbFGF to accelerate healing in chronic wounds.

After the initial success of pioneering the rbFGF clinical application in the world, Professor Li has persevered in the field for the past two decades and continued to make great achievements in both the bioengineering and basic research of FGFs. In recent years, the FGF field has witnessed a major progress by uncovering the metabolic regulatory activities of both endocrine and paracrine FGFs and their underlying mechanisms. Along this line, It is worth mentioning that, Prof. Li proposed the new "FGF axes"theory, which has contributed to theoretical advance of FGF research and will likely have a positive impact on future drug discoveries for the treatment of human diseases. This book collected research results of his group for the past 6 years on tissue repair and regeneration, metabolism, structure, pharmacology, pharmaceutics, engineering of new chimeric FGFs and reviews. I think that this book is very valuable to all researchers in the FGF field.

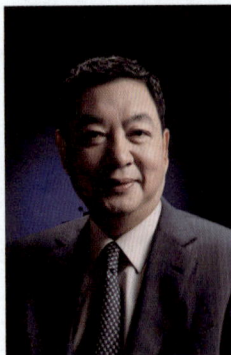

Xiaobing Fu, MD, PhD

Academician, Chinese Academy of Engineering
(Division of Medicine and Health)

Dean of College of Life Sciences
PLA General Hospital and PLA Medical College

Preface

This book is dedicated to the achievements of Prof. Xiaokun Li's group in exploring the function of a family of growth factors called fibroblasts growth factors. These growth factors are involved in every step of our lives, from the control of organogenesis to homeostasis, from metabolic regulation to repair after injury. Trough their regenerative power, they may also hold the key to aging.

When I met Xiaokun, more than 8 years ago, he was already determined to use these growth factors to treat a variety of human diseases. Thanks to his tireless efforts, some of these FGFs are already approved by the Chinese food and drug administration for their beneficial effects in accelerating repair after injury. I met Xiaokun for the first time in 2012, at the occasion of an international FGF meeting that he organized in Wenzhou. I was immediately impressed by his enthusiasm for FGF research and by his vision to bring together a worldwide FGF community. Xiaokun's support, both scientifically and financially, to promote high level international meeting has proven to be unwavering. Some FGF members have emerged to be of particular interest for Xiaokun's team. One of them, called FGF10 (aka Keratinocyte growth factor 2) has proven to be a prime candidate to be used in the future for the repair of many organs, including the lung. If the task of exploring the function of multiple FGFs can be overwhelming for the common scientist, this is not the case for the members of Xiaokun's team. A new generation of internationally trained high-level Chinese scientists, emerging from the core team orchestrated by Prof. Xiaokun will have the fascinating but rewarding task to expand on the important legacy represented by this book.

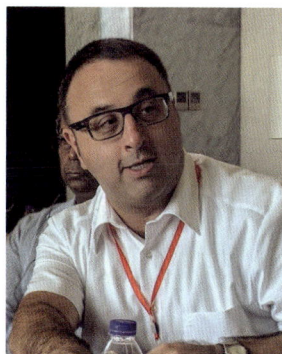

Saverio Bellusci, PhD

Chair for Lung Matrix Remodeling

Excellence Cluster Cardio Pulmonary System
University Justus Liebig Giessen
Giessen, Germany

Preface for first edition

In 1974, Gospodarowicz, Jones and Sato reported the presence of a growth factor for ovarian cells in extracts of pituitary that was subsequently named Fibroblast Growth Factor (FGF) because of its potent mitogenic activity on fibroblasts. The finding led to a potent and essentially ubiquitous tyrosine kinase cell signaling family that is now comprised of 18 receptor-mediated FGF polypeptides and 4 homologues and a myriad of splice variants from four receptor genes controlled by co-factors heparan sulfate and klothos. As members of the signaling family grew, it became apparent that there is unlikely a tissue or biological process where one or more members are not present and at play attracting a growing field of diverse biologists studying details of structure-function to clinical applications. FGF family signaling plays a key role in embryonic development, adult tissue homeostasis and metabolism and its dysfunction of potential importance in related diseases.

Chinese scholars have contributed significantly to our knowledge about the FGF family. Dr. Xiaokun Li was among the first to study FGF in China and has grown to be a driving force in development, application and education in the FGF signaling field within China that extends worldwide. Advancing the field of FGF signaling and its application for benefit of people is his personal passion. I have been fortunate to personally witness this beginning in Wenzhou at the 3rd International Conference on Fibroblast Growth Factors which he hosted. The conference brought together interests from across China and the world.

This book is a collection of research results from Dr. Li's group that spans application of engineered non-mitogenic mutants, structure modification, pathology, physiology, pharmacology, FGF/FGFR inhibitors, bioengineering and drug development to injury repair and regeneration as well as other biological processes. This work should be a helpful primer to scientists and particularly students entering the FGF field with their eye toward applications.

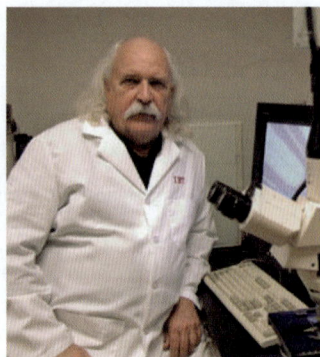

Wallace L. McKeehan

Regents and Distinguished Professor

Institute of Biosciences and Technology, Texas A&M Health Science Center

Preface for first edition

Historically speaking, fibroblast growth factor (FGF) signaling as a research field was conceived in the late 1930s/early 1940s by the observation that bovine pituitary extracts contain mitogenic factors for fibroblast cell lines. Some 30 years later, these mitogens were purified and characterized as FGF1 and FGF2, the founding members of the FGF family. An additional seven FGFs were then discovered either as oncogenes or mitogens using classical functional and biochemical methods and then genomic research added nine more FGFs. The FGF family stands today as one of the largest growth factor families in humans, consisting of 18 members in mammals. Gene knockout in animal models and clinical studies in human patients have attributed pleiotropic functions to FGF family in mammalian development, tissue homeostasis, and metabolism. FGF ligands signal in paracrine and endocrine fashion through four cell-surface FGF receptor (FGFR1-FGFR4) tyrosine kinases and their multiple alternatively spliced isoforms. Ligand binding induces FGFR dimerization enabling tyrosine transphosphorylation of intracellular receptor kinase domains and hence kinase activation. For two decades, several mitogenic, cytoprotective, and angiogenic therapeutic applications of paracrine FGFs have been explored worldwide, and the recent discoveries of the key roles of the endocrine FGFs in energy and mineral homeostasis have expanded the pharmacological potentials of this family. Alongside laboratories in the United States and Western Europe, several Chinese research laboratories have also made valuable contributions to the clinical development of the FGF family.

Notably, Xiaokun Li's group at the Wenzhou Medical College specializes in state-of-art technologies to discover novel FGF-based therapeutics for tissue repair, regeneration, and metabolic disorders. His research efforts has resulted in three A-grade FGF-based drugs and one FGF-containing collagen sponge that have been approved by China SFDA for wound healing and skin repair. This book gives an overview of the basic and applied research conducted in the Xiaokun Li's laboratory and is highly recommended to graduate students and researchers in the FGF field.

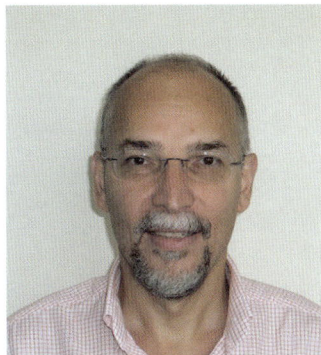

Moosa Mohammadi

Professor

New York University School of Medicine

Contents

The FGF Metabolic Axis

Xiaokun Li

1. Introduction

The fibroblast growth factors (FGFs) are pleiotropic signal molecules for all types of cell and tissue systems in metazoans [1-3]. They share a conserved core structure of β trefoil fold consisting of 12-stranded β-sheets arranged in 3 similar lobes around a central axis, of which 6 strands form an anti-parallel β-barrel [4, 5]. Excluding the 4 FGF-homologous intracrine factors that are functional reminiscent of the ancestor FGF, the FGFs can be classified into mitogenic FGFs and metabolic FGFs on the basis of their distinct functions and endpoint biological effects [6, 7], which overtly regulate cellular proliferation and substrate/energy metabolism, respectively. Both classes of FGFs signal through the same types of transmembrane receptor tyrosine kinases, the FGFR1 to FGFR4 with multiple slicing variants [8]; however, in physiology, the two types of regulatory activities driven by these two classes of FGFs appear to be spatially and temporally segregated. The mitogenic FGFs appear to be incapable of traveling far at a physiological level to other tissues including the metabolic tissues to promote cellular metabolism because of the local trapping after secretion mediated by high affinity binding to the extracellular matrix heparan sulfate. On the other hand, the metabolic FGFs circulate but are inactive for non-metabolic tissues or cells that often undergo active tissue remodeling via renewed cycles of cell proliferation and population growth because of the lack of the critical transmembrane accessory co-receptors. This divergence necessitates a distinction of metabolic axis that the metabolic FGFs drive as we coin hereafter from the mitogenic axis that the mitogenic FGFs drive. The metabolic axis still shares the major aspects of structural coevolution [9, 10] while gaining unique structural and functional divergence with the mitogenic axis within each subfamily, as our recent structural studies have revealed [2, 5, 11]. From the evolutionary standpoint, although these two axes largely parallel and drive differential effects via divergent intracellular mechanisms, they are destined for a common goal of promoting the survival and homeostasis of each cell/tissue system and the organism as a whole, as we have summarized in a previous review [7] (Fig. 1).

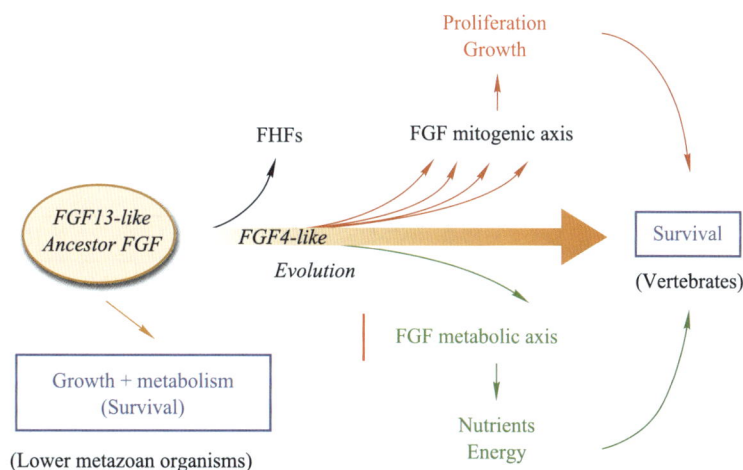

Fig. 1. The evolutionary genesis and specification of the FGF metabolic axis. The FGF family originates from a common FGF13-like ancestor molecule in the early metazoans, and then bifurcates via an FGF4-like molecule into two major functional subfamilies with diverging structural and functional specifications. The so-called autocrine/paracrine FGF subfamily members bind extracellular matrix heparan sulfate and initiate signal axes to promote cell proliferation and population growth, while the endocrine FGF subfamily members including FGF19, 21 and 23 drive signal axes that elucidate broad-spectrum functions in regulating the metabolic homeostasis of bile acid, lipids, glucose, energy, and minerals without apparent direct proliferation-promoting activity. However, both the FGF mitogenic axis and the FGF metabolic axis are designed to promote cell and organismal survival in vertebrates.

2. The mitogenic FGF axis

The classic FGF family consists of seventeen structurally related polypeptides in humans that are secreted and act extracellularly as signaling molecules [1, 3, 7, 12]. For most part of the time since the discovery in late 1970s [13, 14], FGFs are known as a short-range mitogen for a wide variety of cell types in the developing ectoderm, mesoderm, and endoderm. They elicit chemo-attractant activity to promote cell migration and tissue remodeling, as well as anti-apoptotic effect to promote cell survival. FGF1 and 2 are the prototypes initially isolated on the basis of potent mitogenic activity towards fibroblasts or fibroblast-like cells [13, 14]. It was realized early that these mitogenic FGFs bind tightly to the local extracellular matrix heparan sulfate (HS) chains and do not circulate, and accordingly, act in a paracrine or autocrine mode. This heparin/heparan sulfate binding property renders their potent activity temporarily contained but timely released locally upon injury or demand of tissue remodeling [15]. These mitogenic FGFs include 15 members (Table 1), which strongly promote the doubling synthesis of genomic DNA and subsequent cell division and population growth [12, 16, 17], and therefore, play critical roles in the development of multiple tissues/organs [18-20]. They initiate the mitogenic axis through binding to the Ig-like ectodomains of their cognate transmembrane fibroblast growth factor receptors (FGFR) in complex with HS motifs on diverse target cells and tissues in the first step [1, 21, 22]. Subsequent activation of the intracellular kinase domains of FGFRs results in downstream signal relay primarily through the PI3K-AKT, RAS-MAPK and PLCγ-PKC pathways [23-25], as we summarized previously [3]. These HS and FGFR dependent activities driven by the mitogenic FGF axes contributes to not only the regulation of virtually all aspects of development and organogenesis, but also many natural processes of active post-developmental tissue repair, remodeling and homeostasis [26].

The keratinocyte growth factor or FGF7 has the highest specificity for receptor isotypes among the mitogenic FGFs [12, 22, 27]. It only activates the IIIb type isoform of FGFR2. As FGF7 is originated in mesenchyme cells while FGFR2IIIb resides on the epithelial or keratinocyte cells, FGF7 forms a unidirectional paracrine communication axis with FGFR2 from mesenchyme to epithelium compartment within a tissue or organ. On the other hand, epithelial cells secrete FGF1 or FGF9, for an example, which then acts on the mesenchyme cells that harbors FGFR1IIIc within the two-compartmental tissues. These FGF1 and FGF7 driven mutual cell communication axes are, therefore, poised to drive tissue remodeling and maintain tissue homeostasis [28]. Prolonged or abnormal activation of the FGFR-HS binary complexes by the mitogenic FGF axes contributes to an array of cell/tissue-specific developmental diseases and multiple types of cancers [3, 29] (see a brief summary in Table 1). The proliferation and survival promoting activities of the diverse mitogenic FGF axes have been a major focus of utility for a range of regenerative and repair medical settings [30-34]. In the past, we have demonstrated experimentally the benefits of mitogenic FGFs applied to tissue damage complications of diabetic mellitus, including the diabetic cardiomyopathy, nephropathy and neuropathy [35-37], as well as wound healing and spinal cord injury repair [38-40]. On the other hand, the mitogenic FGF mediated cell miscommunication has also been on the menu for developing inhibitors for use in cancer therapy [29, 41, 42].

Table 1. The mitogenic FGF axis

Sub-family	Member of ligands	Physiological function (knockout phenotypes)	Known pathologies	Receptor specificity						
				1b	1c	2b	2c	3b	3c	4
FGF1	FGF1	Adipose tissue homeostasis	Amplification—ovarian cancer	√	√	√	√	√	√	√
	FGF2	Wound healing, angiogenesis	Overexpression—several types of cancers	√	√		√		√	√
FGF4	FGF4	Development of limb bud and heart	Amplification—breast cancer		√		√		√	√
	FGF5	Hair follicle growth & development	Overexpression—glioblastoma		√		√		√	
	FGF6	Muscle development & regeneration	Overexpression—prostate cancer		√		√		√	√

Continued Table

Sub-family	Member of ligands	Physiological function (knockout phenotypes)	Known pathologies	Receptor specificity						
				1b	1c	2b	2c	3b	3c	4
FGF7	FGF3	Inner ear and skeleton development	1. Missense mutation—Michel aplasia, LAMM syndrome 2. Haploinsufficiency—otodental syndrome 3. Amplification—breast cancer	√		√				
	FGF7	Branching morphogenesis	1. Polymorphism—COPD 2. Overexpression—lung adenocarcinoma			√				
	FGF10	1. Lung branching morphogenesis 2. Inner ear development 3. Hair follicle development	1. Polymorphism—myopia 2. Nonsense mutation—Lacrimo-auriculo-dento-digital (LADD) syndrome, Aplasia of the lacrimal and salivary glands (ALSG) 3. Overexpression—breast & prostate cancers	√		√				
	FGF22	Synaptogenesis	Not defined	√		√				
FGF8	FGF8	Development of brain, eye, ear, limb bud, kidney, and heart	1. Missense mutation—cleft lip and palate, holoprosencephaly, craniofacial defects, hypothalamo-pituitary dysfunction 2. Nonsense mutation—familial hypogonadotropic hypogonadism		√		√		√	√
	FGF17	Cerebellum and frontal cortex development	1. Missense mutation—familial hypogonadotropic hypogonadism 2. Overexpression—liver & prostate cancers		√		√		√	√
	FGF18	Lung alveolar and bone, CNS, skeletal, and palate development	1. Polymorphism—cleft lip and palate 2. Overexpression—liver cancer						√	√
FGF9	FGF9	Development of inner ear, gonad, kidney and other organs	1. Promoter mutation—sertoli cell-only syndrome 2. Missense mutation—multisynostosis syndrome 3. Mutations—colorectal & endometrial cancers 4. Overexpression—lung cancer		√		√	√	√	√
	FGF16	Heart development	1. Nonsense mutation—4-5 metacarpal fusion 2. Overexpression—ovarian cancer				√	√	√	√
	FGF20	Kidney, hair, teeth, cochlea, central nervous development,	1. Frame-shift mutation—bilateral renal agenesis 2. Polymorphism—risk of Parkinson's disease		√	√	√	√	√	√

It should be pointed out that although at a physiological level, the mitogenic FGFs are not evolutionarily designed to circulate and target distal tissues or organs for an endocrine effect, at pharmacological or supra-physiological levels they do exert certain regulatory activities beyond promoting cell proliferation and growth. This is likely due to a sufficient concentration accumulation to achieve an effect in distal metabolic tissues where a cognate FGFR isotype is expression. It was shown in the early 1990s that a bonus intravenous injection of FGF1 or FGF2 can target vascular endothelium to decrease arterial blood pressure [43]. FGF16 is expressed in classical brown fat depots during the latter stages of embryonic development, and recombinant FGF16 is a mitogen for adipocytes [44]. Mice overexpressing FGF16 delivered by adeno-associated virus display dramatic weight loss and UCP1 upregulation in inguinal white adipose tissue (WAT) that is a common site for emergent active brown adipose tissue (BAT). These effects are likely a combined result of reduced food and water intake, and abnormal feces replete with lipid and bile acid due to brain, liver and intestinal actions of overexpressed FGF16 [45]. Mice deficient in FGF1 exhibit no significant phenotypes under standard dietary conditions; however, under chronic high-fat diet challenge, they develop an aggressive diabetic phenotype coupled with aberrant adipose phenotypes, including multiple histopathologies in the adipose vasculature network, an accentuated inflammatory response, aberrant adipocyte size distribution and expansion, as well as ectopic expression of pancreatic lipases [46]. In particular, we show by structure-based mutagenesis, FGF1 can be designed to have full metabolic activity of wild-type FGF1 but with reduced proliferative potential both *in vitro* and *in vivo* [47]. These studies underlie an important role of FGF1 in maintaining the local adipose tissue homeostasis, which upon significant tissue perturbations impinges on the metabolic functions that subsequently affect the systemic metabolic state. Taken together, the metabolic effects of some of the mitogenic FGF axes are likely due to either a local function in maintaining the cellular homeostasis that is closely associated with local metabolic state at a physiological concentration, or an induced metabolic response to a supra-physiological concentration from circulation, in the metabolic tissues or organs where an FGFR(s) resides. However, at pharmacological levels, some mitogenic FGFs may also be designed to elicit systemic metabolic effects.

3. The metabolic FGF axis

In contrast to the mitogenic FGFs, the metabolic FGF subfamily contains only three members, namely the FGF19 (mouse FGF15), 21 and 23 [2, 7, 48-51]; however, the metabolic axes of these three FGFs regulate a wide range of metabolic pathways, resulting in tissue and organismal metabolic homeostasis of bile acids, lipid, glucose, energy, and minerals. Although the metabolic FGF axes do not overtly promote DNA doubling synthesis leading to cell proliferation [12, 52, 53], both metabolic and mitogenic FGF axes appear to enhance cell survival and promote an optimal state of homeostasis in target tissues and organisms [7].

Based on the current knowledge, the metabolic FGFs appear to originate from a common FGF13-like ancestor molecule as the mitogenic FGFs, and then bifurcate in early evolution through an FGF4-like molecule from all other mitogenic members through acquiring unique structural and mechanistic properties [5, 10, 11, 54], which lead to specific activities in modulating metabolic states in specific cell and tissue types [2]. Instead of acting locally, they take a hormonal or endocrine route of action by traveling through circulation from the originating tissue far to other peripheral tissues/organs. This endocrine action is attributable to the loss of the structurally conserved HS-binding domain characteristic of the mitogenic FGFs [5]. Both the expression and target tissues of the metabolic FGFs are rather limited to the metabolically active and endocrine organs, such as the liver, intestine, adipose tissue, pancreas, muscle, bone, kidney, heart, parathyroid as well as specific neurons in specific regions of the CNS [55, 56]. In the expression tissues, genes of the metabolic FGFs are subject to direct transcriptional control by several major metabolites-responsive nuclear receptors including FXR, PPARA, PPARG, ChREBP, SREBP1c, RORA, LXRB, and VDR [48-50, 57-65], as well as stress-sensing transcription factors such as ATF4 [66], depending on the location of specific nutrition/energy-sensing cells in specific tissues. In target tissues, the biological effects of the metabolic FGF axes are still mediated by FGFRs, however, in a new binary complex with a new transmembrane non-kinase accessory co-receptor, the α Klotho (KL) or β Klotho (KLB) [5, 11, 55, 67] (Table 2), to which the mitogenic FGFs do not bind. Structurally, the metabolic FGFs coevolve with coreceptor KL/KLB but acquire new structural elements that direct specific contact interacts with KL/KLB and FGFRs, leading to a tethered basic triad complex and subsequent activation of intracellular kinase domains of FGFRs [5, 11]. The C-terminus of metabolic FGFs mimics the interaction mode of a sugar chain that docks into the pseudo glycolytic pocket of KL/KLB while interacting with the FGFR ectodomains through domains that are conserved across the FGF family [5, 68]. On the other hand, the interacting KL/KLB protrudes an "arm" from the membrane-proximal glycosidase domain griping onto the FGFR ectodomain.

Although the FGFRs, in particular the FGFR1, are broadly expressed, the highly restricted expression of KL/KLB as well as the metabolic FGFs, and new structural elements and mutual interaction modes, set the tone for tissue-specific functions of the metabolic FGF axes (Table 2). In addition, the different intracellular molecular constituents in different types of cells, which are tailored to perform specific biological functions, may be also an important limiting factor. For an example, the adult adipocytes are not poised in a normal context to increase population by direct proliferation due to the loss of some key proliferation-controlling pathways, and thus, partly accounting for the inability of the activated FGFR1 by FGF21 to promote adipocyte proliferation. Overall, the metabolic FGFs appear to be in large part inducible stress factors in response to organismal metabolic perturbations [7, 69], and signal distal peripheral tissue(s) through the FGFR-KL/KLB complex to control the due metabolic pathways. In this sense, the metabolic FGFs acts like a key to ignite the FGF-FGFR-KLB/KLB triad complexes, which function similarly as an engine with an axis to drive effects in a tissue-specific manner, leading to beneficial effects that offset the initial adverse metabolic changes and prevent metaflammation and tissue damage not only in the FGF-producing tissue but also systemically [2, 7] (Table 2). Consequently, both the analogs of endocrine FGFs and the agonists of FGF-KL/KLB have been actively pursued clinically for the prevention and treatment of a wide range of metabolic diseases and comorbidities [2, 70-75].

Table 2. The metabolic FGF axis

Sub-family	Member of ligands	Physiological function (knock-out phenotypes)	Known pathologies	Receptor specificity								
				1b	1c	2b	2c	3b	3c	4	KL	KLB
FGF19	FGF19	1. Bile acid metabolism 2. Gall bladder filling 3. Lipid and energy metabolism	1. Bile acid diarrheal, IBD 2. Cholestasis 3. Overexpression—liver cancer		√		√		√	√		√
	FGF21	1. Lipid metabolism—lipolysis, fatty acid oxidation, lipogenesis 2. Energy metabolism—uncoupling thermogenesis 3. Macronutrient preference 4. Starvation response and associated physiology 5. Insulin sensitivity and glucose homeostasis	1. Obesity 2. Diabetes 3. NAFLD 4. Hyperlipidemia 5. Metabolic syndrome 6. Pancreatitis		√				√			√
	FGF23	Phosphate, calcium, sodium, and vitamin D homeostasis	1. Activation mutation—autosomal dominant hypophosphatemic rickets, tumor-induced osteomalacia 2. Inactivation mutation—familial tumoral calcinosis 3. Increase—X-linked dominant hypophosphatemia, CKD 4. Decrease—GALNT3-related familial tumoral calcinosis		√				√	√	√	

4. FGF19 metabolic axis

The FGF19 is a prime controller of diurnal bile acid flux, and the FGF19-driven metabolic axis is a temporal inter-organ cross-talk from the ileum to the liver in response to the rises of postprandial serum and transintestinal flux of bile acids [2, 49] (Fig. 2). This axis serves to negatively control enterohepatic as well as systemic levels of bile acids, which facilitate the uptake and absorption of dietary lipids after a meal but as biodetergent are toxic if the flux is prolonged at elevated levels. The ileal initiation of FGF19 signal is under the transcriptional control of the farnesoid X receptor (FXR), which is stimulated by the enterocyte reabsorbed bile acids as a natural ligand that is originally released from gallbladder and mixed with food traveling down from the duodenum to jejunum and ileum. This enterocyte-derived FGF19 activates the remote FGFR4-KLB complex [67] residing across the membrane of hepatocytes in the liver, resulting in a major feedback termination of the transcription of the rate-limiting enzymes Cyp7A1 and Cyp8b1 in the bile acid biosynthesis pathways [49, 76]. The axis therefore triggers the shut-off of hepatic biosynthesis of new bile acids from cholesterol, as well as the refilling of gallbladder, about 2 hours post the peak of serum bile acids.

In experimental animals, overexpression or administration of FGF19 were shown to elicit other metabolic effects as well [77, 78]. Excessive FGF19 promotes lipolysis, metabolic rate and energy expenditure, and reduces body weight and serum glucose and lipids. The FGFR1-KLB complex on adipose tissues including both the WAT and BAT was suggested, in a large part, to mediate these metabolic effects [79] (Fig. 2). However, the direct metabolic roles of bile acid fluctuation and the bile acid-activated FXR and TGR5 cannot be excluded.

Although there is no evidence on any genetic mutation of FGF19 gene involving in human metabolic diseases, the reduced synthesis and blood levels of FGF19 are suggestive as causative factor of chronic bile acid diarrhea [80, 81] and certain metabolic disorders, such as metabolic syndrome, non-alcoholic fatty liver disease (NAFLD), and insulin resistance. Experimentally, neutralization of FGF19 by specific anti-FGF19 antibodies caused severe diarrhea in monkeys accompanied by increases in bile acid synthesis, serum and fecal total bile acids, specific bile acid transporters, and liver toxicity [82]. In obese patients who undergo Roux-en-Y gastric bypass bariatric surgery, FGF19 increases to normal values, which at least partially underlie the benefits of this approach [83]. On the other hand, high levels of FGF19 expression are found in the livers of patients with extrahepatic cholestasis [84, 85], underlying FGF19 as a therapeutic strategy for this disease.

Recently, FGF19 axis was shown hypertrophic and protective effects on skeletal muscle, presumably through a KLB-FGFR4 dependent mechanism, by increasing myofiber size in the soleus, muscle mass and grip strength [86]. Pharmacological FGF19 ameliorates skeletal muscle atrophy and prevents muscle wasting in mice with glucocorticoid treatment or obesity, as well as sarcopenia. These results highlight a potential treatment strategy for muscle wasting induced by glucocorticoid treatment, obesity, aging as well as cachexia. However, it remains to be determined whether the same

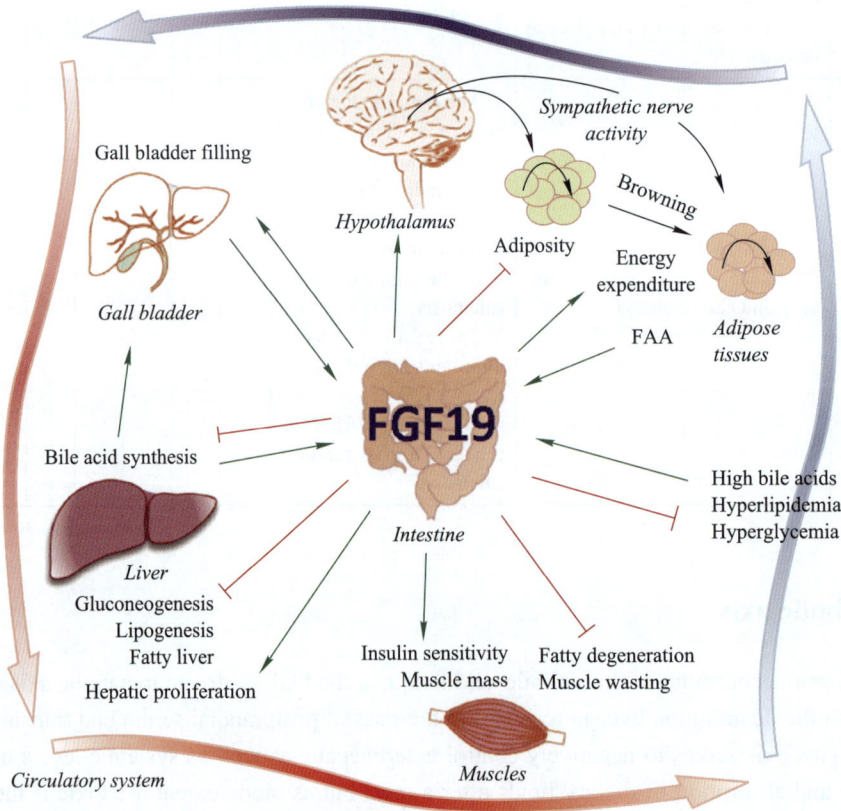

Fig. 2. The FGF19 metabolic axis. The major FGF19 metabolic axis drives a temporal inter-organ cross-talk from the ileum to the liver in response to the rises of postprandial serum and transintestinal flux of bile acids, which serves to discontinue the biosynthesis of new bile acids after sufficient food digestion, and therefore prevent the prolonged exposure of tissues to potential bile acid toxicity. Pharmacological FGF19 may also initiate multiple signal axes to drive effects on multiple tissue/organs, such as promoting (green arrow) energy expenditure in white and brown adipose tissues, increasing muscle mass and insulin sensitivity, and preventing (red long-tailed "T" sign) systemic hyperglycemia and hyperlipidemia. FAA: free fatty acids.

treatment will have a similar adverse effect on the liver, as muscle-specific transgenic mice developed prominent hepatocellular carcinoma [87].

Despite of the tumorigenic concern, the FGF19 analog NGM282 was tested in clinical NASH patients, which markedly reduced liver fat content but with significant side-effects [70]. In a phase 2 trial in patients with type 2 diabetes and chronic idiopathic constipation, NGM282 significantly improved bowel function by accelerating gastric emptying and colonic transit [81]. Furthermore, the NGM282 was further tested in both mouse models and human patients with cholestasis and primary biliary cholangitis, showing efficacy in significantly reducing bile acid levels and improved hepatic inflammatory injury and fibrosis [84, 88, 89].

5. FGF21 metabolic axis

FGF21 is a prime lipid catabolic factor that regulates energy balance, however, the physiological roles and pharmacological effects of FGF21-driven metabolic axes are multifaceted [2, 7, 90] (Fig. 3). FGF21 was discovered as a driver of glucose uptake in adipocytes and a PPARα-dependent hepatic starvation hormone [48, 50, 51]. In mice, its levels are induced when calories are restricted or when glucose is low to allow fats to be burned for energy supply. The rising levels of FGF21 drive diverse aspects of the adaptive starvation response including stimulation of hepatic fatty acid oxidative for ketone body production during prolonged fasting and starvation. Whether this action of FGF21 was autocrine/paracrine in the liver or endocrine in adipose tissues through adipose lipolysis and fatty acid oxidation is a matter of debate. The liver is a major contributor to the circulating FGF21 levels, which is associated with hepatic fat content and adiposity but inversely with serum glucose level [91-93]. The hepatic expression of FGF21 is responsive to not only starvation but also a broad spectrum of cellular, metabolic or pathological changes in the liver as well as systemic metabolic perturbations [7, 69, 94]. As FGF21 is incapable of activating FGFR4-KLB complex [67], which is predominant in the liver in

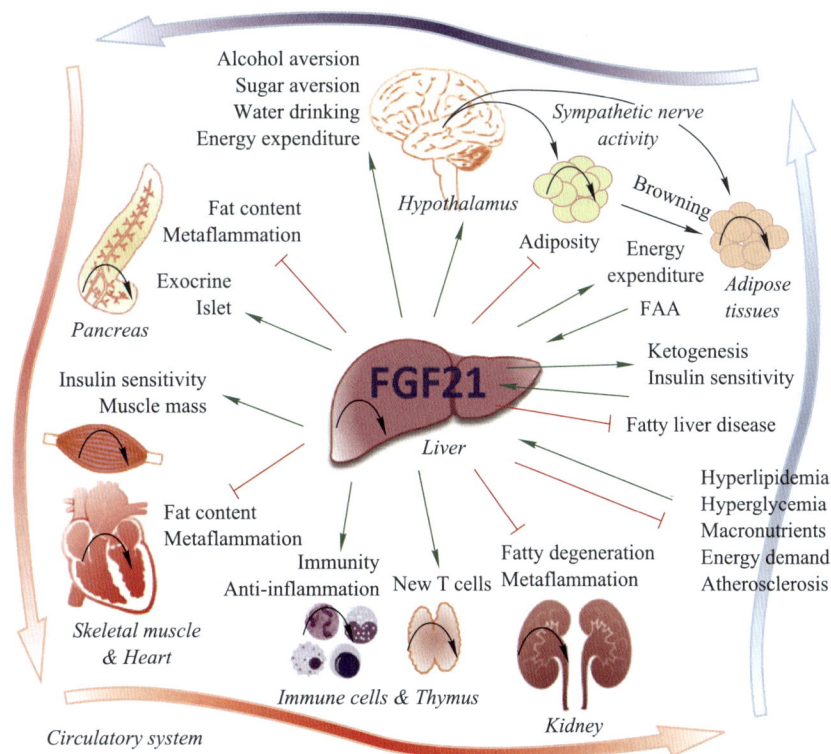

Fig. 3. The FGF21 metabolic axis. The liver is the major organ of origin of endocrine FGF21 in response to a broad spectrum of stress conditions. The hepatic as well as pharmacological FGF21 drives multiple signal axes in multiple tissues/organs, resulting in multifaceted beneficiary metabolic effects, including promoting (green arrow) glucose, lipid and energy homeostasis, offsetting the metabolic derangements, and preventing (red long-tailed "T" sign) metaflammation, inflammatory tissue damage, and tissue-specific pathogenesis, including obesity, type 2 diabetes, fatty liver disease, metabolic syndrome, and associated comorbidities. FAA: free fatty acids. Black semicircular arrows indicate possibility paracrine mode of FGF21 within local tissue environment.

comparison to FGFR1-KLB with low levels, FGF21 acts mainly as an endocrine factor to drive metabolic pathways in peripheral tissues including WAT, BAT, muscle, heart, kidney and CNS that express high levels of FGFR1/2/3-KLB, leading to correction of metabolic derangements and amelioration of metaflammation and stress damage (Fig. 3) [7, 94].

Although the liver is unlikely a major direct target of FGF21, the effects of FGF21 on the liver are prominent. In addition to its role as an regulator of integrated hepatic metabolism in multiple aspects [48, 50, 95-98] including fatty acid oxidation, ketogenesis, gluconeogenesis, and macronutrition preference, FGF21 counteracts hepatic pathologies in response to a number of nutritional and chemical insults, including ketogenic diet, high fat diet, high fructose diet, methionine and choline deficient diet, ethanol supplemented diet, and diethylnitrosamine [99-103]. Under a chronic obesogenic diet, mice deficient of FGF21 developed a spectrum of progressive fatty liver disease including simple hepatosteatosis to NSAH, fibrosis, and HCC, the most lethal complication of this disorder, highlighting the role of FGF21 metabolic axis as a defensive barrier for the deleterious stress damage resulting from metabolic disorders in the liver [104]. Current clinical trials with FGF21 analogs show promising efficacy against NAFLD, NASH and fibrosis without noticeable adverse side effects [73].

Acting on WAT and BAT, the FGF21 axis drives an array of catabolic effects including insulin-independent glucose uptake, lipid droplet expansion inhibition, lipolysis, fatty acid oxidation, white adipocyte beigeing, and thermogenic dissipation of energy [79, 105, 106]. This route of action has been proposed as a major endocrine axis of FGF21 for insulin sensitization, lowering of systemic glucose, triacylglycerol and LDL, fighting against obesity, diabetes, fatty liver diseases, hyperlipidemia and associated comorbidities, and achieving metabolic health [2, 73, 74, 107]. Some of these effects are likely mediated by adipokines, such as CCL11 and adiponectin as we showed in mice [108, 109]. In the cold-induced non-shivering thermogenesis or exercise stress condition, BAT also becomes a source of endocrine FGF21 in a β-adrenergic and cAMP-dependent manner, which in turn facilitates mitochondrial genesis, oxidative capacity, uncoupling and heat generation, leading to adaptation to cold conditions and maintenance of core body temperature [110-112].

In line with the beneficial effects of FGF21 on maintaining metabolic homeostasis during diverse adverse conditions, pharmacological FGF21 markedly extends lifespan in mice by blunting the growth hormone/insulin-like growth factor-1 signaling pathway in the liver, without reducing food intake or affecting longevity-associated markers of NAD+ metabolism, AMP kinase and mTOR signaling pathways [113]. The thymus functions in producing new T cells for the immune system, but with age, it becomes fatty and loses ability to produce sufficient amount of new T cells, which is an important cause of increased risks of infections, obesity, diabetes, certain types of cancers, leading to reduced lifespan in the elderly. FGF21 level in thymic epithelial cells is several fold higher than in the liver. This high level of FGF21 is proposed to protect thymus from the age-related fatty degeneration and to increase the production of new T cells to bolster immune function, thereby, lowering the incidence of diseases and promoting longevity [114].

The acinar cell compartment in the pancreas expresses the highest levels of FGF21 constitutively among tissues, but contributes little to the circulation [56, 115]. Acinar cells appear to be both the dominant source and target (*via* FGFR1-KLB complex) of pancreatic FGF21. The high levels of FGF21 is proposed to act as an exocrine pancreas secretagogue to stimulate pancreatic digestive enzyme secretion and pancreatic juice flow to intestine, thereby relieving potential self-digestion caused proteostasis stress and protecting pancreas from pancreatitis including but not limited to those caused by high-fat diets, pancreatic toxins and alcoholism [116]. Although islets express significantly lower amounts of FGF21, acinar cell derived or endocrine FGF21 helps protect against fatty pancreas, high-fat diet induced islet hyperplasia and inflammatory damage [117-119]. Demyelination in the central nervous system can cause severe neurological deficits such as multiple sclerosis and neurological dysfunction. Pancreatic FGF21 was found to act on the oligodendrocyte precursor cells to promote the remyelination process, leading to better recovery of neurological functions in mice [120].

Exposure to alcohol or sugar induces hepatic FGF21 through ChREBP, which then acts on the hypothalamus reward pathway to suppress the desire for sugar and alcohol in favor of drinking water in mice, depending on the β-adrenergic circuit [97, 98, 121, 122]. This may represent a new hydration pathway that is independent of the classical renin-angiotensin-aldosterone thirsty pathway in the kidney in response to nutritional stress, suggesting a previously underappreciated association of water intake to metabolism through the FGF21 metabolic axis. A human rs838133 allele in FGF21 is associated with higher alcohol as well as sugar intake, higher blood pressure and waist-hip ratio, but lower total body-fat percentage [123]. Comparison of the genomes of more than 105,000 light and heavy social drinkers also identifies a variation in rs11940694 locus of KLB gene in association with the aversion for alcohol [124]. Neuronal cell stress reaction, such as those caused by disturbances of the mitochondria and ER, is an important factor in the development of neurodegenerative diseases. Studies found that the integrated stress response induces neuronal FGF21, which presumably serve to attenuate stress and neural damage [125].

In addition to the liver, pancreas and adipose tissues, cardiac muscle produces FGF21 in response to cardiac stress, cardio exercise, and endurance training [126, 127], which then speeds up glucose uptake, lipid catabolism and energy metabolism, and protects against cardiovascular stress damage, apoptosis and heart dysfunctions, such as cardiac hypertrophy, myopathy, steatosis, ischemic infarction, and atherosclerosis as our results revealed [128-132]. Through a multiorgan crosstalk, hepatic FGF21 drives the expression of angiotensin-converting enzyme 2 in adipocytes and renal cells, which hydrolyzes angiotensin II to active vasodilator angiotensin-(1-7) in the renin–angiotensin system, leading to the alleviation of angiotensin II-associated hypertension and the reversal of vascular damage [133]. Skeletal muscle under bouts of exercise or stress such as mitochondrial myopathies also induces FGF21 expression [134-136]. In turn, FGF21 can act on muscle and adipose tissue to reduce lipid load by increasing lipolysis, fatty acid utilization, energy expenditure and insulin sensitivity, leading to the prevention of diet-induced obesity and insulin resistance [137-140].

Hepatic FGF21 acts on the paraventricular nucleus in the hypothalamus to drive the release of corticotropin-releasing factor, which then stimulates the involuntary sympathetic nerve activity. This leads to the activation of brown adipose tissue to upregulate uncoupling protein-1 (UCP1) and to increase glucose uptake, lipolysis, mitochondrial oxidation of fatty acids and glucose, body heat generation, and weight loss [141, 142]. The increase of corticotropin-releasing factor levels may also stimulate the pituitary to release adrenocorticotrophic hormone and subsequent corticosterone production in adrenal cortex, leading to increased hepatic gluconeogenesis during prolonged fasting to prevent hypoglycemia [143]. Hepatic FGF21 acts on the suprachiasmatic nucleus (SCN) in the hypothalamus to suppress the vasopressin-kisspeptin and gonadotropin-releasing hormone signaling cascade, which then inhibit the proestrus surge in luteinizing hormone from anterior pituitary gland, contributing to female infertility in response to nutritional challenge such as prolonged starvation [144]. The SCN action of FGF21 may also alter circadian behavior [145]. By increasing neuropeptide Y levels and Y1 receptor activation, the hypothalamus action of FGF21 may decrease locomotive activity, metabolic rate and body temperature, leading to torpor under nutrition limitation [146]. There is also a possibility that FGF21 acts on hippocampus to decrease reactive oxygen species and inflammatory damage, thus decreasing brain cell damage and improving cognition [147, 148].

The endocrine FGF21 axes as well as the paracrine FGF21 axes within the local tissue compartments have been shown in many tissues and organs to counteract stress response and attenuate the stress-ensued inflammation and inflammatory damage [7, 104, 117]. Therefore, FGF21 is not only a stress-responsive or stress-induced factor but also an anti-stress and anti-inflammatory factor. The stress-offsetting effects, in particular the anti-inflammatory activities, can be attributable to the metabolic effects of FGF21 axes that prevent fatty degeneration, gluco-lipotoxicity, oxidative and ER stress, and thus, infiltration of inflammatory and immune cells. These metabolic activities may be mediated in part through efficient and durable systemic and local glycemic and lipidemic control, improvement of insulin sensitivity, and promotion of lipid catabolism (lipolysis and fatty acid oxidation), adipose beigeing, and futile energy expenditure in adipose tissues, local adipocytes and brain in both UCP1 dependent and adrenergic sympathetic nervous system dependent mechanisms [79, 105, 106, 141, 149, 150]. As a result, FGF21 effectively reverse hepatic steatosis in obese mice and clinical obese patients [73, 105, 151]. Furthermore, pharmacological FGF21 analogs and FGFR1-KLB agonists have been shown to directly improve the spectrum of adverse components of metabolic syndrome, including central obesity, insulin resistance, elevated fasting glucose, dyslipidemia, systemic hypertension and fatty liver, which are major risk factors for cardiovascular diseases, type 2 diabetes mellitus, chronic kidney disease, and all-cause mortality [2, 7, 73, 74, 107]. The FGF21 axes suppress atherosclerotic plaque by reducing hypercholesterolemia, oxidative stress, and smooth muscle cell proliferation *via* adiponectin dependent and independent mechanisms [129]. FGF21-deficient mice developed significant islet hyperplasia and periductal lymphocytic inflammation upon chronic challenge of an obesogenic high-fat diet, indicating a protective role of FGF21 in compensatory islet hyperplasia and pancreatic inflammation in the obesity conditions [117, 152]. FGF21 directly suppresses triglyceride levels and lipid accumulation in kidney tissues, thereby reducing lipotoxicity, oxidative stress, inflammation, glomerular abnormalities, fibrotic renal injury in diabetic nephropathy, while deficiency of FGF21 aggravates these conditions [153, 154], indicative of a defensive role of FGF21 against kidney pathogenesis associated with obesity and diabetes.

The anti-stress and anti-inflammatory effects of FGF21 may be also attributable to direct action on non-metabolic cells and non-metabolic activities. FGF21 was shown to directly inhibit cardiomyocyte apoptosis, oxidative stress, myocardial injury, thus reducing the risk of pathological cardiac remodeling and dysfunction, cardiac hypertrophy, myocardial ischemia, and heart failure in ischemic heart tissue and diabetic cardiomyopathy [130, 155]. FGF21 protects the pancreas from cerulean and l-arginine induced pancreatitis, acinar cell injury, and fibrosis in mice [118, 119, 156]. FGF21 acts directly on renal mesangial cells to reduce glucose reabsorption and prevent hyperglycemia-induced fibrogenesis in db/db mice [157, 158]. Interestingly, recent evidence supports that FGF21 may directly act on inflammatory and immune cells to attenuate inflammation and inflammatory damage. FGF21 activates THP1 macrophages to promote cholesterol efflux, oxLDL uptake, and foam cell formation and inhibits macrophages inflammatory capacity through the Nrf2 pathway [156, 159, 160]. Adipose tissue is an endocrine organ and plays an active role in inflammation in obesity that can favor CVD and CKD progression by inducing a chronic and low-grade inflammation *via* secreted proinflammatory adipokines. Studies in diet-induced obesity and pancreatitis models indicate that FGF21 promotes anti-inflammatory macrophage polarization in adipose depots and pancreas, as well as white adipose tissue browning and insulin sensitivity, effectively preventing adipose tissue from adopting proinflammatory profiles and the pancreas from inflammatory fibrosis [109, 156, 159, 161]. Interestingly, FGF21 was found highly expressed in neutrophils and monocytes among circulating leukocytes, and stimulates phagocytosis, glucose uptake, and production of reactive oxygen species in a NADPH oxidase dependent manner in the neutrophil-like HL-60 cells and monocytic THP-1 cells [162-164]. In the type II collagen-induced arthritis mouse model, FGF21 acts on the spleen to reduce inflammatory IL-17, TNF-α, IL-1β, IL-6, IL-8, and MMP3, as well as the number of the splenic TH17 cells, thus alleviating arthritis severity [165]. These studies highlight a potential mediator role of FGF21 in innate immunity and inflammatory disorders. It remains to be determined the direct impact of FGF21 on the function of inflammatory and immune cells and the health consequences.

6. FGF23 metabolic axis

FGF23 is a key hormonal regulator of phosphate, vitamin D and calcium metabolism, and its metabolic axes drive a complex interorgan crosstalk network for bone health and systemic mineral balance (Fig. 4) [2, 61, 166-168]. Osteoblastic cells in osseous tissue are the major source of FGF23 in response to the elevated calcitriol, increased phosphate and calcium burdens, increased parathyroid hormone, and active bone remodeling, in a VDR dependent mechanism. Acting on the kidneys that express the FGFR1-KL complex, the FGF23 signal axis represses the expression of NPT2a and NPT2c, the sodium-phosphate cotransporters in the proximal tubule, thereby decreasing the reabsorption and increasing the excretion of phosphate in the renal brush border membrane vesicles. Another important function of this bone to kidney FGF23 signal axis is to suppress the expression of 25-hydroxyvitamin D3-1-α-hydroxylase and to stimulate the expression of 1,25-dihydroxyvitamin D(3) 24-hydroxylase, hence inhibiting the production of active calcitriol in the renal proximal tubules, which subsequently inhibits the expression of NPT2b and phosphate absorption in the apical brush border of small intestine. The bone FGF23 acts on the basolateral FGFR1-KL complex in the renal distal tubules to increase intracellular transport of fully glycosylated TRPV5 from the Golgi apparatus to the plasma membrane, thereby stimulating calcium reabsorption in distal renal tubules and preventing calcium loss [169]. These FGF23-associated axis also directly increases the membrane abundance of the $Na^+:Cl^-$ co-transporter NCC in distal renal tubules, thereby increasing sodium reabsorption, plasma volume, and blood pressure [170]. This may be a new cause of high blood pressure and heart disease under the modern processed phosphate-rich foods.

Bone FGF23 also acts on the parathyroid gland to inhibit the production and secretion of parathyroid hormone (Fig. 4) [171], which then reduces serum calcium through its effects on the bone, kidney, and intestine. High serum FGF23 levels in chronic kidney disease patients decrease calcitriol, thereby contributing to the development of secondary hyperparathyroidism, which has a crucial role in increasing the levels of FGF23, as parathyroid hormone stimulates the expression of FGF23.

Recent studies revealed potential roles of the FGF23 axis in suppressing erythropoiesis in bone marrow. Erythroid progenitor cells highly express FGF23 and FGFR-KL, suggesting that erythroid progenitor cells are both a source and a target of FGF23. Loss of FGF23 or injection of an FGF23 blocking peptide in mice results in increased erythropoiesis, reduced erythroid cell apoptosis, and elevated renal and bone marrow erythropoietin (EPO) expression with increased levels of circulating erythropoietin. On the other hand, the elevated EPO or acute blood loss increases FGF23 expression in the bone marrow with a concomitant increase in serum FGF23 [172, 173]. A recent study suggests that FGF23 may be in-

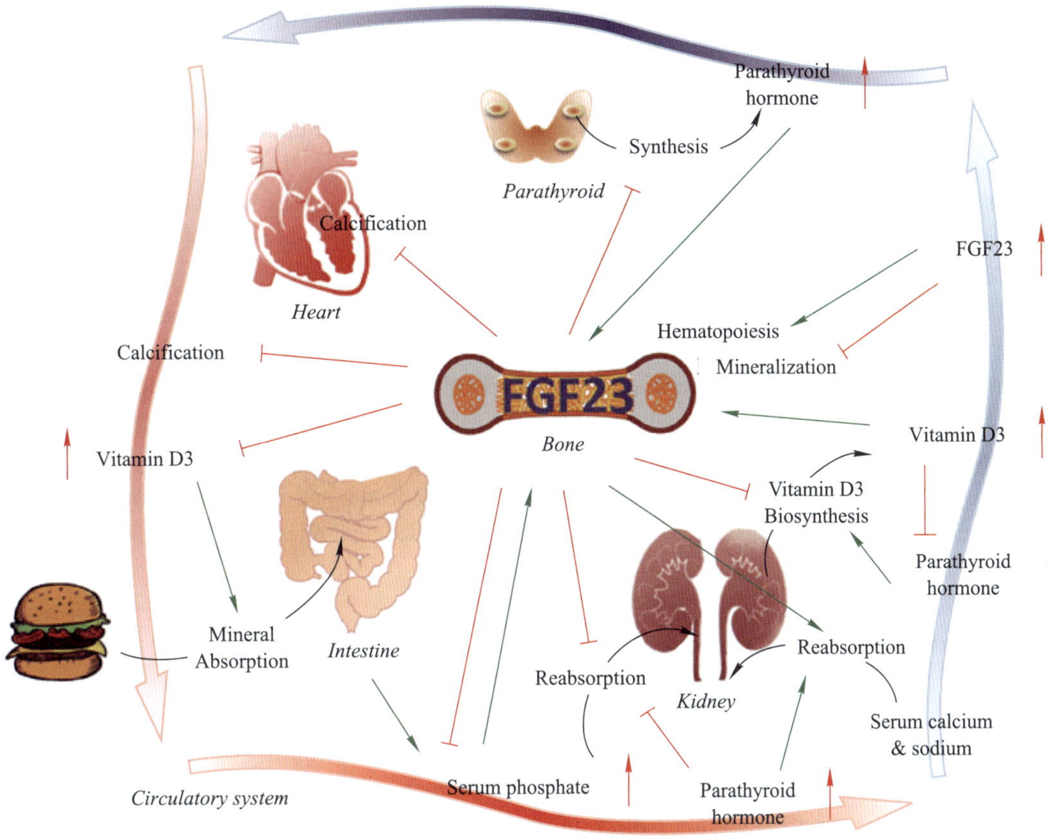

Fig. 4. The FGF23 metabolic axis. The bone-derived FGF23 drives signal axes to promote (green arrows) the metabolic homeostasis of phosphate, vitamin D and calcium through a complex inter-organ crosstalk network for bone health and systemic mineral balance. The bone to the kidney axis of FGF23 is central to the metabolic roles of FGF23, which inhibits (red long-tailed "T" sign) the reabsorption of phosphate and the production of active calcitriol in the renal proximal tubules while increasing the calcium and sodium reabsorption in the renal distal tubules. In addition, the bone to parathyroid axis of FGF23 inhibits the production and secretion of parathyroid hormone that also plays critical roles in mineral and vitamin D balance.

volved in the association between functional iron deficiency and increased EPO levels and death. Further elucidation of the role of the EPO-FGF23 signaling axis in hereditary anemia and chronic hemolytic diseases, chronic kidney disease, and mineralization disorders will add to the understanding of the pathophysiology of these diseases and life expectancy, and will inform new treatment strategies for the diseases.

Current evidence indicates that FGF23 is more structurally unique than FGF19 and FGF21 [5]. The FGF23 contains a conserved furin-sensitive [176]RHTR[179] cleavage site near the C-terminus, which upon cleavage inactivates the intact FGF23, leading to signal attenuation. The biologic importance of this activity control mechanism is demonstrated by point mutations (e.g. R176Q, R179Q and R179W) of this site, which results in cleavage-resistant FGF23 and elevated circulating levels of active FGF23, in autosomal dominant hypophosphatemic and vitamin-D-deficient rickets, characterized by renal phosphate wasting, hypophosphatemia, rickets, osteomalacia, leg deformities, short stature, bone pain and dental abscesses [168, 174, 175]. FGF23 levels are elevated and may play important roles in other hereditable and acquired phosphate wasting disorders, including X-linked dominant hypophosphatemic rickets, autosomal recessive hypophosphatemic rickets, hypophosphatemic rickets associated with McCune-Albright syndrome/fibrous dysplasia of bone, and linear sebaceous nevus syndrome [176, 177]. Raised FGF23 levels are also found in the acquired phosphate wasting disorders in some types of tumors, such as the benign mesenchymal neoplasm phosphaturic mesenchymal tumor, causing tumor-induced osteomalacia, a paraneoplastic syndrome [168].

During posttranslational modification, FGF23 is glycosylated at Thr-178 in the cleavage site by GalNT3, which facilitates the secretion of FGF23 and protects the protein from being broken down, suggesting a novel posttranslational regulatory model of FGF23 involving competing O-glycosylation and proteolytic processing to determines the level of secreted active FGF23 [178]. The importance of this glycosylation modification is demonstrated by inactivating GalNT3 mutations that render FGF23 susceptible to proteolysis [179, 180], thereby reducing circulating intact hormone levels and leading to autosomal recessive familial tumoral calcinosis that manifests with hyperphosphatemic and massive calcium deposits in the skin and subcutaneous tissues throughout the body. Consistently, at least seven mutations in the conserved backbone of FGF23, such as S71G, M96T, S129F and F157L, destabilize the tertiary structure and render FGF23 susceptible to degradation, also resulting in autosomal recessive familial tumoral calcinosis with hyperphosphatemia [2, 5, 181-184].

Patients of chronic kidney disease have elevated serum levels of phosphate as well as FGF23, which lead to increased take up of calcium by the kidneys, resulting in vascular calcification. This explains the cardiovascular disease complications in the chronic kidney disease patients, such as cardiac hypertrophy and congestive heart failure [185, 186]. The inhibition of FGF23 or its axis could be a strategy to bring cardiovascular disease and vascular calcification under control. The level of FGF23 in kidney patients can even indicate their life expectancy. Dysregulation of calcium levels can have an array of serious health consequences. Chronic hypocalcemia can potentially lead to heart failure, nervous system and muscle disorders, and encephalopathy, while hypercalcemia can increase the risk of kidney stones, cause muscle weakness, and worsens psychological issues such as dementia and depression. This may explain some current observations that people with high serum FGF23 may be at risk of dementia, and that mice lacking FGF23 exhibit defective learning and memory problems similar to those seen in the KL deficient mice [187, 188].

7. Conclusion and future perspective

The three members of the metabolic FGFs, including FGF19, 21 and 23, share a conserved core structure of β-trefoil fold but diverge in functions from other mitogenic members of the FGF family during evolution (Fig. 1). They acquire specific structural elements that confer them abilities to function *via* an endocrine mode and to bind different new accessory receptors that have strict expression pattern in metabolic tissues. Although the metabolic FGFs still signal through the transmambrane FGFR tyrosine kinases as the mitogenic FGFs, these new properties divert their functions to metabolic regulation. As such, the FGF19, 21 and FGF23 drive a wide range of diverse metabolic axes that function to maintain the homeostasis of bile acids, glucose, lipids, energy and minerals, offsetting detrimental metabolic derangements, and achieving optimal metabolic health, without an overt effect on cell proliferation and population growth. In this sense, each of the metabolic axes of FGF19, 21 and 23 stands alone as a driver of specific metabolic effects with important physiopathological consequences, and therefore, they constitute the FGF metabolic axis as we start to call out here with broad-spectrum pathophysiological roles and consequences on the quality of survival (Fig. 1).

References

[1] Beenken A, Mohammadi M. The FGF family: biology, pathophysiology and therapy[J]. Nat Rev Drug Discov, 2009, 8(3): 235-253.

[2] Luo Y, Ye S, Li X, *et al*. Emerging structure–function paradigm of endocrine FGFs in metabolic diseases[J]. Trends in Pharmacological Sciences, 40(2): 142-153.

[3] Li X, Wang C, Xiao J, *et al*. Fibroblast growth factors, old kids on the new block[J]. Semin Cell Dev Biol, 2016, 53: 155-167.

[4] Zhang JD, Cousens LS, Barr PJ, *et al*. Three-dimensional structure of human basic fibroblast growth factor, a structural homolog of interleukin 1 beta[J]. Proc Natl Acad Sci U S A, 1991, 88(8): 3446-3450.

[5] Chen G, Liu Y, Goetz R, *et al*. α-Klotho is a non-enzymatic molecular scaffold for FGF23 hormone signalling[J]. Nature, 2018, 553(7689): 461-466.

[6] Degirolamo C, Sabba C, Moschetta A. Therapeutic potential of the endocrine fibroblast growth factors FGF19, FGF21 and FGF23[J]. Nat Rev Drug Discov, 2016, 15(1): 51-69.

[7] Luo Y, Ye S, Chen X, *et al*. Rush to the fire: FGF21 extinguishes metabolic stress, metaflammation and tissue damage[J]. Cytokine Growth Factor Rev, 2017, 38: 59-65.

[8] McKeehan WL, Wang F, Kan M. The heparan sulfate-fibroblast growth factor family: diversity of structure and function[J]. Prog Nucleic Acid Res Mol Biol, 1998, 59: 135-176.

[9] Itoh N, Ornitz DM. Evolution of the Fgf and Fgfr gene families[J]. Trends Genet, 2004, 20(11): 563-569.

[10] Itoh N, Ornitz DM. Fibroblast growth factors: from molecular evolution to roles in development, metabolism and disease[J]. J Biochem, 2011, 149(2): 121-130.

[11] Luo Y, Lu W, Li X. Unraveling Endocrine FGF signaling complex to combat metabolic diseases[J]. Trends in biochemical sciences, 2018, 43(8): 563-566.

[12] Zhang X, Ibrahimi OA, Olsen SK, *et al*. Receptor specificity of the fibroblast growth factor family. The complete mammalian FGF family[J]. Journal of Biological Chemistry, 2006, 281(23): 15694-15700.

[13] Armelin HA. Pituitary extracts and steroid hormones in the control of 3T3 cell growth[J]. Proc Natl Acad Sci U S A, 1973, 70(9): 2702-2706.

[14] Gospodarowicz D. Localisation of a fibroblast growth factor and its effect alone and with hydrocortisone on 3T3 cell growth[J]. Nature, 1974, 249(453): 123-127.

[15] Burgess WH, Maciag T. The heparin-binding (fibroblast) growth

factor family of proteins[J]. Annu Rev Biochem, 1989, 58: 575-606.

[16] Luo Y, Ye S, Kan M, et al. Control of fibroblast growth factor (FGF) 7- and FGF1-induced mitogenesis and downstream signaling by distinct heparin octasaccharide motifs[J]. J Biol Chem, 2006, 281(30): 21052-21061.

[17] Gospodarowicz D, Ill CR, Hornsby PJ, et al. Control of bovine adrenal cortical cell proliferation by fibroblast growth factor. Lack of effect of epidermal growth factor[J]. Endocrinology, 1977, 100(4): 1080-1089.

[18] Mansour SL, Goddard JM, Capecchi MR. Mice homozygous for a targeted disruption of the proto-oncogene int-2 have developmental defects in the tail and inner ear[J]. Development, 1993, 117(1): 13-28.

[19] Guo C, Sun Y, Zhou B, et al. A Tbx1-Six1/Eya1-Fgf8 genetic pathway controls mammalian cardiovascular and craniofacial morphogenesis[J]. J Clin Invest, 2011, 121(4): 1585-1595.

[20] Ornitz DM, Marie PJ. Fibroblast growth factor signaling in skeletal development and disease[J]. Genes Dev, 2015, 29(14): 1463-1486.

[21] Kan M, Wang F, Xu J, et al. An essential heparin-binding domain in the fibroblast growth factor receptor kinase[J]. Science, 1993, 259(5103): 1918-1921.

[22] Ye S, Luo Y, Lu W, et al. Structural basis for interaction of FGF-1, FGF-2, and FGF-7 with different heparan sulfate motifs[J]. Biochemistry, 2001, 40(48): 14429-14439.

[23] Goetz R, Mohammadi M. Exploring mechanisms of FGF signalling through the lens of structural biology[J]. Nat Rev Mol Cell Biol, 2013, 14(3): 166-180.

[24] Kouhara H, Hadari YR, Spivak-Kroizman T, et al. A lipid-anchored Grb2-binding protein that links FGF-receptor activation to the Ras/MAPK signaling pathway[J]. Cell, 1997, 89(5): 693-702.

[25] Huang Z, Marsiglia WM, Roy UB, et al. Two FGF receptor kinase molecules act in concert to recruit and transphosphorylate phospholipase Cγ[J]. Molecular Cell, 2015, 61(1): 98-110.

[26] Dorey K, Amaya E. FGF signalling: diverse roles during early vertebrate embryogenesis[J]. Development, 2010, 137(22): 3731-3742.

[27] Lu W, Luo Y, Kan M, et al. Fibroblast growth factor-10. A second candidate stromal to epithelial cell andromedin in prostate[J]. J Biol Chem, 1999, 274(18): 12827-12834.

[28] Jin C, Wang F, Wu X, et al. Directionally specific paracrine communication mediated by epithelial FGF9 to stromal FGFR3 in two-compartment premalignant prostate tumors[J]. Cancer Res, 2004, 64(13): 4555-4562.

[29] Carter EP, Fearon AE, Grose RP. Careless talk costs lives: fibroblast growth factor receptor signalling and the consequences of pathway malfunction[J]. Trends Cell Biol, 2015, 25(4): 221-233.

[30] Goldberg JD, Zheng J, Castro-Malaspina H, et al. Palifermin is efficacious in recipients of TBI-based but not chemotherapy-based allogeneic hematopoietic stem cell transplants[J]. Bone Marrow Transplant, 2013, 48(1): 99-104.

[31] Uchi H, Igarashi A, Urabe K, et al. Clinical efficacy of basic fibroblast growth factor (bFGF) for diabetic ulcer[J]. Eur J Dermatol, 2009, 19(5): 461-468.

[32] Akita S, Akino K, Imaizumi T, et al. Basic fibroblast growth factor accelerates and improves second-degree burn wound healing[J]. Wound Repair Regen, 16(5): 635-641.

[33] Fu X, Shen Z, Chen Y, et al. Randomised placebo-controlled trial of use of topical recombinant bovine basic fibroblast growth factor for second-degree burns[J]. Lancet, 1998, 352(9141): 1661-1664.

[34] Maddaluno L, Urwyler C, Werner S. Fibroblast growth factors: key players in regeneration and tissue repair[J]. Development, 2017, 144(22): 4047-4060.

[35] Zhao YZ, Zhang M, Wong HL, et al. Prevent diabetic cardiomyopathy in diabetic rats by combined therapy of aFGF-loaded nanoparticles and ultrasound-targeted microbubble destruction

technique[J]. J Control Release, 2016, 223: 11-21.

[36] Liang G, Song L, Chen Z, et al. Fibroblast growth factor 1 ameliorates diabetic nephropathy by an anti-inflammatory mechanism[J]. Kidney Int, 2018, 93(1): 95-109.

[37] Li R, Li Y, Wu Y, et al. Heparin-poloxamer thermosensitive hydrogel loaded with bFGF and NGF enhances peripheral nerve regeneration in diabetic rats[J]. Biomaterials, 2018, 168: 24-37.

[38] Wu J, Zhu J, He C, et al. Comparative study of heparin-poloxamer hydrogel modified bFGF and aFGF for in vivo wound healing efficiency[J]. ACS Appl Mater Interfaces, 2016, 8(29): 18710-18721.

[39] Wu J, Ye J, Zhu J, et al. Heparin-based coacervate of FGF2 improves dermal regeneration by asserting a synergistic role with cell proliferation and endogenous facilitated VEGF for cutaneous wound healing[J]. Biomacromolecules, 2016, 17(6): 2168-2177.

[40] Wang Q, He Y, Zhao Y, et al. A thermosensitive heparin-poloxamer hydrogel bridges aFGF to treat spinal cord injury[J]. ACS Appl Mater Interfaces, 2017, 9(8): 6725-6745.

[41] Katoh M. Therapeutics targeting FGF signaling network in human diseases[J]. Trends Pharmacol Sci, 2016, 37(12): 1081-1096.

[42] Liang G, Liu Z, Wu J, et al. Anticancer molecules targeting fibroblast growth factor receptors[J]. Trends Pharmacol Sci, 2012, 33(10): 531-541.

[43] Cuevas P, Carceller F, Ortega S, et al. Hypotensive activity of fibroblast growth factor[J]. Science, 1991, 254(5035): 1208-1210.

[44] Konishi M, Mikami T, Yamasaki M, et al. Fibroblast growth factor-16 is a growth factor for embryonic brown adipocytes[J]. J Biol Chem, 2000, 275(16): 12119-12122.

[45] Rulifson IC, Collins P, Miao L, et al. In vitro and in vivo analyses reveal profound effects of fibroblast growth factor 16 as a metabolic regulator[J]. J Biol Chem, 2017, 292(5): 1951-1969.

[46] Jonker JW, Suh JM, Atkins AR, et al. A PPARγ-FGF1 axis is required for adaptive adipose remodelling and metabolic homeostasis[J]. Nature, 2012, 485(7398): 391-394.

[47] Huang Z, Tan Y, Gu J, et al. Uncoupling the mitogenic and metabolic functions of FGF1 by tuning FGF1-FGF receptor dimer stability[J]. Cell Rep, 2017, 20(7): 1717-1728.

[48] Huang Z, Tan Y, Gu J, et al. Uncoupling the mitogenic and metabolic functions of FGF1 by tuning FGF1-FGF receptor dimer stability[J]. Cell Rep, 2017, 20(7): 1717-1728.

[49] Inagaki T, Choi M, Moschetta A, et al. Fibroblast growth factor 15 functions as an enterohepatic signal to regulate bile acid homeostasis[J]. Cell Metab, 2005, 2(4): 217-225.

[50] Inagaki T, Dutchak P, Zhao G, et al. Endocrine regulation of the fasting response by PPARα-mediated induction of fibroblast growth factor 21[J]. Cell Metab, 2007, 5(6): 415-425.

[51] Kharitonenkov A, Shiyanova TL, Koester A, et al. FGF-21 as a novel metabolic regulator[J]. J Clin Invest, 2005, 115(6): 1627-1635.

[52] Goetz R, Ohnishi M, Ding X, et al. Klotho coreceptors inhibit signaling by paracrine fibroblast growth factor 8 subfamily ligands[J]. Mol Cell Biol, 2012, 32(10): 1944-1954.

[53] Luo Y, Yang C, Lu W, et al. Metabolic regulator βKlotho interacts with fibroblast growth factor receptor 4 (FGFR4) to induce apoptosis and inhibit tumor cell proliferation[J]. J Biol Chem, 2010, 285(39): 30069-30078.

[54] Itoh M, Nacher JC, Kuma K, et al. Evolutionary history and functional implications of protein domains and their combinations in eukaryotes[J]. Genome Biol, 2007, 8(6): R121.

[55] Kurosu H, Choi M, Ogawa Y, et al. Tissue-specific expression of βKlotho and fibroblast growth factor (FGF) receptor isoforms determines metabolic activity of FGF19 and FGF21[J]. J Biol Chem, 2007, 282(37): 26687-26695.

[56] Fon Tacer K, Bookout AL, Ding X, et al. Research resource: comprehensive expression atlas of the fibroblast growth factor system in adult mouse[J]. Mol Endocrinol, 2010, 24(10): 2050-2064.

[57] Wang H, Qiang L, Farmer SR. Identification of a domain within peroxisome proliferator-activated receptor gamma regulating expression of a group of genes containing fibroblast growth factor 21 that are selectively repressed by SIRT1 in adipocytes[J]. Mol Cell Biol, 2008, 28(1): 188-200.

[58] Iizuka K, Takeda J, Horikawa Y. Glucose induces FGF21 mRNA expression through ChREBP activation in rat hepatocytes[J]. FEBS Lett, 2009, 583(17): 2882-2886.

[59] Wang Y, Solt LA, Burris TP. Regulation of FGF21 expression and secretion by retinoic acid receptor-related orphan receptor alpha[J]. J Biol Chem, 2010, 285(21): 15668-15673.

[60] Uebanso T, Taketani Y, Yamamoto H, et al. Liver X receptor negatively regulates fibroblast growth factor 21 in the fatty liver induced by cholesterol-enriched diet[J]. J Nutr Biochem, 2012, 23(7): 785-790.

[61] Masuyama R, Stockmans I, Torrekens S, et al. Vitamin D receptor in chondrocytes promotes osteoclastogenesis and regulates FGF23 production in osteoblasts[J]. J Clin Invest, 2006, 116(12): 3150-3159.

[62] Kolek OI, Hines ER, Jones MD, et al. 1α,25-Dihydroxyvitamin D3 upregulates FGF23 gene expression in bone: the final link in a renal-gastrointestinal-skeletal axis that controls phosphate transport[J]. Am J Physiol Gastrointest Liver Physiol, 2005, 289(6): G1036-1042.

[63] Zhang Y, Lei T, Huang JF, et al. The link between fibroblast growth factor 21 and sterol regulatory element binding protein 1c during lipogenesis in hepatocytes[J]. Mol Cell Endocrinol, 2011, 342(1-2): 41-47.

[64] Liu TF, Tang JJ, Li PS, et al. Ablation of gp78 in liver improves hyperlipidemia and insulin resistance by inhibiting SREBP to decrease lipid biosynthesis[J]. Cell Metab, 2012, 16(2): 213-225.

[65] Muise ES, Azzolina B, Kuo DW, et al. Adipose fibroblast growth factor 21 is up-regulated by peroxisome proliferator-activated receptor gamma and altered metabolic states[J]. Mol Pharmacol, 2008, 74(2): 403-412.

[66] De Sousa-Coelho AL, Marrero PF, Haro D. Activating transcription factor 4-dependent induction of FGF21 during amino acid deprivation[J]. Biochem J, 2012, 443(1): 165-171.

[67] Yang C, Jin C, Li X, et al. Differential specificity of endocrine FGF19 and FGF21 to FGFR1 and FGFR4 in complex with KLB[J]. PLoS One, 2012, 7(3): e33870.

[68] Lee S, Choi J, Mohanty J, et al. Structures of β-klotho reveal a 'zip code'-like mechanism for endocrine FGF signalling[J]. Nature, 2018, 553(7689): 501-505.

[69] Luo Y, McKeehan WL. Stressed liver and muscle call on adipocytes with FGF21[J]. Front Endocrinol (Lausanne), 2013, 4: 194.

[70] Harrison SA, Rinella ME, Abdelmalek MF, et al. NGM282 for treatment of non-alcoholic steatohepatitis: a multicentre, randomised, double-blind, placebo-controlled, phase 2 trial[J]. Lancet, 2018, 391(10126): 1174-1185.

[71] Hirschfield GM, Chazouilleres O, Drenth JP, et al. Effect of NGM282, an FGF19 analogue, in primary sclerosing cholangitis: A multicenter, randomized, double-blind, placebo-controlled phase II trial[J]. J Hepatol, 2019, 70(3): 483-493.

[72] Harrison SA, Rossi SJ, Paredes AH, et al. NGM282 improves liver fibrosis and histology in 12 weeks in patients with nonalcoholic steatohepatitis[J]. Hepatology, 2019.

[73] Sanyal A, Charles ED, Neuschwander-Tetri BA, et al. Pegbelfermin (BMS-986036), a PEGylated fibroblast growth factor 21 analogue, in patients with non-alcoholic steatohepatitis: a randomised, double-blind, placebo-controlled, phase 2a trial[J]. Lancet, 2019, 392(10165): 2705-2717.

[74] Talukdar S, Zhou Y, Li D, et al. A Long-acting FGF21 molecule, PF-05231023, decreases body weight and improves lipid profile in non-human primates and type 2 diabetic subjects[J]. Cell Metab, 2016, 23(3): 427-440.

[75] Carpenter TO, Imel EA, Ruppe MD, et al. Randomized trial of the anti-FGF23 antibody KRN23 in X-linked hypophosphatemia[J]. J Clin Invest, 2014, 124(4): 1587-1597.

[76] Yu C, Wang F, Kan M, et al. Elevated cholesterol metabolism and bile acid synthesis in mice lacking membrane tyrosine kinase receptor FGFR4[J]. J Biol Chem, 2000, 275(20): 15482-15489.

[77] Fu L, John LM, Adams SH, et al. Fibroblast growth factor 19 increases metabolic rate and reverses dietary and leptin-deficient diabetes[J]. Endocrinology, 2004, 145(6): 2594-2603.

[78] Tomlinson E, Fu L, John L, et al. Transgenic mice expressing human fibroblast growth factor-19 display increased metabolic rate and decreased adiposity[J]. Endocrinology, 2002, 143(5): 1741-1747.

[79] Adams AC, Yang C, Coskun T, et al. The breadth of FGF21's metabolic actions are governed by FGFR1 in adipose tissue[J]. Molecular metabolism, 2013, 2(1): 31-37.

[80] Walters JR, Tasleem AM, Omer OS, et al. A new mechanism for bile acid diarrhea: defective feedback inhibition of bile acid biosynthesis[J]. Clin Gastroenterol Hepatol, 2009, 7(11): 1189-1194.

[81] Oduyebo I, Camilleri M, Nelson AD, et al. Effects of NGM282, an FGF19 variant, on colonic transit and bowel function in functional constipation: a randomized phase 2 trial[J]. Am J Gastroenterol, 2018, 113(5): 725-734.

[82] Pai R, French D, Ma N, et al. Antibody-mediated inhibition of fibroblast growth factor 19 results in increased bile acids synthesis and ileal malabsorption of bile acids in cynomolgus monkeys[J]. Toxicol Sci, 2012, 126(2): 446-456.

[83] Gerhard GS, Styer AM, Wood GC, et al. A role for fibroblast growth factor 19 and bile acids in diabetes remission after Roux-en-Y gastric bypass[J]. Diabetes Care, 2013, 36(7): 1859-1864.

[84] Luo J, Ko B, Elliott M, et al. A nontumorigenic variant of FGF19 treats cholestatic liver diseases[J]. Sci Transl Med, 2014, 6(247): 247ra100.

[85] Schaap FG, van der Gaag NA, Gouma DJ, et al. High expression of the bile salt-homeostatic hormone fibroblast growth factor 19 in the liver of patients with extrahepatic cholestasis[J]. Hepatology, 2009, 49(4): 1228-1235.

[86] Benoit B, Meugnier E, Castelli M, et al. Fibroblast growth factor 19 regulates skeletal muscle mass and ameliorates muscle wasting in mice[J]. Nat Med, 2017, 23(8): 990-996.

[87] Nicholes K, Guillet S, Tomlinson E, et al. A mouse model of hepatocellular carcinoma: ectopic expression of fibroblast growth factor 19 in skeletal muscle of transgenic mice[J]. Am J Pathol, 2002, 160(6): 2295-2307.

[88] Zhou M, Learned RM, Rossi SJ, et al. Engineered fibroblast growth factor 19 reduces liver injury and resolves sclerosing cholangitis in Mdr2-deficient mice[J]. Hepatology, 2016, 63(3): 914-929.

[89] Mayo MJ, Wigg AJ, Leggett BA, et al. NGM282 for Treatment of patients with primary biliary cholangitis: A multicenter, randomized, double-blind, placebo-controlled trial[J]. Hepatol Commun, 2018, 2(9): 1037-1050.

[90] BonDurant LD, Potthoff MJ. Fibroblast growth factor 21: A versatile regulator of metabolic homeostasis[J]. Annu Rev Nutr, 2018, 38: 173-196.

[91] Giannini C, Feldstein AE, Santoro N, et al. Circulating levels of FGF-21 in obese youth: associations with liver fat content and markers of liver damage[J]. J Clin Endocrinol Metab, 2013, 98(7): 2993-3000.

[92] Lin Z, Gong Q, Wu C, et al. Dynamic change of serum FGF21 levels in response to glucose challenge in human[J]. J Clin Endocrinol Metab, 2012, 97(7): E1224-1228.

[93] Yilmaz Y, Eren F, Yonal O, et al. Increased serum FGF21 levels in patients with nonalcoholic fatty liver disease[J]. Eur J Clin Invest, 2010, 40(10): 887-892.

[94] Kliewer SA, Mangelsdorf DJ. A dozen years of discovery: insights

into the physiology and pharmacology of FGF21[J]. Cell Metab, 2019, 29(2): 246-253.

[95] Laeger T, Henagan TM, Albarado DC, et al. FGF21 is an endocrine signal of protein restriction[J]. J Clin Invest, 2014, 124(9): 3913-3922.

[96] Fisher FM, Kim M, Doridot L, et al. A critical role for ChREBP-mediated FGF21 secretion in hepatic fructose metabolism[J]. Mol Metab, 2017, 6(1): 14-21.

[97] von Holstein-Rathlou S, BonDurant LD, Peltekian L, et al. FGF21 mediates endocrine control of simple sugar intake and sweet taste preference by the liver[J]. Cell Metab, 2016, 23(2): 335-343.

[98] Talukdar S, Owen BM, Song P, et al. FGF21 regulates sweet and alcohol preference[J]. Cell Metab, 2016, 23(2): 344-349.

[99] Fisher FM, Chui PC, Nasser IA, et al. Fibroblast growth factor 21 limits lipotoxicity by promoting hepatic fatty acid activation in mice on methionine and choline-deficient diets[J]. Gastroenterology, 2014, 147(5): 1073-1083.e1076.

[100] Huang X, Yu C, Jin C, et al. Forced expression of hepatocyte-specific fibroblast growth factor 21 delays initiation of chemically induced hepatocarcinogenesis[J]. Mol Carcinog, 2006, 45(12): 934-942.

[101] Tanaka N, Takahashi S, Zhang Y, et al. Role of fibroblast growth factor 21 in the early stage of NASH induced by methionine- and choline-deficient diet[J]. Biochim Biophys Acta, 2015, 1852(7): 1242-1252.

[102] Desai BN, Singhal G, Watanabe M, et al. Fibroblast growth factor 21 (FGF21) is robustly induced by ethanol and has a protective role in ethanol associated liver injury[J]. Mol Metab, 2017, 6(11): 1395-1406.

[103] Ye D, Wang Y, Li H, et al. Fibroblast growth factor 21 protects against acetaminophen-induced hepatotoxicity by potentiating peroxisome proliferator-activated receptor coactivator protein-1alpha-mediated antioxidant capacity in mice[J]. Hepatology, 2014, 60(3): 977-989.

[104] Singhal G, Kumar G, Chan S, et al. Deficiency of fibroblast growth factor 21 (FGF21) promotes hepatocellular carcinoma (HCC) in mice on a long term obesogenic diet[J]. Mol Metab, 2018, 13: 56-66.

[105] Ye M, Lu W, Wang X, et al. FGF21-FGFR1 coordinates phospholipid homeostasis, lipid droplet function, and ER stress in obesity[J]. Endocrinology, 2016, 157(12): 4754-4769.

[106] Foltz IN, Hu S, King C, et al. Treating diabetes and obesity with an FGF21-mimetic antibody activating the βKlotho/FGFR1c receptor complex[J]. Sci Transl Med, 2012, 4(162): 162ra153.

[107] Gaich G, Chien JY, Fu H, et al. The effects of LY2405319, an FGF21 analog, in obese human subjects with type 2 diabetes[J]. Cell Metab, 2013, 18(3): 333-340.

[108] Lin Z, Tian H, Lam KS, et al. Adiponectin mediates the metabolic effects of FGF21 on glucose homeostasis and insulin sensitivity in mice[J]. Cell Metab, 2013, 17(5): 779-789.

[109] Huang Z, Zhong L, Lee JTH, et al. The FGF21-CCL11 axis mediates beiging of white adipose tissues by coupling sympathetic nervous system to type 2 immunity[J]. Cell Metab, 2017, 26(3): 493-508.e494.

[110] Lee P, Linderman JD, Smith S, et al. Irisin and FGF21 are cold-induced endocrine activators of brown fat function in humans[J]. Cell Metab, 2014, 19(2): 302-309.

[111] Hondares E, Iglesias R, Giralt A, et al. Thermogenic activation induces FGF21 expression and release in brown adipose tissue[J]. J Biol Chem, 2011, 286(15): 12983-12990.

[112] Ameka M, Markan KR, Morgan DA, et al. Liver derived FGF21 maintains core body temperature during acute cold exposure[J]. Sci Rep, 2019, 9(1): 630.

[113] Zhang Y, Xie Y, Berglund ED, et al. The starvation hormone, fibroblast growth factor-21, extends lifespan in mice[J]. Elife, 2012, 1: e00065.

[114] Youm YH, Horvath TL, Mangelsdorf DJ, et al. Prolongevity hormone FGF21 protects against immune senescence by delaying age-related thymic involution[J]. Proc Natl Acad Sci U S A, 2016, 113(4): 1026-1031.

[115] Adams AC, Coskun T, Cheng CC, et al. Fibroblast growth factor 21 is not required for the antidiabetic actions of the thiazoladinediones [J]. Mol Metab, 2013, 2(3): 205-214.

[116] Coate KC, Hernandez G, Thorne CA, et al. FGF21 is an exocrine pancreas secretagogue[J]. Cell Metab, 2017, 25(2): 472-480.

[117] Singhal G, Fisher FM, Chee MJ, et al. Fibroblast growth factor 21 (FGF21) protects against high fat diet induced inflammation and islet hyperplasia in pancreas[J]. PLoS One, 2016, 11(2): e0148252.

[118] Johnson CL, Mehmood R, Laing SW, et al. Silencing of the fibroblast growth factor 21 gene is an underlying cause of acinar cell injury in mice lacking MIST1[J]. Am J Physiol Endocrinol Metab, 2014, 306(8): E916-E928.

[119] Johnson CL, Weston JY, Chadi SA, et al. Fibroblast growth factor 21 reduces the severity of cerulein-induced pancreatitis in mice[J]. Gastroenterology, 2009, 137(5): 1795-1804.

[120] Kuroda M, Muramatsu R, Maedera N, et al. Peripherally derived FGF21 promotes remyelination in the central nervous system[J]. J Clin Invest, 2017, 127(9): 3496-3509.

[121] Soberg S, Sandholt CH, Jespersen NZ, et al. FGF21 is a sugar-induced hormone associated with sweet intake and preference in humans[J]. Cell Metab, 2017, 25(5): 1045-1053.e1046.

[122] Song P, Zechner C, Hernandez G, et al. The hormone FGF21 stimulates water drinking in response to ketogenic diet and alcohol[J]. Cell Metab, 2018, 27(6): 1338-1347.e1334.

[123] Frayling TM, Beaumont RN, Jones SE, et al. A common allele in FGF21 associated with sugar intake is associated with body shape, lower total body-fat percentage, and higher blood pressure[J]. Cell Rep, 2018, 23(2): 327-336.

[124] Schumann G, Liu C, O'Reilly P, et al. KLB is associated with alcohol drinking, and its gene product β-Klotho is necessary for FGF21 regulation of alcohol preference[J]. Proc Natl Acad Sci U S A, 2016, 113(50): 14372-14377.

[125] Restelli LM, Oettinghaus B, Halliday M, et al. Neuronal mitochondrial dysfunction activates the integrated stress response to induce fibroblast growth factor 21[J]. Cell Rep, 2018, 24(6): 1407-1414.

[126] Planavila A, Redondo I, Hondares E, et al. Fibroblast growth factor 21 protects against cardiac hypertrophy in mice[J]. Nat Commun, 2013, 4: 2019.

[127] Morville T, Sahl RE, Trammell SA, et al. Divergent effects of resistance and endurance exercise on plasma bile acids, FGF19, and FGF21 in humans[J]. JCI Insight, 2018, 3(15):122737

[128] Brahma MK, Adam RC, Pollak NM, et al. Fibroblast growth factor 21 is induced upon cardiac stress and alters cardiac lipid homeostasis[J]. J Lipid Res, 2014, 55(11): 2229-2241.

[129] Lin Z, Pan X, Wu F, et al. Fibroblast growth factor 21 prevents atherosclerosis by suppression of hepatic sterol regulatory element-binding protein-2 and induction of adiponectin in mice[J]. Circulation, 2015, 131(21): 1861-1871.

[130] Liu SQ, Roberts D, Kharitonenkov A, et al. Endocrine protection of ischemic myocardium by FGF21 from the liver and adipose tissue[J]. Sci Rep, 2013, 3: 2767.

[131] Yang H, Feng A, Lin S, et al. Fibroblast growth factor-21 prevents diabetic cardiomyopathy via AMPK-mediated antioxidation and lipid-lowering effects in the heart[J]. Cell Death Dis, 2018, 9(2): 227.

[132] Zhang C, Huang Z, Gu J, et al. Fibroblast growth factor 21 protects the heart from apoptosis in a diabetic mouse model via extracellular signal-regulated kinase 1/2-dependent signalling pathway[J]. Diabetologia, 2015, 58(8): 1937-1948.

[133] Pan X, Shao Y, Wu F, et al. FGF21 prevents angiotensin II-

induced hypertension and vascular dysfunction by activation of ACE2/angiotensin-(1-7) axis in mice[J]. Cell Metab, 2018, 27(6): 1323-1337.e1325.

[134] Kim KH, Jeong YT, Oh H, et al. Autophagy deficiency leads to protection from obesity and insulin resistance by inducing Fgf21 as a mitokine[J]. Nat Med, 2013, 19(1): 83-92.

[135] Lehtonen JM, Forsstrom S, Bottani E, et al. FGF21 is a biomarker for mitochondrial translation and mtDNA maintenance disorders[J]. Neurology, 2016, 87(22): 2290-2299.

[136] Geng L, Liao B, Jin L, et al. Exercise alleviates obesity-induced metabolic dysfunction via enhancing FGF21 sensitivity in adipose tissues[J]. Cell Rep, 2019, 26(10): 2738-2752.e2734.

[137] Pereira RO, Tadinada SM, Zasadny FM, et al. OPA1 deficiency promotes secretion of FGF21 from muscle that prevents obesity and insulin resistance[J]. Embo j, 2017, 36(14): 2126-2145.

[138] Tanimura Y, Aoi W, Takanami Y, et al. Acute exercise increases fibroblast growth factor 21 in metabolic organs and circulation[J]. Physiol Rep, 2016, 4(12). e12828

[139] Lee MS, Choi SE, Ha ES, et al. Fibroblast growth factor-21 protects human skeletal muscle myotubes from palmitate-induced insulin resistance by inhibiting stress kinase and NF-κB[J]. Metabolism, 2012, 61(8): 1142-1151.

[140] Izumiya Y, Bina HA, Ouchi N, et al. FGF21 is an Akt-regulated myokine[J]. FEBS Lett, 2008, 582(27): 3805-3810.

[141] Owen BM, Ding X, Morgan DA, et al. FGF21 acts centrally to induce sympathetic nerve activity, energy expenditure, and weight loss[J]. Cell Metab, 2014, 20(4): 670-677.

[142] Douris N, Stevanovic DM, Fisher FM, et al. Central fibroblast growth factor 21 browns white fat via sympathetic action in male mice[J]. Endocrinology, 2015, 156(7): 2470-2481.

[143] Liang Q, Zhong L, Zhang J, et al. FGF21 maintains glucose homeostasis by mediating the cross talk between liver and brain during prolonged fasting[J]. Diabetes, 2014, 63(12): 4064-4075.

[144] Owen BM, Bookout AL, Ding X, et al. FGF21 contributes to neuroendocrine control of female reproduction[J]. Nat Med, 2013, 19(9): 1153-1156.

[145] Bookout AL, de Groot MH, Owen BM, et al. FGF21 regulates metabolism and circadian behavior by acting on the nervous system[J]. Nat Med, 2013, 19(9): 1147-1152.

[146] Bookout AL, de Groot MH, Owen BM, et al. FGF21 regulates metabolism and circadian behavior by acting on the nervous system[J]. Nat Med, 2013, 19(9): 1147-1152.

[147] Wang Q, Yuan J, Yu Z, et al. FGF21 attenuates high-fat diet-induced cognitive impairment via metabolic regulation and anti-inflammation of obese mice[J]. Mol Neurobiol, 2018, 55(6): 4702-4717.

[148] Yu Y, Bai F, Wang W, et al. Fibroblast growth factor 21 protects mouse brain against D-galactose induced aging via suppression of oxidative stress response and advanced glycation end products formation[J]. Pharmacol Biochem Behav, 2015, 133: 122-131.

[149] Sarruf DA, Thaler JP, Morton GJ, et al. Fibroblast growth factor 21 action in the brain increases energy expenditure and insulin sensitivity in obese rats[J]. Diabetes, 2010, 59(7): 1817-1824.

[150] Veniant MM, Hale C, Helmering J, et al. FGF21 promotes metabolic homeostasis via white adipose and leptin in mice[J]. PLoS One, 2012, 7(7): e40164.

[151] Xu J, Lloyd DJ, Hale C, et al. Fibroblast growth factor 21 reverses hepatic steatosis, increases energy expenditure, and improves insulin sensitivity in diet-induced obese mice[J]. Diabetes, 2009, 58(1): 250-259.

[152] So WY, Cheng Q, Xu A, et al. Loss of fibroblast growth factor 21 action induces insulin resistance, pancreatic islet hyperplasia and dysfunction in mice[J]. Cell Death Dis, 2015, 6: e1707.

[153] Zhang C, Shao M, Yang H, et al. Attenuation of hyperlipidemia- and diabetes-induced early-stage apoptosis and late-stage renal dysfunction via administration of fibroblast growth factor-21 is

associated with suppression of renal inflammation[J]. PLoS One, 2013, 8(12): e82275.

[154] Kim HW, Lee JE, Cha JJ, et al. Fibroblast growth factor 21 improves insulin resistance and ameliorates renal injury in db/db mice[J]. Endocrinology, 2013, 154(9): 3366-3376.

[155] Tang TT, Li YY, Li JJ, et al. Liver-heart crosstalk controls IL-22 activity in cardiac protection after myocardial infarction[J]. Theranostics, 2018, 8(16): 4552-4562.

[156] Wang N, Zhao TT, Li SM, et al. Fibroblast growth factor 21 ameliorates pancreatic fibrogenesis via regulating polarization of macrophages[J]. Exp Cell Res, 2019, 382(1): 111457.

[157] Li S, Guo X, Zhang T, et al. Fibroblast growth factor 21 ameliorates high glucose-induced fibrogenesis in mesangial cells through inhibiting STAT5 signaling pathway[J]. Biomed Pharmacother, 2017, 93: 695-704.

[158] Li S, Wang N, Guo X, et al. Fibroblast growth factor 21 regulates glucose metabolism in part by reducing renal glucose reabsorption[J]. Biomed Pharmacother, 2018, 108: 355-366.

[159] Lin XL, He XL, Zeng JF, et al. FGF21 increases cholesterol efflux by upregulating ABCA1 through the ERK1/2-PPARγ-LXRα pathway in THP1 macrophage-derived foam cells[J]. DNA Cell Biol, 2014, 33(8): 514-521.

[160] Yu Y, He J, Li S, et al. Fibroblast growth factor 21 (FGF21) inhibits macrophage-mediated inflammation by activating Nrf2 and suppressing the NF-κB signaling pathway[J]. Int Immunopharmacol, 2016, 38: 144-152.

[161] Li H, Wu G, Fang Q, et al. Fibroblast growth factor 21 increases insulin sensitivity through specific expansion of subcutaneous fat[J]. Nat Commun, 2018, 9(1): 272.

[162] Li SM, Wang WF, Zhou LH, et al. Fibroblast growth factor 21 expressions in white blood cells and sera of patients with gestational diabetes mellitus during gestation and postpartum[J]. Endocrine, 2015, 48(2): 519-527.

[163] Li JY, Wang N, Khoso MH, et al. FGF-21 elevated IL-10 production to correct LPS-induced inflammation[J]. Inflammation, 2018, 41(3): 751-759.

[164] Wang WF, Ma L, Liu MY, et al. A novel function for fibroblast growth factor 21: stimulation of NADPH oxidase-dependent ROS generation[J]. Endocrine, 2015, 49(2): 385-395.

[165] Li SM, Yu YH, Li L, et al. Treatment of CIA mice with FGF21 down-regulates TH17-IL-17 axis[J]. Inflammation, 2016, 39(1): 309-319.

[166] Saito H, Kusano K, Kinosaki M, et al. Human fibroblast growth factor-23 mutants suppress Na$^+$-dependent phosphate co-transport activity and 1α,25-dihydroxyvitamin D3 production[J]. J Biol Chem, 2003, 278(4): 2206-2211.

[167] Shimada T, Kakitani M, Yamazaki Y, et al. Targeted ablation of Fgf23 demonstrates an essential physiological role of FGF23 in phosphate and vitamin D metabolism[J]. J Clin Invest, 2004, 113(4): 561-568.

[168] Shimada T, Mizutani S, Muto T, et al. Cloning and characterization of FGF23 as a causative factor of tumor-induced osteomalacia[J]. Proc Natl Acad Sci U S A, 2001, 98(11): 6500-6505.

[169] Andrukhova O, Smorodchenko A, Egerbacher M, et al. FGF23 promotes renal calcium reabsorption through the TRPV5 channel[J]. Embo j, 2014, 33(3): 229-246.

[170] Andrukhova O, Slavic S, Smorodchenko A, et al. FGF23 regulates renal sodium handling and blood pressure[J]. EMBO Mol Med, 2014, 6(6): 744-759.

[171] Ben-Dov IZ, Galitzer H, Lavi-Moshayoff V, et al. The parathyroid is a target organ for FGF23 in rats[J]. J Clin Invest, 2007, 117(12): 4003-4008.

[172] Toro L, Barrientos V, Leon P, et al. Erythropoietin induces bone marrow and plasma fibroblast growth factor 23 during acute kidney injury[J]. Kidney Int, 2018, 93(5): 1131-1141.

[173] Rabadi S, Udo I, Leaf DE, *et al*. Acute blood loss stimulates fibroblast growth factor 23 production[J]. Am J Physiol Renal Physiol, 2018, 314(1): F132-F139.

[174] Autosomal dominant hypophosphataemic rickets is associated with mutations in FGF23[J]. Nat Genet, 2000, 26(3): 345-348.

[175] Bowe AE, Finnegan R, Jan de Beur SM, *et al*. FGF-23 inhibits renal tubular phosphate transport and is a PHEX substrate[J]. Biochem Biophys Res Commun, 2001, 284(4): 977-981.

[176] Riminucci M, Collins MT, Fedarko NS, *et al*. FGF-23 in fibrous dysplasia of bone and its relationship to renal phosphate wasting[J]. J Clin Invest, 2003, 112(5): 683-692.

[177] Hoffman WH, Jueppner HW, Deyoung BR, *et al*. Elevated fibroblast growth factor-23 in hypophosphatemic linear nevus sebaceous syndrome[J]. Am J Med Genet A, 2005, 134(3): 233-236.

[178] Kato K, Jeanneau C, Tarp MA, *et al*. Polypeptide GalNAc-transferase T3 and familial tumoral calcinosis. Secretion of fibroblast growth factor 23 requires O-glycosylation[J]. J Biol Chem, 2006, 281(27): 18370-18377.

[179] Ichikawa S, Imel EA, Sorenson AH, *et al*. Tumoral calcinosis presenting with eyelid calcifications due to novel missense mutations in the glycosyl transferase domain of the GALNT3 gene[J]. J Clin Endocrinol Metab, 2006, 91(11): 4472-4475.

[180] Garringer HJ, Fisher C, Larsson TE, *et al*. The role of mutant UDP-N-acetyl-alpha-D-galactosamine-polypeptide N-acetyl-galactosaminyltransferase 3 in regulating serum intact fibroblast growth factor 23 and matrix extracellular phosphoglycoprotein in heritable tumoral calcinosis[J]. J Clin Endocrinol Metab, 2006, 91(10): 4037-4042.

[181] Benet-Pages A, Orlik P, Strom TM, *et al*. An FGF23 missense mutation causes familial tumoral calcinosis with hyperphosphatemia [J]. Hum Mol Genet, 2005, 14(3): 385-390.

[182] Chefetz I, Heller R, Galli-Tsinopoulou A, *et al*. A novel homozygous missense mutation in FGF23 causes familial tumoral calcinosis associated with disseminated visceral calcification[J]. Hum Genet, 2005, 118(2): 261-266.

[183] Araya K, Fukumoto S, Backenroth R, *et al*. A novel mutation in fibroblast growth factor 23 gene as a cause of tumoral calcinosis[J]. J Clin Endocrinol Metab, 2005, 90(10): 5523-5527.

[184] Abbasi F, Ghafouri-Fard S, Javaheri M, *et al*. A new missense mutation in FGF23 gene in a male with hyperostosis-hyperphosphatemia syndrome (HHS)[J]. Gene, 2014, 542(2): 269-271.

[185] Faul C, Amaral AP, Oskouei B, *et al*. FGF23 induces left ventricular hypertrophy[J]. J Clin Invest, 2011, 121(11): 4393-4408.

[186] Mitsnefes MM, Betoko A, Schneider MF, *et al*. FGF23 and left ventricular hypertrophy in children with CKD[J]. Clin J Am Soc Nephrol, 2018, 13(1): 45-52.

[187] McGrath ER, Himali JJ, Levy D, *et al*. Circulating fibroblast growth factor 23 levels and incident dementia: the Framingham heart study[J]. PLoS One, 2019, 14(3): e0213321.

[188] Liu P, Chen L, Bai X, *et al*. Impairment of spatial learning and memory in transgenic mice overexpressing human fibroblast growth factor-23[J]. Brain Res, 2011, 1412: 9-17.

Chapter 1
Growth Factors Reviews

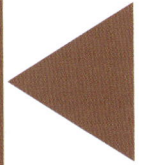

Fibroblast growth factors, old kids on the new block

Xiaokun Li, Cong Wang, Jian Xiao, Wallace L. McKeehan, Fen Wang

It has been gratifying for early basic researchers on fibroblast growth factors (FGF) that their Cinderella in the growth factor arena is now drawing so much attention as a druggable target by pharmaceutical companies and translational researchers. The first two prototype FGFs, FGF1 and FGF2, discovered in the early seventies, were designated acidic and basic FGF (aFGF and bFGF) based on their activity to stimulate fibroblast proliferation and their isoelectric point [1,2]. Subsequently 20 more FGF homologues have been identified as the family members in mammals [3-20]. Genes coding for a large number of FGFs were cloned based on homology in the amino acid sequence. It was soon found that the name "fibroblast growth factor" was not the best name to describe the diverse functions of the family members and their receptors since many FGFs do not even have receptors expressed in fibroblasts and elicit no activity in fibroblasts. In addition, many FGFs induce diverse cellular responses beyond growth promoting signals in different target cells. Despite being misleading to some degrees, the name "fibroblast growth factor" followed by a number (FGF1, 2, 3, 4, etc.) has been preserved and replaced numerous other names used to describe either tissue origin, target, function, or properties of the FGF molecule. FGF signaling has long not been a favorite of pharmaceutical companies largely because of the diversity of both ligands and receptors in the family, its wide range of target cell types, diverse functions, and complexity of FGF signals that intersect either directly or indirectly with multiple pathways. The complexity of the multi-subunit transmembrane FGF signaling complex in both the extracellular and the intracellular portions has also been a major factor. Several cofactors are integral regulatory components of the FGF signaling complex. These include the chemically heterogeneous heparan sulfate (HS) cofactors, and in the case of endocrine FGFs, the Klotho coreceptors. These cofactors and coreceptors not only participate in FGF receptor-binding specificity and affinity, but also in specifying signaling activities. Therefore, a full understanding of the molecular mechanisms underlying the specificity of FGF signaling is important for therapeutic usage of FGFs.

1. FGF signaling axis

1.1 FGFs

The FGFs are single chain polypeptides that are tissue regulatory molecules controlling a broad spectrum of cellular processes in both embryonic and adult tissues. The polypeptides have one conserved domain flanked by non-conserved extensions (Fig. 1A). Most FGFs have an N-terminal signal peptide that facilitates secretion through classical mechanisms. However, several FGFs, including FGF1 and FGF2, do not have a cleavable signal peptide and are secreted in a non-conventional manner. Seven FGF subfamilies have been defined based on their sequence homology and function (Fig. 1B). These FGF subfamilies can also be divided into two general groups, the canonical FGFs comprising paracrine or autocrine-acting FGF1-10, FGF16-18, FGF20, and FGF22 and the endocrine-acting FGFs, FGF15 (mouse)/FGF19 (human), FGF21, and FGF23; and the non-canonical FGFs comprising FGF11-14. The canonical FGFs elicit regulatory functions through high affinity binding to and activating FGF receptors (FGFR). An autocrine canonical FGF acts on the cells of origin as a self-stimulator, and a paracrine

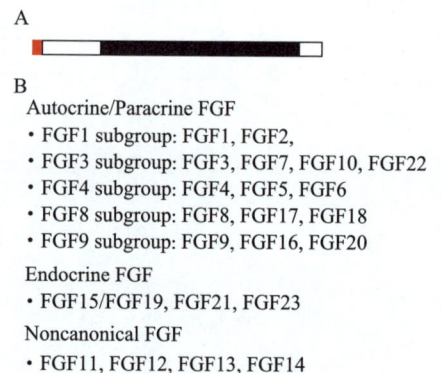

A

B
Autocrine/Paracrine FGF
• FGF1 subgroup: FGF1, FGF2,
• FGF3 subgroup: FGF3, FGF7, FGF10, FGF22
• FGF4 subgroup: FGF4, FGF5, FGF6
• FGF8 subgroup: FGF8, FGF17, FGF18
• FGF9 subgroup: FGF9, FGF16, FGF20

Endocrine FGF
• FGF15/FGF19, FGF21, FGF23

Noncanonical FGF
• FGF11, FGF12, FGF13, FGF14

Fig. 1. The FGF family. (A) Schematic of the FGF. Red box, signal peptide; open boxes, non-conserved, N- and C-terminal domains; solid box, conserved core domain. (B) FGF subfamilies. The 22 FGFs are grouped into 7 subfamilies based on sequence homology and function.

FGF is secreted by one cell and acts on another locally within tissues. In contrast, the endocrine FGF originates at a distal organ site and reaches the target through the blood circulation in a classical endocrine mode of action. The non-canonical FGFs do not bind to the FGFR but elicit their activities intracellularly, such as through interaction with voltage-gated sodium channels and calcium channels [21-23].

1.2 FGFRs

The FGFR is a single chain transmembrane tyrosine kinase that consists of a ligand binding extracellular domain, a single transmembrane domain, and an intracellular tyrosine kinase domain that is separated into two parts by an insertion domain (Fig. 2). The mammalian FGFR is encoded by four highly homologous genes [24-27]. Except for the Fgfr4 gene for which only one splice isoform occurs naturally [28], other three Fgfrs have been found to encode multiple splice variants. These splice variants generate diversity of sequence and function in the ligand-binding extracellular domain and the intracellular substrate-binding and kinase domains [29]. It has been speculated that the combination of FGFR1 splice variation sequences can potentially encode up to 256 splice isoforms [29]. FGFR3 and FGFR4 have 3 immunoglobin (Ig)-like domains in the extracellular domains. As a consequence of alternative splicing, the extracellular domain of both FGFR1 and FGFR2 can contain either 2 or 3 Ig-like loops. The presence of the first Ig-loop modulates the affinity for both FGF and FGFR-binding heparin/heparan sulfate [30-32]. Two major isoforms generated by alternative splicing in the second half of Ig-loop III, namely IIIb and IIIc in FGFR1, FGFR2, and FGFR3 have been reported. This variation defines ligand-binding affinity and specificity of FGFR1-3 [33,34]. Several other splice variations at the extracellular domain have been found in FGFR2, although the functional significance of these variants remains unknown [35]. The role of the alternatively spliced dipeptide VT (valine-threonine) in the intracellular juxtamembrane domain of FGFR is controversial. It has been shown that the presence of VT is required for FGFR to bind FRS2α and FRS2β and therefore contributes to signaling specificity [36,37]. However, other reports show that the dipeptide is dispensable for the binding of FRS2α and FRS2β to FGFR1 even though it enhances the binding affinity between substrate and the receptor kinase [38]. The variations in the kinase domain and C-terminal tail following the kinase domain of FGFRs have only been found in cancer cells [29,39]. Although the kinase domains of the four FGFR isotypes are highly homologous (>80%) in the primary amino acid sequence and share common tyrosine phosphorylation sites (Fig. 2), the four FGFRs elicit receptor-, cofactor-, coreceptor-, and cell type-specific activities in cells [40-43]. Seven major tyrosine autophosphorylation sites have been identified in the FGFR1 kinase domain [44-47]. Y (tyrosine) 653 is predominant in activation (derepression) of the receptor kinase activity [44-47] while Y654 contributes to maximal activation [48]. Phosphorylation of Y766 is required for recruiting phospholipase Cγ (PLCγ) *via* its SH2 domains to the FGFR1 kinase [49-51]. Y463 is a binding site for the adapter proteins CRK and CRK-like [52-54] and phosphorylated Y730 is a binding site for the 85 kDa regulatory subunit alpha of phosphatidylinositol 3-kinase (PI3K) [45,49,55]. The function of other phosphorylation sites, including Y583, and Y585 has not been clearly established, despite some evidence that they contribute to the intensity and extent of FGFR signaling [48]. An FGFR2 splice variant that lacks exon 16 has been reported in prostate epithelial cells, which does not have the PLCγ-binding site [56]. The significance of this splice variant remains to be elucidated.

1.3 Heparan sulfate (HS) cofactors

HS is the glycan component of proteoglycans in the pericellular matrix and on the cell surface. It is a highly heterogeneous glycosaminoglycan [46,57-59]. Variations in degrees and patterns of sulfation on HS motifs affect their interaction with FGFs and FGFRs and have been shown to play a role in determination of ligand-binding and downstream signaling specificity of FGFR complexes [60-65]. Although HS motifs with high affinity for FGFs and FGFRs are normally sulfated,

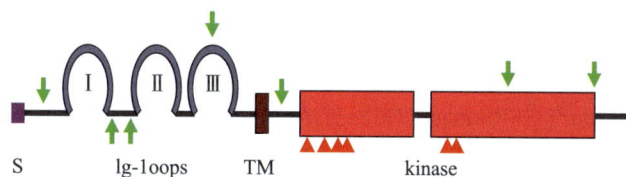

Fig. 2. Topology of a prototypical FGF receptor tyrosine kinase. S, signal peptide; I, II, III, immunoglobulin-like domain 1, 2, and 3; TM, transmembrane domain. Red box, tyrosine kinase domain that is separated by a kinase insertion sequence; green arrows, alternative splice sites; triangles, tyrosine phosphorylation sites.

emerging evidence shows that the affinity is not simply proportional to total charge density and degree of sulfation. Instead, these high-affinity motifs are often less than fully sulfated and have unique sulfation patterns [66,67]. Because of affinity for both FGF and FGFR, HS in the tissue environment largely plays two general roles that impact overall FGFR signaling. Tissue matrix HS acts as an FGFR-independent depot and stabilizes influence for canonical paracrine/autocrine FGFs [68,69]. It limits access of FGF that are generally long-lived and at considerable concentrations in the matrix to cell membrane FGFR except when needed [46]. The second role is as an integral part of the FGF signaling complex through a distinct HS-binding domain in the extracellular domain of FGFR. Motifs within this class of HS are thought to be less abundant and potentially more specific than matrix HS [66,67]. FGFR-bound HS interacts concurrently with both FGFR and FGF within the FGF-FGFR-HS signaling complex.

Both our early models based on protein mutagenesis and in silico modeling [70,71] and the crystal structure [72] of the FGF2-FGFR1c-HS complex show a 2-2-2 complex of FGF-FGFR-HS, in which one single heparan sulfate chain may contact Ig-loop II of one FGFR, the inter-Ig-loop connector sequence and Ig-loop III of the same FGFR, and extend to Ig-loop III of the adjacent FGFR in the FGFR dimer. Ig loops II and III cooperate both within monomers and across dimers with cellular HS to confer cell type-dependent specificity of the FGFR complex for FGF ligands [73]. It is unclear whether FGF stabilizes proximity of random interactions of monomeric units or activates a pre-existing inactive oligomeric complex of HS-FGFR *via* conformation changes [46,61,66,67]. However, emerging data pose that together with HS, the FGFR forms a dimer constitutively in the absence of FGF [70,71,74]. Interaction with HS restrains FGFR dimers in an inactive conformation and FGF binding converts the HS-FGFR complex from the inactive repressed conformation to an active arrangement that allows an initial trans-phosphorylation between the kinase domains of FGFR dimers. Structural studies indicate that trans-phosphorylation of tyrosine 653 and then 654 (in FGFR1) changes conformation of an autoinhibitory loop within the kinase domain that normally restricts access of substrates to the active site of the FGFR kinases [48,75].

1.4 Klothos

Unlike paracrine/autocrine FGFs, the endocrine FGFs, FGF15/FGF19, FGF21, and FGF23 have little or no affinity for HS [76]. This property permits their endocrine circulation and movement through tissue matrices without being trapped and stored prior to reaching distal target cells. The specificity of endocrine FGF signaling at the cellular level is directed by a family of membrane-anchored proteins that include αKlotho (αKL) and βKlotho (KLB). Although endocrine FGFs signal through the same FGFR as canonical FGFs, they have little affinity for FGFR in the absence of Klothos. KLB interacts with FGFR independent of FGF and with FGF independent of FGFR [77-79]. Although αKL binds the extracellular domain of FGFR1, it poorly interacts with FGF23. Instead, binding of αKL with FGFR1 forms a *de novo* site generated at the composite FGFR1c-αKL interface, which binds the C-terminal domain of FGF23 [80]. Thus, the major role of αKL and KLB is to facilitate high affinity binding and subsequent activation of FGFRs by endocrine FGFs. αKL specifically facilitates binding of FGF23 to its receptor and controls mineral metabolism *via* a vitamin D controlled bone to kidney axis where αKL is expressed [81]. Inactivation of αKL induces hyperphosphatemia in mice that highly express FGF23 [82]. The cofactor KLB facilitates high affinity binding and signaling of FGF19 (mouse FGF15) and FGF21 and controls cholesterol/bile acid, lipid, and glucose metabolism in the liver and adipocytes [83].

Expression of neither KLB nor FGFR4 alone affects cell population dynamics in KLB- and FGFR4-deficient cells. However, co-expression of KLB and FGFR4 restricts cell population growth *via* apoptosis in an endocrine FGF19 or FGF1 dependent manner [84]. This indicates that the KLB interaction with the FGFR4 tyrosine kinase complex not only serves to confer high affinity for endocrine FGF19, but also plays a role in directing signaling of the FGFR4 complex independent of the activating FGF [84,85].

1.5 The FGF signaling pathways

The signaling cascade downstream of the transmembrane receptor, including PLC-γ, MAP kinase, and PI3K pathways have been implicated in all four FGFR kinases (Fig. 3). Among them, PLC-γ binds to a specific phosphorylated tyrosine residue at the C-terminal tail of the FGFR kinases [50,51]. However, the MAP kinase and PI3K pathways need to be recruited to the FGFR by a membrane-anchored adaptor protein, FRS2α (FGF receptor substrate 2α), which undergoes an extensive pattern of tyrosine and serine/threonine phosphorylation upon FGFR activation [86-93]. In addition, CRK has also been proposed to serve as a functional adaptor that binds to the FGFR [52], which has been reported to further link the ERK pathway to FGFR1. The activation of the ERK pathway by the FGFR tyrosine kinase is tightly regulated by both positive and negative feedback loops at both transcriptional and post translational levels (Fig. 3). Sprouty (SPRY) proteins, which comprise four conserved members, SPRY1-4, present a feedback regulator of the FGF pathway at the posttranslational level [94]. Tyrosine phosphorylation of SPRY creates a decoy site that binds the docking molecule GRB2 and prevents translocation of SOS to the plasma membrane to activate RAS. SEF (similar expression of FGF) inhibits binding of FRS2α to the FGFR and prevents activation of ERK, and, therefore, negatively regulates the RAS-MAPK pathway [95,96]. Activation of the ERK and PI3K/AKT pathways has been implicated in most FGFR regulatory functions. Deletion of the PLCγ binding site on FGFR1 does not affect FGFR1-elicited cellular responses, which include mitogenesis, neuronal differentiation, mesoderm induction, induction of urokinase-type plasminogen activator, and chemotaxis. However, the PLC-γ binding site is required for FGFR1 to induce benign prostate cancer cells to acquire the proliferative response to FGFR1, although it appears not to be required for the mitogenic response [97]. This suggests that path-

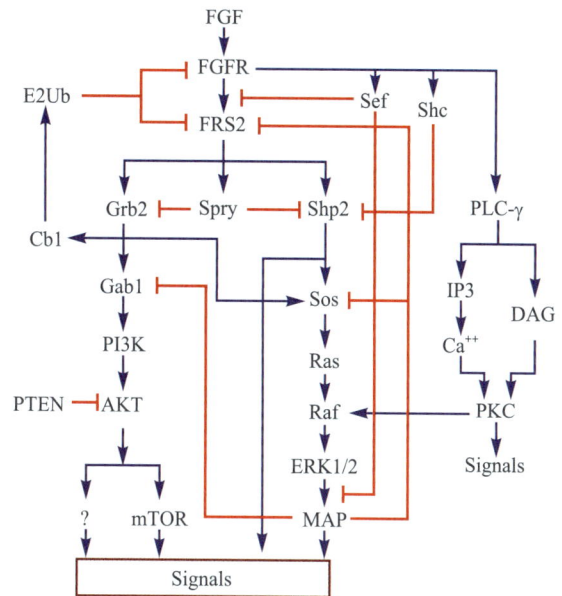

Fig. 3. Signaling pathways downstream of FGFR tyrosine kinase. Shown is a wiring diagram with blue lines indicating positive effects, and red lines indicating negative effects.

ways linked to FGFR1 Y766 contribute to prostate cancer progression rather than playing a direct role in cell cycle and mitogenesis. Experiments with purified recombinant FGFRs *in vitro* or when overexpressed at high levels in cell lines, such as Sf9 insect cells or COS7 mammalian cells, indicate that the four FGFR isotypes exhibit similar if not identical substrate phosphorylation patterns (Wang, unpublished results). However, in the experiments with moderate expression levels in cells, the results are not consistent. In some experimental systems, the four FGFR isotypes elicit similar and redundant effects on cell phenotypes, and in others, exert different effects [40]. Overexpression of the FGFR kinase at levels far beyond the minute normal cellular levels likely homogenizes and masks receptor and cell type specific effects of the different FGFR kinases. More sensitive analytical approaches *in situ* as well as robust and controlled experimental systems that hold promise of revealing and dissecting such differences are needed for developing FGFR isotype- and cell type-specific inhibitors or activators.

The FRS2 family is composed of two highly homologous members, FRS2α and FRS2β, which belong to a category of adaptor proteins that have binding sites for molecules both upstream and downstream of it in signaling networks. It physically presents downstream molecules to the upstream molecules. Depletion of FRS2α abrogates the ability of FGFR kinases to activate the MAP kinase and PI3K/AKT pathways (Wang, unpublished data). Ablation of Frs2α$_z$ in mice causes severe defects in embryonic development and results in early embryonic lethality at E7.0-7.5 [98]. Although it is not clear whether the two FRS2 members are functionally redundant, expression of FRS2β in FRS2α-deficient cells restores the ability of FGFR1 to activate both the MAPK and PI3K/AKT pathways [99]. In addition, FRS2α is also engaged in the feedback regulation of the FGF signaling pathway [100,101]. As illustrated in Fig. 3, FRS2α appears to be the key adaptor protein in the FGFR signaling cascade that mediates multiple downstream pathways of the FGFR, as well as control of the amplitude of the signaling intensity. However, whether FRS2 is also involved in the receptor and cell type specificity of signaling elicited by the FGFR kinases remains to be elucidated.

2. Translational application of the FGFs and their signaling pathways

2.1 Aberrant FGF signaling in diseases

In embryos, the FGF, FGFR kinase, and heparan sulfate components of the FGF signaling complex are expressed in a spatiotemporally- and cell-specific pattern that changes constantly as development proceeds. In adult organs, components of the FGF signaling axis are expressed in a cell type-specific mode and are important in the mediation of external signals and communication within compartments that maintain tissue homeostasis and function. Abnormal expression of FGF and FGFR and aberrant activation of the FGF signaling axis are frequently found associated with various adult tissue-specific pathologies and cause developmental disorders [40,46,53,102-110]. The subversion of the homeostasis-promoting activity of resident epithelial FGFR2 in a variety of tissues [40,41,46,111] and concurrent ectopic expression of normally mesenchymal FGFR1IIIc in epithelial cells [40,112-115] is often found associated with tumor progression. Changes in core protein expression of HS proteoglycans as well as sulfation patterns have been reported to contribute to progression of premalignant tumor cells to malignancy [46]. Currently, extensive efforts have been taken to explore the translational application of manipulation of the FGF signaling activities, both using the FGF directly and chemical agonists or antagonists as in the areas summarized hereafter. As a heparin-binding protein, delivery of heparin-binding FGF through the circulation and the tissue matrix remains a challenging issue. Treating large traumatic tympanic membrane perforation with FGF2 improved closure rates compared with the control group [116]. Recently, new technologies, including multi-walled carbon nanotubes, have been used to deliver FGF2, which improves bone regeneration in animal models [117,118].

2.2 Wound healing

As potent mitogenic factors, both FGF1 and FGF2 have been extensively explored for their potential in wound healing. FGF1 induces cell proliferation in the wounded area and promotes the cells to produce cytokines and other growth factors that induce migration of macrophages and monocytes toward the wounded area to remove damaged or dead cells [119,120]. FGF1 also induces epithelial cells and vessel endothelial cells to migrate toward the healing tissues. True to its original name, FGF promotes growth and differentiation of fibroblasts, and induces cells to release collagenase and plasminogen activators to promote angiogenesis in the wounded tissues [121,122]. In addition, FGF1 also down regulates α I procollagen expression and suppresses collagen production and deposit in fibroblasts and therefore prevents scar formation [123,124].

Recombinant FGF1 and 2 (rFGF1 and rFGF2) have been developed for clinical trials in several countries. Since 1992, recombinant FGF2 has been used in several hospitals in China, and the results show that recombinant FGF2 improves healing in burn trauma, skin flap grafts, intractable cerebrospinal fluid rhinorrhea, intractable skin ulcer, postoperative mastoid cavity problems, pressure ulcers, chronically ischemic tissue and traumatic ulcers, bone fracture, periodontitis-induced damage of human periodontal tissue, diabetic gangrene, diabetes-related chronic ulcers, peripheral artery disease, and gastric ulcers [124-149]. The outcomes of the clinical trials demonstrate that FGF2 can be used as an agent to accelerate the healing of fresh and chronic wounds and improve the quality of healing of wounds of diverse types. In addition, FGF1 has been shown to elicit modest nerve regeneration after spinal cord injury [150]. FGF7 acts exclusively through a subset of FGF receptor isoforms (FGFR2b) and has been developed by Amgen (palifermin) to prevent and speed up the healing of severe sores in the mouth and throat caused by chemotherapy and radiation therapy, which are used to treat cancers of the blood or bone marrow [151-156].

2.3 Cardiac protection

Heart failure also called congestive heart failure or congestive cardiac failure occurs when the heart fails to pump sufficient blood to meet the needs of the body. It remains a major cause of morbidity and mortality and causes critical health problems especially in Western societies. Reduction in the efficiency of the myocardium through overloading or damage leads to cardiac hypertrophy and fibrosis, which subsequently progresses to heart failure. Several members of the FGF family, including FGF1, FGF2, FGF5, FGF16, FGF21, and FGF23 have been shown to play roles in the heart. FGF signaling is essential for cardiomyocyte homeostasis through phosphorylating connexin 43 (Cx43), which is required for the maintenance of gap junctions [157]. FGF1 is released from the myocardial tissue into pericardial fluid during severe myocardial ischemia [158].

Treatment with biodegradable hydrogel microspheres containing FGF2 improved left ventricle function and inhibited left ventricle remodeling by angiogenesis in pigs with chronic myocardial infarction [159]. Intramyocardial injection of FGF-2 plus heparin suppresses the progression of cardiac failure in rat models [160]. Similarly, treating pigs with adenovirus carrying FGF5 cDNA improves wall-thickening and cardiac function [161]. In humans, FGF treatment has likewise shown cardioprotective effects: a single intracoronary infusion of rFGF2 shows trends toward symptomatic improvement of angina and myocardial function in patients with advanced coronary artery disease [162]. Treatment of patients with a bicistronic VEGF/FGF2 plasmid improves cardiac function with respect to exercise tolerance and clinical symptoms [163]. Intracoronary administration FGF-2 in patients with severe ischemic heart disease increases regional wall thickening and reduces the extent of the ischemic area [164]. Treatment with Ad5-FGF4 results in favorable anti-ischemic effects [165]. All these initial small and unblinded studies with FGF proteins or encoding cDNAs were encouraging and demonstrated both clinical improvement and evidence of angiogenesis. However, subsequent double-blind placebo-controlled trials did not confirm the initial high efficacy observed in the small trials [166]. Future larger trials are needed to confirm whether FGF treatment is efficacious, safe, and practical for the heart failure patients.

2.4 Metabolic disorders

The FGFs are best known for their diverse roles in mediating cellular homeostasis through short-range cell-to-cell communication within tissues [167]. However, FGF19 (or mouse FGF15), FGF21, and FGF23, have been identified as endocrine hormones since they originate in tissues distal to the metabolic organs they target and are transported through the circulation [17,168-171]. A diurnal physiologic role of the ileal FGF19-hepatocyte FGFR4 axis in bile acid metabolism during normal feeding has been established [169,172]. FGF21 regulates energy homeostasis mainly through activating the FGFR1/KLB complex in adipocytes [173], and represents a novel target for the development of therapies for the treatment of obesity, diabetes, and cardiovascular diseases.

Expression of FGF21 is controlled by a complex network of transcriptional regulators, which modulate FGF21 expression in response to a wide array of physiological stimuli or pharmacologic agents [174]. The function of FGF21, if any, in normally fed mice is not clear. Generally, the liver FGF21-adipocyte FGFR1 signaling axis appears to come into effect only after prolonged starvation, when it uncouples lipid metabolism between the adipocytes and hepatocytes, prolonging the supply of lipid fuels to maintain life-saving glucose levels as long as possible until a feeding opportunity arises [175]. When administered, both FGF19 and FGF21 dramatically reverse obesity and its associated symptoms, including type 2 diabetes [176-178]. Studies with tissue-specific Fgfr1-knockout animals have revealed that the adipocyte, via FGFR1, is the specific target of FGF19 and FGF21 that alleviates obesity and allied symptoms [173,175,179]. Although several reports show that FGF21 controls ketogenic and triglyceride clearance in the liver [180-183], unlike FGF19, FGF21 is unable to bind FGFR4-KLB complex with affinity comparable to FGFR1-KLB [83,170,184,185]. Therefore, at physiological concentrations, FGF21 is unlikely to signal in the liver where FGFR4-KLB predominantly resides. It has been shown that the metabolic effects of FGF21 on glucose homeostasis and insulin sensitivity are mediated in part by controlling adiponectin production and release in adipocytes [186,187]. More recently, it has been shown that FGF21 is produced by a variety of tissues other than liver under other than extreme metabolic conditions as starvation or obesity [188]. The common features of the conditions that elicit FGF21 in organisms cause diverse tissue and cellular stress. Thus it has been proposed that FGF21 is largely a stress hormone that calls on adipocytes and its metabolic and hormonal secretory products (adipokines) to alleviate diverse tissue stresses [188]. Although numerous reports [189] suggest FGF21, which requires FGFR1-KLB, may directly target other tissues than adipocytes that are very low in KLB, the significance relative to adipocytes on overall FGF21 action remains to be determined.

Endocrine FGF19 and FGF21 act on the same FGFR1 that also mediates the effects of paracrine/autocrine FGFs on cellular homeostasis in developing and mature organs as well as driving numerous proliferative pathologies, such as cancer. However, the canonical cellular activities of FGF19 and FGF21, most prominently their mitogenicity, are prevented by the transmembrane cofactor KLB, which participates directly in the FGFR signaling complex and redirects its output to metabolic signaling [79,84,176]. Co-expression of KLB directs FGFR4 signaling from growth-controlling to apoptosis-promoting, which may explain why FGFR4 elicits specific cellular context control of cell population expansion and tumor suppression rather than tumor promotion [84]. Breast tumor progression in Fgfr4 null mice is delayed rather than accelerated [190]. This correlates with a fortuitous chronic compensatory elevation of ileal FGF19 and an unexpected chronic elevation of circulating FGF21 in the FGFR4-knockout model [191], indicating that persistently elevated FGF19 and FGF21 has a tumor suppressive effect. The persistent elevation of FGF21 in cancer is consistent with its overall role as a stress hormone since cancer is a major source of stress on the organism affecting many tissues.

Obesity and its associated aspects of metabolic syndrome are strong promoters for several cancers, which include breast and prostate cancer. Normally, FGF19/FGF21 serves to maintain normal metabolic homeostasis between adipocytes and other tissues, primarily hepatocytes. Antitumorigenic effects of FGF21 may occur systemically through fat tissues and locally distributed adipocytes, via regulating release of their metabolites and adipokines, which affect tumor cells directly or indirectly by changing the tumor microenvironment (Fig. 4). Although FGF19 directly regulates specific aspects of hepatic contribution to metabolic homeostasis, FGF21 has exquisite specificity for adipocytes *via* FGFR1/KLB without direct effects on hepatic FGFR signaling. This very narrow physiologic role of FGF21 and adipocyte target specificity makes it especially attractive as a pharmacologic antiobesity, antidiabetic, and now antitumor agent for which few side effects are predicted.

2.5 Aberrant FGF signaling in cancer

Ectopic expression of FGF ligand or receptor, as well as mutations in the FGFR that cause activation of the FGF/FGFR signaling axis is common in many epithelial cancers including hepatocellular carcinoma, melanoma, lung, breast, bladder, endometrial, head and neck, and prostate cancers [192]. Point mutations causing constitutive activation of FGFR3 have been detected in more than 60% of non-muscle invasive urothelial

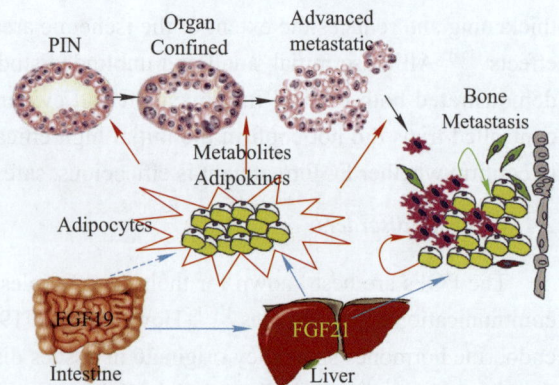

Fig. 4. Endocrine FGFs suppress prostate tumor progression and metastasis by regulating adipokine secretion. FGF21 produced by hepatocyte affects prostate cancer progression *via* controlling adipokine productions in both adipose tissues and local adipocytes in the tumor microenvironment.

carcinomas [193], and a point mutation in the transmembrane domain of Fgfr4 has been reported in human prostate carcinoma [194]. Gene amplification and mutations in the intronic sequence leading to overexpression of FGFR tyrosine kinases is also a mechanism underlying excessive FGF signaling in cancer. For example, amplification of chromosomal region 8p11-12, which encompasses Fgfr1, is frequently found in human prostate carcinoma [195] and approximately 10% of breast carcinomas [192], a point mutation in intron 2 of the Fgfr2 alleles has been found associated with breast cancer [196]. Alternative splicing of FGFR resulting in variants with altered ligand specificities constitutes the third mechanism leading to aberrant FGF signaling in cancer [192]. In addition, downregulation of feed-back controllers of FGF signaling, such as Spry or SEF can also contribute to oncogenic activity of FGF signaling [197].

Aberrant FGF signaling has been implicated in prostate carcinoma development and progression [40,112,198,199]. Elevated production of FGF ligands by prostatic secretory epithelial cells creates an autocrine signaling loop stimulating aberrant epithelial growth and cellular dysplasia and promoting independence from stromal regulation. Upregulation of FGF family members in primary prostate cancer correlates with higher grades of cancer and clinical stage [197,200]. FGF8 is expressed at low levels in normal prostate. However, FGF8 and its cognate receptors are over-expressed in human samples of prostatic intraepithelial neoplasia (PIN) and prostate carcinoma [201-204]. Furthermore, over-expression of FGF8 is associated with decreased patient survival [205]. Exogenous FGF1 induces expression of matrix metalloproteinases and promotes tumor metastasis in prostate carcinoma cells [206]. Overexpression of FGF9 augments reactive stroma formation and promotes cancer progression in mouse models of prostate carcinoma [207]. Attenuating FGF2 activity inhibits cell proliferation, migration, and invasion in cell culture [208,209]. Consistent with this, ablation of FGF2 inhibits prostate tumor progression in the TRAMP transgenic mouse model of prostate cancer [210]. In addition, hyperactivation of the FRS2α-mediated pathway increases tumor angiogenesis and predicts poor outcomes of prostate carcinoma patients [211].

FGFs also have a role in the development of bone metastases, which occur in approximately 80% of patients with advanced prostate cancer [212]. These metastases often abnormally express FGF8 and/or FGF9, which promote osteoblast proliferation/differentiation in culture [213,214]. Forced expression of FGF8 promotes bone growth of prostate carcinoma in a mouse model [215]. Advanced prostate cancer is frequently resistant to castration. Multiple FGFs have been reported to be aberrantly expressed in castration-resistant [205,216,217] or chemotherapy resistant prostate cancer [218,219]. Inhibition of FGF8 and FGF9 signaling has an antitumor effect in mouse models of castrate-resistant prostate cancer [213,220].

Dysregulated expression of FGFRs has also been associated with prostate cancer. Overexpression of FGFR1 has been found in human prostate cancer and accelerates tumor progression of rat premalignant prostate epithelial cells [40,115]. Exposure to aberrant FGFR1 signaling leads to dosage- and time-dependent lesions of prostate, ranging from low-grade PIN to carcinoma *in situ* of the prostate, invasive carcinoma, and metastasis. Forced expression of constitutively active mutants of FGFR1 leads to development of high-grade PIN lesions [221,222]. JOCK-1 is a transgenic mouse model overexpressing an FGFR1 kinase construct, iFGFR1, which contains the membrane anchored FGFR1 intracellular kinase domain in frame fused with a 12 kDa FK506 binding protein (FKBP12) at the C-terminus. Treating the mice with FK506, a dimer inducer to activate the FGFR1 kinase, causes the mice to develop invasive prostate carcinoma and metastasis [223]. On the other hand, deletion of Frs2α or Fgfr1 in prostate epithelial cells inhibits the initiation and progression of prostate cancer in the transgenic adenocarcinoma of the mouse prostate (TRAMP) model [224,225]. Tissue recombination experiments *in vitro* also show that ectopic FGFR1 is required for prostate cancer initiation and progression [226]. Epithelial-mesenchymal transition (EMT) is a process whereby polarized epithelial cells lose epithelial characteristics and acquire mesenchymal features, including enhanced migratory capacity, invasiveness, and elevated resistance to apoptosis [227]. Shifts in alternative splicing of FGFR1 and FGFR2 from IIIb (epithelial) to IIIc (mesenchymal) isoforms are associated with EMT in prostate and other types of cancer [228]. In contrast, downregulation of epithelial cell resident FGFR2 is associated with prostate cancer progression [40,114]. Together, these data suggest that aberrant activation of FGFR1 signaling is sufficient to disrupt prostate tissue homeostasis leading to over-proliferation of prostate cells, and contribute to initiation and progression of the lesion to malignancy in mouse models of prostate cancer.

In contrast to ectopic FGFR isoforms, however, resident FGFR signaling in prostate cells maintains tissue homeostasis, communication with stromal cells, and mediates androgen signaling. The stromal FGF7/FGF10 to epithelial FGFR2 signaling axis maintains prostate tissue homeostasis and mediates androgen signaling in the epithelial cells. Therefore, both FGF7 and FGF10 have been called andromedins [112,199]. Although ablation of Fgfr2 was insufficient to cause full progression to carcinoma, it leads to development of low-grade PIN (Wang and McKeehan, unpublished data). The epithelial FGF9 to stromal FGFR3 signaling axis is engaged in communication between epithelial and stromal cells in the prostate and is lost in advanced prostate cancer. Reinstatement of this signaling axis in advanced rat prostate cancer cells restores the interactions between cancer cells and stromal cells and induces prostate cancer cell differentiation in the Dunning R3327 rat prostate cancer model [216].

2.6 FGF pathway inhibitions in cancer treatment

A number of targeted agents that inhibit FGF/FGFR signaling have been developed, which include tyrosine kinase inhibitors (TKIs), monoclonal antibodies, and FGF ligand traps. The TKIs include both ATP binding site and non ATP binding site molecules. With the exception of AZD4547 that is relatively FGFR specific [229,230], most ATP binding site inhibitors, including dovitinib (TKI258), nintedanib (BIBF 1120), lenvatinib, brivanib, orantinib, and PD173074, cross-inhibit multiple receptor tyrosine kinases [231-237]. Non-ATP binding site inhibitors of FGFR kinase may exhibit a better specificity than the ATP-binding site inhibitors. Several non-ATP binding site inhibitors have been developed, which include L6123, Aea4, Aea25, A114, and A117 [238-240]. All these non-ATP binding site inhibitors exhibit highly FGFR kinase specific inhibitory activities and suppress cancer cell proliferation, migration, and induce cell apoptosis. It remains to be determined, however, whether these non-ATP binding site inhibitors are safe and efficacious for use on cancer patients.

In addition to kinase inhibitors, several strategies have also been developed to block ligand-receptor binding, which includes antibodies against FGF or FGFR, ligand traps, and small peptides that compete with FGF for binding to the receptors. MFGR1877S is a monoclonal antibody against FGFR3 that is currently undergoing phase 1 testing for patients with advanced solid tumors [241]. Both the GP369 antibody that specifically blocks FGFR2 IIIb isoform and the 1A6 antibody that neutralizes FGF19 activities are currently in preclinical development [242,243]. The fusion protein HGS1036 (FP-1039) comprises the extracellular domain of FGFR1c fused with the Fc portion of IgG1, is expected to trap FGF ligands for the FGFR1IIIc isoform and functions as a decoy receptor. It inhibits tumor cell proliferation and blocks angiogenesis and suppresses growth of patient-derived xenograft tumor models of various tissue origins [244]. It has been shown to cause shrinkage of prostate cancer in a phase 1 clinical trial [245]. Two short peptides, P8 (PLLQATAGGGS) that binds to FGF2 and P7 (LSPPRYP) that binds to FGFR1 were identified by screening a phage display library using FGF2 and FGFR1 as the bait, respectively [246,247]. Both peptides exhibit activities to suppress FGF2-FGFR1 binding and block FGF2-induced cell proliferation activity without cytotoxic effect in multiple cell lines. The clinical application of these two peptides in cancer treatment is currently being explored.

3. Perspective

Soon after its discovery in the early seventies, the FGF family was recognized to elicit a broad spectrum of regulatory activities. There are few tissues where no members of this large family are expressed or have an impact on some tissue response marker. Often multiple members of the family, both ligands and receptor isotypes, are co-expressed although they are most commonly cell-specific and compartmented when examined more closely. Cell culture analyses in the absence of physiological restrictions often indicate a considerable redundancy among the family members. However, as FGF family member expression and associated activities have been more closely dissected under physiological conditions, results have indicated an increasing degree of receptor isoform-tissue and cell type contextual specificity. Aberrant and ectopic expression of FGF signaling has been reported as a causal factor for multiple diseases, including cancer. Yet, the determinants of FGF isotype and cell type signaling specificity are poorly understood. It is particularly challenging to understand how the same FGFR isotype can have diverse and often opposing biological endpoints. Sometimes the endpoints are temporally dependent on the point at which activation begins and how long it is sustained. Little is known with respect to kinase-substrate specificity of the FGFR tyrosine kinases, although emerging evidence shows that FGFR elicits isoform-specific activities. The role of co-factors and co-receptors, such as heparan sulfate proteoglycans and Klothos, in FGF signaling specificity should not be ignored. In fact, it has been reported that with or without co-expression of KLB, FGFR4 elicits different activities in 293 cells [84]. In addition, heparan sulfates affect ligand binding specificity of the FGFR, and it remains to be investigated whether heparan sulfates also contribute to signaling specificity at the substrate level. Understanding the signaling specificity of the FGF signaling axis will provide new strategies for developing drugs that will selectively suppress a particular pathway to minimize side effects. As new technologies emerge, unraveling the "gaitou" of FGF signaling specificity is no longer a dream. Therefore, future applications of FGF, the new focus in the pharmaceutical arena, for improving wound healing, alleviating damages of cardiovascular diseases, controlling obesity and diabetes, and suppressing cancer progression and metastasis are visible on the horizon.

References

[1] Armelin H. Pituitary extracts and steroid hormones in the control of 3T3 cell growth[J]. Proceedings of the National Academy of Sciences of the United States of America, 1973, 70(9): 2702-2706.

[2] Gospodarowicz D. Localisation of a fibroblast growth factor and its effect alone and with hydrocortisone on 3T3 cell growth[J]. Nature, 1974, 249(453): 123-127.

[3] Huebner K, Ferrari A, Delli Bovi P, et al. The FGF-related oncogene, K-FGF, maps to human chromosome region 11q13, possibly near int-2[J]. Oncogene research, 1988, 3(3): 263-270.

[4] Taira M, Yoshida T, Miyagawa K, et al. cDNA sequence of human transforming gene hst and identification of the coding sequence required for transforming activity[J]. Proceedings of the National Academy of Sciences of the United States of America, 1987, 84(9): 2980-2984.

[5] Sakamoto H, Mori M, Taira M, et al. Transforming gene from human stomach cancers and a noncancerous portion of stomach mucosa[J]. Proceedings of the National Academy of Sciences of the United States of America, 1986, 83(11): 3997-4001.

[6] Marics I, Adelaide J, Raybaud F, et al. Characterization of the HST-related FGF.6 gene, a new member of the fibroblast growth factor gene family[J]. Oncogene, 1989, 4(3): 335-340.

[7] Rubin JS, Osada H, PW. F, et al. Purification and characterization of a newly identified growth factor specific for epithelial cells[J]. Proceedings of the National Academy of Sciences of the United States of America, 1989, 86(3): 802-806.

[8] Tanaka A, Miyamoto K, Minamino N, et al. Cloning and charac-

terization of an androgen-induced growth factor essential for the androgen-dependent growth of mouse mammary carcinoma cells[J]. Proceedings of the National Academy of Sciences of the United States of America, 1992, 89(19): 8928-8932.

[9] Miyamoto M, Naruo K, C. S, et al. Molecular cloning of a novel cytokine cDNA encoding the ninth member of the fibroblast growth factor family, which has a unique secretion property[J]. Molecular and cellular biology, 1993, 13(7): 4251-4259.

[10] Yamasaki M, Miyake A, S. T, et al. Structure and expression of the rat mRNA encoding a novel member of the fibroblast growth factor family[J]. The Journal of biological chemistry, 1996, 271(27): 15918-15921.

[11] Smallwood PM, Munoz-Sanjuan I, P. T, et al. Fibroblast growth factor (FGF) homologous factors: new members of the FGF family implicated in nervous system development[J]. Proceedings of the National Academy of Sciences of the United States of America, 1996, 93(18): 9850-9857.

[12] Matsubara A, Kan M, S. F, et al. Inhibition of growth of malignant rat prostate tumor cells by restoration of fibroblast growth factor receptor 2[J]. Cancer research, 1998, 58(7): 1509-1514.

[13] Hoshikawa M, Ohbayashi N, Yonamine A, et al. Structure and expression of a novel fibroblast growth factor, FGF-17, preferentially expressed in the embryonic brain[J]. Biochemical and biophysical research communications, 1998, 244(1): 187-191.

[14] Ohbayashi N, Hoshikawa M, Kimura S, et al. Structure and expression of the mRNA encoding a novel fibroblast growth factor, FGF-

18[J]. The Journal of biological chemistry, 1998, 273(29): 18161-18164.

[15] Nishimura T, Utsunomiya Y, Hoshikawa M, et al. Structure and expression of a novel human FGF, FGF-19, expressed in the fetal brain[J]. Biochim. Biophys. Acta, 1999, 1444(1): 148-151.

[16] Powers CJ, McLeskey SW, A. W. Fibroblast growth factors, their receptors and signaling.[J]. Endocrine-related cancer, 2000, 7(3): 165-197.

[17] Nishimura T, Nakatake Y, Konishi M, et al. Identification of a novel FGF, FGF-21, preferentially expressed in the liver[J]. Biochimica et biophysica acta, 2000, 1492(1): 203-206.

[18] Nakatake Y, Hoshikawa M, Asaki T, et al. Identification of a novel fibroblast growth factor, FGF-22, preferentially expressed in the inner root sheath of the hair follicle[J]. Biochimica et biophysica acta, 2001, 1517(3): 460-463.

[19] Yamashita T, Yoshioka M, Itoh N. Identification of a novel fibroblast growth factor, FGF-23, preferentially expressed in the ventrolateral thalamic nucleus of the brain[J]. Biochem. Biophys. Res. Commun., 2000, 277(2): 494-498.

[20] McWhirter JR, Goulding M, Weiner JA, et al. A novel fibroblast growth factor gene expressed in the developing nervous system is a downstream target of the chimeric homeodomain oncoprotein E2A-Pbx1[J]. Development (Cambridge, England), 1997, 124(17): 3221-3232.

[21] Hennessey JA, Wei EQ, Pitt GS. Fibroblast growth factor homologous factors modulate cardiac calcium channels[J]. Circulation research, 2013, 113(4): 381-388.

[22] Wang CJ, Wang C, Hoch EG, et al. Identification of novel interaction sites that determine specificity between fibroblast growth factor homologous factors and voltage-gated sodium channels[J]. The Journal of biological chemistry, 2011, 286(27): 24253-24263.

[23] Olsen SK, Garbi M, Zampieri N, et al. Fibroblast growth factor (FGF) homologous factors share structural but not functional homology with FGFs[J]. The Journal of biological chemistry, 2003, 278(36): 34226-34236.

[24] Lee PL, Johnson DE, Cousens LS, et al. Purification and complementary DNA cloning of a receptor for basic fibroblast growth factor[J]. Science (New York, N.Y.), 1989, 245(4913): 57-60.

[25] Bottaro D, Rubin J, Ron D, et al. Characterization of the receptor for keratinocyte growth factor. Evidence for multiple fibroblast growth factor receptors[J]. The Journal of biological chemistry, 1990, 265(22): 12767-12770.

[26] Keegan K, Johnson DE, Williams LT, et al. Characterization of the FGFR-3 gene and its gene product[J]. Ann. N. Y. Acad. Sci., 1991, 638: 400-402.

[27] Stark KL, McMahon JA, McMahon AP. FGFR-4, a new member of the fibroblast growth factor receptor family, expressed in the definitive endoderm and skeletal muscle lineages of the mouse[J]. Development (Cambridge, England), 1991, 113(2): 641-651.

[28] Takaishi S, Sawada M, Morita Y, et al. Identification of a novel alternative splicing of human FGF receptor 4: soluble-form splice variant expressed in human gastrointestinal epithelial cells[J]. Biochemical and biophysical research communications, 2000, 267(2): 658-662.

[29] Hou JZ, Kan MK, McKeehan K, et al. Fibroblast growth factor receptors from liver vary in three structural domains[J]. Science, 1991, 251(4994): 665-668.

[30] Vaĭnshenker II, Kalinina OV, Nuralova IV, et al. Low-manifest infections in children and adolescents with consequences of perinatal damage of nervous system[J]. Zhurnal Mikrobiologii, Epidemiologii, I Immunobiologii, 2012(5): 77-80.

[31] Wang F, Kan M, Yan G, et al. Alternately spliced NH2-terminal immunoglobulin-like Loop I in the ectodomain of the fibroblast growth factor (FGF) receptor 1 lowers affinity for both heparin and FGF-1[J]. The Journal of biological chemistry, 1995, 270(17): 10231-10235.

[32] Lacher DA, Paolino MJ. Discriminant analysis of laboratory tests in patients admitted to a coronary care unit[J]. Clinical chemistry, 1988, 34(6): 1099-1102.

[33] Zhang X, Ibrahimi OA, Olsen SK, et al. Receptor specificity of the fibroblast growth factor family. The complete mammalian FGF family[J]. The Journal of biological chemistry, 2006, 281(23): 15694-15700.

[34] Luo Y, Lu W, Mohamedali KA, et al. The glycine box: a determinant of specificity for fibroblast growth factor[J]. Biochemistry, 1998, 37(47): 16506-16515.

[35] Yan G, Wang F, Fukabori Y, et al. Expression and transforming activity of a variant of the heparin-binding fibroblast growth factor receptor (flg) gene resulting from splicing of the alpha exon at an alternate 3'-acceptor site[J]. Biochemical and biophysical research communications, 1992, 183(2): 423-430.

[36] Hoch RV, Soriano P. Context-specific requirements for Fgfr1 signaling through Frs2 and Frs3 during mouse development[J]. Development (Cambridge, England), 2006, 133(4): 663-673.

[37] Burgar H, Burns H, Elsden J, et al. Association of the signaling adaptor FRS2 with fibroblast growth factor receptor 1 (Fgfr1) is mediated by alternative splicing of the juxtamembrane domain[J]. The Journal of biological chemistry, 2002, 277(6): 4018-4023.

[38] Zhang Y, McKeehan K, Lin Y, et al. Fibroblast growth factor receptor 1 (FGFR1) tyrosine phosphorylation regulates binding of FGFR substrate 2alpha (FRS2alpha) but not FRS2 to the receptor[J]. Molecular endocrinology (Baltimore, Md.), 2008, 22(1): 167-175.

[39] Hattori Y, Odagiri H, Nakatani H, et al. K-sam, an amplified gene in stomach cancer, is a member of the heparin-binding growth factor receptor genes[J]. Proceedings of the National Academy of Sciences of the United States of America, 1990, 87(15): 5983-5987.

[40] Feng S, Wang F, Matsubara A, et al. Fibroblast growth factor receptor 2 limits and receptor 1 accelerates tumorigenicity of prostate epithelial cells[J]. Cancer research, 1997, 57(23): 5369-5378.

[41] Matsubara A, Kan M, Feng S, et al. Inhibition of growth of malignant rat prostate tumor cells by restoration of fibroblast growth factor receptor 2[J]. Cancer research, 1998, 58(7): 1509-1514.

[42] Luo Y, Yang C, Jin C, et al. Novel phosphotyrosine targets of FGFR2IIIb signaling[J]. Cellular signalling, 2009, 21(9): 1370-1378.

[43] Xian W, Schwertfeger KL, Rosen JM. Distinct roles of fibroblast growth factor receptor 1 and 2 in regulating cell survival and epithelial-mesenchymal transition[J]. Molecular endocrinology (Baltimore, Md.), 2007, 21(4): 987-1000.

[44] Mohammadi M, Dikic I, Sorokin A, et al. Identification of six novel autophosphorylation sites on fibroblast growth factor receptor 1 and elucidation of their importance in receptor activation and signal transduction[J]. Molecular and cellular biology, 1996, 16(3): 977-989.

[45] Powers CJ, McLeskey SW, Wellstein A. Fibroblast growth factors, their receptors and signaling.[J]. Endocrine-related cancer, 2000, 7(3): 165-197.

[46] McKeehan WL, Wang F, Kan M. The heparan sulfate-fibroblast growth factor family: diversity of structure and function[J]. Progress in nucleic acid research and molecular biology, 1998, 59(59): 135-176.

[47] Hou J, Mckeehan K, Kan M, et al. Identification of tyrosines 154 and 307 in the extracellular domain and 653 and 766 in the intracellular domain as phosphorylation sites in the heparin-binding fibroblast growth factor receptor tyrosine kinase (flg)[J]. Protein Science, 1993, 2(1): 86-92.

[48] Lew ED, Furdui CM, Anderson KS, et al. The precise sequence of FGF receptor autophosphorylation is kinetically driven and is disrupted by oncogenic mutations[J]. Science signaling, 2009, 2(58): ra6.

[49] Shi E, Kan M, Xu J, et al. Control of fibroblast growth factor receptor kinase signal transduction by heterodimerization of combinatorial splice variants[J]. Molecular and cellular biology, 1993, 13(7):

3907-3918.

[50] Mohammadi M, Dionne CA, Li W, *et al*. Point mutation in FGF receptor eliminates phosphatidylinositol hydrolysis without affecting mitogenesis[J]. Nature, 1992, 358(6388): 681-684.

[51] Peters KG, Marie J, Wilson E, *et al*. l transduction by fibroblast growth factor receptor[J]. Nature, 1992, 358(6388): 678-681.

[52] Larsson H, Klint P, Landgren E, *et al*. Fibroblast growth factor receptor-1-mediated endothelial cell proliferation is dependent on the Src homology (SH) 2/SH3 domain-containing adaptor protein Crk[J]. The Journal of biological chemistry, 1999, 274(36): 25726-25734.

[53] Klint P, Claesson-Welsh L. Signal transduction by fibroblast growth factor receptors[J]. Frontiers in bioscience : a journal and virtual library, 1999, 4(1-3): D165-177.

[54] Seo JH, Suenaga A, Hatakeyama M, *et al*. Structural and functional basis of a role for CRKL in a fibroblast growth factor 8-induced feed-forward loop[J]. Molecular and cellular biology, 2009, 29(11): 3076-3087.

[55] Francavilla C, Rigbolt KT, Emdal KB, *et al*. Functional proteomics defines the molecular switch underlying FGF receptor trafficking and cellular outputs[J]. Molecular cell, 2013, 51(6): 707-722.

[56] Yan G, McBride G, McKeehan WL. Exon skipping causes alteration of the COOH-terminus and deletion of the phospholipase C gamma 1 interaction site in the FGF receptor 2 kinase in normal prostate epithelial cells[J]. Biochem. Biophys. Res. Commun., 1993, 194(1): 512-518.

[57] Bernfield M, Götte M, Park PW, *et al*. Functions of cell surface heparan sulfate proteoglycans[J]. Annual review of biochemistry, 1999, 68(undefined): 729-777.

[58] Esko JD, Lindahl U. Molecular diversity of heparan sulfate[J]. J. Clin. Invest., 2001, 108(2): 169-173.

[59] Park PW, Reizes O, Bernfield M. Cell surface heparan sulfate proteoglycans: selective regulators of ligand-receptor encounters[J]. J. Biol. Chem., 2000, 275(39): 29923-29926.

[60] Ye S, Luo Y, Lu W, *et al*. Structural basis for interaction of FGF-1, FGF-2, and FGF-7 with different heparan sulfate motifs[J]. Biochemistry, 2001, 40(48): 14429-14439.

[61] Kan M, Wu X, Wang F, *et al*. Specificity for fibroblast growth factors determined by heparan sulfate in a binary complex with the receptor kinase[J]. The Journal of biological chemistry, 1999, 274(22): 15947-15952.

[62] Kreuger J, Salmivirta M, Sturiale L, *et al*. Sequence analysis of heparan sulfate epitopes with graded affinities for fibroblast growth factors 1 and 2[J]. The Journal of biological chemistry, 2001, 276(33): 30744-30752.

[63] Guimond SE, Turnbull JE. Fibroblast growth factor receptor signalling is dictated by specific heparan sulphate saccharides[J]. Current biology : CB, 1999, 9(22): 1343-1346.

[64] Ostrovsky O, Berman B, Gallagher J, *et al*. Differential effects of heparin saccharides on the formation of specific fibroblast growth factor (FGF) and FGF receptor complexes[J]. The Journal of biological chemistry, 2002, 277(4): 2444-2453.

[65] Powell AK, Fernig DG, Turnbull JE. Fibroblast growth factor receptors 1 and 2 interact differently with heparin/heparan sulfate. Implications for dynamic assembly of a ternary signaling complex[J]. The Journal of biological chemistry, 2002, 277(32): 28554-28563.

[66] Luo Y, Ye S, Kan M, *et al*. Control of fibroblast growth factor (FGF) 7- and FGF1-induced mitogenesis and downstream signaling by distinct heparin octasaccharide motifs[J]. The Journal of biological chemistry, 2006, 281(30): 21052-21061.

[67] Luo Y, Ye S, Kan M, *et al*. Structural specificity in a FGF7-affinity purified heparin octasaccharide required for formation of a complex with FGF7 and FGFR2IIIb[J]. Journal of cellular biochemistry, 2006, 97(6): 1241-1258.

[68] Kan M, Shi EG, McKeehan WL. Identification and assay of fibro-

blast growth factor receptors[J]. Meth. Enzymol., 1991, 198: 158-171.

[69] Kan M, DiSorbo D, Hou JZ, *et al*. High and low affinity binding of heparin-binding growth factor to a 130-kDa receptor correlates with stimulation and inhibition of growth of a differentiated human hepatoma cell[J]. J. Biol. Chem., 1988, 263(23): 11306-11313.

[70] Kan M, Wang F, To B, *et al*. Divalent cations and heparin/heparan sulfate cooperate to control assembly and activity of the fibroblast growth factor receptor complex[J]. The Journal of biological chemistry, 1996, 271(42): 26143-26148.

[71] Wang F, Kan M, McKeehan K, *et al*. A homeo-interaction sequence in the ectodomain of the fibroblast growth factor receptor[J]. J. Biol. Chem., 1997, 272(38): 23887-23895.

[72] Schlessinger J, Plotnikov AN, Ibrahimi OA, *et al*. Crystal structure of a ternary FGF-FGFR-heparin complex reveals a dual role for heparin in FGFR binding and dimerization[J]. Molecular cell, 2000, 6(3): 743-750.

[73] Uematsu F, Kan M, Wang F, *et al*. Ligand binding properties of binary complexes of heparin and immunoglobulin-like modules of FGF receptor 2[J]. Biochemical and biophysical research communications, 2000, 272(3): 830-836.

[74] Belov AA, Mohammadi M. Molecular mechanisms of fibroblast growth factor signaling in physiology and pathology[J]. Cold Spring Harbor perspectives in biology, 2013, 5(6): 239-249.

[75] Chen H, Ma J, Lu W, *et al*. A molecular brake in the kinase hinge region regulates the activity of receptor tyrosine kinases[J]. Molecular cell, 2007, 27(5): 717-730.

[76] Goetz R, Beenken A, Ibrahimi OA, *et al*. Molecular insights into the klotho-dependent, endocrine mode of action of fibroblast growth factor 19 subfamily members[J]. Molecular and cellular biology, 2007, 27(9): 3417-3428.

[77] Lin BC, Wang M, Blackmore C, *et al*. Liver-specific activities of FGF19 require Klotho beta[J]. The Journal of biological chemistry, 2007, 282(37): 27277-27284.

[78] Micanovic R, Raches DW, Dunbar JD, *et al*. Different roles of N- and C- termini in the functional activity of FGF21[J]. Journal of cellular physiology, 2009, 219(2): 227-234.

[79] Goetz R, Ohnishi M, Ding X, *et al*. Klotho coreceptors inhibit signaling by paracrine fibroblast growth factor 8 subfamily ligands[J]. Molecular and cellular biology, 2012, 32(10): 1944-1954.

[80] Goetz R, Nakada Y, Hu MC, *et al*. Isolated C-terminal tail of FGF23 alleviates hypophosphatemia by inhibiting FGF23-FGFR-Klotho complex formation[J]. Proceedings of the National Academy of Sciences of the United States of America, 2010, 107(1): 407-412.

[81] Kurosu H, Ogawa Y, Miyoshi M, *et al*. Regulation of fibroblast growth factor-23 signaling by klotho[J]. The Journal of biological chemistry, 2006, 281(10): 6120-6123.

[82] Nakatani T, Ohnishi M, Razzaque MS. Inactivation of klotho function induces hyperphosphatemia even in presence of high serum fibroblast growth factor 23 levels in a genetically engineered hypophosphatemic (Hyp) mouse model[J]. Faseb j., 2009, 23(11): 3702-3711.

[83] Kurosu H, Choi M, Ogawa Y, *et al*. Tissue-specific expression of β Klotho and fibroblast growth factor (FGF) receptor isoforms determines metabolic activity of FGF19 and FGF21[J]. The Journal of biological chemistry, 2007, 282(37): 26687-26695.

[84] Luo Y, Yang C, Lu W, *et al*. Metabolic regulator β Klotho interacts with fibroblast growth factor receptor 4 (FGFR4) to induce apoptosis and inhibit tumor cell proliferation[J]. The Journal of biological chemistry, 2010, 285(39): 30069-30078.

[85] Goetz R, Mohammadi M. Exploring mechanisms of FGF signalling through the lens of structural biology[J]. Nature reviews. Molecular cell biology, 2013, 14(3): 166-180.

[86] McDougall K, Kubu C, Verdi JM, *et al*. Developmental expression patterns of the signaling adapters FRS-2 and FRS-3 during early

embryogenesis[J]. Mechanisms of development, 2001, 103(1): 145-148.

[87] Rabin SJ, Cleghon V, Kaplan DR. SNT, a differentiation-specific target of neurotrophic factor-induced tyrosine kinase activity in neurons and PC12 cells[J]. Molecular and cellular biology, 1993, 13(4): 2203-2213.

[88] Ong SH, Goh KC, Lim YP, et al. Suc1-associated neurotrophic factor target (SNT) protein is a major FGF-stimulated tyrosine phosphorylated 90-kDa protein which binds to the SH2 domain of GRB2[J]. Biochemical and biophysical research communications, 1996, 225(3): 1021-1026.

[89] Arman E, Haffner-Krausz R, Gorivodsky M, et al. Fgfr2 is required for limb outgrowth and lung-branching morphogenesis[J]. Proceedings of the National Academy of Sciences of the United States of America, 1999, 96(21): 11895-11899.

[90] Lin HY, Xu J, Ischenko I, et al. Identification of the cytoplasmic regions of fibroblast growth factor (FGF) receptor 1 which play important roles in induction of neurite outgrowth in PC12 cells by FGF-1[J]. Molecular and cellular biology, 1998, 18(7): 3762-3770.

[91] Kouhara H, Hadari YR, Spivak-Kroizman T, et al. A lipid-anchored Grb2-binding protein that links FGF-receptor activation to the Ras/MAPK signaling pathway[J]. Cell, 1997, 89(5): 693-702.

[92] Xu H, Lee KW, Goldfarb M. Novel recognition motif on fibroblast growth factor receptor mediates direct association and activation of SNT adapter proteins[J]. The Journal of biological chemistry, 1998, 273(29): 17987-17990.

[93] Ong SH, Lim YP, Low BC, et al. SHP2 associates directly with tyrosine phosphorylated p90 (SNT) protein in FGF-stimulated cells[J]. Biochemical and biophysical research communications, 1997, 238(1): 261-266.

[94] Guy GR, Wong ES, Yusoff P, et al. Sprouty: how does the branch manager work?[J]. Journal of cell science, 2003, 116(15): 3061-3068.

[95] Torii S, Kusakabe M, Yamamoto T, et al. Sef is a spatial regulator for Ras/MAP kinase signaling[J]. Developmental cell, 2004, 7(1): 33-44.

[96] Xiong S, Zhao Q, Rong Z, et al. hSef inhibits PC-12 cell differentiation by interfering with Ras-mitogen-activated protein kinase MAPK signaling[J]. The Journal of biological chemistry, 2003, 278(50): 50273-50282.

[97] Wang F, McKeehan K, Yu C, et al. Fibroblast growth factor receptor 1 phosphotyrosine 766: molecular target for prevention of progression of prostate tumors to malignancy[J]. Cancer research, 2002, 62(6): 1898-1903.

[98] Hadari YR, Gotoh N, Kouhara H, et al. Critical role for the docking-protein FRS2 alpha in FGF receptor-mediated signal transduction pathways[J]. Proceedings of the National Academy of Sciences of the United States of America, 2001, 98(15): 8578-8583.

[99] Gotoh N, Laks S, Nakashima M, et al. FRS2 family docking proteins with overlapping roles in activation of MAP kinase have distinct spatial-temporal patterns of expression of their transcripts[J]. FEBS letters, 2004, 564(1): 14-18.

[100] Wong A, Lamothe B, Lee A, et al. FRS2 alpha attenuates FGF receptor signaling by Grb2-mediated recruitment of the ubiquitin ligase Cbl[J]. Proceedings of the National Academy of Sciences of the United States of America, 2002, 99(10): 6684-6689.

[101] Lax I, Wong A, Lamothe B, et al. The docking protein FRS2alpha controls a MAP kinase-mediated negative feedback mechanism for signaling by FGF receptors[J]. Molecular cell, 2002, 10(4): 709-719.

[102] Faham S, Linhardt RJ, Rees DC. Diversity does make a difference: fibroblast growth factor-heparin interactions[J]. Current opinion in structural biology, 1998, 8(5): 578-586.

[103] Ornitz D. FGFs, heparan sulfate and FGFRs: complex interactions essential for development[J]. BioEssays: news and reviews in molecular, cellular and developmental biology, 2000, 22(2): 108-112.

[104] McIntosh I, Bellus GA, Jab EW. The pleiotropic effects of fibroblast growth factor receptors in mammalian development[J]. Cell structure and function, 2000, 25(2): 85-96.

[105] Xu X, Weinstein M, Li C, et al. Fibroblast growth factor receptors (FGFRs) and their roles in limb development[J]. Cell and tissue research, 1999, 296(1): 33-43.

[106] Kannan K, Girol D. FGF receptor mutations: dimerization syndromes, cell growth suppression, and animal models[J]. IUBMB life, 2000, 49(3): 197-205.

[107] Kato S, Sekine K. FGF-FGFR signaling in vertebrate organogenesis[J]. Cellular and molecular biology (Noisy-le-Grand, France), 1999, 45(5): 631-638.

[108] Burke D, Wilkes D, Blundell TL, et al. Fibroblast growth factor receptors: lessons from the genes[J]. Trends in biochemical sciences, 1998, 23(2): 59-62.

[109] Webster MK, Donoghue DJ. FGFR activation in skeletal disorders: too much of a good thing[J]. Trends in genetics : TIG, 1997, 13(5): 178-182.

[110] Muenke M, Schell U. Fibroblast-growth-factor receptor mutations in human skeletal disorders[J]. Trends in genetics : TIG, 1995, 11(8): 308-313.

[111] Kwabi-Addo B, Ropiquet F, Giri D, et al. Alternative splicing of fibroblast growth factor receptors in human prostate cancer[J]. The Prostate, 2001, 46(2): 163-172.

[112] Yan G, Fukabori Y, Nikolaropoulos S, et al. Heparin-binding keratinocyte growth factor is a candidate stromal-to-epithelial-cell andromedin[J]. Molecular endocrinology (Baltimore, Md.), 1992, 6(12): 2123-2128.

[113] Gowardhan B, Douglas DA, Mathers ME, et al. Evaluation of the fibroblast growth factor system as a potential target for therapy in human prostate cancer[J]. British journal of cancer, 2005, 92(2): 320-327.

[114] Freeman KW, Gangula RD, Welm BE, et al. Conditional activation of fibroblast growth factor receptor (FGFR) 1, but not FGFR2, in prostate cancer cells leads to increased osteopontin induction, extracellular signal-regulated kinase activation, and in vivo proliferation[J]. Cancer research, 2003, 63(19): 6237-6243.

[115] Sahadevan K, Darby S, Leung HY, et al. Selective over-expression of fibroblast growth factor receptors 1 and 4 in clinical prostate cancer[J]. The Journal of pathology, 2007, 213(1): 82-90.

[116] Lou Z. Healing large traumatic eardrum perforations in humans using fibroblast growth factor applied directly or via gelfoam[J]. Otology & neurotology : official publication of the American Otological Society, American Neurotology Society [and] European Academy of Otology and Neurotology, 2012, 33(9): 1553-1557.

[117] Hirata E, Ménard-Moyon C, Venturelli E, et al. Carbon nanotubes functionalized with fibroblast growth factor accelerate proliferation of bone marrow-derived stromal cells and bone formation[J]. Nanotechnology, 2013, 24(43): 435101.

[118] Kwan M, Sellmyer M, Quarto N, et al. Chemical control of FGF-2 release for promoting calvarial healing with adipose stem cells[J]. The Journal of biological chemistry, 2011, 286(13): 11307-11313.

[119] Zhang H, Issekutz AC. Down-modulation of monocyte transendothelial migration and endothelial adhesion molecule expression by fibroblast growth factor: reversal by the anti-angiogenic agent SU6668[J]. The American journal of pathology, 2002, 160(6): 2219-2230.

[120] Matuszewska B, Keogan M, Fisher D, et al. Acidic fibroblast growth factor: evaluation of topical formulations in a diabetic mouse wound healing model[J]. Pharmaceutical research, 1994, 11(1): 65-71.

[121] Mellin T, Cashen D, Ronan J, et al. Acidic fibroblast growth factor accelerates dermal wound healing in diabetic mice[J]. The Journal of investigative dermatology, 1995, 104(5): 850-855.

[122] Xie L, Zhang M, Dong B, et al. Improved refractory wound healing with administration of acidic fibroblast growth factor in dia-

betic rats[J]. Diabetes research and clinical practice, 2011, 93(3): 396-403.

[123] Bennett NT, Schultz GS. Growth factors and wound healing: biochemical properties of growth factors and their receptors[J]. American journal of surgery, 1993, 165(6): 728-737.

[124] Ma B, Cheng DS, Xia ZF, et al. Randomized, multicenter, double-blind, and placebo-controlled trial using topical recombinant human acidic fibroblast growth factor for deep partial-thickness burns and skin graft donor site[J]. Wound repair and regeneration : official publication of the Wound Healing Society [and] the European Tissue Repair Society, 2007, 15(6): 795-799.

[125] Akita S, Akino K, Imaizumi T, et al. A basic fibroblast growth factor improved the quality of skin grafting in burn patients[J]. Burns : journal of the International Society for Burn Injuries, 2005, 31(7): 855-858.

[126] Fu X, Shen Z, Chen Y, et al. Randomised placebo-controlled trial of use of topical recombinant bovine basic fibroblast growth factor for second-degree burns[J]. Lancet (London, England), 1998, 352(9141): 1661-1664.

[127] Fu X, Shen Z, Chen Y, et al. Recombinant bovine basic fibroblast growth factor accelerates wound healing in patients with burns, donor sites and chronic dermal ulcers[J]. Chinese medical journal, 2000, 113(4): 367-371.

[128] Nie K, Li P, Zeng X, et al. [Clinical observation of basic fibroblast growth factor combined with topical oxygen therapy in enhancing burn wound healing][J]. Zhongguo xiu fu chong jian wai ke za zhi = Zhongguo xiufu chongjian waike zazhi = Chinese journal of reparative and reconstructive surgery, 2010, 24(6): 643-646.

[129] Akita S, Akino K, Imaizumi T, et al. Basic fibroblast growth factor accelerates and improves second-degree burn wound healing[J]. Wound repair and regeneration : official publication of the Wound Healing Society [and] the European Tissue Repair Society, 2008, 16(5): 635-641.

[130] Akita S, Akino K, Imaizumi T, et al. The quality of pediatric burn scars is improved by early administration of basic fibroblast growth factor[J]. Journal of burn care & research : official publication of the American Burn Association, 2006, 27(3): 333-338.

[131] Akita S, Akino K, Yakabe A, et al. Basic fibroblast growth factor is beneficial for postoperative color uniformity in split-thickness skin grafting[J]. Wound repair and regeneration : official publication of the Wound Healing Society [and] the European Tissue Repair Society, 2010, 18(6): 560-566.

[132] Kubo S, Inui T, Hasegawa H, et al. Repair of intractable cerebrospinal fluid rhinorrhea with mucosal flaps and recombinant human basic fibroblast growth factor: technical case report[J]. Neurosurgery, 2005, 56(3): E627.

[133] Nakada T, Saito Y, Chikenji M, et al. Therapeutic outcome of hyperbaric oxygen and basic fibroblast growth factor on intractable skin ulcer in legs: preliminary report[J]. Plastic and reconstructive surgery, 2006, 117(2): 646-651.

[134] Kakigi A, Sawada S, Takeda T. The effects of basic fibroblast growth factor on postoperative mastoid cavity problems[J]. Otology & neurotology : official publication of the American Otological Society, American Neurotology Society [and] European Academy of Otology and Neurotology, 2005, 26(3): 333-336; discussion 336.

[135] Robson MC, Hill DP, Smith PD, et al. Sequential cytokine therapy for pressure ulcers: clinical and mechanistic response[J]. Annals of surgery, 2000, 231(4): 600-611.

[136] Robson MC, Phillips LG, Lawrence WT, et al. The safety and effect of topically applied recombinant basic fibroblast growth factor on the healing of chronic pressure sores[J]. Annals of surgery, 1992, 216(4): 401-406; discussion 406-408.

[137] Uhl E, Barker J, Bondàr I, et al. Basic fibroblast growth factor accelerates wound healing in chronically ischaemic tissue[J]. The British journal of surgery, 1993, 80(8): 977-980.

[138] Yao C, Yao P, Wu H, et al. Acceleration of wound healing in

traumatic ulcers by absorbable collagen sponge containing recombinant basic fibroblast growth factor[J]. Biomedical materials (Bristol, England), 2006, 1(1): 33-37.

[139] Yamanaka K, Inaba T, Nomura E, et al. Basic fibroblast growth factor treatment for skin ulcerations in scleroderma[J]. Cutis, 2005, 76(6): 373-376.

[140] Kawaguchi H, Oka H, Jingushi S, et al. A local application of recombinant human fibroblast growth factor 2 for tibial shaft fractures: A randomized, placebo-controlled trial[J]. Journal of bone and mineral research : the official journal of the American Society for Bone and Mineral Research, 2010, 25(12): 2735-2743.

[141] Kitamura M, Akamatsu M, Machigashira M, et al. FGF-2 stimulates periodontal regeneration: results of a multi-center randomized clinical trial[J]. Journal of dental research, 2011, 90(1): 35-40.

[142] Asai J, Takenaka H, Ichihashi K, et al. Successful treatment of diabetic gangrene with topical application of a mixture of peripheral blood mononuclear cells and basic fibroblast growth factor[J]. The Journal of dermatology, 2006, 33(5): 349-352.

[143] Richard JL, Parer-Richard C, Daures JP, et al. Effect of topical basic fibroblast growth factor on the healing of chronic diabetic neuropathic ulcer of the foot. A pilot, randomized, double-blind, placebo-controlled study[J]. Diabetes care, 1995, 18(1): 64-69.

[144] Hiroshi UA, I; Kazunori, U;. Clinical efficacy of basic fibroblast growth factor (bFGF) for diabetic ulcer[J]. European journal of dermatology : EJD, 2009, 19(5): 461-468.

[145] Takagi G, Miyamoto M, Tara S, et al. Controlled-release basic fibroblast growth factor for peripheral artery disease: comparison with autologous bone marrow-derived stem cell transfer[J]. Tissue engineering. Part A, 2011, 17: 2787-2794.

[146] Konturek SJ, Brzozowski T, Majka J, et al. Fibroblast growth factor in gastroprotection and ulcer healing: interaction with sucralfate[J]. Gut, 1993, 34(7): 881-887.

[147] Hull MA, Knifton A, Filipowicz B, et al. Healing with basic fibroblast growth factor is associated with reduced indomethacin induced relapse in a human model of gastric ulceration[J]. Gut, 1997, 40(2): 204-210.

[148] Fu X, Shen Z, Chen Y. Basic fibroblast growth factor (bFGF) and wound healing: a multi-centers and controlled clinical trial in 1024 cases[J]. Zhongguo xiu fu chong jian wai ke za zhi = Zhongguo xiufu chongjian waike zazhi = Chinese journal of reparative and reconstructive surgery, 1998, 12(4): 209-211.

[149] Fu XB, Guo ZR, Sheng ZY. Effects of basic fibroblast growth factor on the healing of cutaneous chronic wounds[J]. Zhongguo xiu fu chong jian wai ke za zhi = Zhongguo xiufu chongjian waike zazhi = Chinese journal of reparative and reconstructive surgery, 1999, 13(5): 270-272.

[150] Wu JC, Huang WC, Tsai YA, et al. Nerve repair using acidic fibroblast growth factor in human cervical spinal cord injury: a preliminary Phase I clinical study[J]. Journal of neurosurgery. Spine, 2008, 8(3): 208-214.

[151] Li E, Trovato JA. New developments in management of oral mucositis in patients with head and neck cancer or receiving targeted anticancer therapies[J]. American journal of health-system pharmacy : AJHP : official journal of the American Society of Health-System Pharmacists, 2012, 69(12): 1031-1037.

[152] Finch PW, Rubin JS. Keratinocyte growth factor/fibroblast growth factor 7, a homeostatic factor with therapeutic potential for epithelial protection and repair[J]. Advances in cancer research, 2004, 91: 69-136.

[153] Weigelt C, Haas R, Kobbe G. Pharmacokinetic evaluation of palifermin for mucosal protection from chemotherapy and radiation[J]. Expert opinion on drug metabolism & toxicology, 2011, 7(4): 505-515.

[154] Fliedner M, Baguet B, Blankart J, et al. Palifermin for patients with haematological malignancies: shifting nursing practice from

symptom relief to prevention of oral mucositis[J]. European journal of oncology nursing : the official journal of European Oncology Nursing Society, 2007, 1: S19-26.

[155] Radtke ML, Kolesar JM. Palifermin (Kepivance) for the treatment of oral mucositis in patients with hematologic malignancies requiring hematopoietic stem cell support[J]. Journal of oncology pharmacy practice: official publication of the International Society of Oncology Pharmacy Practitioners, 2005, 11(3): 121-125.

[156] Palifermin: AMJ 9701, KGF-Amgen, recombinant human keratinocyte growth factor, rHu-KGF[J]. Drugs in R&D, 2004, 5(6): 351-354.

[157] Sakurai T, Tsuchida M, Lampe P, et al. Cardiomyocyte FGF signaling is required for Cx43 phosphorylation and cardiac gap junction maintenance[J]. Experimental cell research, 2013, 319(14): 2152-2165.

[158] Iwakura A, Fujita M, Ikemoto M, et al. Myocardial ischemia enhances the expression of acidic fibroblast growth factor in human pericardial fluid[J]. Heart and vessels, 2000, 15(3): 112-116.

[159] Sakakibara Y, Tambara K, Sakaguchi G, et al. Toward surgical angiogenesis using slow-released basic fibroblast growth factor[J]. European journal of cardio-thoracic surgery : official journal of the European Association for Cardio-thoracic Surgery, 2003, 24(1): 105-111; discussion 112.

[160] Yajima S, Ishikawa M, Kubota T, et al. Intramyocardial injection of fibroblast growth factor-2 plus heparin suppresses cardiac failure progression in rats with hypertensive heart disease[J]. International heart journal, 2005, 46(2): 289-301.

[161] Suzuki G, Lee T, Fallavollita J, et al. Adenoviral gene transfer of FGF-5 to hibernating myocardium improves function and stimulates myocytes to hypertrophy and reenter the cell cycle[J]. Circulation research, 2005, 96(7): 767-775.

[162] Simons M, Annex BH, Laham RJ, et al. Pharmacological treatment of coronary artery disease with recombinant fibroblast growth factor-2: double-blind, randomized, controlled clinical trial[J]. Circulation, 2002, 105(7): 788-793.

[163] Kukuła K, Chojnowska L, Dabrowski M, et al. Intramyocardial plasmid-encoding human vascular endothelial growth factor A165/basic fibroblast growth factor therapy using percutaneous transcatheter approach in patients with refractory coronary artery disease (VIF-CAD)[J]. American heart journal, 2011, 161(3): 581-589.

[164] Laham RJ, Chronos NA, Pike M, et al. Intracoronary basic fibroblast growth factor (FGF-2) in patients with severe ischemic heart disease: results of a phase I open-label dose escalation study[J]. Journal of the American College of Cardiology, 2000, 36(7): 2132-2139.

[165] Grines C, Watkins M, Helmer G, et al. Angiogenic Gene Therapy (AGENT) trial in patients with stable angina pectoris[J]. Circulation, 2002, 105(11): 1291-1297.

[166] J. K. Gene therapy and angiogenesis in patients with coronary artery disease[J]. Expert review of cardiovascular therapy, 2010, 8(8): 1127-1138.

[167] Bradshaw RA, Dennis EA. *Handbook of Cell Signaling*: Elsevier Science, 2009.

[168] Itoh N, Ornitz DM. Fibroblast growth factors: from molecular evolution to roles in development, metabolism and disease[J]. Journal of biochemistry, 2011, 149(2): 121-130.

[169] Inagaki T, Choi M, Moschetta A, et al. Fibroblast growth factor 15 functions as an enterohepatic signal to regulate bile acid homeostasis[J]. Cell metabolism, 2005, 2(4): 217-225.

[170] Hotta Y, Nakamura H, Konishi M, et al. Fibroblast growth factor 21 regulates lipolysis in white adipose tissue but is not required for ketogenesis and triglyceride clearance in liver[J]. Endocrinology, 2009, 150(10): 4625-4633.

[171] Urakawa I, Yamazaki Y, Shimada T, et al. Klotho converts canonical FGF receptor into a specific receptor for FGF23[J]. Nature,

2006, 444(7120): 770-774.

[172] Yu C, Wang F, Kan M, et al. Elevated cholesterol metabolism and bile acid synthesis in mice lacking membrane tyrosine kinase receptor FGFR4[J]. The Journal of biological chemistry, 2000, 275(20): 15482-15489.

[173] Foltz IN, Hu S, King C, et al. Treating diabetes and obesity with an FGF21-mimetic antibody activating the βKlotho/FGFR1c receptor complex[J]. Science translational medicine, 2012, 4(162): 162ra153.

[174] Potthoff MJ, Kliewer SA, Mangelsdorf DJ. Endocrine fibroblast growth factors 15/19 and 21: from feast to famine[J]. Genes & development, 2012, 26(4): 312-324.

[175] Yang C, Wang C, Ye M, et al. Control of lipid metabolism by adipocyte FGFR1-mediated adipohepatic communication during hepatic stress[J]. Nutrition & metabolism, 2012, 9(1): 94.

[176] Kharitonenkov A, Shiyanova TL, Koester A, et al. FGF-21 as a novel metabolic regulator[J]. The Journal of clinical investigation, 2005, 115(6): 1627-1635.

[177] Fu L, John LM, Adams SH, et al. Fibroblast growth factor 19 increases metabolic rate and reverses dietary and leptin-deficient diabetes[J]. Endocrinology, 2004, 145(6): 2594-2603.

[178] Kharitonenkov A, Wroblewski VJ, Koester A, et al. The metabolic state of diabetic monkeys is regulated by fibroblast growth factor-21[J]. Endocrinology, 2007, 148(2): 774-781.

[179] Adams AC, Yang C, Coskun T, et al. The breadth of FGF21's metabolic actions are governed by FGFR1 in adipose tissue[J]. Mol Metab, 2012, 2(1): 31-37.

[180] Gälman C, Lundåsen T, Kharitonenkov A, et al. The circulating metabolic regulator FGF21 is induced by prolonged fasting and PPARalpha activation in man[J]. Cell metabolism, 2008, 8(2): 169-174.

[181] Berglund ED, Li CY, Bina HA, et al. Fibroblast growth factor 21 controls glycemia *via* regulation of hepatic glucose flux and insulin sensitivity[J]. Endocrinology, 2009, 150(9): 4084-4093.

[182] Inagaki T, Dutchak P, Zhao G, et al. Endocrine regulation of the fasting response by PPARalpha-mediated induction of fibroblast growth factor 21[J]. Cell metabolism, 2007, 5(6): 415-425.

[183] Potthoff MJ, Inagaki T, Satapati S, et al. FGF21 induces PGC-1alpha and regulates carbohydrate and fatty acid metabolism during the adaptive starvation response[J]. Proceedings of the National Academy of Sciences of the United States of America, 2009, 106(26): 10853-10858.

[184] Yang C, Jin C, Li X, et al. Differential specificity of endocrine FGF19 and FGF21 to FGFR1 and FGFR4 in complex with KLB[J]. PLoS ONE, 2012, 7(3): e33870.

[185] Suzuki M, Uehara Y, Motomura-Matsuzaka K, et al. betaKlotho is required for fibroblast growth factor (FGF) 21 signaling through FGF receptor (FGFR) 1c and FGFR3c[J]. Molecular endocrinology (Baltimore, Md.), 2008, 22(4): 1006-1014.

[186] Lin Z, Tian H, Lam K, et al. Adiponectin mediates the metabolic effects of FGF21 on glucose homeostasis and insulin sensitivity in mice[J]. Cell metabolism, 2013, 17(5): 779-789.

[187] Holland WL, Adams AC, Brozinick JT, et al. An FGF21-adiponectin-ceramide axis controls energy expenditure and insulin action in mice[J]. Cell metabolism, 2013, 17(5): 790-797.

[188] Luo Y, Mckeehan WL. Stressed Liver and Muscle Call on Adipocytes with FGF21[J]. Frontiers in endocrinology, 2013, 4: 194.

[189] Ohta H, Itoh N. Roles of FGFs as Adipokines in Adipose Tissue Development, Remodeling, and Metabolism[J]. Frontiers in endocrinology, 2014, 5: 18.

[190] Fuentes-Mattei E, Velazquez-Torres G, Phan L, et al. Effects of obesity on transcriptomic changes and cancer hallmarks in estrogen receptor-positive breast cancer[J]. Journal of the National Cancer Institute, 2014, 106(7).

[191] Luo Y, Yang C, Ye M, et al. Deficiency of metabolic regulator FGFR4 delays breast cancer progression through systemic and mi-

croenvironmental metabolic alterations[J]. Cancer & metabolism, 2013, 1(1): 21.

[192] Wesche J, Haglund K, Haugsten EM. Fibroblast growth factors and their receptors in cancer[J]. The Biochemical journal, 2011, 437(2): 199-213.

[193] Iyer G, Milowsky MI. Fibroblast growth factor receptor-3 in urothelial tumorigenesis[J]. Urologic oncology, 2013, 31(3): 303-311.

[194] Wang J, Stockton DW, Ittmann M. The fibroblast growth factor receptor-4 Arg388 allele is associated with prostate cancer initiation and progression[J]. Clinical cancer research : an official journal of the American Association for Cancer Research, 2004, 10: 6169-6178.

[195] Taylor BS, Schultz N, Hieronymus H, et al. Integrative genomic profiling of human prostate cancer[J]. Cancer cell, 2010, 18(1): 11-22.

[196] Hunter DJ, Kraft P, Jacobs KB, et al. A genome-wide association study identifies alleles in FGFR2 associated with risk of sporadic postmenopausal breast cancer[J]. Nature genetics, 2007, 39(7): 870-874.

[197] Kwabi-Addo B, Ozen M, Ittmann M. The role of fibroblast growth factors and their receptors in prostate cancer[J]. Endocrine-related cancer, 2004, 11(4): 709-724.

[198] Yan G, Fukabori Y, McBride G, et al. Exon switching and activation of stromal and embryonic fibroblast growth factor (FGF)-FGF receptor genes in prostate epithelial cells accompany stromal independence and malignancy[J]. Molecular and cellular biology, 1993, 13(8): 4513-4522.

[199] Lu W, Luo Y, Kan M, et al. Fibroblast growth factor-10. A second candidate stromal to epithelial cell andromedin in prostate[J]. The Journal of biological chemistry, 1999, 274(18): 12827-12834.

[200] Cotton L, O'Bryan M, Hinton B. Cellular signaling by fibroblast growth factors (FGFs) and their receptors (FGFRs) in male reproduction[J]. Endocrine reviews, 2008, 29(2): 193-216.

[201] Valve EM, Nevalainen MT, Nurmi MJ, et al. Increased expression of FGF-8 isoforms and FGF receptors in human premalignant prostatic intraepithelial neoplasia lesions and prostate cancer[J]. Laboratory investigation; a journal of technical methods and pathology, 2001, 81(6): 815-826.

[202] Leung HY, Dickson C, Robson CN, et al. Over-expression of fibroblast growth factor-8 in human prostate cancer[J]. Oncogene, 1996, 12(8): 1833-1835.

[203] Tanaka A, Furuya A, Yamasaki M, et al. High frequency of fibroblast growth factor (FGF) 8 expression in clinical prostate cancers and breast tissues, immunohistochemically demonstrated by a newly established neutralizing monoclonal antibody against FGF 8[J]. Cancer Res., 1998, 58(10): 2053-2056.

[204] Gnanapragasam VJ, Robinson MC, Marsh C, et al. FGF8 isoform b expression in human prostate cancer[J]. British journal of cancer, 2003, 88(9): 1432-1438.

[205] Dorkin TJ, Robinson MC, Marsh C, et al. FGF8 over-expression in prostate cancer is associated with decreased patient survival and persists in androgen independent disease[J]. Oncogene, 1999, 18(17): 2755-2761.

[206] Udayakumar TS, Nagle RB, Bowden GT. Fibroblast growth factor-1 transcriptionally induces membrane type-1 matrix metalloproteinase expression in prostate carcinoma cell line[J]. The Prostate, 2004, 58(1): 66-75.

[207] Huang Y, Jin C, Hamana T, et al. Overexpression of FGF9 in prostate epithelial cells augments reactive stroma formation and promotes prostate cancer progression[J]. International journal of biological sciences, 2015, 11(8): 948-960.

[208] Wesley UV, McGroarty M, Homoyouni A. Dipeptidyl peptidase inhibits malignant phenotype of prostate cancer cells by blocking basic fibroblast growth factor signaling pathway[J]. Cancer research, 2005, 65(4): 1325-1334.

[209] Yang F, Strand DW, Rowley DR. Fibroblast growth factor-2 me-

diates transforming growth factor-beta action in prostate cancer reactive stroma[J]. Oncogene, 2008, 27(4): 450-459.

[210] Polnaszek N, Kwabi-Addo B, Peterson LE, et al. Fibroblast growth factor 2 promotes tumor progression in an autochthonous mouse model of prostate cancer[J]. Cancer research, 2003, 63(18): 5754-5760.

[211] Liu J, You P, Chen G, et al. Hyperactivated FRS2α-mediated signaling in prostate cancer cells promotes tumor angiogenesis and predicts poor clinical outcome of patients[J]. Oncogene, 2016, 35(14): 1750-1759.

[212] Bubendorf L, Schöpfer A, Wagner U, et al. Metastatic patterns of prostate cancer: an autopsy study of 1,589 patients[J]. Human pathology, 2000, 31(5): 578-583.

[213] Li Z, Mathew P, Yang J, et al. Androgen receptor-negative human prostate cancer cells induce osteogenesis in mice through FGF9-mediated mechanisms[J]. The Journal of clinical investigation, 2008, 118(8): 2697-2710.

[214] Valta MP, Hentunen T, Qu Q, et al. Regulation of osteoblast differentiation: a novel function for fibroblast growth factor 8[J]. Endocrinology, 2006, 147(5): 2171-2182.

[215] Valta MP, Tuomela J, Bjartell A, et al. FGF-8 is involved in bone metastasis of prostate cancer[J]. International journal of cancer, 2008, 123(1): 22-31.

[216] Jin C, Wang F, Wu X, et al. Directionally specific paracrine communication mediated by epithelial FGF9 to stromal FGFR3 in two-compartment premalignant prostate tumors[J]. Cancer research, 2004, 64(13): 4555-4562.

[217] Leung HY, Mehta P, Gray LB, et al. Keratinocyte growth factor expression in hormone insensitive prostate cancer[J]. Oncogene, 1997, 15(9): 1115-1120.

[218] Gan Y, Wientjes MG, Au JL. Expression of basic fibroblast growth factor correlates with resistance to paclitaxel in human patient tumors[J]. Pharmaceutical research, 2006, 23(6): 1324-1331.

[219] Song S, Wientjes MG, Gan Y, et al. Fibroblast growth factors: an epigenetic mechanism of broad spectrum resistance to anticancer drugs[J]. Proceedings of the National Academy of Sciences of the United States of America, 2000, 97(15): 8658-8663.

[220] Maruyama-Takahashi K, Shimada N, Imada T, et al. A neutralizing anti-fibroblast growth factor (FGF) 8 monoclonal antibody shows anti-tumor activity against FGF8b-expressing LNCaP xenografts in androgen-dependent and -independent conditions[J]. The Prostate, 2008, 68(6): 640-650.

[221] Jin C, McKeehan K, Guo W, et al. Cooperation between ectopic FGFR1 and depression of FGFR2 in induction of prostatic intraepithelial neoplasia in the mouse prostate[J]. Cancer research, 2003, 63(24): 8784-8790.

[222] Wang F, McKeehan K, Yu C, et al. Chronic activity of ectopic type 1 fibroblast growth factor receptor tyrosine kinase in prostate epithelium results in hyperplasia accompanied by intraepithelial neoplasia[J]. The Prostate, 2004, 58(1): 1-12.

[223] Acevedo VD, Gangula RD, Freeman KW, et al. Inducible FGFR-1 activation leads to irreversible prostate adenocarcinoma and an epithelial-to-mesenchymal transition[J]. Cancer cell, 2007, 12(6): 559-571.

[224] Zhang Y, Zhang J, Lin Y, et al. Role of epithelial cell fibroblast growth factor receptor substrate 2alpha in prostate development, regeneration and tumorigenesis[J]. Development (Cambridge, England), 2008, 135(4): 775-784.

[225] Yang F, Zhang Y, Ressler SJ, et al. FGFR1 is essential for prostate cancer progression and metastasis[J]. Cancer research, 2013, 73(12): 3716-3724.

[226] Memarzadeh S, Xin L, Mulholland DJ, et al. Enhanced paracrine FGF10 expression promotes formation of multifocal prostate adenocarcinoma and an increase in epithelial androgen receptor[J]. Cancer cell, 2007, 12(6): 572-585.

[227] Kalluri R, Weinberg R. The basics of epithelial-mesenchymal

transition[J]. The Journal of clinical investigation, 2009, 119(6): 1420-1428.

[228] Holzmann K, Grunt T, Heinzle C, *et al*. Alternative Splicing of Fibroblast Growth Factor Receptor IgIII Loops in Cancer[J]. Journal of nucleic acids, 2012, 2012: 950508.

[229] Gavine P, Mooney L, Kilgour E, *et al*. AZD4547: an orally bioavailable, potent, and selective inhibitor of the fibroblast growth factor receptor tyrosine kinase family[J]. Cancer research, 2012, 72(8): 2045-2056.

[230] Xie L, Su X, Zhang L, *et al*. FGFR2 gene amplification in gastric cancer predicts sensitivity to the selective FGFR inhibitor AZD4547[J]. Clinical cancer research : an official journal of the American Association for Cancer Research, 2013, 19(9): 2572-2583.

[231] Trudel S, Li Z, Wei E, *et al*. CHIR-258, a novel, multitargeted tyrosine kinase inhibitor for the potential treatment of t(4;14) multiple myeloma[J]. Blood, 2005, 105(7): 2941-2948.

[232] Hilberg F, Roth G, Krssak M, *et al*. BIBF 1120: triple angiokinase inhibitor with sustained receptor blockade and good antitumor efficacy[J]. Cancer research, 2008, 68(12): 4774-4782.

[233] Okamoto K, Ikemori-Kawada M, Jestel A, *et al*. Distinct binding mode of multikinase inhibitor lenvatinib revealed by biochemical characterization[J]. ACS medicinal chemistry letters, 2015, 6(1): 89-94.

[234] Bhide RS, Cai ZW, Zhang YZ, *et al*. Discovery and preclinical studies of (R)-1-(4-(4-fluoro-2-methyl-1H-indol-5-yloxy)-5-methylpyrrolo[2,1-f][1,2,4]triazin-6-yloxy)propan- 2-ol (BMS-540215), an *in vivo* active potent VEGFR-2 inhibitor[J]. Journal of medicinal chemistry, 2006, 49(7): 2143-2146.

[235] Laird AD, Vajkoczy P, Shawver LK, *et al*. SU6668 is a potent antiangiogenic and antitumor agent that induces regression of established tumors[J]. Cancer Res., 2000, 60(15): 4152-4160.

[236] Daniele G, Corral J, Molife LR, *et al*. FGF receptor inhibitors: role in cancer therapy[J]. Current oncology reports, 2012, 14(2): 111-119.

[237] Mohammadi M, Froum S, Hamby JM, *et al*. Crystal structure of an angiogenesis inhibitor bound to the FGF receptor tyrosine kinase domain[J]. Embo j., 1998, 17(20): 5896-5904.

[238] Xu C, Li W, Qiu P, *et al*. The therapeutic potential of a novel non-ATP-competitive fibroblast growth factor receptor 1 inhibitor on gastric cancer[J]. Anti-cancer drugs, 2015, 26(4): 379-387.

[239] Wu J, Ji J, Weng B, *et al*. Discovery of novel non-ATP competitive FGFR1 inhibitors and evaluation of their anti-tumor activity in non-small cell lung cancer *in vitro* and *in vivo*[J]. Oncotarget, 2014, 5(12): 4543-4553.

[240] Wang Y, Cai Y, Ji J, *et al*. Discovery and identification of new non-ATP competitive FGFR1 inhibitors with therapeutic potential on non-small-cell lung cancer[J]. Cancer letters, 2014, 344(1): 82-89.

[241] Qing J, Du X, Chen Y, *et al*. Antibody-based targeting of FGFR3 in bladder carcinoma and t(4;14)-positive multiple myeloma in mice[J]. The Journal of clinical investigation, 2009, 119(5): 1216-1229.

[242] Bai A, Meetze K, Vo NY, *et al*. GP369, an FGFR2-IIIb-specific antibody, exhibits potent antitumor activity against human cancers driven by activated FGFR2 signaling[J]. Cancer research, 2010, 70(19): 7630-7639.

[243] Pai R, Dunlap D, Qing J, *et al*. Inhibition of fibroblast growth factor 19 reduces tumor growth by modulating beta-catenin signaling[J]. Cancer research, 2008, 68(13): 5086-5095.

[244] Harding TC, Long L, Palencia S, *et al*. Blockade of nonhormonal fibroblast growth factors by FP-1039 inhibits growth of multiple types of cancer[J]. Science translational medicine, 2013, 5(178): 178ra139.

[245] Tolcher A, Papadopoulos. Kyri, Agnew J, *et al*. Abstract A103: Preliminary results of a phase 1 study of FP-1039 (FGFR1:Fc), a novel antagonist of multiple fibroblast growth factor (FGF) ligands, in patients with advanced malignancies[J]. Molecular Cancer Therapeutics, 2009, 8(12 Supplement): A103-A103.

[246] Fan L, Xie H, Chen L, *et al*. A novel FGF2 antagonist peptide P8 with potent antiproliferation activity[J]. Tumour biology : the journal of the International Society for Oncodevelopmental Biology and Medicine, 2014, 35(10): 10571-10579.

[247] Wu X, Huang H, Wang C, *et al*. Identification of a novel peptide that blocks basic fibroblast growth factor-mediated cell proliferation[J]. Oncotarget, 2013, 4(10): 1819-1828.

Pharmacological application of growth factors: basic and clinical

Jian Xiao, Xiaokun Li

Growth factors are signaling molecules that are typically secreted at the site of repair by many different cell types including platelets, stem cells, and fibroblasts. Since Montalcini and Hamburger first described the nerve growth factor (NGF) in 1951, this epoch-making discovery has initiated the detection of a multitude of other growth factors that alter cell growth, cell differentiation, and proliferation, which is essential for wound healing and tissue repair and regeneration. Several growth factors such as fibroblast growth factor (FGF), epidermal growth factor (EGF), and nerve growth factor (NGF) play a key role in brain or spinal cord injury and acute organ injuries. Vascular endothelial growth factor (VEGF) increases vascular permeability, induces angiogenesis, vasculogenesis, which is applied in treatment of ischemic heart disease.

Treatment with growth factors is beginning to gain world-wide prevalence, mainly in plastic and reconstructive surgery. However, the molecular mechanisms of growth factors treatment are still undefined. Thus, further investigations on mechanisms of growth factors in basic and clinical research are urgent. Therefore, we have invited the researchers to contribute few research/review papers to provide evidence that supports the application of growth factor in prevention or treatment of diseases.

In this special issue, we have invited some papers hoping to shed light on some aspects of this very interesting field. We have collected 8 papers by scientists from 4 countries. In the submitted research papers, H. Wang et al. summarize the current understanding of the NGF signaling in retina and the therapeutic implications in the treatment of glaucoma.

NGF offers the promise of actually restoring visual function through acting on the TrkA receptor; however, the future of NGF-dependent treatments in the armamentarium of glaucoma therapy as most of the present studies were in animal models, hence, randomized, controlled glaucoma clinical trials need to be performed to evaluate the therapeutic effect of NGF in the treatment of glaucoma. While M. Ammendola et al. review antitumor and antiangiogenic potential of three agents which are able to inhibit the functions of mast cells (MCs) tryptase: gabexate mesylate, nafamostat mesylate, and tranilast, the authors suggest that future awaited clinical studies aim to evaluate the truly efficacy of the tryptase inhibitors as a novel tumor antiangiogenic therapy. J. Cai et al. concluded the neuroprotective efficacy of neurotrophins (NTs) (NGF, BDNF, FGF-2, IGF, NT3, and NT4/5) in animal models, highlighted outstanding technical challenges, and discussed more recent attempts to harness the neuroprotective capacity of endogenous NTs using small molecule inducers and cell transplantation. On the other hand, J. C. Chen and colleagues demonstrated that NGF exists multiple bioactivity except for the neuronprotective activity. They found NGF accelerates the healing of skin excisional wounds in rats and the fibroblast migration induced by NGF may contribute to this healing process; moreover, the activation of PI3K/Akt, Rac1, JNK, and ERK may be involved in the regulation of NGF-induced fibroblast migration. In two very interesting research papers, Z. G. Feng et al. have shown that tobacco plants express Keratinocyte Growth Factor (KGF1) via Agrobacterium-mediated transformation using a Potato virus X- (PVX-) based vector (pgR107). The plant-derived KGF1 promotes the proliferation of NIH/3T3 cells and significantly stimulates wound healing in the diabetic wounded rat model. This finding indicated that KGF1 from tobacco maintains its biological activity, implying prospective industrial production in a plant bioreactor. While X.S Wang suggested endoplasmic reticulum (ER) stress is the key mechanism for regulating FGF21 in several metabolic diseases. This study showed FGF21 is the target gene for activating transcription factor 4 (ATF4) and CCAAT enhancer binding protein homologous protein (CHOP). ER stress increased the half-life of mRNA of FGF21, which may partly explain the mechanism of increasing FGF21 levels in metabolism disease. In the following papers, H. Nawa et al. discussed neuregulin-1 (NGR1) and EGF to rodent pups, juveniles, and adults and characterized neurobiological and behavioral consequences. The cytokine-driven dopaminergic dysfunction might illustrate some of the psychopathological features of schizophrenia, although it is possible that the responsible factors might be other cytokines other than EGF, NRG1, or virokine. L. J. Xiang et al. investigated the hair growth promoting activities of three approved growth factor drugs, FGF-10, FGF-1, and FGF-2. They observed that FGFs promoted hair growth by inducing the anagen phase in telogenic C57BL/6 mice. FGFs-treated group showed earlier induction of β-catenin and Sonic hedgehog (Shh) in hair follicles, suggesting that FGFs promote hair growth by inducing the anagen phase in resting hair follicles and might be a potential hair growth-promoting agent. Finally, J. Song *et al*. summarized the recent findings on the association between risk factors for vascular dementia and adiponectin including aging, diabetes, hypertension, atherosclerosis, and stroke. The authors suggested that further studies are necessary to examine the role of adiponectin in vascular dementia, and the regulation of adiponectin levels and receptors of adiponectin would be important for the prevention and treatment of vascular dementia.

Cytokines and diabetes research

Jian Xiao, Ji Li, Lu Cai, Subrata Chakrabarti, Xiaokun Li

In recent years, the role of the inflammatory system in the pathogenesis of diabetes has been increasingly investigated. Cytokines, a group of proteins that are expressed by several cell types, act as immune mediators and regulators. Depending on the period of pregnancy, a predominant inflammatory profile is defined by increased production of cytokines. Insulin resistance has been associated with abnormal secretion of proinflammatory cytokines such as tumor necrosis factor-α (TNF-α) and Interleukin-6 (IL-6) and decreased production of anti-inflammatory mediators such as IL-4 and IL-10. Despite some controversies regarding specific cytokine levels, type 2 diabetes mellitus (T2DM) is currently regarded as a chronic inflammatory disease, while type 1 diabetes (T1D) is considered to be a T-helper-(Th)-1 autoimmune disease.

Extensive research in animals and in humans over the last decade has revealed important functions of cytokines in diabetes; adiponectin (APN) and leptin can decrease hepatic gluconeogenesis, resistin (REN) can increase hepatic gluconeogenesis and glycogenolysis, IL-6 can decrease glycogen synthesis, and TNF-α can decrease glucose uptake in liver. Both of them can block hepatic insulin signalling by interfection of insulin receptor signalling and insulin signal transduction. Thus, cytokines are involved in nearly every facet of immunity, inflammation, and development of diabetes.

In this special issue, we have invited some papers hoping to shed light on some aspects of this very interesting field. We have collected 7 papers by scientists from 5 countries. In the submitted research papers, Y. Li et al. summarize recent findings regarding the relationship between adipocytokines and hepatic insulin resistance. Excessive adipose tissue may be detrimental partially through secretion of the following cytokines: TNF-α, IL-6, and resistin. In contrast, the presence of adipose tissues is vital in the prevention of hepatic insulin resistance via secretion of the following cytokines: leptin and adiponectin. While J. Su and colleagues review the relationship between the endoplasmic reticulum (ER) and autophagy, inflammation, and apoptosis in DM to better understand the molecular mechanisms of diabetes, the authors suggest that the ER is therefore an attractive potential therapeutic target, and maintaining or improving ER function appropriately may prevent diabetes. Z. Meng et al. concluded that ethanol causes glucose intolerance by increasing hepatic expression of 11β-hydroxysteroid dehydrogenase type 1 (11β-HSD1) and glucocorticoid receptor (GR), which leads to increased expression of gluconeogenic and glycogenolytic enzymes. In the following papers, J. Liu et al. have shown that uncoupling proteins (UCPs) may affect the development of DM through decreasing mitochondrial membrane potential, increasing energy expenditure especially through glucose and lipid metabolisms, downregulating ROS generation, and gene polymorphisms. In a very interesting research paper, J. Vcelakova et al. have shown, that in T1D patients, important immune response-related pathways were involved. These important immune response-related processes largely included the induction of Th17 and Th22 responses, as well as cytoskeletal rearrangements, MHCII presentation, and the upregulation of CD4, TGF-beta, and STAT3. These findings potentially suggest that these processes could be utilised as predictive markers for the development of T1D or as molecular targets for the repression of specific immunocompetent cell populations for the treatment of diabetes. On the other hand, H. Meng and colleagues demonstrate that amyloid precursor protein 17 peptide (APP17 peptide) has a comprehensive therapeutic effect on diabetic encephalopathy, particularly through improving glycol metabolism. Finally, M. Cui et al. have shown that AMPK activation, which was represented by the level of p-AMPK, did not correlate with the improvement of metabolic conditions in diabetes mice, implying that AMPK activation may not participate in mediating the beneficial effects of chronic caloric restriction (CR) or exercise. However, the autophagy activity might be related to the improved metabolic conditions; thus autophagy may play a role in mediating the effects of chronic CR.

Small molecule inhibition of fibroblast growth factor receptors in cancer

Guang Liang, Xiaokun Li

1. Introduction

Fibroblast growth-factor receptors (FGFRs) form a sub-family of the receptor tyrosine kinase (RTK) superfamily, and they are encoded by four genes (FGFR1, FGFR2, FGFR3, and FGFR4). They are involved in the regulation of organ development, cell proliferation and migration, angiogenesis, and other processes. Recent studies have shown that FGFR-activating mutations and overexpression are closely associated with the development and progression of tumors in humans [1]. FGFR-activating mutations or overexpression can lead to persistent and excessive activation of the FGFR signaling pathway, resulting in carcinogenic functions in the cells, such as excessive proliferation and apoptosis evasion [2]. For example, FGFR-activating mutations in bladder cancer, endometrial carcinomas, multiple myeloma, and rhabdomyosarcoma lead to the development and progression of tumors and a poor prognosis, and they also play an important role in tumor angiogenesis, tumor invasion, and metastasis [2]. In recent years, *in vivo* and *in vitro* studies using FGFR gene knockout and pharmacological inhibition have provided further confirmation that FGFR should be an important target for cancer treatment [2]. Several major pharmaceutical companies and research institutions have designed various types of non-selective and selective FGFR inhibitors, some of which have entered anti-tumor clinical trials and have shown promising clinical effects and application prospects [3]. In this article, we review the key roles of FGFR in tumor development and progression and examine the design, structural characteristics, FGFR-binding mechanisms, and progress of clinical trials of small-molecule FGFR inhibitors.

2. FGFR signaling in cancer

The prototypical FGFR protein consists of an extracellular domain that mediates ligand binding, a single transmembrane helix, and an intracellular domain that possesses tyrosine kinase activity. Classically, the liberated FGFs bind to heparin sulphate proteoglycans (HPSGs) on the surfaces of the cells, which also stabilizes the FGF ligand-receptor interaction, forming a ternary complex with FGFRs [4]. The specificity of the FGF-FGFR interaction was established partly by the differing ligand-binding capacities of the receptor paralogues and alternative splicing of FGFR [5]. FGFRs signal as dimmers, and the ligand-dependent dimerization leads to a conformational shift in the structure of the receptor that activates the intracellular kinase domain, resulting in intermolecular transphosphorylation of the tyrosine kinase domains and the intracellular tail. Phosphorylated tyrosines help facilitate the phosphorylation of the substrate by increasing the proximity of SH2-containing substrates to the kinase. FGFR substrate 2 (FRS2) is a key adapter protein that is directly phosphorylated by FGFR kinase. Phosphorylated FRS2 binds growth factor receptor-bound 2 (Grb2), resulting in the direct binding and activation of the Grb2-associated son of sevenless (SOS), which, in turn, recruits and activates the Ras/mitogen-activated protein kinase (Ras/MAPK) pathway to manifest in cell proliferation and differentiation [6]. Signaling pathways that involve Grb2 are complex, because Grb2 also can bind to Grb2-associated binding protein 1 (GAB1) to recruit PI3K, which activates the AKT signaling pathway to inhibit apoptosis and promote cell survival [7]. Src homology 2 (SH2), which contains phospholipase-Cγ (PLC)γ, associates directly with a phosphorylated tyrosine in the receptor C-terminal tail, facilitating the phosphorylation of PLCγ [8]. Activated PLCγ hydrolyzes phosphatidylinositol-4,5-biphosphate (PIP2) to generate IP3 and diacylglycerol (DAG), the latter of which can activate protein kinase C (PKC) to enhance the level of Raf phosphorylation. In addition, FGFR can activate other signaling molecules, including signal transduction and activation of transcription (STATs) and ribosomal protein S6 kinase 2 (RSK2) [9], which promotes tumor development. The FGFR signaling pathways in carcinogenesis have been reviewed in recent years [1,2,6,10,11].

Three alterations, which include FGFRs-activating mutations, the amplification of receptor genes, and their amplification, lead to the aberrant activation of FGFR signaling pathways in ligand-dependent fashion or in independent fashion in a variety of cancers [6]. In addition, chromosomal translocations involving FGFR genes have been observed in cancer patients [2]. These translocations lead to the amplification of FGFRs, contributing to the initiation, progression, and therapeutic resistance of the disease [2]. Table 1 provides a list that shows the genetic alterations in FGFRs related to cancer.

Table 1.   Genetic alterations in FGFRs related to cancer

Gene	Changes	Sites	Cancer	Refs.
FGFR1	Amplification	8p11-12 amp	Breast cancer (10%)	[14]
			Lung adenocarcinoma (21%)	[16]
			Oral squamous cell carcinoma (17.4%)	[17]
			Prostate cancer (rare)	[18,19]
			Ovarian cancer (~5%)	[20]
			Bladder cancer (3%)	[49]
			Rhabdomyosarcoma (3%)	[21]
	Mutation	N546K/K656E	Glioblastoma (NR[a])	[12,13]
		S125L	Melanoma (rare)	[50]
	Translocation	t(8;13)	Stem cell leukaema (rare)	[23]
		t(8;13)	Lymphoma syndrome (rare)	[23]
		8p11-12 trans	Chronic myeloid leukemia (rare)	[24]
		8p11	Glioblastoma (3.1% with FGFR3 together)	[45]
FGFR2	Amplification	SUM52/MFM233	Breast cancer (~2%)	[28,29]
		SNP[b]	Gastric cancer (10%)	[25]
	Mutation	S252W	Endometrial cancer (12%)	[26]
		W290C	Lung cancer (NR)	[28,32,51]
		K660M	Cervical cancer (NR)	[52]
		I642V	Melanoma (rare)	[53]
		S267P	Stomach (NR)	[54]
FGFR3	Amplification		Bladder cancer (42%)	[43]
	Mutation	S375C/S249C	Bladder cancer (15-20%)	[34,42]
		R248C/S249C/Y375C	Bladder cancer (~50%)	[34,43]
		K650E/K650M/Y373C	Multiple myeloma (~8%)	[37,44]
		K650M	Cervical cancer (5%)	[34]
		S249C/A391E	Prostate cancer (3%)	[55]
		K650E	Spermatocytic seminoma (7%)	[39]
		S249C	Cervix carcinomas (NR)	[34]
		R248C	Seborrheic keratosis (39%)	[40]
		K650T/K650N	Testicular tumor (NR)	[39]
	Translocation	t(4;14) (p16;q32)	Myeloma (15%)	[37,44]
		4p16	Glioblastoma (3.1% with FGFR1 together)	[45]
FGFR4	Mutation	K535/E550	Rhabdomyosarcoma (8%)	[47]
		G388R/Y367C	Breast cancer (NR)	[48,56]

[a] NR, not reported.

[b] SNP, single nucleotide polymorphism.

In patients with glioblastoma, FGFR1 activation can be caused by N546K and K656E mutations [12,13]. FGFR1 amplification is one of the most common focal changes in breast cancer, and it occurs in about 10% of the cases of breast cancer, most of which are estrogen-dependent [14]. An *in vitro* study showed that FGFR1 up-regulation promoted cell proliferation in breast cancer, while FGFR1 down-regulation stimulated apoptosis [15]. Furthermore, recent studies found that the focal amplification of FGFR1 exists in non-small-cell lung cancer, and the results of a small study showed that it occurs in 21% of lung adenocarcinoma [16] cases and 17.4% of oral squamous cell carcinoma cases [17]. FGFR1 is also up-regulated in prostate cancer [18]. Acevedo *et al.* showed that induced FGFR1 overexpression in prostate epithelial cells in a mouse model of prostate cancer can result in epithelial-mesenchymal transition and adenocarcinoma [19]. FGFR1 amplification has been identified in oral squamous cell carcinoma, ovarian cancer, bladder cancer, and sarcoma [17,20-22]. In addition, chromosomal translocation t(8;13) (p11;q11-12) involving the FGFR1 gene has been observed to result in FGFR1 up-regulation in both lymphoma and myeloid leukemia cells from these patients [23,24]. Xiao *et al.* [23] found that the 8p11 translocation breakpoints interrupt intron 8 of the FGFR1 gene, which contributes to diverse oncogenic fusion genes, including FGFR1 with chromosome-13 gene (ZNF198).

FGFR2 mutations are more common than FGFR1 mutations in tumors. Amplification of the FGFR2 gene or missense mutations have been seen in gastric cancer, lung cancer, breast cancer, ovarian cancer, endometrial cancer, and other malignancies [25]. Sequencing analysis showed that FGFR2 mutations occur in 12% of endometrial cancer cases, mostly at S252W [26]. In addition, studies that involved a FGFR2 gene-knockout model or treatment with the FGFR inhibitor PD173074 showed that the activation of FGFR2 has an important role in the development of endometrial cancer, indicating that FGFR2 is a potential target for the treatment of endometrial cancer [27]. FGFR2 amplification loci (SUM52 and MFM233) have been found in 2% of breast cancer cases [28,29], suggesting that FGFR2 can increase the risk of breast cancer [30,31]. In addition, FGFR2 amplification is present in nearly 10% of gastric cancer cases [25], and the FGFR2 mutation W290C has been found in non-small-cell lung cancer [28,32]. FGFR2, as a key regulatory molecule for advanced tumors, is related closely to tumor progression and metastasis [25]. In a recent, population-based, case-controlled study, Marian *et al.* examined the genetic associations of four intronic, FGFR2, single-nucleotide polymorphisms (SNPs) and found that FGFR2 variants were associated significantly with the risk of breast cancer, irrespective of the status of estrogen and progesterone receptors, metastasis, the involvement of lymph nodes, and nuclear grade [33].

Among FGFRs, FGFR3 was the first that was reported to undergo mutations. Over 35% of bladder cancer patients harbor an SNP in the FGFR3 gene [34]. The most common mutations of the FGFR3 gene include R248C, S249C, R248C, and K562E. More than half of the FGFR3 mutations occur in the extracellular domain, leading to the activation of the ligand-independent FGFR receptor [35,36]. Studies of the bladder cancer cell line and xenograft tumor transplantation have demonstrated that anti-bodies and small molecule inhibitors against mutant FGFR3 show remarkable anti-tumor activity [37,38]. Recently, it was found that FGFR3 mutation K650E also occurred in spermatocytic seminoma [39]. FGFR3-activating mutations also have been found in a variety of other cancers, including cervical cancer, testicular tumor, benign seborrheic keratoses, and oral squamous cell carcinoma [34,39-41]. In addition, FGFR3 mutation has been noted in 15%-20% of bladder cancer patients [42,43], and 42% of bladder cancer samples had FGFR3 overexpression [42,43]. In addition to mutation, the t(4;14) translocation is associated with the upregulation of FGFR3 in multiple myeloma [37,44]. Preclinical studies of inhibitors of FGFR3 have shown promise in t(4;14) multiple myeloma, and these studies have led to the initiation of clinical trials. Very recently, it was reported that 3.1% of human glioblastoma harbor oncogenic chromosomal translocations that fuse in-frame the tyrosine kinase coding domains of the FGFR genes (FGFR1 or FGFR3) to the transforming acidic coiled-coil (TACC) coding domains of TACC1 or TACC3, respectively [45].

Of the FGFRs, FGFR4 was the last to be shown to have a role in cancer, and it also has been identified as a target of cancer. FGFR4 gain-of-function mutations have been observed in 8% of patients with rhabdomyosarcoma, and these mutations, which occur at K535 and E550 in the tyrosine kinase domain, can enhance tumor invasion and metastasis [46]. In a breast cancer model, the analyses of single nucleotide polymorphism revealed that the FGFR4 mutation G388R promoted cancer metastasis and was associated with the resistance of breast cancer to chemotherapy [47]. In isolated tumor cells with FGFR4 overexpression, FGFR4 interference was shown to boost the efficacy of chemotherapy significantly [48]. These findings suggest that FGFR4 has an important role in the resistance of breast cancer cells to chemotherapy.

3. Small-molecule inhibitors that target FGFRs

Given the important role of FGFRs in the development and progression of tumors, FGFRs have gradually become the target of cancer treatment in various research institutions and pharmaceutical companies. Based on their modes of action in FGFRs, inhibitors can be divided into two categories, *i.e.*, (1) antibodies or peptides that bind to the extracellular region of FGFRs and neutralize FGF binding, thus inhibiting FGFR dimerization and activation and (2) small-molecule inhibitors that bind to the intracellular kinase domain of FGFRs and inhibit FGFR auto-phosphorylation or its ability to catalyze the phosphorylation of downstream proteins. At present, several small-molecule, FGFR inhibitors are being evaluated in clinical trials to determine their anti-tumor activities. Furthermore, additional, small-molecule inhibitors are being designed and assessed in pre-clinical studies. In this section, we discuss the structural characteristics and structure-activity relationships of the current, small-molecule inhibitors of FGFR in order to identify the patterns that govern their structural design and to better guide the design of drugs.

3.1 Structural features of small-molecule inhibitors bound to the ATP binding site of FGFR (Fig. 1)

The ATP binding pocket of FGFR1 is located in the cleft between the N- and C-lobes and the kinase, and the pocket

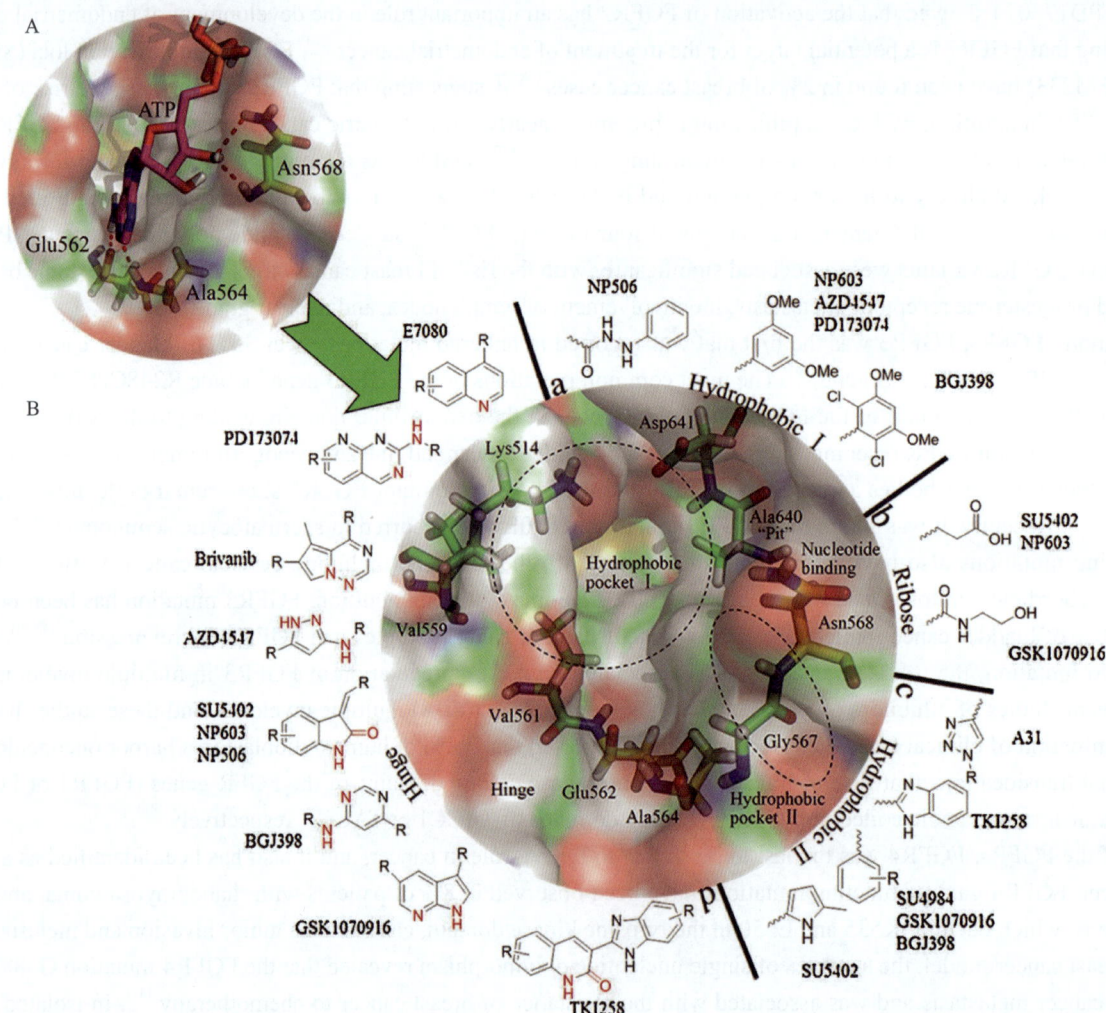

Fig. 1. Structural features of FGFR inhibitors bound to the ATP-binding pocket of FGFR: (A) binding simulation between ATP and FGFR1. The hydrogen bonds are shown using red, dashed lines. (B) Active moieties in current FGFR inhibitors and the structural domain bound to these inhibitors in FGFR. A simulation of the ATP-binding pocket indicates the sites of hydrophobic domain I/II, the nucleotide-binding domain, the hinge region, and the important amino acids inside the pocket. The active moieties of FGFR inhibitors bind to different domains and form different interactions, such as hydrophobic interactions (a, c) and hydrogen bonds (b, d). In domain c, the atoms that form hydrogen bonds with amino acid residues are marked in red.

is composed of residues from the N- and C-lobes, the nucleotide-binding loop, and the hinge region that connects the two lobes (Fig. 1). The adenine ring of ATP is sandwiched between the hydrophobic residues that emanate from both lobes (termed hydrophobic domain I) in the pocket. Hydrophobic domain I is a vast hydrophobic pocket that consists of several hydrophobic amino acid residues, such as Ala640, Val559, and Val561. It forms van der Waals interactions with hydrophobic groups that enter the pocket [57,58], such as the 3,5-dimethoxyphenyl of NP603 [59], AZD4547, and PD173074 [60], the phenylhydrazino group of NP506 [61], and the 2,6-dichloro-3,5-dimethoxy-phenyl of BGJ398 [62]. In addition to van der Waals forces, amino acid residues of the hydrophobic domain form hydrogen bonds with some groups that enter the region. For example, PD173074 has hydrophobic interactions between two methoxy groups on its phenyl ring and Val559 and Val561, as well as with the hydrogen bonds between the oxygen atom in the two methoxy groups and the nitrogen atoms in Lys514 and Asp641 [60]. More importantly, the interaction between Val559 and Val561 and the methoxy groups is considered the primary site for kinase selectivity of FGFR inhibitors. Therefore, NP603, AZD4547, BGJ398, and PD173074 show selectivity for FGFRs [60,63,64]. However, the difference caused by interaction with Val559 and Val561 could not contribute to the selectivity among the highly homologous kinases, such as FGFRs, KDR, and FLT. Very recently, Norman *et al.* defined a new functional site "pit" at Ala640 in hydrophobic domain I *via* protein-ligand crystal structure information, suggesting that compounds that rigidly protruded in an appropriate direction to fill this space might be able to achieve selectivity between FGFR1 and KDR [64]. Accordingly, PD173074 does not protrude into the "pit" at all, and this shows clearly that it is an equipotent inhibitor of FGFR1 and KDR, and AZD4547 showed selectivity of FGFR1 against KDR due to a rigid piperidyl group at the same position.

The hinge region provides key contacts with ATP and small-molecule inhibitors. Almost all FGFR small-molecule inhibitors have a pharmacophore capable of hydrogen bonding with two residues from the hinge region, *i.e.*, Glu562 and Ala564 [57]. Examples of these inhibitors include indolin-2-one of SU5402, NP603, and NP506, amino pyrido pyrimidine of PD173074, quinolinone of TKI258 [65], aza-indole of GSK1070916, pyrrole and triazine of Brivanib [66], quinoline of E7080 [67], aminopyrazole of AZD4547 [68], and aminopyrimidine of BGJ398 [62]. These compounds share two common structural features, *i.e.*, (1) they all contain either a tertiary amino nitrogen atom or a carbonyl oxygen atom that serves as an electron donor, which allows the formation of a hydrogen bond with the amino moiety of kinase and (2) they contain a primary or secondary amino hydrogen atom as the electron acceptor, which bonds with the carbonyl moiety of kinase. These types of bonding mimic the binding mode between adenine in the ATP and this region.

A second hydrophobic pocket located outside of the ATP binding pocket has an important role in binding small molecule inhibitors. It forms van der Waals interactions with some hydrophobic groups, such as methylpyrrol of SU5402 [58], the 3-phenyl ring of SU4984 [58], the 2-phenyl ring of GSK1070916, the phenyl ring on the pyrimidine amino of BGJ398 [62], the phenyl ring on the pyrazol of AZD4547 [68], and the benzimidazolyl of TKI258 [65]. The long-chain, aliphatic amine of PD173074 also interacts with hydrophobic domain II region, but this interaction is very weak as evidenced by the weak electron density for the long-chain, aliphatic amine in the crystals. Jonquoy *et al.* [69] and Le Corre *et al.* [70] replaced the long-chain aliphatic amine with triazole groups and obtained compound A31, which exhibits a greater inhibitory effect against FGFR than PD173074 does. The nucleotide-binding domain is located adjacent to hydrophobic domain II. When ATP binds to the binding site, the hydroxyl in the ribose ring of ATP forms a hydrogen bond with the amino acid residue Asn568 [58]. Not many small-molecule inhibitors involve the nucleotide-binding domain region. Only the long-chain carboxyl of SU5402 and NP603 [70] and the long-chain hydroxyl of GSK1070916 analogs have been reported to interact with this region [71]. In addition, outside the ATP-binding pocket is an active region called the p-loop, which contains a cysteine (Cys486) (Fig. 2A). By forming covalent binding between a Michael acceptor and Cys486, Zhou *et al.* [72] designed and obtained a class of small-molecule, irreversible inhibitors of FGFR1, which is represented by FIIN1 (Fig. 2B).

3.2 Non-ATP-competitive small-molecule inhibitors

Since the ATP binding domain is highly conserved across RTKs, it has a similar three-dimensional structure in almost all RTK family members. As a result, these inhibitors have several shortcomings, including poor specificity, side effects, and multi-drug resistance. In recent years, researchers have begun to investigate non-ATP-competitive inhibitors. In fact, non-ATP-competitive inhibitors also act on the ATP-binding pocket, but they combine with a non-active ATP binding site and induce a conformation shift that is quite different from that of the active ATP binding site. This conformational difference occurs in a D-F-G sequence in the activation loop of the ATP binding pocket. A pocket-inside

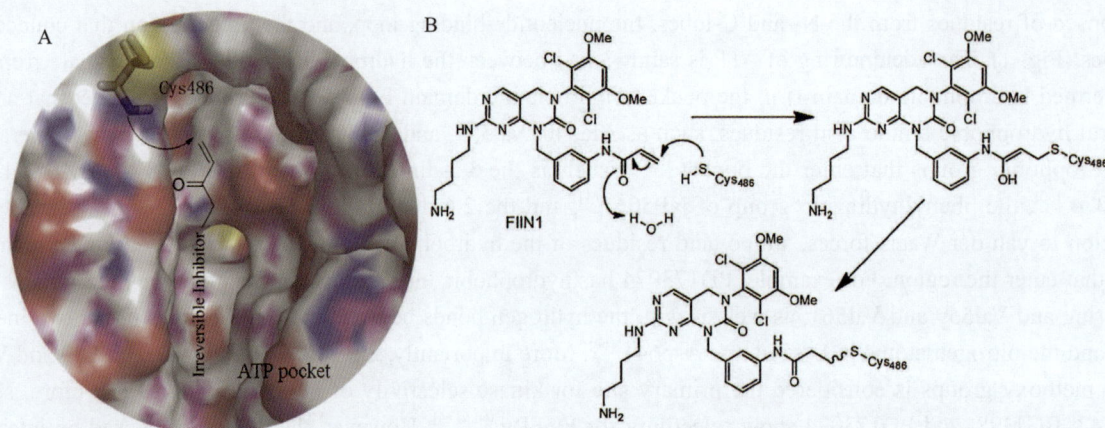

Fig. 2. FGFR-binding mechanism of irreversible FGFR inhibitors: (A) simulation showing the covalent binding between the Michael receptor structure of FGFR inhibitors and Cys486 at the p-loop of the ATP-binding pocket and (B) chemical mechanism by which the thiol group of Cys486 reacts with the acroloyl group in FIIN1, contributing to irreversible, covalent binding.

orientation of the benzene ring of F (Phe) in the DFG sequence causes a non-active ATP-binding site ("DFG-OUT" conformation), while a pocket-outside orientation of this benzene ring forms an active site ("DFG-IN" conformation). This conformational change from "DFG-IN" to "DFG-OUT" causes the kinase to expose an additional hydrophobic pocket known as the allosteric site (Fig. 3). The allosteric site shows considerable sequence variation across different receptor kinases. Therefore, inhibitors designed for this site have favorable kinase selectivity [73-75]. At present, studies of non-ATP-competitive inhibitors of FGFR are still in the early stages. To date, only Eathiraj et al. [74] have reported a class of non-ATP-competitive inhibitors of FGFR, typified by ARQ069, which combine with the "DFG-OUT" conformation, with an inhibitory activity of 0.85 μm for FGFR1 (Fig. 3B). In addition, Krejci et al. [76] reported another class of new Suramin analogs, and the representative compound NF449 also showed non-ATP-competitive inhibition of FGFR3. Nevertheless, its specific binding site remains unclear.

In summary, several studies have placed emphasis on ATP-competitive inhibitors. In an attempt to increase FGFR inhibitor specificity and selectivity to reduce toxic side effects, researches are investigating how inhibitors interact with their protein targets. Based on our analysis of current FGFR inhibitors and their FGFR-binding modes, we suggest that more attention should be paid to the formation of hydrogen bonds between chemicals and amino acids in the hydrophobic domain I. This type of interaction is absent in the binding between ATP and the FGFR ATP-binding pocket, which may increase the selectivity of novel inhibitors. In addition, further exploitation of the nucleotide-binding domain as an

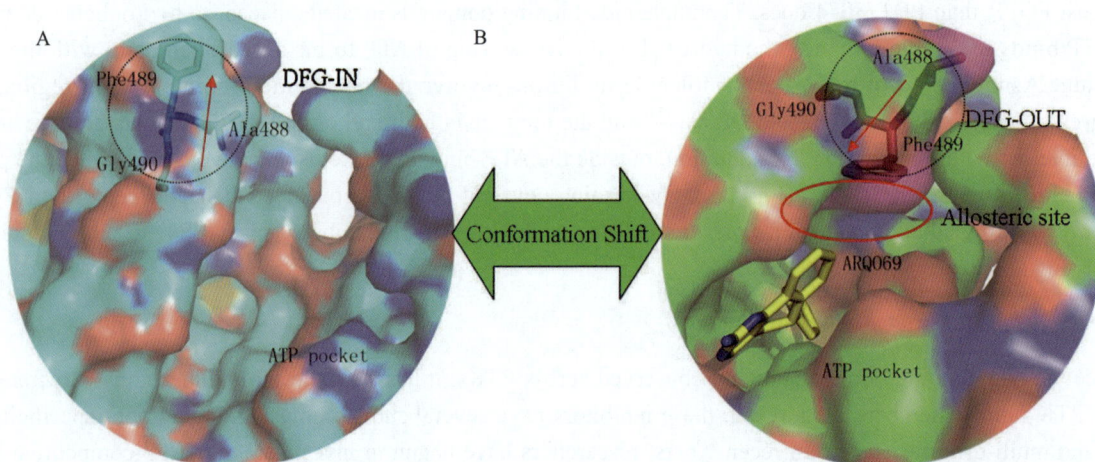

Fig. 3. Conformation shift of DFG that leads to a binding mode of non-ATP-competitive FGFR inhibitors: (A) "DFG-IN" conformation in which the benzene ring in Phe-489 is oriented "pocket-outside" and (B) "DFG-OUT" conformation in which the benzene ring in Phe-489 is oriented "pocket-inside," leading to an allosteric site bound by ARQ069.

important binding site may be an effective way to enhance the inhibitory activity and selectivity of FGFR inhibitors. Conversely, non-ATP competitive inhibitors may emerge as a new research focus for the study of FGFR inhibitors because of their unique strengths and modes of combination.

4. Small-molecule inhibitors of FGFR in clinical trials

Several small-molecule inhibitors of FGFR are being studied in clinical trials. The first generation of small-molecule inhibitors is predominantly ATP-competitive multi-targeted RTK inhibitors that are capable of suppressing a variety of RTKs, including FGFR. However, FGFR may not be their primary target. In recent years, some of the second-generation FGFR-selective inhibitors, which act on FGFR as their primary target, also have entered clinical trials. The results of clinical studies indicate that the latter class of inhibitors represents the developmental trend of FGFR inhibitors. The major FGFR inhibitors, or multi-target FGFR inhibitors, that have entered clinical trials are presented in Table 2.

Brivanib, E-3810, TSU-68, and BIBF1120 are first-generation FGFR inhibitors [66,77-79], and their primary target is the vascular endothelial growth factor receptor (VEGFR). They exert anti-angiogenic and anti-tumor effects through the inhibition of VEGFR. FGFR also has an important role in promoting bFGF-mediated angiogenesis and tumor-cell proliferation, and it can function as a compensation signal for VEGFR. Therefore, the suppression of FGFR by these first-generation inhibitors could attenuate the compensation of FGFR for VEGFR, thereby providing more pronounced anti-tumor effects. In addition, an FGFR3-related phase II clinical study (NCT00866138) is underway to assess the efficacy of masitinib, which targets c-kit, PDGFR, and FGFR3, in patients with multiple myeloma [80]. Although there are several first-generation FGFR inhibitors in clinical trials, their primary target is not FGFRs, and they have only a supporting role in cancer treatment, which precludes our gaining an in-depth understanding of how FGFR may affect clinical efficacy.

Table 2.　Current status of small-molecule FGFR inhibitors currently in clinical development

Drug name	Company	Kinase target	Applications in clinical trials	Comments	Side effects in clinic study	Ref.
Brivanib	Bristol-Myers Squibb	VEFGR, FGFR	Hepatocellular carcinoma (Phase I, NCT01540461); colorectal cancer (Phase II,NCT01367275);	Prodrug hydrolyzed to BMS-540215 *in vivo*; Brivanib in combination with cetuximab fails in Phase III colorectal cancer trial	Fatigue, diarrhea, nausea, vomiting, hypertension, pruritus, and weight loss	[66,83,84]
E-3810	Ethical Oncology Science	VEFGR, FGFR	Solid tumors (Phase I, NCT01283945)	E-3810 is 2 to 5 fold more active in FGF/FGFR-dependent tumor cell lines than FGF/FGFR-independent cells[a]	Not found	[79]
AZD2171	AstraZeneca	VEGFR, FGFR, KIT	Gastrointestinal stromal tumors (Phase II, NCT00385203)	AZD2171 exerted potent anti-tumor activity against gastric cancer xenografts (KATO-III and OCUM2M) overexpressing FGFR2	Fatigue, anorexia, hypertension, and elevated alanine aminotransferase	[85,86]
Ponatinib	Ariad Pharmaceutical	FLT3, FGFR, KIT, PDGFR	Chronic myeloid leukemia (CML) and acute lymphoblastic leukemia (ALL) (Phase II, NCT01207440)	Ponatinib inhibits the *in vitro* kinase activity of all 4 fibroblast growth factor receptors, and cell viability in leukemic cell lines that harbor activating fusions of FGFR1	Rash, dry skin, abdominal pain, headache, fatigue, myalgia, arthralgia, lipase increased, constipation, nausea and asthenia	[87,88]
E-7080	Eisai	VEGFR, FGFR, PDGFR	Endometrial cancer (Phase II, NCT01111461); thyroid cancer (Phase III, NCT01321554)	E7080 inhibits both tumor cell migration and invasion	Hematuria, fatigue, hypertension, AST increased, headache, proteinuria, ALT increased, diarrhea, and lactate dehydrogenase (LDH) increased	[89,90]

Drug name	Company	Kinase target	Applications in clinical trials	Comments	Side effects in clinic study	Ref.
Masitinib	AB Science	KIT, PDGFR, FGFR3	Multiple myeloma (Phase II, NCT00866138)	A selective tyrosine kinase inhibitor targeting KIT, also FGFR3	Nausea, vomiting, rash, diarrhea, peripheral edema, anemia, lymphopenia, thrombocytopenia, pyrexia, neutropenia, asthenia, leucopoenia, and abdominal pain	[80,91]
BIBF 1120	Boehringer Ingelheim Pharmaceuticals	VEGFR, FGFR, PDGFR	Cancer (Phase II, NCT01610869); small cell lung cancer (Phase II, NCT01441297); endometrial	Using BIBF 1120 after chemotherapy for relapsed ovarian cancer, thirty-six-week PFS rates were 16.3% and 5.0% in the BIBF 1120 and placebo groups, respectively	Diarrhea, nausea, vomiting and hepatotoxicity	[92]
TSU-68	Taiho Pharmaceutical	VEGFR, FGFR, PDGFR	Hepatocellular carcinoma (Phase III, NCT01465464)	A phase III trial of TSU-68 combination with transcatheter arterial chemoembolization in patients with unresectable hepatocellular carcinoma	Urinary/feces discoloration, diarrhea, fatigue, anorexia, abdominal/chest pain, and edema	[93]
TKI-258	Novartis	VEGFR, PDGFR, FGFR, FLT3, KIT	Endometrial cancer (Phase II, NCT01379534); urothelial cancer (Phase II, NCT00790426); relapsed or refractory multiple myeloma (Phase II, NCT01058434)	These clinical trials showed the best evidence for physiologically relevant efficacy against activated FGFRs	Fatigue, diarrhea, and nausea	[82]
BGJ398	Novartis	FGFR	Advanced solid tumors (Phase I, NCT01004224)	A potent and selective inhibitor of FGFR3 mutations (K650E, S249C)	Not found	[62]
AZD4547	AstraZeneca	FGFR	Breast cancer (Phase I/II, NCT01202591); advanced gastric or gastro-esophageal junction; cancer (Phase II, NCT01457846)	A selective inhibitor of FGFR1-3	Not found	[68]

ᵃ From http://www.eosmilano.com.

In recent years, second-generation, FGFR-selective inhibitors gradually have entered clinical trials. TKI-258 (also known as dovitinib) is an oral, multi-targeted, RTK inhibitor that was developed by Novartis, and it is now in a clinical trial. However, compared with the aforementioned inhibitors, second-generation inhibitors present a certain degree of FGFR selectivity [81] and target a variety of FGFR-related cancers. In a phase II clinical trial of TKI-258 in FGFR1 amplified and non-amplified metastatic HER2 negative breast cancer patients (NCT00958971), 500 mg of TKI-258 were administered daily on a 5-days-on/2-days-off schedule. Of the 21 female patients, 44% improved. Major adverse events were vomiting, diarrhea, nausea, and weakness [82]. In addition, clinical trials are underway for TKI-258 in FGFR2-mutated, endometrial cancer patients (NCT01379534); multiple myeloma with t(4;14) chromosome translocation patients (NCT01058434); and urothelial carcinoma patients (NCT00790426). BGJ398, another small-molecule FGFR inhibitor developed by Novartis, was more selective for FGFR and showed excellent inhibitory activity in a mouse-tumor model of bladder cancer with FGFR3 mutations and FGFR3 overexpression [62]. Currently, a phase I clinical trial is underway for the treatment of advanced solid tumors with FGFR1 and FGFR2 overexpression and FGFR3 mutations (NCT01004224).

AZD4547 is a selective, small-molecule FGFR inhibitor developed by AstraZeneca. It has an IC50 of 0.2 nM, 2.5

nM and 1.8 nM for FGFR1, FGFR2, and FGFR3, respectively, which is considerably better than its inhibitory activity against other RTKs. In tumor xenograft experiments in nude mice, oral administration of AZD4547 showed potent growth inhibition against FGFR-dependent tumors, but it was ineffective against VEGFR-dependent tumors, indicating that the drug exhibits favorable selectivity *in vivo* as well as *in vitro* [68]. A phase II clinical trial (NCT01457846) to investigate the efficacy of AZD4547 against FGFR2-associated gastric and gastroesophageal junction cancer is ongoing, with taxol serving as the control. Another clinical study is examining the combination of AZD4547 with exemestane for the treatment of ER⁺ breast cancer (NCT01202591); however, the results of these clinical trials of AZD4547 have not been disclosed.

5. Conclusion

In conclusion, FGFR, as a specific target in the treatment of tumors, has drawn increasing attention recently, and several FGFR inhibitors have been identified and have entered clinical trials. However, compared with other RTKs, clinical research on selective inhibitors of FGFR is still in its infancy. Two major problems remain to be resolved. First, adverse reactions and the toxicity of non-selective inhibitors remain as challenges that must be addressed. PD173074 and SU5402 failed to enter phase II clinical trials due to their high toxicity. Other FGFR inhibitors that have entered clinical trials may generate nausea, weakness, elevated blood pressure, and other adverse reactions due to their concurrent inhibition of other RTKs, thereby limiting their clinical efficacy. Adverse reactions also underlie the failure of a clinical trial of brivanib for treating colorectal cancer [83]. Second, FGFR dependence varies dramatically across patients and tumors. Pharmacogenomics and personalized medicine can detect FGFR overexpression and mutation in the tumor prior to administration of FGFR, and these approaches can provide guidance for setting goals and making medication decisions in clinical applications of FGFR inhibitors.

References

[1] Brooks AN, Kilgour E, Smith PD. Molecular pathways: fibroblast growth factor signaling: a new therapeutic opportunity in cancer [J]. Clinical Cancer Research, 2012, 18(7): 1855-1862.

[2] Greulich H, Pollock PM. Targeting mutant fibroblast growth factor receptors in cancer [J]. Trends in molecular medicine, 2011, 17(5): 283-292.

[3] Liang G, Liu Z, Wu J, et al. Anticancer molecules targeting fibroblast growth factor receptors [J]. Trends in pharmacological sciences, 2012, 33(10): 531-541.

[4] Harmer NJ, Ilag LL, Mulloy B, et al. Towards a resolution of the stoichiometry of the fibroblast growth factor (FGF)-FGF receptor-heparin complex [J]. Journal of molecular biology, 2004, 339(4): 821-834.

[5] Zhang X, Ibrahimi OA, Olsen SK, et al. Receptor specificity of the fibroblast growth factor family The complete mammalian fgf family [J]. Journal of Biological Chemistry, 2006, 281(23): 15694-15700.

[6] Wesche J, Haglund K, Haugsten Ellen M. Fibroblast growth factors and their receptors in cancer [J]. Biochemical Journal, 2011, 437(2): 199-213.

[7] Altomare DA, Testa JR. Perturbations of the AKT signaling pathway in human cancer [J]. Oncogene, 2005, 24(50): 7455.

[8] Peters KG, Marie J, Wilson E, et al. Point mutation of an FGF receptor abolishes phosphatidylinositol turnover and Ca²⁺ flux but not mitogenesis [J]. Nature, 1992, 358(6388): 678.

[9] Kang S, Elf S, Dong S, et al. Fibroblast growth factor receptor 3 associates with and tyrosine phosphorylates p90 RSK2, leading to RSK2 activation that mediates hematopoietic transformation [J]. Molecular and cellular biology, 2009, 29(8): 2105-2117.

[10] Turner N, Grose R. Fibroblast growth factor signalling: from development to cancer [J]. Nature Reviews Cancer, 2010, 10(2): 116.

[11] Ahmad I, Iwata T, Leung HY. Mechanisms of FGFR-mediated carcinogenesis [J]. Biochimica et Biophysica Acta (BBA)-Molecular Cell Research, 2012, 1823(4): 850-860.

[12] Network CGAR. Comprehensive genomic characterization defines human glioblastoma genes and core pathways [J]. Nature, 2008, 455(7216): 1061.

[13] Rand V, Huang J, Stockwell T, et al. Sequence survey of receptor tyrosine kinases reveals mutations in glioblastomas [J]. Proceedings of the National Academy of Sciences, 2005, 102(40): 14344-14349.

[14] Gru AA, Allred DC. FGFR1 amplification and the progression of non-invasive to invasive breast cancer. In: BioMed Central, 2012.

[15] Shiang CY, Qi Y, Wang B, et al. Amplification of fibroblast growth factor receptor-1 in breast cancer and the effects of brivanib alaninate [J]. Breast cancer research and treatment, 2010, 123(3): 747-755.

[16] Dutt A, Ramos AH, Hammerman PS, et al. Inhibitor-sensitive FGFR1 amplification in human non-small cell lung cancer [J]. PloS one, 2011, 6(6): e20351.

[17] Freier K, Schwaenen C, Sticht C, et al. Recurrent FGFR1 amplification and high FGFR1 protein expression in oral squamous cell carcinoma (OSCC) [J]. Oral oncology, 2007, 43(1): 60-66.

[18] Murphy T, Darby S, Mathers ME, et al. Evidence for distinct alterations in the FGF axis in prostate cancer progression to an aggressive clinical phenotype [J]. The Journal of Pathology: A Journal of the Pathological Society of Great Britain and Ireland, 2010, 220(4): 452-460.

[19] Acevedo VD, Gangula RD, Freeman KW, et al. Inducible FGFR-1 activation leads to irreversible prostate adenocarcinoma and an epithelial-to-mesenchymal transition [J]. Cancer cell, 2007, 12(6):

559-571.

[20] Gorringe KL, Jacobs S, Thompson ER, *et al.* High-resolution single nucleotide polymorphism array analysis of epithelial ovarian cancer reveals numerous microdeletions and amplifications [J]. Clinical cancer research, 2007, 13(16): 4731-4739.

[21] Missiaglia E, Selfe J, Hamdi M, *et al.* Genomic imbalances in rhabdomyosarcoma cell lines affect expression of genes frequently altered in primary tumors: an approach to identify candidate genes involved in tumor development [J]. Genes, chromosomes and cancer, 2009, 48(6): 455-467.

[22] Simon R, Richter J, Wagner U, *et al.* High-throughput tissue microarray analysis of 3p25 (RAF1) and 8p12 (FGFR1) copy number alterations in urinary bladder cancer [J]. Cancer research, 2001, 61(11): 4514-4519.

[23] Xiao S, Nalabolu SR, Aster JC, *et al.* FGFR1 is fused with a novel zinc-finger gene, ZNF198, in the t (8; 13) leukaemia/lymphoma syndrome [J]. Nature genetics, 1998, 18(1): 84.

[24] Roumiantsev S, Krause DS, Neumann CA, *et al.* Distinct stem cell myeloproliferative/T lymphoma syndromes induced by ZNF198-FGFR1 and BCR-FGFR1 fusion genes from 8p11 translocations [J]. Cancer cell, 2004, 5(3): 287-298.

[25] Katoh Y, Katoh M. FGFR2-related pathogenesis and FGFR2-targeted therapeutics [J]. International journal of molecular medicine, 2009, 23(3): 307-311.

[26] Dutt A, Salvesen HB, Chen TH, *et al.* Drug-sensitive FGFR2 mutations in endometrial carcinoma [J]. Proceedings of the National Academy of Sciences, 2008, 105(25): 8713-8717.

[27] Byron SA, Gartside MG, Wellens CL, *et al.* Inhibition of activated fibroblast growth factor receptor 2 in endometrial cancer cells induces cell death despite PTEN abrogation [J]. Cancer research, 2008, 68(17): 6902-6907.

[28] Bai A, Meetze K, Vo NY, *et al.* GP369, an FGFR2-IIIb–specific antibody, exhibits potent antitumor activity against human cancers driven by activated FGFR2 signaling [J]. Cancer research, 2010, 70(19): 7630-7639.

[29] Heiskanen M, Kononen J, Bärlund M, *et al.* CGH, cDNA and tissue microarray analyses implicate FGFR2 amplification in a small subset of breast tumors [J]. Analytical Cellular Pathology, 2001, 22(4): 229-234.

[30] Vermeulen JF, Kornegoor R, van der Wall E, *et al.* Differential expression of growth factor receptors and membrane-bound tumor markers for imaging in male and female breast cancer [J]. PloS one, 2013, 8(1): e53353.

[31] Zhou L, Yao F, Luan H, *et al.* Three novel functional polymorphisms in the promoter of FGFR2 gene and breast cancer risk: a HuGE review and meta-analysis [J]. Breast cancer research and treatment, 2012, 136(3): 885-897.

[32] Tartaglia M, Valeri S, Velardi F, *et al.* Trp290Cys mutation in exon IIIa of the fibroblast growth factor receptor 2 (FGFR2) gene is associated with Pfeiffer syndrome [J]. Human genetics, 1997, 99(5): 602-606.

[33] Marian C, Ochs-Balcom HM, Nie J, *et al.* FGFR2 intronic SNPs and breast cancer risk: associations with tumor characteristics and interactions with exogenous exposures and other known breast cancer risk factors [J]. International journal of cancer, 2011, 129(3): 702-712.

[34] Cappellen D, De Oliveira C, Ricol D, *et al.* Frequent activating mutations of FGFR3 in human bladder and cervix carcinomas [J]. Nature genetics, 1999, 23(1): 18.

[35] Naski MC, Wang Q, Xu J, *et al.* Graded activation of fibroblast growth factor receptor 3 by mutations causing achondroplasia and thanatophoric dysplasia [J]. Nature genetics, 1996, 13(2): 233.

[36] Di Martino E, L'hôte C, Kennedy W, *et al.* Mutant fibroblast growth factor receptor 3 induces intracellular signaling and cellular transformation in a cell type-and mutation-specific manner [J]. Oncogene, 2009, 28(48): 4306.

[37] Qing J, Du X, Chen Y, *et al.* Antibody-based targeting of FGFR3 in bladder carcinoma and t (4; 14)-positive multiple myeloma in mice [J]. The Journal of clinical investigation, 2009, 119(5): 1216-1229.

[38] Lamont F, Tomlinson D, Cooper PA, *et al.* Small molecule FGF receptor inhibitors block FGFR-dependent urothelial carcinoma growth *in vitro* and *in vivo* [J]. British journal of cancer, 2011, 104(1): 75.

[39] Goriely A, Hansen RM, Taylor IB, *et al.* Activating mutations in FGFR3 and HRAS reveal a shared genetic origin for congenital disorders and testicular tumors [J]. Nature genetics, 2009, 41(11): 1247.

[40] Logie A, Dunois-Larde C, Rosty C, *et al.* Activating mutations of the tyrosine kinase receptor FGFR3 are associated with benign skin tumors in mice and humans [J]. Human molecular genetics, 2005, 14(9): 1153-1160.

[41] Zhang Y, Hiraishi Y, Wang H, *et al.* Constitutive activating mutation of the FGFR3b in oral squamous cell carcinomas [J]. International journal of cancer, 2005, 117(1): 166-168.

[42] van Rhijn BW, van Tilborg AA, Lurkin I, *et al.* Novel fibroblast growth factor receptor 3 (FGFR3) mutations in bladder cancer previously identified in non-lethal skeletal disorders [J]. European Journal of Human Genetics, 2002, 10(12): 819.

[43] Tomlinson D, Baldo O, Harnden P, *et al.* FGFR3 protein expression and its relationship to mutation status and prognostic variables in bladder cancer [J]. The Journal of pathology, 2007, 213(1): 91-98.

[44] Trudel S, Stewart AK, Rom E, *et al.* The inhibitory anti-FGFR3 antibody, PRO-001, is cytotoxic to t (4; 14) multiple myeloma cells [J]. Blood, 2006, 107(10): 4039-4046.

[45] Singh D, Chan JM, Zoppoli P, *et al.* Transforming fusions of FGFR and TACC genes in human glioblastoma [J]. Science, 2012, 337(6099): 1231-1235.

[46] Vi JGT, Cheuk AT, Tsang PS, *et al.* Identification of FGFR4-activating mutations in human rhabdomyosarcomas that promote metastasis in xenotransplanted models [J]. The Journal of clinical investigation, 2009, 119(11): 3395-3407.

[47] Bange J, Prechtl D, Cheburkin Y, *et al.* Cancer progression and tumor cell motility are associated with the FGFR4 Arg388 allele [J]. Cancer research, 2002, 62(3): 840-847.

[48] Roidl A, Berger H-J, Kumar S, *et al.* Resistance to chemotherapy is associated with fibroblast growth factor receptor 4 up-regulation [J]. Clinical Cancer Research, 2009, 15(6): 2058-2066.

[49] Nord H, Segersten U, Sandgren J, *et al.* Focal amplifications are associated with high grade and recurrences in stage Ta bladder carcinoma [J]. International journal of cancer, 2010, 126(6): 1390-1402.

[50] Lin WM, Baker AC, Beroukhim R, *et al.* Modeling genomic diversity and tumor dependency in malignant melanoma [J]. Cancer research, 2008, 68(3): 664-673.

[51] Davies H, Hunter C, Smith R, *et al.* Somatic mutations of the protein kinase gene family in human lung cancer [J]. Cancer research, 2005, 65(17): 7591-7595.

[52] Kawase R, Ishiwata T, Matsuda Y, *et al.* Expression of fibroblast growth factor receptor 2 IIIc in human uterine cervical intraepithelial neoplasia and cervical cancer [J]. International journal of oncology, 2010, 36(2): 331-340.

[53] Gartside MG, Chen H, Ibrahimi OA, *et al.* Loss-of-function fibroblast growth factor receptor-2 mutations in melanoma [J]. Molecular Cancer Research, 2009, 7(1): 41-54.

[54] Jang JH, Shin KH, Park JG. Mutations in fibroblast growth factor receptor 2 and fibroblast growth factor receptor 3 genes associated with human gastric and colorectal cancers [J]. Cancer research, 2001, 61(9): 3541-3543.

[55] Hernández S, De Muga S, Agell L, *et al.* FGFR3 mutations in prostate cancer: association with low-grade tumors [J]. Modern pathology, 2009, 22(6): 848.

[56] Roidl A, Foo P, Wong W, *et al.* The FGFR4 Y367C mutant is a dominant oncogene in MDA-MB453 breast cancer cells [J]. Onco-

gene, 2010, 29(10): 1543.

[57] Mohammadi M, Schlessinger J, Hubbard SR. Structure of the FGF receptor tyrosine kinase domain reveals a novel autoinhibitory mechanism [J]. Cell, 1996, 86(4): 577-587.

[58] Mohammadi M, McMahon G, Sun L, et al. Structures of the tyrosine kinase domain of fibroblast growth factor receptor in complex with inhibitors [J]. Science, 1997, 276(5314): 955-960.

[59] Kammasud N, Boonyarat C, Tsunoda S, et al. Novel inhibitor for fibroblast growth factor receptor tyrosine kinase [J]. Bioorganic & medicinal chemistry letters, 2007, 17(17): 4812-4818.

[60] Mohammadi M, Froum S, Hamby JM, et al. Crystal structure of an angiogenesis inhibitor bound to the FGF receptor tyrosine kinase domain [J]. The EMBO journal, 1998, 17(20): 5896-5904.

[61] Kammasud N, Boonyarat C, Sanphanya K, et al. 5-Substituted pyrido [2, 3-d] pyrimidine, an inhibitor against three receptor tyrosine kinases [J]. Bioorganic & medicinal chemistry letters, 2009, 19(3): 745-750.

[62] Guagnano V, Furet P, Spanka C, et al. Discovery of 3-(2, 6-dichloro-3, 5-dimethoxy-phenyl)-1-{6-[4-(4-ethyl-piperazin-1-yl)-phenylamino]-pyrimidin-4-yl}-1-methyl-urea (NVP-BGJ398), a potent and selective inhibitor of the fibroblast growth factor receptor family of receptor tyrosine kinase [J]. Journal of medicinal chemistry, 2011, 54(20): 7066-7083.

[63] Zhang J, Yang PL, Gray NS. Targeting cancer with small molecule kinase inhibitors [J]. Nature reviews cancer, 2009, 9(1): 28.

[64] Norman RA, Schott AK, Andrews DM, et al. Protein–ligand crystal structures can guide the design of selective inhibitors of the FGFR tyrosine kinase [J]. Journal of medicinal chemistry, 2012, 55(11): 5003-5012.

[65] Renhowe PA, Pecchi S, Shafer CM, et al. Design, structure–activity relationships and in vivo characterization of 4-amino-3-benzimidazol-2-ylhydroquinolin-2-ones: a novel class of receptor tyrosine kinase inhibitors [J]. Journal of medicinal chemistry, 2008, 52(2): 278-292.

[66] Cai Z-w, Zhang Y, Borzilleri RM, et al. Discovery of brivanib alaninate ((S)-((R)-1-(4-(4-fluoro-2-methyl-1 H-indol-5-yloxy)-5-methylpyrrolo [2, 1-f][1, 2, 4] triazin-6-yloxy) propan-2-yl) 2-aminopropanoate), a novel prodrug of dual vascular endothelial growth factor receptor-2 and fibroblast growth factor receptor-1 kinase inhibitor (BMS-540215) [J]. Journal of medicinal chemistry, 2008, 51(6): 1976-1980.

[67] Matsui J, Yamamoto Y, Funahashi Y, et al. E7080, a novel inhibitor that targets multiple kinases, has potent antitumor activities against stem cell factor producing human small cell lung cancer H146, based on angiogenesis inhibition [J]. International journal of cancer, 2008, 122(3): 664-671.

[68] Gavine PR, Mooney L, Kilgour E, et al. AZD4547: an orally bioavailable, potent, and selective inhibitor of the fibroblast growth factor receptor tyrosine kinase family [J]. Cancer research, 2012, 72(8): 2045-2056.

[69] Jonquoy A, Mugniery E, Benoist-Lasselin C, et al. A novel tyrosine kinase inhibitor restores chondrocyte differentiation and promotes bone growth in a gain-of-function Fgfr3 mouse model [J]. Human molecular genetics, 2011, 21(4): 841-851.

[70] Le Corre L, Girard A-L, Aubertin J, et al. Synthesis and biological evaluation of a triazole-based library of pyrido [2, 3-d] pyrimidines as FGFR3 tyrosine kinase inhibitors [J]. Organic & biomolecular chemistry, 2010, 8(9): 2164-2173.

[71] Tsou H-R, MacEwan G, Birnberg G, et al. Discovery and optimization of 2-(4-substituted-pyrrolo [2, 3-b] pyridin-3-yl) methylene-4-hydroxybenzofuran-3 (2H)-ones as potent and selective ATP-competitive inhibitors of the mammalian target of rapamycin (mTOR) [J]. Bioorganic & medicinal chemistry letters, 2010, 20(7): 2321-2325.

[72] Zhou W, Hur W, McDermott U, et al. A structure-guided approach to creating covalent FGFR inhibitors [J]. Chemistry & biology, 2010, 17(3): 285-295.

[73] Liu Y, Gray NS. Rational design of inhibitors that bind to inactive kinase conformations [J]. Nat. Chem. Biol., 2006, 2(7): 358-364.

[74] Eathiraj S, Palma R, Hirschi M, et al. A novel mode of protein kinase inhibition exploiting hydrophobic motifs of autoinhibited Kinases discovery of atp-independent inhibitors of fibroblast growth factor receptor [J]. Journal of Biological Chemistry, 2011, 286(23): 20677-20687.

[75] Pargellis C, Tong L, Churchill L, et al. Inhibition of p38 MAP kinase by utilizing a novel allosteric binding site [J]. Nature Structural & Molecular Biology, 2002, 9(4): 268.

[76] Krejci P, Murakami S, Prochazkova J, et al. NF449 is a novel inhibitor of fibroblast growth factor receptor 3 (FGFR3) signaling active in chondrocytes and multiple myeloma cells [J]. Journal of Biological Chemistry, 2010, 285(27): 20644-20653.

[77] Hilberg F, Roth GJ, Krssak M, et al. BIBF 1120: triple angiokinase inhibitor with sustained receptor blockade and good antitumor efficacy [J]. Cancer research, 2008, 68(12): 4774-4782.

[78] Laird AD, Vajkoczy P, Shawver LK, et al. SU6668 is a potent antiangiogenic and antitumor agent that induces regression of established tumors [J]. Cancer Research, 2000, 60(15): 4152-4160.

[79] Bello E, Colella G, Scarlato V, et al. E-3810 is a potent dual inhibitor of VEGFR and FGFR that exerts antitumor activity in multiple preclinical models [J]. Cancer research, 2011, 71(4): 1396-1405.

[80] Dubreuil P, Letard S, Ciufolini M, et al. Masitinib (AB1010), a potent and selective tyrosine kinase inhibitor targeting KIT [J]. PloS one, 2009, 4(9): e7258.

[81] Lee SH, de Menezes DL, Vora J, et al. In vivo target modulation and biological activity of CHIR-258, a multitargeted growth factor receptor kinase inhibitor, in colon cancer models [J]. Clinical Cancer Research, 2005, 11(10): 3633-3641.

[82] Andre F, Baselga J, Ellis M, et al. Study CTKI258A2202: A multicenter, open-label phase II trial of dovitinib (TKI258) in FGFR1-amplified and nonamplified HER2-negative metastatic breast cancer [J]. Journal of Clinical Oncology, 2010, 28(15_suppl): TPS122-TPS122.

[83] Tuma RS. Brivanib Fails in Phase III Colorectal Cancer Trial [J]. Oncology Times, 2012, 34(4): 28-29.

[84] Finn RS, Kang Y-K, Mulcahy M, et al. Phase II, open-label study of brivanib as second-line therapy in patients with advanced hepatocellular carcinoma [J]. Clinical Cancer Research, 2012, 18(7): 2090-2098.

[85] Takeda M, Arao T, Yokote H, et al. AZD2171 shows potent antitumor activity against gastric cancer over-expressing fibroblast growth factor receptor 2/keratinocyte growth factor receptor [J]. Clinical Cancer Research, 2007, 13(10): 3051-3057.

[86] Laurie SA, Gauthier I, Arnold A, et al. Phase I and pharmacokinetic study of daily oral AZD2171, an inhibitor of vascular endothelial growth factor tyrosine kinases, in combination with carboplatin and paclitaxel in patients with advanced non–small-cell lung cancer: The National Cancer Institute of Canada clinical trials group [J]. Journal of Clinical Oncology, 2008, 26(11): 1871-1878.

[87] Gozgit JM, Wong MJ, Moran L, et al. Ponatinib (AP24534), a multitargeted pan-FGFR inhibitor with activity in multiple FGFR-amplified or mutated cancer models [J]. Molecular cancer therapeutics, 2012, 11(3): 690-699.

[88] Talpaz M, Cortes J, Deininger M, et al. Phase I trial of AP24534 in patients with refractory chronic myeloid leukemia (CML) and hematologic malignancies [J]. Journal of Clinical Oncology, 2010, 28(15_suppl): 6511-6511.

[89] Glen H, Mason S, Patel H, et al. E7080, a multi-targeted tyrosine kinase inhibitor suppresses tumor cell migration and invasion [J]. BMC cancer, 2011, 11(1): 309.

[90] Koyama N, Saito K, Nishioka Y, et al. Pharmacodynamic change in plasma angiogenic proteins: a dose-escalation phase 1 study of the multi-kinase inhibitor lenvatinib [J]. BMC cancer, 2014, 14(1):

530.

[91] Hammel P, Mornex F, Deplanque G, *et al*. Oral tyrosine kinase inhibitor masitinib in combination with gemcitabine in patients with advanced pancreatic cancer: A multicenter phase II study [J]. Journal of Clinical Oncology, 2009, 27(15_suppl): 4617-4617.

[92] Ledermann JA, Hackshaw A, Kaye S, *et al*. Randomized phase II placebo-controlled trial of maintenance therapy using the oral triple angiokinase inhibitor BIBF 1120 after chemotherapy for relapsed ovarian cancer [J]. Journal of Clinical Oncology, 2011, 29(28): 3798-3804.

[93] Ueda Y, Shimoyama T, Murakami H, *et al*. Phase I and pharmacokinetic study of TSU-68, a novel multiple receptor tyrosine kinase inhibitor, by twice daily oral administration between meals in patients with advanced solid tumors [J]. Cancer chemotherapy and pharmacology, 2011, 67(5): 1101-1109.

Research advances in tissue engineering materials for sustained release of growth factors

Haiyang Zhao, Xiaokun Li

1. Introduction

The structure and mechanism of growth factors have been an area of intense research interest as a number of growth factors such as nerve growth factor (NGF) [1], epidermal growth factor (EGF) [2], fibroblast growth factor (FGF) [3], and platelet-derived growth factor (PDGF) [4] have been discovered since the 1950s.

Growth factors are a large class of cytokines that stimulate cell growth and are capable of specifically binding cell membrane receptors seen Table 1. They regulate cell growth, proliferation, migration, and other cellular functions and play important roles in wound healing [5], tissue regeneration [6], and immune regulation [7]. Growth factors cover a broad spectrum of cytokines, including EGFs, NGFs [8], insulin-like growth factors (IGF) [9], FGFs, PDGFs, interleukins, and hematopoietic cell growth factors.

Table 1.　Lists of GFs and their main functions

Type of GFs	Main functions	Reference
bFGF	Promote cell proliferation and regeneration	[42-44]
VEGF	Induce angiogenesis	[45-47]
TGF	Regulation of cell growth, differentiation, and immune function	[48-50]
NGF	An important regulator of neural survival	[51, 52]
IGF	Regulate the somatic growth in an endocrine manner	[53-55]

The study of growth factors has long moved to the molecular level after half a century of research. Some growth factors have now been made into preparations that are used clinically with significant effects. However, growth factors have a short half-life and are prone to burst in the body, often making it difficult to reach ideal drug concentrations. Therefore, how to extend the action time of growth factors in the body and maintain proper drug concentrations has become a new area of research.

Ideal carriers for sustained release of growth factors should meet the following criteria. First, carriers have high drug loading and can maintain sustained release of growth factors to ensure reasonable treatment time and efficacy. Second, the addition of carriers does not undermine the biological activity of growth factors. Third, carriers are biocompatible and their residues or degradation products are not cytotoxic. Numerous materials are currently available as sustained release carriers of growth factors seen in Table 2, which can be divided into organic materials and inorganic materials. Organic materials include collagen, gelatin, hyaluronic acid, chitosan, poly(ethylene argininylaspartate diglyceride) (PEAD) [10], poly-L-lactide (PLLA) [11], and poly-lactic-co-glycolic acid (PLGA) [12]. Inorganic materials include calcium phosphate and hydroxyapatite. Organic materials can also be used in combination with inorganic materials, such as porous hydroxyapatite/collagen composite. This study reviews the characteristics and applications of common sustained release carriers for growth factors in an attempt to provide reference for related research and clinical application.

Table 2.   New material and method for controlled release of varied GFs

Types of GFs	Types of materials	Strategies for loading GFs	*In vitro/in vivo* effect	References
VEGF	PEG-heparin hydrogel	3D porous matrix through photocrosslinker along with the foaming process	Only 34% released over 13 days; more increase in angiogenesis *in vivo*	[56]
bFGF	PMMA-b-PMAETMA	Self-assembled core-shell of heparinized CS/c-PGA nanoparticles	Preserved heparin-bFGF biological activity *in vitro*	[57]
NGF	Iron oxide nanoparticles	Covalently conjugating the factor to iron oxide NP	Significantly promoted neurite outgrowth and increased the complexity of the neuronal branching trees *in vitro*	[58]
IGF-1	Collagen-GAG scaffold	Monitoring the amount of collagen and proteoglycan synthesized by chondrocytes seeded within the scaffolds	Provided an initial therapeutic burst release of IGF-1 which is beneficial in initiating ECM deposition and repair in the *in vitro* model	[59]
TGF-β3	PLCL scaffold	Supercritical CO_2-HFIP cosolvent system	Longterm delivery of TGF-β3 prevented the hypertrophy of differentiated chondrocytes	[60]
VEGF and bFGF	Fibrin-based scaffold	Fibrin-based scaffold containing PLGA nanoparticles loaded with VEGF and bFGF	Complete reepithelialization, with enhanced granulation tissue formation, maturity, and collagen deposition	[61]

2. Organic materials

Organic materials can be divided into natural materials and composite materials according to their sources. Organic materials can be made into sustained release systems in different formulations such as microspheres and nanoparticles according to their different properties. Currently available natural materials, such as gelatin, alginate, and chitosan, are natural polymers, which can associate with growth factors to function as sustained release carriers *in vivo*. Composite materials include widely used PEAD [10], PLLA [11], and PLGA [12].

2.1 Natural materials

Natural materials offer many advantages as sustained release carriers for growth factors, such as reducing rejection and immune stress and having good biodegradability. For example, natural materials such as collagen, hyaluronic acid, and fibrin are naturally occurring in the body, with collagen accounting for nearly one quarter of human proteins by weight. Natural materials from other sources, such as alginate and chitosan, also have many advantages. They can minimize toxicity and chronic inflammation. In addition, they are also highly biocompatible [13], less irritant to the body, and easy to be degraded.

2.1.1 Gelatin

Gelatin is a natural material produced from hydrolysis of collagen at higher temperatures and is often used as a sustained release carrier for growth factors. Depending on the types of gelatin used, gelatin particles may be positively charged or negatively charged [14]. Growth factors can be efficiently encapsulated in the gelatin particles. This strategy does not compromise the biological activity of growth factors and provides sustained release of growth factors by controlling the release rate of growth factors from gelatin particles.

Hori *et al.* [15] designed a sustained release system for ophthalmic application of EGF using cationized gelatin hydrogel (CGH) as the carrier. They placed CGH with incorporated ^{125}I-labelled EGF in the conjunctival sac of mice and measured the residual radioactivity at different times to evaluate EGF release. The results showed that about 60%~67% of EGF applied remained one day after application and about 10%~12% of EGF remained seven days after application. Compared with the topical application of EGF solution or blank CGH membranes alone, CGH membranes with incorporated EGF can reduce corneal epithelial defect and promote significant proliferation of epithelial cells, thereby accelerating ocular wound healing. Oe *et al.* [16] also prepared biodegradable gelatin microspheres using an aqueous solution of glutaraldehyde cross-linked gelatin to encapsulate hepatocyte growth factor (HGF) for its sustained release.

The results revealed that the sustained release carrier improved liver cell function in rats with liver cirrhosis and showed promise as an effective therapy for liver fibrosis.

2.1.2 Alginate and its derivatives

Alginate is a natural linear polysaccharide that can be extracted from the cell walls of seaweed, kelp, and other edible algae. Because of its low toxicity, high biocompatibility, and low price, alginate has been widely used in drug delivery and regenerative medicine [17].

Jeon et al. [18] found that delivery carriers based on photocrosslinked alginic acid and hyaluronic acid have controllable biodegradability [19] and can promote cell adhesion and provide sustained release of growth factors [20]. The researchers grafted heparin to alginate hydrogel and controlled the release of growth factors through heparin in the hydrogel. This hydrogel could provide sustained release of growth factors [transforming growth factor-β (TGF-β1), FGF-2, vascular endothelial growth factor (VEGF), and bone morphogenetic protein (BMP-2)] for up to three weeks, and no initial burst release was observed. Released growth factors could better promote the proliferation of human umbilical vein endothelial cells and alkaline phosphatase activity in osteoblasts. Liu et al. [21] found that alginate microspheres containing single or mixed growth factors (VEGF, FGF, and NGF) could efficiently release a variety of growth factors *in vitro* for more than four weeks. The three growth factors (VEGF, FGF, and NGF) encapsulated in alginate microspheres can generate synergies and better prolong survival of stem cells and promote myogenic differentiation of stem cells while enhancing peripheral nerve regeneration. The results showed that alginate microspheres containing the three growth factors and urine-derived stem cells produced significant effects in an animal model of incontinence. Further studies are needed to develop their potential use in incontinent patients.

2.1.3 Chitosan and its derivatives

Chitosan is a product from deacetylation of chitin and is a natural polymer of sugar monomers. Because of its excellent blood compatibility, biological safety, and microbial degradability, it has been widely used in tissue engineering. Chitosan is a primary derivative of chitin. It is insoluble in water, but soluble in dilute acid, and can be absorbed by the body. Chitosan is a basic cationic polysaccharide polymer and has unique physical, chemical, and bioactive properties. Chitosan-based membranes, sponges, and microspheres encapsulating growth factors have been extensively studied and applied [22]. It has been reported that bFGF-containing chitosan can provide sustained release of bFGF and ensure the sustained release of bFGF over a long period of time [23]. Park et al. [24] designed a porous chondroitin sulfate-chitosan sponge that encapsulated platelet-derived growth factor (PDGF-BB), which provides controlled release of the growth factor by modulating the structure of porous scaffold to increase bone formation rate. Chondroitin sulfate was added to the chitosan solution, which was freeze-dried, cross-linked with tripolyphosphate, and freeze-dried again to yield a porous chondroitin sulfate-chitosan sponge. PDGF-BB solutions at different concentrations were added to the prepared sponge. The sponge was then left to stand at 4 ℃ overnight and freeze-dried to yield the porous chondroitin sulfate-chitosan sponge containing 100, 200, and 400 ng of PDGF-BB, respectively. The chondroitin sulfate-chitosan sponge thus obtained had a pore size of 150-200 microns, providing porous structures needed for cell migration and bone growth. The release rate of PDGF-BB can be controlled by changing the amount of chondroitin sulfate added to the sponge and the initial loading dose of PDGF-BB. The results showed that the application of the chondroitin sulfate-chitosan sponge to provide sustained release of PDGF-BB at the wound site enhanced the adaptability and regenerative potential of osteoblasts.

Platelet lysate is an autologous source of growth factors and contains some bioactive agents capable of acting on bone regeneration. In the study by Santo et al. [25], chondroitin sulfate and chitosan were first prepared into nanoparticles, followed by the addition of platelet lysate; subsequently, polylactic acid foams were used to encapsulate platelet lysate-containing chitosan-chondroitin sulfate nanoparticles using supercritical fluid foaming technology to achieve controlled release of platelet lysate. The results showed that platelet lysate-containing nanoparticles could more quickly stimulate osteoblast differentiation and induce bone regeneration.

2.2 Synthetic materials

Natural materials have been widely used as sustained release carriers for growth factors because of favorable biocompatibility, biodegradability, and low immunogenicity. However, they also suffer from some drawbacks, such as potential contamination in production and sterilization and poor mechanical properties. To overcome these problems, synthetic materials have emerged as an alternative for researchers. The synthetic materials allow greater flexibility in the control of their physical and chemical properties during production. Generally the monomer composition, reaction rate, and the molecular weight of composites can be controlled, which means that molecular weight, monomer species, and reaction rate can be manipulated to improve mechanical strength and change the rate of degradation.

2.2.1 PEAD

Chu et al. [10] prepared PEAD from the polymerization of monomers arginine, aspartic acid, glycerol, and ethylene glycol. In vitro cell culture experiments showed that PEAD was not cytotoxic at a concentration of 1 mg/ml. Meanwhile, subcutaneous injection of 1 mg PEAD did not cause adverse reactions in rats. In addition, potential measurements showed that, like hyaluronic acid, PEAD had high affinity with polyanions such as DNA, which lays the foundation for PEAD to be used as a polymer for modifying protein drugs such as growth factors.

Heparin-binding EGF has been shown to effectively accelerate skin wound healing. Therefore, reducing the amount of growth factors through the use of heparin is very necessary for clinical efficacy. To achieve effective growth factor delivery, Johnson and Wang [26] designed a polymer-growth factor coacervate by using heparin-binding growth factor and attracting growth factor-containing heparin with PEAD through polyvalent charge [27]. In vivo animal experiments showed that the coacervate provided sustained release of the growth factor and significantly accelerated wound healing in 17 days, significantly better than the control group, which used no growth factor, and the heparin-binding growth factor group. This result suggests that the polymer-heparin-growth factor delivery system can improve the biological activity of growth factors and hence accelerate skin wound healing.

2.2.2 PLLA and its derivatives

PLLA membranes have widely been used in controlled drug release systems [11]. Park et al. [28] loaded PDGF-BB to porous PLLA membranes using the atmospheric drying phase inversion technique to provide controlled release of growth factors. PDGF-BB release can be controlled by altering the amount of bovine serum albumin added and the amount of initially loaded PDGF-BB. PLLA membranes encapsulating PDGF-BB significantly promoted new bone formation and completed bone remodeling two weeks after implantation in rats with skull defects. The results showed that PDGF-BB-incorporated PLLA membranes may enhance the guidance of potential tissue regeneration. Wang et al. [29] recently prepared a novel biomodified copolymer, poly(D,L-lactide)-7co-(1,3-trimethylene carbonate) (P (DLLA-co-TMC)), for controlling the release of vascular endothelial cell growth factor (VEGF). The results showed that the release of VEGF did not have a burst effect and that significant therapeutic effects were achieved.

2.2.3 PLGA

PLGA has been widely used as the carrier for growth factors because of its favorable biocompatibility and biodegradability. The use of multiple emulsion technique (water/oil/water) can yield an encapsulation efficiency of up to 42% to 100% for growth factors [30]. The degradation rate of PLGA can be controlled by changing the amount of monomers lactic acid and glycolic acid, thereby controlling the rate of release of growth factors.

Spiller et al. [31] encapsulated IGF-1 in biodegradable PLGA microspheres using the emulsion method, which were then incorporated in polyvinyl alcohol (PVA) hydrogel. In vitro experiments showed that the release of IGF-1 from the hydrogel lasted for more than six weeks. IGF-1 is an important growth factor involved in the regeneration of cartilage. Its sustained release can enhance the formation of cartilage around the hydrogel and promote the integration of cartilage and the hydrogel. The results also demonstrated that the controlled release of growth factors can guide specific tissue regeneration and stem cell differentiation. Wang et al. [32] encapsulated PEGylated EGF in PLGA nanoparticles and erythropoietin (EPO) in PLGA nanoparticles via a poly(sebacic acid) coating to control the release of EGF and EPO. PEGylated EGF and EPO polymeric particles were dispersed in a hyaluronan methylcellulose (HAMC) hydrogel which spatially confines the particles and attenuates the inflammatory response of brain tissue. The results showed that, in a mouse model of stroke, sequential and sustained release of EGF and EPO from the microsphere system could better repair nerve tissue while causing no damage to other accompanying tissues as compared with intracerebroventricular infusion. This technique provides a minimally invasive and effective treatment modality for loss of healthy nerve cells and glial cells as a result of a number of central nervous system disorders such as Alzheimer's disease and spinal cord injury.

3. Inorganic materials

It is well known that organic materials are widely used as sustained release carriers for growth factors, but extensive research efforts are also focused on inorganic materials used alone or in combination with organic materials, particularly in bone repair. Combining growth factors with inorganic materials can also achieve certain sustained release effects. More examples of inorganic materials include calcium phosphate and hydroxyapatite, and there are also various composites of organic and inorganic materials, such as porous hydroxyapatite/collagen (HAp/Col).

3.1　Calcium phosphate

Calcium phosphate scaffolds (*e.g.*, β-tricalcium phosphate [33]) offer favorable biocompatibility, excellent biological activity, and adjustable degradation rate [34, 35], making them an ideal material for bone repair. Calcium phosphate scaffolds used for bone repair often contain human primary cells (such as mesenchymal stem cells, bone cells, and endothelial cells) and growth factors. Growth factors can be encapsulated and embedded within the calcium phosphate scaffolds in a particular way. These factors can then be released into the microenvironment where bone grafting occurs to play a regulatory role by stimulating the expression of relevant genes.

Sun *et al.* [36] examined cell responses induced by the release of growth factors from a biodegradable porous calcium phosphate three-dimensional scaffold. They simulated and reconstructed a three-dimensional system for bone regeneration and assessed the effects of pore size and porosity on bone formation and angiogenesis. The results showed that, compared with pore size, porosity played a leading role in bone formation and angiogenesis and that pore size could adjust the rate of release of growth factors. The model developed by the institute can use specific scaffolds for sustained release of growth factors to predict bone regeneration.

3.2　Hydroxyapatite

Hydroxyapatite features excellent biocompatible and osteoconductive properties and easily combines with other materials [37]. It is an excellent carrier material and is widely used in sustained release of growth factors. It has a composition similar to inorganic bone matrix. Tsurushima *et al.* [38] coated hydroxyapatite ceramic buttons (HAP-CBs) with FGF-2 by precipitation in supersaturated calcium phosphate solution. HAP-CBs coated with high or low doses of FGF-2 were denoted by FGF-H or FGF-L. The release profile and biological activity of FGF-2 released from FGF-H and FGF-L were evaluated. The results showed that FGF-2 could still be detected at day 14 after *in vivo* release and the released growth factor still retained its biological activity. Bone formation is known to require a specific concentration of FGF-2, and this HAP-CB delivery system can release a sufficient amount of FGF-2 to induce bone formation.

The use of inorganic materials in association with various organic materials is more common than the use of inorganic materials alone. For example, although inorganic materials such as ceramics have potential benefits for bone replacement as high compressive strength, biodegradability, and osteoconductivity, they lack intrinsic mechanisms for controlled delivery. In this regard, the design of composite scaffolds is highly advantageous to control the release of growth factors. Fei *et al.* prepared a bone graft composite consisting of rhBMP-2 loaded PLGA microspheres and calcium phosphate cement achieving a controlled release for 28 days [39]. And Maehara *et al.* [40] impregnated porous hydroxyapatite/collagen (HAp/Col) with FGF-2 to repair large cartilage defects in rabbits. The scaffold was composed of hydroxyapatite nanocrystals and type I atelocollagen. The results showed that the FGF-2-incorporated porous hydroxyapatite/collagen effectively enhanced cartilage repair in rabbits. Letic-Gavrilovic *et al.* [41] also coupled collagen/hydroxyapatite (Col/HAp) to nerve growth factor β (NGF-β) for sustained release of the neurotrophin. The results of scanning electron microscopy and histological examination showed that this composite offers a variety of advantages in tissue engineering, such as excellent mechanical strength and biocompatibility, and is very suitable as a biomaterial for filling irregular maxillofacial defects.

4. Conclusions and outlook

Growth factors are a class of versatile regulatory peptides secreted by a variety of cells and regulate important functions such as cell division, proliferation, and migration. Despite their widespread application in the clinic, major challenges remain with the use of growth factors, such as short half-life, susceptibility to inactivation, and rapid dilution and metabolism if used topically. In recent years, notable progress has been made in the research of materials for sustained release of growth factors. The use of natural polymer materials and modification of existing inorganic and organic polymer materials have emerged as an area of intense research for sustained release carriers. Studies have shown that sustained release composite systems can avoid burst release and ensure gradual and stable release of growth factors within certain concentrations. Moreover, it is possible to improve controlled and site-specific drug delivery and therefore enhance the bioavailability of growth factors by harnessing the properties of polymer materials, such as biocompatibility and tissue targeting. This represents a new direction in the research of carriers for sustained release of growth factors.

References

[1] Bella AJ, Lin G, Lin C-S, *et al.* Nerve Growth Factor Modulation of the Cavernous Nerve Response to Injury [J]. Journal Of Sexual Medicine, 2009, 6: 347-352.

[2] Zeng F, Singh AB, Harris RC. The role of the EGF family of ligands and receptors in renal development, physiology and pathophysiology [J]. Experimental Cell Research, 2009, 315(4): 602-610.

[3] Beenken A, Mohammadi M. The FGF family: biology, pathophysiology and therapy [J]. Nature Reviews Drug Discovery, 2009, 8(3): 235-253.

[4] Smith CL, Tallquist MD. PDGF function in diverse neural crest cell populations [J]. Cell Adhesion & Migration, 2010, 4(4): 561-566.

[5] Shi HX, Lin C, Lin BB, *et al.* The anti-scar effects of basic fibroblast growth factor on the wound repair *in vitro* and *in vivo* [J]. Plos One, 2013, 8(4): e59966.

[6] Zhang HY, Zhang X, Wang ZG, *et al.* Exogenous basic fibroblast growth factor inhibits ER stress-induced apoptosis and improves recovery from spinal cord injury [J]. Cns Neuroscience & Therapeutics, 2013, 19(1): 20-29.

[7] Wang ZG, Wang Y, Huang Y, *et al.* bFGF regulates autophagy and ubiquitinated protein accumulation induced by myocardial ischemia/reperfusion *via* the activation of the PI3K/Akt/mTOR pathway [J]. Scientific Reports, 2015, 5: 9287.

[8] Zhang H, Wu F, Kong X, *et al.* Nerve growth factor improves functional recovery by inhibiting endoplasmic reticulum stress-induced neuronal apoptosis in rats with spinal cord injury [J]. Journal Of Translational Medicine, 2014, 12(1): 130.

[9] Sheng MHC, Lau KHW, Baylink DJ. Role of osteocyte-derived insulin-like growth factor I in developmental growth, modeling, remodeling, and regeneration of the bone [J]. Journal of bone metabolism, 2014, 21(1): 41-54.

[10] Chu H, Gao J, Wang Y. Design, synthesis, and biocompatibility of an arginine-based polyester [J]. Biotechnology Progress, 2012, 28(1): 257-264.

[11] Park YJ, Nam KH, Ha SJ, *et al.* Porous poly(L-lactide) membranes for guided tissue regeneration and controlled drug delivery: Membrane fabrication and characterization [J]. Journal Of Controlled Release, 1997, 43(2-3): 151-160.

[12] Yang Y, Zhao Y, Tang G, *et al. In vitro* degradation of porous poly(L-lactide-co-glycolide)/beta-tricalcium phosphate (PLGA/beta-TCP) scaffolds under dynamic and static conditions [J]. Polymer Degradation And Stability, 2008, 93(10): 1838-1845.

[13] Marquis M-E, Lord E, Bergeron E, *et al.* Bone cells-biomaterials interactions [J]. Frontiers In Bioscience-Landmark, 2009, 14: 1023-1067.

[14] Patel ZS, Yamamoto M, Ueda H, *et al.* Biodegradable gelatin microparticles as delivery systems for the controlled release of bone morphogenetic protein-2 [J]. Acta Biomaterialia, 2008, 4(5): 1126-1138.

[15] Hori K, Sotozono C, Hamuro J, *et al.* Controlled-release of epidermal growth factor from cationized gelatin hydrogel enhances corneal epithelial wound healing [J]. Journal Of Controlled Release, 2007, 118(2): 169-176.

[16] Oe S, Fukunaka Y, Hirose T, *et al.* A trial on regeneration therapy of rat liver cirrhosis by controlled release of hepatocyte growth factor [J]. Journal Of Controlled Release, 2003, 88(2): 193-200.

[17] Lu W-N, Lue S-H, Wang H-B, *et al.* Functional Improvement of Infarcted Heart by Co-Injection of Embryonic Stem Cells with Temperature-Responsive Chitosan Hydrogel [J]. Tissue Engineering Part A, 2009, 15(6): 1437-1447.

[18] Jeon O, Powell C, Solorio LD, *et al.* Affinity-based growth factor delivery using biodegradable, photocrosslinked heparin-alginate hydrogels [J]. Journal Of Controlled Release, 2011, 154(3): 258-266.

[19] Jeon O, Bouhadir KH, Mansour JM, *et al.* Photocrosslinked alginate hydrogels with tunable biodegradation rates and mechanical properties [J]. Biomaterials, 2009, 30(14): 2724-2734.

[20] Jeon O, Powell C, Ahmed SM, *et al.* Biodegradable, Photocrosslinked Alginate Hydrogels with Independently Tailorable Physical Properties and Cell Adhesivity [J]. Tissue Engineering Part A, 2010, 16(9): 2915-2925.

[21] Liu G, Pareta RA, Wu R, *et al.* Skeletal myogenic differentiation of urine-derived stem cells and angiogenesis using microbeads loaded with growth factors [J]. Biomaterials, 2013, 34(4): 1311-1326.

[22] Mitra A, Dey B. Chitosan microspheres in novel drug delivery systems [J]. Indian Journal Of Pharmaceutical Sciences, 2011, 73(4): 355-366.

[23] Yang Z, Duan H, Mo L, *et al.* The effect of the dosage of NT-3/chitosan carriers on the proliferation and differentiation of neural stem cells [J]. Biomaterials, 2010, 31(18): 4846-4854.

[24] Park YJ, Lee YM, Lee JY, *et al.* Controlled release of platelet-derived growth factor-BB from chondroitin sulfate-chitosan sponge for guided bone regeneration [J]. Journal Of Controlled Release, 2000, 67(2-3): 385-394.

[25] Santo VE, Duarte ARC, Popa EG, *et al.* Enhancement of osteogenic differentiation of human adipose derived stem cells by the controlled release of platelet lysates from hybrid scaffolds produced by supercritical fluid foaming [J]. Journal Of Controlled Release, 2012, 162(1): 19-27.

[26] Johnson NR, Wang Y. Controlled delivery of heparin-binding EGF-like growth factor yields fast and comprehensive wound healing [J]. Journal Of Controlled Release, 2013, 166(2): 124-129.

[27] Chu H, Johnson NR, Mason NS, *et al.* A polycation:heparin complex releases growth factors with enhanced bioactivity [J]. Journal Of Controlled Release, 2011, 150(2): 157-163.

[28] Park YJ, Ku Y, Chung CP, *et al.* Controlled release of platelet-derived growth factor from porous poly(L-lactide) membranes for guided tissue regeneration [J]. Journal Of Controlled Release, 1998, 51(2-3): 201-211.

[29] Wang Q, Gao Y, Sun X, *et al.* Acceleration of aneurysm healing by P(DLLA-co-TMC)-coated coils enabling the controlled release of vascular endothelial growth factor [J]. Biomedical Materials, 2014, 9(4).

[30] Kirby GTS, White LJ, Rahman CV, *et al.* PLGA-Based Microparticles for the Sustained Release of BMP-2 [J]. Polymers, 2011, 3(1): 571-586.

[31] Spiller KL, Liu Y, Holloway JL, *et al.* A novel method for the direct fabrication of growth factor-loaded microspheres within porous nondegradable hydrogels: Controlled release for cartilage tissue en-

gineering [J]. Journal Of Controlled Release, 2012, 157(1): 39-45.

[32] Wang Y, Cooke MJ, Sachewsky N, *et al.* Bioengineered sequential growth factor delivery stimulates brain tissue regeneration after stroke [J]. Journal Of Controlled Release, 2013, 172(1): 1-11.

[33] Kim CS, Kim JI, Kim J, *et al.* Ectopic bone formation associated with recombinant human bone morphogenetic proteins-2 using absorbable collagen sponge and beta tricalcium phosphate as carriers [J]. Biomaterials, 2005, 26(15): 2501-2507.

[34] Yang YZ, Kim KH, Ong JL. Review on calcium phosphate coatings produced using a sputtering process - an alternative to plasma spraying [J]. Biomaterials, 2005, 26(3): 327-337.

[35] El-Ghannam A. Bone reconstruction: from bioceramics to tissue engineering [J]. Expert Review Of Medical Devices, 2005, 2(1): 87-101.

[36] Sun X, Kang Y, Bao J, *et al.* Modeling vascularized bone regeneration within a porous biodegradable CaP scaffold loaded with growth factors [J]. Biomaterials, 2013, 34(21): 4971-4981.

[37] Kim HW, Knowles JC, Kim HE. Hydroxyapatite/poly(epsilon-caprolactone) composite coatings on hydroxyapatite porous bone scaffold for drug delivery [J]. Biomaterials, 2004, 25(7-8): 1279-1287.

[38] Tsurushima H, Marushima A, Suzuki K, *et al.* Enhanced bone formation using hydroxyapatite ceramic coated with fibroblast growth factor-2 [J]. Acta Biomaterialia, 2010, 6(7): 2751-2759.

[39] Fei Z, Hu Y, Wu D, *et al.* Preparation and property of a novel bone graft composite consisting of rhBMP-2 loaded PLGA microspheres and calcium phosphate cement [J]. Journal Of Materials Science-Materials In Medicine, 2008, 19(3): 1109-1116.

[40] Maehara H, Sotome S, Yoshii T, *et al.* Repair of Large Osteochondral Defects in Rabbits Using Porous Hydroxyapatite/Collagen (HAp/Col) and Fibroblast Growth Factor-2 (FGF-2) [J]. Journal Of Orthopaedic Research, 2010, 28(5): 677-686.

[41] Letic-Gavrilovic A, Piattelli A, Abe K. Nerve growth factor beta(NGF beta) delivery *via* a collagen/hydroxyapatite (Col/HAp) composite and its effects on new bone growth [J]. Journal Of Materials Science-Materials In Medicine, 2003, 14(2): 95-102.

[42] Chu H, Chen CW, Huard J, *et al.* The effect of a heparin-based coacervate of fibroblast growth factor-2 on scarring in the infarcted myocardium [J]. Biomaterials, 2013, 34(6): 1747-1756.

[43] Zhang HY, Wang ZG, Wu FZ, *et al.* Regulation of Autophagy and Ubiquitinated Protein Accumulation by bFGF Promotes Functional Recovery and Neural Protection in a Rat Model of Spinal Cord Injury [J]. Molecular Neurobiology, 2013, 48(3): 452-464.

[44] Wang Z, Wang Y, Ye J, *et al.* bFGF attenuates endoplasmic reticulum stress and mitochondrial injury on myocardial ischaemia/reperfusion *via* activation of PI3K/Akt/ERK1/2 pathway [J]. Journal Of Cellular And Molecular Medicine, 2015, 19(3): 595-607.

[45] Ferrara N. Vascular endothelial growth factor: Basic science and clinical progress [J]. Endocrine Reviews, 2004, 25(4): 581-611.

[46] Aditiawarman. The role of albumin and endoplasmic reticulum in pathogenesis Preeclampsia. Changes of GRP78 and placental VEGF in preeclampsia [J]. Pregnancy hypertension, 2014, 4(3): 247-247.

[47] Deng J, Cui J, Jiang N, *et al.* STAT3 regulation the expression of VEGF-D in HGC-27 gastric cancer cell [J]. American Journal Of Translational Research, 2014, 6(6): 756-767.

[48] Cheng JC, Chang HM, Fang L, *et al.* TGF-beta 1 up-regulates connective tissue growth factor expression in human granulosa cells through smad and ERK1/2 signaling pathways [J]. Plos One, 2015, 10(5).

[49] Gruchlik A, Chodurek E, Dzierzewicz Z. Effect of Gly-His-Lys and its copper complex on TGF-beta 1 secretion in normal human dermal fibroblasts [J]. Acta Poloniae Pharmaceutica, 2014, 71(6): 954-958.

[50] Luo H, Hao Y, Tang B, *et al.* Mouse forestomach carcinoma cells immunosuppress macrophages through TGF-beta 1 [J]. Turkish Journal Of Gastroenterology, 2012, 23(6): 658-665.

[51] Salinas M, Diaz R, Abraham NG, *et al.* Nerve growth factor protects against 6-hydroxydopamine-induced oxidative stress by increasing expression of heme oxygenase-1 in a phosphatidylinositol 3-kinase-dependent manner [J]. Journal Of Biological Chemistry, 2003, 278(16): 13898-13904.

[52] Tang LL, Wang R, Tang XC. Huperzine A protects SHSY5Y neuroblastoma cells against oxidative stress damage *via* nerve growth factor production [J]. European Journal Of Pharmacology, 2005, 519(1-2): 9-15.

[53] Kim MS, Lee DY. Insulin-like growth factor (IGF)-I and IGF binding proteins axis in diabetes mellitus [J]. Annals of pediatric endocrinology & metabolism, 2015, 20(2): 69-73.

[54] Zhang H, Zhang Y, Xu H, *et al.* Olanzapine ameliorates neuropathological changes and increases IGF-1 expression in frontal cortex of C57BL/6 mice exposed to cuprizone [J]. Psychiatry Research, 2014, 216(3): 438-445.

[55] Shih CW, Lin YY, Chang HW, *et al.* Effect of the external field on the soft magnetic properties and microstructure of directly cast Fe75P8.7B5C7Si4.3 nanocrystalline sheets [J]. Journal Of Applied Physics, 2015, 117(17).

[56] Oliviero O, Ventre M, Netti PA. Functional porous hydrogels to study angiogenesis under the effect of controlled release of vascular endothelial growth factor [J]. Acta Biomaterialia, 2012, 8(9): 3294-3301.

[57] Reyes-Ortega F, Rodriguez G, Rosa Aguilar M, *et al.* Encapsulation of low molecular weight heparin (bemiparin) into polymeric nanoparticles obtained from cationic block copolymers: properties and cell activity [J]. Journal Of Materials Chemistry B, 2013, 1(6): 850-860.

[58] Marcus M, Skaat H, Alon N, *et al.* NGF-conjugated iron oxide nanoparticles promote differentiation and outgrowth of PC12 cells [J]. Nanoscale, 2015, 7(3): 1058-1066.

[59] Mullen LM, Best SM, Ghose S, *et al.* Bioactive IGF-1 release from collagen-GAG scaffold to enhance cartilage repair *in vitro* [J]. Journal Of Materials Science-Materials In Medicine, 2015, 26(1).

[60] Kim SH, Kim SH, Jung Y. TGF-beta(3) encapsulated PLCL scaffold by a supercritical CO_2-HFIP co-solvent system for cartilage tissue engineering [J]. Journal Of Controlled Release, 2015, 206: 101-107.

[61] Losi P, Briganti E, Errico C, *et al.* Fibrin-based scaffold incorporating VEGF- and bFGF-loaded nanoparticles stimulates wound healing in diabetic mice [J]. Acta Biomaterialia, 2013, 9(8): 7814-7821.

Minireview: roles of fibroblast growth factors 19 and 21 in metabolic regulation and chronic diseases

Fangfang Zhang, Xiaokun Li, Chi Zhang

The fibroblast growth factor (FGF) family comprises 22 members that are further classified into 7 subfamilies based on their structural similarities and mechanisms of action [1, 2]. Most FGFs bind to and activate cell surface tyrosine kinase FGF receptors (FGFRs) [1- 4] *via* a high-affinity interaction with heparin, and then function in a paracrine/autocrine manner to induce cell proliferation and differentiation [3, 4]. Members of the FGF19 subfamily, including FGF19, FGF21, and FGF23, also function by activating FGFRs. FGF19 activates mainly FGFR4, whereas FGF21 and FGF23 signal predominantly *via* FGFR1c and FGFR2c [5]. Unlike conventional FGFs, FGF19 subfamily members lack a classic heparin-binding domain [6]. This characteristic allows these proteins to avoid capture by local cells; therefore, they are secreted into the bloodstream and function as hormones. However, the FGF19 subfamily has a low affinity for heparin sulfate, another coreceptor named Klotho is required to allow the FGF19 subfamily to exert their biological functions [1, 6]. The klotho gene, named after the spinner, was identified in 1997 as a gene mutated in a mouse strain that exhibited short life span and complex phenotypes resembling human premature aging syndrome. Klotho is a transmembrane protein family that contains α-Klotho, β-Klotho, and lactase-like Klotho [7, 8]. α-Klotho is primarily expressed in the distal convoluted tubules of the kidney and is required for the biological actions of FGF23 [9]. β-Klotho shares 41% amino acid identity with α-Klotho and is required for the biological effects of FGF21 and FGF19 [3, 10]. Members of the FGF19 subfamily function in various biological activities such as regulating the enterohepatic circulation of bile acid, regulating glucose and lipid metabolism, and maintaining phosphate/vitamin D homeostasis [5]. Although FGF19 and FGF21 show only approximately 35% sequence homology, their functions considerably overlap, including maintaining bodyweight and regulating carbohydrate and lipid homeostases [3].

The interaction between carbohydrate and lipid metabolism allows the body to maintain its energy resources, particularly during nutritional stress. Generally, after feeding, glucose may enter any of 4 main metabolic pathways: 1) glucose is decomposed into H_2O and CO_2 or lactate associated with production of ATP through aerobic or anaerobic metabolism pathways, respectively; 2) glucose is decomposed into ribose and reduced nicotinamide adenine dinucleotide phosphate *via* the phosphopentose pathway; 3) excessive glucose is polymerized into glycogen and stored in the liver as an energy source; 4) excessive glucose is transformed to fat and stored in adipose tissues through their common metabolic intermediate product, acetyl-coenzyme A (CoA), which is subsequently transformed into palmitic acid *via* a 4-step reaction of condensation, reduction, dehydration, and reduction. However, during fasting or starvation, the glucose requirement of the body increases. Glucose is thus obtained from food decomposition, glycogenolysis, and glucogenolysis. Gluconeogenesis is derived from fat catabolism. Triglyceride (TG), which is a blood lipid, can be decomposed into glycerol and 3 fatty acids. These products are then transformed into acetyl-CoA, which is the key molecule of gluconeogenesis. In this review, we focus mainly on the metabolic activities of FGF19 and FGF21, with particular emphasis on the similarities and differences between these 2 hormones in terms of maintaining energy homeostasis (glucose and lipid metabolism) and metabolic disorders.

1. Identification of FGF19 and its effect on bile acid hemostasis

In 1999, FGF19 was first discovered in the human brain during embryonic and fetal development, which indicated that it plays an important role in brain development during embryogenesis [11]. Similarly, FGF15, which is an ortholog of FGF19, is expressed in the central nervous system of rodents, where it plays an important role in stimulating the differentiation, but not proliferation, of mature neural cells [12, 13]. Actually, FGF19 and FGF15 are the same protein function in human and rodent, respectively. The nucleotide sequence revealed a complete amino acid sequence of the protein (216 amino acids). The amino sequences of human FGF19 are very similar (~51% amino acid identity) to those of mouse FGF15 (218 amino acids). In adults, however, FGF15/19 is inactive in the neural system and instead, plays an important role in the regulation of bile acid homeostasis [14].

Bile acid is produced by the liver, secreted into the circulation, and then stored mainly in the gallbladder. After each meal, the gallbladder contracts and squeezes bile acids into the intestinal tract to facilitate intestinal absorption and lipid transportation *via* the enterohepatic circulation, which functions not only in feedback inhibition of bile acid synthesis, but also in lipid homeostasis [15]. FGF19 is a negative regulator of bile acid synthesis and transportation. Liver-derived bile acid can bind to farnesoid X receptor in enterocytes, and the resulting heterodimer functions as a transcription factor that induces intestinal FGF19 expression [16]. Then, FGF19 is transported into the liver, where it activates Src homology 2 domain domain-containing protein tyrosine phosphatase-2 signaling in both an autocrine and paracrine manner to inhibit the expression of *Cyp7a1*, which is the rate-limiting enzyme in bile acid synthesis [10]. A number of studies have confirmed the therapeutic potential of FGF19 in the treatment of metabolic disorders using rodent and primate models of obesity and diabetes [3, 10, 17]. However, one major concern relating to the potential use of FGF19 is its mitogenic function, which may facilitate in tumorigenesis [18].

2. FGF21 identification and its general actions

The human *fgf21* gene was first identified by PCR analysis in the liver [19]. Mature FGF21 consists of 209 and 210 amino acids in humans and mice, respectively; the 2 proteins are 75% homologous [19]. Previous studies have shown that FGF21 is predominantly expressed in the liver and adipose tissues, and is also expressed at lower levels in other organs such as skeletal muscle, heart, kidneys, and testes [19-21]. FGF21 had attracted the attention of researchers in 2005, when its metabolic regulatory effects were identified. Specifically, Kharitonenkov *et al* demonstrated that FGF21 increased glucose uptake in both 3T3-L1 adipocytes and human primary adipocytes, and that these effects were mainly due to the up-regulation of glucose transporter (GLUT)-1 but not GLUT-4 [22]. Moreover, FGF21 improves glucose tolerance and insulin sensitivity, as well as decreases blood glucose levels [22]. Similar regulatory effects have been observed in carbohydrates in primate [23]. Unlike insulin, an overdose of FGF21 does not result in hypoglycemia [22]. In addition, FGF21 is not carcinogenic because it lacks a mitogenic function [22]. In the liver, peroxisome proliferator-activated receptor (PPAR)-α is the main mediator of FGF21 expression and function, including the regulation of gluconeogenesis, ketogenesis, torpor, and growth inhibition [3, 24, 25]. Similarly, PPARα-deficiency results in the failure to up-regulate FGF21 expression in the liver, whereas FGF21 deficiency inhibits the biological actions of PPARα [25].

In adipocytes, FGF21 expression is induced by feeding and follows a PPARγ-dependent manner. Mice with the deletion of *fgf21* gene (FGF21-knockout [KO]) fail to display PPARγ activities such decreasing body fat and lipidmia, improving insulin sensitivity, and increasing lipogenesis [26]. In addition, a mechanistic study demonstrated that FGF21 stimulates the transcriptional activity of PPARγ mainly by preventing the sumoylation of PPARγ at K107 [26, 27]. The administration of a PPARα activator induces FGF21 expression in the liver, which is associated with an increase in circulating FGF21 levels. Activation of PPARγ also up-regulates FGF21 expression in adipocytes tissue, although an increase in circulating FGF21 levels was not observed. One possible explanation is that secreted FGF21 from adipocyte tissues is constrained by the white adipocyte tissue (WAT) extracellular matrix [28]. This raises an important question regarding the mechanism by which FGF21 induces adaptive responses to fasting or starvation. Potthoff *et al* demonstrated that PPARγ coactivator protein-1 (PGC-1α) is a key regulator of the biological functions of FGF21, including increased fatty acid oxidation, tricarboxylic acid cycle flux, and gluconeogenesis without increasing glycogenolysis [29]. In addition, Chau *et al* demonstrated that FGF21 regulates mitochondrial activity and enhances the oxidative capacity *via* an AMP-activated protein kinase (AMPK)-sirtuin type 1-PGC-1α-dependent mechanism in adipocytes [30].

Additionally, a large body of studies have indicated that FGF21 expression is up-regulated during different kinds of stresses, including chemicals such as acetaminophen, dioxin, cerulein, and phenylephrine [31-33], environmental stress such as cold, nutritional stress such as starvation (fasting) and overnutrition (obesity), endoplasmic reticulum (ER) stress [34, 35], mitochondria stress [36, 37], and oxidative stress [38, 39]. These facts suggest that FGF21 acts as a key regulator

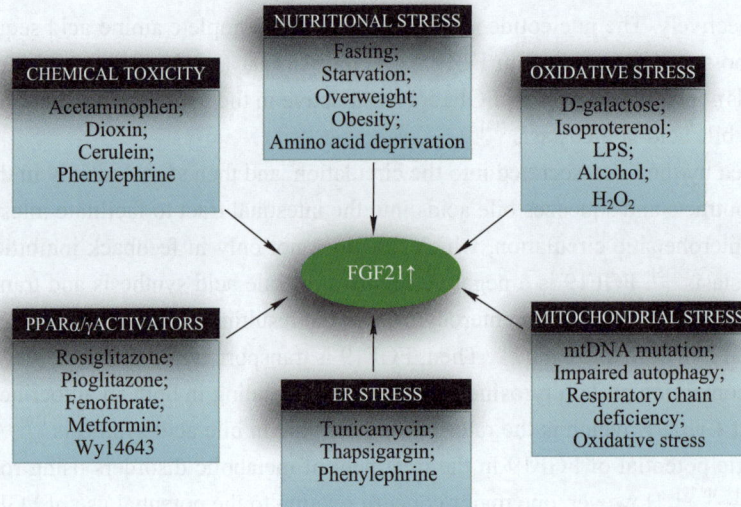

Fig. 1. Summary of FGF21 stimuli. FGF21 is predominantly expressed in the liver, adipocyte tissues, and pancreas in response to multiple stimuli, including chemical toxicity, such as acetaminophen, dioxin, cerulein, and phenylephrine; nutritional stress, such as energy deprivation or overload; activation of PPARα/γ, upstream activators of FGF21; as well as oxidative stress, mitochondrial stress, and ER stress.

in the adaptation of the body or organs to various kinds of stress and may function as a preventive response to limit the progression of stress in these altered conditions (Fig. 1).

3. Role of FGF19 and FGF21 in regulating glucose metabolism

Nutritional status is regulated by multiple factors, including insulin and glucagon, which are early-acting hormones that respond to nutritional stress [40, 41]. In the fed state, insulin production and secretion rapidly increase to maintain carbohydrate homeostasis by enhancing lipogenesis and glycogen synthesis and suppressing gluconeogenesis and protein synthesis [42, 43]. Conversely, in the fasted state, glucagon is the early-acting hormone that induces glucose metabolism, which is characterized by increased glycogenolysis and decreased gluconeogenesis and ketogenesis [3]. In contrast, FGF15/19 and FGF21 are late-acting hormones of the fed and fasted states, respectively; these induce the secretion of insulin and glucagon to regulate glucose homeostasis (Table 1) [3]. A functional study has shown that FGF19 transgenic mice are resistant to high-fat diet (HFD)-induced glucose intolerance and insulin resistance [44]. Similarly, the administration of exogenous FGF19 prevents the development of glucose metabolic disorders in either HFD-fed or *ob/ob* mice [45]. In addition, FGF15-KO mice exhibit impaired glucose tolerance and reduced insulin sensitivity, which is reversed by treatment with recombinant FGF19 [40, 46]. Mechanistic studies have shown that FGF19-maintained glucose homeostasis was attributable not only to the enhancement of glycogen synthesis by increasing glycogen synthase (GS) activity, but also to the suppression of gluconeogenesis *via* activation of the cAMP-response element-binding protein (CREB)/ PGC-1α signaling pathway [47]. Although FGFR4 is generally the main receptor of FGF19, a truncated FGF19 variant lacking the β-Klotho-binding domain could still activate FGFR4 and subsequently regulate bile acid homeostasis, but failed to stimulate glucose uptake in 3T3-L1 adipocytes, suggesting that FGFR4 is not required for the glucose tolerance-improving effects of FGF19 [48]. Additionally, metabolic disorders in FGFR4-KO mice could not be corrected by up-regulating hepatic FGFR4 expression [46], suggesting that other tissues contribute to FGF19-induced glucose homeostasis. In parallel, recent studies further demonstrated that the intracerebroventricular administration of FGF19 induces insulin-independent glucose lowering in *ob/ob* mice and improves insulin sensitivity in HFD-fed rats [49, 50], indicating that the FGF19-induced blood glucose regulatory effect might be due to the action of a central system. The summary of FGF19's function and associated mechanisms are presented in Fig. 2. FGF21 is a metabolic regulator that maintains glucose homeostasis. Unlike FGF19, FGF21 mainly functions at the late stage of fasting [22]. A previous *in vitro* study indicated that FGF21 induces glucose uptake in various cell lines, possibly by enhancing the expression and activity of GLUT-

Table 1.   Function of insulin, FGF19, glucagon, and FGF21 at different nutritional conditions

Nutritional status	Main regulator	Half-life	Functions
Fed	Insulin	≈4 min	Glucose catabolism ↑
			Gluconeogenesis ↓
		Reaches its peak serum level at 1 h after a meal	Lipogenesis ↑
			Protein synthesis ↑
			Glycogen synthesis ↑
After feeding	FGF19	≈30 min	Bile acid synthesis ↓
			Bile acid transportation ↓
		Reaches its peak serum level at 3 h after a meal	Bile acid gallbladder filling ↑
			Glucose catabolism ↑
			Gluconeogenesis ↓
			Protein synthesis ↑
			Glycogen synthesis ↑
Fasted	Glucagon	≈5 min	Glycogenolysis ↑
		Reaches its peak serum level at 3-5 d after a meal	Gluconeogenesis ↑
			Ketogenesis ↑
			Glucose catabolism ↓
Starved	FGF21	≈30 min	Gluconeogenesis ↑
		Reaches its peak serum level at 7 d after a meal	Ketogenesis ↑
			Glucose catabolism ↓
			Lipolysis ↑
			Energy expenditure ↓

1 [51]. Unlike insulin, FGF21 induces glucose uptake *via* a slow-onset pathway that likely requires protein synthesis [22].

However, the combination treatment using insulin and FGF21 induced synergistic effects that further enhanced glucose clearance by activating both GLUT-4 and GLUT-1 in adipocytes [22, 42]. FGF21, which is predominantly expressed in the liver and regulated by hepatic PPARα, induces lipid oxidation, TG clearance, glycolysis, and ketogenesis in the liver [24]. In addition, FGF21 also maintains metabolic homeostasis in other peripheral organs. For example, administration of FGF21 increased the number of islets and insulin content in type 2 diabetic mice, suggesting that the FGF21-induced glucose regulatory effects could be mainly attributed to the preservation of pancreatic β-cells [52]. Moreover, sc administration of FGF21 in diabetic mice significantly decreased fasting insulin and postprandial glucose levels [53]. FGF21 also prevents lipotoxicity- or diabetes-induced insulin resistance in skeletal muscle cells or in kidney tissues [54, 55]. Interestingly, some of these organs mentioned above lack FGFR1 or β-Klotho, which suggests the existence of an indirect action of FGF21. Two recent studies have indicated that FGF21 stimulates the expression of adiponectin, which plays an important role in maintaining glucose and lipid metabolism and homeostasis [56, 57]. Meanwhile, adiponectin-KO mice were refractory to several therapeutic benefits of FGF21 [56, 57]. Therefore, it is possible that adiponectin mediates at least some of the functions of FGF21. Recent studies have demonstrated that FGF21 induces the metabolic regulatory or protective effect on its target organs by fine-tuning cross talk among multiple organs. Xu and coworkers reported that ip administrated FGF21 could be detected in the cerebrospinal fluid, which activates the hypothalamic-pituitary-adrenal axis *via* the FGFR1c/β-klotho-ERK-CREB signaling pathway to release corticosterone and stimulate hepatic gluconeogenesis [58], implying that the central system plays a key role in indirectly mediating FGF21's function (Fig. 3). In addition, we recently demonstrated that FGF21 prevents atherosclerosis *via* integration of the liver, adipocytes tissue, and blood vessels (Fig. 3). Mechanistically, the protective effect of FGF21 on blood vessels against atherosclerosis is attrib-

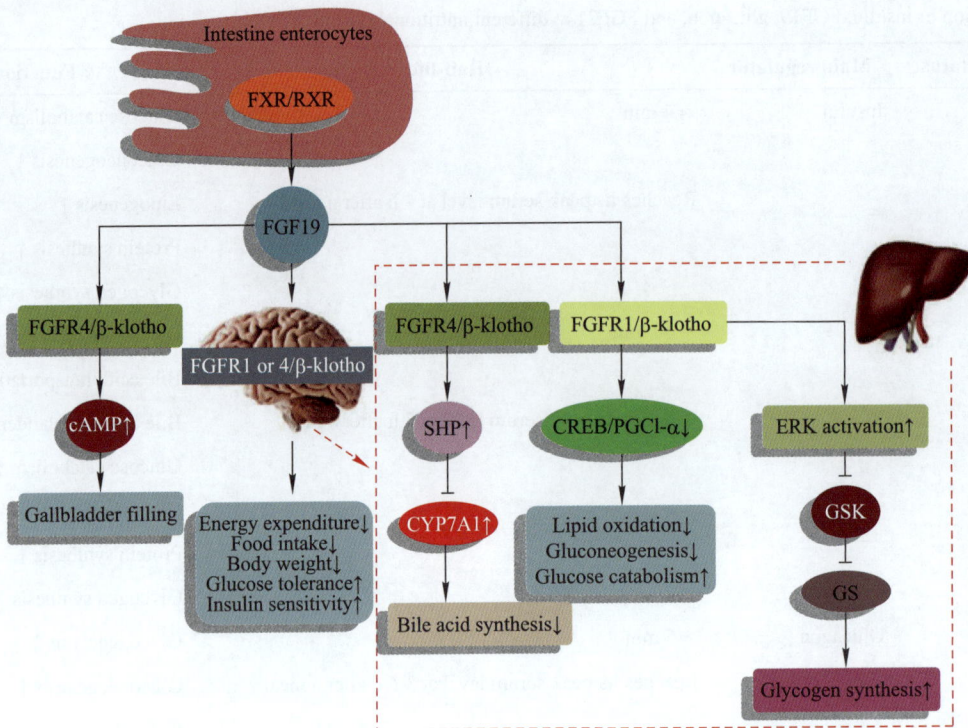

Fig. 2. The functions of FGF19 and the corresponding mechanisms. Endogenous FGF19 expression is induced in intestinal enterocytes by the activation of FXR/RXR heterodimers. Secreted FGF19 mediates multiple metabolic processes. On one hand, FGF19 can bind to FGFR4 in the presence of β-klotho and activation of cAMP, followed by stimulation of bile acid filling into the gallbladder. In addition, liver is another key target organ of FGF19 that activates the SHP/CYP7A1 pathway by binding with FGFR4/β-klotho that negatively regulates bile acid synthesis. On the other hand, by binding with FGFR1/β-klotho, FGF19 mainly regulates glucose metabolism, including suppression of gluconeogenesis and enhancement of glucose catabolism *via* the inhibition of the CREB/PGC-1α pathway, and improvement of glycogen synthesis *via* inhibition of GS kinase (GSK) pathway. CYP7A1, cholesterol 7-a-monooxygenase; FXR, farnesoid X receptor; GSK3, GS kinase-3; RXR, retinoid X receptor; SHP, protein tyrosine phosphatase.

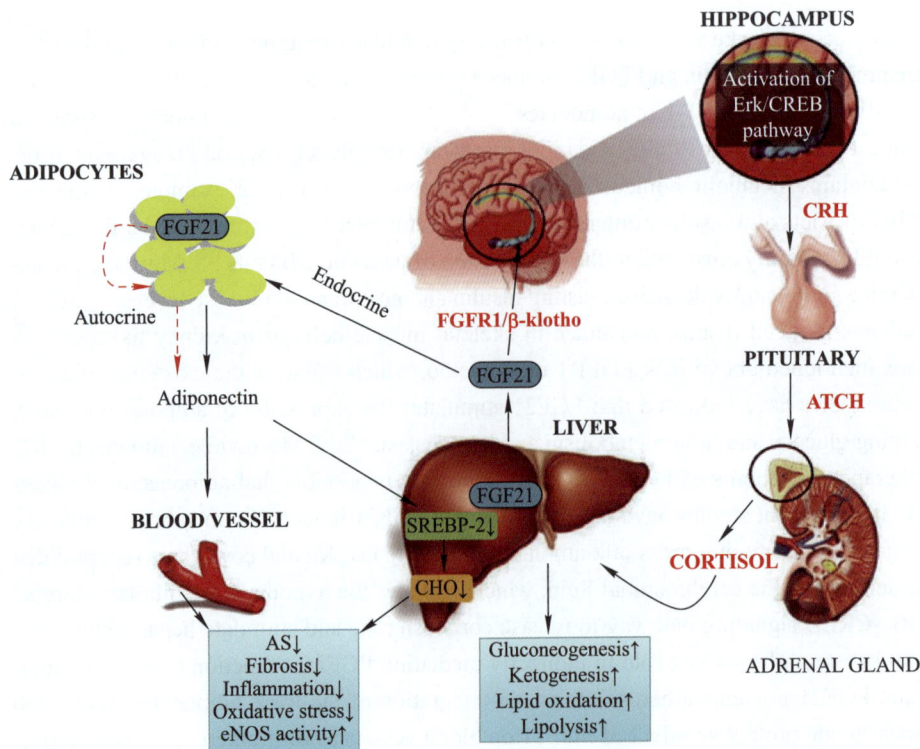

Fig. 3. Pharmacological effect of FGF21 is partly attributed to the interactions among multiple organs. FGF21 was initially regarded as a metabolic regulator that directly acts on the target organs. However, recent studies have revealed that FGF21 also indirectly acts upon target organs. FGF21-induced gluconeogenesis, ketogenesis, and lipolysis are mediated by the activation of hippocampus-pituitary-adrenal gland aix. In addition, FGF21 prevents atherosclerosis by reducing CHO, which is induced by an increase in the production of adiponectin from adipocytes tissue and suppression of SRPBP-2 in the liver

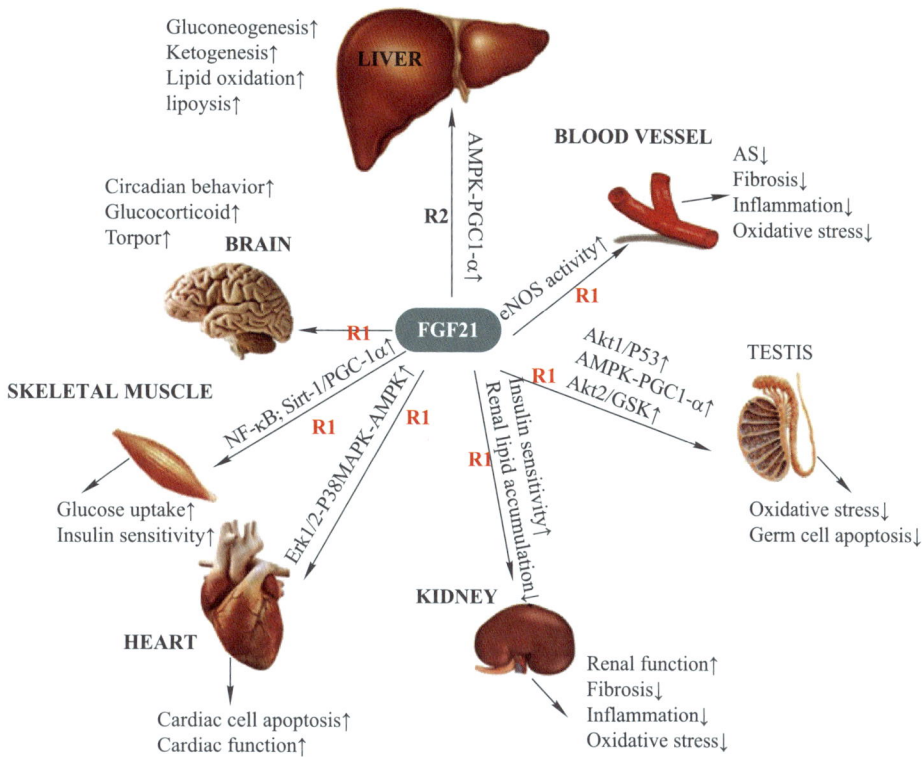

Fig. 4. The functions of FGF21 and the possible mechanism. Secreted FGF21 functions as a metabolic regulator in either endocrine or autocrine manner in multiple organs, including blood vessels, testis, kidney, heart, skeletal muscle, and brain. FGF21 acts on the above organs not only *via* directly binding to FGFRs of these organs in the presence of β-klotho but is also mediated by adiponectin or central neural system. AKT, protein kinase B; AS, atherosclorosis; eNOS, endothelial nitric oxide synthase; NF-κB, nuclear factor-κB; R1, FGFR1; R2, FGFR2; Sirt-1, sirtuin type 1.

utable to the reduction in hypercholesterolemia *via* the induction of adiponectin in adipocytes tissues and suppression of hepatic sterol regulatory element-binding protein (Srebp)-2 in the liver [59].

Unlike FGF19, FGF21 maintains glucose homeostasis in different nutritional states. In the fasted state, FGF21 induces hyperglycemic effects by stimulating lipolysis, ketogenesis, gluconeogenesis, and increasing insulin sensitivity [24]. Interestingly, Inagaki *et al.* indicated that ketogenic effects are comparably enhanced in *fgf21* gene overexpressing transgenic (FGF21-TG) mice and their wildtype (WT) mice during fasting because endogenous FGF21 is sufficient in imparting its biological effects [25]. A similar effect was also observed in FGF21-KO mice, which suggests that most of the effects of FGF21 on glucose metabolism in the liver are due to the pharmacological but not physiological effects of FGF21 [60]. On the other hand, FGF21 induces hypoglycemic effects by stimulating lipogenesis and adipocyte differentiation in the fed state [26]. Therefore, the physiological conditions of these studies assessing the relationship between FGF21 and glucose metabolism should be carefully selected. The summary of the functions and the associated mechanisms of FGF21 are presented in Fig. 4.

4.　Role of FGF19 and FGF21 in regulating lipid metabolism

Bile acids are physiological detergents that mediate the intestinal absorption and transport of lipids. FGF19, a negative regulator of bile acid synthesis and transport, suppresses lipid absorption and hyperlipidemia [15], which indicates that FGF19 plays an important role in regulating lipid metabolism. Clinically, decreased serum FGF19 levels during fasting are associated with the development of nonalcoholic fatty liver disease (NAFLD) in obese adolescents. Tomlinson *et al.* [44] demonstrated that the bodyweight of FGF19 transgenic mice fed on a standard diet significantly decreased and was mainly due to reduced adiposity rather than food intake [44]. In addition, FGF19 transgenic mice are also resistant to HFD-induced obesity and increased fat content. A study conducted by a Japanese group suggested that treating obese mice with recombinant FGF19 decreased the transcription of a series of genes that were closely associated with lipogenesis, including acetyl-CoA carboxylase (*ACC*), *Cd36*, *Srebp-1c*, stearoyl-CoA desaturase 1 (*SCD1*), and *Cyp7a1* (61). A similar negative regulation of lipogenesis was also observed in obese FGF19-TG mice [44]. A mechanistic study revealed that FGF19 inhibits the expression of lipogenic enzymes by activating downstream kinase STAT3, which is an inhibitor of SREBP-1c expression, and decreasing the expression of PGC-1β instead of altering ERK, P38 mitogen-activated protein kinase, or AMPK activity [62]. Interestingly, Wu *et al* reported that treatment using FGF19 increases serum TG and cholesterol levels in diet induced-obese mice [63]. The above findings suggest that FGF19 exerts both lipid-raising and -lowering effects under different conditions. The dual functions of FGF19 could be attributed to different binding receptors and target tissues [63]. For instance, FGF19 induces lipolysis through the activation of FGFR1c, primarily in adipose and other tissues except liver. On the other hand, it induces lipogenesis through the activation of FGFR4 and negatively regulates hepatic bile acid synthesis [48, 63]. Under fasting or starved conditions, the lipolysis-induced production of fatty acids compensates for carbohydrate depletion to provide nearly half of the energy required by the entire body. An *in vitro* study demonstrated that incubating hepatocytes with fatty acids stimulates the secretion of FGF21 [64]. Clinical studies have suggested that serum FGF21 levels are positively correlated with obesity and fatty liver [65, 66]. In addition, a randomize controlled trial showed that lipid infusion increases FGF21 levels [64]. These studies suggest that increased FGF21 levels might be an adaptive protective response to lipotoxicity. Inagaki *et al* reported that the levels of serum and hepatic TGs significantly decreased in FGF21 transgenic mice fed on standard chow compared with WT mice [25]. On the other hand, FGF21 knockdown mice fed on a ketogenic diet showed further enhancement of KD-induced excessive lipid accumulation in the liver [24]. In addition, the size of adipocytes in FGF21 transgenic mice was notably smaller than those in WT mice [25]. A mechanism study demonstrated that FGF21-induced lipolytic effect was due to the up-regulation of various lipases, particularly hormone-sensitive lipase and adipose TG lipase [25]. Besides induction of lipolysis, FGF21 also induces lipid β-oxidation in the liver, as characterized by the increased expression of hydroxyacyl-CoA dehydrogenase, carnitine palmitoyltransferase 1α, acyl-CoA oxidase, and cluster of differentiation 36 (CD36) *via* the AMPK-sirtuin type 1-PGC-1α signaling pathway, which might be mediated by adiponectin [24, 30]. Conversely, another study indicated that FGF21 induces adipocyte differentiation and lipogenesis in obese mice [26]. The observed opposite effect of FGF21 on lipid metabolism suggests that FGF21 has diverse regulatory roles in various nutritional states to maintain lipid homeostasis [67]. FGF21 playing a role in the regulation of the TG/fatty acid cycle might explain why FGF21 could both stimulate and repress lipolysis in white adipocytes [26].

5. Metabolic regulatory effect of FGF21 on carbohydrate and lipid is independent of UCP-1-mediated browning of WAT

Mammalian adipocyte tissue consists of WAT and brown adipocyte tissue (BAT). WAT serves as the main storage tissue of neutral fats. On the other hand, BAT preserves body temperature under cold condition by releasing intracellular BAT lipids during lipolysis and generating heat in mitochondria *via* uncoupling protein (UCP)-1 [68]. UCP-1 imparts a thermogenic effect by eliminating the voltage difference across the mitochondrial membrane and transforming energy to heat instead of generating ATP [69]. However, recent studies have shown that during prolonged exposure to cold condition, WAT can also convert to a "browning-like" state that is characterized by an expansion of its multilocular structure and a decrease in lipid storage [70]. Fisher *et al* demonstrated that FGF21-KO mice displayed an impairment of the ability to adapt to low temperatures with reduced WAT browning. Administration of exogenous FGF21 remarkably enhances the body's defense to chronic cold exposure by inhibiting its regulatory effect on the expressions of UCP-1 and other thermogenic genes in fat tissues [70]. Another mechanistic study demonstrated that FGF21 regulates this process, at least in part, by enhancing adipose tissue PGC-1α protein levels independent of mRNA expression [70]. Do FGF21-induced UCP-1 activity and the browning effect of WAT contribute to the regulation of lipid and carbohydrate metabolism? Two recent publications in *Cell Metabolism* and *Cell Reports* examined the relationship between WAT browning and pharmacological effects of FGF21 on metabolic regulation, and concluded that the therapeutic effects of FGF21 for correcting metabolic disorders of carbohydrate and lipid are, to a large extent, independent of WAT browning [71, 72]. Their studies confirmed that after administration of an FGF21 mimetic, BAT activity and BAT-derived UCP-1 expression were significantly enhanced at both 21℃ and 30℃, whereas the browning effect of WAT was only observed at 21℃. However, exogenous FGF21 or the FGF21 mimetic induced similar results that included an increase in energy expenditure without altering food intake, weight loss, and improvement in glycemic/lipid levels at both temperatures or in both UCP-1-KO and WT mice. These results suggest that WAT browning and UCP-1 are not required in the pharmacological effects of FGF21 treatment on metabolic regulation [71, 72].

6. Effects of FGF19 and FGF21 on metabolic diseases

Metabolic disease pertains to a group of diseases that are caused by metabolic disorders involving carbohydrates, lipids, proteins, and nucleic acids such as obesity, diabetes, hyperlipidemia, gout, and osteoporosis. The prevalence of obesity and diabetes continue to increase around the world, resulting in higher incidence and mortality rates. An epidemiological investigation has shown that more than 600 million people from around the world will be obese in 2013 [73]. The study also confirmed that China has the second largest obese population in the world. Compared with obesity, the development of diabetes is more severe in China. It has been reported that approximately 11.6% of the Chinese population are diabetic, whereas nearly 50% of the population are prediabetic [74]. Furthermore, about 80% of all diabetic patients die from cardiovascular events [75]. Each diabetic patient has as much as a 40% lifetime risk of developing diabetic kidney disease, and it is the single most common cause of end-stage renal disease and diabetic nephropathy. Therefore, finding an ideal preventative measure against metabolic disorders without subsequently generating severe complications is warranted [76].

7. FGF19 and FGF21 in obesity

The evidence described above suggests that FGF19 and FGF21 play important roles in regulating glucose and lipid metabolism. Therefore, extensive research studies have been conducted on the relationship between FGF19/21 and metabolic diseases, especially obesity. A clinical study indicated that plasma FGF19 levels significantly decrease in obese patients compared with healthy control subjects [77]. Similarly, serum FGF19 levels are also lower in obese adolescents with NAFLD compared with healthy control subjects, and are inversely correlated with the probability of nonalcoholic steatohepatitis and fibrosis in children with NAFLD [78]. However, Schreuder et al. showed that insulin resistance did not influence the expression of intestinal FGF19 production in NAFLD patients, although the negative regulatory effects of FGF19 on bile acid synthesis were impaired in NAFLD patients with insulin resistance [79].

The negative correlation between FGF19 and obesity was further confirmed in experimental studies involving animal models. Administration of human recombinant FGF19 to HFD-induced obese mice induced a significant dose-dependent decrease in body mass and blood glucose levels, which were associated with a decrease in the concentrations of TG, as well as increased fatty acid oxidation, brown tissue mass, and insulin sensitivity [45]. FGF15-KO mice exhibited the glucose intolerance and impaired capability of hepatic glycogen storage compared with WT mice [80].

In contrast to FGF19, FGF21 stimulates lipolysis. Obese diabetic db/db mice and obese persons have elevated, rather than reduced, serum FGF21 levels. Similarly, elevated serum FGF21 levels were also observed in NAFLD patients and were positively correlated with intrahepatic TG levels [81]. HFD-induced obese mice also have increased serum FGF21 levels and are insensitive to exogenous FGF21 due to the down-regulation of FGFR1 and β-Klotho, suggesting that obesity is an FGF21-resistant state [82]. However, FGF21 resistance can be reversed by weight loss and lowering blood glucose therapy [83]. Although endogenous FGF21 elevation had no beneficial impact on obesity, administration of exogenous FGF21 resulted in resistance to diet-induced obesity, which was indicative of the potential use of FGF21 as an antiobesity molecule. A similar effect was also observed in FGF21 transgenic mice. The above findings implied that the elevated levels of endogenous FGF21 induced by obesity is still relatively insufficient to induce an antiobesity effect.

8. FGF19 and FGF21 in diabetes

Unlike the defined findings in animal studies, alteration in FGF19 levels in diabetic patients is controversial. Brufau et al. reported similar plasma FGF19 levels between diabetic patients and normal subjects [84]. However, other studies observed reduced plasma FGF19 levels in patients with type 2 diabetes [41]. Similarly, FGF19 levels were also significantly lower in patients with gestational diabetes compared with healthy pregnant females [85]. In addition, plasma FGF19 levels were negatively associated with body mass index, TG/high density lipo-protein-cholesterol (HDL-c), high sensitive-C-reactive protein (CRP), and Hemoglobin A1c in diabetic patients [86]. A functional study demonstrated the antidiabetic effect of exogenous human FGF19 in the *ob/ob* mice, which was characterized by a reduction in hepatic gluconeogenesis and an improvement in glucose utility [50]. A similar antidiabetic effect was also observed in FGF15 transgenic mice [3].

Plasma FGF21 levels are significantly higher in type 2 diabetic patients and are positively correlated with hypertension, hyperglycemia, Hemoglobin A1c insulin resistance, and high sensitive-CRP levels [87]. The above phenomena suggest that FGF21 might be a potential marker for the diagnosis of type 2 diabetes. In a large prospective study involving Chinese subjects, increased plasma FGF21 levels were positively correlated to worsening hyperglycemia and dyslipidemia in prediabetic subjects displaying a normal phenotype [88]. In contrast, serum FGF21 levels were significantly lower in type 1 diabetic and latent autoimmune diabetes in adult patients compared with age- and sex-matched healthy subjects [89]. The lowering effect of circulating FGF21 in type 1 diabetic and latent autoimmune diabetes in adult patients was probably due to the lack of insulin, which acted as an inducer of hepatic FGF21 [90]. Therefore, circulating FGF21 can be regarded as a biomarker not only for subtyping diabetes, but also for predicting the risk of diabetes. A functional study indicated that the administration of exogenous FGF21 to diabetic mice resulted in the amelioration of hyperglycemia and hyperlipidemia, improvement of insulin sensitivity, reduction of body mass, and increase in fat use and energy expenditure [19]. Because reduced plasma FGF19 levels contribute to gestational diabetes mellitus (GDM), significant attention has been paid toward determining the role of FGF21 in these findings. Stein *et al.* reported similar plasma FGF21 levels between GDM patients and healthy pregnant females, but were positively correlated with markers for insulin resistance and dyslipidemia, including TGs, leptin, adiponectin, and HDL [91]. Therefore, the above studies suggest that reduced serum FGF19 levels might play a role in the pathophysiology of GDM, whereas increased serum FGF21 levels might be a compensatory response to this disease. To date, several studies have focused on the relationship between FGF21 and type 2 diabetes.

9. FGF19 and FGF21 in cardiovascular diseases

A recent study involving a Chinese population observed reduced plasma FGF19 levels in patients with coronary artery disease (CAD), which were negatively associated with biomarkers that determine the severity of CAD [92]. An animal study revealed that fgf15-mutant mice exhibited a disorder in the cardiac outflow tract that was likely caused by the aberrant behavior of cardiac neural crest cells [93]. However, studies that have assessed the relationship between FGF19 and cardiovascular disease are limited; therefore, the usefulness of FGF19 as a potential marker for the diagnosis of cardiovascular diseases remains uncertain. Unlike FGF19, patients with CAD exhibit significantly higher plasma FGF21 levels, which were positively associated with serum total cholesterol, TG, and HDL levels [94, 95]. Another study revealed that serum FGF21 levels were higher in patients with carotid atherosclerosis, and were positively correlated with risk factors such as adverse lipid profiles and CRP [96]. An *in vitro* study demonstrated that FGF21 was up-regulated in oxidized LDL-treated cardiac endothelial cells, which was induced by bezafibrate and resulted in the inhibition of oxidized LDL-induced apoptosis in cardiac endothelial cells [97]. In addition, our previous study showed that FGF21 prevents palmitate (a lipotoxic agent)-induced apoptosis in both H9C2 and primary cardiomyocytes *via* ERK1/2-mediated P38 mitogen-activated protein kinase- AMPK signaling, which also mediates the cardiac protection of FGF21 against diabetes-induce cardiac cell death at the early stage and cardiac dysfunction and fibrosis at the late stage [98]. Our research group has also recently revealed that FGF21 deletion-aggravated cardiac lipid accumulation is likely mediated by cardiac nuclear factor erythroid 2 p45 related factor 2-driven CD36 up-regulation, which may contribute to the increase in cardiac oxidative stress and remodeling, and eventual development of diabetic cardiomyopathy [99]. We also showed that FGF21 protected H9c2 cells from ischemia/reperfusion injury *via* an protein kinase B/GS kinase-3β/caspase-3-dependent pathway, as well as prevented oxidative stress and recovered energy supplies [100]. In an *ex vivo* Langendorff system, Patel *et al* showed that FGF21 imparted a cardioprotective effect and restored cardiac function *via* autocrine/paracrine pathways; however, the protective effects were reduced in obese mice [101]. In addition, FGF21-KO mice were more sensitive to isoproterenol-induced cardiac hypertrophy than WT mice, as characterized by an increased heart weight, ventricular dilation, and cardiac dysfunction. These pathological changes were reversed by the administration of recombinant FGF21. We recently revealed that FGF21 provided beneficial effects on the hearts of type 1 diabetic mice. We found that FGF21 prevented type 1 diabetes-induced cardiac cell apoptosis mainly by up-regulating AMPK-mediated pathways [98].

10. FGF19/21 and renal diseases

Stein and Reiche *et al* reported that the serum FGF19 and FGF21 levels were 1.5- and 15-fold higher, respectively, in pa-tients receiving chronic hemodialysis compared with healthy subjects [102,103]. In addition, circulating FGF19 levels were negatively correlated with circulating adiponectin and CRP in patients with chronic hemodialysis [103]. Circulating FGF19 levels are potential predictors of end-stage renal disease [103]. Impaired FGF19 response in mice after feeding was also observed in oxidative stress-associated late-stage chronic kidney disease [104]. The study also confirmed that the abnormal plasma FGF19 levels were corrected by antioxidative therapy [104]. Conversely, recent studies have revealed that serum FGF21 levels were higher in the patients with both chronic and acute renal dysfunction [105]. In addition, Lin *et al* demonstrated that serum FGF21 levels gradually increased with the development of renal disease from the early to late stage [106]. An animal study indicated that FGF21 prevented diabetic nephropathy by improving systematic alterations, including insulin resistance, hyperglycemia, and dyslipidemia, and it had antifibrotic effects [55]. Our previous study also confirmed that FGF21 exhibited beneficial effects on the kidneys of type 1 diabetic mice by preventing oxidative stress, inflammation, apoptosis, and fibrosis [76].

11. Summary

FGF15/19 and FGF21 are key members of the FGF19 subfamily. The expression of both FGF19 and FGF21 is induced by multiple stimuli such as chemical stress, nutritional stress, mitochondrial stress, PPAR activators, oxidative, and ER stress. Due to the absence of a heparin-binding domain, both FGF19 and FGF21 are secreted into the bloodstream and function as endocrine factors that regulate glucose/lipid metabolism and energy homeostasis in multiple target organs, including the liver, heart, skeletal muscle, testis, kidney, blood vessel, and pancreas. A recent study demonstrated that besides its direct action on the target organs, FGF21 can also indirectly induce beneficial or therapeutic effects on target organs by fine-tuning the cross talk among multiple organs. FGF19 acts as a fed-state hormone, whereas FGF21 acts as a fasted-state hormone. Both animal and clinical studies revealed reduced and increased serum FGF19 and FGF21 levels, respectively, in patients with metabolic diseases, including metabolic syndrome, obesity, or type 2 diabetes. The above evidence suggests that FGF19 and FGF21 complement each other and synergistically maintain carbohydrate and lipid metabolism and homeostasis.

Based on the regulatory effects of FGF19 and FGF21, a number of studies have assessed its potential therapeutic value in the treatment of metabolic diseases, which demonstrated that both FGF19 and FGF21 can induce preventive effects on obesity and diabetes, as well as diabetes-induced macrovascular and microvascular complications, specifically the cardiovascular complications and renal complication. However, several bottlenecks have to be resolved before these molecules could be applied to the clinics. One major concern regarding the potential use of FGF19 is its mitogenic function, which may increase the risk of tumorigenesis [18]. Therefore, additional investigations that explore a modified FGF19 to reduce or eradicate its mitogenic ability or analogues that only mimic FGF19-induced metabolic regulatory effect are warranted. Native FGF21 also possesses a few shortcomings, including poor stability and short half-life *in vivo*. To overcome these issues, an analog of FGF21, LY2405319, was designed to induce glucose-, bodyweight-, and lipid-lowering effects that are indistinguishable from native FGF21 [107]. This peptide is suitable for larger-scale production and also for oral administration. For instance, a pharmaceutic agency, Amgen, has developed a modified FGF21 molecules, named fragment crystallizable-FGF21 and polyethylene glycol-modified FGF21, both which can prolong the half-life of FGF21 to 12-30 hours [108, 109]. Alternative analogs such as CVX-343 (Pfizer), mimAb1 (Amgen), and C3201-HAS (Amgen) were also developed as β-Klotho activators [109 -111]. These promising analogs or mimetics will eventually be administered to patients with metabolic syndromes such as obesity, diabetes, and even diabetic complications.

References

[1] Itoh N, Ohta H. Pathophysiological roles of FGF signaling in the heart [J]. Frontiers In Physiology, 2013, 4.

[2] Beenken A, Mohammadi M. The FGF family: biology, pathophysiology and therapy [J]. Nature Reviews Drug Discovery, 2009, 8(3): 235-253.

[3] Potthoff MJ, Kliewer SA, Mangelsdorf DJ. Endocrine fibroblast growth factors 15/19 and 21: from feast to famine [J]. Genes & Development, 2012, 26(4): 312-324.

[4] Kurosu H, Kuro-o M. Endocrine fibroblast growth factors as regulators of metabolic homeostasis [J]. Biofactors, 2009, 35(1): 52-60.

[5] Fukumoto S. Actions and mode of actions of FGF19 subfamily members [J]. Endocrine Journal, 2008, 55(1): 23-31.

[6] Goetz R, Beenken A, Ibrahimi OA, et al. Molecular insights into the klotho-dependent, endocrine mode of action of fibroblast growth factor 19 subfamily members [J]. Molecular And Cellular Biology, 2007, 27(9): 3417-3428.

[7] Kurosu H, Choi M, Ogawa Y, et al. Tissue-specific expression of beta Klotho and fibroblast growth factor (FGF) receptor Isoforms determines metabolic activity of FGF19 and FGF21 [J]. Journal Of Biological Chemistry, 2007, 282(37): 26687-26695.

[8] Kharitonenkov A, Dunbar JD, Bina HA, et al. FGF-21/FGF-21 receptor interaction and activation is determined by beta Klotho [J]. Journal Of Cellular Physiology, 2008, 215(1): 1-7.

[9] Urakawa I, Yamazaki Y, Shimada T, et al. Klotho converts canonical FGF receptor into a specific receptor for FGF23 [J]. Nature, 2006, 444(7120): 770-774.

[10] Cicione C, Degirolamo C, Moschetta A. Emerging role of fibroblast growth factors 15/19 and 21 as metabolic integrators in the liver [J]. Hepatology, 2012, 56(6): 2404-2411.

[11] Nishimura T, Utsunomiya Y, Hoshikawa M, et al. Structure and expression of a novel human FGF, FGF-19, expressed in the fetal brain [J]. Biochimica Et Biophysica Acta-Gene Structure And Expression, 1999, 1444(1): 148-151.

[12] McWhirter JR, Goulding M, Weiner JA, et al. A novel fibroblast growth factor gene expressed in the developing nervous system is a downstream target of the chimeric homeodomain oncoprotein E2A-Pbx1 [J]. Development, 1997, 124(17): 3221-3232.

[13] Gimeno L, Brulet P, Martinez S. Study of Fgf15 gene expression in developing mouse brain [J]. Gene Expression Patterns, 2003, 3(4): 473-481.

[14] Kir S, Kliewer SA, Mangelsdorf DJ. Roles of FGF19 in liver metabolism [J]. Cold Spring Harbor symposia on quantitative biology, 2011, 76: 139-144.

[15] Chiang JYL. Bile acids: regulation of synthesis [J]. Journal Of Lipid Research, 2009, 50(10): 1955-1966.

[16] Pandak WM, Heuman DM, Hylemon PB, et al. Failure of intravenous-infusion of taurocholate to down-regulate cholesterol 7-alpha-hydroxylase in rats with biliary fistulas [J]. Gastroenterology, 1995, 108(2): 533-544.

[17] Jing Z, Ting LH, Chen FQ, et al. Role of fibroblast growth factor 19 in maintaining nutrient homeostasis and disease [J]. Biomedical And Environmental Sciences, 2014, 27(5): 319-324.

[18] Nicholes K, Guillet S, Tomlinson E, et al. A mouse model of hepatocellular carcinoma - Ectopic expression of fibroblast growth factor 19 in skeletal muscle of transgenic mice [J]. American Journal Of Pathology, 2002, 160(6): 2295-2307.

[19] Nishimura T, Nakatake Y, Konishi M, et al. Identification of a novel FGF, FGF-21, preferentially expressed in the liver [J]. Biochimica Et Biophysica Acta-Gene Structure And Expression, 2000, 1492(1): 203-206.

[20] Kharitonenkov A, Shanafelt AB. FGF21: A novel prospect for the treatment of metabolic diseases [J]. Current Opinion In Investigational Drugs, 2009, 10(4): 359-364.

[21] Tacer KF, Bookout AL, Ding X, et al. Research Resource: Comprehensive expression atlas of the fibroblast growth factor system in adult mouse [J]. Molecular Endocrinology, 2010, 24(10): 2050-2064.

[22] Kharitonenkov A, Shiyanova TL, Koester A, et al. FGF-21 as a novel metabolic regulator [J]. Journal Of Clinical Investigation, 2005, 115(6): 1627-1635.

[23] Kharitonenkov A, Wroblewski VJ, Koester A, et al. The metabolic state of diabetic monkeys is regulated by fibroblast growth factor-21 [J]. Endocrinology, 2007, 148(2): 774-781.

[24] Badman MK, Pissios P, Kennedy AR, et al. Hepatic fibroblast growth factor 21 is regulated by PPAR alpha and is a key mediator of hepatic lipid metabolism in ketotic states [J]. Cell Metabolism, 2007, 5(6): 426-437.

[25] Inagaki T, Dutchak P, Zhao G, et al. Endocrine regulation of the fasting response by PPAR alpha-mediated induction of fibroblast growth factor 21 [J]. Cell Metabolism, 2007, 5(6): 415-425.

[26] Dutchak PA, Katafuchi T, Bookout AL, et al. Fibroblast Growth Factor-21 Regulates PPAR gamma Activity and the Antidiabetic Actions of Thiazolidinediones [J]. Cell, 2012, 148(3): 556-567.

[27] Moyers JS, Shiyanova TL, Mehrbod F, et al. Molecular determinants of FGF-21 activity-synergy and cross-talk with PPAR gamma signaling [J]. Journal Of Cellular Physiology, 2007, 210(1): 1-6.

[28] Bae K-H, Kim J-G, Park K-G. Transcriptional Regulation of Fibroblast Growth Factor 21 Expression [J]. Endocrinology And Metabolism, 2014, 29(2): 105-111.

[29] Potthoff MJ, Inagaki T, Satapati S, et al. FGF21 induces PGC-1 alpha and regulates carbohydrate and fatty acid metabolism during the adaptive starvation response [J]. Proceedings Of the National Academy Of Sciences Of the United States Of America, 2009, 106(26): 10853-10858.

[30] Chau MDL, Gao J, Yang Q, et al. Fibroblast growth factor 21 regulates energy metabolism by activating the AMPK-SIRT1-PGC-1 alpha pathway [J]. Proceedings Of the National Academy Of Sciences Of the United States Of America, 2010, 107(28): 12553-12558.

[31] Ye D, Wang Y, Li H, et al. Fibroblast growth factor 21 protects against acetaminophen-induced hepatotoxicity by potentiating peroxisome proliferator-activated receptor coactivator protein-1 alpha-mediated antioxidant capacity in mice [J]. Hepatology, 2014, 60(3): 977-989.

[32] Cheng X, Vispute SG, Liu J, et al. Fibroblast growth factor (Fgf) 21 is a novel target gene of the aryl hydrocarbon receptor (AhR) [J]. Toxicology And Applied Pharmacology, 2014, 278(1): 65-71.

[33] Johnson CL, Weston JY, Chadi SA, et al. Fibroblast Growth Factor 21 Reduces the Severity of Cerulein-Induced Pancreatitis in Mice [J]. Gastroenterology, 2009, 137(5): 1795-1804.

[34] Schaap FG, Kremer AE, Lamers WH, et al. Fibroblast growth factor 21 is induced by endoplasmic reticulum stress [J]. Biochimie, 2013, 95(4): 692-699.

[35] Jiang X, Zhang C, Xin Y, et al. Protective effect of FGF21 on type 1 diabetes-induced testicular apoptotic cell death probably via both mitochondrial- and endoplasmic reticulum stress-dependent pathways in the mouse model [J]. Toxicology Letters, 2013, 219(1): 65-76.

[36] Ji K, Zheng J, Lv J, et al. Skeletal muscle increases FGF21 expression in mitochondrial disorders to compensate for energy metabolic insufficiency by activating the mTOR-YY1-PGC1 alpha pathway

[J]. Free Radical Biology And Medicine, 2015, 84: 161-170.

[37] Ribas F, Villarroya J, Hondares E, *et al.* FGF21 expression and release in muscle cells: involvement of MyoD and regulation by mitochondria-driven signalling [J]. Biochemical Journal, 2014, 463: 191-199.

[38] Yu Y, Bai F, Liu Y, *et al.* Fibroblast growth factor (FGF21) protects mouse liver against D-galactose-induced oxidative stress and apoptosis *via* activating Nrf2 and PI3K/Akt pathways [J]. Molecular And Cellular Biochemistry, 2015, 403(1-2): 287-299.

[39] Planavila A, Redondo-Angulo I, Ribas F, *et al.* Fibroblast growth factor 21 protects the heart from oxidative stress [J]. Cardiovascular Research, 2015, 106(1): 19-31.

[40] Potthoff MJ, Boney-Montoya J, Choi M, *et al.* FGF15/19 regulates hepatic glucose metabolism by inhibiting the CREB-PGC-1 alpha pathway [J]. Cell Metabolism, 2011, 13(6): 729-738.

[41] Schaap FG. Role of fibroblast growth factor 19 in the control of glucose homeostasis [J]. Current Opinion In Clinical Nutrition And Metabolic Care, 2012, 15(4): 386-391.

[42] Li H, Zhang J, Jia W. Fibroblast growth factor 21: a novel metabolic regulator from pharmacology to physiology [J]. Frontiers Of Medicine, 2013, 7(1): 25-30.

[43] Kliewer SA, Mangelsdorf DJ. Fibroblast growth factor 21: from pharmacology to physiology [J]. American Journal Of Clinical Nutrition, 2010, 91(1): 254S-257S.

[44] Tomlinson E, Fu L, John L, *et al.* Transgenic mice expressing human fibroblast growth factor-19 display increased metabolic rate and decreased adiposity [J]. Endocrinology, 2002, 143(5): 1741-1747.

[45] Fu L, John LM, Adams SH, *et al.* Fibroblast growth factor 19 increases metabolic rate I and reverses dietary and leptlin-deficient diabetes [J]. Endocrinology, 2004, 145(6): 2594-2603.

[46] Huang X, Yang C, Luo Y, *et al.* FGFR4 prevents hyperlipidemia and insulin resistance but underlies high-fat diet-induced fatty liver [J]. Diabetes, 2007, 56(10): 2501-2510.

[47] Kir S, Beddow SA, Samuel VT, *et al.* FGF19 as a Postprandial, Insulin-Independent Activator of Hepatic Protein and Glycogen Synthesis [J]. Science, 2011, 331(6024): 1621-1624.

[48] Wu X, Ge H, Lemon B, *et al.* Selective activation of FGFR4 by an FGF19 variant does not improve glucose metabolism in ob/ob mice [J]. Proceedings Of the National Academy Of Sciences Of the United States Of America, 2009, 106(34): 14379-14384.

[49] Ryan KK, Kohli R, Gutierrez-Aguilar R, *et al.* Fibroblast growth factor-19 action in the brain reduces food intake and body weight and improves glucose tolerance in male rats [J]. Endocrinology, 2013, 154(1): 9-15.

[50] Morton GJ, Matsen ME, Bracy DP, *et al.* FGF19 action in the brain induces insulin-independent glucose lowering [J]. Journal Of Clinical Investigation, 2013, 123(11): 4799-4808.

[51] Li K, Li L, Yang M, *et al.* The effects of fibroblast growth factor-21 knockdown and over-expression on its signaling pathway and glucose-lipid metabolism *in vitro* [J]. Molecular And Cellular Endocrinology, 2012, 348(1): 21-26.

[52] Wente W, Efanov AM, Brenner M, *et al.* Fibroblast growth factor-21 improves pancreatic beta-cell function and survival by activation of extracellular signal-regulated kinase 1/2 and Akt signaling pathways [J]. Diabetes, 2006, 55(9): 2470-2478.

[53] Kharitonenkov A, Shanafelt AB. Fibroblast growth factor-21 as a therapeutic agent for metabolic diseases [J]. Biodrugs, 2008, 22(1): 37-44.

[54] Lee MS, Choi S-E, Ha ES, *et al.* Fibroblast growth factor-21 protects human skeletal muscle myotubes from palmitate-induced insulin resistance by inhibiting stress kinase and NF-kappa B [J]. Metabolism-Clinical And Experimental, 2012, 61(8): 1142-1151.

[55] Kim HW, Lee JE, Cha JJ, *et al.* Fibroblast growth factor 21 improves insulin resistance and ameliorates renal injury in db/db mice [J]. Endocrinology, 2013, 154(9): 3366-3376.

[56] Lin Z, Tian H, Lam KSL, *et al.* Adiponectin mediates the metabolic

effects of FGF21 on glucose homeostasis and insulin sensitivity in mice [J]. Cell Metabolism, 2013, 17(5): 779-789.

[57] Holland WL, Adams AC, Brozinick JT, *et al.* An FGF21-adiponectin-ceramide axis controls energy expenditure and insulin action in mice [J]. Cell Metabolism, 2013, 17(5): 790-797.

[58] Liang Q, Zhong L, Zhang J, *et al.* FGF21 Maintains glucose homeostasis by mediating the cross talk between liver and brain during prolonged fasting [J]. Diabetes, 2014, 63(12): 4064-4075.

[59] Lin Z, Pan X, Wu F, *et al.* Fibroblast growth factor 21 prevents atherosclerosis by suppression of hepatic sterol regulatory element-binding protein-2 and induction of adiponectin in mice [J]. Circulation, 2015, 131(21): 1861-1871.

[60] Hotta Y, Nakamura H, Konishi M, *et al.* Fibroblast growth factor 21 regulates lipolysis in white adipose tissue but is not required for ketogenesis and triglyceride clearance in liver [J]. Endocrinology, 2009, 150(10): 4625-4633.

[61] Miyata M, Sakaida Y, Matsuzawa H, *et al.* Fibroblast growth factor 19 treatment ameliorates disruption of hepatic lipid metabolism in farnesoid X receptor (Fxr)-Null Mice [J]. Biological & Pharmaceutical Bulletin, 2011, 34(12): 1885-1889.

[62] Bhatnagar S, Damron HA, Hillgartner FB. Fibroblast growth factor-19, a novel factor that inhibits hepatic fatty acid synthesis [J]. Journal Of Biological Chemistry, 2009, 284(15): 10023-10033.

[63] Wu X, Ge H, Baribault H, *et al.* Dual actions of fibroblast growth factor 19 on lipid metabolism [J]. Journal Of Lipid Research, 2013, 54(2): 325-332.

[64] Mai K, Andres J, Biedasek K, *et al.* Free fatty acids link metabolism and regulation of the insulin-sensitizing fibroblast growth factor-21 [J]. Diabetes, 2009, 58(7): 1532-1538.

[65] Yilmaz Y, Eren F, Yonal O, *et al.* Increased serum FGF21 levels in patients with nonalcoholic fatty liver disease [J]. European Journal Of Clinical Investigation, 2010, 40(10): 887-892.

[66] Zhang X, Yeung DCY, Karpisek M, *et al.* Serum FGF21 levels are increased in obesity and are independently associated with the metabolic syndrome in humans [J]. Diabetes, 2008, 57(5): 1246-1253.

[67] Cuevas-Ramos D, Almeda-Valdes P, Aguilar-Salinas CA, *et al.* The role of fibroblast growth factor 21 (FGF21) on energy balance, glucose and lipid metabolism [J]. Current Diabetes Reviews, 2009, 5(4): 216-220.

[68] Chechi K, Carpentier AC, Richard D. Understanding the brown adipocyte as a contributor to energy homeostasis [J]. Trends In Endocrinology And Metabolism, 2013, 24(8): 408-420.

[69] Nguyen AD, Lee NJ, Wee NK, *et al.* Uncoupling protein-1 is protective of bone mass under mild cold stress conditions [J]. Bone, 2018, 106: 167-178.

[70] Fisher FM, Kleiner S, Douris N, *et al.* FGF21 regulates PGC-1 alpha and browning of white adipose tissues in adaptive thermogenesis [J]. Genes & Development, 2012, 26(3): 271-281.

[71] Samms RJ, Smith DP, Cheng CC, *et al.* Discrete aspects of FGF21 *in vivo* pharmacology do not require UCP1 [J]. Cell Reports, 2015, 11(7): 991-999.

[72] Veniant MM, Sivits G, Helmering J, *et al.* Pharmacologic Effects of FGF21 are independent of the "browning" of white adipose tissue [J]. Cell Metabolism, 2015, 21(5): 731-738.

[73] Ng M, Fleming T, Robinson M, *et al.* Global, regional, and national prevalence of overweight and obesity in children and adults during 1980-2013: a systematic analysis for the Global Burden of Disease Study 2013 [J]. Lancet, 2014, 384(9945): 766-781.

[74] Xu Y, Wang L, He J, *et al.* Prevalence and control of diabetes in chinese adults [J]. Jama-Journal Of the American Medical Association, 2013, 310(9): 948-958.

[75] Coccheri S. Approaches to prevention of cardiovascular complications and events in diabetes mellitus [J]. Drugs, 2007, 67(7): 997-1026.

[76] Zhang C, Shao M, Yang H, *et al.* Attenuation of hyperlipidemia-

and diabetes-induced early-stage apoptosis and late-stage renal dysfunction *via* administration of fibroblast growth factor-21 is associated with suppression of renal inflammation [J]. Plos One, 2013, 8(12).

[77] Gallego-Escuredo JM, Gomez-Ambrosi J, Catalan V, *et al.* Opposite alterations in FGF21 and FGF19 levels and disturbed expression of the receptor machinery for endocrine FGFs in obese patients [J]. International Journal Of Obesity, 2015, 39(1): 121-129.

[78] Wojcik M, Janus D, Dolezal-Oltarzewska K, *et al.* A decrease in fasting FGF19 levels is associated with the development of nonalcoholic fatty liver disease in obese adolescents [J]. Journal Of Pediatric Endocrinology & Metabolism, 2012, 25(11-12): 1089-1093.

[79] Schreuder TCMA, Marsman HA, Lenicek M, *et al.* The hepatic response to FGF19 is impaired in patients with nonalcoholic fatty liver disease and insulin resistance [J]. American Journal Of Physiology-Gastrointestinal And Liver Physiology, 2010, 298(3): G440-G445.

[80] Marcelin G, Jo Y-H, Li X, *et al.* Central action of FGF19 reduces hypothalamic AGRP/NPY neuron activity and improves glucose metabolism [J]. Molecular Metabolism, 2014, 3(1): 19-28.

[81] Li H, Fang Q, Gao F, *et al.* Fibroblast growth factor 21 levels are increased in nonalcoholic fatty liver disease patients and are correlated with hepatic triglyceride [J]. Journal Of Hepatology, 2010, 53(5): 934-940.

[82] Diaz-Delfin J, Hondares E, Iglesias R, *et al.* TNF-alpha represses beta-klotho expression and impairs FGF21 action in adipose cells: involvement of JNK1 in the FGF21 pathway [J]. Endocrinology, 2012, 153(9): 4238-4245.

[83] Reinehr T, Woelfle J, Wunsch R, *et al.* Fibroblast growth factor 21 (FGF-21) and its relation to obesity, metabolic syndrome, and nonalcoholic fatty liver in children: a longitudinal analysis [J]. Journal Of Clinical Endocrinology & Metabolism, 2012, 97(6): 2143-2150.

[84] Brufau G, Stellaard F, Prado K, *et al.* Improved glycemic control with colesevelam treatment in patients with type 2 diabetes is not directly associated with changes in bile acid metabolism [J]. Hepatology, 2010, 52(4): 1455-1464.

[85] Wang D, Zhu W, Li J, *et al.* Serum Concentrations of Fibroblast growth factors 19 and 21 in women with gestational diabetes mellitus: association with insulin resistance, adiponectin, and polycystic ovary syndrome history [J]. Plos One, 2013, 8(11): e81190.

[86] Barutcuoglu B, Basol G, Cakir Y, *et al.* Fibroblast growth factor-19 levels in type 2 diabetic patients with metabolic syndrome [J]. Annals Of Clinical And Laboratory Science, 2011, 41(4): 390-396.

[87] Eto K, Tumenbayar B, Nagashima S-i, *et al.* Distinct association of serum FGF21 or adiponectin levels with clinical parameters in patients with type 2 diabetes [J]. Diabetes Research And Clinical Practice, 2010, 89(1): 52-57.

[88] Chen C, Cheung BMY, Tso AWK, *et al.* High plasma level of fibroblast growth factor 21 is an independent predictor of type 2 diabetes a 5.4-year population-based prospective study in Chinese subjects [J]. Diabetes Care, 2011, 34(9): 2113-2115.

[89] Xiao Y, Xu A, Law LSC, *et al.* Distinct changes in serum fibroblast growth factor 21 levels in different subtypes of diabetes [J]. Journal Of Clinical Endocrinology & Metabolism, 2012, 97(1): E54-E58.

[90] Vienberg SG, Brons C, Nilsson E, *et al.* Impact of short-term high-fat feeding and insulin-stimulated FGF21 levels in subjects with low birth weight and controls [J]. European Journal Of Endocrinology, 2012, 167(1): 49-57.

[91] Stein S, Stepan H, Kratzsch J, *et al.* Serum fibroblast growth factor 21 levels in gestational diabetes mellitus in relation to insulin resistance and dyslipidemia [J]. Metabolism-Clinical And Experimental, 2010, 59(1): 33-37.

[92] Hao Y, Zhou J, Zhou M, *et al.* Serum levels of fibroblast growth factor 19 are inversely associated with coronary artery disease in chinese individuals [J]. Plos One, 2013, 8(8): e72345.

[93] Saitsu H, Shiota K, Ishibashi M. Analysis of fibroblast growth fac-tor 15 cis-elements reveals two conserved enhancers which are closely related to cardiac outflow tract development [J]. Mechanisms Of Development, 2006, 123(9): 665-673.

[94] Shen Y, Ma X, Zhou J, *et al.* Additive relationship between serum fibroblast growth factor 21 level and coronary artery disease [J]. Cardiovascular Diabetology, 2013, 12.

[95] Lin Z, Wu Z, Yin X, *et al.* Serum levels of fgf-21 are increased in coronary heart disease patients and are independently associated with adverse lipid profile [J]. Plos One, 2010, 5(12).

[96] Chow WS, Xu A, Woo YC, *et al.* Serum fibroblast growth factor-21 levels are associated with carotid atherosclerosis independent of established cardiovascular risk factors [J]. Arteriosclerosis Thrombosis And Vascular Biology, 2013, 33(10): 2454-2459.

[97] Lu Y, Liu J-h, Zhang L-k, *et al.* Fibroblast growth factor 21 as a possible endogenous factor inhibits apoptosis in cardiac endothelial cells [J]. Chinese Medical Journal, 2010, 123(23): 3417-3421.

[98] Zhang C, Huang Z, Gu J, *et al.* Fibroblast growth factor 21 protects the heart from apoptosis in a diabetic mouse model *via* extracellular signal-regulated kinase 1/2-dependent signalling pathway [J]. Diabetologia, 2015, 58(8): 1937-1948.

[99] Yan X, Chen J, Zhang C, *et al.* FGF21 deletion exacerbates diabetic cardiomyopathy by aggravating cardiac lipid accumulation [J]. Journal Of Cellular And Molecular Medicine, 2015, 19(7): 1557-1568.

[100] Cong W-T, Ling J, Tian H-S, *et al.* Proteomic study on the protective mechanism of fibroblast growth factor 21 to ischemia-reperfusion injury [J]. Canadian Journal Of Physiology And Pharmacology, 2013, 91(11): 973-984.

[101] Patel V, Adya R, Chen J, *et al.* Novel insights into the cardioprotective effects of FGF21 in lean and obese rat hearts [J]. Plos One, 2014, 9(2).

[102] Stein S, Bachmann A, Loessner U, *et al.* Serum levels of the adipokine FGF21 depend on renal function [J]. Diabetes Care, 2009, 32(1): 126-128.

[103] Reiche M, Bachmann A, Loessner U, *et al.* Fibroblast growth factor 19 serum levels: relation to renal function and metabolic parameters [J]. Hormone And Metabolic Research, 2010, 42(3): 178-181.

[104] Li M, Qureshi AR, Ellis E, *et al.* Impaired postprandial fibroblast growth factor (FGF)-19 response in patients with stage 5 chronic kidney diseases is ameliorated following antioxidative therapy [J]. Nephrology Dialysis Transplantation, 2013, 28: 212-219.

[105] Hindricks J, Ebert T, Bachmann A, *et al.* Serum levels of fibroblast growth factor-21 are increased in chronic and acute renal dysfunction [J]. Clinical Endocrinology, 2014, 80(6): 918-924.

[106] Lin Z, Zhou Z, Liu Y, *et al.* Circulating FGF21 levels are progressively increased from the early to end stages of chronic kidney diseases and are associated with renal function in Chinese [J]. Plos One, 2011, 6(4).

[107] Kharitonenkov A, Beals JM, Micanovic R, *et al.* Rational design of a fibroblast growth factor 21-based clinical candidate, LY2405319 [J]. Plos One, 2013, 8(3).

[108] Hecht R, Li Y-S, Sun J, *et al.* Rationale-based engineering of a potent long-acting FGF21 analog for the treatment of type 2 diabetes [J]. Plos One, 2012, 7(11).

[109] Huang J, Ishino T, Chen G, *et al.* Development of a novel long-acting antidiabetic FGF21 mimetic by targeted conjugation to a scaffold antibody [J]. Journal Of Pharmacology And Experimental Therapeutics, 2013, 346(2): 270-280.

[110] Foltz IN, Hu S, King C, *et al.* Treating diabetes and obesity with an FGF21-mimetic antibody activating the beta klotho/FGFR1c receptor complex [J]. Science Translational Medicine, 2012, 4(162).

[111] Smith R, Duguay A, Bakker A, *et al.* FGF21 can be mimicked *in vitro* and *in vivo* by a novel anti-FGFR1c/beta-klotho bispecific protein [J]. Plos One, 2013, 8(4).

Physiological and pharmacological roles of FGF21 in cardiovascular diseases

Peng Cheng, Xiaokun Li, Chi Zhang

1. Introduction

Cardiovascular diseases (CVDs) are the leading cause of death worldwide composed of heart and blood vessel diseases. In the recent years, the incidence of CVDs has been increasing at a sharp rate globally. According to the World Health Report 2010, CVDs contributed to 17.5 million deaths and these numbers are estimated to increase to 23.3 million by 2030 [1, 2].

Fibroblast growth factor (FGF) is a cytokine superfamily with pleiotropic biological functions including regulating cell growth, differentiation, development, and metabolism [3-7]. Human FGFs contain 22 members which can be divided into 7 subfamilies based on phylogeny and sequence [8-10]. Due to the lack of a heparin binding domain, FGF19 subfamily members (FGF19, FGF21, and FGF23) function in an endocrine manner rather than an autocrine manner as other subfamily members of FGFs [9]. Among them, FGF21 is a polypeptide with 209/210 (human/rodent) amino acid residues that is primarily produced and secreted by the liver, adipose tissue, and thymus [11]. FGF21 expression is mainly regulated by peroxisome proliferator-activated receptor α (PPARα) in the liver [12] and PPARγ in adipocytes [13, 14]. FGF21 was firstly cloned in 2000 [11] and received global attention in recent years due to its outstanding ability on regulating carbohydrate and lipid metabolism including improving insulin sensitivity, lowering blood glucose, reducing hepatic/plasma triglycerides, inducing weight loss by increasing energy expenditure, and reducing fat mass [15-18]. Further studies indicated that FGF21 functions by binding to (FGFR)1c and (FGFR)2c in the presence of coreceptor β-klotho and activation of downstream signaling pathway [19, 20]. Although FGF21 and other members of FGFs share the same FGF receptors, the coreceptors are different (β-klotho for FGF21 and heparin for others) which determined that they have different bioactivity due to activation of various pathways [21, 22]. Unlike traditional insulin therapy in clinics, FGF21 did not cause hypoglycemia [16]. The possible explanation is that FGF21 induces physiological role in healthy condition and pharmacological role under unhealthy condition [23, 24]. Additionally, FGF21 does not lead to carcinogenic event due to lack of mitogenic function which makes it possible to be administrated *in vivo* in clinics [16]. Therefore, FGF21 may hold promise as a clinically therapeutic option due to the abovementioned characters and advantages.

In recent clinical and preclinical studies, CVDs have been closely associated with serum FGF21 which increased in the patients with atherosclerosis, coronary heart disease, myocardial ischemia, cardiac hypertrophy, and diabetic cardiomyopathy [25-27]. Therefore FGF21 has the potential to be considered as a biomarker for the above CVDs.

Whether the increased serum FGF21 level is the basis for CVD pathogenesis or is induced to protect the heart from CVDs is still under discussion. However, growing evidence indicated that administration of exogenous FGF21 induces preventive effects on most of the above CVDs, suggesting that FGF21 not only is a simple marker of cardiovascular risk but also induces a protective effect on the cardiovascular system contributing to a reduction in risk (Table 1). In clinics, serum FGF21 levels were increased in patients with obesity or type 2 diabetes which was associated with high risk of CVDs. The paradoxical phenomenon was supposed to be explained by a compensatory response to induce cardiac protection or resistance to FGF21 which impaired its bioactivity [28, 29]. In animal study, we found that at the early-stage of diabetes serum FGF21 level of mice was sharply increased compared with nondiabetic mice (C57BL/6J), while it was dramatically decreased at the late-stage of diabetes which further confirmed that early-stage increase of serum FGF21 was a compensatory response and induced beneficial effect on the heart; late-stage decrease may be the cause of diabetes-induced cardiac damage [30], since the above CVDs are always attributed to lipid metabolic disorder. Mechanistic studies indicated that FGF21-induced cardiac protection in CVDs is possibly attributed to the suppression of lipotoxicity since the above CVDs are always the consequences of lipotoxicity. This review tries to illuminate the underlying relationship between FGF21 and CVDs and the possible mechanisms.

Table 1. Summary of major pharmacological studies of FGF21 in heart disease

Heart disease	Model	Methods	Outcomes	Ref.
Atherosclerosis	Apolipoprotein E(−/−) mice	Recombinant murine FGF21 was given daily intraperitoneally for 16 weeks	Atherosclerotic lesion area collagen composition ↓	
			Total cholesterol ↓	[63]
			Hypertriglyceridemia ↓	
			Circulating adiponectin ↑	
Coronary heart disease		Mouse FGF21 full length protein was given for 24 or 48 hours	Cell apoptosis ↓	
			Oxidative stress ↓	[55]
			NO production ↑	
			eNOS phosphorylation ↑	
Myocardial ischemia	Coronary artery ligation (ischemia/reperfusion)	Recombinant mouse FGF21 was administered intravenously immediately after myocardial injury every 12 h for 3 days	Activity of caspase-3 ↓	
			Degree of myocardial infarction ↓	[59]
			Left ventricular function ↑	
Cardiac hypertrophy	Isoproterenol infusion-induced cardiac hypertrophy/LPS-induced cardiac hypertrophy	FGF21 was injected intraperitoneally for 7 days or given for 24 hours in neonatal cardiomyocytes	Cardiomyocyte size ↓	
			heart weight/body weight ↓	[64, 65]
			Inflammation ↓	
			Cardiac oxidative stress ↓	
Diabetic cardiomyopathy	Multiple low-dose STZ-induced type 1 diabetes	Knockout FGF21 in type 1 diabetic mouse model	Oxidative stress ↑	
			Lipid accumulation ↑	[66]
			Cardiac dysfunction and remodeling ↑	

2. FGF21 and atherosclerosis and coronary heart disease

Atherosclerosis is a chronic, inflammatory disorder characterized by the deposition of excess lipids in the arterial intima [31]. The accrued evidence indicated that lipid-lowering therapy limits the progression of atherosclerosis and reduces CAD events [32]. Since FGF21 plays an important role in the regulation of lipid metabolism, the effect of FGF21 in atherosclerosis is of interest. Clinical studies showed that increased circulating FGF21 levels were discovered in atherosclerotic patients or the individuals with high risk of developing atherosclerosis [33, 34]. Additionally, an *in vivo* study demonstrated that increased serum FGF21 was observed in aortas of apoE$^{-/-}$ mice (C57BL/6J background)[35] Strong evidence identified that administration of exogenous FGF21 significantly improved lipid metabolic disorders and reduced atherosclerotic plaque areas in these animals [36]. Moreover, Lin *et al.* also reported that FGF21 deficiency enhanced atherosclerotic deterioration and mortality in apoE$^{-/-}$ mice (C57BL/6J background) [35], implying that increased serum FGF21 in patients with atherosclerosis described previously induces beneficial effect rather than the basic for atherosclerotic pathogenesis. Mechanistic study indicated that FGF21-induced prevention of atherosclerosis was associated with suppression of endoplasmic reticulum stress-mediated apoptosis in apoE$^{-/-}$ mice (C57BL/6J background) [37]. Further mechanistic studies revealed that prevention of atherosclerosis by FGF21 was attributed to the fine-tuning of multiorgan cross talk among the liver, adipose tissue, and blood vessels, characterized by suppression of hepatic sterol regulatory element-binding protein-2 and induction of adiponectin in mice with atherosclerosis [35]. Although FGF21 functions in an endocrine manner, whether FGF21 can also induce a direct protection to the blood vessels remains unclear. For decades, lowering levels of low-density lipoprotein (LDL) cholesterol and increasing level of high-density lipoprotein (HDL) have formed the cornerstone of management of patients with atherosclerotic cardiovascular disease.

Strong evidence demonstrated that FGF-21 dramatically improved the condition of atherosclerosis in Wistar rats by decreasing serum LDL levels and increasing serum HDL levels. Moreover, FGF-21-induced antioxidative function is also involved in its therapeutic effect in atherosclerotic Wistar rat characterized by increased levels of superoxide dismutase, reduced glutathione, and reduced malondialdehyde [38].

Along with the development of atherosclerosis, the artery's lining becomes hardened, stiffened, and swollen with all sorts of "gunge," including fatty deposits and abnormal inflammatory cells, to form a plaque and then eventually deteriorate into coronary heart disease [39-41]. Strong evidence indicated that cardiac endothelial cell dysfunction may be an early initiating factor for atherosclerosis which facilitates the development of coronary heart disease [42]. Oxidized LDL (ox-LDL) is a proatherogenic lipoprotein that accumulates in the vascular wall and contributes to vascular dysfunction at the early-stage of atherosclerosis development [43-53]. Enhanced serum ox-LDL and antibodies against its epitopes are predictive for endothelial dysfunction and subsequent coronary heart disease [43]. Previous *in vitro* study indicated that both FGF21 mRNA and protein expressions were increased in response to ox-LDL treatment in cardiac endothelial cells and this was protective against apoptosis caused by ox-LDL [54]. Also, FGF21 has been reported to prevent high glucose induced cell damage and endothelial nitric oxide synthase dysfunction through an AMP-activated protein kinase- (AMPK-) dependent pathway in endothelial cells [55]. Therefore the relationship between FGF21 and coronary heart disease is of interest. Shen *et al.* reported that serum FGF21 level was positively associated with coronary heart disease in clinics [56, 57]. Our previous work confirmed that serum levels of FGF-21 are increased in patients with coronary heart disease independently associated with adverse lipid profiles [33]. In contrast, another study indicated that serum FGF21 has been associated with hypertriglyceridemia, hyperinsulinemia, and pericardial fat accumulation but not associated with coronary heart disease [58]. This paradox may be explained by decreased body mass index of healthy controls compared to patients with coronary heart diseases.

3. FGF21 and myocardial ischemia

Myocardial ischemia, a disorder causing cardiomyocytes injury and myocardial infarction and malfunction, activates adaptive responses enhancing myocardial tolerance to ischemia. Liu *et al.* indicated that, in response to myocardial ischemia in the C57BL/6J mouse, liver- and adipocytes-derived FGF21 was upregulated and secreted into the circulation. After interacting with FGFR1 in cardiomyocytes in the presence of β-klotho, FGF21 activates its downstream kinases and proteins including phosphatidylinositol 3-kinase (PI3K), protein kinase B (PKB/AKT), and Bcl2 antagonist of cell death (BAD), thereby reducing myocardial ischemia-induced apoptosis characterized by reduction of caspase-3 activity [59]. However, the adaptive response was not found in FGF21-deficient mice. Reversely, myocardial ischemic size was significantly smaller in FGF21 transgenic mice than that in wild type mice [59], suggesting that upregulated endogenous FGF21 derived from the liver and adipose tissue in response to myocardial injury induced cardiac protection mediated by activation of FGFR1/β-klotho-PI3K-Akt1-BAD signaling pathway. Although various growth factors and cytokines were upregulated during myocardial ischemia, the expression and secretion of cardiac FGF21 had no alteration, implying FGF21 induces cardiac protection against myocardial ischemia in an endocrine rather than an autocrine manner [59, 60]. To date, a question of whether administration of exogenous FGF21 can also induce cardiac protection during myocardial ischemia and if so whether the protection of exogenous FGF21 against myocardial ischemia can be direct to the heart or cardiomyocytes appears. This question was answered by Patel group [61]. They found that administration of exogenous FGF21 induced significant cardioprotection and restored cardiac function following global ischemia in Langendorff perfused rat hearts. Further study revealed that inhibition of AKT, extracellular signal-regulated kinase (ERK1/2), and AMPK impaired FGF21-induced antimyocardial ischemia effect in the hearts of obese Wistar rats, suggesting that the above kinases are involved in this cardioprotection of FGF21 [61]. Our previous *in vitro* study also confirmed that administration of exogenous FGF-21 attenuated ischemia-reperfusion induced damage in H9c2 cells characterized by inhibition of oxidative stress and apoptosis [62] The mechanistic study revealed that FGF21-induced protection against ischemia-reperfusion injury in cardiac cells mainly depended on the activation of Akt-GSK-3β- caspase-3 signaling pathway by preventing oxidative stress and recovery of the energy supply [62].

4. FGF21 and cardiac hypertrophy

Hypertrophic remodeling characterized by enlarged cardiomyocytes is an adaptive response of the heart to certain stresses. And it is also the leading cause of multiple cardiovascular problems including hypertension, myocardial ischemia, valvular disease, and cardiomyopathy [67-69]. Mature cardiomyocytes are considered to be terminally differentiated cells with no regenerative ability [70-72]. Under stresses, cardiac hypertrophy is characterized by cardiomyocytes enlargement, rather than cells division [73, 74], and this phenomenon is accompanied by the increase of extracellular matrix and fibroblasts inside the heart [75, 76].

Recently, cardiac hypertrophy was reported to induce FGF21 gene expression in the cardiomyocytes of mouse, and this was subjected to transcriptional regulation of the hepatic silent mating type information regulation 2 homolog 1/PPARα pathway [64]. In turn, FGF21 knockout mice had greater heart weights and more severe cardiac dysfunction in response to isoproterenol infusion along with induction of hypertrophic inflammatory markers [64]. However, administration of recombinant FGF21 significantly prevented isoproterenol-induced cardiac hypertrophy damage in mice [25]. Mechanistic studies indicated that FGF21 prevented cardiac hypertrophy by activating mitogen-activated protein kinase (MAPK) signaling *via* activation of FGFR1c/β-klotho [64, 77]. Additionally, FGF21 prevented cardiac hypertrophy by promoting multiple antioxidant genes expressions (*e.g.*, uncoupling proteins 2 and 3, also superoxide dismutase-2) and inhibiting the formation of reactive oxygen species in an autocrine manner [65].

5. FGF21 and diabetic cardiomyopathy

Diabetic patients develop the diabetic cardiomyopathy independent of coronary artery disease and hypertension [78, 79]. Diabetic cardiomyopathy is attributed to multiple pathogenic factors, including hyperglycemia, hyperlipidemia, and inflammation [80-82]. Cardiomyopathy is a late consequence of diabetes-induced early cardiac responses especially the myocardial apoptosis [83, 84]. Thus, treatments to reduce cardiac apoptosis may help control diabetic cardiomyopathy.

Recently, we reported that cardiac FGF21 mRNA expression was positively associated with the development of diabetes in the type 1 diabetic mice, suggesting that the increased cardiac FGF21 expression may be beneficial to the heart in this regard [30]. In the study we also observed cardiac apoptosis in early diabetic mice, which was remarkably prevented by administration of recombinant FGF21 [30]. Similar protection by FGF21 was observed in mice with cardiac lipotoxicity induced by fatty-acid [30]. Mechanistic studies indicated that FGF21-induced antiapoptotic effects *in vitro* and *in vivo* were mediated by ERK1/2-p38-MAPK-AMPK signaling pathway [30]. Thus, FGF21-induced cardioprotection in diabetic mice is mainly attributed to prevention of lipotoxicity by FGF21. Also, long-term treatment of FGF21 prevented diabetic-induced cardiac dysfunction and fibrosis mediated by the same signaling pathway as above [30]. Our work also revealed that FGF21 deletion-aggravated cardiac lipid accumulation is likely mediated by cardiac Nrf2-driven CD36 upregulation in type 1 diabetic mice, which contributes to increased cardiac oxidative stress and remodeling, and eventual development of diabetic cardiomyopathy [66].

6. Summary

CVD includes atherosclerosis, coronary heart disease, myocardial ischemia, cardiac hypertrophy, and diabetic cardiomyopathy which are all closely associated with severe lipid metabolic disorders [85-87]. FGF21, a metabolic regulator of carbohydrates and lipids, has been shown to improve insulin sensitivity and glucose uptake and suppress lipogenesis and lipid oxidation [15-18]. Clinical studies indicated that serum FGF21 changes were positively associated with the development of atherosclerosis, coronary heart disease, myocardial ischemia, cardiac hypertrophy, and diabetic cardiomyopathy, which implies that upregulated endogenous FGF21 may improve CVDs. Specifically, FGF21 prevented atherosclerosis and subsequent coronary heart disease was attributed to multiorgan cross talk among the liver, adipose tissue, and blood vessels and was characterized by suppression of lipid accumulation and increased lipid oxidation [63]. Similarly,

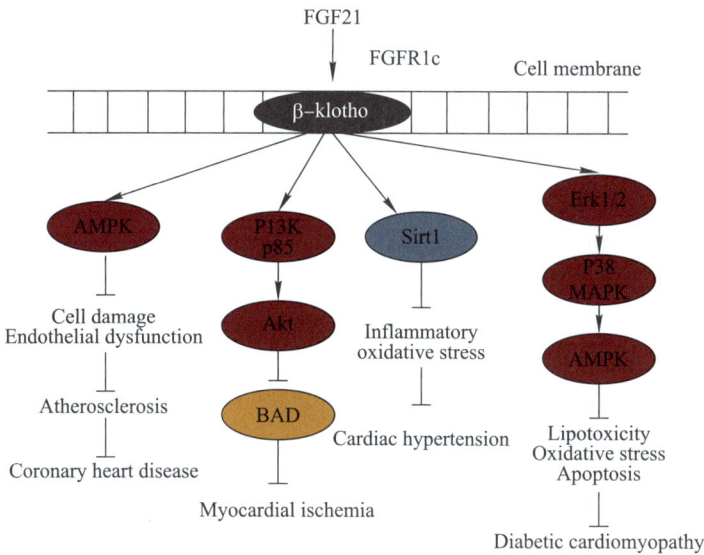

Fig. 1. FGF21 induces preventive effect on CVDs through multiple signaling pathways. As a classical cytokine, FGF21 functions as a metabolic regulator by binding with its receptor FGFR1 or FGFR2 in the presence of β-klotho. Growing studies demonstrated that FGF21 also induced beneficial effects on CVDs probably due to inhibition of glucose or lipid metabolic disorders. For instance, FGF21 prevented atherosclerosis and the subsequent CHD by inhibition of lipogenesis which was also the possible mechanism of FGF21-induced preventive effect on CH. Additionally, FGF21 also prevented MI and DC by activation of Akt- and AMPK-mediated signaling pathway which were usually involved in maintaining glucose and lipid homeostasis.

FGF21 prevented stress-induced CH *via* enhancing lipid oxidation mediated by the ERK1/2-CREB-PGC-1α signaling pathway [64]. FGF21 also prevented myocardial ischemia and diabetic cardiomyopathy *via* Akt- or AMPK-mediated signaling pathways which regulate lipid and glucose metabolisms (Fig. 1). Since serum FGF21 increases in several kinds of CVDs, serum FGF21 levels might be regarded as a potential biomarker not only for diagnosis of metabolic disorders but also for diagnosis of CVD in clinics. And supplementation of exogenous FGF21 might also induce beneficial effect in patients with CVD based on the conclusion of preclinical studies.

References

[1] Yang Y, Duan W, Li Y, *et al.* Novel role of silent information regulator 1 in myocardial ischemia [J]. Circulation, 2013, 128(20): 2232-2240.

[2] Mathers CD, Loncar D. Projections of global mortality and burden of disease from 2002 to 2030 [J]. Plos Medicine, 2006, 3(11).

[3] Burgess WH, Maciag T. The heparin-binding (fibroblast) growth-factor family of proteins [J]. Annual Review Of Biochemistry, 1989, 58: 575-606.

[4] Rifkin DB, Moscatelli D. Recent developments in the cell biology of basic fibroblast growth-factor [J]. Journal Of Cell Biology, 1989, 109(1): 1-6.

[5] Yamaguchi TP, Rossant J. Fibroblast growth-factors in mammalian development [J]. Current Opinion In Genetics & Development, 1995, 5(4): 485-491.

[6] Guillemot F, Zimmer C. From cradle to grave: the multiple roles of fibroblast growth factors in neural development [J]. Neuron, 2011, 71(4): 574-588.

[7] Goldfarb M. Fibroblast growth factor homologous factors: Evolution, structure, and function [J]. Cytokine & Growth Factor Reviews, 2005, 16(2): 215-220.

[8] Bae K-H, Kim J-G, Park K-G. Transcriptional regulation of fibroblast growth factor 21 expression [J]. Endocrinology And Metabolism, 2014, 29(2): 105-111.

[9] Itoh N, Ornitz DM. Evolution of the fgf and fgfr gene families [J]. Trends In Genetics, 2004, 20(11): 563-569.

[10] McKeehan WL, Wang F, Kan M. The heparan sulfate fibroblast growth factor family: diversity of structure and function[A]. In: Progress In Nucleic Acid Research And Molecular Biology, Vol 59 (Moldave K, ed), Vol. 59, 1998: 135-176.

[11] Nishimura T, Nakatake Y, Konishi M, *et al.* Identification of a novel FGF, FGF-21, preferentially expressed in the liver [J]. Biochimica Et Biophysica Acta-Gene Structure And Expression, 2000, 1492(1): 203-206.

[12] Inagaki T, Dutchak P, Zhao G, *et al.* Endocrine regulation of the fasting response by PPAR alpha-mediated induction of fibroblast growth factor 21 [J]. Cell Metabolism, 2007, 5(6): 415-425.

[13] Muise ES, Azzolina B, Kuo DW, *et al.* Adipose fibroblast growth factor 21 is up-regulated by peroxisome proliferator-activated receptor gamma and altered metabolic states [J]. Molecular Pharmacology, 2008, 74(2): 403-412.

[14] Wang H, Qiang L, Farmer SR. Identification of a domain within peroxisome proliferator-activated receptor gamma regulating expression of a group of genes containing fibroblast growth factor 21 that are selectively repressed by SIRT1 in adipocytes [J]. Molecular And Cellular Biology, 2008, 28(1): 188-200.

[15] Kurosu H, Choi M, Ogawa Y, *et al.* Tissue-specific expression of beta Klotho and fibroblast growth factor (FGF) receptor Isoforms determines metabolic activity of FGF19 and FGF21 [J]. Journal Of Biological Chemistry, 2007, 282(37): 26687-26695.

[16] Kharitonenkov A, Shiyanova TL, Koester A, *et al.* FGF-21 as a novel metabolic regulator [J]. Journal Of Clinical Investigation, 2005, 115(6): 1627-1635.

[17] Kharitonenkov A, Dunbar JD, Bina HA, *et al.* FGF-21/FGF-21 receptor interaction and activation is determined by beta Klotho [J]. Journal Of Cellular Physiology, 2008, 215(1): 1-7.

[18] Xu J, Stanislaus S, Chinookoswong N, *et al.* Acute glucose-lowering and insulin-sensitizing action of FGF21 in insulin-resistant mouse models-association with liver and adipose tissue effects [J]. American Journal Of Physiology-Endocrinology And Metabolism, 2009, 297(5): E1105-E1114.

[19] Yie J, Wang W, Deng L, et al. Understanding the physical interactions in the FGF21/FGFR/beta-klotho complex: structural requirements and implications in FGF21 signaling [J]. Chemical Biology & Drug Design, 2012, 79(4): 398-410.

[20] Kharitonenkov A, Adams AC. Inventing new medicines: The FGF21 story [J]. Molecular Metabolism, 2014, 3(3): 221-229.

[21] Suzuki M, Uehara Y, Motomura-Matsuzaka K, et al. beta Klotho is required for fibroblast growth factor (FGF) 21 signaling through FGF receptor (FGFR) 1c and FGFR3c [J]. Molecular Endocrinology, 2008, 22(4): 1006-1014.

[22] Urakawa I, Yamazaki Y, Shimada T, et al. Klotho converts canonical FGF receptor into a specific receptor for FGF23 [J]. Nature, 2006, 444(7120): 770-774.

[23] Li H, Zhang J, Jia W. Fibroblast growth factor 21: a novel metabolic regulator from pharmacology to physiology [J]. Frontiers Of Medicine, 2013, 7(1): 25-30.

[24] Kliewer SA, Mangelsdorf DJ. Fibroblast growth factor 21: from pharmacology to physiology [J]. American Journal Of Clinical Nutrition, 2010, 91(1): 254S-257S.

[25] Kotulak T, Drapalova J, Kopecky P, et al. Increased circulating and epicardial adipose tissue mRNA expression of fibroblast growth factor-21 after cardiac surgery: possible role in postoperative inflammatory response and insulin resistance [J]. Physiological Research, 2011, 60(5): 757-767.

[26] Stanford KI, Middelbeek RJW, Townsend KL, et al. Brown adipose tissue regulates glucose homeostasis and insulin sensitivity [J]. Journal Of Clinical Investigation, 2013, 123(1): 215-223.

[27] Schaap FG, Kremer AE, Lamers WH, et al. Fibroblast growth factor 21 is induced by endoplasmic reticulum stress [J]. Biochimie, 2013, 95(4): 692-699.

[28] Zhang X, Yeung DCY, Karpisek M, et al. Serum FGF21 levels are increased in obesity and are independently associated with the metabolic syndrome in humans [J]. Diabetes, 2008, 57(5): 1246-1253.

[29] Xiao Y, Liu L, Xu A, et al. Serum fibroblast growth factor 21 levels are related to subclinical atherosclerosis in patients with type 2 diabetes [J]. Cardiovascular Diabetology, 2015, 14.

[30] Zhang C, Huang Z, Gu J, et al. Fibroblast growth factor 21 protects the heart from apoptosis in a diabetic mouse model via extracellular signal-regulated kinase 1/2-dependent signalling pathway [J]. Diabetologia, 2015, 58(8): 1937-1948.

[31] Lusis AJ. Atherosclerosis [J]. Nature, 2000, 407(6801): 233-241.

[32] Davignon J. Advances in lipid-lowering therapy in atherosclerosis[A]. In: Diabetes And Cardiovascular Disease: Etiology, Treatment, And Outcomes (Angel A, Dhalla N, Pierce G et al., eds), Vol. 498, 2001: 49-58.

[33] Lin Z, Wu Z, Yin X, et al. Serum levels of FGF-21 are increased in coronary heart disease patients and are independently associated with adverse lipid profile [J]. Plos One, 2010, 5(12): e15534.

[34] Chow WS, Xu A, Woo YC, et al. Serum fibroblast growth factor-21 levels are associated with carotid atherosclerosis independent of established cardiovascular risk factors [J]. Arteriosclerosis Thrombosis And Vascular Biology, 2013, 33(10): 2454-2459.

[35] Lin Z, Pan X, Wu F, et al. Fibroblast growth factor 21 prevents atherosclerosis by suppression of hepatic sterol regulatory element-binding protein-2 and induction of adiponectin in mice [J]. Circulation, 2015, 131(21): 1861-1871.

[36] Wu X, Lu Y, Fu K, et al. Impact of exogenous fibroblast growth factor 21 on atherosclerosis in apolipoprotein E deficient mice [J]. Zhonghua xin xue guan bing za zhi, 2014, 42(2): 126-131.

[37] Wu X, Qi Y-F, Chang J-R, et al. Possible role of fibroblast growth factor 21 on atherosclerosis via amelioration of endoplasmic reticulum stress-mediated apoptosis in apoE(-/-) mice [J]. Heart And Vessels, 2015, 30(5): 657-668.

[38] Zhu W, Wang C, Liu L, et al. Effects of fibroblast growth factor 21 on cell damage in vitro and atherosclerosis in vivo [J]. Canadian

[39] Bhatia SK. Tissue engineering for clinical applications [J]. Biotechnology Journal, 2010, 5(12): 1309-1323.

[40] Faxon DP, Creager MA, Smith SC, et al. Atherosclerotic vascular disease conference-Executive summary-Atherosclerotic vascular disease conference proceeding for healthcare professionals from a special writing group of the American Heart Association [J]. Circulation, 2004, 109(21): 2595-2604.

[41] Akadam-Teker B, Kurnaz O, Coskunpinar E, et al. The effects of age and gender on the relationship between HMGCR promoter-911 SNP (rs33761740) and serum lipids in patients with coronary heart disease [J]. Gene, 2013, 528(2): 93-98.

[42] Rajendran P, Rengarajan T, Thangavel J, et al. The vascular endothelium and human diseases [J]. International Journal Of Biological Sciences, 2013, 9(10): 1057-1069.

[43] Galle J, Hansen-Hagge T, Wanner C, et al. Impact of oxidized low density lipoprotein on vascular cells [J]. Atherosclerosis, 2006, 185(2): 219-226.

[44] Quinn MT, Parthasarathy S, Steinberg D. Lysophosphatidylcholine - a chemotactic factor for human-monocytes and its potential role in atherogenesis [J]. Proceedings Of the National Academy Of Sciences Of the United States Of America, 1988, 85(8): 2805-2809.

[45] Frostegard J, Haegerstrand A, Gidlund M, et al. Biologically modified LDL increases the adhesive properties of endothelial-cells [J]. Atherosclerosis, 1991, 90(2-3): 119-126.

[46] Yui S, Sasaki T, Miyazaki A, et al. Induction of murine macrophage growth by modified LDLs [J]. Arteriosclerosis And Thrombosis, 1993, 13(3): 331-337.

[47] Lindner V, Lappi DA, Baird A, et al. Role of basic fibroblast growth-factor in vascular lesion formation [J]. Circulation Research, 1991, 68(1): 106-113.

[48] Jimi S, Saku K, Uesugi N, et al. Oxidized low-density-lipoprotein stimulates collagen production in cultured arterial smooth-muscle cells [J]. Atherosclerosis, 1995, 116(1): 15-26.

[49] Loidl A, Claus R, Ingolic E, et al. Role of ceramide in activation of stress-associated MAP kinases by minimally modified LDL in vascular smooth muscle cells [J]. Biochimica Et Biophysica Acta-Molecular Basis Of Disease, 2004, 1690(2): 150-158.

[50] Sata M, Walsh K. Oxidized LDL activates fas-mediated endothelial cell apoptosis [J]. Journal Of Clinical Investigation, 1998, 102(9): 1682-1689.

[51] Hardwick SJ, Hegyi L, Clare K, et al. Apoptosis in human monocyte-macrophages exposed to oxidized low density lipoprotein [J]. Journal Of Pathology, 1996, 179(3): 294-302.

[52] Schwartz CJ, Valente AJ, Sprague EA, et al. The pathogenesis of atherosclerosis - an overview [J]. Clinical Cardiology, 1991, 14(2): 1-16.

[53] Li LX, Chen JX, Liao DF, et al. Probucol inhibits oxidized low density lipoprotein-induced adhesion of monocytes to endothelial cells by reducing P-selectin synthesis in vitro [J]. Endothelium-New York, 1998, 6(1): 1-8.

[54] Lu Y, Liu J-h, Zhang L-k, et al. Fibroblast growth factor 21 as a possible endogenous factor inhibits apoptosis in cardiac endothelial cells [J]. Chinese Medical Journal, 2010, 123(23): 3417-3421.

[55] Shao M, Lu X, Cong W, et al. Multiple low-dose radiation prevents type 2 diabetes-induced renal damage through attenuation of dyslipidemia and insulin resistance and subsequent renal inflammation and oxidative stress [J]. Plos One, 2014, 9(3): e92574.

[56] Shen Y, Ma X, Zhou J, et al. Additive relationship between serum fibroblast growth factor 21 level and coronary artery disease [J]. Cardiovascular Diabetology, 2013, 12.

[57] Kim WJ, Kim SS, Lee HC, et al. Association between serum fibroblast growth factor 21 and coronary artery disease in patients with type 2 diabetes [J]. Journal Of Korean Medical Science, 2015, 30(5): 586-590.

[58] Lee Y, Lim S, Hong E-S, et al. Serum FGF21 concentration is asso-

Journal Of Physiology And Pharmacology, 2014, 92(11): 927-935.

ciated with hypertriglyceridaemia, hyperinsulinaemia and pericardial fat accumulation, independently of obesity, but not with current coronary artery status [J]. Clinical Endocrinology, 2014, 80(1): 57-64.

[59] Liu SQ, Roberts D, Kharitonenkov A, et al. Endocrine protection of ischemic myocardium by FGF21 from the liver and adipose tissue [J]. Scientific Reports, 2013, 3.

[60] Liu SQ, Tefft BJ, Roberts DT, et al. Cardioprotective proteins up-regulated in the liver in response to experimental myocardial ischemia [J]. American Journal Of Physiology-Heart And Circulatory Physiology, 2012, 303(12): H1446-H1458.

[61] Patel V, Adya R, Chen J, et al. Novel insights into the cardio-protective effects of fgf21 in lean and obese rat hearts [J]. Plos One, 2014, 9(2).

[62] Cong W-T, Ling J, Tian H-S, et al. Proteomic study on the protective mechanism of fibroblast growth factor 21 to ischemia-reperfusion injury [J]. Canadian Journal Of Physiology And Pharmacology, 2013, 91(11): 973-984.

[63] Lin Z, Pan X, Wu F, et al. Fibroblast growth factor 21 prevents atherosclerosis by suppression of hepatic sterol regulatory element-binding protein-2 and induction of adiponectin in mice [J]. Circulation, 2015, 131(21): 1861-1871.

[64] Planavila A, Redondo I, Hondares E, et al. Fibroblast growth factor 21 protects against cardiac hypertrophy in mice [J]. Nature Communications, 2013, 4.

[65] Planavila A, Redondo-Angulo I, Ribas F, et al. Fibroblast growth factor 21 protects the heart from oxidative stress [J]. Cardiovascular Research, 2015, 106(1): 19-31.

[66] Yan X, Chen J, Zhang C, et al. FGF21 deletion exacerbates diabetic cardiomyopathy by aggravating cardiac lipid accumulation [J]. Journal Of Cellular And Molecular Medicine, 2015, 19(7): 1557-1568.

[67] Nadruz W. Myocardial remodeling in hypertension [J]. Journal Of Human Hypertension, 2015, 29(1): 1-6.

[68] Yamamoto S, Kita S, Iyoda T, et al. New molecular mechanisms for cardiovascular disease: cardiac hypertrophy and cell-volume regulation [J]. Journal Of Pharmacological Sciences, 2011, 116(4): 343-349.

[69] Barry SP, Davidson SM, Townsend PA. Molecular regulation of cardiac hypertrophy [J]. International Journal Of Biochemistry & Cell Biology, 2008, 40(10): 2023-2039.

[70] Shenje LT, Andersen P, Halushka MK, et al. Mutations in Alstrom protein impair terminal differentiation of cardiomyocytes [J]. Nature Communications, 2014, 5.

[71] Lovric J, Mano M, Zentilin L, et al. Terminal differentiation of cardiac and skeletal myocytes induces permissivity to AAV transduction by relieving inhibition imposed by DNA damage response proteins [J]. Molecular Therapy, 2012, 20(11): 2087-2097.

[72] Frohlich ED, Susic D. Pressure overload [J]. Heart Failure Clinics, 2012, 8(1): 21-32.

[73] Grove D, Zak R, Nair KG, et al. Biochemical correlates of cardiac hypertrophy .4. observations on cellular organization of growth during myocardial hypertrophy in rat [J]. Circulation Research, 1969, 25(4): 473-485.

[74] Grove D, Nair KG, Zak R. Biochemical correlates of cardiac hypertrophy .3. changes in DNA content-relative contributions of polyploidy and mitotic activity [J]. Circulation Research, 1969, 25(4): 463-471.

[75] Simko F, Bednarova KR, Krajcirovicova K, et al. Melatonin reduces cardiac remodeling and improves survival in rats with isoproterenol-induced heart failure [J]. Journal Of Pineal Research, 2014, 57(2): 177-184.

[76] Gupta PK, DiPette DJ, Supowit SC. Protective effect of resveratrol against pressure overload-induced heart failure [J]. Food Science & Nutrition, 2014, 2(3): 218-229.

[77] Itoh N, Ohta H. Pathophysiological roles of FGF signaling in the heart [J]. Frontiers In Physiology, 2013, 4.

[78] Sowers JR, Epstein M, Frohlich ED. Diabetes, hypertension, and cardiovascular disease - An update [J]. Hypertension, 2001, 37(4): 1053-1059.

[79] Boudina S, Abel ED. Diabetic cardiomyopathy revisited [J]. Circulation, 2007, 115(25): 3213-3223.

[80] Bugger H, Abel ED. Molecular mechanisms of diabetic cardiomyopathy [J]. Diabetologia, 2014, 57(4): 660-671.

[81] Boudina S, Abel ED. Diabetic cardiomyopathy, causes and effects [J]. Reviews In Endocrine & Metabolic Disorders, 2010, 11(1): 31-39.

[82] Cai L, Kang YJ. Oxidative stress and diabetic cardiomyopathy: a brief review [J]. Cardiovascular toxicology, 2001, 1(3): 181-193.

[83] Acar E, Ural D, Bildirici U, et al. Diabetic cardiomyopathy [J]. Anatolian Journal Of Cardiology, 2011, 11(8): 732-737.

[84] Cai L, Kang YJ. Cell death and diabetic cardiomyopathy [J]. Cardiovascular toxicology, 2003, 3(3): 219-228.

[85] Nabel EG. Cardiovascular disease [J]. New England Journal Of Medicine, 2003, 349(1): 60-72.

[86] Nordestgaard BG, Varbo A. Triglycerides and cardiovascular disease [J]. Lancet, 2014, 384(9943): 626-635.

[87] Chiasson J-L, Le Lorier J. Glycaemic control, cardiovascular disease, and mortality in type 2 diabetes [J]. Lancet, 2014, 384(9958): 1906-1907.

Fibroblast growth factor 21 deficiency exacerbates chronic alcohol-induced hepatic steatosis and injury

Yanlong Liu, Xiaokun Li, Wenke Feng

Alcoholic fatty liver disease (AFLD) is characterized by excessive fat accumulation in the liver, and it may progress to more harmful stages of liver injury, including steatohepatitis, fibrosis, cirrhosis, and even malignancy. Hepatic steatosis has also been observed in patients with obesity and diabetes and in experimental animals fed with a high fat diet. The control of hepatic lipid metabolism is a complex process. Fatty acid synthesis, uptake, oxidation and release are basic regulatory mechanisms responsible for fat accumulation in the liver. Extensive studies have identified key regulators in these processes, including hormones such as insulin and glucagon, transcription factors and regulatory molecules such as peroxisome proliferator-activated receptor α (PPARα)[1], sterol regulatory element-binding protein 1c (SREBP1c)[2], and sirtuin 1(Sirt1)[3]. Chronic alcohol ingestion is believed to cause enhanced hepatic lipogenesis and impaired fatty acid β-oxidation by dysregulation of key hepatic factors such as PPARα, SREBP1c, PPARγ coactivator α (PGC1α), Sirt1 and AMP-activated kinase (AMPK)[4]. During alcohol exposure, production of reactive oxygen species is enhanced due to the up-regulation of cytochrome P450 2E1 (Cyp2e1)[5]. Although profound changes in pancreas-produced insulin and glucagon (known as causative extra-hepatic hormones) have been described, little is known as to whether the paracrine and endocrine signals for metabolic regulation of the liver itself participate in these alcohol-induced alterations in lipid metabolism.

Fibroblast growth factor (FGF21) is a potential metabolic regulator[6]. Unlike typical FGFs, FGF21 lacks heparin binding, and therefore serves as an endocrine factor. FGF21 is activated by binding to FGF receptors and a unique co-receptor, β-Klotho, which is expressed abundantly only in certain metabolic tissues, such as liver, adipose tissue and pancreas[7]. The mechanisms underlying the action of FGF21 in the regulation of hepatic lipid homeostasis have been explored in animals. FGF21 deficient mice display an abnormal lipid response, including attenuated triglyceride clearance and enhanced lipogenesis in the liver during methionine-choline deficient (MCD) diet and high fat diet feeding in mice[8]. Alcoholic liver disease (ALD), in particular in its early stages including AFLD and alcoholic steatohepatitis (ASH), is characterized by hepatic intracellular lipid accumulation. These similarities suggest that FGF21 may be involved in the alcohol-induced hepatic fat accumulation and liver injury. A recent study showing that FGF21 plays a role in alcohol preference in mice further indicates the importance of FGF21 in alcohol related disorders[9]. In the present study, we investigated the role of FGF21 signaling in hepatic lipid regulation and inflammation in ALD. By using global FGF21 knockout (KO), we demonstrate that FGF21 signaling is involved in the development/progression of experimental alcoholic liver disease.

1. Results

1.1 Mice with alcohol-induced steatosis and liver injury have increased serum FGF21

Exposure of 8- to 10-week-old C57BL/6J mice to the Lieber DeCarli liquid diet containing 5% alcohol for 4 weeks resulted in a significant increase in FGF21 expression in the serum and liver (Fig. 1A–C). FGF21 knockout mice served as controls (Fig. 1A,B). FGFR4 and β-Klotho were also markedly elevated in the liver in alcohol-fed mice (Fig. 1D). Alcohol markedly increased FGF21 gene expression in primary hepatocytes isolated from the mice exposed to alcohol (Supplementary Fig. 1A). In contrast, epididymal white adipose tissue isolated from alcohol-exposed mice did not show an alteration in FGF21 gene expression compared to controls (Supplementary Fig. 1B). These results suggest that alco-

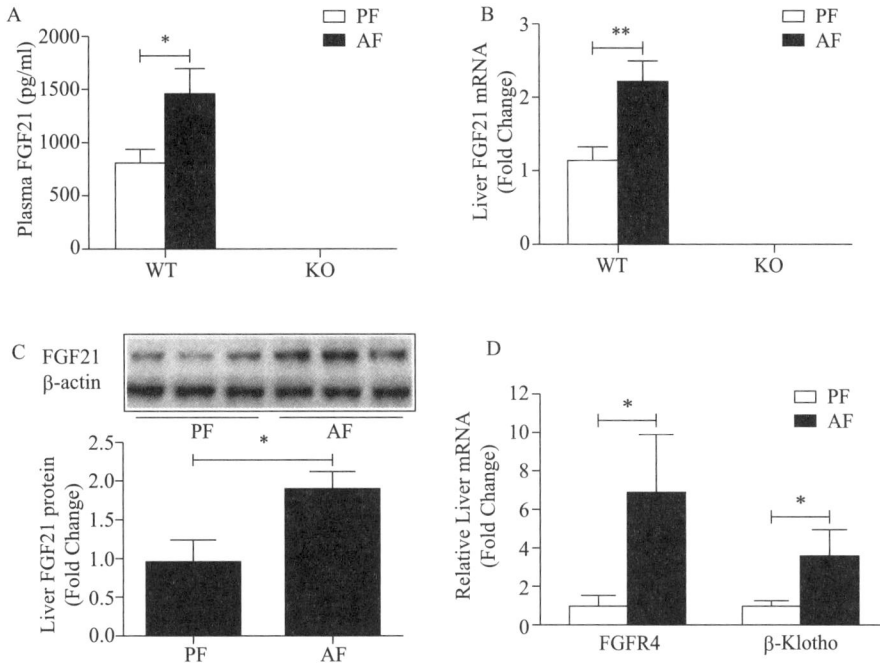

Fig. 1. Alcohol exposure increases FGF21 expression. (A–D): Wild type (WT) and FGF21 KO (KO) mice were treated as described in Material and Methods. (A) Plasma FGF21 concentration. (B) Relative liver mRNA levels of FGF21. (C) Hepatic FGF21 protein levels. (D) Relative liver mRNA levels of β-Klotho and FGFR4.

hol exposure activates FGF21 signaling in hepatocytes.

1.2 Serum FGF21 levels are increased in alcoholic steatohepatitis (ASH) patients

To determine whether humans with ALD have elevated FGF21 levels similar to mice with alcohol-induced hepatic steatosis and liver injury, we measured serum FGF21 concentrations in 24 patients with ASH, in 20 patients with alcoholic cirrhosis (AC) with no fatty liver on ultrasound/CT scan, and in 26 nondrinking healthy subjects with no liver disease. Baseline clinical, biochemical and demographic information is shown in Supplementary Table 1. As shown in Supplementary Fig. 1C, patients with ASH had FGF21 values that were six times greater than those seen in healthy controls, while stable cirrhotics had values that were not significantly different from controls.

1.3 Alcohol feeding increases liver steatosis and injury

The alcohol-fed mice developed fatty liver, as demonstrated by histological analyses of liver sections (Fig. 2A) and hepatic triglyceride (TG) levels (Fig. 2B). Alcohol exposure caused hepatocellular damage, as indicated by elevated plasma alanine aminotransferase (ALT, Fig. 2C) and hepatic apoptosis as determined by TUNEL (terminal deoxynucleotidyl transferase dUTP nick end labeling) staining compared to PF controls (Supplementary Fig. 2).

1.4 FGF21 ablation exacerbates chronic alcohol-induced liver steatosis and injury

Next, we tested whether FGF21 plays a role in the development of ALD. As shown in Supplementary Table 2, alcohol exposure significantly increased liver weight and liver/body weight ratio. These increases were more pronounced in FGF21 KO mice, indicating a likely fat accumulation increase in FGF21 KO mice. Alcohol exposure increased the levels of plasma free fatty acid (FFA) and TG in WT mice. Plasma TG levels were further increased by alcohol exposure in FGF21 KO mice. There were no changes in plasma levels of cholesterol and insulin between WT and FGF21 KO mice. Food intake and blood alcohol concentrations were not different between WT and FGF21 KO mice (data not shown).

However, FGF21 KO mice exhibited a more severe hepatic steatosis (Fig. 2A). Confirming these findings, hepatic TG was markedly increased in FGF21 KO mice (Fig. 2B). Plasma ALT levels were further increased in FGF21 KO mice (Fig. 2C). These findings strongly suggest that FGF21 may be playing a mechanistic role in the hepatic defense to alcohol-induced steatosis and hepatotoxicity.

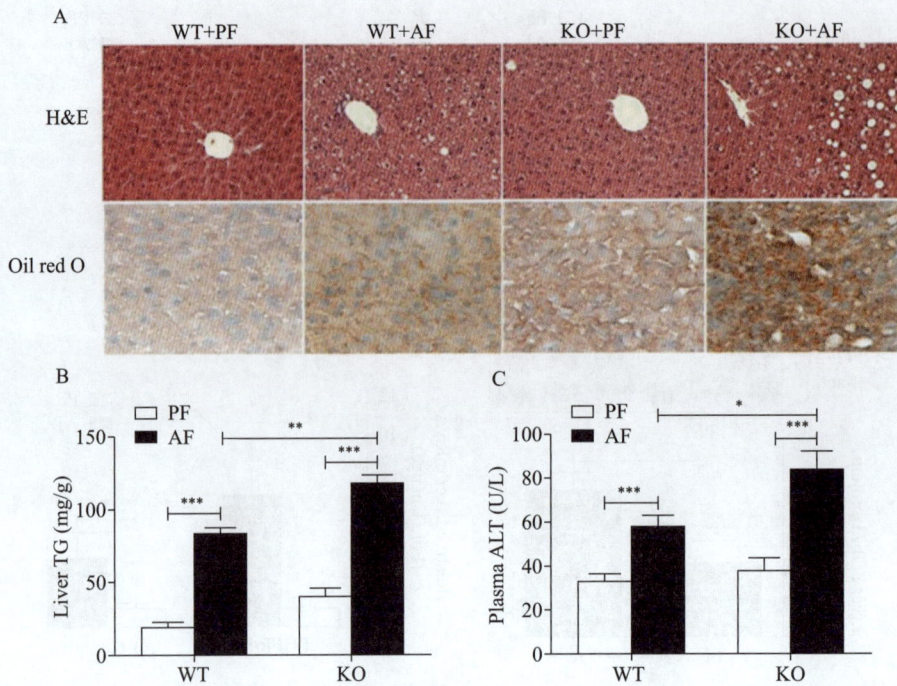

Fig. 2. FGF21 ablation exacerbates chronic alcohol-induced liver steatosis and injury. Mice were treated as described in Material and Methods. (A) Hematoxylin and eosin (H&E, upper panel), and Oil red O (lower panel) staining of liver sections. (B) Liver TG concentrations. (C) Plasma ALT levels.

1.5 FGF21 ablation increases hepatic lipogenesis by alcohol exposure

The control of hepatic lipid metabolism is an intricate process. In both WT and KO mice, chronic alcohol feeding significantly increased the gene expression of cluster of differentiation 36 (CD36), a fatty acid transporter in the liver, but not fatty acid transport protein FATP2 and FATP5 (Supplementary Fig. 3A). There was no change in hepatic expression of the genes responsible for very low-density lipoprotein (VLDL) assembly (Supplementary Fig. 3B).

In agreement with previous studies[2], alcohol exposure increased hepatic gene expression of SREBP1c, a transcription factor which plays a critical role in the control of lipogenic gene expression (Fig. 3A). Accordingly, the gene expression of well-known targets of SREBP1c, fatty acid synthase (FAS), stearoyl-CoA desaturase-1 (SCD1) and acetyl-CoA carboxylase (ACC), was increased by alcohol exposure in the livers of WT mice; and these increases were more pronounced in the KO mice (Fig. 3A). The precursor level of SREBP1c was significantly increased in AF WT mice, but decreased in AF KO mice (Fig. 3B). However, the mature form of SREBP1c tended to be increased in the KO mice resulting in a drastically increased ratio of mature to precursor SREBP1c in AF KO mice, indicating a significant activation of SREBP1c. The levels of the SCD1 protein were markedly increased in the KO mice by AF (Fig. 3C). Furthermore, in the KO mice, alcohol increased SREBP1c protein acetylation level (Fig. 3D), which increases SREBP1c protein stability and activity[10].

Previous studies indicated that Sirt1 is an oxidized nicotinamide adenine dinucleotide (NAD+)-dependent deacetylase, which tightly regulates fatty acid metabolism through multiple nutrient sensors including SREBP1c and PGC-1α[10,11]. Sirt1 activation was impaired more severely in the KO mice. Hepatic Sirt1 transcript expression was significantly decreased in the PF KO mice, and was further decreased in the AF KO mice (Fig. 4A). The reduction was also observed at protein levels (Fig. 4B). We next sought to determine whether FGF21 expression is required in Sirt1 expression. It has been shown that metformin increases Sirt1 expression in hepatocytes[12]. Incubation with metformin for 8 hours resulted in a significant increase in Sirt1 protein expression in primary hepatocytes isolated from WT mice, but the increase was not as great in the KO mice (Supplementary Fig. 4A), indicating a requirement for FGF21 in the metformin induction of Sirt1. Furthermore, rhFGF21 treatment markedly induced Sirt1 nuclear translocation in AML-12 cells (Supplementary Fig. 4B). These results suggest a possible role for FGF21 in the Sirt1-mediated regulation of hepatic lipogenesis induced by chronic alcohol exposure.

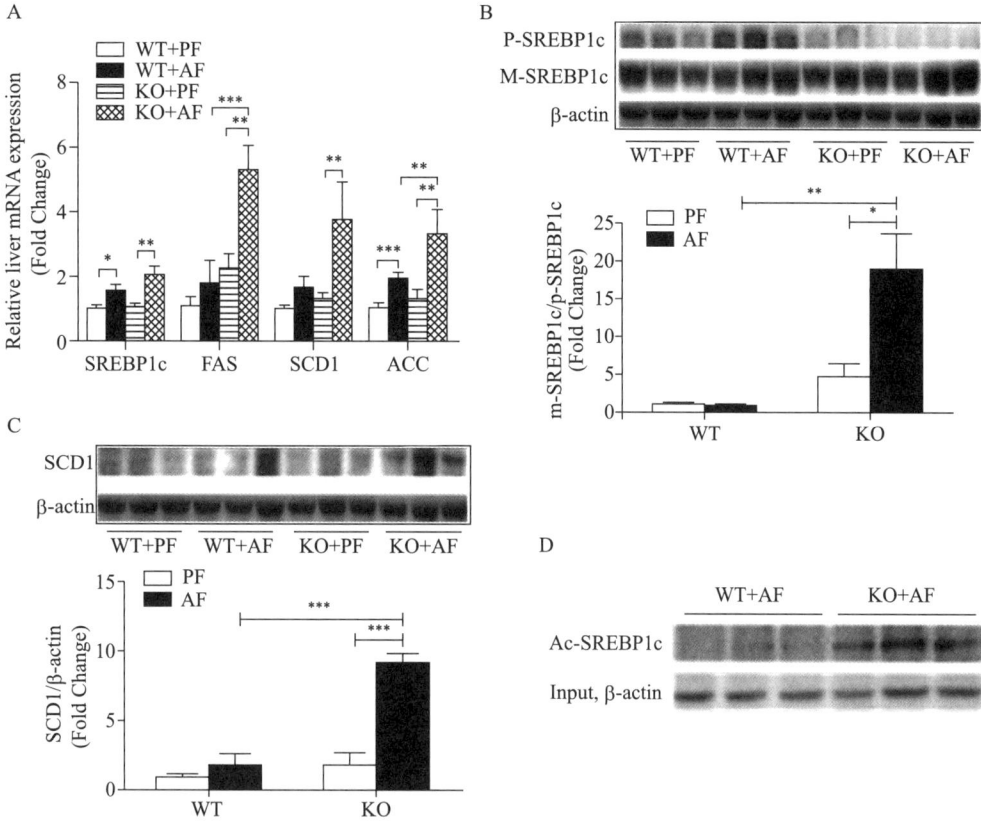

Fig. 3. FGF21 ablation increases hepatic lipogenesis by alcohol exposure. Mice were treated as described in Material and Methods. (A) Relative liver mRNA levels of SREBP1c, FAS, SCD1 and ACC. (B) Hepatic protein levels of precursor (p-SREBP1c) and mature (m-SREBP1c) forms of SREBP1c (upper panel), and the ratio of m-SREBP1c/p-SREBP1c (lower panel). (C) Hepatic SCD1 protein levels. (D) Acetylated SREBP1c levels.

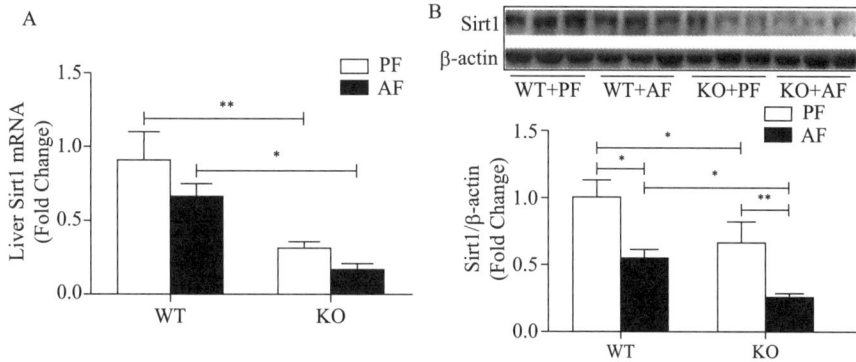

Fig. 4. FGF21 deficiency decreases alcohol-mediated Sirt1 activity. Liver Sirt1 mRNA (A) and protein (B) in the liver of mice treated as described in Material and Methods.

1.6 FGF21 knockout inhibits alcohol-regulated hepatic fatty acid β-oxidation

Alcohol exposure stimulates hepatic fatty acid accumulation *via* inhibition of fat clearance mediated by fatty acid β-oxidation. Therefore, we investigated whether FGF21 is critically involved in fatty acid clearance. Alcohol decreased the transcript levels of genes involved in fatty acid β-oxidation, including PGC1α, PPARα, and carnitine palmitoyltransferase I (CPT1), and these decreases were further exaggerated in the KO mice (Fig. 5A). The mRNA expression of long chain acyl-CoA dehydrogenase (ACADL), a mitochondrial enzyme that catalyzes most fatty acid β-oxidation, was not changed by alcohol in the WT, but significantly decreased in the KO mice (Fig. 5A).

PGC1α is a member of a family of transcription co-activators that play a central role in the regulation of cellular

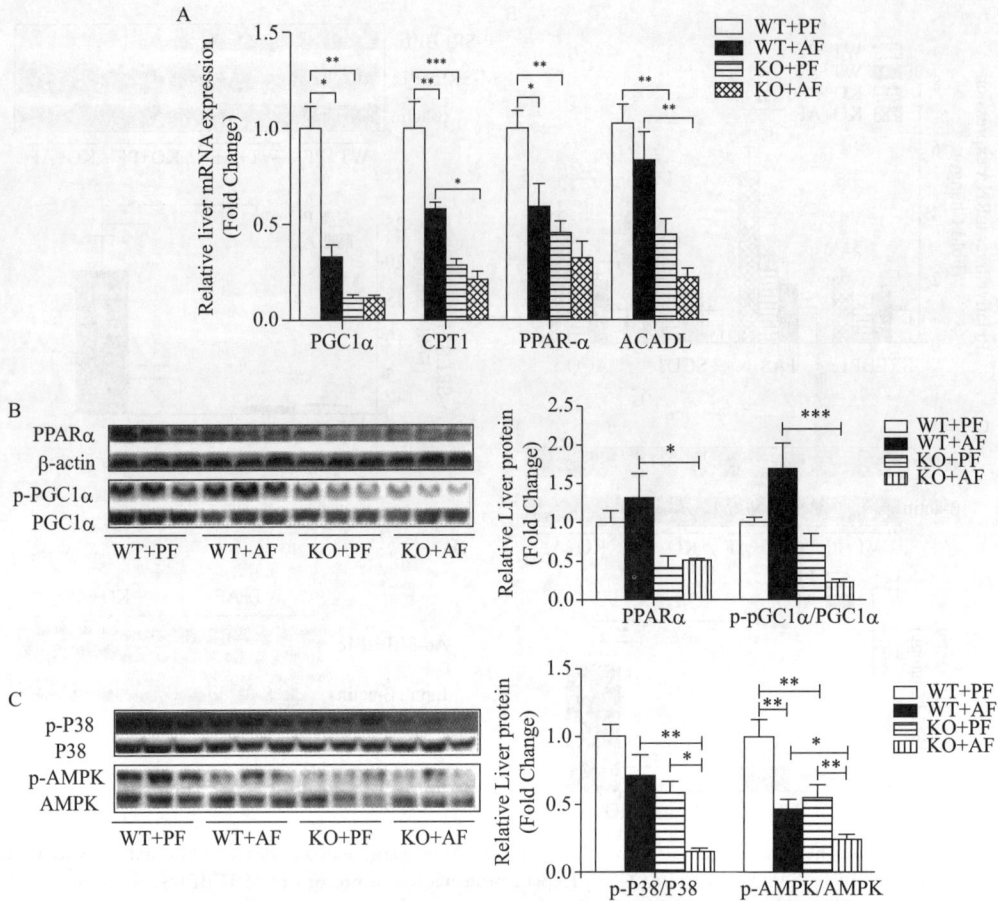

Fig. 5. FGF21 deficiency inhibits alcohol-mediated fatty acid β-oxidation. Mice were treated as described in Material and Methods. (A) Relative liver mRNA levels of PGC1α, CPT1, PPARα, and ACADL. (B) Liver protein levels of PPARα, p-PGC1α and total PGC1α (left panel), and the ratios of PPARα/β-actin and p-PGC1α/PGC1α (right panel). (C) Liver protein levels of p-p38, p-AMPK and total p38, AMPK.

energy metabolism. In the liver, induction of PGC1α stimulates the PPARα-mediated transcription of genes involved in fatty acid oxidation. Alcohol exposure markedly decreased PPARα protein levels in the KO mice (Fig. 5B). Importantly, PGC1α phosphorylation was reduced in the KO mice (Fig. 5B), indicating a decrease in PGC1α activity in the AF KO mice.

PGC1α activation by phosphorylation is mediated by multiple mechanisms. Previous studies demonstrated that p38 MAPK activation directly phosphorylates PGC1α in the liver[13]. Alcohol exposure moderately decreased hepatic p38 phosphorylation in WT mice, but significantly in the KO mice (Fig. 5C). AMPK is a key metabolic master switch which phosphorylates target molecules involved in lipid metabolism in the liver[4]. As expected, alcohol exposure markedly decreased AMPK phosphorylation in WT mice. Importantly, the p-AMPK level was further down-regulated in FGF21 KO mice (Fig. 5C). These results strongly suggest that FGF21 plays a critical role in p38- and AMPK- mediated PGC1α-PPARα activation that regulates the genes involved in fatty acid β-oxidation in response to alcohol exposure.

1.7 FGF21 KO increases chronic alcohol exposure-induced inflammation

Inflammation is a hallmark of alcoholic liver disease. We have previously shown that alcohol exposure increased levels of circulating endotoxin, which activates Kupffer cells in the liver and increases hepatic inflammation[14,15]. The hepatic gene expression of pro-inflammatory cytokines, TNFα (tumor necrosis factor α), IL6 (interleukin 6) and chemokine MCP1 (monocyte chemoattractant protein 1) was significantly elevated in FGF21 KO mice exposed to alcohol compared with WT mice (Fig. 6A). The increase of plasma IL-6 protein (Fig. 6C) and hepatic levels of IL-6 and MCP1 protein was further enhanced in the KO mice (Figs. 6D and 6E). The increase of cytokines and chemokines suggest an enhanced involvement of lymphocyte recruitment in the KO mice fed alcohol. In addition, chronic alcohol exposure also increased neutrophil infiltration in the liver of WT mice, and this increase was further exacerbated in FGF21 KO mice (Fig. 6B). Therefore, the observed effects of alcohol exposure on hepatic inflammation may be mediated, at least

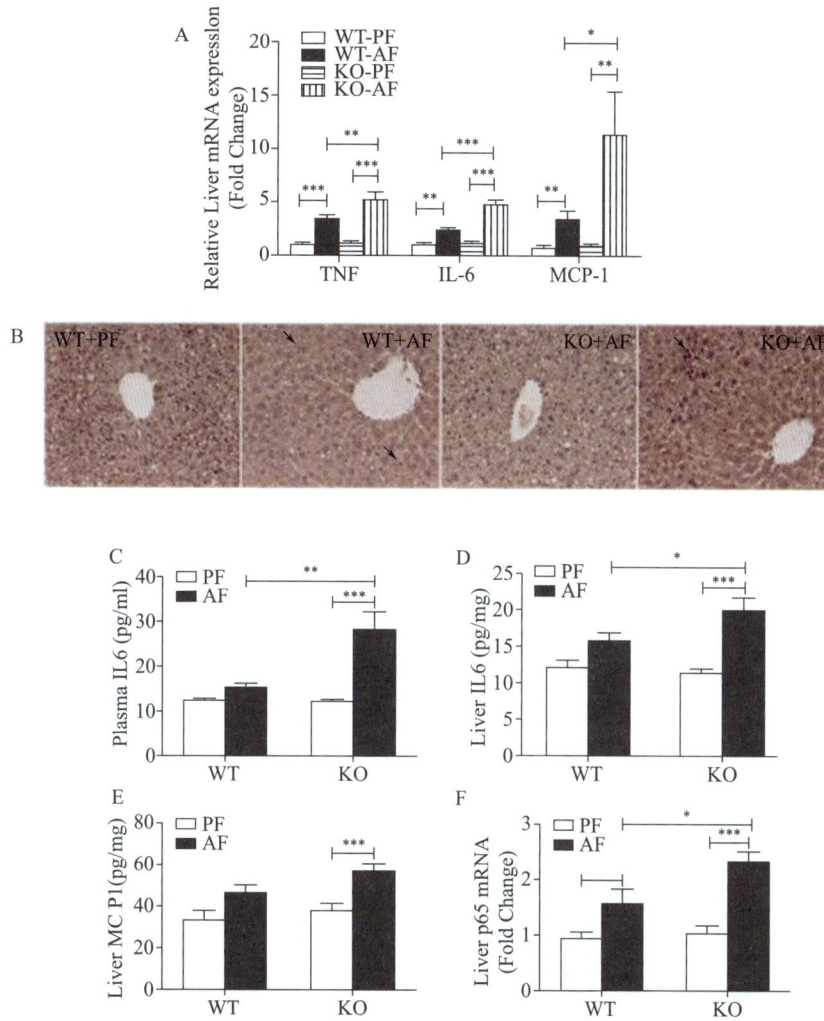

Fig. 6. FGF21 KO increases chronic alcohol exposure-induced inflammation. Mice were treated as described in Material and Methods. (A) Relative liver mRNA levels of TNFα (left panel), IL6 (middle panel) and MCP1 (right panel). (B) Liver inflammation was assessed by CAE staining of liver sections. Arrows denote neutrophil infiltration. (C) Plasma IL6 protein concentrations. Liver IL6 (D) and MCP1 (E) protein levels, expressed in pg/mg total protein. (F) Relative liver mRNA levels of p65.

in part, by FGF21 signaling. In addition, alcohol exposure increased hepatic p65 gene expression, and this increase is further exacerbated in the KO mice (Fig. 6F). This finding indicates that increased hepatic inflammation by chronic alcohol may be mediated through FGF21 signaling.

1.8 Recombinant FGF21 attenuates chronic alcohol-induced hepatic steatosis and injury

Based on above findings, we hypothesized that FGF21 may be beneficial in the treatment of ALD. To test this hypothesis, we injected rhFGF21 once a day at a dose of 4 mg/kg in the last 5 days of alcohol feeding. rhFGF21 treatment significantly attenuated chronic alcohol-induced hepatic fat accumulation (Fig. 7A). This effect was confirmed by the measurement of liver/body weight ratio (Supplementary Fig. 5) and liver TG concentrations (Fig. 7C). Plasma TG concentrations were also significantly decreased by rhFGF21 treatment (Fig. 7B). rhFGF21 treatment resulted in an increase in the gene expression of PGC1α, and a decrease of SCD1 and ACC (Fig. 7D). To evaluate hepatic inflammation, we measured hepatic Myeloperoxidase (MPO) activity and cytokine expression. As expected, hepatic MPO activity (Fig. 7E), TNFα protein levels (Fig. 7F) and plasma IL-6 levels (Fig. 7G) were decreased by rhFGF21 treatment. Lastly, chronic alcohol-induced elevations in plasma levels of ALT and AST (aspartate aminotransferase) were markedly reduced by rhFGF21 treatment (Fig. 7H). These results suggest that FGF21 administration attenuates the chronic alcohol-induced liver steatosis and injury.

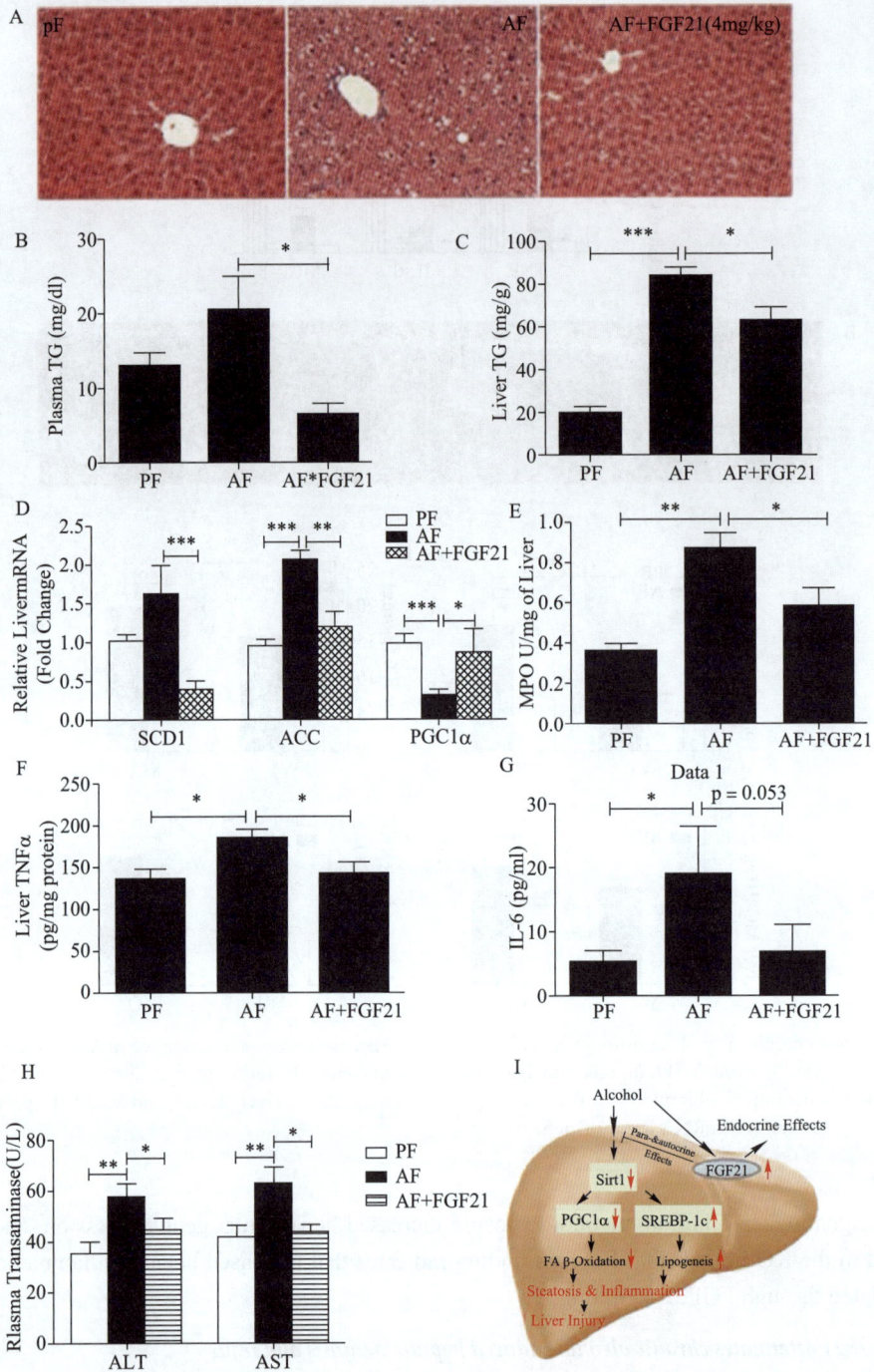

Fig. 7. Recombinant FGF21 treatment attenuates chronic alcohol-induced hepatic steatosis and injury. WT mice were treated as described in Material and Methods. (A) H&E staining of liver sections. (B) Plasma TG levels. (C) Liver TG levels. (D) Relative liver mRNA levels of SCD1, ACC and PGC1α. (E) Liver MPO activity. (F) Liver TNFα protein levels. (G) Plasma IL-6 levels. (H) Plasma ALT and AST levels. (I) Schematic illustration of hypothesized mechanisms. Alcohol exposure increases circulating levels and hepatic expression of FGF21, which inhibit alcohol-induced down-regulation of Sirt1 leading to an increased fatty acid β-oxidation and a decreased lipogenesis mediated by PGC-1α and SREBP-1, respectively, and a reduced inflammation.

2. Discussion

Previous studies have shown that FGF21 is a critical regulator for glucose and lipid metabolism in response to a variety of physiological conditions and pathological challenges. The present study provides evidence for the possible involvement of FGF21 signaling in the development of chronic alcohol-induced hepatic steatosis and injury. Several lines of evidence support this notion. First, we showed that circulating FGF21 levels are increased in patients with alcoholic steatohepatitis and that chronic alcohol exposure resulted in an up-regulation of FGF21 expression in mice. Second, FGF21 KO mice were sensitized to alcohol exposure with regard to hepatic lipogenesis and fatty acid β-oxidation leading to an increased hepatic fat accumulation. Third, FGF21 KO mice also exhibited an enhanced hepatic inflammation in response to alcohol. Fourth, rhFGF21 treatment reversed alcohol-induced hepatic steatosis and liver injury in mice.

Multiple studies suggest that a variety of cell types express FGF21 as an endocrine or paracrine/autocrine hormone with various functions. Serum FGF21 level is positively correlated with hepatic fat content and serum triglyceride concentration[16-18]. Inflammation has been shown to induce hepatic FGF21 expression[19]. Alcohol exposure causes hepatic fat accumulation and inflammation, which are clearly causative factors for FGF21 elevation in steatohepatitis patients and in mice. Although they have severe inflammation, cirrhotic patients have minimum hepatic fat, which may be responsible for the unchanged serum FGF21 level in cirrhotic patients. In addition, our results suggest that the liver is one of the major producing organs for circulating FGF21 induced by alcohol exposure. Liver insufficiency in cirrhotic patients apparently is a major factor for the irresponsibility in FGF21 production.

Hepatic FGF21 expression is under the control of PPARα in response to fasting[20], while adipose expressed FGF21 functions locally, serving as an autocrine factor stimulating peroxisome proliferator-activated receptor γ (PPARγ) activity[21]. However, hepatic protein levels of PPARα are decreased by alcohol exposure, suggesting that PPARα is unlikely to be a major mediator in alcohol-induced hepatic FGF21 expression. Previous studies also identified that FGF21 expression is regulated, either positively or negatively by activating transcription factor 4 (ATF4), liver X receptor (LXR), carbohydrate-responsive element-binding protein (ChREBP) or farnesoid X receptor/retinoid X receptor-α (FXR/RXRα) under multiple pathological or physiological conditions[22]. In particular, application of the endoplasmic reticulum (ER) stressor, tunicamycin, induced hepatic FGF21 expression in mice and a marked elevation of serum FGF21 levels, which can be mimicked by overexpression of ATF4. Studies also indicate that FGF21 expression is induced by ATF4 and C/EBP homologous protein (CHOP)[23], which are two important transcription factors involved in ER stress. Interestingly, previous studies demonstrated that alcohol exposure induces hepatic ER stress in humans[24], experimental animal models[25], and in cultured hepatocytes[26]. It is likely that the alcohol-induced FGF21 expression is regulated by ER stress response in the liver. In fact, the ATF4 DNA binding site has been identified in the FGF21 promoter[23]. Despite the up-regulation of FGF21 expression, treatment with recombinant FGF21 attenuates obesity- and diabetes-induced glucose and lipid dysregulation. Similar to insulin resistance, the enhanced expression of FGF21 has been attributed to a likely "FGF21 resistant state" in obese animals[27]. However, this FGF21 resistant state was not confirmed by other investigators[28], leaving a debate on the nature of FGF21 regulation in the metabolic syndrome. Our results showed that that alcohol exposure and subsequent rhFGF21 treatment enhanced ERK phosphorylation in H4IIE cells (Supplementary Fig. 6), suggesting that alcohol-exposed hepatocytes are not in a FGF21 resistant state. Therefore, exogenous FGF21 could potentially be used as a treatment for alcoholic fatty liver disease.

The enhanced FGF21 expression induced by alcohol is an adaptive response to stimulate cellular defenses against lipid dysregulation. Lack of this adaptive ability in FGF21 KO mice further exacerbated alcohol-induced liver steatosis. These compensatory effects of FGF21 have been demonstrated by others. Up-regulation of FGF21 expression has been shown to protect *ob/ob* mice from toxicity of sepsis[19], and acetaminophen-induced liver injury[29] in mice. A recent study demonstrated that loss of FGF21 induction in general control nonderepressible 2 (GNC2) knockout mice resulted in an exaggerated hepatic steatosis further supporting the notion that FGF21 is important in stimulating cellular defenses against lipid dysregulation[30].

The protective effects of FGF21 in AFLD seem to be closely correlated with *de novo* lipogenesis and fatty acid catabolism. With increased hepatic steatosis, expression and the acetylation levels of hepatic SREBP1c were found to be up-regulated in alcohol exposed FGF21 KO mice leading to enhanced gene expression and activation involved in fatty acid *de novo* synthesis. On the other hand, hepatic PGC1α phosphorylation was severely decreased in FGF21 KO mice exposed to alcohol, leading to a reduction of the expression of genes encoding the molecules responsible for fatty acid β-oxidation. These findings suggest that the loss of FGF21 leads to the dysregulation of lipid metabolism in response to alcohol exposure. Indeed, FGF21 has been shown to regulate these anabolic and catabolic genes at the transcription level in obese and diabetic animals[31]. Phosphorylation of PGC1α increases its ability to interact with PPARα leading to the transcriptional activation[32]. Both AMPK and p38 MAPK phosphorylate PGC1α[13]. We found that phosphor AMPK and p38 levels were severely reduced in FGF21 KO mice exposed to alcohol, indicating a link between FGF21 and

AMPK- and p38-medaited PGC1α activation in alcoholic fatty liver. In addition, high SCD-1 contributes to the suppression of AMPK activity[33]. Therefore, our results can be interpreted to indicate that AMPK and p38 activation mediates the effect of FGF21 on PGC1α activation leading to alteration in fatty acid catabolism in alcoholic fatty liver.

Interestingly, FGF21 ablation markedly decreased the activation of Sirt1 which is a known deacetylase targeting a variety of molecules including SREBP1c and PGC1α. Therefore, it is likely that FGF21 mediates the suppression of hepatic SREBP1c[34,35] and activation of PGC1α[36] through Sirt1 activation in response to alcohol exposure in mice.

A surprising finding was the role of FGF21 in the suppression of alcohol-induced hepatic inflammation. Genetic ablation of FGF21 significantly increased the expression of proinflammatory cytokines in mice exposed to alcohol, suggesting that FGF21 is potentially anti-inflammatory. Our results showed that the anti-inflammatory property of FGF21 was likely mediated by suppression of NFκB activity. Correlating with this finding, a previous study demonstrated that inflammation increases FGF21 expression, which is likely a feedback response to suppress inflammation[19]. Additional studies are needed to evaluate the potential action of FGF21 in the suppression of the activity of NFκB and attenuation of pro-inflammatory cytokines in response to endotoxin and alcohol exposure in Kupffer cells.

The role of FGF21 in ALD appears to be alcohol exposure pattern dependent. Acute alcoholic fatty liver was caused mostly by taking up the mobilized FFAs from adipose tissue[37]; and chronic alcoholic fatty liver involves *in situ* lipogenesis in addition to the increased mobilization of FFAs from adipose tissue[38]. We have demonstrated that chronic-binge alcohol exposure upregulates FGF21 expression which stimulates catecholamine release and enhances adipose tissue lipolysis, leading to increased fat accumulation in the liver[39]. However, in the chronic alcohol exposure model, the enhanced adipose lipolytic effect of FGF21 was overridden by the attenuated *in situ* hepatic lipogeneses and enhanced fatty acid β-oxidation. Further studies dissociating the role of FGF21 in adipose and liver using a tissue specific knock-out strategy in ALD are needed.

A limitation in current study is that the Lieber DeCarli chronic alcohol feeding mouse model induces steatosis with only mild liver injury and inflammation. The protective effects, in particular, the anti-inflammatory effect, of FGF21 need further investigation in more severe rodent models of ALD and in humans to precisely define the potential role of FGF21 in advanced ALD. Unfortunately, there are no experimental models that recapitulate the full progression of ALD in humans.

Regardless this limitation, our findings are relevant to human ALD. Circulating levels of FGF21 are elevated in patients with alcoholic steatohepatitis but not cirrhosis, implying interplay between hepatic fat content and FGF21 expression. Recently, an FGF21 analog, LY2405319, has been developed and used in a randomized, placebo-controlled, double-blind trial in patients with obesity and type 2 diabetes. Patients receiving LY2405319 displayed a significant improvement in dyslipidemia[40], indicating a role of FGF21 in lipid homeostasis in humans. Therefore, FGF21 could potentially be used to treat patients with ALD. Of note, during the submission period, Zhu *et al.* published a paper showing that FGF21 treatment ameliorates ALD in mice[41].

In summary, we demonstrated that loss of FGF21 leads to worsened steatohepatitis in mice chronically exposed to alcohol. Our findings provide novel insights into the functional role of FGF21 in ALD. The effects of FGF21 on AFLD are attributed to multiple factors including the involvement of FGF21 in p38- and AMPK-mediated PGC1α activation in fatty acid catabolism and acetylation of SREBP1c *via* Sirt1 in fatty acid *de novo* synthesis and inflammation (Fig. 7I). The present study suggests that FGF21 treatment reversed the development of experimental ALD and thus prevented the progression of fatty liver to advanced liver disease. Our findings suggest that developing a strategy targeting FGF21 to treat alcoholic steatoheptitis may be warranted.

3. Methods

3.1 *Human studies*

Written informed consent was obtained from all participants. All experiments were conducted in accordance with the guidelines of human research and were approved by Clinical Research Ethics Committees of the University of Louisville and Robley Rex VA Medical Center, Louisville, KY, USA. Samples from patients with alcoholic steatohepatitis (ASH) were selected from a large specimen bank of ASH patients. Patients with severe ASH included in this report all had a liver biopsy during their hospitalization, and a subset of 24 subjects not having underlying cirrhosis was included. All ASH patients had clinical and biochemical evidence of alcoholic hepatitis and further baseline demographic information is provided in Supplementary Table 1. ASH patients were consuming ~46% of total calories (1226 kcal) as alcohol prior to hospitalization, and they had a mean alcohol abuse history of 24 years. Exclusion criteria included: other liver diseases, including viral and metabolic; underlying cancer, and/or active infection. All subjects were active drinking within 1 month of hospitalization.

Twenty patients with alcoholic cirrhosis (AC) had tested supporting a diagnosis of cirrhosis including low platelet count and history or present findings of ascites or esophageal varices, hepatomegaly, history of chronic alcohol intake (>40 g/day for >5 years), as well as exclusion of other causes of cirrhosis, including viral and metabolic. In patients in whom the diagnosis remained uncertain, liver biopsy was performed for histologic confirmation. All subjects were Child-Turcotte-Pugh A or B. Subjects were not actively drinking at the time of study inclusion.

Healthy volunteers were age-, sex-, and BMI-matched to subjects with liver diseases. None of the volunteers had a history of active liver disease.

3.2 Animal studies

Male C57BL/6J mice (wild type, WT) were obtained from Jackson Laboratory (Bar Harbor, Maine). FGF21 KO mice were provided by Dr. Steve Kliewer[42]. All mice were bred in the University of Louisville animal vivarium. The KO mice were back-crossed at least 6 generations onto the C57BL/6 background. Male mice of WT and KO were divided into two groups at 8-10 weeks of age: Lieber DeCarli alcohol diet (alcohol-fed, AF) and isocaloric maltose-dextrin diet (pair-fed, PF) (Bio-Sev, Frenchtown, NJ), as described previous[14]. For the induction of ALD, mice were fed Lieber DeCarli diet with gradually increased alcohol concentration in the first 6 days to reach 5% (w/v) alcohol and were continually on the diet for 28 days. The diet composition was as described as previously[43]. One additional group of alcohol-exposed mice was treated with 4 mg/kg recombinant human FGF21 (rhFGF21)[44] via intraperitoneal injection in the last 5 days. At the end of the experiment, the mice were anesthetized with avertin (2, 2, 2-tribromoethanol). Plasma and tissue samples were collected for assays. All mice were treated according to the protocols reviewed and approved by the Institutional Animal Care and Use Committee of the University of Louisville.

3.3 Blood biochemical assays

Mouse blood samples were centrifuged at 1500 g for 30 min at 4℃ to obtain plasma. Plasma variables were measured using commercial kits closely following the manufacturer's instructions. Alanine aminotransferase (ALT) and aspartate aminotransferase (AST) levels were measured using ALT and AST Assay Kits (Thermo Fisher Scientific Inc., Middletown, VA). Free fatty acids, glycerol, cholesterol and triglyceride levels were quantified using commercial kits (Wako Chemicals, Richmond, VA). IL6 and MCP1 concentrations were measured using commercial kits (Life technologies, Gaithersburg, MD, USA). Mouse blood alcohol concen- trations were measured using a commercial kit (Abcam, Cambridgeshire, UK).

FGF21 concentrations in the plasma of mice and in serum of humans were measured using ELISA kits from Biovendor, Modrice, Czech Republic and R&D, Minneapolis, MN, respectively.

3.4 Liver triglyceride assay

For the liver triglyceride assay, 70-100 mg of liver tissue was homogenized in 1 ml of 50 mM NaCl. Homogenate (500 μl) was mixed with 4 ml of the extraction reagent (methanol:chloroform = 1:2) and incubated overnight at 4℃ before being centrifuged at 1,800 g for 20 min at room temperature. The lower chloroform phase was carefully collected and dried using a Speed Vac, and the pellets were used for triglyceride assay using the Triglyceride Kit (Thermo Fisher Scientific Inc.).

3.5 Determination of hepatic cytokine and chemokine concentration

Fifty to seventy mg liver tissue was homogenized in RIPA buffer (50 mM Tris·HCl, pH 7.4, 150 mM NaCl, 2 mM EDTA, 4 mM Na_3VO_4, 40 mM NaF, 1% Triton X-100, 1 mM phenylmethylsulfonyl fluoride, 1% protease inhibitor cocktail)[14]. TNFα, IL6 and MCP1 protein levels were measured using their respective ELISA kits (BD, Sparks, MD, USA) according to the manufacturer's instructions. The values were expressed in pg/mg total protein.

3.6 Liver histology and fat analyses

The liver sections were fixed in formalin and embedded in paraffin. The sliced liver sections were then stained with H&E as described previously[14]. For hepatic fat visualization, frozen liver sections were processed for staining with Oil red O and then studied by light microscopy[43].

3.7 Liver neutrophil accumulation

Formalin-fixed paraffin-embedded liver sections were deparaffinized and rehydrated. Neutrophils were stained using a naphthol AS-D chloroacetate (Specific Esterase) (CAE) staining kit (Sigma-Aldrich, St. Louis, MO) according to the manufacturer's directions[45].

3.8 TUNEL assay

Formalin-fixed paraffin liver sections were sectioned at 5 μm. The sections were stained for TUNEL with the ApopTag Peroxidase *in situ* Apoptosis Detection Kit (Chemicon, CA, USA). In brief, the slides were deparaffinized and rehydrated, then treated with proteinase K (20 μg/ml) for 15 min at room temperature. Slides were treated with 3% hydrogen peroxide for 5 min to quench endogenous peroxidases, and then incubated with terminal deoxynucleotidyl transferase (TdT) and anti-digoxigenin-peroxidase at 37℃ for 1 h or 30 min respectively. Diaminobenzidine (DAB) was then applied. Hematoxylin was used as counterstaining. Under the microscope, apoptotic cells exhibited a brown nuclear stain as the TUNEL positive and were counted manually.

3.9 Quantitative real time RT-PCR

The mRNA levels were assessed by real-time RT-PCR. In brief, total RNA was isolated with Trizol according to manufacturer's protocol (Invitrogen, Carlsbad, CA) and reverse-transcribed using GenAmp RNA PCR kit (Applied Biosystems, Foster City, CA). The cDNA was amplified in 96-well reaction plates with a SYBR green PCR Master Mix (Applied Biosystems) on an ABI 7500 real-time PCR thermocycler. The sequences of forward and reverse primers are listed in Supplementary Table 2. The relative quantities of target transcripts were calculated from duplicate samples after normalization by a housekeeping gene, β-actin. Dissociation curve analysis was performed after PCR amplification to confirm the specificity of the primers. Relative mRNA expression was calculated using the ΔΔCt method.

3.10 Immunoprecipitation and Western blot analysis

For immunoprecipitation, 1 mg of tissue lysate was incubated with 2 μg of antibody (anti-SREBP1c) at 4℃ overnight. After the addition of 40 μl PureProteome™ Protein A/G Mix Magnetic Beads (Millipore), incubation was continued for an additional 2 h at 4℃. The beads were then collected by magnet and washed three times with washing buffer (PBS containing 0.1% Tween 20). 2× SDS sample buffer was added to the beads and incubated at 95℃ for 10 min, and Western blot was then performed. Acetylated SREBP1c was detected by an anti-acetylated lysine antibody (Cell Signaling, Danvers, MA, USA).

Western blot was performed as described previously[14] to detect precursor and mature forms of SREBP1c (Santa Cruz Biotechnologies, Santa Cruz, CA), pAMPK, AMPK, p-p38, p38, SCD1, Sirt1, acetylated-lysine (Cell Signaling Technologies), FGF21 (Abcam, San Francisco, CA), PPARα, PGC1α, β-actin (Santa Cruz Biotechnology), p-PGC1α (R&D, Minneapolis, MN). Blots were scanned using a Bio-Rad Imaging System (Image Lab™ Upgrade for Chemi-Doc™ XRS + System #170-8299). All specific bands were quantified with the Automated Digitizing System (Image Lab 4.1). Results are representative of three independent experiments.

3.11 Isolation and culture of primary hepatocytes

Hepatocytes were isolated from the WT and FGF21 KO mice by *in situ* digestion of the liver with perfusion of collagenase type IV. Briefly, total liver tissues were perfused with EGTA solution (10 mM HEPES [pH 7.4], 5 mM glucose, 138 mM NaCl, 5.4 mM KCl, 28.3 mM NaHCO$_3$, 0.12 mM Na$_2$HPO$_4$, 0.56 mM NaH$_2$PO$_4$ and 0.5 mM EGTA) into the inferior vena cava. After perfusion, the liver tissues were dissociated into hepatocytes using collagenase solution (10 mM HEPES [pH 7.4], 138 mM NaCl, 5.4 mM KCl, 28.3 mM NaHCO$_3$, 0.12 mM Na$_2$HPO$_4$, 0.56 mM NaH$_2$PO$_4$ supplemented with 0.0857 U/ml type IV collagenase (Roche Diagnostics, Indianapolis, IN) and 3.8 mM CaCl$_2$). Subsequently, the isolated hepatocytes were washed with serum-free Waymouths medium (Gibco BRL, Life Technologies, Inc., Grand Island, NY) and suspended in Waymouths medium supplemented with 10% (*w/v*) fetal bovine serum (FBS) (Gibco BRL, Life Technologies, Inc.), Antibiotic-Antimycotic (Gibco 100 units/mL of penicillin, 100 μg/mL of streptomycin, 0.25 μg/ml of Fungizone) and ITS supplement (VWR). Cell viability was assessed by the trypan blue exclusion test. Isolated hepatocytes were seeded at a density of 3.5×10^5 cells/dish in 35-mm tissue culture dishes and maintained at 37℃ in 5% CO_2. After cell attachment (approximately 4 hours), the culture media were replaced with fresh media for treatment. All cell culture experiments were carried out with the guidelines of biosafety and approved by the Biosafety Committee of the University of Louisville.

3.12 Cell culture and treatment

Mouse AML-12 hepatocytes were provided by Dr. Min You at Northeast Ohio Medical College and were cultured in DMEM/F12 medium (ATCC) supplemented with 10% FBS, 100 μg/ml streptomysin, 100 Unit/mL penicillin, 0.1 μM dexamethasone, and insulin-transferrin-selenium (ITS; Life technologies). Cells were treated with rhFGF21 (1 μg/ml and 3 μg/ml) for 24 hours. Fixed cells were then incubated with anti-Sirt1 antibody (1:100, Cell Signaling) overnight at 4 ℃. Alexa Fluor 488 goat anti-rabbit IgG(H + L) (1 : 500, Life Technologies) was used to visualizing Sirt1 expression. DAPI was used to detect nuclei. Images were obtained with EVOS® FL Cell Imaging System (Life Technologies).

H4IIE cells were purchased from ATCC and maintained in 10% FBS in Eagle's Minimum Essential Medium (ATCC) containing 100 Unit/ml penicillin and 10 μg/ml streptomycin at 37 ℃ under a 5% CO_2 atmosphere. H4IIE cells were exposed to alcohol (100 mM) for 72 hours, and then incubated with rhFGF21 (1 μg/ml) for 5, 10, 20 or 60 minutes, respectively. ERK phosphorylation was detected by Western blot analysis.

3.13 Statistical analysis

Data are expressed as means ± SEM. Two-way ANOVA with Bonferroni post-test, or One-way ANOVA with Tukey post-test, or two-tailed unpaired Student's t-test were used for the determination of statistical significance of the data where they were appropriate. All statistical analyses were performed with GraphPad Prism software Version 5 (GraphPad Software, Inc., San Diego, CA). Differences between groups were considered significant at $^*P < 0.05$, $^{**}P < 0.01$, $^{***}P < 0.001$. For animal study, n = 5-12 per group. For cell culture study, the experiments were performed in duplicate and repeated 3 times.

Additional information

Supplementary information to this article can be found online at http://dx.doi.org/10.1038/srep31026.

References

[1] Bensinger SJ, Tontonoz P. Integration of metabolism and inflammation by lipid-activated nuclear receptors [J]. Nature, 2008, 454(7203): 470-477.

[2] You M, Fischer M, Deeg MA, et al. Ethanol induces fatty acid synthesis pathways by activation of sterol regulatory element-binding protein (SREBP) [J]. Journal Of Biological Chemistry, 2002, 277(32): 29342-29347.

[3] Li Y, Wong K, Giles A, et al. Hepatic sirt1 attenuates hepatic steatosis and controls energy balance in mice by inducing fibroblast growth factor 21 [J]. Gastroenterology, 2014, 146(2): 539-549.

[4] You M, Matsumoto M, Pacold CM, et al. The role of AMP-activated protein kinase in the action of ethanol in the liver [J]. Gastroenterology, 2004, 127(6): 1798-1808.

[5] Leung TM, Nieto N. CYP2E1 and oxidant stress in alcoholic and non-alcoholic fatty liver disease [J]. Journal Of Hepatology, 2013, 58(2): 395-398.

[6] Kharitonenkov A, Shiyanova TL, Koester A, et al. FGF-21 as a nov-

el metabolic regulator [J]. Journal Of Clinical Investigation, 2005, 115(6): 1627-1635.

[7] Tacer KF, Bookout AL, Ding X, et al. Research resource: comprehensive expression atlas of the fibroblast growth factor system in adult mouse [J]. Molecular Endocrinology, 2010, 24(10): 2050-2064.

[8] Tanaka N, Takahashi S, Zhang Y, et al. Role of fibroblast growth factor 21 in the early stage of NASH induced by methionine- and choline-deficient diet [J]. Biochimica et Biophysica Acta (BBA)-Molecular Basis of Disease, 2015, 1852(7): 1242-1252.

[9] Talukdar S, Owen BM, Song P, et al. FGF21 regulates sweet and alcohol preference [J]. Cell Metabolism, 2016, 23(2): 344-349.

[10] You M, Liang X, Ajmo JM, et al. Involvement of mammalian sirtuin 1 in the action of ethanol in the liver [J]. American Journal Of Physiology-Gastrointestinal And Liver Physiology, 2008, 294(4): G892-G898.

[11] Yin H, Hu M, Liang X, et al. Deletion of sirt1 from hepatocytes in

mice disrupts lipin-1 signaling and aggravates alcoholic fatty liver [J]. Gastroenterology, 2014, 146(3): 801-811.

[12] Caton PW, Nayuni NK, Kieswich J, et al. Metformin suppresses hepatic gluconeogenesis through induction of SIRT1 and GCN5 [J]. Journal Of Endocrinology, 2010, 205(1): 97-106.

[13] Puigserver P, Rhee J, Lin JD, et al. Cytokine stimulation of energy expenditure through p38 MAP kinase activation of PPAR gamma coactivator-1 [J]. Molecular Cell, 2001, 8(5): 971-982.

[14] Wang Y, Kirpich I, Liu Y, et al. Lactobacillus rhamnosus GG treatment potentiates intestinal hypoxia-inducible factor, promotes intestinal integrity and ameliorates alcohol-induced liver injury [J]. American Journal Of Pathology, 2011, 179(6): 2866-2875.

[15] Wang Y, Liu Y, Kirpich I, et al. Lactobacillus rhamnosus GG reduces hepatic TNF alpha production and inflammation in chronic alcohol-induced liver injury [J]. Journal Of Nutritional Biochemistry, 2013, 24(9): 1609-1615.

[16] Zhang X, Yeung DCY, Karpisek M, et al. Serum FGF21 levels are increased in obesity and are independently associated with the metabolic syndrome in humans [J]. Diabetes, 2008, 57(5): 1246-1253.

[17] Li H, Fang Q, Gao F, et al. Fibroblast growth factor 21 levels are increased in nonalcoholic fatty liver disease patients and are correlated with hepatic triglyceride [J]. Journal Of Hepatology, 2010, 53(5): 934-940.

[18] Dushay J, Chui PC, Gopalakrishnan GS, et al. Increased fibroblast growth factor 21 in obesity and nonalcoholic fatty liver disease [J]. Gastroenterology, 2010, 139(2): 456-463.

[19] Feingold KR, Grunfeld C, Heuer JG, et al. FGF21 is increased by inflammatory stimuli and protects leptin-deficient ob/ob mice from the toxicity of sepsis [J]. Endocrinology, 2012, 153(6): 2689-2700.

[20] Inagaki T, Dutchak P, Zhao G, et al. Endocrine regulation of the fasting response by PPAR alpha-mediated induction of fibroblast growth factor 21 [J]. Cell Metabolism, 2007, 5(6): 415-425.

[21] Dutchak PA, Katafuchi T, Bookout AL, et al. Fibroblast growth factor-21 regulates PPAR gamma activity and the antidiabetic actions of thiazolidinediones [J]. Cell, 2012, 148(3): 556-567.

[22] Bae K-H, Kim J-G, Park K-G. Transcriptional regulation of fibroblast growth factor 21 expression [J]. Endocrinology And Metabolism, 2014, 29(2): 105-111.

[23] Schaap FG, Kremer AE, Lamers WH, et al. Fibroblast growth factor 21 is induced by endoplasmic reticulum stress [J]. Biochimie, 2013, 95(4): 692-699.

[24] Longato L, Ripp K, Setshedi M, et al. Insulin resistance, ceramide accumulation, and endoplasmic reticulum stress in human chronic alcohol-related liver disease [J]. Oxidative Medicine And Cellular Longevity, 2012.

[25] Galligan JJ, Smathers RL, Shearn CT, et al. Oxidative stress and the er stress response in a murine model for early-stage alcoholic liver disease [J]. Journal Of Toxicology, 2012.

[26] Magne L, Blanc E, Legrand B, et al. ATF4 and the integrated stress response are induced by ethanol and cytochrome P450 2E1 in human hepatocytes [J]. Journal Of Hepatology, 2011, 54(4): 729-737.

[27] Fisher FM, Chui PC, Antonellis PJ, et al. Obesity is a fibroblast growth factor 21 (FGF21)-resistant state [J]. Diabetes, 2010, 59(11): 2781-2789.

[28] Murata Y, Nishio K, Mochiyama T, et al. Fgf21 impairs adipocyte insulin sensitivity in mice fed a low-carbohydrate, high-fat ketogenic diet [J]. Plos One, 2013, 8(7).

[29] Ye D, Wang Y, Li H, et al. Fibroblast growth factor 21 protects against acetaminophen-induced hepatotoxicity by potentiating

peroxisome proliferator-activated receptor coactivator protein-1α-mediated antioxidant capacity in mice [J]. Hepatology, 2014, 60(3): 977-989.

[30] Wilson GJ, Lennox BA, She P, et al. GCN2 is required to increase fibroblast growth factor 21 and maintain hepatic triglyceride homeostasis during asparaginase treatment [J]. American Journal Of Physiology-Endocrinology And Metabolism, 2015, 308(4): E283-E293.

[31] Mai K, Andres J, Biedasek K, et al. Free fatty acids link metabolism and regulation of the insulin-sensitizing fibroblast growth factor-21 [J]. Diabetes, 2009, 58(7): 1532-1538.

[32] Liang H, Ward WF. PGC-1 alpha: a key regulator of energy metabolism [J]. Advances In Physiology Education, 2006, 30(4): 145-151.

[33] Scaglia N, Chisholm JW, Igal RA. Inhibition of StearoylCoA Desaturase-1 Inactivates Acetyl-CoA Carboxylase and Impairs Proliferation in Cancer Cells: Role of AMPK [J]. Plos One, 2009, 4(8).

[34] Ponugoti B, Kim D-H, Xiao Z, et al. Sirt1 deacetylates and inhibits SREBP-1c activity in regulation of hepatic lipid metabolism [J]. Journal Of Biological Chemistry, 2010, 285(44): 33959-33970.

[35] You M, Jogasuria A, Taylor C, et al. Sirtuin 1 signaling and alcoholic fatty liver disease [J]. Hepatobiliary Surgery And Nutrition, 2015, 4(2): 88-100.

[36] Chau MDL, Gao J, Yang Q, et al. Fibroblast growth factor 21 regulates energy metabolism by activating the AMPK-SIRT1-PGC-1 alpha pathway [J]. Proceedings Of the National Academy Of Sciences Of the United States Of America, 2010, 107(28): 12553-12558.

[37] Horning MG, Williams EA, Maling HM, et al. Depot fat as source of increased liver triglycerides after ethanol [J]. Biochemical And Biophysical Research Communications, 1960, 3(6): 635-640.

[38] Muramatsu M, Kuriyama K, Yuki T, et al. Hepatic lipogenesis and mobilization of peripheral fats in the formation of alcoholic fatty liver [J]. Japanese Journal Of Pharmacology, 1981, 31(6): 931-940.

[39] Zhao C, Liu Y, Xiao J, et al. FGF21 mediates alcohol-induced adipose tissue lipolysis by activation of systemic release of catecholamine in mice [J]. Journal Of Lipid Research, 2015, 56(8): 1481-1491.

[40] Gaich G, Chien JY, Fu H, et al. The Effects of LY2405319, an FGF21 analog, in obese human subjects with type 2 diabetes [J]. Cell Metabolism, 2013, 18(3): 333-340.

[41] Zhu S, Ma L, Wu Y, et al. FGF21 treatment ameliorates alcoholic fatty liver through activation of AMPK-SIRT1 pathway [J]. Acta Biochimica Et Biophysica Sinica, 2014, 46(12): 1041-1048.

[42] Potthoff MJ, Inagaki T, Satapati S, et al. FGF21 induces PGC-1 alpha and regulates carbohydrate and fatty acid metabolism during the adaptive starvation response [J]. Proceedings Of the National Academy Of Sciences Of the United States Of America, 2009, 106(26): 10853-10858.

[43] Wang Y, Liu Y, Sidhu A, et al. Lactobacillus rhamnosus GG culture supernatant ameliorates acute alcohol-induced intestinal permeability and liver injury [J]. American Journal Of Physiology-Gastrointestinal And Liver Physiology, 2012, 303(1): G32-G41.

[44] Inagaki T, Lin VY, Goetz R, et al. Inhibition of growth hormone signaling by the fasting-induced hormone FGF21 [J]. Cell Metabolism, 2008, 8(1): 77-83.

[45] Osburn WO, Yates MS, Dolan PD, et al. Genetic or pharmacologic amplification of Nrf2 signaling inhibits acute inflammatory liver injury in mice [J]. Toxicological Sciences, 2008, 104(1): 218-227.

Delivery of growth factor-based therapeutics in vascular diseases: challenges and strategies

Helin Xu, Xiaokun Li, Yingzheng Zhao

1. Introduction

Vascular disease has become the major cause of morbidity and mortality worldwide [1]. Many deleterious factors, including atherosclerosis, the narrowing of the arteries and plaque deposition inside small blood vessels, are the primary cause of this disease. When the blood vessels of the brain, heart and lower limbs are attacked, resulting in vessel occlusion and blockage of blood flow, severe damage and dysfunction of these organs or tissues will subsequently appear because of ischemic injury. Ischemic injury usually includes both acute and chronic conditions. For example, ischemia can manifest as angina, acute coronary syndrome and chronic heart failure in the heart, as stroke in the brain, and as critical limb ischemia in peripheral blood. The prevention and treatment of vascular diseases has been an important subject in modern medicine. Currently, although several treatments for blocked blood vessels have been developed, such as angioplasty, stenting, thrombolysis and surgical bypass, these treatments have inherent drawbacks and do not typically focus on the regeneration of damaged blood vessels or their affiliated organs, which is important for vascular diseases [2].

More attention has been paid to the repair and regeneration of damaged blood vessels or tissues after ischemic injury. Many novel therapeutic strategies for regenerating tissue have been developed. Most focused on the natural mechanism by which blood vessel formation is initiated and neovasculature becomes mature. This process is known as therapeutic angiogenesis, one of the most active areas in tissue engineering. Recently, growth factor- or stem cell-based therapy have been promising because of therapeutic angiogenesis. These growth factors include vascular endothelial growth factor (VEGF), fibroblast growth factor family (FGF), hepatocyte growth factor (HGF), insulin-like growth factor (IGF) and transforming growth factor-β (TGF-β). Although growth factors (both as proteins and genes) have shown promising clinical perspective in CVD treatment, this therapy did not generate consistent benefits as expected. For example, the direct injection of naked plasmids carrying genes is ineffective due to low cellular transfection efficiency. Moreover, virus-based vectors raised safety issues. The random insertion into the host cell genome may also lead to persistent expression of growth factors, which raises the concern for developing pathological angiogenesis or tumorigenesis [3]. Alternatively, using recombinant protein-based growth factors can reduce these safety issues at some level. However, the short circulation half-lives and low stability of these growth factors limit their widespread application in vascular diseases. Multiple injections are required to achieve satisfactory therapeutic effects, which may expose the diseased vascellum to high doses of growth factor, resulting in adverse effects such as hypotension [4], vascular leakage [5] and tissue edema [6].

Another strategy of promoting vascularization is cell-based therapy. Various cell types are known to participate in angiogenesis, including differentiated cells, such as endothelial cells (ECs), and non-differentiated stem cells, such as endothelial progenitor cells (EPCs), adipose-derived stem cells and mesenchymal stem cells. However, due to heterogeneity in both cell phenotypes and genotypes between individuals, as well as low differentiation rates, EC-based therapy has not attracted attention from researchers for tissue engineering and regenerative medicine applications. In contrast, interest has transferred to stem cells or progenitor cells because of their easy availability and multiple differentiations. For example, EPCs can be originated from adipose tissues [7], umbilical cord blood [8] and bone marrow [9]. When transported to the ischemic tissues, these progenitor cells engraft on the ischemic zone, migrate alongside the extracellular matrix, and finally differentiate into mature ECs. Interestingly, despite not being vascellum-derived cells, MSCs also play a vital role in angiogenesis through the paracrine release of angiogenic factors, which have been well documented. Additionally, MSCs are also capable of differentiating into cardiomyocyte-like cells, rendering them suitable for cardiac regeneration [10]. Several routes for delivering cells, including direct intravenous (iv), intracoronary (ic) or epicardial injection, or transplantation to diseased tissues, are available so far, but the low cell survival and lack of precisely targeted localization of cells have become the major bottleneck for their wide application [11-13]. Moreover, the safety of stem cell therapy is also concerning because of their oncologic potential and the possibility of triggering a cancer recurrence. Many factors unique to stem cell-based therapy, such as tissue revascularization, multipotentiality, immunomodulatory effects, and cell homing and migration, are highly correlated with many neoplasias and aid in tumor progression and metastasis, which has been reviewed in an excellent work [14]. Thus, tumorigenesis of cell-based therapy was not the focus of this review and more attention was focused on how to improve cell survival.

In this overview, we focus on recent developments in the field of growth factor-based therapeutics for vascular diseases. First, we provide a summary of various therapeutic strategies related to growth factors. Then, the confronting challenges for these types of therapeutics are reviewed. Lastly, potential strategies are proposed.

2. Therapeutic modes choices based on growth factor therapeutics for vascular diseases

Angiogenesis is a complex process that requires the coordination of multiple cell type and growth factor gradients. Vasculogenesis and angiogenesis are the two main mechanisms for the healing and regeneration of vasculature. During vasculogenesis, *de novo* blood vessels are initially formed, which largely occurs during embryogenesis. Sometimes, under stimuli such as growth factor gradients, vasculogenesis may also occur in the adult through activating EPCs and subsequent differentiation to the vascular lineage, such as mature ECs. These EPCs associated with vasculogenesis, generally having typical stem cell-like phenotypes such as Flk-1, CD34, or CD133 expression, can be originated from bone marrow or peripheral blood [2]. Angiogenesis is the formation of new blood vessels by sprouting from existing vessels, consisting of four chronological steps. ECs play an important role in angiogenesis. First, the quiescent endothelial cells are activated by angiogenic factors. Next, the surrounding capillary basal lamina is degraded by extracellular proteinases, such as matrix metalloproteinases (MMPs), secreted by the activated ECs. Then, capillary sprouting and EC migration occur, and neovascellum forms. Finally, the neovascellum gradually becomes mature under the stimulus of other growth factors, such as angiopoietin-1 or platelet derived growth factor (PDGF).

Because these growth factors associated with angiogenesis, such as FGF, VEGF and PDGF, are effective regulators of cellular signals during the formation of new and stable vascular vessels, their exogenous forms have been proven to be effective therapeutics to treat cardiovascular diseases, including myocardial infarction (MI) and peripheral vascular disease. Although stem cell-based therapy was not included with growth factors, stem cells associated with neovascularization play an important role in vasculogenesis due to their high cell differentiation potential toward mature cells and the paracrine secretion of growth factors. Thus, stem cell-related therapy is also included in this review (Fig. 1).

2.1 Angiogenic growth factor therapy

Growth factor-related therapeutics, such as exogenous growth factor or growth factor-related gene therapy, have played an important role in angiogenesis, and are therefore explored for the prevention and therapy of cardiovascular and peripheral vascular diseases. Of particular note, since their discovery from neural tissue extracts in 1974, fibroblast growth factors (FGFs) have made a significant impact on cardiovascular research because of their potential role in angiogenesis. The functions of the exogenous FGFs and the molecular mechanisms of tissue repair and regeneration after ischemia injury have been the focus of intense research in the field of regenerative medicine. The FGF family is a multigene family of polypeptide/protein-based growth factors that recognize their corresponding cell surface receptors (FGFR) with high affinity to mediate their effects [15]. The biological and molecular aspects of acidic FGF (FGF-1 or aFGF) and basic FGF (FGF-2 or bFGF) have been extensively characterized, and are regarded as the prototypical FGF families [16, 17]. FGF-2 is a multifunctional protein synthesized as high (Hi-) and low (Lo-) molecular weight isoforms. Studies using rodent models showed that Hi- and Lo-FGF-2 exert distinct biological activities. Lo-FGF-2 promoted sustained cardioprotection and angiogenesis after myocardial infarction, while Hi-FGF-2 promoted myocardial hypertrophy and reduced contractile function [18]. Hi-FGF-2 is overexpressed, secreted and localized in human myocardium when exposed to stress stimuli such as oxidative stress and heat shock. Hi-FGF-2 is a potential target for prevention of cardiac remodeling in the human heart [19]. The therapeutic FGF-2 isoform is usually the low-molecular-weight isoform (ca. 18 kDa; Lo-

FGF-2). In the isolated rat heart, the infarct limitation effects were first demonstrated by pretreatment with exogenous FGF-2. Thereafter, in the *in situ* canine heart model, reduced infarct sizes were also observed after intracoronary administration of exogenous FGF-2 (17.3 kDa). Yanagisawa-Miwa *et al.* first demonstrated that the infarct-limiting effect of exogenous FGF-2 was attributed to its angiogenic potential [20]. Several phase I/II human trials are evaluating the benefit of FGF-2 based therapeutics in the form of genes or proteins to improve perfusion in vascular diseases [21, 22]. The other known family members, including FGF-23, FGF-10, FGF-20, FGF-5, FGF-6, and FGF-7/KGF, are effective in tissue repair and regeneration. The detailed therapeutic uses of the FGF family were reviewed in a recent, excellent work [23].

Endogenous VEGF also played a crucial role in angiogenesis *via* cell migration, proliferation, and survival; exogenous VEGF has been examined in clinical trials as a therapeutic strategy in chronic ischemic heart disease [24]. The cardioprotective effect of exogenous VEGF in the acute ischemic animal model was first demonstrated by Luo *et al.* Perfusion of isolated rat hearts with exogenous VEGF improved functional heart recovery and reduced cardiac enzyme release following a sustained period of ischemia-reperfusion injury [25]. Afterward, in a Phase I clinical trial, 178 patients with stable exertional angina were randomly administered with placebo, low-dose (17 ng/kg/min), or high-dose recombinant VEGF (rhVEGF, 50 ng/kg/min) through an intracoronary at day 0, followed by intravenous infusions at days 3, 6, and 9. The high-dose rhVEGF resulted in significant improvement in anginal symptoms at 120 days [26].

HGF, the most potent exogenous angiogenic growth factor identified to date, has multiple effects on cell morphogenesis, migration, proliferation, angiogenesis and anti-inflammation [27]. HGF exerts its effect on angiogenesis *via* regulating either endothelial or vascular smooth muscle cells. HGF binds its C-met receptor on these cell surfaces and subsequently induces activation of Ets-1, which in turn stimulates regional release of angiogenic cytokines, to produce an angiogenic effect [28]. Results of a double-blind and placebo-controlled study using an HGF plasmid have been more encouraging, with significant improvements in limb blood perfusion for patients with critical limb ischemia. In HGF plasmid-treated patients, 100% ulcer healing was observed, and the phase II trial was terminated early; only a 40% improvement of ulcer healing was observed in the placebo-treated groups [29] Additionally, the good safety of the HGF plasmid for IM injections was confirmed by Morishita *et al.* in two phase II trials, which promoted its entrance into phase III clinical trials [30, 31]. Treatment with HGF plasmid to induce overexpression of Ets-1 has been studied in phase III clinical trials [32].

IGF (IGF-I and IGF-II) are widely expressed in the body and are involved in the regulation of cell growth, differentiation, and survival through binding to their tyrosine kinase receptors. Suleiman *et al.* demonstrated that IGF-I reduced myocardial necrosis, apoptosis, and neutrophil accumulation [33]. Afterward, it was found that transgenic mice overexpressing IGF-I exhibited reduced myocardial infarcts and cardiac remodeling, and inhibition of cell apoptosis at seven days post-myocardial in-farction, suggesting the long-term cardioprotective benefits of IGF-I. The cardioprotection of exogenous IGF-1 has also been effective in patients with cardiac failure. A clinical trial enrolled 86 human healthy volunteers and 87 patients with cardiac failure to evaluate therapeutic effect of IGF-1 [34]. After administration of exogenous IGF-I (60 mg/kg) through intramuscular injection, a significant decrease in stroke volume and obvious increase in cardiac output and ejection fraction were observed for patients with cardiac failure. Meanwhile, the blood glucose was less affected.

Transforming growth factor beta (TGF-β) has redundant biological activities, such as angiogenesis, cardiac development and vascular fibrosis [35, 36]. Dysregulated TGF-β signaling is commonly associated with fibrosis, aberrant angiogenesis and accelerated progression into heart failure. TGF-β exists in three different isoforms (1, 2 and 3); the intracellular signaling cascades activated by TGF-β1, TGF-β2, and TGF-β3 have been extensively studied in the process of mediating angiogenesis and heart development. Lefer *et al.* first demonstrated that pretreatment with TGF-β1 could reduce the myocardial injury of rat heart *in vivo* or *ex vivo* [37]. Then, they found that treatment with TGF-β1 after myocardial ischemia and 30 min before myocardial reperfusion decreased the myocardial infarct size of feline heart subjected to 1.5 h ischemia and 4.5 h reperfusion [38]. Moreover, TGF-β1 targeted lethal myocardial reperfusion injury and reduced myocardial infarct size when administered at the time of myocardial reperfusion [39]. Chen *et al.* reported that pretreatment with TGF-β1 improved the cell survival of adult rat cardiomyocytes following ischemia-reperfusion injury [40]. In addition, endothelial-mesenchymal transition, a process involved in heart development, was enhanced by hypoxia in response to TGF-β2 [41]. However, TGF-β1 and TGF-β3 expression was increased in the atria of cardiac disease-affected dogs [42]. Therefore, a potential therapeutic pathway is to modulate TGF-β signaling. However, broad blockage of TGF-β signaling may cause unwanted side effects due to its pivotal role in tissue homeostasis. The specific modulation of TGF-β isoforms involved in the pathogenesis of heart failure has been excellently reviewed [43].

Neuregulin-1 (NRG-1), a member of the neuregulin growth factor family, has been implicated in a number of cellular processes *via* paracrine and juxtacrine signaling during cardiac development, homeostasis, and disease [44]. The discovery of neuregulins was first made in the context of cancer and neural research, and its crucial role in cardiac development was discovered in the late 1990s. NRG-1 regulates cardiovascular homeostasis during development and adulthood by stimulating recruitment and proliferation of cardiac progenitors and cardiomyocytes, as well as inducing angiogenesis, vasculogenesis, and cardiac remodeling [45]. The potential of NRG-1 to be a therapeutic agent throughout this time course from a biostimulant in stem cell therapy to a possible biomarker or drug during cardiac disease was enhanced in recent years.

2.2 Combinational therapy of multiple growth factors

In addition to mediators of angiogenesis, the list of potential therapeutics for cardiac regeneration has continued to grow, and the use of factors involved in cardiac development, stem cell homing, cardiac differentiation/proliferation, or direct cardioprotection could lead to novel approaches for repairing a damaged heart. FGF-1 regulates cardiac remodeling by exerting a protective and proliferative effect on adult cardiomyocytes after MI. On the other hand, neuregulins play crucial roles in the adult cardiovascular system by inducing angiogenesis, cell survival, cell integrity and cell-cell adhesion. The efficacy of combinational delivery of NRG-1 and FGF-1 by using novel microsphere-based delivery was examined by evaluating cardiac function, heart tissue remodeling and revascularization [46]. The combinational therapy led to the inhibition of cardiac remodeling with smaller infarct size, lower fibrosis degree and induction of tissue revascularization.

2.3 Stem cell-based therapy

Cell-based therapy is another strategy of promoting vascularization. Multiple trials have been initiated addressing the transplantation of stem cell populations for cardiac regeneration. Vasculogenesis-related stem cells derived from bone marrow, adipose tissues and umbilical cord blood have been broadly used in the repair or regeneration of angiogenesis due to their high potential capability of differentiation and proliferation [2]. The therapeutic stem cells are easily aspirated from adult bone marrow, a major reservoir for various stem cell populations. The phenotypes of stem cells are diverse, including human mesenchymal stem cells (hMSCs), endothelial progenitor cells, and hematopoietic stem cells. Heterogeneous stem cell populations from bone marrow, e.g. bone marrow aspirate or lineage-unselected bone marrow derived mononuclear cells (BMMNCs), have been used for a significant number of preliminary clinical studies, demonstrating the safety and feasibility of BMMNC administration [47]. Moreover, several studies using heterogeneous populations of bone marrow-derived stem cells have demonstrated that the mixed phenotypes of stem and progenitor cell types could also exert therapeutic effects in ischemia models when these cells are injected locally into the ischemic zone [48, 49].

Recently, bone marrow aspirate has been further purified by phenotypic features into two multipotent cell populations: hMSCs and EPCs. Purified stem cell populations show higher engraftment and can induce endogenous cardiomyogenesis. For example, EPCs can engraft onto the ischemic zone, migrate alongside extracellular matrix, and finally differentiate into mature ECs, while hMSCs induce angiogenesis *via* the paracrine release of some angiogenic factors [50]. In addition, hMSCs are also capable of differentiating into cardiomyocyte-like cells, rendering them suitable for cardiac regeneration [10]. Adipose tissue is also being used as a source of hMSCs. Adipose-derived stem cells (ADSCs) showed similar improvements in cardiac function and increased capillaries in a porcine MI model as bone marrow stem cells [51]. Transplantation of ADSCs in a preclinical model of ischemia/reperfusion also induced a statistically significant long-lasting (three months) improvement in cardiac function and geometry in comparison with control animals [52]. A paracrine-mediated effect of ADSCs dominated in cardiovascular repair and regeneration. Bone marrow aspirate from adults was subjected to isolation of progenitor CD34-positive EPCs using appropriate cell-separation techniques. When CD34-positive EPCs were injected into ischemic muscle, they can adhere to ischemic endothelium and promote new blood vessel formation [113] However, because of the lack of an exclusive cell surface antigen that can accurately isolate a pure population of stem cells from the bone marrow samples, it is not clear whether a stem cell with a pure phenotype is necessary. The details of cell-based therapy in heart infarct have been excellently reviewed in the literature [47].

2.4 Combinational therapy of growth factors and stem cell

The injected stem cells had a low survival rate after transplantation in almost all of these studies. Some growth factors can home to these stem cells and improve their survival rate. Stromal-derived factor-1 (SDF-1) is one of the homing factors used for recruitment of bone marrow stem cells to the area of ischemia [53]. By binding with its associated receptor CXCR4, SDF-1 stimulates cell growth, proliferation, and migration, as well as recruitment and retention, in repair zones such as MI. Delivery of SDF-1 to the ischemic area decreases apoptosis and increases the survival of bone marrow stem cells in the infarct zone [54]. Clinical improvements in CLI (Critical Limb Ischemia) patient symptoms were also reported upon intramuscular injection of both autologous bone marrow mononuclear cells and VEGF plasmids, leading to improved perfusion–ABI (ankle-brachial-index) increased from 0.26 to 0.49–and reduction in rest pain.

A large number of growth factors are involved in cardiac tissue repair through the paracrine effect. They can promote the survival of cardiomyocytes *in vitro* and/or monitor the effect on the damaged myocardium upon delivery *in vivo*. HGF has shown a cardioprotective effect through activation of its canonical receptor (c-Met) in preclinical studies [55]. HGF can reduce infarct size and improve cardiac function in the rat model of ischemic injury. Delivery of MSCs with HGF cDNA-loaded adeno-viruses into infarcted myocardium increased vascular density and reduced ventricular remodeling [56]. HGF was also ectopically expressed in adipose-derived mesenchymal stem cells (ASCs) with lentiviral transduction. The transplantation of HGF-ASCs increased angiogenesis and reduced fibrosis [57].

Studies have shown that the implantation of circulating EPCs in the infarction area is associated with an increased level of VEGF and microvascular density [58-60]. When retrovirally transduced VEGF-ASCs and VEGF-transduced MSCs were implanted, increased vessel density was also observed [61, 62]. Basic fibroblast growth factor (bFGF) can interact with its receptors in endothelial cells and cardiomyocytes to produce multiple biological effects, such as proliferation, survival and migration [63, 64]. Studies have found that bFGF is closely associated with cardiogenic differentiation of human cardiosphere-derived cells, since it significantly promotes the engraftment of these cells [65]. A study has found that bFGF-transduced MSCs exhibited an increased ability to resist hypoxia conditions *in vitro* [65]. Furthermore, in animal models, transplantation of bFGF-MSCs in the myocardial infarcted heart also showed a promising effect on cardiac repair [66]. Platelet-derived growth factor (PDGF) is related to the interaction between cardiac microvascular endothelial cells (CMEC) and neighboring cardiomyocytes [67, 68]. It can exert a cardioprotective effect by fostering bone marrow cell transplantation into an infarcted aging rodent heart [69, 70]. Moreover, PDGF has also been proven to induce bone marrow mesenchymal stem cells to differentiate into beating cardiomyocytes *in vitro* and to foster new contractile cells in the ischemic heart [71].

Other cardioprotective factors, such as insulin-like growth factor-1 (IGF-1)[72], erythropoietin (EPO)[73], stromal cell-derived factor-1[74], and transforming growth factor beta 1 (TGF-β1)[75], have also been reported in the activation of resident stem cells or reduction of cardiomyocyte hypertrophy. Therefore, these growth factors have been included in this review.

3. The therapeutic challenges of growth factors

3.1 The physiochemical challenge of growth factors

Growth factors are effective polypeptide-based biotherapeutics, having broad applications in diverse ailments. Despite being specific and potent, their full clinical potential is limited. Unlike small molecule-based therapeutics, biotherapeutics have unique characteristics such as complex structures, short half-lives, poor stability, and low permeability (as shown in Fig. 1), which raise tremendous challenges in formulation design and wide clinical application [76].

The instability of biotherapeutics is usually caused by either first-structure destruction, such as deamidation, isomerization, hydrolysis and oxidation, or the second or more structural changes such as aggregation and denaturation [77]. The tendency of instability for a biotherapeutic depends on the properties of the protein as well as environmental factors, including exposure to organic solvents, temperature, pH and the ionic strength of the surrounding environment. For example, fibroblast growth factor 23 (FGF23), a regulator of phosphorus and vitamin D, has been found in several diseases of phosphate metabolism. The effects of temperature, storage time, and specimen handling on the stability of FGF23, including intact and C-terminal FGF23 (iFGF23 and cFGF23), have been carefully investigated [78]. When stored at 37 ℃, iFGF23 levels were unstable, showing a steady decline in levels over 48 h. At 37 ℃, its concentration decreased in a time-dependent fashion, with a decrease of 87% for serum and 47% for plasma at 48 h when measured

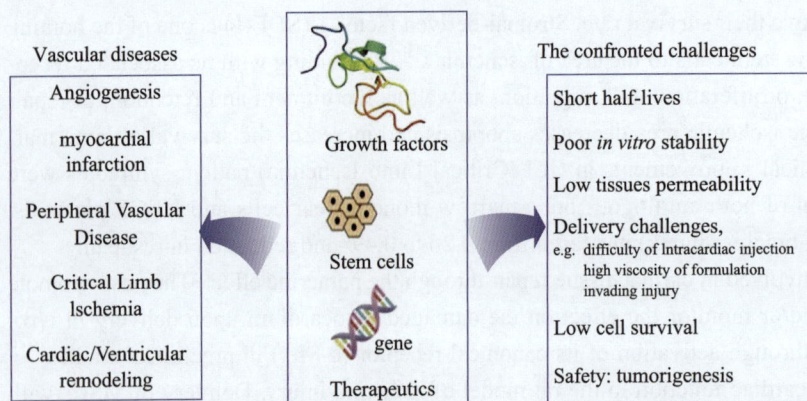

Fig. 1. The potential application of growth factors or stem cells-based therapeutics for vascular diseases and the confronted challenges hindering their clinical transformation from bench to bedside.

using the Kainos assay, and a 90% decline in plasma at 48 h when measured by Immutopics. FGF-1 has a melting temperature (T_m) marginally above physiological temperature, exhibiting poor intrinsic thermodynamic stability [79]. FGF-1 is prone to aggregation and proteolysis when exposed to higher temperature (42°C) or acidic pH environment (pH 3.5). Additionally, thiol-mediated reactions also resulted in the functional instability of FGF-1, because of its three buried free cysteine residues in the structure.

A major limitation of natural growth factors in clinical application is their short effective half-life due to poor stability or fast blood clearance. The half-life of most growth factors *in vivo* was on the order of minutes due to extensive degradation and inactivation [80]. As an example, a functional half-life of FGF-1, with intrinsically low stability, is only one hour in serum at 37°C [81]. As a result, multiple administrations are often required to achieve a therapeutic effect; multiple injections of angiogenic growth factors at the ischemic site may also cause severe side effects, such as hypotension, vascular leakage and tissue edema.

Another challenge for the delivery of growth factors is their poor tissue penetration due to their high molecular sizes. For example, FGF-2 does not cross the blood-brain barrier. Localized delivery is usually required for CNS disease. Local delivery of FGF-2 to the dura and arachnoid mater through intrathecal injection was required to promote functional recovery in a spinal cord injury model [82] FGF-2 delivered from a collagen hydrogel did not penetrate into spinal cord tissue, according to immunohistochemistry analysis.

3.2 Delivery challenge of growth factors

The method of growth factor delivery is partially related to the limited success of the clinical transformation of growth factor-based therapy from bench to bedside in heart vascular diseases [83]. Although several delivery routes, including intravenous, intracoronary, intramyocardial, and perivascular administration, have been tested in animal or patients (Fig. 2), few are successful in wide clinical application [84]. For example, intravenous infusion is considered to be the most popular delivery route because of its practicality, but it usually has a minimal effect on angiogenesis. Systemic exposure to a growth factor raises the potential for unwanted effects such as hypotension. Intracoronary delivery can be easily practiced using catheter-based techniques, and may be effective when adequate doses are used. However, this delivery route may lead to low therapeutic distribution into the myocardium. Only 0.9% of the injected FGF-2 was distributed in the ischemic myocardium at 1 h after intracoronary. In contrast, site-specific delivery, such as intramyo-cardial delivery, is preferred, as it is possible to target the desired areas of the myocardium. Intramyocardial delivery, *e.g.* perivascular delivery either *via* open chest or *via* thoracoscopy, may provide better myocardial dis-

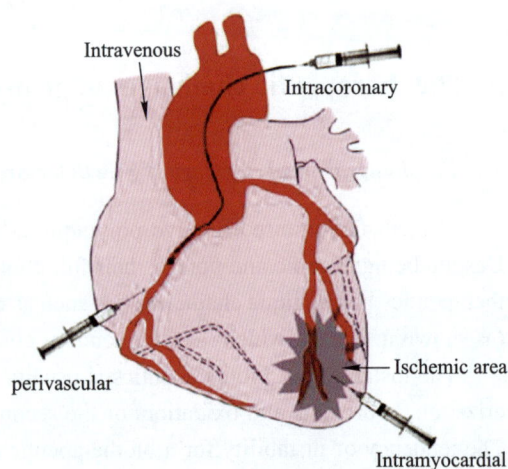

Fig. 2. Current access routes for growth factors or cell-based therapies to the myocardium include intravenous injection, intracoronary perfusion through a specialized catheter, perivascular myocardium delivery *via* open chest or *via* thoracoscopy, and intramyocardial delivery into the border zone of the infarct or the center of the ischemic area. Reproduced with permission from [84].

tribution and retention than intracoronary and intravenous routes. Growth factors can be injected intramyocardially into the border zone of the infarct or the center of the ischemic area. Alternatively, proteins can be intramyocardially targeted by endocardial injection with a specialized intraventricular catheter [84].

Despite these advantages, the invasive injury due to these delivery routes is the most concerning issue. Specifically, how the growth factor-based therapy is delivered can affect the ease of obtaining regulatory approval and the likelihood of the therapy being adopted by hospitals into clinical protocols. For heart disease, needle-based injections are generally considered to be dangerous for patients within the first few days after MI because of the unstable acute infarct wall [85]. A cardiac catheterization procedure may be used to deliver the growth factor-based therapeutics, which is easier to implement after MI than surgically based epicardial injections. Importantly, this procedure can also obviate the need for general anesthesia and therefore reduce the risk to the patient. However, many of the growth factor-based therapeutics that have been tested in rodents are not amenable to cardiac catheters because of their poor compatibility with catheterization-based materials. Therefore, these aspects must be considered when initially designing an injectable formulation of growth factor-based therapeutics. Furthermore, delivery of growth factor-based therapeutics *via* catheter injections is prone to make them leak into the systemic circulation; therefore, hemocompatibility is also concerned.

In peripheral artery disease (PAD), delivery of growth factor-based therapeutics is also confronting its own set of challenges. In many preclinical studies, most groups intramuscularly inject these therapeutics into the site adjacent to femoral artery resection in animal models. In a human patient, the onset of plaque buildup, claudication, and ischemia occurs gradually, and no acute injury site is targeted [86]. Therefore, this delivery procedure may be not applicable. Moreover, the limited distribution of biotherapeutics around the injection sites is also a concern, and the most effective delivery location within the muscle has not been identified. Although endothelial progenitor cells were capable of specifically migrating toward the ischemic zone instead of normal tissue [87], multiple injection sites were usually required and thus raise issues regarding systemic exposure of the therapeutics.

Another issue related to the delivery of biopharmaceutical drugs is the high and variable viscosity of their formulation [88]. Two aspects make them viscous. On one hand, a high protein-based therapeutic dose is required, often reaching hundreds of milligrams for each administration, because the subcutaneous injection of large volumes of formulations in patients was not permitted. This requirement makes formulation difficult as solutions containing multi-hundred milligram per milliliter amounts of protein are very viscous, making them hard to administer [77] On the other hand, polymer-based excipients, which can stabilize growth factors, in the formulation further increase the viscosity of the solutions.

3.3 Poor growth and low survival of stem cell-based therapeutic strategies

Although beneficial effects of stem cell-based strategies on cardiac remodeling and left ventricular function have been obtained in myocardial infarction animal models [89, 90], cell therapy is confronting many issues towards clinical transfer. Insufficient cell retention, poor survival in the damaged site, and uncontrollable cell differentiation are the primary factors hampering the efficiency of stem cell transplantation. Indeed, it was reported that despite the cell type, 90% of transported cells die within 24 h after transporting to the ischemic myocardium [91, 92]. Several factors determined the survival of functional cells after their engraftment. For example, the ischemic microenvironment, the related inflammatory response to exogenous cells, the scarce room to home the transplanted cells, and the transient availability of paracrine and circulating factors have been shown to affect the survival and function of the transported stem cells [93]. These factors affecting the survival of stem cells were excellently reviewed in these publications [2, 14].

4. The strategies to improve the delivery of growth factors

4.1 Hydrogel-based delivery systems

Hydrogels, which are water-swollen, cross-linked polymer networks, have emerged as particularly promising materials for tissue engineering, as they not only act as scaffolding materials but also control the release of biologically active and cell modulating substances *in vivo* [94]. Their unique properties, such as porous structure, high water content and soft nature, mimic biological tissues and make them suitable to accommodate cells and encapsulate and release water-soluble, protein-based or cell-based therapeutics in a controlled fashion. For cardiac tissue engineering, the hydrogel scaffold should mimic the native extracellular matrix (ECM) to reduce injury caused by the hydrogel matrix. Thus, some materials, such as collagen, lyophilized sponges and micropatterned ECM structures, are more suitable for the repair and regeneration of cardiac tissue. Recently, many studies focused on short oligopeptides that self-assemble into nanofibers (NFs), which then self-assemble into nanofibrous gels when mixed with salt solution at physiological pH. These unique properties make NFs not only slowly degradable and low in immunogenicity but also therapeutically potent for the sustained release of a drug or growth factor *via* noncovalent coupling or covalent bonding. The short peptide AcN-RARADADARARADADANH$_2$ could create an intramyocardial microenvironment with prolonged VEGF release to improve post-infarct neovascularization in rats.

Moreover, hydrogels should be degraded in a timely fashion that coincides with the angiogenic process. Many naturally derived or synthesized hydrogel-forming materials have been developed, and some of them have been approved for clinical application. Natural materials include protein-based materials such as silk fibroin, gelatin, and fibrin, and polysaccharide-based materials such as hyaluronan and chitosan. Synthetic materials are commonly polyester-based polymers, including PEG-PLGA, PEG-PLA and PLA-PEG-PEG. Recently, delivery systems combining cells, hydrogel scaffolds and growth factors showed great prospect for the treatment of CVDs. In this part, we review several delivery systems combined with scaffolds, stem cells and growth factors (Fig. 3).

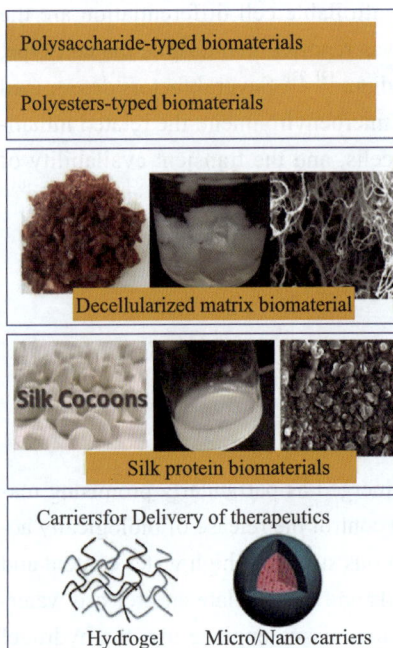

4.1.1 Silk fibroin hydrogel

Silk fibroin (SF) is a fibrous protein that is produced mainly by silkworms and spiders. Recently, its tunable biodegradation rate, unique mechanical properties and the guided differentiation of stem cells toward the endothelial cell lineage have made SF a favorable biomaterial for tissue repair or regeneration. SF possesses a large molecular weight of 200-350 kDa or more and bulky, repetitive, modular hydrophobic domains of GAGAGS, which are interrupted by small hydrophilic groups. The primary structure of SF, originated from *Bombyx mori,* is composed of a heavy (H) and a light (L) chain linked together through a disulfide bond. A glycoprotein with a molecular weight of approximately 25 kDa, named P25, also non-covalently binds to these chains. H-chain, L-chain, and P25 at the ratio of 6:6:1 assembled into mulberry SF, but non-mulberry SF only has the H-chain, and lacks the L-chain and P25. Apart from the primary structure, the secondary organization of silk fibroin dominates its gelatin property. The repeated hydrophobic domains of GAGAGS on the H-chain can form anti-parallel β-sheets, rendering SF solution able to be gelatinized, while the L-chain is hydrophilic in nature, forming an amorphous state and rendering the SF hydrogel relatively elastic.

When responding to external stimuli such as ions, acids, dehydrating agents, and sonication, silk solutions undergo sol-gel transition and form silk hydrogels [95]. The formation of silk hydrogels was attributed to the second configuration

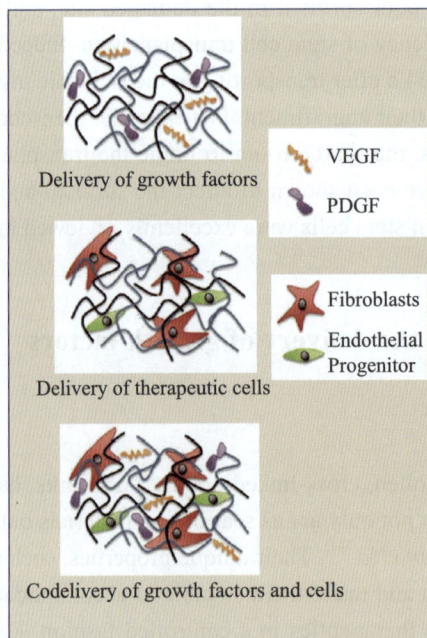

Fig. 3. The potential strategies to overcome the confronted challenges for delivery of growth factors or stem cells include the expertized design of novel biomaterials and construction of suitable delivery carriers.

transition from the coil-like or α-helix into the β-sheet. Silk hydrogels can be useful to control the release of small molecules or macromolecule therapeutics for injectable or noninjectable delivery systems. Vascular endothelial growth factor (VEGF), a key regulator of angiogenesis, was incorporated into sonication-induced silk hydrogels for bone angiogenesis [96]. The slow release of VEGF from these silk gels was observed by ELISA analysis. A larger blood vessel area formed in the administered hydrogel areas for rabbit inflicted sinus floor elevation surgeries.

4.1.2 Polysaccharide-based hydrogels

Heparin, a highly sulfated glycosaminoglycan, has high affinity to a variety of angiogenic growth factors and the capability to sequester them in the extracellular matrix, which makes it the most effective excipient to stabilize growth factors. Interactions between heparin and growth factors occur partly by shape recognition but dominantly through electrostatic attractions between the sulfated residues of heparin and the basic amino acid residues of the growth factors. Heparin-based hydrogels play an important role in sequestering growth factors and controlling their release. Heparin can also stabilize them against degradation by proteinases. A thermo-sensitive graft polymer, poloxamer 188-grafted heparin (HP), was synthesized using poloxamer 188 and heparin as origin materials [97]. HP polymer maintained the temperature-sensitive property of poloxamer 188; that is, when its concentration was more than 0.15 g/ml, the HP solution was a flowable liquid at lower temperature, while the solution rapidly converted to the semisolid hydrogel status as the environmental temperature increased to *ca.* 37℃. Basic fibroblast growth factor (bFGF) was encapsulated into the nanoparticles of HP prepared by the water-in-water technique for diabetic cardiomyopathy (DCM) [98]. The efficient encapsulation and stable bioactivity of bFGF were confirmed *in vitro*. Significant improvements ($P < 0.05$) in both cardiac function and tissue morphology in the DCM rats were observed after treatment with bFGF-NP.

Hyaluronic acid (HA), a component of the extracellular matrix (ECM) of vertebrates, is a non-sulfated glycosaminoglycan (GAG). It consists of repeating disaccharide units (β-1,4-D-glucuronic acid-β-1, 3-*N*-acetyl-D-glucosa-mine) and has molecular weights ranging from *ca.* 100 kDa to 5000 kDa. The high-molecular-weight HA has been reported to inhibit angiogenesis, while the low ones stimulate the proliferation and migration of endothelial cell [99, 100]. Because of the lack of sulfonic groups on HA molecules, its affinity to growth factors is very weak. Recently, chemically modified forms of HA have been successfully constructed to store and release growth factors *in vivo*. The thiolated derivative of HA, HA-DTPH, was synthesized using hydrazide chemistry and formed a hydrogel through crosslinking of disulfide linkage between polymers. In the hydrated hydrogel state, these HA-DTPH hydrogels have an open, highly permeable, sponge-like structure suitable for sequestering exogenous growth factors. Upon transplantation into ischemia mouse models, HA-DTPH hydrogels carrying both VEGF and keratinocyte growth factor (KGF) generated intact beds with well-defined borders from day 7 to day 14 [101]. These microvessels organized into recognizable tubular networks filled with erythrocytes. Moreover, chitosan hydrogel has been used to deliver VEGF and bFGF to induce angiogenesis in myocardial infarction models [102-104].

Chitosan, another polysaccharide-based biomaterial, originates from chitin through partial deacetylation. It has been broadly used as an inert carrier of growth factor for angiogenesis. Chitosan (CS) is a linear polysaccharide consisting of *N*-acetyl-D-glucosamine units. This polymer is well suited as a matrix-based material for the delivery of growth factors due to its biocompatibility and biodegradability. It can be processed into a variety of matrices (e.g. nanoparticles and hydrogels) under mild processing conditions that do not harm sensitive biological therapeutics such as growth factors. For example, bFGF-loaded CS scaffolds (bFGF-CS) were prepared by simply mixing bFGF with CS solution, followed by a lyophilization process. bFGF-CS significantly improved the wound healing of pressure ulcers though angiogenesis in aged mice when compared to a control [105]. In addition to growth factor delivery, chitosan was used as an implantable biomaterial for the delivery of stem cells. One study recently indicated that chitosan solution can not only improve retention of stem cells in the administration site but also promote cardiac differentiation of adipose-derived stem cells and enhance the functional improvements of myocardium in the rat model [106]. To promote the formation of chitosan hydrogel, a water-soluble chitosan derivative has been synthesized [107]. 4-azidobenzoic acid (Az) was conjugated to the available free amine groups of lactose-modified chitosan (CS-LA), synthesizing a novel CS derivate, Az-CS-LA. The viscous Az-CH-LA solution was converted into semisolid hydrogel after exposing to UV irradiation. b-FGF and VEGF were easily encapsulated into the Az-CH-LA hydrogels, effectively inducing vascularization in myocardial infarction models [104].

Alginate, a negatively charged polysaccharide, is composed of the repeated β-D-mannopyranuronosyl-(1→4)-α-L-gulopyranuronosyl-(1→4)-α-L-gulopyranuronate. Alginate hydrogels are easily prepared by addition of aqueous calcium chloride to aqueous sodium alginate. Alginate hydrogels are widely used for the entrapment of enzymes and formation of artificial seeds in plant tissue culture. Alginate hydrogels have been successfully applied to encapsulate cells or growth factors. For example, VEGF and bFGF were encapsulated into alginate hydrogels without additional chemical crosslinking reactions [108]. The prolonged release of VEGF and bFGF from this hydrogel more effectively promoted angiogenesis than did their free solution, reducing side effects of VEGF or bFGF overdoses, such as formation of hemangiomas. Hao *et al.* also used alginate hydrogels to deliver VEGF attached to platelet derived growth factor-BB (PDGF-BB) in the myocardial infarction model to initiate new blood vessel growth and maturation [109]. Recently, stimuli-sensitive hydrogels that can respond to external environmental changes such as pH, temperature, redox potential, ionic strength, and light have been widely used for the delivery of growth factors in the field of tissue engineering [110]. Magnetic stimulation can also be exploited to regulate the release of growth factors and cells from hydrogels in a controlled manner. Alginate was first modified with ethylenediamine, and heparin was then conjugated to the ethylenediamine-modified alginate *via* carbodiimide chemistry, synthesizing a novel alginate-g-heparin polymer [111]. Alginate-based ferrogels containing iron oxide nanoparticles were fabricated *via* ionic cross-linking. TGF-β1 specifically bound to the heparin domain of ferrogels. Under magnetic stimulation, the ferrogels were deformed, which resulted in the sustained release of TGF-β1 from alginate-g-heparin ferrogels.

4.1.3 Acellular matrix scaffold-based hydrogel

Currently, extracellular matrix (ECM) is commonly used for the therapeutic reconstruction and repair of many tissues, including musculotendinous tissues, lower urinary tract, kidney, myocardium, esophagus, peripheral nerve, and central nervous system. For example, ventricular ECM was delivered into the myocardial infarct and border zone *via* transendocardial injections using the NOGA guided Myostar catheter, and then self-assembled into a nanofibrous hydrogel within the heart [112]. This hydrogel mimicked the complex native ECM, increased endogenous cardiomyocyte survival and preserved cardiac function in the rat model. Simultaneously, this hydrogel did not induce arrhythmias, thus demonstrating its clinical potential as a minimally invasive treatment for MI [113].

Acellular matrix scaffold was easily prepared from healthy tissues through simple processing. To create a decellularized matrix scaffold, intact tissues or chopped tissues are continuously agitated in a 1% sodium dodecyl sulfate (SDS) solution. Other decellularization techniques using mechanical, chemical, and enzymatic methods have also been described for the preparation of an acellular matrix scaffold. Because the acellular matrix scaffold retained the sulfated glycosaminoglycan (sGAG) components and exhibited excellent gelation properties *in vitro*, many studies exploited the acellular matrix scaffold as carriers of growth factor-based therapeutics to prolong the release and improve the stability of these therapeutics. For example, when bFGF could bind with an acellular spinal cord scaffold (ASC), the stability of ASC-bound bFGF upon the heating of the solution to above 55 ℃ was significantly improved by the circular dichroism analysis [114]. In addition to electrostatic interactions between bFGF and sGAG components of ASC, receptor-mediated interactions also played an important role, as demonstrated by bFGF receptor staining in the ASC scaffold. These strong interactions between ASC and bFGF also led to the sustained release of bFGF *in vitro*. Sometimes, the weakly bound growth factors were rapidly released within two days. Several strategies have been conceived to enhance the retention of growth factors in acellular scaffolds. For example, anchoring of a VEGF-like peptide on decellularized extracellular matrix (DC-ECM) of HUVECs through"click chemistry" immobilization has been designed, and the enhanced angiogenic responses of the immobilized peptide were observed compared to DC-ECM containing VEGF [115]. Instead of covalent modification, physical encapsulation was a more suitable means to extend the half-life time of VEGF and improve its stability in the administration site. VEGF was encapsulated in nanoparticles of PLGA, exhibiting a significant sustained-release profile *in vitro* [116]. To further reduce the initial burst release, incorporation of VEGF-loaded nanoparticles into bladder acellular matrix allografts (BAMAs) was explored. The burst release was greatly decreased (*ca.* 15% within the first two days) due to the long diffusion pathways of VEGF in the bladder acellular matrix. Additionally, VEGF release from VEGF-loaded nanoparticle-modified BAMAs was only 60% within two months. The long-term sustained release of VEGF significantly enhanced angiogenesis and inhibited graft shrinkage in tissue-engineered bladder [117].

In view of the three-dimensional network of the intact acellular matrix scaffold from healthy tissue, vasculogenesis-related stem cells could adhere to the scaffold, which could be injected into sites near the damaged blood vessel, promoting the regeneration of vascellum. Decellularized adipose tissues (DAT) with adipo-conductive and adipo-inductive properties can provide a highly supportive microenvironment to induce the adipogenic differentiation of human adipose-derived stem/stromal cells (ASCs) [118]. The effects of ASC seeding inside DAT scaffolds on angiogenesis following subcutaneous implantation in an immunocompetent Wistar rat model were systemically investigated. The results indicated that the combination of ASCs and adipose extracellular matrix (ECM) provides an inductive microenvironment for adipose regeneration mediated by angiogenesis [119].

4.1.4 The synthetic polymer-based biomaterials

Hydrogel scaffolds prepared by synthetic materials are the new generation of hydrogel for cardiac tissue engineering. Hydrogel-forming copolymers comprising polyester and PEG blocks are the most common materials used for biomedical applications [120]. For these materials, polyesters blocks are usually biodegradable in the body and biocompatible with biologic tissues. These blocks included poly (lactic acid) (PLA), PLGA, PCL, poly(trimethylene carbonate), and polyanhydrides. Noticeably, by finely controlling the molar ratio of PEG and polyester and designing the copolymer shape, it is easy to construct a thermo-sensitive material. PLGA-based hydrogels are the most biodegradable thermogelling polymers because of their ease of tune/control while formulating, and for their safety profile. The PLGA-based hydrogels were applied to deliver VEGF through anchoring VEGF on alginate beads before its encapsulation into PLGA-based hydrogel [121]. The sustained release of VEGF from PLGA-based hydrogels was obtained and induced the formation of new vascular networks in a rat ischemic hind limb model. Co-delivery of VEGF and PDGF by PLGA-based hydrogels has also been reported [122]. The long lasting retention and delivery of VEGF and PDGF from PLGA-based hydrogels also more efficiently induced the rapid formation of a mature vascular network in a hind limb ischemia model.

4.2 Nano/microcarrier-based delivery systems

The rapid development of nanotechnology in the past two decades has brought about enormous opportunities in the field of biomedical studies and applications. Polymeric nanoparticles have been widely studied for the release of small molecules and proteins. Synthetic poly(lactic-co-glycolic acid) (PLGA) and polyethylene glycol (PEG)-PLGA copolymers have been approved by the FDA for use in humans [123, 124]. Poly-lactide-co-glycolide (PLGA) microspheres emerged as one of the most promising strategies to achieve site-specific drug delivery because of their good biocompatibility and biodegradability. Their potential in cardiac regeneration has been fully assessed in term of their retention in heart tissue after intramyocardial administration [125]. Microspheres with a diameter of 5 μm were the most compatible with intramyocardial administration in terms of injectability through a 29-gauge needle. Particles were present in the heart tissue for up to three months post-implantation, and no particle migration toward other solid organs was observed, demonstrating good myocardial retention. Therefore, biocompatible and biodegradable microspheres may represent a valuable approach to deliver growth factors, and even therapeutic cells, through local implantation in the infarcted myocardium. For example, the use of PLGA microspheres could allow localized and sustained VEGF release and consequently a prolonged biological effect with induction of tissue revascularization in an acute myocardial ischemia-reperfusion model [126]. Neuregulin-1 (NRG) is a growth factor involved in cardiac repair after MI. To avoid problems related to the short half-life of NRG after systemic administration, NRG was successfully encapsulated in PLGA microspheres, with encapsulation efficiencies reaching 92.58% ± 3.84% [127]. NRG maintained its biological activity after the microencapsulation process and was released from PLGA microspheres in a sustained manner. *In vivo* release analysis showed that NRG was also released in a controlled manner throughout the twelve-week study [128] Adipose-derived stem cells (ADSCs), which have shown promising results in cardiac repair, were adhered to PLGA microsphere scaffolds, and their potential for heart administration was assessed in an MI rat model. ADSCs efficiently adhered to particle scaffolds within a few hours. ADSC-microspheres were present in the peri-infarcted tissue for two weeks after implantation [127].

Nanoparticles (NPs) are also widely applied in the delivery of growth factors or genes encoding growth factors. Several NP-based growth factor delivery systems have been developed, including VEGF, insulin growth factor-1 (IGF-1), and tumor growth factor-β3 (TGF-β3). For example, platelet-derived growth factor-BB (PDGF-BB) has previously been encapsulated and released from polymeric nanoparticles. PDGF-AA was encapsulated, with high efficiency, in poly(lactide-co-glycolide) nanoparticles, and its release from the drug delivery system was followed over 21 days [129, 130]. Magnetic gelatin nano-spheres loaded with VEGF plasmid (5-20 nm) were intra-arterially injected and used in a rabbit hind limb ischemia model, resulting in 50% increase in blood vessel density compared to empty nanospheres. Binsalamah *et al.* locally injected proangiogenic and cardioprotective placental growth factor (PlGF)-loaded chitosan-alginate nanoparticles and found a slow, sustained release of PlGF [131]. These NP delivery systems were shown to prevent scar formation and improve left ventricular function behavior in the anti-inflammatory profile of systemic cytokine. Syndecan-4 is an important regulator of bFGF signaling. Liposomal co-delivery of bFGF and syndecan-4 enhanced bFGF uptake, indicating an increased cellular signaling response to bFGF, and improved blood flow up to 1.8-fold compared to liposomal delivery of bFGF alone [132]. Spontaneous coassembly of nanoparticles was fabricated *via* affinity binding of heparin-binding proteins (bFGF, HGF and VEGF) to alginate-sulfate for tissue repair in animal models of severe ischemia [133]. The NPs efficiently encapsulated and protected the proteins from proteolysis. Injection of a combination of NPs encapsulating multiple therapeutic growth factors promoted effective and long-term tissue repair in a murine model of hind limb ischemia and acute myocardial infarction in rats. Similarly, liposomal delivery of VEGF loaded with anti-P-selectin significantly promoted the capillary density of the infarct area in an infarcted model [134].

Temporal control over the release of multiple growth factors is a key factor in cardiac regenerative medicine and particularly in angiogenesis, which remains a challenge for myocardial infarction repair. Angiogenesis is a highly regulated process that is typically driven by the interplay of multiple growth factors. Co-delivery of VEGF and bFGF, followed by the release of PDGF, is considered crucial for guided angiogenesis in an implanted cardiac patch [135]. A bilayer nanoparticle for the simultaneous and/or sequential release of multiple growth factors was fabricated, characterized and biologically assessed. The bilayer nanoparticles featured low burst effect and time-delayed release, and allowed for sequential release of PDGF following co-release of VEGF and bFGF, which promoted angiogenesis.

4.3 Hydrogel-bound micro/nanoparticles

Another promising strategy is a combination of micro/nanoparticles and hydrogel to control release of growth factors and protect them from degradation [136]. Recently, an injectable affinity-binding alginate hydrogel attached to microbeads has been designed to control the release of IGF-1 and HGF and to protect the factors from enzymatic proteolysis [137]. In the first post-infarction phase, sequential release of IGF-1 was shown to protect tissue against cell death and promote survival. In the late phase, release of HGF prevented cardiac remodeling and improved cardiac function. Another hydrogel system prepared by capryol 90-based gelation of VEGF-loaded liposomal nanoparticles in Pluronic F-127 shell was able to sustain VEGF release, promoting neovascularization and improving cardiac function [138].

5. Strategies to overcome the barriers of stem cell therapy for CVDs

5.1 Encapsulation of the therapeutic stem cells in biomaterial-based scaffolds

Recently, stem cell therapy has attracted many scientists in the field of CVD. Although significant progress in stem cell therapy has been achieved in the regeneration of the damaged heart or blood vessels, many challenges remain, such as cell survival, cell fate determination and engraftment after transplantation. Among these problems, the most important is the low rate of cell survival and retention in the administration site.

Biomaterial scaffolds provide a substitutive ECM for the encapsulation of cells, thus enhancing cell survival and improving their retention at the infarct site. Two approaches were generally applied to achieve cellular delivery into the myocardium [139]. One was use of *in situ* hydrogels, which encapsulated therapeutic cells in solution before injection. *In situ* gelation of these biomaterials rapidly occurred when they were exposed to external stimuli confronted in the myocardial wall, forming a three-dimensional network structure to implant the therapeutic cells. When the solution of alginate modified with the cell adhesion peptides RGD and YIGSR is injected *via* a needle into the myocardial infarct, it immediately transits into an *in situ* hydrogel once contacting physiologic calcium ions. Thus, the *in situ* hydrogel can attract growing cells to promote left ventricular remodeling and improve cardiac function in a post-MI rat model [140]. Moreover, this alginate hydrogel implant can provide a temporary physical support for the damaged cardiac tissue by replacing damaged ECM. In addition, cell-preseeded scaffolds are surgically attached to the epicardial surface. Therapeutic stem cells are usually seeded in biomaterial-based scaffolds to create an adequate 3D cell-implanted scaffold, thereby increasing cell survival and even guiding cell differentiation, which was proved to be an effective strategy for MI therapy. The most common application for creating 3D constructs for cell delivery is porous or fibrous preformed scaffolds. A collagen patch was created for delivering human mesenchymal stem cells and human embryonic stem cell-derived mesenchymal cells for cardiac repair [141, 142]. In a recent study, a nanofibrous patch prepared by electrospun poly (ε-caprolactone)/gelatin nanofibers was created as an improved method of cell retention [143]. The grafted MSCs promoted angiogenesis and facilitated cardiac repair. In addition, the nanofibrous PGcell scaffold improved cardiac function, such as increasing fractional shortening and ejection fraction, reducing scar size, and increasing thickness in the infarcted area.

5.2 Co-delivery of therapeutic stem cells and growth factors through matrix scaffolds for CVDs

In cell therapy of CVDs, the lack of an anchorage matrix, the poor maintenance the grafted cells, and the undesirable microenvironment causes massive cell death. Most growth factors benefit myocardial regeneration through improving the survival and proliferation of resident or transplanted stem cells [144, 145]. Some could stimulate the recruitment and differentiation of progenitor/stem cells [146, 147], and some indirectly affect survive and function of the cell therapy *via* promoting both angiogenesis and vasculogenesis [148, 149]. Stem cells combined with scaffolds and growth factors are considered candidates due to the localized and sustained release of growth factors and the unique structure, which provides a beneficial environment for cell differentiation and survival. Therefore, appropriate growth factors combined with functional stem cells are believed to benefit the amelioration of cell engraftment and function.

Indeed, injectable three-dimensional (3D) scaffolds, which not only release drug but also convey stem cells, was conceived by Karam *et al.* [150]. Hepatocyte growth factor (HGF) and insulin-like growth factor (IGF-1) have been encapsulated in poly(lactic-co-glycolic acid) (PLGA) microspheres, while human adipose-derived stem cells (ADSCs) were conveyed on their 3D surface (as depicted in Fig. 4). The sustained release of both IGF-1 and HGF improved stem cell engraftment, survival, homing, and differentiation by inducing the synthesis of the cardiac differentiation markers, GATA4, Nkx2.5, cTnI and CX43, after one week *in vitro*. Recently, hMSCs combined with an injectable thermo-sensitive hydrogel copolymer were shown to continuously release bioactive IGF-1 over two weeks *in vitro*. The cells were grown inside the hydrogel during a seven-day culture, and the IGF-1 significantly accelerated their growth *in vitro* [151]. The BM-derived MSCs and angiogenic cytokine (SCF, SDF-1α) loaded hydrogels were implanted in the MI border zone. The combination of cells, scaffold and cytokines promoted tissue and vasculature regeneration and improved cardiac function [152]. In a mouse infarction model, PEGylated fibrin hydrogel was used to carry covalently bound SDF-1α; 28 days after implantation, the c-kit+ stem cells were enriched in the damaged site, therefore limiting scar expansion and improving cardiac function [153]. This hydrogel was also designed to deliver HGF and BM-derived stem cells to the infarcted heart with beneficial effects on heart function for up to four weeks, thus confirming that combined strategies with controlled release of growth factor and cells can increase the therapeutic potential of stem cells [154]. In other studies, a cardiac patch prepared by a porous collagen scaffold with covalently immobilized VEGF promoted MSC recruitment and engraftment and strengthened the formation of myogenic tissue and blood vessels within the graft [155, 156].

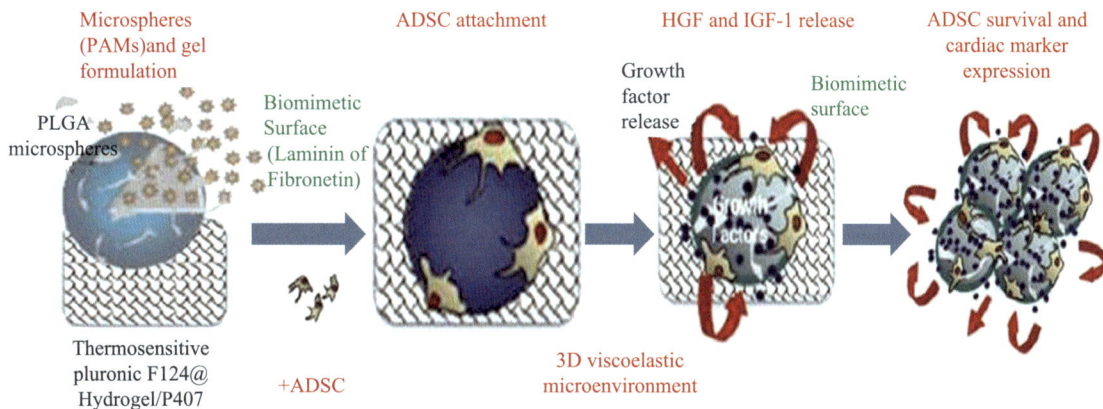

Fig. 4. The scheme of pharmacologically active microcarriers for co-delivery of growth factors and ADSC cells. Growth factors (HGF and IGF-1) were firstly encapsulated inside PLGA microsphere, followed by attachment of ADSC cells on its biomimetic surface through laminin or fibronectin. The sustained release of both IGF-1 and HGF improved the survival and the cardiac differentiation of ADSC cells. Reproduced with permission from [150].

6. Conclusions

Growth factors play an important role in myocardial/ peripheral angiogenesis and even cardiac repair. Although many growth factors have shown promising potential in the treatment of vascular diseases, the short half-lives of growth factors, low cellular transfection efficiency of naked plasmids carrying growth factor genes, and safety issues due to growth factor overdoses remain. Fortunately, novel delivery methods such as the hydrogel, the decellularized matrix and NP-based delivery system can decrease the undesired degradation of growth factors and provide targeted and sustained release of growth factors and genes *in vivo*. Cell-based therapy is another potential strategy of enhancing vascularization. The low survival of stem cells and their uncontrollable differentiation after transportation limit their clinical application. The decellularized matrix scaffolding for cardiac tissue engineering tends to mimic the native ECM and provides an adequate 3D architecture for transplanted cells, thus improving cell survival and guiding cell differentiation *in vivo*. In this way, new biotechnologies combining cells, scaffolds and growth factors were designed for providing a beneficial microenvironment for cell engraftment. Angiogenesis is a complex process that requires the coordination of multiple cell types such as endothelial cells, smooth muscle cells and pericytes with complex signaling regulations. However, existing therapeutic strategies are overly simplistic, mostly delivering just one or two growth factor/genes, which do not recapitulate the natural angiogenesis process. In the future, growth factors and multiple cytokines in spatio-temporal controlled manner by a scaffold transporting stem cells may lead to promising therapy for vascular diseases.

References

[1] Naghavi M, Wang H, Lozano R, *et al.* Global, regional, and national age-sex specific all-cause and cause-specific mortality for 240 causes of death, 1990-2013: a systematic analysis for the Global Burden of Disease Study 2013 [J]. Lancet, 2015, 385(9963): 117-171.

[2] Rufaihah AJ, Seliktar D. Hydrogels for therapeutic cardiovascular angiogenesis [J]. Advanced Drug Delivery Reviews, 2016, 96: 31-39.

[3] Gupta R, Tongers J, Losordo DW. Human studies of angiogenic gene therapy [J]. Circulation Research, 2009, 105(8): 724-736.

[4] Cuevas P, Carceller F, Ortega S, *et al.* Hypotensive activity of fibroblast growth-factor [J]. Science, 1991, 254(5035): 1208-1210.

[5] Thurston G, Suri C, Smith K, *et al.* Leakage-resistant blood vessels in mice transgenically overexpressing angiopoietin-1 [J]. Science, 1999, 286(5449): 2511-2514.

[6] Rissanen TT, Markkanen JE, Arve K, *et al.* Fibroblast growth factor-4 induces vascular permeability, angiogenesis, and arteriogenesis in a rabbit hind limb ischemia model [J]. Faseb Journal, 2002, 16(13): 100-102.

[7] Auxenfans C, Lequeux C, Perrusel E, *et al.* Adipose-derived stem cells (ASCs) as a source of endothelial cells in the reconstruction of endothelialized skin equivalents [J]. Journal Of Tissue Engineering And Regenerative Medicine, 2012, 6(7): 512-518.

[8] Reagan J, Foo T, Watson JT, *et al.* Distinct phenotypes and regenerative potentials of early endothelial progenitor cells and outgrowth endothelial progenitor cells derived from umbilical cord blood [J]. Journal Of Tissue Engineering And Regenerative Medicine, 2011, 5(8): 620-628.

[9] Asahara T, Masuda H, Takahashi T, *et al.* Bone marrow origin of endothelial progenitor cells responsible for postnatal vasculogenesis in physiological and pathological neovascularization [J]. Circulation Research, 1999, 85(3): 221-228.

[10] Minguell JJ, Erices A. Mesenchymal stem cells and the treatment of cardiac disease [J]. Experimental Biology And Medicine, 2006, 231(1): 39-49.

[11] Shi R-Z, Li Q-P. Improving outcome of transplanted mesenchymal stem cells for ischemic heart disease [J]. Biochemical And Biophysical Research Communications, 2008, 376(2): 247-250.

[12] Zhang S, Sun A, Xu D, *et al.* Impact of timing on efficacy and safety of intracoronary autologous bone marrow stem celts transplantation in acute myocardial infarction: a pooled subgroup analysis of randomized controlled trials [J]. Clinical Cardiology, 2009, 32(8): 458-466.

[13] Terrovitis JV, Smith RR, Marban E. Assessment and optimization of cell engraftment after transplantation into the heart [J]. Circulation Research, 2010, 106(3): 479-494.

[14] Tran C, Damaser MS. Stem cells as drug delivery methods: Application of stem cell secretome for regeneration [J]. Advanced Drug Delivery Reviews, 2015, 82-83: 1-11.

[15] Hughes SE, Hall PA. Overview of the fibroblast growth-factor and receptor families: Complexity, functional diversity, and implications for future cardiovascular research [J]. Cardiovascular Research, 1993, 27(7): 1199-1203.

[16] Detillieux KA, Sheikh F, Kardami E, *et al.* Biological activities of fibroblast growth factor-2 in the adult myocardium [J]. Cardiovascular Research, 2003, 57(1): 8-19.

[17] Kardami E, Detillieux K, Ma X, *et al.* Fibroblast growth factor-2 and cardioprotection [J]. Heart Failure Reviews, 2007, 12(3-4): 267-277.

[18] Santiago J-J, Ma X, McNaughton LJ, *et al.* Preferential accumulation and export of high molecular weight FGF-2 by rat cardiac nonmyocytes [J]. Cardiovascular Research, 2011, 89(1): 139-147.

[19] Santiago J-J, McNaughton LJ, Koleini N, *et al.* High molecular weight fibroblast growth factor-2 in the human heart is a potential target for prevention of cardiac remodeling [J]. Plos One, 2014, 9(5).

[20] Yanagisawamiwa A, Uchida Y, Nakamura F, *et al.* Salvage of infarcted myocardium by angiogenic action of basic fibroblast growth-factor [J]. Science, 1992, 257(5075): 1401-1403.

[21] Nikol S, Baumgartner I, Van Belle E, *et al.* Therapeutic angiogen-

esis with intramuscular NV1FGF improves amputation-free survival in patients with critical limb ischemia [J]. Molecular Therapy, 2008, 16(5): 972-978.

[22] McIlwain DW, Zoetemelk M, Myers JD, et al. Coordinated induction of cell survival signaling in the inflamed microenvironment of the prostate [J]. Prostate, 2016, 76(8): 722-734.

[23] Zhang J, Li Y. Therapeutic uses of FGFs [J]. Seminars In Cell & Developmental Biology, 2016, 53: 144-154.

[24] Ahn A, Frishman WH, Gutwein A, et al. Therapeutic angiogenesis a new treatment approach for ischemic heart disease - part I [J]. Cardiology In Review, 2008, 16(4): 163-171.

[25] Luo ZY, Diaco M, Murohara T, et al. Vascular endothelial growth factor attenuates myocardial ischemia-reperfusion injury [J]. Annals Of Thoracic Surgery, 1997, 64(4): 993-998.

[26] Henry TD, Annex BH, McKendall GR, et al. Vascular endothelial growth factor in ischemia for vascular angiogenesis [J]. Circulation, 2003, 107(10): 1359-1365.

[27] Libetta C, Esposito P, Martinelli C, et al. Hepatocyte growth factor (HGF) and hemodialysis: physiopathology and clinical implications [J]. Clinical And Experimental Nephrology, 2016, 20(3): 371-378.

[28] Sala V, Crepaldi T. Novel therapy for myocardial infarction: can HGF/Met be beneficial? [J]. Cellular And Molecular Life Sciences, 2011, 68(10): 1703-1717.

[29] Powell RJ, Simons M, Mendelsohn FO, et al. Results of a double-blind, placebo-controlled Study to Assess the Safety of Intramuscular Injection of Hepatocyte Growth Factor Plasmid to Improve Limb Perfusion in Patients with Critical Limb Ischemia [J]. Circulation, 2008, 118(1): 58-65.

[30] Morishita R, Aoki M, Hashiya N, et al. Safety evaluation of clinical gene therapy using hepatocyte growth factor to treat peripheral arterial disease [J]. Hypertension, 2004, 44(2): 203-209.

[31] Morishita R, Makino H, Aoki M, et al. Phase I/IIa clinical trial of therapeutic angiogenesis using hepatocyte growth factor gene transfer to treat critical limb ischemia [J]. Arteriosclerosis Thrombosis And Vascular Biology, 2011, 31(3): 713-720.

[32] Ko SH, Bandyk DF. Therapeutic angiogenesis for critical limb ischemia [J]. Seminars In Vascular Surgery, 2014, 27(1): 23-31.

[33] Suleiman MS, Singh RJR, Stewart CEH. Apoptosis and the cardiac action of insulin-like growth factor I [J]. Pharmacology & Therapeutics, 2007, 114(3): 278-294.

[34] Filus A, Zdrojewicz Z. Insulin-like growth factor-1 (IGF-1) - structure and the role in the human body [J]. Pediatric endocrinology, diabetes, and metabolism, 2015, 20(4): 161-169.

[35] Hermonat PL, Li D, Yang B, et al. Mechanism of action and delivery possibilities for TGF beta(1) in the treatment of myocardial ischemia [J]. Cardiovascular Research, 2007, 74(2): 235-243.

[36] Ruiz-Ortega M, Rodriguez-Vita J, Sanchez-Lopez E, et al. TGF-beta signaling in vascular fibrosis [J]. Cardiovascular Research, 2007, 74(2): 196-206.

[37] Lefer AM, Tsao P, Aoki N, et al. Mediation of cardioprotection by transforming growth-factor-beta [J]. Science, 1990, 249(4964): 61-64.

[38] Lefer AM, Ma XL, Weyrich AS, et al. Mechanism of the cardioprotective effect of transforming growth factor-beta-1 in feline myocardial-ischemia and reperfusion [J]. Proceedings Of the National Academy Of Sciences Of the United States Of America, 1993, 90(3): 1018-1022.

[39] Baxter GF, Mocanu MM, Brar BK, et al. Cardioprotective effects of transforming growth factor-beta 1 during early reoxygenation or reperfusion are mediated by p42/p44 MAPK [J]. Journal Of Cardiovascular Pharmacology, 2001, 38(6): 930-939.

[40] Chen HJ, Li DY, Saldeen T, et al. TGF-beta(1) modulates NOS expression and phosphorylation of Akt/PKB in rat myocytes exposed to hypoxia-reoxygenation [J]. American Journal Of Physiology-Heart And Circulatory Physiology, 2001, 281(3): H1035-H1039.

[41] Doerr M, Morrison J, Bergeron L, et al. Differential effect of hypoxia on early endothelial-mesenchymal transition response to transforming growth beta isoforms 1 and 2 [J]. Microvascular Research, 2016, 108: 48-63.

[42] Fonfara S, Hetzel U, Tew SR, et al. Myocardial cytokine expression in dogs with systemic and naturally occurring cardiac diseases [J]. American Journal Of Veterinary Research, 2013, 74(3): 408-416.

[43] Weihua S, Xiaomeng W. The role of TGFbeta1 and LRG1 in cardiac remodelling and heart failure [J]. Biophysical Reviews, 2015, 7(1): 91-104.

[44] Rupert CE, Coulombe KLK. The roles of neuregulin-1 in cardiac development, homeostasis, and disease [J]. Biomarker Insights, 2015, 10: 1-9.

[45] Odiete O, Hill MF, Sawyer DB. Neuregulin in cardiovascular development and disease [J]. Circulation Research, 2012, 111(10): 1376-1385.

[46] Formiga FR, Pelacho B, Garbayo E, et al. Controlled delivery of fibroblast growth factor-1 and neuregulin-1 from biodegradable microparticles promotes cardiac repair in a rat myocardial infarction model through activation of endogenous regeneration [J]. Journal Of Controlled Release, 2014, 173: 132-139.

[47] Hastings CL, Roche ET, Ruiz-Hernandez E, et al. Drug and cell delivery for cardiac regeneration [J]. Advanced Drug Delivery Reviews, 2015, 84: 85-106.

[48] Kalka C, Masuda H, Takahashi T, et al. Transplantation of ex vivo expanded endothelial progenitor cells for therapeutic neovascularization [J]. Proceedings Of the National Academy Of Sciences Of the United States Of America, 2000, 97(7): 3422-3427.

[49] Aicher A, Heeschen C, Mildner-Rihm C, et al. Essential role of endothelial nitric oxide synthase for mobilization of stem and progenitor cells [J]. Nature Medicine, 2003, 9(11): 1370-1376.

[50] Pittenger MF, Martin BJ. Mesenchymal stem cells and their potential as cardiac therapeutics [J]. Circulation Research, 2004, 95(1): 9-20.

[51] Valina C, Pinkernell K, Song Y-H, et al. Intracoronary administration of autologous adipose tissue-derived stem cells improves left ventricular function, perfusion, and remodelling after acute myocardial infarction [J]. European Heart Journal, 2007, 28(21): 2667-2677.

[52] Mazo M, Hernandez S, Jose Gavira J, et al. Treatment of reperfused ischemia with adipose-derived stem cells in a preclinical swine model of myocardial infarction [J]. Cell Transplantation, 2012, 21(12): 2723-2733.

[53] Arimitsu N, Shimizu J, Fujiwara N, et al. Role of SDF1/CXCR4 interaction in experimental hemiplegic models with neural cell transplantation [J]. International Journal Of Molecular Sciences, 2012, 13(3): 2636-2649.

[54] Song M, Jang H, Lee J, et al. Regeneration of chronic myocardial infarction by injectable hydrogels containing stem cell homing factor SDF-1 and angiogenic peptide Ac-SDKP [J]. Biomaterials, 2014, 35(8): 2436-2445.

[55] Segers VFM, Lee RT. Protein therapeutics for cardiac regeneration after myocardial infarction [J]. Journal Of Cardiovascular Translational Research, 2010, 3(5): 469-477.

[56] Nakamura T, Mizuno S, Matsumoto K, et al. Myocardial protection from ischemia/reperfusion injury by endogenous and exogenous HGF [J]. Journal Of Clinical Investigation, 2000, 106(12): 1511-1519.

[57] Duan HF, Wu CT, Wu DL, et al. Treatment of myocardial ischemia with bone marrow-derived mesenchymal stem cells overexpressing hepatocyte growth factor [J]. Molecular Therapy, 2003, 8(3): 467-474.

[58] Olsson AK, Dimberg A, Kreuger J, et al. VEGF receptor signalling - in control of vascular function [J]. Nature Reviews Molecular Cell Biology, 2006, 7(5): 359-371.

[59] Hoeben A, Landuyt B, Highley MS, et al. Vascular endothelial

growth factor and angiogenesis [J]. Pharmacological Reviews, 2004, 56(4): 549-580.

[60] Zhou L, Ma W, Yang Z, et al. VEGF(165) and angiopoietin-1 decreased myocardium infarct size through phosphatidylinositol-3 kinase and Bcl-2 pathways [J]. Gene Therapy, 2005, 12(3): 196-202.

[61] Lian F, Xue S, Gu P, et al. The long-term effect of autologous endothelial progenitor cells from peripheral blood implantation on infarcted myocardial contractile force [J]. Journal Of International Medical Research, 2008, 36(1): 40-46.

[62] Melly LF, Marsano A, Frobert A, et al. Controlled angiogenesis in the heart by cell-based expression of specific vascular endothelial growth factor levels [J]. Human Gene Therapy Methods, 2012, 23(5): 346-356.

[63] Yun Y-R, Won JE, Jeon E, et al. Fibroblast growth factors: biology, function, and application for tissue regeneration [J]. Journal Of Tissue Engineering, 2010, 1(1).

[64] Szebenyi G, Fallon JF. Fibroblast growth factors as multifunctional signaling factors[A]. In: International Review Of Cytology-a Survey Of Cell Biology, Vol 185 (Jeon KW, ed), Vol. 185, 1999: 45-106.

[65] Takehara N, Tsutsumi Y, Tateishi K, et al. Controlled delivery of basic fibroblast growth factor promotes human cardiosphere-derived cell engraftment to enhance cardiac repair for chronic myocardial infarction [J]. Journal Of the American College Of Cardiology, 2008, 52(23): 1858-1865.

[66] Song H, Kwon K, Lim S, et al. Transfection of mesenchymal stem cells with the FGF-2 gene improves their survival under hypoxic conditions [J]. Molecules And Cells, 2005, 19(3): 402-407.

[67] Edelberg JM, Cai D, Xaymardan M. Translation of PDGF cardioprotective pathways [J]. Cardiovascular toxicology, 2003, 3(1): 27-35.

[68] Edelberg JM, Aird WC, Wu W, et al. PDGF mediates cardiac microvascular communication [J]. Journal Of Clinical Investigation, 1998, 102(4): 837-843.

[69] Edelberg JM, Tang LL, Hattori K, et al. Young adult bone marrow-derived endothelial precursor cells restore aging-impaired cardiac angiogenic function [J]. Circulation Research, 2002, 90(10): E89-E93.

[70] Edelberg JM, Lee SH, Kaur M, et al. Platelet-derived growth factor-AB limits the extent of myocardial infarction in a rat model - Feasibility of restoring impaired angiogenic capacity in the aging heart [J]. Circulation, 2002, 105(5): 608-613.

[71] Xaymardan M, Tang LL, Zagreda L, et al. Platelet-derived growth factor-AB promotes the generation of adult bone marrow-derived cardiac myocytes [J]. Circulation Research, 2004, 94(5): E39-E45.

[72] McLaren ID, Jerde TJ, Bushman W. Role of interleukins, IGF and stem cells in BPH [J]. Differentiation, 2011, 82(4-5): 237-243.

[73] Lin H, Luo X, Jin B, et al. The effect of EPO Gene overexpression on proliferation and migration of mouse bone marrow-derived mesenchymal stem cells [J]. Cell Biochemistry And Biophysics, 2015, 71(3): 1365-1372.

[74] Wang M, Zou Z. Multiple mechanisms of SDF-1 promoting VEGF-induced endothelial differentiation of mesenchymal stem cells [J]. International Journal Of Cardiology, 2014, 177(3): 1098-1099.

[75] Zhao L, Hantash BM. TGF-beta 1 regulates differentiation of bone marrow mesenchymal stem cells[A]. In: Vitamins And Hormones: Stem Cell Regulators (Litwack G, ed), Vol. 87, 2011: 127-141.

[76] Mitragotri S, Burke PA, Langer R. Overcoming the challenges in administering biopharmaceuticals: formulation and delivery strategies [J]. Nature Reviews Drug Discovery, 2014, 13(9): 655-672.

[77] Vaishya R, Khurana V, Patel S, et al. Long-term delivery of protein therapeutics [J]. Expert Opinion on Drug Delivery, 2015, 12(3): 415-440.

[78] El-Maouche D, Dumitrescu CE, Andreopoulou P, et al. Stability and degradation of fibroblast growth factor 23 (FGF23): the effect of time and temperature and assay type [J]. Osteoporosis International, 2016, 27(7): 2345-2353.

[79] Lee J, Blaber M. The interaction between thermodynamic stability and buried free cysteines in regulating the functional half-life of fibroblast growth factor-1 [J]. Journal Of Molecular Biology, 2009, 393(1): 113-127.

[80] Butko A, Celli GB, Paulson A, et al. Entrapment of basic fibroblast growth factor (bFGF) in a succinylated chitosan nanoparticle delivery system and release profile [J]. Journal Of Biomaterials Science-Polymer Edition, 2016, 27(10): 1045-1057.

[81] Lee J, Blaber M. Increased functional half-life of fibroblast growth factor-1 by recovering a vestigial disulfide bond. [J]. Proteins Proteomics, 2010, 1: 37-42.

[82] Hamann MCJ, Tator CH, Shoichet MS. Injectable intrathecal delivery system for localized administration of EGF and FGF-2 to the injured rat spinal cord [J]. Experimental Neurology, 2005, 194(1): 106-119.

[83] Johnson TD, Christman KL. Injectable hydrogel therapies and their delivery strategies for treating myocardial infarction [J]. Expert Opinion on Drug Delivery, 2013, 10(1): 59-72.

[84] Formiga FR, Tamayo E, Simon-Yarza T, et al. Angiogenic therapy for cardiac repair based on protein delivery systems [J]. Heart Failure Reviews, 2012, 17(3): 449-473.

[85] Ungerleider JL, Christman KL. Concise review: injectable biomaterials for the treatment of myocardial infarction and peripheral artery disease: Translational challenges and progress [J]. Stem Cells Translational Medicine, 2014, 3(9): 1090-1099.

[86] Ouma GO, Jonas RA, Usman MHU, et al. Targets and delivery methods for therapeutic angiogenesis in peripheral artery disease [J]. Vascular Medicine, 2012, 17(3): 174-192.

[87] Agudelo CA, Tachibana Y, Hurtado AF, et al. The use of magnetic resonance cell tracking to monitor endothelial progenitor cells in a rat hindlimb ischemic model [J]. Biomaterials, 2012, 33(8): 2439-2448.

[88] Yadav S, Shire SJ, Kalonia DS. Factors affecting the viscosity in high concentration solutions of different monoclonal antibodies [J]. Journal Of Pharmaceutical Sciences, 2010, 99(12): 4812-4829.

[89] Chugh AR, Beache GM, Loughran JH, et al. Administration of cardiac stem cells in patients with ischemic cardiomyopathy: The SCIPIO trial surgical aspects and interim analysis of myocardial function and viability by magnetic resonance [J]. Circulation, 2012, 126(11): S54-S64.

[90] Makkar RR, Smith RR, Cheng K, et al. Intracoronary cardiosphere-derived cells for heart regeneration after myocardial infarction (CADUCEUS): a prospective, randomised phase 1 trial [J]. Lancet, 2012, 379(9819): 895-904.

[91] Wu KH, Mo XM, Han ZC, et al. Stem cell engraftment and survival in the ischemic heart [J]. Annals Of Thoracic Surgery, 2011, 92(5): 1917-1925.

[92] Segers VFM, Lee RT. Stem-cell therapy for cardiac disease [J]. Nature, 2008, 451(7181): 937-942.

[93] Muscari C, Bonafe F, Martin-Suarez S, et al. Restored perfusion and reduced inflammation in the infarcted heart after grafting stem cells with a hyaluronan-based scaffold [J]. Journal Of Cellular And Molecular Medicine, 2013, 17(4): 518-530.

[94] Censi R, Di Martino P, Vermonden T, et al. Hydrogels for protein delivery in tissue engineering [J]. Journal Of Controlled Release, 2012, 161(2): 680-692.

[95] Kundu B, Rajkhowa R, Kundu SC, et al. Silk fibroin biomaterials for tissue regenerations [J]. Advanced Drug Delivery Reviews, 2013, 65(4): 457-470.

[96] Zhang W, Wang X, Wang S, et al. The use of injectable sonication-induced silk hydrogel for VEGF(165) and BMP-2 delivery for elevation of the maxillary sinus floor [J]. Biomaterials, 2011, 32(35): 9415-9424.

[97] Tian J-L, Zhao Y-Z, Jin Z, et al. Synthesis and characterization of Poloxamer 188-grafted heparin copolymer [J]. Drug Development And Industrial Pharmacy, 2010, 36(7): 832-838.

[98] Zhao Y-Z, Zhang M, Tian X-Q, et al. Using basic fibroblast growth factor nanoliposome combined with ultrasound-introduced technology to early intervene the diabetic cardiomyopathy [J]. International Journal Of Nanomedicine, 2016, 11: 675-686.

[99] Rooney P, Kumar S, Ponting J, et al. The role of hyaluronan in tumor neovascularization (review) [J]. International Journal Of Cancer, 1995, 60(5): 632-636.

[100] Sattar A, Rooney P, Kumar S, et al. Application of angiogenic oligosaccharides of hyaluronan increases blood-vessel numbers in rat skin [J]. Journal Of Investigative Dermatology, 1994, 103(4): 576-579.

[101] Peattie RA, Rieke ER, Hewett EM, et al. Dual growth factor-induced angiogenesis in vivo using hyaluronan hydrogel implants [J]. Biomaterials, 2006, 27(9): 1868-1875.

[102] Obara K, Ishihara M, Fujita M, et al. Acceleration of wound healing in healing-impaired db/db mice with a photocrosslinkable chitosan hydrogel containing fibroblast growth factor-2 [J]. Wound Repair And Regeneration, 2005, 13(4): 390-397.

[103] Fujita M, Ishihara M, Morimoto Y, et al. Efficacy of photocrosslinkable chitosan hydrogel containing fibroblast growth factor-2 in a rabbit model of chronic myocardial infarction [J]. Journal Of Surgical Research, 2005, 126(1): 27-33.

[104] Yeo Y, Geng W, Ito T, et al. Photocrosslinkable hydrogel for myocyte cell culture and injection [J]. Journal Of Biomedical Materials Research Part B-Applied Biomaterials, 2007, 81B(2): 312-322.

[105] Park CJ, Clark SG, Lichtensteiger CA, et al. Accelerated wound closure of pressure ulcers in aged mice by chitosan scaffolds with and without bFGF [J]. Acta Biomaterialia, 2009, 5(6): 1926-1936.

[106] Wang H, Shi J, Wang Y, et al. Promotion of cardiac differentiation of brown adipose derived stem cells by chitosan hydrogel for repair after myocardial infarction [J]. Biomaterials, 2014, 35(13): 3986-3998.

[107] Ono K, Saito Y, Yura H, et al. Photocrosslinkable chitosan as a biological adhesive [J]. Journal Of Biomedical Materials Research, 2000, 49(2): 289-295.

[108] Lee KY, Peters MC, Mooney DJ. Comparison of vascular endothelial growth factor and basic fibroblast growth factor on angiogenesis in SCID mice [J]. Journal Of Controlled Release, 2003, 87(1-3): 49-56.

[109] Hao X, Silva EA, Mansson-Broberg A, et al. Angiogenic effects of sequential release of VEGF-A(165) and PDGF-BB with alginate hydrogels after myocardial infarction [J]. Cardiovascular Research, 2007, 75(1): 178-185.

[110] Lee S-M, Nguyen ST. Smart nanoscale drug delivery platforms from stimuli-responsive polymers and liposomes [J]. Macromolecules, 2013, 46(23): 9169-9180.

[111] Kim H, Park H, Lee JW, et al. Magnetic field-responsive release of transforming growth factor beta 1 from heparin-modified alginate ferrogels [J]. Carbohydrate Polymers, 2016, 151: 467-473.

[112] Christman KL, Singelyn JM, Salvatore M, et al. Catheter-deliverable hydrogel derived from decellularized ventricular extracellular matrix increases cardiomyocyte survival and preserves cardiac function post-myocardial infarction [J]. Journal Of the American College Of Cardiology, 2011, 57(14): E2017-E2017.

[113] Seif-Naraghi SB, Singelyn JM, Salvatore MA, et al. Safety and efficacy of an injectable extracellular matrix hydrogel for treating myocardial infarction [J]. Science Translational Medicine, 2013, 5(173).

[114] Xu HL, Tian FR, Lu CT, et al. Thermo-sensitive hydrogels combined with decellularised matrix deliver bFGF for the functional recovery of rats after a spinal cord injury [J]. Scientific Reports, 2016, 6.

[115] Wang L, Zhao M, Li S, et al. "Click" immobilization of a VEGF-mimetic peptide on decellularized endothelial extracellular matrix to enhance angiogenesis [J]. ACS Applied Materials & Interfaces, 2014, 6(11): 8401-8406.

[116] Geng H, Song H, Qi J, et al. Sustained release of VEGF from PLGA nanoparticles embedded thermo-sensitive hydrogel in full-thickness porcine bladder acellular matrix [J]. Nanoscale Research Letters, 2011, 6.

[117] Jiang X, Xiong Q, Xu G, et al. VEGF-loaded nanoparticle-modified BAMAs enhance angiogenesis and inhibit graft shrinkage in tissue-engineered bladder [J]. Annals Of Biomedical Engineering, 2015, 43(10): 2577-2586.

[118] Omidi E, Fuetterer L, Mousavi SR, et al. Characterization and assessment of hyperelastic and elastic properties of decellularized human adipose tissues [J]. Journal Of Biomechanics, 2014, 47(15): 3657-3663.

[119] Han TTY, Toutounji S, Amsden BG, et al. Adipose-derived stromal cells mediate in vivo adipogenesis, angiogenesis and inflammation in decellularized adipose tissue bioscaffolds [J]. Biomaterials, 2015, 72: 125-137.

[120] Alexander A, Ajazuddin, Khan J, et al. Poly(ethylene glycol)-poly(lactic-co-glycolic acid) based thermosensitive injectable hydrogels for biomedical applications [J]. Journal Of Controlled Release, 2013, 172(3): 715-729.

[121] Sun QH, Chen RR, Shen YC, et al. Sustained vascular endothelial growth factor delivery enhances angiogenesis and perfusion in ischemic hind limb [J]. Pharmaceutical Research, 2005, 22(7): 1110-1116.

[122] Richardson TP, Peters MC, Ennett AB, et al. Polymeric system for dual growth factor delivery [J]. Nature Biotechnology, 2001, 19(11): 1029-1034.

[123] Simon-Yarza T, Formiga FR, Tamayo E, et al. PEGylated-PLGA microparticles containing VEGF for long term drug delivery [J]. International Journal Of Pharmaceutics, 2013, 440(1): 13-18.

[124] Peres C, Matos AI, Conniot J, et al. Poly(lactic acid)-based particulate systems are promising tools for immune modulation [J]. Acta Biomaterialia, 2017, 48: 41-57.

[125] Formiga FR, Garbayo E, Diaz-Herraez P, et al. Biodegradation and heart retention of polymeric micropaticles in a rat model of myocardial ischemia [J]. European Journal Of Pharmaceutics And Biopharmaceutics, 2013, 85(3): 665-672.

[126] Formiga FR, Pelacho B, Garbayo E, et al. Sustained release of VEGF through PLGA microparticles improves vasculogenesis and tissue remodeling in an acute myocardial ischemia-reperfusion model [J]. Journal Of Controlled Release, 2010, 147(1): 30-37.

[127] Diaz-Herraez P, Garbayo E, Simon-Yarza T, et al. Adipose-derived stem cells combined with Neuregulin-1 delivery systems for heart tissue engineering [J]. European Journal Of Pharmaceutics And Biopharmaceutics, 2013, 85(1): 143-150.

[128] Pascual-Gil S, Simon-Yarza T, Garbayo E, et al. Tracking the in vivo release of bioactive NRG from PLGA and PEG-PLGA microparticles in infarcted hearts [J]. Journal Of Controlled Release, 2015, 220: 388-396.

[129] d'Angelo I, Garcia-Fuentes M, Parajo Y, et al. Nanoparticles based on PLGA:Poloxamer blends for the delivery of proangiogenic growth factors [J]. Molecular Pharmaceutics, 2010, 7(5): 1724-1733.

[130] Donaghue IE, Shoichet MS. Controlled release of bioactive PDGF-AA from a hydrogel/nanoparticle composite [J]. Acta Biomaterialia, 2015, 25: 35-42.

[131] Binsalamah ZM, Paul A, Khan AA, et al. Intramyocardial sustained delivery of placental growth factor using nanoparticles as a vehicle for delivery in the rat infarct model [J]. International Journal Of Nanomedicine, 2011, 6: 2667-2678.

[132] Yockman JW, Kastenmeier A, Erickson HM, et al. Novel polymer carriers and gene constructs for treatment of myocardial ischemia and infarction [J]. Journal Of Controlled Release, 2008, 132(3): 260-266.

[133] Ruvinov E, Freeman I, Fredo R, et al. Spontaneous coassembly of biologically active nanoparticles via affinity binding of heparin-

binding proteins to alginate-sulfate [J]. Nano Letters, 2016, 16(2): 883-888.

[134] Scott RC, Rosano JM, Ivanov Z, *et al.* Targeting VEGF-encapsulated immunoliposomes to MI heart improves vascularity and cardiac function [J]. Faseb Journal, 2009, 23(10): 3361-3367.

[135] Izadifar M, Kelly ME, Chen X. Regulation of sequential release of growth factors using bilayer polymeric nanoparticles for cardiac tissue engineering [J]. Nanomedicine, 2016, 11(24): 3237-3259.

[136] Zhu J, Marchant RE. Design properties of hydrogel tissue-engineering scaffolds [J]. Expert Review Of Medical Devices, 2011, 8(5): 607-626.

[137] Ruvinov E, Leor J, Cohen S. The promotion of myocardial repair by the sequential delivery of IGF-1 and HGF from an injectable alginate biomaterial in a model of acute myocardial infarction [J]. Biomaterials, 2011, 32(2): 565-578.

[138] Oh KS, Song JY, Yoon SJ, *et al.* Temperature-induced gel formation of core/shell nanoparticles for the regeneration of ischemic heart [J]. Journal Of Controlled Release, 2010, 146(2): 207-211.

[139] Venugopal JR, Prabhakaran MP, Mukherjee S, *et al.* Biomaterial strategies for alleviation of myocardial infarction [J]. Journal Of the Royal Society Interface, 2012, 9(66): 1-19.

[140] Tsur-Gang O, Ruvinov E, Landa N, *et al.* The effects of peptide-based modification of alginate on left ventricular remodeling and function after myocardial infarction [J]. Biomaterials, 2009, 30(2): 189-195.

[141] Simpson D, Liu H, Fan T-HM, *et al.* A tissue engineering approach to progenitor cell delivery results in significant cell engraftment and improved myocardial remodeling [J]. Stem Cells, 2007, 25(9): 2350-2357.

[142] Simpson DL, Boyd NL, Kaushal S, *et al.* Use of human embryonic stem cell derived-mesenchymal cells for cardiac repair [J]. Biotechnology And Bioengineering, 2012, 109(1): 274-283.

[143] Kai D, Wang Q-L, Wang H-J, *et al.* Stem cell-loaded nanofibrous patch promotes the regeneration of infarcted myocardium with functional improvement in rat model [J]. Acta Biomaterialia, 2014, 10(6): 2727-2738.

[144] Padin-Iruegas ME, Misao Y, Davis ME, *et al.* Cardiac progenitor cells and biotinylated insulin-like growth factor-1 nanofibers improve endogenous and exogenous myocardial regeneration after infarction [J]. Circulation, 2009, 120(10): 876-U115.

[145] Hahn JY, Cho HJ, Kang HJ, *et al.* Pre-treatment of mesenchymal stem cells with a combination of growth factors enhances gap junction formation, cytoprotective effect on cardiomyocytes, and therapeutic efficacy for myocardial infarction [J]. Journal Of the American College Of Cardiology, 2008, 51(9): 933-943.

[146] Forte G, Minieri M, Cossa P, *et al.* Hepatocyte growth factor effects on mesenchymal stem cells: Proliferation, migration, and differentiation [J]. Stem Cells, 2006, 24(1): 23-33.

[147] Srinivas G, Anversa P, Frishman WH. Cytokines and myocardial regeneration a novel treatment option for acute myocardial infarction [J]. Cardiology In Review, 2009, 17(1): 1-9.

[148] Pons J, Huang Y, Arakawa-Hoyt J, *et al.* VEGF improves survival of mesenchymal stem cells in infarcted hearts [J]. Biochemical And Biophysical Research Communications, 2008, 376(2): 419-422.

[149] Muscari C, Giordano E, Bonafe F, *et al.* Strategies affording prevascularized cell-based constructs for myocardial tissue engineering [J]. Stem Cells International, 2014: 222-229.

[150] Karam J-P, Muscari C, Sindji L, *et al.* Pharmacologically active microcarriers associated with thermosensitive hydrogel as a growth factor releasing biomimetic 3D scaffold for cardiac tissue-engineering [J]. Journal Of Controlled Release, 2014, 192: 82-94.

[151] Wang F, Li Z, Khan M, *et al.* Injectable, rapid gelling and highly flexible hydrogel composites as growth factor and cell carriers [J]. Acta Biomaterialia, 2010, 6(6): 1978-1991.

[152] Miyagi Y, Zeng F, Huang XP, *et al.* Surgical ventricular restoration with a cell- and cytokine-seeded biodegradable scaffold [J]. Biomaterials, 2010, 31(30): 7684-7694.

[153] Zhang G, Nakamura Y, Wang X, *et al.* Controlled release of stromal cell-derived factor-1alpha *in situ* increases C-kit(+) cell homing to the infarcted heart [J]. Tissue Engineering, 2007, 13(8): 2063-2071.

[154] Zhang G, Hu Q, Braunlin EA, *et al.* Enhancing efficacy of stem cell transplantation to the heart with a PEGylated fibrin biomatrix [J]. Tissue Engineering Part A, 2008, 14(6): 1025-1036.

[155] Miyagi Y, Chiu LLY, Cimini M, *et al.* Biodegradable collagen patch with covalently immobilized VEGF for myocardial repair [J]. Biomaterials, 2011, 32(5): 1280-1290.

[156] Wang Y, Liu XC, Zhao J, *et al.* Degradable PLGA scaffolds with basic fibroblast growth factor experimental studies in myocardial revascularization [J]. Texas Heart Institute Journal, 2009, 36(2): 89-97.

Fibroblast growth factor 10 in pancreas development and pancreatic cancer

Rodrick Ndlovu, Xiaokun Li, Jinsan Zhang

1. Introduction

The Fibroblast Growth Factor (FGF) family of peptides and the corresponding family of receptor tyrosine kinases (RTKs) collectively constitute one of the most adaptable, complex, and diverse growth factor signaling systems that are involved in many developmental and repair processes in virtually all vertebrate and invertebrate tissues and cells (Goetz and Mohammadi, 2013). Currently, the mammalian FGF nomenclature encompasses FGF1 to FGF23, comprising of secreted signaling proteins that transduce signals *via* their specific FGF receptors (FGFRs), and intracellular FGFs that serve as cofactors for voltage-gated sodium channels. These ligands are divided and grouped into seven subfamilies based on phylogenetic analysis, sequence similarities, and function (Goetz *et al.*, 2009; Ornitz and Itoh, 2015).

FGFR family of RTKs comprises of FGFR1, FGFR2, FGFR3, and FGFR4. As the name suggests, FGFRs bind to members of secreted FGFs along with the sequential formation of complexes with heparin/heparan sulfate (HS) cofactor-proteoglycans to propagate downstream signal transduction pathways, which include activation of PLCγ, MAPK, AKT, and STAT cascades. At the cellular level, paracrine FGF-FGFR-HS signaling engages in vital roles in regulating cell proliferation, migration, survival, and differentiation during the development of the embryo (Kato and Sekine, 1999; Ornitz and Itoh, 2015).

FGF10, a FGF7 subfamily member, is a typical paracrine FGF and chiefly mediates its biological responses by activating FGFR2b. FGF10 is a potent morphogen and plays a crucial role in transmitting mesenchyme signaling to the epithelium. Genetic ablation of FGF10 in mice results in gross developmental defects characterized by agenesis and dysgenesis in a variety of organs and tissues highlighting an essential role of FGF10 signaling for the development of multiple organs including the pancreas (Bellusci *et al.*, 1997; Bhushan *et al.*, 2001; Itoh and Ohta, 2014). Although not as widely explored as in the development field, there is strong evidence suggesting that FGF10 is also involved in the pancreatic carcinogenesis (Nomura *et al.*, 2008). Herein, we summarize the recent information about the involvement of FGF10 in pancreas development and diseases with a focus on pancreatic cancer.

2. FGF10 signaling machinery

Alternative splicing of the extracellular IgIII loop of FGFR1-3 generates IIIb- and IIIc-variants of the receptors. Tissue- and cell-specific expression of these isoforms and modification in binding properties for the FGF ligands confer signaling specificity and functional diversity in regulating interactions in embryonic development, tissue homeostasis, repair, and cancer (Itoh and Ohta, 2014). FGFR2 generates two isoforms *via* alternative splicing, FGFR2b, predominantly expressed in epithelial cells and FGFR2c, chiefly expressed in mesenchymal cells. A distinct feature of the FGF7 subfamily is the preferential binding to their cognate receptor FGFR2b in a HS dependent manner in contrast to most other FGFs predominantly interacting with FGFR2c (Givol and Yayon, 1992; Orr-Urtreger *et al.*, 1993; Lindahl *et al.*, 1998; Holzmann *et al.*, 2012).

Formation of the FGF10-FGFR2b-HS (2:2:2) ternary complex results in the phosphorylation of intracellular tyrosine residues in FGFRs (Fig. 1A). Phosphorylated FGFRs activate FGFR substrate 2α(FRS2α) and phospholipase Cγ (PLCγ1), which mediate cell motility (Zhang *et al.*, 2006; Itoh and Ohta, 2014). FRS2α, in turn, facilitates the activation of RAS-MAPK or PI3K-AKT and PLCγ activates protein kinase C. The RAS-MAPK and PI3K-AKT pathways are pre-

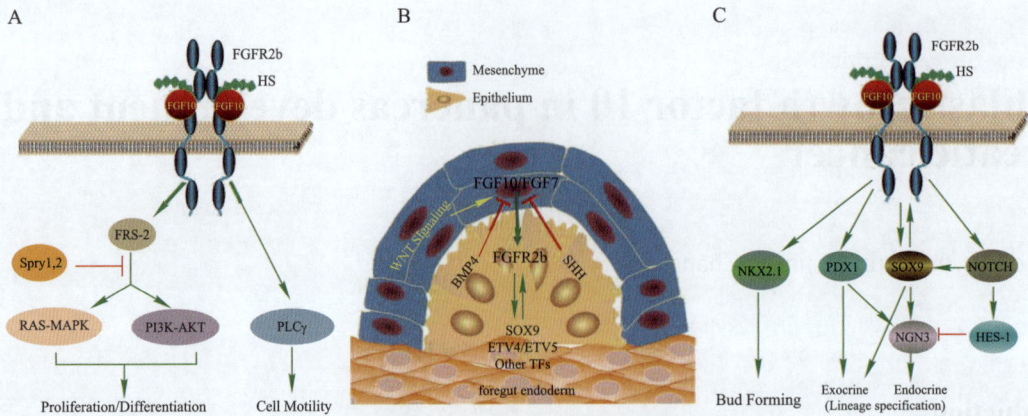

Fig. 1. FGF10 signaling and its key crosstalk during pancreas development. (A) FGF10 is a high affinity ligand for FGFR2b. FGF10 interacts with FGFR2b with HS as cofactor and induces activation of the RAS-MAPK, PI3K-AKT, and PLCγ pathways, which mediate cell differentiation, proliferation, and motility. SPRYs are negative regulators of the RAS-MAPK and PI3K-AKT pathways. (B) FGF10 mediates mesenchyme to epithelial signaling through crosstalk with several key developmental pathways including WNT factors, BMP and SHH, which are important in pancreatic cell fate specification and branching morphogenesis. BMP signaling is required for the normal development of the mesenchyme as well as the epithelium. (C) FGF10 has a crucial role in epithelial branching morphogenesis through crosstalk with several key TFs and regulators for pancreas development. The FGF10/FGFR2b/SOX9 regulatory loop promotes proliferation and maintains pancreatic fate in pancreatic progenitors.

dominantly involved in mitogenic cell responses or cell survival and are subjected to negative regulation by SPRY1 and SPRY2 (Tefft *et al.*, 2002; Zhang *et al.*, 2006). These signaling cascades mediate a diverse range of biological outcomes that define FGF10/FGFR2b dependent signaling (Fig. 1A). The spatiotemporal expression and activity of FGFs and FGFR isoforms is additionally enhanced by the diversity of HS structures, which are also involved in developmental processes, insinuating that tissue-specific HS regulates FGF signaling (Lindahl *et al.*, 1998; Makarenkova *et al.*, 2009).

Interestingly, although FGF7 and FGF10 share a common receptor, expression in mesenchyme and the ability to promote proliferation of embryonic pancreatic epithelial cells *in vitro* (Ye *et al.*, 2005), the phenotypes of their knockout mice are drastically different in that FGF7 null mice are born with no obvious abnormalities (Guo *et al.*, 1996), whereas FGF10 knockout mice die at birth with major defects in multiple organs such as lung agenesis and pancreas dysgenesis (Min *et al.*, 1998; Sekine *et al.*, 1999; Ohuchi *et al.*, 2000; Itoh and Ornitz, 2011). Based on a sophisticated quantitative proteomics approach, Francavilla *et al.* (2013) uncovered a fascinating ligand-dependent mechanism for the control of FGFR2b turnover and signaling outputs. FGF7 stimulation leads to FGFR2b degradation and, ultimately, cell proliferation, whereas FGF10 triggers additional phosphorylation on Y734 of FGFR2b leading to its recruitment of PI3K and SH3BP4 to promote receptor recycling and sustained signaling.

Zinkle and Mohammadi recently proposed a threshold model for RTK signaling specificity and cell fate determination (Makarenkova *et al.*, 2009; Francavilla *et al.*, 2013; Zinkle and Mohammadi, 2018). It is suggested that the intensity and duration of signaling *via* FGFR2b is dependent on the phosphorylation of Y734 within the kinase domain. Higher affinity of FGF10 for binding both FGFR2b and the co-receptor HS (Makarenkova *et al.*, 2009) generates a more robust interaction than FGF7-FGFR2b dimers, therefore propagates more sustained MAPK signal that leads to cell proliferation and migration whilst FGF7 propagates a transient MAPK signal that leads to cell proliferation. It is conceivable that the difference in ligand-induced dimer stability distinguishes FGF7 from FGF10 on the choice and durability of intracellular pathways, which may well contribute to their functional discrepancies on branching morphogenesis during embryonic development.

3. FGF10 in pancreas development

The pancreas is an endoderm-derived glandular organ that partakes in the regulation of glucose homeostasis and nutrient uptake through the concerted functions of its endocrine and exocrine compartments, respectively (Edlund, 1999; Shih *et al.*, 2013). Early mouse pancreas development has two characteristic periods: a primary transition (E9.5-12.5) that is characterized by rapid cell proliferation and histogenesis and a secondary transition (E12,5-birth) after rotation of the gut at E12.5 that is chiefly characterized by cytodifferentiation and formation of the significant intracellular organelles of the adult pancreatic cell (Pictet *et al.*, 1972; Jorgensen *et al.*, 2007; Benitez *et al.*, 2012).

The mesenchyme is critical for the growth of all pancreatic lineages (Landsman *et al.*, 2011). Reports indicate that FGF signaling derived from the surrounding mesenchymal tissue is pivotal for the genesis of specific cellular domains (Hart *et al.*, 2003; Zhou *et al.*, 2007). FGF10, as a mesenchymal factor, has an indispensable role in ensuring the development of the pancreatic epithelium, which gives rise to the functional endocrine and exocrine cell types (Bhushan *et al.*, 2001; Elghazi *et al.*, 2002; Hart *et al.*, 2003; Norgaard *et al.*, 2003). To ascertain the role of FGF10 in pancreas development, Bhushan *et al.* (2001) demonstrated that FGF10 expressed from E9.5 until E11.5 in mice is vital for pancreas growth and differentiation of Pdx1$^+$ epithelial precursor cells. The absence of this mesenchymal protein led to pancreatic hypoplasia (Bhushan *et al.*, 2001). Furthermore, the pancreata of *Fgfr2b*$^{-/-}$ mutant mice were smaller than the wild type littermates with pancreatic duct cell proliferation notably reduced (Miralles *et al.*, 1999; Pulkkinen *et al.*, 2003). FGF10 signaling predominantly targets the adjacent tissue due to its paracrine nature, hence in *Fgf10* null mutant mice, the pancreatic progenitor cells are diminished even before the onset of secondary transition. The few exocrine cells present do undergo differentiation and form acinar structures (Bhushan *et al.*, 2001). Mice deficient in FGFR2b exhibit mild phenotypes comparable to the FGF10 null mice with differentiation of both pancreas compartments and consequent reduction of organ size (Miralles *et al.*, 1999; Pulkkinen *et al.*, 2003).

While many literature sources substantiate the role of FGF10 in epithelial development, the expression levels of the protein decrease to almost unperceivable levels at E13.5 in mice (Bhushan *et al.*, 2001; Elghazi *et al.*, 2002; Kobberup *et al.*, 2010). Explant studies in mice involving pharmacological inhibition of FGF signaling proved that FGF10 is dispensable at later stages of gestation, implying that different epithelial cell types not only depend on FGF10 signals but also on other (same or distinct) mesenchymal factors (Greggio *et al.*, 2013). Possibly, FGF10′s primary role is vital for the initial stage of progenitor growth, then might work in concert with other mesenchymal derived factors or signaling pathways.

4. FGF10 crosstalk with other signaling pathways

The mesenchyme is a source of cell-extrinsic signals that promotes pancreatic specification, yet limits differentiation, so as to allow expansion of the pancreatic epithelium. Besides FGFs, other mesenchymal signals that promote growth of the pancreatic epithelium include WNT factors (Jonckheere *et al.*, 2008), Retinoic Acid (RA) (Stafford *et al.*, 2006), BMP (Ahnfelt-Ronne *et al.*, 2010), and the TGF-β pathway (Crisera *et al.*, 2000; Fig. 1B).

FGFs and WNT factors are known to act in synergy to promote proliferation in a variety of developmental systems (ten Berge *et al.*, 2008; Afelik *et al.*, 2015). Canonical WNT signaling is a mediator of epithelial to mesenchymal signaling, several WNT ligands plus frizzled (FRZ) receptors (*e.g.*, WNT2b, WNT7b, and FRZ2-9) are expressed by both the mesenchyme and pancreatic epithelial cells during organogenesis (Heller *et al.*, 2002; Afelik *et al.*, 2015). Comparable phenotypes are observed between *Pdx1/Frz8CRD* (dominant-negative frizzled 8 receptor) and *Pdx1/Fgf10* null neonates revealing pancreatic hypoplasia, as early as E14, further implying a role for both signaling pathways in pancreatic growth (Papadopoulou and Edlund, 2005; Jonckheere *et al.*, 2008).

RA signaling is also an indispensable mediator of mesenchymal function. In the lung, mesenchyme RA signaling has been implicated in the induction of FGF10 (Desai *et al.*, 2004). Furthermore, absence of RA signaling leads to pancreatic hypoplasia (severe in the dorsal pancreas) (Martin *et al.*, 2005). In an effort to produce functional β cells from endoderm derived human embryonic stem (hES) cells, Mfopou *et al.* (2010) exposed these hES cells to noggin and RA, followed by FGF10 during early stage of induction, and successfully generated pancreatic cells, the majority of them are *Pdx1*$^+$ that coexpressed FOXA2, HNF6, and SOX9.

Unmitigated differentiation of the mesenchyme, which further ensures proper epithelial development, is reliant on many signaling molecules except members of the Hedgehog family from the early pancreatic niche (Kawahira *et al.*, 2005). Ectopic expression of Sonic Hedgehog (SHH) in mice driven by the *Pdx1* promoter results in differentiation of the pancreatic mesenchyme into smooth muscle and the epithelium assumes an intestinal fate with the generation of few early endocrine cell types (Apelqvist *et al.*, 1997). SHH is also implicated in repressing expression of *Fgf10* (Fig. 1B; Bhushan *et al.*, 2001).

5. Transcription factors implicated in FGF10 signaling

Genetic lineage tracing experiments have elucidated that cell clusters committed to adopting the pancreatic lineage express the transcription factor (TF) PDX1 (Pancreatic and duodenal homeobox 1) and PTF1a (Pancreas transcription factor 1). Ablation of either *Pdx1* or *Ptf1a* causes pancreatic agenesis or diabetes and wide gastro-duodenal deformations (Offield *et al.*, 1996; Stoffers *et al.*, 1997; Kawaguchi *et al.*, 2002; Burlison *et al.*, 2008; Fukuda *et al.*, 2008).

After the establishment of the pancreatic anlage, a gene regulatory network is established with *Pdx1* at the focal apex in order to maintain pancreatic identity (Shih *et al.*, 2015). PDX1 exhibits an extensive cross-regulation network between individual TFs and FGFs such as FGF10; however, sustentation of the pancreatic lineage requires high levels of PDX1 (Shih *et al.*, 2015). Augmentation of PDX1 expression levels is supplemented by PTF1a, which binds to enhancer elements of PDX1 (Wiebe *et al.*, 2007), whilst FGF10 is required to maintain the PDX1[+] expressing progenitor cell pool (Fig. 1C; Bhushan *et al.*, 2001).

Genetic lineage tracing has shown that multipotent progenitor cells (MPCs) can be similarly defined by several TFs such as SOX9, HNF6, NKX2.2, HNF1β, HES1, CAP1, and NKX6.1. At this juncture, MPCs not only have the potential to self-renew, but also can differentiate to form exocrine and endocrine progenitors with PDX1 functioning as the central node (Zhou *et al.*, 2007; Pan and Wright, 2011; Seymour, 2014).

The SOX9 interacts with the FGF signaling pathway in concert with PDX1 to maintain both expansion (in a dosage-dependent manner) and organ identity of MPCs (Shih *et al.*, 2013). SOX9 and PDX1 co-regulate the pancreatic *versus* intestinal lineage choice, ablation of both genes causes MPCs to embrace an alternative hepatic fate (Seymour *et al.*, 2012; Shih *et al.*, 2015). In mice, SOX9, FGFR2b, and FGF10 form a feed-forward expression loop; SOX9 cell-autonomously maintains FGFR2b expression, which in turn, augments its epithelial receptivity to FGF10, whilst FGF10 maintains SOX9 expression (Fig. 1C). Hence nullification of any component in this loop leads to pancreatic hypoplasia and loss of both SOX9 plus FGFR2b in FGF10-deficient MPCs leads to hepatic reprogramming (Seymour *et al.*, 2012).

6. FGF10 mediates pancreatic cell fate

Spatial and temporal regulation of gene function is vital in the modeling of specialized cell types from a field of competent cells. FGF10 is known to maintain progenitor cells in an undifferentiated state to allow subsequent proliferation, ectopic expression results in a hyperplastic pancreas. Nascent emergent patterns of budding cells are additionally controlled by conserved developmental pathways such as the NOTCH signaling *via* lateral inhibition/specification in order to integrate terminal differentiation in FGF10 signaling. FGF10-positive progenitor cells express NOTCH1 and NOTCH2, the NOTCH-ligand genes JAG1 and JAG2, as well as the NOTCH target gene HES1 (Murtaugh *et al.*, 2003; Norgaard *et al.*, 2003; Miralles *et al.*, 2006).

During the primary transition, NOTCH and FGF10 signaling are predominantly involved in restricting premature endocrine differentiation and maintenance of the progenitor state. Ablation of Notch target genes such as *Dll1* (Hrabe de Angelis *et al.*, 1997), *Rbp-jk* (Fujikura *et al.*, 2006), or *Hes1* (Jensen *et al.*, 2000) results in an increase of NGN3[+] cells, leading to premature differentiation of the MPCs into glucagon[+]-cells (Apelqvist *et al.*, 1999) and p57-expressing progenitor cells, which undergo premature cell cycle exit evident with the expression of a hypoplastic pancreas (Georgia *et al.*, 2006). This phenotype is comparable to *Fgf10* and *Sox9* null mutant mice. HES1 is known to repress both the transcriptional activation of *Ngn3* and the cyclin kinase inhibitor *P57* (Fig. 1C; Georgia *et al.*, 2006).

SOX9 is a positive regulator of NGN3 in a dosage-dependent manner, and is expressed chiefly in trunk progenitor cells and its depletion results in the reduction of NGN3[+] cells. This suggests that there may exist a complicated but well-organized regulatory system involving FGF10, FGFR2b, NOTCH, HES1, SOX9, and NGN3 that controls endocrine differentiation and maintenance of progenitor cells (Miralles *et al.*, 2006; Kobberup *et al.*, 2010; Gouzi *et al.*, 2011; Afelik and Jensen, 2013; Shih *et al.*, 2015). It can be postulated that both FGF10 and NOTCH signaling pathways are critical for the establishment of two cell lineages:

(i) NGN3$^+$ cells that form the early α-cells.

(ii) NGN3$^+$ that will remain proliferative and available to differentiate to other endocrine cell types (Apelqvist *et al.*, 1999; Jensen *et al.*, 2000; Miralles *et al.*, 2006; Kobberup *et al.*, 2010; Afelik and Jensen, 2013).

Ectopic expression of *Fgf10* from E10.5 to E13.5 leads to nearly complete loss of endocrine and ductal differentiation (Kobberup *et al.*, 2010). This, in turn, favors the exocrine lineage because of the lack of competence to form the endocrine cell lineage. Furthermore, exocrine (acinar) differentiation has been observed to occur in FGF10 null mutant mice implying that FGF10 does not entirely control exocrine differentiation but rather it is permissive toward exocrine lineage fate (Miralles *et al.*, 1999; Bhushan *et al.*, 2001; Kobberup *et al.*, 2010). This is observed with sustained expression of PTF1A in both *Fgf10$^{-/-}$* mutant and wild type mice though reports have indicated that downstream effectors of FGF10, such as *Etv4* and *Etv5,* influence expression of PTF1A (Fig. 1C; Dong *et al.*, 2007; Kobberup *et al.*, 2007, 2010).

Cellular proliferation and differentiation are mutually exclusive events; hence overexpression of FGF10 beyond the primary transition perturbs differentiation of endocrine and ductal cell types. At this stage, progenitor cells typically co-express PDX1, NKX6.1, and PTF1A, failure of endocrine cell formation leads to diabetes in mice (Hart *et al.*, 2003; Petri *et al.*, 2006; Kobberup *et al.*, 2010). FGF10 signaling *via* FGFR2b is at the expense of endocrine cellular differentiation (Celli *et al.*, 1998; Miralles *et al.*, 1999; Pulkkinen *et al.*, 2003). By understanding the exact timing of the competence window toward endocrine fate, FGF10 could be best exploited in cell-based therapeutic strategies to combat diabetes (Madsen and Serup, 2006).

7. FGF10 -FGFR2b in pancreatic ductal adenocarcinoma

Pancreatic ductal adenocarcinoma (PDAC) is the most common exocrine malignancy and represents one of the deadliest diseases with high mortality due to difficulties in its early diagnosis, metastasis and intrinsic resistance to conventional chemoradiotherapy. At a molecular level, cancer cells in PDAC are often characterized by mutations in the KRAS oncogene, SMAD4, and TP53. Several FGFs and FGFRs are expressed in stromal cells scattered around pancreatic cancer cells and their expression levels have been linked to increased cancer motility, proliferation and metastatic invasion (Kalluri and Zeisberg, 2006; Ying *et al.*, 2016). FGF7 and 10 are both expressed in stromal cells surrounding cancer cells. Regardless of the high homology the latter induces cell migration and invasion whilst the former stimulates cell proliferation. FGF10- FGFR2b signaling induces the expression of type1-matrix metalloproteinase and *TGF-β1* genes (Nomura *et al.*, 2008), these genes are related to cell motility (Friess *et al.*, 1993; Seiki, 2003). Moreover, FGF10-FGFR2b signaling induced the secretion of TGF-β1, a crucial regulator of epithelial to mesenchymal transition (Fig. 2; Moustakas and Heldin, 2007; Nomura *et al.*, 2008).

A hallmark genetic alteration of PDAC is the high frequency mutation of *KRAS*. Numerous studies demonstrate that oncogenic KRAS mutations induce Acinar-to-ductal metaplasia (ADM), pancreatic intraepithelial neoplasia (PanIN), and eventually PDAC. Significantly, SOX9 is imperative for KRAS^{G12D}-mediated ADM and PanIN formation (Kopp *et al.*, 2012). A more recent study demonstrated that KRAS can independently induce SOX9 expression and promoted its nuclear translocation and transcriptional activity, which plays a positive role in the proliferation of PDAC cells (Zhou *et al.*, 2018).

Our recent studies further showed that SOX9 could be induced by NFATC1 and NFATC4 in response to EGFR activation and pancreatitis, which promote ADM and PanIN (Chen *et al.*, 2015; Hessmann *et al.*, 2016). In a separate study, SOX9 is reported to

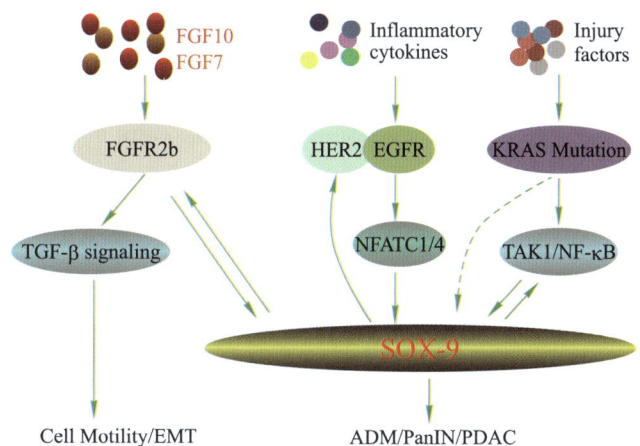

Fig. 2. Crosstalk of FGF10 during pancreatic cancer. Interactions of FGF10 with TGF-β pathway promote EMT and cancer cell invasion. The positive feedback loops between FGF10-SOX9, KRAS/NF-κB-SOX9, and ERBB-SOX9, respectively, are enhanced under inflammatory condition, which contributes to PDAC initiation and progression.

stimulate expression of several members of the ERBB pathway, and is required for ERBB signaling activity to promote pancreatic tumorigenesis (Grimont *et al.*, 2015). These studies further consolidate SOX9 as a central player in pancreatic adenocarcinoma *via* promoting ADM, particularly in the context of oncogenic KRAS and pancreatitis to accelerate development of premalignant lesions and PDAC (Fig. 2). Therefore, three positive feedback loops have emerged from these studies (Fig. 2): (1) FGF10/FGFR2/SOX9 inter-dependent expression is also present in a subset of PDAC patients (Seymour *et al.*, 2012; O'Sullivan *et al.*, 2017); (2) EGFR, *via* activation of NFATC1 and NFATC4, promotes SOX9 expression, whereas activated SOX9 stimulates ERBB2 protein expression (Chen *et al.*, 2015; Grimont *et al.*, 2015; Hessmann *et al.*, 2016); (3) Oncogenic KRAS *via* TAK1/NF-κB promotes SOX9 expression/activation, and SOX9 in turn enhances NF-κB activity (Zhou *et al.*, 2018). These findings open new perspectives for precision therapeutic strategies targeting specific cancer-driven signaling molecules such as ERBB2 or FGFR2.

8. Conclusion and perspective

Animal models lacking each of the secreted FGFs have been developed with diverse phenotypes ranging from mild abnormality in adult physiology to early embryonic lethality. Only three FGFs (FGF9, FGF10, and FGF18) upon knockout result in early postnatal lethality due to severe developmental defects in multiple organs. While *Fgf9* and *Fgf18* are essential for the development of mesenchymal components, numerous studies highlight FGF10 as an indispensable mesenchyme to epithelium signal required for the development of epithelial components in multiple organs. Despite the interesting observations from previous reports, research on FGF10/FGFR2b in the pancreas is lagging behind compared to some other organs such as the lung. There remain some critical questions unanswered regarding how FGF/FGFR2b signaling influence acinar and ductal specification (*e.g.*, further proliferation and differentiation from the progenitor cells), as well as its impact on the endocrine system remain largely unexplored. More elegant and specifically targeted genetic models allowing better spatiotemporal manipulation of gene expression will be essential to better address these questions. During both embryonic development and oncogenic process, FGF10 acquires the ability for unique crosstalk with other pathways as exemplified by its inter-dependent expression with SOX9, which may represent a key knot linking oncogenic KRAS, inflammation and other growth factor signaling. Understanding of FGF10 signaling machinery and its crosstalk with other pathways may provide novel opportunities for PDAC precision therapy and regenerative medicine.

References

[1] Afelik S, Jensen J. Notch signaling in the pancreas: patterning and cell fate specification [J]. Wiley Interdisciplinary Reviews-Developmental Biology, 2013, 2(4): 531-544.

[2] Afelik S, Pool B, Schmerr M, *et al.* Wnt7b is required for epithelial progenitor growth and operates during epithelial-to-mesenchymal signaling in pancreatic development [J]. Developmental Biology, 2015, 399(2): 204-217.

[3] Ahnfelt-Ronne J, Ravassard P, Pardanaud-Glavieux C, *et al.* Mesenchymal bone morphogenetic protein signaling is required for normal pancreas development [J]. Diabetes, 2010, 59(8): 1948-1956.

[4] Apelqvist A, Ahlgren U, Edlund H. Sonic hedgehog directs specialised mesoderm differentiation in the intestine and pancreas [J]. Current Biology, 1997, 7(10): 801-804.

[5] Apelqvist A, Li H, Sommer L, *et al.* Notch signalling controls pancreatic cell differentiation [J]. Nature, 1999, 400(6747): 877-881.

[6] Bellusci S, Grindley J, Emoto H, *et al.* Fibroblast growth factor 10(FGF10) and branching morphogenesis in the embryonic mouse lung [J]. Development, 1997, 124(23): 4867-4878.

[7] Benitez CM, Goodyer WR, Kim SK. Deconstructing pancreas developmental biology [J]. Cold Spring Harbor Perspectives In Biology, 2012, 4(6).

[8] Bhushan A, Itoh N, Kato S, *et al.* Fgf10 is essential for maintaining the proliferative capacity of epithelial progenitor cells during early pancreatic organogenesis [J]. Development, 2001, 128(24): 5109-5117.

[9] Burlison JS, Long Q, Fujitani Y, *et al.* Pdx-1 and Ptf1a concurrently determine fate specification of pancreatic multipotent progenitor cells [J]. Developmental Biology, 2008, 316(1): 74-86.

[10] Celli G, LaRochelle WJ, Mackem S, *et al.* Soluble dominant-negative receptor uncovers essential roles for fibroblast growth factors in multi-organ induction and patterning [J]. Embo Journal, 1998, 17(6): 1642-1655.

[11] Chen N-M, Singh G, Koenig A, *et al.* NFATc1 links EGFR signaling to induction of Sox9 transcription and acinar-ductal transdifferentiation in the pancreas [J]. Gastroenterology, 2015, 148(5): 1024-U1502.

[12] Crisera CA, Maldonado TS, Kadison AS, *et al.* Transforming growth factor-beta 1 in the developing mouse pancreas: a potential regulator of exocrine differentiation [J]. Differentiation, 2000, 65(5): 255-259.

[13] Deangelis MH, McIntyre J, Gossler A. Maintenance of somite borders in mice requires the Delta homologue DlI1 [J]. Nature, 1997, 386(6626): 717-721.

[14] Desai TJ, Malpel S, Flentke GR, *et al.* Retinoic acid selectively

regulates Fgf10 expression and maintains cell identity in the prospective lung field of the developing foregut [J]. Developmental Biology, 2004, 273(2): 402-415.

[15] Dong PDS, Munson CA, Norton W, *et al.* Fgf10 regulates hepatopancreatic ductal system patterning and differentiation [J]. Nature Genetics, 2007, 39(3): 397-402.

[16] Edlund H. Pancreas: how to get there from the gut? [J]. Current Opinion In Cell Biology, 1999, 11(6): 663-668.

[17] Elghazi L, Cras-Meneur C, Czernichow P, *et al.* Role for FGFR2IIIb-mediated signals in controlling pancreatic endocrine progenitor cell proliferation [J]. Proceedings Of the National Academy Of Sciences Of the United States Of America, 2002, 99(6): 3884-3889.

[18] Francavilla C, Rigbolt KTG, Emdal KB, *et al.* Functional proteomics defines the molecular switch underlying FGF receptor trafficking and cellular outputs [J]. Molecular Cell, 2013, 51(6): 707-722.

[19] Friess H, Yamanaka Y, Buchler M, *et al.* Enhanced expression of the type-II transforming growth-factor-beta receptor in human pancreatic-cancer cells without alteration of type-III receptor expression [J]. Cancer Research, 1993, 53(12): 2704-2707.

[20] Fujikura J, Hosoda K, Iwakura H, *et al.* Notch/Rbp-j signaling prevents premature endocrine and ductal cell differentiation in the pancreas [J]. Cell Metabolism, 2006, 3(1): 59-65.

[21] Fukuda A, Kawaguchi Y, Furuyama K, *et al.* Reduction of Ptf1a gene dosage causes pancreatic hypoplasia and diabetes in mice [J]. Diabetes, 2008, 57(9): 2421-2431.

[22] Georgia S, Soliz R, Li M, *et al.* P57 and Hes 1 coordinate cell cycle exit with self-renewal of pancreatic progenitors [J]. Developmental Biology, 2006, 298(1): 22-31.

[23] Givol D, Yayon A. Complexity of FGF receptors: geneticbasis for structural diversity and functional specificity [J]. Faseb Journal, 1992, 6(15): 3362-3369.

[24] Goetz R, Dover K, Laezza F, *et al.* Crystal structure of a fibroblast growth factor homologous factor (FHF) defines a conserved surface on FHFs for binding and modulation of voltage-gated sodium channels [J]. Journal Of Biological Chemistry, 2009, 284(26): 17883-17896.

[25] Goetz R, Mohammadi M. Exploring mechanisms of FGF signalling through the lens of structural biology [J]. Nature Reviews Molecular Cell Biology, 2013, 14(3): 166-180.

[26] Gouzi M, Kim YH, Katsumoto K, *et al.* Neurogenin3 initiates stepwise delamination of differentiating endocrine cells during pancreas development [J]. Developmental Dynamics, 2011, 240(3): 589-604.

[27] Greggio C, De Franceschi F, Figueiredo-Larsen M, *et al.* Artificial three-dimensional niches deconstruct pancreas development *in vitro* [J]. Development, 2013, 140(21): 4452-4462.

[28] Grimont A, Pinho AV, Cowley MJ, *et al.* SOX9 regulates ERBB signalling in pancreatic cancer development [J]. Gut, 2015, 64(11): 1790-1799.

[29] Guo LF, Degenstein L, Fuchs E. Keratinocyte growth factor is required for hair development but not for wound healing [J]. Genes & Development, 1996, 10(2): 165-175.

[30] Hart A, Papadopoulou S, Edlund H. Fgf10 maintains notch activation, stimulates proliferation, and blocks differentiation of pancreatic epithelial cells [J]. Developmental Dynamics, 2003, 228(2): 185-193.

[31] Heller RS, Dichmann DS, Jensen J, *et al.* Expression patterns of Wnts, Frizzleds, sFRPs, and misexpression in transgenic mice suggesting a role for Wnts in pancreas and foregut pattern formation [J]. Developmental Dynamics, 2002, 225(3): 260-270.

[32] Hessmann E, Zhang J-S, Chen N-M, *et al.* NFATc4 Regulates Sox9 Gene Expression in Acinar Cell Plasticity and Pancreatic Cancer Initiation [J]. Stem Cells International, 2016.

[33] Holzmann K, Grunt T, Heinzle C, *et al.* Alternative splicing of fibroblast growth factor receptor IgIII loops in cancer [J]. Journal

Of Nucleic Acids, 2012.

[34] Itoh N, Ohta H. Fgf10: a paracrine-signaling molecule in development, disease, and regenerative medicine [J]. Current Molecular Medicine, 2014, 14(4): 504-509.

[35] Itoh N, Ornitz DM. Fibroblast growth factors: from molecular evolution to roles in development, metabolism and disease [J]. Journal Of Biochemistry, 2011, 149(2): 121-130.

[36] Jensen J, Pedersen EE, Galante P, *et al.* Control sf endodermal endocrine development by Hes-1 [J]. Nature Genetics, 2000, 24(1): 36-44.

[37] Jonckheere N, Mayes E, Shih H-P, *et al.* Analysis of mPygo2 mutant mice suggests a requirement for mesenchymal Wnt signaling in pancreatic growth and differentiation [J]. Developmental Biology, 2008, 318(2): 224-235.

[38] Jorgensen MC, Ahnfelt-Ronne J, Hald J, *et al.* An illustrated review of early pancreas development in the mouse [J]. Endocrine Reviews, 2007, 28(6): 685-705.

[39] Kalluri R, Zeisberg M. Fibroblasts in cancer [J]. Nature Reviews Cancer, 2006, 6(5): 392-401.

[40] Kato S, Sekine K. FGF-FGFR signaling in vertebrate organogenesis [J]. Cellular And Molecular Biology, 1999, 45(5): 631-638.

[41] Kawaguchi Y, Cooper B, Gannon M, *et al.* The role of the transcriptional regulator Ptf1a in converting intestinal to pancreatic progenitors [J]. Nature Genetics, 2002, 32(1): 128-134.

[42] Kawahira H, Scheel DW, Smith SB, *et al.* Hedgehog signaling regulates expansion of pancreatic epithelial cells [J]. Developmental Biology, 2005, 280(1): 111-121.

[43] Kobberup S, Nyeng P, Juhl K, *et al.* VETS-family genes in pancreatic development [J]. Developmental Dynamics, 2007, 236(11): 3100-3110.

[44] Kobberup S, Schmerr M, Dang M-L, *et al.* Conditional control of the differentiation competence of pancreatic endocrine and ductal cells by Fgf10 [J]. Mechanisms Of Development, 2010, 127(3-4): 220-234.

[45] Kopp JL, von Figura G, Mayes E, *et al.* Identification of Sox9-dependent acinar-to-ductal reprogramming as the principal mechanism for initiation of pancreatic ductal adenocarcinoma [J]. Cancer Cell, 2012, 22(6): 737-750.

[46] Landsman L, Nijagal A, Whitchurch TJ, *et al.* Pancreatic mesenchyme regulates epithelial organogenesis throughout development [J]. Plos Biology, 2011, 9(9).

[47] Lindahl U, Kusche-Gullberg M, Kjellen L. Regulated diversity of heparan sulfate [J]. Journal Of Biological Chemistry, 1998, 273(39): 24979-24982.

[48] Madsen OD, Serup P. Towards cell therapy for diabetes [J]. Nature Biotechnology, 2006, 24(12): 1481-1483.

[49] Makarenkova HP, Hoffman MP, Beenken A, *et al.* Differential interactions of FGFs with heparan sulfate control gradient formation and branching morphogenesis [J]. Science Signaling, 2009, 2(88).

[50] Martin M, Gallego-Llamas J, Ribes V, *et al.* Dorsal pancreas agenesis in retinoic acid-deficient Raldh2 mutant mice [J]. Developmental Biology, 2005, 284(2): 399-411.

[51] Mfopou JK, Chen B, Mateizel I, *et al.* Noggin, retinoids, and fibroblast growth factor regulate hepatic or pancreatic fate of human embryonic stem cells [J]. Gastroenterology, 2010, 138(7): 2233-U2285.

[52] Min HS, Danilenko DM, Scully SA, *et al.* Fgf-10 is required for both limb and lung development and exhibits striking functional similarity to Drosophila branchless [J]. Genes & Development, 1998, 12(20): 3156-3161.

[53] Miralles F, Czernichow P, Ozaki K, *et al.* Signaling through fibroblast growth factor receptor 2b plays a key role in the development of the exocrine pancreas [J]. Proceedings Of the National Academy Of Sciences Of the United States Of America, 1999, 96(11): 6267-6272.

[54] Miralles F, Lamotte L, Couton D, *et al.* Interplay between FGF10

and Notch signalling is required for the self-renewal of pancreatic progenitors [J]. International Journal Of Developmental Biology, 2006, 50(1): 17-26.

[55] Moustakas A, Heldin C-H. Signaling networks guiding epithelial-mesenchymal transitions during embryogenesis and cancer progression [J]. Cancer Science, 2007, 98(10): 1512-1520.

[56] Murtaugh LC, Stanger BZ, Kwan KM, et al. Notch signaling controls multiple steps of pancreatic differentiation [J]. Proceedings Of the National Academy Of Sciences Of the United States Of America, 2003, 100(25): 14920-14925.

[57] Nomura S, Yoshitomi H, Takano S, et al. FGF10/FGFR2 signal induces cell migration and invasion in pancreatic cancer [J]. British Journal Of Cancer, 2008, 99(2): 305-313.

[58] Norgaard GA, Jensen JN, Jensen J. FGF10 signaling maintains the pancreatic progenitor cell state revealing a novel role of Notch in organ development [J]. Developmental Biology, 2003, 264(2): 323-338.

[59] Offield MF, Jetton TL, Labosky PA, et al. PDX-1 is required for pancreatic outgrowth and differentiation of the rostral duodenum [J]. Development, 1996, 122(3): 983-995.

[60] Ohuchi H, Hori Y, Yamasaki M, et al. FGF10 acts as a major ligand for FGF receptor 2 IIIb in mouse multi-organ development [J]. Biochemical And Biophysical Research Communications, 2000, 277(3): 643-649.

[61] Ornitz DM, Itoh N. The fibroblast growth factor signaling pathway [J]. Wiley Interdisciplinary Reviews-Developmental Biology, 2015, 4(3): 215-266.

[62] Orr-Urtreger A, Bedford MT, Burakova T, et al. Developmental localization of the splicing alternatives of fibroblast growth-factor receptor-2 (FGFR2) [J]. Developmental Biology, 1993, 158(2): 475-486.

[63] O'Sullivan H, Kelleher FC, Lavelle M, et al. Therapeutic potential for FGFR inhibitors in SOX9-FGFR2 coexpressing pancreatic cancer [J]. Pancreas, 2017, 46(8): E67-E69.

[64] Pan FC, Wright C. Pancreas organogenesis: from bud to plexus to gland [J]. Developmental Dynamics, 2011, 240(3): 530-565.

[65] Papadopoulou S, Edlund H. Attenuated Wnt signaling perturbs pancreatic growth but not pancreatic function [J]. Diabetes, 2005, 54(10): 2844-2851.

[66] Petri A, Ahnfelt-Ronne J, Frederiksen KS, et al. The effect of neurogenin3 deficiency on pancreatic gene expression in embryonic mice [J]. Journal Of Molecular Endocrinology, 2006, 37(2): 301-316.

[67] Pictet RL, Clark WR, Williams RH, et al. Ultrastructural analysis of developing embryonic pancreas [J]. Developmental Biology, 1972, 29(4): 436-467.

[68] Pulkkinen MA, Spencer-Dene B, Dickson C, et al. The IIIb isoform of fibroblast growth factor receptor 2 is required for proper growth and branching of pancreatic ductal epithelium but not for differentiation of exocrine or endocrine cells [J]. Mechanisms Of Development, 2003, 120(2): 167-175.

[69] Seiki M. Membrane-type 1 matrix metalloproteinase: a key enzyme for tumor invasion [J]. Cancer Letters, 2003, 194(1): 1-11.

[70] Sekine K, Ohuchi H, Fujiwara M, et al. Fgf10 is essential for limb and lung formation [J]. Nature Genetics, 1999, 21(1): 138-141.

[71] Seymour PA. Sox9: a master regulator of the pancreatic program [J]. The review of diabetic studies : RDS, 2014, 11(1): 51-83.

[72] Seymour PA, Shih HP, Patel NA, et al. A Sox9/Fgf feed-forward loop maintains pancreatic organ identity [J]. Development, 2012, 139(18): 3363-3372.

[73] Shih HP, Seymour PA, Patel NA, et al. A gene regulatory network cooperatively controlled by Pdx1 and Sox9 governs lineage allocation of foregut progenitor cells [J]. Cell Reports, 2015, 13(2): 326-336.

[74] Shih HP, Wang A, Sander M. Pancreas organogenesis: from lineage determination to morphogenesis[A]. In: *Annual Review Of Cell And Developmental Biology, Vol 29* (Schekman R, ed), Vol. 29, 2013: 81-105.

[75] Stafford D, White RJ, Kinkel MD, et al. Retinoids signal directly to zebrafish endoderm to specify insulin-expressing beta-cells [J]. Development, 2006, 133(5): 949-956.

[76] Stoffers DA, Zinkin NT, Stanojevic V, et al. Pancreatic agenesis attributable to a single nucleotide deletion in the human IPF1 gene coding sequence [J]. Nature Genetics, 1997, 15(1): 106-110.

[77] Tefft D, Lee M, Smith S, et al. mSprouty2 inhibits FGF10-activated MAP kinase by differentially binding to upstream target proteins [J]. American Journal Of Physiology-Lung Cellular And Molecular Physiology, 2002, 283(4): L700-L706.

[78] ten Berge D, Brugmann SA, Helms JA, et al. Wnt and FGF signals interact to coordinate growth with cell fate specification during limb development [J]. Development, 2008, 135(19): 3247-3257.

[79] Wiebe PO, Kormish JD, Roper VT, et al. Ptf1a binds to and activates area III, a highly conserved region of the Pdx1 promoter that mediates early pancreas-wide Pdx1 expression [J]. Molecular And Cellular Biology, 2007, 27(11): 4093-4104.

[80] Ye F, Duvillie B, Scharfmann R. Fibroblast growth factors 7 and 10 are expressed in the human embryonic pancreatic mesenchyme and promote the proliferation of embryonic pancreatic epithelial cells [J]. Diabetologia, 2005, 48(2): 277-281.

[81] Ying H, Dey P, Yao W, et al. Genetics and biology of pancreatic ductal adenocarcinoma [J]. Genes & Development, 2016, 30(4): 355-385.

[82] Zhang X, Ibrahimi OA, Olsen SK, et al. Receptor specificity of the fibroblast growth factor family - The complete mammalian FGF family [J]. Journal Of Biological Chemistry, 2006, 281(23): 15694-15700.

[83] Zhou H, Qin Y, Ji S, et al. SOX9 activity is induced by oncogenic Kras to affect MDC1 and MCMs expression in pancreatic cancer [J]. Oncogene, 2018, 37(7): 912-923.

[84] Zhou Q, Law AC, Rajagopal J, et al. A multipotent progenitor domain guides pancreatic organogenesis [J]. Developmental Cell, 2007, 13(1): 103-114.

[85] Zinkle A, Mohammadi M. A threshold model for receptor tyrosine kinase signaling specificity and cell fate determination [J]. F1000 Research, 2018, 7:872.

Chapter 2
Injury Repair and Regeneration

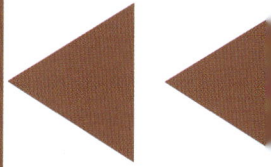

TAT-mediated acidic fibroblast growth factor delivery to the dermis improves wound healing of deep skin tissue in rat

Long Zheng, Xiaokun Li, Xiaojie Wang

1. Introduction

In 2007, deep tissue injury (DTI) was first described by the National Pressure Ulcer Advisory Panel as the newest type of pressure ulcer in the updated staging system [1]. Derived from multiple clinical cases, the definition of DTI was described as "A purple or maroon localized area of discolored intact skin or blood-filled blister due to damage of the underlying soft tissue from pressure and/or shear" [1]. Pressure-related DTI under intact skin in humans may result from a single event of prolonged immobilization, such as a lengthy surgical operation. Studies in animal models have shown that pressure-related ischemia of both subcutaneous tissue and muscle can occur under intact skin [2]; however, there are currently no specific treatments recommended [3].

The fibroblast growth factor (FGF) family regulates developmental processes and tissue homeostasis, including brain patterning, vascular branching morphogenesis and limb development [4]. Fibroblasts are the major mesenchymal cell type in connective tissue and deposit the collagen and elastic fibers of the extracellular matrix (ECM) [5]. Although multiple growth factors, including epidermal growth factor, platelet-derived growth factor, and vascular endothelial growth factor, participate in tissue reconstruction, acidic FGF (aFGF) plays a pivotal role in regulating fibroblasts [6,7], which are central to wound healing in DTI. Previous studies have reported that the administration of aFGF significantly improves wound healing under diabetic conditions [8]. It has been shown that aFGF also enhances local generation of tissue collagen and increases levels of transforming growth factor (TGF)-β1 and proliferating cell nuclear antigen (PCNA) which appear to be involved in the mechanisms underlying wound healing [9]. However, as for many therapeutic proteins, the pharmacological action of aFGF is limited because of low local delivery efficiency. Drug delivery systems such as protein transduction domains, nanoparticles and liposomes have therefore been exploited for the improvement of therapeutic delivery of protein drugs [10,11].

Transactivator of transcription protein (TAT) was discovered by the Frankel and Pabo [12] and Green and Loewenstein [13] groups independently in 1988. It contains a so-called cell-penetrating peptide that mediates the translocation of biological agents from membrane barriers into live cells. This makes TAT a potential vehicle for drug delivery, although the mechanism of its accumulation in cytoplasm is not fully understood [14,15]. The fusion of TAT to metallothionein was shown to enhance metallothionein delivery, thereby inhibiting cell apoptosis, reducing fibrosis and restoring cardiac function in a myocardial ischemia/reperfusion model [16]. Moreover, our previous study demonstrated a potential role for TAT in the delivery of human aFGF$_{19\text{-}154}$ from the surface of the eyeball to the retina in rats [17]. The purpose of this study was to investigate the efficiency of TAT-mediated aFGF delivery in dermal and subcutaneous tissues and evaluate its effectiveness for treating DTI beneath intact skin.

2. Materials and methods

2.1 Delivery gel

Our previous studies showed that the TAT-aFGF fusion protein is stable *in vitro* [18] and that TAT does not affect the bioactivity of aFGF *in vivo* [17]. The delivery gel containing aFGF or TAT-aFGF was prepared as below. Briefly, 0.25 g Carbopol (Sigma-Aldrich, St. Louis, MO) was added to deionized water (45 ml) containing 0.5 ml glycerol (Sigma-Aldrich) and allowed to swell overnight. Methylparaben (0.25 g) and ethylparaben (5 mg) (Sigma-Aldrich) were mixed in 1 ml of phosphate buffered saline (PBS). The pH was immediately adjusted to 7.0 with triethanolamine solution (Sigma-Aldrich). The gel was sterilized for 20 min at 121℃. After the solution was cooled to room temperature, 3 ml of protein solution (15 mg TAT-aFGF or aFGF with 0.5 g of serum albumin) was added to the gel. The gel was then dispensed into aluminum tubes, sealed and stored at 4℃.

2.2 Animals

48 male Sprague-Dawley rats (300–350 g) and 48 male BALB/c mice (18–22 g) (Silaike, Shanghai, China) were maintained in a specific pathogen-free (SPF) animal facility which had controlled temperature and humidity and a 12-hour dark/light cycle. The animals were allowed free access to standard laboratory food and water. All animal protocols were approved by the Institutional Animal Care and Use Committee (IACUC) of Wenzhou Medical University.

2.3 Transdermal delivery of TAT-aFGF proteins in mice

BALB/c mice were anesthetized with chloral hydrate (300 mg/kg, Sigma-Aldrich) and their dorsal hair (3 cm×3 cm) was carefully shaved. Around 24 h later, 50 μl of aFGF or TAT-aFGF solution (60 μg/ml) was topically administrated to the shaved dorsal skin. Blank gel was used as a control solution. At different time points (0, 30 min, 2 h and 8 h), mice were euthanized by cervical dislocation. The skin tissues were harvested and then fixed in 4% paraformaldehyde before embedding for paraffin sections.

2.4 Rat model of pressure ulcers

The model of pressure ulcers was constructed as described previously, but with some modifications [19]. The greater trochanters of the rats were extensively shaved and subsequently pinched between two ceramic disc magnets which were 8 mm in diameter, 4 mm in thickness, 2.4 g in weight and 3,500G in strength. The cycles of ischemia–reperfusion injury were then performed. A single cycle consisted of a dorsal skin magnet pinch for 12 h followed by a rest period of 12 h. This procedure was done consecutively for two days. A single wound with identical size of 0.5 cm in diameter was created in each rat. After the wounds were established, 200 μl of aFGF, TAT-aFGF solution (300 μg/ml) or blank gel was administrated topically. The treatment was repeated daily for 14 days. The ulcers were monitored using digital images which were used to calculate the wound areas using Image Software. Rats were anesthetized with chloral hydrate (300 mg/kg, Sigma-Aldrich) at 0, 3, 7 and 14 days post-treatment. At different time points, the wound contraction was measured quantitatively [20].

2.5 Histopathological evaluation

At time of sacrifice, tissues of skin ulcers (1.5 cm ×1.5 cm) were harvested from rats, followed by fixation in 4% paraformaldehyde and embedding in paraffin. Conventionally, sections were stained with haematoxylin and eosin (HE) and Masson (Sigma-Aldrich). The penetrating effect of TAT-aFGF on the injured skin was evaluated by immunohisto-chemistry, in which the primary antibodies for aFGF, TGF-β1, α-smooth muscle actin (α-SMA), CD68 or PCNA (Santa Cruz, CA) were used accordingly. The CD68 and PCNA levels in each group were quantified using Image-Pro Plus software (Nikon, Tokyo, Japan). The positivity density of α-SMA and TGF-β1 was scored semi-quantitatively as 1 (absent), 2 (low), 3 (medium), 4 (strong), and 5 (very strong) by two observers who were blinded to the grouping [21,22]. Similarly, the HE and Masson-stained sections were semi-quantitatively scored at a range of 0 to 4 according to the level of collagen enrichment.

2.6 Apoptotic DNA fragmentation analysis

The apoptosis ratios of injured tissues were assessed by DNA terminal dUTP nick-end labeling (TUNEL) (Roche, Mannheim, Germany) according to the manufacturer's instructions. The omission of terminal deoxynucleotidyl transfer-ase in tissue sections was used as negative control. The TUNEL index (multiplied by 100) was determined by the ratio of TUNEL-positive nuclei to the total number of nuclei in three random fields under the light microscope.

2.7 Cell culture

The human dermal fibroblast cell line (bought from ATCC, cell line number is PCS-201-012) was a gift from the

Institute of Molecular Pharmacology of Wenzhou Medical University. As described previously [23], cells were cultured in Dulbecco's Modified Eagle's Medium (DMEM) (low glucose) containing 10% fetal bovine serum (FBS) (Gibco, CA) with 0.1% antibiotics. A suspension of 300,000 cells was seeded onto 6-well tissue culture plates. TNF-α (5 ng/ml), TAT-aFGF (10 or 100 ng/ml) or the combination of TNF-α and TAT-aFGF were added into culture media supplemented with 0.1% FBS. Similarly, aFGF was used as a control in cell cultures.

2.8 Western blot analysis

Western blotting was performed as described previously, with some modifications [24]. The α-SMA, TGF-β1 and TGF-βRII proteins were detected in whole lysates of human dermal fibroblasts. Equal amounts of cell lysate protein (70 µg) were separated on 12% SDS-PAGE gels and Western blotting was subsequently performed. The blots were probed with primary antibodies against α-SMA, TGF-β1 or TGF-βRII. Horseradish peroxidase-conjugated secondary antibodies were used accordingly. The membranes were stripped and re-probed with GAPDH antibody as a protein-loading control. Finally, the relative protein levels were quantified by Bio-Rad software.

2.9 Statistical analysis

All data are presented as mean ± standard error of the mean (SEM). A statistical analysis of the difference between triplicate sets of experiments was performed using a Student's t-test in GraphPad Prism Software, assuming a double-sided independent variance with $P < 0.05$ considered significant.

3. Results

3.1 TAT promotes aFGF penetration in skins

Previously, we demonstrated that TAT-conjugated aFGF-His6 (TAT-aFGF-His6) exhibited an efficient penetration into the retina following topical administration to the ocular surface [17]. To further understand its transdermal potential, we topically applied TAT-aFGF to the surface of dorsal skin of BALB/c mice. The results demonstrated positive signals of TAT-aFGF in the skin of TAT-aFGF group from 2 h to 8 h after administration (Fig. 1A). Primarily, TAT-aFGF accumulated in the hair follicles and subcutaneous tissues. These positive signals decreased gradually from 8 h after administration and were undetectable after 24 h (Fig. 1B). In contrast, mice treated with aFGF showed significantly weaker epidermal uptake of aFGF compared with the TAT-aFGF group, with absorption levels similar to that of the control group (Fig. 1A).

To assess the TAT mediation of aFGF accumulation in dermal and subcutaneous tissues, we applied TAT-aFGF, aFGF or blank gels in the rat ulcer model. The results showed that aFGF alone weakly crossed the epidermis and accumulated in hair follicles, whereas higher levels of fluorescence were detected in or around cell nuclei in the epidermis from TAT-aFGF treated mice (Fig. 1C).

3.2 TAT-aFGF enhances wound healing in rats

Pressure loading on the skin has been used to induce deep ulcers [25]. In our study, on day 1 or 3 after pressure-loading in rats, no open ulcer had formed in the skin. However, the injured skin gradually became yellow and hard. On day 10 or 11, the necrotic skins separated from the epidermis and the red open ulcers subsequently formed. During the healing phase, the skin ulcer gradually decreased in size and disappeared from day 14 after treatment (Fig. 2A). There was no visible difference between the three groups before the necrotic skins separated from the epidermis. Moreover, on day 14, the skin ulcers with TAT-aFGF treatment had almost closed. In contrast, the control and aFGF groups still had open wounds (Fig. 2A). The wound contraction rate of TAT-aFGF was higher than the other two groups (Fig. 2B).

The skin ulcers were analyzed histologically, showing that on day 0, there was swelling and necrotic fat cells, blebbing of the vascular wall and early necrosis of follicular units (Fig. 2C). On day 3, although the edema in skins and subcutaneous tissue had decreased, necrosis appeared in the epidermis and follicular units. Prominent polymorphonuclear infiltration and necrosis was found throughout the dermis and subcutaneous tissues (Fig. 2C). On day 7, eschars started to form and the skin tissues started to undergo regeneration. During hypertrophic scar formation, the myofibroblasts

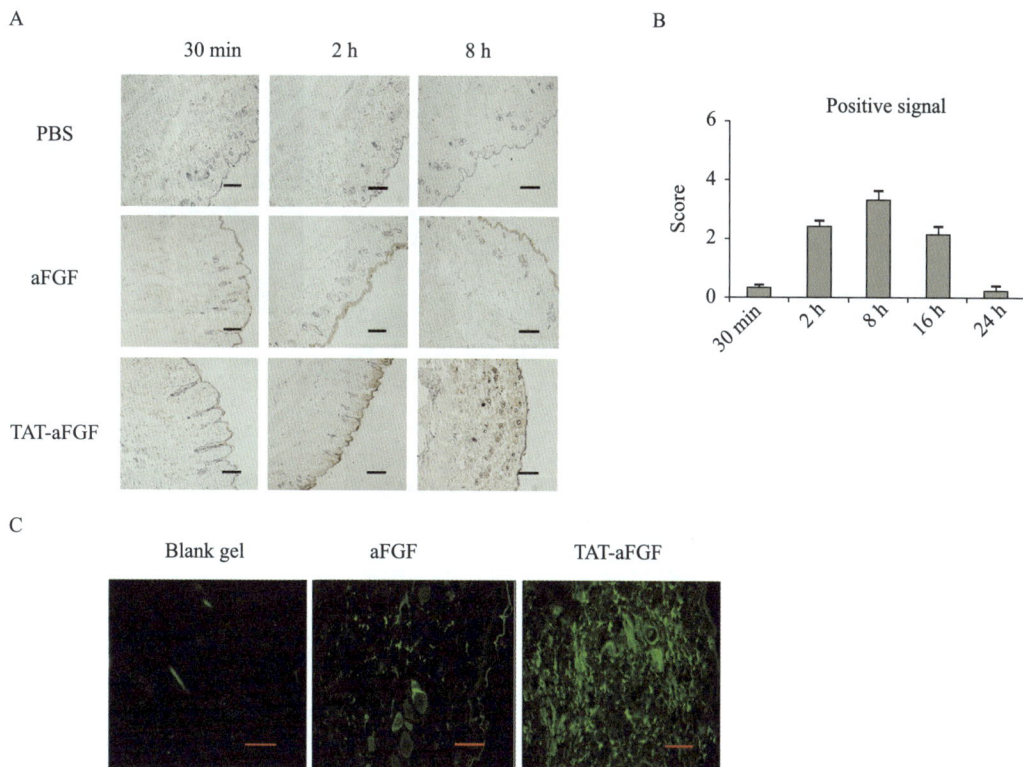

Fig. 1. Effect of TAT on aFGF penetration after topical administration in skin. (A) Under anesthesia, BALB/c mice received topical administration of PBS, aFGF, or TAT-aFGF solutions. Skin tissues were then harvested at the indicated time points. A positive signal of aFGF was detected at 2 h and 8 h in the TAT-aFGF group. Bar = 100 μm. (B) The positive signal for aFGF was scored semi-quantitatively (0 = absent, 1 = low, 2 = medium, 3 = strong, 4 = very strong) and showed gradual reduction of signal in the aFGF group. (C) TAT-aFGF aFGF or blank gel were applied at the end of second loading. Tissues were harvested 5 h later and then processed routinely for embedding. Immunofluoresence was performed to measure aFGF accumulation (green) in the dermal and subcutaneous tissues. In the control and aFGF groups, few cells were stained, except some in corneous and hair follicles, while in the TAT-aFGF group, strongly positive staining was detected under the epidermis. Bar = 100 μm.

continued to remodel the ECM that induces connective-tissue contracture [26]. On day 14, this effect was more pronounced in the control groups than in the TAT-aFGF group (Fig. 2C), suggesting that TAT-aFGF inhibits connective-tissue contracture by enhancing recovery capacity while reducing recovery duration.

Masson staining in the three groups on day 14 showed that all wounds were filled with the newly formed collagen-enriched ECM (Fig. 2D). Wounds in the control and aFGF groups showed deficient collagen deposition and immature tissue organization, whereas a more compact and organized dermis with an abundance of collagen bundles was observed in the TAT-aFGF group (Fig. 2D). Semi-quantitative scoring showed more collagen enrichment in the TAT-aFGF group when compared with the other two groups (Fig. 2E).

3.3 TAT-aFGF transdermal delivery in rats reduces cell apoptosis but enhances proliferation

It has been shown that aFGF prevents the apoptosis of gut epithelial and myocardial cells that is triggered by ischemia-reperfusion injury [27, 28]. This effect contributes to the promotion of the ERK1/2 pathway and cell cycle progression as well as the maintenance of intracellular Ca^{2+} concentrations [28]. In our study, a TUNEL assay revealed that the index of apoptotic nuclear DNA breaks in ulcerated skin tissues (including epidermis, dermis and subcutaneous tissues), decreased significantly upon TAT-aFGF treatment (Fig. 3A, B), suggesting that TAT-aFGF can efficiently penetrate the epidermal barrier and protect cells from apoptosis.

Inflammation was evaluated in skins by staining for CD68 (specific for monocytes/macrophages). Before day 3, there was no significant difference in levels of CD68 between the three groups. However on days 7 and 14 the CD68 level in the TAT-aFGF group had decreased significantly compared with that of the CD68 level in the other two groups (both $P < 0.01$) (Fig. 4A). Immunohistochemical analysis of PCNA showed that proliferation of epidermal cells, especially in the basal layer, was enhanced in the TAT-aFGF group compared to the control or aFGF groups. On days 7 and

A

C

D

E

B

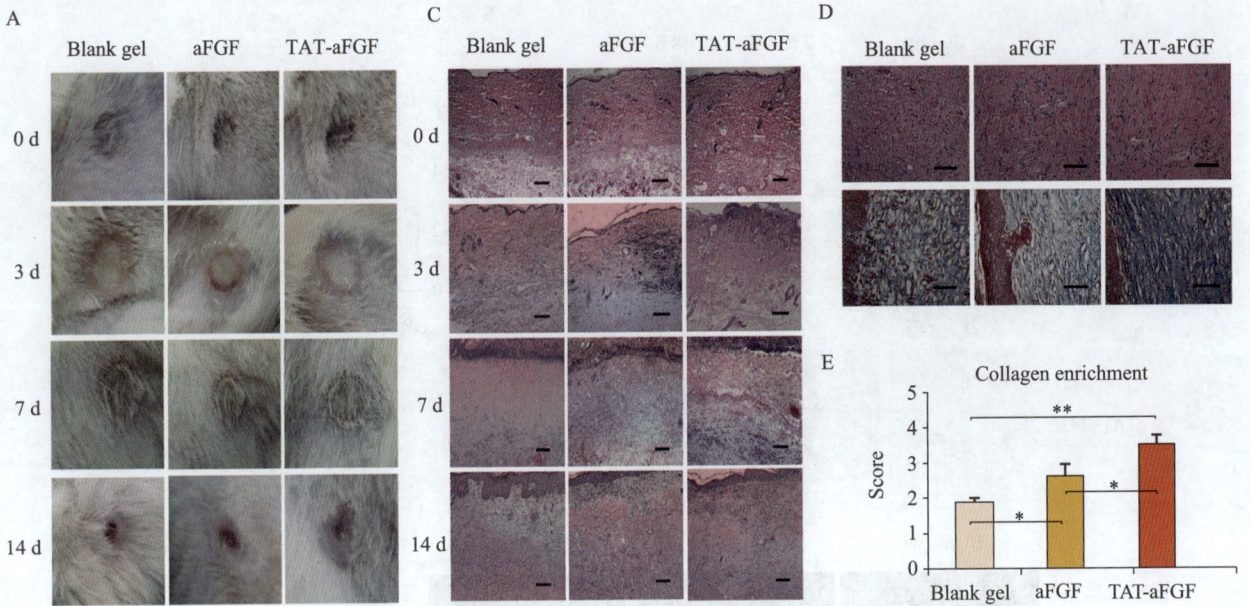

Fig. 2. Evaluation of pressure-induced deep tissue injury. (A) Typical macroscopic views of the TAT-aFGF, aFGF and control groups on days 0, 3, 7, and 14. The red open ulcers remained differentially in the three groups on day 14. (B) Wound contraction was measured quantitatively, showing a higher rate in the TAT-aFGF group on day 14; $^*P < 0.05$, $^{**}P < 0.01$. (C) Typical microscopic views (×100) of hematoxylin and eosin (HE) staining of each group on days 0, 3, 7 and 14. Edema and swelling were obvious on day 0. Bar = 100 μm. (D) HE staining and Masson staining of tissue biopsies on day 14. Bar = 100 μm. (E) Semi-quantitative scoring of sections from mice on day 14. $^*P < 0.05$, $^{**}P < 0.01$.

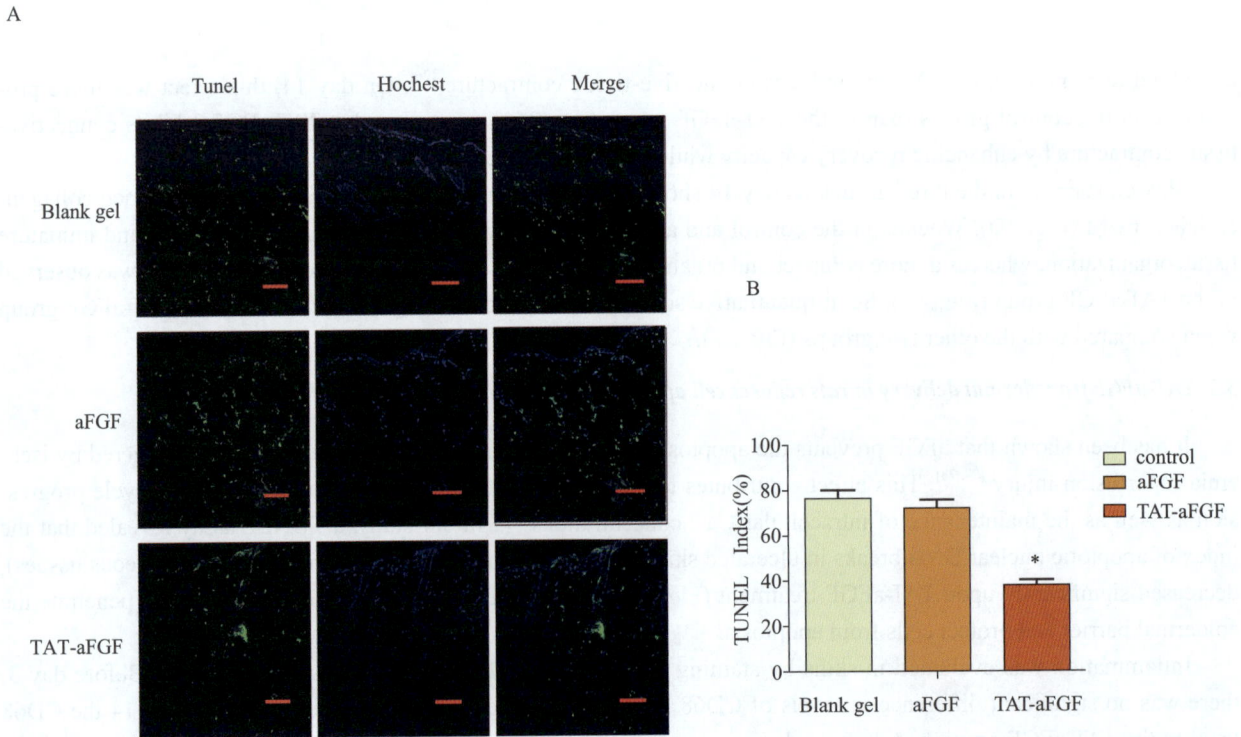

A

B

Fig. 3. TUNEL assay of skins from deep tissue injury models. (A) Terminal dUTP nick-end labeling (TUNEL, green) and DAPI (blue) staining was performed in TAT-aFGF, aFGF and control groups. Skin samples were harvested on day 0. Representative images are shown. Bar = 100 μm. (B) TUNEL index of the three groups. $^*P < 0.05$.

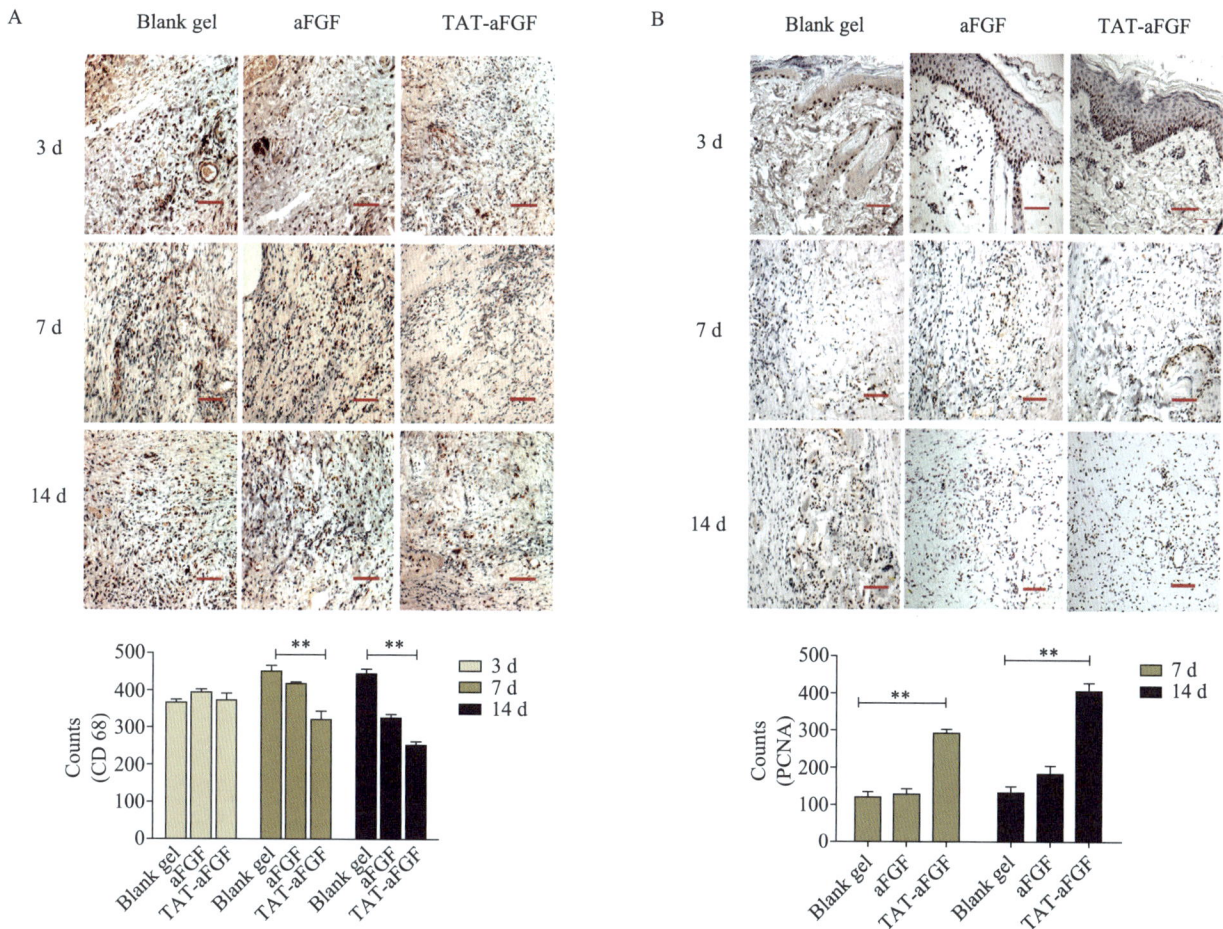

Fig. 4. Effect of TAT-aFGF on CD68 and PCNA expression. (A) The effect of TAT-aFGF, aFGF and control treatments on regional inflammation was assessed by immunohistochemical staining for CD68 (red). Representative images of the three groups on days 3, 7, 14 are shown. Bar = 100 μm. **$P < 0.01$. B: On days 7 and 14, the PCNA expression (red) was detected in the three groups. Representative images were shown. Bar = 100 μm. **$P < 0.01$.

14, the PCNA-positivity also remained higher in TAT-aFGF group compared to the other two groups (Fig. 4B).

TGF-β1 induces α-SMA expression in subcutaneous fibroblasts, both *in vivo* and *in vitro* [29]. On day 3, there was no increase in TGF-β1 in the TAT-aFGF, aFGF or control groups. However, the TAT-aFGF group showed enhanced expression of TGF-β1 on day 7 followed by decreased expression on day 14, when compared with the control group (Fig. 5A). No differences were found between the control and aFGF groups on day 7 or 14 (Fig. 5A). Positive staining of α-SMA was observed underneath the pressure-loading area at the ulcer edge. Vascular smooth muscle cells were found in all groups at day 3 (Fig. 5B). On day 7, myofibroblasts with higher α-SMA expression were observed in the connective tissues from the TAT-aFGF group (Fig. 5B). However, on day 14, fewer α-SMA-positive cells were observed under the recovered neo-epidermis in the TAT-aFGF group compared with the control group (Fig. 5B).

Western blotting revealed that TNF-α treatment decreased α-SMA expression in human dermal fibroblasts (Fig. 6), consistent with data from a previous study [30]. Application of TAT-aFGF reversed the inhibitory effect of TNF-α on α-SMA expression; however, TAT-aFGF alone also decreased α-SMA expression (Fig. 6B). This effect contributed partially to the changes in the levels of TGF-β1 and TGF-βRII (Fig. 6A). In the presence of TNF-α, TAT-aFGF (100 ng/ml) restored TGF-β1 and TGF-βRII expression in human dermal fibroblasts (Fig. 6C, D).

4. Discussion

In this study, we found that TAT facilitated the delivery of aFGF across the cutaneous barrier and the accumulation

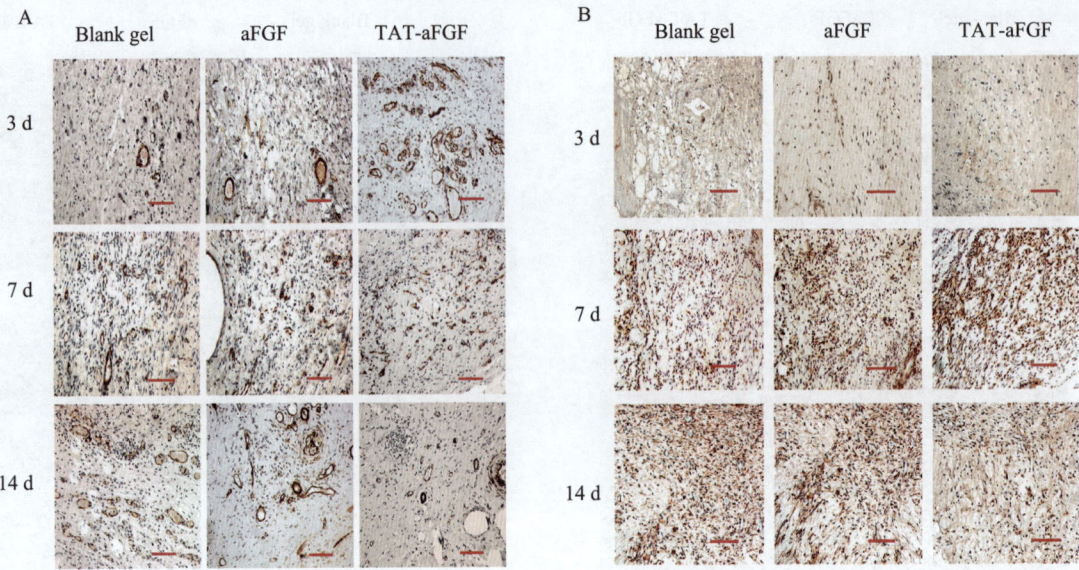

Fig. 5. Effect of TAT-aFGF on TGF-β1 and α-SMA expression. (A) On days 3, 7, and 14, the TGF-β1 expression was detected in TAT-aFGF, aFGF and control treatment groups. Bar = 100 μm. (B) On days 3, 7, and 14, the α-SMA expression was detected in the three groups. Bar = 100 μm.

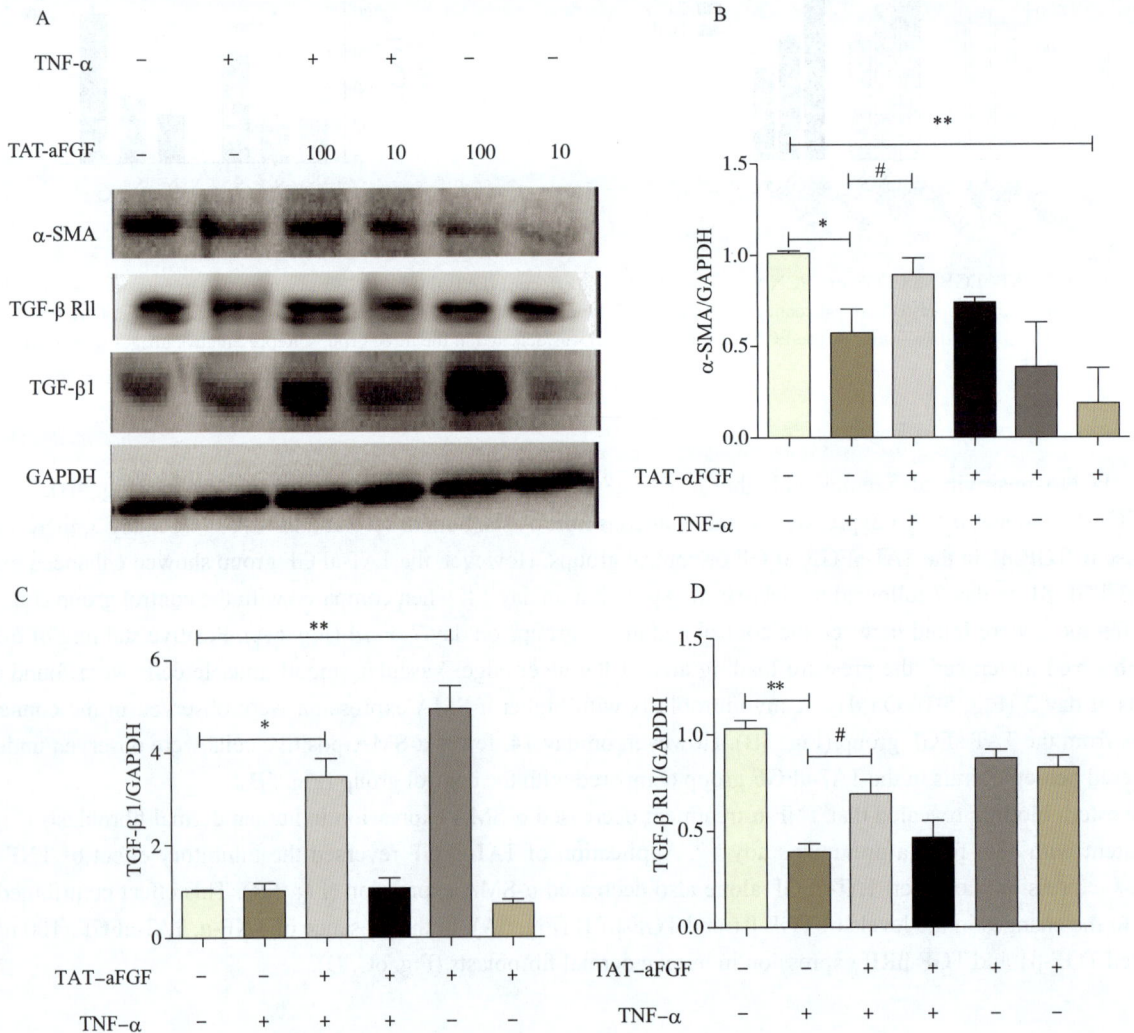

Fig. 6. Western blot analysis of α-SMA, TGF-β1 and TGF-βRII in human dermal fibroblasts. (A) Fibroblasts grown in a monolayer were serum-starved for 24 h before the stimulation of TNF-α (5 ng/ml) or TNF-α plus TAT-aFGF (10 ng/ml or 100 ng/ml). Total protein was extracted at the indicated time points. Western blotting was performed for α-SMA, TGF-β1, and TGF-βRII. (B, C, D) α-SMA, TGF-β1, and TGF-βRII expression was normalized to GAPDH. Data were obtained from 3 independent experiments. *P < 0.05, **P < 0.01.

aFGF in the dermis or subcutaneous tissues. TAT-aFGF enhanced the healing process of deep tissue injury under the skin mediated by aFGF in a rat model. Moreover, TAT-aFGF had higher potential to penetrate the membranes of human dermal fibroblasts *in vitro*, compared with the aFGF alone. In addition, TAT-aFGF reversed the suppressive effect of TNF-α on α-SMA expression and restored TGF-β1 and TGF-βRII expression in dermal fibroblasts. Therefore, our results demonstrate that TAT-aFGF has a favorable therapeutic effect on the healing of deep tissue injury under the skin.

Consistent with a previous report that TAT-aFGF enhance the accumulation of aFGF in the retina following its topical administration to the ocular surface [17], our results show that topical application of TAT-aFGF also enhances aFGF accumulation in both dermis and subcutaneous tissues. In areas of wounded skin, the number of apoptotic cells was significantly reduced with TAT-aFGF treatment, when compared with aFGF or control treatment on day 0 as indicated by the decreased TUNEL index. This finding mirrored the higher penetration efficiency of TAT-aFGF protein in transdermal delivery experiments. In a previous study, we demonstrated that TAT-aFGF-His treatment can reduce cell apoptosis in ischemia–reperfusion rats [17]. Hence, we speculate here that aFGF accumulation in cutaneous tissue ameliorates fibroblast apoptosis. The possible mechanisms underlying such a phenomenon deserve further studies e.g. the effect of aFGF on the activation of FGF receptors in skin tissues.

PCNA is a marker of cell proliferation [31]. We found that PCNA expression was strongly detected in cells within all tissue layers of skin in the TAT-aFGF group. The TAT-aFGF group also showed reduced apoptosis of cells under the epidermis. Hence, the enhanced proliferation and reduced apoptosis of cells which are the main components of skin (such as keratinocytes) could be contributing to the accelerated improvement on pressure ulcer healing, resulting in an early separation of eschar from the skin. Furthermore, enhanced deposition and more complete organization of collagen fibers were observed in the TAT-aFGF group, while the collagen fibers were often irregularly arranged in both the aFGF and control groups. In addition, the contracture of connective tissue was more severe in the control than TAT-aFGF group. These results indicate that TAT-aFGF application leads to better recovery of injured cutaneous tissues and amelioration of chronic scar formation, which was also observed with basic FGF *in vivo* [32].

During wound repair and skin regeneration, myofibroblasts are a specialized subgroup of cells with the features of both fibroblasts and smooth muscle cells [22], the latter of which are characterized by the expression of α-SMA. It has been widely accepted that myofibroblasts numbers correlate not only with wound closure but also with remodeling of the ECM [24]. TNF-α, secreted by inflammatory cells, inhibits ECM synthesis while activating matrix metalloproteinases [33]. A recent study showed that TNF-α suppressed TGF-β1-induced α-SMA expression in human dermal fibroblasts and, furthermore, that JNK phosphorylation and TGF-βRII activation were involved in this process [30, 34]. Although TAT-aFGF showed no detectable effect on the early phase of inflammation in rat skins, α-SMA expression was already significantly higher in this group compared with aFGF alone or controls. Interestingly, α-SMA levels were lower in the TAT-aFGF group than the other two groups on day 14, consistent with a decreased inflammation status in the TAT-aFGF group. Such regulation of α-SMA synthesis by TAT-aFGF not only favors the healing of wounds, but also reduces the formation of scars. These findings further support the opinion that TAT-mediated aFGF delivery efficiently promotes tissue wound remodeling and normally functioning tissue recovery [35]. Finally, our results demonstrate, for the first time, that the upregulation of both TGF-β1 and TGF-βRII is involved in mediating the effect of TAT on aFGF delivery.

5. Conclusion

In summary, our results demonstrate that fusion with TAT enhances the penetration of aFGF through the epidermis and facilitates the healing of DTI in skin. This feature of TAT may be related to its regulation of α-SMA expression and restoration of TGF-β1 and TGF-βRII synthesis by human dermal fibroblasts. Application of TAT-aFGF can be used to developed more efficient and less invasive approaches for the treatment of DTI, such as ulcers resulting from physical damage or the diabetic condition.

References

[1] Black J, Baharestani MM, Cuddigan J, et al. National pressure ulcer advisory panel's updated pressure ulcer staging system[J]. Advances in skin & wound care, 2007, 20(5): 269-274.

[2] Ankrom MA, Bennett RG, Sprigle S, et al. Pressure-related deep tissue injury under intact skin and the current pressure ulcer staging systems[J]. Advances in skin & wound care, 2005, 18(1): 35-42.

[3] Mao CL, Rivet AJ, Sidora T, et al. Update on pressure ulcer management and deep tissue injury[J]. Annals Of Pharmacotherapy, 2010, 44(2): 325-332.

[4] Beenken A, Mohammadi M. The FGF family: biology, pathophysiology and therapy[J]. Nature Reviews Drug Discovery, 2009, 8(3): 235-253.

[5] Driskell RR, Lichtenberger BM, Hoste E, et al. Distinct fibroblast lineages determine dermal architecture in skin development and repair[J]. Nature, 2013, 504(7479): 277-281.

[6] Xie L, Zhang M, Dong B, et al. Improved refractory wound healing with administration of acidic fibroblast growth factor in diabetic rats[J]. Diabetes Research And Clinical Practice, 2011, 93(3): 396-403.

[7] Ma B, Cheng D, Xia Z, et al. Randomized, multicenter, double-blind, and placebo-controlled trial using topical recombinant human acidic fibroblast growth factor for deep partial-thickness burns and skin graft donor site[J]. Wound Repair And Regeneration, 2007, 15(6): 795-799.

[8] Matuszewska B, Keogan M, Fisher DM, et al. Acidic fibroblast growth factor: Evaluation of topical formulations in a diabetic mouse wound healing model[J]. Pharmaceutical Research, 1994, 11(1): 65-71.

[9] Huang Z, Lu M, Zhu G, et al. Acceleration of diabetic-wound healing with PEGylated rhaFGF in healing-impaired streptozocin diabetic rats[J]. Wound Repair And Regeneration, 2011, 19(5): 633-644.

[10] Lee J, Tan CY, Lee S-K, et al. Controlled delivery of heat shock protein using an injectable microsphere/hydrogel combination system for the treatment of myocardial infarction[J]. Journal Of Controlled Release, 2009, 137(3-4): 196-202.

[11] Jin K, Kim Y. Injectable, thermo-reversible and complex coacervate combination gels for protein drug delivery[J]. Journal Of Controlled Release, 2008, 127(3): 249-256.

[12] Frankel AD, Pabo CO. Cellular uptake of the tat protein from human immunodeficiency virus[J]. Cell, 1988, 55(6): 1189-1193.

[13] Green M, Loewenstein PM. Autonomous functional domains of chemically synthesized human immunodeficiency virus tat trans-activator protein[J]. Cell, 1988, 55(6): 1179-1188.

[14] Koren E, Torchilin VP. Cell-penetrating peptides: breaking through to the other side[J]. Trends In Molecular Medicine, 2012, 18(7): 385-393.

[15] Liu L, Venkatraman SS, Yang Y-Y, et al. Polymeric micelles anchored with TAT for delivery of antibiotics across the blood-brain barrier[J]. Biopolymers, 2008, 90(5): 617-623.

[16] Lim KS, Cha M, Kim JK, et al. Protective effects of protein transduction domain-metallothionein fusion proteins against hypoxia- and oxidative stress-induced apoptosis in an ischemia/reperfusion rat model[J]. Journal Of Controlled Release, 2013, 169(3): 306-312.

[17] Wang Y, Lin H, Lin S, et al. Cell-penetrating peptide TAT-mediated delivery of acidic FGF to retina and protection against ischemia-reperfusion injury in rats[J]. Journal Of Cellular And Molecular Medicine, 2010, 14(7): 1998-2005.

[18] Huang Y, Rao Y, Feng C, et al. High-level expression and purification of Tat-haFGF(19-154)[J]. Applied Microbiology And Biotechnology, 2008, 77(5): 1015-1022.

[19] Stadler I, Zhang RY, Oskoui P, et al. Development of a simple, noninvasive, clinically relevant model of pressure ulcers in the mouse[J]. Journal Of Investigative Surgery, 2004, 17(4): 221-227.

[20] Murthy S, Gautam MK, Goel S, et al. Evaluation of in vivo wound healing activity of Bacopa monniera on different wound model in rats[J]. Biomed Research International, 2013.

[21] Tong M, Tuk B, Hekking IM, et al. Stimulated neovascularization, inflammation resolution and collagen maturation in healing rat cutaneous wounds by a heparan sulfate glycosaminoglycan mimetic, OTR4120[J]. Wound Repair And Regeneration, 2009, 17(6): 840-852.

[22] Zhang Y, Yang J, Jiang S, et al. The lupus-derived anti-double-stranded DNA IgG contributes to myofibroblast-like phenotype in mesangial cells[J]. Journal Of Clinical Immunology, 2012, 32(6): 1270-1278.

[23] Yang J, Xia Y, Liu X, et al. Desferrioxamine shows different potentials for enhancing 5-aminolaevulinic acid-based photodynamic therapy in several cutaneous cell lines[J]. Lasers In Medical Science, 2010, 25(2): 251-257.

[24] Zou X, Cheng H, Zhang Y, et al. The antigen-binding fragment of anti-double-stranded DNA IgG enhances F-actin formation in mesangial cells by binding to alpha-actinin-4[J]. Experimental Biology And Medicine, 2012, 237(9): 1023-1031.

[25] Kimura M, Shibahara N, Hikiami H, et al. Traditional Japanese formula Kigikenchuto accelerates healing of pressure-loading skin ulcer in rats[J]. Evidence-Based Complementary And Alternative Medicine, 2011: 1-13.

[26] Tomasek JJ, Gabbiani G, Hinz B, et al. Myofibroblasts and mechano-regulation of connective tissue remodelling[J]. Nature Reviews Molecular Cell Biology, 2002, 3(5): 349-363.

[27] Cuevas P, Reimers D, Carceller F, et al. Fibroblast growth factor-1 prevents myocardial apoptosis triggered by ischemia reperfusion injury[J]. European journal of medical research, 1997, 2(11): 465-468.

[28] Fu X, Li X, Wang T, et al. Enhanced anti-apoptosis and gut epithelium protection function of acidic fibroblast growth factor after cancelling of its mitogenic activity[J]. World Journal Of Gastroenterology, 2004, 10(24): 3590-3596.

[29] Roy SG, Nozaki Y, Phan SH. Regulation of alpha-smooth muscle actin gene expression in myofibroblast differentiation from rat lung fibroblasts[J]. International Journal Of Biochemistry & Cell Biology, 2001, 33(7): 723-734.

[30] Goldberg MT, Han Y-P, Yan C, et al. TNF-alpha suppresses alpha-smooth muscle actin expression in human dermal fibroblasts: An implication for abnormal wound healing[J]. Journal Of Investigative Dermatology, 2007, 127(11): 2645-2655.

[31] Wang S. PCNA: A silent housekeeper or a potential therapeutic target?[J]. Trends In Pharmacological Sciences, 2014, 35(4): 178-186.

[32] Shi H, Lin C, Lin B, et al. The anti-scar effects of basic fibroblast growth factor on the wound repair in vitro and in vivo[J]. Plos One, 2013, 8(4).

[33] Mauviel A, Chen YQ, Dong W, et al. Transcriptional interactions of transforming growth-factor-beta with pro-inflammatory cytokines[J]. Current Biology, 1993, 3(12): 822-831.

[34] Yamane K, Ihn H, Asano Y, et al. Antagonistic effects of TNF-α on TGF-β signaling through down-regulation of TGF-β receptor type II in human dermal fibroblasts[J]. Journal Of Immunology, 2003, 171(7): 3855-3862.

[35] Maltseva O, Folger P, Zekaria D, et al. Fibroblast growth factor reversal of the corneal myofibroblast phenotype[J]. Investigative Ophthalmology & Visual Science, 2001, 42(11): 2490-2495.

Regulation of autophagy and ubiquitinated protein accumulation by bFGF promotes functional recovery and neural protectzion in a rat model of spinal cord injury

Hongyu Zhang, Zhouguang Wang, Fenzan Wu, Xiaoxia Kong, Jie Yang, Beibei Lin, Shiping Zhu, Li Lin, Chaoshi Gan, Xiaobing Fu, Xiaokun Li, Huazi Xu, Jian Xiao

1. Introduction

Spinal cord injury (SCI) is a severe health problem that usually causes lifelong disability, for which few effective treatments exist. The pathology of SCI may usually be divided into two phases: (1) the primary injury, which is the mechanical impact afflicted directly on the spine, and (2) the secondary injury, which involves a complex cascade of molecular events that includes disturbances in ionic homeostasis, local edema, ischemia, focal hemorrhage, free radical stress and inflammatory responses [1]. Previous studies have shown that autophagy plays a key role in secondary injury in both animal models and human tissue by causing progressive degeneration of the spinal cord [2, 3]. Moreover, the molecular pathway of secondary injury and the role of autophagy in the recovery of SCI remain unclear.

Autophagy, literally "self-eating," is essential for survival when cells face metabolic stress and is an intracellular degrading process that has major roles in protein homeostasis. In addition to its role in cellular homeostasis, autophagy may play a cytoprotective role in instances of nutrient starvation [4] or a specific type of programmed cell death [5]. The functional role of autophagy in SCI is currently under intense investigation, and prior studies have characterized this process both *in vitro* and *in vivo*. Interestingly, up-regulation of autophagy has been reported to both contribute as well as to cause cell death in the spine [6, 7]. The ubiquitin-proteasome system (UPS) plays specific roles in the nervous system; it leads to the accumulation of misfolded proteins that may further exacerbate neurological diseases [8]. The ubiquitin-binding protein, p62/SQSTM1 (sequestosome 1) is a multifunctional adaptor protein [9], and the C-terminal of p62 is a ubiquitin-associated domain, which interacts with ubiquitinated proteins and targets them to the microtubule-associated protein 1 light chain 3-II (LC3II), where they are then selectively degraded by autophagy [10, 11]. p62 promotes survival-critical signals, including proliferation, differentiation and induction of anti-apoptotic genes [12, 13]. p62 is considered to be a linking protein between ubiquitinated proteins and autophagosomes; it thus facilitates maintenance of cell homeostasis and survival [14]. The underlying mechanism of recovery in SCI and the role of p62 in this process are not well understood.

Basic fibroblast growth factor (bFGF or FGF-2) is a member of the fibroblast growth factors (FGFs) that regulate a variety of biological functions including proliferation, morphogenesis and suppression of apoptosis during development *via* a complex signal transduction system [15]. bFGF is highly expressed in the nervous system, where it has multiple roles, and it has been previously shown to support the survival and growth of cultured neurons and neural stem cells. Several growth factors have shown neuroprotective effects and improved recovery in SCI; in particular, bFGF transient infusion or transgene therapy may promote axon regeneration and functional recovery [16, 17]. Moreover, recent studies have shown a definite relationship between FGF signals and autophagy through the interaction of the mammalian target rapamycin (mTOR), which is positively regulated by the PI3K/Akt signaling pathway [18, 19]. However, the molecular mechanism of bFGF treatment in recovery in SCI has not been completely defined. Specifically, the relationship between autophagy and ubiquitination and the therapeutic effect of bFGF has not been previously investigated.

In this study, we examined bFGF-mediated effects in neuroprotection, functional recovery, autophagic activity and the accumulation of ubiquitinated proteins and the involvement of downstream signals following SCI through histologic and protein analyses and the application of a traditional BBB functional assessment. To our knowledge, these findings are the first to illustrate a link between bFGF and autophagy-mediated ubiquitinated protein degradation and PI3K/Akt/

mTOR signaling after SCI. Collectively, our results suggest that the investigation of bFGF drug development for nervous system diseases is effective and feasible both *in vivo* and *in vitro*.

2. Materials and methods

2.1 Reagents and antibodies

Recombinant human bFGF was purchased from Grost (Grost Biotechnology, Zhejiang, China). Dulbecco's modified Eagle's medium (DMEM) and fetal bovine serum (FBS) were purchased from Invitrogen (Carlsbad, CA, USA). Anti-Akt and phosphorylated-Akt (Ser473), anti-ubiquitin, anti-p62 and GAPDH antibodies were purchased from Santa Cruz Biotechnology (Santa Cruz, CA, USA). Anti-p-mTOR, anti-mTOR and anti-LC3, goat anti-rabbit and anti-mouse IgG-HRP were purchased from Cell Signaling Technology (Danvers, MA, USA). An enhanced chemiluminescence (ECL) kit was purchased from Bio-Rad (Hercules, CA, USA). Rapamycin (rapa), autophagy inhibitor 3-MA and all of the other reagents were purchased from Sigma-Aldrich (St. Louis, MO, USA) unless otherwise specified.

2.2 Cell culture

PC12 cells were purchased from the Cell Storage Center of Wuhan University (Wuhan, China). Cells were cultured in DMEM (Invitrogen) and supplemented with heat-inactivated 10% FBS (Invitrogen), 5% horse serum, and antibiotics (100 units/ml penicillin, 100 μg/ml streptomycin). They were then incubated in a humidified atmosphere containing 5% CO_2 at 37℃. Based on our previous study, cells were treated with rapamycin (100 nM), bFGF (40 ng/ml), or bFGF compound with rapamycin or the autophagy inhibitor 3-methyladenine (3-MA, 5 mM; Sigma-Aldrich) compound with rapamycin. All experiments were performed in triplicate.

2.3 Procedure for investigating an animal model of spinal cord injury

Adult female Sprague–Dawley rats (220–250 g) were purchased from the Animal Center of the Chinese Academy of Sciences in Shanghai, China. The protocol for animal care and use conformed to the Guide for the Care and Use of Laboratory Animals from the National Institutes of Health and was approved by the Animal Care and Use Committee of Wenzhou Medical College. All animals were housed in standard temperature conditions with a 12 h light/dark cycle and regularly fed with food and water. Following 10% chloralic hydras (3.5 ml/kg, i.p.) anesthesia, rats were positioned on a cork platform. The skin was incised along the midline of the dorsum to expose the vertebral column and to perform a laminectomy carried out at the T9 level. The exposed spinal cord was subjected to crushing injury by compression with a vascular clip (15 g force; Oscar, China). Sham group rats received the same surgical procedure but sustained no impact injury, though the spinal cord was left exposed for 1 min. Postoperative care involved manual urinary bladder emptying twice daily until the return of bladder function and the administration of cefazolin sodium (50 mg/kg, i.p.). Recombinant human bFGF stock solution was diluted with 0.9% NaCl, to achieve a final bFGF concentration of 58.3 μg/ml. Following the spinal cord occlusion, the bFGF solution was injected subcutaneously near the wound to deliver a dose of 80 μg/kg/day until the rats were sacrificed. A different group of rats was treated with 80 μg/kg/day bFGF and 4 μg/kg/day rapamycin at the same time. Following treatment with bFGF or bFGF and rapamycin, animals were treated uniformly until the final analysis of the data. All experimental animals received daily rehabilitation, including passive mobilization of the hind legs twice daily. Subsequently, the rats were sacrificed at 7 days.

2.4 Locomotion recovery assessment

The Basso, Beattie, and Bresnahan (BBB) scores were assessed by two independent examiners who were blinded to treatment to score locomotion recovery in an open field scale at 7 days post-operation. Briefly, the BBB locomotion rating scale scores range from 0 points (complete paralysis) to 21 points (normal locomotion). The scale was developed using the natural progression of locomotion recovery in rats with thoracic SCI.

The inclined plane test was performed *via* a method described previously [20]. In brief, animals were tested in two positions (right side or left side up) on a testing apparatus (i.e., a board covered with a rubber mat containing horizontal ridges that were spaced 3 mm apart). For each position, the maximum angle at which a rat could maintain its position for 5 s without falling was recorded and averaged to obtain a single score for each animal.

2.5 Hematoxylin–Eosin (HE) staining and nissl staining

Sham and SCI rats (n= 5) were deeply re-anesthetized with 10% chloralic hydras (3.5 ml/kg, i.p.) and perfused with 0.9% NaCl, followed by 4% paraformaldehyde in 0.01 M phosphate buffered saline (PBS, pH= 7.4) at 7 days after surgery. The spinal cords from the T7–T10 level around the lesion epicenter were excised, post-fixed in cold 4% para-formaldehyde overnight, and embedded in paraffin. Transverse paraffin sections (5 mm thick) were mounted on poly-L-lysine-coated slides for histopathological examination by HE staining. The sections were also incubated in 1% Cresyl-violet for Nissl staining and examined under a light microscope.

2.6 Western blot analysis

For protein analysis *in vivo*, a spinal cord segment (0.5 cm length) at the contusion epicenter was dissected and rap-idly stored at −80 ℃ for western blotting. For protein extraction, the tissue was homogenized in a modified RIPA buffer (50 mM Tris-HCl, 1% NP-40, 20 mM DTT, 150 mM NaCl, pH= 7.4) containing protease inhibitor cocktail (10 μl/ml, GE Healthcare). The complex was then centrifuged at 12,000 rpm, and the supernatant was obtained for protein assay. PC12 cells used for an *in vitro* model were lysed in RIPA buffer [25 mM Tris-HCl (pH7.6), 150 mM NaCl, 1% Non-idet P-40, 1% sodium deoxycholate, and 0.1% SDS] with protease and phosphatase inhibitors. The extracts above were quantified with bicinchoninic acid (BCA) reagents (Thermo, Rockford, IL, USA). The equivalent of 50 μg protein was separated using 11.5% gel and then transferred onto a PVDF membrane (Bio-Rad). The membrane was blocked with 5% non-fat milk in TBS with 0.05% Tween 20 for 1 h, then incubated with following antibody solutions: Ub (1 ∶ 500), p62 (1 ∶ 600), mTOR, p-mTOR (1 ∶ 1,000), and LC3 (1 ∶ 1,000). The membranes were washed with TBS three times and in-cubated with secondary antibodies for 2 h at room temperature. Signals were visualized using the ChemiDicTM XRS + Imaging System (Bio-Rad), and band densities were quantified with Multi Gauge Software for Science Lab 2006 (Fuji Film Corporation, Japan).

2.7 Immunofluorescence staining

Spinal cord sections were incubated with 10% normal donkey serum for 1 h at room temperature in PBS contain-ing 0.1% Triton X-100. They were then incubated with the appropriate primary antibodies overnight at 4℃ in the same buffer. The nuclei were stained with Hoechst 33258 (0.25 μg/ml) dye. For LC3 and Ub detection, the following pri-mary antibodies were used, based on differing targets: anti-LC3 (1 ∶ 500; Millipore) and anti-Ub (1 ∶ 50; Santa Cruz Biotechnology). After primary antibody incubation, sections were washed for 4× 10 min at room temperature and then incubated with Alexa Fluor 594/647 donkey anti-mouse/rabbit, Alexa-Fluor 488/594 donkey anti-rabbit/mouse, or Alexa Fluor 488/594 donkey anti-goat secondary antibody (1 ∶ 500; Invitrogen) for 1 h at room temperature. Sections were then washed with PBS containing 0.1% Triton X-100 for 4 × 10 min, followed by 3 × 5 min with PBS and then briefly with water. All images were captured on a Nikon ECLIPSE Ti microscope (Nikon, Japan).

2.8 Statistical analysis

Data are expressed as the mean ± SEM. Statistical significance was determined using Student's *t*-test when there were two experimental groups. When more than two groups were compared, statistical evaluation of the data was per-formed using one-way analysis of variance (ANOVA) and Dunnett's *post hoc* test. P values <0.05 were considered sta-tistically significant.

3. Results

3.1 bFGF decreases motor neuron loss and improves functional recovery of SCI in vivo

To evaluate the therapeutic effect of bFGF in SCI, rats were treated with bFGF by injection close to the wound area as described above. As shown in Fig. 1A, the sham group obtained normal BBB scores. At 1 day after contusion, there was no significant difference in BBB scores between the SCI model group and the bFGF treatment group; these values

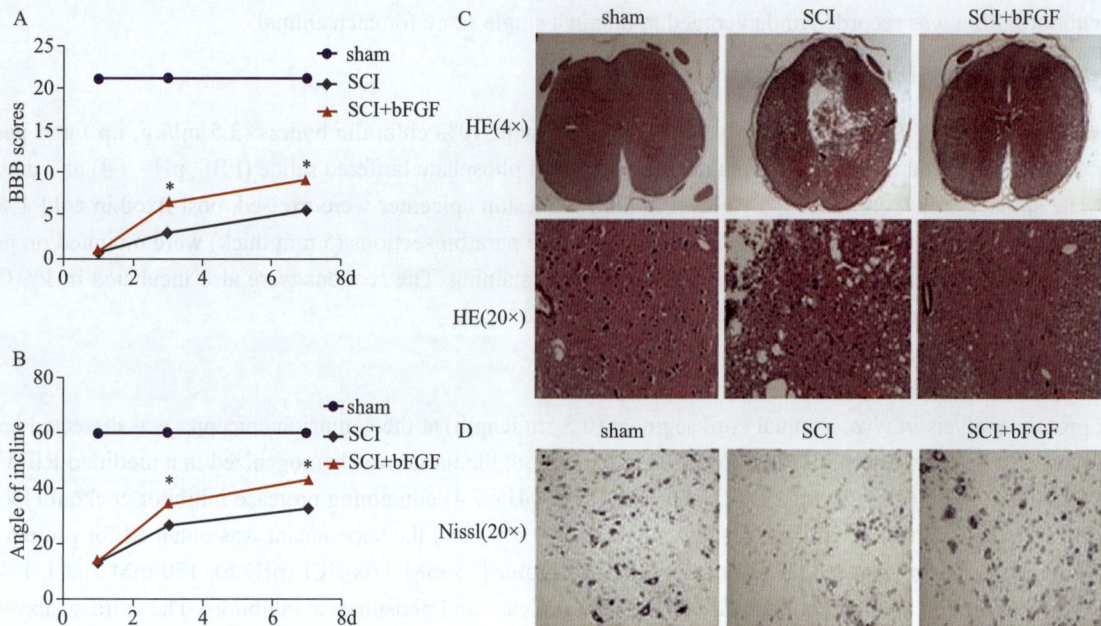

Fig. 1. bFGF treatment improves functional recovery and reduces lesion volume and the loss of motor neurons after SCI. After SCI, bFGF was injected close to the wound area once per day for 1 week, and recovery was assessed *via* BBB scores and the inclined plane test. (A) The BBB scores of the sham, SCI model and SCI model treated with bFGF groups. $P<0.05$ *vs.* the SCI group. (B) The inclined plane test scores of the SCI model group and the SCI model treated with bFGF group. *$P<0.05$ *vs.* the SCI group. (C) HE staining and Nissl staining results for the sham, SCI model and SCI model treated with bFGF groups. (D) Nissl staining results for the sham, SCI model and SCI model treated with bFGF groups.

were 1.1 ± 0.32 and 1.16 ± 0.30, respectively ($P > 0.05$). However, BBB scores increased at 3 days after contusion with bFGF treatment, indicating that locomotor activity was more successfully recovered when compared to the SCI model group ($P < 0.05$). Seven days after contusion, bFGF treatment increased BBB scores to 9.5 ± 0.43; this value is markedly elevated compared with SCI group at 7 days after contusion ($P < 0.05$). The angle of incline test was completed 1 week after injury; values were significantly increased in bFGF-treated rats compared to the vehicle control rats (Fig. 1B). This indicates that bFGF may influence functional improvement of locomotor activity after SCI.

The HE staining results of the sham operation group, SCI group and bFGF treatment model group at 7 days after contusion are shown in Fig. 1C. Compared with the sham group, progressive destruction of the dorsal white matter and central gray matter was found in the SCI group. Compared to the SCI group, bFGF-treated rats showed that there was a significant protective effect of treatment *via* reduced necrosis, karyopyknosis, infiltrated polymorphonuclear leukocytes and macrophages.

The effect of bFGF on the number of motor neurons in the spinal cord was investigated using Nissl staining at 7 days after contusion. As shown in Fig. 1D, SCI mice showed extensive loss of large anterior horn cells. In contrast, motor neurons were remarkably preserved in the anterior horns in mice treated with bFGF when compared to the vehicle control mice. These results further strengthen the idea that bFGF has a neuroprotective effect on motor neurons in SCI rats model *in vivo*.

3.2 The protective effect of bFGF is related to inhibited autophagy in the SCI model mice

It has been reported that autophagy activation is involved in SCI; however, its role has not been clearly defined. In our model, we first detected the level of LC3 protein, which is often used as an indicator of autophagy. Immunofluorescence staining results showed that LC3 positive green dots increased in spinal cord lesions than in the sham surgery group. LC3 positive green dots also decreased in the bFGF-treated group, a result that is consistent with the Western blot results (Fig. 2A).

To further evaluate the effect of bFGF on autophagy, LC3 expression of injured spinal cord tissues was detected *via* Western blot analysis. As shown in Fig. 2B and Figs. S1b and Fig. 2C, the expression of LC3II and the ratio of LC3II/LC3I was significantly greater in SCI model mice than in those in the sham group ($P<0.01$). This effect was clearly inhibited by bFGF treatment at 7 days after contusion.

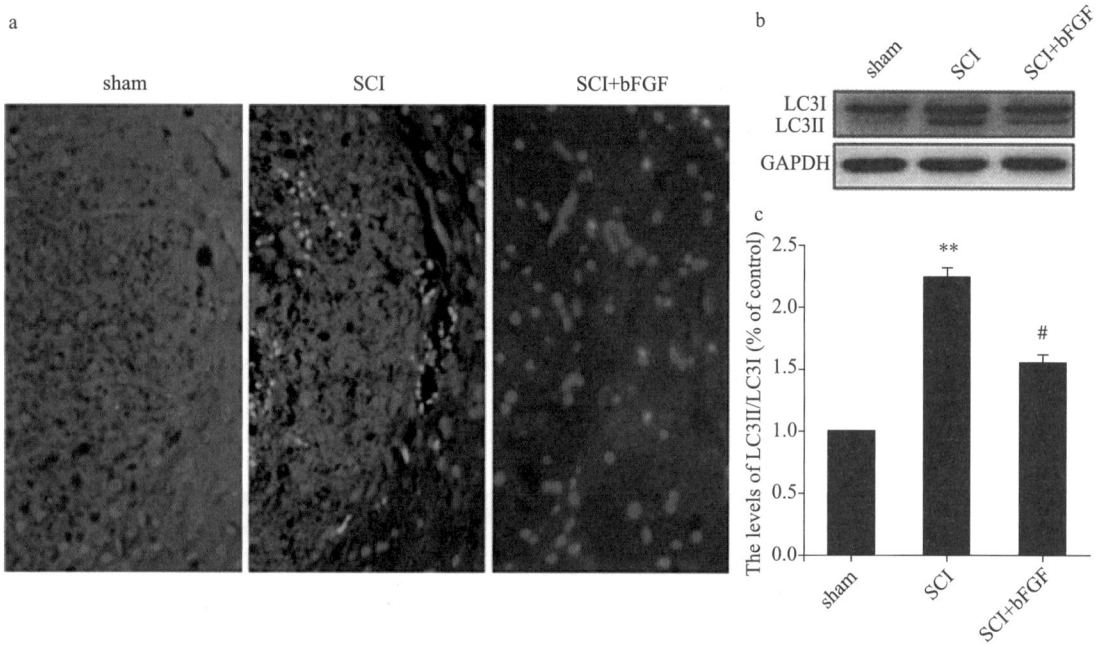

Fig. 2. bFGF administration decreases the level of LC3II/LC3I in spinal cord lesions. (A) Immunofluorescence staining (original magnification× 40) results of LC3 (*green*), nuclei are labeled with Hoechst 33342 (*blue*), and neurons with obvious LC3 signals are identified using *white arrowheads*. (B) Protein expression of LC3 in the sham, SCI model and SCI model treated bFGF groups. (C) The optical density analysis of LC3 protein. **P <0.01 *vs.* the sham group, #P < 0.05 *vs.* the SCI group. Mean values±SEM, n=5.

3.3 Activation of PI3K/Akt/mTOR signaling pathways is involved in the role of bFGF in SCI recovery

Numerous reports have indicated that PI3K/Akt signaling pathways are essential for the role of bFGF in nerve cell proliferation and differentiation. mTOR is upstream signal in the regulation of autophagy which is positively regulated by PI3K/Akt and results in the inhibition of autophagy. Recent studies have demonstrated the effect of Akt/mTOR signaling in the regulation of autophagy in cardiac stem cells [19]; however, whether this mechanism is effective in recovery from SCI has not been discussed. We first detected the activity of Akt/mTOR signaling pathways in our model *in vivo*. Western blot analysis (Fig. 3) demonstrated that the phosphorylation of Akt/mTOR decreased significantly after SCI contusion in rats. Reduced phosphorylation levels of prototypical ratios were recovered after bFGF treatment when compared to the SCI group (P < 0.01). These data demonstrated that recovery from SCI with bFGF treatment may occur in part through the activation of Akt/mTOR signaling and inhibition of autophagy.

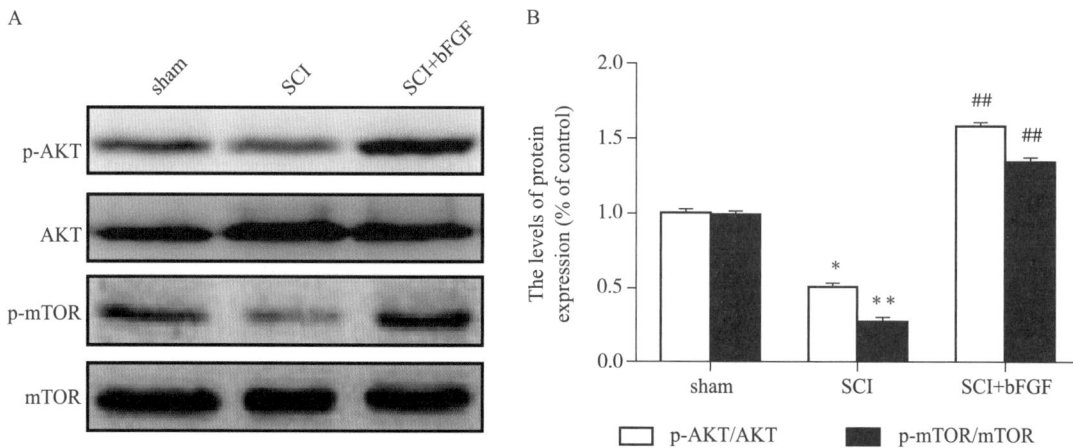

Fig. 3. bFGF administration activates Akt/mTOR signaling pathways in the spinal cord of SCI model mice. a Protein expression of p-Akt/Akt and p-mTOR/mTOR in the sham, SCI model and SCI model mice treated with bFGF groups. (A) The optical density analysis of p-Akt/Akt and p-mTOR/ mTOR proteins. *P< 0.05, **P<0.01 *vs.* the sham group, ##P<0.01 *vs.* the SCI group. Mean values±SEM, n=6.

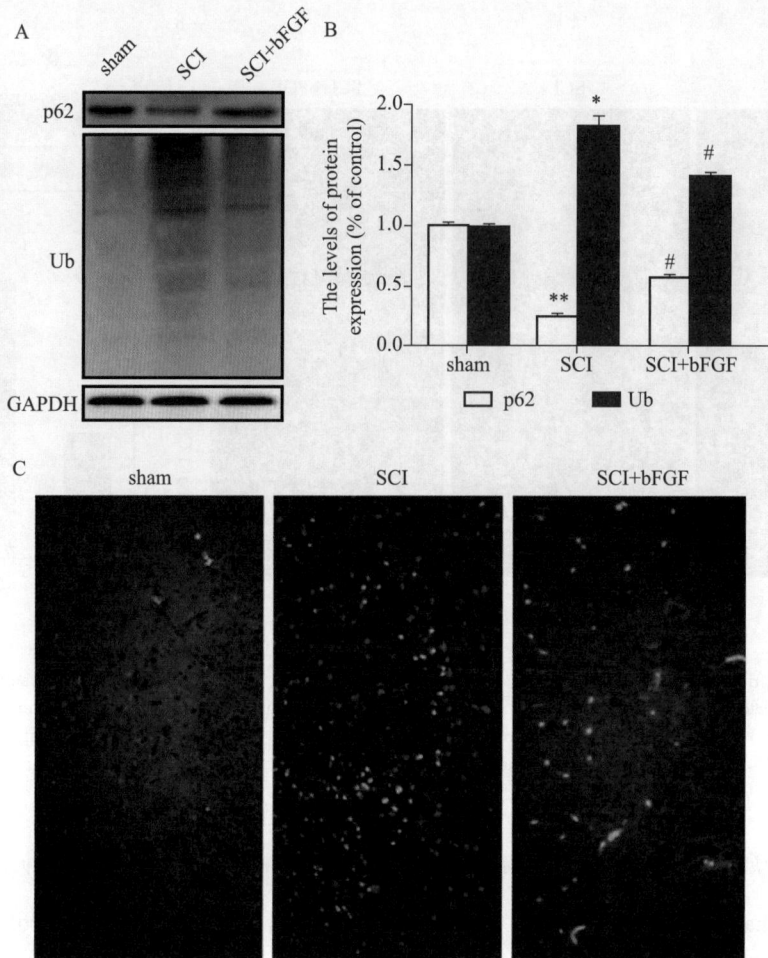

Fig. 4. bFGF administration activates p62 and clears ubiquitinated proteins. (A) Immunofluorescence staining (original magnification×20) results of Ub (*green*), where nuclei are labeled with Hoechst (*blue*). (B) Protein expression of Ub and p62 in the sham, SCI model and SCI model mice treated with bFGF groups. (C) The optical density analysis of Ub and p62 proteins. $^*P < 0.05$, $^{**}P < 0.01$ *vs.* the sham group, $^#P < 0.05$ *vs.* the SCI group. Mean values± SEM, n=6.

3.4 bFGF improves recovery after SCI by autophagic clearance of ubiquitinated protein accumulation

Poly-ubiquitin chains serve as recognition signals for the proteasome, the major regulator of protein abundance in cells, often initiating proteolysis of substrates. p62 is a ubiquitin-binding protein that acts as a shuttling factor that targets poly-ubiquitinated proteins for degradation by either autophagy or proteasome pathways. To evaluate whether bFGF also impacts protein degradation and homeostasis, protein expression of poly-ubiquitinated protein and p62 were determined *via* Western blotting. As shown in Fig. 4A and B, poly-ubiquitinated protein expression increased and p62 decreased after SCI contusion. After bFGF treatment at 7 days post-contusion, the levels of poly-ubiquitinated protein decreased significantly while p62 expression was enhanced ($P < 0.01$). Immunofluorescence staining results (Fig. 4C and Fig. S1C) demonstrated that poly-ubiquitinated protein expression increased significantly in rat spinal cord lesions; bFGF down-regulated the accumulation of poly-ubiquitinated protein. These results suggest that the effect of bFGF in recovery after SCI may also be related to the regulation of autophagic protein degradation that is mediated by p62.

3.5 Combination with the autophagy sensitizer rapamycin partially abolishes the protective effect of bFGF in SCI model rats

To further confirm our hypothesis that inhibition of autophagy is important for the protective effect of bFGF in SCI recovery, a classical autophagy sensitizer, rapamycin, was added to the bFGF solution around the SCI areas. This technique is generally used to induce autophagy both *in vivo* and *in vitro* [21, 22]. BBB scores (Fig. 5A) and the angle of incline test results (Fig. 5B) indicated that, compared to rats treated with bFGF only, bFGF-related recovery in SCI rats was impaired when treatment was combined with rapamycin ($P < 0.05$). HE staining results showed that progressive destruction of the dorsal white matter and central gray matter were aggravated in the SCI group treated with bFGF and rapamycin. This combination significantly increased the deleterious effects; these rats demonstrated greater necrosis, karyopyknosis, infiltrated polymorphonuclear leukocytes and macrophages when compared to the SCI group treated with bFGF alone (Fig. 5C). Nissl staining results also showed that there was an extensive loss of large anterior horn cells in the SCI group treated with bFGF and rapamycin when compared to the bFGF-treated SCI group (Fig. 5D). Moreover, there was no significant effect on cell death in SCI model rats treated with rapamycin alone. These staining results indicate that the addition of rapamycin abolished the effect of exogenous bFGF, which further strengthens the role of bFGF on motor neurons. This observation may be related to the inhibition of autophagy in the SCI model.

Expression of LC3, poly-ubiquitinated protein and p62 was evaluated to address the mechanism of autophagy induction in the neuroprotective effect of bFGF treatment in our SCI model. As shown in Fig. 6A and B, the levels of LC3II/LC3I poly-ubiquitinated protein increased when rapamycin was added to the treatment solution and p62 protein expression was reduced when compared to the bFGF group ($P<0.01$). These findings suggest that rapamycin-induced activation of autophagy played a negative role in recovery from SCI with bFGF treatment; the inhibition of autophagy and clearance of poly-ubiquitinated proteins contributed to the neuroprotective effect of bFGF *in vivo*.

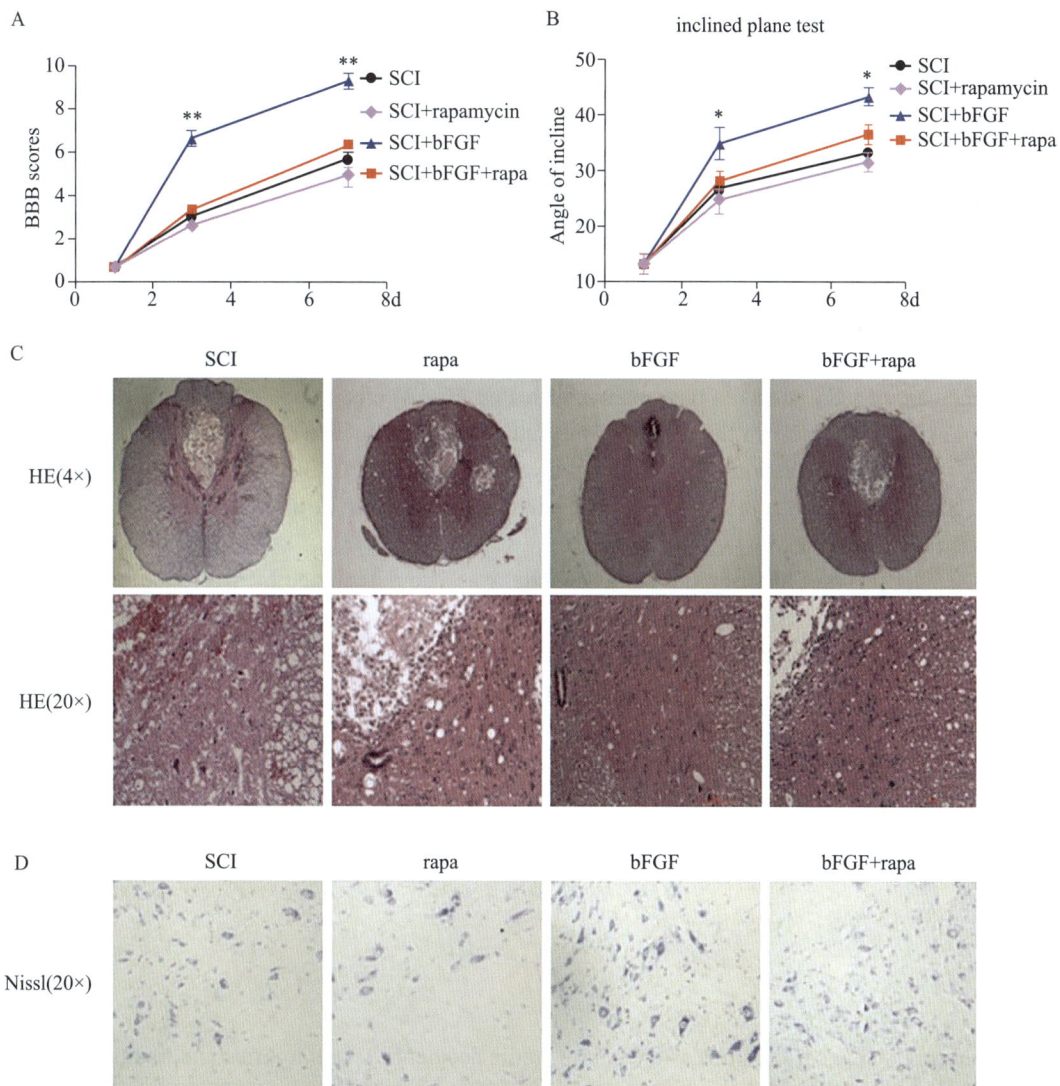

Fig. 5. The protective effect of bFGF in spinal cord injury is inhibited by rapamycin. (A) The BBB scores of SCI rats treated with rapamycin, bFGF and bFGF compound with rapamycin. **$P < 0.01$ *vs.* the SCI group. (B) The inclined plane test results of SCI rats treated with rapamycin, bFGF and bFGF compound with rapamycin. *$P <0.05$ *vs.* the SCI group. (C) HE staining and Nissl staining results of SCI rats treated with rapamycin, bFGF and bFGF compound with rapamycin.

A

B

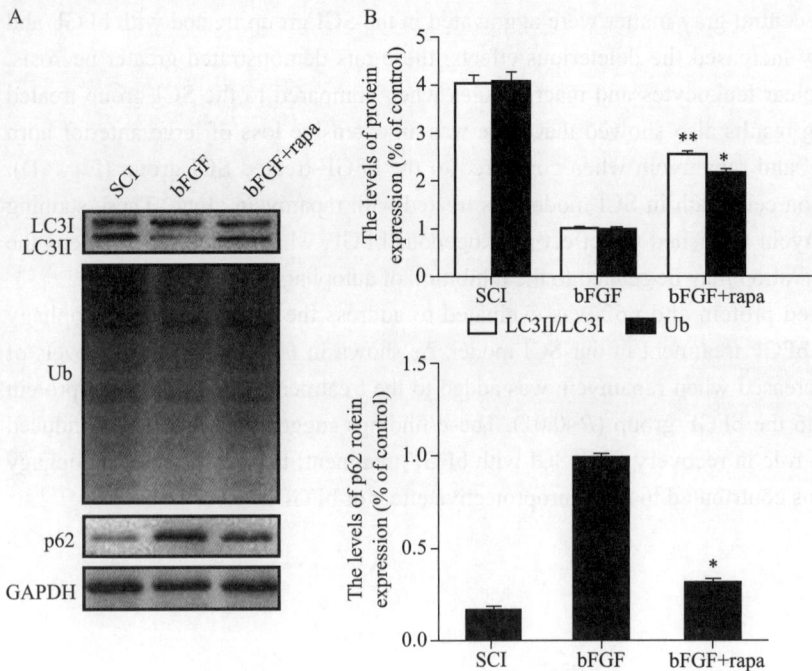

Fig. 6. The effect of autophagy inhibition and ubiquitinated protein clearance by bFGF is reduced by rapamycin. (A) Protein expression of LC3, Ub, and p62 of SCI rats treated with bFGF and bFGF compound with rapamycin. (B) The optical density analysis of LC3, Ub, and p62 of SCI rats treated with bFGF and bFGF compound with rapamycin. $^*P< 0.05$, $^{**}P<0.01$ $vs.$ the bFGF group.

3.6 Exogenous bFGF protects PC-12 cells by inhibition of excessive autophagy in vitro

To further confirm our hypothesis that the effect of bFGF is related to the inhibition of excessive autophagy $in\ vitro$, PC-12 cells were treated with rapamycin or combined with bFGF. In MTT assays, rapamycin-inhibited cell viability was restored after bFGF addition. The same response was detected in the group treated with the autophagy inhibitor 3-MA and rapamycin (Fig. 7A). The effect of bFGF on autophagy was assessed with immunofluorescence staining; our data showed that the increase of LC3 puncta in the rapamycin-treated PC-12 cells group was inhibited when combined with bFGF. This finding was consistent with the results of the autophagy inhibitor 3-MA (Fig. 7B and Fig. S1D). As shown in Fig. 7C and D, rapamycin incubation resulted in significant activation of LC3II, which was previously inhibited by bFGF treatment. These findings illustrate that autophagy inhibition by bFGF is involved in $in\ vitro$ as well as $in\ vivo$ protective effects.

The molecular mechanism of bFGF in our cellular model was also determined by Western blotting. p-Akt/Akt and p-mTOR/mTOR levels were greater in the bFGF-incubated group when compared to the rapamycin group (Fig. 8A and B). This result suggests that the protective role of bFGF in neuronal cell death is partially modulated through PI3K/Akt/mTOR signaling pathways. We then investigated whether exogenous bFGF contributes to cell survival through clearance of poly-ubiquitinated protein accumulation $in\ vitro$. Levels of poly-ubiquitinated proteins and p62 were determined using immunoblotting. As shown in Fig. 8C and D, poly-ubiquitinated protein expression increased with rapamycin and was suppressed by bFGF application. Down-regulation of p62 was also alleviated by bFGF treatment. These data further confirmed that the protective role of bFGF is associated with inhibition of excessive autophagy via PI3K/Akt/mTOR signals and regulation of protein degradation.

4. Discussion

Patients experience spinal cord injuries as a result of traffic accidents, sports injuries and trauma each year, leading to lifelong disability and/or significant economic costs [1]. After crushing SCI, the initial traumatic injury to spinal cord tissue is followed by a long period of secondary damage including oxidative stress, inflammation, necrosis and apoptosis [23, 24]. The loss of neuronal cells is the main contributor interfering with the recovery from secondary damage. Many therapeutic interventions that utilize neurotrophic factors, such as nerve growth factor (NGF), brain-derived neurotroph-

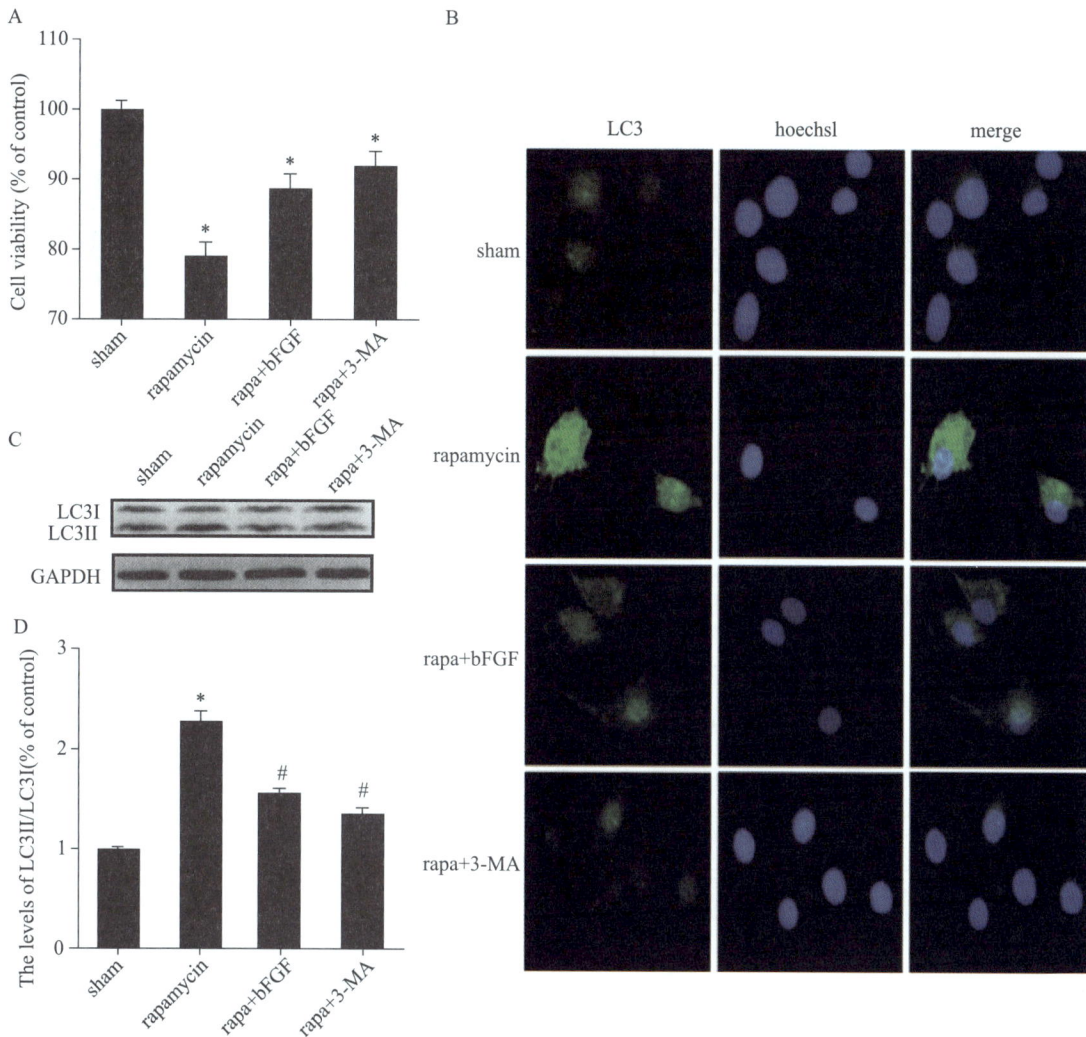

Fig. 7. The neuronal protective effects of bFGF are related to the inhibition of autophagy, which is induced by rapamycin. (A) MTT results of bFGF-trcated PC12 cells induced by rapamycin. (B) Immunofluorescence staining results of LC3 (*green*), where the nuclei are labeled with Hoechst (*blue*). (C) The protein expression of LC3II/LC3I in the sham, SCI model, and SCI model rats treated with bFGF compound with rapamycin and SCI model rats treated with the 3-MA compound with rapamycin. (D) The optical density analysis of LC3II/LC3I in the sham, SCI model, and SCI model rats treated with the bFGF compound with rapamycin and SCI model rats treated with the 3-MA compound with rapamycin. $^{*}P < 0.05$ *vs.* the sham group, $^{#}P < 0.01$ *vs.* the rapamycin group.

ic factor (BDNF) and glial cell line-derived neurotrophic factor (GDNF), have been established to promote functional recovery after SCI [25]. In the present study, we treated SCI rats with recombinant bFGF and demonstrated that the protective effect and molecular mechanism of bFGF recovery after SCI is related to the regulation of autophagy and poly-ubiquitin protein degradation *in vivo*.

Autophagy is an essential process for the maintenance of cellular homeostasis in the central nervous system, both under normal and stress conditions. Autophagy is a key degradation pathway that acts as a quality control sensor that protects myocytes from cytotoxic protein aggregation and dysfunctional organelles by inducing rapid clearance [26]. In contrast, excessive activation of autophagy is detrimental to cells and contributes to the development of pathological conditions. Autophagy may also promote cell death through excessive self-digestion, degradation of essential cellular constituents and/or interaction with apoptotic cascades [27]. Previous studies have demonstrated that autophagy-induced apoptosis was one of the main events in the secondary damage in SCI; however, the underlying mechanism remains unclear [7]. In many circumstances, autophagy and apoptosis can co-occur or occur sequentially [28, 29]. Numerous studies have demonstrated that autophagy is associated with pathologic conditions such as certain neurodegenerative disorders, cardiomyopathies and infectious diseases [30]. More recently, increasing findings suggest that autophagy is involved in SCI. The ratio of LC3II to LC3I was found to be increased in untreated animals 1 day after SCI. Many damaged neu-

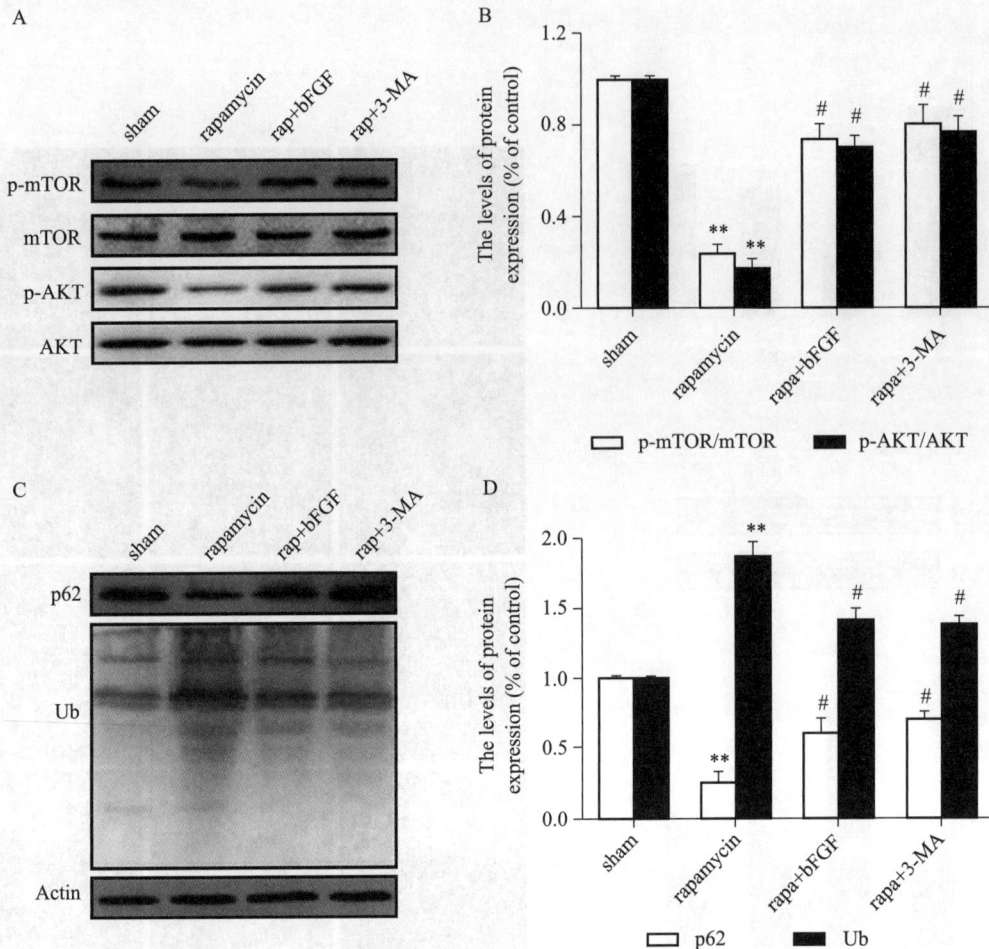

Fig. 8. bFGF administration activates Akt/mTOR signaling pathways and inhibits rapamycin-induced protein ubiquitination in PC12 cells. (A) Protein expression of p-AKT and p-mTOR of the sham, SCI model, and SCI model rats treated with bFGF compound with rapamycin and SCI model rats treated with the 3-MA compound with rapamycin. Ub and p62 in PC12 cells. (B) The optical density analysis of p-AKT and p-mTOR in PC12 cells. (C) The protein expression of Ub and p62 of each group in PC12 cells. (D) The optical density analysis of Ub and p62 in PC12 cells. $^*P < 0.05$, $^{**}P<0.01$ vs. the sham group, $^#P<0.05$ vs. the rapamycin group.

rons exhibited features of autophagic/lysosomal cell death during cervical SCI, such as cytoplasmic autophagic vacuoles and the induction of GFP-LC3 immunofluorescence [24]. bFGF has been shown to be a potential therapeutic treatment for SCI through expression in stem cells or incubation with astrocytes [17, 31]. However, whether these protective effects are related to autophagy regulation has not yet been investigated. In our study, we first reported that bFGF protected the survival of motor neurons and improved recovery from SCI through inhibition of excessive autophagy. It was found that the expression of LC3II protein increased significantly at 7 days after SCI. Immunofluorescence staining results also showed that LC3 puncta were increased in the SCI group compared to the sham injury group and that puncta could be recovered by bFGF treatment. Exogenous bFGF improved locomotor function and recovery of SCI *in vivo*. We also found that bFGF inhibited autophagy induced by the autophagy sensitizer rapamycin and increased viability of a PC-12 cell model *in vitro*. The function of bFGF was compared to that of the classical autophagy inhibitor 3-MA. The results of this comparison further confirmed that the protective effect of bFGF is involved in autophagy regulation.

As the main downstream signal that is activated by bFGF, PI3K/Akt has an essential neurotrophic effect. The PI3K/Akt pathway is particularly important for mediating neuron survival under a wide variety of circumstances. Activation of the PI3K/Akt pathways is essential for neurotrophin-mediated survival; knockdown of Akt expression impairs NGF- and BDNF-mediated H19-7 hippocampal progenitor cell and primary hippocampal neuron survival [32]. Moreover, the downstream signal of PI3K/Akt/mTOR, plays an important role in programmed cell death; phosphorylation of mTOR impairs the process of neuronal cell death in SCI. In particular, previous reports suggest that phosphorylated mTOR provides neuroprotection by reducing autophagy and enhancing recovery in cervical SCI [7]. In our recent report, bFGF was shown to exhibit a neuronal protective effect in an SCI model *via* the activation of both PI3K/Akt and ERK1/2 signals [33]. However, whether the protective effect of bFGF is related to autophagy regulation in SCI remains unclear. In the present study, we demonstrated that autophagy was excessively activated in the early stage of SCI. bFGF treatment stimulated phosphorylation of PI3K/Akt and further enhanced mTOR signals, resulting in autophagy inhibition. As a macrolide anti-biotic, rapamycin is often used to induce autophagy *via* mTOR inhibition [34]. The mTOR signaling pathway is considered a master regulator of multiple interrelated functions and mechanisms relevant to cell growth, proliferation and death [35]. In cerebral ischemia, nicotinamide phosphoribosyltransferase (Nampt, also known as visfatin) promotes neuronal survival through inducing autophagy *via* SIRT1 (sirtuin1)-dependent regulation of the mTOR signaling pathway [36]. In neuron-like PC-12 and SH-SY5Y cells, cadmium induction of ROS signals the Akt/mTOR pathway by activating positive regulators of PI3K; this leads to neuronal apoptosis [37]. Furthermore, mTOR may directly modulate separate mechanisms controlling neuronal death, such as the pro-apoptotic molecules BAD and Bcl-2 [38]. This dual role of mTOR may be based on the level of autophagy activation and/or various activated phases or situations. The mTOR pathway may have opposing effects on neuronal death mechanisms, which depend on the situation and stress level. These factors must be considered in designing potential therapies. In the present study, SCI model rats were treated with bFGF and rapamycin simultaneously and the levels of LC3II/LC3I increased significantly, impairing the neuroprotective function of bFGF. In our PC-12 cell model, rapamycin combined with bFGF or the autophagy inhibitor 3-MA, also showed increased cell viability compared to the rapamycin group. Taken together, these data suggest that the role of bFGF in neuronal cell death and recovery in SCI is related to autophagy inhibition *via* activation of the Akt/mTOR signaling pathway. To our surprise, although rapamycin addition abolished the protective effect of bFGF both *in vivo* and *in vitro*, rapamycin treatment alone did not affect recovery in SCI compared to an untreated group. This finding suggests that a prolonged research trial of up to 3 or 4 weeks of treatment is necessary. When rapamycin treated aloneon SCI models, no significanteffect on cell death was detected, these may related to the over activation of autophagy by acute injury, further stimulation only plays sustaining effect by not aggravation in the early stage of contusions, we suspected that rapamycin treatment may delayed the recovery process of SCI in the prolonged research trial, further investigation is needed. Furthermore, it is notable that as a neurotrophic factor, the function of bFGF on cell proliferation and migration was also impaired by rapamycin, even though the inhibitory effect of autophagy by bFGF was impaired by rapamycin. The molecular mechanism may be related to impaired receptor conjunction or cellular signal transduction; further investigation is needed.

In addition to its central roles in protein quality control, cell cycle regulation, intracellular signaling, DNA damage response and transcription regulation, the UPS plays specific rolcs in the central nervous system. Dysfunction of the UPS is associated with several neurological diseases [39–41]. Excessive accumulation of ubiquitinated protein is also involved in the etiology of SCI which leads to UPS dysfunction. We hypothesized that excessive autophagy may lead to dysfunction of ubiquitinated protein clearance and that bFGF modulates excessive autophagy to a suitable level, contributing to cell homeostasis. Our data showed that bFGF enhanced the clearance of ubiquitinated proteins and significantly increased the expression of p62 in SCI lesions. Recently, it has been demonstrated that clearance of abnormal ubiquitinated protein aggregates by insulin-like growth factor-1 (IGF-1) contributed to neuroprotection against apoptosis following proteasome inhibition [42]. In PC-12 cells treated with the proteasome inhibitor lactacystin, rapamycin pretreatment attenuated lactacystin-induced apoptosis and reduced ubiquitinated protein aggregation. The observed protection was partially blocked by the autophagy inhibitor 3-MA [43]. In the study of type 2 diabetes, extracellular human islet amyloid polypeptide (hIAPP)-induced impairment of the ubiquitin-proteasome pathway led to accumulation of ubiquitinated proteins, which contributed to pancreatic beta-cell and primary cultured human islet apoptosis [44]. These studies suggest that homeostatic regulation by ubiquitinated protein clearance is essential for the survival of neuronal cells. The protective function of bFGF may be involved in the inhibition of excessive autophagic cell death and reversed toxic accumulation of ubiquitinated proteins.

In summary, bFGF significantly reduced the extent of damage caused by spinal cord lesions and improved locomotor recovery in SCI. We first reported that the neuroprotective role of bFGF is related to the inhibition of excessive autophagy and enhanced ubiquitinated protein clearance. Furthermore, activation of the downstream signaling pathways PI3K/Akt/mTOR is essential for the effect of bFGF in neuronal cell death both *in vivo* and *in vitro*. Our study demonstrates that therapeutic strategies using bFGF may be suitable for recovery from central nervous system injury.

Supplementary materials

Supplementary materials to this article can be found in the online version (doi:10.1007/s12035-013-8432-8).

References

[1] Penas C, Guzman M, Verdu E, et al. Spinal cord injury induces endoplasmic reticulum stress with different cell-type dependent response[J]. Journal Of Neurochemistry, 2007, 102(4): 1242-1255.

[2] Chen H, Fong T, Lee A, et al. Autophagy is activated in injured neurons and inhibited by methylprednisolone after experimental spinal cord injury[J]. Spine, 2012, 37(6): 470-475.

[3] Kanno H, Ozawa H, Sekiguchi A, et al. Induction of autophagy and autophagic cell death in damaged neural tissue after acute spinal cord injury in mice[J]. Spine, 2011, 36(22): E1427-E1434.

[4] Katayama M, Kawaguchi T, Berger MS, et al. DNA damaging agent-induced autophagy produces a cytoprotective adenosine triphosphate surge in malignant glioma cells[J]. Cell Death And Differentiation, 2007, 14(3): 548-558.

[5] Criollo A, Maiuri MC, Tasdemir E, et al. Regulation of autophagy by the inositol trisphosphate receptor[J]. Cell Death And Differentiation, 2007, 14(5): 1029-1039.

[6] Sekiguchi A, Kanno H, Ozawa H, et al. Rapamycin promotes autophagy and reduces neural tissue damage and locomotor impairment after spinal cord injury in mice[J]. Journal Of Neurotrauma, 2012, 29(5): 946-956.

[7] Walker CL, Walker MJ, Liu N, et al. Systemic bisperoxovanadium activates Akt/mTOR, reduces autophagy, and enhances recovery following cervical spinal cord injury[J]. Plos One, 2012, 7(1): 315-326.

[8] Chen P, Bhattacharyya BJ, Hanna J, et al. Ubiquitin homeostasis is critical for synaptic development and function[J]. Journal Of Neuroscience, 2011, 31(48): 17505-17513.

[9] Sanchez P, De Carcer G, Sandoval IV, et al. Localization of atypical protein kinase C isoforms into lysosome-targeted endosomes through interaction with p62[J]. Molecular And Cellular Biology, 1998, 18(5): 3069-3080.

[10] Bjorkoy G, Lamark T, Brech A, et al. p62/SQSTM1 forms protein aggregates degraded by autophagy and has a protective effect on huntingtin-induced cell death[J]. Journal Of Cell Biology, 2005, 171(4): 603-614.

[11] Pankiv S, Clausen TH, Lamark T, et al. p62/SQSTM1 binds directly to Atg8/LC3 to facilitate degradation of ubiquitinated protein aggregates by autophagy[J]. Journal Of Biological Chemistry, 2007, 282(33): 24131-24145.

[12] Giorgi C, De Stefani D, Bononi A, et al. Structural and functional link between the mitochondrial network and the endoplasmic reticulum[J]. International Journal Of Biochemistry & Cell Biology, 2009, 41(10): 1817-1827.

[13] Kirkin V, Lamark T, Johansen T, et al. NBR1 cooperates with p62 in selective autophagy of ubiquitinated targets[J]. Autophagy, 2009, 5(5): 732-733.

[14] Komatsu M, Ichimura Y. Physiological significance of selective degradation of p62 by autophagy[J]. Febs Letters, 2010, 584(7): 1374-1378.

[15] Beenken A, Mohammadi M. The FGF family: biology, pathophysiology and therapy[J]. Nature Reviews Drug Discovery, 2009, 8(3): 235-253.

[16] Karimi-Abdolrezaee S, Eftekharpour E, Wang J, et al. Synergistic effects of transplanted adult neural stem/progenitor cells, chondroitinase, and growth factors promote functional repair and plasticity of the chronically injured spinal cord[J]. Journal Of Neuroscience, 2010, 30(5): 1657-1676.

[17] Liu W, Wang Z, Huang Z. Bone marrow-derived mesenchymal stem cells expressing the bFGF transgene promote axon regeneration and functional recovery after spinal cord injury in rats[J]. Neurological Research, 2011, 33(7): 686-693.

[18] Lin X, Zhang Y, Liu L, et al. FRS2 alpha is essential for the fibroblast growth factor to regulate the mTOR pathway and autophagy in mouse embryonic fibroblasts[J]. International Journal Of Biological Sciences, 2011, 7(8): 1114-1121.

[19] Zhang J, Liu J, Liu L, et al. The fibroblast growth factor signaling axis controls cardiac stem cell differentiation through regulating autophagy[J]. Autophagy, 2012, 8(4): 690-691.

[20] Perrin FE, Boniface G, Serguera C, et al. Grafted Human Embryonic Progenitors Expressing Neurogenin-2 Stimulate Axonal Sprouting and Improve Motor Recovery after Severe Spinal Cord Injury[J]. Plos One, 2010, 5(12).

[21] Harada M, Hanada S, Toivola DM, et al. Autophagy activation by rapamycin eliminates mouse Mallory-Denk bodies and blocks their proteasome inhibitor-mediated formation[J]. Hepatology, 2008, 47(6): 2026-2035.

[22] Carloni S, Buonocore G, Longini M, et al. Inhibition of rapamycin-induced autophagy causes necrotic cell death associated with Bax/Bad mitochondrial translocation[J]. Neuroscience, 2012, 203: 160-169.

[23] Cevikbas F, Steinhoff M, Ikoma A. Role of spinal neurotransmitter receptors in itch: new insights into therapies and drug development[J]. Cns Neuroscience & Therapeutics, 2011, 17(6): 742-749.

[24] Moon YJ, Lee JY, Oh MS, et al. Inhibition of inflammation and oxidative stress by Angelica dahuricae radix extract decreases apoptotic cell death and improves functional recovery after spinal cord injury[J]. Journal Of Neuroscience Research, 2012, 90(1): 243-256.

[25] Angelucci F, Aloe L, Iannitelli A, et al. Effect of chronic olanzapine treatment on nerve growth factor and brain-derived neurotrophic factor in the rat brain[J]. European Neuropsychopharmacology, 2005, 15(3): 311-317.

[26] Tanida I. Autophagosome formation and molecular mechanism of autophagy[J]. Antioxidants & Redox Signaling, 2011, 14(11): 2201-2214.

[27] Rubinsztein DC, Codogno P, Levine B. Autophagy modulation as a potential therapeutic target for diverse diseases[J]. Nature Reviews Drug Discovery, 2012, 11(9): 709-730.

[28] Liberski PP, Gajdusek DC, Brown P. How do neurons degenerate in prion diseases or transmissible spongiform encephalopathies (TSEs): neuronal autophagy revisited[J]. Acta Neurobiologiae Experimentalis, 2002, 62(3): 141-147.

[29] Yousefi S, Simon H-U. Apoptosis regulation by autophagy gene 5[J]. Critical Reviews In Oncology Hematology, 2007, 63(3): 241-244.

[30] Cuervo AM. Autophagy: in sickness and in health[J]. Trends In Cell Biology, 2004, 14(2): 70-77.

[31] Cunha JdC, Azevedo Levy BdF, de Luca BA, et al. Responses of reactive astrocytes containing S100 beta protein and fibroblast

growth factor-2 in the border and in the adjacent preserved tissue after a contusion injury of the spinal cord in rats: implications for wound repair and neuroregeneration[J]. Wound Repair And Regeneration, 2007, 15(1): 134-146.

[32] Nguyen TLX, Kim CK, Cho JH, *et al.* Neuroprotection signaling pathway of nerve growth factor and brain-derived neurotrophic factor against staurosporine induced apoptosis in hippocampal H19-7 cells[J]. Experimental And Molecular Medicine, 2010, 42(8): 583-595.

[33] Zhang HY, Zhang X, Wang ZG, *et al.* Exogenous basic fibroblast growth factor inhibits er stress-induced apoptosis and improves recovery from spinal cord injury[J]. Cns Neuroscience & Therapeutics, 2013, 19(1): 20-29.

[34] Gammoh N, Lam D, Puente C, *et al.* Role of autophagy in histone deacetylase inhibitor-induced apoptotic and nonapoptotic cell death[J]. Proceedings Of the National Academy Of Sciences Of the United States Of America, 2012, 109(17): 6561-6565.

[35] Zoncu R, Efeyan A, Sabatini DM. mTOR: from growth signal integration to cancer, diabetes and ageing[J]. Nature Reviews Molecular Cell Biology, 2011, 12(1): 21-35.

[36] Wang P, Guan YF, Du H, *et al.* Induction of autophagy contributes to the neuroprotection of nicotinamide phosphoribosyl transferase in cerebral ischemic stroke[J]. Autophagy, 2012, 8(1): 77-87.

[37] Chen L, Xu B, Liu L, *et al.* Cadmium induction of reactive oxygen species activates the mTOR pathway, leading to neuronal cell death[J]. Free Radical Biology And Medicine, 2011, 50(5): 624-632.

[38] Castedo M, Ferri KF, Kroemer G. Mammalian target of rapamycin (mTOR): Pro- and anti-apoptotic[J]. Cell Death And Differentiation, 2002, 9(2): 99-100.

[39] Chen SM, Ferrone FA, Wetzel R. Huntington's disease age-of-onset linked to polyglutamine aggregation nucleation[J]. Proceedings of the National Academy Of Sciences Of the United States Of America, 2002, 99(18): 11884-11889.

[40] Dohm CP, Kermer P, Baehr M. Aggregopathy in neurodegenerative diseases: Mechanisms and therapeutic implication[J]. Neurodegenerative Diseases, 2008, 5(6): 321-338.

[41] Thorpe JR, Tang H, Atherton J, *et al.* Fine structural analysis of the neuronal inclusions of frontotemporal lobar degeneration with TDP-43 proteinopathy[J]. Journal Of Neural Transmission, 2008, 115(12): 1661-1671.

[42] Cheng B, Maffi SK, Martinez AA, *et al.* Insulin-like growth factor-I mediates neuroprotection in proteasome inhibition-induced cytotoxicity in SH-SY5Y cells[J]. Molecular And Cellular Neuroscience, 2011, 47(3): 181-190.

[43] Pan T, Kondo S, Zhu W, *et al.* Neuroprotection of rapamycin in lactacystin-induced neurodegeneration *via* autophagy enhancement[J]. Neurobiology Of Disease, 2008, 32(1): 16-25.

[44] Casas S, Gomis R, Gribble FM, *et al.* Impairment of the ubiquitin-proteasome pathway is a downstream endoplasmic reticulum stress response induced by extracellular human islet amyloid polypeptide and contributes to pancreatic beta-cell apoptosis[J]. Diabetes, 2007, 56(9): 2284-2294.

The anti-scar effects of basic fibroblast growth factor on the wound repair *in vitro* and *in vivo*

Hongxue Shi, Xiaokun Li, Jian Xiao

1. Introduction

During the repair of a wound proceeds, keloid and hypertrophic scars (HTS) are a common problem. Clinically, they are characterized by excessive deposition of collagen in the dermis and subcutaneous tissues secondary to traumatic. This process is regulated by cytokines and growth factors such as transforming growth factor β (TGF-β), epidermal growth factor (EGF), fibroblast growth factor (FGF) and platelet-derived growth factor (PDGF) [1]. During embryogenesis, FGFs play key roles in regulating cell proliferation, migration, and differentiation. In adult tissues, FGFs have various effects, including mediating angiogenesis and neuroprotection, in addition to their stimulatory effects during wound repair [2,3,4]. Basic fibroblast growth factor (bFGF) is a potent mitogen and chemoattractant for endothelial cells, fibroblasts and keratinocyte. bFGF stimulates the metabolism, growth of the extracellular matrix (ECM), and the movement of mesodermally derived cells [5]. The administration of recombinant bFGF to skin wounds can accelerate acute and chronic wound healing [6,7,8,9]. In addition, bFGF-knockout mice delayed healing of skin wounds [10], which means that bFGF plays a key role for wound healing.

The goal for wound treatment is the fast and scarless healing, although this is quite difficult for adult tissues. The accelerating wound healing may improve the quality of healing and alleviate the scar. The anti-scarring effects of bFGF have been shown in both animal models and clinical use; postoperative administration of bFGF also inhibits hyperplastic scar without side effects [6,11,12,13]. These results suggest that bFGF treatment during wound healing may exert anti-fibrosis effects in keloids. However, little is known about the precise pathological mechanisms of bFGF on the prevention of HTS and keloid formation; thus, the underlying mechanism deserves further investigations.

During the wound healing process, the imbalance of collagen synthesis and degradation resulting in excess accumulation of dermal collagen can lead to the scar complications [14]. Sufficient content of type III collagen may prevent scar tissue formation, while excessive secretion of type I collagen may result in a disorganized fiber structure and hypertrophic scar formation [15]. In addition, α-smooth muscle actin (α-SMA) also plays a major role in the fibrosis, as sustained the myofibroblasts form the granulation tissue [16]. Additionally, TGF-β is particularly important for the fibrosis. Localized increase in the release and activation of TGF-β1 in burn injuries have delayed reepithelialization and enhanced the scarring response [17], TGF-β1 and TGF-β2 induce cuaneous scarring, whereas TGF-β3 seems to inhibit this effect [18,19]. Therefore, collagen distribution, α-SMA expression, and the TGF-β1 mediated signal pathway are analyzed as the mechanisms of anti-scarring effect of bFGF.

This study aims to demonstrate whether bFGF can alleviate or eliminate formed hypertrophic scars in a full-thickness excisional rat model and in the rabbit ear model. To explore the possible mechanism of action, we comparatively evaluated the *in vitro* effects of bFGF on fibroblasts isolated from human HTS and normal skin. Thus, we provide evidence of a new therapeutic strategy: bFGF administration for the treatment of established HTS.

2. Results

2.1 bFGF accelerates acute wound closure in the rat incised injury model

Wound healing of the skin incision was determined by the percentage of wound surface covered by regenerating epidermis. The wounds treated by bFGF recovered much more quickly with better skin appearance (Fig. 1A). After day 8, the wounds treated with bFGF were almost scarless, while the wounds in the control had obvious scars. Thus, bFGF significantly contributed to wound healing, compared to the control group ($P<0.05$; Fig. 1B). After day 14, both the bFGF group and the control group showed wound closure mostly, for natural repair of the rat skin. These wound closure rates made a good match to the results of HE staining and Masson Staining (Fig. 1C). Longer keratinocyte migration tongue and collagen expression was observed on day 14 for bFGF-treated wounds; the results demonstrated the accelerating effect of bFGF on the wound re-epithelization *in vivo*.

Compared with the control group, expression amounts of PCNA and TGF-β1 cell proliferation proteins in the bFGF group significantly increased after establishment of the ulcer model on day 7. On the 14th day, the expression amounts of PCNA were remain increase in bFGF group, while the TGF-β1 levels were decreased in the bFGF group (Fig. 2A and 2C). Inflammatory response is instrumental to supplying growth factor and cytokine signals that orchestrate the cell and tissue movements necessary for repair during wound healing, As a macrophage marker, CD68 belongs to a family of

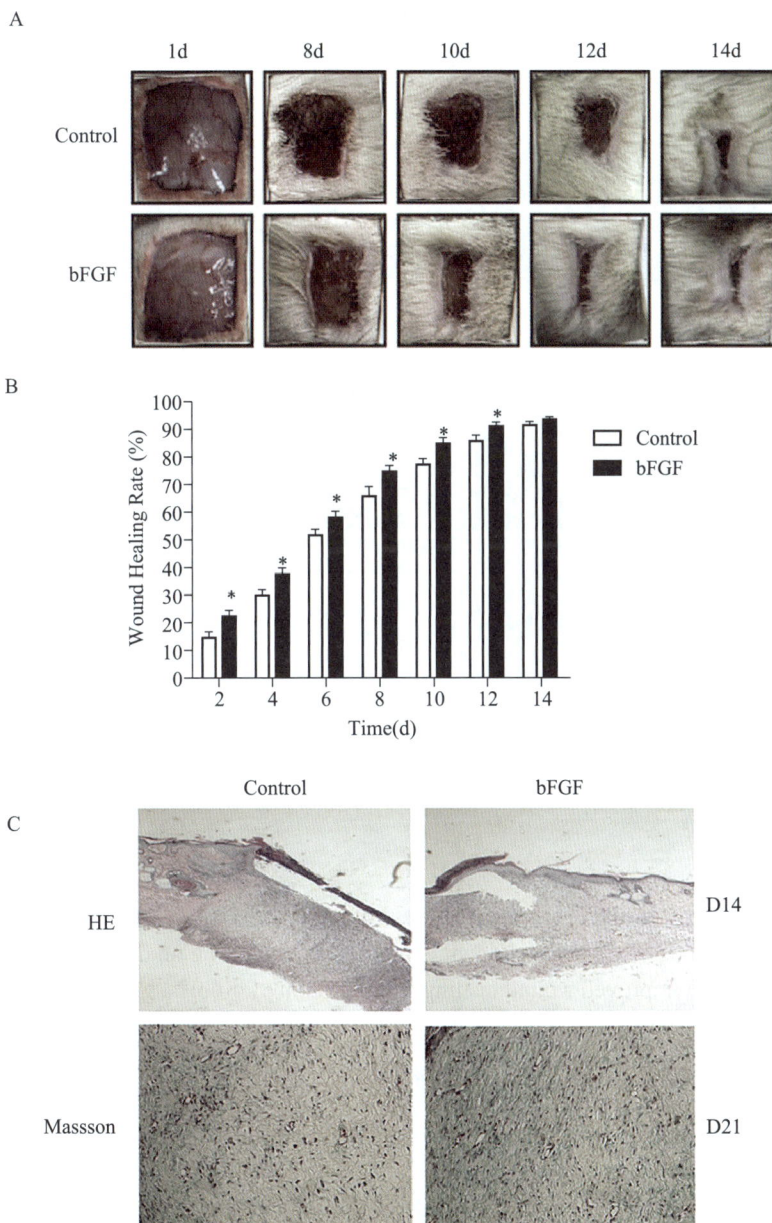

Fig. 1. Wound closure and histopathological characteristics of bFGF treated wound healing in rat. (A) Representative photographs of full-thickness skin wounds at various time points after treatment with or without 1 µg/ml bFGF. (B) The wound healing rates of bFGF. *$P<0.05$ compared to control group, $n = 8$. (C) Histopathological observation and masson staining of collagen in wound healing at day 14 post-wounding (×200).

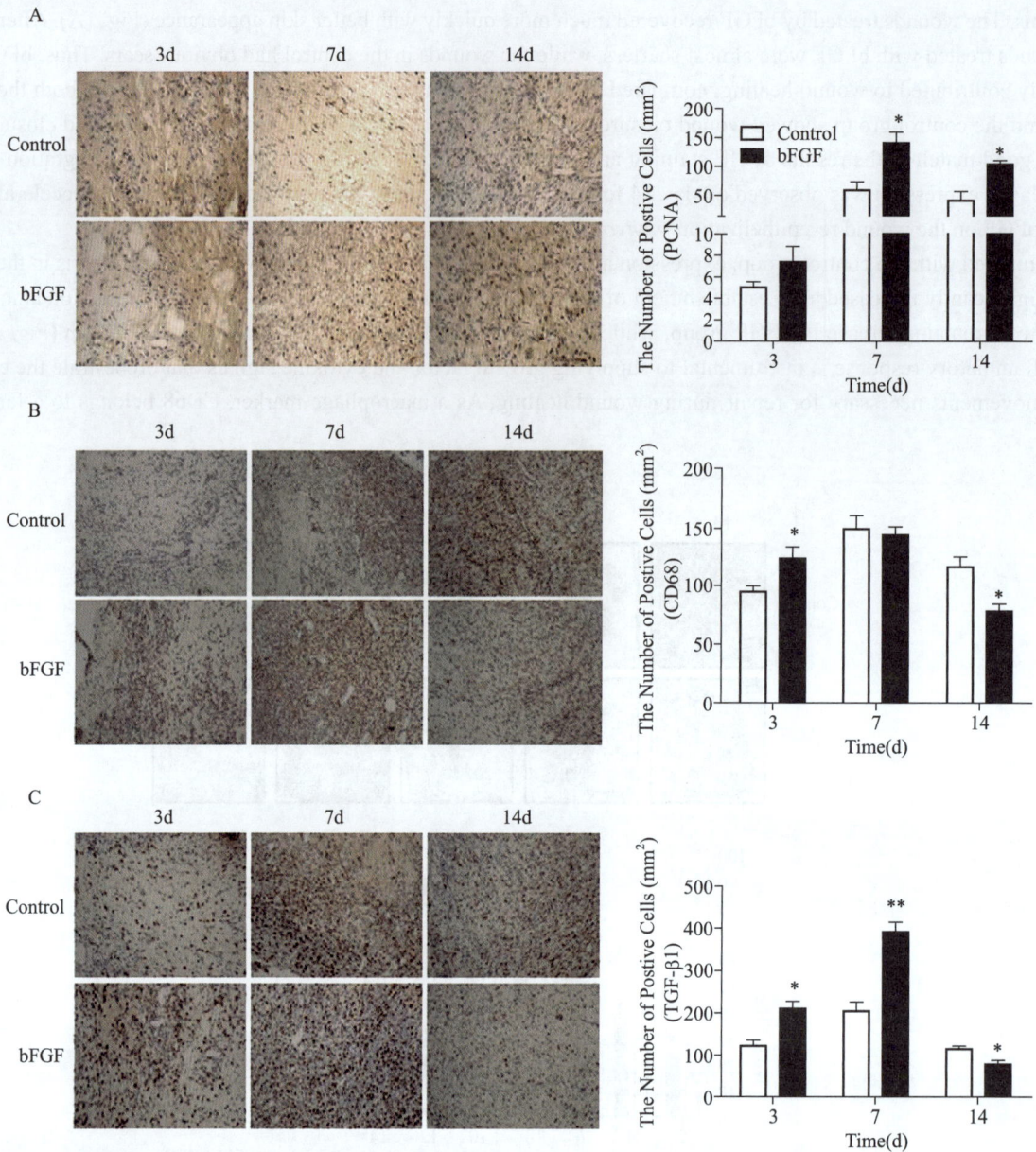

Fig. 2. The expression of PCNA, CD68 and TGF-β1 after bFGF treatment. Immunohistochemistry of (A) PCNA, (B) CD68 and (C) TGF-β1 was performed on the indicated day (×200); the histogram represents the positive cells and optical density of the immunohistochemistry results. *P<0.05 and **P<0.01 compared to control group, n = 8.

acidic, high glucosylated lysosomal glycoproteins (GLPs). Immunohistochemical staining of CD68 indicated upregulated inflammatory response on days 3 and 7 and downregulated the expression on day 14 in the bFGF group (Fig. 2B). These results suggest that bFGF improved wound healing by stimulating fibroblast growth, reducing scar formation, and regulating the inflammation response.

2.2 bFGF alleviates the scar formation in the rabbit ear model

All wounds had adequate scar maturation and showed histologic evidence of scarring. The mean scar thickness (SEI) in the control group was 4.612±0.4152 and 3.369±0.3712, which was higher than that of the bFGF group with 2.939±0.3131, 2.338±0.2446 on days 20 and 40, respectively (Fig. 3A). The mean epidermal thickness (ETI) of the control group was 6.089±0.4744 and 3.758±0.3262 compared with 3.472±0.4232 and 2.490±0.3070 for the bFGF group (P<0.05; Fig. 3B). This represents a significant epidermal thickness reduction in wounds treated with bFGF.

Histologically, the dermis layer of the control scars thickened significantly, and the boundary between the papillary

A

B

C

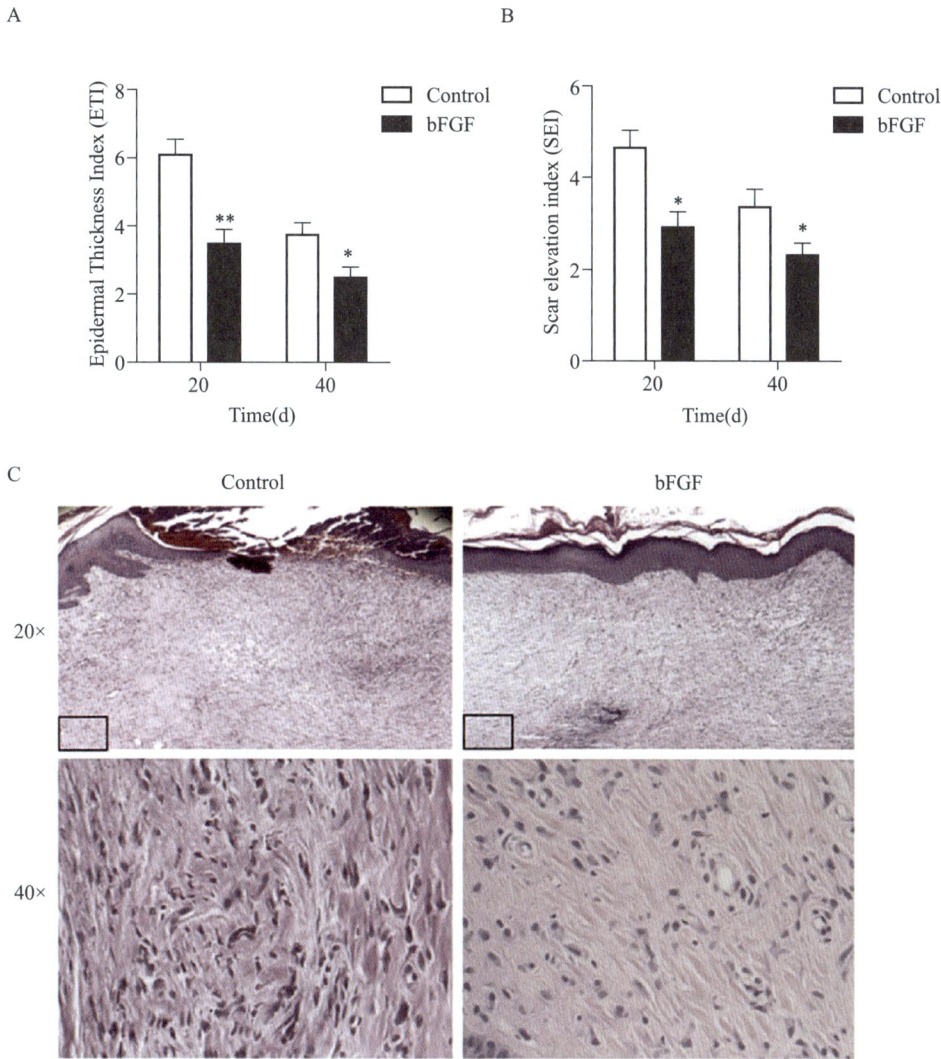

Fig. 3. bFGF alleviated the scar formation in rabbit ear model. (A) The averaged Epidermal Thickness Index (ETI) of the scars. Epidermal hypertrophy was displayed by ETI. ETI>1 depicts a hypertrophic epidermis. (B) The averaged scar elevation index (SEI) of the scars. Dermal hypertrophy is displayed by the SEI, where SEI>1 depicts a hypertrophic scar. $^*P<0.05$, $^{**}P<0.01$ compared to control group, $n = 6$. (C) The microscopic histology of wounds that control or bFGF at day 40, HE stain.

and reticular layers of dermis was obscure; collagen fibers were dense, with derangements in collagen bundles, which were irregularly arranged in the profound dermis and nodular, circular, or whirled in the superficial dermis. The number of cells also increased, while the basal layer of the epidermis in the scars treated with bFGF for 40 day was flattened. The dermis layer was not significantly thickened, and collagen fibers were well arranged, with few cells (Fig. 3C).

2.3 Effect of bFGF on collagen I and collagen III synthesis

In order to evaluate the molecular effects of bFGF on matrix production, we measured protein expression of collagen I and III, which constitute the bulk of the scar ECM. As expected, collagen I expression was significantly decreased on day 20 ($P<0.05$), while collagen I expression was insignificantly decreased on day 40 (Fig. 4A); collagen III significantly reduced on day 40 ($P<0.05$) in the bFGF treated group (Fig. 4B). The collagen density was significantly reduced in wounds treated with bFGF compared with the untreated wounds by immunohistochemical staining of the collagen III on day 40 ($P<0.05$; Fig. 4C and 4D).

2.4 Effect of bFGF on on α-SMA and TGF-β1 expression

The persistent presence of myofibroblasts is a distinctive feature of HTS that contributes to the excessive matrix production. In untreated scars, immunohistochemistry revealed significantly staining for α-SMA. The positive

A

B

C

D

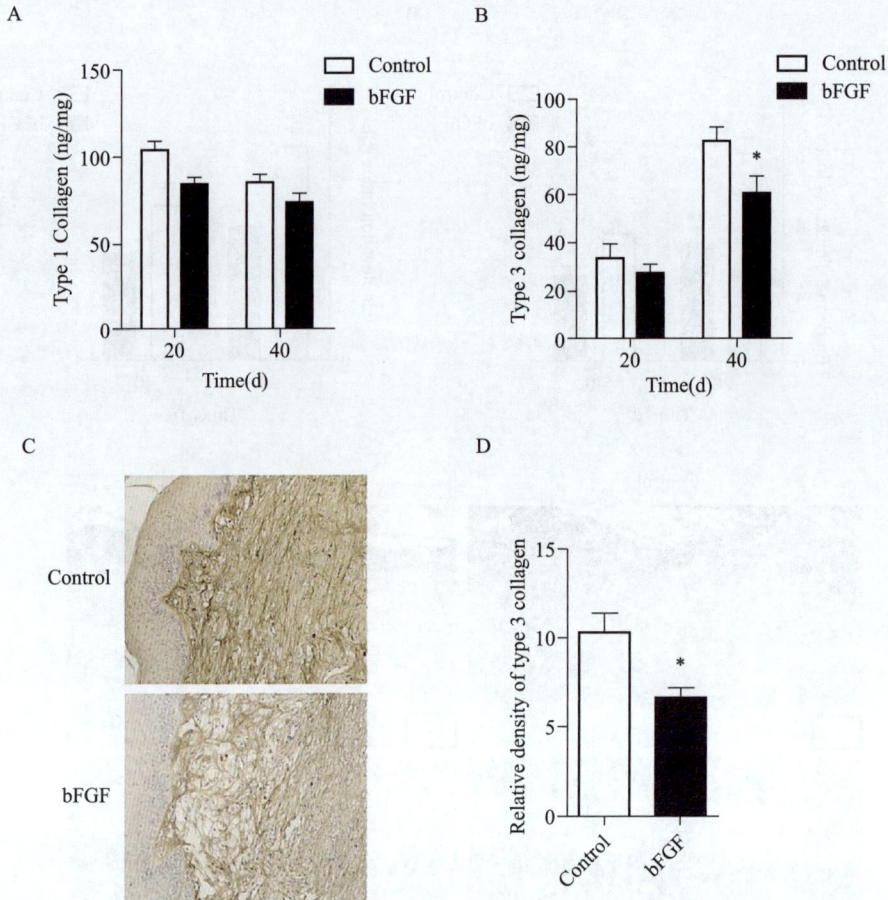

Fig. 4. bFGF decreased collagen I and collagen III synthesis. The levels of expression of (A) collagen I and (B) collagen III in scars treated with saline or bFGF, $^*P<0.05$, $^{**}P<0.01$ compared to control group, $n = 6$. (C) Immunohistochemistry of the expression of collagen III in scars treated with saline or bFGF (×200). (D) Analysis of relative density collagen III, $^*P<0.05$, $^{**}P<0.01$ compared to control group, $n = 6$.

number of α-SMA in the scars treated with bFGF was significant decreased compared with the control group on day 40 (Fig. 5A). Western blot analysis showed that levels of α-SMA expression decreased in the bFGF groups relative to the control group (Fig. 5C and 5E). The expression of TGF-β1 in the scars treated with bFGF decreased compared with the control group after immunohistochemical staining of the TGF-β1 on day 40 (Fig. 5B). Western blot analysis showed that the level of TGF-β1 expression significantly decreased in the bFGF group compared with the control groups on day 40 (Fig. 5C and 5D).

2.5 Effects of bFGF on mRNA expression of HSF

bFGF stimulated cell proliferation of both HTS-derived and normal skin-derived fibroblasts (Data not shown). Real-time PCR indicated that bFGF downregulated FN, collagen I and III, α-SMA, and hydroxylases expression in HTS-derived fibroblasts (Fig. 6A, 6B, 6E, 6J, 6K and 6L). The MMP-1 mRNA expression increased in scar fibroblasts treated with bFGF. As the natural inhibitor of the MMPs, TIMP-1 was downregulated in the bFGF group (Fig. 6F and 6G). Most interestingly, bFGF highly upregulated gene expression of HGF, but downregulated CTGF levels (Fig. 6C and 6D).

2.6 bFGF induces cells apoptosis and inhibits TGF-β1 mediated SMAD signaling

To determine the level of apoptosis in wounds filled with collagen, TUNEL staining was performed. Comparing the TUNEL positive numbers of the bFGF group with those of the control group on day 14, bFGF significantly increased the TUNEL positive numbers (Fig. 7A and 7B). The results suggest that bFGF treatment is a potent stimulator of myofibroblast apoptosis.

A

Control

bFGF

B

Control

bFGF

C

	Control	bFGF
α-SMA		
TGF-β1		
GAPDH		

D

TGF-β1 Levels — Control, bFGF (**)

E

α-SMA Levels — Control, bFGF (**)

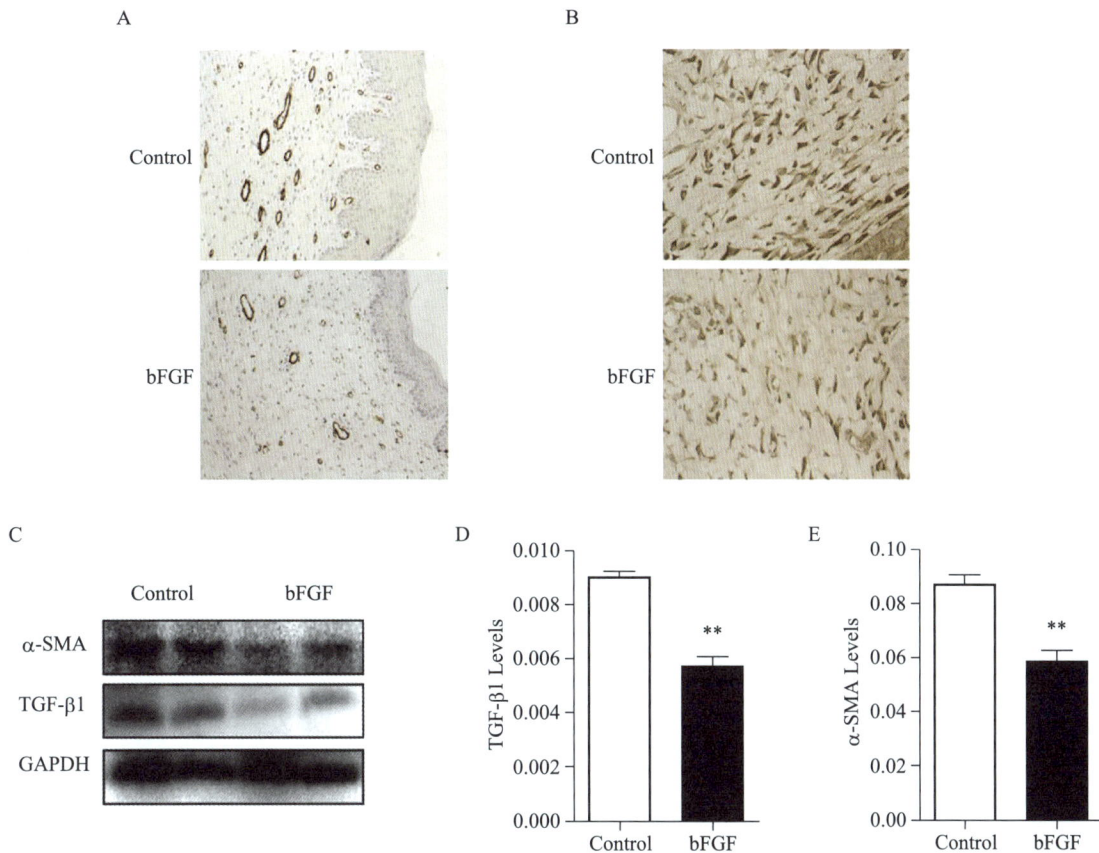

Fig. 5. bFGF decreased α-SMA and TGF-β1 expression in scars. Immunohistochemistry of the expression of (A) α-SMA and (B) TGF-β1 in scars treated with saline or bFGF in scars. (C) The levels of α-SMA and TGF-β1 in scars treated with saline or bFGF by Western blot. Analysis of the relative protein of (D) TGF-β1 and (E) α-SMA was performed. $^{**}P<0.01$ compared to control group.

SMAD proteins as intracellular effectors of TGF-β1 signaling, SMAD7 as the unique negative feedback regulator of TGF-β1 signal pathway prevents SMAD2/3-receptor interactions and subsequent SMAD phosphorylation, and degrade receptor complexes. In this study, gene expression of SMAD7 was markedly upregulated by bFGF in HSF, while the gene expression of SMAD2 was significantly downregulated (Fig. 6H and 6I). Western blot analysis showed that the phosphorylation of SMAD2/3 was upregulated in fibroblasts treated with TGF-β1 (Fig. 7C and 7D), while fibroblasts incubated with TGF-β1 and bFGF showed a significant decrease of phosphorylation of SMAD2/3 (Fig. 7E and 7F), which means that bFGF inhibited the TGF-β/SMAD signal pathway in HTS.

3. Discussion

Scarring is a multifactorial process with different clinical presentations that affects more than 40 million people worldwide [20]. Generally, scars can be classified into two categories, pathological scars and non-pathological scars. There are some preventive and therapeutic measures for exuberant scars, such as silicone, pressure therapy, corticosteroids, laser therapy, cryotherapy, radiation, and surgery [21,22,23,24]. However, there is no consensus about the best treatment for complete and permanent improvement of scars with few side effects.

Funato et al. [25] reported that bFGF is a possible inducer of apoptosis in myofibroblasts during palatal scar formation. Spyrou and Naylor [26] found that treatment with bFGF inhibited the transient phenotypic change of granulation-tissue fibroblasts into myofibroblasts. In order to identify a means to reduce scar formation of the skin after incision, Ono et al. [13] examined the effect of local administration of bFGF in humans. They found that no patient treated with bFGF had hypertrophic scars, while some patients had hypertrophic or very wide scars in the control group; the ratios

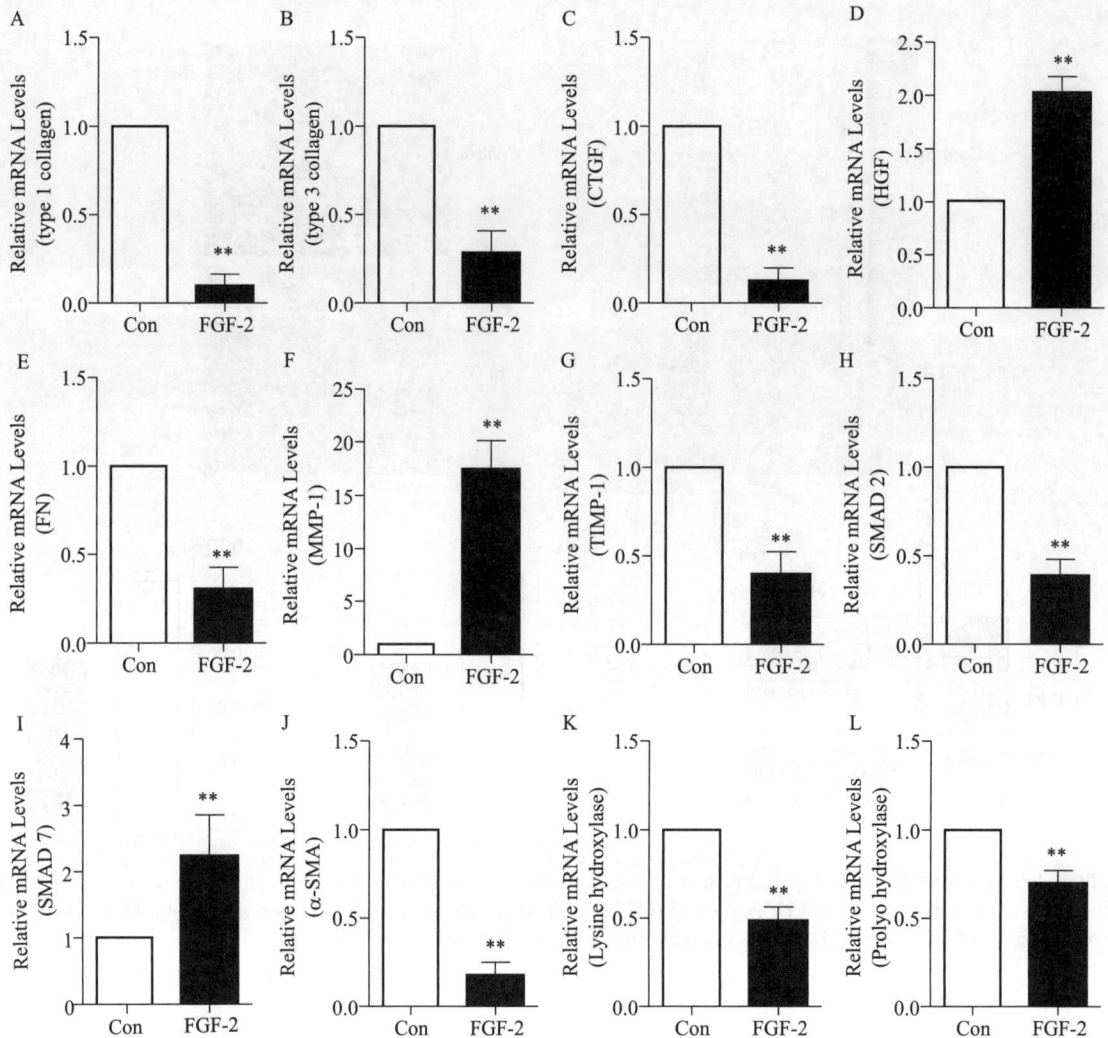

Fig. 6. Effects of bFGF on mRNA levels in HSF. RT-PCR analysis the mRNA levels of type (A) collagen I and (B) collagen III, (C) CTGF, (D) HGF, (E) FN, (F) MMP-1, (G) TIMP-1, (H) SMAD-2, (I) SMAD-7, (J) α-SMA, (K) Lysine hydroxylases and (L) Prolyo hydroxylase in HSF treated with bFGF or saline for 5 days. $^*P<0.05$ compared to control group.

of minimum scarring for the bFGF treatment group were statistically significantly higher than those of control group. In this study, we evalutate the therapeutic potential of bFGF for wound healing and HTS animal model as well as human scar fibroblast cell model and analyze the potential mechanisms. We find that bFGF promoted wound healing and reduced the area of flattened non-pathological scars in rat skin wounds (Fig. 1) as well as the size of hypertrophic scars in the rabbit ear (Fig. 3). In the early stages of incisional-wound healing, bFGF administration has no adverse effect on the tensile strength of the wound and, at later stages, can be attributed to the improved the architecture of the neodermis.

Type I and III collagens are the central components of ECM products. However, the production of collagen can be a double-edged sword: on the one hand, it is necessary for wound healing; on the other hand, excess deposition of collagen can result in scarring [27,28]. Therefore, the appropriate expression of collagen is required for ideal wound healing. Our findings indicate that bFGF can accelerate wound healing with increasing collagen production and subsequent collagen deposition (Fig. 1). The outcome is an improvement in the quality of wound healing. In the rabbit hypertrophic scar model, bFGF resulted in a sparse arrangement of the collagen, similar to normal skin collagen distribution, and reduced type I collagen and type III collagen content, which prevented the formation of nodular structures (Fig. 4). In the HSF, bFGF reduced collagen gene expression (Fig. 6A and 6B). Lysyl hydroxylase and prolyl hydroxylase, as the key enzymes for the formation and stabilization of collagen, also downregulated in bFGF treatment (Fig. 6K and 6L). These results support the alternative effect of bFGF on collagen expression in the different stages of wound healing, which is

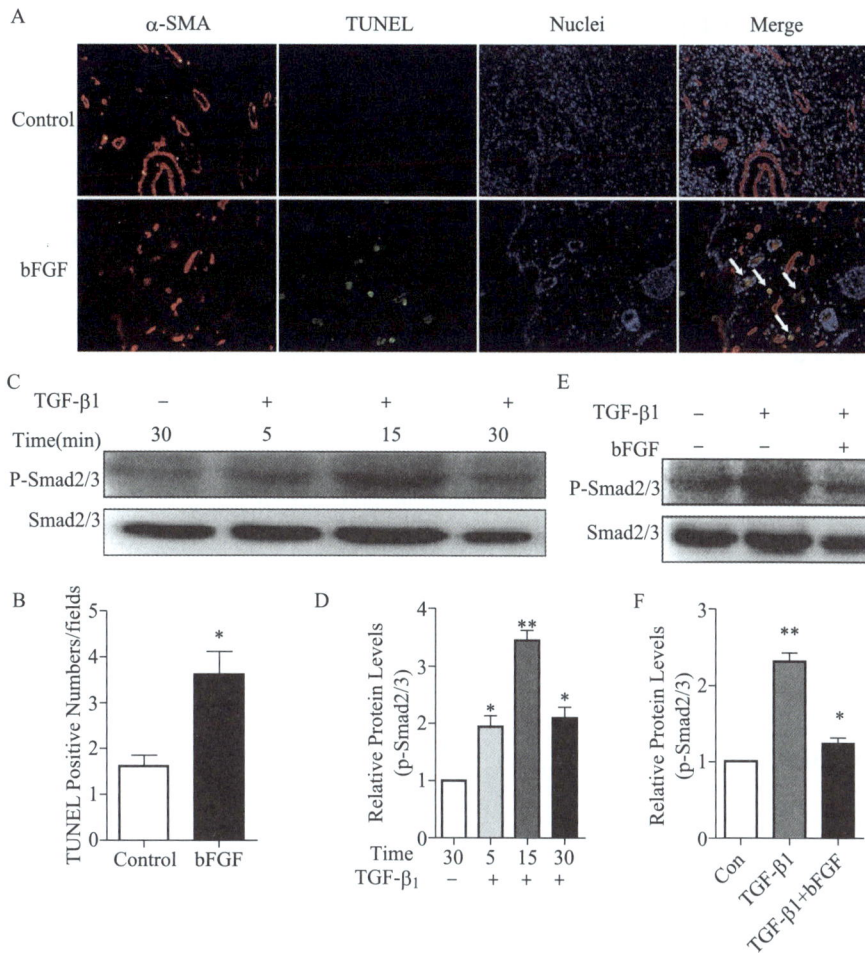

Fig. 7. bFGF induced cells apoptosis and inhibited TGF-β1/SMAD signaling pathway. (A and B) TUNEL staining analysis of the apoptosis cells in rat skin by bFGF or saline in day 14 after wounding. The nuclear was labeled by Hoechst (blue), the myofibroblast was labeled by α-SMA (red), the apoptosis cells was labeled by TUNEL (green). Colocalization of α-SMA and TUNEL indicate apoptosis myofibroblast (white arrow) (6200). *$P<0.05$ compared to control. (C and D) Western blot analysis of the phosphorylation of SMAD2/3 (Ser 423/425) in HSF incubated with TGF-β1 (5 ng/ml). (E and F) Western blot analysis of the phosphorylation of SMAD2/3 in HSF incubated with TGF-β1 and bFGF (10 ng/ml). *$P<0.05$, **$P<0.01$ compared to control group.

beneficial for wound closure and scar diminution. Also, the study by Xie et al. [11] supports the potential of bFGF to accelerate wound healing and improve the quality of scars by regulating the balance of collagen synthesis and degradation.

Consequently, interfering with one or several components of the ECM metabolism could be a potential therapeutic intervention to alleviate scars [1,14]. The amount of ECM in the tissue might be controlled through a balance among ECM production, ECM degradation by MMPs, and inhibition of MMPs by tissue inhibitors of metalloproteinases [14,29]. Our study shows that the stimulation of HSF with bFGF in vitro could result in an upregulation of MMP-1 and decreased TIMP-1 (Fig. 6F and 6G). Fibronectin is one of the most important ingredients of the ECM and plays a particularly important role in wound repair, largely determining the quality of the wound [30,31]. The deposition and/or polymerization of fibronectin into the ECM controls the deposition and stability of other ECM molecules [32,33]. Our data show that bFGF decreased FN gene expression in HSF (Fig. 6E). All of these results indicate that bFGF regulates ECM metabolism to improve wound healing and hypertrophic scarring.

Myofibroblasts, which elaborate matrix proteins and initiate wound contraction, are transiently present in healing wounds. The persistent presence of myofibroblasts is a distinctive feature of HTS and contributes to excessive matrix production [21,34]. Differentiation of fibroblasts into myofibroblasts is closely associated with α-SMA [17,35]. Our results indicate down-regulation of α-SMA expression by bFGF in the HSF and rabbit model (Fig. 5 and 6J). It has been demonstrated that TGF-β1 promoted a-SMA expression [36,37]. The present study also investigated the degree of apoptosis in fibroblastic cells and levels of TGF-β1 expression in scars. Immunofluorescence and western blot show that inclusion of bFGF significantly increased apoptosis in granulation tissue cells of the wound, consistent with other reports [12]. The SMAD2/ SMAD3 signaling system of the TGFβ1/SMAD-dependent pathway is considered an important pathway in scar formation. bFGF treatment also markedly decreased SMAD2/3 phosphorylation in the HSF (Fig. 7). This result indicates that bFGF treatment can increase apoptosis of myofibroblasts, leading to inhibition of scar formation due to inhibition of the TGF-β1 signaling pathway. Taken together, these findings suggest that bFGF reduce scarring and promote wound healing by inhibiting the TGF-β1/SMAD-dependent pathway. Thus bFGF might be applicable as an anti-scarring agent after the surgery of skin or other organs where myofibroblast overgrowth would induce complications for scarring.

In conclusion, we provide evidence of a new therapeutic strategy, bFGF administration for the treatment of HTS. bFGF regulate ECM synthesis and degradation *via* interference in the MMP-1, TIMP-1, lysyl hydroxylase and prolyl hydroxylase gene expression. The efficacy of treatment using bFGF was also demonstrated in animal models and the human cell model. However, it no doubt that the limitations of bFGF in scar therapy still need further investigation and improvement. For example, single a dose of bFGF was treated right after injury, a post-injury treatment of optimal dose and extended time would better evaluate the therapeutic value in the future. It is interesting that although we have tried several concentrations of bFGF in our model *in vivo*, there is no obvious enhancement of the protective effect with the increase of bFGF, which maybe related to the regulation of absorption and metabolism. Nevertheless, the anti-scarring effect of bFGF in the therapy of HTS is confirmative and feasible, to improve the pharmacodynamic action and demonstrate the mechanism underlying is necessary in the following study.

4. Materials and methods

4.1 Ethics statement

All animals were from the Laboratory Animals Center of Wenzhou Medical College, and treated strictly in accordance with international ethical guidelines and the National Institutes of Health Guide concerning the Care and Use of Laboratory Animals. The experiments were carried out with the approval of the Animal Experimentation Ethics Committee of Wenzhou Medical College.

Hypertrophic scar patients were selected according to the Vancouver Scar Scale (VSS) ranging from 10 to 13. All patients were informed of the purpose and procedure of this study and agreed to offer their tissue specimens. Written consent was obtained from all participants involved in this study. All protocols were approved by the Ethics Committee of First Affiliated Hospital of Wenzhou Medical College, Wenzhou, China.

4.2 Animal model

Male Sprague-Dawley rats ($n = 30$), weighing 250 g, were chosen for the experiment. The skin was cleaned with alcohol and two fullthickness wounds (2 cm×2 cm) extending through the panniculus carnosus were made on the dorsum on each side of midline under aseptic conditions. bFGF was obtained from the Key Laboratory of Biotechnology and Pharmaceutical Engineering in Wenzhou Medical College and applied to the wounds of the experimental group (1 ml for each wound) every other day in concentrations of 1 μg/ml (dissolved in 0.9% *w/v* saline), while the control group received equal amounts of 0.9% *w/v* saline treatment for 14 days. Wounds were left uncovered after injury, and wound areas were measured at various time points [9]. The rate of wound closure was calculated using the following formula: Wound closure rate = [(Original wound area-Open area on final day)/Original wound area×100%.

The rabbit ear model of hypertrophic scarring was established as described previously with a minor modification [23]. In brief, 12 Japanese white rabbits (no sex restriction), weighing 2.5 to 3.0 kg, were kept under standard conditions, anesthetized with xylazine (5 mg/kg) and prepared for wounding under sterile conditions. Five 1 cm fullthickness circular wounds were created down to the cartilage on the ventral side of each ear using a 1 cm punch biopsy. The perichondrial membrane was then dissected off the cartilage using a surgical blade. The bFGF solution was applied to the wounds of the experimental group (50 μl to each wound) every day in concentrations of 1.2 μg/ml (dissolved in 0.9% *w/v* saline) for 7 days, while the control group received equal amounts of 0.9% *w/v* saline.

4.3 Histological examination and immunohistochemistry staining

Histological analysis of the skin was performed as previously described [9]. The scar or skin tissues were fixed in 4% paraformaldehyde at 4℃ overnight prior to processing for paraffin embedding, cut in 5 μm sections, and stained with hematoxylin-eosin (HE) or Masson's Trichrome Stain Kit (Sigma-Aldrich, St. Louis, MO). The other half was stored at −80℃ for protein extraction. The scar elevation index (SEI) and epidermal thickness index (ETI) were used for histomorphometric analysis and measured for treated and untreated wounds. The SEI is a ratio of total wound area tissue height to the area of normal tissue below the scar. The height of the normal tissue is determined based on the height of the adjacent unwounded dermis. All measurements were taken within the confines of the wounded area under 40× magnification from the HE stained tissue sections. An SEI of 1 indicates that no newly hypertrophied dermis formed, whereas an index>1 indicates HTS formation. The ETI was used to determine the degree of epidermal hypertrophy and was based on measurements taken from H&E-stained tissue sections at 400× magnification. The ETI is a ratio of averaged epidermal height in scar tissue to the averaged epidermal height in normal uninjured skin. ETI>1 indicates hypertrophic epidermis formation.

The immunohistochemical staining of the PCNA, CD68, TGF-β1, α-SMA and collagen III (Santa Cruz Biotech, Santa Cruz, CA) was conducted by respective antibody. Sections were dewaxed and hydrated; endogenous peroxidase was blocked with 3% hydrogen peroxide for 10 min; nonspecific binding was blocked with 1% BSA for 30 min. Primaries were applied for PCNA (1:100), CD68 (1:100), TGF-β1 (1:150), α-SMA (1:50), and collagen III (1:200) overnight at 4℃. Biotinylated secondary antibodies were then applied at 1:200 for 30 min, followed by incubation with horseradish peroxidase (HRP)-streptavidin at 1:400 for 30 min. Color development was performed with DAB for 3 to 5 min for all samples, followed by haematoxylin counterstaining, dehydration and coverslipping. The immunopositive in fields was counted for per sections using Image-Pro Plus software (Nikon, Tokyo, Japan).

4.4 Terminal deoxynucleotidyl transferase (TdT)-mediated dUTP nick-end labeling (TUNEL) staining

TUNEL was performed using a commercial kit (Roche, Mannheim, Germany) according to the manufacturer's instructions. Negative controls had the TdT substrate omitted from the buffer solution. Following staining by the TUNEL protocol, sections were incubated overnight at 4℃ with rabbit anti-α-SMA at a dilution of 1:200; a secondary antibody were then applied at 1:400 for 60 min at 37℃. Fluorescence was examined using a Nikon microscope (Nikon, Tokyo, Japan) equipped with a reflected light fluorescence device. Negative control experiments, in which anti-α-SMA was replaced by rabbit immunoglobulin at the same final concentration, consistently showed no staining.

4.5 Collagen I and collagen III quantification

The quantification of collagen I and III used an ELISA Kit (R & D Systems Inc., Minneapolis, MN, USA) according to the operation manual. In brief, 100 μl of standards or samples were added to the appropriate well of the antibody pre-coated microtiter plate, followed by 50 μl of conjugate; each well was then covered and incubated for 1 h at 37℃. Next, 50 μl of substrates A and B were added to each well and incubated for 10 min at room temperature (to avoid sunlight). Finally, added 50 μl of the stop solution was added, and the optical density (O.D.) was read at 450 nm using a microtiter plate reader immediately.

4.6 Western blot

Western blotting was performed as previously described [38]. Briefly, the scar tissues or the cells were lysed; then the protein samples were denatured and then separated on 10.6% poly-acrylamide gels, and transferred to the polyvinylidene difluoride membrane. The membranes were incubated in TBS containing 5% nonfat milk and 0.05% Tween-20 for 1 h at room temperature and blotted with primary antibodies (dilution 1:300) at 4℃ overnight. The membranes were washed with TBST for 15 min the next day. Subsequently, the membranes were incubated with horseradish peroxidase-conjugated affinipure goat anti-rabbit antibody (dilution 1:3000) for 1 h at room temperature and washed with TBST for 21 min. The membranes were then detected using ECL. The western blot results were further analyzed with Quantity One software 4.1.1 (Bio-Rad, Hercules, CA).

4.7 Fibroblasts culture

Primary culture of hypertrophic scar fibroblasts (HSF) was established from the patients who had received no previous treatment for burn hypertrophic scar before surgical excision as described [17]. In briefly, the specimens were washed three times in a phosphate-buffered saline (PBS) solution containing 1% penicillin, streptomycin sulfate. Subsequently, the tissues were digested in 0.5% Dispase II overnight at 4℃. The epidermis and subcutaneous tissue were excised from the tissues, which were cut into approximately 1×1×0.5 cm and placed as explants in T25 tissue culture flasks. Dulbecco's modified eagle medium (DMEM) containing 1.0 g/L D-glucose, 10% fetal bovine serum (FBS), 1% penicillin, streptomycin sulfate and 2 mM L-glutamine was used as the growth medium. The medium was replaced every 3 days. The primary fibroblasts were grown at 37℃ in an atmosphere of 5% CO_2 and were passaged every 2 days by trypsinization. Cells were used for experiments at passages three to six.

4.8 Quantitative real-time PCR (RT-PCR)

After HSF was treated with bFGF or saline for 5 days, total RNA from HSF was prepared using Trizol Reagent (Invitrogen, Carlsbad, CA, USA) according to the manufacturer's instructions. cDNA synthesis was conducted according to the RNA PCR kit protocol (Invitrogen, Carlsbad, CA, USA). The primer sequences are shown in Table 1. The reaction conditions were 4 min at 95℃, followed by 40 cycles of 94℃ for 15 s and 60℃ for 25 min. During each extension step, SYBR green fluorescence was monitored and provided the real-time quantitative measurements of the fluorescence. Quantitation was carried out using an external standard curve. Expression levels were calculated by the comparative CT method with glyceraldehyde-3-phosphate dehydrogenase (GAPDH) as an endogenous reference gene.

Table 1.   Primers used for real-time RT-PCR analysis

Gene	Sense	Antisense
Collagen I	AGGGACACAGAGGTTTCAGTGGTT	GCAGCACCAGTAGCACCATCATTT
Collagen III	TATCGAACACGCAAGGCTGTGAGA	GGCCAACGTCCACACCAAATTCTT
CTGF	AGACCTGTGCCTGCCATTA	TGTCTCCGTACATCTTCCTG
HGF	TGCTCCCAAAATTCCAAAC	GCCATTCCCACGATAACAA
FN	AATGCGTTGGTTTGTACTTGTTATG	CTTCAGCTTCAGGTTTACTCTC
MMP-1	TTTGCCGACAGAGATGAAG	AGCCAAAGGAGCTGTAGATG
TIMP-1	CTGTTCCCACTCCCATCTTT	CTGCTGGGTGGTAACTCTT
SMAD2	TGTCGTCCATCTTGCCATT	CCATCCCAGCAGTCTCTT
SMAD7	CTGCTGTGCAAAGTGTTC	CAGAGTCGGCTAAGGTGAT
α-SMA	TTGAGAAGAGTTACGAGTTG	GGACATTGTTAGCATAGAGG
Lysine hydroxylases	GCTGTTGACTTCCCATTGCT	TCTGATCCAGGTGTCTTTACCC
Prolyo hydroxylase	ACAGGCGGATTGGAAGAGCG	CCCATCCCAAAGCAGTCATCC
GAPDH	CGACCACTTTGTCAAGCTCA	AGGGGTCTACATGGCAACTG

4.9 Statistical analysis

The data were expressed as the mean ± SEM. Statistical significance was determined with the student's t-test when there were two experimental groups. For more than two groups, statistical evaluation of the data was performed using one-way analysis of variance (ANOVA), followed by Dunnett's post-hoc test, with values of $P<0.05$ considered significant.

References

[1] Grieb G, Steffens G, Pallua N, et al. Circulating fibrocytes-biology and mechanisms in wound healing and scar formation[A]. In: *International Review Of Cell And Molecular Biology, Vol 291* (Jeon KW, ed), Vol. 291, 2011: 1-19.

[2] Wang W, Lin S, Xiao Y, et al. Acceleration of diabetic wound healing with chitosan-crosslinked collagen sponge containing recombinant human acidic fibroblast growth factor in healing-impaired STZ diabetic rats[J]. Life Sciences, 2008, 82(3-4): 190-204.

[3] Xiao J, Lv Y, Lin S, et al. Cardiac protection by basic fibroblast growth factor from ischemia/reperfusion-induced injury in diabetic rats[J]. Biological & Pharmaceutical Bulletin, 2010, 33(3): 444-449.

[4] Beenken A, Mohammadi M. The FGF family: biology, pathophysiology and therapy[J]. Nature Reviews Drug Discovery, 2009, 8(3): 235-253.

[5] Barrientos S, Stojadinovic O, Golinko MS, et al. Growth factors and cytokines in wound healing[J]. Wound Repair And Regeneration, 2008, 16(5): 585-601.

[6] Akita S, Akino K, Imaizumi T, et al. Basic fibroblast growth factor accelerates and improves second-degree burn wound healing[J]. Wound Repair And Regeneration, 2008, 16(5): 635-641.

[7] Fu XB, Shen ZY, Chen YL, et al. Randomised placebo-controlled trial of use of topical recombinant bovine basic fibroblast growth factor for second-degree burns[J]. Lancet, 1998, 352(9141): 1661-1664.

[8] Tan Y, Xiao J, Huang Z, et al. Comparison of the therapeutic effects recombinant human acidic and basic fibroblast growth factors in wound healing in diabetic patients[J]. Journal Of Health Science, 2008, 54(4): 432-440.

[9] Xiang Q, Xiao J, Zhang H, et al. Preparation and characterisation of bFGF-encapsulated liposomes and evaluation of wound-healing activities in the rat[J]. Burns, 2011, 37(5): 886-895.

[10] Ortega S, Ittmann M, Tsang SH, et al. Neuronal defects and delayed wound healing in mice lacking fibroblast growth factor 2[J]. Procccdings Of the National Academy Of Sciences Of the United States Of America, 1998, 95(10): 5672-5677.

[11] Xie JL, Bian HN, Qi SH, et al. Basic fibroblast growth factor (bFGF) alleviates the scar of the rabbit ear model in wound healing[J]. Wound Repair And Regeneration, 2008, 16(4): 576-581.

[12] Eto H, Suga H, Aoi N, et al. Therapeutic potential of fibroblast growth factor-2 for hypertrophic scars: upregulation of MMP-1 and HGF expression[J]. Laboratory Investigation, 2012, 92(2): 214-223.

[13] Ono I, Akasaka Y, Kikuchi R, et al. Basic fibroblast growth factor reduces scar formation in acute incisional wounds[J]. Wound Repair And Regeneration, 2007, 15(5): 617-623.

[14] Sidgwick GP, Bayat A. Extracellular matrix molecules implicated in hypertrophic and keloid scarring[J]. Journal Of the European Academy Of Dermatology And Venereology, 2012, 26(2): 141-152.

[15] Oliveira GV, Hawkins HK, Chinkes D, et al. Hypertrophic *versus* non hypertrophic scars compared by immunohistochemistry and laser confocal microscopy: type I and III collagens[J]. International Wound Journal, 2009, 6(6): 445-452.

[16] Honardoust D, Ding J, Varkey M, et al. Deep dermal fibroblasts refractory to migration and decorin-induced apoptosis contribute to hypertrophic scarring[J]. Journal Of Burn Care & Research, 2012, 33(5): 668-677.

[17] Colwell AS, Phan TT, Kong W, et al. Hypertrophic scar fibroblasts have increased connective tissue growth factor expression after transforming growth factor-beta stimulation[J]. Plastic And Reconstructive Surgery, 2005, 116(5): 1387-1390.

[18] Chalmers RL. The evidence for the role of transforming growth factor-beta in the formation of abnormal scarring[J]. Int Wound J, 2011, 8(3): 218-223.

[19] Kryger ZB, Roy NK, Lu L, et al. Temporal expression of the transforming growth factor-beta pathway on the rabbit ear model of wound healing and scarring[J]. Journal Of the American College Of Surgeons, 2007, 205(1): 78-88.

[20] Bloemen MCT, van der Veer WM, Ulrich MMW, et al. Prevention and curative management of hypertrophic scar formation[J]. Burns, 2009, 35(4): 463-475.

[21] Aarabi S, Longaker MT, Gurtner GC. Hypertrophic scar formation following burns and trauma: New approaches to treatment[J]. Plos Medicine, 2007, 4(9): 1464-1470.

[22] Niessen FB, Spauwen PHM, Robinson PH, et al. The use of silicone occlusive sheeting (Sil-K) and silicone occlusive gel (epiderm) in the prevention of hypertrophic scar formation[J]. Plastic And Reconstructive Surgery, 1998, 102(6): 1962-1972.

[23] Ward RS. Pressure Therapy for the control of hypertrophic scar formation after burn injury[J]. Journal of Burn Care and Rehabilitation, 1991, 12(3): 257-262.

[24] van der Veer WM, Ferreira JA, de Jong EH, et al. Perioperative conditions affect long-term hypertrophic scar formation[J]. Annals Of Plastic Surgery, 2010, 65(3): 321-325.

[25] Funato N, Moriyama K, Shimokawa H, et al. Basic fibroblast growth factor induces apoptosis in myofibroblastic cells isolated from rat palatal mucosa[J]. Biochemical And Biophysical Research Communications, 1997, 240(1): 21-26.

[26] Spyrou GE, Naylor IL. The effect of basic fibroblast growth factor on scarring[J]. British Journal Of Plastic Surgery, 2002, 55(4): 275-282.

[27] Verhaegen PD, van Marle J, Kuehne A, et al. Collagen bundle morphometry in skin and scar tissue: a novel distance mapping method provides superior measurements compared to Fourier analysis[J]. Journal Of Microscopy, 2012, 245(1): 82-89.

[28] Verhaegen PD, Schouten HJ, Tigchelaar-Gutter W, et al. Adaptation of the dermal collagen structure of human skin and scar tissue in response to stretch: An experimental study[J]. Wound Repair And Regeneration, 2012, 20(5): 658-666.

[29] Imaizumi R, Akasaka Y, Inomata N, et al. Promoted activation of matrix metalloproteinase (MMP)-2 in keloid fibroblasts and increased expression of MMP-2 in collagen bundle regions: implications for mechanisms of keloid progression[J]. Histopathology, 2009, 54(6): 722-730.

[30] Shi F, Sottile J. MT1-MMP regulates the turnover and endocytosis of extracellular matrix fibronectin[J]. Journal Of Cell Science, 2011, 124(23): 4039-4050.

[31] Singh P, Reimer CL, Peters JH, et al. The spatial and temporal expression patterns of integrin alpha 9 beta 1 and one of its ligands, the EIIIA segment of fibronectin, in cutaneous wound healing[J]. Journal Of Investigative Dermatology, 2004, 123(6): 1176-1181.

[32] Martino MM, Tortelli F, Mochizuki M, et al. Engineering the growth factor microenvironment with fibronectin domains to promote wound and bone tissue healing[J]. Sci Transl Med, 2011, 3(100): 100ra189.

[33] Haines P, Samuel GH, Cohen H, et al. Caveolin-1 is a negative regulator of MMP-1 gene expression in human dermal fibroblasts *via* inhibition of Erk1/2/Ets1 signaling pathway[J]. Journal Of Dermatological Science, 2011, 64(3): 210-216.

[34] Nedelec B, Shankowsky H, Scott PG, et al. Myofibroblasts and apoptosis in human hypertrophic scars: The effect of interferon-

alpha 2b[J]. Surgery, 2001, 130(5): 798-808.

[35] El Kahi CG, Atiyeh BS, Hussein IAH, *et al.* Modulation of wound contracture alpha-smooth muscle actin and multispecific vitronectin receptor integrin alpha v beta 3 in the rabbit's experimental model[J]. International Wound Journal, 2009, 6(3): 214-224.

[36] Satish L, Gallo PH, Baratz ME, *et al.* Reversal of TGF-beta(1) stimulation of alpha-smooth muscle actin and extracellular matrix components by cyclic AMP in Dupuytren's - derived fibroblasts[J]. Bmc Musculoskeletal Disorders, 2011, 12.

[37] Dabiri G, Campaner A, Morgan JR, *et al.* A TGF-β1-dependent autocrine loop regulates the structure of focal adhesions in hypertrophic scar fibroblasts[J]. Journal Of Investigative Dermatology, 2006, 126(5): 963-970.

[38] Zhang HY, Zhang X, Wang ZG, *et al.* Exogenous basic fibroblast growth factor inhibits ER stress-induced apoptosis and improves recovery from spinal cord injury[J]. CNS Neurosci Ther, 2013, 19(1): 20-29.

Exogenous basic fibroblast growth factor inhibits ER Stress-induced apoptosis and improves recovery from spinal cord injury

Hongyu Zhang, Xiaokun Li, Jian Xiao

1. Introduction

Spinal cord injury (SCI) is a severe health problem that usually causes lifelong disability for a patient. The pathology of SCI is divided into two phases: the primary injury is the mechanical impact afflicted directly on the spine, and the secondary injury is a complex cascade of molecular events including disturbances in ionic homeostasis, local edema, ischemia, focal hemorrhage, free radical stress, and inflammatory response [1]. Studies have shown that apoptosis plays a key role in secondary damage in animal models and human tissue by causing progressive degeneration of the spinal cord [2,3]. Although the exact molecular pathway of this secondary injury is still controversial, therapeutic strategies that inhibit or delay apoptosis and cell death may contribute to SCI recovery.

The endoplasmic reticulum (ER) is an important intracellular organelle that is responsible for proper protein folding [4]. Various exogenous stressors, including glucose deprivation [5], depletion of ER Ca^{2+} stores [6], exposure to free radicals [7], and accumulation of unfolded or misfolded proteins [8], disrupt the proper function of the ER and trigger the unfolded protein response (UPR), which plays an important role in regulating cell growth, differentiation and apoptosis to cope with this adverse situation. ER stress-induced apoptosis is related to the activation of the glucose-regulated protein 78 (GRP78), the transcription activation of the C/ EBP homologous transcription factor (CHOP), and the activation of ER-associated caspase-12 [9]. During SCI, prolonged ER stress without successful cellular protective mechanisms by the UPR eventually results in neural apoptosis [10,11]. It has been proven that ER stress is involved in cell apoptosis after SCI, especially in neurons and oligodendrocytes but not astrocytes [1]. The latest study indicated that deletion of pro-apoptotic CHOP did not result in improvement of locomotor function after severe contusive spinal cord injury [12]. The role of ER stress-induced apoptosis and related proteins in spinal cord injuries needs further investigation.

As an extensively expressed protein family, fibroblast growth factor can share receptors and affect a variety of biological functions, including proliferation, morphogenesis, and suppression of apoptosis during development *via* a more complex signal transduction system [13–15]. Basic fibroblast growth factor (bFGF), also named FGF2, is highly expressed in the nervous system and has multiple roles. bFGF is a differentiation factor in the hippocampus and has neurotrophic activities, such as supporting the survival and growth of cultured neurons and neural stem cells [16,17]. In neural stem/progenitor cell transplant treatment after spinal cord injury in rats, bFGF transient infusion or transgene can promote axon regeneration and functional recovery [18,19]. Several growth factors, such as nerve growth factor (NGF) and brain-derived neurotrophic factor (BDNF), show neuroprotective effects and improve SCI recovery [20,21]. However, the molecular mechanism of bFGF treatment in SCI recovery is still undefined. In this study, we investigated the mechanism of ER stress-induced apoptosis as well as the protective action of bFGF both *in vivo* and *in vitro*.

2. Materials and methods

2.1 Cell culture and viability assay

PC12 cells were purchased from the Cell Storage Center of Wuhan University. Cells were cultured in DMEM, incubated in a humidified atmosphere containing 5% CO_2 at 37℃, and supplemented with heat-inactivated 10% fetal bovine serum and 5% horse serum. PC12 cells were seeded on 96-well plates and treated with different doses of the ER stress activator, thapsigargin (TG) for 12 h. Based on our previous study, cells were also pretreated with recombinant bFGF (40 ng/ml) for 2 h [22]. Cell viability was assessed using the MTT assay. To further evaluate the effect of PI3K/Akt and ERK1/2 activation on oxidative injury, cells were pretreated for 2 h with specific inhibitors, LY294002 (20 μM) and U0126 (20 μM), before the addition of bFGF, as previously described [22,23]. All experiments were performed in triplicate.

2.2 Procedure of the animal model of spinal cord injury

Young adult female Sprague-Dawley rats (220–250 g) were purchased from the Animal Center of the Chinese Academy of Sciences. The animal use and care protocol conformed to the Guide for the Care and Use of Laboratory Animals from the National Institutes of Health and was approved by the Animal Care and Use Committee of Wenzhou Medical College. All animals were housed in standard conditions of temperature and 12-h light/dark cycle and fed with food and water. Rats were positioned on a cork platform after being anesthetized with 10% chloralic hydras (3.5 ml/kg, i.p.). For each rat, the skin was incised along the midline of the back, and the vertebral column was exposed. A laminectomy was performed at the T9 level. The exposed spinal cord was subjected to crushed injury compressing with a vascular clip (15 g forces, Oscar, China). Sham groups received the same surgical procedure but sustained no impact injury. Their spinal cords were exposed for 1 min. Postoperative care involved manually emptying the urinary bladder twice a day (until the return of bladder function) and administration of cefazolin sodium (50 mg/kg, i.p.). Recombinant human bFGF was purchased from Sigma (Sigma-Aldrich, St. Louis, MO, USA). Following the spinal cord occlusion, the bFGF solution was injected subcutaneously near the back wound at a dose of 80 μg/kg/day until the animal was executed.

2.3 Locomotion recovery assessment

Two blind independent examiners scored the locomotion recovery in an open field, according to the Basso, Beattie and Bresnahan (BBB) scale during the 7-day postoperative period. Briefly, the BBB locomotion rating scale ranges from 0 points (complete paralysis) to 21 points (normal locomotion). The scale is based upon the natural progression of locomotion recovery in rats with thoracic spinal cord injuries.

2.4 Hematoxylin–eosin staining and immunohistochemistry

The rats were deeply anesthetized with 10% chloralic hydras and perfused transcardially with saline and buffered 4% para-formaldehyde at 1, 3 and 7 days. The spinal cords T7–T10 around the lesion epicenter were excised, the transverse paraffin sections were mounted in Poly-L-Lysine-coated slides for histopathological examination by Hematoxylin-eosin (HE) staining. The transverse paraffin sections were also incubated in 3% H_2O_2 and 80% carbinol for 30 min and then in blocking solution for 1 h at room temperature. Subsequently, the sections were incubated at 4℃ overnight with the following primary antibodies:CHOP (1:150), GRP78 (1:200), and caspase-12 (1:600, Santa Cruz Biotech, Santa Cruz, CA, USA). After triple washing in PBS, the sections were incubated with horseradish peroxidase-conjugated secondary antibodies for 2 h at 37℃. The reaction was stopped with 3, 3′-diaminobenzidine (DAB). The results were imaged at a magnification of 400 using a Nikon ECLPSE 80i (Nikon, Tokyo, Japan). The optical densities and positive neuron numbers of CHOP, GRP78 and caspase-12 were counted at 5 randomly selected fields per sample.

2.5 Western blot analysis

Total proteins were purified using protein extraction reagents for the spinal cord segment and PC12 cells. The equivalent of 50 μg of protein was separated by 11.5% gel and then transferred onto a PVDF membrane. After blocking with 5% fat-free milk, the membranes were incubated with the following antibodies:CHOP (1:500), GRP78 (1:200), and caspase-12 (1:600) overnight. The membranes were washed with TBS and treated with horseradish peroxidase-conjugated secondary antibodies for 2 h at room temperature. The signals were visualized with the ChemiDicTM XRS+Imaging System (Bio-Rad Laboratories, Hercules, CA, USA), and the band densities were quantified with Multi Gauge Software of Science Lab 2006 (FUJIFILM Corporation, Tokyo, Japan).

2.6 Apoptosis assay

DNA fragmentation *in vivo* was detected by the one step TUNEL Apoptosis Assay KIT (Roche, Mannheim, Germany). The images were captured with a Nikon ECLIPSE Ti microscope (Nikon, Japan). The apoptotic rates of the PC12 cells treated with TG and bFGF were measured using a PI/Annexin V-FITC kit (Invitrogen, Carlsbad, CA, USA) and then analyzed by a FACScan flow cytometer (Becton Dickinson, Franklin Lakes, NJ, USA) as the manual description.

2.7 Immunofluorescence staining

The sections were incubated with 10% normal donkey serum for 1 h at room temperature in PBS. They were then incubated with the appropriate primary antibodies overnight at 4 ℃ in the same buffer. The nuclei were stained with Hoechst 33258 (0.25 μg/ml) dye. For neurons and GAP43 detection, the following primary antibodies were used based on different targets: anti-NeuN (1:500, Millipore), anti-GAP43 (1:50), and antistathmin (1:50). After primary antibody incubation, the sections were washed and then incubated for 1 h with secondary antibody (1:500). All images were captured on Nikon ECLIPSE Ti microscope.

2.8 Statistical analysis

The data were expressed as the mean ± SEM. Statistical significance was determined with Student's t-test when there were two experimental groups. For more than two groups, statistical evaluation of the data was performed using the one-way analysis of variance (ANOVA) test, followed by Dunnett's $post\ hoc$ test with values of $P < 0.05$ considered significant.

3. Results

3.1 ER stress–induced apoptosis is involved in the early stages of SCI

To evaluate the role of ER stress in SCI, we performed the animal model as described previously (Fig. 1A). Animals subjected to spinal cord contusions showed dramatic and bilateral hindlimb paralysis with no movement at all or only slight movements of a joint from the first 1-h postinjury. At 1 day after injury, the BBB scale score of the SCI group was 2.33 ± 0.67, which corresponds to slight and/or extensive movement of two or three joints. The locomotor scores increased progressively during the experimental period. At 3 and 7 days after contusion, the BBB scores were 3.67 ± 0.88 ($P < 0.05$) and 8.00 ± 0.58 ($P < 0.001$), which corresponds to occasional plantar step placement with weight support (Fig. 1B). Compared with the sham operation group (1-d post-trauma), the gray matter of the SCI group exhibited large hemorrhages, which were most pronounced in the central and dorsal horn of the lesioned spinal cords. Progressive destruction of the dorsal white matter and central gray matter tissue was found 3-day postinjury. The lesion segments displayed hemorrhagic necrosis, neuron loss, karyopyknosis, and infiltrated polymorpho-nuclear leukocytes and macrophages. In the segments collected at 7-day postinjury, there was minimal hemorrhaging and some neuron regeneration, but demyelination appeared as well as numerous cavities (Fig. 1C). The cell apoptosis in the spinal lesions were detected by TUNEL staining; the bright green dots were deemed apoptosis-positive cells in the lesions. There is no apoptosis-positive cell in the sham group. The numbers of TUNEL-positive cells increased significantly 1 day after injury and were maximal at 3 days (Fig. 1D,E).

Immunohistochemistry staining was used to investigate the molecular mechanism of ER stress–induced apoptosis in SCI. We found that GRP78, CHOP, caspase-12-positive cells were expressed in both gray matter and white matter, and the staining was more intense in the gray matter than white matter (Fig. 2A). The numbers of CHOP, GRP78, caspase-12-positive gray and white matter cells and the optical densities increased significantly; all were maximal at 3 days. After this time, the numbers of positive cells and optical densities gradually decreased but were still observed 7 days after the contusions (Fig. 2B,C). The protein expressions of GRP78, CHOP, caspase-12 were also determined by Western blot analysis. The levels of GRP78, CHOP, caspase-12 increased 1 day after injury. The maximal induction of all proteins occurred at 3 days and decreased later, 7 days after contusion (Fig. 2D,E), which is consistent with the results of immunohistochemistry staining.

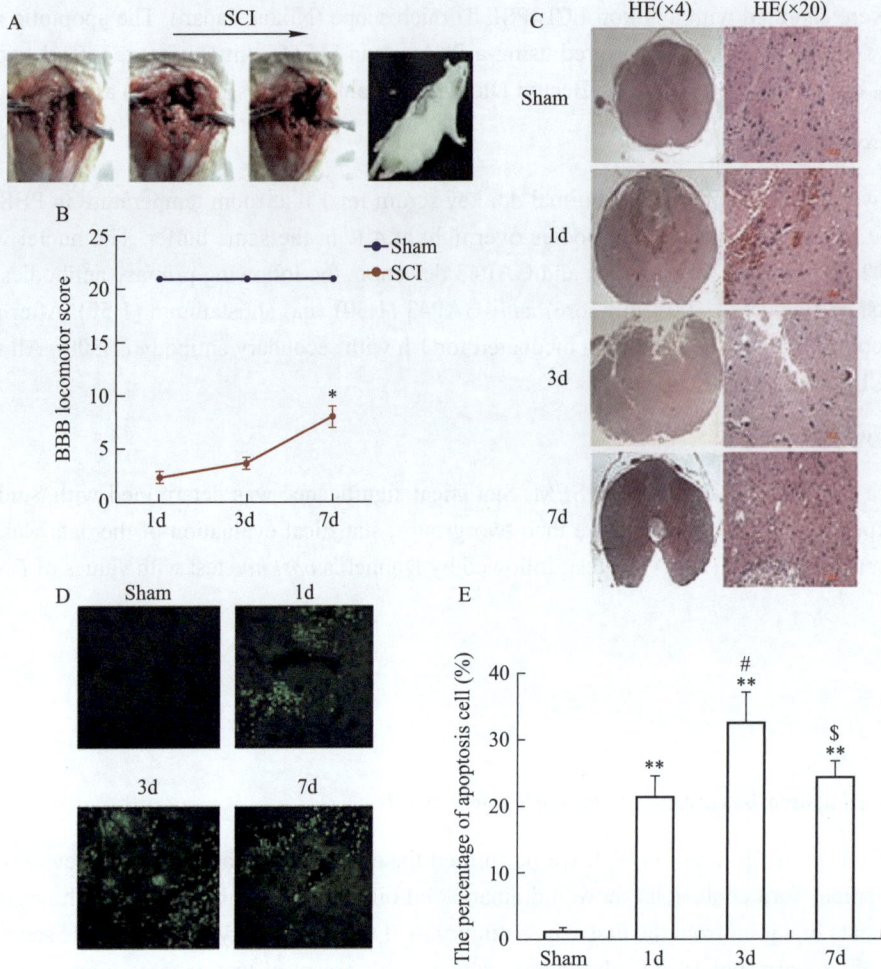

Fig. 1. The procedure and assessment of spinal cord injury (SCI) model rat. (A) The procedure of the SCI model from left to right, as shown by arrow head. (B) The Basso, Beattie and Bresnahan (BBB) scores of SCI model rat at 1, 3 and 7 days after contusion. The score of the sham group was 21 points (meaning normal locomotion). *represents $P < 0.05$ vs. the sham group. Data are the mean values ± SEM, $n = 6$. One-way ANOVA with Dunnett's *post hoc* test was performed for statistical evaluation. (C) H and E staining results of SCI rat at 1, 3 and 7 days after contusion. (D) TUNEL apoptosis assay of model rat spinal cord lesions. Immunofluorescence results of the TUNEL assay. Bright green dots were deemed positive apoptosis cell, magnification was 20× (E) The analysis of apoptosis cell 1, 3 and 7 days after spinal cord injury lesions. The percentage of apoptosis was counted from 3 random 1×1 mm² areas. **represents $P < 0.01$ vs. the sham group, #represents $P < 0.05$ vs. the 1 day group, and $represents $P < 0.05$ vs. the 3 days group. Data are the mean values ± SEM, $n = 6$.

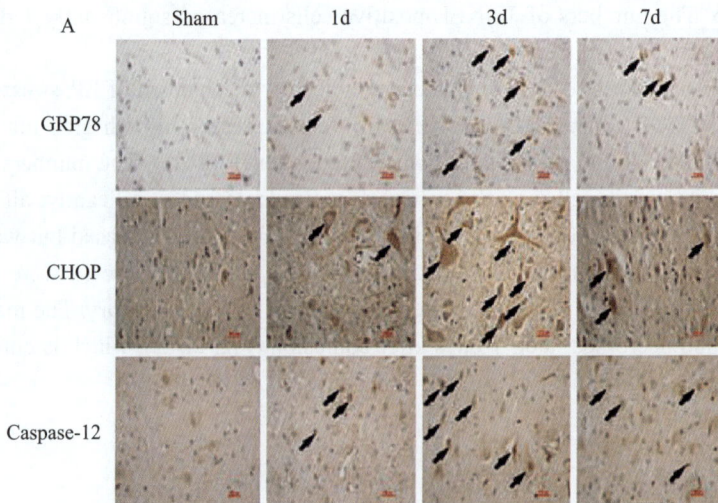

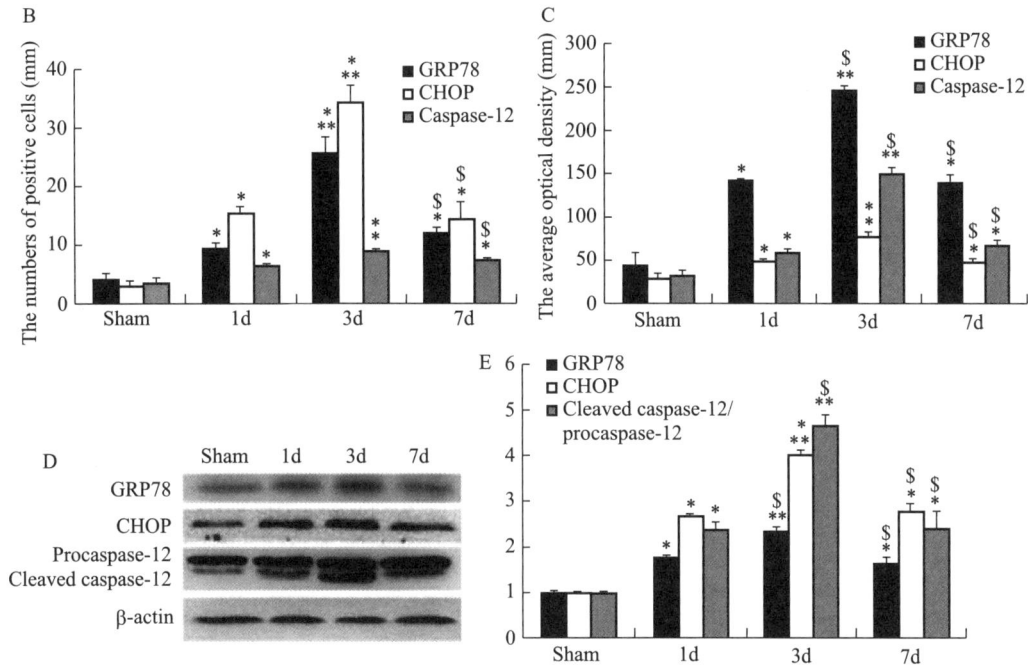

Fig. 2. ER stress–induced apoptosis was involved in the early stage of spinal cord injury (SCI). (A) Immunohistochemistry for GRP78, CHOP and caspase-12 in sham, 1, 3 and 7 days after spinal cord injury lesions groups (B) Analysis of the positive cells and optical density (C) of the immunohistochemistry results. *represents $P < 0.05$ vs. the sham group, **represents $P < 0.01$ vs. the sham group, #represents $P < 0.05$ versus the 1 day group, and $represents $P < 0.05$ vs. the 3 days group. Data are the mean values ± SEM, $n = 6$. (D) Protein expressions of GRP78, CHOP and caspase-12 in the spinal cord segment at the contusion epicenter. β-actin was used as the loading control and for band density normalization. (E) The optical density analyses of GRP78, CHOP, and caspase-12 protein. *represents $P < 0.05$ vs. the sham group, **represents $P < 0.01$ vs. the sham group, #represents $P < 0.05$ vs. the 1 day group, and $represents $P < 0.05$ vs. the 3 days group. Data are the mean values ± SEM, $n = 6$.

3.2 bFGF increased the survival of neurons and improved SCI recovery

Model rat were treated with bFGF injections close to the wound areas to evaluate the therapeutic effect of bFGF on SCI. The sham group showed normal BBB scores. At 1 day after contusion, there was no significant difference in the BBB scores between SCI model and bFGF treatment groups. However, the BBB scores of the bFGF treatment group increased 3 days after contusion, indicating that the locomotor activity was recovered compared with the SCI group. At 7 days after contusion, the BBB scores of the bFGF treatment group increased to 14.3 ± 1.76, which is markedly increased compared with the SCI group ($P < 0.05$, Fig. 3A). Progressive destruction of the dorsal white matter and central gray matter tissue was found in the 7 days SCI group compared with the sham operation group. Compared with the SCI group, the bFGF treatment group showed significant protective effects, such as less necrosis and karyopyknosis and fewer infiltrated polymorphonuclear leukocytes and macrophages (Fig. 3B).

To further confirm the protective effect of bFGF, we investigated the survival of neurons directly by immunofluorescence staining. Spinal cord neurons in both white and gray matter tissue were marked by the neuronal marker, NeuN. The number of positively stained cells decreased significantly 7 days after SCI and increased in the bFGF treatment group (Fig. 3B,C). Our data indicated that bFGF administration has a protective effect and significantly improves the SCI recovery.

3.3 bFGF-inhibited ER stress–induced apoptosis and up-regulated the neuroprotective factors

The protein expressions of ER stress–induced apoptosis were detected by immunohistochemistry staining and Western blot. The ER stress-induced apoptosis protein (CHOP, GRP78 and caspase-12) positive cells and optical density gradually decreased with bFGF administration 7 days after contusion (Fig. 4A,B). We found the levels of the CHOP, GRP78 and caspase-12 proteins decreased after bFGF treatment as compared with the SCI group, 7 days after contusion (Fig. 4C,D).

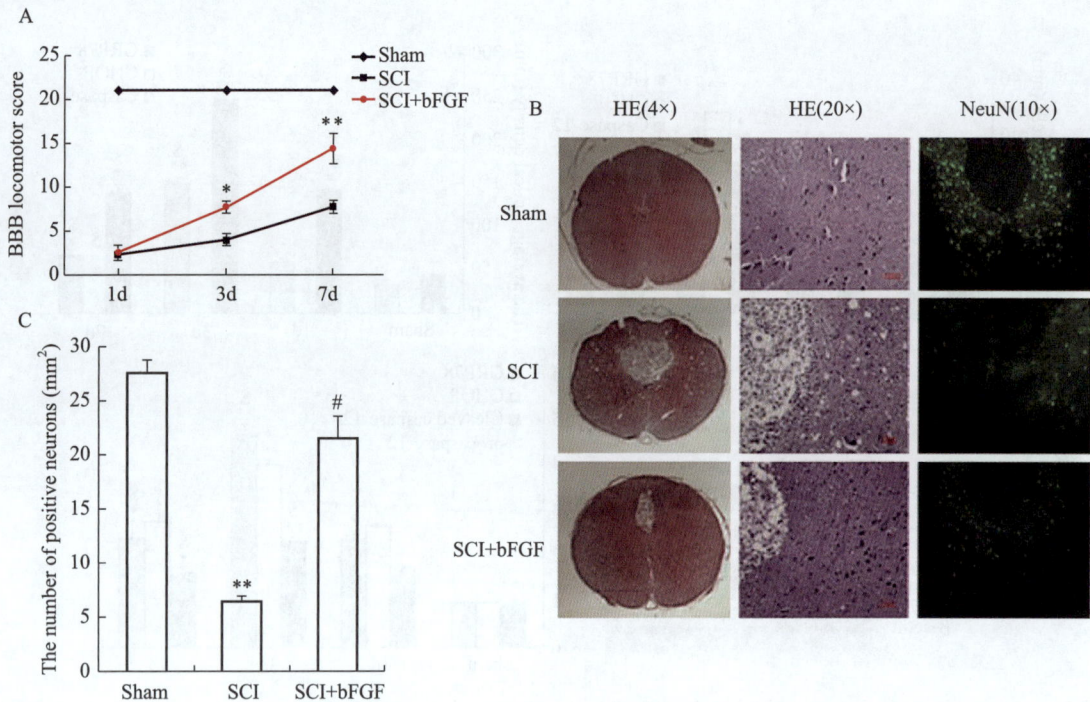

Fig. 3. Basic fibroblast growth factor (bFGF) improves the recovery of spinal cord injury (SCI) rat and the survival of neurons. (A) The Basso, Beattie and Bresnahan (BBB) scores of sham, SCI group and SCI rat treated with bFGF group. *represents $P < 0.05$ vs. the SCI group, and **represents $P < 0.01$ vs. the SCI group, $n = 6$. (B) H and E staining and NeuN staining results of the sham, SCI group and SCI rat treated with bFGF group. The bright green dots in the right column are positive staining neurons. (C) Analysis of the positive neurons of the NeuN staining results. **represents $P < 0.01$ vs. the sham group, and #represents $P < 0.05$ vs. the SCI group, $n = 6$.

GAP43 is expressed in developing and regenerating neurons, and this protein is often used to score the condition of neural regeneration. We found that the positive red fluorescence signal in the cytoplasm was enhanced in the bFGF administration group but not in the SCI group 7 days after contusion (Fig. 5A). Western blot analysis of the GAP43 protein also demonstrated that the expression of GAP43 was greater in the bFGF treatment group than the SCI group 7 days after contusion (Fig. 5B,C). This result was consistent with the results of the immunofluorescence staining analysis.

3.4 The protective role of bFGF was related to the activation of PI3K/Akt and ERK1/2

The PI3K/Akt and ERK1/2 pathways are the main downstream signals that are activated by bFGF. These two pathways are related to the cell survival, differentiation and migration [24,25]. We determined that the protective effect of bFGF in SCI recovery was partially through the activation of these two signal pathways. Western blot analysis demonstrated decreases in the expressions of the phosphorylations of Akt, ERK1/2 and GSK-3β (downstream of Akt signal) after SCI contusion. The phosphorylation decreases were reversed in the bFGF treatment group at 7 days (Fig. 6A, B). These data indicated that both the PI3K/Akt and ERK1/2 signals were involved in the role of bFGF in SCI recovery.

To further confirm the role of bFGF in ER stress-induced apoptosis in vitro, we used TG-treated PC12 cells (TG is an ER stress activator) to replicate the apoptosis model [26,27]. Cell viability decreased as TG concentration increased, while bFGF combination partially increased cell viability compared with that of the TG group (Fig. 6C,D). Cell apoptosis rate was analyzed by flow cytometer, and the results showed that bFGF-inhibited apoptosis induced by TG in PC12 cells, compared with the TG group (Fig. 6E,F). These data indicated that bFGF also had a protective effect in the cell death model.

To demonstrate the molecular mechanism of bFGF in the ER stress-induced cell apoptosis model, two classic signal inhibitors, LY294002 for PI3K/Akt and U0126 for ERK1/2 were added into the cell stress model. Both of these inhibitors have no effect on cell death when used [22,28]. The activation of CHOP by TG treatment was inhibited by bFGF addition, but the protective effect of bFGF was abolished by LY294002 and U0126. The expression of CHOP increased significantly with the combination of inhibitors, compared with the bFGF treatment group. The levels of p-Akt, p-ERK1/2

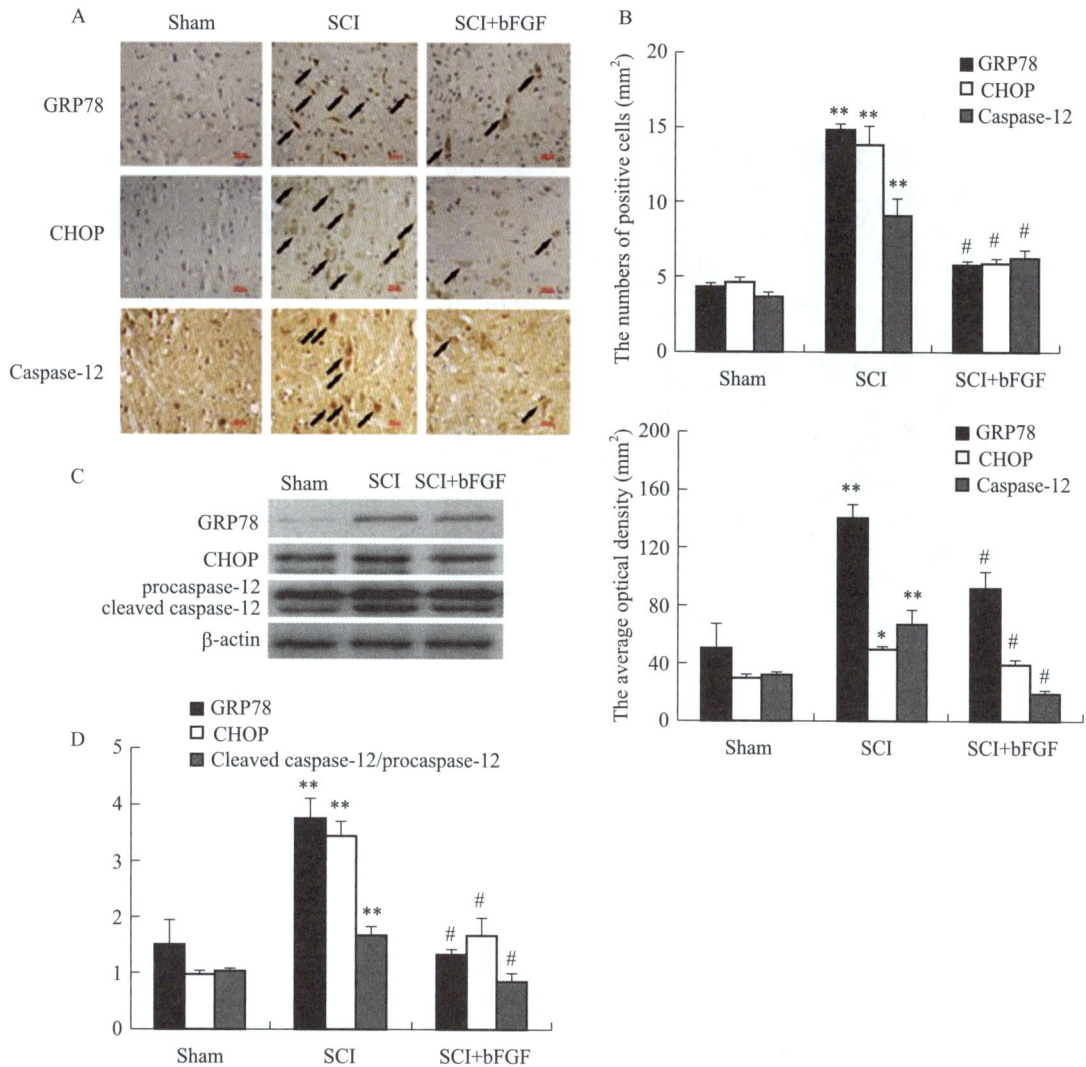

Fig. 4. Basic fibroblast growth factor (bFGF) administration inhibits the expressions of ER stress–induced apoptosis response proteins, GRP78, CHOP and caspase-12. Immunohistochemistry for GRP78, CHOP and caspase-12 in the sham, 7 days after spinal cord injury lesion and bFGF treatment 7 days after injury groups (A) Analysis of the positive cells and optical density (B) of the immunohistochemistry results. *Represents P < 0.05 *vs.* the sham group, **represents P < 0.01 *vs.* the sham group, #represents P < 0.05 *vs.* the spinal cord injury (SCI) group, Data are the mean values ± SEM, n = 6. (C) Protein expressions of GRP78, CHOP and caspase-12 for the sham, SCI and bFGF treatment groups. β-actin was used as the loading control and for band density normalization. (D) The optical density analysis of GRP78, CHOP, and caspase-12 protein. **represents P < 0.01 *vs.* the sham group, #represents P < 0.05 *vs.* the 1 day group. Data are the mean values ± SEM, n = 6.

and p-GSK-3β increased with bFGF treatment and decreased with the addition of the inhibitors (Fig. 6G,H). All of these data demonstrated that the protective role of bFGF in ER stress-induced apoptosis is related to the activation of downstream signals, PI3K/Akt and ERK1/2, both *in vitro* and *in vivo*.

4. Discussion

Spinal cord crushed injuries have devastating consequences of lifelong disability and significant economic costs. Vertebral impact injury is clinically common, and this type of injury may be caused by traffic accidents, sports injuries or tumors in spinal cords. After a spinal cord crushed injury, the initial traumatic injury to spinal cord tissues is followed by a long period of secondary damages, including oxidative stress, inflammation, necrosis and apoptosis [29,30]. The loss of neuronal cells is the main factor that interferes with recovery from the secondary damage. Many therapeutic interventions using neurotrophic factors have been established to promote functional SCI recovery, such as NGF, BDNF and glial cell line-derived neurotrophic factor (GDNF) [31,32]. In the present study, we treated SCI rat with bFGF and demon-

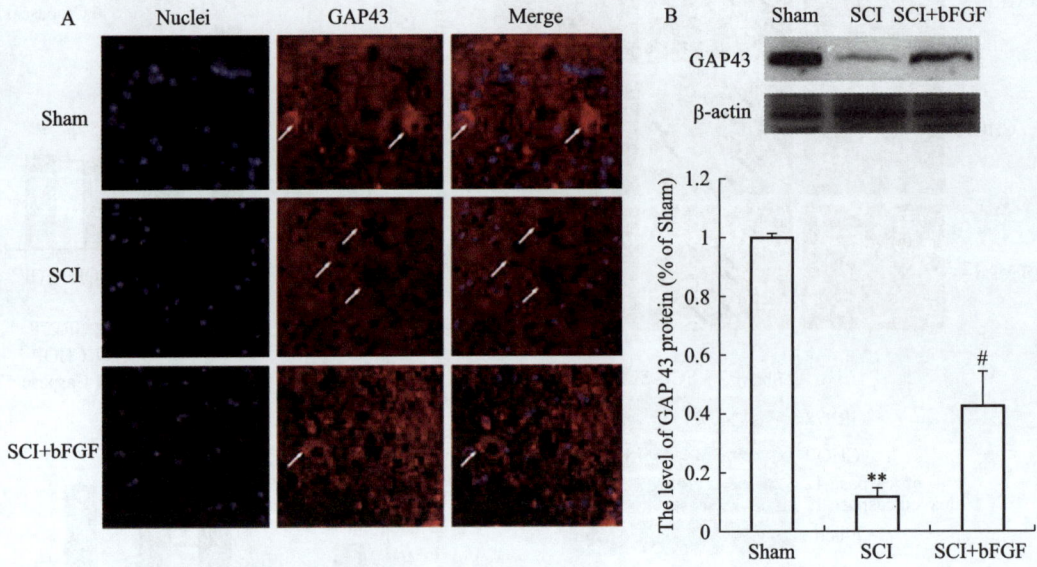

Fig. 5. Basic fibroblast growth factor (bFGF) administration increases the level of GAP43 in spinal cord lesions. (A) Immunofluorescence staining results of GAP43; the nuclear is labeled by Hoechst (blue), the neurons with obvious GAP43 signals are labeled with white arrow heads, magnification was 20×. (B) The protein expressions of GAP43 in the sham, spinal cord injury (SCI) rat and SCI rat treated with bFGF groups. (C) The optical density analysis of GAP43 protein. **represents $P < 0.01$ vs. the sham group, and #represents $P < 0.05$ vs. the SCI group. Data are the mean values ± SEM, $n = 6$.

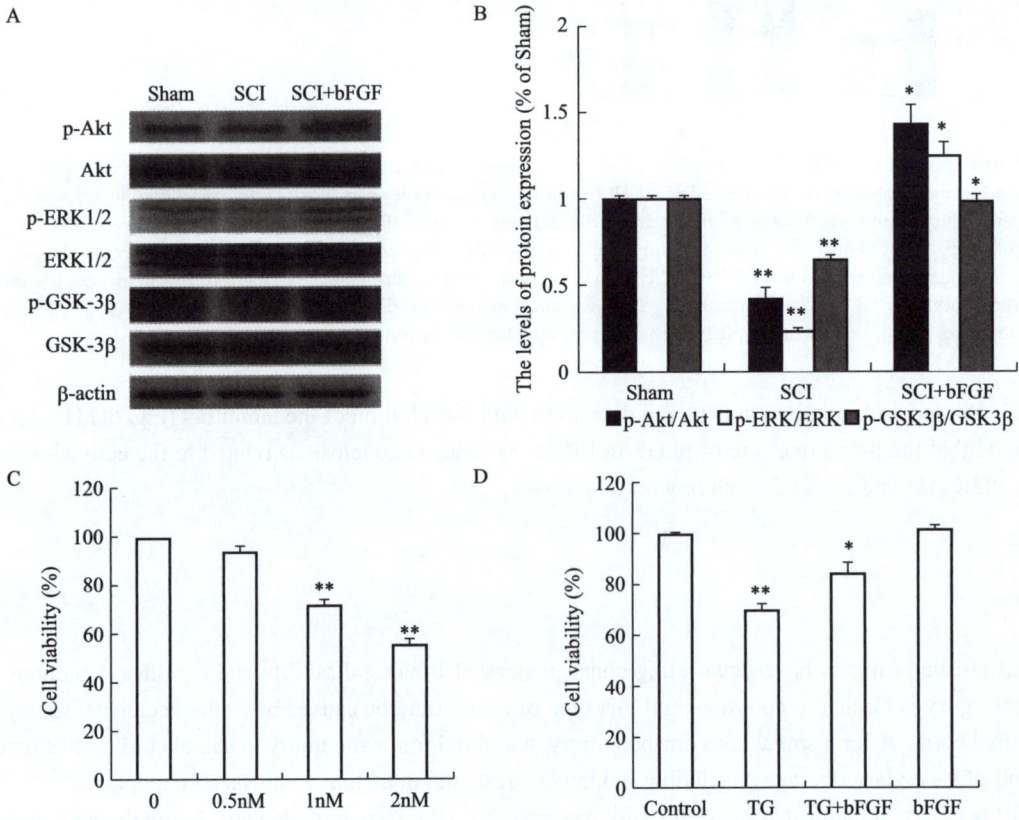

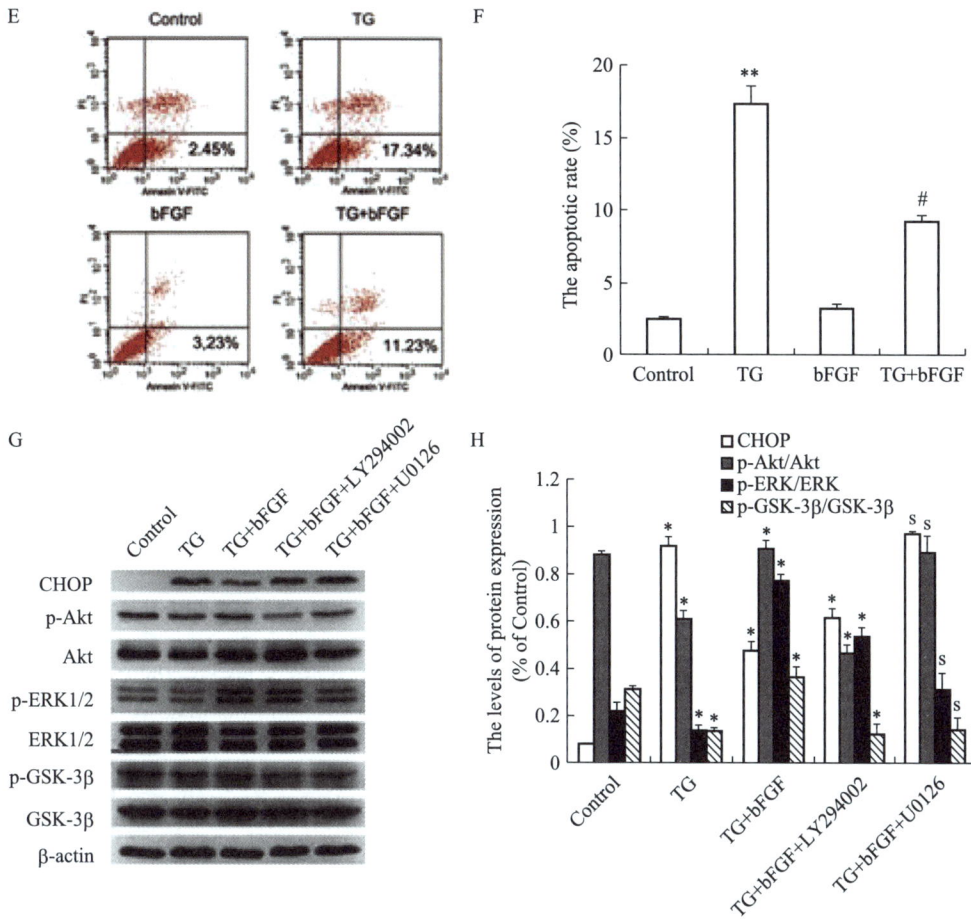

Fig. 6. PI3K/Akt/GSK-3β and ERK1/2 signal pathways are involved in the protective effect of basic fibroblast growth factor (bFGF) both in the spinal cord of spinal cord injury (SCI) rat and PC12 cells under stress. (A) The protein expressions of p-Akt/Akt, p-ERK/ERK, p-GSK-3β/GSK-3β in the sham, SCI model and SCI rat treated with bFGF groups. (B) The optical density analysis of p-Akt/Akt, p-ERK/ERK, p-GSK-3β/GSK-3β protein. **represents $P < 0.01$ vs. the sham group, and #represents $P < 0.05$ vs. the SCI group. Data are the mean values ± SEM, $n = 6$. (C) MTT results of the different concentrations of thapsigargin (TG)-treated PC12 cells. (D) MTT result of bFGF-treated PC12 cells induced by TG. (E) FACScan result of PI/Annexin V-FITC staining for cell apoptosis analysis. (F) Statistical result of apoptosis rate in PC12 cells treated with TG and bFGF. **represents $P < 0.01$ vs. the control group, and #represents $P < 0.05$ vs. the TG group. Data are the mean values ± SEM, $n = 3$. (G) The protein expressions of CHOP, GRP78, p-Akt, p-ERK1/2, p-GSK-3β in ER stress-induced apoptosis PC12 cells treated with bFGF and different inhibitors. β-actin was used as the loading control and for band density normalization. (H) The optical density analysis of CHOP, GRP78, p-Akt, p-ERK1/2 and p-GSK-3β protein. *represents $P < 0.05$ vs. the control group, #represents $P < 0.01$ vs. the TG group, $represents $P < 0.05$ vs. the TG+bFGF group. Data are the mean values ± SEM, $n = 3$.

strated the protective effect and molecular mechanism of bFGF in ER stress-induced apoptosis both *in vivo* and *in vitro*.

The ER stress pathway was first identified as a cellular response induced by the accumulation of unfolded proteins in the ER to preserve the organelle function. The ER stress pathway is also activated by various cellular stress processes that may induce apoptosis to remove damaged cells [33]. Previous studies have demonstrated that ER stress-induced apoptosis was one of the main events in secondary damages of a spinal cord injury [5,11]. The increased production and nuclearization of the pro-apoptotic factor, CHOP, coincides with activation of caspase-12. In WT and CHOP null mice that received moderate T9 contusive injuries, deletion of CHOP led to an overall attenuation of the UPR after contusive SCI. Furthermore, analyses of hindlimb locomotion demonstrated a significant functional recovery that correlated with an increase in white matter sparing, transcript levels of myelin basic protein and decreased oligodendrocyte apoptosis in CHOP null mice compared with WT animals. This result indicates the important role of CHOP in cell death caused by SCI [11]. Therefore, CHOP and caspase 12-mediated ER stress-induced cell death seems to be the major mediator of apoptotic neuronal death after SCI. This result also implies that CHOP and caspase 12-mediated ER stress might be a potential therapeutic target to stop the apoptotic course after injury. Moreover, GRP78 is also involved in ER stress-induced apoptosis in serious spinal cord injuries [1,34]. In our study, the levels of these ER stress-induced apoptosis proteins after spinal cord contusions were detected to investigate the molecular mechanism of bFGF in SCI recovery. We found that the expressions of GRP78, CHOP and caspase-12 increased significantly the first day after SCI. Exogenous bFGF treatment after contusion decreased the levels of ER stress-induced apoptosis proteins and improved locomotor function and SCI recovery. These results indicated the role of bFGF in SCI therapy is related to the inhibition of ER stress response proteins. In addition, protein-folding stress at the ER is a salient feature of specialized secretory cells and is also involved in the pathogenesis of diseases. ER stress is buffered by the activation of the UPR, and failure to adapt to ER stress results in apoptosis [35]. Further study is needed to determine whether inhibition of ER stress-induced apoptosis by bFGF also leads to a reversal of the UPR and subsequently reactivates the innate immunity, metabolism and cell differentiation.

The main downstream signals activated by bFGF, the PI3K/Akt and ERK1/2 pathways are essential for the neurotropic effect. The PI3K/Akt pathway is particularly important for mediating neuronal survival under a wide variety of circumstances [14,36]. Akt acts before the release of cytochrome c by regulating Bcl-2 family member activity and mitochondrial function as well as components of the apoptosome [37,38]. For instance, Akt phosphorylates the pro-apoptotic Bcl-2 family member BAD, which inhibits BAD pro-apoptotic functions [39]. In addition to its effects on the cytoplasmic apoptotic machinery, the PI3K/Akt pathway also regulates apoptosis by suppressing the expression of death genes, such as the forkhead box transcription factor by phosphorylating FOXOs (Forkhead box, group O), which is also related to the ERK1/2 signal [36,40]. However, in the neuronal cell death of CNS diseases, it has been reported that PI3K/Akt partially mediates BDNF-mediated survival. This reveals that neuroprotection by BDNF is also partially dependent on ERK1/2 signaling [41,42]. Activation of the PI3K/Akt pathway is essential for neurotrophin-mediated survival. Overexpression of Akt not only blocks DNA fragmentation but also suppresses caspase-3 substrate PARP degradation under growth factor stimulation. Knockdown of Akt expression impairs NGF and BDNF-mediated H19-7 hippocampal progenitor cell and primary hippocampal neurons survival [43]. As the downstream signal of PI3K/Akt, GSK-3β also plays an important role in cell death. Phosphorylated GSK-3β inhibits the opening of mitochondrial permeability transition pores (mPTP), which results in the release of cytochrome c to the cytoplasm [44]. In particular, a previous study suggested that phosphorylated GSK-3β provides cardioprotection against myocardial I/R injury [45]. In our recent study, bFGF shows a neuronal protective effect in stroke rat model *via* the activation of both the PI3K/Akt and ERK1/2 signals [22]. Similarly to our results, Xia also reported that BDNF prevented phencyclidine-induced apoptosis in the developing brain by the activation of both the PI3K/Akt and ERK1/2 pathways [46]. In this study, we demonstrated that the role of bFGF in SCI recovery is also related to the activation of both the PI3K/Akt and ERK1/2 signals *in vivo*. To further confirm that these two pathways are essential for the protective effect of bFGF, we used ER stress inducer, TG, treated PC12 cells (combined with PI3K/ Akt inhibitor LY294002 or ERK1/2 inhibitor U0126) to show that the apoptosis induced by TG was inhibited by bFGF treatment and further abolished by this combination of inhibitors.

However, there is no doubt that the limitations of bFGF in SCI therapy still need for further study and investigation. For example, a single dose of bFGF was treated right after injury, postinjury treatment of optimal dose and extended time would better evaluate the therapeutic value in the future. In this study, 7-day outcome may not be long enough, which needs to be further investigated on the longterm neurological outcome, such as 2–3 weeks or longer period. Moreover, PC12 cell used *in vitro* is informative, future tests in spinal cord neuron cultures would be more persuasive. Nevertheless, the neuroprotective effect of bFGF following spinal cord contusion injury is confirmed and feasible to improve the pharmacodynamic actions and demonstrate the underlying mechanisms is necessary in the further studies.

In summary, administration of bFGF significantly reduced damage to spinal cord lesions and improved locomotor SCI recovery, which is related to the inhibition of ER stress-induced cell apoptosis. Our study demonstrates the possibility that bFGF therapy may be suitable for recovery from central nervous system injury diseases.

References

[1] Penas C, Guzman M-S, Verdu E, *et al.* Spinal cord injury induces endoplasmic reticulum stress with different cell-type dependent response[J]. Journal Of Neurochemistry, 2007, 102(4): 1242-1255.

[2] Dasari VR, Veeravalli KK, Tsung AJ, *et al.* Neuronal apoptosis is inhibited by cord blood stem cells after spinal cord injury[J]. Journal Of Neurotrauma, 2009, 26(11): 2057-2069.

[3] Beattie MS. Inflammation and apoptosis: linked therapeutic targets in spinal cord injury[J]. Trends In Molecular Medicine, 2004,

10(12): 580-583.

[4] Jing G, Wang JJ, Zhang SX. ER Stress and Apoptosis: A new mechanism for retinal cell death[J]. Experimental Diabetes Research, 2012.

[5] Badiola N, Penas C, Minano Molina A, et al. Induction of ER stress in response to oxygen-glucose deprivation of cortical cultures involves the activation of the PERK and IRE-1 pathways and of caspase-12[J]. Cell Death & Disease, 2011, 2.

[6] Zha BS, Zhou H. ER stress and lipid metabolism in adipocytes[J]. Biochemistry Research International, 2012.

[7] Ding W, Yang L, Zhang M, et al. Reactive oxygen species-mediated endoplasmic reticulum stress contributes to aldosterone-induced apoptosis in tubular epithelial cells[J]. Biochemical And Biophysical Research Communications, 2012, 418(3): 451-456.

[8] Liu X, Ko S, Xu Y, et al. Transient aggregation of ubiquitinated proteins is a cytosolic unfolded protein response to inflammation and endoplasmic reticulum stress[J]. Journal Of Biological Chemistry, 2012, 287(23): 19687-19698.

[9] Zhang Z, Tong N, Gong Y, et al. Valproate protects the retina from endoplasmic reticulum stress-induced apoptosis after ischemia-reperfusion injury[J]. Neuroscience Letters, 2011, 504(2): 88-92.

[10] Valenzuela V, Collyer E, Armentano D, et al. Activation of the unfolded protein response enhances motor recovery after spinal cord injury[J]. Cell Death & Disease, 2012, 3.

[11] Ohri SS, Maddie MA, Zhao Y, et al. Attenuating the endoplasmic reticulum stress response improves functional recovery after spinal cord injury[J]. Glia, 2011, 59(10): 1489-1502.

[12] Ohri SS, Maddie MA, Zhang Y, et al. Deletion of the pro-apoptotic endoplasmic reticulum stress response effector CHOP does not result in improved locomotor function after severe contusive spinal cord injury[J]. Journal Of Neurotrauma, 2012, 29(3): 579-588.

[13] Itoh N, Ornitz DM. Fibroblast growth factors: from molecular evolution to roles in development, metabolism and disease[J]. Journal Of Biochemistry, 2011, 149(2): 121-130.

[14] Beenken A, Mohammadi M. The FGF family: biology, pathophysiology and therapy[J]. Nature Reviews Drug Discovery, 2009, 8(3): 235-253.

[15] Xiao J, Lv Y, Lin S, et al. Cardiac protection by basic fibroblast growth factor from ischemia/reperfusion-induced injury in diabetic rats[J]. Biological & Pharmaceutical Bulletin, 2010, 33(3): 444-449.

[16] Abe K, Saitoh H. Effects of basic fibroblast growth factor on central nervous system functions[J]. Pharmacological Research, 2001, 43(4): 307-312.

[17] Yu Y, Gu S, Huang H, et al. Combination of bFGF, heparin and laminin induce the generation of dopaminergic neurons from rat neural stem cells both *in vitro* and *in vivo*[J]. Journal Of the Neurological Sciences, 2007, 255(1-2): 81-86.

[18] Liu WG, Wang ZY, Huang ZS. Bone marrow-derived mesenchymal stem cells expressing the bFGF transgene promote axon regeneration and functional recovery after spinal cord injury in rats[J]. Neurological Research, 2011, 33(7): 686-693.

[19] Karimi-Abdolrezaee S, Eftekharpour E, Wang J, et al. Synergistic effects of transplanted adult neural stem/progenitor cells, chondroitinase, and growth factors promote functional repair and plasticity of the chronically injured spinal cord[J]. Journal Of Neuroscience, 2010, 30(5): 1657-1676.

[20] Kishi S, Shimoke K, Nakatani Y, et al. Nerve growth factor attenuates 2-deoxy-D-glucose-triggered endoplasmic reticulum stress-mediated apoptosis *via* enhanced expression of GRP78[J]. Neuroscience Research, 2010, 66(1): 14-21.

[21] de Oliveira MR, da Rocha RF, Stertz L, et al. Total and mitochondrial nitrosative stress, decreased brain-derived neurotrophic factor (BDNF) Levels and Glutamate Uptake, and Evidence of Endoplasmic Reticulum Stress in the Hippocampus of Vitamin A-Treated Rats[J]. Neurochemical Research, 2011, 36(3): 506-517.

[22] Wang Z, Zhang H, Xu X, et al. bFGF inhibits ER stress induced by ischemic oxidative injury *via* activation of the PI3K/Akt and ERK1/2 pathways[J]. Toxicology Letters, 2012, 212(2): 137-146.

[23] Jameson MJ, Beckler AD, Taniguchi LE, et al. Activation of the insulin-like growth factor-1 receptor induces resistance to epidermal growth factor receptor antagonism in head and neck squamous carcinoma cells[J]. Molecular Cancer Therapeutics, 2011, 10(11): 2124-2134.

[24] Echeverria V, Zeitlin R. Cotinine: A potential new therapeutic agent against alzheimer's disease[J]. Cns Neuroscience & Therapeutics, 2012, 18(7): 517-523.

[25] Pisanti S, Picardi P, Prota L, et al. Genetic and pharmacologic inactivation of cannabinoid CB1 receptor inhibits angiogenesis[J]. Blood, 2011, 117(20): 5541-5550.

[26] Shimoke K, Kishi S, Utsumi T, et al. NGF-induced phosphatidylinositol 3-kinase signaling pathway prevents thapsigargin-triggered ER stress-mediated apoptosis in PC12 cells[J]. Neuroscience Letters, 2005, 389(3): 124-128.

[27] Szegezdi E, Herbert KR, Kavanagh ET, et al. Nerve growth factor blocks thapsigargin-induced apoptosis at the level of the mitochondrion viaregulation of Bim[J]. Journal Of Cellular And Molecular Medicine, 2008, 12(6A): 2482-2496.

[28] Xu R, Chen J, Cong X, et al. Lovastatin protects mesenchymal stem cells against hypoxia- and serum deprivation-induced apoptosis by activation of PI3K/Akt and ERK1/2[J]. Journal Of Cellular Biochemistry, 2008, 103(1): 256-269.

[29] Cevikbas F, Steinhoff M, Ikoma A. Role of spinal neurotransmitter receptors in Itch: new insights into therapies and drug development[J]. Cns Neuroscience & Therapeutics, 2011, 17(6): 742-749.

[30] Moon YJ, Lee JY, Oh MS, et al. Inhibition of inflammation and oxidative stress by Angelica dahuricae radix extract decreases apoptotic cell death and improves functional recovery after spinal cord injury[J]. Journal Of Neuroscience Research, 2012, 90(1): 243-256.

[31] Gelfo F, Tirassa P, De Bartolo P, et al. NPY intraperitoneal injections produce antidepressant-like effects and downregulate BDNF in the rat hypothalamus[J]. Cns Neuroscience & Therapeutics, 2012, 18(6): 487-492.

[32] Zhang L, Ma Z, Smith GM, et al. GDNF-enhanced axonal regeneration and myelination following spinal cord injury is mediated by primary effects on neurons[J]. Glia, 2009, 57(11): 1178-1191.

[33] Appenzeller-Herzog C, Hall MN. Bidirectional crosstalk between endoplasmic reticulum stress and mTOR signaling[J]. Trends In Cell Biology, 2012, 22(5): 274-282.

[34] Yamauchi T, Sakurai M, Abe K, et al. Impact of the endoplasmic reticulum stress response in spinal cord after transient ischemia[J]. Brain Research, 2007, 1169: 24-33.

[35] Hetz C. The unfolded protein response: controlling cell fate decisions under ER stress and beyond[J]. Nature Reviews Molecular Cell Biology, 2012, 13(2): 89-102.

[36] Brunet A, Bonni A, Zigmond MJ, et al. Akt promotes cell survival by phosphorylating and inhibiting a forkhead transcription factor[J]. Cell, 1999, 96(6): 857-868.

[37] Yuan Y, Xue X, Guo R, et al. Resveratrol enhances the antitumor effects of temozolomide in glioblastoma *via* ROS-dependent AMPK-TSC-mTOR signaling pathway[J]. Cns Neuroscience & Therapeutics, 2012, 18(7): 536-546.

[38] Zhang H, Kong X, Kang J, et al. Oxidative stress induces parallel autophagy and mitochondria dysfunction in human glioma U251 Cells[J]. Toxicological Sciences, 2009, 110(2): 376-388.

[39] Datta SR, Dudek H, Tao X, et al. Akt phosphorylation of BAD couples survival signals to the cell-intrinsic death machinery[J]. Cell, 1997, 91(2): 231-241.

[40] Roy SK, Srivastava RK, Shankar S. Inhibition of PI3K/AKT and MAPK/ERK pathways causes activation of FOXO transcription factor, leading to cell cycle arrest and apoptosis in pancreatic

cancer[J]. Journal of molecular signaling, 2010, 5: 10-10.

[41] Meyer Franke A, Wilkinson GA, Kruttgen A, *et al.* Depolarization and cAMP elevation rapidly recruit TrkB to the plasma membrane of CNS neurons[J]. Neuron, 1998, 21(4): 681-693.

[42] Yoshii A, Constantine Paton M. BDNF induces transport of PSD-95 to dendrites through PI3K-AKT signaling after NMDA receptor activation[J]. Nature Neuroscience, 2007, 10(6): 702-711.

[43] Nguyen TLX, Kim CK, Cho JH, *et al.* Neuroprotection signaling pathway of nerve growth factor and brain-derived neurotrophic factor against staurosporine induced apoptosis in hippocampal H19-7 cells[J]. Experimental And Molecular Medicine, 2010, 42(8):

583-595.

[44] Juhaszova M, Zorov DB, Yaniv Y, *et al.* Role of glycogen synthase kinase-3 beta in cardioprotection[J]. Circulation Research, 2009, 104(11): 1240-1252.

[45] Miura T, Miki T. GSK-3 beta, a Therapeutic target for cardiomyocyte protection[J]. Circulation Journal, 2009, 73(7): 1184-1192.

[46] Xia Y, Wang CZ, Liu J, *et al.* Brain-derived neurotrophic factor prevents phencyclidine-induced apoptosis in developing brain by parallel activation of both the ERK and PI-3K/Akt pathways[J]. Neuropharmacology, 2010, 58(2): 330-336.

FGF10 protects against renal ischemia/reperfusion injury by regulating autophagy and inflammatory signaling

Xiaohua Tan , Xiaokun Li, Jinsan Zhang

1. Introduction

Acute kidney injury is a global health concern. AKI is mainly caused by renal I/R injury, sepsis, and nephrotoxicant (such as cisplatin, cyclosporine and aristolochic acid) (Paller *et al.*, 1984; Thadhani *et al.*, 1996; Zuk and Bonventre, 2016). The primary characteristic of AKI is the rapid decline in kidney function as measured by detection of GFR (Bonventre and Yang, 2011; Havasi and Borkan, 2011). Despite advances in therapeutic strategies and nursing measures, including dialysis and kidney transplantation, the mortality of patients after AKI remains very high (Ueda *et al.*, 2000; Chertow *et al.*, 2005). In the past decades, AKI has been extensively studied both in clinic and experimental animal settings. The disease mechanisms underlying the etiology and pathogenesis of AKI are complex and include mitochondrial dysfunction, ROS, ER stress, autophagy, inflammation, apoptosis and necrosis (Basile *et al.*, 2012; Tan *et al.*, 2013, 2017; He *et al.*, 2014; Kaushal and Shah, 2016; Xu *et al.*, 2016). To date, there are no satisfying strategies or drugs for the therapy of patients with AKI.

A number of recent studies have demonstrated the crucial role of autophagy in animal models of AKI induced by I/R injury and nephrotoxic agents (Mizushima and Komatsu, 2011; Basile *et al.*, 2012; Jiang *et al.*, 2012; He *et al.*, 2014; Guan *et al.*, 2015; De Rechter *et al.*, 2016; Lenoir *et al.*, 2016). Autophagy is a highly conserved eukaryotic cellular recycling process by which cytoplasmic components are engulfed and degraded in the lysosome (Mizushima and Komatsu, 2011). Generally, autophagy is thought to be highly inducible under stress conditions such as ischemia, hypoxia, nutrient deprivation, genotoxic stress, infection, UPR, and other insults, all of which participate in the pathogenesis of AKI (Mizushima and Komatsu, 2011; Basile *et al.*, 2012; He *et al.*, 2014; De Rechter *et al.*, 2016; Kaushal and Shah, 2016; Zuk and Bonventre, 2016). Whether autophagy is protective or damaging in AKI remains controversial. Renoprotective effects of autophagy in AKI have been reported in several studies (Pallet *et al.*, 2008; Jiang *et al.*, 2012). However, excessive activation of autophagy results in widespread cell death predominantly in RTCs due to extensive degradation of essential materials and organelles (Chien *et al.*, 2007; Suzuki *et al.*, 2008; Inoue *et al.*, 2010). Therefore, activation of autophagy has dual roles in regulating cell survival or cell death in AKI.

Inflammatory response is another important component in the initiation and exacerbation of AKI. Although inflammation is an essential element of the body's defense system, excessive activation of inflammatory cells and cytokine secretion impose severe damage to renal parenchyma cells (Jang and Rabb, 2009; Shibutani *et al.*, 2015). High-mobility group box 1 is a member of the high-mobility group (HMG) protein family and one of the highly conserved and abundantly expressed proteins in almost all types of eukaryotic cells (Lotze and Tracey, 2005; Kang *et al.*, 2014). Recently, the pathophysiological role of HMGB1 in human diseases has been extensively studied. In healthy circumstances, HMGB1 is localized in the nuclei of cells and participates in multiple cellular processes including DNA repair, transcription, and cell differentiation. However, HMGB1 can be released into the extracellular space and function as a signaling molecule in various biological processes such as inflammatory response (Tang *et al.*, 2010a; Xu *et al.*, 2014; Ouyang *et al.*, 2016). Circulating HMBG1 is capable of engaging with toll-like receptors (TLRs), particularly TLR2 and TLR4, to activate the expression of multiple pro-inflammatory cytokines such as TNF-α, IL-1β and IL-6. Studies demonstrate that HMGB1 plays an important role in the interaction of autophagy and apoptosis/necrosis in various disorders including AKI (Nikoletopoulou *et al.*, 2013; Kim *et al.*, 2014; Chen *et al.*, 2016).

Fibroblast growth factor 10, also known as Keratinocyte growth factor 2, is a typical paracrine FGF family member and signals through interactions with its high affinity receptor FGFR2-IIIb splicing isoform. FGF10 is a multifunctional growth factor playing crucial roles in the development of many organs and tissues including the kidney (Beenken and Mohammadi, 2009; Itoh, 2015). Deletion of either *Fgf10* or its receptor *Fgfr2-IIIb* in mice led to kidney dysgenesis characterized by fewer collecting ducts and nephrons (Bates, 2007). Overexpression of a dominant negative receptor isoform in transgenic mice has revealed more striking defects including renal aplasia or severe dysplasia (Bates, 2007). Recent studies have reported the protective effect of FGF10 on spinal cord injury, cerebral ischemia injury and acute lung injury *via* inhibiting inflammation, activating PI3K/AKT signaling pathway or mobilization of stem cells (Li *et al.*, 2016; Tong *et al.*, 2016; Chen *et al.*, 2017). Currently, there are no published reports regarding whether exogenous FGF10 can promote the recovery of AKI. In the present work, we tested the hypothesis that FGF10 administration might protect renal cells exposed to I/R injury through regulating autophagy and inflammation.

2. Materials and methods

2.1 Reagents and antibodies

Recombinant human FGF10 was acquired from Zhejiang Grost Biotechnology (Wenzhou). Antibodies against mTOR, LC3, SQSTM1, Beclin-1 and GAPDH were purchased from Santa Cruz Biotechnology (Santa Cruz, CA, United States). Antibodies against cleaved Caspase-3, HMGB1, phospho-FGFR, TNF-α and Caspase-9 were bought from Cell Signaling Technology (Beverly, MA, United States). TGF-β antibody was purchased from Abcam (Cambridge, MA, United States). The autophagy inhibitor chloroquine, autophagy activator rapamycin and 4′, 6-diamidino-2-phenylindole (DAPI) were purchased from Sigma-Aldrich (St Louis, MO, United States) and Invitrogen (Carlsbad, CA, United States), respectively.

2.2 Animals

Adult male Sprague Dawley (SD) rats (8–12 weeks old) were supplied by Shanghai SLAC Laboratory Animal Co., Ltd., and housed in SPF facility of Wenzhou Medical University. The protocols for all animal experiments were approved by the institutional Animal Care and Use committee. Rats were anesthetized with intra-peritoneal injection of 4% pentobarbital sodium (50 mg/kg, Merck, Germany) and underwent right nephrectomy followed by ischemia for 60 min with renal artery clamping. SD rats were randomly divided into four groups: (I) Sham group: the left kidney was exposed with an unrestricted renal artery; (II) I/R group: the left kidneys were subjected to 60 min of ischemia by renal artery clamping followed by reperfusion (Kalogeris *et al.*, 2012; Tan *et al.*, 2017); (III) I/R-FGF10 group: a single dose of FGF10 (0.5 mg/kg) was injected into the abdominal cavity 30 min before the 60 min exposure to ischemia; (IV) RAPA group: a single dose of rapamycin (10 mg/kg, intramuscular injection, i.m) was injected followed by the injection of FGF10 same with I/R-FGF10 group, and then the left kidneys were subjected to 60 min of ischemia. For combined treatment with chloroquine (I/R-CL group): a single dose of chloroquine (60 mg/kg) was injected into the abdominal cavity 30 min before the 60 min exposure to ischemia. Animals were sacrificed at indicated time points after reperfusion upon surgical operation and kidneys were harvested for further experiment.

2.3 Renal function and histopathology

Serum creatinine and BUN were used to assess changes of renal function after AKI. The levels of SCr and BUN were determined by the Creatine and the Urease colorimetry methods, respectively, which were performed at the Medical Laboratory Center of the First Affiliated Hospital, Wenzhou Medical University. For renal histology analysis, Kidneys were dissected and fixed with 10% formaldehyde for 48 h, then embedded in paraffin. To access the severity of renal injury after AKI, sections (5 μm) were stained with H&E to observe the changes of the renal morphology.

Immunohistochemistry and immunofluorescent staining. The slides were incubated with antibodies against cleaved-Capase-3, p-FGFR, SQSTM1 and TNF-α at 4℃ overnight and stained with Diaminobenzidine (DAB) and counterstained with hematoxylin. The slides were then subjected to gradient ethanol dehydration, dimethyl benzene transparent, and mounted with Neutral resin cover slides. Images were captured using a Nikon ECLPSE 80i. For immunofluorescent staining, 5 μm sections were incubated at 4℃ overnight with primary antibody against LC3, Beclin-1 and HMGB1, respectively. The slides were then TABLE 1 | Primer sequences used to amplify rat cDNAs. incubated with donkey anti-rabbit secondary antibodies (Abcam, MA, United States) or donkey anti-mouse IgG-PE secondary antibodies (Santa

Cruz, CA, United States) for 1 h at room temperature. The images were captured using a laser confocal microscope (Nikon, Ti-E&A1 plus).

2.4　Apoptosis assay

To measure the apoptosis rates after I/R injury, DNA fragmentation *in vivo* was detected using a one-step TUNEL Apoptosis Assay KIT (Roche, Mannheim, Germany) as previously described (Tan *et al.*, 2017). The images were captured with a Nikon ECLPSE Ti microscope (Nikon, Japan).

2.5　Western blot analysis

Tissue protein samples were prepared with protein extraction reagents from renal tissues. Protein concentrations were measured with a Pierce BCA Protein Assay Kit (Thermo Fisher Scientific). Samples with equal amount of proteins were separated with SDS-PAGE and then transferred onto a PVDF membrane for Western blot analysis with specified antibodies. The ChemiDic TM XRS imaging system (Bio-Rad Laboratories, Hercules, United States) was used to analyze the signals and the band densities were quantified with Multi Gauge software of science Lab 2010 (FUJIFILM Corporation, Tokyo, Japan).

2.6　Real-time quantitative RT-PCR

Total RNA from kidney tissues was extracted using RNeasy column (QIAGEN), and reverse transcription was performed using Prime Script TM RT reagent Kit (TaKaRa) according to the manufacturer's instructions. Real-time RT-PCR was performed using the SYBR Green gene expression assays (TaKaRa) to access mRNA expression. The target values were normalized to GAPDH (Tan *et al.*, 2017). The PCR primers used for mRNA expression analysis of *Tlr2, Tlr4, Il-1β, Il-6*, and *Gapdh* are summarized in Table 1.

Table 1.　Primer sequences used to amplify rat cDNAs

Gene	GenBank	Primer sequences
GAPDH	NM_012675	5'- GACATGCCGCCTGGAGAAAC-3'
		5'-AGCCCAGGATGCCCTTTAGT-3'
IL-1β	NM_031512	5'-TGCAGGCTTCGAGATGAAC-3'
		5'-GGGATTTTGTCGTTGCTTGTC-3'
IL-6	NM_012589	5'-AAGCCAGAGTCATTCAGAGC-3'
		5'-GTCCTTAGCCACTCCTTCTG-3'
TLR2	NM_198769	5'-ATGAACACTAAGACATACCTGGAG-3'
		5'-CAAGACAGAAACAGGGTGGAG-3'
TLR4	NM_019178	5'-CATGACATCCCTTATTCAACCAAG-3'
		5'-GCCATGCCTTGTCTTCAATTG-3'
TNFα	NM_012675	5'-CTTCTCATTCCTGCTCGTGG-3'
		5'-TGATCTGAGTGTGAGGGTCTG-3'

GAPDH: Glyceraldehyde 3-phosphate dehydrogenase; IL-1β: interleukin-1β; IL-6: interleukin-6; TLR2: Toll-like receptor-2; TLR4: Toll-like receptor-4; TNFα: tumor necrosis factor-α.

2.7　Statistical analysis

Data is expressed as the mean SEM of independent experiments ($n \geqslant 5$). Statistical significance was determined using Student's *t*-test when there were two experimental groups. When more than two groups were compared, statistical evaluation of the data was performed using one-way analysis of variance (ANOVA). *$P < 0.05$, **$P < 0.01$, ***$P < 0.001$, P-values < 0.05 was regarded as statistically significant.

3. Results

3.1 FGF10 ameliorates I/R-induced renal dysfunction and histological damage

We employed an I/R injury rat model to investigate the potential effect of FGF10 on AKI at 24, 48, and 72 h, respectively. Renal histological changes were assessed by H&E staining, no apparent damage was observed in the kidney of sham group, whereas the rats in I/R group and RAPA group showed swelling of RTCs, intraluminal necrotic cellular debris, interstitial congestion and luminal narrowing characteristic of I/R-induced tubular epithelial injury at each time point after reperfusion (Fig. 1A). Significantly, Pre-administration of FGF10 markedly attenuated the degree of renal damages and largely preserved the normal tissue architecture and integrity. Renal function was assessed by measuring SCr and BUN at 48 h after reperfusion. As expected, the levels of SCr and BUN were both increased significantly in I/R rats compared to Sham group (Fig. 1C,D). Notably, the levels of SCr and BUN in I/R-FGF10 group were significantly lower compared to that of I/R group ($P < 0.001$), whereas Rapamycin largely abolished the protective effect of FGF10 against I/R injury. To investigate the association between FGF10/FGFR signaling pathway and I/R injury, we detected the activation of FGFR by immunohistochemistry (IHC) staining with p-FGFR antibody. As shown in Fig. 1B, few p-FGFR positive cells were detected in kidneys of sham group, whereas the number of p-FGFR positive cells was increased in I/R group at 48 h after reperfusion. However, both the number of p-FGFR positive renal tubular cells (RTCs) and the staining intensity were noticeably increased in kidneys of I/R-FGF10 group or RAPA group compared to I/R group.

3.2 FGF10 reduced apoptosis of RTCs via regulation of pro-apoptotic proteins

TUNEL staining was carried out to assess the apoptosis in RTCs. As shown in Fig. 2A, compared to the sham group, the number of TUNEL-positive cells in I/R rats was dramatically increased ($P < 0.001$). Significantly, the proportion of TUNEL-positive cells was much lower in I/R-FGF10 group ($P < 0.001$). However, this apparent effect of FGF10 against I/R-induced apoptosis was mostly antagonized by rapamycin treatment (Fig. 2A). The number of TUNEL-positive cells was strikingly increased in RAPA group compared to the IR-FGF10 group. Quantification analysis of TUNEL staining revealed that the average percentage of apoptotic cells were 2.40% (24 h), 2.64% (48 h) and 1.92% (72 h) in sham group; 11.8% (24 h), 40.34% (48 h), 32.8% (72 h) in I/R group; 8.14% (24 h), 13.22% (48 h), 12.38% (72 h) in I/R-FGF10 group and 13.2% (24 h), 32.9% (48 h), 34.28% (72 h) in RAPA group, respectively (Fig. 2B). The results indicated that FGF10 treatment protected RTCs from I/R-induced apoptosis based on TUNEL staining. However, the protective role of FGF10 against apoptosis was diminished by rapamycin.

To understand the protective mechanism of FGF10 against I/R-induced RTC apoptosis, we examined the expression of pro-apoptotic proteins involved in regulation of cell apoptosis (BCL-2, BAX) and cleaved-Caspase-3 by IHC staining (Fig. 3A) and western blot (Figs. 3B–E), respectively. The expression of BAX and cleaved-Caspase-3 were significantly increased upon I/R injury, whereas BCL2 expression was decreased. Significantly, FGF10 treatment inhibited the pro-apoptotic expression/activation of Bax/BCL2 and cleaved-Caspase-3, respectively. Consistent with the results of apoptosis, the effect of FGF10 was largely inhibited by co-treatment with rapamycin. Together, the results suggest that FGF10 protects RTCs from I/R-induced apoptosis *via* regulation of pro-apoptotic proteins. However, rapamycin inhibited the role of FGF10 and thus the expression of pro-apoptotic proteins was increased.

3.3 The protective effect of FGF10 is related to the regulation of autophagy via mTOR pathway

Autophagy is known to play a crucial role in the etiology of AKI caused by renal I/R injury. The fact that rapamycin, a well-established allosteric mTOR kinase inhibitor and agonist of autophagy, mostly reduced the protective effect of FGF10 against I/R-induced renal damage apoptosis of RTCs prompted us to further examine the involvement of autophagy in mediating protective effect of FGF10.

Detection of LC3I to LC3II conversion and expression of Beclin-1 and SQSTM1/p62 (SQSTM1 is used hereafter) remains the most reliable methods to gauge autophagic activity. We therefore examined the expression of LC3, Beclin-1 and SQSTM1 at tissue and protein levels by immunofluorescence staining and immunoblot, respectively. The confocal

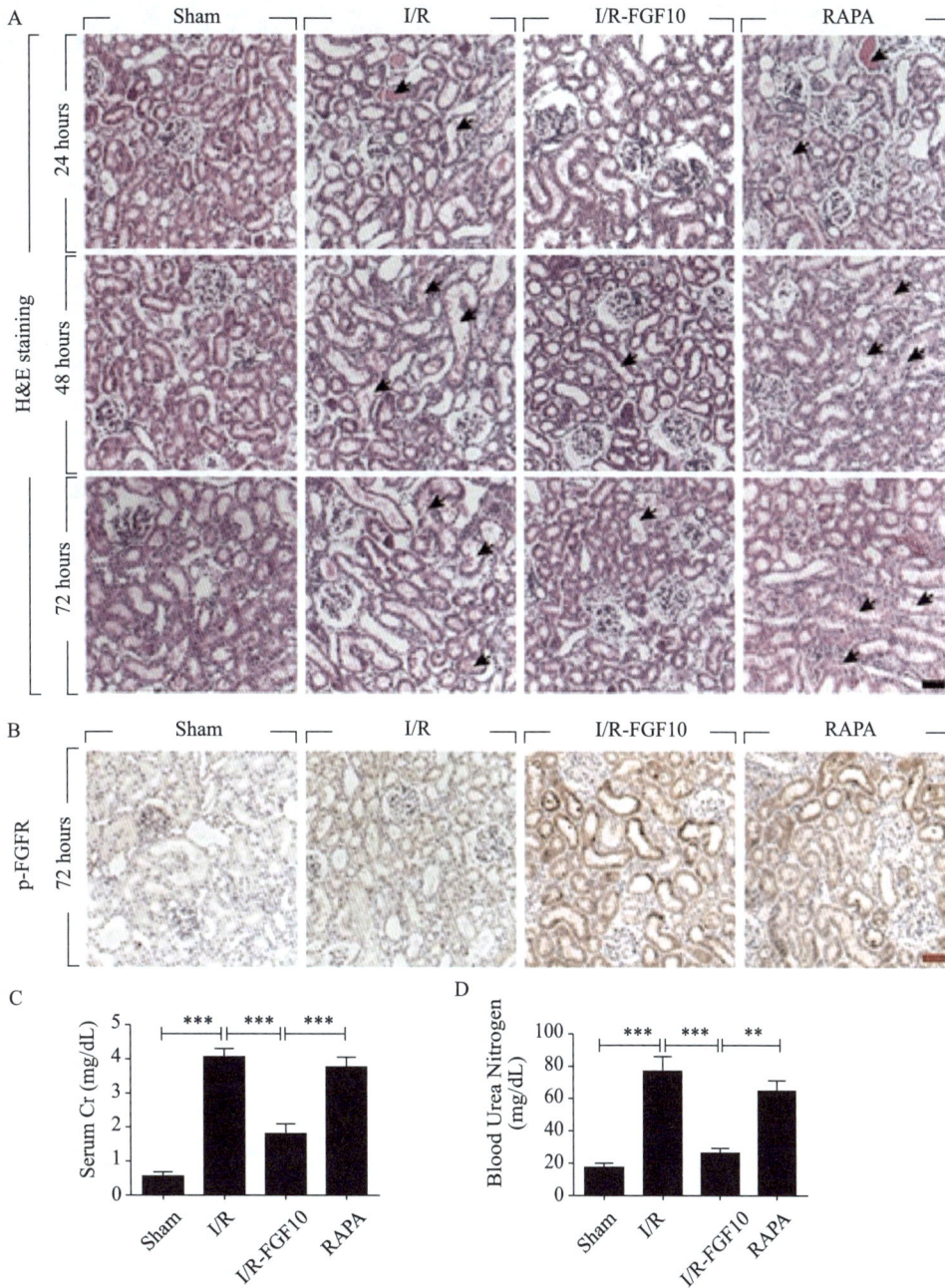

Fig. 1. FGF10 protects against renal histological and function damage after I/R injury. (A) Histological changes of kidneys detected by H&E staining at 24, 48, and 72 h, respectively, after reperfusion. Animals were randomly assigned into 4 groups: namely, Sham group, I/R group, I/R-FGF10 group and RAPA group. The details of operations and treatment animals received were described in the materials and methods. Arrows show intraluminal necrotic cells. Scale bars = 50 μm. (B) IHC staining for p-FGFR in renal tissue sections of indicated groups. Scale bars = 50 μm. (C,D) Determination of SCr and BUN levels in the above grouped rats at 2 days after reperfusion (mean ± SEM; $n = 5$). [**]$P < 0.01$, [***]$P < 0.001$.

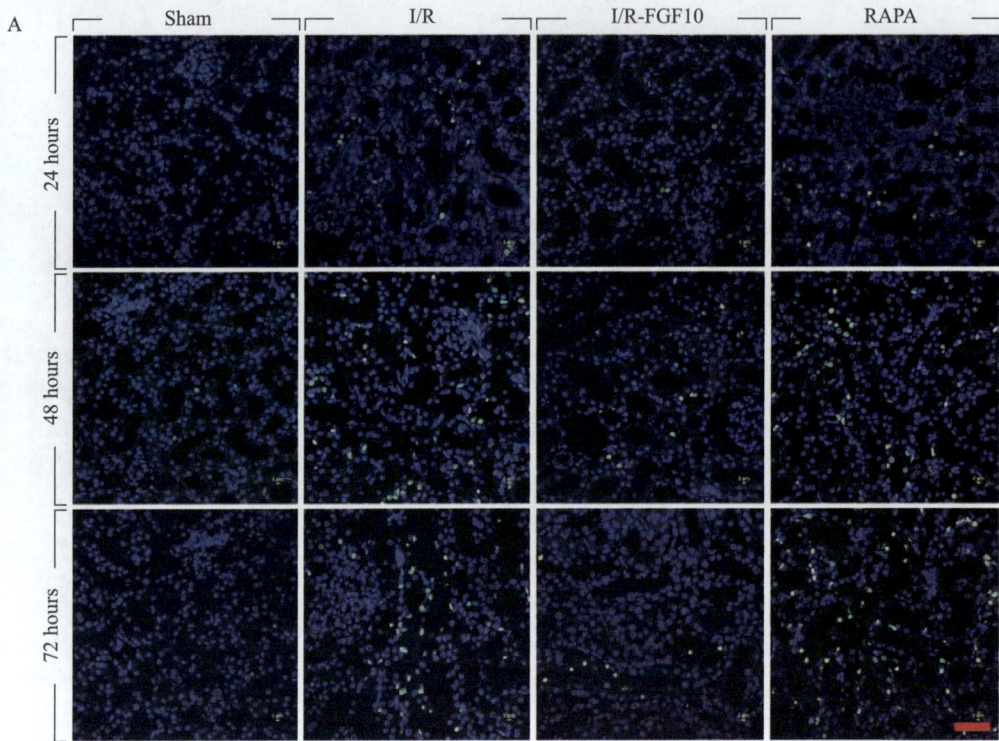

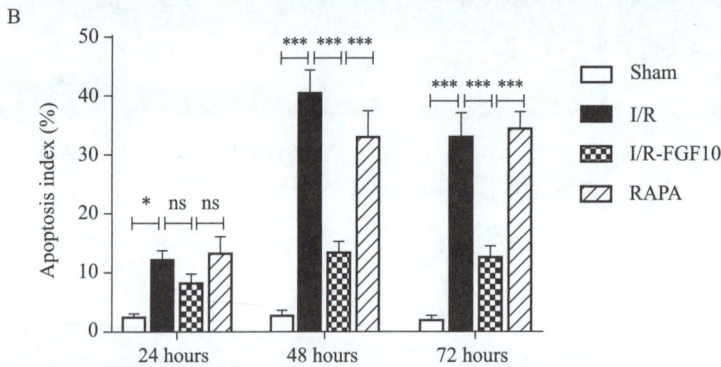

Fig. 2. FGF10 protects against I/R induced apoptosis in RTCs. (A) Representative sections of nuclear DNA fragmentation staining were performed using TUNEL in different groups at 24, 48, and 72 h, respectively, after reperfusion. Scale bars = 50 μM. (B) Quantitative analysis of the number of TUNEL-positive RTCs. Data are presented as the mean ± SD ($n = 5$). $^{*}P < 0.05$, $^{***}P < 0.001$. The percentage of positive cells was analyzed with 5 individual magnification × 400 fields per group.

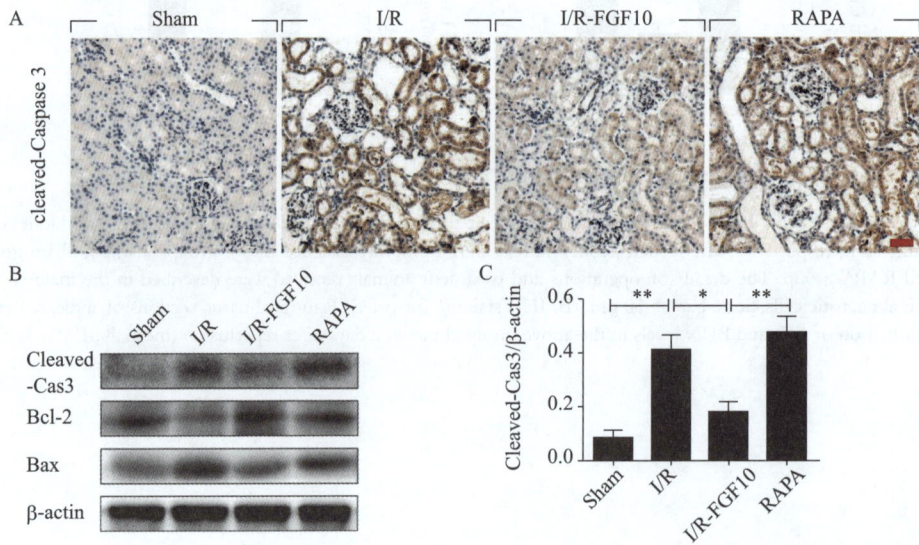

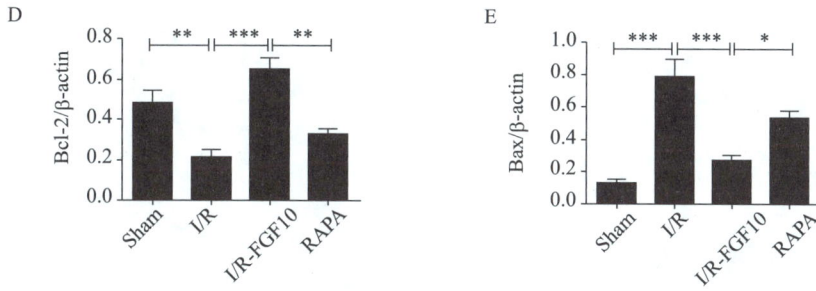

Fig. 3. FGF10 reduces the expression of pro-apoptotic proteins IHC staining and Western blot analyses were performed at 2 days after reperfusion. (A) IHC staining for cleaved caspase-3 in kidneys of indicated groups. Scale bars = 50 μm. (B) The expression of cleaved Caspase-3, Bcl-2 and Bax were detected by Western blot with β-actin as loading control. (C–E) The optical density analysis of cleaved Caspase-3, Bcl-2 and Bax (mean ± SEM; n = 5). $^*P < 0.05$, $^{**}P < 0.01$, $^{***}P < 0.001$.

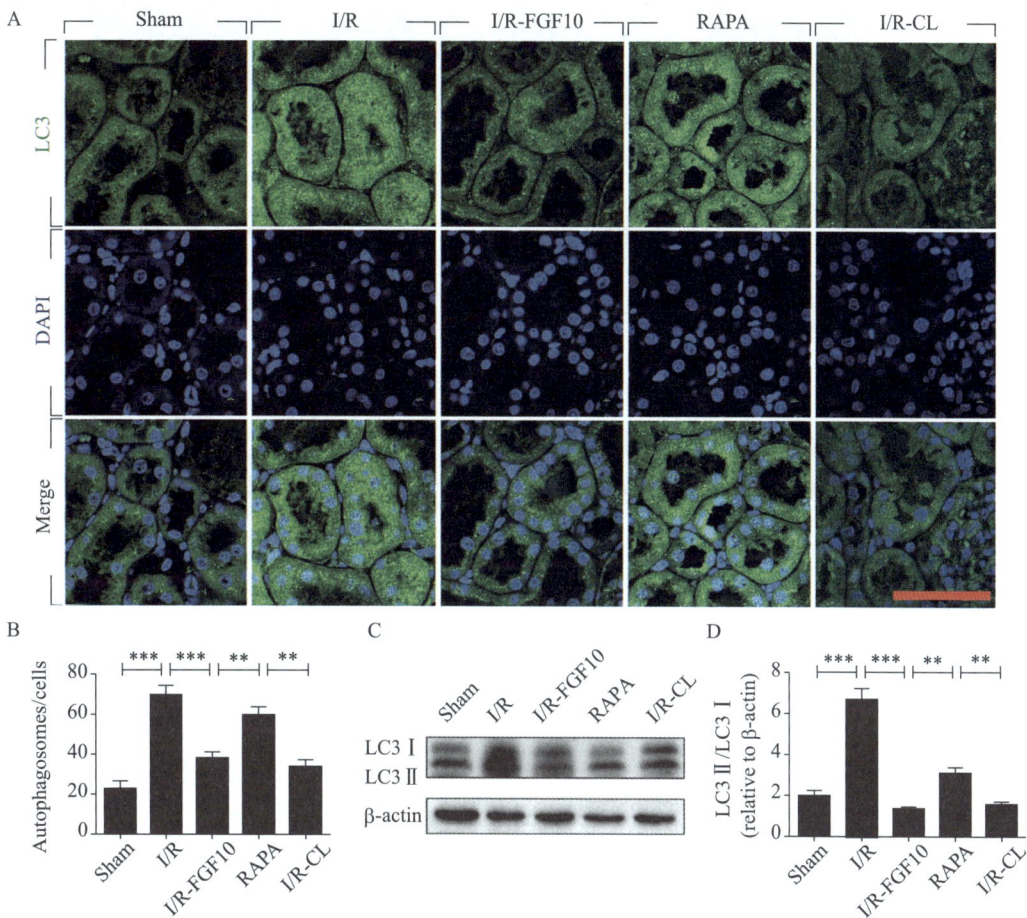

Fig. 4. FGF10 reduces the formation of autophagosome and the expression of LC3II. (A) Immunofluorescence staining of LC3 (green) was performed at 48 h after reperfusion. Nuclei were labeled with DAPI (blue). Scale bars = 50 μm. (B) Statistic analysis of the number of autophagosomes in RTCs with 5 randomly selected images in each group. (C) The protein expression of LC3II/LC3I in renal tissue was determined by Western blot and the optical densities were quantified (D). Data are presented as the mean ± SEM (n = 5). $^*P < 0.05$, $^{**}P < 0.01$, $^{***}P < 0.001$.

imaging in Fig. 4A shows that the number of LC3 positive dots (autophagosomes) were dramatically increased in the I/R group compared to sham group, but greatly reduced by FGF10. Rapamycin treatment effectively abolished the effect of FGF10 in this setting. However, chloroquine, as a specific autophagy inhibitor, markedly reduced the number of autophagosomes in RTCs caused by I/R injury. The statistical analysis about the number of autophagosomes in each group was shown in Fig. 4B. This result is confirmed with immunoblot analysis showing that I/R induced LC3II was partially prevented by FGF10 treatment (Fig. 4C, and quantification result in Fig. 4D). Co-detection of Beclin-1 and LC3 by im-

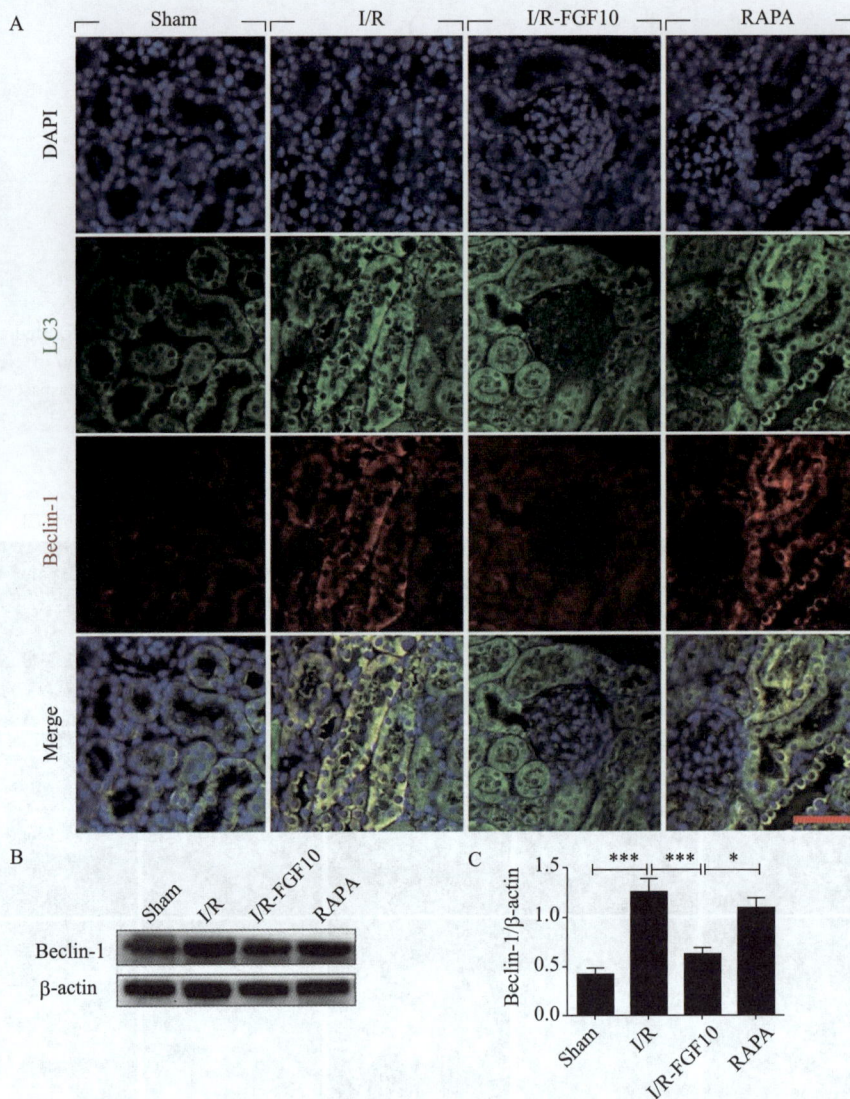

Fig. 5. FGF10 reduces the expression of Beclin-1. (A) Immunofluorescence staining and confocal images for LC3 (Green) and Beclin-1 (red) at 2 days after reperfusion. Nuclei were labeled with DAPI (blue). Scale bars = 50 μm. (B) Representative western blotting result for Beclin-1 expression. (C) Optical density analysis of protein bands. Data are presented as the mean ± SEM (n = 5). *P < 0.05, ***P < 0.001.

munofluorescence staining also revealed that increased expression of Beclin-1 in I/R tissues was largely prevented by FGF10, an effect also reversed by treatment with rapamycin (Fig. 5A). Western blot detection and quantification analysis on Beclin-1 expression (shown in Fig. 5B,C) revealed a similar trend of alteration to LC3II (Fig. 4C,D), and was consistent with confocal image analysis (Fig. 4A, 5A).

Besides LC3II and Beclin-1, we also examined the expression of SQSTM1, a selective autophagic receptor and substrate. As shown in Fig. 6A, SQSTM1 was expressed in the cytoplasm of RTCs, which was significantly decreased in I/R group. It was evident that FGF10 not only reversed I/R-induced decrease of SQSTM1, but further increased its expression above the one observed for the sham control (Fig. 6B,C), this effect again was abolished by rapamycin. To determine whether the mTOR pathway is subjected to FGF10 regulation, we examined the phosphorylation of mTOR by immunoblot. As shown in Fig. 6B, the changes in phosphorylation of mTOR highly resembled that of SQSTM1, which was decreased in I/R group, but became markedly increased in FGF10 treated group, an effect mostly inhibited by co-treatment with rapamycin (Fig. 6D).

3.4 FGF10 inhibited the release of HMGB1 in response to renal I/R injury

HMGB1 is a major DAMP protein, which can be activated by renal I/R and participates in inflammatory response (Wu *et al.*, 2010). We therefore examined the expression and localization of HMGB1 by Immunofluorescence stain-

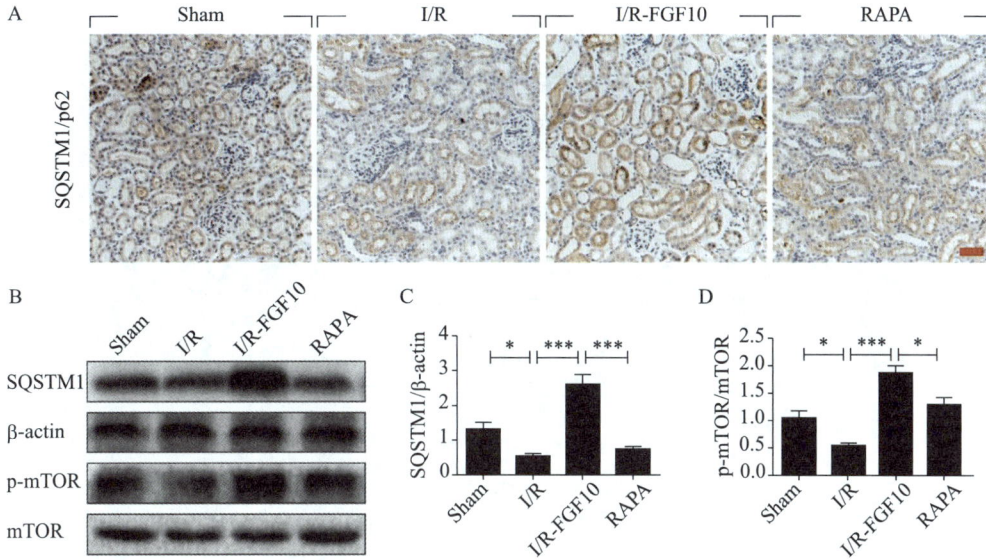

Fig. 6. FGF10 increases the expression of SQSTM1 and p-mTOR in I/R rats. (A) IHC staining was performed at 2 days after reperfusion for SQSTM1 in kidney tissues from indicated animal groups. Scale bars = 50 μm. (B) The expression of SQSTM1, p-mTOR and mTOR were detected by western blotting (mean ± SEM; n = 5). β-actin was used as control. $^*P < 0.05$, $^{***}P < 0.001$. (C,D) Optical density analysis for SQSTM1 and p-mTOR, which were normalized to β-actin and mTOR, respectively.

ing and confocal imaging analyses. As expected, HMGB1 was predominantly localized in the nuclei of RTCs in sham control. Following I/R injury, the level of HMGB1 appeared to be decreased in nuclei, but increased in the cytoplasmic domain. Strikingly, FGF10 almost completely prevented the decrease of nuclear HMGB1 and concomitant increase in the cytoplasm, an effect abolished by rapamycin treatment (Fig. 7A). To confirm the nucleus to cytoplasm shuttling and extracellular release of HMGB1, we further examined the levels of nuclear as well as serum HMGB1 by western blot and ELISA, respectively (Fig. 7B–D). The expression of HMGB1 in the nuclear fraction was significantly decreased, whereas the serum HMGB1 was significantly increased in I/R group compared with sham group. FGF10 treatment completely prevented the I/R-induced decrease of nuclear HMGB1 (Fig. 7B,C), and largely abolished the increase in serum HMGB1 (Fig. 7D). Extracellular HMGB1 is known to signal through TLRs, particularly TLR2 and TLR4, to activate pro-inflammatory response. Indeed, we found that the level of *Tlr2* mRNA expression was increased nearly threefold against sham-operated rats (Fig. 7E). Importantly, FGF10 treatment mostly obliterated I/R-induced *Tlr2* expression, an effect partially reversed by rapamycin treatment. The effect of FGF10 on the mRNA expression of *Tlr4* was similar to that of *Tlr2* (Fig. 7F). These results provide evidence that FGF10 could inhibit the release of HMGB1 from the nucleus to the extracellular matrix thereby preventing the HMGB1-mediated inflammatory response *via* the TLR2/TLR4 signaling pathway.

3.5 FGF10 inhibited the expression of inflammatory cytokines after I/R injury

The ability of FGF10 to prevent I/R induced HMGB1 nuclear to cytoplasmic shuttling and releases, as well as TLR2 induction in response to I/R injury suggests that FGF10 may inhibit the expression of pro-inflammatory cytokines such as TNF-α. We therefore examined the expression of TNF-α in kidneys by IHC staining (Fig. 8A) and western blot (Fig. 8B,C). The serum TNF-α was also examined by ELISA (Fig. 8D). I/R-induced TNF-α expression was mostly prevented by FGF10, but such effect, was largely obliterated by rapamycin treatment. We next performed RT-qPCR to determine the mRNA expression of two other inflammatory cytokines *Il-1β* and *Il-6* in renal tissues. These results also demonstrated that I/R-induced expression of these cytokines could be effectively inhibited by FGF10, but not in the presence of rapamycin (Fig. 8E,F).

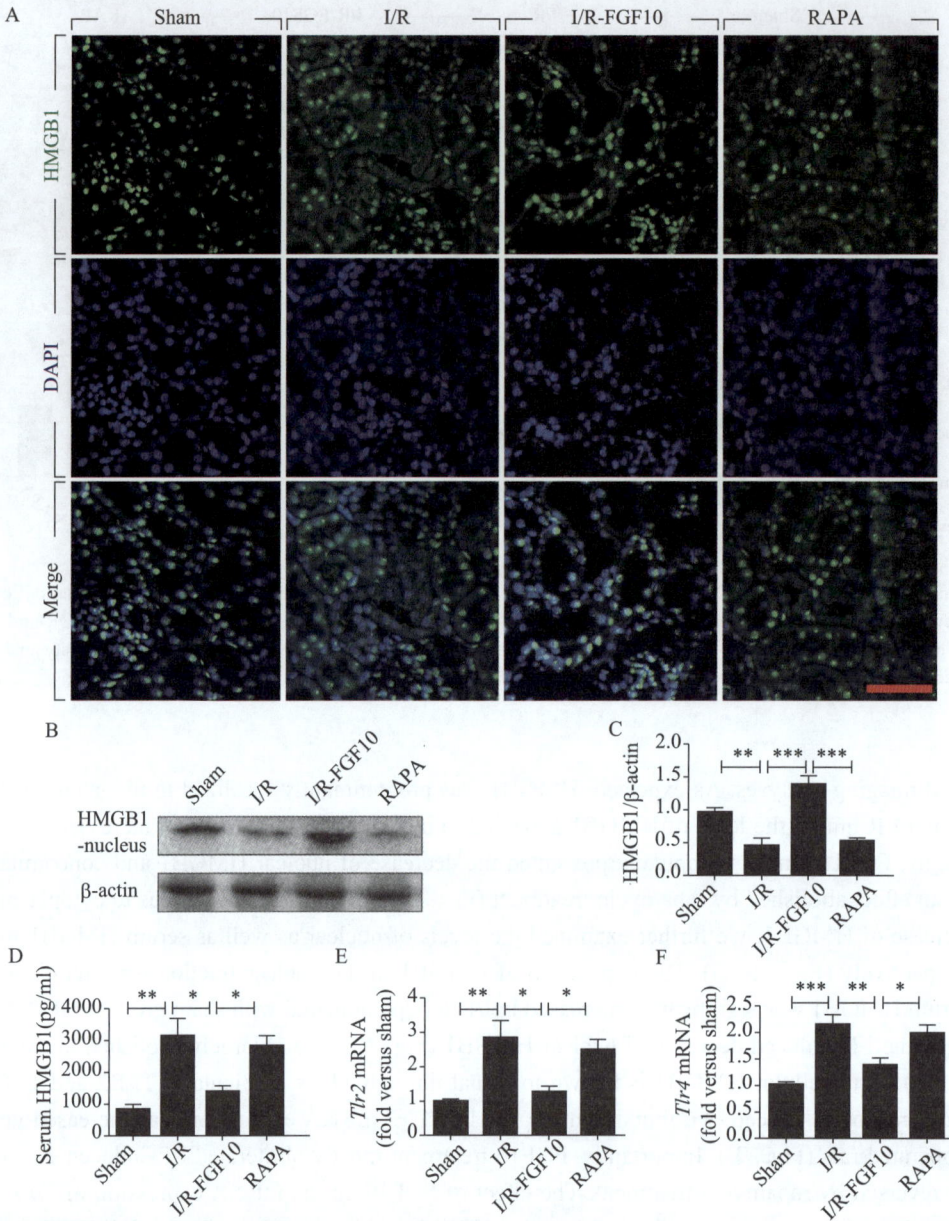

Fig. 7. FGF10 inhibits the release of nuclear HMGB1 to the serum and regulates the TLR mRNA expression. (A) Immunofluorescence staining of HMGB1 at 2 days after reperfusion. Nuclei were labeled with DAPI (blue). Scale bars = 50 μm. (B,C) Protein expression of HMGB1 in the nuclear fraction of renal tissues by Western blot and optical density analysis with β-actin as loading control (mean ± SEM; $n = 5$). $^{**}P < 0.01$, $^{***}P < 0.001$. (D) Level of serum HMGB1 was determined by ELISA (mean ± SEM; $n = 5$). $^{*}P < 0.05$, $^{**}P < 0.01$. (E,F) Expression of Tlr2 and Tlr4 mRNA in the kidney were examined by RT-qPCR and normalized to Gapdh. $^{*}P < 0.05$, $^{**}P < 0.01$, $^{***}P < 0.001$.

4. Discussion

FGF10, a multifunctional growth factor, is crucial in transmitting mesenchymal to epithelial signaling in organ development and regenerative medicine (Itoh, 2016). The role of FGF10 in cerebral ischemia injury, pulmonary fibrosis and wound healing, has been extensively researched (Li *et al.*, 2016; Tong *et al.*, 2016; Chao *et al.*, 2017; Chen *et al.*, 2017; El Agha *et al.*, 2017). As a typical paracrine growth factor, FGF10 and its predominant receptor FGFR2-IIIb play crucial roles in the development of kidney. However, the potential effect of FGF10 on AKI has not been reported so far. We herein used a well-established renal I/R model to investigate the potential protection effect of FGF10 against I/R injury. We confirmed that I/R rats were associated with increased SCr and BUN indicating a decline in the GFR. The current work provided experimental evidence that FGF10 administration effectively alleviated I/R-induced functional

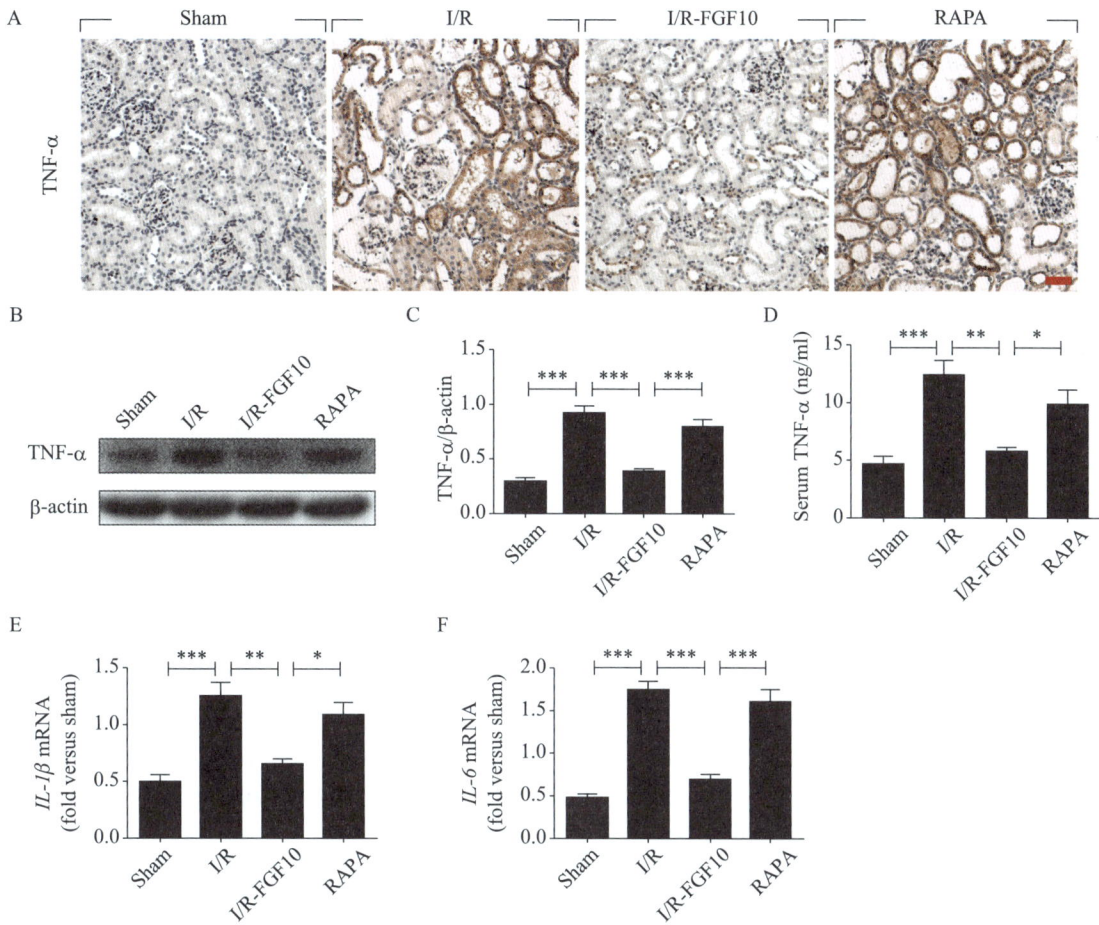

Fig. 8. FGF10 regulates the expression of inflammatory cytokines. (A) IHC staining for TNF-α in kidney tissues from indicated groups. Scale bars = 50 μm. (B,C) The expression of TNF-α was detected by western blot using TNF-α specific antibody. Optical density analyses (mean ± SEM; n = 5) with β-actin as control.(D) Levels of serum TNF-α were determined by ELISA (mean ± SEM; n = 5). $^*P$ < 0.05, $^{**}P$ < 0.01, $^{***}P$ < 0.001. (E,F) The mRNA expression of Il-1β and Il-6 in the kidney was examined by RT-qPCR and normalized to Gapdh. $^*P$ < 0.05, $^{**}P$ < 0.01, $^{***}P$ < 0.001.

impairment as well as histological damage of the kidney. Mechanistically, besides curbing apoptosis induction in RTCs, administration of FGF10 effectively alleviated the excessive autophagy, a common phenotype in RTCs exposed to I/R injury. HMGB1 is a damage-associated molecule that is rapidly released from nucleus to extracellular matrix and acts as a crucial molecule in the mediation of apoptosis and inflammation. We here demonstrated that FGF10 can inhibit the translocation of HMGB1 and thus attenuates RTC apoptosis upon I/R injury. Therefore, FGF10 treatment appears to protect kidneys from AKI *via* the regulation of autophagy and HMGB1 mediated inflammatory signaling pathways.

Extensive research has demonstrated that death of renal parenchyma cells, including apoptosis and necrosis, is the major mechanism underlying the pathogenesis of the AKI, as well as inflammation (Oberbauer *et al.*, 2001). The RTCs detached from basement membrane, along with other cellular debris, enter and obstruct the tubular lumen, thereby decrease GFR. Upon examining multiple parameters of cell death including TUNEL assays which detects both apoptosis and necrosis, as well as crucial mitochondrial regulators, we conclude that FGF10 treatment ameliorates the pro-apoptotic alteration of Bax/Bcl-2 as well Caspase-3, therefore RTC apoptosis following I/R injury. The results are in line with our previous studies showing that FGF2, another FGF family member, protects against renal I/R injury through attenuating mitochondrial damage (Tan *et al.*, 2017). Two recent studies suggested that neuron and microglia or macrophage-derived FGF10 participates in activation of PI3K/AKT/mTOR, which contributes to either ameliorate cerebral ischemia injury or improve functional recovery after spinal cord injury (Li *et al.*, 2016; Chen *et al.*, 2017). Further studies will be required to delineate the molecular mechanisms underlying FGF10 mediated protection against renal I/R injury.

A number of reports have established the involvement of autophagy in I/R-induced AKI in various animal models. In a myocardial I/R model, FGF2 is shown to improve heart function recovery and survival of cardiomyocytes through inhibition of excessive autophagy and increased ubiquitinated protein clearance *via* the activation of PI3K/AKT/mTOR signaling (Wang *et al.*, 2015). Under normal physiological conditions, basal autophagy is required to maintain homeostasis in both visceral epithelial cells (podocytes) and RTCs. So far, both the beneficial and detrimental effects of autophagy have been reported after renal I/R injury in animal experiments (Decuypere *et al.*, 2015; Kaushal and Shah, 2016; Lenoir *et al.*, 2016). Autophagy has been reported to have a protective role in cell survival by degrading misfolded/unfolded proteins, damaged organelles and generate necessary nutrient substance during AKI in some reports (Kimura *et al.*, 2011; Guan *et al.*, 2015; Xie *et al.*, 2018), whereas in others, it also causes apoptosis through excessive degradation of essential proteins and digestion of organelles (Shintani and Klionsky, 2004; Thorburn, 2008). Therefore, the role of autophagy in the pathogenesis and resolution of AKI injuries remains controversial, and is likely affected by the cellular context and also the extent of injury (Huber *et al.*, 2012).

Given that rapamycin, an mTOR inhibitor and agonist of autophagy, impaired the protective effect of FGF10 on renal function, we therefore further examined several well-established autophagy parameters by immunoblot, immunofluorescence staining and associated autophagic phenotypes. LC3 is a crucial cytoplasmic protein required for the formation and elongation of autophagosome. LC3 positive punctate formation and the conversation of LC3I to LC3II are often used to examine the induction of autophagy. Our immunofluorescent analysis of LC3 indicated that FGF10 treatment could prevent I/R-induced conversion of LC3I to LC3II and inhibited the formation of autophagic vacuoles and autophagosome. More strikingly, the effect of FGF10 on I/R-induced autophagy was nearly completely antagonized by rapamycin therefore establishing a role of autophagy in the protective effect of FGF10 again I/R injury. Consistent results were observed with the expression of Beclin-1, a marker of autophagosome as well as SQSTM1, an ubiquitously expressed protein which directly interacts with LC3 and subsequently degraded in autophagosome (Johansen and Lamark, 2011; Weidberg *et al.*, 2011). The decreased expression of SQSTM1 upon I/R injury was partially restored by FGF10 treatment. The data collectively suggest that FGF10 treatment could reduce autophagosome formation and inhibit excessive autophagy in RTCs after I/R injury *via* mTOR pathway.

Although both apoptosis and autophagy are rapidly induced in RTCs during AKI, but the role of autophagy in AKI is not as clear as apoptosis, and the interaction between apoptosis and autophagy in response to stimuli is complex and poorly defined. It is generally accepted that moderate autophagy may enhance the cellular ability to cope with stress response and thus promotes cell survival. Several studies have reported the renoprotective effect of autophagy in AKI caused by 25–40 min of renal ischemia-reperfusion (Kimura *et al.*, 2011; Jiang *et al.*, 2012; Xie *et al.*, 2018). Once the autophagy is exacerbated due to severe injury, the program of apoptosis would be activated and eliminate the irreversibly damaged cells. Our results clearly indicate that FGF10 treatment could alleviate the excessive autophagy induced by 60 min of I/R exposure and thus protects RTCs from apoptosis. Therefore the extent of renal injury may render autophagy to either alleviate or augment the I/R injury. However, no study has shown a definite demarcation point to distinguish the dual roles of autophagy on damaged cells. The regulatory mechanism between autophagy and apoptosis in response to I/R injury should be a focus of future studies.

The innate immune response is another integral pathological mechanism with AKI and the subsequent CKD. Emerging evidence suggests that the relationship between autophagy and inflammation is far more complicated than previously appreciated (Leventhal *et al.*, 2014). Both autophagy and immune response play crucial roles in the pathogenesis of AKI. Immune responses can affect the activation and perpetuation of autophagy in RTCs after reperfusion. Autophagy is identified a modulator that can both regulate and be regulated by immune responses in many diseases (Kaushal and Shah, 2016; Kimura *et al.*, 2017). Further research is needed to clarify the precise effects of autophagy on inflammation.

Many studies reported the multiple roles of HMGB1 in the pathogenesis of various diseases. However, the crosstalk between HMGB1 and apoptosis is complicated and requires further elucidation. HMGB1 shows dual roles in the regulation of apoptosis. Intracellular HMGB1 is generally an anti-apoptosis molecule, whereas overexpression of extracellular HMGB1 promotes apoptosis (Kang *et al.*, 2014). The two-way interaction between HMGB1 and autophagy has been wildly studied. Autophagy participates in various physiological and pathological processes including the release and degradation of HMGB1 (Thorburn *et al.*, 2009; Dupont *et al.*, 2011). Autophagy is regulated by HMGB1 which involves many molecules such as heat shock protein β-1 (HSPB1), Bcl-2 and Beclin-1 (Tang *et al.*, 2010b; Zhao *et al.*, 2011). Studies with HMGB1 knockout mice suggest that loss of HMGB1 leads to autophagy deficiency, whereas increased extracellular HMGB1 promotes autophagy through binding to Receptor for advanced glycation end products

(RAGE), a negative regulator of apoptosis (Tang *et al.*, 2010a; Yanai *et al.*, 2013). HMGB1 participates in the formation of renal fibrosis in the development of CKD through binding to TLR2 and RAGE. Therefore, future studies are warranted to explore the effect of FGF10 on CKD.

In summary, the present study demonstrates for the first time that exogenously administered recombinant FGF10 protects against I/R-induced functional and tissue damage to the kidney. The potent protective effect is attributed to its ability to attenuate several I/R-induced pro-apoptotic alteration of BCL2/BAX expression and Caspase-3 activation, therefor apoptotic cell death of renal parenchyma cells. The present work also indicates that protective effect of FGF10 against I/R injury is related to its down-regulation of excessive autophagy as well as release of HMGB1, Which in turn regulates pro-inflammatory immune response *via* TLR2/TLR4 signaling pathway. Apoptosis and autophagy are both rapidly activated upon renal I/R injury, which may interact with each other to govern the pathological and recovery processes of AKI. Our study suggests that FGF10 may provide a potential therapeutic option for treating AKI.

References

[1] Basile DP, Anderson MD, Sutton TA. Pathophysiology of acute kidney injury[J]. Comprehensive Physiology, 2012, 2(2): 1303-1353.

[2] Bates CM. Role of fibroblast growth factor receptor signaling in kidney development[J]. Pediatric Nephrology, 2007, 22(3): 343-349.

[3] Beenken A, Mohammadi M. The FGF family: biology, pathophysiology and therapy[J]. Nature Reviews Drug Discovery, 2009, 8(3): 235-253.

[4] Bonventre JV, Yang L. Cellular pathophysiology of ischemic acute kidney injury[J]. Journal Of Clinical Investigation, 2011, 121(11): 4210-4221.

[5] Chao CM, Yahya F, Moiseenko A, *et al.* FGF10 deficiency is causative for lethality in a mouse model of bronchopulmonary dysplasia[J]. Journal Of Pathology, 2017, 241(1): 91-103.

[6] Chen J, Wang Z, Zheng Z, *et al.* Neuron and microglia/macrophage-derived FGF10 activate neuronal FGFR2/PI3K/Akt signaling and inhibit microglia/macrophages TLR4/NF-kappa B-dependent neuroinflammation to improve functional recovery after spinal cord injury[J]. Cell Death & Disease, 2017, 8.

[7] Chen Q, Guan X, Zuo X, *et al.* The role of high mobility group box 1 (HMGB1) in the pathogenesis of kidney diseases[J]. Acta Pharmaceutica Sinica B, 2016, 6(3): 183-188.

[8] Chertow GM, Burdick E, Honour M, *et al.* Acute kidney injury, mortality, length of stay, and costs in hospitalized patients[J]. Journal Of the American Society Of Nephrology, 2005, 16(11): 3365-3370.

[9] Chien CT, Shyue SK, Lai MK. Bcl-xL augmentation potentially reduces ischemia/reperfusion induced proximal and distal tubular apoptosis and autophagy[J]. Transplantation, 2007, 84(9): 1183-1190.

[10] de Rechter S, Decuypere JP, Ivanova E, *et al.* Autophagy in renal diseases[J]. Pediatric Nephrology, 2016, 31(5): 737-752.

[11] Decuypere JP, Ceulemans LJ, Agostinis P, *et al.* Autophagy and the kidney: implications for ischemia-reperfusion injury and therapy[J]. American Journal Of Kidney Diseases, 2015, 66(4): 699-709.

[12] Dupont N, Jiang S, Pilli M, *et al.* Autophagy-based unconventional secretory pathway for extracellular delivery of IL-1 beta[J]. Embo Journal, 2011, 30(23): 4701-4711.

[13] el Agha E, Moiseenko A, Kheirollahi V, *et al.* Two-way conversion between lipogenic and myogenic fibroblastic phenotypes marks the progression and resolution of lung fibrosis[J]. Cell Stem Cell, 2017, 20(2): 261-273.

[14] Guan X, Qian Y, Shen Y, *et al.* Autophagy protects renal tubular cells against ischemia/reperfusion injury in a time-dependent manner[J]. Cellular Physiology And Biochemistry, 2015, 36(1): 285-298.

[15] Havasi A, Borkan SC. Apoptosis and acute kidney injury[J]. Kidney International, 2011, 80(1): 29-40.

[16] He L, Livingston MJ, Dong Z. Autophagy in acute kidney injury and repair[J]. Nephron Clinical Practice, 2014, 127(1-4): 56-60.

[17] Huber TB, Edelstein CL, Hartleben B, *et al.* Emerging role of autophagy in kidney function, diseases and aging[J]. Autophagy, 2012, 8(7): 1009-1031.

[18] Inoue K, Kuwana H, Shimamura Y, *et al.* Cisplatin-induced macroautophagy occurs prior to apoptosis in proximal tubules *in vivo*[J]. Clinical And Experimental Nephrology, 2010, 14(2): 112-122.

[19] Itoh N. FGF10: A multifunctional mesenchymal-epithelial signaling growth factor in development, health, and disease[J]. Cytokine & Growth Factor Reviews, 2016, 28: 63-69.

[20] Jang HR, Rabb H. The innate immune response in ischemic acute kidney injury[J]. Clinical Immunology, 2009, 130(1): 41-50.

[21] Jiang M, Wei Q, Dong G, *et al.* Autophagy in proximal tubules protects against acute kidney injury[J]. Kidney International, 2012, 82(12): 1271-1283.

[22] Johansen T, Lamark T. Selective autophagy mediated by autophagic adapter proteins[J]. Autophagy, 2011, 7(3): 279-296.

[23] Kalogeris T, Baines CP, Krenz M, *et al.* Cell biology of ischemia/reperfusion injury[A]. In: *International Review Of Cell And Molecular Biology, Vol 298* (Jeon KW, ed), Vol. 298, 2012: 229-317.

[24] Kang R, Chen R, Zhang Q, *et al.* HMGB1 in health and disease[J]. Molecular Aspects Of Medicine, 2014, 40: 1-116.

[25] Kaushal GP, Shah SV. Autophagy in acute kidney injury[J]. Kidney International, 2016, 89(4): 779-791.

[26] Kim HJ, Park SJ, Koo S, *et al.* Inhibition of kidney ischemia-reperfusion injury through local infusion of a TLR2 blocker[J]. Journal Of Immunological Methods, 2014, 407: 146-150.

[27] Kimura T, Isaka Y, Yoshimori T. Autophagy and kidney inflammation[J]. Autophagy, 2017, 13(6): 997-1003.

[28] Kimura T, Takabatake Y, Takahashi A, *et al.* Autophagy protects the proximal tubule from degeneration and acute ischemic injury[J]. Journal Of the American Society Of Nephrology, 2011, 22(5): 902-913.

[29] Lenoir O, Tharaux PL, Huber TB. Autophagy in kidney disease and aging: lessons from rodent models[J]. Kidney International, 2016, 90(5): 950-964.

[30] Leventhal JS, He JC, Ross MJ. Autophagy and immune response in kidneys[J]. Seminars In Nephrology, 2014, 34(1): 53-61.

[31] Li YH, Fu HL, Tian ML, *et al.* Neuron-derived FGF10 ameliorates cerebral ischemia injury *via* inhibiting NF-kappa B-dependent neuroinflammation and activating PI3K/Akt survival signaling pathway in mice[J]. Scientific Reports, 2016, 6.

[32] Lotze MT, Tracey KJ. High-mobility group box 1 protein (HMGB): Nuclear weapon in the immune arsenal[J]. Nature Reviews Immu-

nology, 2005, 5(4): 331-342.

[33] Mizushima N, Komatsu M. Autophagy: Renovation of cells and tissues[J]. Cell, 2011, 147(4): 728-741.

[34] Nikoletopoulou V, Markaki M, Palikaras K, *et al.* Crosstalk between apoptosis, necrosis and autophagy[J]. Biochimica Et Biophysica Acta-Molecular Cell Research, 2013, 1833(12): 3448-3459.

[35] Oberbauer R, Schwarz C, Regele HM, *et al.* Regulation of renal tubular cell apoptosis and proliferation after ischemic injury to a solitary kidney[J]. Journal Of Laboratory And Clinical Medicine, 2001, 138(5): 343-351.

[36] Ouyang F, Huang H, Zhang M, *et al.* HMGB1 induces apoptosis and EMT in association with increased autophagy following H/R injury in cardiomyocytes[J]. International Journal Of Molecular Medicine, 2016, 37(3): 679-689.

[37] Paller MS, Hoidal JR, Ferris TF. Oxygen free-radicals in ischemic acute-renal-failure in the rat[J]. Journal Of Clinical Investigation, 1984, 74(4): 1156-1164.

[38] Pallet N, Bouvier N, Legendre C, *et al.* Autophagy protects renal tubular cells against cyclosporine toxicity[J]. Autophagy, 2008, 4(6): 783-791.

[39] Shibutani ST, Saitoh T, Nowag H, *et al.* Autophagy and autophagy-related proteins in the immune system[J]. Nature Immunology, 2015, 16(10): 1014-1024.

[40] Shintani T, Klionsky DJ. Autophagy in health and disease: A double-edged sword[J]. Science, 2004, 306(5698): 990-995.

[41] Suzuki C, Isaka Y, Takabatake Y, *et al.* Participation of autophagy in renal ischemia/reperfusion injury[J]. Biochemical And Biophysical Research Communications, 2008, 368(1): 100-106.

[42] Tan X, Zhang L, Jiang Y, *et al.* Postconditioning ameliorates mitochondrial DNA damage and deletion after renal ischemic injury[J]. Nephrology Dialysis Transplantation, 2013, 28(11): 2754-2765.

[43] Tan XH, Zheng XM, Yu LX, *et al.* Fibroblast growth factor 2 protects against renal ischaemia/reperfusion injury by attenuating mitochondrial damage and proinflammatory signalling[J]. Journal Of Cellular And Molecular Medicine, 2017, 21(11): 2909-2925.

[44] Tang D, Kang R, Livesey KM, *et al.* Endogenous HMGB1 regulates autophagy[J]. Journal Of Cell Biology, 2010, 190(5): 881-892.

[45] Tang D, Lotze MT, Zeh HJ, *et al.* The redox protein HMGB1 regulates cell death and survival in cancer treatment[J]. Autophagy, 2010, 6(8): 1181-1183.

[46] Thadhani R, Pascual M, Bonventre JV. Medical progress-Acute renal failure[J]. New England Journal Of Medicine, 1996, 334(22): 1448-1460.

[47] Thorburn A. Apoptosis and autophagy: regulatory connections between two supposedly different processes[J]. Apoptosis, 2008, 13(1): 1-9.

[48] Thorburn J, Frankel AE, Thorburn A. Regulation of HMGB1 release by autophagy[J]. Autophagy, 2009, 5(2): 247-249.

[49] Tong L, Zhou J, Rong L, *et al.* Fibroblast growth factor-10 (FGF-10) mobilizes lung-resident mesenchymal stem cells and protects against acute lung injury[J]. Scientific Reports, 2016, 6.

[50] Ueda N, Kaushal GP, Shah SV. Apoptotic mechanisms in acute renal failure[J]. American Journal Of Medicine, 2000, 108(5): 403-415.

[51] Wang Z, Wang Y, Ye J, *et al.* bFGF attenuates endoplasmic reticulum stress and mitochondrial injury on myocardial ischaemia/reperfusion *via* activation of PI3K/Akt/ERK1/2 pathway[J]. Journal Of Cellular And Molecular Medicine, 2015, 19(3): 595-607.

[52] Weidberg H, Shvets E, Elazar Z. Biogenesis and cargo selectivity of autophagosomes[A]. In: *Annual Review Of Biochemistry, Vol 80* (Kornberg RD, Raetz CRH, Rothman JE *et al.*, eds), Vol. 80, 2011: 125-156.

[53] Wu H, Ma J, Wang P, *et al.* HMGB1 contributes to kidney ischemia reperfusion injury[J]. Journal Of the American Society Of Nephrology, 2010, 21(11): 1878-1890.

[54] Xie Y, Xu F, Li D, *et al.* Efficient message authentication scheme with conditional privacy-preserving and signature aggregation for vehicular cloud network[J]. Wireless Communications & Mobile Computing, 2018.

[55] Xu W, Jiang H, Hu X, *et al.* Effects of high-mobility group box 1 on the expression of Beclin-1 and LC3 proteins following hypoxia and reoxygenation injury in rat cardiomyocytes[J]. International Journal Of Clinical And Experimental Medicine, 2014, 7(12): 5353-5357.

[56] Xu Y, Guo M, Jiang W, *et al.* Endoplasmic reticulum stress and its effects on renal tubular cells apoptosis in ischemic acute kidney injury[J]. Renal Failure, 2016, 38(5): 831-837.

[57] Yanai H, Matsuda A, An J, *et al.* Conditional ablation of HMGB1 in mice reveals its protective function against endotoxemia and bacterial infection[J]. Proceedings Of the National Academy Of Sciences Of the United States Of America, 2013, 110(51): 20699-20704.

[58] Zhao M, Yang M, Yang L, *et al.* HMGB1 regulates autophagy through increasing transcriptional activities of JNK and ERK in human myeloid leukemia cells[J]. Bmb Reports, 2011, 44(9): 601-606.

[59] Zuk A, Bonventre JV. Acute kidney injury[A]. In: *Annual Review Of Medicine, Vol 67* (Caskey CT, ed), Vol. 67, 2016: 293-307.

Reduction of cellular stress is essential for Fibroblast growth factor 1 treatment for diabetic nephropathy

Yanqing Wu, Xiaokun Li, Jian Xiao

1. Introduction

Diabetes mellitus (DM) is one kind of lifelong metabolic diseases characterized by multiple causes of hyperglycemia, leading to a series of complications with diabetic retinopathy, diabetic neuropathy, and diabetic nephropathy (DN).[1] DN is one of the most common and serious complications of diabetic patients. The patho-mechanism of DN is multifactorial and complicated. Free fatty acids, advanced glycated end products (AGEs), autophagy, and angiotensin II receptor pathway are known to be participated in the development of DN.[2] With a rising prevalence of diabetes, it is greatly important to illuminate molecular mechanism underlying DN and seek the proper and effective treatment strategies to reduce patient morbidty and financial burden due to DN.

Cellular stress is a component of the development of various kidney diseases.[3,4] Our mechanism studies have revealed that elevated oxidative stress and ER stress are the causal events for diabetes-related complications.[5,6] Oxidative stress is a condition in which generation of reactive oxygen species (ROS) exceeds the capacity of the antioxidant defense system, caused by increased ROS production and impaired antioxidant capacity.[7] Subsequent studies have also implicated that the NADPH oxidases (NOX) family of enzymes as major cytosolic sources of superoxide, and it is now appreciated that several sources exist within the cell that contribute to the increased oxidative stress accompanying diabetes.[4] It has been demonstrated hyperglycemia induces oxidative and nitrosative stress, and increases renal functional impairment *via* nuclear factor erythroid-2 related factor 2 (Nrf2) signalling.[8,9] Evidence suggests that ER stress not only contributes to the pathogenesis of acute kidney diseases, but also has a role in the progression to chronic kidney diseases. Treatment with 4-PBA (an ER stress inhibitor) attenuates the increases of renal ER stress markers, α-smooth muscle actin (α-SMA), connective tissue growth factor, tubulointerstitial fibrosis and apoptosis.[3,10]

Fibroblast growth factor 1 (FGF1) is an autocrine/paracrine regulator and known to act on cells from a variety of tissue origins including the liver, vasculature, and skin, exerting classic mitogenic activity [11] and neuroprotective role.[12] Our previous study had demonstrated that FGF1 treatment ameliorated diabetes-induced nephropathy by inhibiting inflammation *via* JNK/NF-κB signalling pathway.[13] But there are no studies to focus on the effect of FGF1 on cellular stress during FGF1 treatment for DN. It is well known that hyperglycemia resulting in glucotoxicity is the main factor for diabetes-induced complications.[5,6] As an insulin sensitizer, FGF1 is also capable of impinging on multiple pathways mediating homeostatic control of normal glycemia.[14,15] FGF1 reduces the level of oxidative stress in high glucose treated H9c2 cells and HMVECs.[16] Our previous study had also demonstrated that FGF1 treatment blocks ER stress and consequently apoptosis of DA neuron during development of Parkinson's disease (PD).[17] Moreover, FGF23, the FGF family, has also an anti-oxidative stress activity.[18,19] Thus, we hypothesized that FGF1-associated glucose decreases and subsequent reduction of cellular stress is the another potential cellular molecule mechanisms mediating FGF1 treatment for DN.

In present study, we had further confirmed the protective role of FGF1 on DN with attenuation of renal fibrosis and glomerulosclerosis. Moreover, it was found that FGF1 administration blocked diabetes-induced oxidative stress though NOX2-ROS-Nrf2 signalling, and elevated ER stress evidencing with induction of ER stress makers in kidney. Current study suggests that reduction of cellular stress is the another potential molecular mechanism underlying FGF1 treatment for DN, which further replenishes the molecular mechanism underlying FGF1 treatment for DN.

2. Materials and methods

2.1 Animal and experimental design

12-week old male db/db (C57BLKS/J-leprdb/leprdb) mice and their nondiabetic db/m littermates were purchased from the Model Animal Research Center of Nanjing University (Nanjing, China). The animals were maintained under a 14-h light/10-h dark condition. After arrived, the animals were acclimatized to animal house before use. The db/db mice were divided into two groups and intraperitoneally (i.p.) injected either with FGF1 (0.5 mg/kg body weight) or physiologic saline every other day for 4 weeks. After 4 weeks, blood glucose level and body weight were measure. The serum was used for detection the levels of MDA (Beyotime, Shanghai, China), SOD (Beyotime) and AOC (Beyotime) using assay kits. The kidneys from mice were collected for biochemical and molecular analyses.

2.2 H & E staining and immunohistochemistry

The kidneys were collected and fixed with 4% paraformaldehyde in phosphate-buffered saline (PBS). Kidneys were dehydrated in alcohol and embedded with paraffin. After that, 5-μm sections were dewaxed and hydrated, then stained with hematoxylin and eosin (H&E) and observed under light microscope. After dewaxing and hydration, the sections were also incubated in 3% H_2O_2 for 15 minutes and then in blocking solution for 45 minutes. Subsequently, the sections were incubated at 4℃ over-night with the following primary antibodies: α-SMA (1:500; Abcam, Cambridge, UK), Collagen I(1:500; Abcam), Collagen III (1:500; Abcam), SOD2 (1:500; Santa Cruz Biotechnology, Santa Cruz, CA, USA) and HO-1 (1:200; Santa Cruz Biotechnology). After washing in PBS three times, the sections were incubated with horseradish peroxidase-conjugated secondary antibodies for 2 hours at 37℃. Then, the sections were reacted with 3, 3-diaminobenzidine (DAB). The results were imaged using a Nikon ECLPSE 80i (Nikon, Tokyo, Japan).

2.3 Immunofluorescence staining

The kidneys were collected and fixed with 4% paraformaldehyde in phosphate-buffered saline (PBS). Kidneys were dehydrated in alcohol and embedded with paraffin. After dewaxing, rehydrating and washing in PBS, the 5-μm sections were respectively incubated with 5% bovine serum albumin (BSA) in 37℃ oven for 0.5 hours. Then, the sections were incubated with mouse anti-IgM (1:400; Abcam) as primary antibody in 4℃ overnight. After triple washing in PBS at room temperature, the sections were once again incubated with donkey anti-mouse TR (1:1000; Abcam) as secondary antibody for 4 h. Fluorescence images were captured using a Nikon ECLPSE 80i.

2.4 Masson staining and PAS staining

Briefly, the kidneys were collected and fixed with 4% paraformaldehyde in phosphate-buffered saline (PBS). After dewaxing, rehydrating, and washing in PBS, 5-μm thick paraffin-embedded cardiac tissue sections were stained using standard masson trichrome staining kits (Solarbio Science & Technology, Beijing, China, G1340) and PAS staining kits (Solarbio Science & Technology, G1280) according to the manufacturer's instructions. Digital pictures were captured using a Nikon ECLPSE 80i.

2.5 Immunoblotting

Immunoblotting was performed as previously described. Briefly, the kidneys from different experimental groups were sonicated in the lysis buffer, containing a protease inhibitor cocktail (Sigma, St Louis, MO). Equal amounts of protein and the Precision Plus Protein Standards (Bio-Rad, Hercules, CA, USA) were resolved by SDS-PAGE electrophoresis and transferred onto PVDF membranes. Membranes were incubated in 5% nonfat milk for 45 min and then incubated for 18 hours at 4℃ with the primary antibodies at dilution of 1:1000 in 5% non-fat milk. To test whether equivalent amounts of protein were loaded among all samples, membranes were stripped and incubated with a mouse antibody against GADPH (Abcam) to generate a signal used as a loading control. Using the Super Signal West Femto Maximum Sensitivity Substrate kit (Thermo Scientific, Rockford, IL, USA), chemiluminescence emitted from the bands was directly captured using a UVP Bioimage EC3 system. Densitometric analysis of chemiluminescence signals was performed using VisionWorks LS software. The quantitative analysis of protein was calculated as the densitometric value of phosphorylated protein level/the densitometric value of unphosphorylated protein. All experiments were repeated in triplicate with the use of independently prepared tissue lysates.

2.6 Dihydroethidium (DHE) staining

Dihydroethidium staining was used to detect superoxide. DHE reacts with superoxide that is bound to cellular components including protein and DNA and exhibits bright red fluorescence. The kidneys were fixed in 4% paraformaldehyde (PFA) for 30 minutes, washed three times with PBS (5 minutes per wash), and then embedded in OCT. 10-mm frozen embryonic sections were incubated with 1.5 mmol/L DHE for 5 minutes at room temperature, and then washed three times with PBS for 5 minutes per wash. Sections were counterstained with DAPI and mounted with aqueous mounting medium (Sigma).

2.7 Statistical analyses

Data were presented as means ± SEM. Experiments were repeated at least three times, and kidneys from each replicate were from different mice. Statistical differences were determined by one-way analysis of variance (ANOVA) using SigmaStat 3.5 software. In one-way ANOVA analysis, Turkey test was used to estimate the significance of the results ($P < 0.05$).

3. Results

3.1 FGF1 treatment ameliorated diabetes-induced renal injury

Here, we had confirmed that FGF1 significantly ameliorated diabetes-induced nephropathy. We found that FGF1 treatment significantly downregulated the blood glucose level of db/db mice (Fig. 1A). The ratio of kidney/body weight in db/db mice is significantly lower than that in db/m mice with remarkable nephrarctia in db/db group, which is reversed by FGF1 treatment (Fig. 1B, C). Morphological analysis showed significant renal interstitial fibrosis and glomerular damage in kidneys from db/db mice as indicated by glomerular mesangial expansion with hypercellularity, capillary collapse, and fibrous deposition in glomeruli and interstitial, which is significantly attenuated by FGF1 treatment (Fig. 1D). Additionally, the IgM was dispersively deposited in glomerular mesangium in db/db mice's kidney. FGF1 treatment significantly blocked IgM deposition in kidney (Fig. 1D). Taken together, above data further confirmed that FGF1 treatment ameliorated diabetes-induced renal dysfunction.

3.2 FGF1 treatment remitted diabetes-induced renal interstitial fibrosis

The expression levels of collagen and α-SMA in the outer medulla was used as the index of interstitial injury. We found that the positive staining areas of α-SMA and collagen I were significantly larger in the kidneys from db/db mice, but not collagen III, which were reversed by FGF1 treatment (Fig. 2A–D). Consistence with the immunohistochemical results, further quantitation of collagen I and α-SMA expression in kidneys by Western blot analyses also showed that the protein levels of α-SMA and collagen I in kidneys from db/db mice were significantly upregulated, but much lower in the FGF1 treatment group (Fig. 2E,F). These results suggested that FGF1 treatment remitted diabetes-induced renal interstitial fibrosis by abolishing the increases of collagen accumulation and α-SMA expressions in kidneys.

3.3 FGF1 treatment reduced diabetes-induced oxidative stress and nitrosative stress in kidney

Oxidative stress is the major molecular mechanism that involves in diabetic complication.[20,21] Here, we try to determine whether FGF1 treatment reverses diabetes-induced oxidative stress and subsequently ameliorates renal dysfunction. Oxidative stress markers and nitrosative stress markers were detected and presented in Fig. 3. It was found that lipid peroxidation (LPO) (MDA/mg protein), antioxidant biomarker (superoxide dismutase, SOD) in serum was significantly upregulated in kidney from db/db group (Fig. 3A, B), and the total antioxidant capacity (AOC) levels in diabetic kidney was significantly less than those in control group (Fig. 3C). Although the SOD level in serum was upregulated, SOD1 and SOD2 expression levels in kidney were significantly downregulated in db/db mice when compared with those in

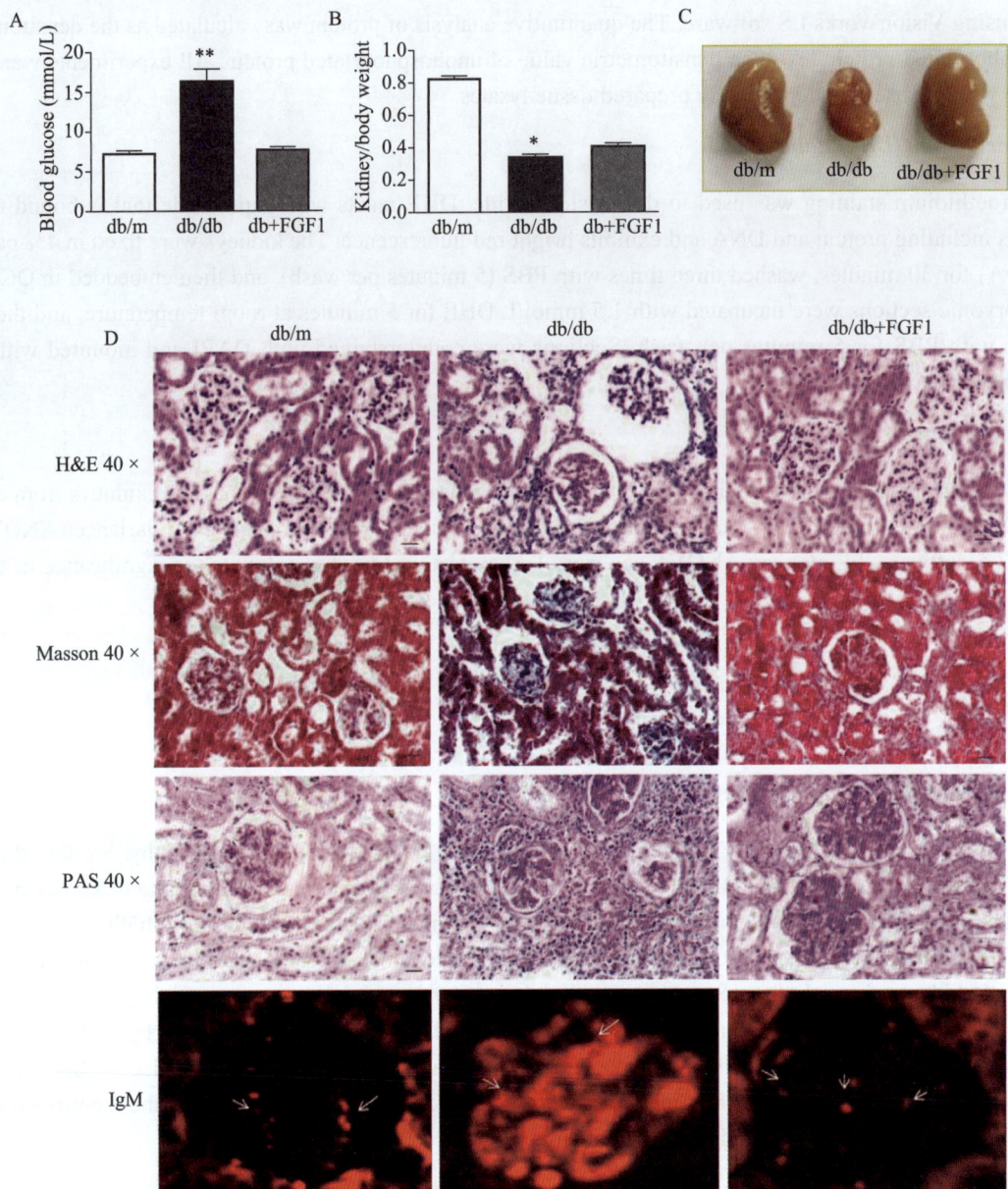

Fig. 1. FGF1 treatment ameliorated diabetes-induced renal injury. (A) Blood glucose level of mice from db/m, db/db and db+FGF1 group after fasting for 16 h; (B) The ratio of kidney/body weight of mice from db/m, db/db and db+FGF1 group; (C) Morphological appearance of kidney from db/m, db/db and db+FGF1 group; (D) The H&E, Masson staining, PAS staining and IgM staining of kidney from db/m, db/db and db+FGF1 group. All data are presented as the mean ± SEM, $n = 3$. $^{*}P < 0.05$ and $^{**}P < 0.01$ vs. the db/m group and db+FGF1 group.

db/m group and FGF1 treatment group (Fig. 3F–H). Elevated level of nitrotyrosine modified protein is indicative of nitrosative stress. Level of nitrotyrosine modified protein in diabetic kidney was significantly higher than that in control group (Fig. 3D). NOX activity is increased in different animal models of renal injury, which participates in the generation of superoxide and/or hydrogen peroxide. Here, we found that FGF1 administration significantly suppressed diabetes-induced overexpression of NOX2 in kidney (Fig. 3E). The positive signalling of DHE staining in kidney from db/m group and FGF1 treatment group (Fig. 3G, I). Moreover, FGF1 treatment suppressed diabetes-induced down-regulation of Nrf2 expression (Fig. 4A, B). However, the expression level of HO-1 level was upregulated (Fig. 4A–D). Taken together, FGF1 treatment reversed diabetes-induced oxidative stress and nitrosative stress in kidney.

3.4 FGF1 treatment suppressed diabetes-induced ER stress and up-regulation of Bax in kidney

To detect whether FGF1 treatment inhibited diabetes-induced ER stress in kidney, we had detected the expression

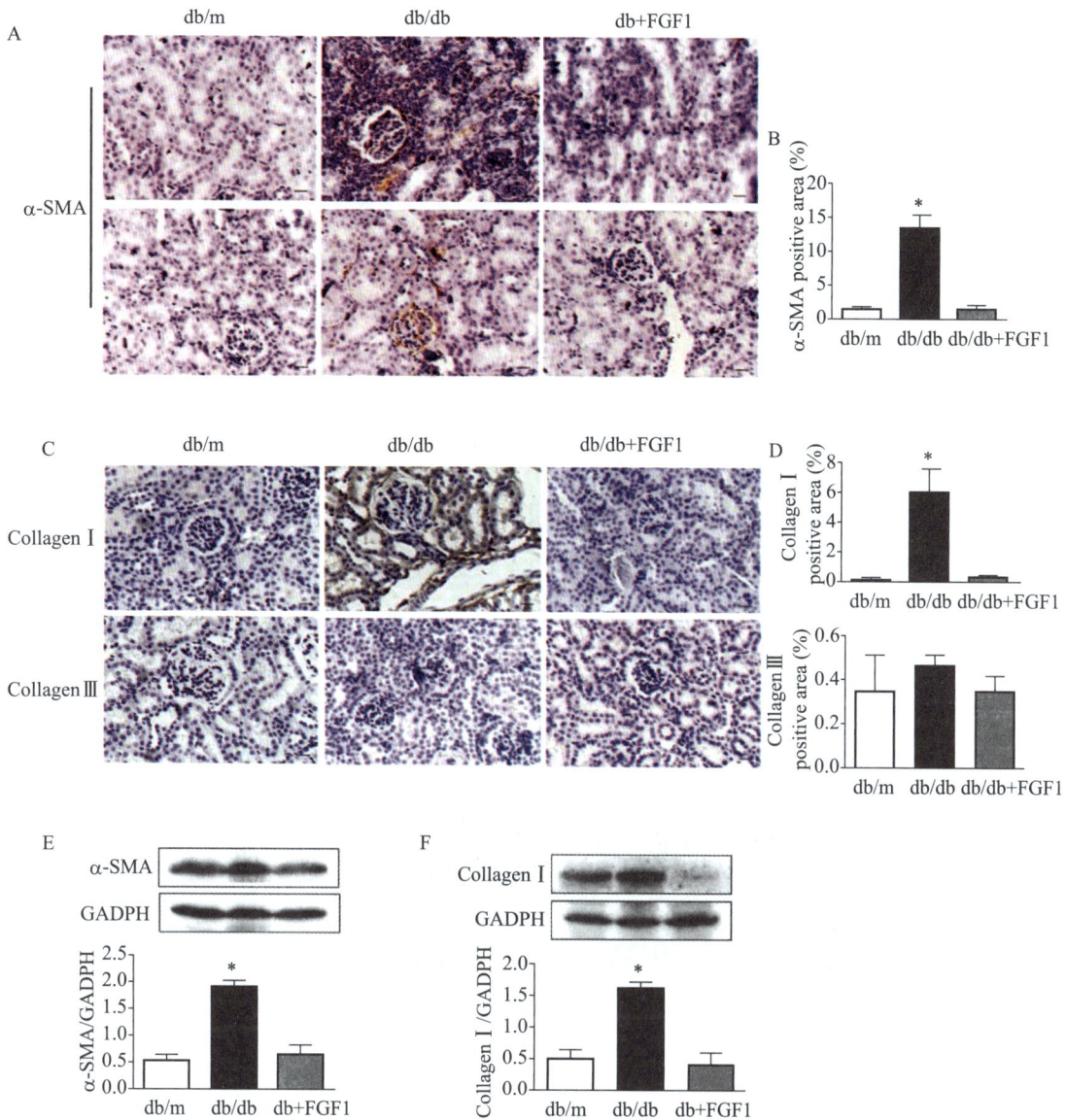

Fig. 2. FGF1 treatment remitted diabetes-induced renal interstitial fibrosis. (A–D), Immunohistochemical staining of α-SMA, collagen I and collagen III of kidney from db/m, db/db and db+FGF1 group (scale bars = 30 μm); (E, F) The protein expression of α-SMA and collagen I of kidney from db/m, db/db and db+FGF1 group. All data are presented as the mean ± SEM, $n = 3$. *$P < 0.05$ vs. the db/m group and db+FGF1 group.

levels of ER stress markers. The protein levels of phosphorylated protein kinase RNA-like ER kinase (p-PERK), phosphorylated inositol-requiring protein-1α (p-IRE1α), activating transcription factor 6 (ATF6), glucose regulated protein 78 (GRP78) and C/EBP-homologous protein(CHOP) in kidney were significantly induced by diabetes (Fig. 5A, B). FGF1 treatment significantly suppressed diabetes-induced ER stress (Fig. 5A, B). Consistence with Western blotting results, the fluorescence intensity of CHOP was up-regulated in kidney from db/db mice (Fig. 5D, E). Moreover, elevated expression level of Bax was observed in kidneys from db/db mice (Fig. 5C). Our current results suggest that ER stress may be involved in the FGF1 administration-mediated attenuation of DN.

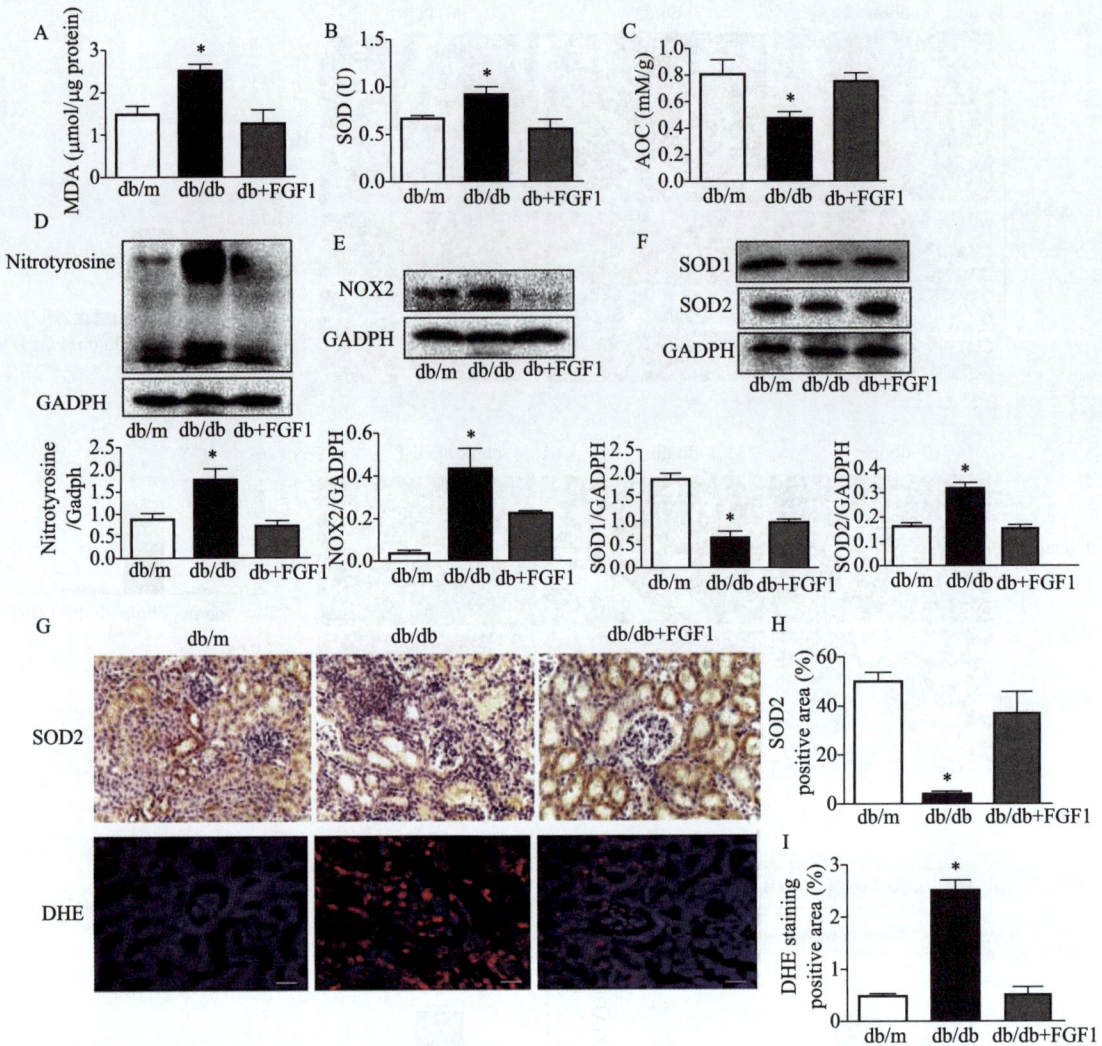

Fig. 3. FGF1 treatment reduced diabetes-induced oxidative stress and nitrosative stress in kidney. (A–C) The levels of MDA, SOD and AOC of serum from db/m, db/db and db+FGF1 group; (D–F) The protein expression of nitrotyrosine, NOX2, SOD1 and SOD2 of kidney from db/m, db/db and db+FGF1 group; (G, H) Immunohistochemical staining of SOD2 of kidney from db/m, db/db and db+FGF1 group (scale bars = 30 μm); (G, I) DHE staining of kidney from db/m, db/db and db+FGF1 group (scale bars = 30 μm). All data are presented as the mean ± SEM, $n = 3$. *$P < 0.05$ *vs.* the db/m group and db+FGF1 group.

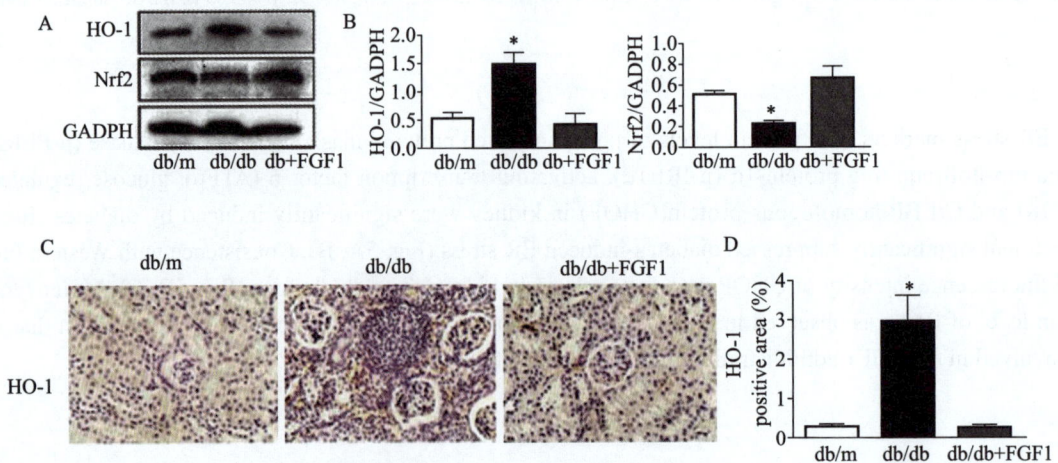

Fig. 4. The effect of Nrf2/HO-1 signalling during FGF1 administration for diabetes-induced oxidative stress and nitrosative stress in kidney. (A, B) The protein expression of HO-1 and Nrf2 of kidney from db/m, db/db and db+FGF1 group; (C, D) Immunohistochemical staining of HO-1 of kidney from db/m, db/db and db+FGF1 group (scale bars = 30 μm). All data are presented as the mean ± SEM, $n = 3$. *$P < 0.05$ *vs.* the db/m group and db+FGF1 group.

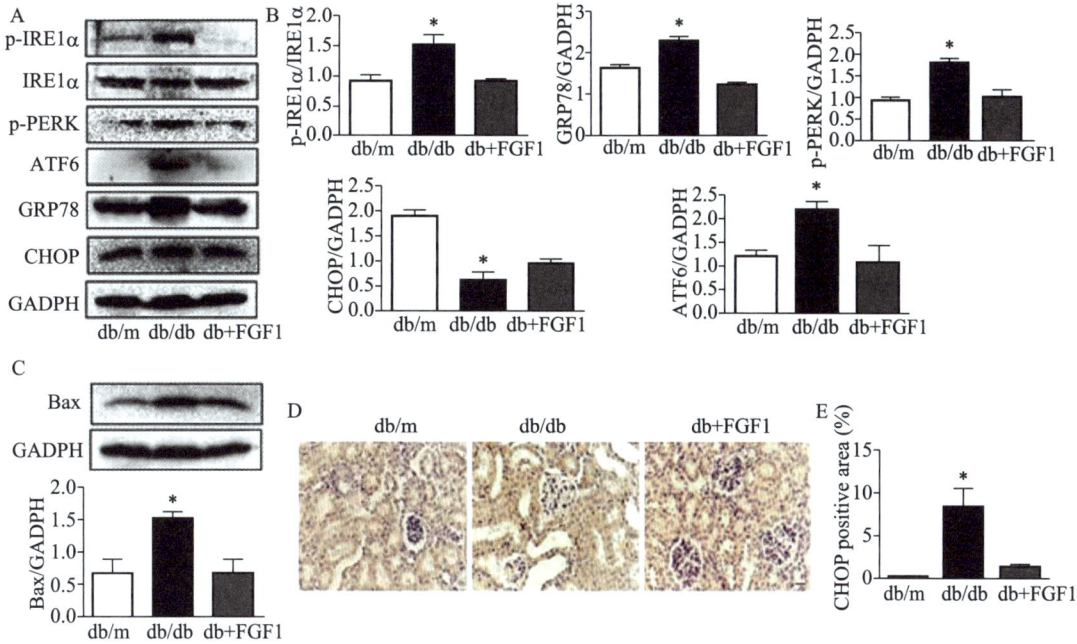

Fig. 5. FGF1 treatment suppressed diabetes-induced ER stress and up-regulation of Bax in kidney. (A) The protein expression of p-PERK, p-IRE1α, ATF6, GRP78 and CHOP of kidney from db/m, db/db and db+FGF1 group; (B) Intensities of p-IRE1α normalized to IRE1α, p-PERK, ATF6, CHOP and GRP78 normalized to GADPH; (C) The protein expression of Bax of kidney from db/m, db/db and db+FGF1 group; (D, E), Immunohistochemical staining of CHOP of kidney from db/m, db/db and db+FGF1 group (scale bars = 30 μm). All data are presented as the mean ± SEM, $n = 3$. $^*P < 0.05$ vs. the db/m group and db+FGF1 group.

4. Discussion

DN is a serious and common complication of diabetes, which leads to end-stage kidney disease,[4,22] and therefore, it is important to illuminate the mechanisms and explore the effective therapeutic strategy for DN. Specific treatment of patients with diabetic nephropathy can be divided into 4 major arenas: cardiovascular risk reduction, glycemic control, blood pressure control, and inhibition of the reninangiotensin system (RAS).[1] Our previous studies have demonstrated that FGF1 administration protected against renal injury by reducing inflammation.[13] Based on previous study, our current study had further confirmed that FGF1 administration ameliorated diabetes-induced glomerular damage and interstitial fibrosis. Mechanistic studies had found that the induction of cellular stress in diabetic kidneys was blocked by FGF1 treatment, indicating that reduction of cellular stress is another potential crucial molecular mechanism during FGF1 treatment for DN.

Our current study had demonstrated that FGF1 treatment blocked diabetes-associated α-SMA overexpression and collagen accumulation. Histologically, progressive kidney disease is marked by renal fibrosis and glomerulosclerosis.[4,23] It is well known that α-SMA is the marker of cell transdifferentiation, including epithelial–mesenchymal transition (EMT) and fibroblast activation into myofibroblast, which importantly contributes to the progression of CKD.[24,25] Our results suggest that FGF1 treatment may be involved in the relatively early stage of pathogenic process of DN via ameliorating tubulointerstitial damage.

Our current study had verified the important regulatory effect of FGF1 for cellular stress during DN. Previous studies had reported that FGF1 suppressed the oxidative stress and consequently blocked diabetes-induced cardiomyopathy.[16] Our current study has found that FGF1 treatment blocked the diabetes-induced oxidative stress during DN. It was widely regarded that elevated cellular stress is a major causal event of diabetes-associated the onset of complications.[6,26] Diabetes significantly induces oxidative stress [27] and ER stress.[28] Hemodialysis and CKD patients manifest impaired mitochondrial respiration indicative of dysregulated aerobic metabolism and increased oxidative stress.[29] NADPH oxidases (NOX) family has been significantly induced during renal injury, and reduced NOX activity is associated with renal protection in pre-clinical models of CKD.[30,31] Nox1, Nox2, and Nox4, which are expressed in both human and rodent kidneys, have a central role in mediating oxidative stress in CKD.[32] These studies suggest that oxidative stress, involving various reactive oxygen and nitrogen species, exerts a promoted role in the progress of CKD development.[4]

Consistence with prior studies, we found that diabetes significantly triggered oxidative stress evidencing with the upregulated expression of nitrotryosine and NOX2, and reduction of SODs expression and AOC activity in kidney from db/db mice. FGF1 treatment blocked the dysfunction of oxidability and antioxidant ability in kidney.

Nrf2 signalling regulates expression of many genes that oppose inflammatory and oxidative damage, including HO-1, SODs, and NQO1, which is protective in various models of renal disease. In current study, diabetes significantly induced down-regulation of Nrf2 expression and SODs, but the expression level of HO-1 level was upregulated. It was well known that the Nrf2 signalling may compensatorily increase for responding to acute stress. In our study, the mice were under hyperglycemia condition for a long time, which exceeds the compensatory capacity and leads to the down-regulation of Nrf2 and SODs. We speculate that the expression of HO-1 will also decrease as time gone on. These data indicated that FGF1 treatment ameliorated hyperglycemia and subsequently oxidative stress during DN *via* NOX2-ROS-Nrf2 signalling.

Multiple studies have shown that induction of ER stress are responsible for the pathogenetic progression of DN.[3,33] ER stress occurs when misfolded proteins accumulate in the ER lumen and cause ER dysfunction, which is known as unfolded protein response (UPR).[34,35] The UPR is mediated by the activation of three major sensors: IRE1, PERK and ATF6, which are suppressed by binding to GRP78. Upon ER stress is activated, GRP78 is released from the combination of IRE1, PERK and ATF6 to bind accumulated dysfunctional proteins.[36] Our data are consistent with the prior finding where it was shown that diabetes significantly triggered ER stress markers expression in kidney, which was blocked by FGF1 treatment.

FGF1, is an autocrine/paracrine regulator whose binding to heparan sulphate proteoglycans, plays a role on proliferation, neuroprotection and effectively normalizing hyperglycemia in T2D mice. Previous studies had found that pharmacologically relevant FGF1 doses (0.5 mg/kg) to T2D mouse models (ie, ob/ob or db/db) with impaired insulin sensitivity led to impressive changes in several measures of metabolism in which blood glucose was nearly normalized and long-lasting (35 days).[14] Our results expanded on this notion by showing that FGF1 blocked the hyperglycemia in db/db mice. Although type 2 diabetes is a complex metabolic disorder, hyper-glycemia with resulting glucotoxicity is a major mediator of diabetes-induced complications. The kidney is the main target organ involved in the major complications caused by diabetes mellitus.[1,37] Based on above results, we can conclude that FGF1 normalized the metabolic activity and subsequently blocked cellular stress, finally ameliorated kidney complications in diabetes.

An interesting finding in present study was verified that reduction of oxidative stress and ER stress contributes to the FGF1 treatment for DN. However, there are some limitations in present study. It has been postulated that ER stress is involved in redox homeostasis *via* activation of Nrf2.[8] But the causal relationship between oxidative stress and ER stress during DN is still unknown. Moreover, although our and other's studies have demonstrated that both cellular stress and inflammation are the potential mechanism contributing for FGF1 treatment for DN, whether cellular stress is mutually regulated with inflammation during DN still isn't elucidated. The present study did not further provide the evidence of the relationship between cellular stress and inflammation. Therefore, it is interesting to further explore the causal relationship between oxidative stress and ER stress, cellular stress, and inflammation during DN.

In summary, our current study has further confirmed the protective role of FGF1 on DN with attenuation of renal fibrosis and glomerulosclerosis, and demonstrated that FGF1 administration blocked diabetes-induced oxidative stress level through NOX2-ROS-Nrf2 signalling, and elevated ER stress (**Fig. 6**), suggesting that reduction of cellular stress

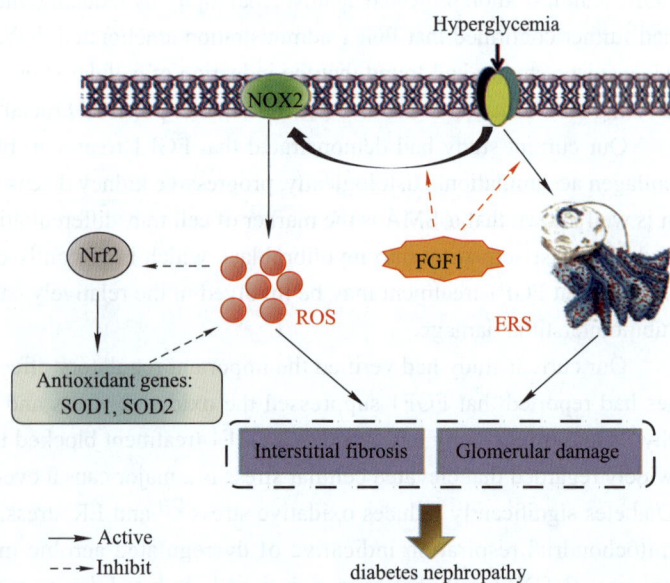

Fig. 6. A Schematic showing the effect of cellular stress during FGF1 treatment for Diabetic nephropathy. FGF1 treatment blocked hyperglycemia-induced oxidative stress though NOX2-ROS-Nrf2 signalling, and elevated ER stress in kidney, which ameliorated interstitial fibrosis and glomerular damage.

is another potential mechanism underlying FGF1 treatment for DN. These findings suggest that FGF1 also plays a potential renal protective effect for DN *via* exerting the effective glucose control function and subsequently reducing the cellular stress in kidney.

References

[1] Umanath K, Lewis JB. Update on Diabetic Nephropathy: Core curriculum 2018[J]. Am J Kidney Dis, 2018, 71(6): 884-895.

[2] Dadras F, Khoshjou F. Endoplasmic reticulum and its role in diabetic nephropathy[J]. Iran J Kidney Dis, 2015, 9(4): 267-272.

[3] Cybulsky AV. Endoplasmic reticulum stress, the unfolded protein response and autophagy in kidney diseases[J]. Nat Rev Nephrol, 2017, 13(11): 681-696.

[4] Lv W, Booz GW, Fan F, et al. Oxidative stress and renal fibrosis: recent insights for the development of novel therapeutic strategies[J]. Front Physiol, 2018, 9: 105.

[5] Wu Y, Reece EA, Zhong J, et al. Type 2 diabetes mellitus induces congenital heart defects in murine embryos by increasing oxidative stress, endoplasmic reticulum stress, and apoptosis[J]. Am J Obstet Gynecol, 2016, 215(3): 366.e361-366.e310.

[6] Wu Y, Wang F, Fu M, et al. Cellular Stress, Excessive apoptosis, and the effect of metformin in a mouse model of Type 2 diabetic embryopathy[J]. Diabetes, 2015, 64(7): 2526-2536.

[7] Wilcox CS. Oxidative stress and nitric oxide deficiency in the kidney: a critical link to hypertension?[J]. Am J Physiol Regul Integr Comp Physiol, 2005, 289(4): R913-935.

[8] Cullinan SB, Diehl JA. PERK-dependent activation of Nrf2 contributes to redox homeostasis and cell survival following endoplasmic reticulum stress[J]. J Biol Chem, 2004, 279(19): 20108-20117.

[9] Yoh K, Hirayama A, Ishizaki K, et al. Hyperglycemia induces oxidative and nitrosative stress and increases renal functional impairment in Nrf2-deficient mice[J]. Genes Cells, 2008, 13(11): 1159-1170.

[10] Yum V, Carlisle RE, Lu C, et al. Endoplasmic reticulum stress inhibition limits the progression of chronic kidney disease in the Dahl salt-sensitive rat[J]. Am J Physiol Renal Physiol, 2017, 312(1): F230-F244.

[11] Wu J, Zhu J, He C, et al. Comparative study of heparin-Poloxamer Hydrogel Modified bFGF and aFGF for *in Vivo* Wound Healing Efficiency[J]. ACS Appl Mater Interfaces, 2016, 8(29): 18710-18721.

[12] Wang Q, He Y, Zhao Y, et al. A Thermosensitive heparin-poloxamer hydrogel bridges aFGF to treat spinal cord injury[J]. ACS Appl Mater Interfaces, 2017, 9(8): 6725-6745.

[13] Liang G, Song L, Chen Z, et al. Fibroblast growth factor 1 ameliorates diabetic nephropathy by an anti-inflammatory mechanism[J]. Kidney Int, 2018, 93(1): 95-109.

[14] Suh JM, Jonker JW, Ahmadian M, et al. Corrigendum: Endocrinization of FGF1 produces a neomorphic and potent insulin sensitizer[J]. Nature, 2015, 520(7547): 388.

[15] Crunkhorn S. Metabolic disease: FGF1 stops diabetes in its tracks[J]. Nat Rev Drug Discov, 2016, 15(7): 456.

[16] Zhang C, Zhang L, Chen S, et al. The prevention of diabetic cardiomyopathy by non-mitogenic acidic fibroblast growth factor is probably mediated by the suppression of oxidative stress and damage[J]. PLoS One, 2013, 8(12): e82287.

[17] Wei X, He S, Wang Z, et al. Fibroblast growth factor 1attenuates 6-hydroxydopamine-induced neurotoxicity: an *in vitro* and *in vivo* investigation in experimental models of parkinson's disease[J]. Am J Transl Res, 2014, 6(6): 664-677.

[18] Ohta J, Rakugi H, Ishikawa K, et al. Klotho gene delivery suppresses oxidative stress *in vivo*[J]. Geriatrics & Gerontology International, 2007, 7: 293-299.

[19] Deng M, Luo Y, Li Y, et al. Klotho gene delivery ameliorates renal hypertrophy and fibrosis in streptozotocin-induced diabetic rats by suppressing the Rho-associated coiled-coil kinase signaling pathway[J]. Molecular medicine reports, 2015, 12(1): 45-54.

[20] Ruiz S, Pergola PE, Zager RA, et al. Targeting the transcription factor Nrf2 to ameliorate oxidative stress and inflammation in chronic kidney disease[J]. Kidney Int, 2013, 83(6): 1029-1041.

[21] Yang P, Reece EA, Wang F, et al. Decoding the oxidative stress hypothesis in diabetic embryopathy through proapoptotic kinase signaling[J]. Am J Obstet Gynecol, 2015, 212(5): 569-579.

[22] Bai X, Li X, Tian J, et al. A new model of diabetic nephropathy in C57BL/6 mice challenged with advanced oxidation protein products[J]. Free Radic Biol Med, 2018, 118: 71-84.

[23] Liu Y. Cellular and molecular mechanisms of renal fibrosis[J]. Nat Rev Nephrol, 2011, 7(12): 684-696.

[24] Strutz FM. EMT and proteinuria as progression factors[J]. Kidney Int, 2009, 75(5): 475-481.

[25] Zeisberg M, Kalluri R. The role of epithelial-to-mesenchymal transition in renal fibrosis[J]. J Mol Med (Berl), 2004, 82(3): 175-181.

[26] Wu Y, Wang F, Reece EA, et al. Curcumin ameliorates high glucose-induced neural tube defects by suppressing cellular stress and apoptosis[J]. American Journal Of Obstetrics And Gynecology, 2015, 212(6).

[27] Brownlee M. Biochemistry and molecular cell biology of diabetic complications[J]. Nature, 2001, 414(6865): 813-820.

[28] Wang F, Reece EA, Yang P. Superoxide dismutase 1 overexpression in mice abolishes maternal diabetes-induced endoplasmic reticulum stress in diabetic embryopathy[J]. American Journal Of Obstetrics And Gynecology, 2013, 209(4).

[29] Granata S, Zaza G, Simone S, et al. Mitochondrial dysregulation and oxidative stress in patients with chronic kidney disease[J]. Bmc Genomics, 2009, 10.

[30] Baltanás A, Miguel-Carrasco JL, San José G, et al. A synthetic peptide from transforming growth factor-β1 type III receptor inhibits NADPH oxidase and prevents oxidative stress in the kidney of spontaneously hypertensive rats[J]. Antioxidants & Redox Signaling, 2013, 19(14): 1607-1618.

[31] Holterman CE, Read NC, Kennedy CRJ. Nox and renal disease[J]. Clinical Science, 2015, 128(8): 465-481.

[32] Decleves AE, Sharma K. Novel targets of antifibrotic and anti-inflammatory treatment in CKD[J]. Nature Reviews Nephrology, 2014, 10(5): 257-267.

[33] Guo J, Zhu J, Ma L, et al. Chronic kidney disease exacerbates myocardial ischemia reperfusion injury: role of endoplasmic reticulum stress-mediated apoptosis[J]. Shock, 2018, 49(6): 712-720.

[34] Schroder M, Kaufman RJ. The mammalian unfolded protein response[J]. Annual Review Of Biochemistry, 2005, 74: 739-789.

[35] Hetz C. The unfolded protein response: controlling cell fate decisions under ER stress and beyond[J]. Nature Reviews Molecular Cell Biology, 2012, 13(2): 89-102.

[36] Lai E, Teodoro T, Volchuk A. Endoplasmic reticulum stress: Signaling the unfolded protein response[J]. Physiology, 2007, 22: 193-201.

[37] Tang L, Wu Y, Tian M, et al. Dapagliflozin slows the progression of the renal and liver fibrosis associated with type 2 diabetes[J]. Am J Physiol Endocrinol Metab, 2017, 313(5): E563-E576.

Chapter 3
Endocrinology and Metabolism

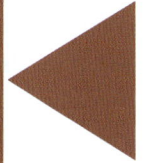

Fibroblast growth factor 21 (FGF21) therapy attenuates left ventricular dysfunction and metabolic disturbance by improving FGF21 sensitivity, cardiac mitochondrial redox homoeostasis and structural changes in pre-diabetic rats

Pongpan Tanajak, Xiaokun Li, Nipon Chattipakorn

Long-term consumption of a high-fat diet (HFD) causes obesity–insulin resistance (Pratchayasakul *et al.*, 2011; Pipatpiboon *et al.*, 2012) and fibroblast growth factor 21 (FGF21) resistance (Fisher *et al.*, 2010; Hale *et al.,* 2012; Patel *et al.,* 2014), leading to metabolic disturbance (Pratchayasakul *et al.*, 2011; Pipatpiboon *et al.*, 2012; Pintana *et al.*, 2014), impaired cardiac autonomic regulation and left ventricular (LV) dysfunction (Ouwens *et al.*, 2005, Apaijai *et al.*, 2012, 2013, 2014). Growing evidence demonstrates that FGF21 plays an important role in the regulation of energy metabolism (Chau *et al.*, 2010, Planavila *et al.*, 2013) and may exert cardioprotection (Patel *et al.*, 2014, Joki *et al.*, 2015, Yan *et al.*, 2015) in several pathological states such as cardiac ischaemia (Patel *et al.*, 2014) and cardiac hypertrophy (Planavila *et al.*, 2013). These benefits of FGF21 have been demonstrated to occur *via* its activation of the β-Klotho/ FGFR1c receptor complex on the cell surface membrane (Cong *et al.*, 2013, Planavila *et al.*, 2013, 2014, Patel *et al.*, 2014, Joki *et al.*, 2015, Tanajak *et al.*, 2015, Yan *et al.*, 2015, Yu *et al.*, 2015, Zhang *et al.*, 2015). FGF21 resistance was reported for the first time in 2010 by Fisher *et al.*. They found that HFD-induced obesity led to significantly increased FGF21 levels, and the heart responded poorly to the endogenous FGF21 levels and exogenous FGF21 administration in acute therapy, thus giving rise to the term 'FGF21 resistance' (Fisher *et al.*, 2010). Recently, (Patel *et al.*, 2014) demonstrated that short-term pre-treatment with FGF21 following cardiac ischaemia–reperfusion (I/R) injury in diet-induced obese rats responds poorly to exogenous FGF21 administration, indicating FGF21 resistance in the heart. Although short-term administration has been shown to be ineffective in cardioprotection (Fisher *et al.*, 2010, Patel *et al.*, 2014), the potential long-term FGF21 therapeutic benefits on FGF21 sensitivity, cardiac autonomic regulation, cardiac mitochondrial redox homoeostasis and structural changes and LV function in obesity–insulin resistance have not been investigated.

In this study, we tested the hypothesis that long-term FGF21 administration improves FGF21 sensitivity by increasing cardiac mitochondrial fatty acid β-oxidation (FAO) and cardiac anti-apoptotic signalling pathways and attenuating cardiac mitochondrial redox dyshomoeostasis and structural changes, leading to the improvement of cardiometabolic regulation and LV function in HFD-induced obese, insulin-resistant rats.

1. Materials and methods

1.1 Ethical approval

All experiments in this study were approved by the Faculty of Medicine, Chiang Mai University Institutional Animal Care and Use Committee (Permit No. 16/2558), were in compliance with NIH guidelines and were in accordance with the ARRIVE guidelines for reporting experiments involving animals (Kilkenny *et al.*, 2010).

1.2 Animals and diet

Eighteen adult male Wistar rats weighing 180–200 g were purchased from the National Animal Center, Salaya Campus, Mahidol University, Bangkok, Thailand. All rats were housed in a temperature- and humidity-controlled housing unit with a light–dark cycle of 12 : 12 h with controlled temperature (25℃). Rats were divided into two groups and received either a normal diet (ND) that contained 19.77% energy from fat or a HFD that contained 59.28% energy from fat for 12 weeks (Pratchayasakul *et al.*, 2011).

1.3 Drugs and vehicle

Recombinant human FGF21 (rhFGF21) was produced using *Escherichia coli* and purified to be endotoxin-free (Wang *et al.*, 2010). The rhFGF21 was obtained from Prof. Dr. Xiao Kun Li, Zhejiang Provincial Key Laboratory of Biopharmaceuticals, Wenzhou Medical College, Wenzhou, Zhejiang 325035, China. One vial (3.84 mg/vial; powder) was diluted in 10 ml 0.9% normal saline solution (NSS) to give a final concentration of 0.384 mg/ml. For a vehicle, 0.9% NSS was used in an equal volume to rhFGF21 (Apaijai *et al.*, 2012, 2014). Rats were injected intraperitoneally with vehicle or rhFGF21 (0.1 mg/kg) once a day for 28 days.

1.4 Experiment protocol

After acclimatization for 1 week, all rats were divided into two groups and received either a ND ($n = 6$) or a HFD ($n = 12$) for 12 weeks. Then, rats in the ND group continued to receive ND food, whereas rats in the HFD group were divided into two subgroups and receive one of the following treatments: vehicle (HFV; $n = 6$) or rhFGF21 (HFF; $n = 6$) for another 4 weeks. The body weight, food intake, heart rate variability (HRV), blood pressure (BP) and echocardiography were recorded at week 12 and at the end of the experiments. Metabolic parameter measurements including plasma glucose, insulin, high-density lipoprotein cholesterol (HDL-C), low-density lipoprotein cholesterol (LDL-C), total cholesterol (TC) and triglyceride (TG) were determined at week 12 and at the end of the experiments. Blood chemistry parameters including serum adiponectin, serum TNF-α and plasma FGF21 levels were also determined. To determine the insulin sensitivity, an oral glucose tolerance test (OGTT) was also carried out. At the end of the treatment protocol, the pressure–volume (P-V) loop was used to determine the LV function. Finally, the hearts were removed and used to determine the cardiac mitochondrial redox homoeostasis and structural changes, serum and cardiac tissue malondialdehyde (MDA) levels and cardiac FGF21 signalling cascade protein expression including β-Klotho, FGFR1, p-FGFR1, ERK1/2, p-ERK1/2, Bax, Bcl-2, cleaved caspase-3, PGC-1α and CPT-1 using Western blot analysis.

1.5 Metabolic parameter assessments

The plasma HDL-C level was determined using a commercial colorimetric assay kit (BioVision, Milpitas, CA, USA) (Apaijai *et al.*, 2013). The plasma glucose, TC and TG levels were determined using a colorimetric assay kit (ERBA Mannheim, Mannheim, Germany) (Pratchayasakul *et al.*, 2011, Apaijai *et al.*, 2014). The Friedewald equation was used to determine the plasma LDL-C level after plasma HDL-C, TC and TG were determined (Friedewald *et al.*, 1972, Apaijai *et al.*, 2014). The plasma insulin levels were determined using a commercial sandwich ELISA kit (LINCO Research, St. Charles, MO, USA) (Apaijai *et al.*, 2013, 2014). Finally, the homoeostasis model assessment (HOMA) index was calculated using the following formula: HOMA index = [Fasting plasma insulin (μU/ml)] × [fasting plasma glucose (mmol/L)/22.5]. Increased HOMA index indicates a higher degree of insulin resistance (Pipatpiboon *et al.*, 2012).

1.6 Serum TNF-α, adiponectin and plasma FGF21 assessments

Serum TNF-*α* level and serum adiponectin level were determined using an ELISA kit (Invitrogen, Life Technologies, Carlsbad, CA, USA). Plasma FGF21 levels were determined using the quantitative sandwich enzyme immunoassay technique for mouse/rat FGF21, the ELISA kit (R&D Systems, Minneapolis, MN, USA; Yan *et al.*, 2015).

1.7 Tail-cuff BP measurement

Non-invasive BP was determined using the volume–pressure recording (VPR) tail-cuff method CODA 2 (Kent Scientific Corporation, Torrington, CT, USA; Feng *et al.*, 2008). The BP was recorded at week 12 and at the end of the study. The animal warming platform was set at a controlled temperature of 32–35 ℃. The rats were placed into the holder, and the thumb nut was tightened to allow the tail of the animal to extend out of the rear of the holder. The cuff was attached onto the rat's tail using the occlusion cuff, placing it near the base, while the VPR cuff was placed at the distal end. An average of the BP was taken from 20 cycles of measurement.

1.8 Heart rate variability

Heart rate variability was determined from lead II ECG using PowerLab (ADInstruments, Colorado Springs, CO,

USA) equipped with the CHART 5.0 program for 20 min. The stable ECG that was displayed was used to determine the relationship between the RR interval and the beat numbers (tachogram) using a MATLAB program (Pratchayasakul *et al.*, 2011; Apaijai *et al.*, 2012, 2013). Power spectra of RR interval variability were obtained using the fast Fourier transform algorithm. The high-frequency (HF; 0.6–3 Hz) band, low-frequency (LF; 0.2–0.6 Hz) band and very low-frequency (VLF; below 0.1 Hz) band were detected. Each spectral component was calculated as integrals under the respective part of the power spectral density function and was presented in absolute units (ms^2) (Chattipakorn *et al.*, 2007). To minimize the effect of changes in total power on the LF and HF bands, LF and HF were expressed as normalized units by dividing the reading by the total power minus VLF (Chattipakorn *et al.*, 2007). The increase in the LF/HF ratio indicates an increase in sympathetic activity or depressed of HRV (Pongchaidecha *et al.*, 2009; Apaijai *et al.*, 2012, 2013).

1.9 Echocardiography for LV function assessment

The M-mode of echocardiography (Vivid i; GE Medical Systems, Aurora, OH, USA) was used to determine % fractional shortening (%FS) and was performed at the papillary muscle levels. The papillary muscle level was used as the positional landmark and the probe was adjusted to give the best image view. Then, the %FS was determined using the LV function mode. An increase in %FS was considered to be an indicator of increased LV function (Apaijai *et al.*, 2012, 2013).

1.10 P-V loop assessment

Rats were anaesthetized with Zoletil (50 mg/kg BW) and xylazine (0.15 mg/kg BW) *via* intramuscular injection before starting the P-V loop protocol. The right common carotid artery was identified, and a P-V loop catheter (Sciences, London, ON, Canada) was inserted into it. After that, the systolic BP (SBP) and diastolic BP were determined with the catheter staying in the ascending aorta. LV function including heart rate (HR), end-systolic pressure (ESP), end-diastolic pressure (EDP), dP/dt_{max}, dP/dt_{min} and stroke volume (SV), was determined when the catheter was advanced into the LV chamber. P-V loop data analysis was carried out using an analytical software program (LAB-SCRIBE2; iWorx System, Dover, NH, USA) (Apaijai *et al.*, 2013; Chinda *et al.*, 2014).

1.11 Measurements of cardiac mitochondrial redox homoeostasis and structural changes

The rats hearts were perfused with 10 ml of 0.9% NSS and removed rapidly. The hearts were then homogenized in ice-cold 7.2-pH buffer which contained 300 mM sucrose, 0.2 mM EGTA and 5 mM TES in 8 ml. The homogenates were centrifuged at 800 g, 4 ℃ for 5 min, and after that, the supernatant was kept and centrifuged at 8800 g, 4℃ for 5 min. The mitochondrial pellet was resuspended in 8 ml of isolation buffer and centrifuged at 8800 g, 4℃ for 5 min. The mitochondrial pellet from the last method was collected and resuspended in the respiration buffer in 2 ml per each buffer, and the protein concentration was determined using the UV-Vis spectrophotometer (UV-1700 series; BioSurplus, San Diego, CA, USA).

The cardiac mitochondrial reactive oxygen species (ROS) production was determined by incubating the mitochondria with 2 M DCFH-DA dye at 25 ℃ for 20 min, and the fluorescent intensity of the solution was detected by a fluorescent microplate reader with excitation wavelength at 485 nm and emission wave-length at 530 nm (BioTek Instruments, Winooski, VT, USA). An increase in the fluorescent intensity indicated an increased mitochondrial ROS production (Thummasorn *et al.*, 2011; Apaijai *et al.*, 2012, 2013; Chinda *et al.*, 2013).

The cardiac mitochondrial membrane potential change ($\Delta\psi$) was determined using 5 μM JC-1 dye and incubating the mitochondria with JC-1 at 37 ℃ for 30 min (Thummasorn *et al.*, 2011; Apaijai *et al.*, 2013, 2014). The changes in cardiac mitochondrial membrane potential were detected using a fluorescent microplate reader. The JC-1 monomer form concentration is represented by the green fluorescence and is excited by a wavelength of 485 nm, and the emission is detected at 590 nm. The aggregate form of JC-1 is represented by the red fluorescence and is excited at a wavelength of 485 nm, and the emission is detected at 530 nm. A decrease in the red/green fluorescent intensity ratio indicates an increase in cardiac mitochondrial membrane depolarization (Thummasorn *et al.*, 2011; Apaijai *et al.*, 2012, 2013; Chinda *et al.*, 2013).

The cardiac mitochondrial swelling was determined by incubating cardiac mitochondria with 1.5 mM respiration buffer. The absorbance was determined using a spectrophotometer. A decreased absorbance indicated increased cardiac mitochondrial swelling (Thummasorn *et al.*, 2011; Apaijai *et al.*, 2012, 2013; Chinda *et al.*, 2013).

The cardiac mitochondria were collected during the cardiac mitochondrial redox homoeostasis assessment and fixed by 2.5% glutaraldehyde in a 0.1 M phosphate buffer overnight. After that, they were fixed in a 1% cacodylate buffer–osmium tetroxide for 2 h, and a graded series of ethanols were used to dehydrate them. A diamond knife was used to cut the cardiac mitochondria embedded in Epon–Araldite and stained with uranyl acetate. Finally, the cardiac mitochondrial morphology was observed using a transmission electron microscope (Thummasorn *et al.*, 2011; Apaijai *et al.*, 2014).

1.12   Plasma and cardiac MDA by HPLC assay

The fresh cardiac tissues and serum were used to determine the MDA concentration levels by HPLC-based assay (Thermo Scientific, Bangkok, Thailand). Plasma and cardiac MDA levels were mixed with H_3PO_4 and thiobarbituric acid (TBA) to produce TBA-reactive substances (TBARS). The plasma and cardiac TBARS concentrations were determined directly from a standard curve and reported as equivalent to the MDA concentration (Apaijai *et al.*, 2012, 2013).

1.13   Western blot analysis

Fresh heart tissues from the LV apex were obtained for the determination of the FGF21 signalling pathways at the end of experiments, as described in the previous studies (Palee *et al.*, 2013; Surinkaew *et al.*, 2013). The FGF21 signalling protein expression and phosphorylation were determined, including FGFR1 and p-FGFR1 as a dilution of 1 : 200 (Sigma-Aldrich, Singapore, Singapore), β-Klotho, PGC-1α, and CPT-1 as a 1 : 200 dilution (Santa Cruz Biotechnology, Dallas, TX, USA), ERK1/2, p-ERK1/2, Bax, cleaved caspase-3 as a 1 : 1000 dilution (Santa Cruz Biotechnology, Dallas, TX, USA), β-actin as a 1 : 2000 dilution (Santa Cruz Biotechnology, Dallas, TX, USA) and Bcl-2 as a 1 : 1000 dilution (Cell Signaling Technology, Danvers, MA, USA).

The horse anti-mouse IgG conjugate HRP-linked antibody in a 1:2,000 dilution (Cell Signaling Technology, Danvers, MA, USA) was used to detect the β-actin (Surinkaew *et al.*, 2013); the rabbit anti-goat IgG conjugate HRP-linked antibody in a 1 : 2000 dilution (Santa Cruz Biotechnology, Dallas, TX, USA) was used to detect the for β-Klotho; and goat anti-rabbit IgG conjugate HRP-linked antibody in a 1 : 2000 dilution (Cell Signaling Technology, Danvers, MA, USA) was used to detect the following proteins: FGFR1, p-FGFR1, ERK1/2, p-ERK1/2, Bax, Bcl-2, cleaved caspase-3, PGC-1α and CPT-1. The ChemiDoc touch imaging system (Bio-Rad Laboratories, Hercules, CA, USA) was used to expose the membrane using the Chemiluminescence mode (Besic *et al.*, 2015; Kmiecik *et al.*, 2015; Liu *et al.*, 2015; Tor *et al.*, 2015). Finally, the ImageJ program was used to determine the densitometry which was normalized with β-actin (Chinda *et al.*, 2014).

1.14   Statistical analysis

Data were expressed as mean ± SEM. A one-way ANOVA followed by LSD *post hoc* test was used to test the difference between the groups. $P < 0.05$ was considered statistically significant.

2.   Results

2.1   FGF21 restores the metabolic disturbance, lipid peroxidation and blood chemistry

At 16 weeks after HFD feeding, the results showed that the body weight, visceral fat, plasma insulin, plasma TC, plasma LDL-C, serum MDA levels, serum TNF-α, the area under the curve (AUCg) by OGTT and HOMA index were increased in the HFD rats, compared with the NDV group (Table 1). Our results showed that the heart weight was not different between groups. However, the heart weight/body weight ratio was lower in the HFV rats, whereas this parameter was increased in the HFF rats (Table 1). This is due to the fact that the body weight was markedly increased in the HFV group, whereas the body weight was significantly decreased in the HFF rats. Moreover, serum adiponectin and plasma HDL-C were decreased in the HFD group, compared with the NDV group. The FGF21 therapy significantly decreased the body weight, visceral fat, plasma insulin, plasma TC, plasma HDL-C, serum and tissue MDA levels, serum TNF-α, AUCg and HOMA index, compared with the HFV group. Moreover, serum adiponectin and plasma HDL-C were increased in the HFF group, compared with the HFV group (Table 1).

Table 1.   Effects of FGF21 treatment on metabolic parameters in HFD-induced obese, insulin-resistant rats

Parameters	Groups		
	NDV	HFV	HFF
Body weight (g)	440 ± 22	672 ± 15*	595 ± 20*,†
Visceral fat (g)	19 ± 2	66 ± 1*	56 ± 3*,†
Heart weight (g)	1.23 ± 0.02	1.25 ± 0.02	1.25 ± 0.01
HW/BW ratio (g/kg)	2.69 ± 0.09	1.86 ± 0.06*	2.10 ± 0.07*,†
Food intake (g/day)	28 ± 1	30 ± 1	29 ± 1
Plasma glucose (mg/dl)	124 ± 3	137 ± 6	132 ± 4
Plasma TC (mg/dl)	78 ± 3	113 ± 8*	86 ± 1†
Plasma TG (mg/dl)	62 ± 6	55 ± 2	55 ± 2
Plasma LDL-C (mg/dl)	38 ± 3	64 ± 7*	41 ± 5†
Plasma HDL-C (mg/dl)	35 ± 1	25 ± 2*	36 ± 2†
Serum adiponectin (μg/ml)	24.2 ± 3.7	8.7 ± 2.9*	25.7 ± 2.8†
Serum TNF-α (pg/ml)	0.6 ± 0.1	2.6 ± 0.5*	1.6 ± 0.3†
Plasma insulin (ng/ml)	2.5 ± 0.1	4.6 ± 0.6*	2.9 ± 0.3†
HOMA index	15.2 ± 0.9	33.2 ± 8.6*	17.7 ± 1.9†
Serum MDA (μmol/ml)	1.36 ± 0.03	3.36 ± 1.05*	1.15 ± 0.17†
AUCg (mg/dl × min × 10^4)	49 252 ± 2330	67 362 ± 4643*	53 578 ± 3050†

HFD, high-fat diet; NDV, normal diet treated with vehicle; HFV, high-fat diet treated with vehicle; HFF, high-fat diet treated with FGF21; TC, total cholesterol; TG, triglyceride; LDL-C, low-density lipoprotein cholesterol; HDL-C, high-density lipoprotein cholesterol; TNF-α, tumour necrosis factor-alpha; HOMA, homoeostasis model assessment; MDA, malondialdehyde; AUCg, area under the curve.

*$P < 0.05$ vs. NDV, †$P < 0.05$ vs. HFV.

2.2 FGF21 restores the BP and LV function impaired by HFD

At 16 weeks after HFD feeding, the results showed that the HFD significantly increased SBP, mean arterial pressure (MAP) and HR, compared with the NDV. However, rats in the HFF group had significantly decreased SBP, MAP and HR, compared with the HFV group (Table 2). Regarding LV function, the P-V loop results showed that there was a significant increase in EDP, and a decrease in ESP, TdP/dt and SV in the HFV group, compared with the NDV group (Table 2). In the HFF group, there was a significant decrease in EDP, and an increase in ESP, TdP/dt and SV, compared with the HFV group (Table 2).

Table 2.   Effects of FGF21 treatment on blood pressure and left ventricular function in high-fat diet-induced obese, insulin-resistant rats

Parameters	Groups		
	NDV	HFV	HFF
SBP (mmHg)	129 ± 5	153 ± 2*	139 ± 3†
DBP (mmHg)	85 ± 3	85 ± 3	86 ± 5
MAP (mmHg)	100 ± 4	115 ± 1*	102 ± 5†
HR (beats/min)	393 ± 6	416 ± 6*	398 ± 5†
ESP (mmHg)	132 ± 5	116 ± 1*	126 ± 1†
EDP (mmHg)	19 ± 1	35 ± 1*	21 ± 1†
+dP/dt (mmHg s^{-1})	8290 ± 36	6029 ± 184*	8816 ± 294†
−dP/dt (mmHg s^{-1})	−5627 ± 198	−4040 ± 165*	−5813 ± 246†
SV (ml/gBW)	1.02 ± 0.04	0.74 ± 0.08*	1.05 ± 0.03†

SBP, systolic blood pressure; DBP, diastolic blood pressure; MAP, mean arterial pressure; HR, heart rate; ESP, end-systolic pressure; EDP, end-diastolic pressure; SV, stroke volume.

*$P < 0.05$ vs. NDV, †$P < 0.05$ vs. HFV.

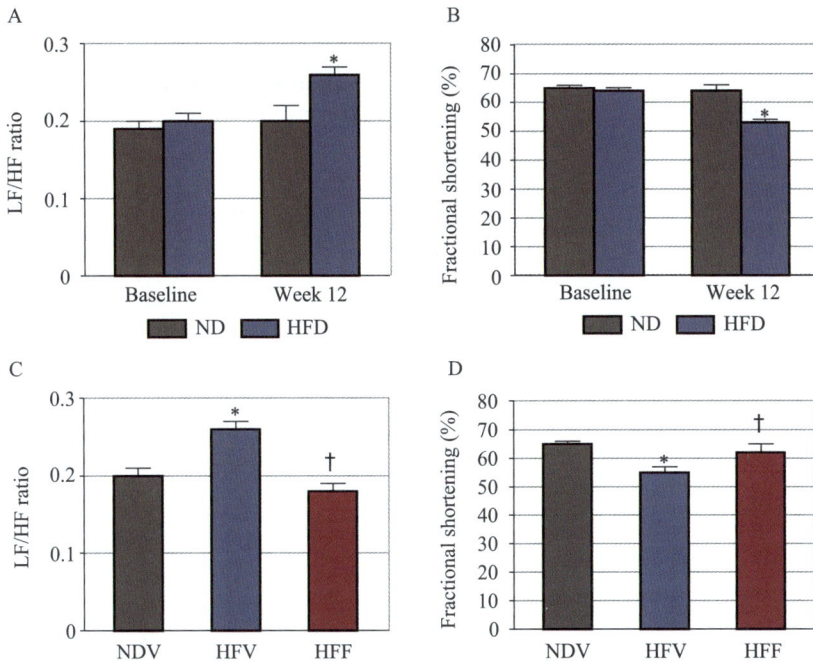

Fig. 1. Effects of HFD consumption and FGF21 treatment on HRV and echocardiographic parameters. (A) HRV and (B)% fractional shortening (%FS) in ND and HFD rats at baseline and week 12. *$P < 0.05$ vs. ND. (C) HRV and (D)% FS in ND and HFD rats treated with vehicle and FGF21. *$P < 0.05$ vs. NDV, †$P < 0.05$ vs. HFV. HRV, heart rate variability; HFD, high-fat diet; ND, normal diet; NDV, normal diet treated with vehicle; HFV, high-fat diet treated with vehicle; HFF, high-fat diet treated with FGF21.

2.3 FGF21 restores the HRV impaired by HFD

For the HRV, the results showed that HFD significantly increased the LF/HF ratio since week 12 in the HFD rats, compared with the ND (Fig. 1A). In the same way, it was found that %FS was significantly decreased at week 12 in the HFD group, compared with the ND group (Fig. 1B). After 16 weeks of HFD feeding, there was still a significant increase in the LF/HF ratio in the HFV rats, compared with the NDV group. However, the LF/HF ratio was significantly decreased after FGF21 administration in the HFF group, compared with the HFV group (Fig. 1C). Moreover, %FS also significantly decreased in the HFV group, compared with the NDV group. The %FS also significantly increased after FGF21 treatment in the HFF rats, compared with the HFV group (Fig. 1D).

2.4 FGF21 restores the FGF21 sensitivity by increased FGFR1 phosphorylation in the heart

The levels of plasma FGF21 were significantly higher in the HFD group, compared to the ND rats at week 12 of HFD feeding (Fig. 2A). Plasma FGF21 levels at week 16 were also significantly increased in the HFV group, compared with the NDV group (Fig. 2B). However, the plasma FGF21 levels were significantly increased in the HFF (894.9 ± 64.1 pg/ml) group, compared with the HFV and NDV groups (Fig. 2B).

The FGF21 receptor complex in the heart was significantly altered after HFD feeding. At 16 weeks after HFD feeding, there were significantly decreased levels of FGFR1 phosphorylation (p-FGFR1) (Fig. 2C) and the p-FGFR1/t-FGFR1 ratio (Fig. 2E) in the HFV rats, compared with the NDV group. FGF21 treatment significantly increased the levels of p-FGFR1/β-actin (Fig. 2C) and the p-FGFR1/t-FGFR1 ratio (Fig. 2E) in the HFF rats, compared with the HFV group. However, no difference was found in total FGFR1 (t-FGFR1) (Fig. 2D) and β-Klotho levels (Fig. 2F) between groups.

2.5 FGF21 restores the secondary messenger ERK1/2, antiapoptotic and mitochondrial FAO signalling pathways in the heart

Our results showed that there was no significant difference in the levels of p-ERK1/2 (Fig. 3A) and t-ERK1/2 (Fig. 3B) between the NDV, HFV and HFF rats. However, a significant decrease in the p-ERK1/2/ t-ERK1/2 ratio was observed in the HFV rats (Fig. 3C), compared with the NDV group. Moreover, a significant increase in the p-ERK1/2/t-ERK1/2 ratio (Fig. 3C) was also observed in the HFF rats, compared with the HFV group.

Regarding apoptosis, a significant increase in Bax level (Fig. 4A), Bax/Bcl-2 ratio (Fig. 4C) and the cleaved caspase-3/t-caspase-3 ratio (Fig. 4D) was found in the HFV rats, compared with the NDV group. In addition, a significant increase in Bcl-2 (Fig. 4B), PGC-1α (Fig. 4E) and CPT-1 (Fig. 4F) was found in the HFV rats, compared with the NDV group. However, no significant difference in the levels of t-caspase-3 was found between all groups (Fig. 4D).

In the HFF rats, a significant decrease in the levels of Bax (Fig. 4A), Bax/Bcl-2 ratio (Fig. 4C) and the cleaved cas-

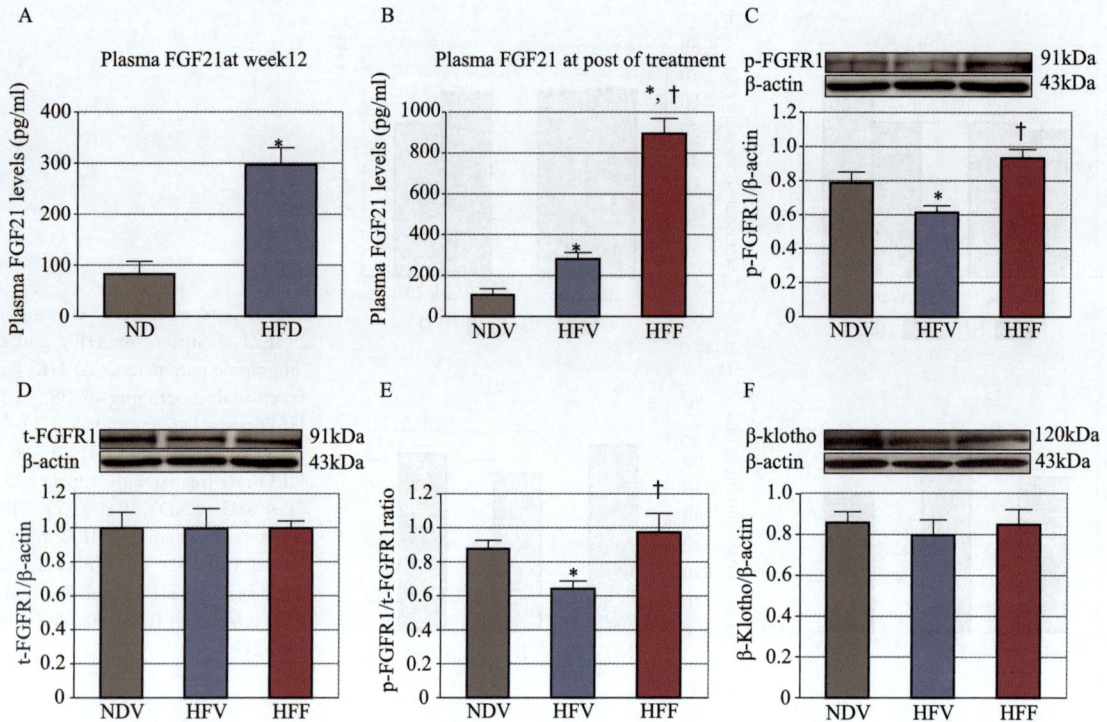

Fig. 2. Effects of HFD consumption and FGF21 treatment on plasma FGF21 levels and FGFR1/β-klotho receptors complex. (A) Plasma FGF21 levels at week 12, (B) plasma FGF21 levels post-treatment, (C) p-FGFR1, (D) t-FGFR1, (E) p-FGFR1/t-FGFR1 and (F) β-klotho in ND and HFD rats treated with vehicle and FGF21. $^*P < 0.05$ *vs.* NDV, $^{†}P < 0.05$ *vs.* HFV. HFD, high-fat diet; ND, normal diet; NDV, normal diet treated with vehicle; HFV, high-fat diet treated with vehicle; HFF, high-fat diet treated with FGF21; FGFR1, fibroblast growth factor receptor 1.

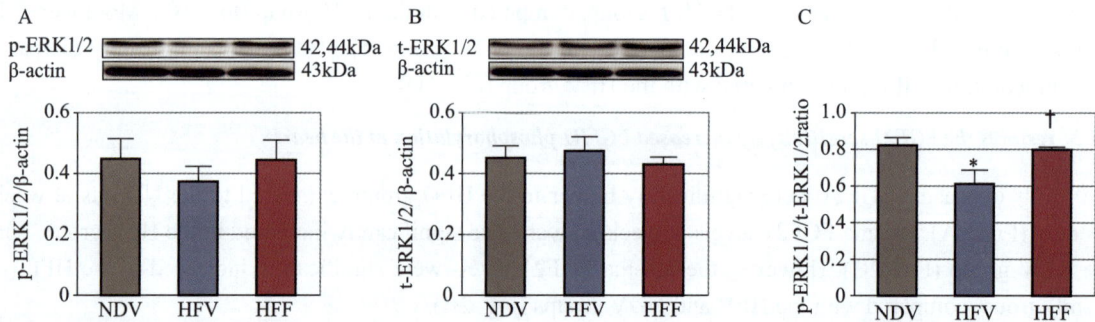

Fig. 3. Effects of HFD consumption and FGF21 treatment on the ERK1/2 expression and phosphorylation. (A) p-ERK1/2, (B) t-ERK1/2 and (C) p-ERK1/2/t-ERK1/2 ratio in ND and HFD rats treated with vehicle and FGF21. $^*P < 0.05$ *vs.* NDV, $^{†}P < 0.05$ *vs.* HFV. HFD, high-fat diet; ND, normal diet; NDV, normal diet treated with vehicle; HFV, high-fat diet treated with vehicle; HFF, high-fat diet treated with FGF21; ERK1/2, extracellular signal regulated protein kinases 1 and 2.

pase-3/t-caspase-3 ratio was observed (Fig. 4D), compared with the HFV group. Moreover, a significant increase in the levels of Bcl-2 (Fig. 4B), PGC-1α (Fig. 4E) and CPT-1 was found (Fig. 4F) in the HFF rats, when compared to the HFV group.

2.6 FGF21 restores cardiac mitochondrial redox homoeostasis, structural changes and lipid peroxidation

In the HFV rats, there was a significant increase in cardiac mitochondrial ROS production (Fig. 5A), cardiac mitochondrial depolarization (Fig. 5B) and cardiac mitochondrial swelling (Fig. 5C), compared with the NDV group. However, after FGF21 treatment, the cardiac mitochondrial ROS production (Fig. 5A) was significantly decreased in the HFF rats, compared with the HFV group. In addition, cardiac mitochondrial depolarization (Fig. 5B), cardiac mitochondrial swelling (Fig. 5C) and cardiac lipid peroxidation (Fig. 5E) were significantly decreased in the HFF rats, compared with the HFV group. The representative electron micrographs illustrate the cardiac mitochondrial morphology with unfolded cristae in the heart of the HFV rat indicating mitochondrial swelling, and the FGF21 treatment attenuated the swelling as indicated by increased folded cristae in the mitochondria (Fig. 5D).

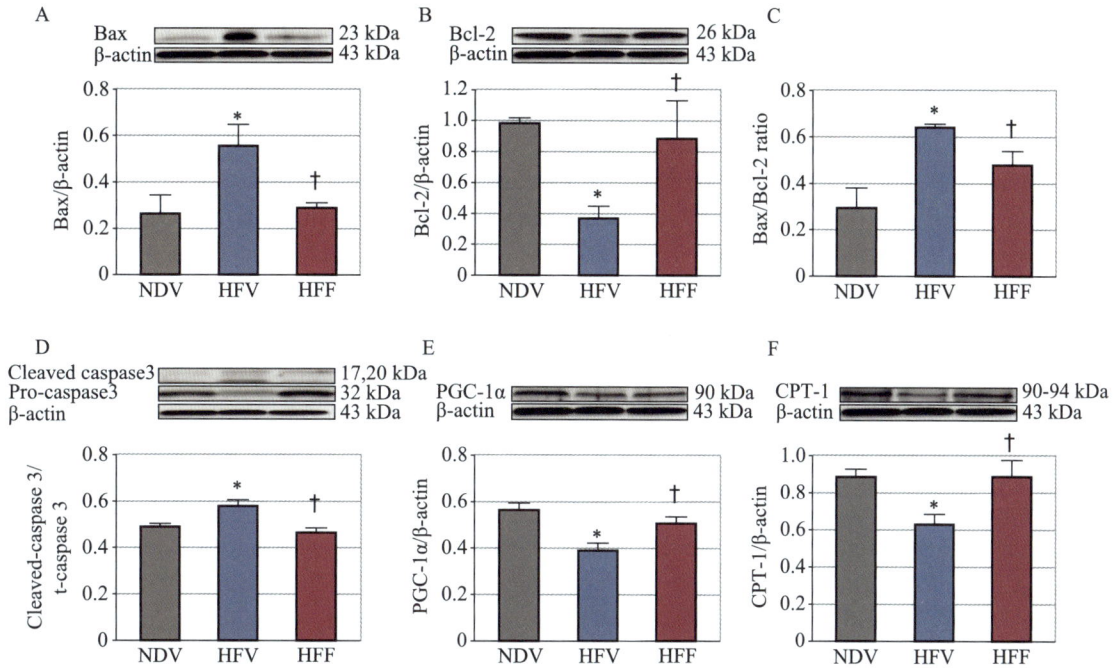

Fig. 4. Effects of HFD consumption and FGF21 treatment on cardiac FGF21 signalling pathways. (A) Bax, (B) Bcl-2, (C) Bax/ Bcl-2 ratio, (D) cleaved caspase-3/t-caspase-3 ratio, (E) PGC-1α and (F) CPT-1 in ND and HFD rats treated with vehicle and FGF21. *P < 0.05 vs. NDV, †P < 0.05 vs. HFV. HFD, high-fat diet, ND, normal diet; NDV, normal diet treated with vehicle; HFV, high-fat diet treated with vehicle; HFF, high-fat diet treated with FGF21.

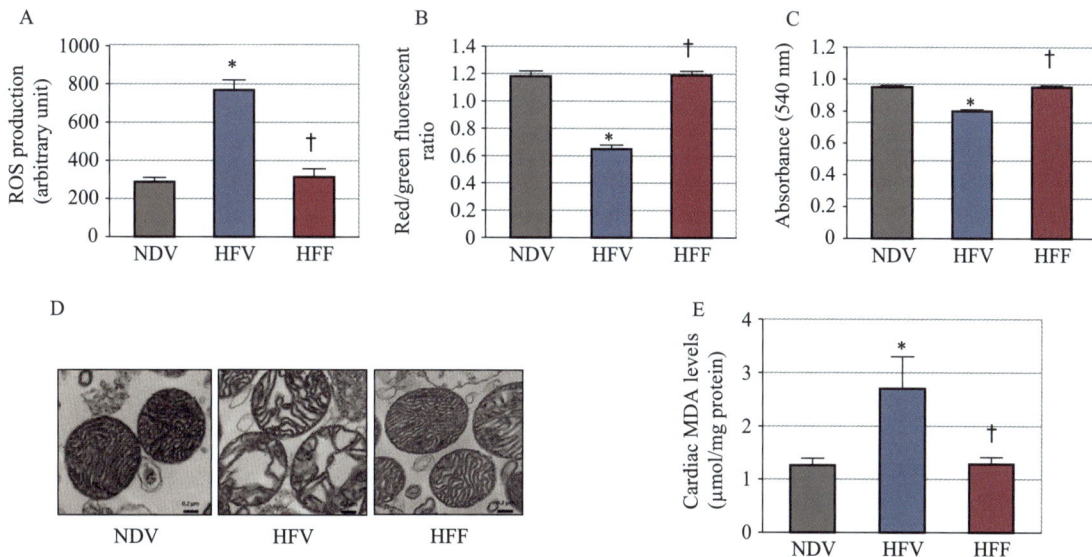

Fig. 5. Effects of HFD consumption and FGF21 treatment on cardiac mitochondrial redox homoeostasis, structural changes and lipid peroxidation. (A) Cardiac mitochondrial ROS production, (B) red/green fluorescent intensity ratio, (C) cardiac mitochondrial swelling and (D) cardiac mitochondrial morphology by transmission electron microscope (TEM) and (E) cardiac lipid peroxidation in ND and HFD rats treated with vehicle and FGF21. *P < 0.05 vs. NDV, †P < 0.05 vs. HFV. HFD, high-fat diet; ND, normal diet; NDV, normal diet treated with vehicle; HFV, high-fat diet treated with vehicle; HFF, high-fat diet treated with FGF21.

3. Discussion

The major findings of this study are as follows. First, long-term HFD consumption causes metabolic disturbance, progressive insulin resistance, activation of the systemic and cardiac oxidative stress processes, activation of the pro-inflammatory cytokines, increased BP, cardiac mitochondrial redox dyshomoeostasis and structural changes, progressive FGF21 resistance and decreased HRV; all of these lead to LV dysfunction. Secondly, long-term FGF21 administration can reverse the adverse effects of HFD consumption by decreasing metabolic disturbance, systemic and cardiac oxidative stress and cardiac mitochondrial redox dyshomoeostasis and structural changes. It also leads to decreased pro-inflammatory cytokines, reduced BP and increased HRV, thus attenuating FGF21 resistance in the heart, and finally leading to restoration of LV function. However, the high levels of plasma FGF21 observed in the HFF group were due to the exogenous FGF21 administration that we continuously performed in those rats. Moreover, the exogenous FGF21 administration has been shown to cause an upregulation of the FGF21 synthesis, which might even lead to a further increase in the FGF21 levels (Planavila *et al.*, 2013; Tanajak *et al.*, 2015).

Obesity–insulin resistance due to consumption of a HFD has been shown to cause metabolic disturbance, leading to cardiac mitochondrial redox dyshomoeostasis and structural changes and impaired LV function (Apaijai *et al.*, 2012, 2013, 2014). Our results also demonstrated that HFD consumption increased the serum levels of pro-inflammatory cytokine TNF-α and decreased serum adiponectin levels. TNF-α plays an important role in the inflammation process and has been shown to contribute to both heart and vascular damage (Kubota *et al.*, 2000). In this study, long-term HFD consumption increased plasma TNF-α and cardiac mitochondrial ROS production, indicating an increase in inflammation and oxidative stress respectively. Increasing inflammation and oxidative stress are known to cause the impairment of endothelial nitric oxide synthesis and activity, leading to endothelial dysfunction and increased BP (Rees *et al.*, 1989; Cai and Harrison, 2000).

FGF21 resistance has been shown to affect metabolic regulation and cardiac function (Hale *et al.*, 2012; Patel *et al.*, 2014). In the obese, insulin-resistant rats, obesity being caused by long-term HFD consumption, increased plasma FGF21 levels were observed. Moreover, abnormal FGF21 signalling was also found in the heart of these rats despite the increased plasma FGF21 level. This was shown by decreased FGFR1 phosphorylation and decreased response of its downstream signalling pathways in the heart including p-ERK1/2/t-ERK1/2 ratio, Bcl-2, PGC- 1α and CPT-1, while there were increases in Bax, Bax/ Bcl-2 ratio and cleaved caspase-3 expression. These findings indicated FGF21 resistance in the heart of these obese, insulin-resistant rats. The decrease in FGF21 signalling cascades has been shown to interrupt the cardioprotective effects of FGF21 by reducing its anti-apoptosis (Cong *et al.*, 2013; Zhang *et al.*, 2015), antioxidative stress (Planavila *et al.*, 2014), antihypertrophy and remodelling effects (Planavila *et al.*, 2013; Joki *et al.*, 2015), and also acceleration of the development of diabetic cardiomyopathy (Yan *et al.*, 2015; Zhang *et al.*, 2015). From these findings, the FGF21-resistant state has been suggested as a limitation to FGF21 treatment to take action on the cells and leads to low efficiency or ineffective short-term FGF21 therapy. This is supported by the findings that acute FGF21 treatment by giving FGF21 for 10 min prior to I/R injury failed to decrease myocardial infarct size and was unable to improve cardiac function in diet-induced obesity models with FGF21 resistance as indicated by no improvement of a reduced response of the FGF21 receptor complex and FGF21 signalling cascade (Patel *et al.*, 2014).

The FGF21-resistant state could be represented by a decrease in both primary receptors (FGFR1c and FGFR2c) and the coreceptor β-Klotho (Fisher *et al.*, 2010), or a decrease in the β-Klotho expression without an alteration in the FGFR1c expression (Patel *et al.*, 2014). In this study, FGF21 resistance was characterized by increased plasma FGF21 levels and decreased p-FGFR1 and p-FGFR1/t-FGFR1 ratio, whereas β-Klotho expression remained unaltered. However, the downstream signalling cascades including p-ERK1/2/t-ERK1/2 ratio were also decreased. Moreover, FGF21 resistance found in this study could contribute to a decreased cardiac mitochondrial FAO as indicated by decreased levels of PGC-1α and CPT-1 expression in the heart of obese, insulin-resistant rats.

Long-term FGF21 administration can reverse the adverse effects of long-term HFD consumption on inflammation as shown by the effective decrease in the serum TNF-α levels, suggesting it has the ability to decrease inflammation (Planavila *et al.*, 2013). FGF21 also increased serum adiponectin levels, an adipokine secreted from adipocytes regulating glucose and lipid metabolism (Kadowaki *et al.*, 2006). In the cardiovascular system, adiponectin has been shown to play an important role in improving endothelial dysfunction (Wang *et al.*, 2009), atherosclerosis (Ewart *et al.*, 2008) and hypertension (Yamawaki *et al.*, 2011). The improved BP found in this study could be due to the protective effect of adiponectin. Moreover, the exogenous FGF21 has been shown to increase the expression of the antioxidant genes, leading to a decrease in the ROS production in neonatal cardiac myocytes (Planavila *et al.*, 2014). Our study demonstrated that long-term exogenous FGF21 therapy effectively decreased ROS production in cardiac mitochondria, leading to improved cardiac mitochondrial redox homoeostasis and structural changes. In addition, this study also demonstrated that long-term FGF21 therapy could increase the anti-apoptosis signalling pathways by increasing Bcl-2 expression and also decreased Bax and cleaved caspase-3 expression.

As FGF21 plays an important role in regulating the mitochondrial FAO metabolism, where the majority of ATP is generated in the heart (Neely *et al.*, 1972; Neely and Morgan, 1974), long-term FGF21 therapy in our study could effectively increase the PGC-1α and CPT-1 expression, hence promoting increased FAO and ATP synthesis in the heart. Although most studies regarding HFD-induced obesity and/or insulin resistance demonstrated the increased fatty acid oxidation (FAO) in the heart (Aasum *et al.*, 2003; Mazumder *et al.*, 2004; Alrob *et al.*, 2014), inconsistent findings exist (Young *et al.*, 2002; Atkinson *et al.*, 2003; Gupte *et al.*, 2013; Neves *et al.*, 2014). It has been shown that FAO was not altered in insulin-resistant model (Atkinson *et al.*, 2003) and HFD-induced obesity model (Gupte *et al.*, 2013). Moreover, decreased FAO in HFD-induced obesity model (Neves *et al.*, 2014) and obese model (Young *et al.*, 2002) has been demonstrated. These findings indicate a complicate relationship between these two parameters. In the present study, the changes in PGC-1α and CPT-1 protein expression could be influenced by multiple factors which may explain these results. Firstly, FGF21 has been shown to regulate PGC-1α and CPT-1 mRNA and protein expression in the heart (Planavila *et al.*, 2013). Additionally, several studies reported that long-term HFD consumption could induce FGF21 resistance, which could impair FGF21 receptor function (Fisher *et al.*, 2010; Patel *et al.*, 2014). An impairment of FGF21 receptor function could reduce FGF21's downstream signalling cascades including PGC-1α and CPT-1 (Planavila *et al.*, 2013). These findings suggest that FGF21 induced by long-term HFD consumption could lead to reduced PGC-1α and CPT-1 levels as observed in our study. Secondly, the effect of obesity–insulin resistance and diabetes on the relationship between FAO and CPT-1 is still unclear. Although it has been shown that FAO levels were increased in obese, insulin-resistant rats and this was associated with an increase in CPT-1 expression (Neves *et al.*, 2014), several studies reported that FAO and CPT-1 levels were unchanged in obese, insulin-resistant animals, when compared to healthy controls (Atkinson *et al.*, 2003). Moreover, a previous study has reported a decrease in FAO in obese Zucker rats' hearts (Young *et al.*, 2002). These findings suggest that changes (either decrease or increase) in PGC-1α and CPT-1 protein expression do not always reflect changes in the FAO in the heart. A summary of the cardioprotective effects of long-term FGF21 therapy in HFD-induced obese, insulin-resistant rats is shown in Fig. 6.

4. Conclusions

Long-term FGF21 therapy attenuates FGF21 resistance by increasing FGF21 sensitivity and also improves insulin resistance by increasing insulin sensitivity in this model. Long-term FGF21 therapy not only activates anti-apoptotic pathways and improves cardiac mitochondrial redox homoeostasis and structural changes, but also activates mitochondrial FAO pathways in the heart, leading to improved cardiac function in obese, insulin-resistant rats with FGF21 resistance.

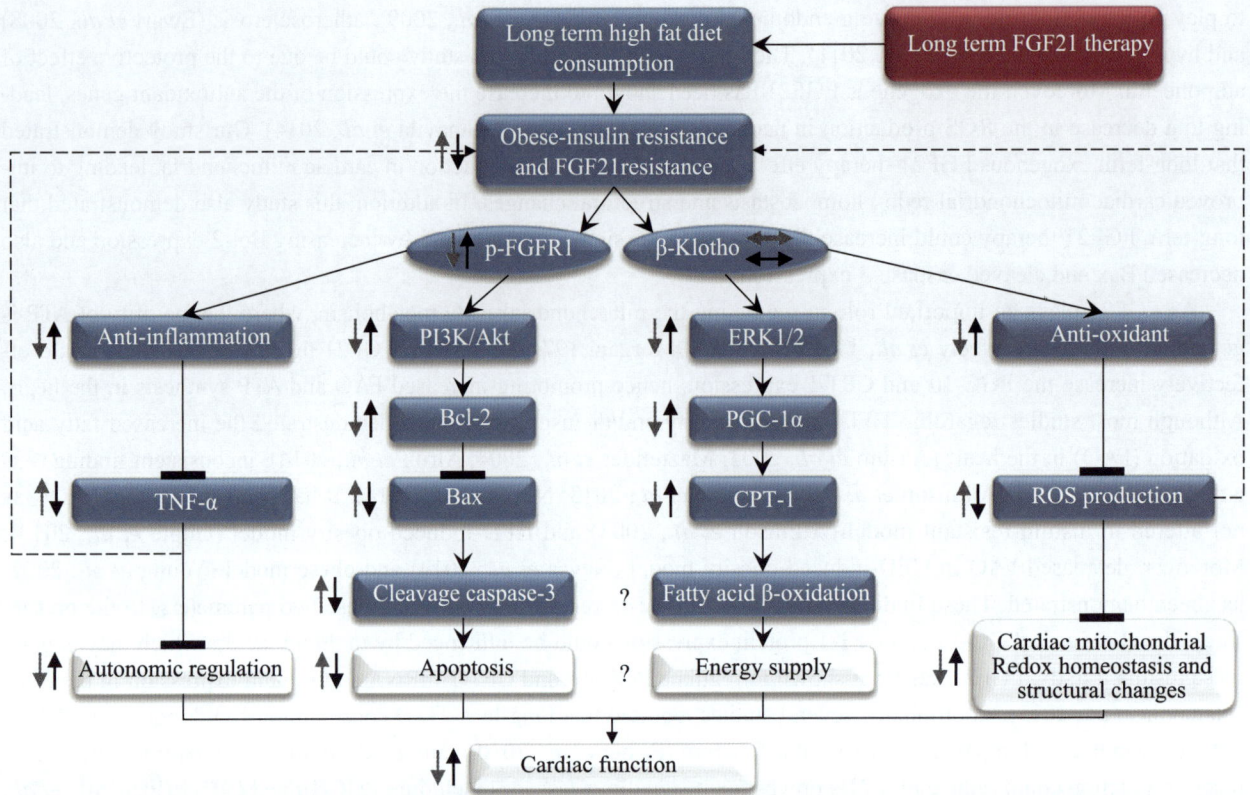

Fig. 6. Effects of short-term and long-term FGF21 therapy on cardiac function in high-fat diet (HFD)-induced obese, insulin-resistant rats. Long-term consumption of a HFD decreases response of p-FGFR1 which contributes to inflammation, oxidative stress, apoptosis and impaired cardiac mitochondrial fatty acid β-oxidation (FAO). It also leads to impaired cardiac autonomic regulation, cardiac mitochondrial redox homoeostasis and structural changes and affected cardiac function. FGF21, fibroblast growth factor 21; p-FGFR1, fibroblast growth factor receptor 1 phosphorylation; TNF-α, tumour necrosis factor-alpha; PI3K, phosphatidylinositol-3-kinase; Akt, protein kinase B (PKB); ERK1/2, extracellular signal regulated protein kinases 1 and 2; PGC-1α, peroxisome proliferator-activated receptor gamma coactivator 1-alpha; CPT-1, carnitine palmitoyltransferase I; ?, unclear effects/association with the FAO and cardiac function.

References

[1] Aasum E, Hafstad AD, Severson DL, *et al.* Age-dependent changes in metabolism, contractile function, and ischemic sensitivity in hearts from db/db mice[J]. Diabetes, 2003, 52(2): 434-441.

[2] Alrob OA, Sankaralingam S, Ma C, *et al.* Obesity-induced lysine acetylation increases cardiac fatty acid oxidation and impairs insulin signalling[J]. Cardiovascular Research, 2014, 103(4): 485-497.

[3] Apaijai N, Pintana H, Chattipakorn SC, *et al.* Cardioprotective effects of metformin and vildagliptin in adult rats with insulin resistance induced by a high-fat diet[J]. Endocrinology, 2012, 153(8): 3878-3885.

[4] Apaijai N, Pintana H, Chattipakorn SC, *et al.* Effects of vildagliptin *versus* sitagliptin, on cardiac function, heart rate variability and mitochondrial function in obese insulin-resistant rats[J]. Br J Pharmacol, 2013, 169(5): 1048-1057.

[5] Apaijai N, Chinda K, Palee S, *et al.* Combined vildagliptin and metformin exert better cardioprotection than monotherapy against ischemia-reperfusion injury in obese-insulin resistant rats[J]. PLoS One, 2014, 9(7): e102374.

[6] Atkinson LL, Kozak R, Kelly SE, *et al.* Potential mechanisms and consequences of cardiac triacylglycerol accumulation in insulin-re-

sistant rats[J]. Am J Physiol Endocrinol Metab, 2003, 284(5): E923-930.

[7] Besic V, Shi H, Stubbs RS, *et al.* Aberrant liver insulin receptor isoform a expression normalises with remission of type 2 diabetes after gastric bypass surgery[J]. PLoS One, 2015, 10(3): e0119270.

[8] Cai H, Harrison DG. Endothelial dysfunction in cardiovascular diseases: the role of oxidant stress[J]. Circ Res, 2000, 87(10): 840-844.

[9] Chattipakorn N, Incharoen T, Kanlop N, *et al.* Heart rate variability in myocardial infarction and heart failure[J]. Int J Cardiol, 2007, 120(3): 289-296.

[10] Chau MD, Gao J, Yang Q, *et al.* Fibroblast growth factor 21 regulates energy metabolism by activating the AMPK-SIRT1-PGC-1alpha pathway[J]. Proc Natl Acad Sci U S A, 2010, 107(28): 12553-12558.

[11] Chinda K, Palee S, Surinkaew S, *et al.* Cardioprotective effect of dipeptidyl peptidase-4 inhibitor during ischemia-reperfusion injury[J]. Int J Cardiol, 2013, 167(2): 451-457.

[12] Chinda K, Sanit J, Chattipakorn S, *et al.* Dipeptidyl peptidase-4 inhibitor reduces infarct size and preserves cardiac function *via* mitochondrial protection in ischaemia-reperfusion rat heart[J]. Diab

Vasc Dis Res, 2014, 11(2): 75-83.

[13] Cong WT, Ling J, Tian HS, *et al.* Proteomic study on the protective mechanism of fibroblast growth factor 21 to ischemia-reperfusion injury[J]. Can J Physiol Pharmacol, 2013, 91(11): 973-984.

[14] Ewart MA, Kohlhaas CF, Salt IP. Inhibition of tumor necrosis factor alpha-stimulated monocyte adhesion to human aortic endothelial cells by AMP-activated protein kinase[J]. Arterioscler Thromb Vasc Biol, 2008, 28(12): 2255-2257.

[15] Feng M, Whitesall S, Zhang Y, *et al.* Validation of volume-pressure recording tail-cuff blood pressure measurements[J]. Am J Hypertens, 2008, 21(12): 1288-1291.

[16] Fisher FM, Chui PC, Antonellis PJ, *et al.* Obesity is a fibroblast growth factor 21 (FGF21)-resistant state[J]. Diabetes, 2010, 59(11): 2781-2789.

[17] Friedewald WT, Levy RI, Fredrickson DS. Estimation of the concentration of low-density lipoprotein cholesterol in plasma, without use of the preparative ultracentrifuge[J]. Clin Chem, 1972, 18(6): 499-502.

[18] Gupte AA, Minze LJ, Reyes M, *et al.* High-fat feeding-induced hyperinsulinemia increases cardiac glucose uptake and mitochondrial function despite peripheral insulin resistance[J]. Endocrinology, 2013, 154(8): 2650-2662.

[19] Hale C, Chen MM, Stanislaus S, *et al.* Lack of overt FGF21 resistance in two mouse models of obesity and insulin resistance[J]. Endocrinology, 2012, 153(1): 69-80.

[20] Joki Y, Ohashi K, Yuasa D, *et al.* FGF21 attenuates pathological myocardial remodeling following myocardial infarction through the adiponectin-dependent mechanism[J]. Biochem Biophys Res Commun, 2015, 459(1): 124-130.

[21] Kadowaki T, Yamauchi T, Kubota N, *et al.* Adiponectin and adiponectin receptors in insulin resistance, diabetes, and the metabolic syndrome[J]. J Clin Invest, 2006, 116(7): 1784-1792.

[22] Kilkenny C, Browne W, Cuthill IC, *et al.* Animal research: reporting *in vivo* experiments: the ARRIVE guidelines[J]. Br J Pharmacol, 2010, 160(7): 1577-1579.

[23] Kmiecik AM, Pula B, Suchanski J, *et al.* Metallothionein-3 increases triple-negative breast cancer cell invasiveness *via* induction of metalloproteinase expression[J]. PLoS One, 2015, 10(5): e0124865.

[24] Kubota T, Bounoutas GS, Miyagishima M, *et al.* Soluble tumor necrosis factor receptor abrogates myocardial inflammation but not hypertrophy in cytokine-induced cardiomyopathy[J]. Circulation, 2000, 101(21): 2518-2525.

[25] Liu S, Niger C, Koh EY, *et al.* Connexin43 mediated delivery of ADAMTS5 targeting siRNAs from mesenchymal stem cells to synovial fibroblasts[J]. PLoS One, 2015, 10(6): e0129999.

[26] Mazumder PK, O'Neill BT, Roberts MW, *et al.* Impaired cardiac efficiency and increased fatty acid oxidation in insulin-resistant ob/ob mouse hearts[J]. Diabetes, 2004, 53(9): 2366-2374.

[27] Neely JR, Morgan HE. Relationship between carbohydrate and lipid metabolism and the energy balance of heart muscle[J]. Annu Rev Physiol, 1974, 36: 413-459.

[28] Neely JR, Rovetto MJ, Oram JF. Myocardial utilization of carbohydrate and lipids[J]. Prog Cardiovasc Dis, 1972, 15(3): 289-329.

[29] Neves FA, Cortez E, Bernardo AF, *et al.* Heart energy metabolism impairment in Western-diet induced obese mice[J]. J Nutr Biochem, 2014, 25(1): 50-57.

[30] Ouwens DM, Boer C, Fodor M, *et al.* Cardiac dysfunction induced by high-fat diet is associated with altered myocardial insulin signalling in rats[J]. Diabetologia, 2005, 48(6): 1229-1237.

[31] Palee S, Weerateerangkul P, Chinda K, *et al.* Mechanisms responsible for beneficial and adverse effects of rosiglitazone in a rat model of acute cardiac ischaemia-reperfusion[J]. Exp Physiol, 2013, 98(5): 1028-1037.

[32] Patel V, Adya R, Chen J, *et al.* Novel insights into the cardio-protective effects of FGF21 in lean and obese rat hearts[J]. PLoS One,

2014, 9(2): e87102.

[33] Pintana H, Sripetchwandee J, Supakul L, *et al.* Garlic extract attenuates brain mitochondrial dysfunction and cognitive deficit in obese-insulin resistant rats[J]. Appl Physiol Nutr Metab, 2014, 39(12): 1373-1379.

[34] Pipatpiboon N, Pratchayasakul W, Chattipakorn N, *et al.* PPARγ agonist improves neuronal insulin receptor function in hippocampus and brain mitochondria function in rats with insulin resistance induced by long term high-fat diets[J]. Endocrinology, 2012, 153(1): 329-338.

[35] Planavila A, Redondo I, Hondares E, *et al.* Fibroblast growth factor 21 protects against cardiac hypertrophy in mice[J]. Nature communications, 2013, 4: 2019.

[36] Pongchaidecha A, Lailerd N, Boonprasert W, *et al.* Effects of curcuminoid supplement on cardiac autonomic status in high-fat-induced obese rats[J]. Nutrition (Burbank, Los Angeles County, Calif.), 2009, 25: 870-878.

[37] Pratchayasakul W, Kerdphoo S, Petsophonsakul P, *et al.* Effects of high-fat diet on insulin receptor function in rat hippocampus and the level of neuronal corticosterone[J]. Life Sci, 2011, 88(13-14): 619-627.

[38] Rees DD, Palmer RM, Moncada S. Role of endothelium-derived nitric oxide in the regulation of blood pressure[J]. Proc Natl Acad Sci U S A, 1989, 86(9): 3375-3378.

[39] Surinkaew S, Kumphune S, Chattipakorn S, *et al.* Inhibition of p38 MAPK during ischemia, but not reperfusion, effectively attenuates fatal arrhythmia in ischemia/reperfusion heart[J]. J Cardiovasc Pharmacol, 2013, 61(2): 133-141.

[40] Tanajak P, Chattipakorn SC, Chattipakorn N. Effects of fibroblast growth factor 21 on the heart[J]. J Endocrinol, 2015, 227(2): R13-30.

[41] Thummasorn S, Kumfu S, Chattipakorn S, *et al.* Granulocyte-colony stimulating factor attenuates mitochondrial dysfunction induced by oxidative stress in cardiac mitochondria[J]. Mitochondrion, 2011, 11(3): 457-466.

[42] Tor YS, Yazan LS, Foo JB, *et al.* Induction of apoptosis in MCF-7 cells *via* oxidative stress generation, mitochondria-dependent and caspase-independent pathway by ethyl acetate extract of dillenia suffruticosa and Its chemical profile[J]. PLoS One, 2015, 10(6): e0127441.

[43] Wang P, Xu TY, Guan YF, *et al.* Perivascular adipose tissue-derived visfatin is a vascular smooth muscle cell growth factor: role of nicotinamide mononucleotide[J]. Cardiovasc Res, 2009, 81(2): 370-380.

[44] Wang H, Xiao Y, Fu L, *et al.* High-level expression and purification of soluble recombinant FGF21 protein by SUMO fusion in Escherichia coli[J]. BMC Biotechnol, 2010, 10: 14.

[45] Yamawaki H, Kuramoto J, Kameshima S, *et al.* Omentin, a novel adipocytokine inhibits TNF-induced vascular inflammation in human endothelial cells[J]. Biochem Biophys Res Commun, 2011, 408(2): 339-343.

[46] Yan X, Chen J, Zhang C, *et al.* FGF21 deletion exacerbates diabetic cardiomyopathy by aggravating cardiac lipid accumulation[J]. J Cell Mol Med, 2015, 19(7): 1557-1568.

[47] Young ME, Guthrie PH, Razeghi P, *et al.* Impaired long-chain fatty acid oxidation and contractile dysfunction in the obese Zucker rat heart[J]. Diabetes, 2002, 51(8): 2587-2595.

[48] Yu Y, Bai F, Liu Y, *et al.* Fibroblast growth factor (FGF21) protects mouse liver against D-galactose-induced oxidative stress and apoptosis *via* activating Nrf2 and PI3K/Akt pathways[J]. Mol Cell Biochem, 2015, 403(1-2): 287-299.

[49] Zhang C, Huang Z, Gu J, *et al.* Fibroblast growth factor 21 protects the heart from apoptosis in a diabetic mouse model *via* extracellular signal-regulated kinase 1/2-dependent signalling pathway[J]. Diabetologia, 2015, 58(8): 1937-1948.

NMR-based metabolomics reveal a recovery from metabolic changes in the striatum of 6-OHDA-induced rats treated with basic fibroblast growth factor

Hong Zheng, Xiaokun Li, Hongchang Gao

1. Introduction

Parkinson's disease (PD), as a neurodegenerative disorder, is second only to Alzheimer disease and is affecting hundreds of millions of people around the world [1]. The development of PD is caused by a selective loss of nigrostriatal dopamine neurons and a decrease of striatal dopamine [2]. Since these neurons regulate and control voluntary movements, PD results in rest tremor, postural imbalance, muscular rigidity, and slowness of movements [3]. The pathogenic cause underlying PD is multifactor including genetic factors [4], environmental toxins [4], mitochondrial dysfunction [5], oxidative stress [6], neuro-inflammation [7], and aldehyde dehydrogenase inhibition [8]. In addition, aging is also an influence factor, which has been associated with an increase in dopaminergic neurons degeneration [9]. Hence, it is a great challenge to treat PD for physicians. So far, treatment strategies mainly include gene therapy [10], cell therapy [11], medications [12], and neurostimulation [13]. However, it is still of great interest and importance to develop new effective treatment strategies of PD.

Basic fibroblast growth factor (bFGF), also known as FGF-2, is one of members in the FGF family. bFGF has been reported to increase the survival and growth of dopaminergic (DA) neurons *in vitro* [14, 15]. Ratzka *et al.* [16] found that bFGF also regulate the development of DA neurons *in vivo*. An increase in striatal and nigral neurogenesis was reported after FGF-2 treatment in the 1-methyl-4-phenyl-1,2,3,6-tetrahydropyridine (MPTP)-induced PD mouse model [17]. Timmer *et al.* [18] reported that FGF-2 prevented against DA neuronal death in 6-hydroxydopamine (6-OHDA)-induced mouse model, while the number of DA neurons was regulated by FGF-receptor-3. In addition, Shults *et al.* [19] found that FGF-2-producing fibroblasts implanted in the striatum of mice can protect the nigrostriatal DA system. Therefore, due to the neurotrophic and protective effect of bFGF on DA neurons, it has been considered as a potential candidate for the treatment of PD. However, the potential metabolic mechanisms of bFGF administration on PD are still unknown.

Metabolomics attempts to comprehensively analyze the metabolic changes in biological samples and has been considered as a promising tool in research area of PD. For instance, the predictive models of PD have been successfully developed on the basis of the metabolic profile of urine [20] and cerebrospinal fluid [21]. Roede *et al.* [22] used serum metabolomics to distinguish between slow and fast progression PD and found the change in polyamine metabolism may be associated with rapidly progressing PD. Using a metabolomic approach, increased levels in several amino acids, pyroglutamate, and 2-oxoisocaproate and reduced levels in C16–C18 saturated and unsaturated fatty acids were observed in plasma of PD patients [23]. In cerebrospinal fluid, they found that PD decreased 3-hydroxyisovaleric acid, tryptophan, and creatinine levels. Moreover, metabolomics results from Hatano *et al.* [24] showed that PD patients had lower levels of tryptophan, caffeine, bilirubin, and ergothioneine and higher concentrations of levodopa metabolites and biliverdin as compared with healthy subjects. However, metabolomics should be further proceeded to better elucidate metabolic mechanisms related to PD diagnosis and treatment. Nuclear magnetic resonance (NMR) spectroscopy is an attractive technique used in metabolomic research due to several advantages, such as simple sample preparation, high reproducibility, and fast analysis. Considering the role of striatum in the development of PD [2], therefore, through NMR-based metabolomics, the aims of the present study were (1) to examine the metabolic changes in striatum of 6-OHDA-induced PD mice and (2) to investigate the potential metabolic mechanisms underlying PD treatment using bFGF.

2. Materials and methods

2.1 Animals

Male Sprague–Dawley rats weighing 220±15 g (8 weeks of age) were purchased from the SLAC Laboratory Animal Co., Ltd. (Shanghai, China) and housed in a specific pathogen-free colony with controlled temperature and humidity and 12-h light–dark cycle (lights on at 8:00 a.m.) at the Laboratory Animal Center of Wenzhou Medical University (Wenzhou, China). All rats were given ad libitum access to standard rat chow and tap water. All animals received care in accordance to the "Guide For the Care and Use of Laboratory Animals." Procedures using mice were approved by the Institutional Animal Care and Use Committee of Wenzhou Medical University (document number: wydw2012-0083).

2.2 Brain stereotaxic 6-OHDA lesions

Animals were weighted and randomly divided into control and lesion groups. 6-OHDA was prepared at a concentration of 1.5 µg/µl in 0.9% NaCl, containing 0.2% ascorbic acid to avoid oxidation. Then, rats were intraperitoneally anesthetized with 10% chloral hydrate (3 ml/kg body weight) and immobilized in a stereotaxic frame. The first hole was drilled for placing a skull screw used as anchors for dental acrylic. The second hole over the dorsal striatum was drilled to place a cannula at the coordinates (mm): AP0+0.7, ML0+3.0, and V0−5.5. Then, 6-OHDA was injected into the right striatum of rats using microsyringes at a rate of 0.6 µl/min, and the injection volume for each rat is 10 µl. The cannula was kept for 10 min in order to achieve sufficient diffusion of 6-OHDA. The control rats were performed with identical surgical treatment, but injected the same volume of saline containing 0.2% ascorbic acid.

2.3 Rotational test for lesion verification

After a 4-week recovery period, 6-OHDA-induced lesions were confirmed with apomorphine-induced rotation test. Apomorphine is a dopamine receptor agonist, which can induce contralateral turning by stimulating supersensitive dopamine receptors in untreated striatum. The number of 360° turns was recorded, and 20 rats with at least 7 turns/min to apomorphine (0.05 mg/kg) were selected for further study.

2.4 Treatment of bFGF

Twenty lesion rats were weighted and randomly assigned into PD and bFGF groups with 10 rats per group. The same surgical procedure with 6-OHDA injection was conducted. The rats in the bFGF group were administrated with 15 µg of bFGF (1.5 µg/µl) using microsyringes at a rate of 1.0 µl/ min, and the cannula was kept for 5 min. In addition, the rats in the control and PD groups were injected the same volume of normal saline. Treatments were continued for 7 days.

2.5 Tyrosine hydroxylase immunohistochemistry

Rats (n=3 for each group) were perfused transcardially with normal saline followed by a fixing solution containing 4% paraformaldehyde for 30 min. The substantia nigra tissues were rapidly dissected, fixed in 10% buffered formalin overnight, and embedded in paraffin. Then, paraffin sections were subjected to tyrosine hydroxylase (TH) immunohistochemical staining for examining dopamine neuron death following the manufacturer's protocol. The images were captured with a Nikon ECLIPSE 80i (Nikon, Japan).

2.6 Sample preparation

The remaining rats were sacrificed by decapitation at 24 h after a 7-day bFGF treatment. Striatum samples were dissected immediately, frozen in liquid nitrogen, and stored at −80 ℃ until analysis. The frozen tissue was weighed into an Eppendorf tube, and then, ice-cold methanol (4 ml/g) and distilled water (0.85 ml/g) were first added into the tube. The mixture was homogenized at 4 ℃ after thawing and mixed by vortex. Then, ice-cold chloroform (2 ml/g) and distilled water (2 ml/g) were consecutively added into the tube and mixed again. The mixture was kept on ice for 15 min and centrifuged at 10,000g for 15 min at 4 ℃. The supernatant was transferred to a fresh Eppendorf tube and lyophilized for around 24 h. The dried extract was stored at −80 ℃ until NMR analysis. The dried sample was redissolved in 0.6 ml of 99.5% D_2O containing 0.05% sodium trimethylsilyl propionate-d_4 (TSP) and transferred to a 5-mm NMR tube for metabolomic analysis.

2.7 NMR measurement

^1H NMR spectra were acquired using a 600.13 MHz on a Bruker AVANCE III 600 MHz NMR spectrometer with a 5-mm TXI probe (Bruker BioSpin, Rheinstetten, Germany). The ^1H NMR spectra were recorded by a standard single-pulse experiment with water signal pre-saturation, Zgprn (Bruker BioSpin, Gmbh, Rheinstetten, Germany) at 37℃. The main acquisition parameters included data points, 64 K; relaxation delay, 2 s; spectral width, 12,000 Hz; and acquisition time, 2.65 s per scan.

2.8 NMR data preprocessing

All spectra were preprocessed using auto-phase and auto-baseline corrections and referenced to TSP peak at 0 ppm in the Topspin software (v2.1 pl4, Bruker BioSpin, Germany). The Icoshift procedure was performed to align NMR spectra in MATLAB (R2012a, The MathWorks Inc., Natick, MA, USA) [25]. The spectral region from 0.5 to 4.6 ppm was subdivided with a size of 0.01 ppm and integrated to binning data. Finally, prior to multivariate data analysis, the binned data of each NMR spectrum were normalized to the corresponding tissue weight in order to estimate the relative concentrations of metabolites.

2.9 Multivariate data analysis

Partial least squares-discriminant analysis (PLS-DA) was carried out on Pareto-scaled data using SIMCA 12.0 software (Umetrics, Umeå, Sweden). A leave-one-out cross-validation (LOOCV) method was performed, and meanwhile, two parameters were calculated to assess model performance: R^2Y, the explained variance in the Y matrix, and Q^2, the predictive capability of the model. Generally, these two parameters close to 1.0 represent an excellent model. The significance of variables in PLS-DA was evaluated using the variable importance in the projection (VIP) method, and those variables were considered important when VIP scores above 2.0. Then, the NMR signals with VIP>2.0 were assigned according to our previous paper [26] and HMDB [27]. The relative concentrations of identified metabolites were calculated on the basis of their peak areas relative to the internal standard TSP concentration.

2.10 Statistical analysis

Analysis of variance (ANOVA) was conducted using Student's t test with Bonferroni correction for multiple comparisons in SAS 9.2 (SAS Institute Inc, Cary, NC), and a Bonferroni-adjusted P value <0.05 was considered as a statistically significant difference.

3. Results

3.1 NMR-based metabolic profile in the striatum of rats

Fig. 1A illustrates a typical ^1H NMR spectrum of the rat striatum and a total of 12 identified metabolites including neurotransmitters (glutamate (Glu), glutamine (Gln), and γ-aminobutyric acid (GABA)), antioxidants and osmolytes (taurine (Tau) and myoinositol (Myo)), energy metabolism (lactate (Lac), alanine (Ala), succinate (Suc), creatine (Cre), and ethanol (Eth)), and myelination and membrane metabolism (choline (Cho) and N-acetyl aspartate (NAA)). In the present study, NMR spectra were normalized to the corresponding tissue weight to evaluate the relative content of metabolite extracted and binned to reduce data dimension for further metabolomic analyses, as shown in Fig. 1B. It can be seen that the intensities of NMR spectra recorded from the PD group were higher than those from the control and bFGF groups, which is also demonstrated from PLS-DA score plot that the PD group was separated from the other two groups along PLS1 (Fig. 1C).

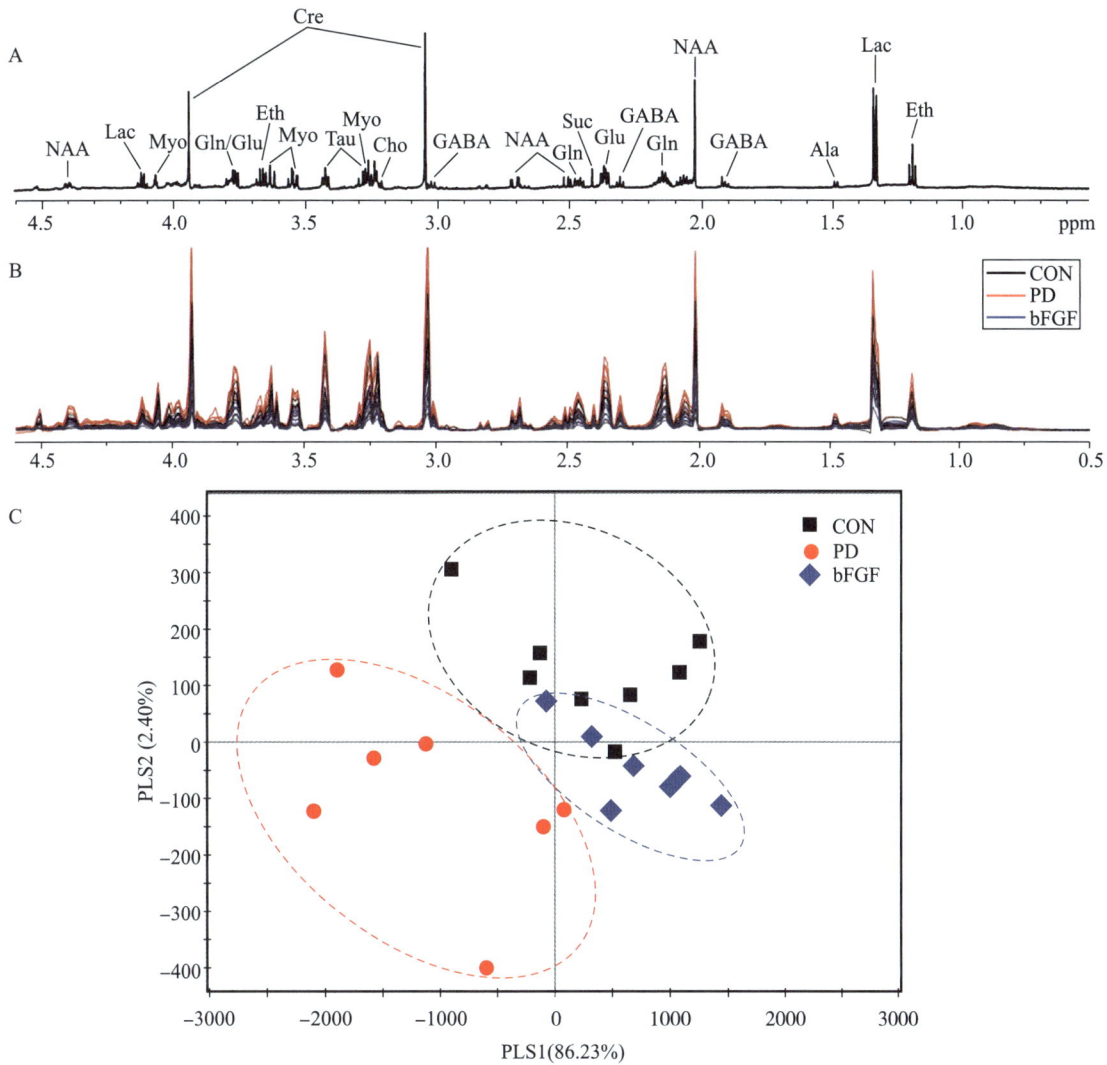

Fig. 1. A representative 600 MHz ^{1}H NMR spectrum of the rat striatum (A) normalized spectra obtained from the control (CON), 6-OHDA-induced (PD), and bFGF-treated (bFGF) groups (B) and PLS-DA classification based on the normalized spectra (C).

3.2　Metabolic differences in the striatum of PD rats treated with bFGF

PLS-DA was used to identify metabolic differences between any two groups in the present study, and the performance parameters of PLS-DA are listed in Table 1. Interestingly, no reliable model can be developed between the control and bFGF groups ($Q^2 = 0.05$), indicating that the metabolic difference between them was negligible. Table 1 also shows that PLS-DA model parameters between the PD and bFGF groups ($R^2Y = 0.89$, $Q^2 = 0.78$) were higher than those between the control and PD groups ($R^2Y = 0.65$, $Q^2 = 0.46$). In this study, VIP statistics (VIP> 2.0) were used to identify

Table 1.　Summary of model quality parameters of PLS-DA

Model	PLS	R^2Y	Q^2
CON[a] *vs.* PD[b]	2	0.65	0.46
CON *vs.* bFGF[c]	2	0.44	0.05
PD *vs.* bFGF	2	0.89	0.78

[a] Control group.

[b] 6-OHDA-induced group.

[c] bFGF-treated group.

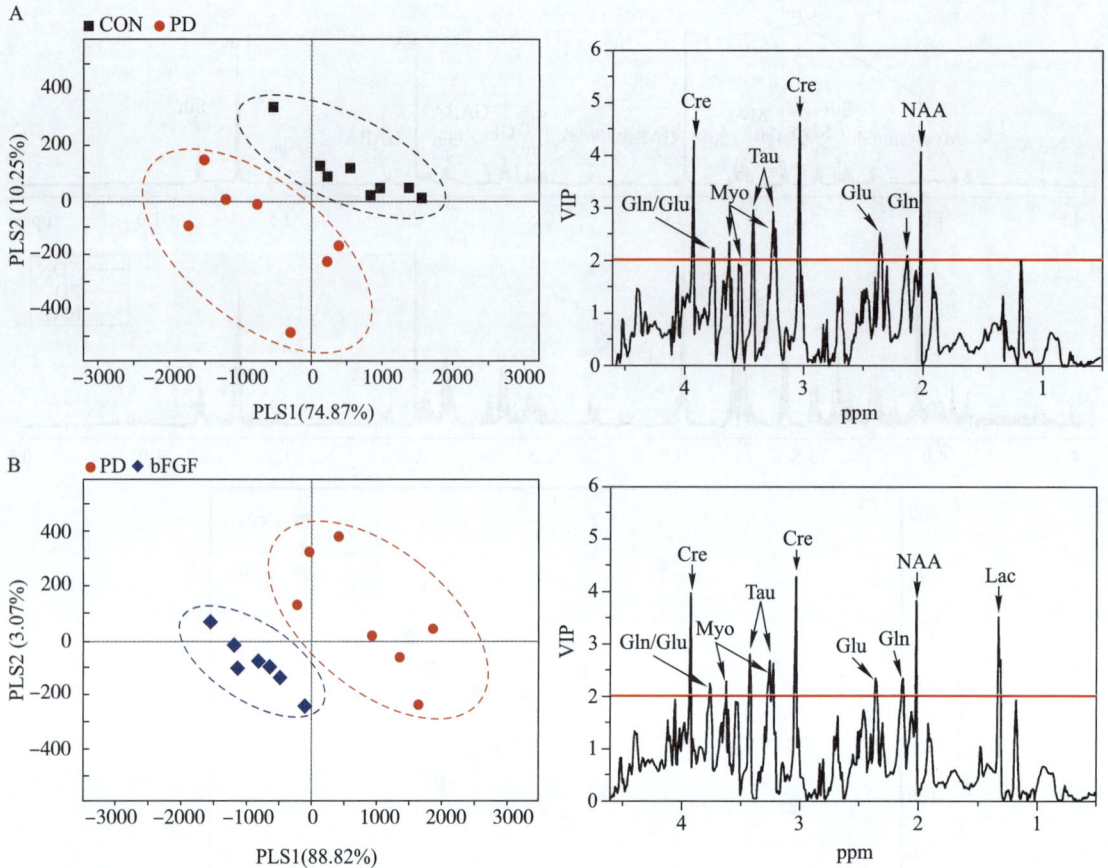

Fig. 2. PLS-DA score and VIP plots obtained from NMR-based metabolomics of the rat striatum in the control (CON), 6-OHDA-induced (PD), and bFGF-treated (bFGF) groups: (A) CON *vs.* PD and (B) PD *vs.* bFGF. The corresponding model parameters are listed in Table 1. Metabolite assignment: lactate (Lac), 1.32 ppm; N-acetylaspartate (NAA), 2.03 ppm; glutamine (Gln), 2.14 and 3.76 ppm; glutamate (Glu), 2.46 and 3.76 ppm; creatine (Cre), 3.04 and 3.93 ppm; taurine (Tau), 3.25 and 3.42 ppm; myo-inositol (Myo), 3.26, 3.52 and 3.62 ppm.

metabolites that mainly contributed to the separations between two groups. The corresponding score and VIP plots are shown in Fig. 2. It can be seen from the VIP plots that NAA, Glu, Gln, Cre, Tau, and Myo were the common contributive metabolites in these two models. Moreover, Lac had VIP values above 2.0 in the model between the PD and bFGF groups (Fig. 2B).

3.3 Changes in metabolites and TH neuronal contents in PD rats treated with bFGF

Fig. 3 shows that all identified metabolites were significantly increased in the striatum of PD rats relative to normal rats (the control group), while increased levels of metabolites were reduced to normal levels after treatment of bFGF. It is worth noting that disturbances of the Gln/Glu-GABA cycle induced by PD can be recovered to normal by bFGF treatment (Fig. 3E). In addition, stereological analyses using tyrosine hydroxylase (TH) staining of dopamine neurons expectedly show that the number of TH-positive neurons was obviously decreased in the substantia nigra of PD rats as compared with the control rats (Fig. 3F). However, most interestingly, bFGF treatment can effectively recover the lost TH-positive neurons, as shown in Fig. 3F.

4. Discussion

PD, as a neurodegenerative disease, is seriously affecting quality of human life [28], so it is an urgent need to develop more effective treatment strategies. Ferreira *et al.* [12] summarized the treatment recommendations for early and late PD by medications. It is worth noting that bFGF as a potential drug candidate is increasingly attracting attention. In the present study, the underlying therapeutic effects and metabolic mechanisms were investigated in 6-OHDA-induced PD

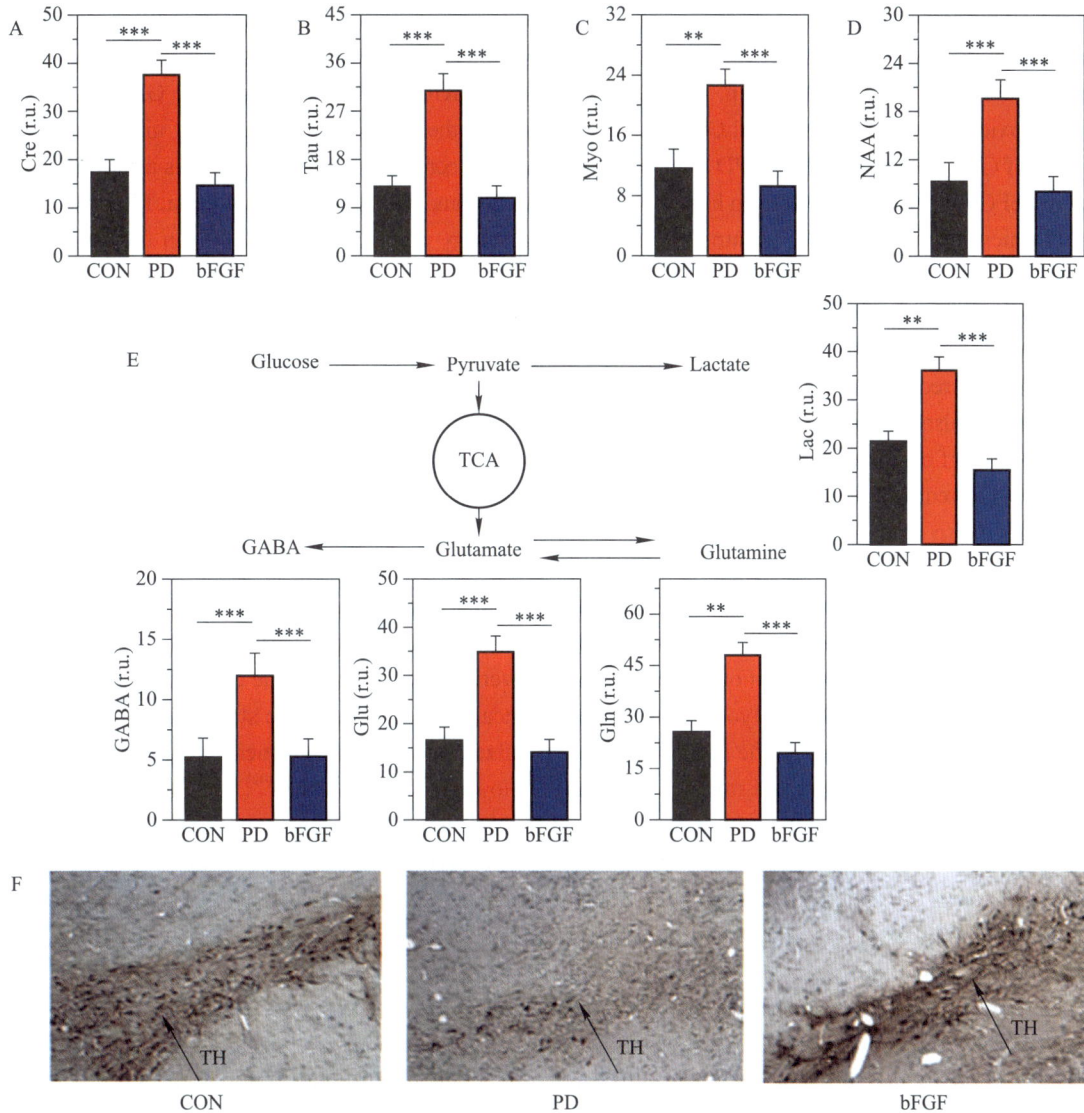

Fig. 3. Changes in metabolite levels and tyrosine hydroxylase (TH) immunohistochemistry among the control (CON), 6-OHDA-induced (PD), and bFGF-treated (bFGF) groups: (A) creatine, (B) taurine, (C) myo-inositol, (D) N-acetylaspartate, (E) the glutamine/glutamate-GABA cycle and lactate, and (F) TH immunohistochemistry. *r.u.* relative unit. Significant level: **$P<0.01$; ***$P<0.001$.

rats after treatment of bFGF.

The degeneration of dopaminergic neurons in the substantia nigra is well known as a main cause of development of PD [2]. Tyrosine hydroxylase (TH) is a rate-limiting enzyme in dopamine production, which can catalyze the conversion of L-tyrosine to L-3,4-dihydroxyphenylalanine [29]. Therefore, to be expected, a reduction in the number of TH-positive neurons was observed in the substantia nigra of PD rats, which results in dopamine deficiency and in turn induces PD symptoms [3]. However, we surprisingly found that the treatment of bFGF can increase TH-positive neurons, indicating a recovery of dopamine neuron loss and a promising therapeutic role for PD.

Metabolomics demonstrates that bFGF treatment may engage in neurochemical homeostasis regulation, which is critical for maintaining normal brain function. The Gln/Glu-GABA cycle (GGC) between astrocytes and neurons has been known to be involved in central nervous system (CNS) function [30]. Disturbance of the GGC results in changes in glutamatergic and GABA ergic neurotransmitter pathways and is associated with the development of PD [26]. In the present study, we found significant increases in Glu, Gln, and GABA levels in the striatum of 6-OHDA-induced PD rats compared with normal rats, suggesting an upregulation of the GGC. Podell *et al.* [31] and Chassain *et al.* [32] also reported that both Glu and Gln levels were increased in the striatum of PD feline and mouse models, respectively. In addition, an increased level of striatal GABA level has been observed in PD patients [33] as well as in mouse [32] and rat [34] models of PD. In the GGC, Gln is an amino acid that couples ammonia metabolism to directly synthesize the excitatory neurotransmitter, Glu, and then indirectly generate the inhibitory neurotransmitter, GABA. Thus, the increased Gln/Glu can directly lead to a higher GABA production. The major role of the GGC is to regulate synaptic Glu levels and in turn prevent excitotoxicity and maintain normal CNS function. However, the most interesting finding in this study is that increased levels of Gln, Glu, and GABA in PD rats were significantly decreased to be normal levels after bFGF treatment, indicating that bFGF can contribute to keep homeostasis of the GGC and thereby prevent and treat PD.

Metabolomics reveals that bFGF treatment also involves energy metabolism regulation in the striatum. Lactate has been reported as an alternative energy substrate in brain [35]. In the present study, we found a significant increase in lactate level in the striatum of 6-OHDA-induced PD rats relative to normal rats. Besides, an increased lactate was also observed in the striatum of MPTP-treated mice and has been attributed to the loss of nigrostriatal dopamine neurons [36]. Thus, bFGF-induced reduction of lactate may be due to the recovery of dopamine neuron loss after bFGF treatment. In addition, creatine also plays a certain role in brain energy homeostasis [37]. As in our previous study [26], we again observed that the level of creatine was increased in the striatum of 6-OHDA-induced rats, while its level was reduced and not significantly different from normal rats after bFGF administration.

Metabolomics also shows that bFGF treatment may affect osmoregulation in astrocytes. Both Myo and Tau have been used as a marker for astrocytic activity and play a key role in osmoregulation of astrocytes [38, 39]. We found that the level of Myo was increased in the striatum of 6-OHDA-induced rats, which is in agreement with the finding in MPTP-treated PD mice model [40]. Moreover, a similar result was also obtained in Tau level. Thus, the increased Myo and Tau levels may indicate that microglial activation and inflammation were caused by dopamine cell death. After bFGF administration, however, we found that both Myo and Tau were significantly decreased in the striatum of PD rats, suggesting that bFGF may have a potential role in the inhibition of brain inflammation. NAA is generally considered as a neuronal marker since it is mainly synthesized and stored in neurons [41]. However, Jenkins et al. [42] and Demougeot et al. [43] suggested it as a marker of neuronal dysfunction rather than neuronal density. NAA does not engage in neurophysiological effects, while it plays an important role in the neuron, such as an acetyl donor and a carbon transfer source via the mitochondrial membrane [44]. In addition, NAA can be released to the interstitial space as an osmolytes during osmotic stress [45]. Our results show that after bFGF administration, the level of NAA in the striatum of 6-OHDA-induced PD rats can be recovered as that in normal rates.

NMR-based metabolomics has been proposed as a great potential for exploring important issues about PD treatment and diagnosis [46]. To our knowledge, however, this is the first study addressing the metabolic changes in the striatum of PD rats after bFGF treatment by an NMR-based metabolomic approach. Our metabolomic results reveal that bFGF treatment may regulate PD-induced metabolic changes to be a metabolic status in normal rats. Moreover, we also found that the loss of TH-positive neurons can be recovered in the substantia nigra of PD rats after bFGF treatment. However, the detailed metabolic mechanisms after bFGF administration still need further studies for promoting its clinical development and application. On the one hand, more sensitive techniques such as LC-MS and GC-MS are recommended to detect more metabolites for drawing the more detailed metabolic pathways. On the other, metabolomics coupled with other omics techniques, for instance, genomics and proteomics, will advance understanding of the mechanisms of bFGF on PD treatment.

References

[1] de Lau LM, Breteler MM. Epidemiology of Parkinson's disease[J]. Lancet Neurol, 2006, 5(6): 525-535.

[2] Hornykiewicz O. The discovery of dopamine deficiency in the parkinsonian brain[J]. J Neural Transm Suppl, 2006, (70): 9-15.

[3] Dauer W, Przedborski S. Parkinson's disease: mechanisms and models[J]. Neuron, 2003, 39(6): 889-909.

[4] Warner TT, Schapira AHV. Genetic and environmental factors in the cause of Parkinson's disease[J]. Annals of Neurology, 2003, 53(S3): S16.

[5] Hauser DN, Hastings TG. Mitochondrial dysfunction and oxidative stress in Parkinson's disease and monogenic parkinsonism[J]. Neurobiol Dis, 2013, 51: 35-42.

[6] Hwang O. Role of oxidative stress in Parkinson's disease[J]. Exp Neurobiol, 2013, 22(1): 11-17.

[7] More SV, Kumar H, Kim IS, et al. Cellular and molecular mediators of neuroinflammation in the pathogenesis of Parkinson's disease[J]. Mediators Inflamm, 2013, 2013: 952375.

[8] Fitzmaurice AG, Rhodes SL, Lulla A, et al. Aldehyde dehydrogenase inhibition as a pathogenic mechanism in Parkinson disease[J]. Proc Natl Acad Sci U S A, 2013, 110(2): 636-641.

[9] Obeso JA, Rodriguez-Oroz MC, Goetz CG, et al. Missing pieces in the Parkinson's disease puzzle[J]. Nat Med, 2010, 16(6): 653-661.

[10] Butcher J. Parkin gene therapy could treat Parkinson's disease[J]. Lancet Neurol, 2005, 4(2): 82.

[11] Lindvall O, Bjorklund A. Cell therapy in Parkinson's disease[J]. NeuroRx, 2004, 1(4): 382-393.

[12] Ferreira JJ, Katzenschlager R, Bloem BR, *et al.* Summary of the recommendations of the EFNS/MDS-ES review on therapeutic management of Parkinson's disease[J]. Eur J Neurol, 2013, 20(1): 5-15.

[13] Deuschl G, Agid Y. Subthalamic neurostimulation for Parkinson's disease with early fluctuations: balancing the risks and benefits[J]. Lancet Neurol, 2013, 12(10): 1025-1034.

[14] Mena MA, Casarejos MJ, Gimenez-Gallego G, *et al.* Fibroblast growth factors: structure-activity on dopamine neurons *in vitro*[J]. J Neural Transm Park Dis Dement Sect, 1995, 9(1): 1-14.

[15] Sanchez-Pernaute R, Lee H, Patterson M, *et al.* Parthenogenetic dopamine neurons from primate embryonic stem cells restore function in experimental Parkinson's disease[J]. Brain, 2008, 131(Pt 8): 2127-2139.

[16] Ratzka A, Baron O, Stachowiak MK, *et al.* Fibroblast growth factor 2 regulates dopaminergic neuron development *in vivo*[J]. J Neurochem, 2012, 122(1): 94-105.

[17] Peng J, Xie L, Jin K, *et al.* Fibroblast growth factor 2 enhances striatal and nigral neurogenesis in the acute 1-methyl-4-phenyl-1,2,3,6-tetrahydropyridine model of Parkinson's disease[J]. Neuroscience, 2008, 153(3): 664-670.

[18] Timmer M, Cesnulevicius K, Winkler C, *et al.* Fibroblast growth factor (FGF)-2 and FGF receptor 3 are required for the development of the substantia nigra, and FGF-2 plays a crucial role for the rescue of dopaminergic neurons after 6-hydroxydopamine lesion[J]. J Neurosci, 2007, 27(3): 459-471.

[19] Shults CW, Ray J, Tsuboi K, *et al.* Fibroblast growth factor-2-producing fibroblasts protect the nigrostriatal dopaminergic system from 6-hydroxydopamine[J]. Brain Res, 2000, 883(2): 192-204.

[20] Poliquin PO, Chen J, Cloutier M, *et al.* Metabolomics and in-silico analysis reveal critical energy deregulations in animal models of Parkinson's disease[J]. PLoS One, 2013, 8(7): e69146.

[21] Lewitt PA, Li J, Lu M, *et al.* 3-hydroxykynurenine and other Parkinson's disease biomarkers discovered by metabolomic analysis[J]. Mov Disord, 2013, 28(12): 1653-1660.

[22] Roede JR, Uppal K, Park Y, *et al.* Serum metabolomics of slow *vs.* rapid motor progression Parkinson's disease: a pilot study[J]. PLoS One, 2013, 8(10): e77629.

[23] Trupp M, Jonsson P, Ohrfelt A, *et al.* Metabolite and peptide levels in plasma and CSF differentiating healthy controls from patients with newly diagnosed Parkinson's disease[J]. J Parkinsons Dis, 2014, 4(3): 549-560.

[24] Hatano T, Saiki S, Okuzumi A, *et al.* Identification of novel biomarkers for Parkinson's disease by metabolomic technologies[J]. J Neurol Neurosurg Psychiatry, 2016, 87(3): 295-301.

[25] Savorani F, Tomasi G, Engelsen SB. icoshift: A versatile tool for the rapid alignment of 1D NMR spectra[J]. J Magn Reson, 2010, 202(2): 190-202.

[26] Gao HC, Zhu H, Song CY, *et al.* Metabolic changes detected by ex vivo high resolution 1H NMR spectroscopy in the striatum of 6-OHDA-induced Parkinson's rat[J]. Mol Neurobiol, 2013, 47(1): 123-130.

[27] Wishart DS, Jewison T, Guo AC, *et al.* HMDB 3.0--The Human Metabolome Database in 2013[J]. Nucleic Acids Res, 2013, 41(Database issue): D801-807.

[28] Schrag A, Jahanshahi M, Quinn N. How does Parkinson's disease affect quality of life? A comparison with quality of life in the general population[J]. Mov Disord, 2000, 15(6): 1112-1118.

[29] Nakashima A, Hayashi N, Kaneko YS, *et al.* Role of N-terminus of tyrosine hydroxylase in the biosynthesis of catecholamines[J]. J Neural Transm (Vienna), 2009, 116(11): 1355-1362.

[30] Sidoryk-Wegrzynowicz M, Aschner M. Manganese toxicity in the central nervous system: the glutamine/glutamate-gamma-aminobutyric acid cycle[J]. J Intern Med, 2013, 273(5): 466-477.

[31] Podell M, Hadjiconstantinou M, Smith MA, *et al.* Proton magnetic resonance imaging and spectroscopy identify metabolic changes in the striatum in the MPTP feline model of parkinsonism[J]. Exp Neurol, 2003, 179(2): 159-166.

[32] Chassain C, Bielicki G, Keller C, *et al.* Metabolic changes detected *in vivo* by 1H MRS in the MPTP-intoxicated mouse[J]. NMR Biomed, 2010, 23(6): 547-553.

[33] Emir UE, Tuite PJ, Oz G. Elevated pontine and putamenal GABA levels in mild-moderate Parkinson disease detected by 7 tesla proton MRS[J]. PLoS One, 2012, 7(1): e30918.

[34] Coune PG, Craveiro M, Gaugler MN, *et al.* An in vivo ultrahigh field 14.1 T (1) H-MRS study on 6-OHDA and alpha-synuclein-based rat models of Parkinson's disease: GABA as an early disease marker[J]. NMR Biomed, 2013, 26(1): 43-50.

[35] Belanger M, Allaman I, Magistretti PJ. Brain energy metabolism: focus on astrocyte-neuron metabolic cooperation[J]. Cell Metab, 2011, 14(6): 724-738.

[36] Koga K, Mori A, Ohashi S, *et al.* H MRS identifies lactate rise in the striatum of MPTP-treated C57BL/6 mice[J]. Eur J Neurosci, 2006, 23(4): 1077-1081.

[37] Lowe MT, Kim EH, Faull RL, *et al.* Dissociated expression of mitochondrial and cytosolic creatine kinases in the human brain: a new perspective on the role of creatine in brain energy metabolism[J]. J Cereb Blood Flow Metab, 2013, 33(8): 1295-1306.

[38] Isaacks RE, Bender AS, Kim CY, *et al.* Osmotic regulation of myo-inositol uptake in primary astrocyte cultures[J]. Neurochem Res, 1994, 19(3): 331-338.

[39] Strange K, Emma F, Paredes A, *et al.* Osmoregulatory changes in myo-inositol content and Na+/myo-inositol cotransport in rat cortical astrocytes[J]. Glia, 1994, 12(1): 35-43.

[40] Bagga P, Chugani AN, Varadarajan KS, *et al. In vivo* NMR studies of regional cerebral energetics in MPTP model of Parkinson's disease: recovery of cerebral metabolism with acute levodopa treatment[J]. J Neurochem, 2013, 127(3): 365-377.

[41] Baslow MH. N-acetylaspartate in the vertebrate brain: metabolism and function[J]. Neurochem Res, 2003, 28(6): 941-953.

[42] Jenkins BG, Klivenyi P, Kustermann E, *et al.* Nonlinear decrease over time in N-acetyl aspartate levels in the absence of neuronal loss and increases in glutamine and glucose in transgenic Huntington's disease mice[J]. J Neurochem, 2000, 74(5): 2108-2119.

[43] Demougeot C, Garnier P, Mossiat C, *et al.* N-Acetylaspartate, a marker of both cellular dysfunction and neuronal loss: its relevance to studies of acute brain injury[J]. J Neurochem, 2001, 77(2): 408-415.

[44] Tsai G, Coyle JT. N-acetylaspartate in neuropsychiatric disorders[J]. Prog Neurobiol, 1995, 46(5): 531-540.

[45] Davies SE, Gotoh M, Richards DA, *et al.* Hypoosmolarity induces an increase of extracellular N-acetylaspartate concentration in the rat striatum[J]. Neurochem Res, 1998, 23(8): 1021-1025.

[46] Lei S, Powers R. NMR Metabolomics Analysis of Parkinson's Disease[J]. Curr Metabolomics, 2013, 1(3): 191-209.

FGF21 mediates alcohol-induced adipose tissue lipolysis by activation of systemic release of catecholamine in mice

Cuiqing Zhao, Xiaokun Li, Wenke Feng

Adipose tissue is a specialized connective tissue that functions as the major storage site for fat in the form of TGs. Serving as an energy reservoir, adipose tissue synthesizes TGs when energy intake exceeds energy output. During fasting or in response to stress, adipose tissue mobilizes FFAs and glycerol (lipolysis), providing other tissues with metabolites and energy substrates [1, 2]. While lipolysis is a physiological response to metabolic changes, excess lipolysis may lead to increased circulating FFA levels, which is a risk factor for insulin resistance and fatty liver. Clinical and experimental animal studies showed that white adipose tissue (WAT) hyperlipolysis was associated with increased hepatic fat accumulation in alcoholic liver disease (ALD) [3, 4]. Reducing lipolysis by dietary supplementation decreased fatty liver in mice with ALD [5, 6].

Although alcohol-associated adipose tissue lipolysis contributes to the development and progression of ALD in patients and in animal models, the underlying mechanisms are not yet clear. Fibroblast growth factor (FGF)21 is an FGF family member produced by the liver and other metabolic tissues that plays an important role in energy homeostasis and glucose and lipid metabolism [7]. Systemic administration of FGF21 alters lipid profiles in animal models [8, 9], in part, by regulating lipolysis in WAT. However, the exact action of FGF21 on WAT lipolysis remains elusive. The phenotypes of FGF21 transgenic mice suggest that FGF21 stimulates adipose tissue lipolysis[10], while other studies showed that FGF21 attenuates hormone-stimulated lipolysis in both human and murine adipocytes [11]. A recent study suggests that the role of FGF21 in adipose tissue lipolysis is metabolic state dependent; FGF21 stimulates lipolysis in the WAT during normal feeding but inhibits it during fasting [12].

To elucidate the roles of FGF21 in alcohol-induced adipose tissue lipolysis, we exposed FGF21 KO mice to alcohol using a chronic-binge model. Absence of FGF21 attenuates alcohol-induced lipolysis in WAT, which is likely mediated by sympathetic nervous system (SNS) activation.

1. Materials and methods

1.1 Animal experiments

Male C57BL/6J mice (WT) and FGF21 KO mice [13] were used for this study. Alcohol-fed (AF) groups were allowed free access to the liquid diet (Lieber DeCarli; Research Diets, Inc., New Brunswick, NJ) containing 5% (m/v) alcohol for 12 days, and control groups were pair-fed (PF) with the isocaloric maltose dextrin[14] in the following groups: WT+PF, WT+AF, KO+PF, and KO+AF. The mice in the PF groups were given the same amount of food consumed by the mice in AF groups in the previous day. On the last day of the experiment, mice were gavaged with a single dose of alcohol (5 g/kg body weight) or isocaloric maltose dextrin. Mice were euthanized 6 h later. One group of alcohol-exposed FGF21 KO mice was treated with 4 mg/kg recombinant human FGF21 (rhFGF21) (KO+AF+rhFGF21) [15] via intraperitoneal injection during the last 5 days. rhFGF21 was produced in *Escherichia coli* and purified to be endotoxin free [16]. The treatment schedule is illustrated in supplementary Fig. 1. At the end of the experiment, the mice were anesthetized with Avertin (2,2,2-tribromoethanol) and plasma and tissue samples were collected for assays. All mice were housed under controlled lighting (6:00 AM to 6:00 PM light cycle/6:00 PM to 6:00 AM dark cycle). All mice were treated according to the protocols reviewed and approved by the Institutional Animal Care and Use Committee of the University of Louisville.

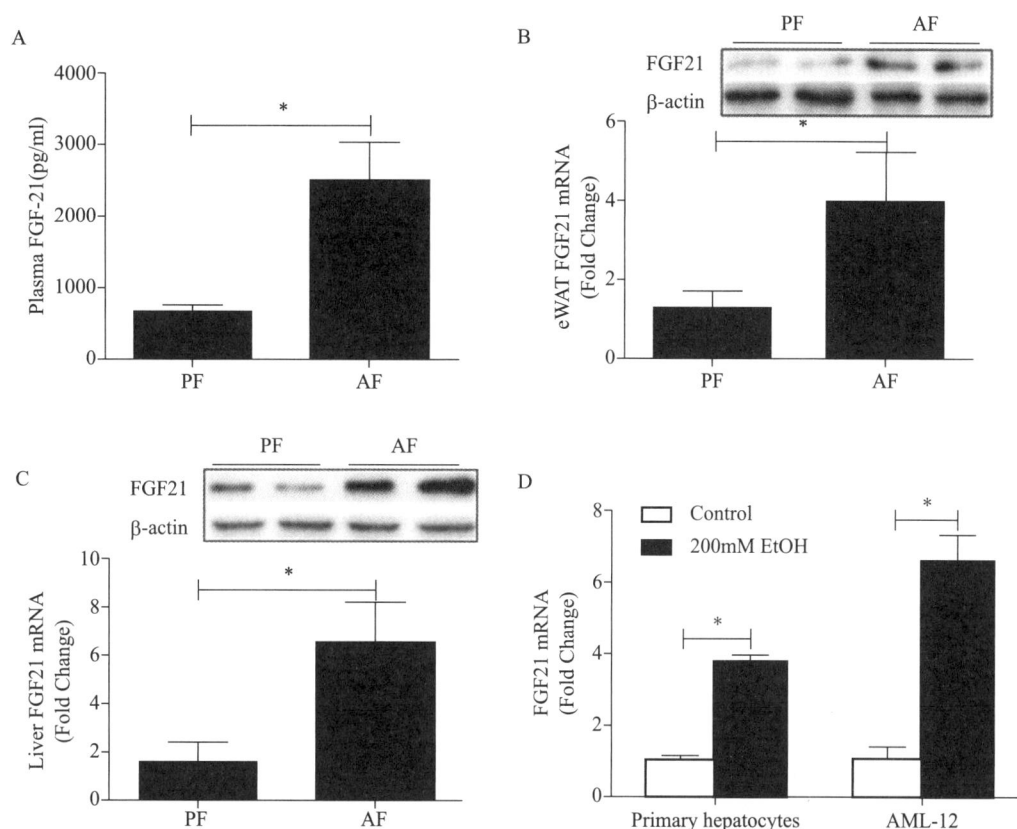

Fig. 1. Effects of alcohol on FGF21 expression. C57BL/6 J mice were fed Lieber DeCarli liquid diet containing 5% alcohol (AF) or pair-fed iso-caloric maltose dextrin diet (PF) as described in the Materials and Methods. On the last day of the experiment, AF and PF mice were gavaged with a single dose of alcohol (5 g/kg body weight) or isocaloric maltose dextrin, respectively, and euthanized 6 h later. (A) Plasma FGF21 protein levels. (B) FGF21 protein (top) and mRNA (bottom) levels in eWAT. (C) FGF21 protein (top) and mRNA (bottom) levels in liver. (D) mRNA levels of FGF21 in primary hepatocytes isolated from WT mice and in AML-12 cells after 200 mM ethanol treatment for 4 h.

1.2 Statistical analysis

Two-way ANOVA with Bonferroni's *post hoc* test, one-way ANOVA with Tukey's *post hoc* test, or two-tailed un-paired Student's *t*-test were used for the determination of statistical significance of the data where they were appropriate. All statistical analyses were performed with GraphPad Prism software version 5 (GraphPad Software, Inc., San Diego, CA). For animal studies, each experimental group had seven mice. For cell culture studies, experiments were repeated three times in triplicate for each experiment. Results are expressed as mean ± SEM. Differences between groups were considered significant at $*P < 0.05$, $**P < 0.01$, and $***P < 0.001$.

Additional methods are described in the supplementary Materials and Methods.

2. Results

2.1 Alcohol exposure increases FGF21 expression

The liver is considered the main source for the production of FGF21. Extrahepatic tissues, including white and brown adipose tissue, also express FGF21 [17]. To determine whether alcohol exposure affects FGF21 expression, we exposed 8- to 10-week-old mice to alcohol in a chronic-binge exposure model as described in the Materials and Methods. Chronic-binge alcohol exposure increased plasma FGF21 concentration by 4-fold approximately (Fig. 1A). A marked increase in FGF21 gene expression and protein concentration in both liver and epididymal WAT (eWAT) was observed, as shown in Fig. 1B, C. Furthermore, to determine whether the hepatocyte responds to alcohol for FGF21 expres-sion, we incubated mouse primary hepatocytes and AML-12 (a hepatocyte cell line) cells with 200 mM ethanol for 4 h

(200 mM shown here. Positive dose-response starting at 50 mM, data not shown). FGF21 mRNA levels were increased nearly 4 and 7 times in primary hepatocytes and AML-12 cells, respectively, after alcohol exposure (Fig. 1D).

2.2 FGF21 deficiency markedly reduces chronic-binge alcohol exposure-induced eWAT lipolysis

FGF21 KO mice have similar eWAT size compared with WT mice. Chronic-binge alcohol exposure markedly reduced eWAT weight in WT mice. Surprisingly, this eWAT weight loss was significantly reduced in FGF21 KO mice (Fig. 2A). The ratio of eWAT to total body weight was reduced approximately 62% in WT mice by alcohol exposure, but only a 22% reduction was observed in FGF21 KO mice (Fig. 2B). In addition, adipocyte size was reduced about 50% in WT mice, but unchanged in FGF21 KO mice, as measured by hematoxylin and eosin staining of eWAT (Fig. 2C, D). These observations indicate that FGF21 KO mice are resistant to alcohol-induced lipolysis in eWAT. To further characterize the role of FGF21 in alcohol-mediated adipose tissue lipolysis, we measured glycerol and NEFA levels in the circulation. Chronic-binge alcohol exposure significantly increased plasma glycerol and NEFA concentrations in WT mice, but not in FGF21 KO mice (Fig. 2E, F).

To further understand the role of FGF21 in adipose tissue, we analyzed the mRNA and protein levels, and the activation of a set of genes known to regulate lipolysis in eWAT. Alcohol exposure did not change the mRNA expression

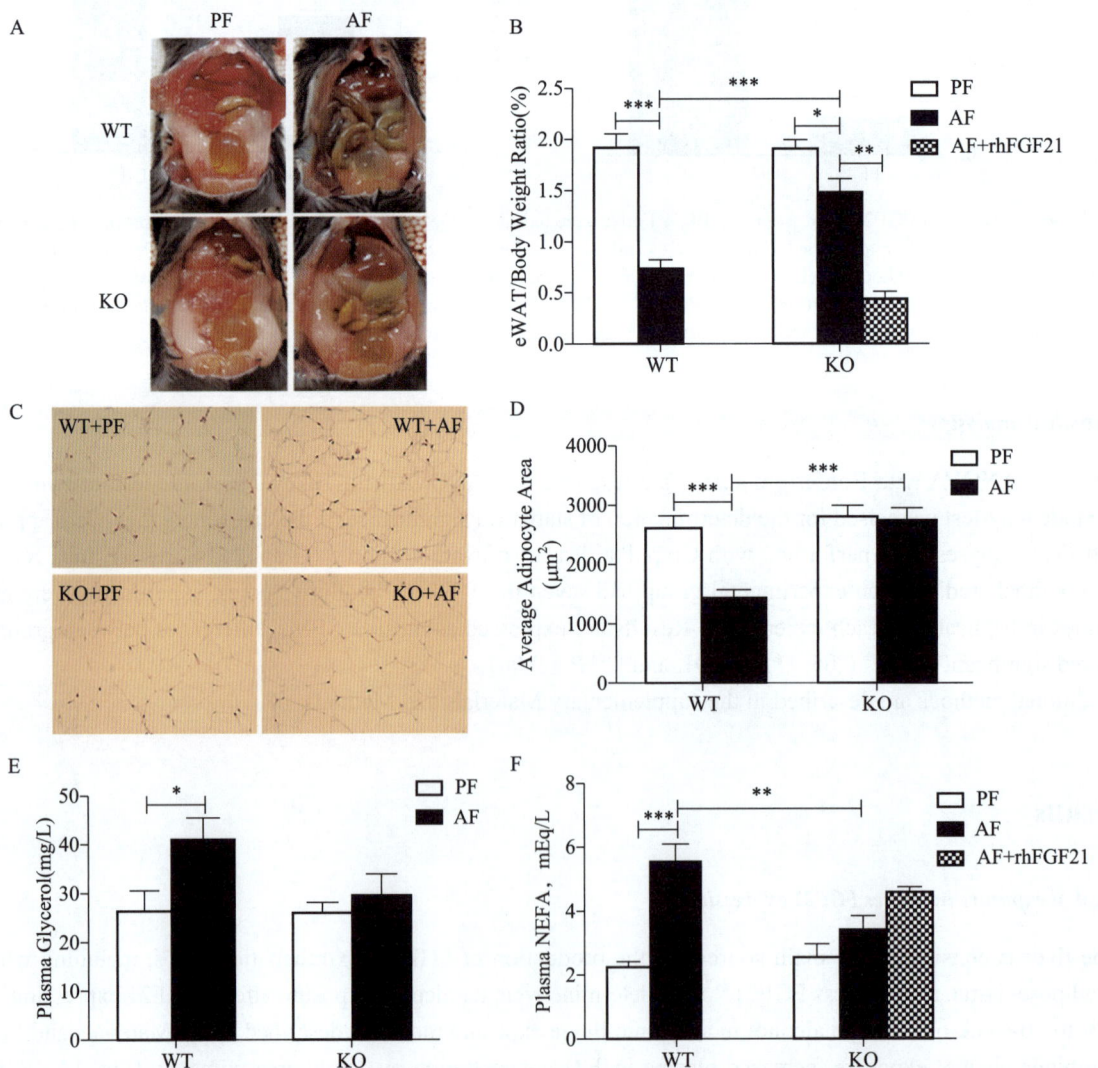

Fig. 2. FGF21 deficiency markedly reduces chronic-binge alcohol exposure-induced eWAT lipolysis. FGF21 KO mice and their WT controls were treated as described in the Materials and Methods. The mice in the KO+AF group were injected intraperitoneally with rhFGF21 at a dose of 4 mg/kg body weight once a day for the last 5 days. (A) Epididymal adipose tissue image. (B) Epididymal adipose tissue/body weight ratio. (C) Histopathology of eWAT depots (200×). (D) Quantification of adipocyte size. (E) Plasma glycerol concentrations. (F) Plasma NEFA concentrations.

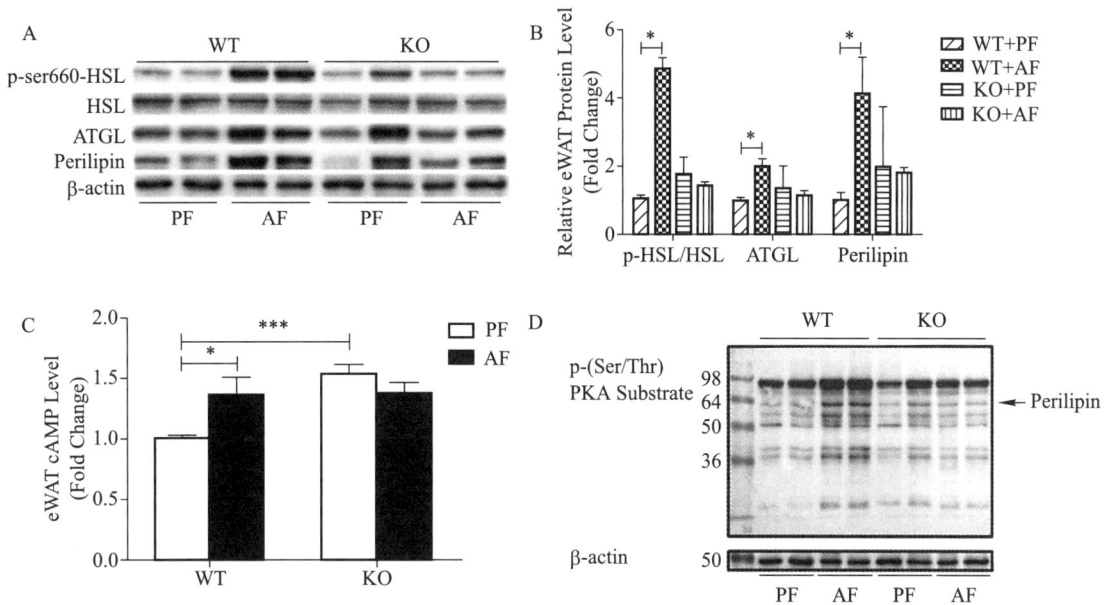

Fig. 3. FGF21 KO mice have reduced expression and activity of proteins involved in adipose tissue lipolysis. Mice were fed as described in the Materials and Methods. Proteins in eWAT were analyzed by Western blotting. (A) Levels of p-HSL, ATGL, and PLIN. (B) The quantification of protein bands in (A) by densitometry analysis; β-actin levels served as loading controls. (C) Epididymal adipose tissue cAMP concentrations. (D) The p-(Ser/Thr) PKA substrate levels; β-actin levels as loading controls.

of hormone sensitive lipase (HSL), adipose tissue TG lipase (ATGL), and perilipin (PLIN) in either WT or FGF21 KO mice (data not shown), but markedly increased HSL-ser660 phosphorylation and ATGL and PLIN protein levels (Fig. 3A, B). It is known that HSL phosphorylation is regulated by protein kinase A (PKA) activation, which is mediated by adipose cAMP. eWAT cAMP levels were markedly increased in WT mice compared with KO mice in response to alcohol exposure (Fig. 3C). PLIN is a coating protein on the lipid droplets in adipocytes. PKA phosphorylates PLIN, exposing the lipid droplet to HSL-mediated lipolysis. We used anti-p-(Ser/Thr) PKA substrate antibody to detect adipose PKA substrates, including PLIN, which were significantly phosphorylated by alcohol exposure in the eWAT of WT mice, while they were inhibited in the KO mice (Fig. 3D). This approach has been used in previous studies to determine PKA-mediated PLIN phosphorylation[18].

The effects of alcohol exposure models were also examined. Chronic alcohol consumption (4 weeks) markedly reduced the eWAT/body weight ratio in WT mice, but not in the KO mice (Fig. 4A). Similarly, acute alcohol exposure (one gavage of 5 g/kg alcohol) induced changes in circulating glycerol, and NEFAs were more pronounced in the WT mice than in the KO mice (Fig. 4B). Thus, FGF21 KO mice are consistently resistant to adipose lipolysis in three different alcohol-exposure models. In the following studies, we focused on the chronic-binge alcohol exposure model.

2.3 Insulin signaling is not associated with alcohol-induced adipose lipolysis in FGF21 KO mice

Insulin is well-known as a major antilipolytic hormone acting to limit release of fatty acids from adipose tissue, and insulin signaling pathways are also targets of alcohol [19]. To determine the role of insulin in the regulation of lipolysis by FGF21 in response to alcohol exposure, we analyzed insulin and Akt activation. Plasma insulin levels did not differ between mouse groups of PF and AF in WT and FGF21 KO mice (Fig. 5A). Alcohol exposure increased Akt phosphorylation, which is known to be a downstream target of insulin, in both WT and FGF21 KO mice (Fig. 5B). To determine whether FGF21 directly activates Akt signaling, we incubated fully differentiated 3T3-L1 adipocytes with rhFGF21. Western blot analysis showed that FGF21, indeed, increased phosphorylation levels of Akt in adipocytes (Fig. 5C). Due to the antilipolytic effect of insulin, the increased insulin signaling would attenuate alcohol-induced adipose tissue lipolysis. As mentioned above, however, alcohol exposure increased eWAT lipolysis, indicating that insulin signaling is unlikely to be the major causative factor in alcohol-induced lipolysis.

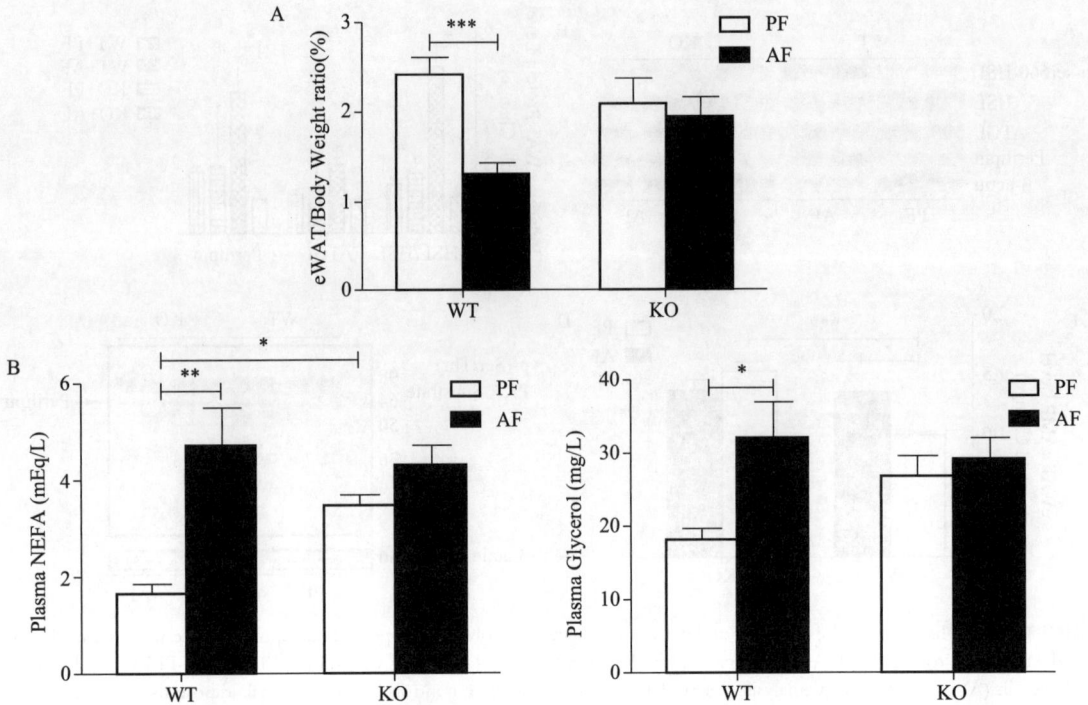

Fig. 4. FGF21 KO mice display attenuated eWAT lipolysis by chronic or acute alcohol exposure. For chronic alcohol exposure, C57BL/6 J and FGF21 KO mice were fed Lieber DeCarli liquid diet containing 5% alcohol (AF) or pair-fed isocaloric maltose dextrin diet (PF) for 4 weeks. (A) eWAT/body weight ratio. For acute alcohol exposure, C57BL/6 J mice and FGF21 KO mice were gavaged in the early morning with a single dose of alcohol (5 g/kg body weight (AF) or isocaloric maltose dextrin (PF)). Blood was collected 6 h later. (B) Plasma NEFA and glycerol concentrations.

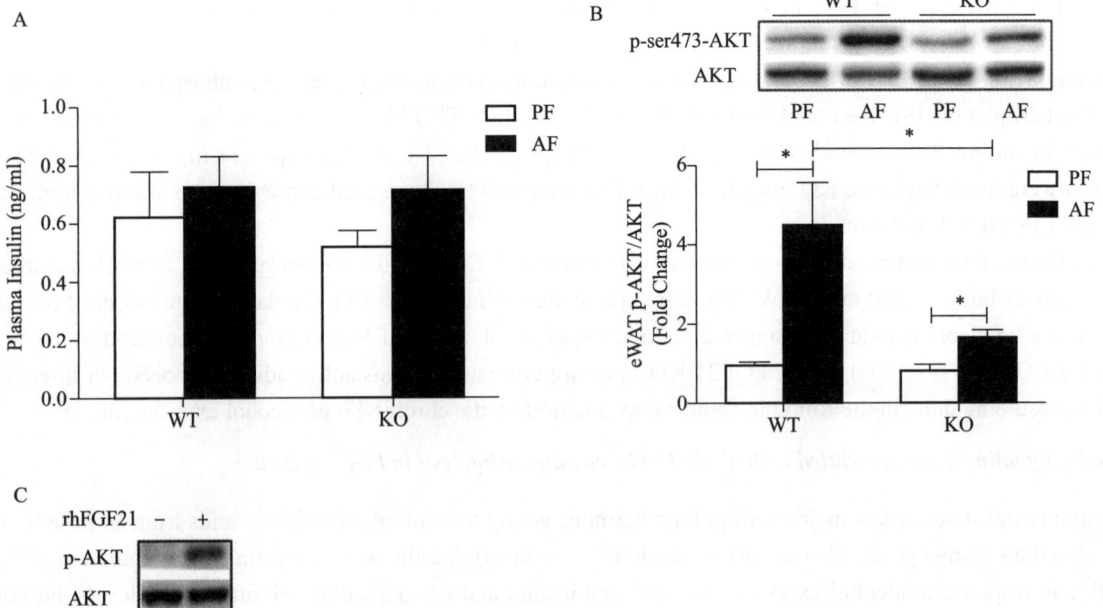

Fig. 5. Insulin is not correlated with alcohol-induced adipose dysfunction. Mice were fed as described in the Materials and Methods. (A) Plasma insulin levels. (B) Immunoblot analysis of eWAT phospho-AKT ser-473, AKT protein levels (top), quantification of the immunoblot bands (bottom). (C) 3T3-L1 adipocytes were treated with vehicle or 1 μg/ml rhFGF21 for 5 min. Cell lysates were immunoblotted for phospho-AKT ser-473 or total AKT as indicated.

2.4 The adipocyte does not respond to FGF21 and alcohol to induce lipolysis

To further investigate the mechanisms of FGF21 and alcohol-mediated lipolysis in adipocytes, we measured the median glycerol concentration in fully differentiated 3T3- L1 cells and primary mouse adipocytes exposed to alcohol or rhFGF21. As shown in supplementary Fig. 2A, differentiated 3T3-L1 cells responded to rhFGF21, as evidenced by the increased phosphorylation of ERK. Isoproterenol, a synthetic catecholamine, significantly increased median glycerol concentrations in both primary adipocytes and fully differentiated 3T3-L1 adipocytes. A sympatholytic non-selective β-blocker (propranolol) inhibited isoproterenol-induced lipolysis in primary adipocytes. However, alcohol and rhFGF21 had no lipolytic effect in either cell type (supplementary Fig. 2B, C), indicating that neither alcohol nor FGF21 directly acts on adipocytes to induce lipolysis. The effects of alcohol, rhFGF21, and isoproterenol on glycerol release were similar in the primary adipocytes isolated from WT and FGF21 KO mice (supplementary Fig. 2B), further suggesting that local action of FGF21 does not affect adipose lipolysis.

2.5 FGF21 mediates alcohol-enhanced catecholamine release

Next, we investigated the effects of alcohol exposure on catecholamine release. Epinephrine (EP) and norepinephrine (NE), secreted through SNS innervation, have been acknowledged as the principal initiators of lipolysis [20–22]. To explore the mechanisms by which alcohol stimulates lipolysis, plasma EP and NE were measured. Alcohol exposure lead to about a 4-fold increase in EP release (Fig. 6A), and about a 2-fold increase in NE release (Fig. 6B) in WT mice. However, in FGF21-deficient mice, alcohol induced only about a 2-fold increase in EP release and virtually no change for NE (Fig. 6A, B). The plasma EP concentrations were positively correlated with the mRNA levels of phenyl-ethanolamine N- methyltransferase (PNMT), which is a major enzyme involved in EP synthesis in the adrenal gland (Fig. 6C). As PNMT activity is largely regulated by adrenal glucocorticoids, we measured plasma corticosterone levels. Alcohol exposure significantly increased plasma corticosterone levels in both WT and KO mice. However, the elevation in the KO mice was less significant than in WT mice (data not shown). EP and NE stimulate lipolysis through promoting β-adrenergic receptor (β-AR) activation [23, 24]. β-ARs have three subtypes, $β_1$-, $β_2$-, and $β_3$-AR. As shown in supplementary Fig. 3A, $β_3$-AR had the highest expression level in eWAT ($^\Delta$Ct values). However, no difference was found in

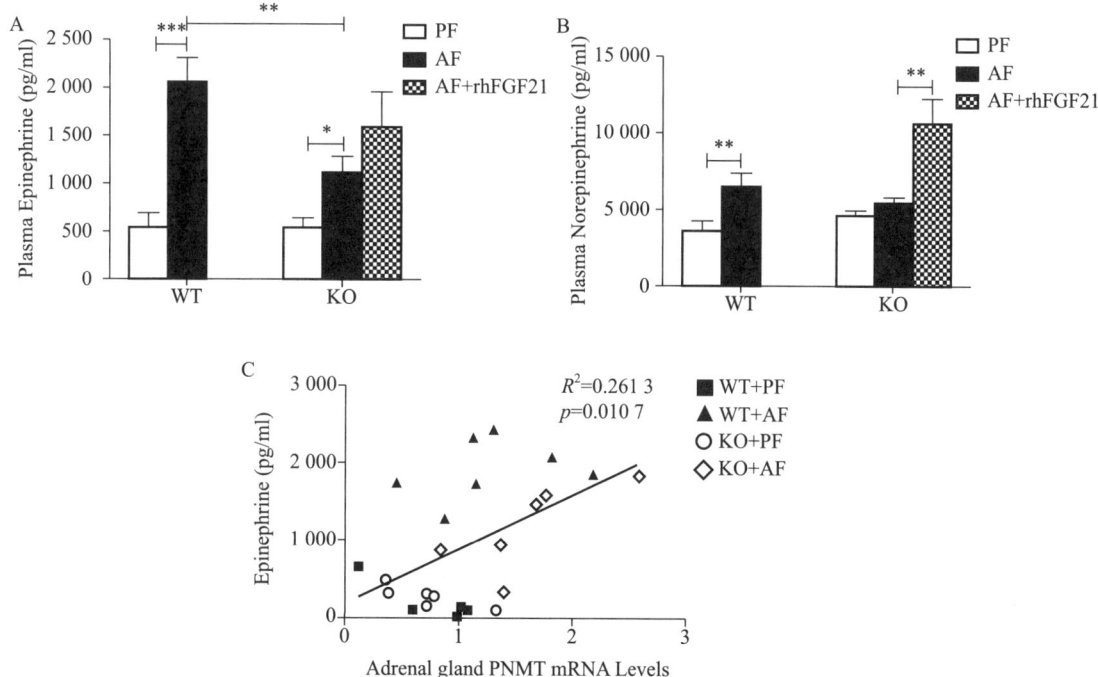

Fig. 6. FGF21 KO mice have reduced plasma levels of EP and NE in response to alcohol exposure. Mice were fed as described in the Materials and Methods, the mice in KO+AF group were injected intraperitoneally with rhFGF21 at a dose of 4 mg/kg body weight once a day for the last 5 days. (A) Plasma EP levels. (B) Plasma NE levels. (C) Linear correlation of the adrenal gland PNMT mRNA expression and plasma EP level.

chronic-binge alcohol exposure-induced β-AR expression between eWAT in WT and KO mice (supplementary Fig. 3B–D).

2.6 Exogenous FGF21 administration exacerbates chronic-binge alcohol exposure-induced lipolysis

Based on the above findings, we hypothesized that FGF21 may enhance chronic-binge alcohol exposure-induced eWAT lipolysis through the regulation of systemic catecholamine release. To test this hypothesis, one group of alcohol-exposed FGF21 KO mice (KO+AF+FGF21) was treated with 4 mg/kg/day rhFGF21 *via* intraperitoneal injection for the last 5 days. As expected, rhFGF21 treatment significantly increased eWAT weight loss. Compared with the alcohol exposure group, the ratio of eWAT to total body weight was decreased 71% after rhFGF21 treatment in KO mice (Fig. 2B). Interestingly, the decrease in eWAT by rhFGF21 administration was accompanied by an increase in EP and NE in the plasma (Fig. 6A, B). The increased lipolysis in the KO mice by rhFGF21 was further supported by the increased plasma NEFA levels (Fig. 2F), although the change did not reach statistical significance.

2.7 Effects of FGF21 deletion on chronic-binge alcohol-induced hepatic steatosis and injury

Adipose tissue lipolysis contributes to chronic-alcohol-induced hepatic steatosis [4]. To determine whether FGF21-mediated adipose lipolysis is involved in the chronic-binge alcohol exposure-induced fatty liver, the hepatic steatosis index and liver markers of injury were measured. Alcohol exposure significantly increased liver/body weight ratios in both WT and FGF21 KO mice, and the change in FGF21 KO mice was smaller than in WT mice (Fig. 7A). Similarly, there were significant changes in liver TG concentrations by alcohol exposure in both WT and KO mice (Fig. 7B). Notably, chronic-binge alcohol exposure increased liver TG levels by about 6-fold in the WT mice, but only by about 2-fold in the KO mice. These results indicate that the KO mice are less sensitive to chronic-binge alcohol exposure in hepatic fat accumulation (Fig. 7B). A baseline increase in TG levels in the KO+PF mice may contribute to the reduced sensitivity to chronic-binge alcohol exposure, but insignificantly. Confirming the biochemical assays, the histological examinations showed a reduced fat accumulation in the livers of the KO mice in response to alcohol exposure (Fig. 7C). Alcohol exposure significantly increased plasma alanine aminotransferase (ALT) and aspartate aminotransferase (AST) levels (Fig. 7D, E) in WT mice, and these elevations tended to be reduced in the KO mice, indicating a likely reduction of liver injury by chronic-binge alcohol exposure in the KO mice.

3. Discussion

Alcohol-induced hepatic fat accumulation is considered to be the earliest pathological alteration in ALD. Clinical and experimental studies have demonstrated that a reduction of *in situ* liver lipogenesis and an increase of lipid β-oxidation prevent hepatic steatosis and slow or halt the progression of ALD [25, 26]. On the other hand, alcohol-induced fatty liver disease is associated with reverse transport of FFAs derived from adipose lipoatrophy by alcohol ingestion. The mechanisms by which alcohol disrupts adipose tissue homeostasis to contribute to alcoholic fatty liver disease are not fully understood. In the current study, we demonstrated that chronic-binge alcohol exposure significantly reduced epididymal adipose fat mass, but this reduction was inhibited in the FGF21 KO mice. Supplementation of the rhFGF21 to the FGF21 KO mice further exacerbated alcohol-induced adipose lipolysis. Importantly, we showed that the function of FGF21 was associated with elevation of circulating catecholamine concentrations due to alcohol exposure.

Adipose tissue lipolysis is an exquisitely controlled process [27, 28]. cAMP signaling represents the principal prolipolytic pathway in WAT. cAMP activation stimulates PKA activation, which mediates the activation of HSL by phosphorylation. PLIN is a coating protein that binds to the surface of lipid droplets and appears to be essential for lipid degradation [29]. PKA activation promotes HSL phosphorylation at Ser 660, which is crucial for its activation and translocation to PLIN-containing droplets[30, 31], where HSL catalyzes the hydrolysis of diglycerides to monoglycerides [32, 33]. Recently, another lipase, ATGL, has been identified. ATGL favors TG substrates and is a rate-determining enzyme for lipolysis in adipose tissue [34, 35]. ATGL is not a direct substrate for PKA [35] and its activity depends on PLIN activation [36]. These concepts were supported by our current study, which showed that the levels of ATGL, PLIN, and p-HSL were increased in the eWAT by chronic-binge alcohol exposure.

Adipose lipid metabolism is known to be affected by hormones [37]. Lipolysis is negatively regulated by insulin and positively regulated by catecholamine [38]. Insulin exerts its influence by stimulating the phosphoinositide 3-kinase-Akt

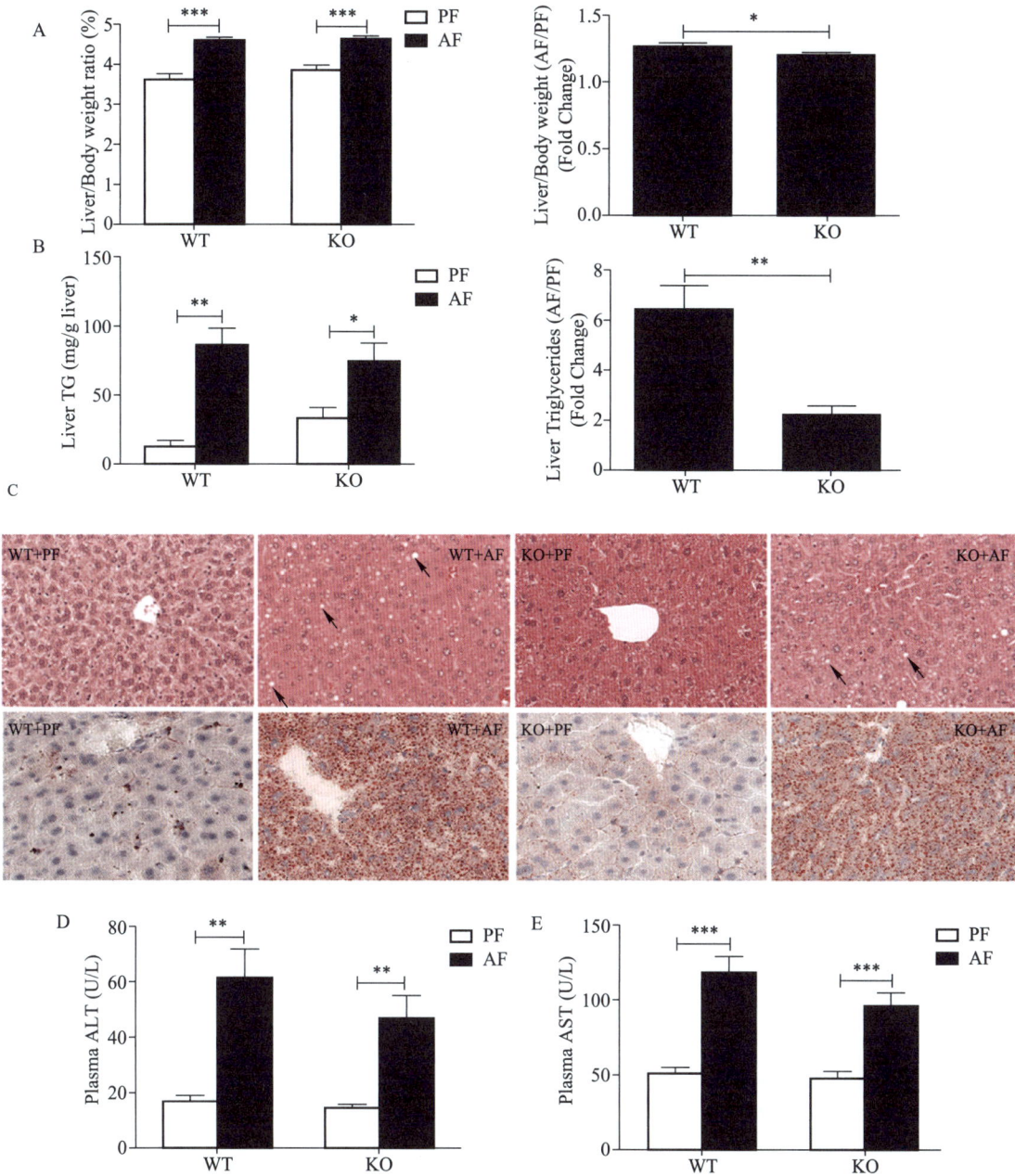

Fig. 7. Effects of FGF21 deletion on chronic-binge alcohol-induced hepatic steatosis and injury. Mice were fed as described in the Materials and Methods. (A) Liver to body weight ratios. (B) Liver TG concentrations. (C) Hematoxylin and eosin (upper) and Oil Red O (below) staining of hepatic tissues (arrows indicate lipid droplets). (D) Plasma ALT concentrations. (E) Plasma AST concentrations.

pathway in the adipose tissue. Earlier studies showed that insulin-induced tyrosine phosphorylation of phosphoinositide 3-kinase and phosphorylation of Akt were affected by chronic alcohol feeding [3, 39], leaving the effect of alcohol on insulin signaling in adipose tissue elusive. It is, however, an important issue because cross-talk between insulin and FGF21 has been demonstrated [40–42]. Exogenous FGF21 administration increased insulin sensitivity in several animal models of metabolic diseases [8, 43, 44]. We showed that plasma insulin levels were not affected, but phosphorylation of Akt was increased by alcohol exposure, indicating an activation of insulin action. Our observations are different than a previous study in which an inhibition of insulin action by chronic alcohol exposure was demonstrated [4]. The differences may be due to the various alcohol exposure models. In fact, the chronic and binge alcohol exposure models produced remarkable differences in the reverse transport of FFAs derived from adipose lipolysis into the liver in animal models[45, 46]. Nevertheless, adipose lipolysis is increased by both chronic and acute alcohol exposure. Thus, the potentially increased insulin action observed in chronic-binge alcohol groups might inhibit lipolysis, but this inhibition may be overridden by other stimulatory factors.

A major extra-adipose signaling pathway for adipose lipolysis is catecholamine signaling. Catecholamines (EP and NE) [47], the end mediators of the sympatho-adrenergic system, are secreted mainly from the adrenal medulla by SNS activation and have been implicated as important modulators of lipolytic activity. Catecholamines are known to act physiologically *via* binding to β-ARs (subtypes β$_{1-3}$-ARs). β$_1$-AR is found predominantly in the brain and heart [48], β$_2$-AR is widely expressed [49], and β$_3$-AR is mainly expressed in adipose tissue [50]. Binding to adipose tissue β-ARs, catecholamines activate Gs protein and enhance intracellular cAMP concentration and stimulate cAMP-dependent PKA activation, leading to the phosphorylation and activation of HSL [51]. Chronic-binge alcohol exposure does not act directly on the adipose tissue to stimulate lipolysis. Instead, we showed that alcohol exposure increased SNS activity and stimulated the release of NE and EP in the circulation to activate β-AR. This agrees with the clinical observation that alcohol ingestion elevates blood catecholamine levels [52].

The most important finding in the current study is that FGF21 mediates catecholamine release in response to alcohol exposure. We showed that chronic-binge alcohol-induced adipose tissue lipolysis was inhibited in FGF21 KO mice. Intra-adipose lipolysis signaling exhibited a resistance phenotype in the KO mice, evidenced by the reduced response to ATGL and PLIN expression and p-HSL levels. However, FGF21 does not act directly on adipocytes to stimulate lipolysis. Using primary adipocytes and differentiated 3T3-L1 cells, we showed that alcohol did not increase median glycerol levels, and this lack of response was FGF21 independent. Rather, we demonstrated that the alcohol-induced catecholamine elevation is significantly attenuated in FGF21 KO mice. In addition, treatment of FGF21 KO mice with rhFGF21 significantly elevated the plasma NE. Taken together, our findings support the concept that FGF21 increases SNS activity to increase the release of catecholamine, which mediates the stimulatory effect on alcohol-induced lipolysis.

The role of FGF21 on adipose lipolysis is still elusive. While some studies suggested that FGF21 stimulates glycerol secretion from adipocytes [10], other studies showed that FGF21 was likely a negative factor in adipose lipolysis [11]. Upon binding to the FGF receptors, FGF21 activates ERK by phosphorylation, which has been shown to contribute to adipose tissue lipolysis [53, 54]. However, our *in vitro* experiment using adipocytes does not support this notion in response to alcohol. Our results unambiguously demonstrate that FGF21 promotes adipose lipolysis under conditions of chronic-binge alcohol exposure. This stimulatory effect is likely mediated by global SNS activation. Although this hypothesis is further supported by a novel finding that FGF21 can stimulate SNS activity in brown adipose tissue [55], additional experiments are needed to confirm this direct effect on SNS activation.

Multiple studies have demonstrated that FGF21 plays a critical role in hepatic lipid accumulation [9, 56]. In a parallel study, we showed that lack of FGF21 exacerbated chronic alcohol exposure-induced fatty liver through SIRT-1-mediated fatty acid β-oxidation (unpublished observations). However, in the chronic-binge alcohol exposure model, hepatic fat accumulation tended to decrease in FGF21 KO mice. The discrepancy clearly indicates diverse roles of FGF21 in different alcohol exposure models. Multiple studies have shown the complexity of FGF21 in metabolic disease. The different roles of FGF21 may depend on the expression and activation of FGF receptors and the cofactor, β-klotho, involved in different forms metabolic stress [57]. Accumulation of hepatic fat due to alcohol ingestion is derived from two major sources: *in situ* hepatic events for lipid handling, including lipogenesis and fat clearance; and adipose events characterized by lipolysis. A lack of FGF21 would increase fat synthesis and decrease the clearance in the liver, but would decrease adipose fat degradation and fatty acid reverse transport into the liver. Our findings support the concept that, in global FGF21 KO mice, *in situ* hepatic events are dominant for chronic alcohol-induced liver fat increase, while adipose tissue lipolysis significantly compensates for the hepatic events in the chronic-binge exposure model.

It has to be noted that although there is protection on hepatic fat accumulation, there are minimal alterations in serum ALT and AST levels in FGF21 KO mice under the condition of chronic-binge alcohol exposure. The fact that most alcoholics develop fatty liver, but do not experience hepatitis and cirrhosis, has led to a second-hit hypothesis in ALD[58]. Hepatic fat accumulation, as the first hit, sensitizes the liver to the second or multiple hit(s). The increased adipose tissue lipolysis and the likely increased reverse fatty acid transport into the liver by chronic-binge alcohol exposure may serve as the first hit and sensitize the liver to the second hit, which could be excessive intake of alcohol or other environmental challenges [58].

In conclusion, as depicted in Fig. 8, the present study indicates that FGF21 plays a pivotal role in alcohol-induced adipose tissue lipolysis through global catecholamine regulation. Although studies have described the protective role of FGF21 in diet-induced liver lipid metabolism, its relevance to various human diseases and underlying mechanisms

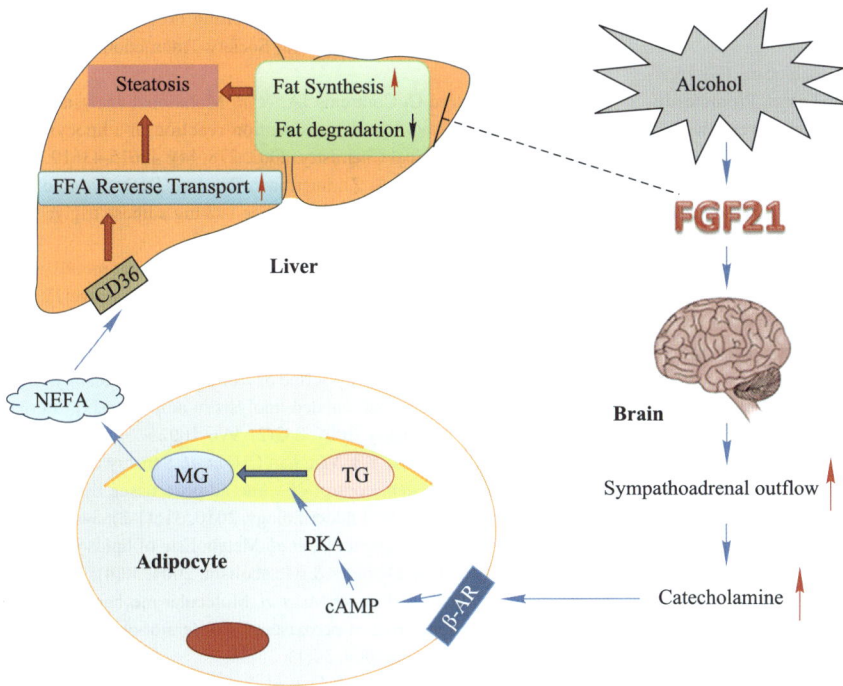

Fig. 8. A working model of how FGF21 mediates alcohol-induced adipose tissue lipolysis by activation of the systemic release of catecholamine in mice. Alcohol exposure increases systemic FGF21 level which activates SNS to release catecholamine in the circulation. Catecholamine increases adipose tissue fat degradation by binding to β-AR leading to increased circulating NEFA concentration, which increases NEFA reverse transport into the liver and hepatic steatosis. CD36, cluster of differentiation 36; MG, monoacylglycerol.

is not fully understood. We have demonstrated that anti-FGF21 may be beneficial for the reduction of alcohol-induced excess-lipolysis. Therefore, strategies targeting the SNS activation to block FGF21-mediated excess-adipose lipolysis might be developed to prevent/treat acute alcohol-induced fatty liver disease.

Supplemental materials

Supplemental materials can be found at http://www.jlr.org/content/suppl/2015/06/19/jlr.M058610.DC1.html.

References

[1] Raclot T, Groscolas R. Selective mobilization of adipose tissue fatty acids during energy depletion in the rat[J]. J Lipid Res, 1995, 36(10): 2164-2173.

[2] Halliwell KJ, Fielding BA, Samra JS, et al. Release of individual fatty acids from human adipose tissue in vivo after an overnight fast[J]. J Lipid Res, 1996, 37(9): 1842-1848.

[3] Kang L, Chen X, Sebastian BM, et al. Chronic ethanol and triglyceride turnover in white adipose tissue in rats: inhibition of the anti-lipolytic action of insulin after chronic ethanol contributes to increased triglyceride degradation[J]. J Biol Chem, 2007, 282(39): 28465-28473.

[4] Zhong W, Zhao Y, Tang Y, et al. Chronic alcohol exposure stimulates adipose tissue lipolysis in mice: role of reverse triglyceride transport in the pathogenesis of alcoholic steatosis[J]. Am J Pathol, 2012, 180(3): 998-1007.

[5] Dou X, Xia Y, Chen J, et al. Rectification of impaired adipose tissue methylation status and lipolytic response contributes to hepatoprotective effect of betaine in a mouse model of alcoholic liver disease[J]. Br J Pharmacol, 2014, 171(17): 4073-4086.

[6] Zhou Z, Wang L, Song Z, et al. Zinc supplementation prevents alcoholic liver injury in mice through attenuation of oxidative stress[J]. Am J Pathol, 2005, 166(6): 1681-1690.

[7] Badman MK, Koester A, Flier JS, et al. Fibroblast growth factor 21-deficient mice demonstrate impaired adaptation to ketosis[J]. Endocrinology, 2009, 150(11): 4931-4940.

[8] Kharitonenkov A, Shiyanova TL, Koester A, et al. FGF-21 as a novel metabolic regulator[J]. J Clin Invest, 2005, 115(6): 1627-1635.

[9] Xu J, Lloyd DJ, Hale C, et al. Fibroblast growth factor 21 reverses hepatic steatosis, increases energy expenditure, and improves insulin sensitivity in diet-induced obese mice[J]. Diabetes, 2009, 58(1): 250-259.

[10] Inagaki T, Dutchak P, Zhao G, et al. Endocrine regulation of the fasting response by PPAR alpha-mediated induction of fibroblast growth factor 21[J]. Cell Metabolism, 2007, 5(6): 415-425.

[11] Arner P, Pettersson A, Mitchell PJ, et al. FGF21 attenuates lipolysis in human adipocytes - A possible link to improved insulin sensitivity[J]. Febs Letters, 2008, 582(12): 1725-1730.

[12] Hotta Y, Nakamura H, Konishi M, et al. Fibroblast Growth Factor 21 Regulates Lipolysis in White Adipose Tissue But Is Not Required for Ketogenesis and Triglyceride Clearance in Liver[J]. Endocrinology, 2009, 150(10): 4625-4633.

[13] Potthoff MJ, Inagaki T, Satapati S, et al. FGF21 induces PGC-1 alpha and regulates carbohydrate and fatty acid metabolism during the adaptive starvation response[J]. Proceedings of the National

Academy of Sciences of the United States of America, 2009, 106(26): 10853-10858.

[14] Wang Y, Kirpich I, Liu Y, et al. Lactobacillus rhamnosus GG Treatment Potentiates Intestinal Hypoxia-Inducible Factor, Promotes Intestinal Integrity and Ameliorates Alcohol-Induced Liver Injury[J]. American Journal of Pathology, 2011, 179(6): 2866-2875.

[15] Inagaki T, Lin VY, Goetz R, et al. Inhibition of growth hormone signaling by the fasting-induced hormone FGF21[J]. Cell Metabolism, 2008, 8(1): 77-83.

[16] Plotnikov AN, Hubbard SR, Schlessinger J, et al. Crystal structures of two FGF-FGFR complexes reveal the determinants of ligand-receptor specificity[J]. Cell, 2000, 101(4): 413-424.

[17] Muise ES, Azzolina B, Kuo DW, et al. Adipose fibroblast growth factor 21 is up-regulated by peroxisome proliferator-activated receptor gamma and altered metabolic states[J]. Molecular Pharmacology, 2008, 74(2): 403-412.

[18] Fernandez-Galilea M, Perez-Matute P, Prieto-Hontoria PL, et al. Effects of lipoic acid on lipolysis in 3T3-L1 adipocytes[J]. Journal of Lipid Research, 2012, 53(11): 2296-2306.

[19] Stumvoll M, Wahl HG, Loblein K, et al. A novel use of the hyperinsulinemic-euglycemic clamp technique to estimate insulin sensitivity of systemic lipolysis[J]. Hormone and Metabolic Research, 2001, 33(2): 89-95.

[20] Prigge WF. Effects of glucagon, epinephrine and insulin on in-vitro lipolysis of adipose tissue from mammals ind birds[J]. Comparative Biochemistry and Physiology B, 1971, 39(1): 69-82.

[21] Froesch ER, Burgi H, Bally P, et al. Insulin inhibition of spontaneous adipose tissue lipolysis and effects upon fructose and glucose metabolism[J]. Molecular Pharmacology, 1965, 1(3): 280-296.

[22] Goodridg AG, Ball EG. Studies on metabolism of adipose tissue.18. in vitro effects of insulin epinephrine and glucagon on lipolysis and glycolysis in pigeon adipose tissue[J]. Comparative Biochemistry and Physiology, 1965, 16(4): 367-381.

[23] Lafontan M, Berlan M. Fat-cell adrenergic-receptors and the control of white and brown fat-cell function[J]. Journal of Lipid Research, 1993, 34(7): 1057-1091.

[24] Lafontan M. Differential recruitment and differential regulation by physiological amines of fat-cell beta-1, beta-2 and beta-3 adrenergic-receptors expressed in native fat-cells and in transfected[J]. Cellular Signalling, 1994, 6(4): 363-392.

[25] Siler SQ, Neese RA, Hellerstein MK. De novo lipogenesis, lipid kinetics, and whole-body lipid balances in humans after acute alcohol consumption[J]. American Journal of Clinical Nutrition, 1999, 70(5): 928-936.

[26] Ji C, Chan C, Kaplowitz N. Predominant role of sterol response element binding proteins (SREBP) lipogenic pathways in hepatic steatosis in the murine intragastric ethanol feeding model[J]. Journal of Hepatology, 2006, 45(5): 717-724.

[27] Fiorenza CG, Chou SH, Mantzoros CS. Lipodystrophy: pathophysiology and advances in treatment[J]. Nature Reviews Endocrinology, 2011, 7(3): 137-150.

[28] Kolditz C-I, Langin D. Adipose tissue lipolysis[J]. Current Opinion in Clinical Nutrition and Metabolic Care, 2010, 13(4): 377-381.

[29] Miyoshi H, Souza SC, Zhang H-H, et al. Perilipin promotes hormone-sensitive lipase-mediated adipocyte lipolysis via phosphorylation-dependent and -independent mechanisms[J]. Journal of Biological Chemistry, 2006, 281(23): 15837-15844.

[30] Londos C, Brasaemle DL, Schultz CJ, et al. On the control of lipolysis in adipocytes[A]. In: The Metabolic Syndrome X: Convergence of Insulin Resistance, Glucose Intolerance, Hypertension, Obesity, and Dyslipidemias-Searching for the Underlying Defects (Hansen BC, Saye J, Wennogle LP, eds), Vol. 892, 1999: 155-168.

[31] Moore HPH, Silver RB, Mottillo EP, et al. Perilipin targets a novel pool of lipid droplets for lipolytic attack by hormone-sensitive lipase[J]. Journal of Biological Chemistry, 2005, 280(52): 43109-43120.

[32] Holm C. Molecular mechanisms regulating hormone-sensitive lipase and lipolysis[J]. Biochemical Society Transactions, 2003, 31: 1120-1124.

[33] Su CL, Sztalryd C, Contreras JA, et al. Mutational analysis of the hormone-sensitive lipase translocation reaction in adipocytes[J]. Journal of Biological Chemistry, 2003, 278(44): 43615-43619.

[34] Haemmerle G, Lass A, Zimmermann R, et al. Defective lipolysis and altered energy metabolism in mice lacking adipose triglyceride lipase[J]. Science, 2006, 312(5774): 734-737.

[35] Zimmermann R, Strauss JG, Haemmerle G, et al. Fat mobilization in adipose tissue is promoted by adipose triglyceride lipase[J]. Science, 2004, 306(5700): 1383-1386.

[36] Miyoshi H, Perfield JW, II, Souza SC, et al. Control of adipose triglyceride lipase action by serine 517 of perilipin A globally regulates protein kinase A-stimulated lipolysis in adipocytes[J]. Journal of Biological Chemistry, 2007, 282(2): 996-1002.

[37] Bartness TJ, Shrestha YB, Vaughan CH, et al. Sensory and sympathetic nervous system control of white adipose tissue lipolysis[J]. Molecular and Cellular Endocrinology, 2010, 318(1-2): 34-43.

[38] Large V, Peroni O, Letexier D, et al. Metabolism of lipids in human white adipocyte[J]. Diabetes & Metabolism, 2004, 30(4): 294-309.

[39] Crabb DW, Galli A, Fischer M, et al. Molecular mechanisms of alcoholic fatty liver: role of peroxisome proliferator-activated receptor alpha[J]. Alcohol, 2004, 34(1): 35-38.

[40] Semba RD, Sun K, Egan JM, et al. Relationship of Serum Fibroblast Growth Factor 21 with Abnormal Glucose Metabolism and Insulin Resistance: The Baltimore Longitudinal Study of Aging[J]. Journal of Clinical Endocrinology & Metabolism, 2012, 97(4): 1375-1382.

[41] Dutchak PA, Katafuchi T, Bookout AL, et al. Fibroblast Growth Factor-21 Regulates PPARγ Activity and the Antidiabetic Actions of Thiazolidinediones[J]. Cell, 2012, 148(3): 556-567.

[42] Kliewer SA, Mangelsdorf DJ. Fibroblast growth factor 21: from pharmacology to physiology[J]. American Journal of Clinical Nutrition, 2010, 91(1): 254S-257S.

[43] Camporez JPG, Jornayvaz FR, Petersen MC, et al. Cellular Mechanisms by Which FGF21 Improves Insulin Sensitivity in Male Mice[J]. Endocrinology, 2013, 154(9): 3099-3109.

[44] Lin Z, Tian H, Lam KSL, et al. Adiponectin Mediates the Metabolic Effects of FGF21 on Glucose Homeostasis and Insulin Sensitivity in Mice[J]. Cell Metabolism, 2013, 17(5): 779-789.

[45] Horning MG, Williams EA, Maling HM, et al. Depot fat as source of increased liver triglycerides after ethanol[J]. Biochemical and Biophysical Research Communications, 1960, 3(6): 635-640.

[46] Lee R, Feinbaum R, Ambros V. A short history of a short RNA[J]. Cell, 2004, S116(2): S89-S92.

[47] Zouhal H, Jacob C, Delamarche P, et al. Catecholamines and the effects of exercise, training and gender[J]. Sports Medicine, 2008, 38(5): 401-423.

[48] Frielle T, Collins S, Daniel KW, et al. Cloning of the cdna for the human beta-1-adrenergic receptor[J]. Proceedings of the National Academy of Sciences of the United States of America, 1987, 84(22): 7920-7924.

[49] Dixon RAF, Kobilka BK, Strader DJ, et al. Cloning of the gene and cdna for mammalian beta-adrenergic-receptor and homology with rhodopsin[J]. Nature, 1986, 321(6065): 75-79.

[50] Emorine LJ, Marullo S, Briendsutren MM, et al. Molecular characterization of the human beta-3-adrenergic receptor[J]. Science, 1989, 245(4922): 1118-1121.

[51] Lafontan M. Kidney, adipose tissue, adipocytes - what's new?[J]. Nephrologie & Therapeutique, 2011, 7(2): 69-79.

[52] Ireland MA, Vandongen R, Davidson L, et al. Acute effects of moderate alcohol-consumption on blood-pressure and plasma-catecholamines[J]. Clinical Science, 1984, 66(6): 643-648.

[53] Jager J, Gremeaux T, Gonzalez T, et al. Tpl2 Kinase Is Upregulated in Adipose Tissue in Obesity and May Mediate Interleukin-1 beta

and Tumor Necrosis Factor-alpha Effects on Extracellular Signal-Regulated Kinase Activation and Lipolysis[J]. Diabetes, 2010, 59(1): 61-70.

[54] Zhang HH, Halbleib M, Ahmad F, *et al.* Tumor necrosis factor-alpha stimulates lipolysis in differentiated human Adipocytes through activation of extracellular signal-related kinase and elevation of intracellular cAMP[J]. Diabetes, 2002, 51(10): 2929-2935.

[55] Owen BM, Ding X, Morgan DA, *et al.* FGF21 Acts Centrally to Induce Sympathetic Nerve Activity, Energy Expenditure, and Weight Loss[J]. Cell Metabolism, 2014, 20(4): 670-677.

[56] Badman MK, Pissios P, Kennedy AR, *et al.* Hepatic fibroblast growth factor 21 is regulated by PPAR alpha and is a key mediator of hepatic lipid metabolism in ketotic states[J]. Cell Metabolism, 2007, 5(6): 426-437.

[57] Kurosu H, Choi M, Ogawa Y, *et al.* Tissue-specific expression of beta Klotho and fibroblast growth factor (FGF) receptor Isoforms determines metabolic activity of FGF19 and FGF21[J]. Journal of Biological Chemistry, 2007, 282(37): 26687-26695.

[58] Tsukamoto H, Machida K, Dynnyk A, *et al.* "Second Hit" Models of Alcoholic Liver Disease[J]. Seminars in Liver Disease, 2009, 29(2): 178-187.

Fibroblast growth factor 21 deletion aggravates diabetes-induced pathogenic changes in the aorta in type 1 diabetic mice

Xiaoqing Yan, Xiaokun Li, Yi Tan

1. Introduction

Diabetic vascular complications, including macroangiopathy, microangiopathy and peripheral vascular complications, are the most common diabetic complications in both type 1 [1] and type 2 [2] diabetes mellitus and make major contributions to diabetic mortality and morbidity [2]. Diabetic microvascular disease is a leading cause of blindness, renal failure and nerve damage. Furthermore, diabetic macroangiopathy and peripheral vascular complications lead to increased risk of myocardial infarction, stroke and limb amputation [3]. About 80% of all diabetic patients die from cardiovascular events. Of which, 75% are due to coronary heart disease and the remaining 25% are attributed to cerebrovascular, peripheral or other macrovascular disease [4].

Even though the exact mechanism for accelerated vascular disease in diabetes is not yet fully clear, existing research has defined numerous risk factors involved in diabetes, such as oxidative stress [5, 6], dyslipidemia [4, 5], advanced glycation [7], decline in nitric oxide production, activation of the reninangiotensin aldosterone system, and endothelial inflammation [4]. All contribute to the development of diabetic vascular complications.

Fibroblast growth factor 21 (FGF21), a newly-defined member of the FGF family [8], has been identified as a potent metabolic regulator with specific effects on glucose and lipid metabolism [9]. FGF21 can stimulate glucose uptake in adipocytes [10], and enhance glucose clearance by enhancing the browning of white adipose tissues [11]. In response to fasting, FGF21 can regulate lipolysis in adipocytes [12]. FGF21 also shows beneficial effects on lipid profiles as demonstrated by lower circulating lipids in both rodent [13] and primate [14] diabetic models following FGF21 administration. FGF21 treatment also enhanced expression and secretion of the down stream effector, adiponectin, in adipocytes, which in turn further improved fatty acid oxidation and lipid clearance in the liver and skeletal muscle [15]. Moreover, FGF21 has an insulin-sensitizing ability [15] and can ameliorate glucose tolerance [16] by reducing hepatic glucose production and stimulating glucose uptake in adipocytes.

Because of its ability to regulate glucose and lipid metabolism, FGF21 has shown therapeutic potential in treating diabetes [17]. FGF21 transgenic mice were lean and resistant to age-associated or diet-induced obesity and insulin resistance [13]. Both acute [18] and chronic [14] administration of FGF21 can ameliorate the metabolic state of diabetes. FGF21 treatment resulted in rapid decline of blood glucose levels and immediate improvement of glucose tolerance and insulin sensitivity in both *ob/ob* and diet-induced obese mice [18, 19] over the short term and ameliorated fasting hyperglycemia in both *ob/ob* mice [19] and diabetic monkeys [14] over the long term treatment. In addition, the level of serum FGF21 is reported to be positively associated with coronary artery disease [20] and higher risk of cardiovascular events in patients with type 2 diabetes [21], which might indicate a compensatory response. However, the direct effects of FGF21 on diabetic complications still remain largely unknown.

Almost all specific risk factors of diabetic vascular complications are directly related to hyperglycemia [1] and/or hyperlipidemia [2]. Ameliorating glucose and lipid metabolism is still a major preventive and assistive therapeutic strategy for diabetic vascular complications. Considering the anti-hyperglycemic and anti-hyperlipidemic effects of FGF21 on diabetes, and the fact that its preferred receptor, fibroblast growth factor receptor 1c (FGFR1c), and coreceptor, β-klotho, are highly-expressed in aorta [22], FGF21 is indicated to be involved in pathogenic changes in the aorta under diabetic conditions. Therefore, we investigated the role of FGF21 in the development and progression of pathogenic changes in the aorta in a streptozotocin (STZ)-induced type 1 diabetic model using FGF21 knockout (FGF21KO) mice.

2. Materials and methods

2.1 Ethic statement

This study was carried out in strict accordance with the recommendations in the Guide for the Care and Use of Laboratory Animals of the National Institutes of Health. The protocol was approved by the Animal Policy and Welfare Committee of Wenzhou Medical University and the Institutional Animal Care and Use Committee of the University of Louisville. All surgeries were performed under anesthesia induced by intraperitoneal injection of 1.2% 2,2,2-Tribromo-ethanol (Avertin) at the dose of 300 mg/kg body weight and all efforts were made to minimize suffering.

2.2 Animal model

The present study used male FGF21KO mice with C57 BL/6 J background (gifted by Dr. Steve Kliewer, University of Texas Southwestern Medical Center) [23] and wild type (WT) C57 BL/6 J mice purchased from Jackson Laboratory (Bar Harbor, Maine). The type 1 diabetes model was induced in 10 week-old male FGF21KO mice and age-matched WT mice by intraperitoneal injection of 6 consecutive doses of STZ (60 mg/kg body weight, Sigma, St. Louis, MO) in 10 mM sodium citrate buffer, pH 4.5. FGF21KO and WT mice control groups (Ctrl) received citrate buffer alone. Seven days after the last STZ injection, whole blood glucose obtained from the mouse tail vein was assayed using a SureStep complete blood glucose monitor (LifeScan, Milpitas, CA). Animals with blood glucose levels greater than 250 mg/dL were considered diabetic. At 1, 2 and 4 months following diabetes onset, mice were sacrificed and aorta tissue was collected.

In FGF21 treatment experiment, an acute type 1 diabetic model was induced in 10 week-old male FGF21KO mice and age-matched WT mice as described above. FGF21KO and WT mice control groups (Ctrl) received citrate buffer alone. FGF21KO diabetic mice in FGF21 treatment group received intraperitoneal injection of FGF21 (100 µg/kg body weight per day) for 2 months. Thereafter, mice were sacrificed and aorta tissue was collected.

2.3 Aorta sample preparation and histopathological examination

Under anesthesia, thoracotomies were performed on mice and the descending thoracic aortas were carefully harvested and fixed in 10% buffered formalin. Next, aorta tissues were cut into ring segments (2–3 mm in length), dehydrated in graded alcohol, cleared with xylene, and finally embedded in paraffin. Sections (5 µm thickness) were cut for pathological and immunohistochemical staining. Histological changes in the aorta were evaluated by hematoxylin and eosin (H&E) staining using Image Pro Plus 6.0 software for measuring the means of the tunica media width as the thickness of aortic tunica media.

2.4 Sirius-red staining for collagen

Aortic fibrosis was evaluated by Sirius-red staining, as described previously [24]. Briefly, 5 µm tissue sections were stained with 0.1% Sirius-red F3BA and 0.25% Fast Green FCF and assessed for the proportion of collagen using a Nikon Eclipse E600 microscopy system.

2.5 TUNEL staining

Terminal deoxynucleotidyl-transferase-mediated dUTP nick-end labeling (TUNEL) staining was performed on formalin-fixed, paraffin-embedded sections with Peroxidase In Situ Apoptosis Detection Kit (Millipore, Billerica, MA) according to the manufacturer's instructions and nuclei were stained using methyl green (FD Neurotechnologies, Columbia, MD). Positively stained apoptotic cells were counted randomly in a minimum of five microscopic fields in each of the three slides per aorta under light microscopy. The percentage of TUNEL positive cells relative to 100 nuclei was presented.

2.6 Immunohistochemical staining

Formalin-fixed, paraffin-embedded aorta sections were dewaxed using xylene and rehydrated by serial washes in graded alcohol and a final wash in dH$_2$O for 15 min. After balanced with phosphate buffered saline (PBS), aorta sections were incubated in Target Retrieval buffer (DAKO, Carpinteria, CA) at 95 ℃, and endogenous peroxidase was quenched by incubating in 3% H$_2$O$_2$ at room temperature for 10 min. After washing with PBS 3 times, sections were blocked in 5% bovine serum albumin (BSA) for 30 min, then incubated with primary antibody against mice tumor necrosis factor α (TNF-α), connective tissue growth factor (CTGF), transforming growth factor β (TGF-β), 3-nitrotyrocine (3-NT), 4-Hydroxynonenal (4-HNE), nuclear factor E2-related factor-2 (Nrf2) or phosphorylated endothelial nitric oxide synthase (p-eNOS, Ser 1177) over-night at 4℃. Sections incubated with PBS were used as negative controls. After washing, sections were incubated with corresponding secondary antibodies at room temperature for 1 h. For the development of color, sections were treated with peroxidase substrate DAB kit (Vector Laboratories, Inc. Burlingame, CA) and counter stained with hematoxylin. Quantitative analysis was carried out using Image J software.

2.7 Enzyme linked immunosorbent assay (ELISA)

Whole blood was collected in a lithium heparin tube (BD, Franklin Lakes, NJ) and centrifuged at 2000 rpm for 20 min. Plasma was used for interleukin- 6 (IL-6) assay using a mouse IL-6 ELISA kit (Invitrogen, Frederick, MD) according to the manufacturer's instructions.

2.8 Statistical analysis

Data were collected from several animals (n=5–9) and presented as means ± SD. Image Pro Plus 6.0 software was used to measure pathological changes as described above. Comparisons were performed by one-way ANOVA for the different groups, followed by *post hoc* pairwise repetitive comparisons using Tukey's test. Statistical analysis was done using Origin 7.5 Lab data analysis and graphing software. Statistical significance was considered as $P < 0.05$.

3. Results

3.1 FGF21 deletion accelerated diabetes-induced aortic thickening

Thickening is one of the major pathologic changes in diabetic aorta [24]. At 1, 2 and 4 months after diabetes onset, aortic thickening was evaluated by H&E staining and thickness was measured using Image J software. Under non-diabetic conditions, FGF21KO mice did not show marked alterations in aortic wall thickness compared to the WT controls. Both WT and FGF21KO diabetic mice showed aortic wall thickness changes. However, WT diabetic mice only exhibited aortic wall thickening at the 4th month after diabetes onset, while FGF21KO diabetic mice developed aortic wall thickening at the 2nd month after diabetes onset with more severe aortic wall thickening than WT diabetic mice at the 4th

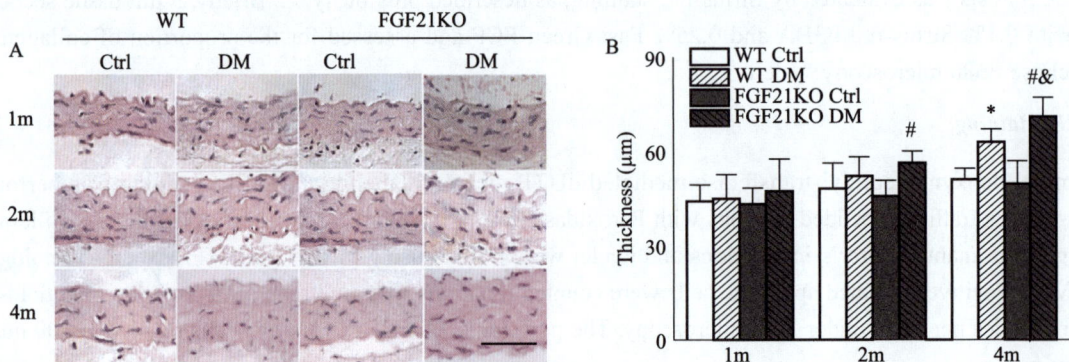

Fig. 1. FGF21 deletion accelerated and aggravated diabetes-induced aortic thickening. At indicated time points after diabetes onset, histological change of aorta was evaluated by H&E staining (A) and aorta thickness was measured using Image Pro Plus 6.0 software (B). Data are presented as means ± SD, $n \geqslant 5$ for each group. $^*P < 0.05$ *vs.* WT Ctrl group; $^\#P < 0.05$ *vs.* FGF21KO Ctrl group; $^\&P < 0.05$ *vs.* WT DM group. Bar = 50 μm. Ctrl: control; DM: diabetes mellitus; WT: wild type; FGF21KO: FGF21 knockout; m: month(s).

month after diabetes onset (Fig. 1A, B).

3.2 FGF21 deletion aggravated diabetes-induced aortic fibrosis

Fibrosis is another major pathologic change in diabetic macroangiopathy [24–26]. Sirius red staining demonstrated that FGF21 deletion did not increase collagen accumulation under non-diabetic conditions compared to the WT control (Fig. 2). WT diabetic mice did not show obvious collagen accumulation until the 4th month after diabetes onset. But diabetes significantly accelerated and aggravated collagen accumulation in FGF21KO mice at 2 months after diabetes onset (Fig. 2A, B).

The aggravated fibrosis was also confirmed by immunohistochemical staining for the fibrotic mediator, CTGF. It was demonstrated that diabetes significantly up-regulated CTGF expression in both WT and FGF21KO diabetic mice at 4 months compared to their corresponding controls. This was significantly higher in FGF21KO diabetic mice than in WT diabetic mice (Fig. 2C, D). However, FGF21 deletion had no significant effect on CTGF expression under non-diabetic conditions compared to WT control mice at all 3 time points.

3.3 FGF21 deletion exacerbated diabetes-induced aortic inflammation

Inflammation is an important cause of the pathologic changes in aorta under diabetic conditions [25]. Immunohisto-chemical staining showed a significant increase in inflammatory markers TGF-β and TNF-α expression in aortic tunica media of diabetic mice (Fig. 3). Both WT and FGF21KO diabetic mice had elevated TGF-β expression at the 4th month compared to their corresponding control mice, and the aortic expression of FGF21KO in diabetic mice was significantly higher than that of WT diabetic mice (Fig. 3A, B). TNF-α expression was also elevated in WT diabetic mice at the 4th month after diabetes onset compared to WT control mice. Furthermore, its expression was up-regulated at the 2nd month after diabetes onset in FGF21KO mice and was much higher than that of WT diabetic mice at the 4th month after diabetes onset (Fig. 3C, D). Under non-diabetic conditions, both TGF-β and TNF-α expression maintained their low levels and no differences between FGF21KO and WT mice were observed. In addition, FGF21 deletion dramatically up-regulated plasma IL-6 content under diabetic conditions (Fig. 3E), which indicated an aggravated systemic inflammation in

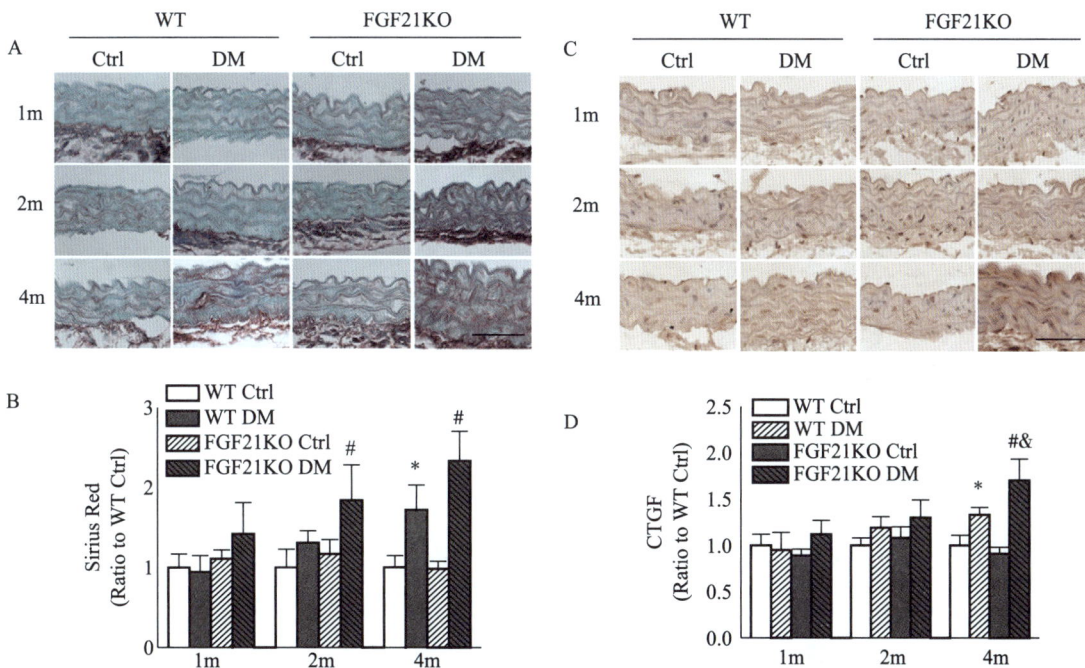

Fig. 2. FGF21 deletion accelerated and aggravated diabetes-induced aortic fibrosis. At indicated time points after diabetes onset, aortic fibrosis was evaluated by Sirius Red staining of collagen accumulation (A, B) and immunohistochemical staining of CTGF expression (C, D). Data are presented as means ± SD, $n \geqslant 5$ for each group. *$P<0.05$ vs. WT Ctrl group; #$P<0.05$ vs. FGF21KO Ctrl group; &$P < 0.05$ vs. WT DM group. Bar = 50 μm. Abbreviations are the same as the Fig. 1.

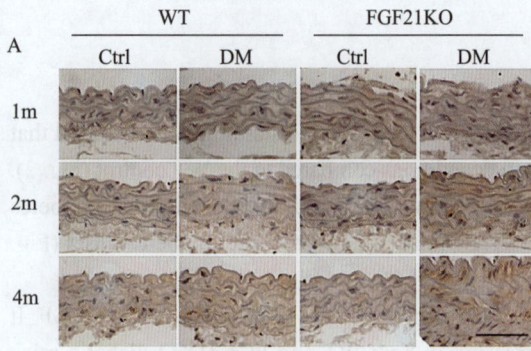

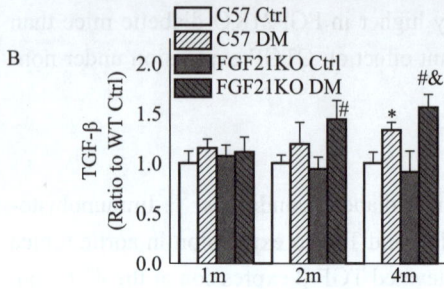

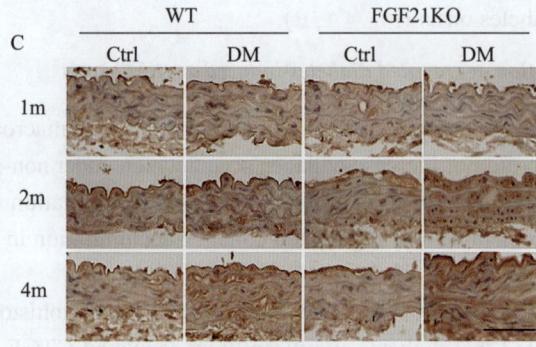

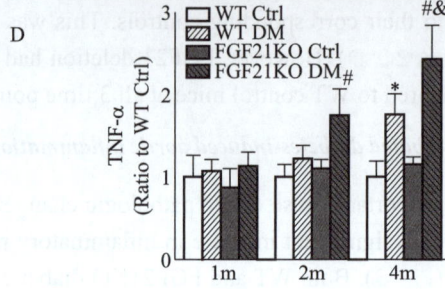

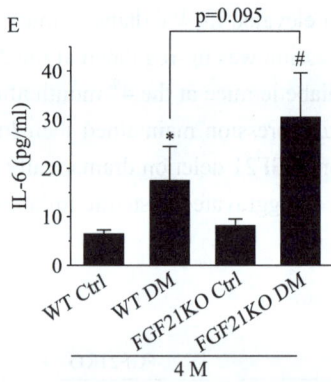

Fig. 3. FGF21 deficiency aggravated diabetes-induced inflammation. At indicated time points after diabetes onset, aortic inflammation was evaluated by immunohistochemical staining of TGF-β expression (A, B) and TNF-α (C, D). Plasma IL-6 was detected by ELISA (E). Data are presented as means ± SD, $n \geq 5$ for each group. $^{*}P < 0.05$ vs. WT Ctrl group; $^{#}P < 0.05$ vs. FGF21KO Ctrl group; $^{&}P < 0.05$ vs. WT DM group. Bar = 50 μm. Abbreviations are the same as the Fig. 1.

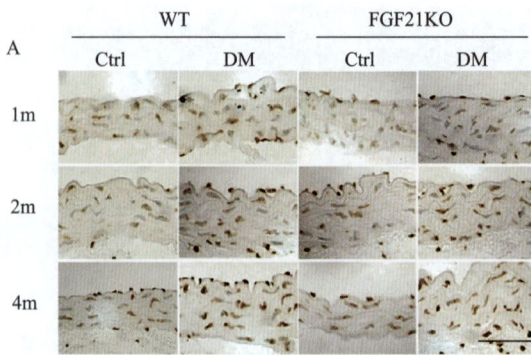

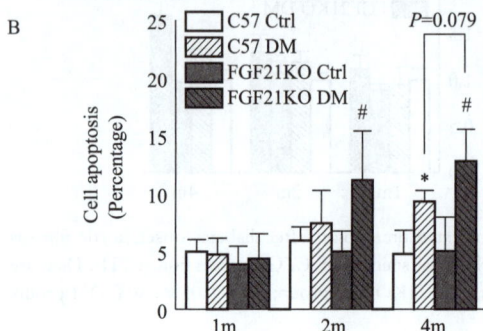

Fig. 4. FGF21 deficiency accelerated diabetes-induced cell apoptosis. At indicated time points after diabetes onset, cell apoptosis was evaluated by TUNEL staining (A, B). Data are presented as means ± SD, $n \geq 5$ for each group. $^{*}P < 0.05$ vs. WT Ctrl group; $^{#}P < 0.05$ vs. FGF21KO Ctrl group. Bar = 50 μm. Abbreviations are the same as the Fig. 1.

FGF21KO diabetic mice.

3.4 FGF21 deletion aggravated diabetes-induced aortic cell apoptosis

Effect of FGF21 deletion on aortic cell apoptosis was evaluated by TUNEL staining. Obvious aortic cell apoptosis was observed in tunica intima and media in both WT and FGF21KO diabetic mice (Fig. 4). WT diabetic mice showed significant aortic cell apoptosis at the 4th month after diabetes onset compared to the WT control mice. This phenomenon was observed in FGF21KO diabetic mice at the 2nd month after diabetes onset. At the 4th month after diabetes onset, FGF21KO diabetic mice showed aggravated aortic cell apoptosis when compared to WT diabetic mice ($P = 0.079$). However, FGF21 deficiency did not induce aortic cell apoptosis under non-diabetic conditions (Fig. 4A, B).

3.5 FGF21 deletion exacerbated diabetes-induced aortic oxidative stress

Excessive oxidative stress is considered a critical cause of aortic cell apoptosis and inflammation [25, 27]. Aortic oxidative stress was evaluated by measuring the accumulation of 3-NT and 4-HNE. FGF21KO mice did not show marked alterations in 3-NT accumulation under non-diabetic conditions (Fig. 5). Significant elevation of 3-NT accumulation was observed at the 4th month in WT diabetic mice, and from the 2nd month after diabetes onset in FGF21KO diabetic mice. Moreover, the aortic 3-NT accumulation in FGF21KO diabetic mice was significantly higher than that of WT diabetic mice at 2 and 4 months after diabetes onset (Fig. 5A, B). A similar pattern was observed in 4-HNE accumulation (Fig. 5C, D). The accumulation of 4-HNE in both WT and FGF21KO diabetic mice elevated since the 2nd month after diabetes onset compared to the corresponding control mice. FGF21 deletion obviously exacerbated aortic 4-HNE accumulation at the 4th month after diabetes onset compared to that of the WT diabetic mice ($P = 0.062$).

Nrf2, a transcription factor in regulation of various antioxidative and cytoprotective responses, has been shown to play an important role in cellular prevention against oxidative stress and damage in vitro and in vivo [25]. In FGF21KO diabetic mice, the aortic Nrf2 expression was significantly up-regulated, especially at the 4th month (Fig. 5E, F), indicating an adaptive response to the aggravated oxidative stress.

3.6 FGF21 deletion exacerbated diabetes-induced impairment of eNOS activation

Nitric oxide synthase (NOS) is the pivotal enzyme in the production of nitric oxide (NO), which plays an essential role in vascular homeostasis as the elusive endothelium-derived relaxing factor [28]. eNOS is one of the major isoform of NOS existing in endothelium. eNOS-derived NO serves important functions including the regulation of vascular tone and regional blood flow, suppression of vascular smooth muscle cell proliferation, modulation of leukocyte endothelial

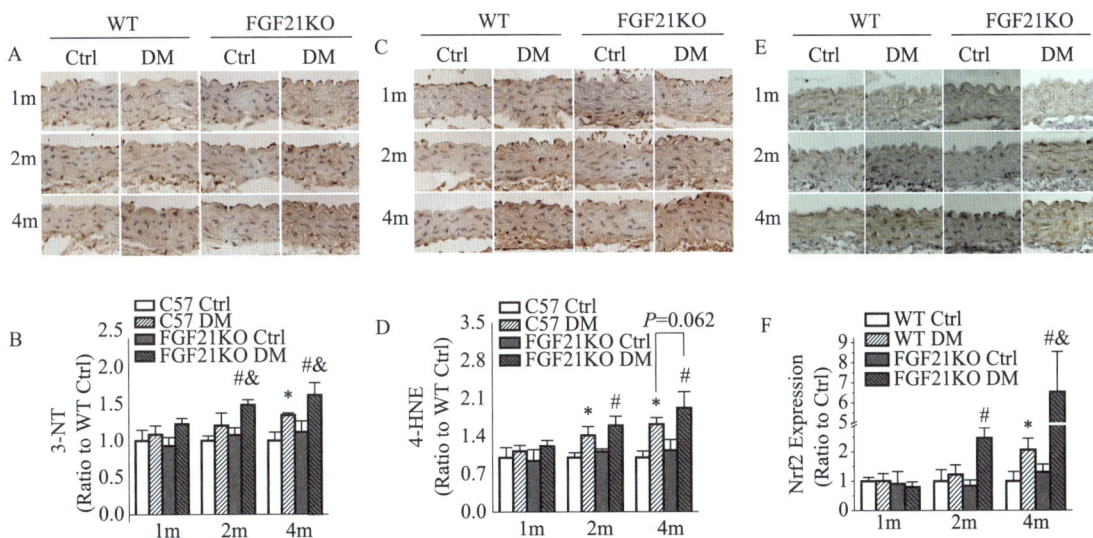

Fig. 5. FGF21 deficiency accelerated and aggravated diabetes-induced oxidative stress. At indicated time points after diabetes onset, oxidative stress was evaluated by immunohistochemical staining of 3-NT (A, B) and 4-HNE (C, D). Antioxidative response was also evaluated by immunohistochemical staining of transcription factor Nrf2 (E, F). Data are presented as means ± SD, $n \geq 5$ for each group. $^*P < 0.05$ vs. WT Ctrl group; $^\#P < 0.05$ vs FGF21KO Ctrl group; $^\&P < 0.05$ vs. WT DM group. Bar = 50 μm. Abbreviations are the same as the Fig. 1.

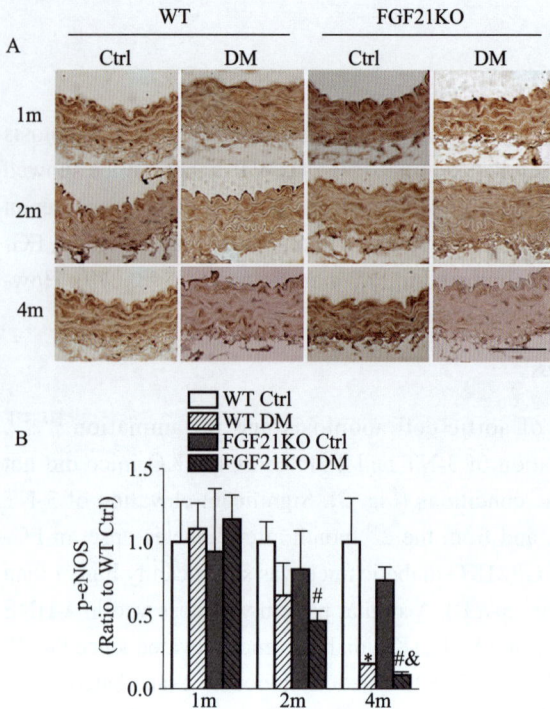

Fig. 6. FGF21 deficiency accelerated and aggravated the impairment of eNOS activation in diabetes. At indicated time points after diabetes onset, eNOS activation was evaluated by immunohistochemical staining of p-eNOS (Ser-1177) (A, B). Data are presented as means ± SD, $n \geqslant 5$ for each group. *$P < 0.05$ vs. WT Ctrl group; #$P < 0.05$ vs. FGF21KO Ctrl group; &$P < 0.05$ vs. WT DM group. Bar = 50 μm. Abbreviations are the same as the Fig. 1.

interactions and thrombosis [29]. The activity of eNOS is promoted by phosphorylation at Ser-615, Ser-633 or Ser-1177, but inhibited by phosphorylation at Thr-495 [30]. Herein, we found that diabetes significantly inhibited aortic eNOS phosphorylation at Ser-1177 in WT diabetic mice at the 4th month, and from the 2nd month after diabetes onset in FGF21KO diabetic mice. Moreover, FGF21 deletion further attenuated the aortic eNOS function in FGF21KO diabetic mice compared to that of WT diabetic mice at 2 and 4 months after diabetes onset (Fig. 6).

3.7 FGF21 administration ameliorated diabetes induced aorta dysfunction

FGF21 deficiency aggravated aorta dysfunction induced by diabetes, and then we investigated whether FGF21 administration can reverse this process. In an acute type1 diabetes model, we found that FGF21 administration can ameliorate aortic thickening (Fig. 7A) and fibrosis (Fig. 7B) in FGF21KO diabetic mice. FGF21 treatment can also reverse cell apoptosis in FGF21KO diabetic mice. Moreover, cell apoptosis in the aorta of FGF21 treated FGF21KO diabetic mice was even lower than that in WT diabetic mice (Fig. 7C).

4. Discussion

The therapeutic effect of FGF21 on diabetes and diabetic complications has been widely appreciated [13, 14]. But its effect on diabetic vasculopathy remains largely unknown. High level expression of the preferred receptor, FGFR1c, and co-receptor, β-klotho, in the aorta [22] indicates that aorta is a potential target tissue of FGF21. By using the FGF21KO mouse model, we provided the first experimental evidence to show that FGF21 deletion further accelerated and aggravated diabetes-induced aortic thickening, fibrotic remodeling, inflammation, cell apoptosis and oxidative stress, and FGF21 administration can reverse the pathologic changes in FGF21KO diabetic mice.

FGF21 has been considered as a potent regulator in glucose and lipid metabolism. The fact that blood glucose and lipid levels are comparable in WT and FGF21KO diabetic mice [31] and that FGF21 deletion further aggravates of the aortic thickening (Fig. 1), fibrosis (Fig. 2), inflammation (Fig. 3), cell apoptosis (Fig. 4) and oxidative stress (Fig. 5), suggests that the detrimental effect of FGF21 deletion on the aorta is most likely mediated by its direct action in aortic tissues rather than secondary actions such as manipulating systemic glucose and/or lipid metabolism.

The endothelium, which consists of a metabolically active monolayer of endothelial cells covering the entire lumi-

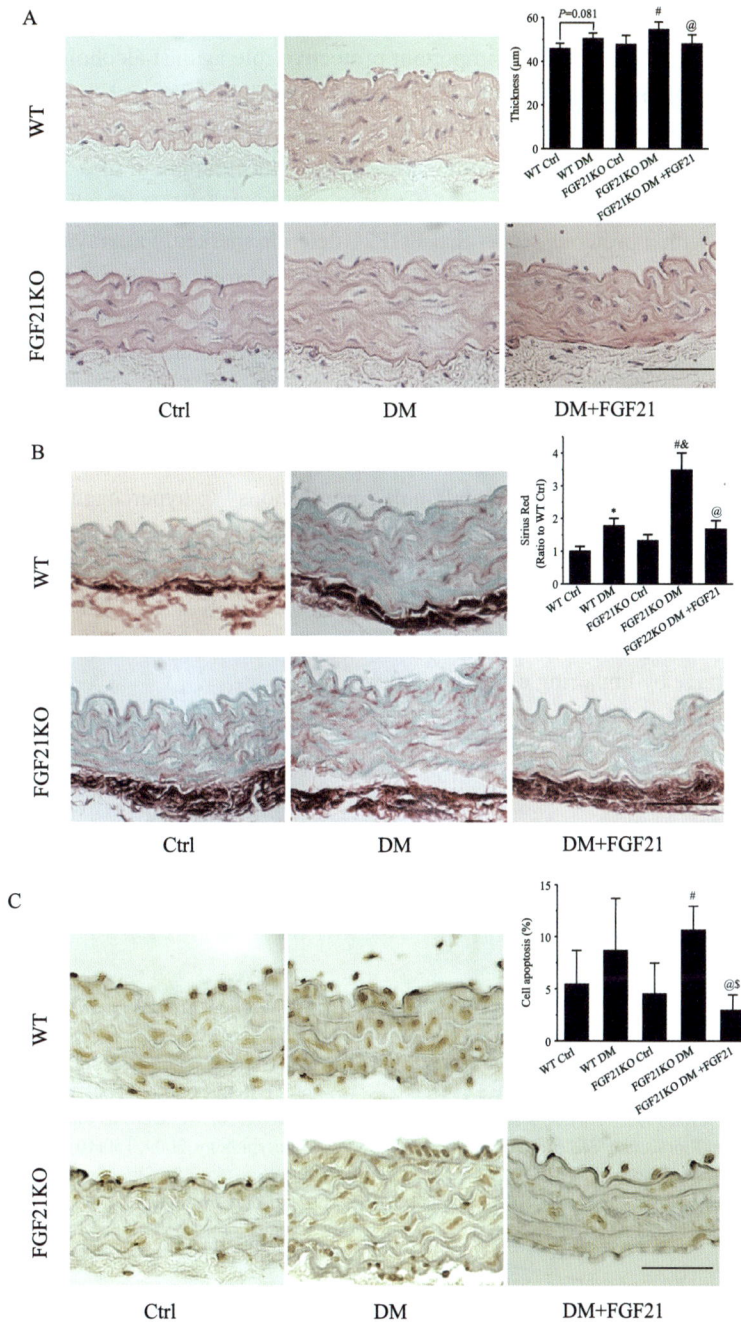

Fig. 7. FGF21 administration reversed pathologic changes in the aorta of FGF21KO DM mice. In a type 1 diabetes model, FGF21 administration reversed aortic thickening (A), fibrosis (B) and cell apoptosis (C) in the aorta of FGF21KO DM mice. Data are presented as means ± SD, $n \geqslant 5$ for each group. $^*P < 0.05$ vs. WT Ctrl group; $^\#P < 0.05$ vs. FGF21KO Ctrl; $^@P < 0.05$ vs. FGF21KO DM; $^\$P < 0.05$ vs. WT DM. Bar = 50 μm. Abbreviations are the same as the Fig. 1. FGF21KO DM + FGF21: FGF21KO DM mice received FGF21 administration.

nal surface of blood vessels, plays a fundamental role in maintaining vascular homeostasis. Endothelial dysfunction was considered as a starting point for macroangiopathy and microangiopathy in both type1 and type 2 diabetes which would trigger the development of diabetic vasculopathy [4]. Cell apoptosis was assessed as an initial step of endothelial dysfunction [32]. In the present study, we found that FGF21 deletion accelerated and aggravated diabetes-induced aortic cell apoptosis (Fig. 4). These results are consistent with recent studies that FGF21 inhibits endothelial cell apoptosis induced by oxidized low density lipoprotein [33] or high glucose [34], enhances cell viability and decreases the apoptotic cell death in human umbilical vein endothelial cells (HUVECs) caused by H_2O_2 stress induction *in vitro*, while improves the condition of atherosclerotic rats *in vivo* [35, 36].

Chronic inflammation and oxidative stress play important roles in the development and progression of various chronic vascular pathological changes, including endothelial remodeling and apoptotic cell death under diabetic conditions [37]. It has been shown that FGF21 plays an important protective role against alcoholic fatty liver disease [38], drug-induced hepatotoxicity [39], atherosclerosis [35] and diabetic nephropathy [40] through its anti-oxidative stress and/ or anti-inflammatory actions. Herein we found that FGF21 deletion aggravated diabetes-induced oxidative stress, inflammation and fibrotic remodeling in aortas, reflected in the exacerbated accumulation of 3-NT and 4-HNE (Fig. 5 A–D), expression of TGF-β and TNF-α (Fig. 3), and accumulation of collagen and CTGF expression (Fig. 2), respectively. These results are consistent with a previous report that FGF21 deletion markedly aggravated acetaminophen overdose-induced liver damage, which was accompanied by increased oxidative stress and impaired antioxidant capacities. The replenishment of recombinant FGF21 largely reversed acetaminophen-induced hepatic oxidative stress and liver injury in FGF21KO mice [39], and are concurrent with our previous studies that demonstrated FGF21 administration attenuates diabetes-induced oxidative stress and inflammation in testis [27] and kidney [41].

One possible cause for the aggravated pathological changes of the aorta in FGF21KO diabetic mice is the dysfunction of eNOS. eNOS gene deficiency resulted in hypertension [42], increased vascular smooth muscle cell proliferation in response to vessel injury [43], increased leukocyte-endothelial interactions [44], hypercoagulability [45] and increased diet-induced atherosclerosis [46]. Recently, an *in vitro* study [34] showed that eNOS phosphorylation at Ser-1177 and Ser-633 in HUVECs was impaired under diabetic conditions, which can be rescued by FGF21 administration in an AMP-activated protein kinase-dependent manner. In present study, phosphorylation of eNOS at Ser-1177 was further down-regulated in FGF21KO diabetic mice than that in WT diabetic mice (Fig. 6), which indicated that FGF21 deficiency may contribute to the aggravated aortic damage by impairing eNOS activation.

In conclusion, we found that FGF21 deletion accelerates and aggravates diabetes-induced aortic pathological changes reflected by exacerbated aortic thickening, collagen accumulation and fibrotic remodeling, which is most likely due to FGF21 deficiency-induced aggravation of aortic oxidative stress, inflammation, and cell apoptosis, and FGF21 administration can reverse those pathologic changes in FGF21KO diabetic mice.

References

[1] Schnell O, Cappuccio F, Genovese S, *et al.* Type 1 diabetes and cardiovascular disease[J]. Cardiovascular Diabetology, 2013, 12.

[2] Laight DW, Carrier MJ, Anggard EE. Endothelial cell dysfunction and the pathogenesis of diabetic macroangiopathy[J]. Diabetes-Metabolism Research and Reviews, 1999, 15(4): 274-282.

[3] Brownlee M. Biochemistry and molecular cell biology of diabetic complications[J]. Nature, 2001, 414(6865): 813-820.

[4] Coccheri S. Approaches to prevention of cardiovascular complications and events in diabetes mellitus[J]. Drugs, 2007, 67(7): 997-1026.

[5] Laight DW, Carrier MJ, Anggard EE. Antioxidants, diabetes and endothelial dysfunction[J]. Cardiovascular Research, 2000, 47(3): 457-464.

[6] Gaertner V, Eigentler TK. Pathogenesis of diabetic macro- and microangiopathy[J]. Clinical Nephrology, 2008, 70(1): 1-9.

[7] Gugliucci A. Glycation as the glucose link to diabetic complications[J]. Journal of the American Osteopathic Association, 2000, 100(10): 621-634.

[8] Nishimura T, Nakatake Y, Konishi M, *et al.* Identification of a novel FGF, FGF-21, preferentially expressed in the liver[J]. Biochimica Et Biophysica Acta-Gene Structure and Expression, 2000, 1492(1): 203-206.

[9] Adams AC, Kharitonenkov A. FGF21: The Center of a Transcriptional Nexus in Metabolic Regulation[J]. Current Diabetes Reviews, 2012, 8(4): 285-293.

[10] Iglesias P, Selgas R, Romero S, *et al.* Biological role, clinical significance, and therapeutic possibilities of the recently discovered metabolic hormone fibroblastic growth factor 21[J]. European Journal of Endocrinology, 2012, 167(3): 301-309.

[11] Fisher FM, Kleiner S, Douris N, *et al.* FGF21 regulates PGC-1 alpha and browning of white adipose tissues in adaptive thermogenesis[J]. Genes & Development, 2012, 26(3): 271-281.

[12] Hotta Y, Nakamura H, Konishi M, *et al.* Fibroblast Growth Factor 21 Regulates Lipolysis in White Adipose Tissue But Is Not Required for Ketogenesis and Triglyceride Clearance in Liver[J]. Endocrinology, 2009, 150(10): 4625-4633.

[13] Kharitonenkov A, Shiyanova TL, Koester A, *et al.* FGF-21 as a novel metabolic regulator[J]. Journal of Clinical Investigation, 2005, 115(6): 1627-1635.

[14] Kharitonenkov A, Wroblewski VJ, Koester A, *et al.* The metabolic state of diabetic monkeys is regulated by fibroblast growth factor-21[J]. Endocrinology, 2007, 148(2): 774-781.

[15] Lin Z, Tian H, Lam KSL, *et al.* Adiponectin Mediates the Metabolic Effects of FGF21 on Glucose Homeostasis and Insulin Sensitivity in Mice[J]. Cell Metabolism, 2013, 17(5): 779-789.

[16] Sarruf DA, Thaler JP, Morton GJ, *et al.* Fibroblast Growth Factor 21 Action in the Brain Increases Energy Expenditure and Insulin Sensitivity in Obese Rats[J]. Diabetes, 2010, 59(7): 1817-1824.

[17] Zhao Y, Dunbar JD, Kharitonenkov A. FGF21 as a therapeutic reagent[A]. In: *Endocrine Fgfs and Klothos* (KuroO M, ed), Vol. 728, 2012: 214-228.

[18] Xu J, Lloyd DJ, Hale C, *et al.* Fibroblast growth factor 21 reverses hepatic steatosis, increases energy expenditure, and improves insulin sensitivity in diet-induced obese mice[J]. Diabetes, 2009, 58(1): 250-259.

[19] Berglund ED, Li CY, Bina HA, *et al.* Fibroblast Growth Factor 21 Controls Glycemia *via* Regulation of Hepatic Glucose Flux and Insulin Sensitivity[J]. Endocrinology, 2009, 150(9): 4084-4093.

[20] Shen Y, Ma X, Zhou J, *et al.* Additive relationship between serum fibroblast growth factor 21 level and coronary artery disease[J].

Cardiovascular Diabetology, 2013, 12.

[21] Ong K-L, Januszewski AS, O'Connell R, *et al.* The relationship of fibroblast growth factor 21 with cardiovascular outcome events in the Fenofibrate Intervention and Event Lowering in Diabetes study[J]. Diabetologia, 2015, 58(3): 464-473.

[22] Tacer KF, Bookout AL, Ding X, *et al.* Research Resource: Comprehensive Expression Atlas of the Fibroblast Growth Factor System in Adult Mouse[J]. Molecular Endocrinology, 2010, 24(10): 2050-2064.

[23] Potthoff MJ, Inagaki T, Satapati S, *et al.* FGF21 induces PGC-1 alpha and regulates carbohydrate and fatty acid metabolism during the adaptive starvation response[J]. Proceedings of the National Academy of Sciences of the United States of America, 2009, 106(26): 10853-10858.

[24] Miao X, Wang Y, Sun J, *et al.* Zinc protects against diabetes-induced pathogenic changes in the aorta: roles of metallothionein and nuclear factor (erythroid-derived 2)-like 2[J]. Cardiovascular Diabetology, 2013, 12.

[25] Miao X, Cui W, Sun W, *et al.* Therapeutic Effect of MG132 on the Aortic Oxidative Damage and Inflammatory Response in OVE26 Type 1 Diabetic Mice[J]. Oxidative Medicine and Cellular Longevity, 2013.

[26] Bai Y, Tan Y, Wang B, *et al.* Deletion of angiotensin II type 1 receptor gene or scavenge of superoxide prevents chronic alcohol-induced aortic damage and remodelling[J]. Journal of Cellular and Molecular Medicine, 2012, 16(10): 2530-2538.

[27] Jiang X, Zhang C, Xin Y, *et al.* Protective effect of FGF21 on type 1 diabetes-induced testicular apoptotic cell death probably *via* both mitochondrial- and endoplasmic reticulum stress-dependent pathways in the mouse model[J]. Toxicology Letters, 2013, 219(1): 65-76.

[28] Ignarro LJ, Buga GM, Wood KS, *et al.* Endothelium-derived relaxing factor produced and released from artery and vein is nitric-oxide[J]. Proceedings of the National Academy of Sciences of the United States of America, 1987, 84(24): 9265-9269.

[29] Huang PL. eNOS, metabolic syndrome and cardiovascular disease[J]. Trends in Endocrinology and Metabolism, 2009, 20(6): 295-302.

[30] Kukreja RC, Xi L. eNOS phosphorylation: A pivotal molecular switch in vasodilation and cardioprotection?[J]. Journal of Molecular and Cellular Cardiology, 2007, 42(2): 280-282.

[31] Yan X, Chen J, Zhang C, *et al.* FGF21 deletion exacerbates diabetic cardiomyopathy by aggravating cardiac lipid accumulation[J]. J Cell Mol Med, 2015, 19(7): 1557-1568.

[32] Dimmeler S, Zeiher AM. Vascular repair by circulating endothelial progenitor cells: the missing link in atherosclerosis?[J]. Journal of Molecular Medicine, 2004, 82(10): 671-677.

[33] Lu Y, Liu J, Zhang L, *et al.* Fibroblast growth factor 21 as a possible endogenous factor inhibits apoptosis in cardiac endothelial cells[J]. Chinese Medical Journal, 2010, 123(23): 3417-3421.

[34] Wang X-M, Song S-S, Xiao H, *et al.* Fibroblast Growth Factor 21 Protects Against High Glucose Induced Cellular Damage and Dysfunction of Endothelial Nitric-Oxide Synthase in Endothelial Cells[J]. Cellular Physiology and Biochemistry, 2014, 34(3): 658-671.

[35] Zhu W, Wang C, Liu L, *et al.* Effects of fibroblast growth factor 21 on cell damage *in vitro* and atherosclerosis *in vivo*[J]. Canadian Journal of Physiology and Pharmacology, 2014, 92(11): 927-935.

[36] Lin Z, Pan X, Wu F, *et al.* Fibroblast Growth Factor 21 Prevents Atherosclerosis by Suppression of Hepatic Sterol Regulatory Element-Binding Protein-2 and Induction of Adiponectin in Mice[J]. Circulation, 2015, 131(21): 1861-1871.

[37] Insull W, Jr. The Pathology of Atherosclerosis: Plaque Development and Plaque Responses to Medical Treatment[J]. American Journal of Medicine, 2009, 122(1): S3-S14.

[38] Zhu S, Ma L, Wu Y, *et al.* FGF21 treatment ameliorates alcoholic fatty liver through activation of AMPK-SIRT1 pathway[J]. Acta Biochimica Et Biophysica Sinica, 2014, 46(12): 1041-1048.

[39] Ye D, Wang Y, Li H, *et al.* Fibroblast Growth Factor 21 Protects Against Acetaminophen-Induced Hepatotoxicity by Potentiating Peroxisome Proliferator-Activated Receptor Coactivator Protein-1 alpha-Mediated Antioxidant Capacity in Mice[J]. Hepatology, 2014, 60(3): 977-989.

[40] Kim HW, Lee JE, Cha JJ, *et al.* Fibroblast Growth Factor 21 Improves Insulin Resistance and Ameliorates Renal Injury in db/db Mice[J]. Endocrinology, 2013, 154(9): 3366-3376.

[41] Zhang C, Shao M, Yang H, *et al.* Attenuation of Hyperlipidemia-and Diabetes-Induced Early-Stage Apoptosis and Late-Stage Renal Dysfunction *via* Administration of Fibroblast Growth Factor-21 Is Associated with Suppression of Renal Inflammation[J]. Plos One, 2013, 8(12).

[42] Huang PL, Huang ZH, Mashimo H, *et al.* Hypertension in mice lacking the gene for endothelial nitric-oxide synthase[J]. Nature, 1995, 377(6546): 239-242.

[43] Moroi M, Zhang L, Yasuda T, *et al.* Interaction of genetic deficiency of endothelial nitric oxide, gender, and pregnancy in vascular response to injury in mice[J]. Journal of Clinical Investigation, 1998, 101(6): 1225-1232.

[44] Lefer DJ, Jones SP, Girod WG, *et al.* Leukocyte-endothelial cell interactions in nitric oxide synthase-deficient mice[J]. American Journal of Physiology-Heart and Circulatory Physiology, 1999, 276(6): H1943-H1950.

[45] Freedman JE, Sauter R, Battinelli EM, *et al.* Deficient platelet-derived nitric oxide and enhanced hemostasis in mice lacking the NOSIII gene[J]. Circulation Research, 1999, 84(12): 1416-1421.

[46] Kuhlencordt PJ, Gyurko R, Han F, *et al.* Accelerated atherosclerosis, aortic aneurysm formation, and ischemic heart disease in apolipoprotein E/endothelial nitric oxide synthase double-knockout mice[J]. Circulation, 2001, 104(4): 448-454.

Additive protection by LDR and FGF21 treatment against diabetic nephropathy in type 2 diabetes model

Minglong Shao, Xiaokun Li, Yi Tan, Lu Cai

Diabetic nephropathy (DN) is a severe complication of diabetes and the leading cause of end-stage renal disease [38]. DN initiates with the thickening of the glomerular basement membrane, which is followed by mild and moderate mesangial expansion, capillary collapse in the renal tubule, epithelial cell degeneration, and a gradual increase in proteinuria, and finally leads to renal fibrosis and kidney failure [43, 56]. Hyperglycemia, hyperlipidemia, and subsequent insulin resistance are the initial and systemic pathogeneses of DN, which is also associated with renal pathogeneses, such as oxidative stress, inflammation, and fibrosis. There are currently multiple therapies to treat patients with DN, including reducing blood sugar levels, lowering lipid levels, enhancing insulin sensitivity, and reducing oxidative stress, inflammation, or fibrosis [1, 19, 50]. However, most of these treatments just slow rather than arrest the progression toward DN, since blocking any single pathway is not sufficient to prevent the development of DN [8, 19]. Therefore, identifying a treatment that inhibits both the systemic and renal pathogeneses will prevent the development of DN efficiently.

Fibroblast growth factor (FGF)-21 is a novel member of the FGF family that functions as an endocrine hormone rather than regulating cellular proliferation and differentiation [3, 29]. FGF21 acts on multiple tissues to regulate carbohydrate and lipid metabolism. Large amounts of evidence have demonstrated that FGF21 also induces beneficial effects in diabetes and its related complications by lowering blood glucose levels, stimulating lipid β-oxidation, and enhancing insulin sensitivity [25, 26]. In addition, FGF21 protects the heart against oxidative stress-induced damage in two different mice models [isoproterenol-induced cardiac hypertrophy[40] and the LPS-induced proinflammatory pathway [7] by inducing the expression of antioxidant proteins, including uncoupling proteins and SOD-2 [41]]. FGF21 also protects the liver from D-gal-induced oxidative stress by activating Nrf2 and subsequent antioxidant genes [54]. Moreover, Kim et al [27]. demonstrated that FGF21 protects the kidneys in a mouse model of type 2 diabetes by improving insulin sensitivity. Our previous study[56] also demonstrated the beneficial effect of FGF21 on type 1 diabetes-induced renal damage.

Low-dose radiation (LDR) generally refers to radiation at a dose less than 100 mGy for low linear energy transfer (LET) [32], which induces beneficial effects, including stimulating DNA/RNA repair, increasing the cellular antioxidant capacity, prolonging life span, and activating immune functions [13, 14]. These cellular hormetic effects of LDR protect cells *in vitro* or tissues *in vivo* against gene mutations, DNA damage, and the chromosomal aberrations caused by subsequent large doses of radiation or toxic chemicals *via* an adaptive response [9, 10, 12]. Increasing evidence has suggested that LDR reduces the incidence of diabetes and also exerts beneficial effects on diabetic complications such as DN [35, 45]. In addition, our previous studies [43] showed that exposure to LDR greatly prevented type 2 diabetes-induced renal injury and also inhibited renal oxidative stress, inflammation, and fibrosis without altering blood glucose levels. We [51, 57] further demonstrated that LDR could increase Akt phosphorylation and the expression of Nrf2 and its downstream antioxidants significantly.

Taken together, the evidence above suggests that both FGF21 and LDR induce beneficial effects on DN. FGF21 might mainly suppress the systemic pathogenesis, whereas LDR might protect the kidneys from diabetes mainly *via* anti-inflammatory, antioxidative, and antifibrotic mechanisms[51, 56, 57]. Therefore, the aim of the present study was to investigate whether the combination treatment with LDR and FGF21 could exert additive effects on the prevention of DN *via* both systemic and renal mechanisms.

1. Materials and methods

1.1 Ethics statement

Eight-week-old male C57BL/6J mice (weighting 18–22 g) were purchased from the Experimental Animal Center of Beijing University of Medical Science (Beijing, China) and allowed to acclimate for 2 wk. All mice were housed in the Experimental Animal Center of Jilin University at 22℃ with 12:12-h light-dark cycles and free access to rodent chow and tap water. The animal production license is No. SCXK 2007-0003. All animal procedures were approved by the University Animal Care and Use Committee (permit number 2007-0011), which is certified by the Chinese Association of Accreditation of Laboratory Animal Care.

1.2 Animals and type 2 diabetes model

The high-fat diet (HFD)/ streptozotocin (STZ) protocol was applied to establish the model of type 2 diabetes [34, 43, 49]. Mice were fed a HFD (40% of calories from fat; Shanghai SLAC Laboratory Animal, Shanghai, China) for12 wk to induce metabolic syndrome, characterized by obesity, abnormal glucose tolerance, and insulin resistance. Age-matched nondiabetic mice were fed a standard diet (SD, 10% of calories from fat; Shanghai SLAC Laboratory Animal). The obese mice were divided randomly into two groups: one group was given a single injection of 50 mg/kg body wt STZ ip to induce hyperglycemia and the onset of type 2 diabetes, whereas the other group was given an ip injection of an equivalent volume of citrate buffer (Con). Mice were considered diabetic when their blood glucose exceeded 12 mmol/l. Subsequently, the diabetic mice were divided into four subgroups: diabetes mellitus (DM) plus LDR treatment (DM/LDR), DM plus FGF21 treatment (DM/FGF21), and DM plus the combination of LDR and FGF21 treatment (DM/Com).

1.3 Whole body LDR and FGF21 treatment

A 180-kVp X-ray generator (Model XSZ-Z20/20, China) was used to deliver radiation at a dose rate of 12.5 mGy/min (120 kv, 13 mA). Diabetic mice in the DM/LDR and DM/Com groups received whole body irradiation every 2 days at a dose of 50 mGy/day for 4 wk, based on our previous observations [56]. Mice in the DM/FGF21 or DM/Com groups were given intraperitoneal (ip) injections of 1.5 mg/kg FGF21 daily for 8 wk. Therefore, the DM/Com group received both LDR and FGF21 treatment for 4 wk followed by an additional 4 wk of FGF21 treatment alone.

1.4 Glucose and insulin tolerance tests

To evaluate glucose tolerance, mice were given an injection of D-glucose (1.5 g/kg ip) after an overnight fast (12 h) with free access to water. Venous blood was collected 30 min before the injection of glucose (*time 0*), as well as 15, 30, 60, and 120 min after injection from the tail of each mouse, and glucose levels were measured using a OneTouch SureStep complete blood glucose monitor (LifeScan, Milpitas, CA). To evaluate insulin tolerance, a single dose of 0.5 U/kg Novolin R regular insulin (Novo Nordisk, Bagsvaerd, Denmark) was administered ip after a 4-h fast with free access to water, and the blood glucose levels were measured as described above.

1.5 Measuring renal function

Mice were placed in metabolic cages individually with free access to tap water on the day before euthanasia to collect 24-h urine samples. Total urinary protein (UP), urinary microalbumin (mAlb), and urinary creatinine (U-Cre) contents were measured as parameters of renal function using enzyme-linked immunosorbent assay (ELISA) kits purchased from R&D Systems (Itasea, MN) according to the manufacturer's instructions.

1.6 Measuring serum and renal lipid profiles

Mice were euthanized after being anesthetized, and blood was collected by cardiac puncture and centrifuged at 2,000 *g* for 20 min at 4℃ to prepare serum. Serum triglycerides (TG), total cholesterol (CHO), high-density lipoprotein (HDL)-cholesterol, and low-density lipoprotein (LDL)-cholesterol levels were determined using an Olympus Au800 automatic biochemical analyzer (Olympus, Japan).

To measure TG and free fatty acid (FFA) contents in the kidney,~80 mg of kidney tissue from each mouse was homogenized in 250 µl of buffer containing 150 mM NaCl and 10 mM Tris (pH 7.5), and then extracted using 200 µl of methanol and 400 µl of chloroform, as described by Bligh and Dyer[6]. The rest of the procedure was same as that described above, using an Olympus Au800 automatic biochemical analyzer.

1.7 Total protein extraction and Western blotting

Renal tissues were homogenized in lysis buffer (Santa Cruz Biotechnology, Santa Cruz, CA), and the supernatants were collected by centrifugation at 12,000 g and 4 ℃. After determination of the total protein concentration, equal amounts of each sample were run on 10% SDS-polyacrylamide gel electrophoresis and then transferred to nitrocellulose membranes. After blocking with nonfat milk for 1 h at room temperature, the membranes were incubated overnight at 4 ℃ with the following primary antibodies: nuclear factor E2-related factor 2 (Nrf-2, 1:1,000), superoxide dismutase-1 (SOD-1, 1:2,000), NAD(P)H:quinone oxidoreductase-1 (NQO-1, 1:1,000), heme oxygenase-1 (HO-1, 1:2,000), 3-nitrotyrosine (3-NT, 1:1,000), intercellular adhesion molecule 1 (ICAM-1, 1:2,000), plasminogen activator inhibitor 1 (PAI-1, 1:2,000), connective tissue growth factor (CTGF, 1:2,000), tumor necrosis factor-α (TNF-α, 1:1,000), and β-actin (1:2,000). All antibodies were purchased from Abcam (Cambridge, MA), except for β-actin (Cell Signaling Technology, Danvers, MA). After three washes in Tris-buffered saline containing 0.05% Tween 20, the membranes were incubated with horseradish peroxidase-conjugated secondary antibodies for 1 h at room temperature. Antigen-antibody complexes were then visualized using an enhanced chemiluminescence kit (Amersham, Piscataway, NJ), and the intensity of the protein bands was quantified using Quantity One software (v. 4.6.2; Bio-Rad, Hercules, CA).

1.8 Histological examination

Kidney tissues were fixed in 10% formalin at room temperature for 48 h. After dehydration, the tissue blocks were embedded in paraffin and cut into 4-mm-thick sections. They were then stained with hematoxylin and eosin (H&E) for general morphological examination, periodic acid-Schiff (PAS) for glomerulosclerosis evaluation, and Masson's Trichrome staining for interstitial expansion assessment, as described previously [24, 44, 56]. Five different fields were selected randomly from each slice, each containing at least 50 glomeruli. The degree of glomerulosclerosis was divided into five grades from 0 to 4 according to the number of sclerotic lesions in each glomerulus (grade 0, normal glomerulus; grade 1, sclerotic area of 1%–25%; grade 2, sclerotic area of 26%–50%; grade 3, sclerotic area of 51%–75%; grade 4, sclerotic area of 76%–100%). The glomerulosclerosis index (GSI) was calculated using following formula:

$$\text{GSI} = [(N_1 \times 1) + (N_2 \times 2) + (N_3 \times 3) + (N_4 \times 4)]/N_{\text{total}}$$

where N represents the number of the corresponding degree of glomerulosclerosis and N_{total} is the total number of glomeruli. Similarly, the extent of interstitial expansion was quantified by calculating the tubular interstitial collagen-positive area (blue) of Masson's Trichrome staining using Image-Pro Plus 6.0 software (Media Cybernetics, Silver Spring, MD). Twenty consecutive glomeruli were examined for each section, and the mean percentage of collagen-positive lesions was calculated for each mouse.

1.9 Assaying lipid oxidation

A thiobarbituric acid (TBA) assay was used to measure relative malondialdehyde (MDA) production as an index of lipid peroxidation, as described previously [11]. Briefly, tissue proteins were collected by centrifuging at 12,000 g at 4 ℃ for 15 min, and the protein concentrations were measured using Bradford assays. Then, 50 µl of sample was mixed with 20 µl of 8.1% sodium dodecyl sulfate (SDS), 150 µl of 20% acetic acid, and 210 µl of 0.0571% TBA and was incubated at 90 ℃ for 70 min. Samples were centrifuged at 4,000 rpm for 15 min at 4 ℃, harvested, and transferred to 96-well plates, and the optical density was read at 540 nm.

1.10 Statistical analysis

Data were collected from nine mice in each group, and the results are presented as means ± SE. Statistical analyses were performed using one-way or two-way ANOVA, followed by *post hoc* multiple comparisons using Bonferroni's tests. All analyses were performed using GraphPad Prism 5.0 (GraphPad Software, San Diego, CA). Statistical significance was defined as $P < 0.05$.

2. Results

2.1 Type 2 diabetic mouse model

Clinically, the major features of type 2 diabetes are insulin resistance together with obesity, hyperlipidemia, and hyperglycemia. Therefore, in the current study mice were fed a HFD to induce obesity, hyperlipidemia, and insulin resistance and were then treated using a single injection of STZ to induce hyperglycemia and establish a model of type 2 diabetes. As shown in Fig. 1, there was a significant increase in their body weight starting 4 wk after HFD feeding compared with SD feeding (Con), and the difference between the two groups increased gradually in a time-dependent manner (Fig. 1A). In the glucose tolerance test (GTT), the blood glucose level in the HFD-fed mice after glucose infusion was greater than that in the SD-fed mice at 30 min, suggesting that the HFD-fed mice were glucose intolerant (Fig. 1B). In addition, the blood glucose level in the HFD-fed mice remained higher than that in the SD-fed mice until the final measurement, although there were no statistically significant differences between the two groups (Fig. 1B). Furthermore, blood glucose levels during the insulin tolerance test (ITT) were significant higher in HFD-fed mice than in SD-fed mice at all time points (Fig. 1C). The results above suggested that the mice fed a HFD for 12 wk had already developed glucose intolerance and insulin resistance (Fig. 1B and C). A single injection of STZ induced a significant increase in blood glucose compared with both HFD-fed alone and SD-fed (Con) groups. But no significant difference was observed between SD- and HFD-fed groups (Fig. 1D).

2.2 The combination of LDR and FGF21 improved insulin sensitivity in type 2 diabetic mice significantly compared with treatment of either alone

Diabetic mice were fed a HFD in the presence of FGF21 alone, LDR alone, or the combination of both treatments. At the end of experiment, FGF21 and the combination treatment, not LDR alone, decreased blood glucose levels significantly compared with the DM group (Fig. 2A). Although the blood glucose levels in the combination group were decreased slightly compared with FGF21 treatment alone, the difference was not statistically significant (Fig. 2A). In addition, both LDR and FGF21 significantly ameliorated diabetes-induced insulin resistance (Fig. 2B); how-

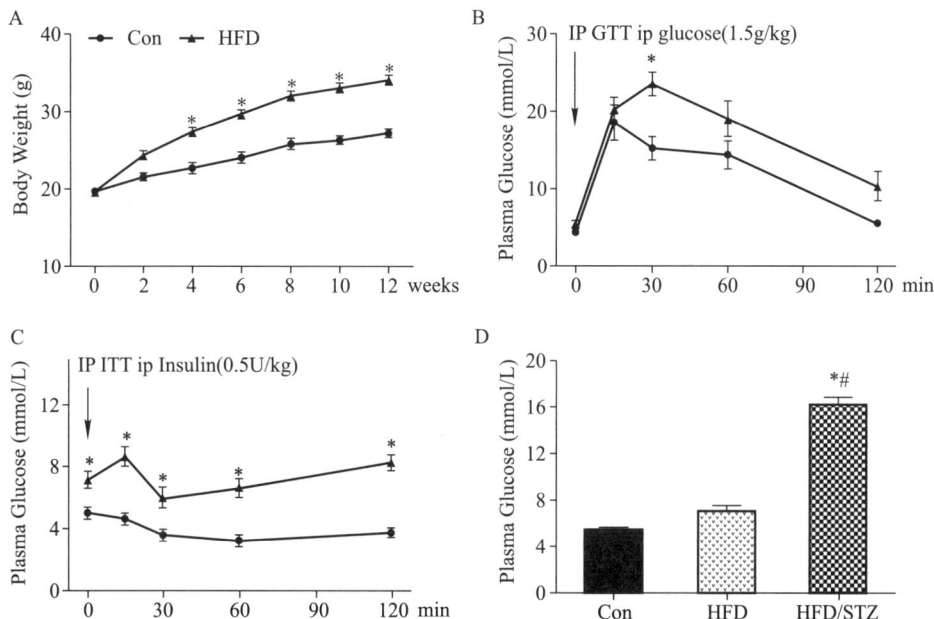

Fig. 1. Establishing a type 2 diabetic mouse (DM) model using the HFD/STZ (high-fat diet/streptozotocin) model. C57BL/6J. mice were fed a HFD (40% of calories from fat) for 12 wk to induce obesity. Body weight (A), glucose tolerance (B), and insulin sensitivity (C) were examined. Three days after injection of STZ, blood glucose was measured (D). Mice were regarded as diabetic once hyperglycemia was observed (>12 mmol/l). Data are presented as means ± SE; $n = 9$ per group. GTT, glucose tolerance test; ITT, insulin tolerance test. $^{*}P < 0.05$ vs. HFD group; $^{\#}P < 0.05$ vs. DM group.

A

B

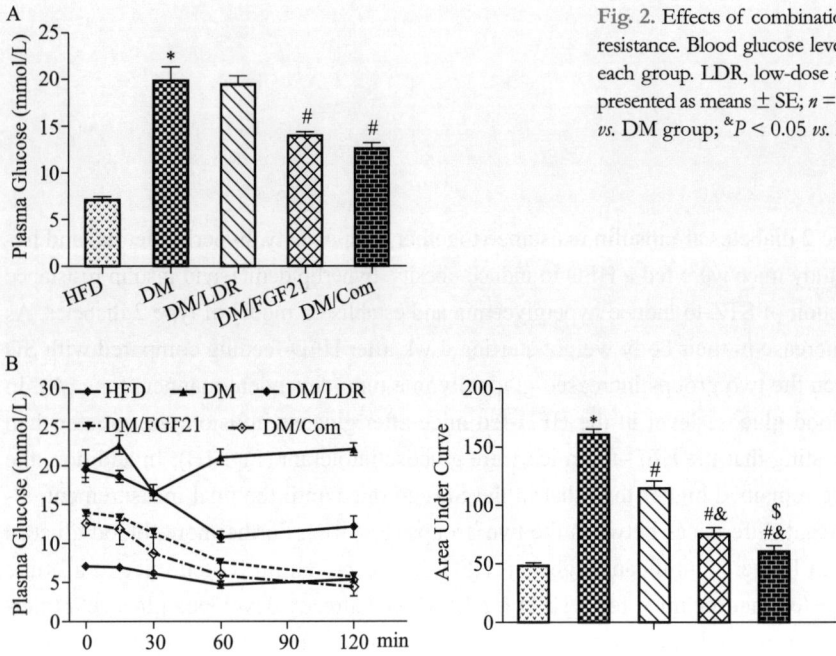

Fig. 2. Effects of combination treatment strategy on hyperglycemia and insulin resistance. Blood glucose levels (A) and insulin tolerance (B) were examined in each group. LDR, low-dose radiation; FGF, fibroblast growth factor. Data are presented as means ± SE; $n = 9$ per group. *$P < 0.05$ vs. HFD group; #$P < 0.05$ vs. DM group; &$P < 0.05$ vs. LDR group; $P < 0.05$ vs. FGF21 group.

ever, the combination treatment improved insulin sensitivity additively compared with either single treatment alone (Fig. 2B).

2.3 Effects of the different treatments on renal dysfunction in diabetic mice

Diabetes increased the levels of UP and mAlb significantly, indicating the induction of renal dysfunction (Table 1). However, FGF21 treatment prevented diabetes-induced renal dysfunction significantly, as shown by reduced UP and mAlb and increased U-Cre levels. Exposure to LDR also reduced UP and mAlb significantly but did not affect U-Cre levels. Renal dysfunction, which is reflected by increased UP and mAlb levels, was diminished further in mice that received the combination treatment compared with either treatment alone. Both FGF21 alone and the combination treatment, but not LDR alone, increased U-Cre excretion significantly compared with the DM group (Table 1).

Table 1.   Renal function of mice fed a HFD with or without additional treatments

Parameters	HFD	DM	DM/LDR	DM/FGF21	DM/Com
Urine protein, µg/day	120.9 ± 10.5	985.4 ± 25.9*	750.5 ± 30.2#	664.2 ± 34.0#	480.2 ± 30.6#&$
Urine mAlb, µg/day	17.8 ± 4.7	305.2 ± 24.7*	184.8 ± 21.2#	138.8 ± 23.1#	102.5 ± 20.3#&$
Urine creatinine	33.8 ± 2.0	31.2 ± 1.0	35.5 ± 1.2	37.6 ± 1.5#	38.3 ± 1.4#

Data are presented as means ± SE; $n = 9$/group. mAlb, microalbumin; HFD, high-fat diet; DM, diabetes mellitus; LDR, low-dose radiation; FGF, fibroblast growth factor; Com, combination LDR + FGF21. *$P < 0.05$ vs. HFD group; #$P < 0.05$ vs. DM group; &$P < 0.05$ vs. LDR group; $P < 0.05$ vs. FGF21 group.

2.4 Effects of the different treatments on diabetes-induced renal hypertrophy and pathological changes

Generally, renal dysfunction reflects pathological changes in the kidney. Consistent with the functional findings (Table 1), mesangial cell proliferation, capillary wall thickness, capillary collapse, tubular dilation, and epithelial cell degeneration were all obvious in diabetic kidneys after H&E staining (Fig. 3A). These pathological changes were suppressed significantly by LDR or FGF21 treatment alone (Fig. 3A), and to a greater extent by the combination treatment.

Next, the kidney tissues were stained with PAS to detect glomerulosclerosis. As shown in Fig. 3, B and D, the GSI was increased significantly in diabetic mice, which was prevented significantly by treatment with either LDR or FGF21 alone and to a greater extent by the combination treatment.

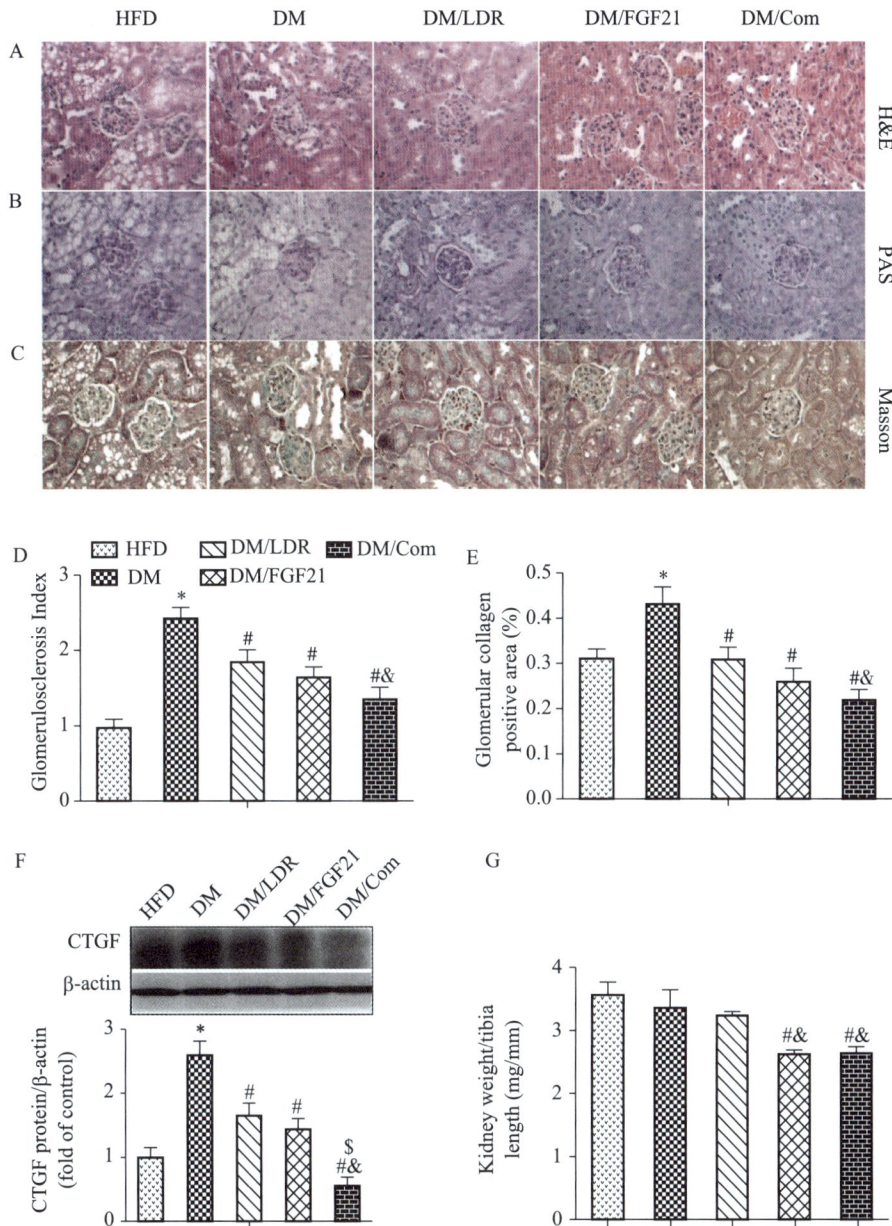

Fig. 3. Effects of combination treatment strategy on diabetes-induced histopathological changes in the kidneys of mice. Representative images of hematoxylin and eosin (A, H and E) staining, periodic acid-Schiff (B, PAS) staining, and Masson's Trichrome staining (C, Masson) to detect renal pathological changes, glomerulosclerosis, and collagen deposition, respectively. Magnification × 400. Glomerulosclerosis and collagen accumulation were examined in PAS- or Masson's-stained slices, respectively, and quantified using Image-Pro Plus 6.0 software (D and E). Renal connective tissue growth factor (CTGF) expression was measured using Western blotting (F). Renal hypertrophy was examined by assessing the change in the kidney weight-to-tibia length ratio (G). Data are presented as means ± SE; $n = 9$ per group. $^*P < 0.05$ vs. HFD group; $^#P < 0.05$ vs. DM group; $^&P < 0.05$ vs. LDR group.

Masson's Trichrome staining revealed significant collagen accumulation in the kidneys of diabetic mice, indicating that interstitial fibrosis had developed (Fig. 3C and E). Treatment with either LDR or FGF21 alone prevented these pathological changes significantly, and the preventive effects were additive in the combination treatment group. To confirm these observations, we assessed CTGF expression in the kidneys as a classical molecular marker of fibrosis using western blotting. Consistent with the results of Masson's staining, renal CTGF expression was increased significantly in the DM group which was remarkably suppressed by treatment with wither LDR and FGF21 alone. Furthermore a additive suppression was observed in the combination treatment group (Fig. 3F).

Diabetes-induced kidney injury is always associated with renal hypertrophy, which is characterized by an increased kidney weight to tibia length ratio. The ratio decreased slightly after exposure to LDR compared with DM and HFD groups. In contrast, treatment with FGF21 alone or in combination with LDR decreased the ratio significantly compared with the DM group (Fig. 3G).

2.5 Effects of the different treatments on systemic and renal dyslipidemia in type 2 diabetic mice

In addition to hyperglycemia, dyslipidemia is a crucial systemic pathogenesis of DN. As shown in Table 2, hyperlipidemia was evident in the DM groups, as shown by increased serum TG levels. Consistent with the serum profiles, kidney tissue H&E staining revealed an increased number of fat vacuoles in the kidney (Fig. 3A); the renal TG and FFA levels were also increased significantly in the diabetic mice (Table 2). These results suggest that renal lipid accumulation was increased in the DM group. However, treatment with FGF21 normalized all of the above abnormal profiles remarkably. Similar effects were observed in the DM/ LDR mice, except that there was no change in CHO levels compared with the DM group. Importantly, the combination treatment normalized serum and renal TG, serum LDL, and renal FFA levels (Table 2) and significantly reduced the number of renal fat vacuoles (Fig. 3A).

Table 2.   Serum and renal lipid metabolic parameters in mice fed a HFD with or without additional treatments

Parameters	HFD	DM	DM/LDR	DM/FGF21	DM/Com
Serum TG, mmol/l	1.39 ± 0.17	6.58 ± 0.70*	4.28 ± 0.72#	3.60 ± 0.65#	3.06 ± 0.48#&$
Serum CHO, mmol/l	4.41 ± 0.47	4.70 ± 0.38	4.58 ± 0.34	3.83 ± 0.68#	3.65 ± 0.37#
Serum HDL, mmol/l	1.95 ± 0.25	1.65 ± 0.24	2.35 ± 0.28#	2.42 ± 0.17#	2.47 ± 0.21#
Serum LDL, mmol/l	0.45 ± 0.07	0.66 ± 0.16	0.53 ± 0.07	0.50 ± 0.08#	0.35 ± 0.07#&$
Renal TG, mg/g tissue	6.17 ± 1.20	9.82 ± 1.42*	6.20 ± 1.13#	4.45 ± 1.20#	3.52 ± 1.50#&$
Renal FFA, mg/g tissue	9.58 ± 1.72	16.25 ± 1.64*	10.46 ± 1.55#	8.20 ± 1.69#	7.15 ± 1.82#&$

Data are presented as means ± SE; n = 9/group. TG, triglycerides; CHO, cholesterol; HDL, high-density lipoprotein; LDL, low-density lipoprotein; FFA, free fatty acids. *P < 0.05 vs. HFD group; #P < 0.05 vs. DM group. &P < 0.05 vs. LDR group; $$P$ < 0.05 vs. FGF21 group.

2.6 Effects of the different treatments on diabetes-induced renal oxidative stress and inflammation

As markers of nitrosative or oxidative damage, respectively, renal 3-NT (Fig. 4A) and MDA (Fig. 4B) levels were increased significantly in the DM group but not in the DM/LDR, DM/FGF21, and DM/Com groups (Fig. 4, A and B). To confirm these observations, Western blotting was used to examine the levels of classic inflammatory factors in the kidney, including ICAM-1 (Fig. 5A), TNF-α (Fig. 5B), and PAI-1 (Fig. 5C). Consistent with the above results, diabetes increased the expression of these inflammatory factors in the kidney significantly. However, the increase was prevented by treatment with LDR or FGF21 alone and to an even greater extent by the combination treatment.

2.7 Effects of the different treatments on the renal expression of antioxidants in diabetic mice

Next, we measured the renal expression of multiple antioxidants in treated and untreated diabetic mice. Western blotting revealed that the expression of SOD-1 (Fig. 6A), NQO-1 (Fig. 6B), and HO-1 (Fig. 6C) was decreased significantly in the kidneys of DM mice and DM/ FGF21 mice. Interestingly, exposure to LDR reversed, but FGF21 treatment

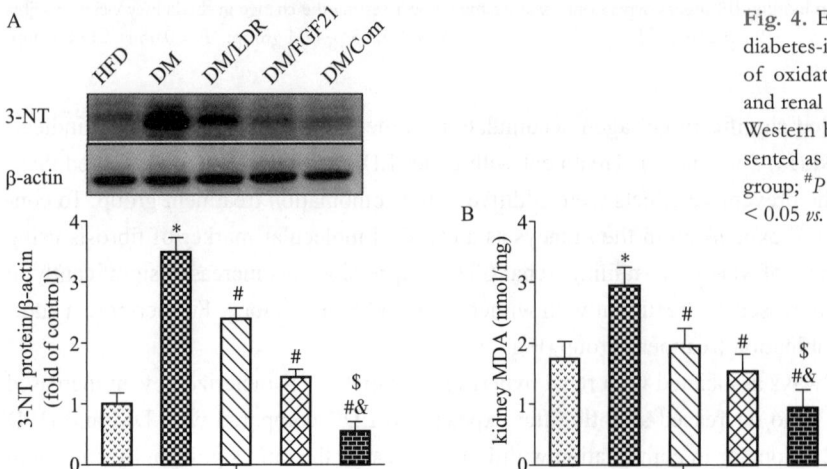

Fig. 4. Effects of combination treatment strategy on diabetes-induced oxidative stress in kidneys. Expression of oxidative damage markers 3-nitrotyrosine (3-NT; A) and renal malondialdehyde (MDA; B) were measured using Western blotting and ELISA, respectively. Data are presented as means ± SE; n = 9 per group. *P < 0.05 vs. HFD group; #P < 0.05 vs. DM group; &P < 0.05 vs. LDR group; $$P$ < 0.05 vs. FGF21 group.

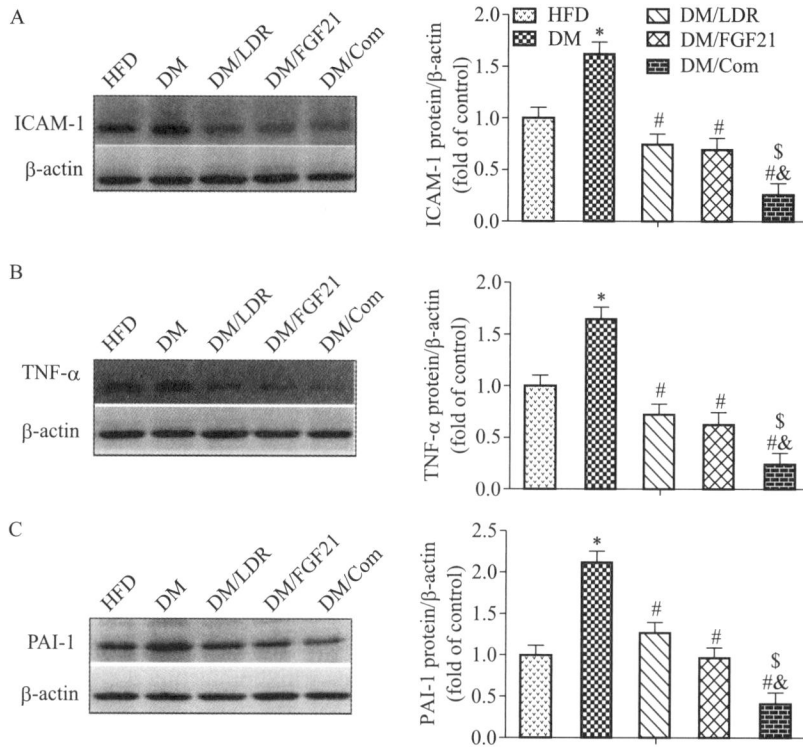

Fig. 5. Effects of combination treatment strategy on renal inflammation in type 2 diabetic mice. Renal tissues were collected from the different groups at the indicated times, and intercellular adhesion molecule 1 (ICAM-1), tumor necrosis factor-α (TNF-α), and plasminogen activator inhibitor 1 (PAI-1) expression was measured using Western blotting (A–C). Data are presented as means ± SE; n = 9 per group. $^*P$ < 0.05 $vs.$ HFD group; $^\#P$ < 0.05 $vs.$ DM group; $^\&P$ < 0.05 $vs.$ LDR group; $^\$P$ < 0.05 $vs.$ FGF21 group.

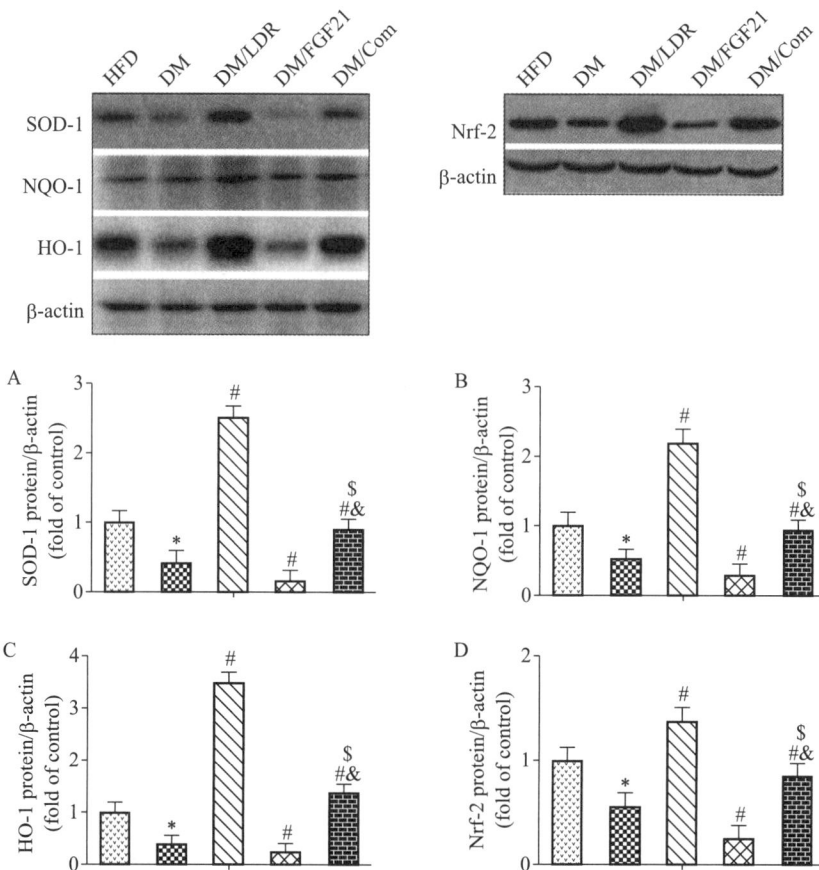

Fig. 6. Effects of combination treatment strategy on expression of renal nuclear factor E2-related factor 2 (Nrf-2) and its downstream targets in type 2 diabetic mice. Renal tissues were collected from the different groups at indicated times, and superoxide dismutase-1 (SOD-1), NAD(P)H:quinone oxidoreductase-1 (NQO-1), heme oxygenase-1 (HO-1), and Nrf-2 expression was measured using Western blotting (A–D). Data are presented as means ± SE; n = 9 per group. $^*P$ < 0.05 $vs.$ HFD group; $^\#P$ < 0.05 $vs.$ DM group; $^\&P$ < 0.05 $vs.$ LDR group; $^\$P$ < 0.05 $vs.$ FGF21 group.

further enhanced the diabetes-induced suppression of these antioxidants significantly, and the expression of these anti-oxidants was much higher in the DM/LDR group than in the DM group (Fig. 6A–C). The expression of the antioxidants was similar in DM/Com and control mice. These results suggest that LDR, but not FGF-21, increased renal antioxidant levels significantly under diabetic conditions.

2.8 Expression of the above-mentioned antioxidants is regulated positively by the transcription factor Nrf2

We demonstrated previously that Nrf2 is upregulated in diabetic mice exposed to LDR [51, 57]. Therefore, we next determined whether the altered antioxidant expression in the DM/LDR and DM/Com groups was due to altered renal Nrf2 levels (Fig. 6D). As expected, the pattern of Nrf2 expression was similar to the antioxidant expression in the different groups, suggesting that diabetes downregulated and LDR upregulated renal antioxidant levels mainly by altering Nrf2 expression.

3. Discussion

The kidney is the main target organ of diabetes, which leads to the development of DN. DN is characterized by renal dysfunction and pathological changes such as renal hypertrophy, fibrosis, and glomerulosclerosis [18, 21, 33]. The pathogenesis of DN is highly complex and is the consequence of both systemic and renal pathogeneses. Therefore, we hypothesized that improving the systemic pathogenesis of diabetes while protecting the kidney from diabetes-induced damage might additively prevent the development of DN.

FGF21 is a member of the FGF family, which exerts systemic therapeutic effects to improve hyperglycemia, dys-lipidemia, and insulin resistance [2, 16]. Serum FGF21 levels were increased significantly in humans with both acute and chronic renal dysfunction during early- to end-stage kidney disease, which might be an adaptive response to diabetes to confer protective effects [30]. FGF21 suppresses diabetes-induced inflammation, oxidative stress, and fibrosis in multiple organs, which could be attributed to its effects on maintaining glucose and lipid homeostasis and improving insulin resistance [22, 27, 56]. Similarly, renal protective effects of FGF21 were also observed in our recent study performed in an acute lipotoxic model of type 1 diabetes [56].

High doses of ionizing radiation (HDR) induce a variety of harmful effects, including acute death and late carcinogenesis. Although LDR was also considered dangerous according to the linear no-threshold (LNT) hypothesis [32], increasing evidence has suggested that LET radiation at dose levels <100 mGy could induce beneficial effects, including extending life span, enhancing immunity, and improving DNA repair [17, 23, 36]. Epidemiological surveys have analyzed individuals exposed to <100 mGy radiation. Generally, there was *1*) no increase or even a reduced risk of the incidence of solid cancer, *2*) no increase in the incidence of leukemia, and *3*) no increase in cardiovascular diseases [5, 15, 28, 31, 37]. A study supported by the Radiation Effects Research Foundation showed that the dose-response relationship supported the LNT model in principle in the dose range 0–150 mGy; however, the dose-response relationship <100 mGy tends to fluctuate, which limits statistical significance in the increase in the incidence of cancer at lower doses [42]. Our recent studies demonstrated that LDR also induces beneficial effects on diabetes and its associated complications [43, 56, 57]. The available data suggest that preexposure to LDR reduces the incidence of alloxan-induced diabetes and also delays the onset of hyperglycemia in diabetes-prone nonobese diabetic mice [46, 48]. This protection is associated with the prevention of oxidative damage [51–53, 57]. Our previous study revealed that, in addition to antioxidative effects, LDR also prevents inflammation to protect against DN [43, 51, 55, 56]. Patients with DN have poor renal function; however, most drugs used to treat DN are excreted through the kidney, which further increases the renal working load in diabetic patients. Therefore, the use of LDR as a noninvasive approach has been investigated to prevent chronic renal diseases [4, 47]. In the present study, we combined LDR and FGF21 as a therapeutic strategy for the first time to explore whether simultaneously blocking the systemic and renal pathogeneses could further prevent the development of DN.

We developed a human-like type 2 diabetic model using a HFD/STZ protocol. After the model of type 2 diabetes was established successfully, the mice were exposed to LDR (50 mGy/day, every other day for 4 wk) with and without FGF21 (1.5 mg/kg, daily for 8 wk) based on doses optimized in our previous studies [43].

In the early stage of DN, some abnormalities are frequently associated with enlarged kidneys. We evaluated renal hypertrophy by calculating the kidney weight-to-tibia length ratio. The HFD- and diabetes-induced increase in this ratio was suppressed slightly by LDR and significantly by FGF21 alone and the combination treatment. In addition to renal hypertrophy, morphological analysis revealed obvious glomerular basement membrane thickening, mesangial cell proliferation, mesangial matrix expansion, glomerulosclerosis, and fibrosis in the diabetic kidneys. Diabetes also caused severe renal dysfunction, as characterized by increased UP levels and mAlb excretion. These pathological and functional diabetic changes were reduced by each single-treatment strategy and suppressed further by the combination treatment. Taken together, these findings suggest that the combination of LDR and FGF21 exerts additive renal protective effects in a model of diabetes.

Next, we assessed whether the combination treatment could be attributed to preventing both systemic and renal pathogenic changes. First, we examined blood glucose levels and serum lipid profiles as global indicators of diabetes. Our data revealed that FGF21, but not LDR, treatment lowered blood glucose levels significantly. The combination treatment exhibited a similar lowering effect on blood glucose to FGF21 treatment alone, suggesting that the hypoglycemic activity of the combination treatment could be attributed completely to FGF21. Hyperglycemia is always correlated positively with insulin resistance in patients with type 2 diabetes. As expected, FGF21 treatment improved insulin sensitivity significantly, which was enhanced further by the combination treatment. However, LDR also improved insulin sensitivity, implying that there must be other mechanisms by which LDR contributes to the improved insulin sensitivity. Strong evidence suggests that dyslipidemia is a key cause of insulin resistance. Excessive levels of fatty acids and their derivatives function as signaling molecules that activate protein kinases [20]. These kinases can then impair insulin signaling, finally leading to insulin resistance [39, 43]. Since our animal model was characterized by obesity and insulin resistance [43], we next examined whether the different therapeutic strategies exerted beneficial effects to correct the abnormal lipid profiles in diabetic mice. Consistent with our hypothesis, obvious dyslipidemia was observed in diabetic mice, as characterized by increased serum TG levels. TG and FFA levels were also upregulated in diabetic kidneys. Treatment with either LDR or FGF21 alone corrected the diabetes-induced abnormal lipid profiles greatly, which was enhanced further by the combination treatment. Therefore, it is likely that the additive effects of LDR and FGF21 on insulin sensitivity were due mainly to correction of the abnormal lipid profile.

Next, we assessed whether the combination strategy also afforded local renal protection at the cellular and molecular levels, in addition to the above-mentioned systemic effects. Large bodies of evidence have demonstrated that oxidative stress, inflammation, and subsequent fibrosis are the main pathogeneses of diabetes in the kidney [1, 19, 50]. In the current study, we confirmed that diabetes increased the levels of 3-NT and MDA significantly as markers of nitrosative and oxidative damage and decreased the expression of multiple antioxidants and their upstream transcription factor Nrf2. Moreover, inflammatory cell infiltration and increased levels of multiple inflammatory factors such as ICAM-1, TNF-α, and PAI-1 were also observed in diabetic kidneys. Fibrosis, which reflects late-stage pathological damage, was also observed in the kidneys of diabetic mice, as determined using renal CTGF expression and Masson's Trichrome staining. Consistent with our hypothesis, all these pathological changes were suppressed significantly by either LDR or FGF21 treatment, and the combination treatment further protected the kidneys from in jury. Therefore, the combination of LDR and FGF21 could confer protection against renal damage.

In summary, the present study has shown that exposing mice to the combination of LDR and FGF21 exerted additive effects to further protect against type 2 diabetes-induced renal damage. These effects were exerted by blocking hyperglycemia, dyslipidemia, renal oxidative stress, inflammation, and fibrosis. In addition, FGF21 regulates carbohydrate and lipid metabolism without inducing hypoglycemia and cell growth. Meanwhile, since whole body exposure to LDR is easy to perform, is noninvasive, and does not increase the kidney workload, this combination strategy might provide a novel therapeutic approach for diabetic patients in the near future.

References

[1] Steffes MW, Chavers BM, Molitch ME, *et al.* Sustained effect of intensive treatment of type 1 diabetes mellitus on development and progression of diabetic nephropathy - The epidemiology of diabetes interventions and complications (EDIC) study[J]. Jama-Journal of the American Medical Association, 2003, 290(16): 2159-2167.

[2] Alisi A, Panera N, Nobili V. Commentary: FGF21 holds promises for treating obesity-related insulin resistance and hepatosteatosis[J]. Endocrinology, 2014, 155(2): 343-346.

[3] Antonellis PJ, Kharitonenkov A, Adams AC. Physiology and endocrinology symposium: FGF21: Insights into mechanism of action from preclinical studies[J]. Journal of Animal Science, 2014, 92(2): 407-413.

[4] Aunapuu M, Pechter U, Gerskevits E, *et al.* Low-dose radiation modifies the progression of chronic renal failure[J]. Annals of Anatomy-Anatomischer Anzeiger, 2004, 186(3): 277-282.

[5] Averbeck D. Does scientific evidence support a change from the LNT model for low-dose radiation risk extrapolation? [J]. Health Physics, 2009, 97(5): 493-504.

[6] Bligh EG, Dyer WJ. A rapid method of total lipid extraction and purification [J]. Canadian Journal of Biochemistry and Physiology, 1959, 37(8): 911-917.

[7] Bocharov AV, Baranova IN, Vishnyakova TG, *et al.* Targeting of scavenger receptor class B type I by synthetic amphipathic alpha-helical-containing peptides blocks lipopolysaccharide (LPS) uptake and LPS-induced pro-inflammatory cytokine responses in THP-1 monocyte cells[J]. Journal of Biological Chemistry, 2004, 279(34): 36072-36082.

[8] Brenner BM, Cooper ME, de Zeeuw D, *et al.* Effects of losartan on renal and cardiovascular outcomes in patients with type 2 diabetes and nephropathy[J]. New England Journal of Medicine, 2001, 345(12): 861-869.

[9] Cai L. Research of the adaptive response induced by low-dose radiation: where have we been and where should we go?[J]. Human & Experimental Toxicology, 1999, 18(7): 419-425.

[10] Cai L, Jiang J, Wang B, *et al.* IInduction of an adaptiveresponse to dominant lethality and to chromosome damage of mouse germcells by low dose radiation [J]. Mutation Research, 1993, 303(4): 157-161.

[11] Cai L, Wang JX, Li Y, *et al.* Inhibition of superoxide generation and associated nitrosative damage is involved in metallothionein prevention of diabetic cardiomyopathy[J]. Diabetes, 2005, 54(6): 1829-1837.

[12] Cai L, Wang P. Induction of a cytogenetic adaptive response in germ cells of irradiated mice with very low-dose rate of chronic gamma-irradiationand its biological influence on radiation-induced DNA or chromosomaldamage and cell killing in their male offspring [J]. Mutagenesis, 1995, 10(2): 95-100.

[13] Calabrese EJ. Hormesis: changing view of the dose-response, a personal account of the history and current status[J]. Mutation Research-Reviews in Mutation Research, 2002, 511(3): 181-189.

[14] Calabrese EJ, Baldwin LA. Hormesis: The dose-response revolution[J]. Annual Review of Pharmacology and Toxicology, 2003, 43: 175-197.

[15] Cuttler JM, Pollycove M. Nuclear energy and health and the benefits of low-dose Radiation Hormesis[J]. Dose-Response, 2009, 7(1): 52-89.

[16] Emanuelli B, Vienberg SG, Smyth G, *et al.* Interplay between FGF21 and insulin action in the liver regulates metabolism[J]. Journal of Clinical Investigation, 2014, 124(2): 515-527.

[17] Farooque A, Mathur R, Verma A, *et al.* Low-dose radiation therapy of cancer: role of immune enhancement[J]. Expert Review of Anticancer Therapy, 2011, 11(5): 791-802.

[18] Franceschini N, Shara NM, Wang H, *et al.* The association of genetic variants of type 2 diabetes with kidney function[J]. Kidney International, 2012, 82(2): 220-225.

[19] Furukawa M, Gohda T, Tanimoto M, *et al.* Pathogenesis and novel treatment from the mouse model of type 2 diabetic nephropathy[J]. Scientific World Journal, 2013.

[20] Harjai KJ. Potential new cardiovascular risk factors: Left ventricular hypertrophy, homocysteine, lipoprotein(a), triglycerides, oxidative stress, and fibrinogen[J]. Annals of Internal Medicine, 1999, 131(5): 376-386.

[21] Heerspink HJL, de Zeeuw D. The kidney in type 2 diabetes therapy[J]. The review of diabetic studies : RDS, 2011, 8(3): 392-402.

[22] Iglesias P, Selgas R, Romero S, *et al.* Biological role, clinical significance, and therapeutic possibilities of the recently discovered metabolic hormone fibroblastic growth factor 21[J]. European Journal of Endocrinology, 2012, 167(3): 301-309.

[23] James SJ, Enger SM, Makinodan T. DNA strand breaks and DNA repairresponse in lymphocytes after chronic *in vivo* exposure to very low dosesof ionizing radiation in mice [J]. Mutation Research, 1991, 249(1): 255-263.

[24] Ji H, Pesce C, Zheng W, *et al.* Sex differences in renal injury and nitric oxide production in renal wrap hypertension[J]. American Journal of Physiology-Heart and Circulatory Physiology, 2005, 288(1): H43-H47.

[25] Kharitonenkov A, Adams AC. Inventing new medicines: The FGF21 story[J]. Molecular Metabolism, 2014, 3(3): 221-229.

[26] Kharitonenkov A, Shiyanova TL, Koester A, *et al.* FGF-21 as a novel metabolic regulator[J]. Journal of Clinical Investigation, 2005, 115(6): 1627-1635.

[27] Kim HW, Lee JE, Cha JJ, *et al.* Fibroblast Growth Factor 21 Improves Insulin Resistance and Ameliorates Renal Injury in db/db Mice[J]. Endocrinology, 2013, 154(9): 3366-3376.

[28] Koana T, Tsujimura H. A U-shaped dose-response relationship between X radiation and sex-linked recessive lethal mutation in male germ cells of drosophila[J]. Radiation Research, 2010, 174(1): 46-51.

[29] Li H, Zhang J, Jia W. Fibroblast growth factor 21: a novel metabolic regulator from pharmacology to physiology[J]. Frontiers of Medicine, 2013, 7(1): 25-30.

[30] Lin Z, Zhou Z, Liu Y, *et al.* Circulating FGF21 levels are progressively increased from the early to end stages of chronic kidney diseases and are associated with renal function in Chinese[J]. Plos One, 2011, 6(4).

[31] Little MP. Cancer and non-cancer effects in Japanese atomic bomb survivors[J]. Journal of Radiological Protection, 2009, 29(2A): A43-A59.

[32] Liu G, Gong P, Bernstein LR, *et al.* Apoptotic cell death induced by low-dose radiation in male germ cells: Hormesis and adaptation[J]. Critical Reviews in Toxicology, 2007, 37(7): 587-605.

[33] Meguro S, Tomita M, Kabeya Y, *et al.* Factors associated with the decline of kidney function differ among eGFR strata in subjects with type 2 diabetes mellitus[J]. International Journal of Endocrinology, 2012.

[34] Mu J, Woods J, Zhou Y, *et al.* Chronic inhibition of dipeptidyl peptidase-4 with a sitagliptin analog preserves pancreatic beta-cell mass and function in a rodent model of type 2 diabetes[J]. Diabetes, 2006, 55(6): 1695-1704.

[35] Nomura T, Li X-H, Ogata H, *et al.* Suppressive effects of continuous low-dose-rate gamma irradiation on diabetic nephropathy in type II diabetes mellitus model mice[J]. Radiation Research, 2011, 176(3): 356-365.

[36] Nomura T, Sakai K, Ogata H, *et al.* Prolongation of life span in the accelerated aging klotho mouse model, by low-dose-rate continuous gamma irradiation[J]. Radiation Research, 2013, 179(6): 717-724.

[37] Ogura K, Magae J, Kawakami Y, *et al.* Reduction in mutation frequency by very low-dose gamma irradiation of drosophila melanogaster germ cells[J]. Radiation Research, 2009, 171(1): 1-8.

[38] Parving HH, Lehnert H, Brochner-Mortensen J, *et al.* The effect of irbesartan on the development of diabetic nephropathy in patients with type 2 diabetes[J]. New England Journal of Medicine, 2001, 345(12): 870-878.

[39] Petersen KF, Shulman GI. Etiology of insulin resistance[J]. American Journal of Medicine, 2006, 119(5): 10S-16S.

[40] Planavila A, Iglesias R, Giralt M, *et al.* Sirt1 acts in association with PPAR alpha to protect the heart from hypertrophy, metabolic dysregulation, and inflammation[J]. Cardiovascular Research, 2011, 90(2): 276-284.

[41] Planavila A, Redondo-Angulo I, Ribas F, *et al.* Fibroblast growth factor 21 protects the heart from oxidative stress[J]. Cardiovasc Res, 2015, 106(1): 19-31.

[42] Preston DL, Ron E, Tokuoka S, *et al.* Solid cancer incidence in atomic bomb survivors: 1958-1998[J]. Radiation Research, 2007, 168(1): 1-64.

[43] Shao M, Lu X, Cong W, *et al.* Multiple low-dose radiation prevents type 2 diabetes-induced renal damage through attenuation of dyslipidemia and insulin resistance and subsequent renal inflammation and oxidative stress[J]. Plos One, 2014, 9(3).

[44] Song Y, Li C, Cai L. Fluvastatin prevents nephropathy likely through suppression of connective tissue growth factor-mediated extracellular matrix accumulation[J]. Experimental and Molecular Pathology, 2004, 76(1): 66-75.

[45] Takahashi M, Kojima S, Yamaoka K, *et al.* Prevention of type I diabetes by low-dose gamma irradiation in NOD mice[J]. Radiation Research, 2000, 154(6): 680-685.

[46] Takehara Y, Yamaoka K, Hiraki Y, *et al.* Protection against alloxan diabetes by low-dose Co-60 gamma irradiation before alloxan administration[J]. Physiological Chemistry and Physics and Medical Nmr, 1995, 27(3): 149-159.

[47] van Kleef EM, Zurcher C, Oussoren YG, *et al.* Long-term effects of total-body irradiation on the kidney of Rhesus monkeys[J]. International Journal of Radiation Biology, 2000, 76(5): 641-648.

[48] Wang G, Li X, Sakai K, *et al.* Low-dose radiation and its clinical implications: diabetes[J]. Human & Experimental Toxicology, 2008, 27(2): 135-142.

[49] Watts LM, Manchem VP, Leedom TA, *et al.* Reduction of hepatic and adipose tissue glucocorticoid receptor expression with antisense oligonucleotides improves hyperglycemia and hyperlipidemia in diabetic rodents without causing systemic glucocorticoid antagonism[J]. Diabetes, 2005, 54(6): 1846-1853.

[50] Sustained effect of intensive treatment of type 1 diabetes mellitus on development and progression of diabetic nephropathy: the Epidemiology of Diabetes Interventions and Complications (EDIC) study[J]. Jama, 2003, 290(16): 2159-2167.

[51] Xing X, Zhang C, Shao M, *et al.* Low-dose radiation activates Akt and Nrf2 in the kidney of diabetic mice: A potential mechanism to prevent diabetic nephropathy[J]. Oxidative Medicine and Cellular Longevity, 2012.

[52] Yamaoka K, Kojima S, Nomura T. Changes of SOD-like substances in mouse organs after low-dose X-ray irradiation[J]. Physiological Chemistry and Physics and Medical NMR, 1999, 31(1): 23-28.

[53] Yamaoka K, Mori S, Nomura T, *et al.* Elevation of antioxidant potency in mice brain by low-dose X-ray irradiation and its effect on Fe-NTA-induced brain damage[J]. Physiological Chemistry and Physics and Medical NMR, 2002, 34(2): 119-132.

[54] Yu Y, Bai F, Liu Y, *et al.* Fibroblast growth factor (FGF21) protects mouse liver against D-galactose-induced oxidative stress and apoptosis *via* activating Nrf2 and PI3K/Akt pathways[J]. Mol Cell Biochem, 2015, 403(1-2): 287-299.

[55] Zhang C, Jin S, Guo W, *et al.* Attenuation of diabetes-induced cardiac inflammation and pathological remodeling by low-dose radiation[J]. Radiation Research, 2011, 175(3): 307-321.

[56] Zhang C, Shao M, Yang H, *et al.* Attenuation of hyperlipidemia- and diabetes-induced early-stage apoptosis and late-stage renal dysfunction *via* administration of fibroblast growth factor-21 is associated with suppression of renal inflammation[J]. Plos One, 2013, 8(12).

[57] Zhang C, Xing X, Zhang F, *et al.* Low-dose radiation induces renal SOD1 expression and activity in type 1 diabetic mice[J]. International Journal of Radiation Biology, 2014, 90(3): 224-230.

FGF21 deletion exacerbates diabetic cardiomyopathy by aggravating cardiac lipid accumulation

Xiaoqing Yan, Xiaokun Li, Yi Tan

1. Introduction

Diabetic cardiomyopathy (DCM) is one of the most severe diabetic complications. It has been defined as ventricular dysfunction that occurs independently of coronary artery disease and hypertension [1]. The pathogenesis of DCM is multifactorial [2]. Altered myocardial substrate and energy metabolism has emerged as an important contributor to the development of DCM [3]. Despite an increase in fatty acid use in diabetic hearts, fatty acid uptake likely exceeds its oxidation rate, thereby resulting in cardiac lipid accumulation that promotes cardiac lipotoxicity [4]. Thus, targeting to correct diabetes-induced abnormal substrate metabolism in the heart will potentially lower the prevalence of DCM, thereby improve long-term survival of the patients with diabetes.

Fibroblast growth factor 21 (FGF21), a novel member of the FGF family, encoded by the *fgf21* gene located in chromosome 19 in human [5] and chromosome 7 in mice, has been identified as a potent metabolic regulator with specific effects on glucose and lipid metabolism [6]. FGF21 is preferentially expressed in the liver [5]. But other tissues, such as pancreas [7], white [8] and brown [9] adipose tissues, skeletal muscle [10] and heart [7] also express FGF21. FGF21 stimulates glucose uptake in adipocytes *via* the induction of glucose transporter-1, which is additive and independent of insulin [11]. Under hypothermic conditions, FGF21 can induce browning of white adipose tissues to up-regulate thermogenic activity, which could, at least in part, lead to a greater clearance of glucose [12]. Moreover, FGF21 has shown beneficial effects on lipid profiles in animal models [13, 14]. FGF21 can also regulate lipolysis in adipocytes in response to fasting [15]. Treatment with FGF21 enhances the expression and secretion of downstream effector adiponectin in adipocytes which in turn further improves fatty acid oxidation and lipid clearance in the liver and skeletal muscle [16].

Since its benefits in regulating glucose and lipid metabolism, FGF21 has shown therapeutic potential in treating diabetes [17]. FGF21 has insulin-sensitizing ability [16] and can ameliorate glucose tolerance [18] by reducing hepatic glucose production and stimulating glucose uptake in adipocytes. Acute FGF21 treatment suppressed hepatic glucose production, increased liver glycogen, lowered glucagon and improved glucose clearance in *ob/+* mice, while chronic FGF21 treatment ameliorated fasting hyperglycaemia in *ob/ob* mice *via* increased glucose disposal and improved hepatic insulin sensitivity [19]. Besides those insulin-mimetic properties, FGF21 does not induce mitogenicity, hypoglycaemia or weight gain at any dose tested in diabetic or healthy animals or when overexpressed in transgenic mice [13]; therefore, FGF21 shows a promise as an effective treatment of diabetes.

To date, the function of FGF21 has been extensively investigated, but most studies focused on the liver, adipose tissue [20] and skeletal muscle [10, 16]. The effect of FGF21 on the heart has been neglected. FGF21 activity depends on its binding to the fibroblast growth factor receptor 1 (FGFR1), especially FGFR1c, and co-factor β-klotho [21]. The existence of FGFR1c, β-klotho [22] and FGF21 [7] in the heart suggests that FGF21 may play certain roles in the physiological and pathophysiological aspects of the heart. Recently, FGF21 was found to have cardio-protective effects against myocardial ischaemia/reperfusion injury [23] and isoproterenol-induced cardiac hypertrophy [24]. However, its effect on DCM has not been characterized. In this study, we investigated the effect of FGF21 deletion on the development of DCM in a FGF21 knockout (FGF21KO) mouse model. We found that mice lacking the *fgf21* gene are more prone to develop DCM, which is likely because of the overexpression of CD36-mediated cardiac lipid accumulation.

2. Materials and methods

2.1 Ethics statement

This study was carried out in strict accordance with the recommendations in the Guide for the Care and Use of Laboratory Animals of the National Institutes of Health. The protocol was approved by the Animal Policy and Welfare Committee of Wenzhou Medical University and the Institutional Animal Care and Use Committee of the University of Louis-ville. All surgeries were performed under anaesthesia induced by intraperitoneal injection of 1.2% 2,2,2-Tribromoethanol (avertin) at the dose of 300 mg/kg bw and all efforts were made to minimize suffering.

2.2 Animal model

Male FGF21KO mice with C57 BL/6J background (gift from Dr. Steve Kliewer, University of Texas Southwestern Medical Center) and wildtype (WT) C57 BL/6J mice purchased from Jackson Laboratory (Bar Harbor, ME, USA) were used in this study. Type 1 diabetic mouse model was induced in 10 week-old male FGF21KO mice and age-matched WT mice by intraperitoneal (i.p.) injection of six doses of streptozotocin (STZ, Sigma-Aldrich, St. Louis, MO, USA in 10 mM sodium citrate buffer, pH 4.5) at 60 mg/kg bw daily. Control group (Ctrl) of FGF21KO and WT mice received citrate buffer alone. Seven days after the last STZ injection, whole blood glucose obtained from the mouse tail vein was detected using a SureStep complete blood glucose monitor (LifeScan, Milpitas, CA, USA), and animals with blood glucose levels greater than 250 mg/dl were considered diabetic. At 1, 2 and 4 months after diabetes onset, heart function and blood pressure were measured and mice were then killed.

2.3 Echocardiography

At 1, 2 and 4 months after diabetes onset, heart function was evaluated by transthoracic echocardiography (ECHO). ECHO was performed on mice using a Visual Sonics Vevo 770 high-resolution imaging system (Visual Sonics, Toronto, ON, Canada) and equipped with a RMV 707B High-Frame-Rate Scanhead (focal length 12.7 mm, frequency 30.0 MHz), as described previously [25]. Under sedation with avertin (300 mg/kg bw), mice were placed in a supine position on a heating pad to maintain body temperature at 36 – 37℃ that was continuously monitored using a rectal thermometer probe. Under these conditions, the animal's heart rate ranged between 400 and 550 beats/min. Two-dimensional and M-mode ECHO were used to assess wall motion, chamber dimensions and cardiac function.

2.4 Blood pressure measurement

Blood pressure was measured using a CODA™ mouse/rat tail-cuff system (Kent scientific, Torrington, CT, USA) following our previous published protocol [25].

2.5 Plasma FGF21 assay

Whole blood was collected in a lithium heparin tube (BD, Franklin Lakes, NJ, USA), and centrifuged at 2000 rpm for 20 min. Then, plasma was collected for FGF21 assay using a FGF21 Quantikine Elisa kit (R&D systems, Minneapolis, MN, USA) according to the manufacturer's instructions.

2.6 Plasma and cardiac triglyceride assay

Triglyceride concentrations were measured using a triglyceride assay kit (Cayman Chemicals, Ann Arbor, MI, USA) according to the manufacture's protocol. For plasma triglyceride assay, plasma from diabetic mice was diluted 1:1 with standard diluent assay reagent, while the plasma from control mice was not diluted. For cardiac triglyceride assay, 10 – 20 mg heart tissue was minced into small pieces and then homogenized in standard diluent assay reagent (10 μl/mg tissue). Tissue homogenate was centrifuged at 10,000 × g for 10 min. at 4℃, and 10 μl supernatant was used for triglyceride assay.

2.7 Histopathological examination

Paraffin sections (5 μm) from cardiac tissue dissected from mice were stained with haematoxylin and eosin and observed under light microscopy as described before [26].

2.8 Oil Red O staining

Lipid accumulation was evaluated by Oil Red O staining as described previously [27]. Cryosections (10 μm thick) from heart tissue embedded in optimal cutting temperature medium (Tissue-Tek® O.C.T™ Compound, Sakura, Torrance, CA, USA) were fixed in 10% buffered formalin for 30 min at room temperature and stained with Oil Red O for 1 h. After washing with 60% isopropanol, the sections were then counter-stained with haematoxylin (DAKO, Carpinteria, CA, USA) for 30 sec. A Nikon Eclipse E600 microscope (Nikon, Melville, NY, USA) was used to capture the Oil Red O-stained tissue sections at 40 × magnification.

2.9 Sirius Red staining

Sirius Red staining for collagen deposition was used to determine cardiac fibrosis as described previously [25]. Briefly, 5 μm paraffin-embedded heart tissue sections were stained with 0.1% Sirius Red F3BA and 0.25% Fast Green FCF. The proportion of collagen in Sirius Red-stained sections was then evaluated using a Nikon Eclipse E600 microscopy system.

2.10 Real-time quantitative polymerase chain reaction (RT-qPCR)

Total RNA was extracted from heart tissue using TRIzol reagent (Invitrogen, Carlsbad, CA, USA). After quantified using a Nanodrop ND-1000 spectrophotometer, 1 μg total RNA was used to synthesize first-strand complimentary DNA (cDNA) using reverse transcription kit (Promega, WI, USA) as described before [28]. RT-qPCR was carried out with the ABI 7 300 real-time PCR system (Applied Biosystems, Grand Island, NY, USA) in a 20 μl reaction system containing 10 μl of TaqMan Universal PCR Master Mix, 1 μl of primers, 6 μl ddH$_2$O and 3 μl of cDNA (1:4 dilution with nuclease-free water). Primers for mouse glyceraldehyde 3-phosphate dehydrogenase (GAPDH) and FGFR1 (Invitrogen) were used for RT-qPCR assay.

2.11 Western blot

Total proteins from heart tissue were fractionated on 10% SDS-PAGE gels and transferred to a nitrocellulose membrane. The membrane was blocked with 5% non-fat milk for 1 h, and incubated overnight at 4℃ on a rocking platform with the following primary antibodies: anti-phosphor-AMP-activated protein kinase (AMPK) a (Thr172), anti-AMPKa (Cell Signaling, Danvers, MA, USA), anti-CD36, anti-peroxisome proliferator-activated receptor gamma co-activator 1alpha (PGC1α; Abcam, MA, USA), anti-connective tissue growth factor (CTGF), anti-hexokinase II (HKII), anti-nuclear factor (erythroid-derived 2)-like 2 (Nrf2) and anti-GAPDH (Santa Cruz Biotechnology, Dallas, TX, USA). After unbound antibodies were washed out with tris-buffered saline (pH 7.2) containing 0.05% Tween20, membranes were incubated with corresponding secondary antibody for 1 h at room temperature. Antigen-antibody complexes were visualized with an enhanced chemiluminescence detection kit (Thermo Scientific, Waltham, MA, USA). Quantitative densitometry was performed on the identified bands by using a computer-based measurement system as performed in previous studies [25, 29].

2.12 Statistical analysis

Data were collected from five or more mice per group and presented as mean ± SD. One-way ANOVA was used to determine general difference, followed by a *post hoc* Turkey's test for the difference between groups, using Origin 7.5 laboratory data analysis and graphing software. Statistical significance was considered as $P < 0.05$.

3. Results

3.1 FGF21 expression decreased under type 1 diabetes conditions

Wild-type and FGF21KO diabetic mice showed similar, persistent increases in whole blood glucose and plasma triglyceride levels up until organ harvested 4 months after STZ-induced diabetes onset (Fig. 1A, B). To elucidate the relationship between FGF21 and DCM, we measured the plasma levels of FGF21 and the cardiac mRNA levels of its preferred receptor FGFR1 in both WT and FGF21KO mice under diabetic and non-diabetic conditions. Plasma FGF21 level in WT diabetic mice significantly decreased at 1, 2 and 4 months after diabetes onset (Fig. 1C), which was accompanied by obvious trend of cardiac FGFR1 mRNA level up-regulation at 1 and 2 months after DM onset (Fig. 1D), indicating that type 1 diabetes systematically down-regulation of FGF21 resulted in its receptor compensative up-regulation in cardiac tissue. No obvious FGF21 expression was observed under diabetic and non-diabetic conditions in FGF21KO mice, as expected (Fig. 1C). The deletion of FGF21 was accompanied by a slight compensative up-regulation of cardiac FGFR1 mRNA under basal conditions, which was significantly amplified by diabetes in FGF21KO mice (Fig. 1D).

3.2 FGF21 deletion-aggravated diabetes-induced cardiac dysfunction

The role of FGF21 in the development of DCM was investigated by determining the effect of FGF21 deletion on cardiac structure and function in diabetic mice. Under basal conditions, FGF21KO mice did not show marked alterations in heart weight (Fig. S1), cardiac structure and function (Fig. 2 and Table S1). However, both WT and FGF21KO diabetic mice showed heart weight decrease at 1, 2, and 4 months after diabetes onset (Fig. S1). WT diabetic mice did

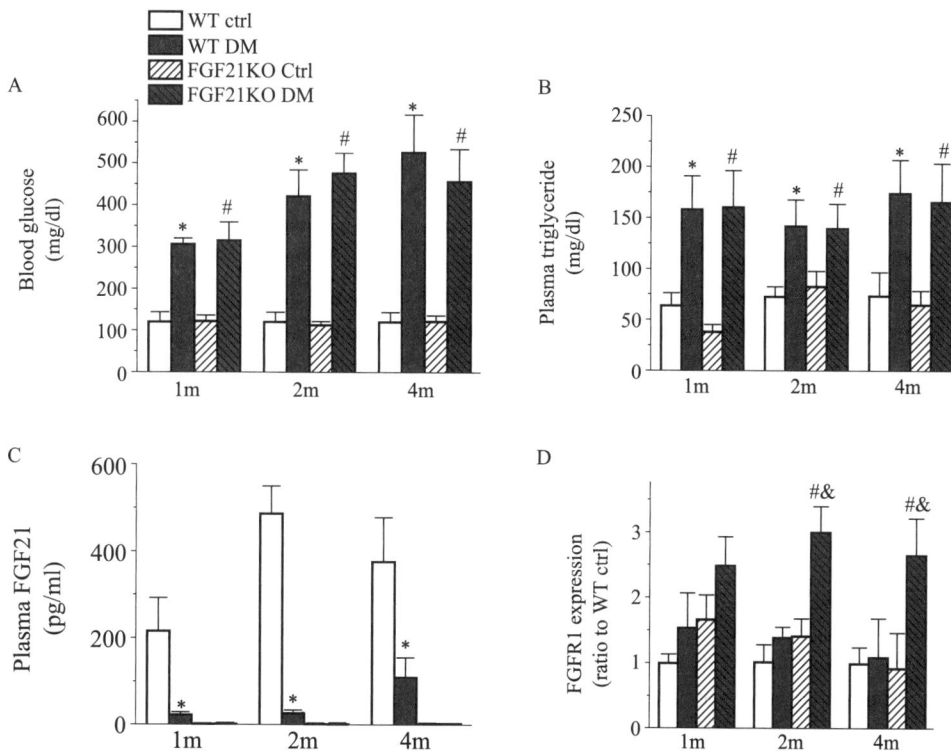

Fig. 1. Diabetes-induced high blood glucose and triglyceride levels, and FGF21 deficiency. At indicated time-points after diabetes onset, fasting blood glucose was detected using a SureStep complete blood glucose monitor (A), plasma triglyceride level was measured using a triglyceride assay kit (B), and plasma FGF21 was assayed using a FGF21 Quantikine Elisa kit (C). The expression of cardiac FGFR1 mRNA was detected by RT-qPCR and GAPDH was used as the loading control. Three duplications were set for each sample (D). Data are presented as means ± SD ($n \geqslant 5$ for each group). $^{*}P < 0.05$ *vs.* WT Ctrl group; $^{#}P < 0.05$ *vs.* FGF21KO Ctrl group; $^{&}P < 0.05$ *vs.* WT DM group. Ctrl: control; DM: diabetes mellitus; WT: wild-type; FGF21KO: FGF21 knockout; m: month(s).

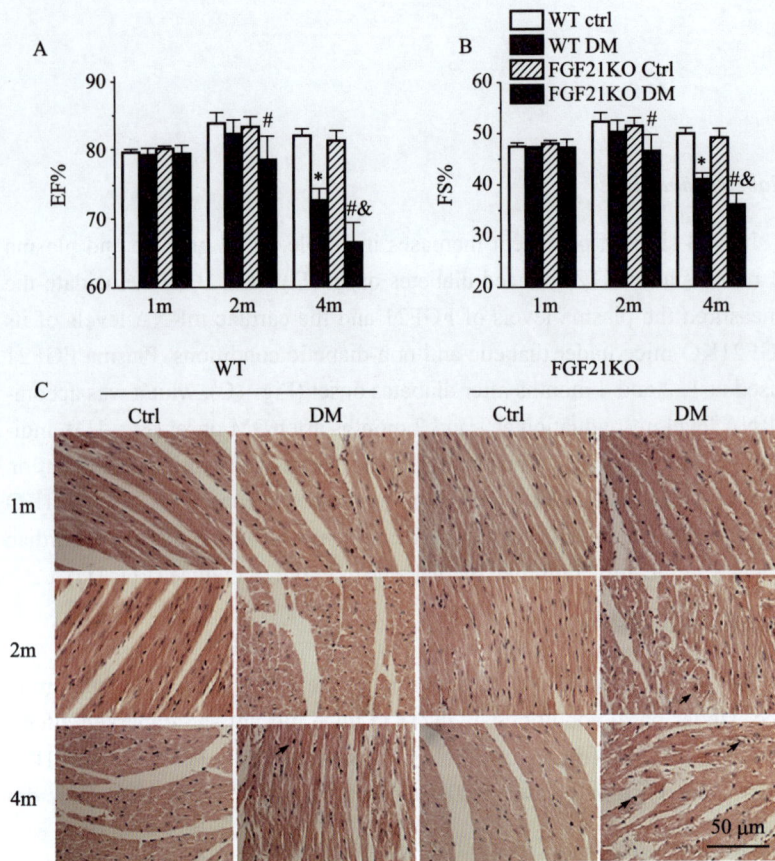

Fig. 2. FGF21 deletion-aggravated diabetes-induced cardiac dysfunction. At indicated time-points after diabetes onset, cardiac function was evaluated by transthoracic echocardiography and expressed as LV ejection fraction (EF%, A) and fraction shortening (FS%, B). Myocardial structural damage indicated by haematoxylin and eosin staining (C). Paraffin-embedded heart tissue was stained with haematoxylin and eosin and examined under light microscope. Arrows indicate cardiac cell death with karyorrhexis, pyknosis and/or karyolysis. Magnification = 400 ×. Data are presented as means ± SD ($n \geq 5$ for each group). $^{*}P < 0.05$ vs. WT Ctrl group; $^{\#}P < 0.05$ vs. FGF21KO Ctrl group; $^{\&}P < 0.05$ vs. WT DM group. The abbreviations are same as in Fig. 1.

not exhibit cardiac dysfunction until 4 months after diabetes, reflected by decreased ejection fraction and fraction shortening (Fig. 2). FGF21KO diabetic mice developed cardiac dysfunction at 2 months after diabetes onset; at 4 months, FGF21KO diabetic mice showed more severe cardiac functional impairment than WT diabetic mice (Fig. 2). Parameters of cardiac structure showed similar patterns of change (Table S1). At 4 months, WT diabetic mice showed decrease in diastolic and systolic LVPW and systolic LVID, and an increase in systolic LV volume compared to WT control mice, and FGF21KO diabetic mice showed decrease in systolic and diastolic IVS and LVPW, and an increase in diastolic LVID and systolic LVID. Moreover, FGF21KO diabetic mice had dramatically lower systolic IVS and diastolic and systolic LVPW, and higher systolic LVID and diastolic and systolic LV volume than WT diabetic mice (Table S1). These results demonstrate that the cardiac dysfunction developed in FGF21KO diabetic mice was earlier and more severe than that in WT diabetic mice, indicating that deletion of FGF21 aggravated the development of DCM.

Histological examination revealed severe pathological changes in the hearts of FGF21KO diabetic mice in comparison with that of FGF21KO control and WT diabetic mice. As shown in Fig. 2C, both FGF21KO and WT control hearts had regular and intact myocardial arrangements and clearly visible nuclei, and WT diabetic hearts showed certain irregularity of the myocardial fibres, especially at 4 months after diabetes onset, while FGF21KO diabetic hearts exhibited large areas of irregular myocardial arrangements, myofibrillar discontinuation and cell death (karyorrhexis, pyknosis and/or karyolysis).

Blood pressure was detected using a CODA™ mouse tail-cuff system, and no significant changes in systolic and diastolic pressure were observed in both WT and FGF21KO mice under diabetic and non-diabetic conditions (Fig. S2), which indicated that FGF21 deletion did not affect blood pressure under basal and experimental diabetic conditions. The above-mentioned diabetes-induced cardiac dysfunction was independent of blood pressure changes.

3.3 FGF21 deletion accelerated diabetes-induced cardiac remodelling

FGF21KO mice did not show marked cardiac fibrosis compared to WT mice under normal conditions, but diabetes-induced significant cardiac remodelling. Collagen accumulation (Fig. 3A) and expression of fibrotic mediator CTGF

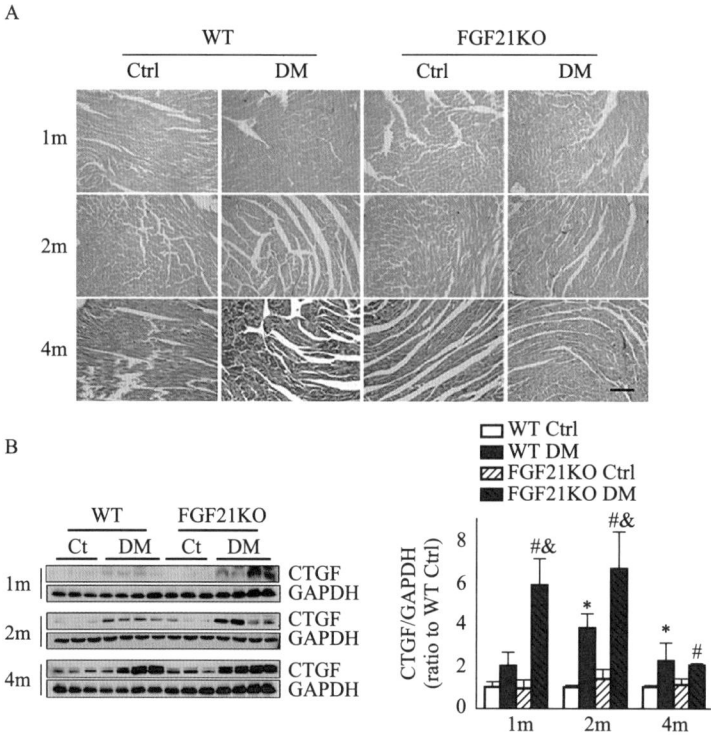

Fig. 3. FGF21 deletion accelerated diabetes-induced cardiac remodelling. At indicated time-points after diabetes onset, cardiac fibrosis was evaluated by Sirius Red staining of collagen accumulation (A) and Western blot of CTGF expression (B). Data are presented as means ± SD ($n \geqslant$ 5 for each group). *P < 0.05 vs. WT Ctrl group; #P < 0.05 vs. FGF21KO Ctrl group; &P < 0.05 vs. WT DM group; bar = 100 μm. The abbreviations are same as in Fig. 1.

(Fig. 3B) were significantly increased in the heart of WT diabetic mice from 2 months, and FGF21KO diabetic mice from 1 month after diabetes onset. The elevation of collagen accumulation and CTGF expression was higher in FGF21KO diabetic mice than that in WT diabetic mice at 2 months after diabetes (Fig. 3A, B), indicating that FGF21 deletion accelerated and aggravated diabetes-induced cardiac fibrotic remodelling.

3.4 FGF21 deletion-exacerbated diabetes-induced cardiac oxidative stress

Diabetic hyperglycaemia- and hyperlipidaemia-induced oxidative stress plays a critical role in the development of DCM [29]. Consequently, cardiac oxidative status was evaluated by the expression of 3-NT and 4-HNE as in our previous report [30]. The expression of 3-NT remained unchanged in FGF21KO mice under basal conditions, but was elevated under diabetic conditions (Fig. 4A). It was elevated only at 4 months in WT diabetic mice, but at both 2 and 4 months after diabetes onset in FGF21KO diabetic mice (Fig. 4A). Moreover, the 3-NT expression in FGF21KO diabetic mice was significantly higher than that of WT diabetic mice at 2 and 4 months after diabetes onset (Fig. 4A). The expression of 4-HNE showed similar change pattern with that of 3-NT, both FGF21KO and WT diabetic mice exhibited higher 4-HNE expression than their controls at 2 and 4 months after diabetes onset, but FGF21KO diabetic mice had higher 4-HNE

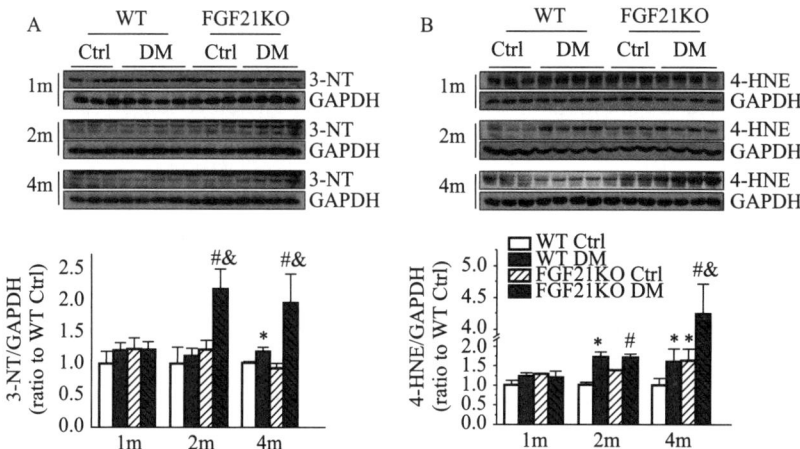

Fig. 4. FGF21 deletion-exacerbated diabetes-induced cardiac oxidative stress. At indicated time-points after diabetes onset, the markers of cardiac oxidative stress including 3-NT (A) and 4-HNE (B) were evaluated by Western blot. Data are presented as means ± SD ($n \geqslant$ 5 for each group). *P < 0.05 vs. WT Ctrl group; #P < 0.05 vs. FGF21KO Ctrl group; &P < 0.05 vs. WT DM group. The abbreviations are same as in Fig. 1.

250 ▶▶ Fibroblast Growth Factors, Second Edition

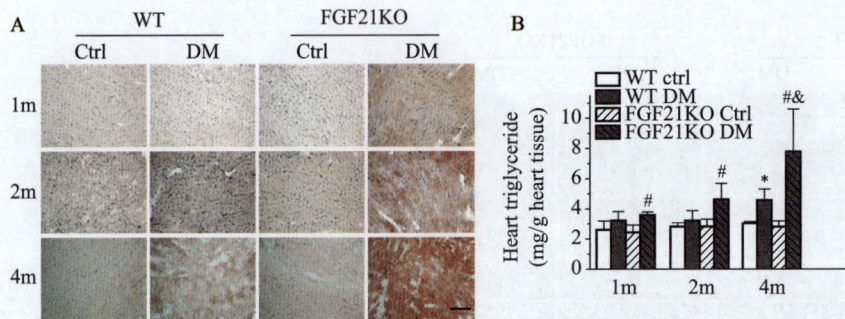

Fig. 5. FGF21 deletion-aggravated diabetes-induced cardiac lipid accumulation. At indicated time-points after diabetes onset, cardiac lipid accumulation was evaluated by Oil Red O staining (A) and triglyceride content (B). Data are presented as means ± SD ($n \geqslant 5$ for each group). $^*P < 0.05$ vs. WT Ctrl group; $^\#P < 0.05$ vs. FGF21KO Ctrl group; $^\&P < 0.05$ vs. WT DM group; bar = 100 μm. The abbreviations are same as in Fig. 1.

expression than WT diabetic mice at 4 months after diabetes onset (Fig. 4B).

3.5 FGF21 deletion-aggravated diabetes-induced cardiac lipid accumulation

Fibroblast growth factor 21 was identified as a potent metabolic regulator for lipid metabolism in several organs [6]. We therefore quantified cardiac lipid accumulation by Oil Red O staining (Fig. 5A) and triglyceride assay (Fig. 5B). No obvious cardiac lipid accumulation was observed in both WT and FGF21KO mice under basal conditions (Fig. 5A and B). Diabetes-induced significant cardiac lipid accumulation in WT mice only at 4 months, but in the FGF21KO mice starting from 1 month until 4 months after diabetes onset (Fig. 5A and B). Moreover, FGF21KO diabetic mice exhibited more severe cardiac lipid accumulation at 2 and 4 months after diabetes onset than WT diabetic mice (Fig. 5A and B). These results demonstrate that FGF21 deletion accelerated and exacerbated cardiac lipid accumulation under diabetic conditions.

3.6 FGF21 deletion accelerated diabetes-induced cardiac CD36 and Nrf2 up-regulation and PGC1α down-regulation

To uncover how FGF21 deletion affects cardiac lipid accumulation, the expression of CD36, a critical regulator of fatty acid transport [31], was detected by Western blot. FGF21 deletion had no obvious effects on cardiac CD36 expression under basal conditions, but diabetes significantly up-regulated CD36 expression in both WT and FGF21KO hearts (Fig. 6A). Cardiac CD36 expression was elevated from 2 months in WT diabetic mice and from 1 month in FGF21KO diabetic mice after diabetes onset. At 4 months after diabetes onset, cardiac CD36 expression in FGF21KO diabetic mice was significantly higher than that of WT diabetic mice (Fig. 6A). Reportedly, Nrf2-mediated CD36 up-regulation plays critical role in lipid metabolism in macrophage, aorta and liver tissues [32–34]. So, we detected cardiac Nrf2 expression by Western blot (Fig. 6B). We found that cardiac Nrf2 expression showed no difference between FGF21KO mice and WT mice under basal conditions (Fig. 6B). Under diabetic conditions, Nrf2 expression was slightly, but not significantly, elevated in WT mice; but progressively increased from 1 to 4 months after diabetes onset in FGF21KO mice (Fig. 6B). These results indicate that FGF21 deletion-exacerbated diabetes-induced cardiac Nrf2 and CD36 up-regulation.

PGC1α, an essential regulator of fatty acid oxidation [35], was also detected by Western blot. The cardiac PGC1α expression was not affected by FGF21 deletion under basal conditions, but was significantly attenuated by diabetes in FGF21KO diabetic mice at 4 months after diabetes onset (Fig. 6C). No significant changes of cardiac PGC1α expression were observed under either diabetic or non-diabetic conditions in WT mice (Fig. 6C). The elevation of Nrf2 and CD36, and decline of PGC1α expression imply that FGF21 deletion increased lipid uptake and decreased lipid oxidation leading to suboptimal cardiac lipid metabolism under diabetic conditions, which resulted in aggravated cardiac lipid accumulation in FGF21KO diabetic mice.

3.7 FGF21 deletion accelerated diabetes-induced cardiac glucose metabolism impairment

In addition to lipid, glucose metabolism is another important source of energy for heart contraction. Reportedly, FGF-21 is also a potent glucose metabolic regulator in several organs including the heart [6], and AMPK is a sensor of energy homoeostasis and a regulator of glucose uptake and fatty acid β-oxidation [36]. So, glucose metabolism in cardiac tissue was also investigated to evaluate the effect of FGF21 deletion. FGF21KO mice did not show marked alterations

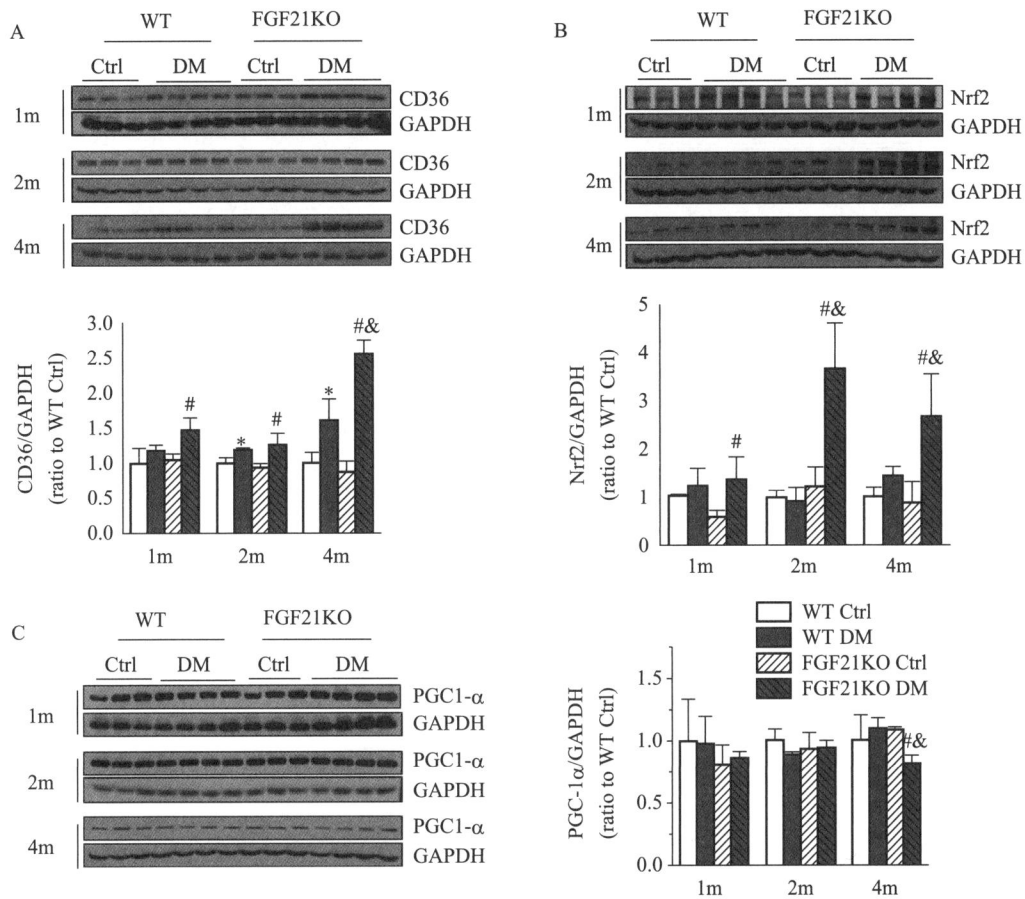

Fig. 6. FGF21 deletion accelerated diabetes-induced cardiac CD36 and Nrf2 up-regulation and PGC1α down-regulation. At indicated time-points after diabetes onset, the expression of CD36 (A), Nrf2 (B) and PGC1α (C) were detected by Western blot. Data are presented as means ± SD ($n \geq 5$ for each group). $^*P < 0.05$ vs. WT Ctrl group; $^\#P < 0.05$ vs. FGF21KO Ctrl group; $^\&P < 0.05$ vs. WT DM group. The abbreviations are same as in Fig. 1.

in phosphorylation of AMPK under basal conditions (Fig. 7A). Significant down-regulation of cardiac AMPK phosphorylation was observed from 2 months in WT diabetic mice, and from 1 month after diabetes onset in FGF21KO diabetic mice. Moreover, the cardiac AMPK phosphorylation in FGF21KO diabetic mice was significantly lower than that of WT diabetic mice at 1 and 4 months after diabetes onset (Fig. 7A). The expression of HKII, an enzyme that catalyses the first step of glycolysis by conversion of glucose to glucose-6-phosphate, was also detected. The cardiac HKII expression was not affected by FGF21 deletion under basal conditions, but was significantly impaired by diabetes in FGF21KO diabetic mice at 2 and 4 months after diabetes onset (Fig. 7B). No significant changes of cardiac HKII expression were observed under both diabetic and non-diabetic conditions in WT mice (Fig. 7B). These results indicate that FGF21 deletion-aggravated diabetes-induced impairment of cardiac glucose metabolism and cardiac energy metabolic balance in FGF21KO diabetic mice.

4. Discussion

Fibroblast growth factor 21 is a newly discovered metabolic hormone. In addition to its essential roles in regulating glucose and lipid metabolism through pleiotropic actions in liver and adipocyte tissues, FGF21 also plays critical role in cardiac pathogenesis. In this study, for the first time we established that FGF21 deletion is susceptible to develop DCM in STZ-induced type 1 diabetic mice, which is predominantly attributed to the exacerbated cardiac lipid accumulation *via* Nrf2 up-regulation of CD36-mediated cardiac fatty acid accumulation.

In STZ-induced type 1 diabetes in this study, circulating FGF21 reduced from 1 month to the experimental termi-

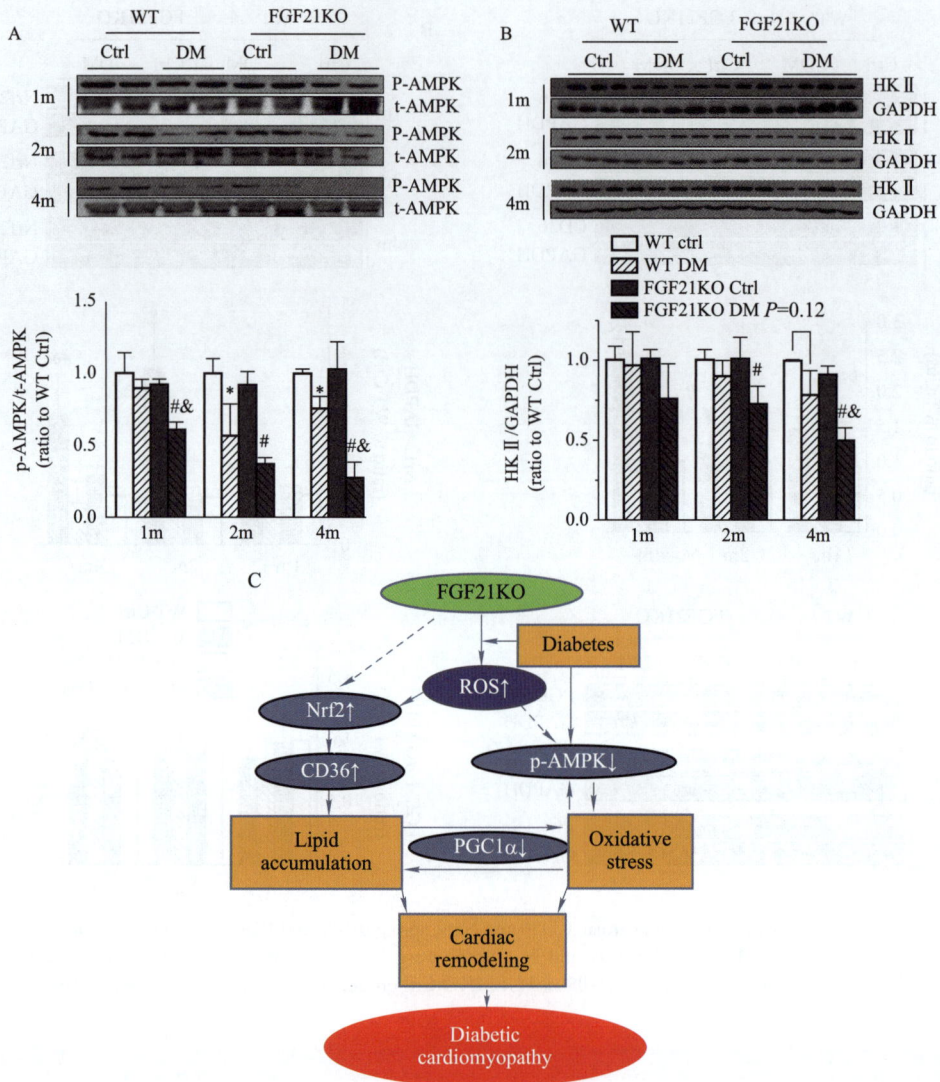

Fig. 7. FGF21 deletion accelerated diabetes-induced cardiac glucose metabolism impairment. At indicated time-points after diabetes onset, cardiac AMPK phosphorylation (A) and HKII expression (B) were detected by Western blot. Data are presented as means ± SD ($n \geq 5$ for each group). [*]$P < 0.05$ *vs.* WT Ctrl group; [#]$P < 0.05$ *vs.* FGF21KO Ctrl group; [&]$P < 0.05$ *vs.* WTDM group. The proposed mechanism of FGF21 deletion leading to aggravated DCM is schematically described (C): FGF21 deletion aggravates the ROS accumulation induced by diabetes, which in turn increases Nrf2 expression. Nrf2 up-regulation elevates CD36 expression, and induces fatty acid over-uptake and cardiac lipid accumulation. In addition, FGF21 deletion-mediated diabetic ROS accumulation attenuates the phosphorylation of AMPK, which leads to impairment of cardiac glucose metabolism and cardiac energy metabolic balance and further aggravates cardiac oxidative stress. The elevated cardiac lipid accumulation and oxidative stress synergistically down-regulate PGC1α function and induce cardiac remodelling, and eventually accelerate the development of DCM.

nation at 4 months after diabetes onset (Fig. 1C), which was consistent with a previous report that serum FGF21 levels were significantly lower in type 1 diabetic patients than that of control subjects [37]. It was also found that decreased FGF21 levels were accompanied by significant cardiac dysfunction, remodelling and oxidative stress at 4 months after diabetes onset in WT diabetic mice, while FGF21 complete deletion significantly accelerated and aggravated the above-mentioned cardiac structural, functional and oxidative stress changes in FGF21KO diabetic mice (Figs. 2–4 and Table S1), which indicate that FGF21 plays a critical role in protecting the heart against the development of DCM under experimental type 1 diabetic conditions.

Since diabetic down-regulation of plasma FGF21 levels (Fig. 1C) was accompanied by an obvious trend of compensatory up-regulation of cardiac FGFR1 mRNA levels in WT mice (Fig. 1D), while the deletion of FGF21 was also accompanied by a slight compensatory up-regulation of cardiac FGFR1 mRNA levels under basal conditions, which was significantly amplified under diabetic condition in FGF21KO mice (Fig. 1D). These results imply that the exacerbation of DCM by the *fgf21* gene deletion might directly attribute to the dysfunction of FGF21/FGFR1 axis.

Fibroblast growth factor 21 was reported to have anti-hyperglycemic and anti-hyperlipidemic properties in diabetic rodent [13] and monkey [14] models, and hyperglycaemia and hyperlipidaemia were thought to be the major contributors to DCM [2]. Thus, we assumed that FGF21 deletion might further elevate plasma glucose and triglyceride levels, contributing to the accelerated and aggravated development of DCM in FGF21KO diabetic mice. Unexpectedly, both FGF21KO and WT diabetic mice have typically diabetic hyperglycaemia and hyperlipidaemia, no significant differences were observed in plasma glucose (Fig. 1A) and triglyceride (Fig. 1B) levels between FGF21KO and WT diabetic mice. This implies that the dramatic diabetes-induced down-regulation of plasma FGF21 levels in WT type 1 diabetic mice (Fig. 1C) were comparable to FGF21 deletion in FGF21KO diabetic mice with respect to the whole body glucose and lipid metabolic regulation by FGF21. The elevated serum FGF21 was reported to associate with hypertension [38]. But in the present study, FGF21KO mice did not exhibit alteration in blood pressure under either basal or diabetic conditions (Fig. S2).

Cardiac lipid accumulation plays a causative role in the development of DCM [39]. FGF21 was also reported to regulate lipid homoeostasis in liver [40], adipose tissue [41] and kidney [27]. In the present study, we observed that FGF21 deletion significantly aggravated cardiac lipid accumulation (Fig. 5), which was time-dependently associated with diabetes-accelerated cardiac dysfunction (Fig. 2) and remodelling (Fig. 3) in FGF21KO diabetic mice, indicating that FGF21 plays a critical role in cardiac protection from the development of DCM by regulation of cardiac lipid metabolism under type 1 diabetic conditions.

CD36 is a pivotal lipid transport protein that mediates fatty acid transport and utilization in the heart [42]. CD36 is believed to play a critical role in intramyocardial lipid accumulation, fatty acid and glucose oxidation and in the subsequent deterioration in cardiac ATP supply in age-induced cardiomyopathy in mice [43]. Under physiological conditions, increased cardiac CD36 expression can compensate for the decreased supply of long-chain fatty acid [44]; but under diabetic conditions, the elevated cardiac CD36 expression mediates excess uptake of fatty acid leading to cardiac lipid accumulation [31]. In the present study, cardiac CD36 expression was further up-regulated in FGF21KO diabetic mice (Fig. 6A), which was time-dependently associated with excess cardiac lipid accumulation (Fig. 5A, B). Meanwhile, cardiac AMPK phosphorylation (Fig. 7A), an indicator of energy homoeostasis, and HKII expression (Fig. 7B), an indicator of glucose utilization, were also time-dependently further decreased in FGF21KO diabetic mice. Moreover, PGC1α, a critical regulator of fatty acid β-oxidation and a key mediator of FGF21 regulation of lipid metabolism [45] was significantly decreased only in the heart of FGF21KO diabetic mice at the late stage of DCM (Fig. 6C). These results imply that FGF21 deletion-induced excess cardiac lipid uptake and lipid accumulation might impair cardiac lipid and glucose utilization and energetic balance, which further exacerbated lipid accumulation and impaired lipid β-oxidation, contributing to the accelerated DCM in FGF21KO diabetic mice.

CD36 expression was strictly regulated in the heart tissue [46]. Accumulating evidence indicate that Nrf2 up-regulation of CD36-mediated lipid uptake and excess accumulation in macrophages and smooth muscle cells play critical roles in the development of atherosclerosis [32–34]. Consistent with these previous studies, cardiac Nrf2 expression was also found to be largely elevated in FGF21KO diabetic mice, but not in WT diabetic mice (Fig. 6B), which were time-dependently associated with the up-regulation of cardiac CD36 expression (Fig. 6A) and cardiac lipid accumulation (Fig. 5A, B) in the present study. Even though there was one report that has identified Nrf2 as a novel regulator repressing FGF21 expression in liver and adipose tissue under long-term high-fat diet-induced obese conditions [47], further study to dissect the mechanism of FGF21 deletion-mediated up-regulation of cardiac Nrf2-driven CD36 expression and lipid accumulation under type 1 diabetic conditions is warranted.

Among diabetic patients, 90%–95% suffer from type 2 diabetes [48, 49]. A limitation of the present study is the lack of the relevance to type 2 diabetes. It has been generally accepted that DCM has similar pathological mechanisms in both type 1 and type 2 diabetes [50], but FGF21 has been demonstrated to have different changing patterns of serum level increase in type 2 diabetes and decrease in type 1 diabetes [37]. To ensure a greater clinical relevance, whether FGF21 plays a similar role in the development of DCM in type 1 and type 2 diabetes really needs to be comparatively studied in the future.

In conclusion, FGF21 deletion up-regulation of Nrf2-driven CD36 expression exacerbates cardiac lipid uptake and accumulation, which in turn impairs cardiac lipid and glucose utilization and cardiac energy balance, and aggravates cardiac oxidative stress, eventually accelerating the development of DCM (Fig. 7C). FGF21 deletion-aggravated DCM indicates that FGF21 may be a therapeutic target for the treatment of diabetic cardiovascular complications.

Supporting imformation

Additional supporting information may be found in the online version of this article (doi:10.1111/jcmm.12530).

References

[1] Rubler S, Yuceoglu YZ, Kumral T, et al. New type of cardiomyopathy associated with diabetic glomerulosclerosis[J]. American Journal of Cardiology, 1972, 30(6): 595-602.

[2] Boudina S, Abel ED. Diabetic cardiomyopathy revisited[J]. Circulation, 2007, 115(25): 3213-3223.

[3] Taegtmeyer H, McNulty P, Young ME. Adaptation and maladaptation of the heart in diabetes: Part I General concepts[J]. Circulation, 2002, 105(14): 1727-1733.

[4] McGavock JM, Victor RG, Unger RH, et al. Adiposity of the heart*, revisited[J]. Annals of Internal Medicine, 2006, 144(7): 517-524.

[5] Nishimura T, Nakatake Y, Konishi M, et al. Identification of a novel FGF, FGF-21, preferentially expressed in the liver[J]. Biochimica et Biophysica Acta-Gene Structure and Expression, 2000, 1492(1): 203-206.

[6] Adams AC, Kharitonenkov A. FGF21: The center of a transcriptional nexus in metabolic regulation[J]. Current Diabetes Reviews, 2012, 8(4): 285-293.

[7] Tacer KF, Bookout AL, Ding X, et al. Research resource: Comprehensive expression atlas of the fibroblast growth factor system in adult mouse[J]. Molecular Endocrinology, 2010, 24(10): 2050-2064.

[8] Muise ES, Azzolina B, Kuo DW, et al. Adipose fibroblast growth factor 21 is up-regulated by peroxisome proliferator-activated receptor gamma and altered metabolic states[J]. Molecular Pharmacology, 2008, 74(2): 403-412.

[9] Hondares E, Iglesias R, Giralt A, et al. Thermogenic activation induces FGF21 expression and release in brown adipose tissue[J]. Journal of Biological Chemistry, 2011, 286(15): 12983-12990.

[10] Kim KH, Jeong YT, Oh H, et al. Autophagy deficiency leads to protection from obesity and insulin resistance by inducing FGF21 as a mitokine[J]. Nature Medicine, 2013, 19(1): 83-92.

[11] Iglesias P, Selgas R, Romero S, et al. Biological role, clinical significance, and therapeutic possibilities of the recently discovered metabolic hormone fibroblastic growth factor 21[J]. European Journal of Endocrinology, 2012, 167(3): 301-309.

[12] Fisher FM, Kleiner S, Douris N, et al. FGF21 regulates PGC-1 alpha and browning of white adipose tissues in adaptive thermogenesis[J]. Genes & Development, 2012, 26(3): 271-281.

[13] Kharitonenkov A, Shiyanova TL, Koester A, et al. FGF-21 as a novel metabolic regulator[J]. Journal of Clinical Investigation, 2005, 115(6): 1627-1635.

[14] Kharitonenkov A, Wroblewski VJ, Koester A, et al. The metabolic state of diabetic monkeys is regulated by fibroblast growth factor-21[J]. Endocrinology, 2007, 148(2): 774-781.

[15] Hotta Y, Nakamura H, Konishi M, et al. Fibroblast growth factor 21 regulates lipolysis in white adipose tissue but is not required for ketogenesis and triglyceride clearance in liver[J]. Endocrinology, 2009, 150(10): 4625-4633.

[16] Lin Z, Tian H, Lam KSL, et al. Adiponectin mediates the metabolic effects of FGF21 on glucose homeostasis and insulin sensitivity in mice[J]. Cell Metabolism, 2013, 17(5): 779-789.

[17] Zhao Y, Dunbar JD, Kharitonenkov A. FGF21 As a therapeutic reagent[A]. In: Endocrine FGFs and Klothos (KuroO M, ed), Vol.

728, 2012: 214-228.

[18] Sarruf DA, Thaler JP, Morton GJ, et al. Fibroblast growth factor 21 action in the brain increases energy expenditure and insulin sensitivity in obese rats[J]. Diabetes, 2010, 59(7): 1817-1824.

[19] Berglund ED, Li CY, Bina HA, et al. Fibroblast growth factor 21 controls glycemia via regulation of hepatic glucose flux and insulin sensitivity[J]. Endocrinology, 2009, 150(9): 4084-4093.

[20] Mraz M, Bartlova M, Lacinova Z, et al. Serum concentrations and tissue expression of a novel endocrine regulator fibroblast growth factor-21 in patients with type 2 diabetes and obesity[J]. Clinical Endocrinology, 2009, 71(3): 369-375.

[21] Suzuki M, Uehara Y, Motomura-Matsuzaka K, et al. beta Klotho is required for fibroblast growth factor (FGF) 21 signaling through FGF receptor (FGFR) 1c and FGFR3c[J]. Molecular Endocrinology, 2008, 22(4): 1006-1014.

[22] Kurosu H, Choi M, Ogawa Y, et al. Tissue-specific expression of beta Klotho and fibroblast growth factor (FGF) receptor Isoforms determines metabolic activity of FGF19 and FGF21[J]. Journal of Biological Chemistry, 2007, 282(37): 26687-26695.

[23] Liu SQ, Roberts D, Kharitonenkov A, et al. Endocrine protection of ischemic myocardium by FGF21 from the liver and adipose tissue[J]. Scientific Reports, 2013, 3.

[24] Planavila A, Redondo I, Hondares E, et al. Fibroblast growth factor 21 protects against cardiac hypertrophy in mice[J]. Nature Communications, 2013, 4.

[25] Zhou G, Li X, Hein DW, et al. Metallothionein suppresses angiotensin II-Induced nicotinamide adenine dinucleotide phosphate oxidase activation, nitrosative stress, apoptosis, and pathological remodeling in the diabetic heart[J]. Journal of the American College of Cardiology, 2008, 52(8): 655-666.

[26] Tan Y, Li Y, Xiao J, et al. A novel CXCR4 antagonist derived from human SDF-1 beta enhances angiogenesis in ischaemic mice[J]. Cardiovascular Research, 2009, 82(3): 513-521.

[27] Zhang C, Shao M, Yang H, et al. Attenuation of hyperlipidemia- and diabetes-induced early-stage apoptosis and late-stage renal dysfunction via administration of fibroblast growth factor-21 is associated with suppression of renal inflammation[J]. Plos One, 2013, 8(12).

[28] Miao X, Wang Y, Sun J, et al. Zinc protects against diabetes-induced pathogenic changes in the aorta: roles of metallothionein and nuclear factor (erythroid-derived 2)-like 2[J]. Cardiovascular Diabetology, 2013, 12.

[29] Tan Y, Ichikawa T, Li J, et al. Diabetic downregulation of Nrf2 activity via ERK contributes to oxidative stress-induced insulin resistance in cardiac cells in vitro and in vivo[J]. Diabetes, 2011, 60(2): 625-633.

[30] Bai Y, Cui W, Xin Y, et al. Prevention by sulforaphane of diabetic cardiomyopathy is associated with up-regulation of Nrf2 expression and transcription activation[J]. Journal of Molecular and Cellular Cardiology, 2013, 57: 82-95.

[31] Greenwalt DE, Scheck SH, Rhinehartjones T. Heart CD36 expression is increased in murine models of diabetes and in mice fed

a high-fat diet[J]. Journal of Clinical Investigation, 1995, 96(3): 1382-1388.

[32] Bozaykut P, Karademir B, Yazgan B, et al. Effects of vitamin E on peroxisome proliferator-activated receptor gamma and nuclear factor-erythroid 2-related factor 2 in hypercholesterolemia-induced atherosclerosis[J]. Free Radical Biology and Medicine, 2014, 70: 174-181.

[33] Ishii T, Itoh K, Ruiz E, et al. Role of Nrf2 in the regulation of CD36 and stress protein expression in murine macrophages - Activation by oxidatively modified LDL and 4-hydroxynonenal[J]. Circulation Research, 2004, 94(5): 609-616.

[34] More VR, Xu J, Shimpi PC, et al. Keap1 knockdown increases markers of metabolic syndrome after long-term high fat diet feeding[J]. Free Radical Biology and Medicine, 2013, 61: 85-94.

[35] Wang Y, Feng W, Xue W, et al. Inactivation of GSK-3 beta by metallothionein prevents diabetes-related changes in cardiac energy metabolism, inflammation, nitrosative damage, and remodeling[J]. Diabetes, 2009, 58(6): 1391-1402.

[36] Hardie DG, Ross FA, Hawley SA. AMPK: a nutrient and energy sensor that maintains energy homeostasis[J]. Nature Reviews Molecular Cell Biology, 2012, 13(4): 251-262.

[37] Xiao Y, Xu A, Law LSC, et al. Distinct changes in serum fibroblast growth factor 21 levels in different subtypes of diabetes[J]. Journal of Clinical Endocrinology & Metabolism, 2012, 97(1): E54-E58.

[38] Semba RD, Crasto C, Strait J, et al. Elevated serum fibroblast growth factor 21 is associated with hypertension in community-dwelling adults[J]. Journal of Human Hypertension, 2013, 27(6): 397-399.

[39] Goldberg IJ, Trent CM, Schulze PC. Lipid metabolism and toxicity in the heart[J]. Cell Metabolism, 2012, 15(6): 805-812.

[40] Badman MK, Pissios P, Kennedy AR, et al. Hepatic fibroblast growth factor 21 is regulated by PPAR alpha and is a key mediator of hepatic lipid metabolism in ketotic states[J]. Cell Metabolism, 2007, 5(6): 426-437.

[41] Muise ES, Souza S, Chi A, et al. Downstream signaling pathways in mouse adipose tissues following acute in vivo administration of fibroblast growth factor 21[J]. Plos One, 2013, 8(9).

[42] Koonen DPY, Glatz JFC, Bonen A, et al. Long-chain fatty acid uptake and FAT/CD36 translocation in heart and skeletal muscle[J]. Biochimica Et Biophysica Acta-Molecular and Cell Biology of Lipids, 2005, 1736(3): 163-180.

[43] Koonen DPY, Febbraio M, Bonnet S, et al. CD36 expression contributes to age-induced cardiomyopathy in mice[J]. Circulation, 2007, 116(19): 2139-2147.

[44] Luiken J, Coort SLM, Koonen DPY, et al. Regulation of cardiac long-chain fatty acid and glucose uptake by translocation of substrate transporters[J]. Pflugers Archiv-European Journal of Physiology, 2004, 448(1): 1-15.

[45] Potthoff MJ, Inagaki T, Satapati S, et al. FGF21 induces PGC-1 alpha and regulates carbohydrate and fatty acid metabolism during the adaptive starvation response[J]. Proceedings of the National Academy of Sciences of the United States of America, 2009, 106(26): 10853-10858.

[46] Chen M, Yang Y-K, Loux TJ, et al. The role of hyperglycemia in FAT/CD36 expression and function[J]. Pediatric Surgery International, 2006, 22(8): 647-654.

[47] Chartoumpekis DV, Ziros PG, Psyrogiannis AI, et al. Nrf2 represses FGF21 during long-term high-fat diet-induced obesity in mice[J]. Diabetes, 2011, 60(10): 2465-2473.

[48] Georgescu A. Vascular dysfunction in diabetes: The endothelial progenitor cells as new therapeutic strategy[J]. World Journal of Diabetes, 2011, 2(6): 92-97.

[49] Yan J, Tie G, Park B, et al. Recovery from hind limb ischemia is less effective in type 2 than in type 1 diabetic mice: Roles of endothelial nitric oxide synthase and endothelial progenitor cells[J]. Journal of Vascular Surgery, 2009, 50(6): 1412-1422.

[50] Bugger H, Abel ED. Rodent models of diabetic cardiomyopathy[J]. Disease Models & Mechanisms, 2009, 2(9-10): 454-466.

Fibroblast growth factor 21 prevents atherosclerosis by suppression of hepatic sterol regulatory element-binding protein-2 and induction of adiponectin in mice

Zhuofeng Lin, Xiaokun Li, Aimin Xu

Fibroblast growth factor (FGF) 21 is a member of the endocrine FGF subfamily that is produced predominantly in the liver[1]. Physiologically, FGF21 plays a key role in mediating the metabolic responses to fasting/starvation by enhancing fatty acid oxidation and ketogenesis and inducing growth hormone resistance.[2,3]. Pharmacologically, therapeutic intervention with recombinant FGF21 has been shown to counteract obesity and its related metabolic disorders in both rodents and nonhuman primates, including reduction of adiposity and amelioration of hyperglycemia, hyperinsulinemia, insulin resistance, dyslipidemia, and fatty liver disease[4,5]. Furthermore, FGF21 is the downstream target of both peroxisome proliferator-activated receptor (PPAR) α and PPARγ, and a growing body of evidence suggest that the glucose-lowering and insulin-sensitizing effects of the PPARγ agonists (thiazolidinediones)and the therapeutic benefits of the PPARα agonists (fenofibrates) on lipid profiles are mediated in part by induction of FGF21[6].

FGF21 exerts its metabolic actions by binding to the complex receptor between the FGF receptor (FGFR) and β-klotho, a single transmembrane protein that is highly expressed in adipose tissue, liver, pancreas, and hypothalamus[4,7,8]. Adipocytes are the primary target of FGF21, where it increases glucose uptake, modulates lipolysis[9], enhances mitochondrial oxidative capacity, enhances PPARγ activity[10], and promotes browning of white adipose tissue[11]. Furthermore, therapeutic administration of FGF21 has been shown to increase the production of adiponectin[12,13], an adipocyte-secreted hormone with insulin-sensitizing, anti-inflammatory, and vascular protective activity. Adiponectin knockout mice are resistant to the effects of FGF21 on alleviation of insulin resistance, hyper glycemia, dyslipidemia, and fatty liver disease associated with dietary or genetic obesity[12], suggesting that adiponectin acts as an obligatory downstream mediator of FGF21 on energy metabolism and insulin sensitivity. In addition, FGF21 has also been shown to exert its direct actions on the pancreas, hypothalamus, heart, and liver[14-18], acting as a mediator to coordinate the multiorganic crosstalk under various patho physiological conditions.

Although the metabolic functions of FGF21 are well characterized, little is known about its pathophysiological roles in atherosclerosis, a chronic inflammatory disease intimately associated with metabolic syndrome. A number of clinical studies have observed an increased circulating level of FGF21 in patients with atherosclerosis or those individuals who are at high risk of developing this disease[19,20]. In both rhesus monkeys and humans with obesity and diabetes mellitus, chronic administration of FGF21 decreases low-density lipoprotein (LDL) cholesterol and increases high-density lipoprotein cholesterol[5,21,22]. However, whether such a beneficial effect of FGF21 on lipid profiles is sufficient to render a protection against atherosclerotic diseases has not been explored. To address this issue, we investigated the impact of both FGF21 deficiency and replenishment on the pathogenesis of atherosclerosis in apolipoprotein (apo) E$^{-/-}$ mice. Our results showed a markedly aggravated atherosclerotic phenotype of FGF21 knockout mice, which can be reversed by replenishment of FGF21. Therefore, we further investigated the mechanisms whereby FGF21 protects atherosclerosis via its multiple actions in both adipose tissue and liver.

1. Methods

Additional details of mice and experimental procedures are included in the online-only Data Supplement. All of the animal studies were approved by the animal research ethics committees of Wenzhou Medical University and the University of Hong Kong.

Statistical analysis was performed using either the Mann-Whitney U test or the Kruskal-Wallis test when more than 2 experimental conditions were compared. When the global Kruskal-Wallis test was significant, pairwise comparisons were performed with the Dunn-Sidak procedure for multiple corrections. Repeated-measure ANOVA was used to compare circulating FGF21 levels between wild-type and apoE$^{-/-}$ mice at different time points, as well as serum levels of FGF21 and adiponectin in FGF21 and apoE$^{-/-}$ double deficiency (DKO) mice at different time points after administration with FGF21 or adiponectin. The survival of mice was compared using Kaplan-Meier survival analysis with a log-rank test. All of the statistical analyses were performed with IBM SPSS version 20.0 (IBM Corporation, Armonk, NY). A value of $P<0.05$ was considered statistically significant.

2. Results

2.1 FGF21 deficiency accelerates atherosclerotic plaque formation in ApoE$^{-/-}$ mice

Several clinical studies have observed a significantly elevated serum level of FGF21 in patients with atherosclerosis[19,20]. Consistently, both circulating levels of FGF21 and its hepatic mRNA expression were progressively elevated in apoE$^{-/-}$ mice with spontaneous development of hypercholesterolemia and atherosclerosis (Fig. I in the online-only Data Supplement). To explore the pathophysiological roles of FGF21 in atherosclerosis, we generated DKO mice by backcrossing FGF21 knockout mice into apoE$^{-/-}$ mice in C57BL/J background for more than 10 generations. DKO mice were confirmed by both polymerase chain reaction analysis and Western blot analysis of the liver tissue (Fig. II in the online-only Data Supplement). There were no obvious differences in food intake and body weight between apoE$^{-/-}$ mice and DKO mice on standard chow (Fig. IIIA in the online-only Data Supplement). However, the atherosclerotic lesion area in DKO, as determined by oil red O staining of the entire aorta, was 1.6-fold and 1.8-fold greater at 24 weeks and 52 weeks than age- and sex-matched apoE$^{-/-}$ mice ($P<0.01$; Fig. 1A). Additional histological evaluation showed that the plaque areas in the aortic sinus and brachiocephalic artery of 24-week-old DKO mice were 2.1-fold and 2.9-fold greater than in apoE$^{-/-}$ mice (Fig. 1B, 1C). Likewise, both macrophage infiltration and smooth muscle proliferation in the atherosclerotic lesion area of the aortic sinus in DKO mice were significantly higher than in apoE$^{-/-}$ mice (Fig. 1D, E). Cholesterol ester contents extracted from the brachiocephalic artery of DKO mice were also much higher than those in apoE$^{-/-}$ mice (Fig. 1F), suggesting that FGF21 deficiency renders apoE$^{-/-}$ mice more susceptible to atherosclerosis.

To investigate whether accelerated atherosclerosis in DKO mice decreases longevity, we monitored DKO ($n=20$) and apoE$^{-/-}$ mice ($n=20$) on standard chow for 18 months. The surviving rate of DKO was decreased to ~45%, which was significantly lower than that in apoE$^{-/-}$ mice (80%; Fig. 1G).

2.2 DKO mice display exacerbated hyperlipidemia and augmented inflammation

Because FGF21 is an important metabolic regulator, we next investigated whether the atherosclerosis-prone phenotype of DKO mice is attributed to impaired glucose or lipid metabolism. Glucose and insulin levels were comparable between DKO and apoE$^{-/-}$ mice (Fig. IIIB in the online-only Data Supplement). A glucose tolerance test showed a similar glucose excursion in response to intraperitoneal glucose challenge (Fig. IIIC and IIID in the online-only Data Supplement). On the other hand, DKO mice exhibited a 1.5-fold and 2.1-fold increase in plasma levels of total triglyceride and cholesterol, respectively (Fig. 2A, B). Additional analysis of lipoprotein compositions demonstrated a significantly increased LDL and very LDL but decreased high-density lipoprotein levels in DKO mice as compared with apoE$^{-/-}$ controls (Fig. 2C–2E).

Quantitative real-time polymerase chain reaction analysis demonstrated a significantly increased expression of the adhesion molecules intercellular adhesion molecule-1 and vascular cell adhesion protein-1 and the proinflammatory cytokines monocyte chemotactic protein-1 and tumor necrosis factor-α in aortic tissues of DKO mice as compared with apoE$^{-/-}$ mice (Fig. 2F). Likewise, the circulating levels of these proinflammatory chemokines and cytokines in DKO mice were much higher than those in apoE$^{-/-}$ mice (Fig. 2G–J), suggesting that FGF21 deficiency exacerbates both local inflammation in atherosclerotic lesions and systemic inflammation.

Similar to the above findings in chow-fed mice, high-fat, high-cholesterol-induced atherosclerotic plaque formation, hypertriglyceridemia, hypercholesterolemia, and production of the proinflammatory cytokines were significantly

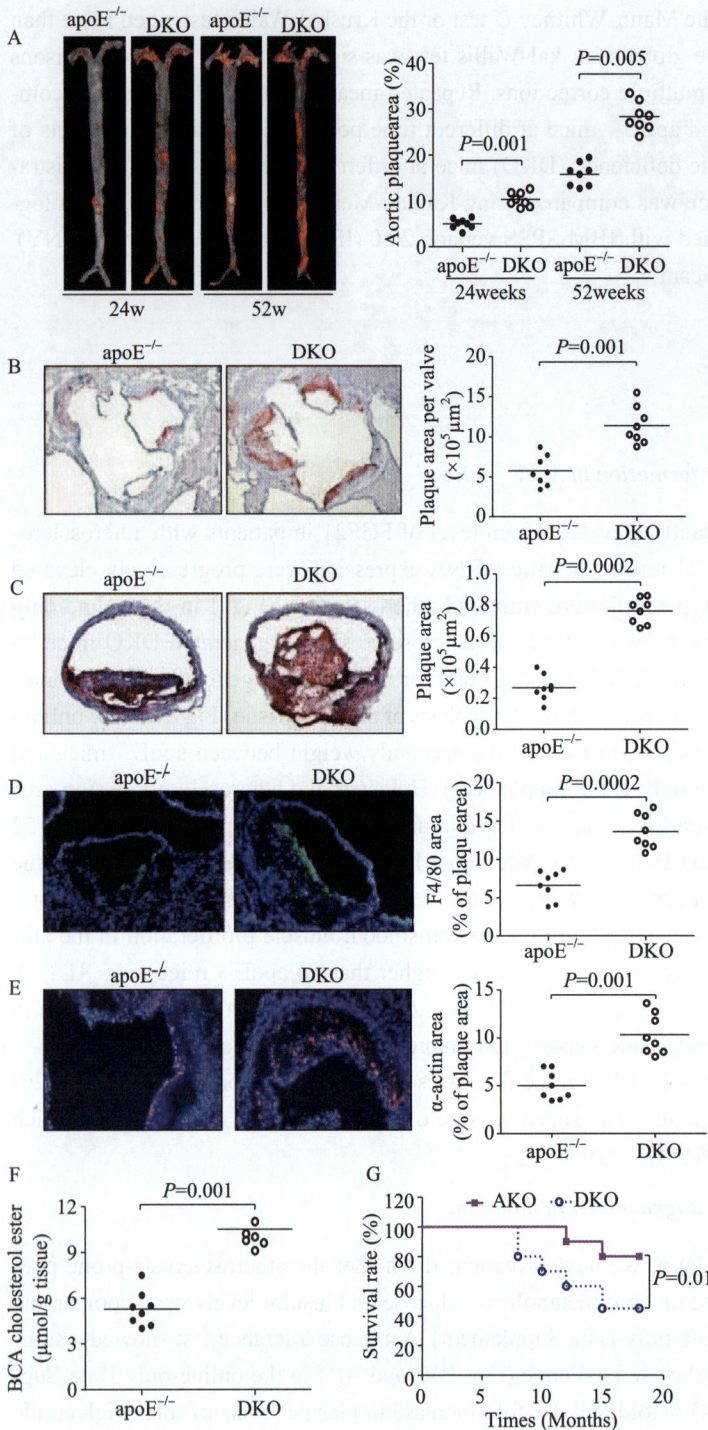

Fig. 1. Apolipoprotein (apo) E$^{-/-}$ mice with fibroblast growth factor (FGF) 21 deficiency exhibit exacerbated atherosclerosis and premature death. Aortas were dissected from 24- and 52-week-old apoE$^{-/-}$ mice and apoE$^{-/-}$FGF21$^{-/-}$ (DKO) mice. n=8 in each group. (A) *En face* staining of entire aortas of 24-week-old mice with oil red O. (B) and (C), Cross-sections of aortic sinuses and brachiocephalic arteries of 24-week-old mice, respectively. (D) and (E), Macrophage infiltration and smooth muscle proliferation in aortic sinus as determined by immunostaining for F4/80 and α-actin, respectively. (F) Cholesterol ester levels in brachiocephalic arteries (BCA) of 24-week-old mice. (G) The surviving rate of apoE$^{-/-}$ mice (n=20) and DKO mice (n=20) on standard chow was monitored for 18 months. Data are presented as dot plots with the line indicating the median. The Mann-Whitney U test was used for 2-group comparisons (A–F); the survivals of mice were compared using Kaplan-Meier survival analysis with the log-rank test (G).

exacerbated in DKO mice as compared with apoE$^{-/-}$ mice (Fig. IV in the online-only Data Supplement), suggesting that FGF21 is also an important protector against Western diet-induced dyslipidemia and atherosclerosis in mice.

2.3 FGF21 exerts its antiatherosclerotic effects via both adiponectin-dependent and -independent mechanisms

Adipocytes are the primary target of FGF21, where it induces FGF21 are mediated by adiponectin[12,13], we next investigated whether FGF21 exerts its antiatherosclerotic activities *via* induction of adiponectin. As expected, both circulating levels of adiponectin and its mRNA expression in different adipose depots, including epididymal, subcutaneous, perivascular, and perirenal adipose tissues, were significantly reduced in DKO mice as compared with apoE$^{-/-}$ mice

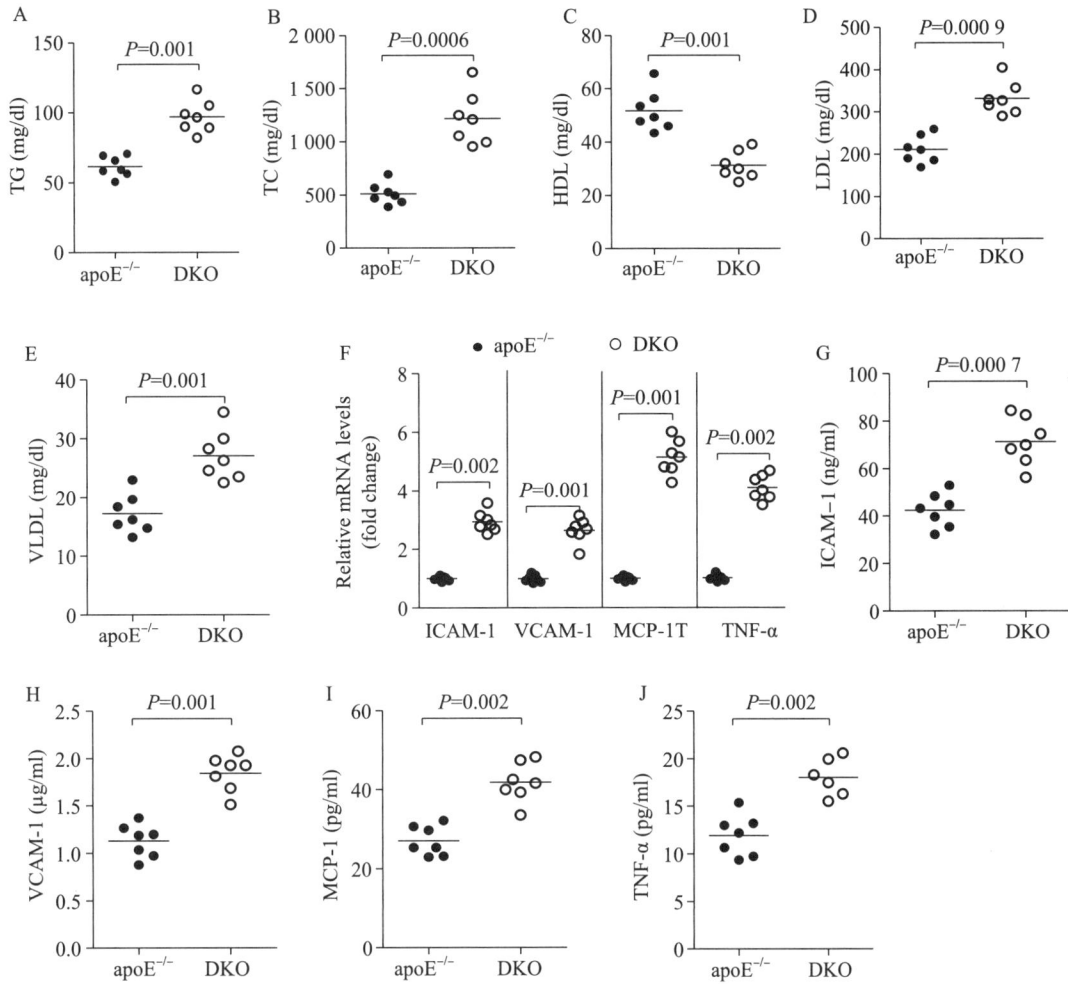

Fig. 2. Fibroblast growth factor (FGF) 21 deficiency worsens lipid profiles and exacerbates inflammation in apolipoprotein (apo) E$^{-/-}$ mice. ApoE$^{-/-}$FGF21$^{-/-}$ (DKO) and apoE$^{-/-}$ mice fed with standard chow were euthanized at 24 weeks after birth. Plasma samples were collected for measurement of triglycerides (TG; A), totalcholesterol (TC; B), high-density lipoprotein (HDL; C), low-density lipoprotein (LDL; D), and very LDL (VLDL; E). (F) The mRNA expression of intercellular adhesion molecule-1 (ICAM-1) vascular cell adhesion protein-1 (VCAM-1), tumor necrosis factor-α (TNFα), and monocyte chemotactic and cytokines, were measured with real-time polymerase chain reaction and ELISA, respectively. n=6 to 7. Data are presented as dot plots with the line indicating the median. The Mann-Whitney U test was used for comparison of 2 groups.

(Fig. 3A, B). Daily administration of recombinant mouse FGF21 (rmFGF21) for a period of 16 weeks led to higher circulating levels of adiponectin in DKO mice (Fig. VA and VB in the online-only Data Supplement), which was accompanied by a significant reduction of atherosclerotic lesion area, as determined by both oil red O staining of the entire aorta and histological quantification of plaque areas between the sinus aorta and brachiocephalic arteries (Fig. 3C–E). Chronic administration of recombinant mouse adiponectin (Fig. VC in the online-only Data Supplement) also alleviated atherosclerotic plaque formation in DKO mice, whereas the magnitude of reduction in atherosclerosis by adiponectin was significantly smaller than that by rmFGF21.

Further histological analysis demonstrated that rmFGF21 and adiponectin caused a similar degree of decrease in collagen composition, smooth muscle proliferation, and macrophage infiltration (Fig. 4A). The magnitude of reduction in expression of proinflammatory chemokines intercellular adhesion molecule-1 and vascular cell adhesion protein-1 and cytokines tumor necrosis factor-α and monocyte chemotactic protein-1 was also comparable between rmFGF21- and adiponectin-treated DKO mice (Fig. 4B–F). However, in adiponectin-treated DKO mice, cholesterol ester contents in brachiocephalic arteries were reduced only by 22%, which was significantly lower than rmFGF21-mediated reduction (56%; Fig. 4G). Notably, whereas rmFGF21 decreased total cholesterol in DKO mice to a level comparable with apoE$^{-/-}$ mice, adiponectin had no effect on hypercholesterolemia

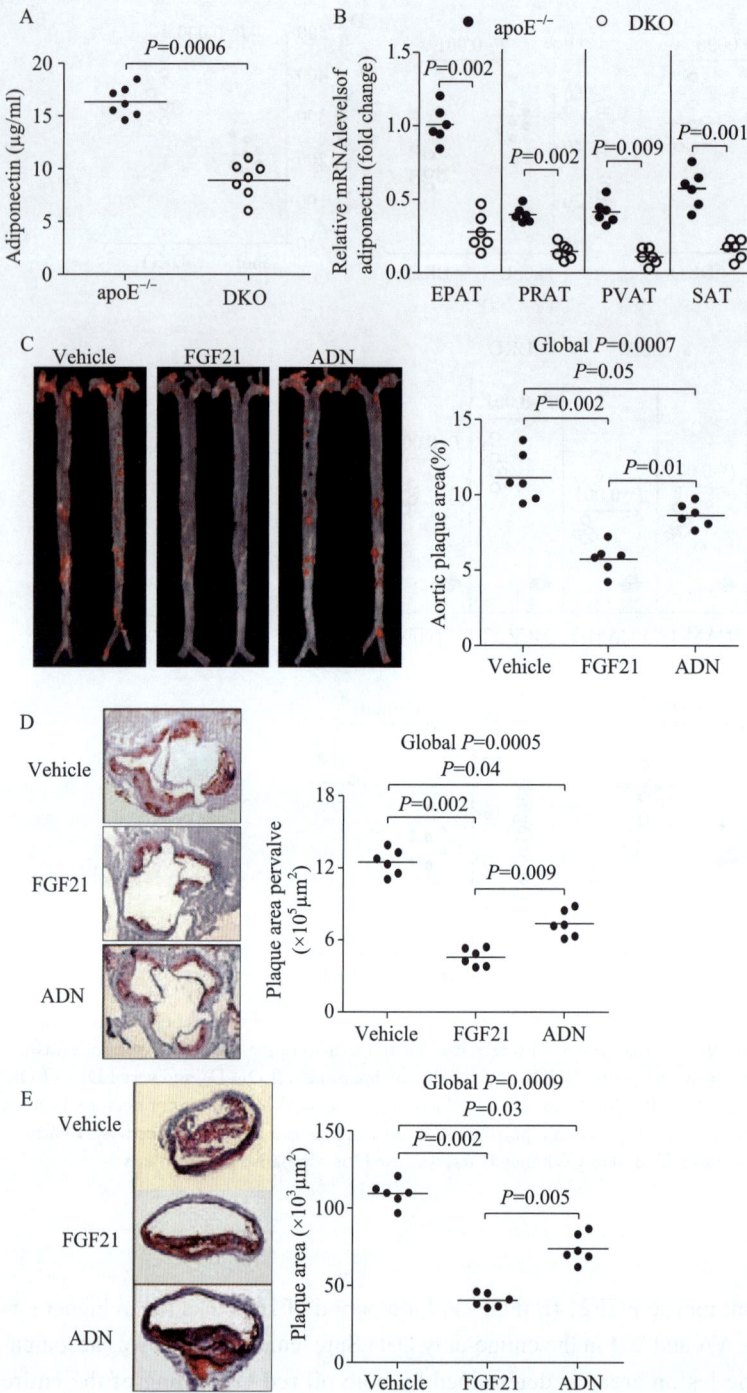

Fig. 3. Recombinant mouse fibroblast growth factor (FGF) 21 and adiponectin (ADN) attenuate the atherosclerotic plaque formation in apolipoprotein E$^{-/-}$ FGF21$^{-/-}$ (DKO) mice. Eight-week- old DKO mice were treated with recombinant mouse FGF21 (0.1 mg/kg per day), adiponectin (10 mg/kg per day), or vehicle by daily intraperitoneal injection for a period of 16 weeks. (A) and (B), Plasma levels of adiponectin and its mRNA expression in epididymal adipose tissues (EPAT), subcutaneous (SAT), perivascular (PVAT), and perirenal (PRAT) adipose tissues. (C) En face staining of entire aortas with oil red O. (D) and (E), Cross-section analysis of aortic sinuses and brachiocephalic arteries with oil red O, respectively. n=6 to 7. Data are presented as dot plots with the line indicating the median. The Mann-Whitney U test was used to compare 2 groups (A and B). The global significance among 3 groups was determined by Kruskal-Wallis test, followed by pairwise comparisons with the Dunn-Sidak procedure (C–E).

caused by FGF21 deficiency (Fig. 4H), despite that both rmFGF21 and adiponectin had a similar potency in decreasing the expression and secretion of adiponectin, an adipokine with insulin-sensitizing, anti-inflammatory, and antiatherosclerotic activities[23-25]. Because the insulin-sensitizing actions of hypertriglyceridemia in DKO mice (Fig. 4I).

We next compared the direct effects of adiponectin and rmFGF21 in several types of blood vessel cells. Consistent with previous reports[26,27], recombinant adiponectin directly inhibited platelet-derived growth factor-induced proliferation and migration of human smooth muscle cells (Fig. VIA and VIB in the online-only Data Supplement) and also reduced the uptake of acetylated LDL in peritoneal macrophages (Fig. VIC in the online-only Data Supplement). However, rmFGF21 had no direct effect on these cells.

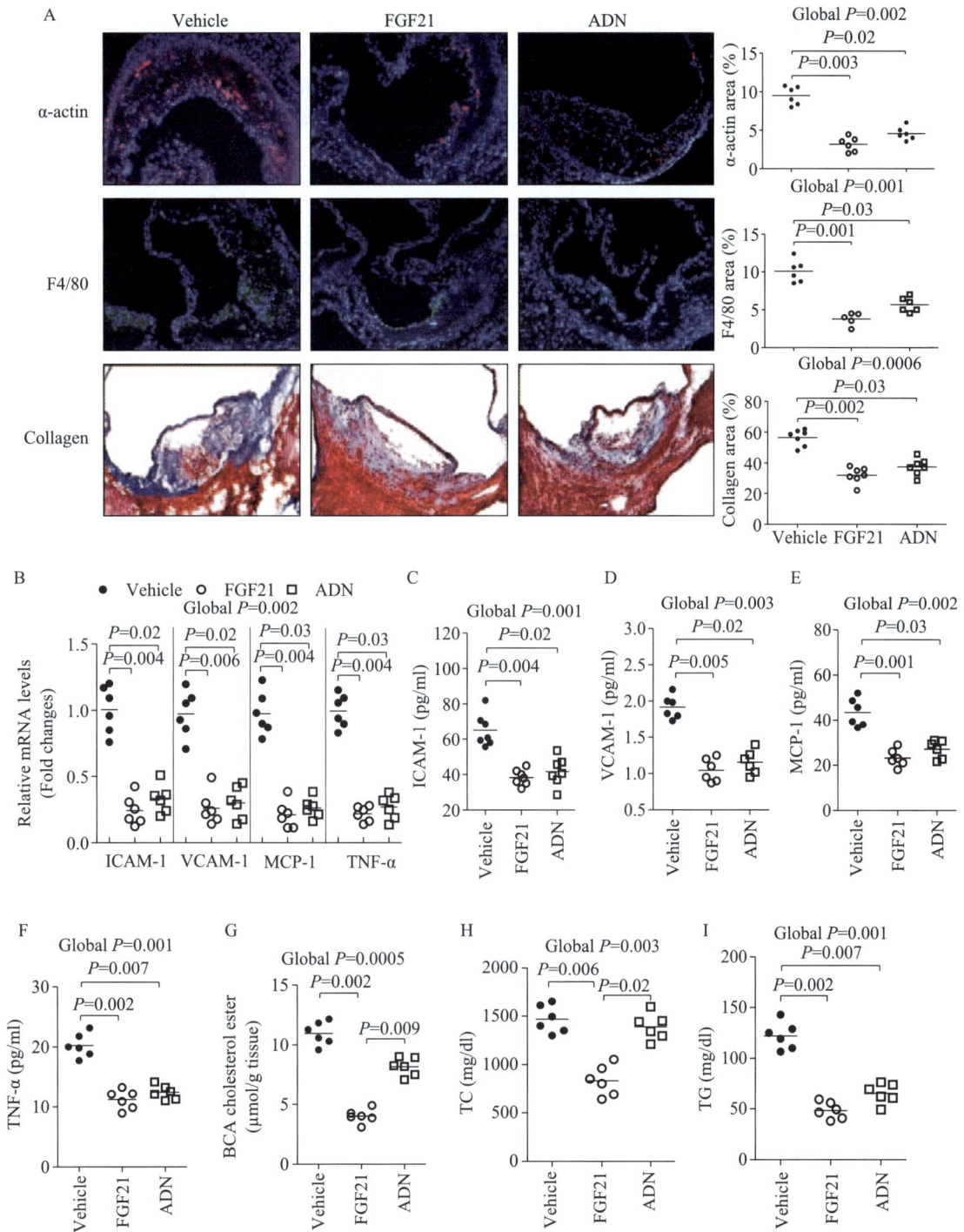

Fig. 4. Differential effects of fibroblast growth factor (FGF) 21 and adiponectin on lipid profiles and atherosclerotic plaque composition in apolipoprotein E$^{-/-}$FGF21$^{-/-}$ (DKO) mice. DKO mice were treated with recombinant mouse FGF21, adiponectin (ADN), or vehicle for 16 weeks as in Fig. 3. (A) Immunohistological analysis of atherosclerotic lesion areas in aortic sinuses with antibodies against the smooth muscle marker α-actin, the macrophage marker F4/80, or with Masson trichrome staining for the collagen composition as indicated. (B–F), The mRNA expression of several proinflammatory chemokines and cytokines in the aortic sinus and their plasma levels as determined by real-time polymerase chain reaction and ELISA, respectively. (G) Cholesterol ester content in the brachiocephalic arteries. (H, I) Plasma cholesterol and triglyceride levels in DKO mice treated with recombinant mouse (rm) FGF21, ADN, or vehicle, respectively. n=5 to 7. Data are presented as dot plots with the line indicating the median. The global significance among 3 groups was determined by Kruskal-Wallis test, followed by pairwise comparisons with the Dunn-Sidak procedure.

2.4 FGF21 suppresses cholesterol biosynthesis and enhances cholesterol efflux in mice

Because our data suggest that the cholesterol-lowering effects of rmFGF21 are independent of adiponectin, we further explored the mechanisms by which FGF21 modulates cholesterol metabolism in mice. The intestinal absorption of cholesterol, as measured by the fecal dual isotope ratio of $^{14}C:^{3}H$ in feces, was comparable between apoE$^{-/-}$ mice and DKO mice and was not affected by treatment with either rmFGF21 or adiponectin (Fig. 5A). There was a modest but significant decrease in cholesterol contents in the feces of DKO mice, and this change was reversed by treatment with rmFGF21 but not adiponectin (Fig. 5B). On the other hand, the excretion of bile acids into the feces was not altered by either FGF21 deficiency or replenishment with rmFGF21 (Fig. 5C). The *de novo* biosynthesis of cholesterol in the liver, as measured with the amount of $[1-^{14}C]$-acetate incorporated into sterols in liver, was markedly increased by 1.49-fold in DKO mice as compared with apoE$^{-/-}$ mice, and this augmented cholesterol synthesis was completely rectified by replenishment with rmFGF21 but not adiponectin (Fig. 5D). Likewise, hepatic cholesterol accumulation was elevated by FGF21 deficiency but was suppressed by treatment with rmFGF21 (Fig. 5E).

We next evaluated the impact of FGF21 on the expression of key genes involved in cholesterol metabolism in the liver. In DKO mice, hepatic expression of 3-hydroxy-3-methylglutaryl-CoA reductase (a rate-limiting enzyme involved in cholesterol synthesis) and several other cholesterologenic genes was significantly elevated when compared with apoE$^{-/-}$ mice, whereas this elevation in DKO mice was inhibited by administration of rmFGF21 but not adiponectin

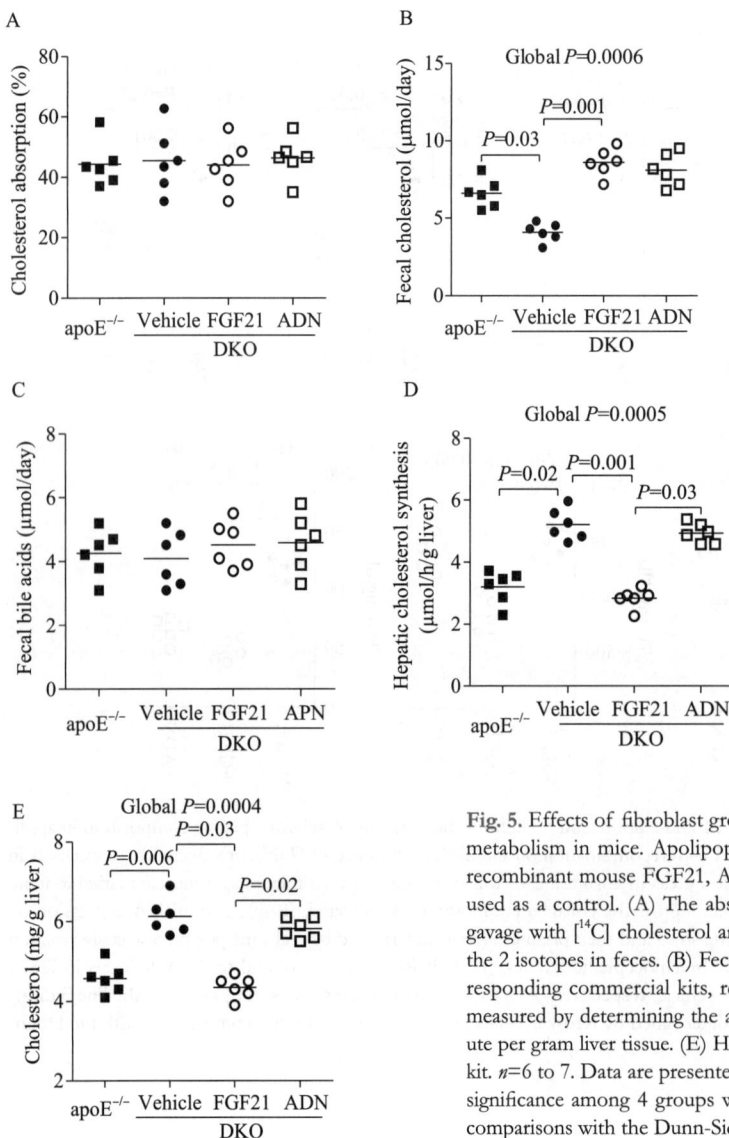

Fig. 5. Effects of fibroblast growth factor (FGF) 21 and adiponectin (ADN) on cholesterol metabolism in mice. Apolipoprotein (apo) E$^{-/-}$FGF21$^{-/-}$ (DKO) mice were treated with recombinant mouse FGF21, ADN, or vehicle for 4 weeks as in Fig. 4. ApoE$^{-/-}$ mice were used as a control. (A) The absorption rate of dietary cholesterol was determined by oral gavage with $[^{14}C]$ cholesterol and $[^{3}H]$ sitostanol, followed by measurement of the ratio of the 2 isotopes in feces. (B) Fecal cholesterol and (C) bile acids were measured with the corresponding commercial kits, respectively. (D) The rate of *de novo* cholesterol synthesis as measured by determining the amount of $[1-^{14}C]$-acetate incorporated into sterols per minute per gram liver tissue. (E) Hepatic cholesterol contents determined by a cholesterol assay kit. *n*=6 to 7. Data are presented as dot plots with the line indicating the median. The global significance among 4 groups was determined by Kruskal-Wallis test, followed by pairwise comparisons with the Dunn-Sidak procedure.

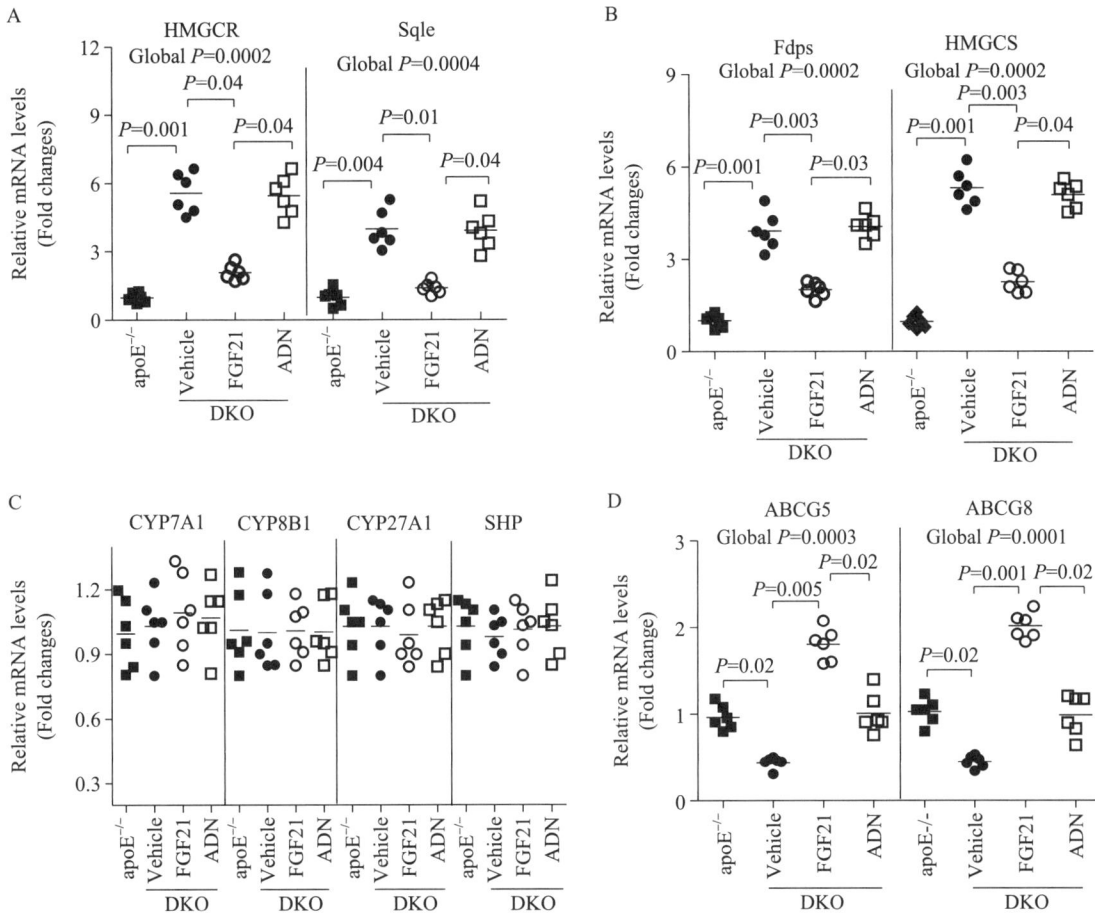

Fig. 6. Fibroblast growth factor (FGF) 21, but not adiponectin (ADN), alters hepatic expression of the key genes involved in cholesterol biosynthesis and transport. Total RNA extracted from the liver of apolipoprotein (apo) E$^{-/-}$ mice or apoE$^{-/-}$FGF21$^{-/-}$ (DKO) mice treated with recombinant mouse FGF21, ADN, or vehicle as in Fig. 4 was subjected to real-time polymerase chain reaction analysis. Figure shows the relative mRNA expression levels of genes involved in cholesterol synthesis, including 3-hydroxy-3-methylglutaryl-CoA reductase (HMGCR), 3-hydroxy-3-methylglutaryl-CoA synthetase (HMGCS), squalene synthase (Sqle), and farnesyl diphosphate synthetase (Fdps; A and B) genes involved in bile acids metabolism including cholesterol 7-α-monooxygenase (CYP7A1), sterol 12-α-hydroxylase (CYP8B1), sterol 27-hydroxylase (CYP27A1), and small heterodimer partner (SHP; C), as well as genes involved in cholesterol transports including ABCG5 and ABCG8 (D). n=5 to 7. Data are presented as dot plots with the line indicating the median. The global significance among 4 groups was determined by Kruskal-Wallis test, followed by pairwise comparisons with the Dunn-Sidak procedure.

(Fig. 6A, B). On the other hand, the expression levels of key genes involved in bile acid metabolism and secretion, including cholesterol 7-α-monooxygenase, sterol 27-hydroxylase, sterol 12-α-hydroxylase, and small heterodimer partner, were not altered by either FGF21 deficiency or administration (Fig. 6C). DKO mice exhibited a modest elevation in the expression of ABCG5 and ABCG8 (Fig. 6D), the 2 ATP-binding cassette transporters that promote cholesterol secretion[28]. The reduced expression of ABCG5 and ABCG8 was reversed by replenishment with rmFGF21 but not adiponectin.

2.5 FGF21 inhibits cholesterol biosynthesis via suppression of sterol regulatory element-binding protein-2

Cholesterol homeostasis is orchestrated by a number of transcriptional factors, including sterol regulatory element-binding protein (Srebp)-1a, -1c, and -2; liver X receptors; and farnesoid X receptor[29,30]. We next investigated whether FGF21 modulates cholesterol metabolism *via* these transcription factors. There was no obvious difference in either mRNA or protein expression of liver X receptor α, farnesoid X receptor, and Srebp-1 between DKO mice and apoE$^{-/-}$ mice (Fig. 7A, B). In contrast, DKO mice exhibited a marked elevation in both mRNA and protein expression of Srebp-2, and this change was reversed by administration of rmFGF21 but not adiponectin (Fig. 7C, D). Consistently, the transcriptional activity of nuclear Srebp-2 in the liver of DKO mice was ~2.9-fold higher than in apoE$^{-/-}$ mice, as

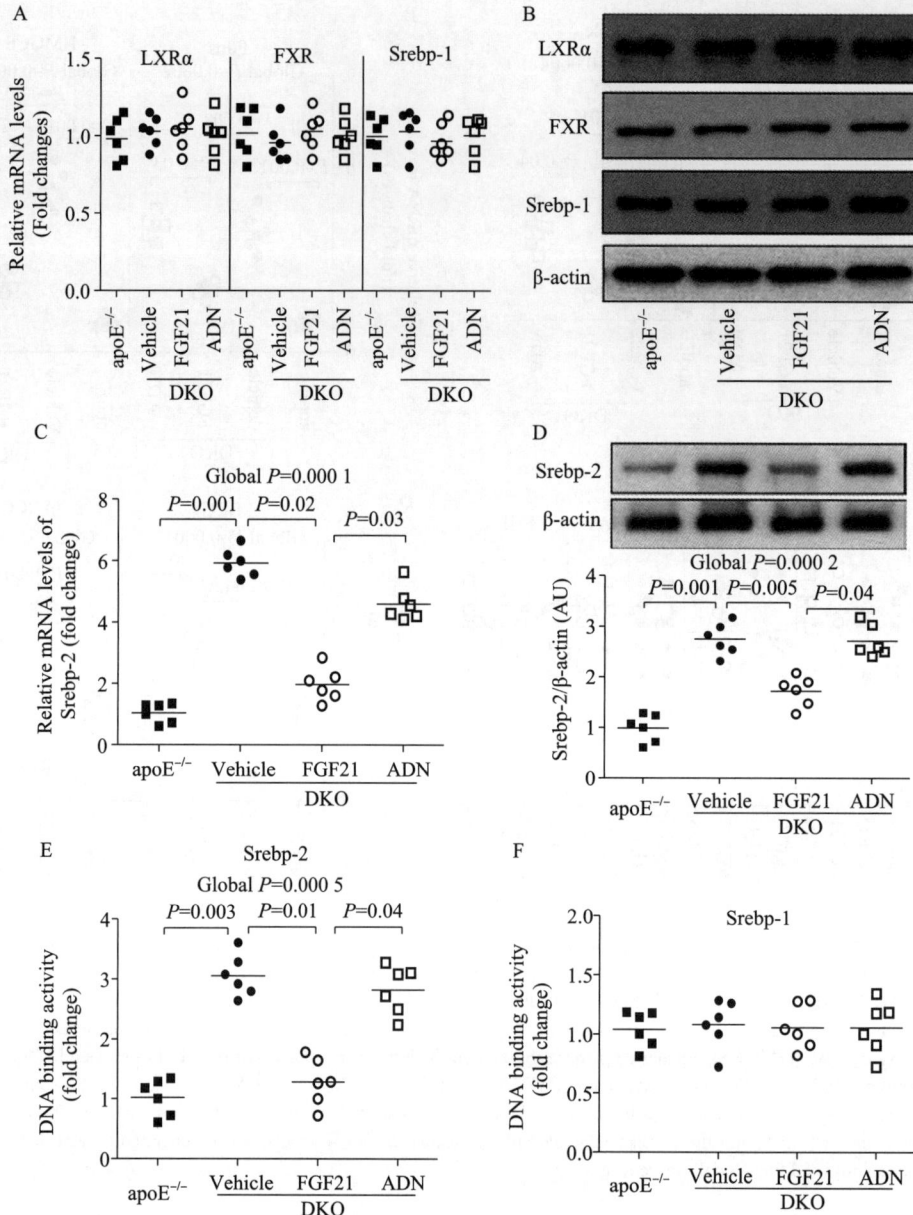

Fig. 7. Effects of fibroblast growth factor (FGF) 21 and adiponectin (ADN) on several key transcription factors involved in cholesterol metabolism. The liver samples from apolipoprotein (apo) E$^{-/-}$ mice or apoE$^{-/-}$ FGF21$^{-/-}$ (DKO) mice treated with recombinant mouse FGF21, ADN, or vehicle as in Fig. 4 were subjected to real-time polymerase chain reaction or Western blot analysis. (A) and (B), The relative mRNA and protein expression levels of liver X receptor (LXR) α, farnesoid X receptor (FXR), and sterol regulatory element-binding protein (Srebp)-1. (C) and (D), The relative mRNA and protein expression of Srebp-2. (E) and (F), The DNA binding activities of Srebp-1 and Srebp-2 in the nuclear extracts of liver tissues. n=5 to 7. Data are presented as dot plots with the line indicating the median. The global significance among 4 groups was determined by Kruskal-Wallis test, followed by pairwise comparisons with the Dunn-Sidak procedure.

determined by the binding of Srebp-2 in the nuclear extracts to the specific DNA sequences (Fig. 7E). Elevated transcriptional activity of Srebp-2 in DKO mice was largely reversed by treatment with rmFGF21 but not adiponectin. On the other hand, the transcriptional activity of nuclear Srebp-1 in the liver was not altered by either FGF21 deficiency or supplementation (Fig. 7F).

To explore whether FGF21 lowers cholesterol *via* inhibition of Srebp-2, adenovirus delivery system was used to knock down or overexpress Srebp-2 in the liver. After tail-vein injection of recombinant adenovirus encoding Srebp-2–specific small interfering RNA, an obvious reduction in Srebp-2 expression was observed at 2 days postinfection (data not shown), and its expression continued to decline to a level comparable with apoE$^{-/-}$ mice at days 6 and 12 after adenoviral Srebp-2 small interfering RNA infection (Fig. 8A, B). Notably, suppression of Srebp-2 expression reversed

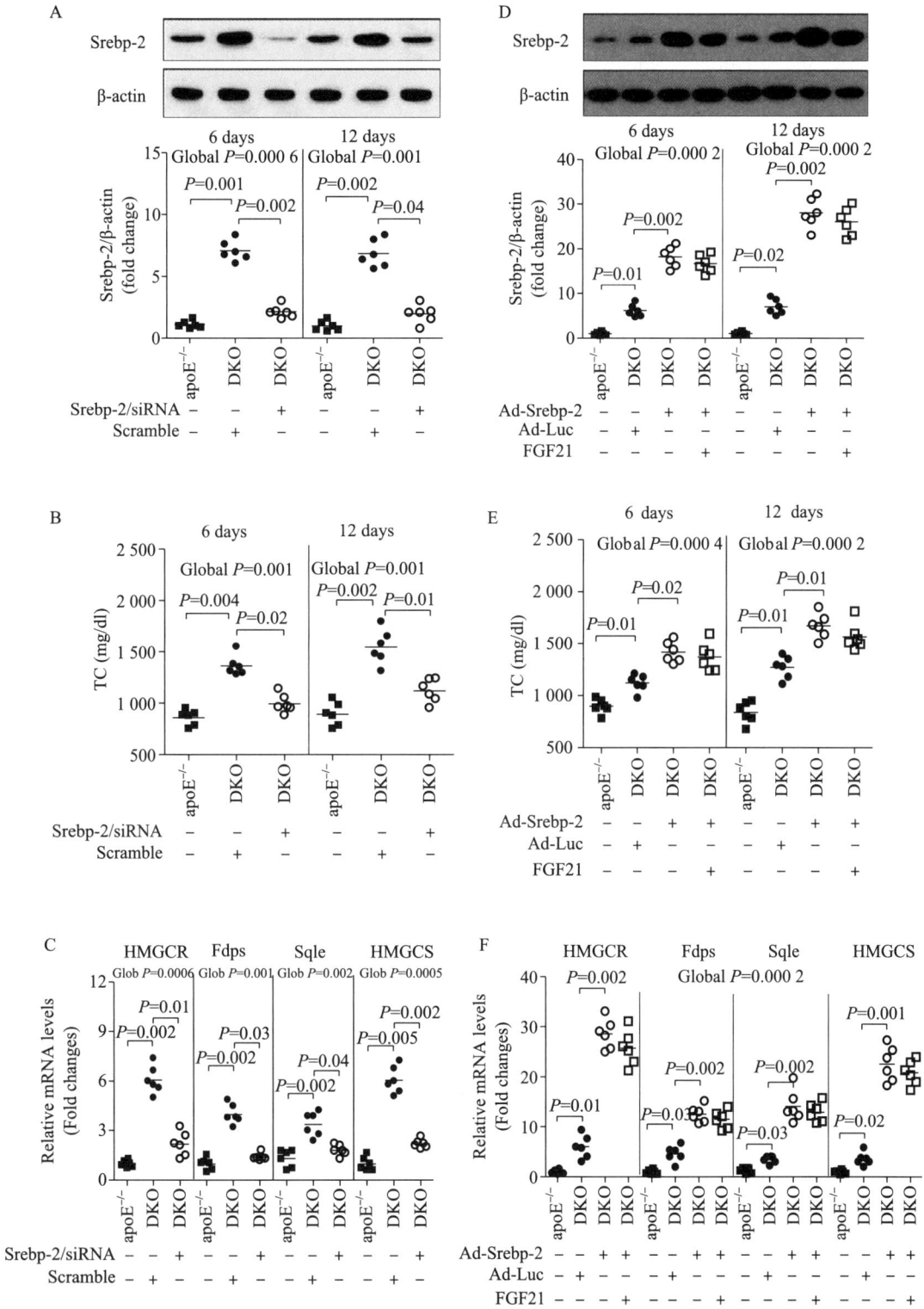

Fig. 8. Fibroblast growth factor (FGF) 21 decreases hypercholesterolemia *via* inhibition of hepatic sterol regulatory element-binding protein (Srebp)-2. (A–C), Apolipoprotein (apo) E$^{-/-}$FGF21$^{-/-}$ (DKO) mice were infected with adenovirus encoding small interfering RNA (siRNA) specific to Srebp-2 or scrambled control (5×10^8 plaque-forming units per mouse) for various periods. Age-matched apoE$^{-/-}$ mice were used as a control. (A) Protein expression levels of hepatic Srebp-2 at day 6 and day 12 after adenoviral infection. (B) Circulating levels of total cholesterol (TC) and (C) the expression levels of cholesterologenic genes determined by real-time polymerase chain reaction analysis at day 12 (n=6). (D) and (E), DKO mice were infected with adenovirus encoding Srebp-2 (Ad-Srebp-2) or luciferase (Ad-Luc) for 6 days (as control), followed by treatment with daily intraperitoneal injection of recombinant mouse (rm) FGF21 (0.1 mg/kg per day) for another 6 days. (D) The protein expression levels of Srebp-2 in the liver and (E) serum levels of total cholesterol. (F) The mRNA expression of cholesterologenic genes at 12 days after adenoviral infection (n=6). Data are presented as dot plots with the line indicating the median. The global significance among 3 groups was determined by Kruskal-Wallis test, followed by pairwise comparisons with the Dunn-Sidak procedure.

hypercholesterolemia in DKO mice caused by FGF21 deficiency and concurrently reduced the expression of several cholesterologenic genes, including 3-hydroxy-3-methylglutaryl-CoA reductase, farnesyl diphosphate synthetase, squalene synthase, and 3-hydroxy-3-methylglutaryl-CoA synthetase, which are all well-known downstream targets of Srebp-2 (Fig. 8C). Conversely, the effects of rmFGF21 administration on the alleviation of hypercholesterolemia and suppression of cholesterologenic gene expression were abrogated by adenovirus- mediated expression of Srebp-2 (Fig. 8D–F).

2.6 Suppressive effects of FGF21 on cholesterol biosynthesis are mediated by β-klotho and FGFR2 in the liver

FGF21 exerts its actions by binding to FGFR and its coreceptor β-klotho, the latter of which is highly expressed in the liver[31]. To determine whether the regulatory effects of FGF21 on cholesterol homeostasis are attributed to its direct hepatic actions, we generated the β-klotho liver-specific knockout (β-klotho-LKO) mice by intravenous injection of adenovirus-associated virus encoding Cre recombinase into β-klotho-floxed mice (Fig. VIIA and VIIB in the online-only Data Supplement). Daily administration of FGF21 significantly decreased high-fat, high-cholesterol diet-induced hypercholesterolemia, which was accompanied by decreased expression of Srebp-2 and several cholesterologenic genes in β-klotho-floxed mice injected with AAV encoding green fluorescent protein as wild-type control, whereas these effects of FGF21 were largely abrogated in β-klotho-LKO mice. By contrast, the stimulatory effects of FGF21 on adiponectin production were comparable between β-klotho-LKO mice and β-klotho-floxed mice, suggesting that hepatic β-klotho mediates the effects of FGF21 on lowering cholesterol but not on elevating adiponectin levels (Fig. VIIC through VIIH in the online-only Data Supplement).

Among 4 major subtypes of FGFRs, FGFR1 plays a key role in mediating the FGF21 actions in adipose tissues.[31] However, hepatic expression levels of FGFR1 were hardly detectable (Fig. VIIIA in the online-only Data Supplement). Instead, FGFR4 and FGFR2 were abundantly present in the liver, followed by FGFR3[31]. We next explored the role of these FGFRs in mediating the hepatic actions of FGF21 on cholesterol metabolism using adenovirus-mediated knockdown of their expression. Notably, the inhibitory effects of FGF21 on the expression of Srebp-2 and cholesterologenic genes and hypercholesterolemia were significantly compromised in mice with reduced hepatic expression of FGFR2 (Fig. VIIIB through VIIIG in the online-only Data Supplement). By contrast, these FGF21 actions on cholesterol metabolism were little affected by knocking down the expression of the other 3 FGFRs despite >70% knocking down efficiency (data not shown). Taken together, these findings suggest that the regulatory effects of FGF21 on cholesterol homeostasis are mediated at least in part by the FGFR2-β-klotho complex.

3. Discussion

Despite intensive research on metabolic functions of FGF21, its role in the cardiovascular system has scarcely been explored. This study provides novel evidence that FGF21 deficiency causes a marked exacerbation of atherosclerosis and increased mortality of apoE$^{-/-}$ mice, suggesting that FGF21 is a physiological protector against vascular diseases. In this connection, elevated circulating FGF21 levels in patients and rodents with atherosclerosis may represent the defense mechanism of the body to prevent vascular damage. In support of this notion, upregulated FGF21 has been shown to act as a compensatory mechanism to protect against cerulein-induced pancreatitis[15], endotoxin-induced sepsis[32], and acetaminophen-induced acute liver injury[33].

Atherosclerosis is a chronic inflammatory disease involving multiple cell types at various stages of plaque formation, including endothelial cells, lymphocytes, monocytes/macrophages, and smooth muscle cells[34]. Our histological and immunologic analysis demonstrated that depletion of FGF21 in apoE$^{-/-}$ mice causes a markedly increased endothelial activation (as determined by expression of endothelial adhesion molecules), augmented macrophage infiltration and foam cell formation, exacerbated smooth muscle cell proliferation, and collagen deposition, all of which can be reversed by the replenishment of exogenous rmFGF21, suggesting that FGF21 is able to inhibit almost every key pathogenic event of atherosclerosis. However, these antiatherosclerotic effects of FGF21 are not attributed to its direct actions on the vascular walls but attributed to the ability of FGF21 in the induction of adiponectin in adipocytes and reduction of cholesterol biosynthesis in the liver. In support of this notion, the expression of β-klotho, an obligatory coreceptor of FGF21, is hardly detectable in any type of blood vessel cells (Z.L. and A.X., unpublished data, 2014), despite its high abundance in adipose tissue and liver[7,8].

Recent studies have demonstrated the effects of FGF21 on the elevation of circulating adiponectin in both rodents and humans[12,13]. In adipocytes, FGF21 can stimulate the gene expression, as well as the protein secretion, of adiponectin in a PPARγ-dependent manner[12]. Adiponectin possesses potent anti-inflammatory and antiatherosclerotic activities *via* its multiple actions on blood vessels[35]. In humans, hypoadiponectinemia is an independent risk factor for vascular inflammation and atherosclerosis[36]. In contrast, elevation of circulating adiponectin by either pharmacological or genetic intervention can decrease neointima formation and atherosclerosis in both rodents and rabbits[24,37]. Adiponectin accumulates in the atherosclerotic lesion area, where it protects the vascular endothelium by promoting nitric oxide and alleviating oxidative stress, suppresses smooth muscle cell proliferation and migration, inhibits macrophage infiltration and foam cell formation, and ameliorates the collagen deposition[35]. In line with these reports, our results demonstrated that adiponectin, but not FGF21, suppresses platelet-derived growth factor-induced proliferation and migration of smooth muscle cells and blocks LDL uptake and cholesterol accumulation in macrophages. On the other hand, the exacerbated smooth muscle proliferation and macrophage infiltration in the atherosclerotic plaques of DKO mice can largely be reversed by replenishment with adiponectin. Taken together, these findings suggest that the effects of FGF21 on smooth muscle cells and macrophages in the vessel walls are indirect, mediated in part by the induction of adiponectin.

Dyslipidemia, especially elevated LDL cholesterol, is a major contributor to atherosclerotic plaque formation. The cholesterol-lowering drugs, such as statins, have been used clinically to reduce the risk of coronary heart disease. Therapeutic administration of FGF21 has been shown to alleviate dyslipidemia in rodents[4], obese monkeys[22], and patients with type 2 diabetes mellitus[38], including reductions in total and LDL cholesterol and triglycerides, elevations in high-density lipoprotein cholesterol, and a shift to a less atherogenic apolipoprotein profile. Consistent with these pharmacological studies, our present study showed that FGF21 deficiency in apoE[−/−] mice causes a further aggravation of hypercholesterolemia and a shift of apolipoprotein profiles from high-density lipoprotein to LDL. Notably, the severe hypercholesterolemia in DKO mice is accompanied by augmented *de novo* cholesterol biosynthesis and increased expression of several cholesterologenic genes in the liver, suggesting that endogenous FGF21 is a physiological suppressor of hepatic cholesterol production. However, whereas adiponectin replenishment reverses hypertriglyceridemia, it has little effect on hypercholesterolemia and augmented hepatic cholesterogenesis in DKO mice, suggesting that the cholesterol-lowering activity of FGF21 is independent of adiponectin. Given that hepatic FGF21 expression is progressively elevated with the development of hypercholesterolemia in apoE[−/−] mice, it is possible that FGF21 acts as a sensor of cholesterol overload, which in turn prevents further worsening of hypercholesterolemia *via* its autocrine inhibition of hepatic cholesterogenesis.

Srebps, which structurally belong to the basic helix-loop-helix-leucine zipper transcription factor family, are the principal regulator of lipid synthesis[29]. Unlike other members of this class of transcription factor, Srebps are synthesized as membrane-bound precursors that require cleavage by a 2-step proteolytic process to release their amino-terminal transactivation domain into the nucleus to bind to a specific DNA sequence (sterol regulatory element) and activate their target genes[29]. Hepatic expression and activity of Srebps are tightly regulated at both transcriptional and post-translational levels by metabolic hormones and nutritional factors[29]. Srebp-1a and 1c preferably activate transcription of genes involved in fatty acid synthesis, whereas Srebp-2 displays strong specificity for genes involved in cholesterol biosynthesis[39,40]. Our present study demonstrated that the expression and transcriptional activity of Srebp-2, but not Srebp-1, is significantly enhanced by FGF21 deficiency but is markedly suppressed by FGF21 treatment. Furthermore, adenovirus-mediated silencing of hepatic Srebp-2 expression is sufficient to counteract exacerbation of hypercholesterolemia and augmentation of hepatic cholesterol biosynthesis caused by FGF21 deficiency, whereas the therapeutic benefits of systemic FGF21 administration on the inhibition of hepatic cholesterogenesis and reduction of hypercholesterolemia are abrogated by overexpression of Srebp-2. Thus, our study identifies hepatic Srebp-2 as a key intracellular mediator conferring the regulatory effects of FGF21 on cholesterol homeostasis.

Although the precise signaling pathways whereby FGF21 selectively suppresses hepatic Srebp-2 remain unclear, differential regulation of Srebp-1 and Srebp-2 has been reported in several previous studies[41,42]. A high-carbohydrate diet induces the mRNA and protein expression of Srebp-1 but not Srebp-2[41], whereas dietary cholesterol enhances the expression of Srebp-2 and Srebp-1c but not Srebp-1a[42]. The NAD[+]-dependent deacetylase sirtuin (Sirt) 6 and FOXO3 suppress the transcriptional activation of the *Srebp-2* gene without any obvious effect on Srebp-1[43]. Notably, FGF21 has been shown to form a regulatory loop with Sirt1 to reduce diet-induced fatty liver disease[44]. Additional investigation is warranted to interrogate the role of the sirtuin family members in mediating FGF21-induced suppression of hepatic Srebp-2.

There are several limitations in our study. First, our observations are solely based on rodent models. In light of the fact that there is a difference in lipid metabolism and cardiovascular structure between rodents and humans, the pathophysiological relevance of our findings remains to be confirmed in humanoid large animals (eg, pigs) and in clinical studies. Second, although our data demonstrated the obligatory role of β-klotho and FGFR2 in mediating the cholesterol-lowering effects of FGF21 *via* suppression of Srebp-2 in the liver, the signaling pathways that link the FGF21 receptor with its regulation of cholesterol metabolism need further investigation.

In summary, our present study uncovers the protective effects of FGF21 against atherosclerosis *via* the induction of adiponectin in adipose tissue, reduction of hypercholesterolemia by suppression of hepatic Srebp-2, and augmentation of cholesterol efflux possibly by increasing ABCG5/8 expression (Fig. IX in the online-only Data Supplement). Consistent with our animal data, a recent clinical trial in obese patients with type 2 diabetes mellitus showed that chronic administration of a long-acting form of FGF21 causes a marked elevation of adiponectin and an obvious reduction in total and LDL cholesterol but has little effect on hyperglycemia[38]. Therefore, our present study, together with these clinical data, raises the possibility that FGF21 or its agonists might be more effective for the treatment of atherosclerosis, instead of diabetes mellitus.

Supplementary data

Supplementary data is available with this article at http://circ.ahajournals.org/lookup/suppl/doi:10.1161/CIRCULATIONAHA.115.015308/-/DC1.

References

[1] Kharitonenkov A, Shiyanova TL, Koester A, *et al.* FGF-21 as a novel metabolic regulator[J]. Journal of Clinical Investigation, 2005, 115(6): 1627-1635.

[2] Badman MK, Pissios P, Kennedy AR, *et al.* Hepatic fibroblast growth factor 21 is regulated by PPAR alpha and is a key mediator of hepatic lipid metabolism in ketotic states[J]. Cell Metabolism, 2007, 5(6): 426-437.

[3] Potthoff MJ, Inagaki T, Satapati S, *et al.* FGF21 induces PGC-1 alpha and regulates carbohydrate and fatty acid metabolism during the adaptive starvation response[J]. Proceedings of the National Academy of Sciences of the United States of America, 2009, 106(26): 10853-10858.

[4] Coskun T, Bina HA, Schneider MA, *et al.* Fibroblast growth factor 21 corrects obesity in mice[J]. Endocrinology, 2008, 149(12): 6018-6027.

[5] Kharitonenkov A, Wroblewski VJ, Koester A, *et al.* The metabolic state of diabetic monkeys is regulated by fibroblast growth factor-21[J]. Endocrinology, 2007, 148(2): 774-781.

[6] Li H, Gao Z, Zhang J, *et al.* Sodium butyrate stimulates expression of fibroblast growth factor 21 in liver by inhibition of histone deacetylase 3[J]. Diabetes, 2012, 61(4): 797-806.

[7] Ito S, Kinoshita S, Shiraishi N, *et al.* Molecular cloning and expression analyses of mouse ss klotho, which encodes a novel Klotho family protein[J]. Mechanisms of Development, 2000, 98(1-2): 115-119.

[8] Adams AC, Cheng CC, Coskun T, *et al.* FGF21 Requires beta klotho to act *in vivo*[J]. Plos One, 2012, 7(11).

[9] Chen W, Hoo RL, Konishi M, *et al.* Growth hormone induces hepatic production of fibroblast growth factor 21 through a mechanism dependent on lipolysis in adipocytes[J]. Journal of Biological Chemistry, 2011, 286(40): 34559-34566.

[10] Murata Y, Konishi M, Itoh N. FGF21 as an Endocrine Regulator in Lipid Metabolism: From Molecular Evolution to Physiology and Pathophysiology[J]. J Nutr Metab, 2011, 2011: 981315.

[11] Fisher FM, Kleiner S, Douris N, *et al.* FGF21 regulates PGC-1 alpha and browning of white adipose tissues in adaptive thermogenesis[J]. Genes & Development, 2012, 26(3): 271-281.

[12] Lin Z, Tian H, Lam KSL, *et al.* Adiponectin mediates the metabolic effects of FGF21 on glucose homeostasis and insulin sensitivity in mice[J]. Cell Metabolism, 2013, 17(5): 779-789.

[13] Holland WL, Adams AC, Brozinick JT, *et al.* An FGF21-adiponectin-ceramide axis controls energy expenditure and insulin action in mice[J]. Cell Metabolism, 2013, 17(5): 790-797.

[14] Xu J, Lloyd DJ, Hale C, *et al.* Fibroblast growth factor 21 reverses hepatic steatosis, increases energy expenditure, and improves insulin sensitivity in diet-induced obese mice[J]. Diabetes, 2009, 58(1): 250-259.

[15] Johnson CL, Weston JY, Chadi SA, *et al.* Fibroblast growth factor 21 reduces the severity of cerulein-induced pancreatitis in mice[J]. Gastroenterology, 2009, 137(5): 1795-1804.

[16] Planavila A, Redondo I, Hondares E, *et al.* Fibroblast growth factor 21 protects against cardiac hypertrophy in mice[J]. Nature Communications, 2013, 4.

[17] Berglund ED, Li CY, Bina HA, *et al.* Fibroblast growth factor 21 controls glycemia *via* regulation of hepatic glucose flux and insulin sensitivity[J]. Endocrinology, 2009, 150(9): 4084-4093.

[18] Wente W, Efanov AM, Brenner M, *et al.* Fibroblast growth factor-21 improves pancreatic beta-cell function and survival by activation of extracellular signal-regulated kinase 1/2 and Akt signaling pathways[J]. Diabetes, 2006, 55(9): 2470-2478.

[19] Lin Z, Wu Z, Yin X, *et al.* Serum levels of FGF-21 are increased in coronary heart disease patients and are independently associated with adverse lipid profile[J]. Plos One, 2010, 5(12).

[20] Chow WS, Xu A, Woo YC, *et al.* Serum fibroblast growth factor-21 levels are associated with carotid atherosclerosis independent of established cardiovascular risk factors[J]. Arteriosclerosis Throm-

bosis and Vascular Biology, 2013, 33(10): 2454-2459.

[21] Adams AC, Halstead CA, Hansen BC, *et al.* LY2405319, an engineered FGF21 variant, improves the metabolic status of diabetic monkeys[J]. Plos One, 2013, 8(6).

[22] Veniant MM, Komorowski R, Chen P, *et al.* Long-acting FGF21 has enhanced efficacy in diet-induced obese mice and in obese rhesus monkeys[J]. Endocrinology, 2012, 153(9): 4192-4203.

[23] Yamauchi T, Kamon J, Waki H, *et al.* The fat-derived hormone adiponectin reverses insulin resistance associated with both lipoatrophy and obesity[J]. Nature Medicine, 2001, 7(8): 941-946.

[24] Okamoto Y, Kihara S, Ouchi N, *et al.* Adiponectin reduces atherosclerosis in apolipoprotein E-deficient mice[J]. Circulation, 2002, 106(22): 2767-2770.

[25] Xu AM, Wang Y, Keshaw H, *et al.* The fat-derived hormone adiponectin alleviates alcoholic and nonalcoholic fatty liver diseases in mice[J]. Journal of Clinical Investigation, 2003, 112(1): 91-100.

[26] Wang Y, Lam KSL, Xu JY, *et al.* Adiponectin inhibits cell proliferation by interacting with several growth factors in an oligomerization-dependent manner[J]. Journal of Biological Chemistry, 2005, 280(18): 18341-18347.

[27] Ouchi N, Kihara S, Arita Y, *et al.* Adipocyte-derived plasma protein, adiponectin, suppresses lipid accumulation and class A scavenger receptor expression in human monocyte-derived macrophages[J]. Circulation, 2001, 103(8): 1057-1063.

[28] Yu LQ, Li-Hawkins J, Hammer RE, *et al.* Overexpression of ABCG5 and ABCG8 promotes biliary cholesterol secretion and reduces fractional absorption of dietary cholesterol[J]. Journal of Clinical Investigation, 2002, 110(5): 671-680.

[29] Brown MS, Goldstein JL. The SREBP pathway: Regulation of cholesterol metabolism by proteolysis of a membrane-bound transcription factor[J]. Cell, 1997, 89(3): 331-340.

[30] Calkin AC, Tontonoz P. Transcriptional integration of metabolism by the nuclear sterol-activated receptors LXR and FXR[J]. Nature Reviews Molecular Cell Biology, 2012, 13(4): 213-224.

[31] Fisher FM, Estall JL, Adams AC, *et al.* Integrated regulation of hepatic metabolism by fibroblast growth factor 21 (FGF21) *in vivo*[J]. Endocrinology, 2011, 152(8): 2996-3004.

[32] Feingold KR, Grunfeld C, Heuer JG, *et al.* FGF21 is increased by inflammatory stimuli and protects leptin-deficient ob/ob mice from the toxicity of sepsis[J]. Endocrinology, 2012, 153(6): 2689-2700.

[33] Ye D, Wang Y, Li H, *et al.* Fibroblast growth factor 21 protects against acetaminophen-induced hepatotoxicity by potentiating per-

oxisome proliferator-activated receptor coactivator protein-1 alpha-mediated antioxidant capacity in mice[J]. Hepatology, 2014, 60(3): 977-989.

[34] Libby P. Inflammation in atherosclerosis[J]. Nature, 2002, 420(6917): 868-874.

[35] Hui X, Lam KSL, Vanhoutte PM, *et al.* Adiponectin and cardiovascular health: an update[J]. British Journal of Pharmacology, 2012, 165(3): 574-590.

[36] Shioji K, Moriguchi A, Moriwaki S, *et al.* Hypoadiponectinemia implies the development of atherosclerosis in carotid and coronary arteries[J]. Journal of cardiology, 2005, 46(3): 105-112.

[37] Kurosu H, Choi M, Ogawa Y, *et al.* Tissue-specific expression of beta klotho and fibroblast growth factor (FGF) receptor isoforms determines metabolic activity of FGF19 and FGF21[J]. Journal of Biological Chemistry, 2007, 282(37): 26687-26695.

[38] Gaich G, Chien JY, Fu H, *et al.* The effects of LY2405319, an FGF21 analog, in obese human subjects with type 2 diabetes[J]. Cell Metabolism, 2013, 18(3): 333-340.

[39] Shimano H, Horton JD, Shimomura I, *et al.* Isoform 1c of sterol regulatory element binding protein is less active than isoform 1a in livers of transgenic mice and in cultured cells[J]. Journal of Clinical Investigation, 1997, 99(5): 846-854.

[40] Horton JD, Shimomura I, Brown MS, *et al.* Activation of cholesterol synthesis in preference to fatty acid synthesis in liver and adipose tissue of transgenic mice overproducing sterol regulatory element-binding protein-2[J]. Journal of Clinical Investigation, 1998, 101(11): 2331-2339.

[41] Horton JD, Bashmakov Y, Shimomura I, *et al.* Regulation of sterol regulatory element binding proteins in livers of fasted and refed mice[J]. Proceedings of the National Academy of Sciences of the United States of America, 1998, 95(11): 5987-5992.

[42] Field FJ, Born E, Murthy S, *et al.* Regulation of sterol regulatory element-binding proteins in hamster intestine by changes in cholesterol flux[J]. Journal of Biological Chemistry, 2001, 276(20): 17576-17583.

[43] Tao R, Xiong X, DePinho RA, *et al.* Hepatic SREBP-2 and cholesterol biosynthesis are regulated by FoxO3 and Sirt6[J]. Journal of Lipid Research, 2013, 54(10): 2745-2753.

[44] Lee J, Hong S-W, Park SE, *et al.* Exendin-4 regulates lipid metabolism and fibroblast growth factor 21 in hepatic steatosis[J]. Metabolism-Clinical and Experimental, 2014, 63(8): 1041-1048.

Attenuation of hyperlipidemia and diabetes-induced early-stage apoptosis and late-stage renal dysfunction *via* administration of fibroblast growth factor-21 is associated with suppression of renal inflammation

Chi Zhang, Xiaokun Li, Lu Cai

1. Introduction

Diabetes mellitus is a fatal disease whose incidence is increasing rapidly worldwide [1]. Complications associated with diabetes can be severe, and include diabetic kidney disease (DKD). Each diabetic patient has as much as a 40% lifetime risk of developing DKD, and it is the single most common cause of end-stage renal disease and diabetic nephropathy [2]. DKD begins as an early renal response to the acute pathogenic stresses of diabetes [3–6]. In these early stages, lipotoxicity (the accumulation of lipid intermediates) is considered a key instigator of diabetic renal damage and dysfunction [7–12].

Renal lipotoxicity is characterized by excessive intracellular free fatty acids (FFAs), which leads to the accumulation of potentially toxic metabolites such as diacylglycerol and ceramides [13]. Renal injury induced by lipotoxicity occurs through several mechanisms, including the generation of reactive oxygen species and release of proinflammatory and pro-fibrotic factors [14,15]. All of these interact and finally contribute to renal apoptosis and chronic tubule damage with subsequent renal dysfunction and nephropathy [16]. To prevent early-stage renal cell death and halt the further development of DKD, an appropriate therapy must be found to simultaneously suppress lipid accumulation, inflammation, oxidative stress, and fibrotic factors during the early stages of diabetes.

Fibroblast growth factor (FGF)21, a member of the FGF family, is a lipid metabolic regulator which has beneficial effects against dyslipidemia and lipotoxicity [17,18]. There is increasing evidence that FGF21 is involved in suppression of inflammation, oxidative stress, and the fibrotic effect. For example, serum FGF21 levels were elevated under inflammatory conditions [19]. Another study also confirmed that a deficiency of FGF21 enhanced inflammation induced by isoproterenol and lipopolysaccharide *via* inhibition of NF-κB (nuclear factor kappa-light-chain-enhancer of activated B cells) [20]. The same study found that FGF21 was associated with an anti-oxidative effect in cardiac cells, as evidenced by suppression of reactive oxygen species production [20]. Results of a recent study suggest that important biofunctions of FGF21 include anti-fibrotic effects. FGF21 significantly prevented the type 1 diabetes-induced gene expression of pro-fibrotic cytokines, including type IV collagen, plasminogen activator inhibitor-1 (PAI-1) and transforming growth factor (TGF)-β1 in the kidney [21].

To date, the study of FGF21 has focused on its effects in liver and adipose tissue [22]; kidney has relatively low levels of FGF21 [23]. Recently we demonstrated a significant and positive association between serum FGF21 and the progression of renal disease, from early- to end-stage chronic kidney disease [24]. Other research groups have also reported a close association between FGF21 levels and renal dysfunction and insulin resistance in end-stage renal disease patients [25,26]. Altogether, the evidence suggests that lipotoxicity is crucially involved in the development of DKD, associated as it is with the suppression of the pathological mechanisms of hyperlipidemia, inflammation, oxidative stress and fibrotic effects. The present study investigated whether FGF21 has a renal protective function under lipotoxic and diabetic conditions, and the possible protective mechanism.

2. Materials and methods

2.1 Ethics statement

This study was carried out in strict accordance with the recommendations of the Guide for the Care and Use of Laboratory Animals of the National Institutes of Health. The Institutional Animal Care and Use Committee of the University of Louisville (IACUC #: 09018, 10102) approved the protocol. All surgery was performed under anesthesia induced by intraperitoneal injection of 1.2% 2,2,2-tribromoethanol (Avertin) at a dose of 0.2 ml/10 g body weight and all efforts were made to minimize suffering.

2.2 Experimental animals

Male friend virus B-type (FVB) mice, 9 weeks old (18–22 g of body weight), were obtained from Jackson Laboratory (Bar Harbor, Maine). FGF21 knock-out (FGF21-KO) mice, 9 weeks old (18–22 g of body weight) with a C57BL/6J genetic background were given as a gift from Dr. Steve Kliewer, University of Texas Southwestern Medical Center. Age-matched C57BL/6J mice for controls were obtained from Jackson Laboratory. All mice were housed at 22 ℃ with a 12:12-h light-dark cycle with free access to rodent chow and tap water. Animals were kept under these conditions for 2 weeks before the experiments.

Mouse model of hyperlipidemia. FVB mice were given a daily intraperitoneal injection of bovine serum albumin (BSA) with FFAs (BSA-FA; A4503, Sigma-Aldrich, St. Louis, MO) or essentially FFA-free BSA (BSA; A6003, Sigma) at 10 mg/g body weight, or sham-injected with the same volume of saline ($n = 6$). Albumin solutions were prepared using sterile saline (150 mM NaCl) as a diluent [27]. The albumin concentration of the solutions was assayed and solutions were diluted to 33%. The pH of the BSA-FA solution was 6.5, and that of the BSA solution was 6.9 [28]. The BSA preparations tested negative for endotoxin [29]. The BSA-FA and BSA treated mice were intraperitoneally given FGF21 (100 μg/kg, synthetized in our laboratory by gene engineering [30]) or the same volume saline as well as the FFA treatment for 10 days.

Type 1 diabetic mouse model. Type 1 diabetes was induced in FVB, C57BL/6J, and FGF21-KO mice with a single intraperitoneal injection of streptozotocin (STZ) at 150 mg/kg, since acute b cell damage due to STZ rapidly increases tissue lipid accumulation [31]. In addition, the mice treated with same dose STZ, which unsuccessfully developed hyperglycemia were used to identify whether diabetes, but STZ, was the only reason to cause the subsequent pathological changes. After hyperglycemia was diagnosed, diabetic mice were treated with or without FGF21 ($n = 6$) for 10 days. Then the mice were euthanized after collection of blood plasma and 24-h serum urea.

2.3 Measurements for renal function

Blood urea nitrogen (BioAssay Systems, Hayward, CA) were assayed in accordance with the manufacturers' instructions in the kits. Mouse urine was collected before the animals were euthanized. Urine albumin (Bethyl Laboratories, Montgomery, TX) and urinary creatinine (BioAssay Systems) were measured in accordance with the manufacturers' instructions. Urinary total protein-to-creatinine (PCR) and urinary albumin-to-creatinine ratio (ACR) were calculated.

2.4 Plasma and renal triglyceride (TG) assay

Plasma TG concentrations were measured using a TG assay kit (Cayman Chemicals, Ann Arbor, MI). For the renal TG assay, mouse kidneys were homogenized in $1 \times$ phosphate buffer saline (PBS). Tissue lipids were extracted with methanol: chloroform (1:2), dried in an evaporating centrifuge, and resuspended in 1% Triton X-100. A colorimetric assessment of renal TG levels was carried out using Triglyceride Assay Reagent (Thermo Fisher Scientific). Values were normalized to protein in homogenate before extraction, determined by the Bradford assay (Bio-Rad Laboratories, Hercules, CA).

2.5 Oil Red O staining for lipid accumulation

Cryosections from optimal cutting temperature medium (OCT)-embedded tissue samples of the kidney (10-mm thick) were fixed in 10% buffered formalin for 5 min at room temperature, stained with Oil Red O for 1 h, washed with 10% isopropanol, and then counterstained with hematoxylin (DAKO, Carpinteria, CA) for 30 s. A Nikon microscope (Nikon, Melville, NY) was used to capture the Oil Red O-stained tissue sections at 40 × magnification.

2.6 Terminal deoxynucleotidyl transferase-mediated dUTP nick end labeling (TUNEL) assay

Kidney tissue was fixed in 10% formalin and embedded in paraffin. Fixed kidney tissues were cut into 3-mm-thick blocks. The tissue blocks were embedded in paraffin and cut into 5-μm slices. After deparaffinization (using xylene and ethanol dilutions) and rehydration the sections were stained for TUNEL with an ApopTag Peroxidase *In Situ* Apoptosis Detection Kit (Chemicon, CA, USA), as described in previous studies [32]. Briefly, each slide was deparaffinized and rehydrated, and treated with proteinase K (20 mg/L) for 15 min. The endogenous peroxidase was inhibited with 3% hydrogen peroxide for 5 min, and then incubated with the TUNEL reaction mixture containing terminal deoxynucleotidyl transferase (TdT) and digoxigenin-11-dUTP for 1 h. The TdT reaction was carried out in a humidified chamber at 37 ℃, and then 3,3-diaminobenzidine chromogen was applied. Hematoxylin was used as counterstaining. For the negative control, TdT was omitted from the reaction mixture. Apoptotic cell death was quantitatively analyzed by counting the TUNEL-positive cells selected randomly from 10 fields, at 40 × magnification. Results were presented as the number of TUNEL-positive cells per 10^3 cells.

2.7 Western blot assays

Western blot assays were performed as described previously [33]. Briefly, renal tissues were homogenized in lysis buffer. Proteins were collected by centrifuging at 12 000 × g at 4 ℃. A sample of total protein was subjected to electrophoresis in a 10% SDS-PAGE gel. After electrophoresis of the gel and transferring the proteins to a nitrocellulose membrane, these membranes were rinsed briefly in tris-buffered saline, blocked in blocking buffer (5% milk and 0.5% BSA) for 1 h, and washed three times with tris-buffered saline containing 0.05% Tween 20 (TBST). The membranes were incubated serially with different primary antibodies (below) overnight at 4 ℃, washed with TBST and incubated with secondary horseradish peroxidase-conjugated antibody for 1 h at room temperature. Antigen-antibody complexes were then visualized using an enhanced chemiluminescence kit (Amersham, Piscataway, NJ). The intensity of protein bands on blots was quantified by densitometric scanning (Epson perfection V700 photo, Epson) and analyzed by Quantity One software (Bio Rad).

The primary antibodies were against 3-nitrotyrosine (3-NT; 1:1000, Chemicon), 4-hydroxynonenal (4-HNE; 1:2000; Calbiochem, San Diego, CA), intercellular adhesion molecule-1 (ICAM- 1; 1:500; Santa Cruz Biotechnology, Santa Cruz, CA), anti-connective tissue growth factor (CTGF), β-actin (1:1000; Santa Cruz), plasminogen activator inhibitor type 1 (PAI-1; 1:2000, BD Biosciences, Sparks, MD), and tumor necrosis factor (TNF-α, 1:500, Cell Signaling Technology, Danvers, MA).

2.8 Statistical analyses

Data were collected from 6 mice per group and presented as mean ± standard deviation (SD). One-way ANOVA was used to determine general differences, followed by a *post-hoc* Tukey's test for the difference between groups, using Origin 7.5 software for laboratory data analysis and graphing. Statistical significance was considered $P<0.05$.

3. Results

3.1 FGF21 prevented hyperlipidemia-induced renal damage

3.1.1 FGF21 prevented acute hyperlipidemia-induced renal dysfunction

FVB mice were injected intraperitoneally BSA-FA (10 mg/g) with or without simultaneous administration of FGF21 (100 μg/kg) for 10 days (Table 1). The ratio of kidney weight to tibia length (KW/TL) and renal function were calculated. The results showed that the mean KW/TL was significantly higher in the mice of the BSA-FA group than in the BSA and control groups. In addition, FFA induced renal dysfunction characterized by higher ratio of urinary total protein to creatinine (PCR), and the ratio of urinary albumin-to-creatinine ratio (ACR). Although BUN of both BSA and BSA-FA treated mice tended to be higher compared to the mice in control group, the difference were not statistically significant respectively (Table 1). The rises of BUN, PCR and ACR were further enhanced inBSA-FFA treated mice. In contrast, administration of FGF21 significantly prevented lipotoxicity induced kidney weight increase (a feature of renal hypertrophy) and renal dysfunction (Table 1).

Table 1.   Effect of FGF21 on lipotoxicity-induced renal hypertrophy and dysfunction

	Control	FGF21	BSA	BSA-FA	BSA-FA/FGF21
KW/TL (mg/mm)	17.55 ± 3.53	17.64 ± 2.71	21.42 ± 5.53	$23.97 \pm 2.13^{*}$	$18.98 \pm 2.57^{\$}$
PCR (mg/mg)	24.45 ± 3.52	25.56 ± 4.37	$79.33 \pm 6.23^{*}$	$247.12 \pm 12.21^{*\#}$	$114.76 \pm 9.26^{\$}$
BUN (mg/dl)	34.11 ± 5.67	37.83 ± 7.36	45.33 ± 16.23	52.18 ± 15.49	37.16 ± 6.25
ACR (μg/mg)	107.43 ± 11.23	116.58 ± 12.35	$16471.76 \pm 179.11^{*}$	$36188.34 \pm 198.97^{*\#}$	$10079.21 \pm 106.72^{\$}$

$^{*}P < 0.05$ compared with control; $^{\#}P < 0.05$ compared with BSA group; $^{\$}P < 0.05$ compared with BSA-FA group.

3.1.2 FGF21 prevented lipotoxicity induced renal apoptosis.

Renal dysfunction always initiates with apoptosis, which can be caused by lipotoxicity [16]. We tried to identify whether FGF21 had a protective effect against renal apoptosis upon injection of excess lipid. TUNEL staining showed larger numbers of apoptotic cells in the BSA-FA treated mice but not in either the FGF21 or BSA groups (Fig. 1). However, administration of FGF21 significantly prevented FFA-induced renal apoptosis. In addition, the combined results of 3 independent experiments observing TUNEL-positive cells revealed that FGF21 almost completely prevented FFA-induced renal apoptosis (Fig. 1B).

3.1.3 FGF21 prevented FFA induced lipid accumulation in the kidney

Excessive lipid accumulation is the principle instigator of renal damage caused by lipotoxicity. We found that the administration of FGF21 significantly prevented lipotoxicity-induced renal apoptosis and dysfunction. Therefore, we tried to identify whether the renal protection provided by FGF21 was associated with suppression of renal lipid accumulation. We detected plasma and renal TG levels as well as lipid accumulation in the kidneys of the mice of the treatment groups. The results showed that under normal conditions, neither FGF21 nor BSA had any impact on plasma or renal TG levels, but these were significantly higher after 10 days of BSA-FFA treatments (Fig. 2A, B). FGF21 remarkably lowered FFA-induced renal TG levels but had no impact on plasma TG levels although a decrease tendency was observed (Fig. 2B). In addition, Oil Red O staining also confirmed that FFA significantly increased lipid accumulation in the kidney, which was strongly attenuated by FGF21 treatment (Fig. 2C).

3.1.4 FGF21 prevented lipotoxicity induced inflammation, oxidative stress and fibrotic effect

Inflammation is a principal pathological consequence of lipotoxicity, characterized by the release of multiple inflammatory factors. Results of a recent study suggested that FGF21 prevented cardiac hypertrophy via suppression of inflammation [20]. Thus, we next determined whether the renal protective effect associ-

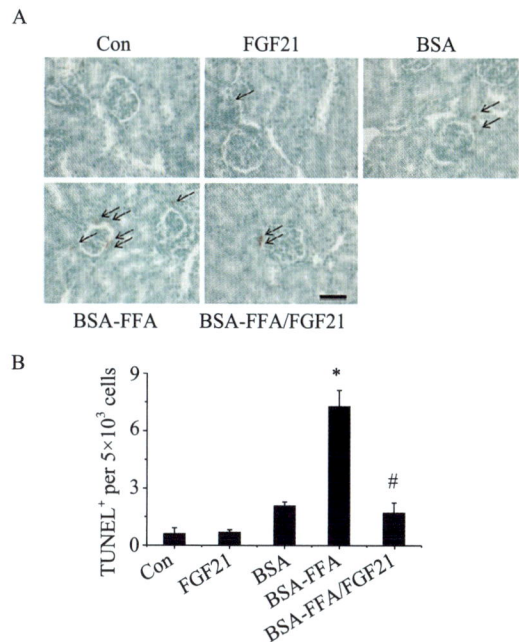

Fig. 1. FGF21 prevents FFA-induced renal apoptosis. FVB mice were intraperitoneal injection with FFA (10 mg/g) with and without FGF21 (100 μg/kg) for 10 days. Renal apoptosis was examined with TUNEL staining (A) and semi-quantitative analysis for apoptotic examination was scored (B). Data are presented as mean ± SD ($n = 6$ at least in each group). $^{*}P < 0.05$ compared with control. $^{\#}P < 0.05$ compared with BSA-FFA.

ated with FGF21 against lipotoxicity was directly anti-inflammatory. The protein levels of the classic inflammatory factors ICAM-1, TNF-α, and PAI-1 were detected *via* Western blot assay. The results revealed that FFA strongly upregulated the expressions of ICAM-1, TNF-α, and PAI-1 in the kidney (Fig. 3A–C), but these effects were not observed in either the FGF21 or BSA groups (Fig. 3A–C). Administration of FGF21 almost completely reversed the FFA-induced upregulation of renal ICAM-1 expression from the baseline (Fig. 3A) and significantly attenuated both TNF-α and PAI-1 expression in the kidney (Fig. 3B, C).

Renal inflammatory responses are always associated with oxidative stress and pro-fibrotic effects [34–40]. *Via* Western blot, we determined the effect of FGF21 on lipotoxicity-induced oxidative stress by measuring 3-NT as an index of nitrosative damage (Fig. 3D) and 4-HNE (lipid peroxide) as an index of oxidative damage (Fig. 3E); CTGF, an index of fibrosis, was considered a reflection of the fibrotic effect (Fig. 3F). The results indicated that FFA strongly upregulated 3-NT, 4-HNE, and CTGF expression in the kidney, which were significantly suppressed by FGF21 treatment. However, under normal conditions, neither FGF21 nor BSA had any impact on renal 3-NT, 4-HNE, or CTGF expression (Fig. 3).

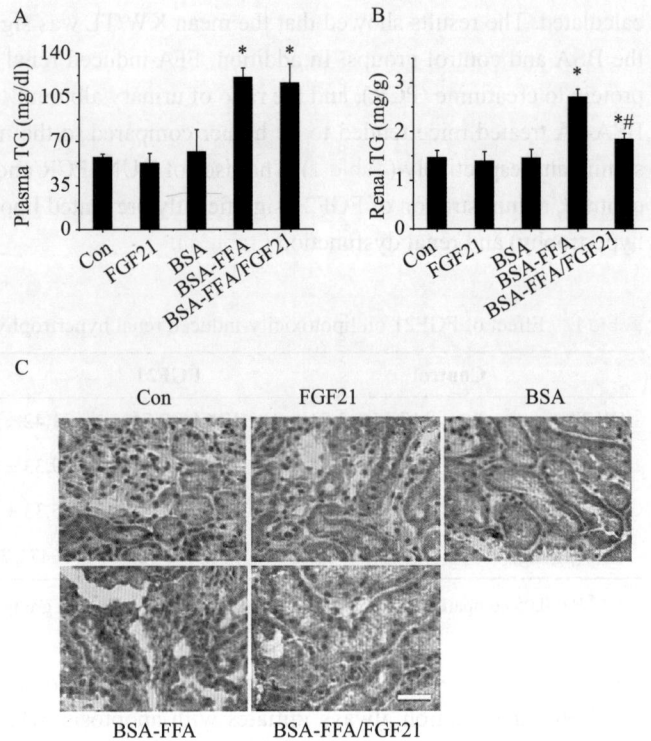

Fig. 2. FGF21 prevents FFA-induced renal lipid accumulation. The FFA injection mouse models were prepared as in Fig. 1. The plasma and renal tissue were collected. Plasma TG (A) and renal TG (B) were examined by ELISA kits and TG reagent respectively. Renal lipid accumulation was examined by Oil Red O staining (C, 40 ×). Data are presented as mean ± SD ($n = 6$ at least in each group). $^*P < 0.05$ compared with control. $^\#P < 0.05$ compared with BSA-FFA.

3.2 FGF21 prevented diabetes induced kidney disease

3.2.1 FGF21 prevented renal dysfunction under diabetic conditions

There is much evidence to support that lipotoxicity is a key component in the pathogenesis of DKD [7–9,41–43]. Thus, we next determined whether FGF21 had protective effect against diabetes-induced renal pathological changes, and if so, whether the possible protective mechanism was attributable to an anti-lipotoxic role. FVB mice were intraperitoneally injected with a single high dose of STZ (150 mg/kg) to induce type 1 diabetes. Then diabetic mice and age-matched non-diabetic mice were further stratified into groups with and without treatment of FGF21 (100 μg/kg) daily for 10 days. KW/TL and renal function were determined (Table 2). The results showed that the mouse diabetic model had slightly but not significantly higher KW/TL, PCR, BUN, and ACR compared to the control group. After treatment with FGF21, the tendencies toward higher levels of these indices were no longer present, but all were at normal levels (Table 2). However, under normal conditions, FGF21 had no impact on the kidney weight or renal function.

Table 2. Effect of FGF21 on diabetes-induced renal hypertrophy and dysfunction

	Control	FGF21	DM	DM/FGF21
KW/TL (mg/mm)	17.63 ± 4.11	17.25 ± 3.07	21.73 ± 4.46	18.98 ± 4.54
PCR (mg/mg)	25.55 ± 4.98	25.65 ± 3.47	27.12 ± 5.21	25.55 ± 4.17
BUN (mg/dl)	36.43 ± 4.23	37.38 ± 5.64	39.49 ± 4.98	37.61 ± 5.15
ACR (mg/mg)	103.3 ± 68.55	107.64 ± 7.17	113.09 ± 10.71	109.12 ± 10.33

Note: DM means diabetes mellitus.

3.2.2 FGF21 prevented renal apoptosis under diabetic conditions

Diabetes-induced renal damage usually initiates with tubular cell apoptosis [44]. Thus, we next determined whether

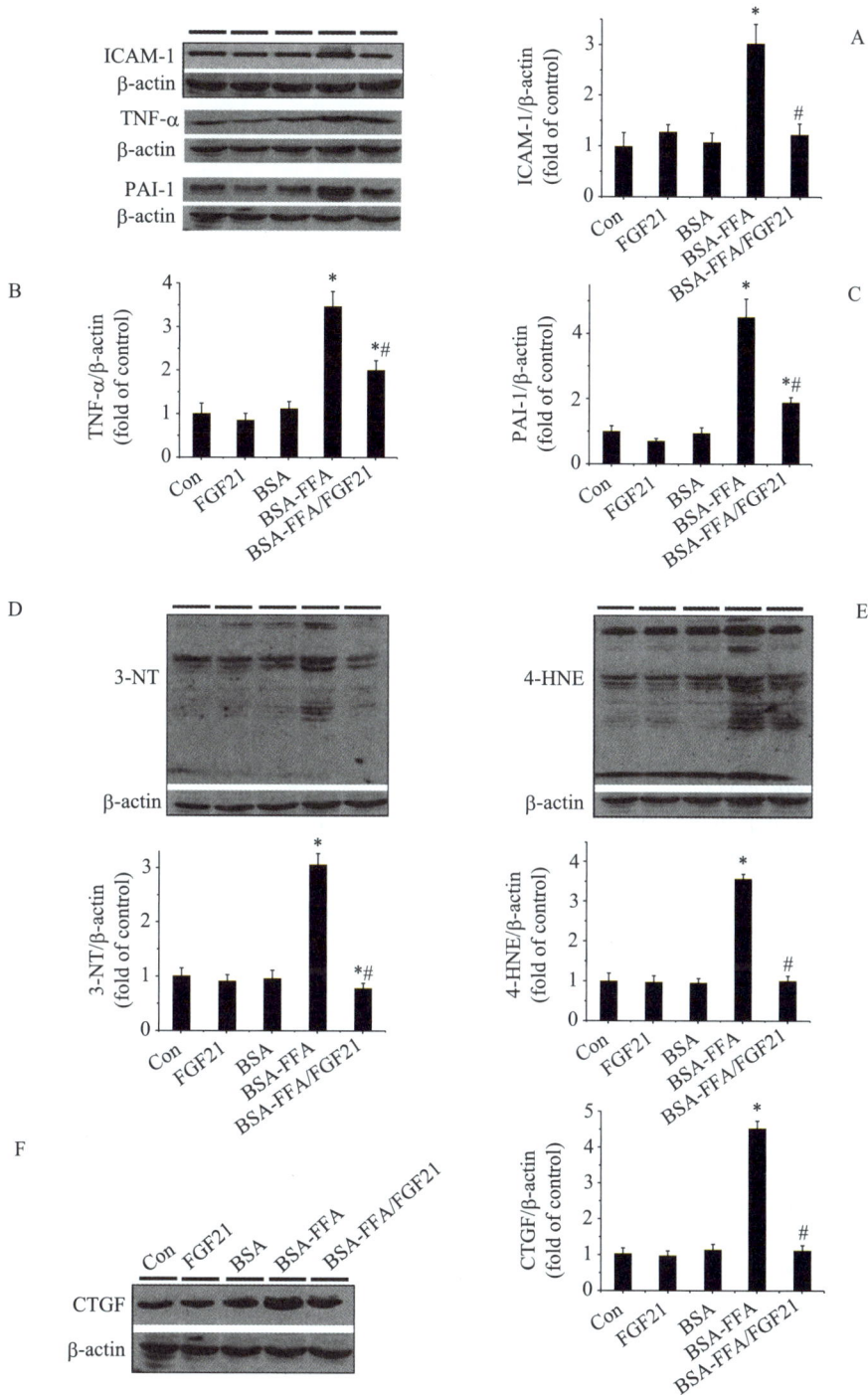

Fig. 3. FGF21 prevented FFA-induced inflammation oxidative damage and fibrotic effect. Renal expression of inflammatory factors, including ICAM -1 (A), TNF-α (B), and PAI -1 (C) was examined by Western blotting. Renal oxidative damage was examined by Western blot for the expression of 3-NT as an index of protein nitration (D) and 4-HNE as an index of lipid peroxidation (E). Renal fibrotic effect was measured by Western blot for the expression of CTGF (F). Data are presented as mean ± SD ($n = 6$ at least in each group). *$P < 0.05$ compared with control. #$P < 0.05$ compared with BSA-FFA.

FGF21 can protect renal cells from apoptosis induced by diabetes. TUNEL staining was performed in renal tissues of the mice from each group (Fig. 4). Increased positive staining for apoptosis was observed in the kidney of diabetic mice, which was significantly prevented by FGF21 treatment. The combined results of TUNEL-positive cells from 3 independent experiments are quantitatively summarized in Fig. 4B, which shows that FGF21 remarkably prevented diabetes-induced renal apoptosis.

3.2.3 FGF21 prevented diabetes induced lipid accumulation in the kidney

Compared to the untreated diabetic model, mice treated with FFA is more likely to cause renal lipotoxicity and further amplify the damage signal. Although the renal function of the diabetic mice was only slightly impaired, we still found that FGF21 had a protective effect. Thus whether FGF21 can decrease lipid accumulation in the kidney needed to be determined. We detected the plasma and renal TG levels, and lipid accumulation in the kidneys, of the mice in the different groups. In control group, FGF21 had no impact on either plasma or renal TG levels (Fig. 5A, B), but these were significantly higher in the diabetic mice (Fig. 5A, B). Although FGF21 slightly suppressed diabetes-induced plasma TGs, there was no significant difference between the untreated diabetic model mice and diabetic mice treated with FGF21 (Fig. 5A). In contrast, FGF21 significantly suppressed diabetes-induced elevations in renal TG levels (Fig. 5B). In addition, Oil Red O staining revealed that diabetes strongly increased lipid accumulation in the kidney, which was significantly attenuated by FGF21 treatment (Fig. 5C).

3.2.4 FGF21 prevented diabetes induced inflammation, oxidative stress and fibrotic effect

Based on our finding that FGF21 prevented lipotoxicity-induced renal inflammation, oxidative stress, and fibrosis we next examined whether FGF21 had a beneficial effect against DKD. The Western blot assay revealed that in normal mice, FGF21 had no influence on the expression of renal ICAM-1, TNF-α, or

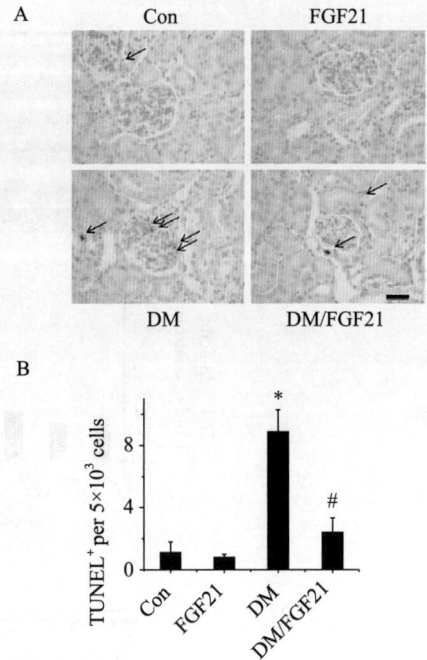

Fig. 4. FGF21 prevents diabetes-induced cardiac apoptosis. Type 1 diabetes was induced with STZ (150 mg/kg). Diabetic and age-matched control mice were administered daily intraperitoneal injections of FGF21 (100 μg/kg) or PBS for 10 days. Renal apoptosis was examined with TUNEL staining (A) and semi-quantitative analysis for apoptotic examination was scored (B). Data are presented as mean ± SD ($n = 6$ at least in each group). *$P<0.05$ compared with control. #$P<0.05$ compared with diabetes (DM).

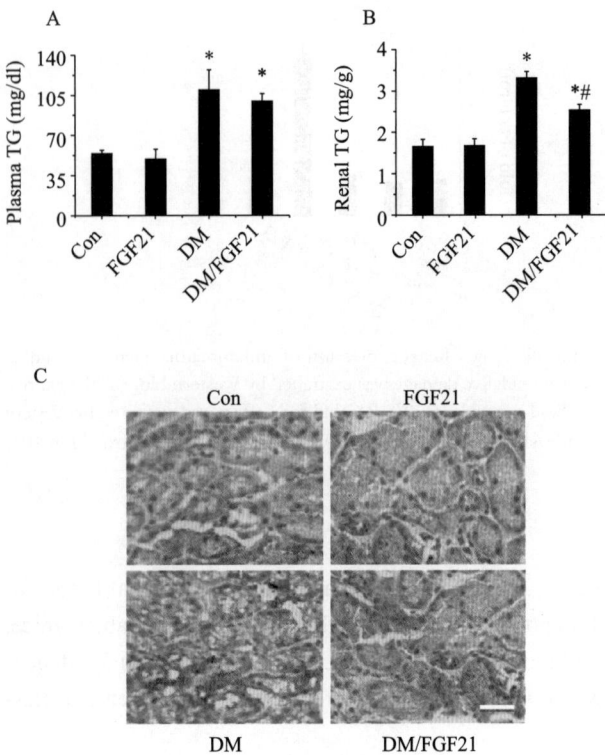

Fig. 5. FGF21 prevents diabetes-induced renal lipid accumulation. The diabetic mouse models were prepared as in Fig. 4. The plasma and renal tissue were collected. Plasma TG (A) and renal TG (B) were examined by ELISA kits and TG reagent respectively. Renal lipid accumulation was examined by Oil Red Staining (C, 40×). Data are presented as mean ± SD ($n = 6$ at least in each group). *$P<0.05$ compared with control. #$P<0.05$ compared with diabetes (DM).

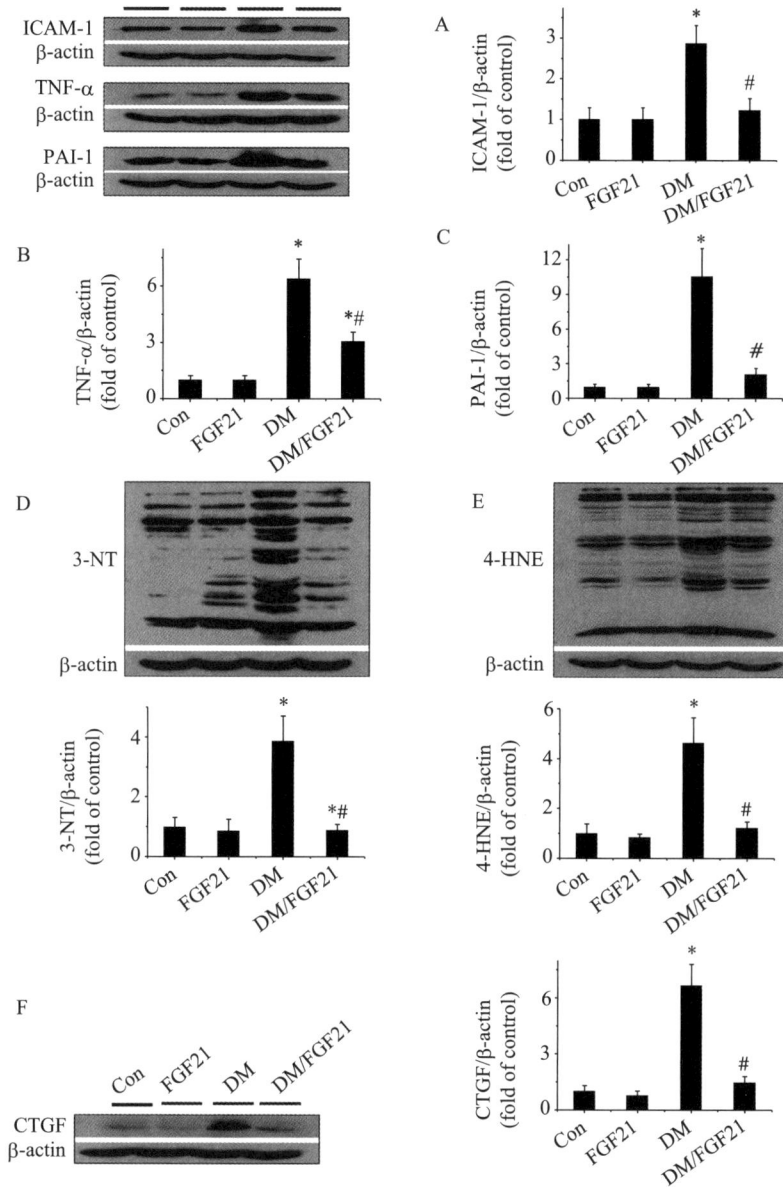

Fig. 6. FGF21 prevented diabetes-induced inflammation, oxidative damage and fibrotic effect. Renal expression of inflammatory factors, including ICAM -1 (A), TNF-α (B), and PAI -1 (C) was examined by Western blotting. Renal oxidative damage was examined by Western blotting assay for the expression of 3-NT as an index of protein nitration (D) and 4-HNE as an index of lipid peroxidation (E). Renal fibrotic effect was measured by Western-blotting for the expression of CTGF (F). Data are presented as mean ± SD (n = 6 at least in each group). $^{*}P<0.05$ compared with control. $^{#}P<0.05$ compared with diabetes (DM).

PAI-1, levels of which were strongly elevated in diabetic mice (Fig. 6A–C). However, administration of FGF21 almost completely suppressed the increased expression of all these inflammatory factors induced by diabetes in the kidney (Fig. 6A–C). Additionally we found that diabetes increased renal 3-NT, 4-HNE, and CTGF expression, which were also significantly suppressed by FGF21 treatment (Fig. 6D–F).

3.3 Deficiency of FGF21 enhanced diabetes induced pathological changes in the kidney

3.3.1 Deficiency of FGF21 aggravated diabetes-induced chronic renal dysfunction

In the present study, type 1 diabetes was induced in both C57BL/6J and FGF21-KO mice. Diabetic mice and age-matched non-diabetic mice were divided into groups with and without treatment of FGF21 (100 µg/kg) daily for either 10 days or 3 months. The results showed that diabetes significantly induced kidney weight increase and dysfunction in FGF21-KO mice at the early-stage of diabetes, which was not found in C57BL/6J mice (Table 3). In C57BL/6J mice,

278 ▶▶ Fibroblast Growth Factors, Second Edition

a slight increase in KW/TL, PCR, BUN, and ACR became significant at 80 days with diabetes, which was further enhanced in FGF-KO mice (Table 3). However, administration of FGF21 remarkably prevented diabetes-induced renal dysfunction and hypertrophy.

Table 3. Renal function under diabetic condition in both C57BL/6J and FGF21-KO mice

		KW/TL (mg/mm)		PCR (mg/mg)		BUN (mg/dl)		ACR (μg/mg)	
		10 d	80 d	10 d	80 d	10 d	80 d	10 d	80 d
Control	C57BL/6J	18.06 ± 3.91	18.55 ± 4.14	25.65 ± 4.32	24.32 ± 4.28	37.83 ± 3.58	31.69 ± 4.39	106.96 ± 5.15	112.97 ± 10.49
	FGF21-KO	18.44 ± 3.79	19.86 ± 4.13	24.14 ± 3.98	24.73 ± 4.45	36.99 ± 4.87	31.64 ± 3.36	107.12 ± 5.64	110.92 ± 9.47
DM	C57BL/6J	21.66 ± 3.21	27.15 ± 2.92	28.46 ± 3.23	201.44 ± 14.32	39.14 ± 5.15	49.93 ± 5.75	114.77 ± 7.64	21324.32 ± 121.68
	FGF21-KO	26.13 ± 3.59	35.65 ± 1.35^{a,b}	103.44 ± 9.85	253.43 ± 15.38^{a,b}	47.92 ± 4.61	61.11 ± 9.58^{a,b}	10986.36 ± 98.91	28974.13 ± 115.67^{a,b}
STZ	C57BL/6J	18.54 ± 4.14	18.64 ± 1.52	24.75 ± 4.87	24.84 ± 3.19	37.11 ± 5.19	31.43 ± 3.54	104.63 ± 7.72	114.45 ± 9.64
	FGF21-KO	18.87 ± 3.19	19.51 ± 4.6	25.12 ± 4.33	23.39 ± 4.69	36.23 ± 3.97	31.65 ± 4.38	106.05 ± 5.07	113.44 ± 12.79
DM/ FGF21	FGF21-KO	19.64 ± 4.01	21.89 ± 2.79^c	25.35 ± 3.71	101.32 ± 10.79^{a,c}	37.31 ± 5.41	41.16 ± 4.29^{a,c}	108.15 ± 9.04	18008.33 ± 126.47^{a,c}

$^a P < 0.05$ compared with corresponding control; $^b P < 0.05$ compared with DM in C57BL/6J mice; $^c P < 0.05$ compared with corresponding DM.

3.3.2 Deficiency of FGF21 aggravated diabetes induced renal lipid accumulation and apoptosis

Renal apoptosis and lipid accumulation were examined and compared between C57BL/6J and FGF21-KO mice under either the normal or diabetic condition. We found in the C57BL/6J mice that diabetes, but not STZ, strongly induced renal apoptosis, which was further enhanced in FGF21-KO mice. Administration of FGF21 significantly protected renal cells from apoptosis induced by diabetes (Fig. 7A, B). Furthermore, we found that the diabetes, rather than STZ, significantly increased both plasma and renal TG levels in C57BL/6J mice, which was further aggravated in FGF21-KO mice (Fig. 7C, D). Administration of FGF21 had no influence on plasma TG levels (Fig. 7C), but showed great lowering effect on renal TG levels (Fig. 7D). Oil Red O staining confirmed that deficiency of FGF21 further enhanced diabetes-induced lipid accumulation in the kidney, which was significantly attenuated by administration of FGF21 (Fig. 7E).

3.3.3 Deficiency of FGF21 aggravated diabetes-induced inflammation, oxidative stress, and fibrotic effect

Western-blot assay revealed that diabetes, but not STZ significantly upregulated ICAM-1, TNF-α, and PAI-1 expression in the kidneys of C57BL/6J mice, which were further increased in FGF21-KO mice (Fig. 8A–C). Deficiency of FGF21 also further enhanced diabetes-induced oxidative stress and fibrotic effect by upregulation of the expression of renal 3-NT/4HNE and CTGF (Fig. 8 D–F). Administration of FGF21 greatly attenuated diabetes- induced renal inflammation, oxidative stress, and fibrotic effect in FGF21-KO mice (Fig. 8A–F).

4. Discussion

In the present study, the lipotoxic mouse model was induced by intraperitoneal injection of FFA bound to BSA (10 mg/g) as described previously [27,28]. In this model, FFA bound to albumin had a role in the generation of tubulointerstitial disease associated with the release of inflammatory factors, which in turn enhanced tubulointerstitial damage. In the present study, acute injection of FFA induced renal dysfunction, characterized by an increase in PCR and ACR. Furthermore, the kidney weight increased in FFA-treated mice, which was a sign of renal hypertrophy. These renal pathological changes indicated that the lipotoxic mouse model was successfully established (Table 1). We also found that administration of FGF21 significantly prevented lipotoxicity induced renal hypertrophy and dysfunction. It is generally accepted that renal dysfunction always initiates with apoptosis [44]. Thus, in the present study we determined whether the renal beneficial effect induced by FGF21 against lipotoxicity was attributed to anti-apoptosis. TUNEL staining showed that FFA injection significantly induced apoptosis in the kidney, but a similar phenomenon was not found in BSA-treated mice, and this apoptosis was remarkably attenuated by administration of FGF21. This result confirmed that FGF21-induced renal protection against lipotoxicity was due to an anti-apoptotic effect.

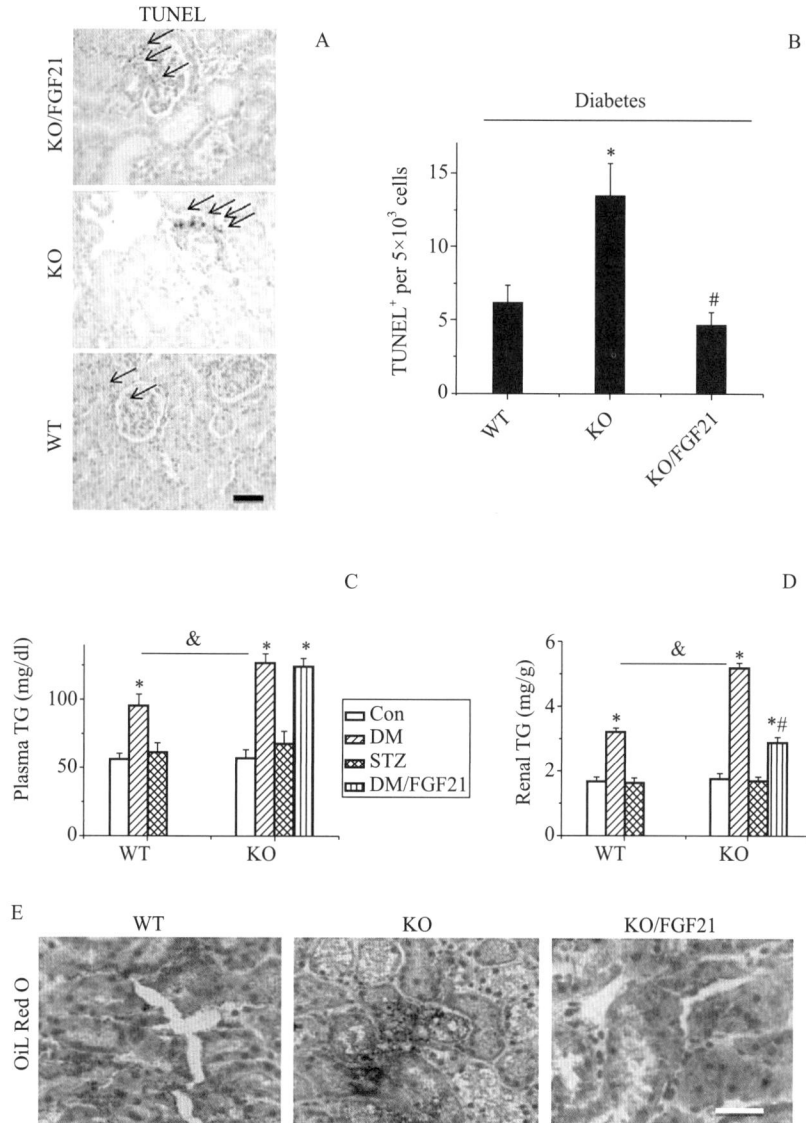

Fig. 7. FGF21-KO mice were more sensitive to diabetes-induced cardiac apoptosis and lipid accumulation. FGF21-KO and C57BL/6J (C57BL/6J) mice were induced as diabetic with STZ (200 mg/kg) and treated with FGF21 (100 μg/kg) for 10 days. Renal apoptosis was detected with TUNEL staining (A). Quantitative data presented as (B) The plasma and renal tissue were collected. Plasma TG (C) and renal TG (D) were examined by ELISA kits and TG reagent respectively. Renal lipid accumulation was examined by Oil Red Staining (E, 40 ×). Data are presented as mean ± SD ($n = 6$ at least in each group). [*]$P < 0.05$ compared with corresponding control. [#]$P < 0.05$ compared with corresponding diabetes (DM). [&]$P < 0.05$ compared with DM in wild type group.

In the present study, we found for the first time that FGF21 has a crucial role in renal protection against lipotoxicity by preventing renal apoptosis and dysfunction. Subsequent to this finding, we attempted to determine the underlying mechanisms of this protective effect. Previously we found that FGF21 lowered cellular lipid accumulation through enhancement of fatty acid oxidation and lipolysis. Therefore we had to identify whether the lipid-lowering effect attributed to FGF21 induced renal protection. We determined the renal TG levels and lipid accumulation among the treatment groups, and found FFA significantly increased lipid accumulation and TG levels in kidney tissues, which was remarkably suppressed by administration of FGF21. However, no similar phenomenon was found in plasma TG levels. This implies that FGF21-induced renal protection was specifically due to a lipid-lowering effect in the kidney rather than through systematic lipid metabolism. Simultaneously we found that FGF21 significantly, but not completely, lowered renal lipid accumulation, suggesting that FGF21 induced renal protection only partially by lessening renal lipid accumulation. Other protective mechanisms are probable.

The inflammatory response is considered one of the major mechanisms by which lipotoxicity causes renal oxidative injury, fibrosis, and dysfunction [45-48]. This process includes diverse inflammatory molecules, for example, increases in

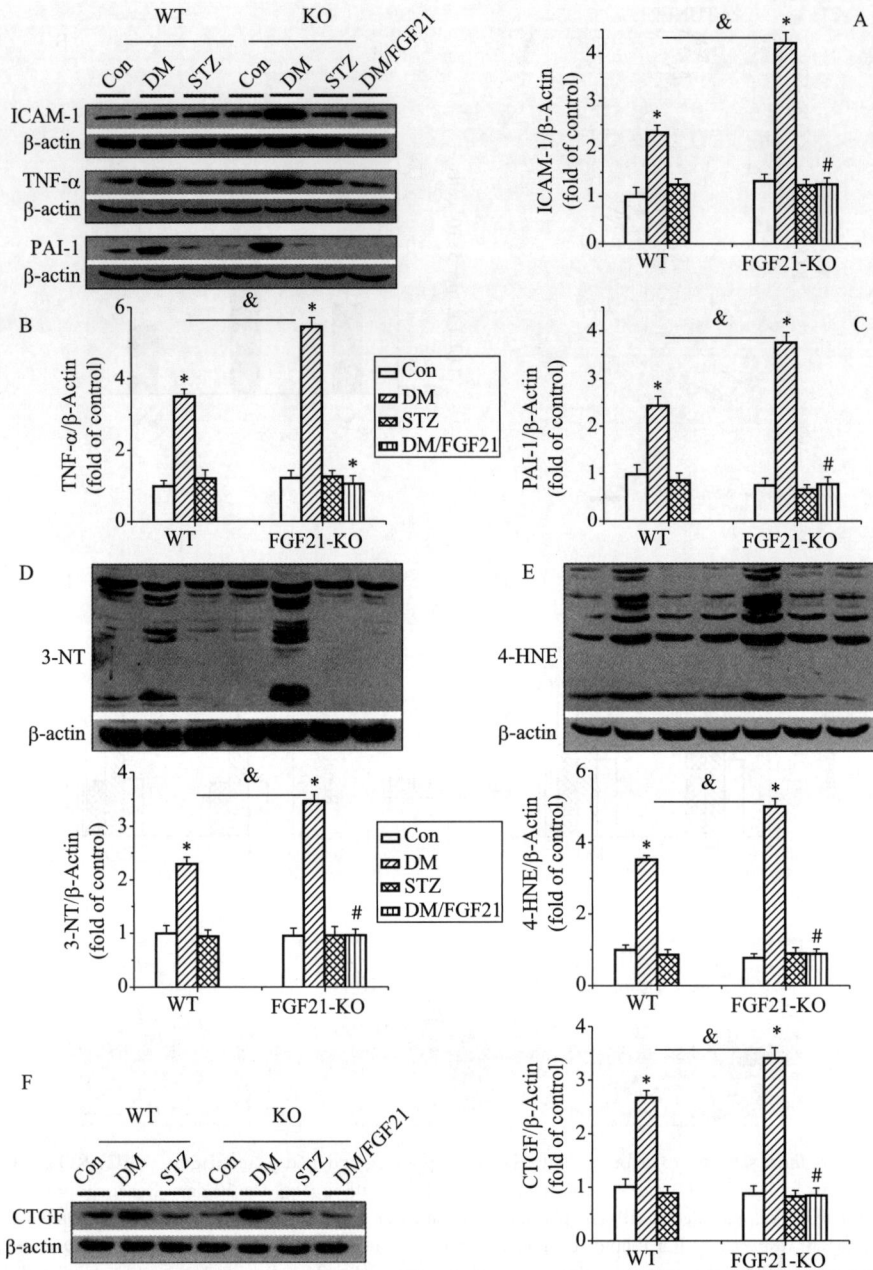

Fig. 8. FGF-21 KO further enhances diabetes induced renal inflammation, oxidative damge and fibrotic effect. Renal expression of inflammatory factors, including ICAM-1 (A), TNF-α (B), and PAI-1 (C) was examined by Western blotting. Renal oxidative damage was examined by Western blotting assay for the expression of 3-NT as an index of protein nitration (D) and 4-HNE as an index of lipid peroxidation (E). Renal fibrotic effect was measured by Western-blotting for the expression of CTGF (F). Data are presented as mean ± SD (n = 6 at least in each group). $^{*}P$ < 0.05 compared with corresponding control. $^{#}P$ < 0.05 compared with corresponding diabetes (DM). $^{&}P$ < 0.05 compared with DM in wild type group.

ICAM-1 lead to inflammatory cell migration in renal inflammatory pathogenesis [49]. TNF-α contributes significantly to sodium retention and renal hypertrophy and alters the barrier function of the glomerular capillary wall, resulting in an enhanced albumin permeability [34,35,49].

In our study, we found significant increases in the renal expression of the proinflammatory cytokines ICAM-1, TNF-α, and PAI-1 induced by FFA injection. A consequence of the inflammatory response is the overgeneration of reactive oxygen species that induces oxidative and nitrosative damage character ized by increased renal accumulation of 3-NT and 4-HNE [50,51]. Our study also confirmed that FFA strongly upregulated the expressions of renal 3-NT and 4-HNE. Moreover, since PAI-1 also promotes collagen deposition by stimulating migration of leukocytes and collagen-producing cells into damaged tissues finally leading to fibrosis [38,52], it is also considered a fibrotic factor. Analysis of another fibrotic marker, CTGF, in the kidney also proved that lipotoxicity strongly induced fibrosis as well as elevating inflammation and oxidative stress. However, all the above pathological changes induced by lipotoxicity were significantly prevented by FGF21 treatment. This suggests that FGF21-induced renal protection against acute lipotoxicity was not only due to lowering lipid accumulation but also to the inhibition of subsequent inflammation, oxidative stress, and fibrotic effect in the kidney.

The kidney is one of the main organs damaged by diabetes, leading to DKD and subsequent diabetic nephropathy, and accompanied by an increased risk of cardiovascular disease [53], decreased quality of life, increases in financial costs to the patient and society, and shortened life span [53]. Since lipotoxicity is a key pathogenic cause of DKD [7-9,41], we investigated whether FGF21 can induce similar renal protection in a diabetic model as in the FFA injection model, and if so, whether this protection was associated with attenuation of diabetic lipotoxicity and subsequent inflammation, oxidative stress, and fibrotic effect. To answer these questions, type 1 diabetic mice induced by STZ and age-matched non-diabetic mice were treated with or without FGF21 for either 10 days or 80 days. We found at the early stage (10 days) that, although renal hypertrophy and dysfunction was not observed, diabetes significantly induced renal apoptosis and an increase of lipid accumulation and subsequent inflammation, oxidative stress, and fibrotic effect, which were remarkably prevented by FGF21 treatment. In contrast, at 80 days renal hypertrophy and dysfunction were observed in the diabetic mice, evidenced by increases in BUN, PCR and ACR. Administration of FGF21 significantly prevented renal damage-induced diabetes. This indicates that FGF21 induced renal protection against early-stage renal apoptosis and late-stage renal dysfunction due to diabetes, through prevention of lipid accumulation and subsequent inflammation, oxidative stress, and fibrotic effect.

We also found that diabetes induced renal lipotoxicity, and the subsequent pathological changes were further enhanced in FGF21-KO mice. Similar phenomena were not found in STZ-treated mice which unsuccessfully developed hyperglycemia. Administration of FGF21 significantly prevented renal damage induced by diabetes. This suggests that all the pathological changes were induced by diabetes, and not by STZ *per se*. In addition, FGF21-KO mice were more sensitive to diabetes- induced renal injury, which was remarkably prevented by FGF21 treatment through the mechanism of lowering lipid accumulation, and by anti-inflammation, anti-oxidation, and anti-fibrosis effects.

Mechanistically the beneficial effect of FGF21 against oxidative stress, inflammation and fibrosis may related to the activation of adenosine 5′-monophosphate-activated protein kinase (AMPK) induced signaling pathway [54]. AMPK is a crucial kinase in eukaryotes, which induced multiple bio-functions by activation of the downstream Sirtuin (SirT)1-peroxisome proliferator activated receptor co-activator (PGC) 1α signaling pathway [7,54]. Increasing evidence showed that activation of AMPK-SirT1-PGC1α pathway prevented inflammation and oxidative stress through inhibiting NF-κB function and promoting fatty-acid β-oxidation as well as antioxidant expressions [55–60]. Moreover, it is reported that AMPK also participated in anti-fibrosis by inhibiting TGF-β1 to ameliorate renal fibrosis and structure alterations [61]. Reportedly AMPK signaling pathway can be activated by FGF21 through up-regulating the expression of AMPK activator liver kinase B1 (LKB1) [62], which implied that AMPK may be the mediator for FGF21-induced anti-oxidative stress, anti-inflammation, and anti-fibrosis in the kidney under diabetic conditions.

In summary, we report for the first time that administration of FGF21 can significantly prevent lipotoxicity- and diabetes-induced early-stage renal apoptosis, hypertrophy, and dysfunction, and significantly prevent renal lipid accumulation and subsequent inflammation, oxidative damage and fibrotic effect. Deficiency of FGF21 (in FGF21-KO mice) enhanced lipotoxicity and diabetes-induced renal damages, which were significantly prevented by intraperitoneal injection of FGF21. Therefore, our study suggests that FGF21 is a potential candidate for therapeutic application against DKD.

References

[1] Hakim FA, Pflueger A. Role of oxidative stress in diabetic kidney disease[J]. Medical Science Monitor, 2010, 16(2): RA37-RA48.

[2] Osterby R, Parving HH, Hommel E, *et al.* Glomerular structure and function in diabetic nephropathy. Early to advanced stages[J]. Diabetes, 1990, 39(9): 1057-1063.

[3] Wu J, Guan T-j, Zheng S, *et al.* Inhibition of inflammation by pento-

san polysulfate impedes the development and progression of severe diabetic nephropathy in aging C57B6 mice[J]. Laboratory Investigation, 2011, 91(10): 1459-1471.

[4] Min D, Lyons JG, Bonner J, *et al.* Mesangial cell-derived factors alter monocyte activation and function through inflammatory pathways: possible pathogenic role in diabetic nephropathy[J]. American

Journal of Physiology-Renal Physiology, 2009, 297(5): F1229-F1237.

[5] Kim HW, Lee JE, Cha JJ, et al. Fibroblast growth factor 21 improves insulin resistance and ameliorates renal injury in db/db mice[J]. Endocrinology, 2013, 154(9): 3366-3376.

[6] Vlassara H, Uribarri J, Cai W, et al. Effects of sevelamer on HbA1c, inflammation, and advanced glycation end products in diabetic kidney disease[J]. Clinical Journal of the American Society of Nephrology, 2012, 7(6): 934-942.

[7] Kim MY, Lim JH, Youn HH, et al. Resveratrol prevents renal lipotoxicity and inhibits mesangial cell glucotoxicity in a manner dependent on the AMPK-SIRT1-PGC1 alpha axis in db/db mice[J]. Diabetologia, 2013, 56(1): 204-217.

[8] Shapiro H, Theilla M, Attal-Singer J, et al. Effects of polyunsaturated fatty acid consumption in diabetic nephropathy[J]. Nature Reviews Nephrology, 2011, 7(2): 110-121.

[9] Murea M, Freedman BI, Parks JS, et al. Lipotoxicity in diabetic nephropathy: The potential role of fatty acid oxidation[J]. Clinical Journal of the American Society of Nephrology, 2010, 5(12): 2373-2379.

[10] Moorhead JF, Elnahas M, Chan MK, et al. Lipid nephrotoxicity in chronic progressive glomerular and tubulo-interstitial disease[J]. Lancet, 1982, 2(8311): 1309-1311.

[11] Ruan XZ, Varghese Z, Moorhead JF. An update on the lipid nephrotoxicity hypothesis[J]. Nature Reviews Nephrology, 2009, 5(12): 713-721.

[12] Wahba IM, Mak RH. Obesity and obesity-initiated metabolic syndrome: Mechanistic links to chronic kidney disease[J]. Clinical Journal of the American Society of Nephrology, 2007, 2(3): 550-562.

[13] Bobulescu IA. Renal lipid metabolism and lipotoxicity[J]. Current Opinion in Nephrology and Hypertension, 2010, 19(4): 393-402.

[14] Wang XX, Jiang T, Shen Y, et al. The farnesoid X receptor modulates renal lipid metabolism and diet-induced renal inflammation, fibrosis, and proteinuria[J]. American Journal of Physiology-Renal Physiology, 2009, 297(6): F1587-F1596.

[15] Proctor G, Jiang T, Iwahashi M, et al. Regulation of renal fatty acid and cholesterol metabolism, inflammation, and fibrosis in Akita and OVE26 mice with type 1 diabetes[J]. Diabetes, 2006, 55(9): 2502-2509.

[16] Weinberg JM. Lipotoxicity[J]. Kidney International, 2006, 70(9): 1560-1566.

[17] Adams AC, Kharitonenkov A. FGF21: The center of a transcriptional nexus in metabolic regulation[J]. Current Diabetes Reviews, 2012, 8(4): 285-293.

[18] Cuevas-Ramos D, Almeda-Valdes P, Aguilar-Salinas CA, et al. The role of fibroblast growth factor 21 (FGF21) on energy balance, glucose and lipid metabolism[J]. Current Diabetes Reviews, 2009, 5(4): 216-220.

[19] Feingold KR, Grunfeld C, Heuer JG, et al. FGF21 is increased by inflammatory stimuli and protects leptin-deficient ob/ob mice from the toxicity of sepsis[J]. Endocrinology, 2012, 153(6): 2689-2700.

[20] Planavila A, Redondo I, Hondares E, et al. Fibroblast growth factor 21 protects against cardiac hypertrophy in mice[J]. Nature Communications, 2013, 4.

[21] Mraz M, Bartlova M, Lacinova Z, et al. Serum concentrations and tissue expression of a novel endocrine regulator fibroblast growth factor-21 in patients with type 2 diabetes and obesity[J]. Clinical Endocrinology, 2009, 71(3): 369-375.

[22] Tacer KF, Bookout AL, Ding X, et al. Research resource: Comprehensive expression atlas of the fibroblast growth factor system in adult mouse[J]. Molecular Endocrinology, 2010, 24(10): 2050-2064.

[23] Lin Z, Zhou Z, Liu Y, et al. Circulating FGF21 levels are progressively increased from the early to end stages of chronic kidney diseases and are associated with renal function in Chinese[J]. Plos One, 2011, 6(4).

[24] Crasto C, Semba RD, Sun K, et al. Serum fibroblast growth factor 21 is associated with renal function and chronic kidney disease in community-dwelling adults[J]. Journal of the American Geriatrics Society, 2012, 60(4): 792-793.

[25] Han SH, Choi SH, Cho BJ, et al. Serum fibroblast growth factor-21 concentration is associated with residual renal function and insulin resistance in end-stage renal disease patients receiving long-term peritoneal dialysis[J]. Metabolism-Clinical and Experimental, 2010, 59(11): 1656-1662.

[26] Thomas ME, Harris KPG, Walls J, et al. Fatty acids exacerbate tubulointerstitial injury in protein-overload proteinuria[J]. American Journal of Physiology-Renal Physiology, 2002, 283(4): F640-F647.

[27] Kamijo A, Kimura K, Sugaya T, et al. Urinary free fatty acids bound to albumin aggravate tubulointerstitial damage[J]. Kidney International, 2002, 62(5): 1628-1637.

[28] Thomas ME, Brunskill NJ, Harris KPG, et al. Proteinuria induces tubular cell turnover: A potential mechanism for tubular atrophy[J]. Kidney International, 1999, 55(3): 890-898.

[29] Wang H, Xiao Y, Fu L, et al. High-level expression and purification of soluble recombinant FGF21 protein by SUMO fusion in Escherichia coli[J]. Bmc Biotechnology, 2010, 10.

[30] Kewalramani G, An D, Kim MS, et al. AMPK control of myocardial fatty acid metabolism fluctuates with the intensity of insulin-deficient diabetes[J]. Journal of Molecular and Cellular Cardiology, 2007, 42(2): 333-342.

[31] Cai L, Wang Y, Zhou G, et al. Attenuation by metallothionein of early cardiac cell death via suppression of mitochondrial oxidative stress results in a prevention of diabetic cardiomyopathy[J]. Journal of the American College of Cardiology, 2006, 48(8): 1688-1697.

[32] Zhao Y, Tan Y, Dai J, et al. Exacerbation of diabetes-induced testicular apoptosis by zinc deficiency is most likely associated with oxidative stress, p38 MAPK activation, and p53 activation in mice[J]. Toxicology Letters, 2011, 200(1-2): 100-106.

[33] DiPetrillo K, Coutermarsh B, Gesek FA. Urinary tumor necrosis factor contributes to sodium retention and renal hypertrophy during diabetes[J]. American Journal of Physiology-Renal Physiology, 2003, 284(1): F113-F121.

[34] DiPetrillo K, Coutermarsh B, Soucy N, et al. Tumor necrosis factor induces sodium retention in diabetic rats through sequential effects on distal tubule cells[J]. Kidney International, 2004, 65(5): 1676-1683.

[35] Giunti S, Barit D, Cooper ME. Diabetic nephropathy: from mechanisms to rational therapies[J]. Minerva medica, 2006, 97(3): 241-262.

[36] Ichinose K, Kawasaki E, Eguchi K. Recent advancement of understanding pathogenesis of type 1 diabetes and potential relevance to diabetic nephropathy[J]. American Journal of Nephrology, 2007, 27(6): 554-564.

[37] Lee HB, Ha H. Plasminogen activator inhibitor-1 and diabetic nephropathy[J]. Nephrology, 2005, 10: S11-S13.

[38] Lin J, Glynn RJ, Rifai N, et al. Inflammation and progressive nephropathy in type 1 diabetes in the diabetes control and complications trial[J]. Diabetes Care, 2008, 31(12): 2338-2343.

[39] Navarro-Gonzalez JF, Mora-Fernandez C. The role of inflammatory cytokines in diabetic nephropathy[J]. Journal of the American Society of Nephrology, 2008, 19(3): 433-442.

[40] Dominguez J, Wu P, Packer CS, et al. Lipotoxic and inflammatory phenotypes in rats with uncontrolled metabolic syndrome and nephropathy[J]. American Journal of Physiology-Renal Physiology, 2007, 293(3): F670-F679.

[41] Rutkowski P, Klassen A, Sebekova K, et al. Renal disease in obesity: The need for greater attention[J]. Journal of Renal Nutrition, 2006, 16(3): 216-223.

[42] Leung RKK, Wang Y, Ma RCW, et al. Using a multi-staged strategy based on machine learning and mathematical modeling to pre-

dict genotype-phenotype risk patterns in diabetic kidney disease: a prospective case-control cohort analysis[J]. Bmc Nephrology, 2013, 14.

[43] Habib SL. Diabetes and renal tubular cell apoptosis[J]. World Journal of Diabetes, 2013, 4(2): 27-30.

[44] Savary S, Trompier D, Andreoletti P, et al. Fatty acids - Induced lipotoxicity and inflammation[J]. Current Drug Metabolism, 2012, 13(10): 1358-1370.

[45] Carroll WX, Kalupahana NS, Booker SL, et al. Angiotensinogen gene silencing reduces markers of lipid accumulation and inflammation in cultured adipocytes[J]. Frontiers in endocrinology, 2013, 4: 10-10.

[46] Zhang G, Li Q, Wang L, et al. The effects of inflammation on lipid accumulation in the kidneys of children with primary nephrotic syndrome[J]. Inflammation, 2011, 34(6): 645-652.

[47] Leite JO, DeOgburn R, Ratliff J, et al. Low-carbohydrate diets reduce lipid accumulation and arterial inflammation in guinea pigs fed a high-cholesterol diet[J]. Atherosclerosis, 2010, 209(2): 442-448.

[48] Rivero A, Mora C, Muros M, et al. Pathogenic perspectives for the role of inflammation in diabetic nephropathy[J]. Clinical Science, 2009, 116(5-6): 479-492.

[49] Zhang C, Lu X, Tan Y, et al. Diabetes-induced hepatic pathogenic damage, inflammation, oxidative stress, and insulin resistance was exacerbated in zinc deficient mouse model[J]. Plos One, 2012, 7(12).

[50] Zhang C, Tan Y, Guo W, et al. Attenuation of diabetes-induced renal dysfunction by multiple exposures to low-dose radiation is associated with the suppression of systemic and renal inflammation[J]. American Journal of Physiology-Endocrinology and Metabolism, 2009, 297(6): E1366-E1377.

[51] Rerolle JP, Hertig A, Nguyen G, et al. Plasminogen activator inhibitor type 1 is a potential target in renal fibrogenesis[J]. Kidney International, 2000, 58(5): 1841-1850.

[52] Stanton RC. Oxidative stress and diabetic kidney disease[J]. Current Diabetes Reports, 2011, 11(4): 330-336.

[53] Chang C-C, Chang C-Y, Wu Y-T, et al. Resveratrol retards progression of diabetic nephropathy through modulations of oxidative stress, proinflammatory cytokines, and AMP-activated protein kinase[J]. Journal of Biomedical Science, 2011, 18.

[54] Fang F, Liu GC, Kim C, et al. Adiponectin attenuates angiotensin II-induced oxidative stress in renal tubular cells through AMPK and cAMP-Epac signal transduction pathways[J]. American Journal of Physiology-Renal Physiology, 2013, 304(11): F1366-F1374.

[55] Salminen A, Hyttinen JMT, Kaarniranta K. AMP-activated protein kinase inhibits NF-kappa B signaling and inflammation: impact on healthspan and lifespan[J]. Journal of Molecular Medicine-Jmm, 2011, 89(7): 667-676.

[56] Jung JE, Lee JW, Ha JH, et al. 5-Aminoimidazole-4-carboxamide-ribonucleoside enhances oxidative stress-induced apoptosis through activation of nuclear factor-kappa B in mouse neuro 2a neuroblastoma cells[J]. Neuroscience Letters, 2004, 354(3): 197-200.

[57] Barroso E, Astudillo AM, Balsinde J, et al. PPAR beta/delta Activation prevents hypertriglyceridemia caused by a high fat diet. Involvement of AMPK and PGC-1 alpha-Lipin 1-PPAR alpha pathway[J]. Clinica E Investigacion En Arteriosclerosis, 2013, 25(2): 63-73.

[58] Ramjiawan A, Bagchi RA, Blant A, et al. Roles of histone deacetylation and AMP kinase in regulation of cardiomyocyte PGC-1 alpha gene expression in hypoxia[J]. American Journal of Physiology-Cell Physiology, 2013, 304(11): C1064-C1072.

[59] Kitada M, Kume S, Imaizumi N, et al. Resveratrol improves oxidative stress and protects against diabetic nephropathy through normalization of Mn-SOD dysfunction in AMPK/SIRT1-independent Pathway[J]. Diabetes, 2011, 60(2): 634-643.

[60] Satriano J, Sharma K, Blantz RC, et al. Induction of AMPK activity corrects early pathophysiological alterations in the subtotal nephrectomy model of chronic kidney disease[J]. American Journal of Physiology-Renal Physiology, 2013, 305(5): F727-F733.

[61] Chau MDL, Gao J, Yang Q, et al. Fibroblast growth factor 21 regulates energy metabolism by activating the AMPK-SIRT1-PGC-1 alpha pathway[J]. Proceedings of the National Academy of Sciences of the United States of America, 2010, 107(28): 12553-12558.

The prevention of diabetic cardiomyopathy by non-mitogenic acidic fibroblast growth factor is probably mediated by the suppression of oxidative stress and damage

Chi Zhang, Xiaokun Li, Lu Cai

1. Introduction

Diabetic cardiomyopathy was considered to be associated with oxidative stress and DNA damage which are regarded as main incentives to initiate ventricular remodeling, characterized by cardiac hypertrophy and fibrosis and heart dysfunction [1-3]. Therefore, attenuation of diabetes-induced oxidative damage and the subsequent cardiac hypertrophy and fibrosis are expected to exert beneficial effects and may be a potential novel therapeutic strategy for diabetic cardiomyopathy.

Fibroblast growth factor (FGF) is a super family including at least 23 members. As the earliest found, the acidic FGF (aFGF or FGF-1) and basic FGF (bFGF or FGF-2) are regarded as the representatives of the FGF family, which are characterized by a high affinity to heparin and play critical role in cell proliferation [4-6]. It is reported that aFGF is highly expressed in the heart and stimulates angiogenesis [7,8]. Cardiac aFGF participates in heart development and stimulates both cardiomyocyte proliferation and subsequent capillary angiogenesis [9-11]. In addition, expression of aFGF by adult cardiomyocyte can maintain cell survival by induction of DNA synthesis and regulation of gene expression [12]. Some studies mentioned that intracoronary, intrapericardial, or myocardial administration of aFGF or bFGF into ischemic canine and porcine hearts significantly minimized infarct size and improved cardiac function [13-15].

Diabetes was found to impair the expression of endogenous FGFs [16]. Some studies reported that administration of aFGF greatly improved wound healing under diabetic condition [17-19]. To date, whether aFGF can offer beneficial effect in the heart under diabetic condition is still unknown. However, growing evidence demonstrates that as an analogue of aFGF, bFGF induces significant cardio-protective effect under various pathological conditions [8,20-22]. It was reported that bFGF prevented lipopolysaccharide-induced cardiac apoptosis through suppression of iNOS pathway [20,21]. bFGF also protected against myocardial dysfunction and infarction induced by ischemia/reperfusion [22]. Our in vivo studies also confirmed that bFGF induced protection from ischemia/reperfusion induced cardiac injury in streptozotocin (STZ) induced type 1 diabetic rats [8]. Furthermore, a recent study also mentioned that aFGF improved cardio-protective effect in ischemic myocardium with ultrasound-mediated cavitation of heparin modified microbubbles [15].

Therefore, the present study was to test the hypothesis that aFGF can have a similar cardiac protection from diabetes-induced oxidative damage and subsequently remodeling. Considering that native FGF has the potential tumorigenic ability due to its nonspecific stimulation of cell growth, we have modified the native aFGF by gene engineering to generate a non-mitogenic aFGF (nm-aFGF) that only loses the potential to stimulate cell proliferation with all other functions compared to native aFGF [23,24]. To these ends, we applied STZ-induced type 1 diabetic mouse model with chronic treatment of nm-aFGF at the dose of 10 mg/kg body weight, based on previous studies [23,24]. In addition, we also used in vitro cultures of cardiomyocytes, cardiac and endothelial cell lines, in combination of using in vivo cardiac tissues treated with and without nm-aFGF to perform mechanistic studies. We found that chronic administration of nm-aFGF can indeed protect the diabetes-induced cardiac dysfunction, which may be attributed to the suppression of cardiac oxidative damage, hypertrophy, and fibrosis.

2. Materials and methods

2.1 Ethics statement

All experimental procedures for the animal usage were approved by the Institutional Animal Care and Use Committee of the University of Louisville, which is compliant with the Guide for the Care and Use of Laboratory Animals published by the US National Institutes of Health (NIH Publication No. 85–23, revised 1996). The protocol was approved by the Institutional Animal Care and Use Committee of the University of Louisville (IACUC #: 10155). All surgery was performed under sodium avertin anesthesia, and all efforts were made to minimize suffering.

2.2 Cell culture

Cardiomyoblasts (H9C2 cell line) were maintained in Dulbecco's modified Eagle's medium (DMEM) with 10% heat-inactivated fetal bovine serum, penicillin 100 IU/ml, and streptomycin 10 μg/ml. Cells were grown and maintained in 60 mm cell culture dishes at 37℃ in a 5% CO_2 humidified incubator. Glucose incubation (25 mmol/L) was performed for 48 hours with 200 ng/ml nm-aFGF pretreatment of cells in morphometric analysis mRNA expression detection.

Dermal-derived human microvascular endothelial cells (HMVECs) were obtained from Lonza Walkersville (Walkersville, USA). The culture conditions have been previously described [25]. Briefly, HMVECs were grown in EBM-2 (Lonza Walkersville) containing 1‰ human epidermal growth factor, 0.4‰ hydrocortisone, 1‰ gentamicin, 10% fetal bovine serum, 1‰ vascular endothelial growth factor, 4‰ human bFGF, 1‰ long R3 insulin-like growth factor 1, and 1‰ ascorbic acid. In both EBM and EBM-2, the glucose concentration was 5 mmol/L. Cells were grown in 25 cm^2 tissue culture flasks and maintained in a humidified atmosphere containing 5% CO_2 at 37℃. Cells at 80% confluence were growth-arrested by incubation in serum-free medium overnight before incubation with glucose (25 mmol/L). All experiments were carried out after 48 hours of glucose incubation with or without 1 hour pretreatment of nm-aFGF (200 ng/ml).

Neonatal rat cardiomyocytes were isolated from newborn Harlan Sprague-Dawley rat heart ventricles, as described previously [26]. Isolated primary cardiomyocytes were plated onto 6 cm cell culture dishes (Primaria Tissue Culture Dish; Becton Dickinson) at a density of 3.0×10^4 cells/cm^2 and were maintained for 48 hours in Dulbecco's Modified Eagle's Medium-Ham's F-12 supplemented with 10% fetal bovine serum, 10 μg/ml transferrin, 10 μg/ml insulin, 10 ng/ml selenium, 50 units/ml penicillin, 50 mg/ml streptomycin, 2 mg/ml bovine serum albumin, 5 μg/ml linoleic acid, 3 mM pyruvic acid, 0.1 mM minimum essential medium (MEM) nonessential amino acids, 10% MEM vitamin, 0.1 mM bromodeoxyuridine, 100 μM L-ascorbic acid, and 30 mM HEPES (pH 7.1). The cells were serum starved overnight prior to all experiments. Unless otherwise stated, all chemicals were of reagent grade quality and were purchased from Sigma Chemical (Sigma, Oakville, ON, Canada). All experiments were carried out after 48 hours of 25 mmol/L glucose incubation with or without nm-aFGF (200 ng/ml) pretreatment for 1 hour.

2.3 Cellular reactive oxygen species levels

Intracellular reactive oxygen species (ROS) generation was assessed using an intracellular ROS assay kit from Cell Biolabs (San Diego, CA, USA) according to the manufacturer's instructions.

2.4 Immunofluorescence

HMVECs and H9C2 cells were plated on eight-chamber tissue culture slides and incubated for 48 hours with the presence of glucose (25 mmol/L) and nm-aFGF (200 ng/ml), and then these cells were fixed with ethanol for staining with 8-OHdG antibody (Santa Cruz Biotehnology). Goat IgG labeled with FITC (Vector Laboratories, Burlingame, CA) was used for detection of the fluorescence. Slides were mounted in Vectashield fluorescence mounting medium with 4,6-diamidino-2-phenylindole (DAPI; Vector Laboratories) for nuclear staining. Microscopic observation was performed by an examiner unaware of the identity of the sample, using a Zeiss LSM 410 inverted laser scan microscope equipped with fluorescein, rhodamine, and DAPI filters (Carl Zeiss Canada, North York, ON, Canada)

2.5 Morphometric analysis

Cell surface areas were determined to assess cellular hypertrophy. Cells were visualized with a Leica inverted microscope, and images were captured at × 20 magnification. Cell area was determined using Mocha Software (SPSS). Cell surface area was determined from 50 randomly selected cells per petri dish and expressed as micrometers squared.

2.6 Animals

To keep consistence with our previous study [27], male FVB mice, 8–10 weeks of age, were purchased from the Jackson Laboratory (Bar Harbor, Maine) and housed in the University of Louisville Research Resources Center at 22 °C with a 12-h light/ dark cycle and free access to standard rodent chow and tap water. For induction of the type 1 diabetes, mice were injected intraperitoneally with multiple-STZ [Sigma-Aldich, St. Louis, MO, dissolved in 0.1 M sodium citrate (pH 4.5)] at 50 mg/kg body weight daily for 5 consecutive days while age-matched control mice were received multiple injections of the same volume of sodium citrate buffer. Five days after the last injection of STZ, mice with hyperglycemia (blood glucose levels ⩾250 mg/dl) were defined as diabetic as described previously [27]. Both diabetic and non-diabetic mice were treated with or without nm-aFGF treatment. Nm-aFGF (produced by our group using gene engineering approach) was intraperitoneally given at a dose of 10 μg/kg body weight daily for 1 and 6 months.

2.7 Non-invasive blood pressure

Blood pressure (BP) was measured by tail-cuff manometry using a CODATM non-invasive BP monitoring system (Kent Scientific Corporation, Torrington, CT) at each time point. Mice were kept warm on the heating pad to ensure sufficient blood flow to the tail. Mice were restrained in a plastic tube restrainer. Occlusion and volume-pressure recording cuffs were placed over the tail. Each mouse was allowed to adapt to the restrainer for 5 min prior to BP measurement. The BP was measured for 10 acclimation cycles followed by 20 measurement cycles. After three days of training for the BP measurement, formal measurements for the unanesthetized BP and heart rate (HR) were collected (Table 1), as described previously [3].

Table 1. Effect of nm-aFGF on diabetes-induced unanesthetized blood pressure and heart rate

	Control	nm-aFGF	DM	DM/nm-aFGF
1 month				
HR (beats/min)	667.71 ± 46.63	647.97 ± 59.62	644.1 ± 29.21	589.62 ± 49.98
Diastolic BP (mm Hg)	70.75 ± 7.19	67.81 ± 3.66	73.81 ± 6. 42	71.44 ± 5. 41
Systolic BP (mm Hg)	114.18 ± 4.55	111.34 ± 8.86	119.05 ± 8.13	112.52 ± 8.22
Mean BP (mm Hg)	94.52 ± 5.46	89.63 ± 2.791	90.42 ± 4.57	91.82 ± 8.29
6 months				
HR (beats/min)	645.45 ± 23.45	641.76 ± 39.79	654.1 ± 35.15	639.62 ± 44.88
Diastolic BP (mm Hg)	83.68 ± 5.43	83.39 ± 3.02	97.83 ± 3.11*	73.44 ± 8.33*#
Systolic BP (mm Hg)	113. 57 ± 5.32	106. 48 ± 5.62	129.14 ± 8.34*	102.21 ± 8.26*#
Mean BP (mm Hg)	94.25 ± 5.61	89.63 ± 4.18	104.42 ± 4.03*	82.82 ± 5.93*#

Notes: Data were presented as means ± SEM. HR = heart rate; BP = blood pressure. *$P < 0.05$ vs. control. #$P < 0.05$ vs. DM group.

2.8 Echocardiography

Transthoracic echocardiography (Echo) was performed for Avertin anesthetized mice at rest using a high-resolution imaging system for small animals (Vevo 770, VisualSonics, Canada), equipped with a high-frequent ultrasound probe (RMV-707B). All hair was removed from the chest using a chemical hair remover and the aquasonic clear ultrasound gel (Parker Laboratories, Fairfield, NJ) without bubbles and was applied to the thorax surface to optimize the visibility of the cardiac chambers. Parasternal long-axis and short-axis views were acquired. Left ventricular (LV) dimensions and wall thicknesses were determined from parasternal short axis M-mode images. The anesthetized HR was collected. Meanwhile, ejection fraction (EF), fractional shortening (FS), and LV mass were calculated by Vevo770 software (Table 2). The final data represent averaged values of 10 cardiac cycles [28].

2.9 Sirius Red staining of collagen

Tissue sections at 5 mm were used for Sirius Red staining of collagen with 0.1% Sirius Red F3BA and 0.25% Fast Green FCF. The sections stained for Sirius Red then were assessed for the proportion of fibrosis (collagen) using a computer-assisted image analysis system as described in our previous study [29].

2.10 RNA extraction and real-time PCR

Trizol reagent (Invitrogen, Burlington, Canada) was used to isolate RNA as previously described [30]. RNA was extracted with chloroform followed by centrifugation to separate the sample into aqueous and organic phases. RNA was recovered from the aqueous phase by isopropyl alcohol precipitation and suspended in diethylpyrocarbonate-treated water. Total RNA (2 μg) was used for cDNA synthesis with high capacity cDNA reverse transcription kit (Applied Biosystems, Foster City, USA). The resulting cDNA products were stored at −20℃. Real-time RT-PCR was performed by using the LightCycler (Roche Diagnostics Canada, Laval, Canada), as previously described [31]. For a final reaction volume of 20 μl, the following reagents were added: 10 μl SYBR Advantage qPCR Premix (Clontech, Mountain View, USA), 1 μl each of forward and reverse 10 μmol/L primers, 7 μl H$_2$O, and 1 μl cDNA template. The mRNA levels were quantified by using the standard curve method. Standard curves were constructed by using a serially diluted standard template. The data was normalized to 18S ribosomal RNA or β-actin RNA to account for differences in reverse transcription efficiencies and the amount of template in the reaction mixtures.

2.11 Statistical analysis

Data is presented as mean ± standard error. Statistical significance of differences between groups was tested with Student's t test or one-way ANOVA followed by *post hoc* analysis, as appropriate. A *P*-value of 0.05 or less was considered to be significant. All calculations were performed with SPSS version 15.0 software.

3. Results

3.1 Chronic administration of nm-aFGF did not impact on diabetes-induced body weight loss and blood glucose increase, but significantly prevented diabetes-induced high blood pressure and cardiac dysfunction

FVB mice were intraperitoneally injected with multiple low-dose STZs (50 mg/kg) to induce type 1 diabetes. Diabetic mice and age-matched non-diabetic mice were divided into groups with and without treatment of nm-aFGF (10 μg/kg daily) for 1 and 6 months. The body weight and blood glucose of the mice in each group were detected at each time point. Results showed that the body weight of the four groups were equal at 1 month after treatment (Fig. 1A). Meanwhile, blood glucose was significantly up-regulated in DM and DM/nm-aFGF groups (Fig. 1B). However, the body weight of DM mice greatly decreased at 6 months. Administration of nm-aFGF had no impact on the body weight loss and blood glucose levels (Fig. 1).

Unanesthetized BP and HR of these mice were examined by tail-cuff manometry. Diastolic, systolic, and averaged BPs were significantly increased at 6 months in DM group, which were not found at 1 month (Table 1). Chronic administration of nm-aFGF almost completely attenuated diabetes induced BPs increase. There was no significant difference

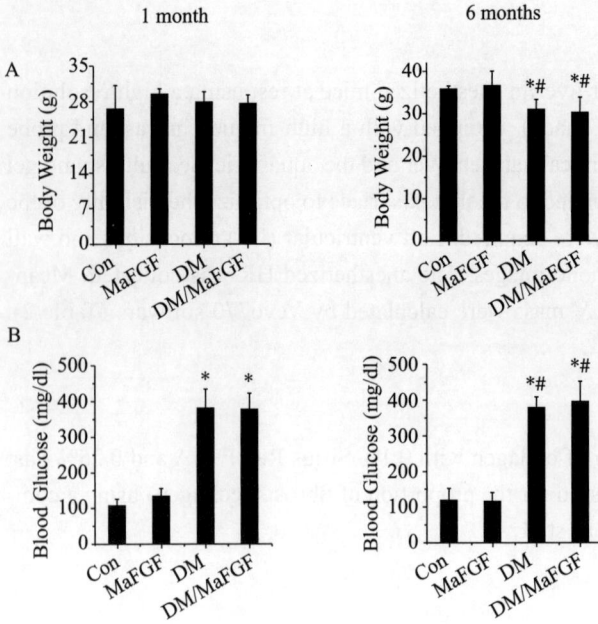

Fig. 1. Effects of nm-aFGF on body weight, blood glucose levels in non-diabetic and diabetic mice. STZ induced type 1 diabetic FVB mice were intraperitoneally treated with or without nm-aFGF (10 μg/kg) treatment daily for either 1 or 6 months. The body weights (A) and blood glucose level (B) were monitored weekly and presented at indicated time points. Data are presented as means ± SD ($n = 8$). $^{*}P < 0.05$ $vs.$ control; $^{\#}P < 0.05$ $vs.$ DM (diabetic) group.

of HR among groups at either 1 or 6 months (Table 1). The HRs of anesthetized mice, detected by Echo examination (Table 2), were lower than that of unanesthetized mice (Table 1), but were equal among groups at each time point. In addition, cardiac function was significantly impaired under diabetic condition at 6 months, rather than 1 month, with the characteristics of progressive increases in IVS;d, LVPW;d, LVID and LV Vol as well as progressive decreases in IVS;s, LVPW;s,%EF and%FS (Table 2). Administration of nm-aFGF almost completely prevented these cardiac dysfunctions in diabetic mice by reversing all the indices back to a normal level.

Table 2.　Effect of nm-aFGF on diabetes-induced cardiac dysfunction and anesthetized heart rate

		Control	nm-aFGF	DM	DM/nm-aFGF
	HR (beats/min)	454 ± 41.33	464.7 ± 30.24	432.5 ± 40.51	431.2 ± 23.93
	LVID;d (mm)	3.31 ± 0.09	3.34 ± 0.11	3.37 ± 0.12	3.29 ± 0.14
	LVID;s (mm)	1.34 ± 0.04	1.32 ± 0.11	1.45 ± 0.07	1.298 ± 0.09
	IVS;d (mm)	0.72 ± 0.01	0.71 ± 0.02	0.72 ± 0.01	0.73 ± 0.03
	IVS;s (mm)	1.03 ± 0.02	1.06 ± 0.05	0.99 ± 0.08	0.95 ± 0.06
	LVPW;d (mm)	0.83 ± 0.01	0.79 ± 0.04	0.85 ± 0.05	0.84 ± 0.05
	LVPW;s (mm)	1.6 ± 0.047	1.62 ± 0.09	1.523 ± 0.07	1.59 ± 0.12
1 month	LV Vol;d (μL)	44.48 ± 2.92	45.7 ± 3.46	46.39 ± 4.06	43.98 ± 4.36
	LV Vol;s (μL)	4.62 ± 0.38	4.57 ± 0.76	6.51 ± 0.73	4.28 ± 0.75
	%EF (%)	89.69 ± 0.14	90.15 ± 1.65	87.98 ± 1.32	89.95 ± 0.85
	% FS (%)	59.61 ± 1.12	60.49 ± 2.39	56.97 ± 1.84	59.72 ± 1.23
	LV mass (mg)	82.49 ± 3.76	81.08 ± 4.05	83.13 ± 6.76	83.09 ± 9.52
	LVMC (mg)	65.99 ± 3.01	64.87 ± 3.24	66.5 ± 5.41*	66.39 ± 7.46
	HR (beats/min)	454.71 ± 29.56	469.29 ± 30.14	456.5 ± 30.18	430.4 ± 31.56
	LVID;d (mm)	3.55 ± 0.24	3.43 ± 0.19	4.52 ± 0.54*	3.49 ± 0.13$^{*\#}$
	LVID;s (mm)	1.55 ± 0.06	1.61 ± 0.05	2.55 ± 0.08*	1.62 ± 0.07$^{*\#}$
	IVS;d (mm)	0.77 ± 0.05	0.78 ± 0.04	0.92 ± 0.04*	0.82 ± 0.02$^{*\#}$
	IVS;s (mm)	1.05 ± 0.03	1.07 ± 0.05	0.82 ± 0.03*	1.03 ± 0.04$^{*\#}$
	LVPW;d (mm)	0.89 ± 0.08	0.93 ± 0.09	1.24 ± 0.06*	0.96 ± 0.06$^{*\#}$

Continued Table

		Control	nm-aFGF	DM	DM/nm-aFGF
6 months	LVPW;s (mm)	1.7 ± 0.07	1.65 ± 0.06	1.16 ± 0.04*	1.64 ± 0.08*#
	LV Vol;d (μL)	58.1 ± 1.89	48.3 ± 5.76	66.74 ± 5.68*	50.7 ± 4.36*#
	LV Vol;s (μL)	8.07 ± 0.48	7.36 ± 0.53	23.42 ± 0.46*	7.41 ± 0.36*#
	%EF (%)	86.11 ± 4.68	85.29 ± 5.54	67.02 ± 5.96*	84.76 ± 4.36*#
	% FS (%)	54.84 ± 4.12	53.72 ± 3.67	35.03 ± 6.45*	52.87 ± 4.34*#
	LV mass (mg)	114.8 ± 5.28	100.76 ± 7.91	146.45 ± 8.1*	109.62 ± 4.31*#
	LVMC (mg)	91.84 ± 5.02	80.61 ± 6.33	117.16 ± 6.48*	87.7 ± 3.45*#

Notes: Data were presented as means ± SEM. LVID;d = LV end-diastolic diameter; LVID;s = LV end-systolic diameter; LVPW = LV posterior wall; IVS = interventricular septum; FS = fractional shortening; EF = ejection fraction; LVMC = LV mass corrected. $^*P < 0.05$ vs. control. $^#P < 0.05$ vs. DM group.

3.2 In vitro mechanistic study on the preventive effect of nm-aFGF on high glucose induced oxidative stress, DNA oxidative damage, and the hypertrophic and fibrotic gene expression

3.2.1 Nm-aFGF prevented high glucose-induced oxidative stress and damage

Strong evidence demonstrated that the development of diabetic cardiomyopathy is related to the induction of cardiac oxidative stress, characterized by production of ROS, leading to subsequent cell death, hypertrophy, and fibrosis. Therefore, we investigated whether the nm-aFGF induced cardiac protection by against diabetes was attributed to the suppression of oxidative stress. In our present study, we treated the H9c2 cells with high glucose (25 mmol/L) for 48 hours to mimic in vivo diabetic condition. Nm-aFGF was dissolved in PBS and added to a subset of cells with the working concentration of 200 ng/ml at 1 hour before and during high glucose treatment for 15 hours. We detected ROS level and the mRNA expression of endothelial nitric oxide synthase (eNOS) in both H9c2 cells and HMVECs. The results showed that high glucose increased cellular ROS level (Fig. 2A,C) and the mRNA expression of eNOS (Fig. 2B,D) in

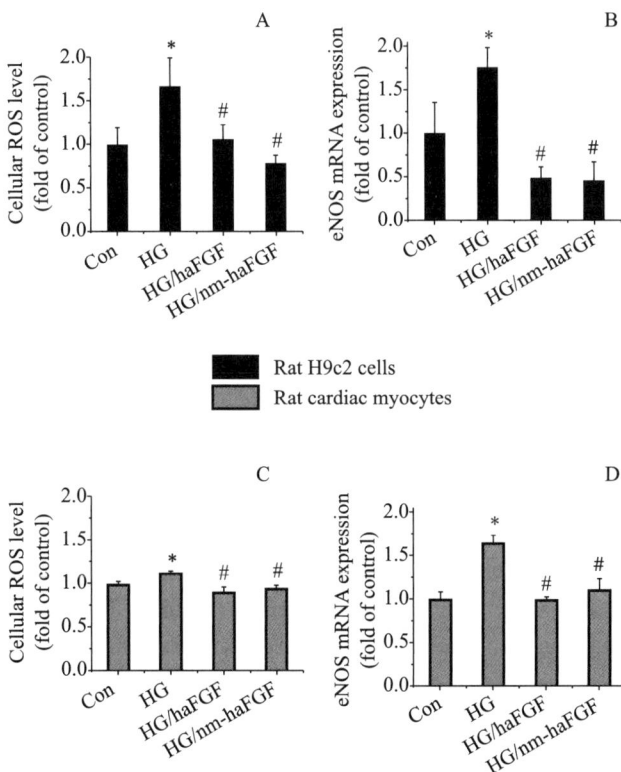

Fig. 2. Effect of native aFGF or nm-aFGF on high glucose induced oxidative stress in cardiac cells. Pre-treatment of H9C2 cells and Rat cardiac myocytes with both native or nm-aFGF (200 ng/ml) for 1 hour followed by 48 hours treatment with both high glucose (25 mmol/L) and two types of aFGF. Both native aFGF and nm-aFGF prevented high glucose induced up-regulation of cellular ROS level (A) and eNOS mRNA expression (B) in either H9c2 or cardiac myocytes. Data were presented as means ± SD. All in vitro data were obtained from at least 3 independent experiments. $^*P < 0.05$ vs. control. $^#P < 0.05$ vs. high glucose (HG).

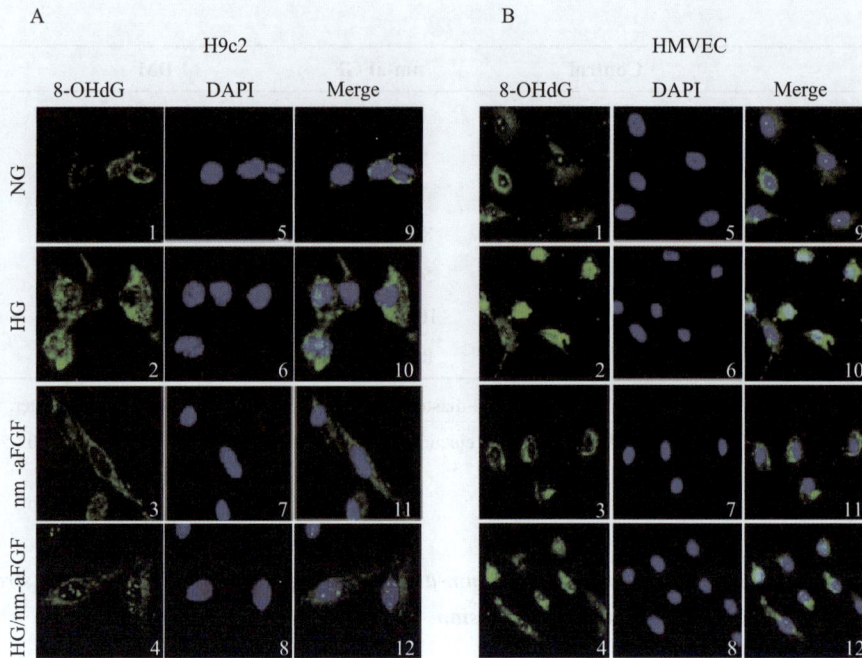

Fig. 3. Effect of nm-aFGF on high glucose induced DNA oxidative damage in both H9c2 cells and HMVECs. Cells were exposed to nm-aFGF (200 ng/ml) for 1 hour prior to combination treatment of both high glucose (25 mmol/L) and nm-aFGF for 48 hours. After harvesting, cells were fixed for immunocytochemistry analysis of 8-OHdG (FITC A1-4, B1-4) and nuclear morphology (DAPI A5-8, B5-8) using fluorescence microscopy. DAPI staining is pseudocolored blue and 8-OHdG is shown in green. Images were merged and showed in A9-12 and B9-12. Each image is representative of at least 3 separate experiments.

both H9c2 cells and HMVECs, which were significantly suppressed by both native and nm-aFGF treatments (Fig. 2) without significant difference between native aFGF-treated and nm-aFGF treated groups.

Oxidative DNA damage was measured by immunofluorescent staining for 8-OHdG as the most sensitive approach. In line with the overgeneration of ROS (Fig. 2), the oxidative DNA damage positive staining increased in both cardiac H9c2 cells and HMVECs after 48-hour high glucose treatment (Fig. 3A,B, green), which was co-localized with that of nuclear dye DAPI (blue). The increased 8-OHdG stain in the nucleus induced by exposure to high glucose was significantly attenuated by treatment with nm-aFGF (200 ng/ml).

3.2.2 Nm-aFGF prevented high glucose-induced hypertrophic effect

Oxidative stress has been considered one of the key contributors in the development of cardiac hypertrophy with the characteristic of cardiac cell size increase [32–34]. Therefore, the effect of nm-aFGF on cardiac cell size under high glucose conditions was investigated. We found that nm-aFGF had no impact on cell size under normal condition, but exposure to high glucose significantly increased the cell size (Fig. 4A), that was about 2 fold larger than the normal cell size (Fig. 4B). The cardiac cell hypertrophic effect induced by exposure to high glucose was almost completely prevented by nm-aFGF treatment.

To further explore the hypertrophic effect of cardiac cells induced by high glucose, we examined the mRNA expression of hypertrophic cytokines atrial natriuretic peptide (ANP) and angiotensinogen (ANG) [35–37]. High glucose significantly increased the mRNA expression of ANP and ANG in H9c2 cells (Fig. 4C,D) and rat cardiomyocytes (Fig. 4E,F), which was dramatically attenuated by native aFGF and nm-aFGF, respectively, without significant difference between two forms of FGFs.

3.2.3 Nm-aFGF prevented fibrotic response induced by high glucose

Fibrosis plays a critical role in cardiac remodeling [38,39]; therefore, we also examined fibrosis-related gene fibronectin (FN) expression under high glucose condition, with or without native/modified aFGF treatment in cardiac H9c2 cells and rat cardiomyocytes. We found FN mRNA expression was significantly upregulated after 48-hour exposure to high glucose (Fig. 5). Both native aFGF and nm-aFGF had significantly inhibitive effect on FN mRNA expression in H9c2 cells (Fig. 5A) and rat cardiomyocytes (Fig. 5B).

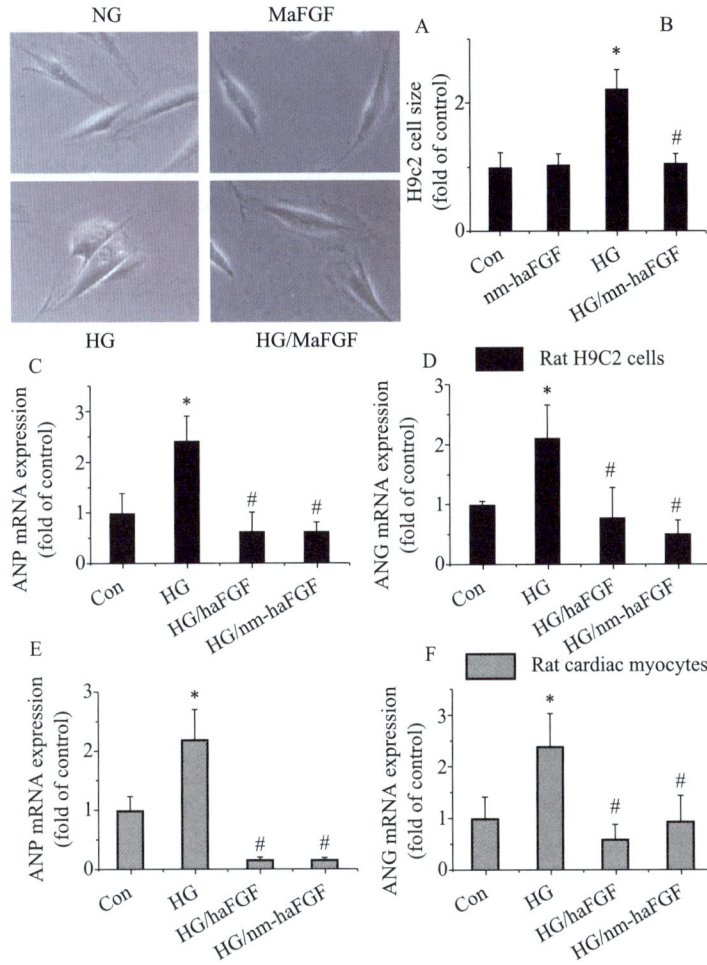

Fig. 4. Both native aFGF and nm-aFGF showed preventive effect on high glucose induced cardiac cell hypertrophy *in vitro*. H9c2 cells and rat cardiomyocytes were treated as the same condition described in Fig. 2. Cells were visualized with a Leica inverted microscope, and images were captured at × 20 magnification (A). Cell area was determined using Mocha software (B). Cell surface area was determined from 50 randomly selected cells per petri dish and expressed as micrometers squared. After harvesting, cardiac hypertrophic markers ANP mRNA (C, E) and ANG mRNA (D, F) expression in H9c2 and Rat cardiac myocytes were measured by real-time qPCR. Data were presented as means ± SD. All *in vitro* data were obtained from at least 3 independent experiments. *$P < 0.05$ vs. control. #$P < 0.05$ vs. high glucose (HG).

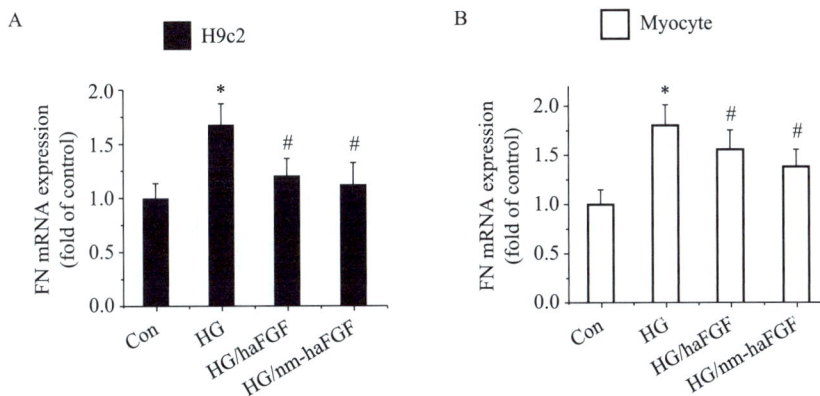

Fig. 5. Both native aFGF and nm-aFGF showed preventive effect on high glucose induced mRNA expression upregulation of fibrotic markers *in vitro*. H9c2 cells, rat cardiomyocytes, and HMVECs were treated as described in Fig. 2. After harvesting, fibrotic markers FN mRNA expression in H9c2 cells (A) and rat cardiomyocytes (B) were measured by real-time PCR. Data were presented as means ± SD. All *in vitro* data were obtained from at least 3 independent experiments. *$P < 0.05$ vs. control. #$P < 0.05$ vs. high glucose (HG).

3.3 Chronic administration of nm-aFGF prevented diabetes induced cardiac hypertrophy and fibrosis

Our *in vitro* study revealed that nm-aFGF prevented high glucose-induced upregulation of ANP and ANG mRNA expression; therefore, we tested whether nm-aFGF plays a similar anti-hypertrophic role *in vivo*. Results from Table 2 showed that diabetes induced a significant increase of LV mass at 6 months, suggesting the possible induction of cardiac hypertrophy. This was confirmed by the ratio of the heart weight to tibia length of diabetic mice at 6 months (Fig. 6B) which was not found at 1 month (Fig. 6A).

Furthermore, molecular hypertrophy markers ANP, ANG and β-MHC were also significantly increased at mRNA level in the heart of diabetic mice 6 months after diabetes onset (Fig. 6D). Although diabetes-induced hypertrophy was not found at 1month according to the Echo data, the pathological changes already initiated at molecular level (Fig. 6C). Administration of nm-aFGF significantly prevented the hypertrophic changes at both 1 and 6 months (Table 2, Fig. 6).

We also examined the fibrotic effect of diabetes on the heart by Sirius-Red staining for collagen (Fig. 7A). Diabetes induced a significant amount of collagen accumulation, predominantly in interstitial, but also included the perivascular area, which was increased at 6 months. Nm-aFGF treatment completely prevented the collagen accumulation. DM-

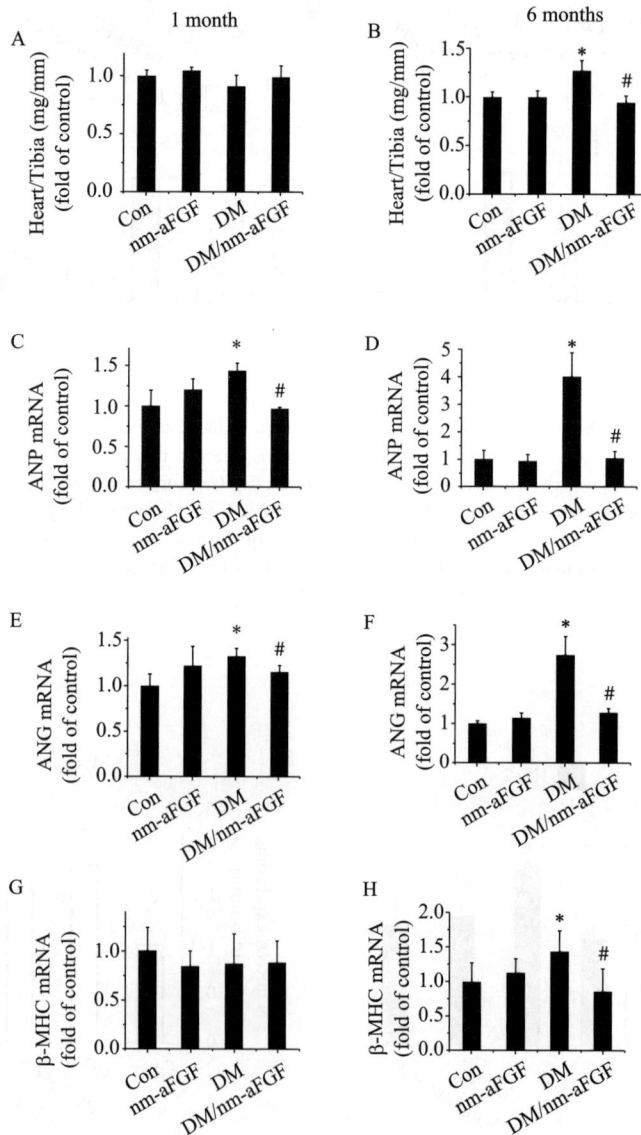

Fig. 6. Prevention by nm-aFGF of diabetes-induced cardiac hypertrophy *in vivo*. Diabetic and age-matched mice were intraperitoneally injected with nm-aFGF at 10 μg/kg daily for 1 and 6 months. The ratio of the heart weight to tibia length (A, B) were measured and calculated after mice were sacrificed. Cardiac mRNA expression of the hypertrophic markers ANP mRNA (C, D), ANG mRNA (E, F) and β-MHC mRNA (G, H) expression was measured by real-time qPCR. Data are presented as means ± SD ($n = 8$). *$P < 0.05$ *vs.* control; #$P < 0.05$ *vs.* DM (diabetic) group.

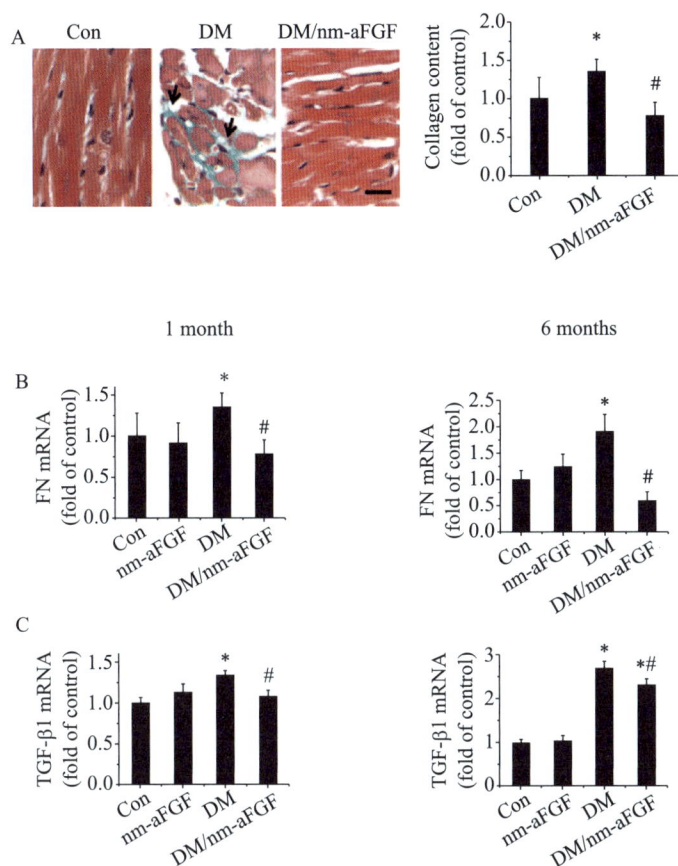

Fig. 7. Prevention by nm-aFGF of diabetes-induced cardiac fibrosis *in vivo*. Mice were treated as described in Fig. 6. Cardiac sections were subject to Sirius-Red staining with 0.1% Sirius-Red F3BA and 0.25% Fast green FCF for collagen accumulation and quantization by collagen content analysis (A). To further confirm the anti-fibrosis effect of nm-aFGF, the mRNA expression of fibrotic markers, including FN (B) and TGF-β1 (C) was measured by real-time PCR assay. Data are presented as means ± SD ($n = 8$). $^*P < 0.05$ *vs*, control; $^\#P < 0.05$ *vs*, DM (diabetic) groups.

induced cardiac fibrosis was further confirmed by increased cardiac FN and TGF-β1 mRNA expressions (Fig. 7B, C) at both 1 and 6 months. Administration of nm-aFGF completely attenuated most of the fibrotic changes. For TGF-β1 mRNA at 6 months, although the therapeutic group was higher than normal mice, there was a slightly (but statistically different) decrease compared with non-treated diabetic group (Fig. 7).

4. Discussion

Diabetes is a serious global issue nowadays, which leads to many kinds of fatal complications such as diabetic cardiomyopathy. Therefore, it is urgent to find a proper way to prevent oxidative stress and the consequently pathological changes in the heart.

We know that aFGF, highly expressed in the heart, is a specific well-defined angiogenic stimulant for the heart development. Cardiomyocyte-derived aFGF functions to increase the fetal ventricular cardiomyocyte population in absolute number as well as to facilitate the subsequent increase in capillary angiogenesis that occurs during cardiomyocyte maturation and ventricular remodeling [11]. As described above, the decrease of serum bFGF appears in infarction, stroke and peripheral vascular disease associated with diabetes [16]. Our previous study revealed that bFGF protected the heart in type 1 diabetes model [8]. We proposed that as an analogue of bFGF, aFGF may induce similar beneficial effect in the diabetic heart. In order to abrogate the oncogenicity of native aFGF, the nm-aFGF was applied in our present study to define whether nm-aFGF showed protection on diabetic cardiomyopathy.

In the present study using multiple-STZ-induced type 1 diabetic mouse model, the diabetic cardiomyopathy was successfully established at 6 months, shown by significantly cardiac dysfunction, including great increases in BPs,

IVS;d, LVPW;d, LVID, LV Vol and LV mass along with significant decreases in LV EF and FS. We reported for the first time that chronic administration of nm-aFGF significantly prevented diabetes-induced hypertension and cardiac dysfunction at 6 months. It should be mentioned that there was no preventive effect of nm-aFGF on diabetic heart at the time of 1 month after diabetes since there was no significant manifestation of diabetic pathological changes.

From onset of diabetes to the development of diabetic cardiomyopathy, there are several pathological developing steps. Accumulated evidence indicates that oxidative stress may play a key role in the etiology of diabetic cardiomyopathy [40]. Under physiological conditions, ROS are continuously produced in cardiac cells, but the levels of ROS are regulated by a number of enzymes and antioxidants, so normally there is a physiological balance between ROS and antioxidants. However, under pathological conditions such as diabetes, hyperglycemia can destroy the balance with overproduction of ROS, leading to oxidative stress condition. As a result, oxidative stress will initiate harmful effect on cardiac cells, resulting in myocardial cell death and consequent hypertrophy and fibrosis, finally leading to diabetic dysfunction (cardiomyopathy) [41]. Some studies mentioned that the expression of aFGF was up-regulated by oxidative stress, implying that the increase of aFGF expression was an adaptive response and may show a protective effect against oxidative stress [42–44]. Since hyperglycemia is the predominant trigger of diabetic complications, the mechanistic studies here were performed with the H9c2 cells exposed to high glucose for mimicking diabetic hyperglycemia in vitro. For these studies we added native or modified aFGF into the medium of H9c2 cell culture to investigate whether aFGF can induce anti-oxidative effect in the H9c2 cells under high glucose conditions. The level of ROS and eNOS were examined in this study. We found that both ROS and eNOS levels were increased under high glucose condition, which were significantly attenuated by either native aFGF or nm-aFGF treatment. This implies that anti-oxidative function of aFGF might be the mechanism to prevent diabetic cardiac dysfunction and cardio-myopathy.

It is worthy to mention that nm-aFGF exhibited an equal anti-oxidation capacity to native aFGF even though nm-aFGF does not have mitogenic effect as we have demonstrated before [45,46]. Therefore, nm-aFGF will have no oncogenic effect compared to the native aFGF, suggesting that nm-aFGF has more potential for clinical implications. In order to ensure the general protection by nm-aFGF from high glucose-induced oxidative stress in other cells, HMVECs were also applied in this study, which showed similar results: both native and modified aFGF significantly prevented high glucose-induced increases in cellular ROS level and cardiac eNOS mRNA expression.

Oxidative stress-induced cardiac cell death is attributed to DNA damage, including chromatin cross-linking, chromosome deletion, DNA strand breaks and base oxidation [47]. We know that aFGF plays a key role in the stimulation of cell proliferation and the prevention of cell death [45]. Cultured cells in the medium without FGF showed slow cell proliferation with cell death [48]. Therefore, in the present study we also tried to determine whether nm-aFGF could protect oxidative DNA damage of cardiac cells exposed to high glucose. Both H9c2 cells and HMVECs were treated as mentioned above, which showed that under normal conditions, the staining of oxidative DNA damage marker 8-OHDG was very low in both cell types. Treatment of normal cells with nm-aFGF had no impact on 8-OHDG staining; however, 8-OHDG staining was dramatically increased in the cells exposed to high glucose, but not in the cells exposed to both high glucose and nm-aFGF treatment. Therefore, nm-aFGF protects high glucose-induced oxidative DNA damage in cardiac cells.

Cardiac hypertrophy is characterized by enlargement of the heart caused by an increased myocyte size, which is generally associated with numerous side effects, including depressed LV ER%, heart failure and overall mortality [32,49]. In term of its mechanism, a growing body of evidence revealed that oxidative stress plays a key role in the development of cardiac hypertrophy [32]. In cultured cardiomyocytes, hypertrophy induced by angiotensin II, endothelin 1, tumor necrosis factor-α or pulsatile mechanical stretch has been shown to be associated with the increase of intracellular ROS production [50]. Another study reported that ROS production contributed to the development of LV hypertrophy during chronic pressure overload [51]. The most widely recognized effect of increased oxidative stress is the oxidation and damage of macromolecules, membranes, DNA and enzymes involved in cellular function and homeostasis [52]. In the present study we demonstrated that nm-aFGF showed almost equal beneficial effects to the native aFGF on the prevention of high glucose-induced oxidative stress and oxidative DNA damage.

Due to the close relationship between oxidative stress and cardiac cell hypertrophy, we also tried to identify whether nm-aFGF showed protection of high glucose-induced cardiac cell hypertrophy, by examining cardiac cell size and mRNA expression of hypertrophic cytokines. Under normal conditions, nm-aFGF had no impact on cardiac H9c2 cell shape and size. However, the cells were significantly enlarged under high glucose condition. In the cells exposed to high glucose with nm-aFGF, there was no hypertrophic effect. In addition, high glucose up-regulated mRNA expression of ANP and ANG in both H9c2 cells and rat myocytes, which were significantly attenuated by treatment with either native aFGF or nm-aFGF. These *in vitro* findings were confirmed by *in vivo* animal studies, e.g.: administration of nm-aFGF significantly prevented diabetes-induced ratio increase of heart weight to tibia length. Although there was a significant difference for the ratio of heart weight to tibia length only at 6 month, rather than at 1 month, the significantly increased mRNA expression of the molecular hypertrophic markers, ANP, ANG and β-MHC in the heart were observed at 1 month, suggesting the process of hypertrophy has started at molecular level from 1 month of diabetes. Treatment with nm-aFGF could protect diabetes-induced molecular levels of cardiac damage at the early-stage, resulting in a prevention of cardiac hypertrophy.

We also demonstrated the up-regulation of FN mRNA expression in the both *in vitro* cultured cells exposed to high glucose and *in vivo* diabetic mouse model at 6 month after diabetes onset. Using the *in vitro* model we also detected the mRNA expression of fibrosis markers FN and TGF-β. During the study we found high glucose significantly increased FN mRNA expression in H9c2 cells, HMVECs and rat myocytes, which was remarkably prevented by both native and modified aFGF treatment. The anti-fibrotic effect of nm-aFGF was equal to native aFGF. The *in vitro* finding was also confirmed during the *in vivo* study. Sirius red staining showed that at 6 months after diabetes onset there was a clear fibrotic response in the heart, which was significantly inhibited by nm-aFGF treatment. Moreover, administration of nm-aFGF to diabetic mice also prevented mRNA expression of fibrotic markers including FN and TGF-β1 in diabetic heart.

5. Conclusions

In summary, diabetic cardiomyopathy is a clinical problem that develops in diabetes, and potentially involves oxidative stress and the subsequent cardiac myocytes death, hypertrophy and fibrosis. These pathogenic changes may contribute to compromised ventricular dysfunction in diabetes, which is the leading cause of death in the world today. In our present study, we found that nm-aFGF significantly protected cardiac cell death, hypertension, cardiac dysfunction and prevented cardiomyopathy in diabetic heart. By *in vitro* mechanistic study, we identified the protective mechanism of nm-aFGF against diabetic cardiomyopathy. We demonstrated that nm-aFGF has a similar cardiac protection to native aFGF, from diabetes. Considering that the modified nm-aFGF only losses its mitogenetic effect, but preserves all other bio-effects such as anti-apoptosis effect and cardio-protection [7], nm-aFGF maybe a potential candidate for the therapeutic application against diabetic cardiomyopathy in clinics due to its lack of oncogenic potential.

References

[1] Wang Y, Sun W, Du B, et al. Therapeutic effect of MG-132 on diabetic cardiomyopathy is associated with its suppression of proteasomal activities: roles of Nrf2 and NF-kappa B[J]. American Journal of Physiology-Heart and Circulatory Physiology, 2013, 304(4): H567-H578.

[2] Guan S, Ma Z, Wu Y, et al. Long-term administration of fasudil improves cardiomyopathy in streptozotocin-induced diabetic rats[J]. Food and Chemical Toxicology, 2012, 50(6): 1874-1882.

[3] Tan Y, Li X, Prabhu SD, et al. Angiotensin II plays a critical role in alcohol-induced cardiac nitrative damage, cell death, remodeling, and cardiomyopathy in a protein kinase C/nicotinamide adenine dinucleotide phosphate oxidase-dependent manner[J]. Journal of the American College of Cardiology, 2012, 59(16): 1477-1486.

[4] Tacer KF, Bookout AL, Ding X, et al. Research resource: Comprehensive expression atlas of the fibroblast growth factor system in adult mouse[J]. Molecular Endocrinology, 2010, 24(10): 2050-2064.

[5] Turner CA, Watson SJ, Akil H. The fibroblast growth factor family: Neuromodulation of affective behavior[J]. Neuron, 2012, 76(1): 160-174.

[6] Krejci P, Prochazkova J, Bryja V, et al. Molecular pathology of the fibroblast growth factor family[J]. Human Mutation, 2009, 30(9):

1245-1255.

[7] Shen H, MacDonald R, Bruemmer D, et al. Zinc deficiency alters lipid metabolism in LDL receptor-deficient mice treated with rosiglitazone[J]. Journal of Nutrition, 2007, 137(11): 2339-2345.

[8] Xiao J, Lv Y, Lin S, et al. Cardiac protection by basic fibroblast growth factor from ischemia/reperfusion-induced injury in diabetic rats[J]. Biological & Pharmaceutical Bulletin, 2010, 33(3): 444-449.

[9] Vlodavsky I, Fuks Z, Ishaimichaeli R, et al. Extracellular matrix-resident basic fibroblast growth factor: implication for the control of angiogenesis[J]. Journal of Cellular Biochemistry, 1991, 45(2): 167-176.

[10] Ingber DE, Folkman J. How does extracellular matrix control capillary morphogenesis?[J]. Cell, 1989, 58(5): 803-805.

[11] Engelmann GL, Dionne CA, Jaye MC. Acidic fibroblast growth factor and heart development. Role in myocyte proliferation and capillary angiogenesis[J]. Circulation Research, 1993, 72(1): 7-19.

[12] Speir E, Tanner V, Gonzalez AM, et al. Acidic and basic fibroblast growth factors in adult rat heart myocytes. Localization,regulation in culture, and effects on DNA synthesis[J]. Circulation Research, 1992, 71(2): 251-259.

[13] Detillieux KA, Sheikh F, Kardami E, et al. Biological activities of

fibroblast growth factor-2 in the adult myocardium[J]. Cardiovascular Research, 2003, 57(1): 8-19.

[14] Waltenberger J. Modulation of growth factor action - Implications for the treatment of cardiovascular diseases[J]. Circulation, 1997, 96(11): 4083-4094.

[15] Zhao Y, Lu C, Li X, et al. Improving the cardio protective effect of aFGF in ischemic myocardium with ultrasound-mediated cavitation of heparin modified microbubbles: preliminary experiment[J]. Journal of Drug Targeting, 2012, 20(7): 623-631.

[16] Yeboah J, Sane DC, Crouse JR, et al. Low plasma levels of FGF-2 and PDGF-BB are associated with cardiovascular events in type II diabetes mellitus (diabetes heart study)[J]. Disease Markers, 2007, 23(3): 173-178.

[17] Mellin TN, Cashen DE, Ronan JJ, et al. Acidic fibroblast growth factor accelerates dermal wound healing in diabetic mice[J]. Journal of Investigative Dermatology, 1995, 104(5): 850-855.

[18] Matuszewska B, Keogan M, Fisher DM, et al. Acidic fibroblast growth factor: evaluation of topical formulations in a diabetic mouse wound healing model[J]. Pharmaceutical Research, 1994, 11(1): 65-71.

[19] Xie L, Zhang M, Dong B, et al. Improved refractory wound healing with administration of acidic fibroblast growth factor in diabetic rats[J]. Diabetes Research and Clinical Practice, 2011, 93(3): 396-403.

[20] Iwai-Kanai E, Hasegawa K, Fujita M, et al. Basic fibroblast growth factor protects cardiac myocytes from iNOS-mediated apoptosis[J]. Journal of Cellular Physiology, 2002, 190(1): 54-62.

[21] Suzuki YJ. Growth factor signaling for cardioprotection against oxidative stress-induced apoptosis[J]. Antioxidants & Redox Signaling, 2003, 5(6): 741-749.

[22] House SL, Bolte C, Zhou M, et al. Cardiac-specific overexpression of fibroblast growth factor-2 protects against myocardial dysfunction and infarction in a murine model of low-flow ischemia[J]. Circulation, 2003, 108(25): 3140-3148.

[23] Chen W, Yu M, Wang Y, et al. Non-mitogenic human acidic fibroblast growth factor reduces retinal degeneration induced by sodium iodate[J]. Journal of Ocular Pharmacology and Therapeutics, 2009, 25(4): 315-319.

[24] Wu X, Su Z, Li X, et al. High-level expression and purification of a nonmitogenic form of human acidic fibroblast growth factor in Escherichia coli[J]. Protein Expression and Purification, 2005, 42(1): 7-11.

[25] Chen SL, Mukherjee S, Chakraborty C, et al. High glucose-induced, endothelin-dependent fibronectin synthesis is mediated via NF-kappa B and AP-1[J]. American Journal of Physiology-Cell Physiology, 2003, 284(2): C263-C272.

[26] Gan XT, Chakrabarti S, Karmazyn M. Increased endothelin-1 and endothelin receptor expression in myocytes of ischemic and reperfused rat hearts and ventricular myocytes exposed to ischemic conditions and its inhibition by nitric oxide generation[J]. Canadian Journal of Physiology and Pharmacology, 2003, 81(2): 105-113.

[27] Cai L, Wang J, Li Y, et al. Inhibition of superoxide generation and associated nitrosative damage is involved in metallothionein prevention of diabetic cardiomyopathy[J]. Diabetes, 2005, 54(6): 1829-1837.

[28] Basu R, Oudit GY, Wang X, et al. Type 1 diabetic cardiomyopathy in the Akita (Ins2(WT/C96Y)) mouse model is characterized by lipotoxicity and diastolic dysfunction with preserved systolic function[J]. American Journal of Physiology-Heart and Circulatory Physiology, 2009, 297(6): H2096-H2108.

[29] Zhou G, Li X, Hein DW, et al. Metallothionein suppresses angiotensin II-Induced nicotinamide adenine dinucleotide phosphate oxidase activation, nitrosative stress, apoptosis, and pathological remodeling in the diabetic heart[J]. Journal of the American College of Cardiology, 2008, 52(8): 655-666.

[30] Chen JW, Ledet T, Orskov H, et al. A highly sensitive and specific assay for determination of IGF-I bioactivity in human serum[J]. American Journal of Physiology-Endocrinology and Metabolism, 2003, 284(6): E1149-E1155.

[31] Khan ZA, Cukiernik M, Gonder JR, et al. Oncofetal fibronectin in diabetic retinopathy[J]. Investigative Ophthalmology & Visual Science, 2004, 45(1): 287-295.

[32] Maulik SK, Kumar S. Oxidative stress and cardiac hypertrophy: a review[J]. Toxicology Mechanisms and Methods, 2012, 22(5): 359-366.

[33] Chong ZZ, Maiese K. Mammalian target of rapamycin signaling in diabetic cardiovascular disease[J]. Cardiovascular Diabetology, 2012, 11.

[34] Feng B, Chen S, George B, et al. miR133a regulates cardiomyocyte hypertrophy in diabetes[J]. Diabetes-Metabolism Research and Reviews, 2010, 26(1): 40-49.

[35] Akazawa H, Komuro I. Roles of cardiac transcription factors in cardiac hypertrophy[J]. Circulation Research, 2003, 92(10): 1079-1088.

[36] Chung CY, Bien H, Sobie EA, et al. Hypertrophic phenotype in cardiac cell assemblies solely by structural cues and ensuing self-organization[J]. Faseb Journal, 2011, 25(3): 851-862.

[37] Horio T, Nishikimi T, Yoshihara F, et al. Inhibitory regulation of hypertrophy by endogenous atrial natriuretic peptide in cultured cardiac myocytes[J]. Hypertension, 2000, 35(1): 19-24.

[38] Conrad CH, Brooks WW, Hayes JA, et al. Myocardial fibrosis and stiffness with hypertrophy and heart failure in the spontaneously hypertensive rat[J]. Circulation, 1995, 91(1): 161-170.

[39] Gunstad J, Lhotsky A, Wendell CR, et al. Longitudinal examination of obesity and cognitive function: Results from the Baltimore longitudinal study of aging[J]. Neuroepidemiology, 2010, 34(4): 222-229.

[40] Mezzetti A, Cipollone F, Cuccurullo F. Oxidative stress and cardiovascular complications in diabetes: isoprostanes as new markers on an old paradigm[J]. Cardiovascular Research, 2000, 47(3): 475-488.

[41] Watanabe K, Thandavarayan RA, Harima M, et al. Role of differential signaling pathways and oxidative stress in diabetic cardiomyopathy[J]. Current Cardiology Reviews, 2010, 6(4): 280-290.

[42] Ito JI, Nagayasu Y, Hoshikawa M, et al. Enhancement of FGF-1 release along with cytosolic proteins from rat astrocytes by hydrogen peroxide[J]. Brain Research, 2013, 1522: 12-21.

[43] Hicks KK, Shin JT, Opalenik SR, et al. Molecular mechanisms of angiogenesis: experimental models define cellular trafficking of FGF-1[J]. Puerto Rico health sciences journal, 1996, 15(3): 179-186.

[44] Cassina P, Pehar M, Vargas MR, et al. Astrocyte activation by fibroblast growth factor-1 and motor neuron apoptosis: implications for amyotrophic lateral sclerosis[J]. Journal of Neurochemistry, 2005, 93(1): 38-46.

[45] Fu X, Li X, Wang T, et al. Enhanced anti-apoptosis and gut epithelium protection function of acidic fibroblast growth factor after cancelling of its mitogenic activity[J]. World Journal of Gastroenterology, 2004, 10(24): 3590-3596.

[46] Li H, Fu X, Sun T, et al. Non-mitogenic acidic fibroblast growth factor reduces intestinal dysfunction induced by ischemia and reperfusion injury in rats[J]. Journal of Gastroenterology and Hepatology, 2007, 22(3): 363-370.

[47] Agarwal A, Said TM. Oxidative stress, DNA damage and apoptosis in male infertility: a clinical approach[J]. Bju International, 2005, 95(4): 503-507.

[48] Miao J, Zhao B, Li H, et al. Effect of safrole oxide on vascular endothelial cell growth and apoptosis induced by deprivation of fibroblast growth factor[J]. Acta Pharmacologica Sinica, 2002, 23(4): 323-326.

[49] Levy D, Garrison RJ, Savage DD, et al. Prognostic implications

of echocardiographically determined left ventricular mass in the Framingham Heart Study[J]. New England Journal of Medicine, 1990, 322(22): 1561-1566.

[50] Cave A, Grieve D, Johar S, *et al.* NADPH oxidase-derived reactive oxygen species in cardiac pathophysiology[J]. Philosophical Transactions of the Royal Society B-Biological Sciences, 2005, 360(1464): 2327-2334.

[51] Takimoto E, Champion HC, Li M, *et al.* Oxidant stress from nitric oxide synthase-3 uncoupling stimulates cardiac pathologic remodeling from chronic pressure load[J]. Journal of Clinical Investigation, 2005, 115(5): 1221-1231.

[52] Suematsu N, Tsutsui H, Wen J, *et al.* Oxidative stress mediates tumor necrosis factor-alpha-induced mitochondrial DNA damage and dysfunction in cardiac myocytes[J]. Circulation, 2003, 107(10): 1418-1423.

Pancreatic fibroblast growth factor 21 protects against type 2 diabetes in mice by promoting insulin expression and secretion in a PI3K/Akt signaling-dependent manner

Yingying Pan, Xiaokun Li, Xuebo Pan

1. Introduction

Type 2 diabetes mellitus (T2DM) is the predominant form of diabetes and is characterized by insulin resistance and pancreatic β-cell failure, which lead to abnormally high blood glucose levels (hyperglycaemia)[1,2]. Impaired function of β-cells, which are responsible for the production and secretion of insulin, is a critical contributing factor for the progression from prediabetes to diabetes[3,4]. The loss of responding β-cells in pancreatic islets has been found in genetically diabetic (db/db) mice[5]. Although previous studies have reported that the β-cell-specific transcription factors pancreatic duodenal homeobox 1 (PDX-1) and v-Maf musculoaponeurotic fibrosarcoma oncogene family, protein A (MafA) play key roles in the maintenance of β-cell function and the production of insulin[6,7], the precise molecular mechanisms underlying β-cell function and insulin expression remain largely unknown, thus greatly limiting the development of effective therapeutic strategies against T2DM.

Fibroblast growth factor 21 (FGF21) is a member of the FGF subfamily but lacks mitogenic activity[8]. Increasing evidence has shown that FGF21 is overexpressed in response to fasting/starvation and mediates fatty acid metabolism, ketogenesis and growth hormone resistance[9-11]. In addition, administration or ectopic overexpression of FGF21 protects against obesity and obesity-associated metabolic disorders in both rodent and nonhuman primate models[12-14]. Mechanistically, FGF21 functions through activating FGF receptor 1/β-klotho complex, which is abundant in adipose tissue as well as the liver, pancreas and hypothalamus[12,15,16]. FGF21 has been shown to play important roles in cellular processes in adipocytes, including glucose uptake, lipolysis[17], mitochondrial fatty acid oxidation[18], peroxisome proliferator-activated receptor-γ activation[19] and white adipose browning[20].

On the other hand, FGF21 also has significant effects on hepatic glucose homeostasis and hepatic insulin sensitivity in T2DM mice[12]. Moreover, FGF21 has a high basal expression in pancreatic islets of mice[21-23] as well as enhances β-cell function and survival in diabetic mice[24,25]. Importantly, exogenous FGF21 replenishment has been shown to increase insulin secretion and content in pancreatic islets isolated from diabetic rodents[25]. However, the role of pancreatic FGF21 in the maintenance of pancreatic islet morphology and function remains obscure. In this study, we investigated the expression pattern and role of FGF21 in pancreatic islets using a T2DM mouse model and proposed the underlying regulatory mechanism.

2. Materials and methods

2.1 Animal study

FGF21-knockout mice using the C57BL/6J genetic background were generated as described previously[26]. Ten-week-old male T2DM BKS.Cg-Dock7^m+/+Lepr^{db}/J mice (BKS-db/db mice) and lean controls were purchased from The Jackson Laboratory (#000642; Bar Harbor, ME, USA). The mice were housed in clean cages with a regular 12-hour dark/light cycle and had free access to food and water. The animal experiments were carried out in accordance with Wenzhou Medical University Guidelines for the Care and Use of Laboratory Animals (wydw2015-0096). Adeno-associated viral (AAV, serotype 5) vector encoding green fluorescent protein (GFP) driven by the modified mouse insulin promoter and the AAV helper vector were purchased from Viraltherapy Technologies (Viraltherapy Technologies, Hubei, China). To determine the effect of FGF21 on insulin synthesis and secretion in β-cells, 16-week-old db/db mice were treated with AAV-GFP or AAV-FGF21 carrying the mouse insulin promoter by tail intravenous injection at a final dose of 1×10^{11} vg/mouse in a total volume of 100 μl. The intraperitoneal glucose tolerance test was performed at 4 weeks after the treatment. Mice were fasted overnight (17:00 to 9:00) prior to the intraperitoneal injection of 1.0 g/kg body weight of glucose. Blood glucose levels were measured using a glucometer (B. Braun, Germany) loaded with a small drop of blood (~5 μl) from the tail tip at 15, 30, 45, 60, 75, 90 and 120 minutes after the administration of glucose. After the intraperitoneal glucose tolerance test, the animals were killed and the following experiments were performed.

2.2 Pancreatic islet isolation and primary culture

The animals were dissected, and the pancreatic tissue was exposed, followed by perfusion with 2 ml of type IV collagenase (2 mg/ml; Sigma) *via* the bile duct. The tissue was then digested by shaking gently for 10 minutes at 37℃. Digestion was terminated by perfusion with 30 ml of Hank's solution, and then the islets were hand-picked under a stereo microscope and maintained in RPMI-1640 culture medium (Gibco, Life Technologies) supplemented with 10% foetal bovine serum (Gibco, Life Technologies) and 100 U/ml penicillin–0.1 mg/ml streptomycin (Invitrogen, VIC, Australia) overnight. The isolated islets were washed twice and pre-incubated in Krebs-Ringer bicarbonate buffer containing 0.1% fatty acid-free bovine serum albumin and 3 mmol/L glucose for 1 hour, followed by stimulation with 16.7 mmol/L glucose for 1 hour. Insulin secretion in each fraction was measured using an insulin enzyme-linked immunosorbent assay (ELISA) kit (Antibody and Immunoassay Services, The University of Hong Kong). For signaling studies, the freshly isolated islets were serum-starved for 8 hours and then treated with 1 mmol/L palmitate for 48 hours.

2.3 Cell viability assay

Islet viability was detected by fluorescein diacetate/propidium iodide staining. Fluorescein diacetate (Sigma Aldrich, St. Louis, MO, USA) stains living cells, exhibiting green fluorescence; while propidium iodide (Sigma Aldrich) stains dead cells, exhibiting red fluorescence. Islets were incubated with fluorescein diacetate for 2 minutes, followed by incubation with propidium iodide for 30 seconds. Then, the islets were washed three times with phosphate-buffered saline and observed under a fluorescence microscope (Nikon Eclipse TE 200-S, Chiyoda-Ku, Japan) at 200× magnification.

2.4 Immunofluorescence and immunohistochemistry

Mouse pancreatic tissues were collected, fixed in paraformaldehyde, dehydrated and then embedded in paraffin. Five-micrometer thick sections were prepared for immunofluorescence staining. Briefly, after deparaffinization and rehydration, sections were blocked in 5% bovine serum albumin, followed by incubation with primary antibodies overnight at 4℃, and then with FITC- or TRITC-conjugated secondary antibodies (Santa Cruz) for 60 minutes at 37℃. The sections were washed with phosphate-buffered saline–Tween 20 three times, then mounted with DAPI (Abcam) for nuclear staining. For immuno-histochemical staining, horseradish peroxidase-conjugated anti-rabbit secondary antibodies were used, and the staining was visualized using diaminobenzidine, followed by counterstaining with haematoxylin. The following primary antibodies were used: anti-amylase (sc-46657; Santa Cruz), anti-insulin (sc-9168; Santa Cruz), anti-insulin (ab6995; Abcam), anti-glucagon (sc-13091; Santa Cruz), anti-FGF21 (ab64857; Abcam), anti-syntaxin-1 (STX-1) (sc-12736; Santa Cruz), anti-SNAP25 (ab41455; Abcam), anti-VAMP2 (ab3347; Abcam) and anti-cleaved caspase-3 (9664; Cell Signaling Technology).

2.5 Biochemical measurements

Blood glucose levels were measured using a standard automated glucose monitor (B. Braun, Germany). Plasma insulin levels were determined using a high-sensitive mouse-insulin ELISA Kit (Antibody and Immunoassay Services, The University of Hong Kong). FGF21 levels were measured using a mouse-FGF21 ELISA Kit (Antibody and Immunoassay Services, The University of Hong Kong).

2.6 Western blot

Briefly, tissues or islets were homogenized and lysed with RIPA buffer supplemented with a Complete Mini Protease Inhibitor Cocktail (Roche, Basel, Switzerland) and phosphatase inhibitors. Lysates were obtained, and protein concentrations were determined using a bicinchoninic acid protein assay. Protein samples (20 μg) were loaded, separated by sodium dodecyl sulfate–polyacrylamide gel electrophoresis and transferred onto a nitrocellulose membrane. The membrane was blocked with 5% non-fat dry milk in Tris-buffered saline–Tween 20, then incubated with primary antibodies overnight at 4℃ and finally incubated with horseradish peroxidase-conjugated secondary antibody for 1 hour at 37℃. Detection was performed with enhanced chemiluminescence reagents (Advansta). The antibodies used were as follows: anti-MafA (sc-66958; Santa Cruz), anti-MafB (sc-10022; Santa Cruz), anti-PDX-1 (sc-14662; Santa Cruz), anti-STX-1 (sc-12736; Santa Cruz), anti-FGF21 (ab171941; Abcam), anti-SNAP25 (ab41455; Abcam), anti-VAMP2 (ab3347; Abcam), anti-cleaved caspase-3 (9664; Cell Signaling Technology), anti-caspase-3 (9662; Cell Signaling Technology), anti-phospho-phosphatidylinositol 3-kinase (PI3K) at Tyr458/Tyr199 (4228; Cell Signaling Technology), anti-total PI3K (4249; Cell Signaling Technology), anti-phospho-Akt at Ser-473 (4060; Cell Signaling Technology), anti-total Akt (4685; Cell Signaling Technology) and anti-GAPDH (AB-P-R001; GoodHere Technology).

2.7 Real-time PCR analysis

Total RNA was extracted from tissue or isolated islets using TRIzol reagent (Invitrogen). cDNA was synthesized from 0.5 μg of total RNA using a supermix consisting of oligo (dT), random hexamer primers and reverse transcriptase (Invitrogen). Relative gene expression levels were determined by reverse transcription–polymerase chain reaction (PCR) (Applied Biosystems, Foster City, CA, USA) using SYBR Green with normalization to GAPDH. The primers used are listed in Table S1.

2.8 Apoptosis analysis

A TUNEL assay was performed to detect apoptosis using a TMR green *in situ* cell death detection kit (Roche Applied Science), according to the manufacturer's instructions. The fluorescence was detected under a fluorescence microscope at 400× magnification.

2.9 Statistical analysis

Data were analysed using Microsoft Excel 2016 and GraphPad Prism 6.0 software (San Diego, CA, USA) and are presented as means ± SEM. The one-way ANOVA test was performed, and $P < 0.05$ was considered statistically significant.

3. Results

3.1 Low FGF21 expression is associated with islet β-cell dysfunction in vivo

To investigate the possible role of FGF21 in maintaining pancreatic islet function, we first examined the expression pattern of FGF21 in pancreatic islets of db/db mice. As shown in Fig. 1A and B and Fig. S1A, FGF21 was highly expressed in pancreas and specifically expressed in pancreatic islets of lean mice where insulin was produced (Fig. 1A) and was down-regulated in the islets of db/db mice, compared with that in lean controls (Fig. 1B). These findings were further confirmed by quantitative PCR and western blot analyses (Fig. 1C, D). Notably, however, we found significantly increased circulating FGF21 levels and hepatic FGF21 expression in db/db mice (Fig. S1B–D), consistent with a previous study that plasma FGF21 is mainly liver driving[27]. In addition, we found that the development of islet β-cells was impaired in db/db mice, as demonstrated by the decreased population of islet β-cells specifically expressing insulin and the increased population of islet α-cells specifically expressing glucagon, compared with the levels in the lean controls (Fig. 1E). Consistently, the rate of apoptosis was significantly higher in the islet β-cells of db/db mice (Fig. 1F), compared to that in lean controls. Collectively, these data suggest that pancreatic FGF21 is inhibited in db/ db mice, which may be correlated with islet β-cell dysfunction in T2DM.

3.2 Pancreatic FGF21 is essential for islet β-cell function ex vivo

As low FGF21 expression in islets may be associated with islet β-cell dysfunction as described above, we next in-

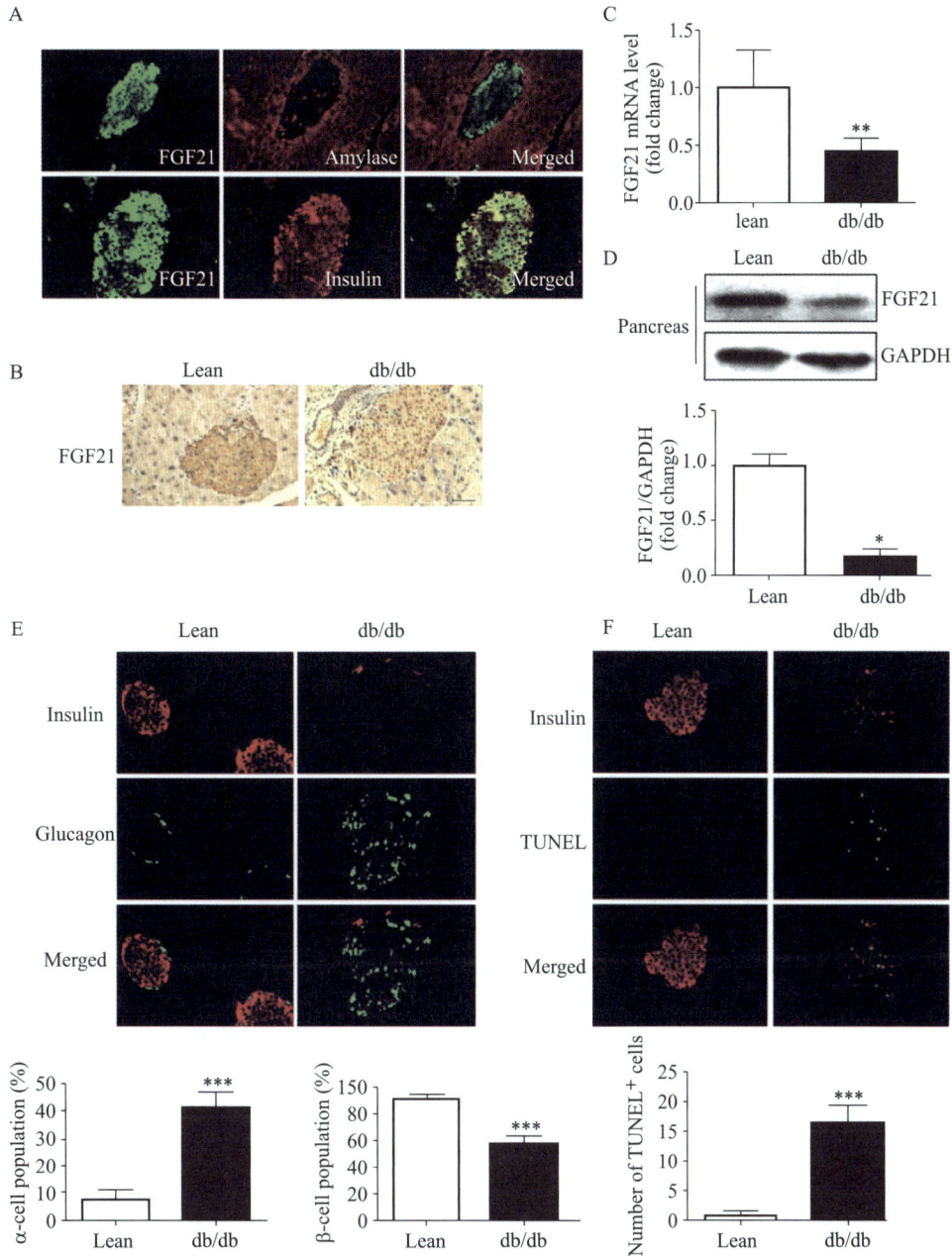

Fig. 1. Low FGF21 expression was associated with islet β-cell dysfunction in db/db mice. (A) Immunofluorescence staining of FGF21 (green), amylase (red) and insulin (red) in pancreatic tissues of 8-week-old lean mice. (B) Immunohistochemical staining of FGF21 in pancreatic tissues of 8-week-old lean mice and db/db mice. (C) Quantitative PCR analysis of FGF21 mRNA expression. (D) Western blot analysis of FGF21 protein expression, normalized to GAPDH. (E) Immunofluorescence staining of insulin (red) and glucagon (green) in pancreatic sections and quantification of insulin- or glucagon-positive cells. (F) Immunofluorescence staining of insulin (red) and TUNEL (green) staining in pancreatic sections as well as quantification of TUNEL-positive β-cells. $^{*}P < 0.05$, $^{**}P < 0.01$. Scale bar = 50 μm. (A–C) $n = 5$. (D) $n = 3$

vestigated whether FGF21 plays a role in maintaining islet β-cell function using a loss-of-function assay. As shown in Fig. 2A, palmitate induced the failure of cultured wild-type islets along with the significant down-regulation of FGF21 in wild-type islets; whereas FGF21 knockout further exacerbated the adverse effects of palmitate on the islets, as demonstrated by stronger propidium iodide staining in FGF21-deficient islets than that in wild-type islets (Fig. S2), suggesting the positive role of FGF21 in islets. To further examine the effect of lack of FGF21 on β-cell defect, we assessed glucose-stimulated insulin secretion (GSIS) of isolated islets. As expected, there was a marked increase in palmitate-induced inhibition of GSIS under high-glucose conditions (16.7 mmol/L) in islets from FGF21 knockout mice, compared with that in islets from wild-type mice (Fig. 2B). Taken together, these results suggest that FGF21 is important for

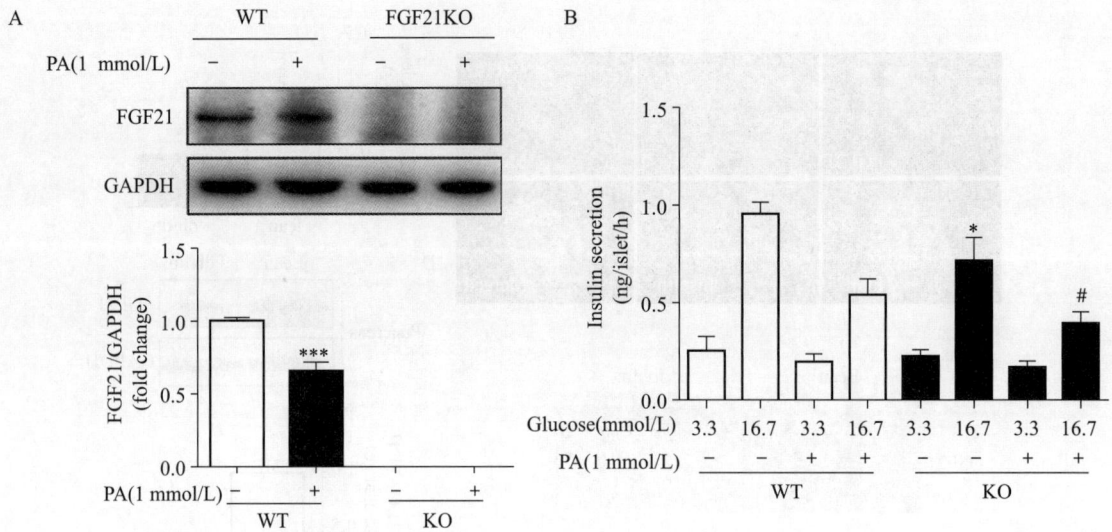

Fig. 2. FGF21 deficiency exacerbated palmitate (PA)-induced islet β-cell failure. Isolated islets from wild-type (WT) mice or FGF21 knockout (KO) mice were exposed to 1 mmol/L PA for 48 h followed by (A) western blot assay ($^{***}P < 0.001$ vs. the blank WT group), and (B) the glucose-stimulated insulin secretion (GSIS) test ($^*P < 0.05$ vs. the WT group stimulated with 16.7 mmol/L glucose, $^\#P < 0.05$ vs. the KO group stimulated with 16.7 mmol/L glucose). ($n = 4$–5).

the maintenance of islet β-cell function.

3.3 Overexpression of pancreatic FGF21 improves islet β-cell function and lipid metabolism disorder in vivo

Overexpression of FGF21 in islets by AAV-FGF21 was confirmed by immunohistochemistry (Fig. 3A). Western blot analysis also showed that the treatments with AAV-FGF21 increased FGF21 protein expression in islet of db/db mice (Fig. 3B). In addition, AAV-FGF21 further increased plasma FGF21 levels significantly in db/db mice (Fig. 3C). The beneficial effect of FGF21 on islet β-cells was further confirmed by our findings that AAV-FGF21 treatment attenuated hyperglycaemia (Fig. 3D, E) and ameliorated glucose intolerance in db/db mice (Fig. 3F, G). However, β-cell-specific delivery of FGF21 did not affect the body weights significantly in db/db mice (Fig. S3A). The AAV-FGF21 significantly increased the serum adiponectin and decreased the lipid profiles (Fig. S3B–F) and attenuated fat accumulation both in the liver and pancreas in diabetic mice at weeks 4 after gene treatment (Fig. S3G). These data demonstrate that FGF21 plays a protective role against diabetes, which is likely as a result of the improvement of islet β-cell function by FGF21.

To further investigate the role of FGF21 in maintaining islet β-cell function, a gain-of-function assay was performed in db/db mice. The results showed that administration of AAV-FGF21 effectively promoted insulin production in the islets, improved the distorted islet morphology, and alleviated islet hyperplasia (Fig. 4A) as well as increased the islet β-cell population and decreased the islet α-cell population in db/db mice (Fig. 4B), compared with the AAV-GFP group. Furthermore, AAV-F21 also suppressed islet β-cell apoptosis, as demonstrated by the reduction in both the number of TUNEL-positive cells and the expression level of cleaved caspase-3 in the islets of db/db mice (Fig. 4C, D). Taken together, these results suggest that pancreatic FGF21 may have a beneficial effect on islet β-cells in vivo.

3.4 FGF21 promotes insulin expression and secretion as well as the expression of insulin gene transcription factors and soluble N-ethylmaleimide-sensitive factor activating protein receptor proteins

To explore the mechanisms underlying the role of FGF21 in islet β-cells, we investigated the effect of FGF21 on insulin and insulin-regulating transcription factors like MafA, MafB and PDX-1 in islets of db/db mice. As shown in Fig. 5A–D, the mRNA expression of these four genes was inhibited in islets of db/db mice, compared with that in islets of lean controls. The inhibited expression was significantly restored by overexpression of FGF21, which was consistent with the protein expression patterns of these four genes(Fig. 5E–G, Fig. S4). These data suggest that the protective effect of FGF21 may be attributable to collective up-regulation of insulin and insulin-regulating transcription factors.

As soluble N-ethylmaleimide-sensitive factor attachment protein receptor (SNARE) proteins are the main regula-

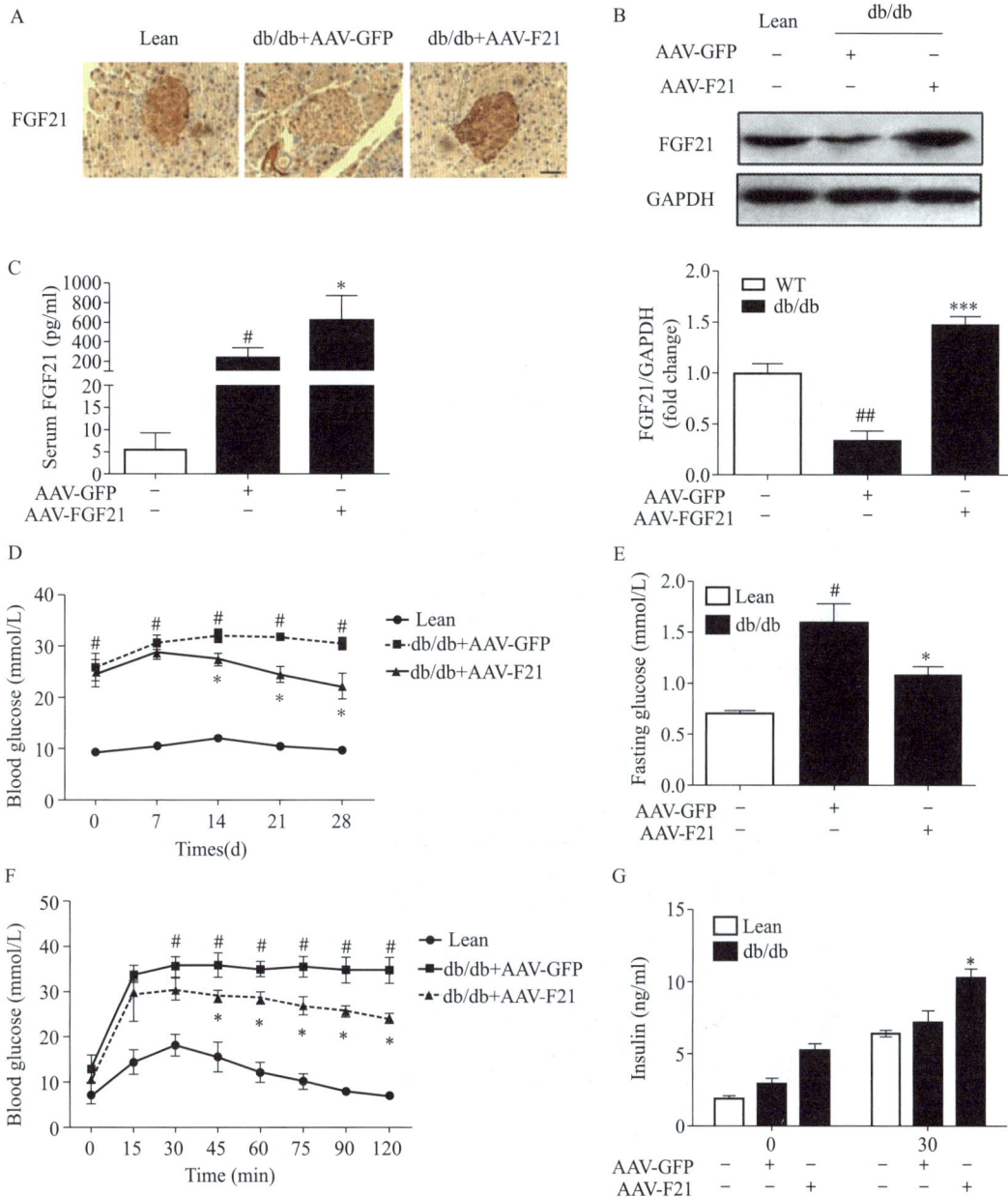

Fig. 3. Overexpression of FGF21 ameliorated hyperglycaemia and glucose intolerance in db/db mice. Sixteen-week-old db/db mice were intra-peritoneally injected with AAV-FGF21. Serum samples at the indicated time points were collected to determine the blood glucose and circulating FGF21 levels. Age-matched lean mice with the same genetic background were injected with AAV-GFP, which served as controls. (A) Immunohis-tochemical staining of FGF21. (B) Western blot analysis of FGF21 protein expression in islets. (C) Serum FGF21 after 4 weeks of gene delivery in the fed state. (E) Fasting glucose levels after treatment with AAV-FGF21. (D) Time course of blood glucose levels. (F) GTT results after gene treatment. (G) Plasma insulin levels at 0 and 30 min after intraperitoneal glucose injection were quantified by ELISA. $^{#}P < 0.05$ vs. the lean con-trols, $^{*}P < 0.05$ vs. db/db mice treated with AAV-GFP. Scale bar = 50 μm ($n = 5$)

tors of insulin secretion[28], we next determined whether FGF21 is also involved in the regulation of insulin secretion and insulin secretion-related SNARE proteins. As shown in Fig. 6A and B, both the plasma insulin levels and GSIS were significantly elevated in db/db mice following AAV-FGF21 treatment. In addition, AAV-FGF21 treatment restored the mRNA and protein expression of three SNARE proteins (STX-1, SNAP25 and VAMP2) in db/db mice (Fig. 6C–H, Fig. S5). These data suggest that FGF21 may function through promoting insulin secretion and up-regulating the expression of SNARE proteins in islets.

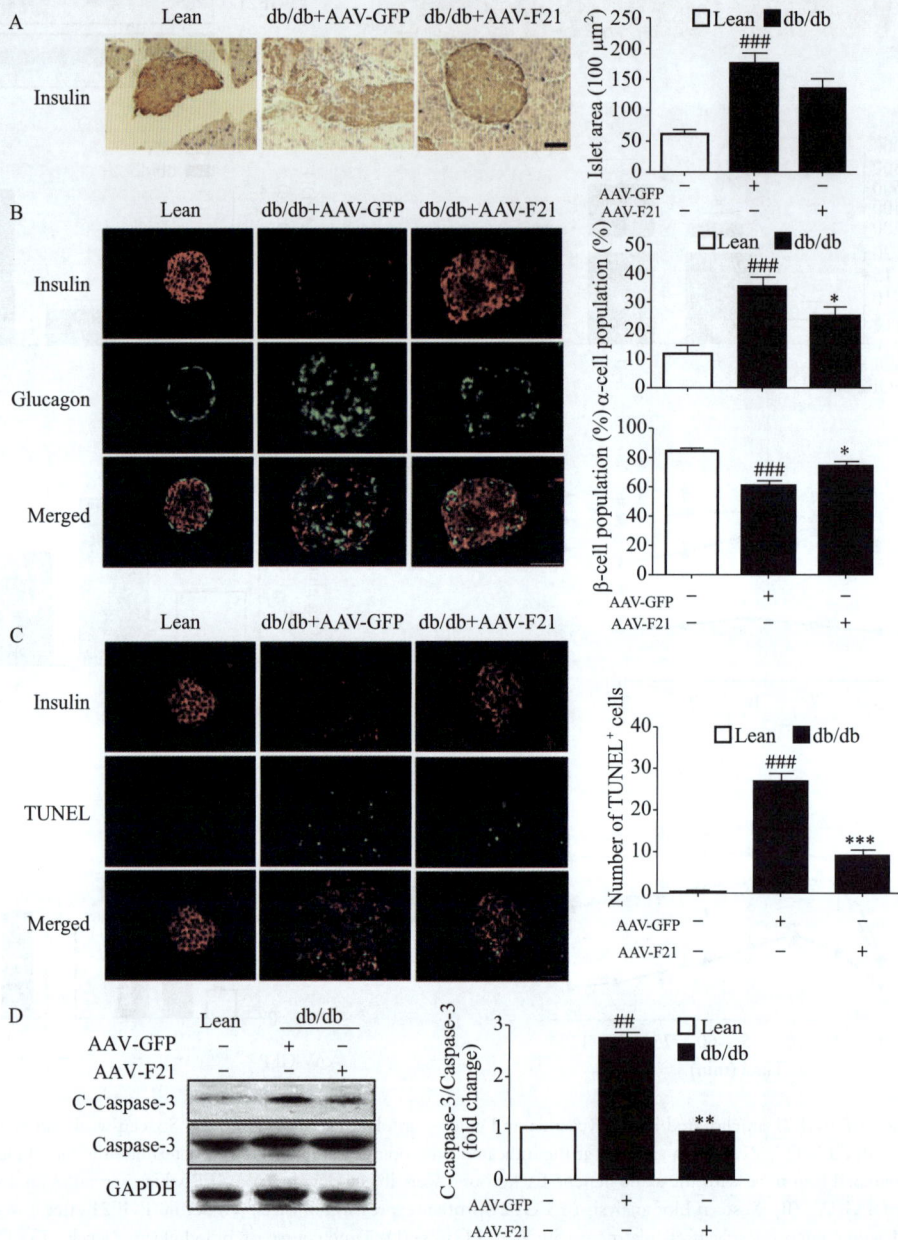

Fig. 4. FGF21 improved islet β-cell function *in vivo*. Sixteen-week-old db/db mice and their lean controls were intraperitoneally injected with AAV-F21 or AAV-GFP. Mice were killed at 4 weeks after the AAV injection. (A) Immunohistochemical staining of insulin and measurement of the islet area in pancreatic sections. (B) Immunofluorescence staining of insulin and glucagon in pancreatic sections and quantification of insulin- or glucagon-positive cells. (C) Immunofluorescence staining of insulin and TUNEL in pancreatic sections as well as quantification of TUNEL-positive β-cells. (D) Western blot analysis of cleaved and total caspase-3 expression in the islets isolated from db/db mice, normalized to GAPDH expression. ###$P < 0.001$ *vs.* the lean controls, *$P < 0.05$, **$P < 0.01$, and ***$P < 0.00$ *vs.* db/db mice treated with AAV-GFP. Scale bar = 50 μm. (A–C) $n = 5$. (D) $n = 3$

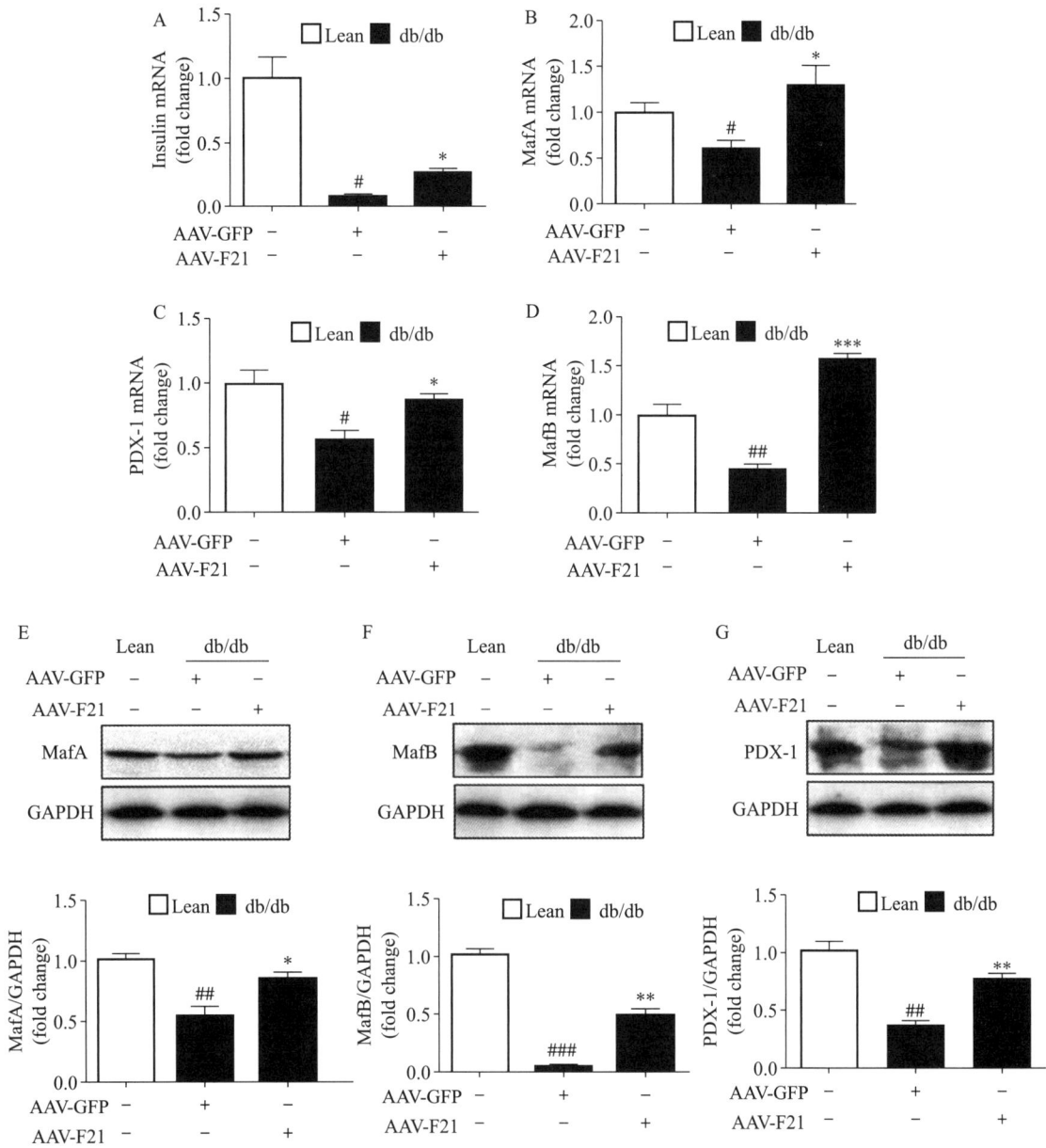

Fig. 5. FGF21 promoted insulin secretion along with up-regulation of insulin gene transcription factors. Sixteen-week-old db/db mice and their lean controls were intraperitoneally injected with AAV-F21 or AAV-GFP and analysed 4 weeks later. (A–D) Quantitative PCR analysis of insulin, MafA, MafB and PDX1 mRNA expression in the islets. (E–G) Western blot analysis of insulin, MafA, MafB and PDX1 protein expression in the islets. $^{#}P < 0.05$ and $^{##}P < 0.01$ vs. the lean controls; $^{*}P < 0.05$, $^{**}P < 0.01$ and $^{***}P < 0.001$ vs. db/db mice treated with AAV-GFP (n = 3-5 for each group)

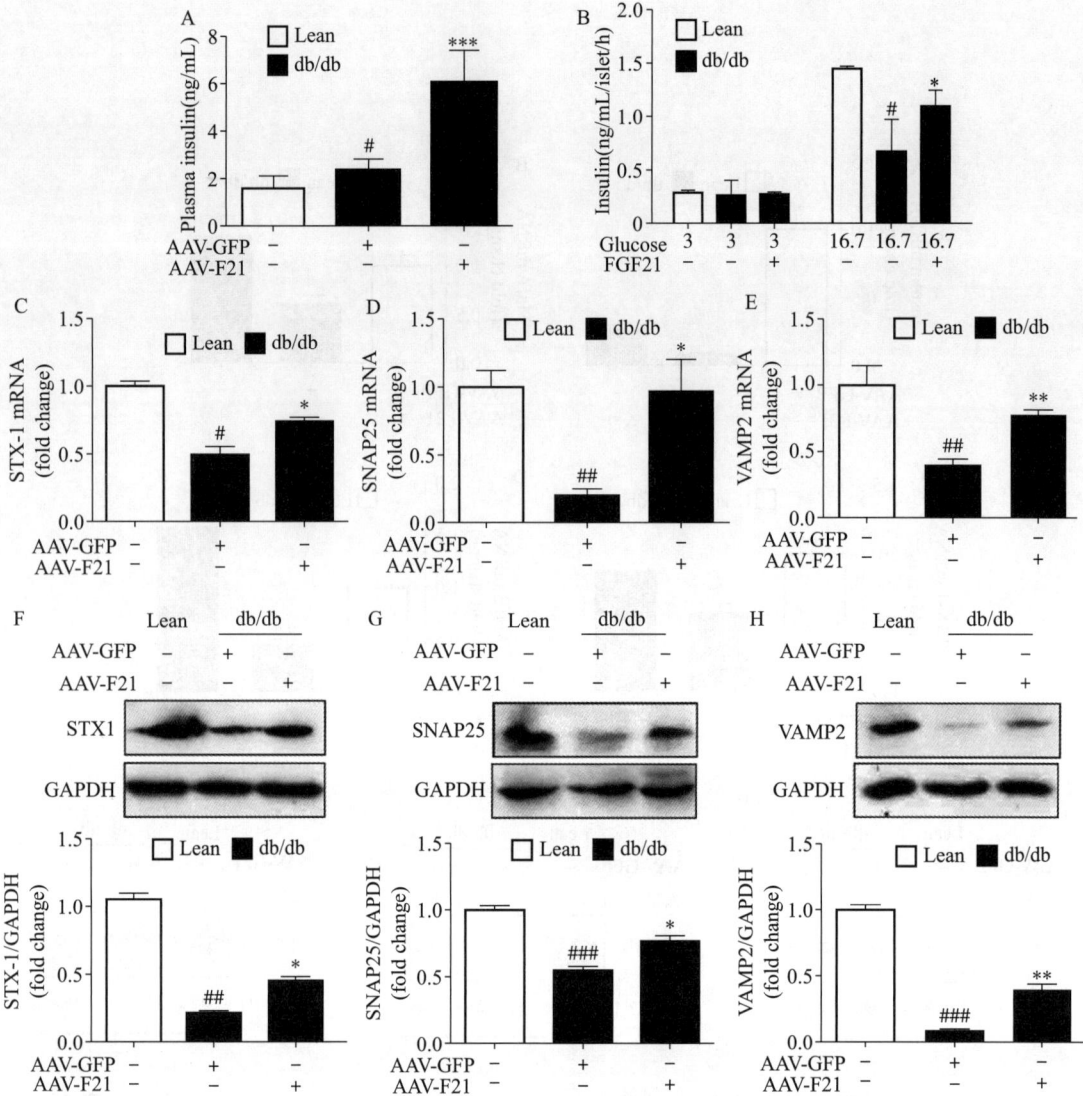

Fig. 6. FGF21 promoted insulin secretion along with up-regulation of SNARE proteins. Sixteen-week-old db/db mice and their lean controls were intraperitoneally injected with AAV-F21 or AAV-GFP and killed 4 weeks later. (A) The plasma insulin levels were measured immediately following the killing. (B) Static glucose-stimulated insulin secretion (GSIS) in isolated islets was measured at 1 h after 16.7 mmol/L glucose stimulation. (C–E) Quantitative PCR analysis of STX1, SNAP25 and VAMP2 in isolated islets. (F–H) Western blot analysis of STX1, SNAP25 and VAMP2 in isolated islets. [#]$P < 0.05$, [##]$P < 0.01$ and [###]$P < 0.001$ vs. the lean controls; [*]$P < 0.05$ and [**]$P < 0.01$ vs. db/db mice treated with AAV-GFP. (A) $n = 5$. (B–H) $n = 3$-5.

3.5 FGF21 functions in a PI3K/Akt signaling-dependent manner

Izumiya et al[29] proved that FGF21 secreted from muscle is regulated by an Akt1 signaling pathway-dependent mechanism. In addition, numerous studies have implicated that the PI3K/Akt signaling cascade plays a pivotal role in the regulation of insulin secretion[30,31], we sought to examine whether the promotive effects of FGF21 on insulin expression and secretion are dependent on the PI3K/Akt signaling pathway. FGF21 effect results from activation of β-klotho. AAV-FGF21-induced up-regulation of β-klotho in db/db mice was shown in Fig. 7A. As shown in Fig. 7B and C, the activity of PI3K and Akt was significantly suppressed in the islets of db/db mice, compared with lean controls, whereas the suppressive effects were markedly reversed by replenishment of FGF21. Importantly, pharmaceutical inhibition of PI3K/Akt signaling in islets by GDC-0941 and MK-2206 significantly inhibited FGF21-induced insulin expression and secretion in cultured islets (Fig. 7D–G), suggesting that PI3K/Akt signaling is essential for the effects of FGF21 on insulin expression and secretion.

Next, we sought to investigate whether FGF21 regulates insulin gene transcription factors and SNARE proteins via

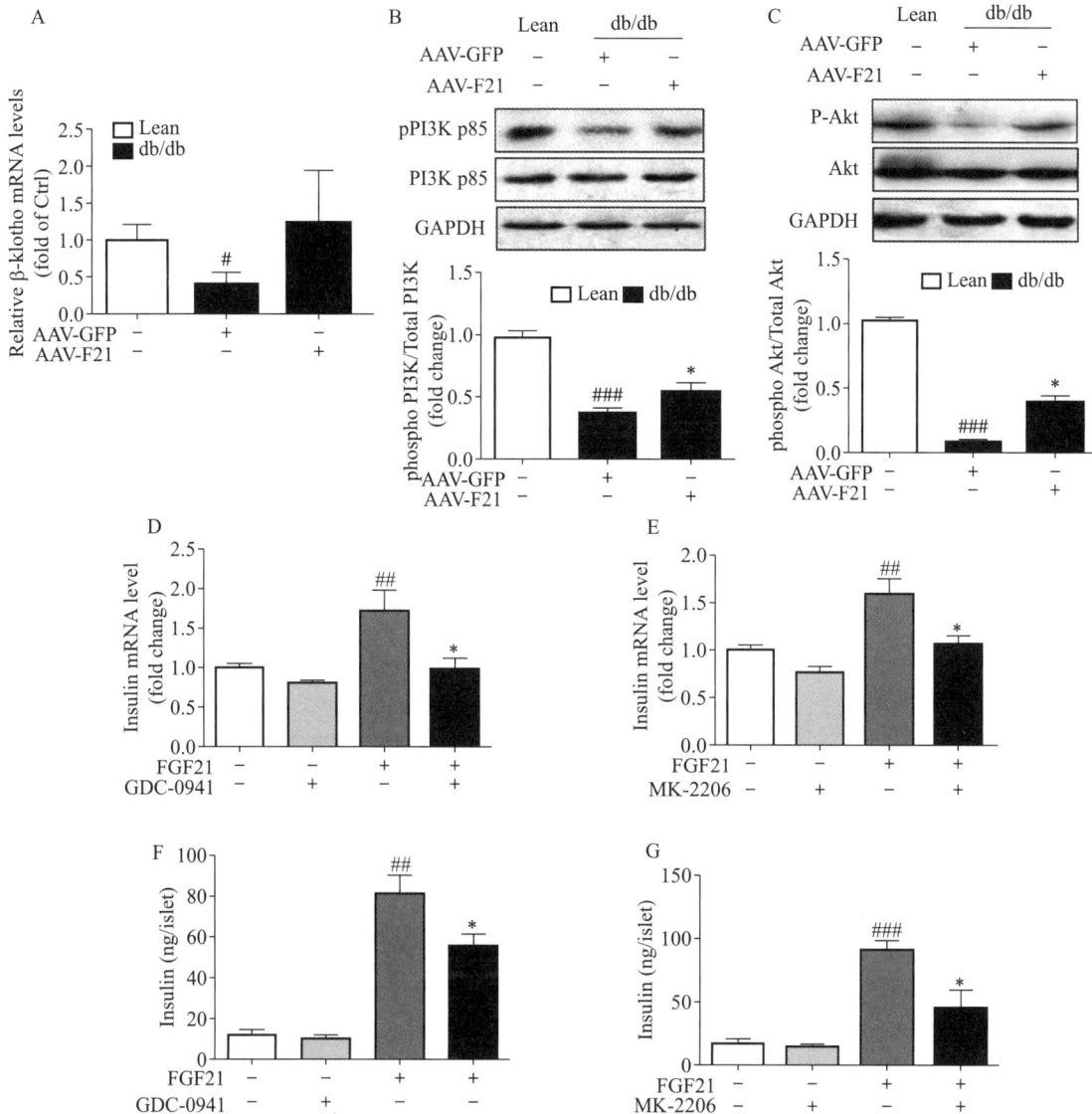

Fig. 7. FGF21 regulated insulin expression and secretion in islets *via* PI3K/Akt signaling pathways. (A) Quantitative PCR analysis of β-klotho mRNA expression in islet. (B and C) Sixteen-week-old db/db mice and their lean controls were intraperitoneally injected with AAV-F21 or AAV-GFP and analysed 4 weeks later. Western blot analysis of phosphorylated and total PI3K and Akt protein expression. $^{###}P < 0.001$ *vs.* the lean controls, $^{*}P < 0.05$ *vs.* db/db mice treated with AAV-GFP ($n = 3$). (D-G) Islets were isolated from 12-week-old lean mice and then treated with 100 ng/ml FGF21 in the absence or presence of PI3K inhibitor (GDC-0941, 5 μmol/L) or Akt inhibitor (MK-2206, 1 μmol/L) for 12 h. (D and E) Quantitative PCR analysis of insulin mRNA levels in islets after the treatment. (F and G) Static insulin secretion in isolated islets. $^{##}P < 0.01$ and $^{###}P < 0.001$ *vs.* the vehicle group; $^{*}P < 0.05$ *vs.* the FGF21 group without GDC-0941 or MK-2206 ($n = 5$)

PI3K/Akt signaling as well. As shown in Fig. 8A–D, the PI3K/Akt signaling inhibitors GDC-0941 and MK-2206 dramatically inhibited the FGF21-induced expression of insulin gene transcription factors and SNARE proteins. These data suggest that the role of FGF21 in regulating insulin expression and secretion-related factors is dependent on the PI3K/Akt signaling cascade.

4. Discussion

Substantial β-cell failure occurs at the early stage of T2DM[32] and serves as a major contributing factor of the pathogenesis of T2DM[33]. In this study, we demonstrated that FGF21 expression was decreased dramatically in pancreatic islets of db/db mice and that pancreatic islet-specific overexpression of FGF21 by AAV-FGF21 significantly improved glycolipid metabolism and alleviated the development of diabetes in db/db mice. On the other hand, our ex vivo

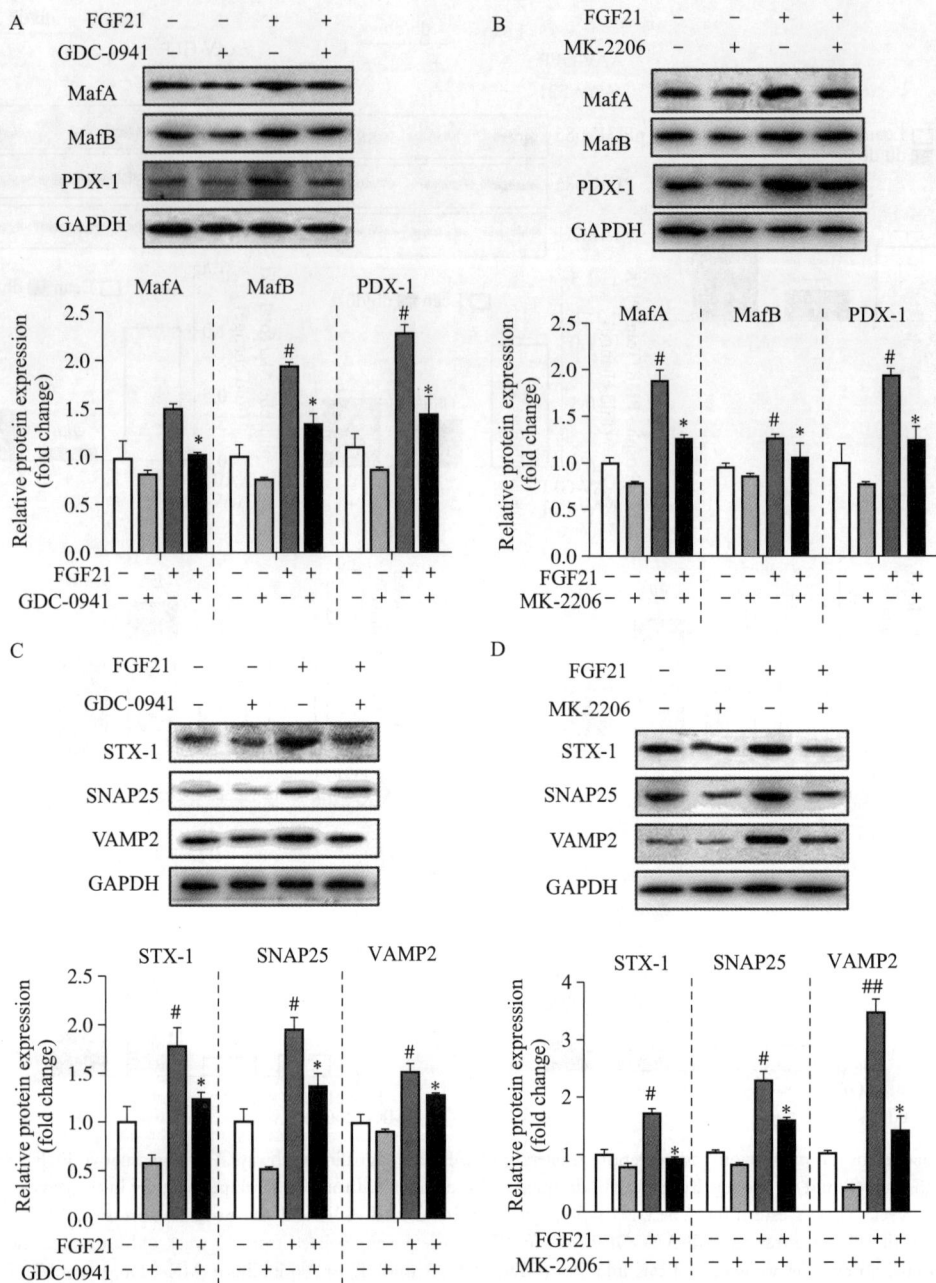

Fig. 8. FGF21 regulated insulin gene transcription factors and SNARE proteins *via* PI3K/Akt signaling pathways. Islets were isolated from 12-week-old lean mice and then treated with 100 ng/ml FGF21 in the absence or presence of PI3K inhibitor (GDC-0941, 5 μmol/L) or Akt inhibitor (MK-2206, 1 μmol/L) for 12 h. (A and B) Western blot analyses of MafA, MafB and PDX-1 in islets after the treatment. (C and D) Western blot analyses of SNARE protein expression in islets after the treatment. $^{#}P < 0.05$ and $^{##}P < 0.01$ *vs.* the vehicle group; $^{*}P < 0.05$ *vs.* the FGF21 group without GDC-0941 or MK-2206 ($n = 4$)

studies also indicated that FGF21 deficiency accelerated palmitate-induced islet injury in cultured islets and attenuated islet function, as demonstrated by the decreased insulin expression and secretion. Collectively, these findings suggest that pancreatic FGF21 is important for promoting insulin expression and secretion, which in turn protect against the progression of diabetes.

Previous studies indicate that FGF21 is a metabolic hormone preferentially expressed in liver tissue with multiple functions[34,35]. In addition to the liver, FGF21 is highly expressed in adipose tissue and the hypothalamus. Recent studies have shown that FGF21 is also abundant in the pancreas[36] and plays an anti-inflammatory role in pancreatitis in mice[37]. Furthermore, exogenous administration of FGF21 can improve islet transplant success as well as protect islets from glucolipotoxicity and cytokine-induced apoptosis[23,25]. A recent study has suggested that FGF21 is highly expressed in exocrine pancreas and functions as an exocrine pancreas secretagogue[38], which is not consistent with our findings that the majority of pancreatic FGF21 is synthesized in the islets of C57/BL6 mice at the basal state. Furthermore, another report stated that FGF21[23] is highly expressed in pancreatic islets, supporting out data, and pancreatic islet and liver may be major sources of systemic FGF21 since chemical ablation of pancreatic β-cells by streptozotocin and liver-specific FGF21 KO both result in a dramatic reduction in circulating FGF21[27]. Our data showed that pancreatic FGF21 expression was extremely weak in db/db mice, along with a decrease in the number of β-cells as well as islet insulin-synthesizing and -secreting function. Interestingly, hepatic and circulating FGF21 levels were increased in db/db mice along with the decrease in β-klotho in islets, suggesting that pancreatic β-cells may have been resistant to hepatic and circulating FGF21 because of the loss of β-klotho. These findings were consistent with previous works[39,40] showing that mice lacking β-klotho are unresponsive to FGF21 stimulation. What is more, the changes of hepatic and pancreatic FGF21 in db/db mice also suggest that the liver is a main source of serum FGF21. In addition, hepatic FGF21 has been found to regulate fatty acid metabolism and improve fatty liver disease in db/db mice[41,42]. These results suggest that pancreatic FGF21 may be involved in the pathogenesis of diabetes. In support of this observation, AAV-mediated FGF21 expression in islets significantly decreased the glucose levels and improved glucose tolerance in db/db mice.

It is well established that insulin expression is mediated by MafA, MafB and PDX-1[43] and that insulin secretion is mediated by SNARE proteins in β-cells[28]. Under diabetic conditions, the expression of MafA, MafB and PDX-1 is markedly decreased in β-cells, leading to suppressed insulin biosynthesis and secretion. Meanwhile, the secretory vesicle (v) SNAREs (VAMP2) interact with the target membrane SNARE proteins (STX-1 and SNAP25) to form a stable heterotrimeric complex to facilitate membrane fusion[44-46], and their deficiency is responsible, in part, for the impaired insulin secretion in both human T2DM and animal models of T2DM[5,47]. Consistent with these findings, SNARE proteins as well as MafA, MafB and PDX-1 were found to be significantly decreased in db/db mice. Importantly, AAV-mediated β-cell-specific overexpression of FGF21 significantly increased the mRNA and protein expression levels of MafA, MafB and PDX-1 as well as SNARE proteins in the islets of mice. Functionally, overexpression of FGF21 attenuated hyperglycaemia and insulin storage, improved glucose tolerance and preserved islet β-cells from apoptosis. Consistently, our data also indicate that insulin was significantly up-regulated along with increased GSIS in isolated islets from db/db mice after AAV-FGF21 treatment. These results suggest that FGF21 may protect against T2DM in mice through promoting insulin expression and secretion as a result of collective up-regulation of MafA, MafB and PDX-1 as well as SNARE proteins in islets of db/db mice.

Growing evidence has shown that PI3K/Akt signaling plays a critical role in the regulation of β-cell function[30,48] and that inactivation of PI3K/Akt signaling in β-cells leads to glucose intolerance and decreases insulin secretion in response to glucose challenge as a result of down-regulation of SNARE complex proteins[48]. Consistently, we demonstrated for the first time that PI3K/Akt signaling was significantly inhibited in the islets of db/db mice, whereas AAV-FGF21 significantly promoted the phosphorylation of PI3K and Akt, in parallel with an increase in insulin expression and a decrease in β-cell apoptosis. On the other hand, our ex vivo data also indicated that treatment with FGF21 protein also increased insulin expression and activated PI3K/Akt signaling in cultured islets. However, this effect was partially reversed in the presence of PI3K/Akt signaling inhibitors, indicating that other pathways may be involved in the FGF21-mediated signal transduction. We also found that mTOR is hyperactivated in diabetic islets and FGF21 up-regulation inhibits mTOR activity while promoting insulin secretion in db/db mouse islets (data not shown). Taken together, these data suggest that the beneficial effects of FGF21 on insulin synthesis and secretion may be at least partially attributed to activation of PI3K/Akt signaling.

In summary, our findings demonstrate that pancreatic FGF21 protects β-cells from T2DM-induced injury through promoting insulin synthesis and secretion, which are mediated by PI3K/Akt signaling-dependent up-regulation of MafA, MafB and PDX-1 as well as SNARE proteins. In future studies, the protective role of pancreatic FGF21 in T2DM needs to be further confirmed using a β-cell-specific knockout FGF21 mouse model.

References

[1] Ors D, Altinova AE, Yalcin MM, et al. Fibroblast growth factor 21 and its relationship with insulin sensitivity in first-degree relatives of patients with type 2 diabetes mellitus[J]. Endokrynologia Polska, 2016, 67(3): 260-264.

[2] Alejandro EU, Gregg B, Blandino-Rosano M, et al. Natural history of beta-cell adaptation and failure in type 2 diabetes[J]. Molecular Aspects of Medicine, 2015, 42: 19-41.

[3] Leahy JL, Hirsch IB, Peterson KA, et al. Targeting beta-cell function early in the course of therapy for type 2 diabetes mellitus[J]. Journal of Clinical Endocrinology & Metabolism, 2010, 95(9): 4206-4216.

[4] Do OH, Gunton JE, Gaisano HY, et al. Changes in beta cell function occur in prediabetes and early disease in the Lepr(db) mouse model of diabetes[J]. Diabetologia, 2016, 59(6): 1222-1230.

[5] Do OH, Low JT, Gaisano HY, et al. The secretory deficit in islets from db/db mice is mainly due to a loss of responding beta cells[J]. Diabetologia, 2014, 57(7): 1400-1409.

[6] Gannon M, Ables ET, Crawford L, et al. pdx-1 function is specifically required in embryonic cells to generate appropriate numbers of endocrine cell types and maintain glucose homeostasis[J]. Developmental Biology, 2008, 314(2): 406-417.

[7] Arcidiacono B, Iiritano S, Chiefari E, et al. Cooperation between HMGA1, PDX-1, and MafA is essential for glucose-induced insulin transcription in pancreatic beta cells[J]. Frontiers in Endocrinology, 2015, 5.

[8] Kharitonenkov A, Shiyanova TL, Koester A, et al. FGF-21 as a novel metabolic regulator[J]. Journal of Clinical Investigation, 2005, 115(6): 1627-1635.

[9] Badman MK, Pissios P, Kennedy AR, et al. Hepatic fibroblast growth factor 21 is regulated by PPAR alpha and is a key mediator of hepatic lipid metabolism in ketotic states[J]. Cell Metabolism, 2007, 5(6): 426-437.

[10] Inagaki T, Dutchak P, Zhao G, et al. Endocrine regulation of the fasting response by PPAR alpha-mediated induction of fibroblast growth factor 21[J]. Cell Metabolism, 2007, 5(6): 415-425.

[11] Potthoff MJ, Inagaki T, Satapati S, et al. FGF21 induces PGC-1 alpha and regulates carbohydrate and fatty acid metabolism during the adaptive starvation response[J]. Proceedings of the National Academy of Sciences of the United States of America, 2009, 106(26): 10853-10858.

[12] Coskun T, Bina HA, Schneider MA, et al. Fibroblast growth factor 21 corrects obesity in mice[J]. Endocrinology, 2008, 149(12): 6018-6027.

[13] Kharitonenkov A, Wroblewski VJ, Koester A, et al. The metabolic state of diabetic monkeys is regulated by fibroblast growth factor-21[J]. Endocrinology, 2007, 148(2): 774-781.

[14] Xu J, Lloyd DJ, Hale C, et al. Fibroblast growth factor 21 reverses hepatic steatosis, increases energy expenditure, and improves insulin sensitivity in diet-induced obese mice[J]. Diabetes, 2009, 58(1): 250-259.

[15] Ito S, Kinoshita S, Shiraishi N, et al. Molecular cloning and expression analyses of mouse ss klotho, which encodes a novel Klotho family protein[J]. Mechanisms of Development, 2000, 98(1-2): 115-119.

[16] Adams AC, Cheng CC, Coskun T, et al. FGF21 Requires beta klotho to Act In Vivo[J]. Plos One, 2012, 7(11).

[17] Chen W, Hoo RL-c, Konishi M, et al. Growth hormone induces hepatic production of fibroblast growth factor 21 through a mechanism dependent on lipolysis in adipocytes[J]. Journal of Biological Chemistry, 2011, 286(40): 34559-34566.

[18] Chau MDL, Gao J, Yang Q, et al. Fibroblast growth factor 21 regulates energy metabolism by activating the AMPK-SIRT1-PGC-1 alpha pathway[J]. Proceedings of the National Academy of Sciences of the United States of America, 2010, 107(28): 12553-12558.

[19] Yusuke M, Morichika K, Nobuyuki I. FGF21 as an Endocrine Regulator in Lipid Metabolism: From Molecular Evolution to Physiology and Pathophysiology[J]. Journal of Nutrition and Metabolism,2011,(2011-01-13), 2011, 2011(2090-0724): 981315.

[20] Fisher FM, Kleiner S, Douris N, et al. FGF21 regulates PGC-1 alpha and browning of white adipose tissues in adaptive thermogenesis[J]. Genes & Development, 2012, 26(3): 271-281.

[21] Sun MY, Yoo E, Green BJ, et al. Autofluorescence imaging of living pancreatic islets reveals fibroblast growth factor-21 (FGF21)-induced metabolism[J]. Biophysical Journal, 2012, 103(11): 2379-2388.

[22] Chen XY, Li GM, Dong Q, et al. miR-577 inhibits pancreatic beta-cell function and survival by targeting fibroblast growth factor 21 (FGF-21) in pediatric diabetes[J]. Genetics and Molecular Research, 2015, 14(4): 15462-15470.

[23] Omar BA, Andersen B, Hald J, et al. Fibroblast growth factor 21 (FGF21) and glucagon-like peptide 1 contribute to diabetes resistance in glucagon receptor-deficient mice[J]. Diabetes, 2014, 63(1): 101-110.

[24] Mu J, Pinkstaff J, Li Z, et al. FGF21 analogs of sustained action enabled by orthogonal biosynthesis demonstrate enhanced antidiabetic pharmacology in rodents[J]. Diabetes, 2012, 61(2): 505-512.

[25] Wente W, Efanov AM, Brenner M, et al. Fibroblast growth factor-21 improves pancreatic beta-cell function and survival by activation of extracellular signal-regulated kinase 1/2 and Akt signaling pathways[J]. Diabetes, 2006, 55(9): 2470-2478.

[26] Lin Z, Pan X, Wu F, et al. Fibroblast growth factor 21 prevents atherosclerosis by suppression of hepatic sterol regulatory element-binding protein-2 and induction of adiponectin in mice[J]. Circulation, 2015, 131(21): 1861-1871.

[27] Markan KR, Naber MC, Ameka MK, et al. Circulating FGF21 is liver derived and enhances glucose uptake during refeeding and overfeeding[J]. Diabetes, 2014, 63(12): 4057-4063.

[28] Ostenson CG, Gaisano H, Sheu L, et al. Impaired gene and protein expression of exocytotic soluble N-ethylmaleimide attachment protein receptor complex proteins in pancreatic islets of type 2 diabetic patients[J]. Diabetes, 2006, 55(2): 435-440.

[29] Izumiya Y, Bina HA, Ouchi N, et al. FGF21 is an Akt-regulated myokine[J]. Febs Letters, 2008, 582(27): 3805-3810.

[30] Hakonen E, Ustinov J, Eizirik DL, et al. In vivo activation of the PI3K-Akt pathway in mouse beta cells by the EGFR mutation L858R protects against diabetes[J]. Diabetologia, 2014, 57(5): 970-979.

[31] Bernal-Mizrachi E, Wen W, Stahlhut S, et al. Islet beta cell expression of constitutively active Akt1/PKB alpha induces striking hypertrophy, hyperplasia, and hyperinsulinemia[J]. Journal of Clinical Investigation, 2001, 108(11): 1631-1638.

[32] Butler AE, Janson J, Bonner-Weir S, et al. beta-cell deficit and increased beta-cell apoptosis in humans with type 2 diabetes[J]. Diabetes, 2003, 52(1): 102-110.

[33] Mb SEK. The importance of the beta-cell in the pathogenesis of type 2 diabetes mellitus[J]. American Journal of Medicine, 2000, 108 Suppl 6a(6): 2-8.

[34] Xu J, Stanislaus S, Chinookoswong N, et al. Acute glucose-lowering and insulin-sensitizing action of FGF21 in insulin-resistant mouse models-association with liver and adipose tissue effects[J]. American Journal of Physiology-Endocrinology and Metabolism, 2009, 297(5): E1105-E1114.

[35] Tacer KF, Bookout AL, Ding X, et al. Research resource: Comprehensive expression atlas of the fibroblast growth factor system in adult mouse[J]. Molecular Endocrinology, 2010, 24(10): 2050-2064.

[36] Hale C, Chen MM, Stanislaus S, et al. Lack of overt FGF21 resistance in two mouse models of obesity and insulin resistance[J]. Endocrinology, 2012, 153(1): 69-80.

[37] Shenoy VK, Beaver KM, Fisher FM, et al. Elevated serum fibroblast growth factor 21 in humans with acute pancreatitis[J]. Plos One, 2016, 11(11).

[38] Coate KC, Hernandez G, Thorne CA, et al. FGF21 is an exocrine pancreas secretagogue[J]. Cell Metabolism, 2017, 25(2): 472-480.

[39] Ding X, Boney-Montoya J, Owen BM, et al. beta klotho is required for fibroblast growth factor 21 effects on growth and metabolism[J]. Cell Metabolism, 2012, 16(3): 387-393.

[40] So WY, Cheng Q, Chen L, *et al.* High glucose represses beta-klotho expression and impairs fibroblast growth factor 21 action in mouse pancreatic islets involvement of peroxisome proliferator-activated receptor gamma signaling[J]. Diabetes, 2013, 62(11): 3751-3759.

[41] Fisher FM, Chui PC, Nasser IA, *et al.* Fibroblast growth factor 21 limits lipotoxicity by promoting hepatic fatty acid activation in mice on methionine and choline-deficient diets[J]. Gastroenterology, 2014, 147(5): 1073-1083.

[42] Zhu S, Ma L, Wu Y, *et al.* FGF21 treatment ameliorates alcoholic fatty liver through activation of AMPK-SIRT1 pathway[J]. Acta Biochimica Et Biophysica Sinica, 2014, 46(12): 1041-1048.

[43] Kaneto H, Miyatsuka T, Kawamori D, *et al.* PDX-1 and MafA play a crucial role in pancreatic beta-cell differentiation and maintenance of mature beta-cell function[J]. Endocrine Journal, 2008, 55(2): 235-252.

[44] Takahashi N, Hatakeyama H, Okado H, *et al.* SNARE conformational changes that prepare vesicles for exocytosis[J]. Cell Metabolism, 2010, 12(1): 19-29.

[45] Torrejon-Escribano B, Escoriza J, Montanya E, *et al.* Glucose-dependent changes in SNARE protein levels in pancreatic beta-cells[J]. Endocrinology, 2011, 152(4): 1290-1299.

[46] Zhu D, Koo E, Kwan E, *et al.* Syntaxin-3 regulates newcomer insulin granule exocytosis and compound fusion in pancreatic beta cells[J]. Diabetologia, 2013, 56(2): 359-369.

Chapter 4
Structure and Modification

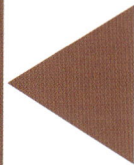

α-Klotho is a non-enzymatic molecular scaffold for FGF23 hormone signalling

Gaozhi Chen, Guang Liang, Xiaokun Li, Moosa Mohammadi

Endocrine FGF23 regulates phosphate and vitamin D homeostasis by reducing the cell surface expression of sodium phosphate co-transporters and by repressing transcription of rate-limiting enzymes for vitamin D biosynthesis[1,2] in the kidney. FGF23 exerts its metabolic functions by binding and activating FGFR tyrosine kinases[3] in an α-klotho co-receptor dependent fashion. The extracellular domain of a prototypical FGFR consists of three immunoglobulin-like domains: D1, D2 and D3. The membrane proximal portion comprising D2, D3 and the D2–D3 linker (FGFR^{ecto}) is both necessary and sufficient for FGF ligand binding[4,5]. Tissue-specific alternative splicing in the D3 domain of FGFR1–FGFR3 generates "b" and "c" isoforms, each with distinct ligand-binding specificity[5,6]. α-klotho, fortuitously discovered as an ageing-suppressor gene[7], is a single-pass transmembrane protein with an extracellular domain composed of two tandem domains (KL1 and KL2), each with notable homology to family 1 glycosidases[8] (Extended Data Fig. 1A). Membrane-bound α-klotho (α-klotho^{TM}) associates with cognate FGFRs of FGF23, namely the "c" splice isoforms of FGFR1 and FGFR3 (FGFR1c and FGFR3c) and FGFR4[9-12]. This enables them to bind and respond to FGF23[9,11,12]. α-klotho^{TM} is predominantly expressed in the kidney distal tubules, the parathyroid gland, and the brain choroid plexus[7,13], and this is considered to determine the target tissue specificity of FGF23[11,12]. Cleavage of α-klotho^{TM} by ADAM proteases[14-15] in kidney distal tubules sheds the α-klotho ectodomain (α-klotho^{ecto}; Extended Data Fig. 1A) into body fluids, for example, serum, urine and cerebrospinal fluid[16-19]. α-Klotho^{ecto} is thought to lack co-receptor activity and act as a circulating anti-ageing hormone independently of FGF23[20,21]. A plethora of activities has been attributed to shed α-klotho^{ecto}, the bulk of which require a purported intrinsic glycosidase activity[22-25].

Here we show that circulating α-klotho^{ecto} is an on-demand bona fide co-receptor for FGF23, and determine its crystal structure in complex with FGFR1c^{ecto} and FGF23. The structure reveals that α-klotho serves as a non-enzymatic scaffold that simultaneously tethers FGFR1c and FGF23 to implement FGF23–FGFR1c proximity and hence stability. Surprisingly, heparan sulfate (HS), a mandatory cofactor for paracrine FGFs, is still required as an ancillary cofactor to promote the formation of a symmetric 2:2:2:2 FGF23–FGFR1c–klotho-HS quaternary signalling complex.

1. Soluble α-klotho^{ecto} acts as a co-receptor for FGF23

To determine whether soluble α-klotho^{ecto} can support FGF23 signalling, α-klotho-deficient HEK293 cells, which naturally express FGFRs, were incubated with a concentration of α-klotho^{ecto} sufficient to drive all available cell-surface cognate FGFRs into binary complexed form. After brief rinses with PBS, the cells were stimulated with increasing concentrations of FGF23. In parallel, a HEK293 cell line that overexpresses membrane-bound α-klotho (HEK293-α-klotho^{TM}) was treated with increasing concentrations of FGF23. The dose–response for FGF23-induced ERK phosphorylation in α-klotho^{ecto}- pretreated untransfected HEK293 cells was similar to that observed in HEK293-α-klotho^{TM} cells (Extended Data Fig. 1B, top), suggesting that α-klotho^{ecto} can serve as a co-receptor for FGF23. Pre-treatment of HEK293-α-klotho^{TM} cells with α-klotho^{ecto} did not result in any further increase in FGF23 signalling, indicating that all cell-surface FGFRs in this cell line were in binary FGFR–α-klotho^{TM} form (Extended Data Fig. 1B, bottom). We conclude that soluble and transmembrane forms of α-klotho possess a similar capacity to support FGF23 signalling. Consistent with these results, injection of wild-type mice with α-klotho^{ecto} protein led to an increase in renal phosphate excretion and a decrease in serum phosphate (Extended Data Fig. 1C). Notably, it also led to a 1.5-fold increase in *Egr1* transcripts in the kidney (Extended Data Fig. 1D), demonstrating that α-klotho^{ecto} can serve as a bona fide co-receptor to

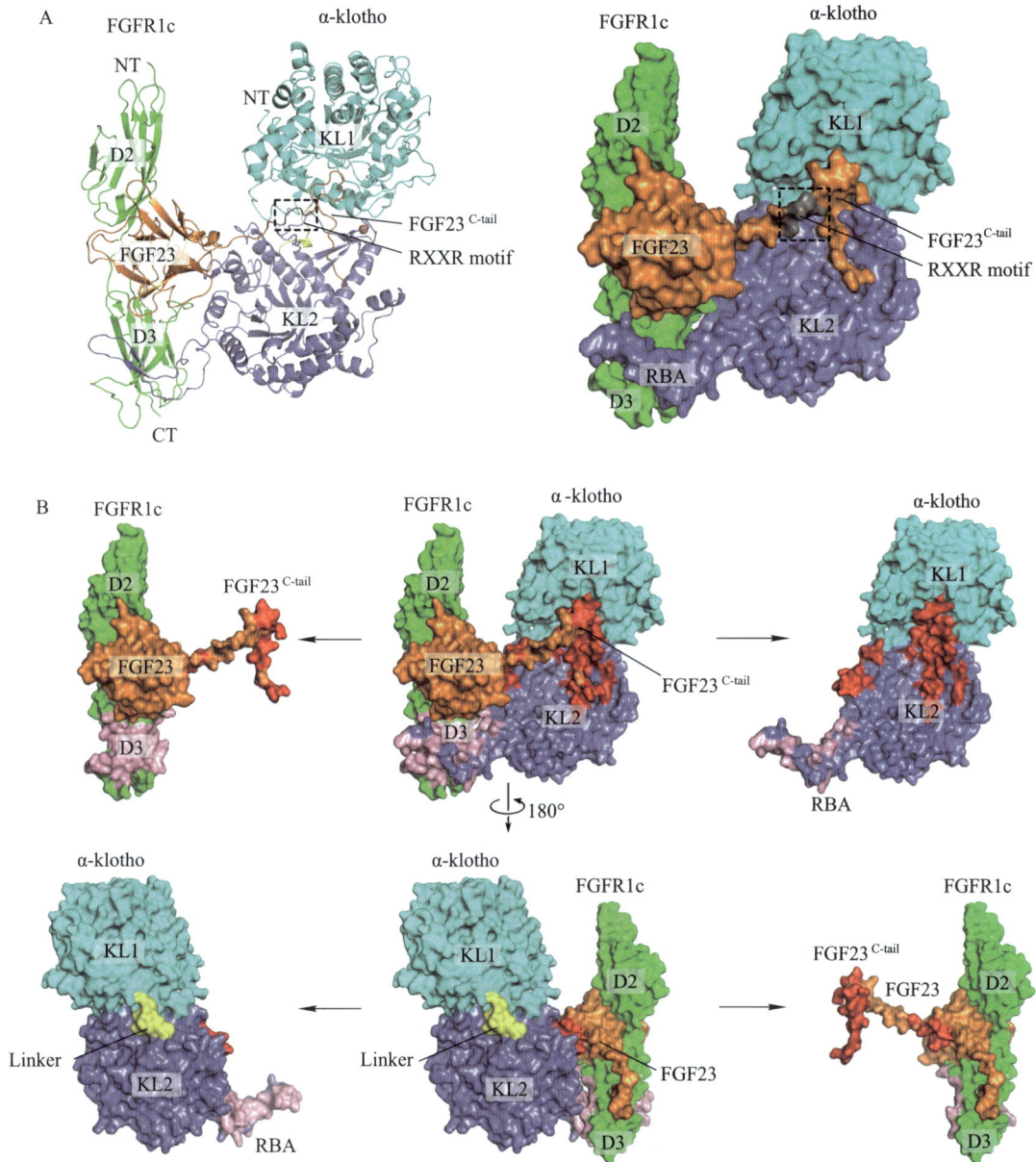

Fig. 1. Overall topology of the FGF23–FGFR1c^ecto–α-klotho^ecto complex. (A) Cartoon (left) and surface representation (right) of the ternary complex structure. The α-klotho KL1 (cyan) and KL2 (blue) domains are joined by a short proline-rich linker (yellow; not visible in the surface presentation). FGF23 is in orange with its proteolytic cleavage motif in grey. FGFR1c is in green. CT, C terminus; NT, N terminus. (B) Binding interfaces between α-klotho^ecto and the FGF23–FGFR1c^ecto complex. The ternary complex (centre) is shown in two different orientations related by a 180° rotation along the vertical axis. FGF23–α-klotho^ecto (red) and FGFR1c^ecto–α-klotho^ecto (pink) interfaces are visualized by pulling α-klotho^ecto and the FGF23–FGFR1c^ecto complex away from each other. The separated components are shown to the left and right of the ternary complex.

support FGF23 signalling in renal proximal tubules. In light of these data, we propose that the pleiotropic anti-ageing effects of α-klotho are all dependent on FGF23.

2. Structural basis of α-klotho co-receptor function

We solved the crystal structure of a human 1:1:1 FGF23–FGFR1c^ecto–α-klotho^ecto ternary complex at 3.0 Å resolution (Extended Data Table 1). In this complex, α-klotho^ecto serves as a massive scaffold, tethering both FGFR1c and FGF23 to itself. In doing so, α-klotho^ecto enforces FGF23– FGFR1c proximity and thus augments FGF23–FGFR1c binding affinity (Fig. 1). The overall geometry of the ternary complex is compatible with its formation on the cell surface (Extended Data Fig. 2A).

The binary FGF23–FGFR1c[ecto] complex adopts a canonical FGF– FGFR complex topology, in which FGF23 is bound between the D2 and D3 domains of the receptor, engaging both these domains and a short interdomain linker (Extended Data Fig. 3A). However, compared to paracrine FGFs, FGF23 makes fewer or weaker contacts with the D3 domain and D2–D3 linker, explaining the inherently low affinity of FGF23 for FGFR1c (Extended Data Fig. 3B, C). Notably, analysis of the binding interface between FGF23 and FGFR1c D3 in the crystal structure reveals specific contacts between FGF23 and a serine residue uniquely present in the "c" splice isoforms of FGFR1–FGFR3 and in FGFR4

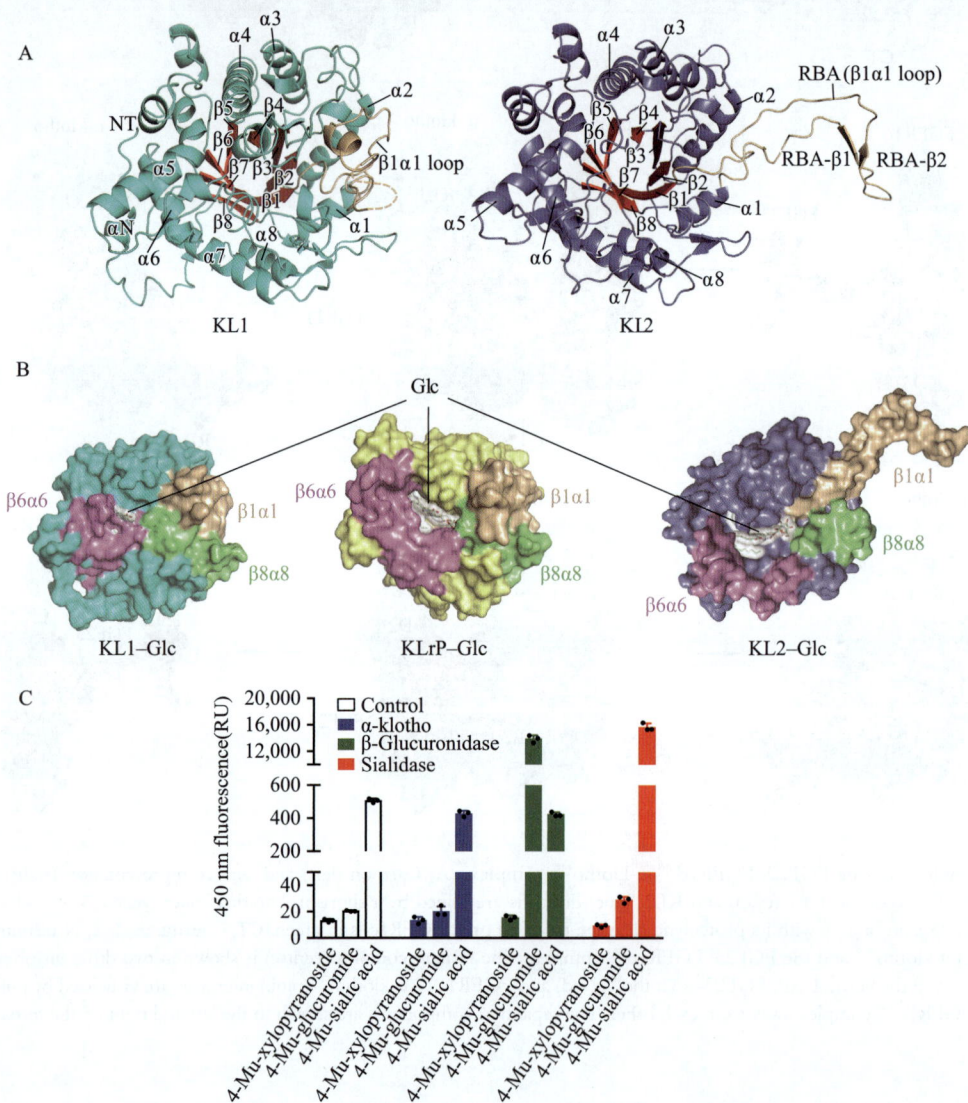

Fig. 2. α-Klotho is a non-enzymatic molecular scaffold. (A) Triosephosphate isomerase (TIM) barrel topology of the α-klotho KL1 and KL2 domains. KL1 is in the same orientation as in Fig. 1A, whereas KL2 has been superimposed onto KL1 and has thus been reoriented. The eight alternating β-strands (red) and α-helices (cyan/blue) that define the TIM barrel are labelled according to the standard nomenclature for the TIM fold[8]. KL1 and KL2 differ markedly in the conformation of the β1α1 loop (wheat). In KL2, this loop protrudes away from the TIM barrel and serves as a receptor binding arm (RBA; Fig. 1). (B) Molecular surfaces of KLrP–glucosylceramide (Glc) (centre; KLrP in yellow), KL1–Glc (left; KL1 in cyan) and KL2–Glc (right; KL2 in blue). Binding of Glc to KL1 and KL2 was simulated by superimposing KL1 and KL2 onto KLrP–Glc. In all cases, Glc is shown as pale grey sticks or surface. The divergent conformation of the β6α6 loop (pink) in KL1 almost seals off the entrance to the catalytic pocket, while the divergent conformations of the β1α1 (RBA; wheat), β6α6 (pink) and β8α8 (green) loops in KL2 leave the central barrel cavity in KL2 in a more solvent-exposed state that is less capable of ligating substrate (see also Extended Data Fig. 5). (C) Glycosidase activity of α-klotho[ecto], sialidase and β-glucuronidase. Data are mean and s.d. Dots denote individual data points; $n = 3$ independent experiments. RU, relative units.

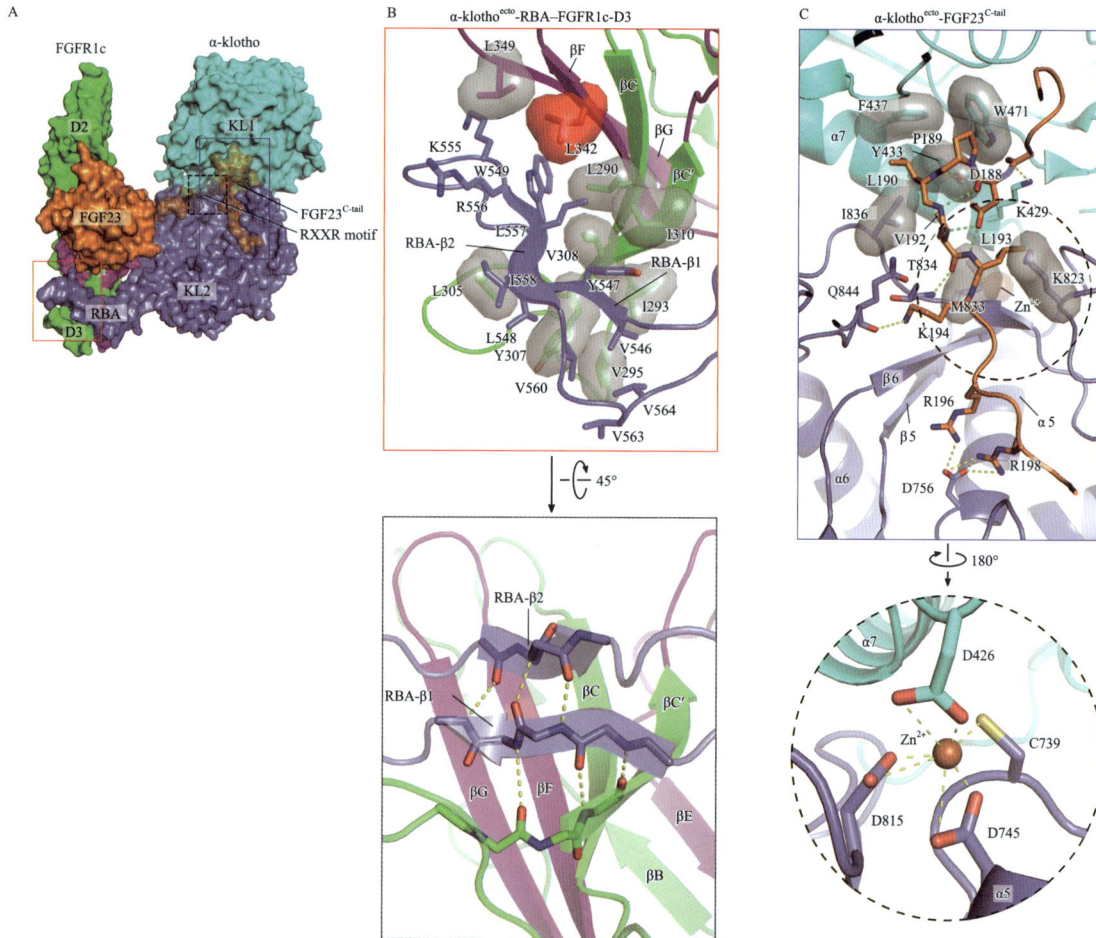

Fig. 3. α-Klotho simultaneously tethers FGFR1c by its D3 domain and FGF23 by its C-terminal tail. (A) Ternary complex structure in surface representation. Colouring is as in Fig. 1A, except that the alternatively spliced region of FGFR1c is highlighted in purple. Red box denotes perimeter of interface between distal tip of α-klotho RBA and the hydrophobic FGFR1c D3 groove. Blue box denotes the perimeter of α-klotho−FGF23[C-tail] interface. (B) RBA stretches out of the KL2 domain of α-klotho[ecto] and latches onto the FGFR1c D3 domain. Top, interface between the distal tip of RBA and the D3 groove detailing hydrophobic interactions (grey transparent surfaces). Note that Leu342 (red) from the spliced region of the D3 groove is strictly conserved in "c" splice isoforms of FGFR1–FGFR3 and FGFR4 and is mutated in Kallmann syndrome[36]. Bottom, close-up view of the extended β-sheet between the RBA-β1:RBA-β2 strand pair and the four-stranded β-sheet in D3 (βC'-βC-βF-βG). This structure forms *via* hydrogen bonding (dashed yellow lines) between backbone atoms of RBA-β1 and D3-βC'. (C) Both KL domains of α-klotho[ecto] participate in tethering of the flexible C-terminal tail of FGF23 (FGF23[C-tail]). FGF23[C-tail] residues Asp188–Thr200 thread through the KL1–KL2 cleft and the β-barrel cavity of KL2. Of these residues, Asp188–Leu193 adopt a cage-like conformation that is partially stabilized by intramolecular hydrogen bonds (dashed green lines). Dashed yellow lines denote intermolecular hydrogen bonds; grey transparent surfaces denote hydrophobic interactions. Note that Tyr433 from the KL1 α7 helix deep inside the KL1–KL2 cleft has a prominent role in tethering the cage-like structure in the FGF23[C-tail] formed by Asp188–Leu193. Dashed circle (shown at greater magnification below) denotes the KL1−KL2 interface where residues from both α-klotho domains jointly coordinate a Zn^{2+} ion (orange sphere).

(Extended Data Fig. 4A). Indeed, replacing this "c"-isoform- specific serine residue with a "b"-isoform-specific tyrosine impaired FGF23 signalling (Extended Data Fig. 4B, C). We conclude that the FGFR binding specificity inherent to FGF23 operates alongside that of α-klotho (Extended Data Fig. 4D, E) to restrict FGF23 signalling to the "c" splice isoforms and FGFR4[11,12].

In the ternary complex, α-klotho[ecto] exists in an extended conformation. Consistent with their sequence homology to the Lin glycoside hydrolase A clan[8], the α-klotho KL1 (Glu34 to Phe506) and KL2 (Leu515 to Ser950) domains each assume a $(\beta\alpha)_8$ triosephosphate isomerase (TIM) barrel fold consisting of an inner eight-stranded parallel β-barrel and eight surrounding α-helices (Fig. 2A, Extended Data Fig. 5A). The two KL domains are connected by a short, proline-rich and hence stiff linker (Pro507 to Pro514) (Fig. 1A, B). KL1 sits atop KL2, engaging it *via* a few interdomain contacts involving the N terminus preceding the β1 strand and the α7 helix of KL1, and the β5α5 and β6α6 loops and α7 helix of KL2 (Extended Data Fig. 2B). Notably, one of the interdomain contacts is mediated by a Zn^{2+} ion (Fig. 3C the

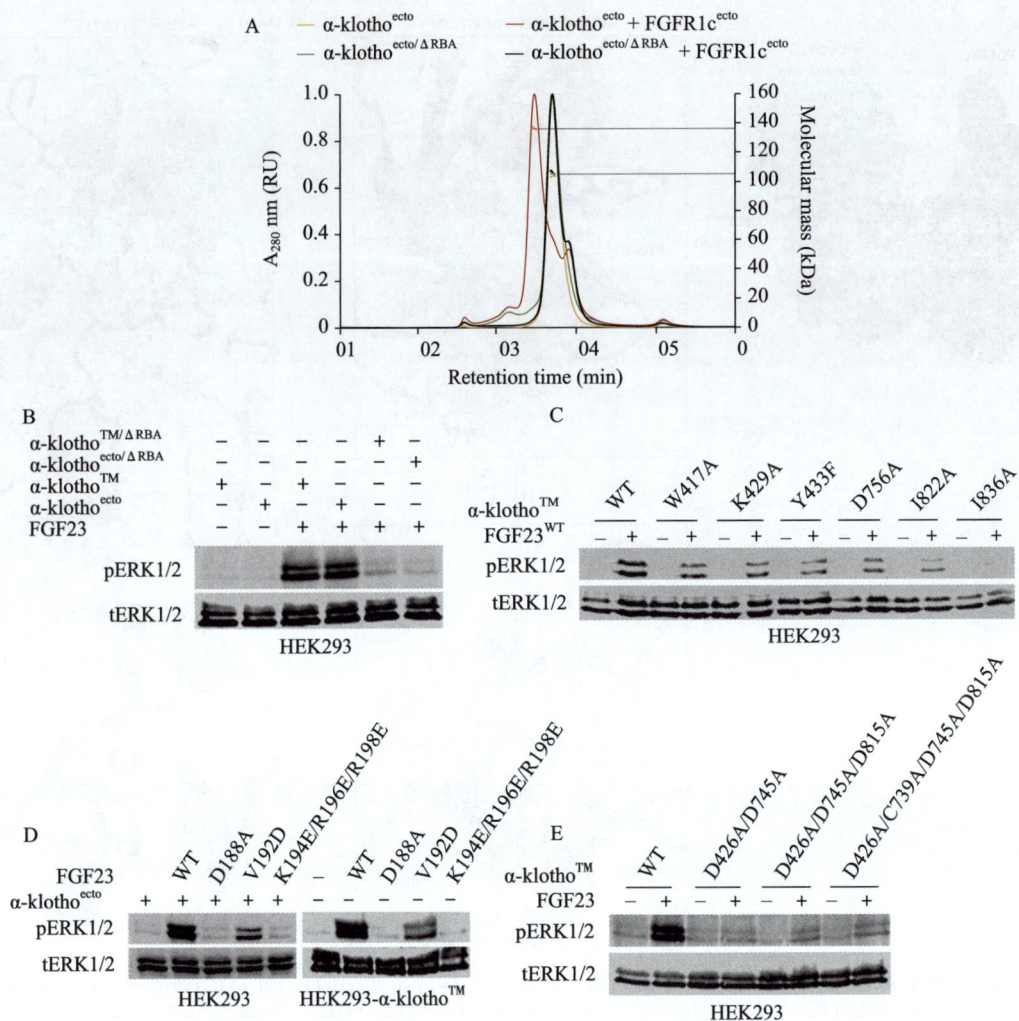

Fig. 4. Mutagenesis experiments validate the crystallographically deduced mode of ternary complex formation. (A) Size exclusion chromatography–multi-angle light scattering (SEC–MALS) analysis of FGFR1c^{ecto} interaction with wild-type α-klotho^{ecto} or its RBA deletion mutant. (B–E) Representative immunoblots of phosphorylated ERK (pERK1/2; top) and total ERK (tERK1/2; bottom; sample loading controls) in total HEK293 cell lysates ($n = 3$ independent experiments for each panel). (B) Analysis of the effects of RBA deletion on the co-receptor activity of α-klotho^{ecto} and α-klotho^{TM} isoforms. (C) Analysis of mutations in the α-klotho binding pocket that engages the FGF23^{C-tail}. WT, wild type. (D) Analysis of mutations in the FGF23^{C-tail} that disrupt α-klotho–FGF23^{C-tail} interaction. (E) Analysis of mutations of the four Zn^{2+}-coordinating amino acids in α-klotho.

FGF23–FGFR1c^{ecto} complex away from each other. The separated and Extended Data Fig. 2B, C). These contacts stabilize the observed elongated conformation of α-klotho^{ecto}, creating a deep cleft between the two KL domains. This merges with a wide-open central β-barrel cavity in KL2, and forms a large binding pocket that tethers the distal C-terminal tail of FGF23 past the 176-Arg-His-Thr-Arg-179 proteolytic cleavage site (Fig. 1B). Meanwhile, the long β1α1 loop of KL2 (Fig. 2A) protrudes as much as 35 Å away from the KL2 core to latch onto the FGFR1c D3 domain, thus anchoring the receptor to α-klotho (Fig. 1B). Accordingly, we have named this KL2 loop the receptor binding arm (RBA; residues 530–578; Extended Data Fig. 5A).

We superimposed the TIM barrels of KL1 and KL2 onto that of klotho-related protein (KLrP, also known as GBA3), the cytosolic member of the klotho family with proven glycosylceramidase activity[26]. This comparison revealed major conformational differences in the loops surrounding the entrance to the catalytic pocket in KL1 and KL2 (Fig. 2B, Extended Data Fig. 5B–D). Moreover, both KL domains lack one of the key catalytic glutamates deep within the putative catalytic pocket. These substantial differences are incompatible with an intrinsic glycosidase activity for α-klotho[22-25]. Indeed, α-klotho^{ecto} failed to hydrolyse substrates for both sialidase and β-glucuronidase in vitro (Fig. 2C). Together, our data define α-klotho as the only known example of a TIM barrel protein that serves purely as a non-enzymatic molecular scaffold.

3. Binding interface between α-klotho and FGFR1c

The interface between α-klotho RBA and FGFR1c D3 (Fig. 3A) buries over 2,200 Å^2 of solvent-exposed surface area, which is consistent with the high affinity of α-klotho binding to FGFR1c (dissociation constant (K_d) = 72 nM)[10]. At the distal tip of the RBA, residues 547-Tyr-Leu-Trp-549 and 556-Ile-Leu-Arg-558 form a short β-strand pair (RBA-β1:RBA-β2) as their hydrophobic side chains are immersed in a wide hydrophobic groove between the four-stranded βC′-βC-βF-βG sheet and the βC-βC′ loop of FGFR1c D3 (Fig. 3B, top). The RBA- β1:RBA-β2 strand pair forms an extended β-sheet with the βC′-βC-βF-βG sheet of D3 as the backbone atoms of RBA-β1 and D3 βC′ make three hydrogen bonds that further augment the interface (Fig. 3B, bottom). Residues at the proximal end of the RBA engage a second smaller binding pocket at the bottom edge of D3 next to the hydrophobic groove (Extended Data Fig. 6A, B). Both α-klotho binding pockets in the receptor D3 domain differ between "b" and "c" splice isoforms. Leu342, for example, is strictly conserved in the "c" splice isoforms of FGFR1–FGFR3 and FGFR4. This explains the previously described binding selectivity of α-klotho for this subset of FGFRs[9,11,12](Extended Data Fig. 4A).

Consistent with the crystal structure, soluble α-klotho lacking the RBA (α-klotho$^{ecto/ΔRBA}$) failed to form a binary complex with FGFR1cecto in solution (Fig. 4A) and hence could not support FGF23 signalling (Fig. 4B). Likewise, membrane-bound α-klotho lacking the RBA (α-klotho$^{TM/ΔRBA}$) was also disabled in acting as a FGF23 co-receptor (Fig. 4B). Importantly, α-klotho$^{ecto/ΔRBA}$ did not exhibit any phosphaturic activity *in vivo* (Extended Data Fig. 7A). On the contrary, the α-klotho$^{ecto/ΔRBA}$ mutant antagonized the activity of native α-klotho by sequestering FGF23 into functionally inactive binary complexes, that is, by acting as an FGF23 ligand trap (Extended Data Fig. 7). These data refute the concept that α-klotho^{ecto} functions as an FGF23-independent phosphaturic enzyme[24]. Our conclusion is supported by a gene knockout study that compared the phenotypes of mice with knockout of FGF23 (*Fgf23$^{-/-}$*), mice with knockout of α-klotho (*Kl$^{-/-}$*) and double-knockout mice (*Fgf23$^{-/-}$Kl$^{-/-}$*)[27].

4. Binding interface between α-klotho and FGF23

Regions from both KL domains act together to recruit FGF23 (Fig. 1B), thus explaining why only an intact α-klotho ectodomain is capable of supporting FGF23 signalling[12,28]. The interactions between FGF23 and α-klotho result in the burial of a large amount of solvent-exposed surface area (2 732 Å^2), of which nearly two-thirds (1 961 Å^2) are buried between the FGF23 C-terminal tail and α-klotho, and the remaining one-third is buried between the FGF23 core and α-klotho (Fig. 3A). At the interface between α-klotho and the FGF23 C-terminal tail, FGF23 residues 188-Asp-Pro-Leu-Asn-Val-Leu-193 adopt an unusual cage-like conformation (Fig. 3A, C), which is tethered by residues from both KL domains *via* hydrogen bonds and hydrophobic contacts deep inside the KL1–KL2 cleft (Fig. 3C). Further downstream, the side chains of Lys194, Arg196 and Arg198 of the FGF23 C-terminal tail dip into the central barrel cavity of KL2, making hydrogen bonds with several α-klotho residues (Fig. 3C). At the interface between the FGF23 β-trefoil core and α-klotho, residues from the β5β6 turn and the αC helix of FGF23 make hydrogen bonds and hydrophobic contacts with residues in the short β7α7 and β8α8 loops at the upper rim of the KL2 cavity (Extended Data Fig. 6A, C).

To test the biological relevance of the observed contacts between α-klotho and the FGF23 C-terminal tail, we introduced several mutations into α-klotho^{TM} and FGF23 to disrupt α-klotho–FGF23 binding (Fig. 4C). Consistent with our structure-based predictions, all α-klotho^{TM} mutants showed an impaired ability to support FGF23 signalling (Fig. 4C). The FGF23 mutants also exhibited a reduced ability to signal, regardless of whether soluble or membrane-bound α-klotho served as co-receptor (Fig. 4D). Remarkably, the FGF23(D188A) mutant (which eliminates the intramolecular hydrogen bonds that support cage conformation) was totally inactive, underscoring the importance of the cage-like conformation in the tethering of FGF23 to α-klotho. Notably, tethering of this cage-like structure requires precise alignment of residues from both KL domains deep within the KL1–KL2 cleft (Fig. 3C), indicating that their correct apposition is critically important for α-klotho co-receptor activity. These structural observations suggest that the bound Zn^{2+} ion serves as a prosthetic group in α-klotho by minimizing interdomain flexibility and hence promoting co-receptor activity. Consistent with such a role, mutants of membrane-anchored α-klotho[TM] carrying alanine in place of two, three or all four Zn^{2+} coordinating amino acids (Fig. 3C) showed a reduced ability to support FGF23 signalling (Fig. 4E). Together with our data on the effect of RBA deletion, these results corroborate the biological relevance of the crystallographically deduced mode by which α-klotho implements FGF23–FGFR1c proximity and thus confers high binding affinity.

5. FGF23 signalling is α-klotho and HS-dependent

Both FGF23 and FGFR1c have a measurable (albeit weak) binding affinity for HS. Because HS is ubiquitously expressed, we wondered whether it participates in the apparent α-klotho[ecto]-mediated FGF23– FGFR dimerization in our cell-based and *in vivo* experiments. We therefore analysed the molecular mass of the ternary complex in the absence and presence of increasing molar equivalents of homogenously sulfated heparin hexasaccharide (HS6). Consistent with our previous observations, in the absence of HS6, the ternary complex migrated as a monomeric species[10] with an apparent molecular mass of 150 kDa, in good agreement with the theoretical value for a 1:1:1 complex (160 kDa) (Fig. 5A). With increasing molar ratios of HS6 to ternary complex, the peak for monomeric ternary complex diminished, while a new peak with a molecular mass of 300 kDa (corresponding to a 2:2:2 FGF23–FGFR1c[ecto]–α-klotho[ecto]dimer) appeared and increased in prominence. Excess HS6 beyond a 1:1 molar ratio of HS6 to ternary complex did not lead to any further increase in the amount of dimer complex formed, as judged by the integrated area of the dimer complex peak (Fig. 5A). We conclude that HS is required for the dimerization of 1:1:1 FGF23–FGFR1c[ecto]-α-klotho[ecto] complexes, and that at least a 1:1 molar ratio of HS6 to ternary complex is required for complete dimerization of the complex in solution (Fig. 5A). To confirm the dependency of dimerization on HS, we introduced mutations into the HS-binding[ΔHBS] sites of FGFR1c (K160Q/K163Q, FGFR1c, and K207Q/R209Q, FGFR1c[ΔHBS']) and FGF23 (R140A/R143A, FGF23[ΔHBS]). Neither mutating the HS-binding site in FGFR1c nor mutating that site in FGF23 affected the formation of a monomeric 1:1:1 FGF23–FGFR1c–α-klotho complex in solution, demonstrating that α-klotho-mediated stabilization of the FGF23–FGFR complex is independent of HS. However, ternary complexes containing any of these three mutants failed to dimerize in the presence of HS6 (Fig. 5B).

Reconstitution experiments in the context of BaF3 cells (an FGFR, α-klotho and HS triple-deficient cell line[29]) showed that both soluble α-klotho[ecto] and membrane-bound α-klotho[TM] required HS to support FGF23-mediated FG-FR1c activation in a more physiological context (Fig. 5C). We also examined the impact of the HS-binding site mutations in FGFR1c and FGF23 on FGFR1c activation by FGF23 in BaF3 cells (Fig. 5D). In agreement with our solution binding data, activation by FGF23 of HS-binding site mutants of FGFR1c in BaF3 cells was markedly impaired, regardless of whether soluble or membrane-bound α-klotho served as the co-receptor (Fig. 5D). Similarly, the binding site mutant of FGF23 showed a markedly reduced ability to activate FGFR1c (Fig. 5E). These *in vitro* and cell-based analyses unequivocally demonstrate that whereas HS fulfils a dual role in paracrine FGF signalling—enhancing 1:1 FGF–FGFR binding and promoting 2:2 FGF–FGFR dimerization—it shares this task with α-klotho in FGF23 signalling. Thus, α-klotho primarily acts to promote 1:1 FGF23–FGFR1c binding, whereas HS induces the dimerization of the resulting FGF23–FGFR1c–α-klotho complexes.

On the basis of the crystallographically deduced 2:2:2 [Protein Data Bank (PDB) code 1FQ9][4] and 2:2:1 (PDB code 1E0O)[30] paracrine FGF–FGFR–HS dimerization models, two distinct HS-induced 2:2:2 endocrine FGF23–FG-FR1c–α-klotho quaternary dimers can be predicted that differ markedly in the composition of the dimer interface (Extended Data Fig. 8). Specifically, in the 2:2:2:1 model, there would be no protein–protein contacts between the two 1:1:1 FGF23–FGFR1c–α-klotho protomers (Extended Data Fig. 8A). By contrast, in the 2:2:2:2 model, FGF23 and FGFR1c from one 1:1:1 FGF23–FGFR1c–α-klotho protomer would interact with the D2 domain of FGFR1c in the adjacent 1:1:1 FGF23–FGFR1c–α-klotho protomer across a two-fold dimer interface (Extended Data Fig. 8B). On the basis of the fundamental differences in the composition of the dimer interface between these two models, we introduced mutations into the secondary-receptor-binding site (SRBS) in FGF23 (M149A/N150A/P151A; FGF23[ΔSRBS]) and into the corresponding secondary-ligand-binding site (SLBS) in FGFR1c D2 (I203E, FGFR1c[ΔSLBS], and V221D, FGFR1c[ΔSLBS']), both of which are unique to the 2:2:2:2 quaternary dimer model. The direct receptor– receptor binding site (RRBS) in FGFR1c D2 (A171D; FGFR1c[ΔRRBS]), another binding site unique to the 2:2:2:2 model, was also mutated (Extended Data Fig. 8B). Although all of these FGF23 and FGFR1c mutants were able to form ternary complexes with α-klotho[ecto], the ternary

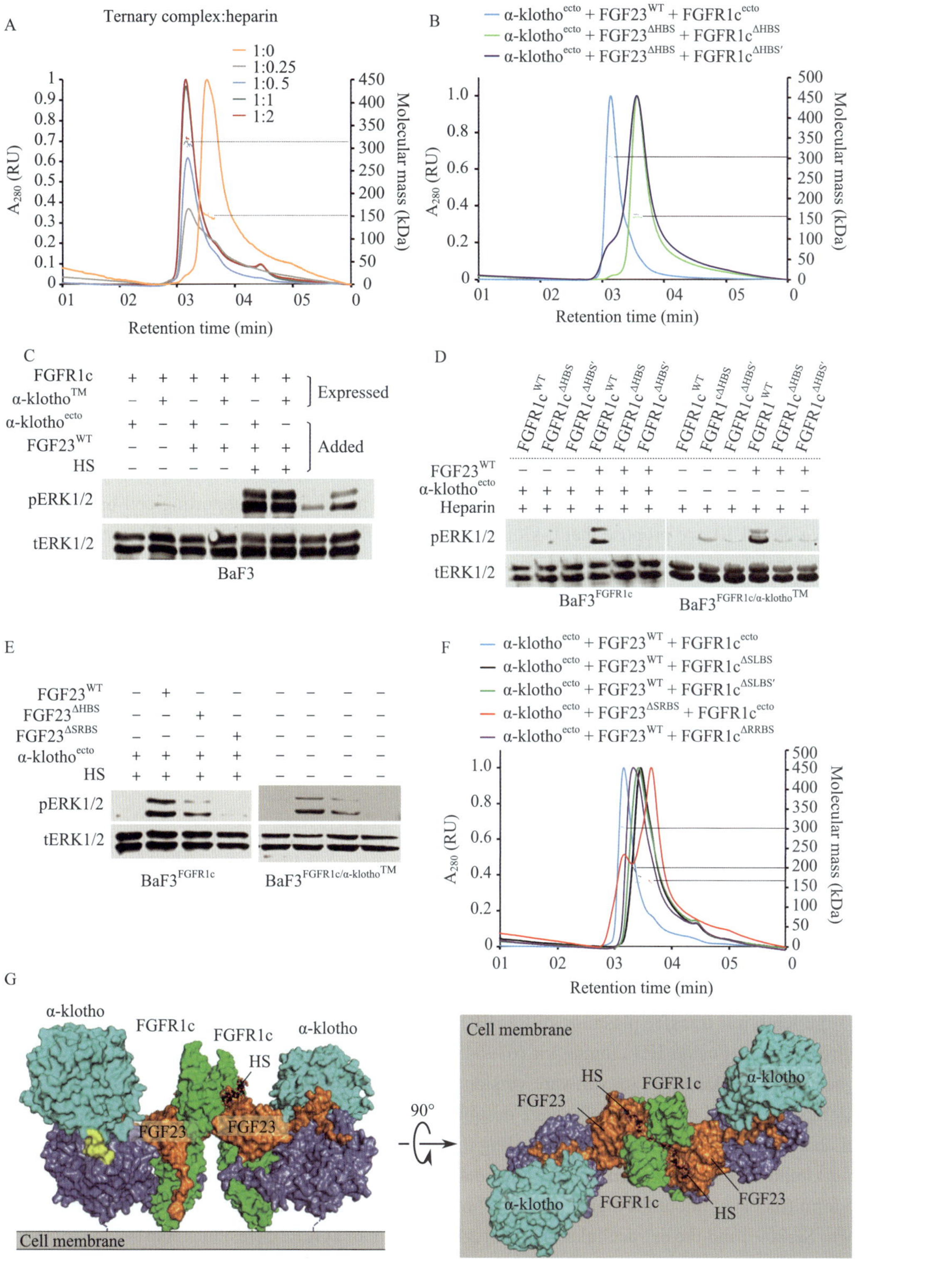

Fig. 5. Heparan sulfate dimerizes two 1:1:1 FGF23–FGFR1c–α-klotho complexes into a symmetric 2:2:2:2 FGF23–FGFR1c–α-klotho–HS signal transduction unit. (A) SEC–MALS analysis of the FGF23–FGFR1c^{ecto}–α-klotho^{ecto} complex in the absence or presence of increasing molar amounts of heparin hexasaccharide (HS6). (B) SEC–MALS analysis of the FGF23–FGFR1c^{ecto}–α-klotho^{ecto} complexes containing HS-binding site mutations of FGF23 and FGFR1c. (C–E) Representative immunoblots of phosphorylated ERK (top) and total ERK (bottom; sample loading controls) in total BaF3 cell lysates (n = 3 independent experiments for each panel). (C) Analysis of HS dependency of FGF23 signalling. (D, E) Analysis of mutations in the HS-binding site of FGFR1c (D) and in the HS-binding site or secondary receptor-binding site of FGF23 (E). (F) SEC–MALS analysis of FGF23–FGFR1c^{ecto}–α-klotho^{ecto} complexes containing a secondary receptor-binding site mutation in FGF23, a secondary ligand-binding site mutation in FGFR1c, or a direct receptor–receptor-binding site mutation in FGFR1c. In (B) and (F), wild-type ternary complex served as controls. (G) Molecular surface of a 2:2:2:2 FGF23–FGFR1c–α-klotho–HS dimer in two orientations related by a 90° rotation around the horizontal axis: a side-view looking parallel to the plane of a cell membrane (left) and a bird's-eye view looking down onto the plane of a cell membrane (right). HS molecules are shown as black sticks.

complexes containing any of the mutated proteins were impaired in their ability to dimerize in the presence of HS6 in solution (Fig. 5F). Moreover, the FGF23ΔSRBS mutant showed a markedly diminished ability to activate FGFR1c in BaF3 cells (Fig. 5E). The loss-of-function effects of these mutations are consistent with a 2:2:2:2 quaternary dimer model (Extended Data Fig. 8B). Hence, we envision that HS engages the HS-binding sites of FGFR1c and FGF23 in two stabilized 1:1:1 FGF23–FGFR1c–α-FGF23–FGFR1c–α-klotho–HS dimer (Fig. 5G). In doing so, HS enhances reciprocal interactions of FGFR1c D2 and FGF23 from one ternary complex with FGFR1c D2 in the other ternary complex, thereby buttressing the dimer (Extended Data Fig. 8B). This replicates the role that HS has in paracrine FGF signalling[4]. In contrast to HS, α-klotho molecules do not directly participate in the dimer interface (Fig. 5G), but rather indirectly support HS-induced dimerization by enhancing 1:1 FGF23–FGFR1c binding affinity. Hence, FGF23 seems to strike a fine balance between losing a large amount of HS-binding affinity to enable its endocrine mode of action and retaining sufficient HS-binding affinity to allow HS-mediated dimerization of two 1:1:1 FGF23– FGFR1c–α-klotho complexes. These considerations do not formally exclude the possibility that 2:2:2:2 and 2:2:2:1 quaternary dimers might co-exist as a higher order cluster on the cell surface, as has been proposed previously for paracrine 2:2:2 and 2:2:1 FGF–FGFR1–HS dimers[31].

FGF19 and FGF21, the other two endocrine FGFs, both require β-klotho as an obligate co-receptor to bind and activate cognate FGFRs[32,33] so as to mediate effects that regulate, for example, metabolic pathways involved in bile acid biosynthesis or fatty acid oxidation. On the basis of the structural analysis and supporting cell-based data shown in Extended Data Fig. 9 and 10, we propose that β-klotho, similar to α-klotho, functions as a non-enzymatic molecular scaffold to promote signalling by these two FGF hormones.

Online Content Methods, along with any additional Extended Data display items and Source Data, are available in the online version of the paper; references unique to these sections appear only in the online paper.

klotho ternary complexes to promote the formation of a two-fold symmetric 2:2:2:2 Supplementary Information is available in the online version of the paper.

6. Methods

No statistical methods were used to predetermine sample size. The experiments were not randomized and, except for the data shown in Extended Data Fig. 7A, B, investigators were not blinded to allocation during experiments and outcome assessment.

6.1 DNA expression constructs

cDNA fragments encoding full-length human α-klotho, β-klotho and FGFR1c were amplified by PCR and subcloned into the lentiviral transfer plasmids pEF1α-IRES-hygro (α-/β-klotho) or pEF1α-IRES-Neo (FGFR1c) using a ligation-independent In-Fusion HD cloning kit (639648, Clontech Laboratories). PCR primers for *FGFR1* "c" isotype were designed using NEBaseChanger software version 1.2.6 (New England Biolabs) and primers for *KL* and *KLB* (encoding α-klotho and β-klotho, respectively) were designed using the primer design tool for the In-Fusion HD cloning kit (Clontech Laboratories). A cDNA fragment encoding the entire extracellular domain of human α-klotho (residues Met1 to Ser981; α-klotho[ecto]) was subcloned into the mammalian expression plasmid pEF1α/myc-His A. DNA fragments for the mature form (that is, without the signal sequence) of human FGF23 (residues Tyr25 to Ile251), human FGF21 (residues His29 to Ser209), and the extracellular D2–D3 region of human FGFR1c (residues Asp142 to Arg365; FGFR1c[ecto]), which is both necessary and sufficient for FGF binding, were amplified by PCR and ligated into the cloning sites of the bacterial expression plasmids pET-30a and pET-28a, respectively. Single/multiple site mutations, loop deletions and truncations were introduced into expression constructs encoding the wild-type proteins using a Q5 Site-Directed Mutagenesis Kit (E0554S, New England Biolabs). The integrity of each expression construct was confirmed by restriction enzyme digestion and DNA sequencing. Information on the constructs is provided in the Supplementary Tables 1 and 2.

6.2 Recombinant protein expression and purification

N-acetylglucosaminyltransferase I (GnTI) deficient HEK293S cells (CRL-3022, American Type Culture Collection (ATCC)) were transfected by calcium phosphate co-precipitation with the expression construct encoding α-klotho[ecto].

G418-resistant colonies were selected for α-klotho^{ecto} expression using 0.5 mg/ml G418 (6483, KSE Scientific). The clone with the highest expression level was propagated in DME/F12 medium (SH30023.02, HyClone) supplemented with 10% fetal bovine serum (FBS) (35-010-CV, CORNING), 100 U/ml penicillin plus 100 μg/ml streptomycin (15140-122, Gibco), and 0.5 mg/ml G418. For protein production, $1×10^6$ cells were seeded in 25 cm cell culture dishes in 20 ml DME/F12 medium containing 10% FBS and grown for 24 h. Thereafter, the medium was replaced with 25 mL DME/F12 medium containing 1% FBS. Three days later, secreted α-klotho^{ecto} from two litres of conditioned medium was captured on a 5 ml heparin affinity HiTrap column (GE Healthcare) and eluted with a 100 ml linear NaCl gradient (0–1.0 M). Column fractions containing α-klotho^{ecto} were pooled and diluted tenfold with 25 mM Tris pH 8.0 buffer, and the diluted protein sample was loaded onto an anion exchange column (SOUCRE Q, GE Healthcare) and eluted with a 280 ml linear NaCl gradient (0–0.4 M). As a final purification step, SOURCE Q fractions containing α-klotho^{ecto} were concentrated and applied to a Superdex 200 column (GE Healthcare). α-Klotho^{ecto} protein was eluted isocratically in 25 mM HEPES pH 7.5 buffer containing 500 mM NaCl and 100 mM $(NH_4)_2SO_4$. A mutant of α-klotho^{ecto} lacking the receptor binding arm (α-klotho$^{ecto/ΔRBA}$) was expressed and purified similarly as the wild-type counterpart.

Human wild-type FGF23 and its mutants were expressed in *Escherichia coli* BL21 DE3 cells. Inclusion bodies enriched in misfolded insoluble FGF23 protein were dissolved in 6 M guanidinium hydrochloride and FGF23 proteins were refolded by dialysis for 2 days at 4℃ against buffer A (25 mM HEPES pH 7.5, 150 mM NaCl, 7.5% glycerol) followed by buffer B (25 mM HEPES pH 7.5, 100 mM NaCl, 5% glycerol). Correctly folded FGF23 proteins were captured on a 5 ml heparin affinity HiTrap column (GE Healthcare) and eluted with a 100 ml linear NaCl gradient (0–2.0 M). Final purification of FGF23 proteins was achieved by cation exchange chromatography (SOURCE S, GE Healthcare) with a 280 ml linear NaCl gradient (0–0.4 M). Human FGFR1c^{ecto} and its mutants were also expressed as inclusion bodies in *E. coli* BL21 DE3 and refolded *in vitro* by slow dialysis at 4℃ against the following buffers: buffer A (25 mM Tris pH 8.2, 150 mM NaCl, 7.5% glycerol), buffer B (25 mM Tris pH 8.2, 100 mM NaCl, 5% glycerol), and buffer C (25 mM Tris pH 8.2, 50 mM NaCl, 5% glycerol); dialysis against each buffer was for minimally 12 h. Properly folded FGFR1c proteins were purified by heparin affinity chromatography followed by size-exclusion chromatography as described above. All column chromatography was performed at 4℃ on an AKTA pure 25 l system (GE Healthcare).

6.3　Crystallization and X-ray crystal structure determination

To facilitate crystallization of the FGF23–FGFR1c^{ecto}–α-klotho^{ecto} complex, we used a proteolytically and structurally more stable FGF23 protein variant, which lacked 46 residues from the FGF23 C-terminus (Cys206 to Ile251) and carried Arg-to-Gln mutations at positions 176 and 179 of the 176-Arg-His-Thr-Arg-179 proteolytic cleavage motif in FGF23. The Arg-to-Gln mutations occur naturally in patients with autosomal dominant hypophosphatemic rickets (ADHR)[37], and deletion of C-terminal residues Cys206 to Ile251 has no effect on the phosphaturic activity of FGF23 in mice or its signalling potential in α-klotho^{TM}-expressing cultured cells[10]. Thus, the first 26 amino acids (Ser180 to Ser205) of the 72-amino-acid-long C-terminal tail of FGF23, defined as the region past the 176-Arg-His-Thr-Arg-179 proteolytic cleavage site, comprise the minimal region of the FGF23 C-terminal tail for binding the FGFR1c^{ecto}–α-klotho^{ecto} complex[10]. To prepare the FGF23–FGFR1c^{ecto}–α-klotho^{ecto} complex, its purified components were mixed at a molar ratio of 1.2:1.2:1 and spin-concentrated using an Amicon Ultra-15 concentrator (UFC901024, Merck Millipore). The concentrated sample was applied to a Superdex 200 column (GE Healthcare) and eluted isocratically in 25 mM HEPES pH 7.5 buffer containing 500 mM NaCl and 100 mM $(NH_4)_2SO_4$. Column peak fractions were analysed by SDS-PAGE and peak fractions containing the ternary complex were concentrated to 7 mg/ml. Concentrated ternary complex was screened for crystallization by sitting drop vapour diffusion. A range of commercially available crystallization screen kits was used: Protein Complex Suite (130715), Classics Suite (130701), Classics Ⅱ Suite (130723), and Classics Lite Suite (130702) from Qiagen; Crystal Screen (HR2-110), Crystal Screen 2 (HR2-112), Crystal Screen Lite (HR2-128), PEG/Ion Screen (HR2-126), and PEGRx1 (HR2-082) from Hampton Research; and PEG Grid Screening Kit (36436) and Crystallization Cryo Kit (75403) from Sigma-Aldrich. Drops consisting of 100 nl reservoir solution and 100 nl protein complex solution were equilibrated against 100 μl well volume set up in 96-well plates (Fisher Scientific) using a Mosquito crystallization robot (TTP Labtech). Plates were stored at 18℃ and automatically imaged by Rock Imager 1000 (Formulatrix). Image data were collected and managed using Rock Maker software version 3.1.4.0 (Formulatrix). One crystal hit was obtained after 7 days of plate incubation at 18℃ and one crystallization condition from the Protein Complex Suite (130715, Qiagen) was chosen for optimization using the Additive Screen (HR2-428) from

Hampton Research. Crystals were confirmed as protein crystals by UV imaging using Rock Imager 1000 (Formulatrix). Crystal growth in optimized conditions was scaled up in 24-well VDXm plates (Hampton Research) where crystals were grown by hanging drop vapour diffusion. Larger crystals (80 μm × 76 μm × 35 μm) were obtained within 28 days by mixing 1 μl of protein complex and 1 μl of crystallization solution. Some of those crystals were dissolved in Lämmli sample buffer after thorough rinsing, and analysed by SDS-PAGE and staining with Coomassie blue to confirm the presence of all three proteins in the ternary complex.

Crystals of ternary complex were briefly soaked in cryo-protective solution consisting of mother liquor supplemented with 25% (w/v) glycerol. These were then mounted on CryoLoops (Hampton Research) and flash-frozen in liquid nitrogen. Crystal screening for X-ray diffraction and diffraction data collection were performed at 100 K on one of the NE-CAT beam lines at the Advanced Photon Source synchrotron of Argonne National Laboratory. X-ray images were recorded with an ADSC Quantum 315 CCD detector with primary oscillations at 100 K, a wavelength of 0.97918 Å, and a crystal-to-detector distance of 420 mm. Crystals of the ternary complex belong to the monoclinic space group C2, and contain one ternary complex molecule in the asymmetric unit. X-ray diffraction data sets were collected to 3.0 Å from native protein crystals, integrated, and scaled using XDS[38] and SCALA[39] from the CCP4 software suite[40].

A clear molecular replacement solution was found for both KL domains using the Phaser module of PHENIX[41] and homology models of KL1 and KL2, which were built with Rosetta software available through the ROBETTA Protein Structure Prediction Server (http://robetta.bakerlab.org). However, the FGF23– FGFR1c component of the ternary complex could not be found even after fixing the coordinates of the partial solution found for the KL domains. Through careful inspection of the crystal lattice and the $F_o - F_c$ difference and $2F_o - F_c$ composite maps generated using the partial model, we succeeded in manually placing an FGF23–FGFR1c D2 portion of the FGF23–FGFR1c complex. This was created using the experimental crystal structures of SOS-bound FGF23[42] (PDB code 2P39) and the FGF2-bound FGFR1c^{ecto} domain[43] (PDB code 1CVS). After a few rounds of refinements, FGFR1c D3 could also be placed manually. Iterative rounds of model building and refinement were carried out using Coot[44] and the Phenix. Refine module of PHENIX[41].

The structure has been refined to 3.0 Å resolution with working and free R-factors of 23.46 and 28.26%, respectively, and good Ramachandran plot statistics. X-ray diffraction data collection and structure refinement statistics are summarized in Extended Data Table 1. The final model comprises residues Glu34 to His977 of human α-klotho^{ecto}, residues Met149 to Ala361 of human FGFR1c^{ecto} and residues Tyr25 to Thr200 of human FGF23. Owing to insufficient electron density, the following residues of the ternary complex could not be built: (1) Leu98 to Ser115 (β1α1 loop) of α-klotho^{ecto} KL1, (2) Glu957 to Glu960 (an ADAM protease cleavage site) at the junction between the rigid core of α-klotho^{ecto} KL2 and the flexible extracellular juxtamembrane linker that connects KL2 to the transmem brane helix of α-klotho, (3) the last four residues of the extracellular juxtamembrane linker (Thr978 to Ser981) of α-klotho^{ecto}, (4) the last five C-terminal residues of FGF23 (Pro201 to Ser205), (5) Asp142 to Arg148 N-terminal to the D2 domain of FGFR1c^{ecto}, and (6) Leu362 to Arg365 C-terminal to the D3 domain of FGFR1c^{ecto}. Ordering of the first six N-terminal residues of FGF23 (Tyr25 to Pro30) is influenced by crystal lattice contacts.

6.4 SEC–mALS

The SEC–MALS instrument setup consisted of a Waters Breeze 2 HPLC system (Waters), a miniDAWN-TREOS 18-angle static light scattering detector with built-in 658.0 nm wavelength laser (Wyatt Technology Corp.), and an Optilab rEX refractive index detector (Wyatt Technology Corp.). A Superdex 200 10/300 GL column (GE Healthcare) was placed in-line between the HPLC pump (Waters 1525) and the HPLC UV (Waters 2998 Photodiode Array), laser light scattering, and refractive index detectors. Light scattering and refractive index detectors were calibrated following the manufacturer's guidelines. The refractive index increment (dn/dc), in which n is the refractive index and c is the concentration of the mixture of DDM and CHS in 20 mM Tris-HCl pH 8.0 buffer containing 300 mM NaCl, was determined offline using an Optilab T-rEX refractive index detector. Monomeric bovine serum albumin (23210, Thermo Scientific) was used as part of routine data quality control.

At least 60 ml of 25 mM HEPES pH 7.5 buffer containing 150 mM NaCl were passed through the system at a flow rate of 0.5 ml/min to equilibrate the Superdex 200 10/300 GL column and establish stable baselines for light scattering and refractive index detectors. Purified α-klotho^{ecto}, FGFR1c^{ecto} (wild type or mutant), and FGF23 (wild type or mutant) proteins were mixed at a molar ratio of 1:1:1 and concentrated to 12.5 μM. Protein samples (50 μl) with a molar equivalent of a heparin hexasaccharide (HO06, Iduron) were injected onto the gel filtration column, and the column eluent was continuously monitored for 280 nm absorbance, laser light scattering, and refractive index. In a separate set of experiments, 50 μl of 1:1:1 FGF23–FGFR1c^{ecto}–α-klotho^{ecto} ternary complex at 12.5 μM concentration was mixed with heparin hexasaccharide at molar ratios of 1:0.25, 1:0.5, 1:1 or 1:2, and the mixtures were injected onto the gel filtration column. As a control, 50 μl of ternary complex without added heparin hexasaccharide were run on the column. In yet another set of experiments, α-klotho^{ecto} (wild type or mutant) and FGFR1c^{ecto} were mixed at a molar ratio of 1:1, and 50 μl of concentrated protein mixtures were injected onto the gel filtration column. 50 μl of concentrated α-klotho^{ecto} (wild type or mutant) alone were run as a control in these experiments. The analyses were performed at ambient temperature. Data were collected every second at a flow rate of 0.5 ml/min. Laser light scattering intensity and eluent refractive index (concentration) data were adjusted manually for the volume delay of UV absorbance at 280 nm, and were processed using ASTRA software (Wyatt Technology Corp.). A protein refractive index increment (dn/dc value) of 0.185 ml/g was used for molecular mass calculations.

6.5 Cell line culture and stimulation and analysis of protein phosphorylation

HEK293 cells (a gift from A. Mansukhani, identified by morphology check under microscope, mycoplasma negative in DAPI) were maintained in DMEM medium (10-017-CV, CORNING) supplemented with 10% FBS, 100 U/ml of penicillin and 100 μg/ml streptomycin. HEK293 cells naturally express multiple FGFR isoforms including FGFR1c, FGFR3c and FGFR4, but lack α-klotho or β-klotho co-receptors. BaF3 cells (a gift from S. Byron, identified by morphology check under microscope, mycoplasma negative in DAPI), an IL-3-dependent haematopoietic pro B cell line, were cultured in RPMI 1640 medium (10-040-CV, CORNING) supplemented with 10% FBS, 100 U/ml of penicillin, 100 μg/ml streptomycin and 5 ng/ml mouse IL-3 (#GFM1, Cell Guidance Systems). BaF3 cells do not express FGFRs, α-/β-klotho co-receptors, or HS cofactors, and hence are naturally non-responsive to FGFs. However, *via* controlled ectopic expression of FGFRs and klotho co-receptors and exogenous supplementation with soluble HS, these cells can be forced to respond to FGF stimulation. As such, the BaF3 cell line has served as a powerful tool for reconstituting FGF–FGFR cell surface signal transduction complexes to dissect the molecular mechanisms of paracrine and endocrine FGF signalling[29,45,46].

Stable or transient expression of full-length (transmembrane) human α-klotho, β-klotho, FGFR1c, and mutants of these proteins in HEK293 or BaF3 cells was achieved using lentiviral vectors. To generate lentiviral expression vectors, HEK293 cells were seeded at a density of about 8×10^5 in 10 cm cell culture dishes and co-transfected by calcium phosphate co-precipitation with 8 μg of lentiviral transfer plasmid encoding wild-type or mutant α-klotho, β-klotho or FGFR1c, 1.6 μg of pMD2.G envelope plasmid, and 2.5 μg of psPAX2 packaging plasmid. Fresh medium was added to the cells for a 3-day period after transfection. Cell culture supernatant containing recombinant lentivirus particles was collected and used to infect 2×10^5 HEK293 or BaF3 cells in the presence of polybrene (5 μg/ml; 134220, Santa Cruz Biotechnology). Stable transfectants were selected using hygromycin (1 mg/ml, ant-hg-1, *In vivo* Gen) or G418 (0.5 mg/ml, 6483, KSE Scientific). For transient protein expression, 2×10^5 HEK293 cells were plated in 6-well cell culture dishes and on the following day, the cells were infected with recombinant lentivirus in the presence of polybrene (16 μg).

For cell stimulation studies, unmodified and stably transfected HEK293 cells were seeded in 6-well cell culture plates at a density of 4×10^5 cells per well and maintained for 24 h in cell culture medium without FBS. In the case of transiently transfected HEK293 cells, medium containing lentivirus particles was removed from the cells after incubation for approximately 12 h, and the cells were also serum-starved for 24 h. Stably transfected BaF3 cells were seeded in 10 cm cell culture dishes at a density of 6×10^6 cells and serum-starved for 6 h. Unmodified HEK293 cells were stimulated for 10 min with wild-type or mutant FGF23 both in the presence and absence of wild-type or mutant α-klotho^{ecto}. HEK293 cells stably or transiently expressing wild-type α-klotho^{TM} or its mutants were stimulated with wild-type or mutant FGF23 alone. In one set of experiments, HEK293 cells expressing wild-type α-klotho^{TM} were pretreated with α-klotho^{ecto} for 10 min before stimulation with wild-type FGF23. BaF3 cells expressing wild-type or mutant FGFR1c were stimulated with wild-type or mutant FGF23 in the presence or absence of α-klotho^{ecto} and heparin. BaF3 cells co-expressing wild-type α-klotho^{TM} and wild-type or mutant FGFR1c were stimulated with wild-type or mutant FGF23 in the presence of heparin. BaF3 cells co-expressing wild- type FGFR1c and wild-type or mutant β-klotho^{TM} were stimulated with wild-type FGF21 in the presence or absence of heparin.

After stimulation, cells were lysed, and lysate samples containing approximately 30 μg total cellular protein were electrophoresed on 12% SDS-PAGE and electrotransferred onto a nitrocellulose membrane. The membrane was blocked for 1 h at ambient temperature in Tris-buffered saline pH 7.6 containing 0.05% Tween-20 and 5% BSA (BP1600-100, Fisher BioReagents). Rabbit monoclonal antibodies to phosphorylated ERK1/2 (4370, Cell Signaling Technology) and total (phosphorylated and unphosphorylated) ERK1/2 (4695, Cell Signaling Technology) were diluted 1:2 000 and 1:1 000, respectively, in blocking buffer. After overnight incubation at 4℃ with one of these diluted antibodies, the blot was washed with Tris-buffered saline pH 7.6 containing 0.05% Tween-20, and then incubated at ambient temperature for 30 min with 1:10 000-diluted IRDye secondary antibody [926-32211 (goat anti-rabbit), LI-COR]. After another round of washing with Tris-buffered saline pH 7.6 containing 0.05% Tween-20, the blot was imaged on an Odyssey Fc Dual-mode Imaging System (LI-COR).

6.6 α-Klotho treatment of mice and serum, urinary phosphate analysis

Mice of the strain 129/Sv (Charles River Laboratories) were housed in a room with a temperature of $22℃ ± 1℃$ and a 12 h:12 h light/dark cycle, and had ad libitum access to tap water and Teklad global 16% rodent diet (Envigo). Ten female and ten male 6-week-old mice of each gender were assigned to receive either recombinant α-klotho^{ecto} protein diluted in isotonic saline (0.1 mg/kg body weight) or protein diluent only (buffer control). Mice were placed in metabolic cages for a one-day acclimation, and returned to the cages for 24 h urine collection after intraperitoneal injection of α-klotho^{ecto} protein or buffer control. After urine collection, mice were placed under isofluorane anaesthesia, and blood was drawn from the retro-orbital sinus and transferred into tubes containing a few drops of sterile solution of heparin (Sagent Pharmaceuticals). After centrifugation at 3 000 g at 4℃ for 5 min, supernatant plasma was taken out of the tubes and stored at −80℃. Blood and urine samples were also collected before injection of α-klotho^{ecto} or buffer control. Phosphate and creatinine concentrations in plasma and urine were measured using a Vitros Chemistry Analyzer (Ortho-Clinical Diagnosis) and a P/ACE MDQ Capillary Electrophoresis System equipped with a photodiode detector (Beckman-Coulter), respectively. The Mouse Metabolic Phenotyping Core Facility at UT Southwestern Medical Center carried out the measurements of these analytes.

In a separate set of experiments, 10- to 12-week-old mice were given an intraperitoneal injection of wild-type α-klotho^{ecto} (0.1 mg/kg body weight), RBA deletion mutant, α-klotho$^{ecto/ΔRBA}$ (0.1 mg/kg body weight), or protein diluent only (three female and three male mice per group), and blood and urine samples were collected for measurement of phosphate and creatinine as described above. In yet another set of experiments, 10- to 12-week-old mice were injected intraperitoneally with 0.1 mg/kg body weight of wild-type α-klotho^{ecto} (two female and one male mice), mutant α-klotho$^{ecto/ΔRBA}$ (two female and two male mice), or protein diluent only (two female and one male mice), and kidneys were obtained from the mice under isofluorane anaesthesia four hours after the injection. Total RNA was extracted from the kidneys using RNAeasy kit (Qiagen), and *Egr1* mRNA levels were quantified by quantitative PCR (qPCR) with cyclophilin (also known as *Ppia*) as a control. Template cDNA for the PCR was generated using SuperScript Ⅲ First Strand Synthesis System (Invitrogen) and oligo-(dT) primers. PCR primers for *Egr1* were 5′-GAGGAGATGAT-GCTGCTGAG-3′ and 5′-TGCTGCTGCTGCTATTACC-3′. PCR primers for cyclophilin were 5′-GTCTCTTTTCGC-CGCTTGCT-3′ and 5′-TCTGCTGTCTTTGGAACTTTGTCTG-3′. qPCR was performed in triplicate for each kidney RNA sample. Except for *Egr1* expression analysis, data were analysed by paired Student's *t*-test. All studies in mice were approved by the Institutional Animal Care and Use Committee at the University of Texas Southwestern Medical Center and conducted following the National Institutes of Health Guide for the Care and Use of Laboratory Animals.

6.7 Enzymatic assay

To examine α-klotho^{ecto} for glycoside-hydrolase activity, 4-methylumbelliferyl-β-d-xylopyranoside (M7008, Sigma-Aldrich), 4-methylumbelliferyl-β-d-glucuronide (474427, Sigma-Aldrich) and 4-methylumbelliferyl-α-d-*N*-acetylneuraminic acid (69587, Sigma-Aldrich) were selected as substrates and commercially available recombinant neuraminidase (#10269611001, Roche Diagnostics GmbH) and β-glucuronidase (#G0251, Sigma-Aldrich) were used as positive controls. 20 μg of α-klotho^{ecto} or the control enzymes were added into reaction buffer (0.1 M sodium citrate buffer, pH 5.6, 0.05 M NaCl, 0.01% Tween 20) containing 0.5 mM substrate at a final volume of 100 μl, and the reaction mixtures were incubated at 37℃ for 2 h. Enzymatic activity was assessed by quantifying fluorescence intensity of released 4-methylumbelliferone at an excitation wavelength of 360 nm and an emission wavelength of 450 nm using a FlexStation 3 Multi-Mode Microplate Reader (Molecular Devices).

6.8 Fluorescence dye-based thermal shift assay

SYPRO Orange dye (S6650, Thermo Fisher Scientific) was used as the fluorescent probe. 15 μl of 20 μM solutions of protein samples (wild-type and mutated forms of FGF23; α-klotho^{ecto} or α-klotho$^{ecto/\Delta RBA}$ alone; 1:1 mixtures of α-klotho^{ecto} or α-klotho$^{ecto/\Delta RBA}$ with FGF23 C-terminal tail peptide) were mixed with 5 μl of working dye solution (1:25 dilution) in duplicate in PCR strips. A temperature gradient from 4 ℃ to 100 ℃, at 1 ℃ per min increment was carried out with a CFX96 Touch Real-Time PCR Detection System (Bio-Rad). Fluorescence was recorded as a function of temperature in real time. The melting temperature (T_m) was calculated with Step One software v2.2 as the maximum of the derivative of the resulting SYPRO Orange fluorescence curves.

6.9 Statistics and reproducibility

Glycoside-hydrolase activity of α-klotho^{ecto}, neuraminidase and β-glucuronidase was measured in triplicate; one triplicate representative of three independent experiments is shown in Fig. 2C. Each set of immunoblot experiments (data shown in Fig. 4B–E, 5C–E and Extended Data Fig. 1B, 4C, 7E and 10B, C) was independently repeated three times. Renal mRNA levels of mouse *Egr1* and cyclophilin were each measured in triplicate, and mean values of relative *Egr1* mRNA concentrations from three independent samples for buffer control, three independent samples for α-klotho^{ecto} treatment, and four independent samples for α-klotho$^{ecto/\Delta RBA}$ treatment are shown in Extended Data Fig. 1D and 7B, respectively. Protein elution profiles from size-exclusion columns shown in Fig. 4A, 5A, B, f and Extended Data Fig. 7C are each representative of three independent experiments.

6.10 Data availability

Atomic coordinates and structure factors for the crystal structure of the FGF23–FGFR1c^{ecto}–α-klotho^{ecto} ternary complex are accessible at the RCBS Protein Data Bank (PDB) under accession code 5W21. Requests for *in vivo* datasets should be directed to O.W.M. Requests for all other reagents and datasets, including recombinant proteins, engineered cell lines and cell-based data, should be made to M.M.

Supplementary information

Extended data to this article can be found in the online version (doi:10.1038/nature 25451).

References

[1] Shimada T, Kakitani M, Yamazaki Y, *et al.* Targeted ablation of Fgf23 demonstrates an essential physiological role of FGF23 in phosphate and vitamin D metabolism[J]. Journal Of Clinical Investigation, 2004, 113(4): 561-568.

[2] Gattineni J, Bates C, Twombley K, *et al.* FGF23 decreases renal NaPi-2a and NaPi-2c expression and induces hypophosphatemia *in vivo* predominantly *via* FGF receptor 1[J]. American Journal Of Physiology-Renal Physiology, 2009, 297(2): F282-F291.

[3] Lemmon MA, Schlessinger J. Cell Signaling by Receptor Tyrosine Kinases[J]. Cell, 2010, 141(7): 1117-1134.

[4] Schlessinger J, Plotnikov AN, Ibrahimi OA, *et al.* Crystal structure of a ternary FGF-FGFR-heparin complex reveals a dual role for heparin in FGFR binding and dimerization[J]. Molecular Cell, 2000, 6(3): 743-750.

[5] Mohammadi M, Olsen SK, Ibrahimi OA. Structural basis for fibroblast growth factor receptor activation[J]. Cytokine & Growth Factor Reviews, 2005, 16(2): 107-137.

[6] Goetz R, Mohammadi M. Exploring mechanisms of FGF signalling through the lens of structural biology[J]. Nature Reviews Molecular Cell Biology, 2013, 14(3): 166-180.

[7] Kuroo M, Matsumura Y, Aizawa H, *et al.* Mutation of the mouse klotho gene leads to a syndrome resembling ageing[J]. Nature, 1997, 390(6655): 45-51.

[8] Henrissat B, Davies G. Structural and sequence-based classification of glycoside hydrolases[J]. Current Opinion In Structural Biology, 1997, 7(5): 637-644.

[9] Goetz R, Ohnishi M, Ding X, *et al.* Klotho coreceptors inhibit signaling by paracrine fibroblast growth factor 8 subfamily ligands[J]. Molecular And Cellular Biology, 2012, 32(10): 1944-1954.

[10] Goetz R, Nakada Y, Hu MC, *et al.* Isolated C-terminal tail of FGF23 alleviates hypophosphatemia by inhibiting FGF23-FGFR-Klotho complex formation[J]. Proceedings Of the National Academy Of Sciences Of the United States Of America, 2010, 107(1): 407-412.

[11] Urakawa I, Yamazaki Y, Shimada T, *et al.* Klotho converts canonical FGF receptor into a specific receptor for FGF23[J]. Nature, 2006, 444(7120): 770-774.

[12] Kurosu H, Ogawa Y, Miyoshi M, *et al.* Regulation of fibroblast growth factor-23 signaling by Klotho[J]. Journal Of Biological Chemistry, 2006, 281(10): 6120-6123.

[13] Li SA, Watanabe M, Yamada H, *et al.* Immunohistochemical localization of Klotho protein in brain, kidney, and reproductive organs

of mice[J]. Cell Structure And Function, 2004, 29(4): 91-99.

[14] van Loon EPM, Pulskens WP, van der Hagen EAE, *et al.* Shedding of klotho by ADAMs in the kidney[J]. American Journal Of Physiology-Renal Physiology, 2015, 309(4): F359-F368.

[15] Lindberg K, Amin R, Moe OW, *et al.* The kidney is the principal organ mediating klotho effects[J]. Journal Of the American Society Of Nephrology, 2014, 25(10): 2169-2175.

[16] Chen CD, Podvin S, Gillespie E, *et al.* Insulin stimulates the cleavage and release of the extracellular domain of klotho by ADAM10 and ADAM 17[J]. Proceedings Of the National Academy Of Sciences Of the United States Of America, 2007, 104(50): 19796-19801.

[17] Imura A, Iwano A, Tohyama O, *et al.* Secreted Klotho protein in sera and CSF: implication for post-translational cleavage in release of Klotho protein from cell membrane[J]. Febs Letters, 2004, 565(1-3): 143-147.

[18] Matsumura Y, Aizawa H, Shiraki-Iida T, *et al.* Identification of the human klotho gene and its two transcripts encoding membrane and secreted klotho protein[J]. Biochemical And Biophysical Research Communications, 1998, 242(3): 626-630.

[19] Shiraki-Iida T, Aizawa H, Matsumura Y, *et al.* Structure of the mouse klotho gene and its two transcripts encoding membrane and secreted protein[J]. Febs Letters, 1998, 424(1-2): 6-10.

[20] Kurosu H, Yamamoto M, Clark JD, *et al.* Suppression of aging in mice by the hormone Klotho[J]. Science, 2005, 309(5742): 1829-1833.

[21] Hu MC, Shiizaki K, Kuro-o M, *et al.* Fibroblast growth factor 23 and klotho: physiology and pathophysiology of an endocrine network of mineral metabolism[A]. In: *Annual Review Of Physiology, Vol 75* (Julius D, ed), Vol. 75, 2013: 503-533.

[22] Chang Q, Hoefs S, van der Kemp AW, *et al.* The β-glucuronidase klotho hydrolyzes and activates the TRPV5 channel[J]. Science, 2005, 310(5747): 490-493.

[23] Cha SK, Ortega B, Kurosu H, *et al.* Removal of sialic acid involving klotho causes cell-surface retention of TRPV5 channel *via* binding to galectin-1[J]. Proceedings Of the National Academy Of Sciences Of the United States Of America, 2008, 105(28): 9805-9810.

[24] Hu MC, Shi M, Zhang J, *et al.* Klotho: a novel phosphaturic substance acting as an autocrine enzyme in the renal proximal tubule[J]. Faseb Journal, 2010, 24(9): 3438-3450.

[25] Imura A, Tsuji Y, Murata M, *et al.* alpha-klotho as a regulator of calcium homeostasis[J]. Science, 2007, 316(5831): 1615-1618.

[26] Hayashi Y, Okino N, Kakuta Y, *et al.* Klotho-related protein is a novel cytosolic neutral beta-glycosylceramidase[J]. Journal Of Biological Chemistry, 2007, 282(42): 30889-30900.

[27] Andrukhova O, Bayer J, Schueler C, *et al.* Klotho lacks an FGF23-independent role in mineral homeostasis[J]. Journal Of Bone And Mineral Research, 2017, 32(10): 2049-2061.

[28] Wu X, Lemon B, Li X, *et al.* C-terminal tail of FGF19 determines its specificity toward klotho co-receptors[J]. Journal Of Biological Chemistry, 2008, 283(48): 33304-33309.

[29] Ornitz DM, Yayon A, Flanagan JG, *et al.* Heparin is required for cell-free binding of basic fibroblast growth-factor to a soluble receptor and for mitogenesis in whole cells[J]. Molecular And Cellular Biology, 1992, 12(1): 240-247.

[30] Pellegrini L, Burke DF, von Delft F, *et al.* Crystal structure of fibroblast growth factor receptor ectodomain bound to ligand and heparin[J]. Nature, 2000, 407(6807): 1029-1034.

[31] Harmer NJ, Ilag LL, Mulloy B, *et al.* Towards a resolution of the stoichiometry of the fibroblast growth factor (FGF)-FGIF receptor-Heparin complex[J]. Journal Of Molecular Biology, 2004, 339(4): 821-834.

[32] Ogawa Y, Kurosu H, Yamamoto M, *et al.* β-Klotho is required for metabolic activity of fibroblast growth factor 21[J]. Proceedings

Of the National Academy Of Sciences Of the United States Of America, 2007, 104(18): 7432-7437.

[33] Kurosu H, Choi M, Ogawa Y, *et al.* Tissue-specific expression of beta Klotho and fibroblast growth factor (FGF) receptor Isoforms determines metabolic activity of FGF19 and FGF21[J]. Journal Of Biological Chemistry, 2007, 282(37): 26687-26695.

[34] Holt JA, Luo GZ, Billin AN, *et al.* Definition of a novel growth factor-dependent signal cascade for the suppression of bile acid biosynthesis[J]. Genes & Development, 2003, 17(13): 1581-1591.

[35] Potthoff MJ, Inagaki T, Satapati S, *et al.* FGF21 induces PGC-1 alpha and regulates carbohydrate and fatty acid metabolism during the adaptive starvation response[J]. Proceedings Of the National Academy Of Sciences Of the United States Of America, 2009, 106(26): 10853-10858.

[36] Pitteloud N, Quinton R, Pearce S, *et al.* Digenic mutations account for variable phenotypes in idiopathic hypogonadotropic hypogonadism[J]. Journal Of Clinical Investigation, 2007, 117(2): 457-463.

[37] White KE, Evans WE, O'Riordan JLH, *et al.* Autosomal dominant hypophosphataemic rickets is associated with mutations in FGF23[J]. Nature Genetics, 2000, 26(3): 345-348.

[38] Kabsch W. XDS[J]. Acta Crystallographica Section D-Biological Crystallography, 2010, 66: 125-132.

[39] Evans P. Scaling and assessment of data quality[J]. Acta Crystallographica Section D-Structural Biology, 2006, 62: 72-82.

[40] Winn MD, Ballard CC, Cowtan KD, *et al.* Overview of the CCP4 suite and current developments[J]. Acta Crystallographica Section D-Biological Crystallography, 2011, 67: 235-242.

[41] Adams PD, Afonine PV, Bunkoczi G, *et al.* PHENIX: a comprehensive Python-based system for macromolecular structure solution[J]. Acta Crystallographica Section D-Biological Crystallography, 2010, 66: 213-221.

[42] Goetz R, Beenken A, Ibrahimi OA, *et al.* Molecular insights into the klotho-dependent, endocrine mode of action of fibroblast growth factor 19 subfamily members[J]. Molecular And Cellular Biology, 2007, 27(9): 3417-3428.

[43] Plotnikov AN, Schlessinger J, Hubbard SR, *et al.* Structural basis for FGF receptor dimerization and activation[J]. Cell, 1999, 98(5): 641-650.

[44] Emsley P, Cowtan K. Coot: model-building tools for molecular graphics[J]. Acta Crystallographica Section D-Biological Crystallography, 2004, 60: 2126-2132.

[45] Suzuki M, Uehara Y, Motomura-Matsuzaka K, *et al.* β-Klotho is required for fibroblast growth factor (FGF) 21 signaling through FGF receptor (FGFR) 1c and FGFR3c[J]. Molecular Endocrinology, 2008, 22(4): 1006-1014.

[46] Ornitz DM, Herr AB, Nilsson M, *et al.* FGF Binding and FGF receptor activation by synthetic heparan-derived disaccharides and trisaccharides[J]. Science, 1995, 268(5209): 432-436.

[47] Liu Y, Ma J, Beenken A, *et al.* Regulation of Receptor Binding Specificity of FGF9 by an Autoinhibitory Homodimerization[J]. Structure, 2017, 25(9): 1325-1336.

[48] Belov AA, Mohammadi M. Molecular mechanisms of fibroblast growth factor signaling in physiology and pathology[J]. Cold Spring Harbor Perspectives In Biology, 2013, 5(6).

[49] Beenken A, Eliseenkova AV, Ibrahimi OA, *et al.* Plasticity in Interactions of Fibroblast Growth Factor 1 (FGF1) N Terminus with FGF Receptors Underlies Promiscuity of FGF1[J]. Journal Of Biological Chemistry, 2012, 287(5): 3067-3078.

[50] Olsen SK, Li JYH, Bromleigh C, *et al.* Structural basis by which alternative splicing modulates the organizer activity of FGF8 in the brain[J]. Genes & Development, 2006, 20(2): 185-198.

[51] Robinson CJ, Harmer NJ, Goodger SJ, *et al.* Cooperative dimerization of fibroblast growth factor 1 (FGF1) upon a single heparin saccharide may drive the formation of 2 : 2 : 1 FGF1 center dot

FGFR2c center dot heparin ternary complexes[J]. Journal Of Biological Chemistry, 2005, 280(51): 42274-42282.

[52] Goodger SJ, Robinson CJ, Murphy KJ, *et al.* Evidence that heparin saccharides promote FGF2 mitogenesis through two distinct mechanisms[J]. Journal Of Biological Chemistry, 2008, 283(19):

13001-13008.

[53] Dunshee DR, Bainbridge TW, Kljavin NM, *et al.* Fibroblast activation protein cleaves and inactivates fibroblast growth factor 21[J]. Journal Of Biological Chemistry, 2016, 291(11): 5986-5996.

Comparative study of heparin-poloxamer hydrogel modified bFGF and aFGF for *in vivo* wound healing efficiency

Jiang Wu, Xiaokun Li, Jian Xiao

1. Introduction

Wound healing therapy remains a great clinical challenge,[1–3] because wound healing is a remarkably dynamic, complex, and interactive process, typically involving three overlapped stages of inflammatory phase, cell proliferation phase, and extracellular matrix remodeling phase.[4,5] It is well-known that the angio-genesis growth factors (GFs) are critically important for regulating the wound repair process,[6,7] including cell migration and proliferation, extracellular matrix deposition, angiogenesis, and remodeling.[8,9] Thus, significant efforts have been made to develop a wide variety of biocompatible materials (e.g., chitosan, collagen, alginate, peptide, and polyurethane) to incorporate GFs for maximizing their bioactivity in the wound bed.[10–12] However, these common materials usually have application of growth factors to accelerate wound healing still remains largely unknown.[16]

Hydrogels, containing 80% – 90% water and 3D porous structure, are considered as promising dressing materials to load and deliver GFs for wound treatments.[17–20] In general, different hydrogels have been developed to contain some functional groups for specifically interacting with the loaded molecules to realize its control-release behaviors *in vitro* and *in vivo*.[21–26] Such surface modifications facilitate binding specificity and affinity between modified groups with GFs and help to remedy the biochemical properties of the conjugated biomolecules, such as water-solubility, bioavailability, selectivity, and even toxicity.[27–29] Among these, heparin is often used as a bridge to modify GFs to achieve their combinatorial several limitations, including poor anti-infective properties, low hydration environment, and frequent dressing exchanges,[13–15] any of which would delay a whole wound healing process. Moreover, the fundamental understanding of the topicalivity.[30–32] Briefly, heparin is a negative linear polysaccharide[33] that can easily bind to GFs domains (namely, heparin-binding GFs[34]) containing rich positively charged lysine and arginine residues.[35,36] Such heparin-GFs binding helps to not only stabilize GFs[37] but also enhance GFs binding affinity to cell-surface receptors to initiate more intracellular signaling[38] pathways. Hence, the use of heparin-based hydrogels to incorporate different growth factors and cytokines through their heparin-binding domain is the most possible, efficient way to form a (multi)functional complex.[37,39] Several heparin-GF hydrogel systems have been reported as proof-of-concept models for wound healings, including a star PEG-heparin 3D hydrogel with both bFGF and VEGF,[40,41] chitosan/pluronic hydrogel containing heparin/bFGF,[42,43] heparin-alginate bFGF hydrogels,[44] and NGF loaded thermosensitive heparin-poloxamer (HP) hydrogel.[45,46]

Since all these heparin-GF hydrogels exhibit different degrees of wound healing improvement *in vivo* or *in vitro*, it appears to be a common opinion that, regardless of different GFs, the same heparin-based materials can always interact with GFs and load GFs into heparin host materials due to the presence of heparin binding domain.[47–49] However, in our opinion, it is expected that the heparin binding domain of the GFs, as well as different GFs of different structural properties (surface charge intensity changes, hydrophobicity, and hydrophilicity[50]), would affect the binding and releasing behaviors of GFs in host materials. Not much attention has been paid to the structural-dependent effect of different GFs on their binding/release behaviors in host materials, as well as their consequences on wound healing. For instance, aFGF and bFGF are the two most commonly used heparin binding GFs, both of which show similar chemical structures but a major difference in isoelectric point (IP). aFGF has 140 amino acids, 15.8 kDa in molecular mass, and 5.6 of IP, showing acidity in saline,[51] while bFGF has 146 amino acids, 16.4 kDa in molecular mass, and 9.6 of IP, showing alkalinity in saline.[52,53] This totally different acid-base property between aFGF and bFGF will lead to different surface charges,[54] especially when loading into heparin-based hydrogels in physiological saline solution. It is reasonable to speculate that aFGF and bFGF will have different interactions with heparin-based materials in physiological saline solution, probably leading to different GF-induced wound healing effects *via* different binding and release behaviors between GFs and host heparin-based materials.

To examine this hypothesis, here we synthesized heparin-poloxamer (HP) hydrogels, followed by modification of HP hydrogels with different aFGF and bFGF to better understand different GFs/hydrogel-induced wound healing effects *in vivo*. Particularly, we focused on the investigation and comparison of different GFs/hydrogel-induced wound healing effects between free aFGF and bFGF, between HP-aFGF and HP-bFGF, and between a/bFGFs and the corresponding HP-a/bFGFs. *In vivo* wound efficacy was assessed by C57BL/6 mice using the full-thickness wound. While all FGF-based dressings stimulated and improved wound healing *in vivo*, wound healing efficiency was largely different. Specifically, both HP-GF hydrogels exhibited superior wound healing activity as compared to free a/bFGF in terms of wound closure, granulation formation, reepithelization, and blood vessel density. Moreover, HP-aFGF out-performed HP-bFGF to achieve the better wound-healing capacity because aFGF can be efficiently released from HP hydrogels. The results suggest that this rationally designed construct is critical for better understanding biomaterial mediated wound healing and rational design of wound healing biomaterials.

2. Materials and methods

2.1 Preparation of HP-aFGF hydrogels and HP-bFGF

Hydrogels. Heparin–poloxamer conjugate was prepared according to the EDC/NHS method reported in a previous paper.[55] HP-aFGF hydrogels and HP-bFGF hydrogels containing different amounts of HP and aFGF/bFGF were prepared using the cold method.[56] In brief, lyophilized HP powder was mixed with aFGF/bFGF (the Key Laboratory of Biotechnology and Pharmaceutical Engineering, Wenzhou Medical University, China) at 4 ℃ under gentle stirring. The mixture was kept in a refrigerator at 4 ℃ overnight, and finally, a clear solution was obtained.

2.2 Micromorphology of hydrogel system

The micro-morphology of the dehydrated HP, HP-bFGF, and HP-aFGF hydrogels was observed on a scanning electron microscope (SEM; Hitachi, H-7500, Japan). The hydrogels were frozen and lyophilized with a vacuum freeze-dryer for 24 h. The dehydrated specimens were cross-sectioned and sputtered with gold, and their surface of solid was observed by scanning electron microscopy.

2.3 Rheological behavior of HP and HP-GFs hydrogels

Rheological measurements of the HP, HP-aFGF, and HP-bFGF were carried out using the rheometer (TA-AR-G2) at different temperatures from 10 to 40 ℃. The elastic modulus and viscous shear modulus were measured using the flat plates (12 mm), and shear frequency was set to 10 rad/s; shear strain was set to 1%.

2.4 Releasing profile of aFGF/bFGF from HP-aFGF/HP-bFGF

HP-GFs were prepared as before. At each time point (0 h, 6 h, 12 h, 24 h, 3 day, 8 day, 14 day, and 17 day), GFs were collected through the supernatant and then replaced with fresh solution. The released GFs were analyzed by a specific GF enzyme-linked immunosorbent assay kit (ELISA, Westang system, Shanghai, China). The amount of released GFs was normalized through the former and final concentrations. The GFs release system was carried out at 37 ℃. This trend of the release profile was maintained up to the end of the experiment.

2.5 In vivo wound healing model

6–7 week old male C57BL/6 mice were purchased from the Animal Center of Chinese Academy of Sciences, Shanghai, China. The experiments were carried out according to the National Institutes of Health Guide Concerning the Care and Use of Laboratory Animals. All animal experiments were performed in accordance with the guidelines approved by the Animal Experimentation Ethics Committee of Wenzhou Medical University, Wenzhou, China. Mice were maintained for at least 7 days before the experiment on a standard diet and water was provided freely available. Temperature (23~25 ℃), humidity (35%~60%), and photoperiod (12 h light/dark cycle) were kept constant.

All the animals were anaesthetized by an intraperitoneal injection of 4% chloral hydrate (0.1 ml/10 g), and the dorsal area was shaved. 0.5 mm-thick silicone donut-shaped splints (external diameter of 16 mm, internal diameter of 8 mm) were fixed on either side of the dorsalmidline using a 6−0 Prolene suture. Two full-thickness cutaneous wounds were made using a 6 mm round skin biopsy punch (Acuderminc., Ft Lauderdale, FL, USA). The forty-two C57BL/6 mice were randomly selected for each group. Saline, vehicle alone, or 1.6 µg of free aFGF/bFGF or HP-aFGF/bFGF hydrogels was administered to wounds ($n = 7$ animals/14 wounds per group) as a 10 µl solution. To avoid cross-contamination, all wounds received the same treatment. The wounds of the treated animals were applied a Tegaderm transparent dressing (3 M Health Care, Germany) and wrapped with self-adhesive wrap to deter chewing of the splints. All the animals were fed in individual cages with food and water *ad libitum* and watched every day during the total period of the experiment. At days 0, 7, 10, 14, and 17 post-treatments, the wound closure rate was determined by measuring the wound area by Image-Pro plus to trace the wound margin (wound closure rate (%) = (wound area$_{day0}$ − wound area$_{day\#}$) × 100%/wound area$_{day0}$). At day 3 or 17 postsurgery, C57BL/6 mice were sacrificed, and wounds with surrounding tissue were harvested for histological evaluation.

2.6 Histological analysis

For histological preparation, the skin was fixed in 4% paraformaldehyde in 0.01 M phosphate buffered saline (PBS, pH = 7.4) overnight and paraffin embedded. Skin tissue was sectioned into 5 µm thickness slices for Hematoxylin and Eosin (H&E) (Beyotime Institute of Biotechnology, China) staining and for collagen formation by Masson's trichrome staining (Beyotime), using standard procedures. Sections were analyzed, and images were captured using a Nikon ECLPSE 80i (Nikon, Japan).

2.7 Immunohistochemical staining

Wound sections were fixed with 4% paraformaldehyde solution for 24 h and dehydrated in graded ethanol series and then embedded in paraffin. Skin tissue sections, prepared by a microtome to 5 µm thickness, were deparaffinized and rehydrated and then immersed in 3% H_2O_2 and 80% carbinol for 15 min at room temperature to block the endogenous peroxidase activity. The tissue sections were heated to antigen recovery in 10 mM sodium citrate buffer (pH 6.0), and after washing, the samples were blocked using 5% bovine serum albumin (BSA) (Beyotime) for 30 min at room temperature. Primary antibody rabbit polyclonal anticytokeratin (ab9377, 1:75, Abcam), mouse monoclonal anti-PCNA (sc25280, 1:200, Santa Cruz Biotech, CA, USA), rabbit polyclonal anticollagen III (ab7778, 1:300, Abcam), rabbit polyclonal anticollagen I (ab21286, 1:300, Abcam), and tagged secondary antibody goat antimouse or goat antirabbit were used. The tissue was treated with a DAB chromogen kit (ZSGB-BIO, Beijing, China) and then counterstained with hematoxylin (Beyotime Institute of Biotechnology, China) for 5 min. Day 17 skin sections were stained with rabbit polyclonal anti-CD31 (ab28364, 1:200, Abcam) followed by goat antirabbit IgG Alexa Fluor 647-conjugated secondary antibody (ab150083, 1:1500, Abcam) and nuclei with DAPI (Beyotime). All fluorescent images were taken using a Nikon confocal laser microscope (Nikon, A1 PLUS, Tokyo, Japan).

2.8 Statistical analysis

All statistical data are expressed as means ± standard deviation (SD). Statistical analysis of all data was performed: one-way analysis of variance (ANOVA) followed by Tukey's test with GraphPad Prism 5 software (GraphPad Software Inc., La Jolla, CA, USA). For all comparisons, P values <0.05 were considered to be statistically significant.

3. Results and discussion

Considering that the wound-healing process generally involves three overlapping stages, the inflammatory stage, the proliferative stage, and the remodeling phase, here we systematically tested our hydrogel dressings on wound closure, granulation formation with collagen deposition, re-epithelialization, and neovascularization as well as protein related cell proliferation and collagen I and collagen III synthesis upon the wound.

3.1 Characterization of HP-aFGF and HP-bFGF hydrogels

Since copolymer heparin-poloxamer (HP) ex-hibited a thermal-sensitive sol-gel phase transition achieved by po-loxamer's PEO−PEG ratio, HP was used as smart biomaterials to load and deliver both aFGF and bFGF for wound regeneration tests. As shown in Fig. 1A, HP formed hydrogels upon heating to a body temperature of 37℃, while melting to sols when cooling down to 4℃. This sol-gel transition first allows GFs to well mix in HP solution at 4℃. Then, when applying the GF-HP solution to the *in vivo* wound bed at 37℃, HP gelation occurs, allowing GFs to be successfully loaded into HP hydrogels (namely, as hydrogels thereafter). Rheology tests were conducted to reveal the gelation process of HP-based hydrogels by varying temperatures (Fig. 1B). When a hydrogel exhibits viscoelastic behaviors, the storage (G') and loss (G'') moduli are used to measure its elastic and viscous components. Fig. 1B showed that all HP-based hydrogels, regardless of loading of GFs, displayed a similar sol-to-gel transition at around 27℃. When temperatures were above 27℃, both G' and G'' values of the HP-based hydrogels increased rapidly. The transition temperature of 27℃ is close to room temperature as well, making HP-based hydrogels suitable for biomedical applications. Similar rheol_ogcial results among different HP-based hydrogels also indicate that loading of GFs into HPs does not significantly change the rheological properties of HP-based hydrogels. Fig. 1C shows the micromorphology of HP, HP-aFGF, and HP-bFGF hydrogels by SEM. SEM images did not show any obvious differences in porous structures of HP hydrogels in the absence and presence of loaded GFs. This is because within the scale of hundreds of micrometers in SEM images, a very small loading of GFs (~1.6 μg) into HP hydrogels (~1 800 μg) will not cause significant changes in porous structures of HP hydrogels. Moreover, inside all HP-based hydrogels, there existed many sponge-like structures interconnected with each other, which allow growth factors to diffuse through these 3D network structures and realize release. It should be noted that all HP-based dressings can attach easily to the wounds with no need for biological adhesives, due to the gelation structure and high water content (>80%) of HP hydrogels, thus allowing the wound to stay desirably hydrated. In addition, we also tested the biocompatibility of HP hydrogels using the 3T3 fibroblast cell line, which is the most commonly used cell line for wound treatment. Light microscope images (Fig. S1A) showed that, at 0.1 and 1 wt% HP concentration, fibroblast cells were able to retain their healthy morphologies similar to those in the control group. Consistently, Fig. S1B quantitatively showed that HP hydrogels of 0.1 and 1 wt% were not toxic to cells, with >100% cell viability, indicating the excellent biocompatibility and safety of HP hydrogels *in vitro*.

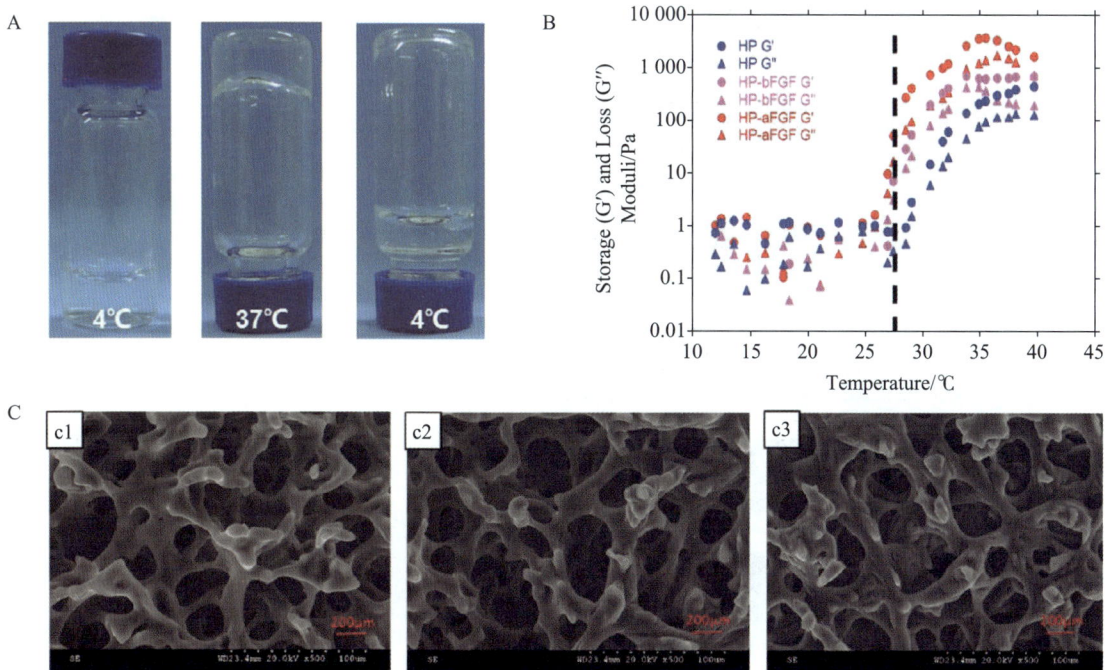

Fig. 1. (A) Temperature-sensitive characteristics of HP hydrogels at 4, 37, and 4℃. (B) Storage (G') and loss (G'') moduli of different HP-based gels as a function of temperature from 40 to 10℃. (C) SEM images of HP (c1), HP-aFGF (c2), and HP-bFGF (c3). Scale bars in c1−c3 are 200 μm.

3.2 HP-GFs accelerate wound closure in mice

To evaluate the effect of HP-GFs in the skin wound regeneration process, aFGF, bFGF, HP-aFGF, and HP-bFGF dressings were applied to the full-thickness cutaneous C57BL/6 mice model, in comparison to saline and HP dressings as controls. Fig. 2A shows the side-by-side comparison of different GF-treated wounds on days 7, 10, 14, and 17, respectively. Visual inspection of the wound closure in mice revealed that, unlike the negative control that exhibited almost no reduction in wound size during the whole treatment period (17 days), all of the other tested dressings displayed noticeable reductions in the wound sizes on days 14 and 17. Particularly, the wound closure was greatly enhanced with HP-bFGF and HP-aFGF dressings. Quantitatively, Fig. 2B presents the wound closure rate for each case, as sampled from at least six replicates of the wounds. Consistent with visual inspection of wound closure in Fig. 2A, HP-aFGF showed the highest wound closure rate at every time point and achieved a final wound closure rate of 96.1% ± 6.4% on day 17, as compared to the wound closure rate of the other dressings in decreasing order: HP-bFGF (91.3% ± 10.9%), bFGF (72.9% ± 11.8%), aFGF (68.8% ± 9.3%), HP (65.8 ± 13.6), and control (60.8 ± 18.4). More importantly, upon addition of aFGF or bFGF to HP, the healing efficiencies of both HP-aFGF and HP-bFGF were increased as compared to those of pure aFGF and bFGF in the absence of HP, and such an HP-enhanced wound healing effect became more pronounced in the case of HP-aFGF (Fig. 2C). It was also reported that aFGF alone is 10−100-fold less potent than bFGF in inducing wound related cell proliferation.[57] These data indicate that synergetic interactions between HP and aFGF offer the more efficient suturing effect at the wound site, thus promoting wound closure during the early stage of the wound-healing process.

3.3 HP-GFs improve granulation formation

Granulation tissue formation generally starts to appear at the wound site in 2−5 days after injury.[58] Fig. 3 shows the H&E staining of wound histology sections treated with HP, HP-aFGF, and HP-bFGF dressings. At day 7, no obvious neoepidermis was observed underneath the eschar of all groups. While the length of wound closure for all groups showed no significant difference, the thickness of the granulation was significantly different between all groups. Both control and HP groups had the thinnest granulation layers (Fig. 3A,B). HP-GFs (Fig. 3D,F) had far thicker and more

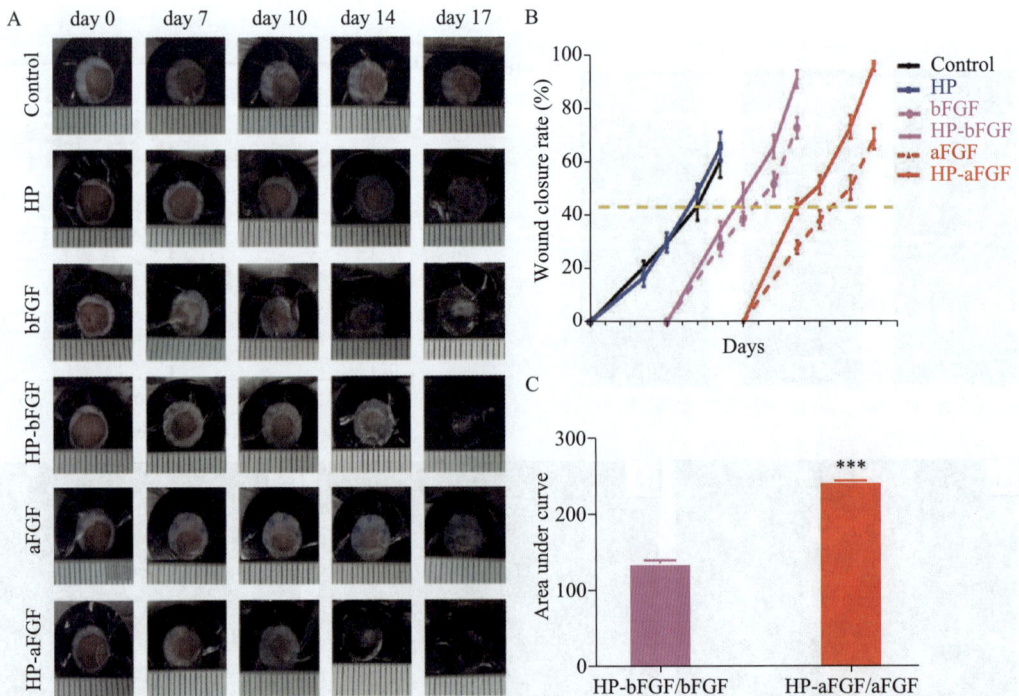

Fig. 2. HP-GFs accelerate wound closure. (A) Wound closure in C57BL/6 mice treated with normal saline, HP, bFGF, HP-bFGF, aFGF, and HP-aFGF at day 0, 7, 10, 14, and 17. Unit is mm. (B) Wound closure rates of control, free aFGF and bFGF, and HP-aFGF and HP-bFGF groups. (C) HP-induced wound closure increment as calculated by the difference between the area under curve of HP-aFGF and aFGF vs. HP-bFGF and bFGF. Bars indicate means ± SD; ***P < 0.001.

continuous layers of granulation across the entire wound gap than GFs alone (Fig. 3C,E), indicating that the incorporation of GFs into HP hydrogels improves the granulation formation. At day 17, neoepidermis formation was observed in all groups, though both HP and control groups still retained the larger unclosure areas at the wound site. The thickness of the neoepidermis followed the same order (from the thickest to the thinnest): HP-GFs groups (Fig. 3J,L) > GFs groups (Fig. 3I,K) > control groups (Fig. 3G,H). Consistently, the HP-aFGF group showed a thicker epidermis than the HP-bFGF group.

3.4 HP-GFs enhance collagen deposition

Collagen deposition is a critical factor to determine the strength and appearance of the scar that has formed.[59-61] Fig. 4 shows collagen deposition in the dermis of regenerated skin for all six groups at day 7 and 17 using Masson Trichrome Staining (MTS). At day 7, all six groups showed different amounts of *collagen deposition*, among which HP-GFs-treated wounds exhibited the highest collagen deposition (as indicated by the strongest blue staining intensity of regenerated collagens, Fig. 4D,F), while two control groups had the least collagen deposition (Fig. 4A,B). At day 17, difference in collagen deposition became even more pronounced. HP-aFGF-treated wounds had the most densely packed collagen fibers running in a parallel arrangement in all groups (Fig. 4L), while HP-bFGF-treated wounds took second place in collagen deposition with a similar parallel arrangement (Fig. 4J). Compared to HP-GFs groups, the other four groups appeared to have loosely packed collagen fibers running in irregular arrangements (Fig. 4G–I,K). Consistently, among six groups, the HP-GF dressings have promoted mature granulation tissue formation with dense collagen deposition, where HP-aFGF shows relatively higher uniform collagen alignment than HP-bFGF.

3.5 HP-GFs activate cytokeratin expression related to re-epithelialization

Furthermore, immunohistochemical staining of re-epithelialization related cytokeratin was performed to evaluate the re-epithelialization of wound regeneration. HP-aFGF (Fig. 5F,L) and HP-bFGF (Fig. 5D,J) groups exhibited faster re-epithelization than GFs (Fig. 5C,E,I,K) and control groups (Fig. 5A,G) on 7 and 17 days, as evidenced by the early

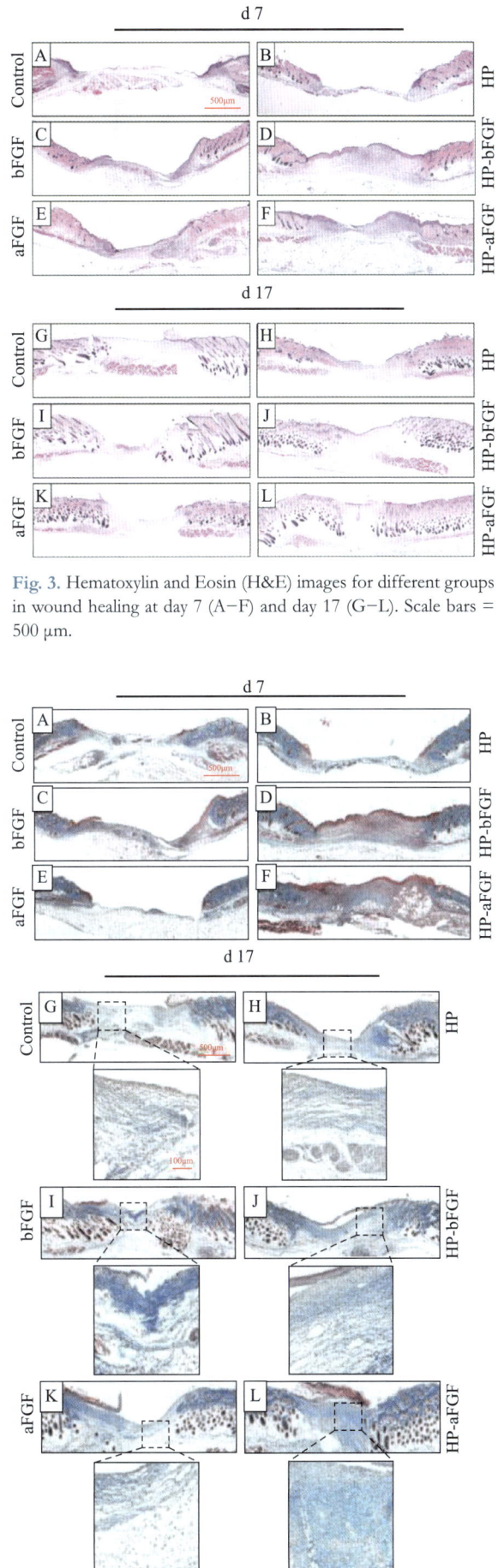

Fig. 3. Hematoxylin and Eosin (H&E) images for different groups in wound healing at day 7 (A–F) and day 17 (G–L). Scale bars = 500 μm.

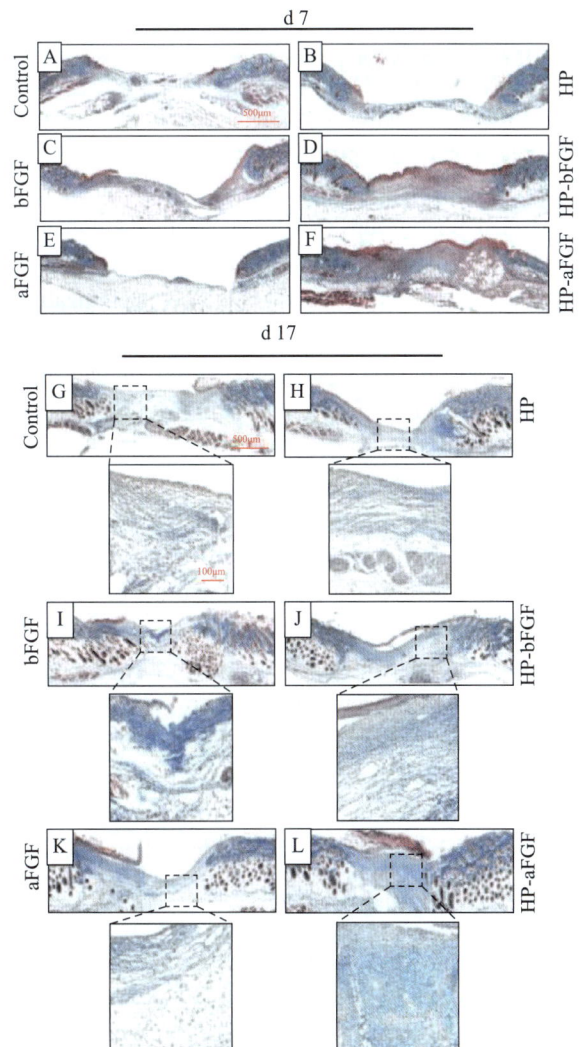

Fig. 4. Histochemical staining of collagens during postwounding at day 7 (A–F) and day 17 (G–L). Tissue sections are stained with Masson's trichrome (blue = collagen; red = cytoplasm and muscle fibers). The nucleus was counterstained with hematoxylin (violet). Rectangles refer to the close-up areas. Original scale bar = 500 μm, and close-up scale bar = 100 μm.

expression of more cytokeratin in the thicker epidermis. While both HP-GFs groups promoted the formation of skin appendages from day 7 to day 17, HP-aFGF-treated wounds exhibited a much higher number of skin appendages and thicker epithelial layers than HP-bFGF-treated wounds (Fig. 5J,L). Additionally, a close-up visualization also revealed the regeneration of hair follicles in the wounds treated with HP-GFs groups, demonstrating the fast healing effect of HP-GFs on the re-epithelization of wounds *in vivo*. On the other hand, GFs groups actually did not show large differences from control groups regarding the formation of epithelization and epidermis. Thus, the epithelization of wound incisions increased in the order of HP-aFGF and HP-bFGF > GFs > control. Taken together, both sustaining release of aFGF and bFGF are known to promote wound healing. When incorporating GFs into HP hydrogels, HP hydrogels not only retain and prolong the bioactivities of GFs but also offer a hydrated environment to greatly accelerate the wound healing process, as demonstrated by fast wound closure, earlier formation of granulation tissue, epithelization, thicker epidermis, and dense and uniform collagen deposition.

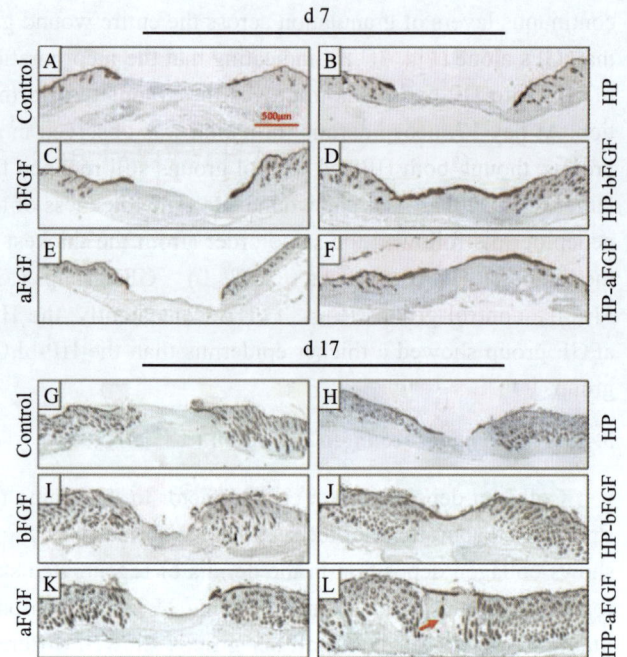

Fig. 5. Representative light microscopy images of wound center sections stained immunohistochemically for cytokeratin (IHC-Cytokeratin, a marker of epithelial cells) at day 7 (A–F) and day 17 (G–L). Arrows indicate newly formed dermal appendages and hair follicles within granulation tissues. Bar = 500 μm.

3.6 HP-GFs induce cell proliferative activities and collagen synthesis

In order to better understand wound healing mechanisms, here we mainly used immunohistochemistry of tissue sections to study the proliferative activities of cells by detecting the expression level of cell nuclear antigen (PCNA) as a biomarker. It can be seen that HP-GFs groups had up-regulated the more PCNA positive keratinocytes at the wound edge than other groups at day 7, indicating a higher cellular proliferation of HP-GFs (Fig. 6A, HP-aFGF, $P < 0.001$ and HP-bFGF, $P < 0.01$). Additionally, HP-GFs (HP-aFGF = 40.62 ± 4.91, HP-bFGF = 28.08 ± 5.34) always had the higher degree of PCNA expression in both re-epithelialization tongues and dermis than the corresponding GFs (aFGF = 14.75 ± 2.79, bFGF = 15.20 ± 4.30) (Fig. 6B), and this confirms that HP can indeed promote the level of PCNA. PCNA results are agreeable to H&E, MTS, and cytokeratin data above, explaining that the better wound healing efficiency of HP-GFs is stimulated and enhanced by the formation of a larger amount of collagen and ECM substrates secreted by the higher cellular proliferation.

Since collagen I and III play an important role in formation of new capillaries at wound sites,[62,63] further immunechemical staining of the newly formed extracellular matrix by collagen I and III was quantified and shown in Fig. 7. As expected, both collagen I and III expressions in all six groups retained the same trend as collagen deposition (Fig. 7B,D), as evidenced by a decreasing order of HP-aFGF (1139.5 ± 118.9 for collagen I, 155.1 ± 2.4 for collagen III) > HP-bFGF (881.0 ± 74.9 for collagen I, 125.2 ± 11.8 for collagen III) > bFGF (565.7 ± 109.8 for collagen I, 73.3 ± 6.7 for collagen III) > aFGF (550.2 ± 56.6 for collagen I, 66.6 ± 8.5 for collagen III) > HP (251.2 ± 119.6 for collagen I, 21.3 ± 5.2 for collagen III) and control (252.8 ± 67.5 for collagen I, 18.9 ± 3.4 for collagen III). The enhanced granulation formation as shown in H&E and MTS was mainly attributed to the collagen synthesis at the early stage of the wound regeneration process. These results reveal that the sustained release of GFs from HP hydrogels plays a continuous role in stimulating the protein expression of PCNA and collagen I/III at wound sites, which in turn promotes the formation of new provisional ECM for cell proliferation and cell migration.

3.7 HP-GFs boost angiogenesis

Proper wound healing requires angiogenesis of newly generated dermis. To evaluate neovascularization of the wounds, the newly formed vessels at both wound bed and edge were characterized by CD31 (cluster of differentiation 31) staining, a vascular endothelial cells marker on day 17,[64] from which the average vessel density is quantified in Fig. 8.

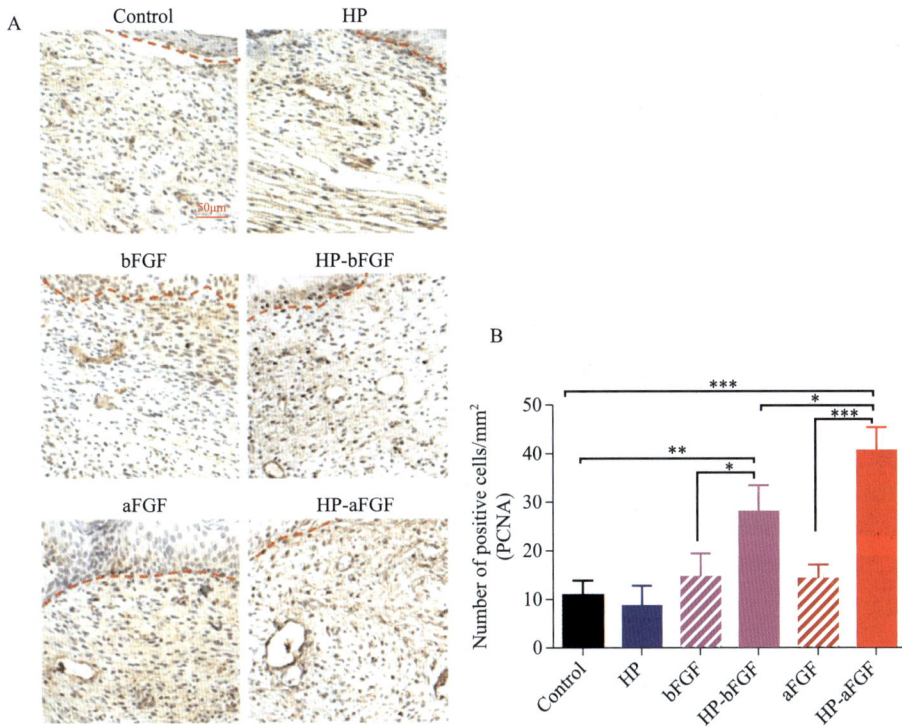

Fig. 6. (A) Representative images of PCNA immunohistochemistry staining on day 7 of postwounding in mice, showing enhanced cellular proliferation as evidenced by increased expression of PCNA. Red dotted lines are used to separate the epidermis and the dermis. Scale bar = 50 μm. (B) Quantitative analysis of relative density of PCNA at day 7 after surgery; $^{***}P < 0.001$; $^{**}P < 0.01$; $^{*}P < 0.05$; $n = 3$.

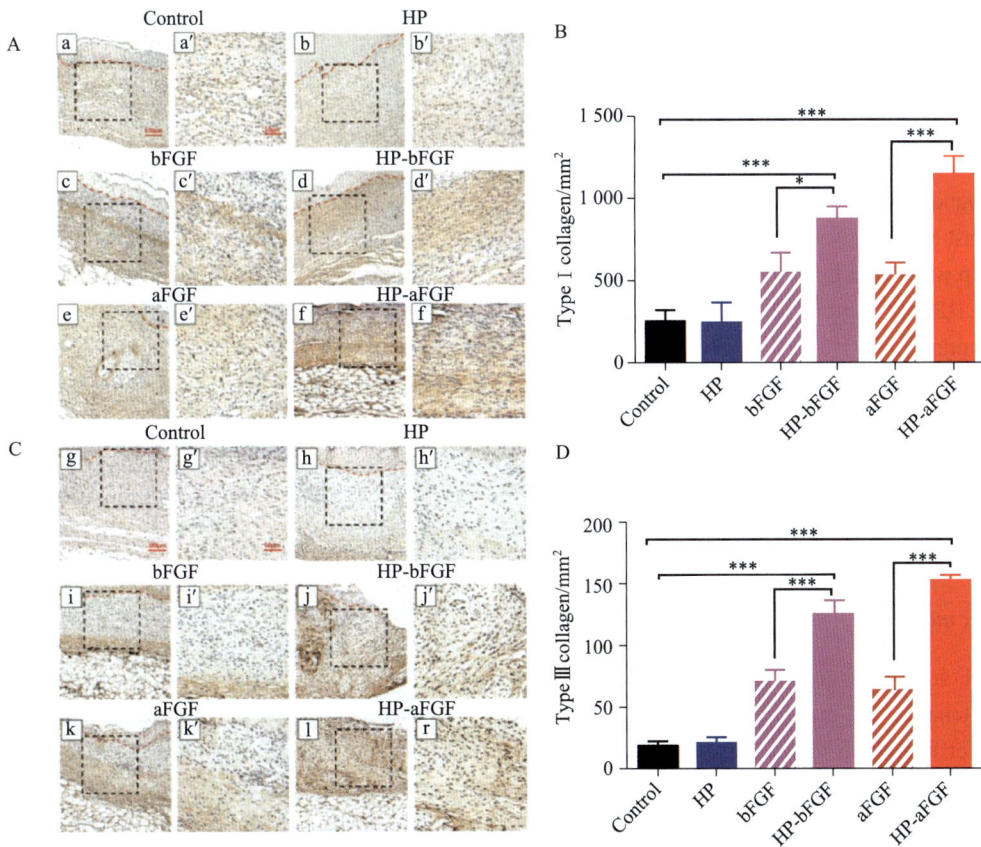

Fig. 7. Immunohistochemistry staining images for (A) collagen I and (C) collagen III on day 7 of postwounding in mice. Red dotted lines are used to separate the epidermis and the dermis. Scale bar = 100 μm; magnification scale bar = 50 μm. Quantitative analysis of relative density of (B) collagen I and (D) collagen III at day 7 after surgery. $^{***}P < 0.001$; $^{**}P < 0.01$; $^{*}P < 0.05$; $n = 3$.

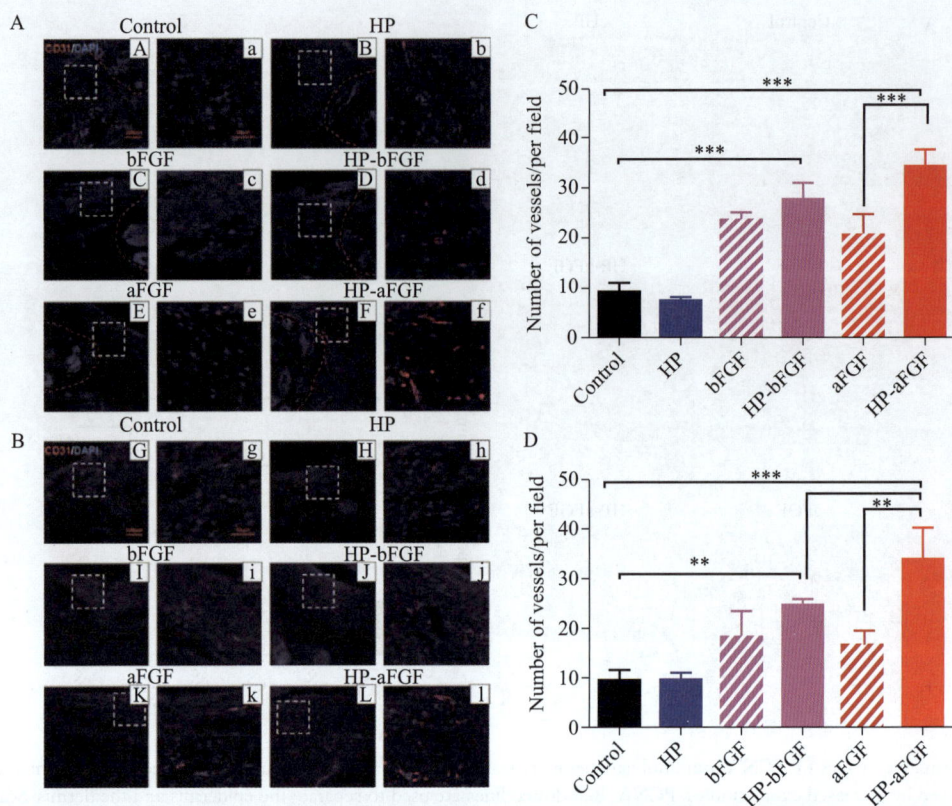

Fig. 8. New blood vessels stained with CD31 (red) and DAPI (blue) in (A) wound edge and (B) wound bed at day 17 postoperative. Scale bar = 100 μm; magnification scale bar = 50 μm. Quantitative analysis of number of vessels per field at day 17 after surgery in (C) wound edge and (D) wound bed. ***$P < 0.001$; **$P < 0.01$; *$P < 0.05$; $n = 3$.

Visual inspection of immunofluorescence of CD31 and DAPI on wound bed and wound edge (Fig. 8A,B) confirmed the large amount of newly formed vessels in HP-GFs groups (Fig. 8D,F,J,L), but only a little or no CD31 expression of vascular cells was found in the control (Fig. 8A,L), HP (Fig. 8B,H), and GFs groups, suggesting that HP-GFs boost angiogenesis and lead to a fast healing. Quantitatively, the average vessel density was quantified in Fig. 8C, and the vessel density of the HP-aFGF group was found to be the highest (36.7 ± 2.5 per field in wound edge, 34.3 ± 5.9 per field in wound bed), higher than that of the HP- bFGF group (26.3 ± 3.3 per field in wound edge, 24.7 ± 1.2 per field in wound bed), bFGF group (24.1 ± 1 per field in wound edge, 18.7 ± 4.7 per field in wound bed), and aFGF group (22.3 ± 3.5 per field in wound edge, 16.7 ± 2.2 per field in wound bed). Moreover, the vessel densities of both HP-GFs groups were always significantly higher than those other groups.

Both control and HP groups had almost undetectable CD31 at day 17. These results further confirm that incorporation of GFs into HP hydrogels has a large positive effect on vessel generation. Additionally, the HP-aFGF group was also found to have more active CD31 expression than HP-bFGF, demonstrating a better effect of HP-aFGF on neovascularization than HP-bFGF.

3.8 Mechanistic model of HP modifying aFGF versus bFGF

Both aFGF and bFGF are well-known important classes of growth factors, which act as a crucial extrinsic cue for stem cell maintenance and differentiation, possessing angiogenesis and neuroprotective properties. However, aFGF and bFGF also suffer from their low stability caused by enzymatic degradation that greatly limits their use in clinical applications. Since HP contains specific binding sites for FGF, which stabilizes this protein within the ECM, we developed the HP hydrogel to load and stabilize aFGF and bFGF and performed a series comparative study of their wound healing efficiency *in vivo*. Collective data have shown that GF-loaded HP hydrogels are extremely more effective than free GFs, due to the protection of the HP hydrogel matrix. More importantly, while both GF-loaded HP hydrogels can achieve fast wound closure, granulation tissue formation, collagen deposition, and re-epithelialization due to the higher PCNA expression with specific collagen synthesis and angiogenesis, it is interesting to observe an opposite trend in overall wound healing efficiency between free aFGF and bFGF hydrogel and between HP-aFGF and HP-bFGF hydrogels. In the absence of HP hydrogels, free aFGF has lower wound healing efficiency than free bFGF, but when incorporating a/bFGF into the HP hydrogels, HP-aFGF showed a higher wound healing efficiency than HP-bFGF. Such a sharp difference has not been studied before, so on the basis of our findings, we proposed a mechanistic model to interpret the wound healing differences between free FGFs and HP- loaded FGFs (Fig. 9).

Free aFGF and bFGF have very similar structures but different surface charge in physiological saline solution due to different isoelectric points (IPaFGF = 5.6 and IPbFGF = 9.6),[54] resulting in aFGF being negatively charged and bFGF being positively charged on the surface. HP itself is negatively charged due to the presence of heparin. Thus, it is clear that the loading of a/bFGF into HP hydrogels would change the interactions between a/bFGF and HP and the release rate of a/bFGF from HP. As illustrated in Fig. 9A, during the formation of HP-GF hydrogels in stage I, bFGF can bind stronger and easier to HP than aFGF due to favorable electrostatic interactions. However, such strong binding between bFGF and HP, in turn, causes difficulty in the release of bFGF from HP during the release stage II. Fig. 9B clearly shows a substantial difference in the release profiles from the two HP-GFs systems. While both HP-GFs hydrogels demonstrate a sustained release of a/bFGF for over 10 days, more aFGF (42.8%) is released from HP-aFGF than bFGF (24.3%) released from HP-bFGF, confirming that binding of different FGFs to heparin modulates their release from the heparin-containing hydrogels. To better understand the release behavior of GFs from HP hydrogels, we designed two different experiments to examine the degradation of HP hydrogels by either immersing whole hydrogels into bulk water or having the bottom face of the hydrogel in contact with water. Within 10 days, no obvious degradation was observed in both cases, but slight gel dissolution occurred at the hydrogel-water interface (Fig. S2). We should mention that the degradation of HP hydrogels is unlikely to occur at the wound interface, simply because the water content at the hydrogel-wound interface would be much less than that in the bulk water we tested. Thus, the release of GFs from HP hydrogels is mainly caused by a combined release behavior of GF diffusion and gel dissolution but not by HP degradation.

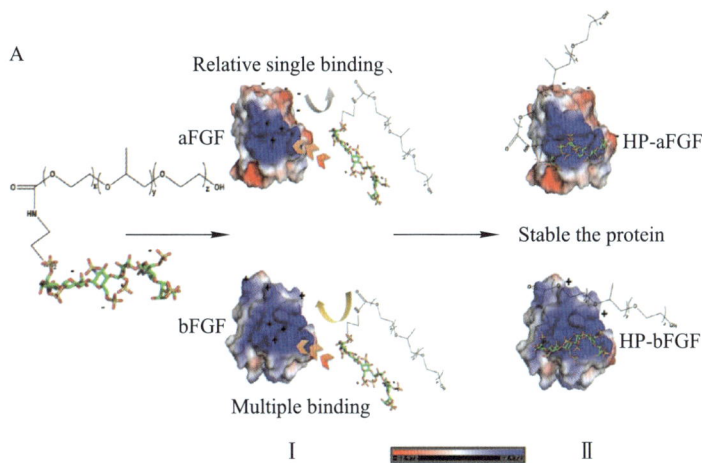

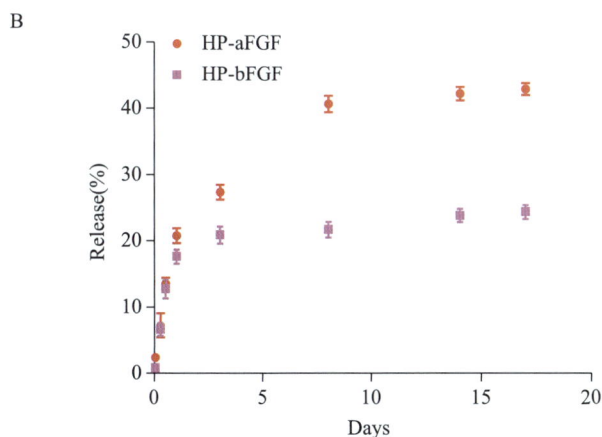

Fig. 9. (A) Scheme of different interactions between HP-aFGF and HP-bFGF. Positively charged bFGF binds stronger to negatively charged HP than negatively charged aFGF due to favorable electrostatic interactions caused by different PIs of aFGF and bFGF. (B) Release profiles of aFGF from HP-aFGF hydrogels and bFGF from HP-bFGF hydrogels.

Different a/bFGF surface properties in saline solution lead to different binding and release behaviors in HP hydrogels, which are attributed to different wound healing efficiencies.

4. Conclusions

In this work, HP-GF hydrogels were designed and synthesized to demonstrate their improved wound healing capacity *in vivo*. Upon incorporation of aFGF and bFGF into HP hydrogels, *in vivo* wound healing results showed that both HP-GF hydrogels accelerated the wound closure of full-thickness excisional wounds of mice with enhanced granulation tissue formation during initial stages of healing and stimulated angiogenesis and re-epithelization through the proliferation stage. Furthermore, both HP-GF hydrogels prompted expression of cell proliferation and collagen synthesis, all of which are beneficial for vascularization. Moreover, due to the different surface charge properties between aFGF and bFGF, positively charged bFGF had the stronger interactions with negatively charged HP than negatively charged aFGF, which makes bFGF difficult to be released from HP hydrogels leading to less wound healing efficiency. Such different interaction modes between aFGF-HP and bFGF-HP hydrogels influence not only the FGF binding and releasing behaviors but also FGF-induced wound healing effect. Irrespective of the mechanistic details, enhancement of wound healing by HP-GF-based materials is likely to be the combination of (i) a GF that can recognize and interact with specific GF receptors to stimulate wound healing, (ii) a biocompatible HP platform that provides solid supports to stabilize loaded proteins and facilitate GF binding, and (iii) a synergetic healing effect of GF-HP materials. While many studies have reported that FGFs stimulate angiogenesis and wound healing, this work reveals the possible structural-dependent interactions between different FGF and HP on wound healing effect, and hopefully, this information will be carefully considered for future development of heparin-based polymers with GFs for wound healing applications. In addition, other structural properties should also be considered for the future design of GFs for wound healing, including ionic property, surface charges, surface hydrophobicity, surface modification ratio, and cytokine activation/binding sites with GFs receptors upon modification. Hopefully, this work will lead to the structural-based design for new GF-based materials for wound healing.

Supporting information

Supporting information to this article can be found on the ACS publications website (doi:10.1021/acsami.6b06047).

References

[1] Franz MG, Robson MC, Steed DL, *et al.* Guidelines to aid healing of acute wounds by decreasing impediments of healing[J]. Wound Repair And Regeneration, 2008, 16(6): 723-748.

[2] Sarhan WA, Azzazy HME, El-Sherbiny IM. Honey/Chitosan Nanofiber Wound Dressing Enriched with Allium sativum and Cleome droserifolia: Enhanced Antimicrobial and Wound Healing Activity[J]. Acs Applied Materials & Interfaces, 2016, 8(10): 6379-6390.

[3] Gurtner GC, Werner S, Barrandon Y, *et al.* Wound repair and regeneration[J]. Nature, 2008, 453(7193): 314-321.

[4] Sun L, Huang Y, Bian Z, *et al.* Sundew-Inspired Adhesive Hydrogels Combined with Adipose-Derived Stem Cells for Wound Healing[J]. Acs Applied Materials & Interfaces, 2016, 8(3): 2423-2434.

[5] Fonder MA, Lazarus GS, Cowan DA, *et al.* Treating the chronic wound: A practical approach to the care of nonhealing wounds and wound care dressings[J]. Journal Of the American Academy Of Dermatology, 2008, 58(2): 185-206.

[6] Barrientos S, Stojadinovic O, Golinko MS, *et al.* Growth factors and cytokines in wound healing[J]. Wound Repair And Regeneration, 2008, 16(5): 585-601.

[7] Guan J, Stankus JJ, Wagner WR. Biodegradable elastomeric scaffolds with basic fibroblast growth factor release[J]. Journal Of Controlled Release, 2007, 120(1-2): 70-78.

[8] Hajimiri M, Shahverdi S, Esfandiari MA, *et al.* Preparation of hydrogel embedded polymer-growth factor conjugated nanoparticles as a diabetic wound dressing[J]. Drug Development And Industrial Pharmacy, 2016, 42(5): 707-719.

[9] Yu H, Peng J, Xu Y, *et al.* Bioglass Activated skin tissue engineering constructs for wound healing[J]. Acs Applied Materials & Interfaces, 2016, 8(1): 703-715.

[10] Johnson NR, Wang Y. Coacervate delivery of HB-EGF accelerates healing of type 2 diabetic wounds[J]. Wound Repair And Regeneration, 2015, 23(4): 591-600.

[11] Fujita M, Ishihara M, Simizu M, *et al.* Vascularization *in vivo* caused by the controlled release of fibroblast growth factor-2 from an injectable chitosan/non-anticoagulant heparin hydrogel[J]. Biomaterials, 2004, 25(4): 699-706.

[12] Kalaji N, Deloge A, Sheibat-Othman N, *et al.* Controlled release carriers of growth factors FGF-2 and TGF beta 1: Synthesis, characterization and kinetic modelling[J]. Journal Of Biomedical Nanotechnology, 2010, 6(2): 106-116.

[13] Baum CL, Arpey CJ. Normal cutaneous wound healing: Clinical correlation with cellular and molecular events[J]. Dermatologic Surgery, 2005, 31(6): 674-686.

[14] Goldman R. Growth factors and chronic wound healing: past, present, and future[J]. Advances in skin & wound care, 2004, 17(1): 24-35.

[15] Singer AJ, Clark RAF. Mechanisms of disease - Cutaneous wound healing[J]. New England Journal Of Medicine, 1999, 341(10): 738-746.

[16] Behm B, Babilas P, Landthaler M, et al. Cytokines, chemokines and growth factors in wound healing[J]. Journal Of the European Academy Of Dermatology And Venereology, 2012, 26(7): 812-820.

[17] Awada HK, Johnson NR, Wang Y. Dual delivery of vascular endothelial growth factor and hepatocyte growth factor coacervate displays strong angiogenic effects[J]. Macromolecular Bioscience, 2014, 14(5): 679-686.

[18] Wilgus TA. Immune cells in the healing skin wound: Influential players at each stage of repair[J]. Pharmacological Research, 2008, 58(2): 112-116.

[19] Schreml S, Szeimies RM, Prantl L, et al. Wound healing in the 21st century[J]. Journal Of the American Academy Of Dermatology, 2010, 63(5): 866-881.

[20] Gong C, Qi T, Wei X, et al. Thermosensitive polymeric hydrogels as drug delivery systems[J]. Current Medicinal Chemistry, 2013, 20(1): 79-94.

[21] Wang F, Li Z, Khan M, et al. Injectable, rapid gelling and highly flexible hydrogel composites as growth factor and cell carriers[J]. Acta Biomaterialia, 2010, 6(6): 1978-1991.

[22] Vermonden T, Censi R, Hennink WE. Hydrogels for Protein Delivery[J]. Chemical Reviews, 2012, 112(5): 2853-2888.

[23] Xie Z, Aphale NV, Kadapure TD, et al. Design of antimicrobial peptides conjugated biodegradable citric acid derived hydrogels for wound healing[J]. Journal Of Biomedical Materials Research Part A, 2015, 103(12): 3907-3918.

[24] Jeffords ME, Wu J, Shah M, et al. Tailoring material properties of cardiac matrix hydrogels to induce endothelial differentiation of human mesenchymal stem cells[J]. Acs Applied Materials & Interfaces, 2015, 7(20): 11053-11061.

[25] Gong C, Wu Q, Wang Y, et al. A biodegradable hydrogel system containing curcumin encapsulated in micelles for cutaneous wound healing[J]. Biomaterials, 2013, 34(27): 6377-6387.

[26] Shin K, Lee S, Song W-Y, et al. Genetic Identification of ACC-resistant2 reveals involvement of lysine histidine transporter1 in the uptake of 1-aminocyclopropane-1-carboxylic acid in arabidopsis thaliana[J]. Plant And Cell Physiology, 2015, 56(3): 572-582.

[27] Brandl F, Hammer N, Blunk T, et al. Biodegradable hydrogels for time-controlled release of tethered peptides or proteins[J]. Biomacromolecules, 2010, 11(2): 496-504.

[28] Yamamoto M, Ikada Y, Tabata Y. Controlled release of growth factors based on biodegradation of gelatin hydrogel[J]. Journal Of Biomaterials Science-Polymer Edition, 2001, 12(1): 77-88.

[29] Meyvis T, De Smedt S, Stubbe B, et al. On the release of proteins from degrading dextran methacrylate hydrogels and the correlation with the rheologic properties of the hydrogels[J]. Pharmaceutical Research, 2001, 18(11): 1593-1599.

[30] Liang Y, Kiick KL. Heparin-functionalized polymeric biomaterials in tissue engineering and drug delivery applications[J]. Acta Biomaterialia, 2014, 10(4): 1588-1600.

[31] Kharkar PM, Kiick KL, Kloxin AM. Designing degradable hydrogels for orthogonal control of cell microenvironments[J]. Chemical Society Reviews, 2013, 42(17): 7335-7372.

[32] Xu X, Jha AK, Duncan RL, et al. Heparin-decorated, hyaluronic acid-based hydrogel particles for the controlled release of bone morphogenetic protein 2[J]. Acta Biomaterialia, 2011, 7(8): 3050-3059.

[33] Rabenstein DL. Heparin and heparan sulfate: structure and

[34] function[J]. Natural Product Reports, 2002, 19(3): 312-331.

[34] Burgess WH, Maciag T. The heparin-binding (fibroblast) growth-factor family of proteins[J]. Annual Review Of Biochemistry, 1989, 58: 575-606.

[35] Klagsbrun M. The affinity of fibroblast growth factors (FGFs) for heparin; FGF-heparan sulfate interactions in cells and extracellular matrix[J]. Current Opinion In Cell Biology, 1990, 2(5): 857-863.

[36] Gospodarowicz D, Cheng J. Heparin protects basic and acidic FGF from inactivation[J]. Journal Of Cellular Physiology, 1986, 128(3): 475-484.

[37] Tian J-L, Zhao Y-Z, Jin Z, et al. Synthesis and characterization of Poloxamer 188-grafted heparin copolymer[J]. Drug Development And Industrial Pharmacy, 2010, 36(7): 832-838.

[38] Rapraeger AC, Krufka A, Olwin BB. Requirement of heparan-sulfate for bfgf-mediated fibroblast growth and myoblast differentiation[J]. Science, 1991, 252(5013): 1705-1708.

[39] Chu H, Johnson NR, Mason NS, et al. A polycation:heparin complex releases growth factors with enhanced bioactivity[J]. Journal Of Controlled Release, 2011, 150(2): 157-163.

[40] Zieris A, Chwalek K, Prokoph S, et al. Dual independent delivery of pro-angiogenic growth factors from starPEG-heparin hydrogels[J]. Journal Of Controlled Release, 2011, 156(1): 28-36.

[41] Zieris A, Prokoph S, Levental KR, et al. FGF-2 and VEGF functionalization of starPEG-heparin hydrogels to modulate biomolecular and physical cues of angiogenesis[J]. Biomaterials, 2010, 31(31): 7985-7994.

[42] Choi JS, Yoo HS. Chitosan/pluronic hydrogel containing bFGF/heparin for encapsulation of human dermal fibroblasts[J]. Journal Of Biomaterials Science-Polymer Edition, 2013, 24(2): 210-223.

[43] Ishihara M, Obara K, Ishizuka T, et al. Controlled release of fibroblast growth factors and heparin from photocrosslinked chitosan hydrogels and subsequent effect on in vivo vascularization[J]. Journal Of Biomedical Materials Research Part A, 2003, 64A(3): 551-559.

[44] Jeon O, Powell C, Solorio LD, et al. Affinity-based growth factor delivery using biodegradable, photocrosslinked heparin-alginate hydrogels[J]. Journal Of Controlled Release, 2011, 154(3): 258-266.

[45] Zhao YZ, Lv HF, Lu CT, et al. Evaluation of a novel thermosensitive heparin-poloxamer hydrogel for improving vascular anastomosis quality and safety in a rabbit model[J]. Plos One, 2013, 8(8).

[46] Zhao YZ, Jiang X, Xiao J, et al. Using NGF heparin-poloxamer thermosensitive hydrogels to enhance the nerve regeneration for spinal cord injury[J]. Acta Biomaterialia, 2016, 29: 71-80.

[47] Chu H, Chen CW, Huard J, et al. The effect of a heparin-based coacervate of fibroblast growth factor-2 on scarring in the infarcted myocardium[J]. Biomaterials, 2013, 34(6): 1747-1756.

[48] Johnson NR, Wang Y. Controlled delivery of heparin-binding EGF-like growth factor yields fast and comprehensive wound healing[J]. Journal Of Controlled Release, 2013, 166(2): 124-129.

[49] Chu H, Gao J, Chen CW, et al. Injectable fibroblast growth factor-2 coacervate for persistent angiogenesis[J]. Proceedings Of the National Academy Of Sciences Of the United States Of America, 2011, 108(33): 13444-13449.

[50] Dephillips P, Lenhoff AM. Relative retention of the fibroblast growth factors FGF-1 and FGF-2 on strong cation-exchange sorbents[J]. Journal Of Chromatography A, 2004, 1036(1): 51-60.

[51] Chen CH, Poucher SM, Lu J, et al. Fibroblast growth factor 2: From laboratory evidence to clinical application[J]. Current Vascular Pharmacology, 2004, 2(1): 33-43.

[52] Dephillips P, Lenhoff AM. Relative retention of the fibroblast growth factors FGF-1 and FGF-2 on strong cation-exchange sorbents[J]. Journal Of Chromatography A, 2004, 1036(1): 51-60.

[53] Karey KP, Sirbasku DA. Glutaraldehyde fixation increases retention of low-molecular weight proteins (growth-factors) transferred to nylon membranes for western blot analysis[J]. Analytical Bio-

chemistry, 1989, 178(2): 255-259.

[54] Klagsbrun M, Shing Y. Heparin affinity of anionic and cationic capillary endothelial cell-growth factors - analysis of hypothalamus-derived growth-factors and fibroblast growth-factors[J]. Proceedings Of the National Academy Of Sciences Of the United States Of America, 1985, 82(3): 805-809.

[55] Chung TW, Yang J, Akaike T, et al. Preparation of alginate/galactosylated chitosan scaffold for hepatocyte attachment[J]. Biomaterials, 2002, 23(14): 2827-2834.

[56] Yong CS, Choi JS, Quan QZ, et al. Effect of sodium chloride on the gelation temperature, gel strength and bioadhesive force of poloxamer gels containing diclofenac sodium[J]. International Journal Of Pharmaceutics, 2001, 226(1-2): 195-205.

[57] Albert C. Gene expression in the central nervous system[J]. Elsevier: New York, 1995, 105.

[58] Yu H, Peng J, Xu Y, et al. Bioglass activated skin tissue engineering constructs for wound healing[J]. Acs Applied Materials & Interfaces, 2016, 8(1): 703-715.

[59] Leivonen SK, Hakkinen L, Liu D, et al. Smad3 and extracellular signal-regulated kinase 1/2 coordinately mediate transforming growth factor-beta-induced expression of connective tissue growth factor in human fibroblasts[J]. Journal Of Investigative Dermatology, 2005, 124(6): 1162-1169.

[60] Brem H, Kodra A, Golinko MS, et al. Mechanism of sustained release of vascular endothelial growth factor in accelerating experimental diabetic healing[J]. Journal Of Investigative Dermatology, 2009, 129(9): 2275-2287.

[61] Werner S, Krieg T, Smola H. Keratinocyte-fibroblast interactions in wound healing[J]. Journal Of Investigative Dermatology, 2007, 127(5): 998-1008.

[62] Clark RAF. Basics of cutaneous wound repair[J]. Journal Of Dermatologic Surgery And Oncology, 1993, 19(8): 693-706.

[63] Merkel JR, Dipaolo BR, Hallock GG, et al. Type-I and type-III collagen content of healing wounds in fetal and adult-rats[J]. Proceedings Of the Society for Experimental Biology And Medicine, 1988, 187(4): 493-497.

[64] Sun G, Zhang X, Shen YI, et al. Dextran hydrogel scaffolds enhance angiogenic responses and promote complete skin regeneration during burn wound healing[J]. Proceedings Of the National Academy Of Sciences Of the United States Of America, 2011, 108(52): 20976-20981.

Fibroblast growth factor-21 restores insulin sensitivity but induces aberrant bone microstructure in obese insulin-resistant rats

Narattaphol Charoenphandhu, Xiaokun Li, Siriporn Chattipakorn

1. Introduction

As a major cause of metabolic disturbance with high global prevalence, long-term consumption of a high-fat diet (HF) is detrimental to the body, leading to obesity, insulin resistance, and metabolic disease. Besides insulin, other endocrine factors such as adipokines and certain members of fibroblast growth factor (FGF), play a role in protecting against abnormal fat metabolism. FGF-21 in particular could be a major anti-diabetic agent since it potently enhances adipocyte glucose uptake, decreases circulating glucose and triglyceride levels, and improves insulin sensitivity in obese and diabetic animals [1, 2]. Since mesenchymal stem cells, osteoblast precursor cells, and osteoblasts themselves also abundantly express several subtypes of FGF receptors (FGFRs), e.g., FGFR1 and FGFR2, it is possible that systemic FGF-21 is capable of altering bone microstructure, bone mineral density (BMD), and bone mechanical properties in rodents.

Most members of the FGF family exert their functions locally because they have a strong interaction with extracellular matrix. On the other hand, FGF21 is generally recognized as a member of the endocrine family of FGF as it lacks the heparin-binding domain, which is required for binding most FGFs to the extracellular matrix of their target tissue [3, 4]. Several tissues, such as liver, pancreas, and adipose tissue itself, are the most important sources of circulating FGF21 in rodents [5–7]. After being released into the circulation, FGF21 binds to certain subtypes of FGFRs, especially FGFR1 and FGFR2, together with a co-receptor called β-klotho before activating various intracellular signaling pathways, e.g., ERK1/2, AMPK, and peroxisome proliferator-activated receptor (PPAR)-γ [8]. At the systemic level, FGF21 is considered a starvation hormone that increases energy expenditure and fat utilization [8].

High circulating levels of FGF-21 induced by high-dose injections (1 mg/kg/day) or gain-of-function mutation have previously been shown to induce bone loss and skeletal fragility [9]. FGF-21 has also been reported to strongly induce the sumoylation of PPAR-γ, thereby prolonging the action of this transcription factor which is known to modulate not only the function of adipocytes but also osteoblasts and osteoclasts causing bone loss and fracture through inhibition of osteoblast function [10]. Hence, FGF-21-induced bone loss could be due to its activation of PPAR-γ. Interestingly, bone is a dynamic tissue and long bone was found to be slightly more resistant to fracture with increased body weight. Therefore, it was unclear whether obese rats treated with FGF-21 as part of early treatment for insulin resistance or diabetes might, on the other hand, exhibit bone loss with impaired bone mechanical properties.

In the present study, obesity with insulin resistance was induced by treating rats with HF, as reported previously [11, 12]. FGF-21 was administered to demonstrate whether FGF-21 could restore metabolic parameters in obese insulin-resistant rats. The principal objective of this study was to evaluate bone mechanical property and bone microstructure in HF-fed rats treated with low-dose FGF-21 (0.1 mg/ kg/day), which appeared to effectively alleviate insulin resistance.

2. Materials and methods

2.1 Animals

Six-week old male Wistar rats were obtained from the National Laboratory Animal Center, Mahidol University, Thailand. Rats were individually housed in a temperature and humidity-controlled room with a 12 h light/12 h dark cycle. This study was approved by the Institutional Animal Care and Use Committee, Faculty of Medicine, Chiang Mai University, Thailand.

2.2 Experimental design

Rats were randomly divided into 3 groups ($n = 4$–6/ group)—vehicle (normal saline)-treated normal diet (ND)-fed rats, vehicle-treated HF-fed rats, and FGF-21-treated HF-fed rats. The ND and HF contained 19.77 and 59.28% energy from fat, respectively. The rats were fed ND or HF for 12 weeks prior to FGF-21 administration. Recombinant FGF-21 (kindly provided by School of Pharmaceutical Sciences, Wenzhou Medical University, Wenzhou, Zhejiang, China) was injected subcutaneously (s.c.) once daily at 0.1 mg/kg of body weight for 4 weeks. Body weight and food intake were recorded weekly throughout the experiment. After 16 weeks of HF and/or FGF-21 treatments, all the rats were killed by isoflurane, and bone, visceral fat, and plasma samples were collected. Bone specimens were evaluated for microstructural defect and mechanical properties, while plasma samples were used to determine levels of glucose, cholesterol, triglyceride, insulin, homeostatic model assessment (HOMA; an index of insulin resistance), and the area under the curve of plasma glucose (AUCg). Serum levels of FGF-21 were determined using a commercial enzyme immunoassay kit (MF 2100; R&D Systems, Minneapolis, MN, USA). The experimental protocol is depicted in Fig. 1A.

2.3 Analysis of bone mechanical properties using the 3-point bending test

The right tibiae were dissected, cleaned of adhering tissue, and kept moist until analysis using 3-point bending apparatus (model 5943; Instron, Norwood, MA, USA). After measuring the anteroposterior midshaft diameter of the tibiae, each tibia was placed with anterior part facing down on two rounded supporting bars with a distance of 18 mm. A preload of 2 N was applied at the midshaft with a dis- placement rate of 2 mm/min until failure. From the force-

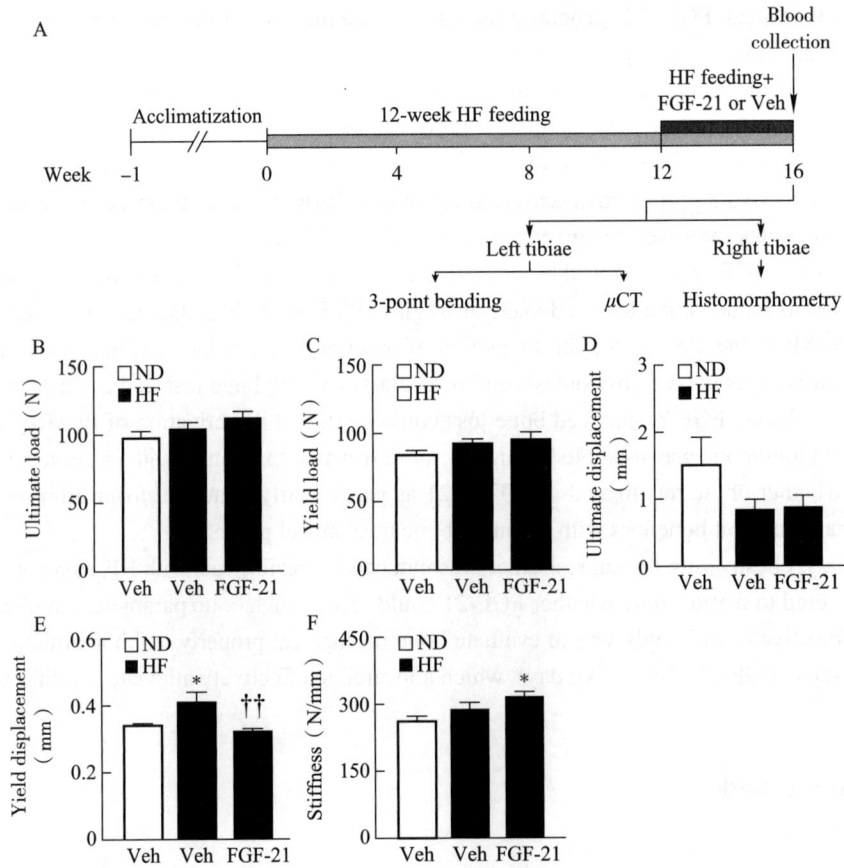

Fig. 1. (A) Timeline of the present experiment. (B–F) Mechanical properties of tibial midshaft in rats fed high-fat diet (HF) or normal diet (ND). Twelve rats were fed HF for 12 weeks prior to 4-week FGF-21 administration (0.1 mg/kg body weight, s.c.) or vehicle (Veh). Total duration for ND or HF treatment was 16 weeks. Values are mean ± standard error ($n = 4$–6 per group). $^{*}P < 0.05$ compared with vehicle-treated ND rats; $^{\dagger\dagger}P < 0.01$ compared with vehicle-treated HF rats.

displacement curve, the mechanical parameters were determined using Bluehill 3 software. The measured parameters included ultimate load, yield load, ultimate displacement, yield displacement, and stiffness.

2.4　Analysis of bone microstructure using microcomputed tomography (μCT)

The right tibiae were dissected and wrapped in moist gauze to prevent tissue drying during scanning, and placed in a horizontal position on a polystyrene supporter. Images were acquired by a μCT (model Skyscan 1178; Bruker MicroCT, Kontich, Belgium) at 65 kV, 615 μA with rotation angle of 0.54°, and voxel resolution of 85 μm. There-after, images were reconstructed by NRecon software (version 1.6.4.8) with a ring artifact and hardening correction of 10% and 30%, respectively. CTAn software (version 1.14.4) was used to analyze volumetric BMD (vBMD) and cortical microstruc-ture. Trabecular vBMD and cortical vBMD were analyzed at 1.360–5.610 and 14.110–18.360 mm, respectively, distal to the proximal growth plate. Microstructural indices of cortex included cortical thickness (mm), cortical area (mm^2), periosteal perimeter (mm), endosteal perimeter (mm), moment of inertia (MMI; mm^4) in x- and y-axes, and polar MMI.

2.5　Bone histomorphometric analysis of bone trabecular structure

The proximal part of each left tibia (approximately 1.5 mm long) was cleaned of connective tissue, dehydrated in graded ethanol (i.e., 70%, 95% and absolute ethanol for 3, 3 and 2 days, respectively), and embedded in methyl meth-acrylate resin. As described previously [13], embedded bone samples were sliced to obtain frontal sections of 7 μm thick-ness using a semi-automated rotary microtome (model RM2255; Leica, Nussloch, Germany). Each section was mounted on a standard microscopic slide. After drying, bone sections were stained with Goldner's trichrome. Microstructural analyses of cancellous bone were obtained under a light microscope (model eclipse NiU; Nikon) using the OsteoMea-sure system version 4.10 (OsteoMetrics, Atlanta, GA, USA). Trabecular microstructure was analyzed at a location 1 mm distal to the epiphyseal plate (i.e., secondary spongiosa). Microstructural parameters included trabecular bone volume normalized by tissue volume (also known as bone volume fraction, %), trabecular thickness (μm), trabecular separation (μm), trabecular number (mm^{-1}), osteoblast surface normalized by bone surface (%), osteoclast surface (%), and adipo-cyte number normalized by tissue area (mm^{-2}).

2.6　Biochemical analyses of blood compositions and HOMA index

Plasma glucose and cholesterol levels were determined by colorimetric assay (Biotech, Bangkok, Thailand). Plasma insulin levels were determined using a sandwich ELISA kit (Linco Research, St. Charles, MO, USA). Peripheral insulin resistance was assessed using HOMA, as described in previous studies [14, 15].

2.7　Oral glucose tolerance test (OGTT) and AUCg

OGTT was performed as described previously [16]. Briefly, rats were starved overnight before the test and received 2 g/kg body weight of glucose solution *via* oral gavage. Blood samples were collected from the tail vein at 0, 15, 30, 60, 90 and 120 min after glucose administration. AUCg was then calculated to evaluate glucose tolerance.

2.8　Statistical analysis

Two groups of data were analyzed by unpaired Student's t test, while multiple groups of data were compared by oneway analysis of variance (ANOVA). All statistical tests were performed by GraphPad Prism 6 for Mac OS X. The level of significance was $P < 0.05$.

3.　Results

The effects of FGF-21 on body weight, visceral fat, and biochemical parameters in plasma are shown in Table 1. The vehicle-treated HF-fed rats had a significantly increased body weight, visceral fat, plasma cholesterol level, plasma insulin level, and HOMA index compared to the vehicle-treated ND-fed rats ($P < 0.05$). FGF-21 significantly decreased plasma cholesterol level, plasma insulin level and HOMA index in HF-fed rats ($P < 0.05$). Regarding the glucose toler-ance test, the AUCg of the vehicle-treated HF group was significantly greater than that of the vehicle-treated ND group (Table 1). The administration of FGF-21 also decreased the AUCg in HF-fed rats ($P < 0.05$). Meanwhile, HF also elevated the plasma FGF-21 levels by ~2.5-fold, suggesting the presence of FGF-21 resistance in obese rats, whereas exogenous FGF- 21 administration markedly increased FGF-21 levels by approximately eight-fold (Table 1).

Table 1. Effects of high-fat diet and FGF-21 administration on the body weight, visceral fat, food intake, metabolic parameters, and plasma FGF-21 levels

Parameters	NDV	HFV	HFF
Body weight (kg)	500.83 ± 9.17	$640.00 \pm 18.44^*$	$570.00 \pm 30.87^{*\dagger}$
Visceral fat (g)	23.79 ± 1.71	$61.68 \pm 3.65^*$	$51.62 \pm 1.95^{*\dagger}$
Food intake (g/day)	20.88 ± 0.76	22.54 ± 1.00	20.30 ± 1.47
Plasma glucose (mg/dl)	128.62 ± 1.65	130.49 ± 6.54	130.35 ± 3.87
Cholesterol (mg/dl)	79.31 ± 4.18	$112.23 \pm 4.32^*$	$88.47 \pm 3.59^{\dagger}$
Triglyceride (mg/dl)	55.53 ± 3.92	55.68 ± 1.95	56.02 ± 2.20
Insulin (ng/ml)	2.65 ± 0.20	$4.43 \pm 0.46^*$	$2.80 \pm 0.29^{\dagger}$
HOMA index	17.50 ± 1.49	$32.47 \pm 5.23^*$	$17.32 \pm 1.77^{\dagger}$
AUCg (mg/dl × min × 10^4)	5.20 ± 0.33	$6.89 \pm 0.68^*$	$5.38 \pm 0.32^{\dagger}$
Plasma FGF-21 (pg/ml)	96.73 ± 27.95	$244.00 \pm 52.41^*$	$743.09 \pm 117.99^{*\dagger}$

Values are mean ± standard error, n=6/group. Rats were treated with normal diet (ND) or high-fat diet (HF) for 16 weeks. At week 13, HF rats were injected s.c. with FGF-21 (HFF) or vehicle (HFV) for 4 weeks. Vehicle-treated ND rats (NDV).

HOMA homeostatic model assessment for insulin resistance, AUCg area under the curve of plasma glucose *P < 0.05 compared with vehicle-treated ND rats, $^{\dagger}P$ < 0.05 compared with vehicle-treated HF rats.

The 3-point bending test revealed that tibiae of HF rats increased the yield displacement, which was used as an indicator of ability to be deformed without losing toughness (Fig. 1; values are presented in Supplemental Table S1). Other mechanical properties, i.e., ultimate load, yield load, ultimate displacement, and stiffness, were not altered by HF treatment (Fig. 1). In addition, 16-week HF treatment did not alter vBMD, cortical thickness, cortical bone area, periosteal perimeter, endosteal perimeter, or moment of inertia (Fig. 2).

However, FGF-21 attenuated the HF-associated increase in yield displacement (Fig. 1E), and increased bone stiffness compared to ND-fed rats (Fig. 1F). Although μCT analysis of tibiae from FGF-21-treated HF-fed rats (Fig. 2) did not show changes in cortical parameters compared to vehicle-treated HF-fed rats, trabecular vBMD was significantly lower in the FGF-21-treated HF-fed rats than vehicle-treated HF-fed rats (Fig. 2A). Mineralized tissues (green color in Goldner's trichrome-stained section; Fig. 3A) were apparently diminished after FGF-21 treatment, while marrow fats (white spots in bone marrow, as indicated by arrow heads; Fig. 3A) were conspicuously increased, consistent with the hypothesis that FGF-21 can direct mesenchymal stem cells toward adipocytes rather than osteoblasts [8]. Further bone histomorpho metric study thus demonstrated that HF-fed rats treated with FGF-21 had less trabecular bone volume, trabecular thickness, and osteoblast surface with no changes in trabecular separation, trabecular number, or osteoclast surface when compared with those treated with vehicle (Figs. 3B–E, 4A, B). Adipocyte number was also greater in FGF-21-treated HF rats than vehicle-treated HF rats (Fig. 4C).

4. Discussion

Long-term HF consumption is detrimental to body metabolism, leading to visceral fat accumulation, dyslipidemia, and insulin resistance [16, 17]. FGF-21 administration has been proposed as an efficient therapeutic approach to correct these metabolic disorders, especially at their early stages, e.g., insulin resistance with euglycemia and prediabetes [1, 18]. In the present study, FGF-21 clearly mitigated metabolic disturbance in HF-fed rats by reducing body weight, visceral fat, blood cholesterol, and insulin resistance compared to control HF-fed rats. Furthermore, we elaborated that a relatively low dose of FGF-21 (i.e., 0.1 mg/kg/day), which appeared to effectively alleviate insulin resistance, could eventu-

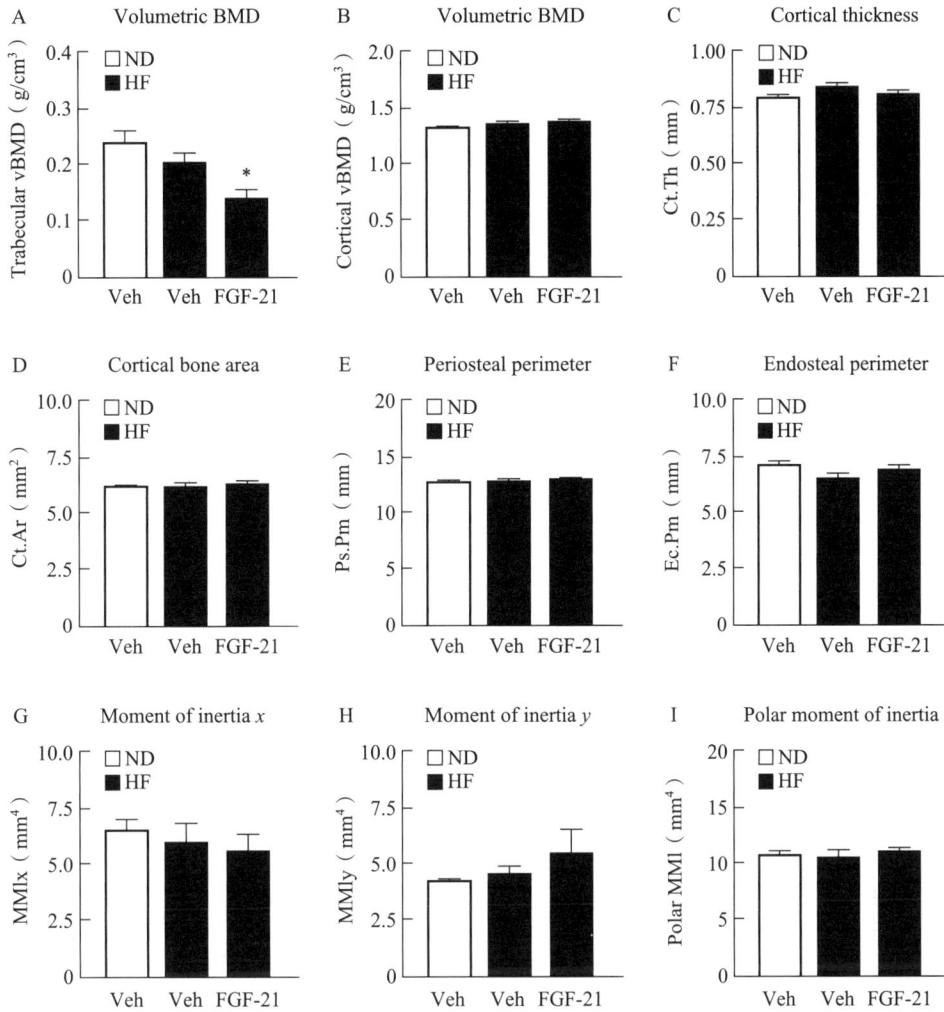

Fig. 2. Three-dimensional analyses of tibial microstructure by μCT in rats fed high-fat diet (HF) or normal diet (ND). During treatment, HF rats were subcutaneously injected once daily with 0.1 mg/kg FGF-21 or vehicle (Veh). The measured parameters are trabecular (A) and cortical (B) volumetric bone mineral density (vBMD), cortical thickness (Ct.Th; C), cortical bone area (Ct.Ar; D), periosteal perimeter (Ps.Pm; E), endosteal perimeter (Ec.Pm; F), moment of inertia in x- and y-axes (MMIx and MMIy; G, H), and polar moment of inertia (polar MMI; I). Values are mean standard error ($n = 4$ per group). $^{*}P < 0.05$ compared with vehicle-treated ND rats. $^{\dagger}P < 0.05$ compared with vehicle-treated HF rats.

ally induce bone loss in obese rats. This led us to draw a conclusion that FGF-21 was indeed very useful for alleviation of insulin resistance and perhaps prediabetes. However, bone health should be regularly evaluated during FGF-21 treatment since this low-dose FGF-21 administration was able to impair bone microstructure and its mechanical properties.

FGF-21 has been reported to act *via* a number of mechanisms to reduce body weight and insulin resistance. For example, Xu *et al.* [19] provided evidence that FGF-21 increased whole-body energy expenditure and physical activity, in part, by inducing the mRNA expression of uncoupling protein-1 and -2 in brown adipocytes. Moreover, it also enhanced the expression of glucose transporter-1 for glucose uptake in adipose tissue as well as the insulin-induced suppression of hepatic glucose output and insulin sensitivity in the heart and skeletal muscle [19, 20]. Glucose uptake in adipocytes was markedly stimulated by FGF-21 [1]. Under certain conditions, such as during cold exposure, FGF-21 was also capable of promoting the browning of white fat for thermogenesis [8].

Although FGF-21 showed several positive effects on metabolic parameters, its administration led to deterioration of bone mechanical property and microstructure. Specifically, HF was associated with an increase in yield displacement (Fig. 1), making bone more ductile, which could be an adaptive change in response to overweight. This higher yield displacement therefore indicated more work required to make a permanent damage to the bone structure under HF conditions. After FGF-21 treatment, bone became more susceptible to permanent damage (plastic deformation) as the FGF-21-treated HF rats with inappropriately reduced yield displacement still had greater body weight than ND rats. In other

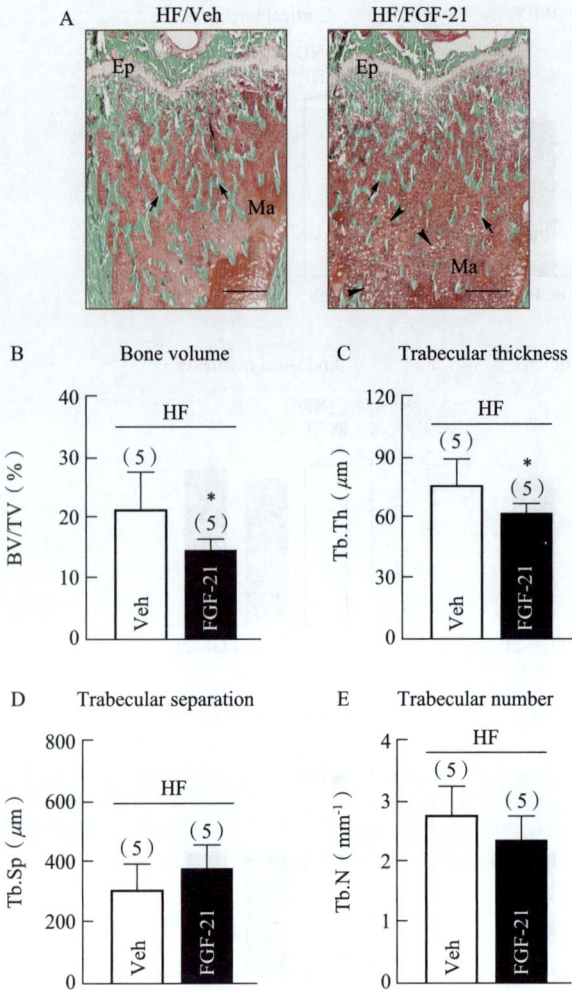

Fig. 3. Microstructural analyses of proximal tibial metaphyses by bone histomorphometry. (A) Representative Goldner's trichrome-stained photomicrographs of the tibial metaphyses. *Scale bars* 1 000 µm; Ep, epiphyseal plate; Ma, bone marrow. Arrows and arrow heads indicate bone trabeculae (green) and marrow fat (i.e., white spots in bone marrow), respectively. Quantitative parameters are bone volume fraction (BV/TV; B), trabecular thickness (Tb.Th; C), trabecular separation (Tb.Sp; D), and trabecular number (Tb.N; E). Rats were fed high fat diet (HF) for 16 weeks and were injected s.c. once daily with 0.1 mg/kg FGF-21 or vehicle (Veh) for 4 weeks. Results are mean standard deviation ($n=5$ per group). *$P < 0.05$ compared with vehicle-treated rats.

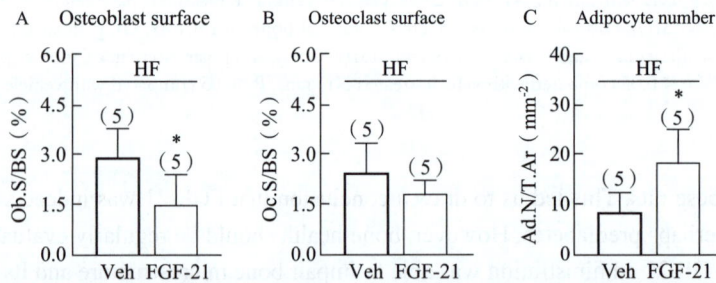

Fig. 4. Osteoblast surface normalized by bone surface (Ob.S/BS; A), osteoclast surface (Oc.S/BS; B), and adipocyte number normalized by tissue area (Ad.N/T.Ar; C) as determined by static bone histomorphometry. Rats were fed high fat diet (HF) for 16 weeks and were injected s.c. once daily with 0.1 mg/kg FGF-21 or vehicle (Veh) for 4 weeks. Results are mean ± standard deviation ($n=5$ per group).*$P < 0.05$ compared with vehicle-treated rats.

words, FGF-21-treated HF rats should maintain yield displacement above the level of ND rats to accommodate ~70 g extra body weight (body weights of vehicle-treated ND rats and FGF-21-treated HF rats were ~500 and 570, respectively). Furthermore, although stiffness often represented how much force to elastically deform bone, an increase in stiffness was not necessary a protective factor against bone deformation. Rigid or highly mineralized bone with increased stiffness was apparently brittle and sometimes required less-than-normal energy to fracture. Taken together, after FGF-21 treatment, the HF-associated increase in yield displacement completely disappeared and inappropriate bone stiffness was observed which, in turn, might make bone more susceptible to fracture. Indeed, these signs of impaired mechanical properties occurred despite no change in cortical parameter, e.g., cortical thickness, cortical bone area, or moment of inertia, as evaluated by μCT.

Meanwhile, the trabecular portion of long bone was apparently more vulnerable to FGF-21 administration. Results showed that the tibial trabecular vBMD was significantly decreased by FGF-21 compared to vehicle-treated HF-fed rats. Further investigation of the tibial secondary spongiosum, a trabecula-rich area of the long bone, consistently revealed decreases in bone volume and trabecular thickness without change in trabecular separation or number. The observed negative effects of FGF-21 on bone of HF-fed rats could be explained based on the previous finding that FGF-21 was a potent stimulator of PPAR-γ activity [9]. This transcription factor plays its salient role in deciding whether mesenchymal stem cells will differentiate into adipocytes or osteoblast [21]. Therefore, its upregulation could lead to inhibition of osteo-blastogenesis from mesenchymal stem cells, thereby suppressing bone formation[9]. Other activators of PPAR-γ known as thiazolidinediones, e.g., the anti-diabetic drug rosiglitazone, also induced bone loss by a similar mechanism[10, 22]. Hence, an increase in adipocyte number and a decrease in osteoblast surface well confirmed the aforementioned PPAR-γ hypothesis. Nevertheless, since mature osteoblasts abundantly expressed FGFRs [23], it was tempting to postulate that FGF-21 could also directly suppress osteoblast function. In addition to suppression of bone formation, the FGF-21-induced decreases in trabecular bone volume and thickness might have resulted from PPAR-γ-mediated osteoclastogenesis [24, 25]. Wan *et al.* [24] clearly showed that activation of PPAR-γ promoted osteoclast differentiation through the c-Fos-dependent pathway, leading to osteoclast-mediated bone resorption and osteoporosis. However, osteoclast surface was not altered in the present study, perhaps due to the use of low-dose FGF-21 administration; however, more investigations are required to directly determine osteoclast activity and circulating levels of osteoclastogenic markers, such as receptor activator of nuclear factor κB ligand (RANKL).

In conclusion, FGF-21 altered bone mechanical properties and reduced trabecular vBMD as well as trabecular bone volume and thickness in the tibial metaphysis of HF-fed rats. Although further experiments are required to demon-strate the underlying cellular and molecular mechanisms of FGF-21, related bone biomarkers (e.g., osteocalcin, osterix, RANKL, and osteoprotegerin), and contributions of other obesity-related osteoregulatory endocrine factors (particularly leptin) [26] in obese animals, FGF-21 can be used to improve metabolic disturbance and insulin resistance caused by HF consumption. However, bone change should be closely monitored during long-term administration.

Supplementary material

Supplementary material to this article can be found in the online version (doi:10.1007/s00774-016-0745-z).

References

[1] Kharitonenkov A, Shiyanova TL, Koester A, *et al.* FGF-21 as a nov-el metabolic regulator[J]. Journal Of Clinical Investigation, 2005, 115(6): 1627-1635.

[2] Kharitonenkov A, Wroblewski VJ, Koester A, *et al.* The metabolic state of diabetic monkeys is regulated by fibroblast growth factor-21[J]. Endocrinology, 2007, 148(2): 774-781.

[3] Goetz R, Beenken A, Ibrahimi OA, *et al.* Molecular insights into the klotho-dependent, endocrine mode of action of fibroblast growth factor 19 subfamily members[J]. Molecular And Cellular Biology, 2007, 27(9): 3417-3428.

[4] Zhang X, Ibrahimi OA, Olsen SK, *et al.* Receptor specificity of the fibroblast growth factor family - The complete mammalian FGF family[J]. Journal Of Biological Chemistry, 2006, 281(23): 15694-15700.

[5] Nishimura T, Nakatake Y, Konishi M, *et al.* Identification of a novel FGF, FGF-21, preferentially expressed in the liver[J]. Biochimica Et Biophysica Acta-Gene Structure And Expression, 2000, 1492(1): 203-206.

[6] Wente W, Efanov AM, Brenner M, *et al.* Fibroblast growth fac-tor-21 improves pancreatic beta-cell function and survival by activa-tion of extracellular signal-regulated kinase 1/2 and Akt signaling

pathways[J]. Diabetes, 2006, 55(9): 2470-2478.

[7] Muise ES, Azzolina B, Kuo DW, *et al.* Adipose fibroblast growth factor 21 is up-regulated by peroxisome proliferator-activated recep-tor gamma and altered metabolic states[J]. Molecular Pharmacology, 2008, 74(2): 403-412.

[8] Canto C, Auwerx J. FGF21 Takes a fat bite[J]. Science, 2012, 336(6082): 675-676.

[9] Wei W, Dutchak PA, Wang X, *et al.* Fibroblast growth factor 21 promotes bone loss by potentiating the effects of peroxisome proliferator-activated receptor gamma[J]. Proceedings Of the Na-tional Academy Of Sciences Of the United States Of America, 2012, 109(8): 3143-3148.

[10] Ali AA, Weinstein RS, Stewart SA, *et al.* Rosiglitazone causes bone loss in mice by suppressing osteoblast differentiation and bone formation[J]. Endocrinology, 2005, 146(3): 1226-1235.

[11] Apaijai N, Pintana H, Chattipakorn SC, *et al.* Cardioprotective ef-fects of metformin and vildagliptin in adult rats with insulin resis-tance induced by a high-fat diet[J]. Endocrinology, 2012, 153(8): 3878-3885.

[12] Pintana H, Apaijai N, Pratchayasakul W, *et al.* Effects of metformin on learning and memory behaviors and brain mitochondrial func-

tions in high fat diet induced insulin resistant rats[J]. Life Sciences, 2012, 91(11-12): 409-414.

[13] Suntornsaratoon P, Krishnamra N, Charoenphandhu N. Positive long-term outcomes from presuckling calcium supplementation in lactating rats and the offspring[J]. American Journal Of Physiology-Endocrinology And Metabolism, 2015, 308(11): E1010-E1022.

[14] Appleton DJ, Rand JS, Sunvold GD. Basal plasma insulin and homeostasis model assessment (HOMA) are indicators of insulin sensitivity in cats[J]. Journal Of Feline Medicine And Surgery, 2005, 7(3): 183-193.

[15] Haffner SM, Miettinen H, Stern MP. The homeostasis model in the San Antonio Heart Study[J]. Diabetes Care, 1997, 20(7): 1087-1092.

[16] Pipatpiboon N, Pintana H, Pratchayasakul W, et al. DPP4-inhibitor improves neuronal insulin receptor function, brain mitochondrial function and cognitive function in rats with insulin resistance induced by high-fat diet consumption[J]. European Journal Of Neuroscience, 2013, 37(5): 839-849.

[17] Pipatpiboon N, Pratchayasakul W, Chattipakorn N, et al. PPAR gamma Agonist Improves Neuronal Insulin Receptor Function in Hippocampus and Brain Mitochondria Function in Rats with Insulin Resistance Induced by Long Term High-Fat Diets[J]. Endocrinology, 2012, 153(1): 329-338.

[18] Huang J, Ishino T, Chen G, et al. Development of a novel long-acting antidiabetic FGF21 mimetic by targeted conjugation to a scaffold antibody[J]. Journal Of Pharmacology And Experimental Therapeutics, 2013, 346(2): 270-280.

[19] Xu J, Lloyd DJ, Hale C, et al. Fibroblast growth factor 21 reverses hepatic steatosis, increases energy expenditure, and improves insulin sensitivity in diet-induced obese mice[J]. Diabetes, 2009, 58(1): 250-259.

[20] Berglund ED, Li CY, Bina HA, et al. Fibroblast growth factor 21 controls glycemia via regulation of hepatic glucose flux and insulin sensitivity[J]. Endocrinology, 2009, 150(9): 4084-4093.

[21] Lecka-Czernik B, Moerman EJ, Grant DF, et al. Divergent effects of selective peroxisome proliferator-activated receptor-gamma 2 ligands on adipocyte versus osteoblast differentiation[J]. Endocrinology, 2002, 143(6): 2376-2384.

[22] Rzonca SO, Suva LJ, Gaddy D, et al. Bone is a target for the antidiabetic compound rosiglitazone[J]. Endocrinology, 2004, 145(1): 401-406.

[23] Caverzasio J, Thouverey C. Activation of FGF receptors is a new mechanism by which strontium ranelate induces osteoblastic cell growth[J]. Cellular Physiology And Biochemistry, 2011, 27(3-4): 243-250.

[24] Wan Y, Chong LW, Evans RM. PPAR-γ regulates osteoclastogenesis in mice[J]. Nature Medicine, 2007, 13(12): 1496-1503.

[25] Wan Y. Bone marrow mesenchymal stem cells: Fat on and blast off by FGF21[J]. International Journal Of Biochemistry & Cell Biology, 2013, 45(3): 546-549.

[26] Chen XX, Yang T. Roles of leptin in bone metabolism and bone diseases[J]. Journal Of Bone And Mineral Metabolism, 2015, 33(5): 474-485.

Two FGF receptor kinase molecules act in concert to recruit and transphosphorylate phospholipase Cγ

Zhifeng Huang, Xiaokun Li, Moosa Mohammadi

1. Introduction

Receptor tyrosine kinase (RTK) signaling plays essential roles in human biology and pathology (Hunter, 2000; Lemmon and Schlessinger, 2010). Ligand-induced dimerization of the extracellular domains of RTKs juxtaposes the cytoplasmic kinase domains to enable kinase *trans*-tyrosine phosphorylation (Chen *et al.*, 2008; Goetz and Mohammadi, 2013; Hubbard, 2004; Hunter, 2002; Jura *et al.*, 2011; Lemmon and Schlessinger, 2010). Phosphorylation of tyrosines in the regulatory kinase A-loop elevates the intrinsic kinase activity in an allosteric fashion (Chen *et al.*, 2007; Pellicena and Kuriyan, 2006; Rajakulendran and Sicheri, 2010). In contrast, phosphorylation on tyrosines in the juxtamembrane region, kinase insert, or C-terminal tail creates specific recruitment sites for Src Homology 2 (SH2)—or phos photyrosine binding (PTB)—containing intracellular substrates including enzymes and adaptor proteins (Lemmon and Schlessinger, 2010; Pawson, 2004; Schlessinger and Lemmon, 2003) to facilitate their phosphorylation, which then triggers activation of specific intracellular signaling pathways leading to distinct biological responses (Rotin *et al.*, 1992; Schlessinger and Lemmon, 2003). For example, phosphorylation of a conserved tyrosine in the C-terminal tail of FGFRs creates a docking site for Phospholipase Cg1 (PLCγ1), a tandem SH2-containing substrate (Eswarakumar *et al.*, 2005; Mohammadi *et al.*, 1991; Peters *et al.*, 1992). This recruitment plays a dual role in the activation of the PLCγ pathway: (1) it facilitates phosphorylation of PLCγ that relieves PLCγ autoinhibition, resulting in upregulation of the lipase activity of the enzyme (Bunney *et al.*, 2012; Hajicek *et al.*, 2013; Poulin *et al.*, 2005), and (2) it translocates PLCγ to the vicinity of its substrate phosphatidylinositol 4,5-bisphosphate (PIP2) in the plasma membrane, where the activated enzyme can hydrolyze PIP2 leading to the generation of the second messengers DAG and IP3 (Ellis *et al.*, 1998; Schlessinger, 1997).

There is a major gap in our understanding of the molecular mechanism by which SH2- or PTB-mediated recruitment/phosphorylation of substrates takes place. The recent elucidation of the crystal structure of 1:1 complex of the activated FGFR1 kinase with the tandem nSH2-cSH2 domain fragment of PLCγ (PDB: 3GQI) (Bae *et al.*, 2009) has been the closest attempt to address this fundamental process in RTK signaling. In this structure, the tyrosine phosphorylated C-tail of FGFR1 kinase binds the nSH2 domain of PLCγ, but none of the three PLCγ phosphorylation sites included in the tandem SH2 construct are engaged by the active site of the FGFR1 kinase, leaving it uncertain as to how SH2-mediated recruitment facilitates substrate phosphorylation.

Here, we used an assortment of X-ray crystallography, nuclear magnetic resonance (NMR) spectroscopy, mass spectrometry, and other biophysical and cell-based experiments to show how two FGFR kinases act cooperatively to recruit and phosphorylate PLCγ, thus overturning the current paradigm that recruitment and phosphorylation of the substrates are carried out by the same receptor (*i.e.*, in *cis*). In addition, our data unravel the molecular basis by which the phosphorylated substrate is disembarked from the FGFR, allowing for next cycles of recruitment and phosphorylation to ensue.

2. Results and discussion

2.1 C-terminal SH2 domain of PLCγ mediates the recruitment and phosphorylation of PLCγ by FGFR, EGFR, PDGFR, and VEGFR in living cells

PLCγ is a key signaling protein for a number of RTKs including FGFRs, EGFRs, PDGFRs, VEGFRs, and NG-

FRs (Kim *et al.*, 1991; Lemmon and Schlessinger, 2010; Liu *et al.*, 2012; Pascal *et al.*, 1994). PLCγ possesses tandem SH2 domains, an N-terminal SH2 (nSH2), and a C-terminal SH2 (cSH2), which share about 35% sequence identity. To test the roles of the two SH2 domains in the recruitment and phosphorylation of PLCγ by RTKs in living cells, we ablated the phosphotyrosine (pTyr) binding function of the nSH2 and cSH2 domains individually or in combination by mutating the arginine from the SH2 domaininvariant FLVR motif (Bae *et al.*, 2009; Hidaka *et al.*, 1991) within the pTyr binding pocket (Arg-586 of nSH2 and Arg-694 of cSH2) to alanine (Fig. 1A) and transiently transfected the wild-type or mutated PLCγ constructs into *PLCγ1⁻/⁻* mouse embryonic fibroblasts (MEFs) (Ji *et al.*, 1997). Conveniently, $PLC\gamma 1^{-/-}$ MEF endogenously expresses FGFR1, EGFR, and PDGFR, obviating the need for transfecting these three RTKs into these cells. However, since $PLC\gamma 1^{-/-}$ MEFs do not express VEGFR2, a stable cell line overexpressing VEGFR2 was established. Transfected cells were stimulated with FGF1, EGF, PDGF, or VEGF, and phosphorylation on Tyr-783, one of the three major phosphorylation sites of PLCγ, was analyzed. Inactivation of the cSH2 domain alone (N^+C^-) or of both SH2 domains (N^-C^-) abrogated the ability of all four RTKs to phosphorylate PLCγ, whereas inactivation of the nSH2 domain alone (N^-C^+) had no effect (Fig. 1B). Consistent with the PLCγ phosphorylation data, the PLCγ construct with ablated cSH2 domain (N^+C^-) failed to co-precipitate with the activated FGFR1, whereas the PLCγ construct with disabled nSH2 domain (N^-C^+) co-precipitated with FGFR1 as efficiently as the wild-type PLCγ did (Fig. 1C). Moreover, cells transfected with PLCγ devoid of a functional cSH2 domain failed to respond to FGF1 with an increase in IP3 production, whereas FGF1 treatment of cells transfected with PLCγ lacking a functional nSH2 domain gave rise to similar level of IP3 release as cells transfected with wild-type PLCγ (Fig. 1D). These data demonstrate that the cSH2 domain of PLCγ mediates recruitment and phosphorylation of PLCγ by FGFR, VEGFR, EGFR, and PDGFR in living cells.

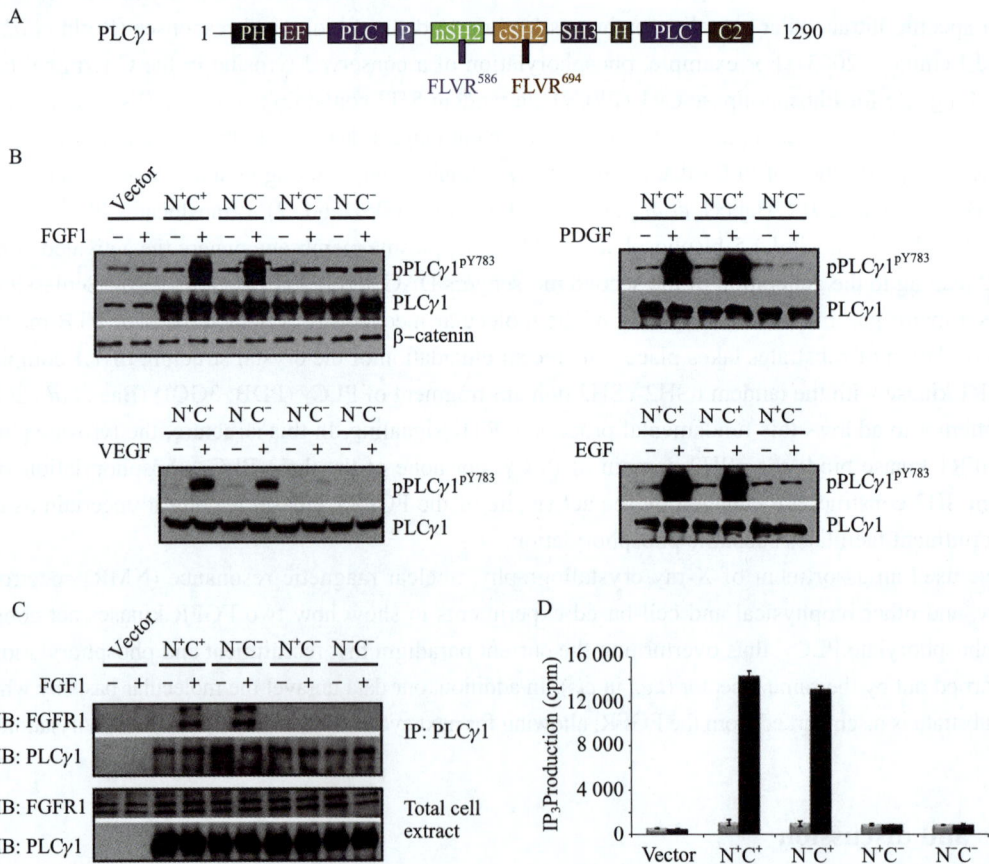

Fig. 1. The cSH2 domain of PLCγ Is necessary and sufficient for PLCγ phosphorylation by FGFR, EGFR, PDGFR, and VEGFR in living cells. (A) Domain organization of full-length PLCγ. The FLVR motifs in the nSH2 and cSH2 domains are labeled in blue and red, respectively. (B) Immunoblotting analysis of PLCγ phosphorylation by FGFR, EGFR, VEGFR2, and PDGFR in living cells. (C) Co-immunoprecipitation assay using wild-type and mutated PLCγ constructs in living cells. $PLC\gamma 1^{-/-}$ MEF were transfected with the indicated PLCγ constructs and stimulated with FGF1. FGF-induced PI hydrolysis in $PLC\gamma 1^{-/-}$ MEF cells transfected with the indicated wild-type and mutated PLCγ constructs. Data are represented as mean ± SEM (*n* = 3). See also Fig. S1.

2.2 cSH2 of PLCγ is sufficient and necessary for the recruitment of PLCγ by the FGFR kinase in vitro

Next, we sought to confirm the requirement for the cSH2 domain in recruitment of PLCγ by FGFR kinase *in vitro*. To this end, recombinant wild-type tandem SH2 fragment of PLCγ (nSH2-cSH2) and the corresponding three mutated fragments (nSH2[R586A]-cSH2, nSH2-cSH2[R694A], and nSH2[R586A]-cSH2[R694A]) were made (Fig. 2A). As for the recombinant FGFR kinase, the kinase domain of FGFR2, including C-terminal Tyr-769, whose phosphorylation is required for PLCγ recruitment and phosphorylation, was made. To generate a homogeneously phosphorylated kinase sample, all of the autophosphorylation sites of FGFR2 kinase except for Tyr-769 were mutated to non-phosphorylatable residues. To drive the kinase into the active state conformation in the absence of A-loop tyrosine phosphorylation, two pathogenic gain-of-function mutations, Glu565Ala (E565A) and Lys659Glu (K659E) (Chen *et al.*, 2007, 2013; Naski *et al.*, 1996), were introduced into the kinase (Fig. 2A).

Binding of wild-type or mutated tandem nSH2-cSH2 fragments of PLCγ (nSH2-cSH2, nSH2[R586A]-cSH2, nSH2-cSH2[R694A], and nSH2[R586A]-cSH2[R694A]) to the activated FGFR2 kinase, which is mono-phosphorylated on Tyr-769 (FGFR2K[pY769]), was studied using isothermal titration calorimetry (ITC), surface plasmon resonance (SPR) spectroscopy (Fig. 2B–E), size exclusion chromatography (SEC), and native gel electrophoresis (Fig. S1A–H). In ITC experiments, the nSH2[R586A]-cSH2 construct bound FGFR2K[pY769] with a comparable affinity as the wild-type nSH2-cSH2 construct did whereas both nSH2-cSH2[R694A], and nSH2[R586A]-cSH2[R694A] failed to bind FGFR2K[pY769] (Fig. 2B–E). Consistent with the

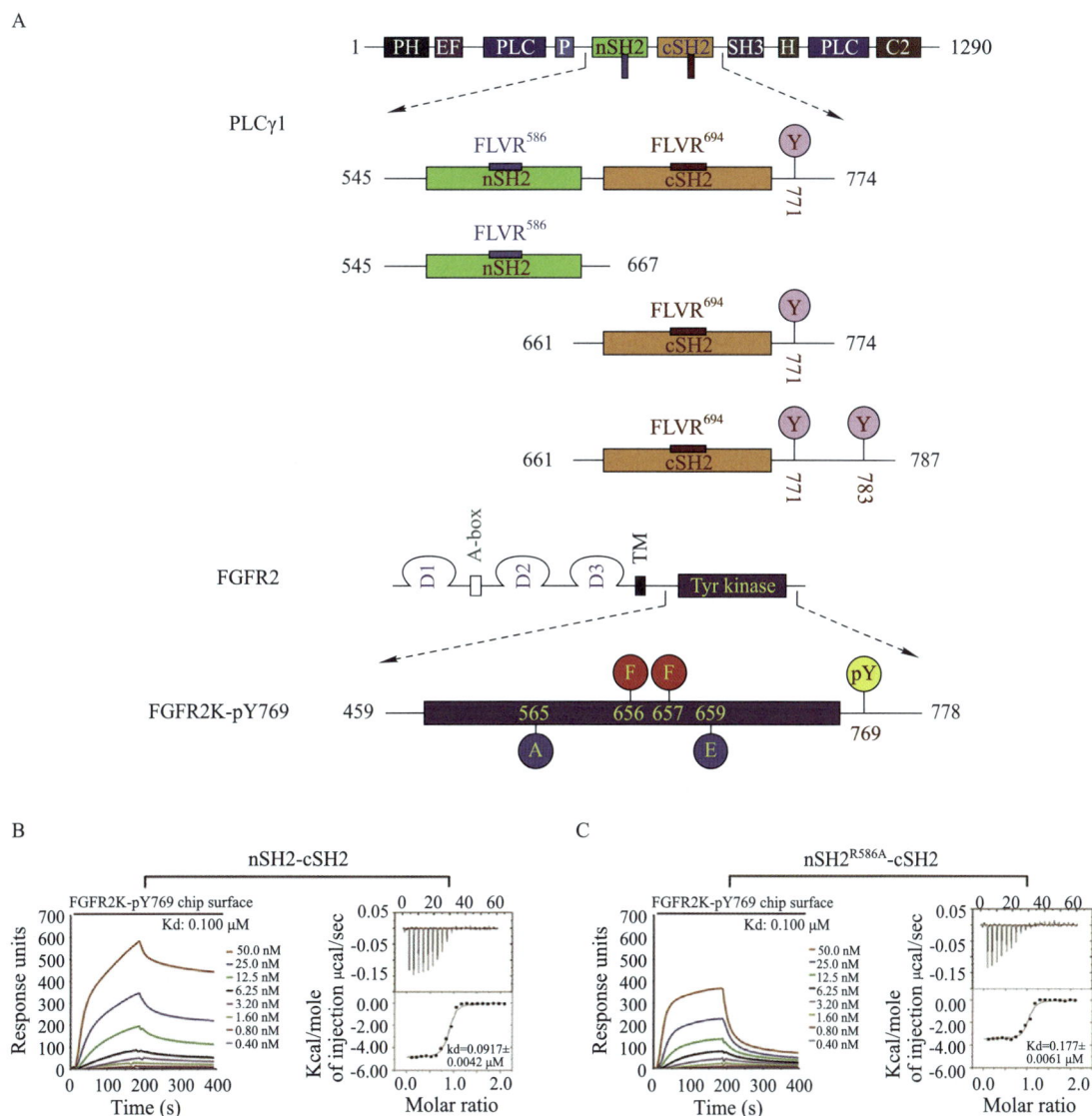

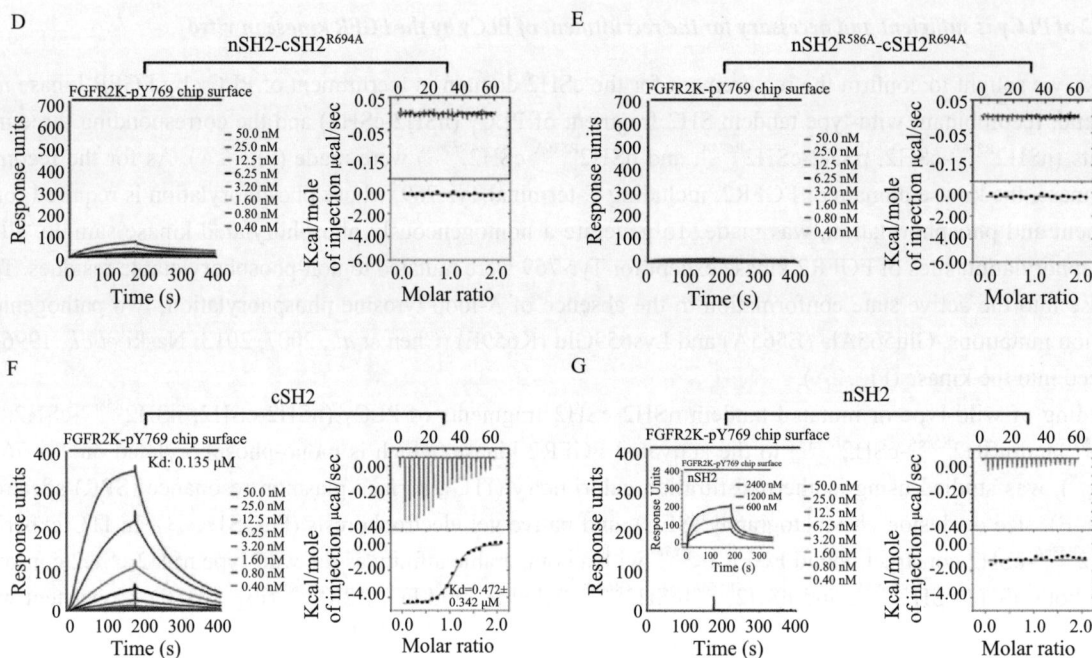

Fig. 2. The cSH2 domain of PLCγ mediates the recruitment of PLCγ by FGFR kinase *in vitro*. (A) Domain organization of PLCγ and FGFR2 as well as the design of the engineered PLCγ and FGFR2 fragments used in this study. Tyrosine phosphorylation sites included in the tandem SH2 and isolated cSH2 fragments are marked with pink circles. The phosphorylation sites in the A-loop of FGFR2 kinase (Tyr-656 and Tyr-657), which were mutated to phenylalanine, are indicated with red circles. The location of the two gain-of-function mutations introduced to force the kinase into the active state is indicated with blue circles. Tyr-769, the single remaining phosphorylation site in the FGFR2K is highlighted with a yellow circle. (B–G) Analysis by SPR and ITC of the recruitment of wild-type tandem nSH2-cSH2 fragment of PLCγ (B), nSH2^{R586A}-cSH2 (C), nSH2-cSH2^{R694A} (D), nSH2^{R586A}-cSH2^{R694A} (E), cSH2 domain (F), and nSH2 domain (G) of PLCγ by activated FGFR2K^{pY769}. Inset of (G) is SPR binding analysis of nSH2 domain at high concentrations with activated FGFR2K^{pY769}. See also Fig. S1.

ITC data, SPR experiments showed that inactivation of nSH2 had a subtle effect on the binding of tandem SH2 to the immobilized FGFR2K^{pY769}, whereas the cSH2-inactivated nSH2-cSH2^{R694A} construct showed a major loss in binding to the immobilized FGFR2K^{pY769} (Fig. 2B–E). To further corroborate these data, binding interactions of FGFR2K^{pY769} with the individual nSH2 and cSH2 domains were also studied. As shown in Fig. 2F, cSH2 domain bound FGFR2K^{pY769} with a comparable affinity as the wild-type tandem nSH2-cSH2 construct whereas only weak binding of nSH2 domain could be observed at very high concentrations (Fig. 2G, inset panel). Lastly, we also examined binding interactions of the individual SH2 domains with FGFR2K^{pY769} using solution NMR spectroscopy. Uniformly ^{15}N-labeled nSH2 and cSH2 domains were prepared and their HSQC spectra in the absence and presence of 0.5, 1, and 2 molar equivalents of unlabeled FGFR2K^{pY769} were acquired (Fig. S1I, J). Titration of cSH2 domain with a 0.5 molar equivalent of FGFR2K^{pY769} led to major chemical shift perturbations in the cSH2 domain and resulted in the appearance of a new set of peaks representing the complexed form (i.e., slow chemical exchange) (Fig. S1I). Upon further addition of FGFR2K^{pY769} to give a 1:1 molar ratio, only the peaks corresponding to the bound form of cSH2 were observed, which shows that cSH2 domain and FGFR2K^{pY769} form a tight 1:1 complex in solution. To the contrary, FGFR2K^{pY769} did not induce any new peaks in the spectrum for the nSH2 domain when titrated at 1:1 molar ratio (Fig. S1J). Only reductions in peak intensity and insignificant chemical shift perturbations were observed for some of the resonances, which likely stemmed from intermediate and fast exchange, respectively, indicative of poor binding affinity between nSH2 domain and FGFR2K^{pY769} relative to the cSH2 domain.

To exclude the possibility that the presence of the gain-of-function mutations may have biased the binding of FGFR2K^{pY769} toward cSH2 domain, we also analyzed binding interactions of phosphorylated wild-type FGFR2K with wild-type and mutated tandem nSH2-cSH2 fragments using native gel electrophoresis (Fig. S1L). This analysis showed that the phosphorylated wild-type FGFR2K also binds selectively to the cSH2 domain. Lastly, we also tested whether cSH2-mediated recruitment of PLCγ is applicable to all FGFRs by analyzing the binding interactions of phosphorylated wild-type FGFR1, FGFR3, and FGFR4 kinases with wild-type or mutated tandem nSH2-cSH2 fragments using native gel electrophoresis. The results clearly show that all four human FGFRs recruit PLCγ *via* its cSH2 domain (Fig. S1K–S1N).

2.3 Crystal structure of FGFR2K^{pY769} in complex with the PLCγ cSH2 domain reveals a 2:1 FGFR-PLCγ stoichiometry

Having demonstrated that the cSH2 domain is necessary and sufficient for the recruitment and phosphorylation of PLCγ, we then solved the crystal structure of FGFR2K^{pY769} in complex with a PLCγ cSH2 fragment consisting of residues Asn-661 to Leu-774 in the presence of a non-hydrolyzable ATP analog (AMP-PCP) at 2.6Å resolution (Figs. 3, 4; Table 1). This cSH2 construct includes the cSH2 domain and Tyr-771, the first phosphorylation site of PLCγ past the cSH2 domain.

The asymmetric unit of the crystal contains a 1:1 FGFR2K^{pY769}-PLCγ cSH2 complex mediated by contacts between the phosphorylated C-tail of FGFR2K^{pY769} and the pTyr binding pocket of the PLCγ cSH2 domain (Fig. 3A). Despite lacking the A-loop tyrosines, FGFR2K^{pY769} adopts the active state conformation and contains an AMP-PCP molecule in its ATP binding cleft, demonstrating that the E565A and K659E gain-of-function mutations have forced the kinase into active state without A-loop tyrosine phosphorylation (Fig. S2). Surprisingly, however, the phosphorylatable Y771 of the PLCγ cSH2 domain is not bound in *cis* into the active site of the kinase in the 1:1 complex (Fig. 3A). Instead, Y771 binds in *trans* into the active site of the neighboring kinase in the crystal lattice where it is poised to be phosphorylated

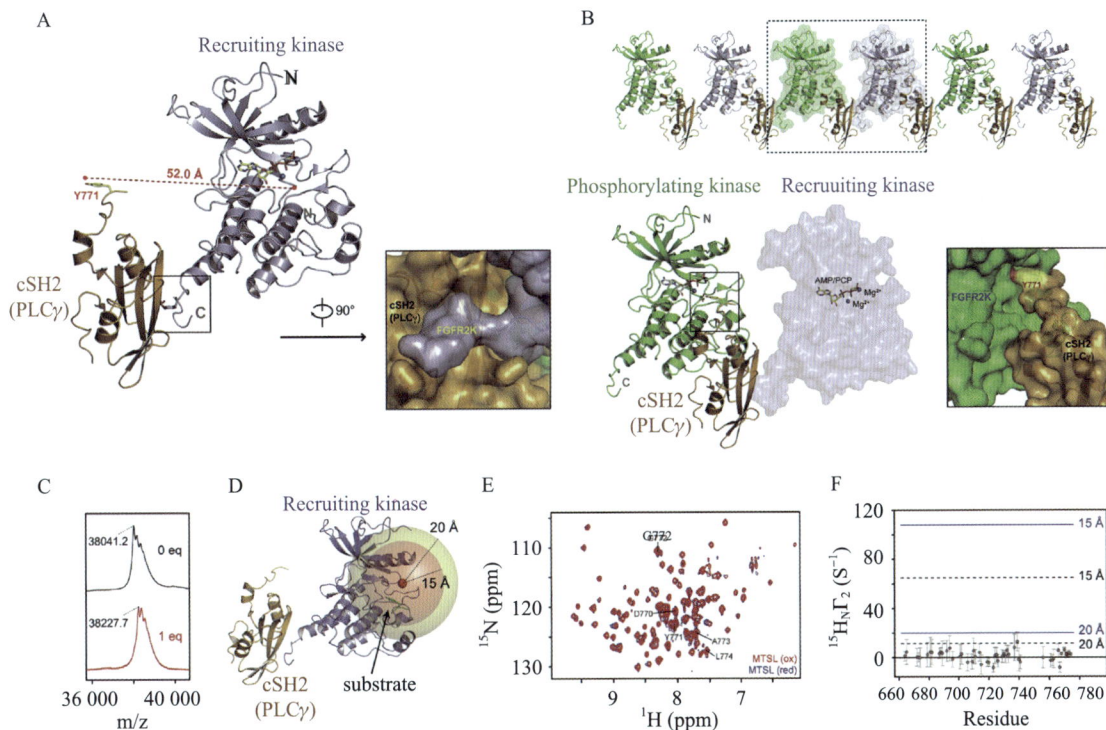

Fig. 3. Recruitment and phosphorylation of cSH2 cannot be accomplished by the same kinase in *cis*. (A) Ribbon diagram of the crystal structure of the complex between mutationally activated monophosphorylated FGFR2K^{pY769} in complex with PLCγ cSH2 domain. Surface representation showing insertion of phosphorylated C-terminal tail of recruiting kinase into the phosphotyrosine binding pocket of the PLCγ cSH2 domain. (B) 2:1 FGFR2 kinase-PLCγ cSH2 complex is observed in the crystal lattice. Surface representation showing insertion of Tyr-771 phosphorylation site from the PLCγ cSH2 domain into the active site of the phosphorylating kinase. The phosphorylating kinase and the recruiting kinase are colored green and light blue, respectively. The PLCγ cSH2 domain is colored orange. The ATP analog (AMP-PCP) and magnesium ions are rendered as sticks and blue spheres, respectively. (C) MALDI-TOF results of MTSL labeling of Cys-491 in the glycine-rich loop of FGFR2K^{pY769} (FGFR2K-pY769^{MTSL}). The observed mass/charge difference uponlabeling with MTSL was 186.5, which agrees closely with the expected value of 186.3. (D) Crystal structure of recruiting FGFR2K^{pY769} bound to cSH2 showing the C$_\beta$ of Cys-491 (red sphere) and two spheres of 15 Å and 20 Å surrounding this site. A bound substrate tyrosine in the catalytic pocket, shown in green color stick, would be expected to lie within the 15 Å sphere. (E) ^{1}H/^{15}N TROSY spectra of 1:1 samples of cSH2:FGFR2K-pY769^{MTSL} before (intact MTSL; red) and after treatment with ascorbic acid (reduced MTSL; blue). The cSH2 samples were 70% deuterated. (F) ^{1}H relaxation enhancement (Γ_2) due to the presence of the MTSL spin label probed using a two-point TROSY method where the difference in the relaxation delays was 10 ms (Iwahara *et al.*, 2007). Y771 is shown as a red circle. Distances of 15 Å and 20 Å between the spin label and amide proton are shown on the plot using correlation times of 15 ns (black, dotted line) and 25 ns (blue, solid line). A G$_2$ value close to zero indicates a distance >~25 Å from the spin label. Based on the crystal structures of FGFR kinases-substrate complexes, the distance between the tyrosine to be phosphorylated and adjacent residues ranges from 10 to 13 Å. See also Fig. S2–S4 and S6.

Table 1. X-ray data collection and refinement statistics

Construct	FGFR2K-PLCγ[cSH2]
Data Collection	
X-ray wavelength	0.97907
Space group	C2
Unit Cell Dimensions	
a, b, c (Å)	79.609, 53.231, 127.660
α, β, γ (°)	90.00, 100.11, 90.00
Resolution (Å)	50–2.60 (2.64–2.60)[a]
No. measured reflections	105,439
No. unique reflections	15981 (788)
Data redundancy	6.6 (4.9)
Data completeness (%)	98.2 (93.5)
R^{sym} (%)[b]	9.3 (25.6)
I/sig	27.9 (5.9)
Refinement	
Resolution (Å)	37.90–2.60 (2.69–2.60)
No. unique reflections	15,973
No. Reflections (R_{free})[c]	1,597
R_{work}/R_{free}	18.41/23.59
Number of atoms	
Protein	3,323
Ligand/Ion	33
Solvent	48
R.m.s. deviations	
Bond length (Å)	0.009
Bond angle (°)	1.235
Average B factors (Å^2)	
Protein	35.3
Ligand/Ion	35.6
Solvent	30.2
Ramachandran plot	
Outliers (%)	0.73
Allowed (%)	2.20
Favored (%)	97.07
Rotamer outliers (%)	0.56
No. C-Beta Deviations	0
All-Atom Clashscore	4.66

[a]Values in parenthsy are fortro highest resolution shell. [b]Rsym $=\Sigma|I - <I>|/\Sigma I$. where I is the observed intensity of a reflection and $<I>$ is the average intensity of all the symmetry related reflections. [c]For R_{free} calculation, 10% of reflections were randomly excluded from the refinement.

(Fig. 3B). Hence, the FGFR2K^{pY769}-PLCγ cSH2 complex structure implies that PLCγ recruitment and phosphorylation involves a 2:1 receptor-substrate complex wherein one receptor acts as "recruiter" and the other receptor serves as "phosphorylater." In fact, structural analysis (Figs. 3A, 4) shows that due to spatial constraints, recruitment and phosphorylation of the PLCγ cSH2 domain cannot be carried out by the same kinase, that is, in *cis*. Tyr-771 is only five residues away from the end of the rigid core of PLCγ cSH2 domain, which is not enough to provide sufficient flexibility for Tyr-771 to reach the active site of the kinase. Like-wise, Tyr-769 of FGFR2 is only two residues away from the end of the aI helix, which also does not provide enough C-terminal flexibility to position the cSH2 domain closer to the active site of the FGFR kinase such that phosphorylation of Tyr-771 can occur in *cis*. Nevertheless, to rule out the possibility that crystal packing contacts may have hindered binding in *cis* of Tyr-771 into the active site of the recruiting kinase, we performed para-magnetic relaxation enhancement (PRE) experiments to obtain proximity information between Tyr-771 of the cSH2 domain and the substrate tyrosine binding pocket of FGFR2K^{pY769}. For this purpose, we attached an MTSL, a commonly used nitroxide paramagnetic spin label, to Cys-491 in the Gly-rich loop of the FGFR2K^{pY769} (Fig. 3C, D). Conveniently, this naturally occurring cysteine is about 10 Å away from the catalytic base of the kinase, which is well within the PRE transfer range of MTSL (Fig. 3D). Following a series of triple resonance experiments to assign the backbone amide ^{1}H/^{15}N resonances of the cSH2 domain (Fig. 3E), a 1:1 complex of 70% deuterated, ^{15}N-labeled cSH2 with the spin-labeled FGFR2K-pY769^{MTSL} was prepared and ^{1}H T$_2$ relaxation enhancements in the cSH2 domain was probed using a two-point TROSY method (Iwahara *et al.*, 2007) where the difference in the relaxation delays was 10 ms. Following collection of the data on the paramagnetically labeled FGFR2K-pY769^{MTSL}, ascorbic acid was added to reduce the nitroxide allowing us to measure relaxation rates in the absence of the paramagnetic state. As shown in Fig. 3F, the corresponding ^{1}H PRE G$_2$ rates for C-terminal residues 760–773 of cSH2, which include the phosphorylatable tyrosine 771, are close to zero. Moreover, there are no discernable spectral differences between ^{15}N-HSQC paramagnetic and diamagnetic spectra or spectra of the native complex prepared in the absence of MTSL incorporation. Taken together, these NMR PRE data show that Tyr-771 of cSH2 and its surrounding sequences are more than ~20 Å away from the spin label. To ensure that our PRE assay is capable of detecting spectral changes/rate enhancements within ~20 Å range, we performed a control PRE experiment wherein the minimal kinase domain of FGFR2 (residues 459 to 768; FGFR2K^{short}) was isotopically enriched with ^{15}N and subsequently labeled with MTSL on Cys-491 in the same manner as FGFR2K^{pY769}. A comparison of paramagnetic and diamagnetic spectra of this construct shows several missing peaks in the former consistent with the distance-dependent perturbation by the spin label on the Gly-rich loop (Fig. S3). Taken together, these PRE experiments support the crystal structure showing that recruitment and phosphorylation cannot be accomplished by the same kinase in *cis*.

2.4 Interactions at the interfaces between cSH2 and the recruiting and phosphorylating FGFR2 kinases

The interface between the cSH2 molecule and the recruiting kinase molecule buries a total of 967 Å^2 of solvent exposed surface area (Fig. 4A, B). At this interface, the phosphorylated Tyr-769 (pTyr-769) and the following Leu-770 and Leu-772 of the recruiting kinase plug into the pTyr binding pocket of the cSH2 domain using the canonical "two-prong in socket" mechanism with pTyr-769 engaging the hydrophilic hole, and Leu-770 and Leu-772 engaging the hydrophobic hole of the socket (Fig. 4C, D). pTyr-769 engages in a total of seven hydrogen bonds: two each with both Arg-675 and Arg-696 and three with Arg-694 of the PLCγ cSH2 domain. In addition, backbone atoms of Glu-768 and Leu-770 of the recruiting kinase molecule make hydrogen bonds with the side chain of Arg-675 and backbone carbonyl oxygen of His-714 of the PLCγ cSH2 domain. Another notable contact at this hydrophilic hole of the socket is the π-cation interaction between the phenyl ring of pTyr-769 and Arg-716 of the PLCγ cSH2 domain (Fig. 4D). In the second hydrophobic hole of the socket, Leu-770 and Leu-772 of the recruiting kinase are immersed in hydrophobic contacts with Phe-706, Cys-715, Leu-726, Tyr-741, Leu-746, and Tyr-747 of the PLCγ cSH2 domain (Fig. 4D).

The interface between the cSH2 molecule and the phosphorylating kinase molecule buries a total of 1,246 Å^2 of solvent exposed surface area (Fig. 4A, B) and harbors several canonical kinase-substrate contacts at the enzyme active site (Fig. 4C, E). The hydroxyl moiety of Tyr-771 makes two short hydrogen bonds with the catalytic base (Asp-626) of the kinase and is also engaged in a π-cation interaction with Arg-664 from the A-loop of the phosphorylater kinase. In addition to these canonical contacts proximal to the enzyme active site, the phosphorylating kinase and the PLCγ cSH2 domain engage each other in six hydrogen bonding contacts away from the enzyme active site. These distal contacts include the bidentate hydrogen bonds between Glu-762 of PLCγ and Arg-580 of the kinase, two hydrogen bonds between

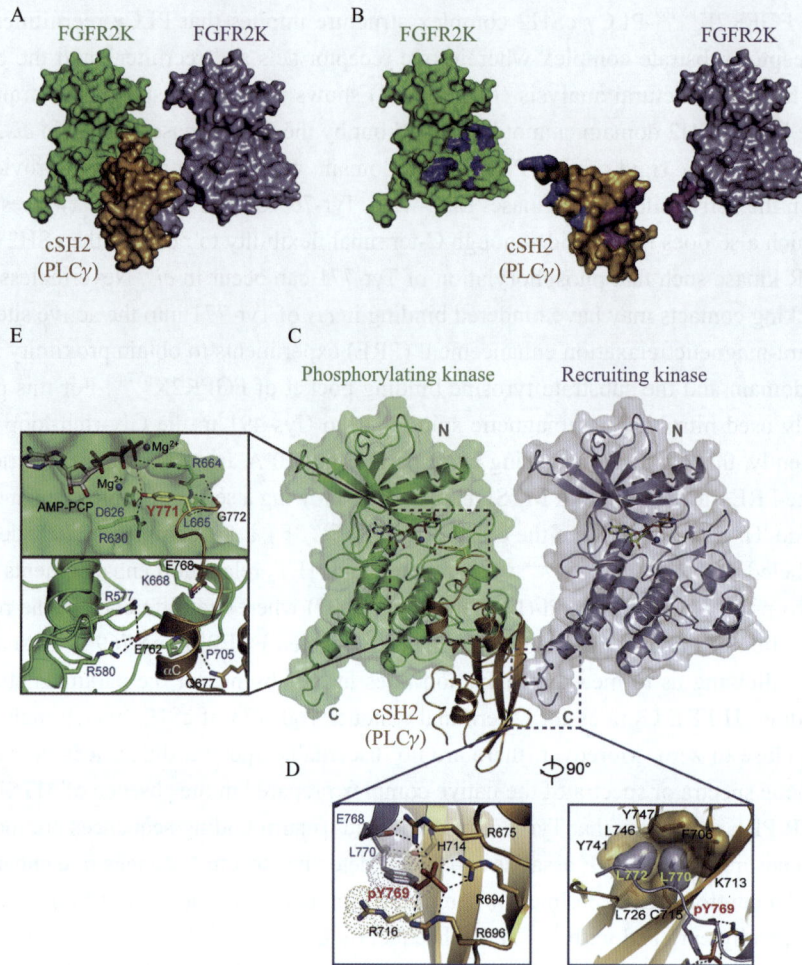

Fig. 4. Crystal structure of 2:1 FGFR2 kinase-PLCγ cSH2 complex. (A) Whole view of the 2:1 FGFR2 kinase-PLCγ cSH2 complex. (B) The binding interfaces between the cSH2 domain and the recruiting kinase are colored magenta, and those between the cSH2 domain and the phosphorylating kinase are colored blue. (C) The PTB pocket of the PLCγ cSH2 domain (in orange) is engaged by the phosphorylated tyrosine (pTyr-769) at the C-terminal tail of the recruiting kinase (in lightblue) while Tyr-771 of PLCγ is docked into the active site of the phosphorylating kinase (in green). (D) Close-up views of the interactions between the recruiting kinase and the cSH2 domain. (E) Close-up views of the interactions between the phosphorylating kinase and the PLCγ cSH2 domain. In (D) and (E), side chains of key interacting residues are shown as sticks. Hydrogen bonds are shown as dashed lines. Oxygen atoms are colored red and nitrogen atoms are colored blue. The ATP analog (AMP-PCP) and magnesium ions are rendered as sticks and blue spheres, respectively. See also Fig. S2, S4, and S6.

Glu-768 of PLCγ and Lys-668 of the kinase, and one hydrogen bond between Gln-677 of PLCγ and the kinase backbone oxygen of Pro-705 (Fig. 4E). Harmonious with the requirement for the cSH2 domain in mediating PLCγ phosphorylation by FGFR kinase, Gln-677, Glu-762, and Glu-768 are fully conserved among the PLCγ orthologs across species (Fig. S4A).

2.5 The cSH2 recruitment by FGFR2K^{pY769} induces a conformational change at the C-tail of cSH2

Based on the structure, we inferred that the engagement of pTyr binding pocket of the cSH2 domain by the recruiting kinase might induce conformational changes in the cSH2 that facilitate its phosphorylation on Tyr-771 by the phosphorylating kinase. Hence, we employed NMR spectroscopy to probe the conformational changes of the cSH2 domain upon recruitment. To this end, chemical shift perturbation of perdeuterated, ^{15}N-labeled cSH2 in the presence of FGFR2K^{pY769} were calculated and plotted as function of residue (Fig. 5A). Mapping the perturbed residues onto the crystal structure revealed three clusters of residues in the cSH2 domain that incur significant chemical shifts/signal attenuation in the presence of FGFR2K^{pY769} (Fig. 5B–D). One cluster is comprised of residues within/or close to the pTyr binding pocket that binds the phosphorylated C-terminal tail of the recruiting kinase in the crystal structure. Two other regions with significant chemical shift perturbations included the core and C-terminal tail of cSH2 domain that face the phosphorylating kinase opposite to the pTyr binding pocket. Interestingly, we observed a new set of resonances for the C-terminal residues of cSH2 domain including Tyr-771 (Fig. 5B, C), indicating that the C terminus of the cSH2 domain undergoes a conformational change when the pTyr pocket of cSH2 is engaged by the phosphorylated C-tail of FGFR2K^{pY769}.

To functionally test this possible conformational rearrangement in the cSH2 domain, we compared phosphorylation of the wild-type cSH2 and the cSH2^{R694A} mutant on Tyr-783 by FGFR2K^{pY769} *in vitro* (Fig. 5E, F, H, I). The cSH2^{R694A}

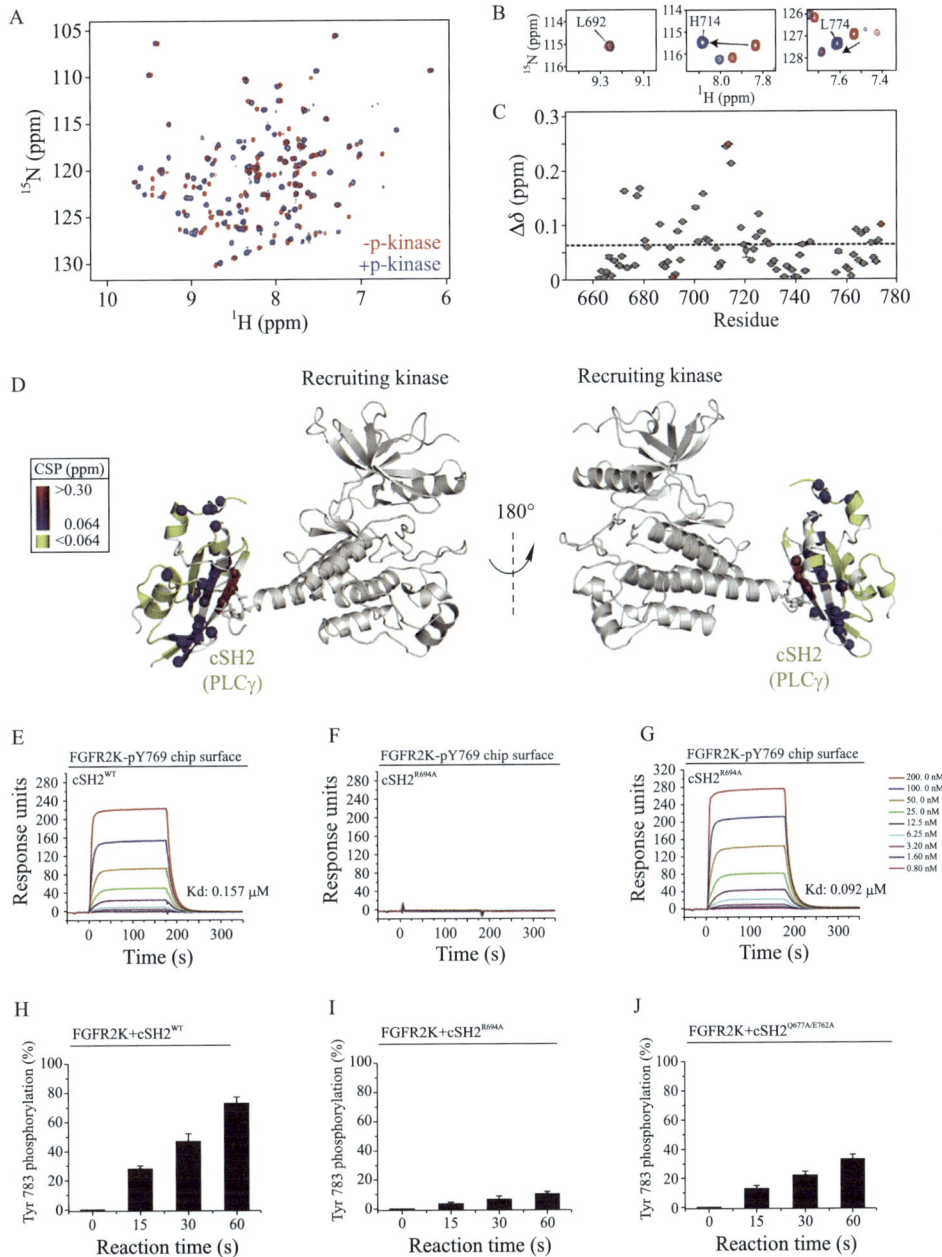

Fig. 5. Upon recruitment *via* its pTyr binding pocket to the phosphorylated tail of FGFR2K^{pY769}, the cSH2 domain experience global conformational changes that facilitate the phosphorylation of C-Terminal Tyr-771 and Tyr-783 of cSH2 by another FGFR2K^{pY769} in *Trans*. (A) Overlay of ^{1}H/^{15}N TROSY spectra of free cSH2 and a 1:1 complex of cSH2:FGFR2K^{pY769}. (B) Examples of specific residues experiencing chemical shift perturbations from (A). (C) Combined chemical shift perturbation plot showing the difference between free and bound cSH2 as a function of residue. The red circles correspond to the three residues shown in (B). (D) Chemical shift perturbations from (C) mapped onto the structure. (E–G) Comparison of binding interactions of wild-type cSH2 domain and mutants thereof harboring R694A single and Q677A/E762A double mutations by SPR. (H–J) Comparison of phosphorylation of wild-type cSH2 domain and mutants thereof harboring R694A single and Q677A/E762A double mutations using *in vitro* kinas assay. In (H)–(J), wild-type and mutated cSH2 domains were offered as substrate to the FGFR2K^{pY769} in the presence of ATP:MgCl2, and phosphorylation of cSH2 domain on Tyr-783 was quantitated using mass spectrometry. Data are represented as mean ± SEM (*n* = 3). See also Fig. S5.

mutant harbors an alanine in place of the critical arginine from the FLVR motif, which disables cSH2 domain from binding to FGFR2K^{pY769}, as determined by SPR (Fig. 5F). Compared to the wild-type cSH2, the cSH2^{R694A} mutant was phosphorylated to a significantly lower amount (Fig. 5I), supporting our NMR data that recruitment of cSH2 domain to one kinase molecule facilitates the *trans*-phosphorylation of the tyrosine located in the C-terminal tail of cSH2 domain by another kinase.

To provide further evidence for the 2:1 FGFR2K^{pY769}-cSH2 complex in solution, we studied the impact of Glu-762-Ala and Gln-677-Ala mutations on the recruitment and *trans*-phosphorylation of the cSH2 domain on Tyr-783 by the FGFR2K^{pY769} *in vitro*. As these two residues interact with the "phosphorylater" kinase (Fig. 4), we reasoned that their mutations should impair phosphorylation of the cSH2 domain on its tail tyrosine without impacting recruitment of cSH2 domain to FGFR2K^{pY769}. Consistent with the crystal structure, binding analysis by SPR spectroscopy shows that the cSH2$^{Q677A/E762A}$ mutant binds with comparable affinity to the FGFR2K^{pY769} as the wild-type cSH2 does (Fig. 5G). Despite retaining the full capacity to be recruited, the cSH2$^{Q677A/E762A}$ mutant was phosphorylated to a much lesser degree than the wild-type cSH2 domain (Fig. 5J). Lastly, we also devised an *in vitro* kinase complementation to demonstrate that phosphorylation of cSH2 domain on tyrosines occurs in *trans*. In this experiment, which is shown schematically in Fig. S5, an enzymatically dead but recruitment-able version of FGFR2K harboring the K514M mutation was monophosphorylated on Tyr-769 (pY769-FGFR2K^{dead}) by an FGFR2K lacking Tyr-769 (FGFR2K^{short}) in *trans*, which was subsequently complexed with either wild-type cSH2 domain or the cSH2$^{Q677A/E762A}$. Purified 1:1 pY769-FGFR2K^{dead}:cSH2 and pY769-FGFR2K^{dead}:cSH2$^{Q677A/E762A}$ complexes were then mixed with the recruitment-deficient FGFR2K^{short,} and time-dependent phosphorylation on Tyr-771 of cSH2 was quantitated by mass spectrometry and expressed as % total tryptic peptide containing Tyr-771. As shown in Fig. S5, the cSH2$^{Q677A/E762A}$ mutant was phosphorylated to a much lesser degree than the wild-type cSH2 domain. Taken together with the NMR results, these data provide functional evidence for formation of an allosteric 2:1 FGFR2K^{pY769}-cSH2 complex that is necessary for phosphorylation of cSH2 domain on tyrosine in solution.

2.6 Cell-based experiments validate the structurally deduced 2:1 RTK-PLCγ phosphorylation model

To test the biological relevance of our structurally deduced 2:1 RTK-substrate phosphorylation model (Fig. 6A), we also examined the impact of mutating Glu-762 and Gln-677 of PLCγ to alanine on the phosphorylation of PLCγ by activated RTKs in living cells. Consistent with the results of *in vitro* transphosphorylation, phosphorylation of PLCγ$^{Q677A/E762A}$ in cells was also significantly reduced even though PLCγ$^{Q677A/E762A}$ was effectively co-precipitated with the activated RTKs such as FGFR2, PDGFR, and VEGFR2 (Fig. 6B–D). Our ability to uncouple recruitment and phosphorylation of PLCγ from one another both *in vitro* and in living cells provides strong evidence in support of the 2:1 RTK-substrate model whereby PLCγ is engaged by two RTKs with one receptor serving as "recruiter" and the other acting as the "enzyme."

To further validate the 2:1 RTK-PLCγ recruitment/phosphorylation model, we devised a complementation assay in living cells. In this assay, two full-length RTK mutants are made as follows: one containing mutation of the lysine from the ATP binding cleft and another carrying mutation of the C-terminal tyrosine, whose phosphorylation is necessary for PLCγ recruitment, to phenylalanine. Both mutants are defective in PLCγ phosphorylation either due to lack of phosphotransfer activity ("kinase-dead") or inability to recruit PLCγ. We reasoned that if our 2:1 model holds true, then these receptor mutants should be able to complement each other in phosphorylating PLCγ when co-expressed on the surface of cells and treated with ligand. Specifically, ligand treatment should induce heterodimerization between half of these mutants (the other half being inactive mutant homodimers) allowing the enzymatically active but recruitment-deficient RTK to phosphorylate the "kinase-dead" on the C-terminal tyrosine, thereby creating a docking site for the cSH2 domain of PLCγ on the "kinase-dead" RTK. The phosphorylated "kinase-dead" RTK would then recruit PLCγ offering the substrate for phosphorylation in *trans* to the recruitment-deficient but kinase active RTK in the context of heterodimer (Fig. 7A). We chose to test this using FGFR1 and VEGFR2 as examples. A lentiviral expression system was used to express the FGFR1 mutants in BaF3 cells, which lack endogenous FGFR expression. Indeed, as shown in Fig. 7B, treatment of cells co-infected with both constructs resulted in phosphorylation of PLCγ, whereas no PLCγ phosphorylation was observed in cells infected with either of the two FGFR1 mutants individually. As predicted from our 2:1 model, the phosphorylation level of PLCγ in the co-transfected cells was about 50% of that observed in cells transfected with wild-type FGFR1 (Fig. 7B, C). As for VEGFR2, porcine aortic endothelial (PAE) cell lines stably expressing

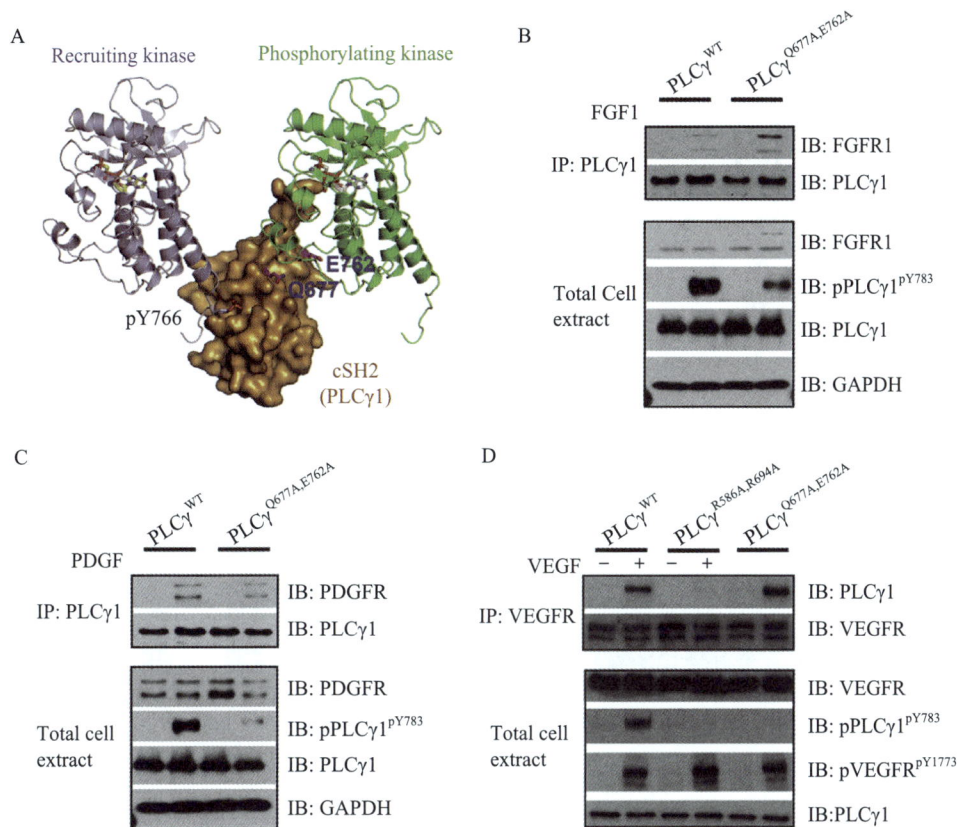

Fig. 6. Mutations of PLCγ residues that interface with the "phosphorylating" kinase impair PLCγ phosphorylation without impacting PLCγ recruitment to the FGFR, PDGFR, and VEGFR. (A) Gln-677 and Glu-762 of PLCγ and the phos-photyrosine binding pocket of cSH2 domain lie on the opposing faces of cSH2 domain. (B–D) PLCγ-null fibroblasts were transfected with expression vectors for wild-type PLCγ and the indicated PLCγ mutants. Following cell stimulation with 50 ng/ml FGF1, PDGF, or VEGF, cell lysates were blotted with the indicated antibodies. See also Fig. S5.

kinase-dead (VEGFR2^{K866R}) or recruitment-deficient (VEGFR2^{Y1173F}) VEGFR2 mutants were made. The VEGFR2^{Y1173F}-expressing cells were then used to infect with retrovirus expression vector for recruitment-deficient VEGFR2^{K866R}. Upon treatment with VEGF, there was no detectable phosphorylation of PLCγ in the VEGFR2^{K866R} or VEGFR2^{Y1173F} cells. In contrast, in VEGFR2^{Y1173F} cells infected with retroviral vector for VEGFR2^{K866R}, phosphorylation of PLCγ was induced upon ligand treatment (Fig. 7D, E). These cell-based data unambiguously demonstrate that substrate phosphorylation occurs in the context of an FGFR or VEGFR dimer wherein one receptor monomer serves as the recruiter and the other acts as the phosphorylating enzyme.

Our identification of cSH2 domain as the principal mediator of PLCγ recruitment to FGFR2 is diametrically opposed to the previously reported crystal structure of the activated FGFR1 kinase complexed with the tandem nSH2-cSH2 domain fragment of PLCγ (PDB: 3GQI) (Bae *et al.*, 2009) showing that this tandem construct is recruited *via* nSH2 domain. Notably, 3GQI does not provide a satisfactory explanation as to how the nSH2-mediated recruitment would facilitate PLCγ phosphorylation, as none of the phosphorylation sites that follow the cSH2 domain are engaged by the FGFR1 kinase. In fact, the PLCγ phosphorylation site (Tyr-771) is over 60 Å away from the active site of FGFR1 kinase (Bae *et al.*, 2009) (Fig. S6). These disparities prompted us to carefully inspect the 3GQI (Bae *et al.*, 2009) structure. Upon close inspection, it appears that the presence of decavanadate complex ions in the crystallization conditions together with crystal packing contacts (Fig. S6) have contributed to non- physiological binding of the nSH2 domain of PLCγ to the activated FGFR1 kinase.

Insights into the preferential binding of FGFR and other RTKs to the cSH2 domain of PLCγ can be gleaned through sequence alignment of PLCγ recruitment sites from several RTKs that utilize PLCγ as their common intracellular substrate. Relative to cSH2, the hydrophobic hole of the socket in nSH2 appears narrower due to insertion of three residues in the loop between aB helix and bG strand (Fig. S4A, B). Additionally, substitution of Arg-696 of cSH2 domain with

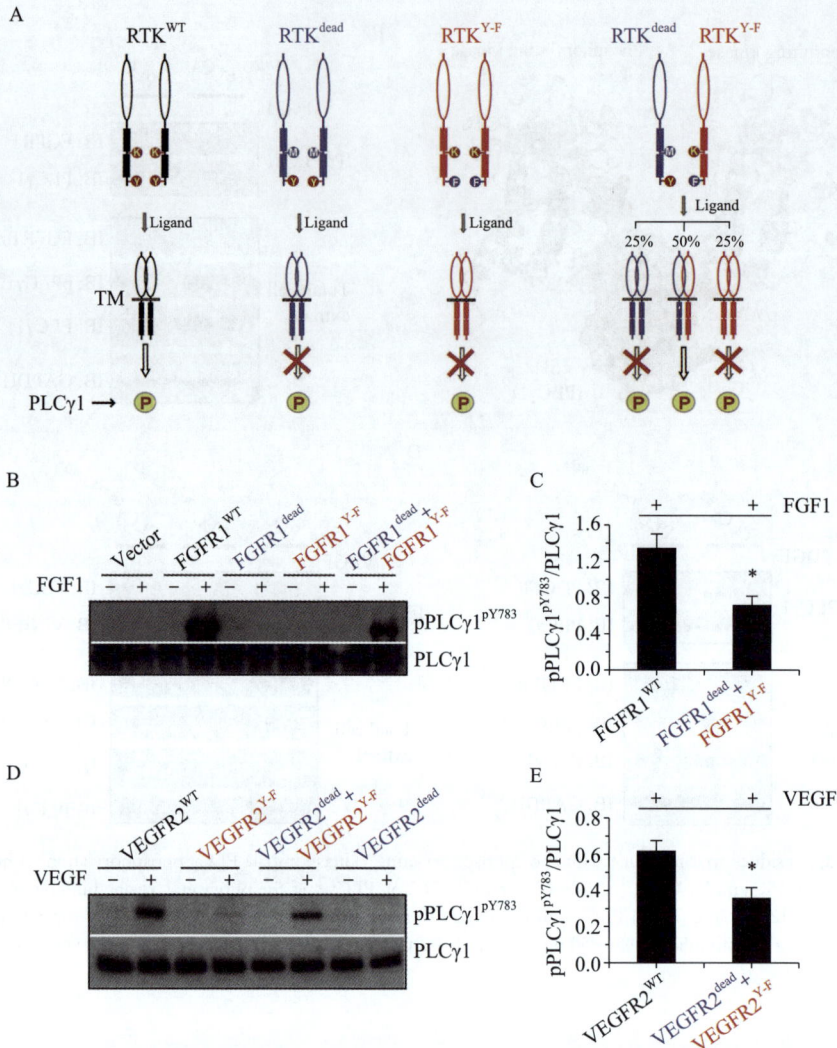

Fig. 7. Receptor complementation experiment confirms the validity of the 2:1 RTK-substrate model in living cells. (A) Schematic of the receptor complementation experiment used to validate the 2:1 RTK-substrate model in living cells. RTK^{dead} is devoid of kinase activity and hence cannot phosphorylate PLCγ. RTKY-F is catalytically active but is also defective in phosphorylating PLCγ as it cannot recruit PLCγ. (B and C) FGFR1^{Dead}(FGFR1^{K514M}) and FGFR1^{Y-F}(FGFR1^{Y766F}) receptors complement each other in phosphorylating PLCγ. BaF3 cells were infected with lentiviral expression vectors for FGFR1^{WT}, FGFR1^{K514M}, and FGFR1^{Y766F} individually or co-infected with FGFR1K514M and FGFR1^{Y766F}. Cells were stimulated with FGF1, and cell lysates were analyzed by western blotting with the indicated antibodies (B). Semi-quantitation of the phosphorylation level of PLCγ was from western blotting result (C). Data are represented as mean ± SEM (n = 3), *P < 0.01. (D and E) VEGFR2^{dead}(VEGFR2^{K866R}) and VEGFR2Y-F(VEGFR2^{Y1173F}) receptors complement each other in phosphorylating PLCγ. Cells were stimulated with VEGF, and cell lysates derived from PAE cells stably expressing wild-type VEGFR2, VEGFR-2^{Y1173F} alone, or co-expressing VEGFR2^{Y1173F} with kinase-dead receptor, and VEGFR2^{K866R} alone, were blotted for total PLCγ1 and phospho-PLCγ1 (D). Semiquantitation of the phosphorylation level of PLCγ was from western blotting result (E). Data are represented as mean ± SEM (n = 3), *P < 0.01. See also Fig. S5 and S7.

Ser-588 in nSH2 domain in the hydrophilic hole of socket should also reduce the overall affinity of nSH2 domain for pTyr containing peptides. As shown in Fig. 4D, Arg-696 of cSH2 domain, which makes two tight hydrogen bonds with phosphate moiety of pTyr-769, is not conserved in the nSH2 domain of PLCγ (Ser-588 in nSH2) (Fig. S4A). Interestingly, in all RTKs, the PLCγ recruitment sites maps to the C-terminal tail of the receptor not too far from the aI helix, the last secondary structure element of the kinase domain. In fact, in FGFRs, VEGFRs, TRKs, C-KIT, CSF1R, and RET the recruitment sites are nearly equidistant from the predicted end of kinase domain (Fig. S4C). Based on these observations, it is likely that additional selectivity for cSH2 domain may be achieved due to steric factors in the quaternary structure that are more permissible for cSH2 than nSH2 domain.

2.7 Structural basis for the post-phosphorylation dissociation step of PLCγ from RTKs

Once phosphorylation of PLCγ is completed, the phosphorylated PLCγ must dissociate from the recruiting receptor kinase so that the next cycle of recruitment and phosphorylation can ensue. Phosphorylated Tyr-783 has been shown to fold over and bind in *cis* to the cSH2 domain of PLCγ (Bunney *et al.*, 2012; DeBell *et al.*, 2007; Poulin *et al.*, 2005). This intramolecular interaction induces a major structural rearrangement in PLCγ, which relieves PLCγ autoinhibition, thereby elevating the lipase activity of the enzyme (Bunney *et al.*, 2012; Poulin *et al.*, 2000, 2005). According to our structure, such a *cis* interaction would compete with binding of pTyr-769 of the recruiting FGFR2 kinase to the cSH2 domain, thus forcing the phosphorylated PLCγ to come off the recruiting receptor. To test this hypothesis, we prepared cSH2 domain phosphorylated on Tyr783 (pY783-cSH2) and examined its interaction with FGFR2K^{pY769} using SPR spectroscopy. As shown in Fig. S7A, pY783-cSH2 failed to bind FGFR2K^{pY769}, supporting the model that the intramolecular interaction between phosphorylated Tyr-783 and the cSH2 domain of PLCγ competes with pTyr-769 of the FGFR2 kinase for binding to the cSH2 domain. Hence, our data provide a plausible molecular basis for how PLCγ is disengaged from the activated FGFR once phosphorylation of PLCγ is completed (Fig. S7B). Notably, our structural data expose the presence of an elegant coupling mechanism between phosphorylation-induced disengagement of PLCγ from FGFR and phospholipase activation of PLCγ.

In summary, the structural and biochemical data presented in this manuscript clearly establish that the recruitment and phosphorylation of SH2-containing substrates, a fundamental process in RTK signaling, is achieved in the context of a receptor dimer wherein one monomer recruits the substrate and offers it to the second monomer that acts as the "enzyme". Thus, our findings overturn the current paradigm that SH2-mediated recruitment and phosphorylation are carried out by the same receptor (i.e., in *cis*). Moreover, our 2:1 *trans* model suggests that SH2 binding specificity is achieved at the quaternary level within an RTK dimer, thus challenging the current view regarding determinants of specificity of substrate recognition by an RTK. Our data identify an unprecedented role for receptor dimerization in substrate phosphorylation in addition to its canonical role in kinase activation. In addition to providing the molecular basis for one of the fundamental steps in RTK signaling, our data will have major impact on future drug discovery efforts in the RTK field. Essentially all of the current RTK inhibitors target the ATP binding pockets and often are cross-reactive between RTKs due to the significant sequence conservation of ATP binding pockets among RTKs. In addition, these inhibitors indiscriminately block all the pathways downstream of RTKs, including those that may not be involved in a particular disease. Based on our model, it would be now possible to discover drugs that interfere with binding of PLCγ to the "phosphorylating" FGFR. Such drugs would selectively inhibit the PLCγ pathway in human diseases such as myeloproliferative syndrome, where PLCγ signaling has been shown to be a critical downstream effector of the ZNF198-FGFR1 fusion gene (Roumiantsev *et al.*, 2004).

3. Experimental procedures

3.1 Cell culture and immunoblotting experiments

Transient transfection of *PLCγ1*$^{-/-}$ mouse embryo fibroblasts (MEFs) (generous gift from Dr. Graham Carpenter) with pRK5 expression vectors for PLCγ1 (N$^+$C$^+$), PLCγ1^{R586A} (N$^-$C$^+$), PLCγ1^{R694A} (N$^+$C$^-$), and PLCγ1^{R586A,R694A} (N$^-$C$^-$) was done using lipofectamine 2000 according to manufacturer's protocol. The FUCRW lentiviral vector (Memarzadeh *et al.*, 2007) was used to express wild-type and mutated FGFR2 and VEGFR2 molecules in BaF3 and PAE cell lines, respectively, for receptor complementation experiments. Full details are described in Supplemental Experimental Procedures.

3.2 Phosphatidylinositol hydrolysis assay in PLCγ1$^{-/-}$ MEF cells

IP3 formation was measured as previously described (Everett *et al.*, 2009) and detailed in Supplemental Experimental Procedures.

3.3 Protein expression and purification

All the wild-type and mutated FGFR kinases, wild-type and mutated tandem nSH2-cSH2 domains, and individual nSH2 and cSH2 domains, including the isotopically enriched cSH2 (U-^{15}N, U-^{15}N/^{13}C, U-^{2}H/^{15}N), were expressed in *coli* (BL21) and purified as described in Supplemental Experimental Procedures.

3.4 In vitro binding assays

The ITC, SPR spectroscopy, SEC, native gel electrophoresis, and NMR spectroscopy were used to determine the binding selectivity of the PLCγ SH2 domains toward FGFR2K^{pY769}. For full experimental details, please refer to the Supplemental Experimental Procedures.

3.5 PRE experiments

Prior to incorporation of the spin label, FGFR2K^{pY769} was treated with 20 mM DTT for 15 min in a buffer containing 20 mM Tris-HCl (pH 7.5) and 150 mM NaCl. The protein was then exchanged into a buffer containing 20 mM Tris-HCl (pH 6.5) and 150 mM NaCl and diluted to a concentration of 40 mM. A 150 mM solution of S-(1-oxyl-2,2,5,5-tetramethyl-2,5-dihydro-1H-pyrrol-3-yl) methyl methanesulfonothioate (MTSL) in acetonitrile was added in half-molar equivalent portions every 10 min on ice. The progress of the reaction was monitored using a Bruker ultrafleXtreme^{TM} MALDI-TOF. Fully labeled FGFR2K^{pY769} was buffer exchanged into 25 mM HEPES (pH 7.5), 150 mM NaCl 0.1% NaN$_3$, and 5% D2O and added to a sample of 70% deuterated cSH2 to give a final molar ratio of 1.4:1, FGFR2K-pY769:cSH2. A two-point ^{1}H/^{15}N TROSY method was used to calculate ^{1}HN T2 relaxation enhancement values (G$_2$) as previously described (Iwahara et al., 2007) and detailed in Supplemental Experimental Procedures.

3.6 Crystallization and structure determination

Crystals of FGFR2K^{pY769}-cSH2 complex were grown by hanging drop vapor diffusion at 4℃ using crystallization buffer composed of 25 mM HEPES (pH 7.5), PEG 20000 (12%–18%), and 2% (w/v) Benzamidine hydrochloride. Diffraction data were processed using HKL2000 Suite (Otwinowski and Minor, 1997). Molecular replacement solutions for the FGFR2 kinase and the cSH2 domain were found by the program Phaser in CCP4 Suite (Collaborative Computational Project Number 4, 1994) using the crystal structure of FGFR2 kinase (PDB: 2PVY) (Chen et al., 2007) and the crystal structure of cSH2 domain (PDB: 3GQI) (Bae et al., 2009) as the search model, respectively. Model building was carried out using Coot (Emsley and Cowtan, 2004), and iterative positional and B-factor refinements were done using PHENIX (Adams et al., 2002). The refined structure shows good geometry and Ramachandran statistics. Data collection and structure refinement statistics are listed in Table 1. Full details are described in Supplemental Experimental Procedures.

Supplemental information

Supplemental information to this article can be found online at http://dx.doi.org/10.1016/j.molcel.2015.11.010.

References

[1] Adams PD, Grosse-Kunstleve RW, Hung LW, et al. PHENIX: building new software for automated crystallographic structure determination[J]. Acta Crystallographica Section D-Biological Crystallography, 2002, 58: 1948-1954.

[2] Bae JH, Lew ED, Yuzawa S, et al. The selectivity of receptor tyrosine kinase signaling is Controlled by a Secondary SH2 Domain Binding Site[J]. Cell, 2009, 138(3): 514-524.

[3] Bailey S. The CCP4 suite-programs for protein crystallography[J]. Acta Crystallographica Section D-Biological Crystallography, 1994, 50: 760-763.

[4] Bunney TD, Esposito D, Mas-Droux C, et al. Structural and functional integration of the PLC gamma interaction domains critical for regulatory mechanisms and signaling deregulation[J]. Structure, 2012, 20(12): 2062-2075.

[5] Chen H, Huang Z, Dutta K, et al. Cracking the molecular origin of intrinsic tyrosine kinase activity through analysis of pathogenic gain-of-function mutations[J]. Cell Reports, 2013, 4(2): 376-384.

[6] Chen H, Ma J, Li W, et al. A molecular brake in the kinase hinge region regulates the activity of receptor tyrosine kinases[J]. Molecular Cell, 2007, 27(5): 717-730.

[7] Chen H, Xu CF, Ma J, et al. A crystallographic snapshot of tyrosine trans-phosphorylation in action[J]. Proceedings Of the National Academy Of Sciences Of the United States Of America, 2008, 105(50): 19660-19665.

[8] DeBell K, Graham L, Reischl I, et al. Intramolecular regulation of phospholipase C-gamma 1 by its C-terminal Src homology 2 domain[J]. Molecular And Cellular Biology, 2007, 27(3): 854-863.

[9] Ellis MV, James SR, Perisic O, et al. Catalytic domain of phosphoinositide-specific phospholipase C (PLC) -Mutational analysis of residues within the active site and hydrophobic ridge of PLC delta 1[J]. Journal Of Biological Chemistry, 1998, 273(19): 11650-11659.

[10] Emsley P, Cowtan K. Coot: model-building tools for molecular graphics[J]. Acta Crystallographica Section D-Biological Crystallography, 2004, 60: 2126-2132.

[11] Eswarakumar VP, Lax I, Schlessinger J. Cellular signaling by fibroblast growth factor receptors[J]. Cytokine & Growth Factor Reviews, 2005, 16(2): 139-149.

[12] Goetz R, Mohammadi M. Exploring mechanisms of FGF signalling through the lens of structural biology[J]. Nature Reviews Molecular Cell Biology, 2013, 14(3): 166-180.

[13] Hidaka M, Homma Y, Takenawa T. Highly conserved 8 amino-acid-sequence in SH2 is important for recognition of phosphotyrosine site[J]. Biochemical And Biophysical Research Communications, 1991, 180(3): 1490-1497.

[14] Hubbard SR. Juxtamembrane autoinhibition in receptor tyrosine kinases[J]. Nature Reviews Molecular Cell Biology, 2004, 5(6): 464-470.

[15] Hunter T. Signaling-2000 and beyond[J]. Cell, 2000, 100(1): 113-127.

[16] Hunter T. Tyrosine phosphorylation in cell signaling and disease[J]. Keio Journal of Medicine, 2002, 51(2): 61-71.

[17] Iwahara J, Tang C, Clore GM. Practical aspects of H-1 transverse paramagnetic relaxation enhancement measurements on macromolecules[J]. Journal Of Magnetic Resonance, 2007, 184(2): 185-195.

[18] Ji QS, Winnier GE, Niswender KD, et al. Essential role of the tyrosine kinase substrate phospholipase C-gamma 1 in mammalian growth and development[J]. Proceedings Of the National Academy Of Sciences Of the United States Of America, 1997, 94(7): 2999-3003.

[19] Jura N, Zhang X, Endres NF, et al. Catalytic control in the EGF receptor and its connection to general kinase regulatory mechanisms[J]. Molecular Cell, 2011, 42(1): 9-22.

[20] Kim HK, Kim JW, Zilberstein A, et al. PDGF stimulation of inositol phospholipid hydrolysis requires plc-gamma-1 phosphorylation on tyrosine residues 783 and 1254[J]. Cell, 1991, 65(3): 435-441.

[21] Lemmon MA, Schlessinger J. Cell signaling by receptor tyrosine kinases[J]. Cell, 2010, 141(7): 1117-1134.

[22] Liu BA, Engelmann BW, Jablonowski K, et al. SRC homology 2 domain binding sites in insulin, IGF-1 and FGF receptor mediated signaling networks reveal an extensive potential interactome[J]. Cell Communication And Signaling, 2012, 10.

[23] Memarzadeh S, Xin L, Mulholland DJ, et al. Enhanced paracrine FGF10 expression promotes formation of multifocal prostate adenocarcinoma and an increase in epithelial androgen receptor[J]. Cancer Cell, 2007, 12(6): 572-585.

[24] Mohammadi M, Honegger AM, Rotin D, et al. A tyrosine-phosphorylated carboxy-terminal peptide of the fibroblast growth-factor receptor (flg) is a binding-site for the SH2 domain of phospholipase c-gamma-1[J]. Molecular And Cellular Biology, 1991, 11(10): 5068-5078.

[25] Naski MC, Wang Q, Xu JS, et al. Graded activation of fibroblast

growth factor receptor 3 by mutations causing achondroplasia and thanatophoric dysplasia[J]. Nature Genetics, 1996, 13(2): 233-237.

[26] Otwinowski Z, Minor W. Processing of X-ray diffraction data collected in oscillation mode[J]. Macromolecular Crystallography, Pt A, 1997, 276: 307-326.

[27] Pascal SM, Singer AU, Gish G, et al. Nuclear-magnetic-resonance structure of an SH2 domain of phospholipase C-gamma-1 complexed with a high-affinity binding peptide[J]. Cell, 1994, 77(3): 461-472.

[28] Pawson T. Specificity in signal transduction: From phosphotyrosine-SH2 domain interactions to complex cellular systems[J]. Cell, 2004, 116(2): 191-203.

[29] Pellicena P, Kuriyan J. Protein-protein interactions in the allosteric regulation of protein kinases[J]. Current Opinion In Structural Biology, 2006, 16(6): 702-709.

[30] Peters KG, Marie J, Wilson E, et al. Point mutation of an fgf receptor abolishes phosphatidylinositol turnover and Ca^{2+} flux but not mitogenesis[J]. Nature, 1992, 358(6388): 678-681.

[31] Poulin B, Sekiya F, Rhee SG. Differential roles of the Src homology 2 domains of phospholipase C-gamma 1 (PLC-gamma 1) in platelet-derived growth factor-induced activation of PLC-gamma 1 in intact cells[J]. Journal Of Biological Chemistry, 2000, 275(9): 6411-6416.

[32] Poulin B, Sekiya F, Rhee SG. Intramolecular interaction between phosphorylated tyrosine-783 and the C-terminal Src homology 2 domain activates phospholipase C-gamma 1[J]. Proceedings Of the National Academy Of Sciences Of the United States Of America, 2005, 102(12): 4276-4281.

[33] Rajakulendran T, Sicheri F. Allosteric Protein kinase regulation by pseudokinases: insights from STRAD[J]. Science Signaling, 2010, 3(111).

[34] Rotin D, Honegger AM, Margolis BL, et al. Presence of SH2 domains of phospholipase-C-gamma-1 enhances substrate phosphorylation by increasing the affinity toward the epidermal growth-factor receptor[J]. Journal Of Biological Chemistry, 1992, 267(14): 9678-9683.

[35] Roumiantsev S, Krause DS, Neumann CA, et al. Distinct stem cell myeloproliferative/T lymphoma syndromes induced by ZNF198-FGFR1 and BCR-FGFR1 fusion genes from 8p11 translocations[J]. Cancer Cell, 2004, 5(3): 287-298.

[36] Schlessinger J. Phospholipase C gamma activation and phosphoinositide hydrolysis are essential for embryonal development[J]. Proceedings Of the National Academy Of Sciences Of the United States Of America, 1997, 94(7): 2798-2799.

[37] Schlessinger J, Lemmon MA. SH2 and PTB domains in tyrosine kinase signaling[J]. Science's STKE : signal transduction knowledge environment, 2003, 2003(191): RE12-RE12.

A solid-phase PEGylation strategy for protein therapeutics using a potent FGF21 analog

Lintao Song, Xiaokun Li , Zhifeng Huang

1. Introduction

Fibroblast growth factors (FGFs) are widely expressed in fetal and adult tissues [1], and play critical roles in multiple physiological functions, including angiogenesis, mitogenesis, pattern formation, cell differentiation, metabolic regulation and tissue injury repair [2]. The 209-amino acid fibroblast growth factor 21 (FGF21) is predicted to be a structural homolog to FGF19 and FGF23 [3], which together comprise the FGF19 subfamily. Due to their atypical b-trefoil fold, FGF19 subfamily members exhibit poor heparin sulfate (HS) binding affinity. This enables FGF19 members to diffuse away from the extracellular matrix and into the plasma, allowing them to act in tissues far from their source of secretion and production, and thus justifying their classification as endocrine-acting FGFs [4-6]. Coexpression of β-klotho, and FGFR c-isoforms dictate the tissue-specific activity of FGF21 [7], which has been shown to be active in adipose tissue, pancreatic and liver organs, without apparent mitogenicity in a number of cell types [8]. Since the initial identification of FGF21 as an important metabolic regulator, this protein has become the focus of intense research in the area of glucose and lipid homeostasis and is an important target for drug development initiatives [4].

As the type 2 diabetic (T2D) patient population is expected to increase dramatically [9], developing treatments of metabolic disorders associated with T2D has become critical. The pathobiology of T2D is typically referred to as an "insulin-resistant" state, whereby the body is unable to regulate its blood glucose by a failure of insulin uptake [10,11]. FGF21 was originally identified in a screen for molecules modulating glucose uptake in 3T3-L1 adipocytes [4], and has since been examined for its potential use in the treatment of T2D [12-15]. Administration of recombinant human FGF21 in preclinical animal models lowered blood glucose, insulin, as well as circulating triglycerides and cholesterol levels, improved insulin sensitivity, energy expenditure, and obesity [4,13,16]. In diabetic rhesus monkeys, treatment also resulted in a significant improvement of lipoprotein profiles, which included reduced low-density cholesterol and increased high-density cholesterol, and the loss of body weight [16]. Furthermore, transgenic mice over-expressing FGF21 are lean and insulin-sensitive, whereas FGF21 knockout mice are mildly obese and insulin-resistant [17,18].

It has become clear that native FGF21 has pharmaceutical limitations, such as short serum half-life and low bioavailability, which has diminished its attraction for clinical testing and has forestalled its development [14,16]. Recent clinical trials of an FGF21 variant, LY2405319 (LY), have shown promising effects in regulating triglyceride and fasting insulin levels. However, glucose levels post-treatment were not significantly affected, perhaps due to the proteins' short serum half-life, despite its increased thermostability *in vitro* [19,20].

Polyethylene glycol (PEG) modification is regarded as one of the most successful strategies employed to modify native proteins to obtain an increase in body-residence time, protein stability and a decrease in immunogenicity [21]. It has been previously reported that PEGylated interleukin-2 (IL-2) [22], monoclonal antibody A7 [23], interferon α-2α [24] and immunotoxin [25], exhibited superior clinical properties compared to corresponding non-PEGylated molecules. PEGylation delays serum drug accumulation and prolongs its half-life, which improves the patients' compliance by greatly reducing the frequency of drug administration [26]. However, the lack of site-specific modification and multiple attachments of PEG to protein targets commonly cause a dramatic decrease in *in vitro* bioactivity, thus partially limiting the practical application of liquid-phase PEGylation. As the PEG-maleimides (PEG-MAL) react rapidly with reduced thiol (eSH groups) cysteines forming a stable thioether [27], a site-specific and wellcontrolled mono-PEGylation strategy utilizing introduced cysteine residues would increase the homogeneity of the products, and potentially improve their clinical application.

In this study, we hypothesized that the pharmacological properties of FGF21 can be improved by stabilizing the protein. To achieve this, stabilizing cysteine substitutions were introduced into FGF21 based on the FGF19 structure and sequence. Further stabilization of ligand was obtained by conjugating the FGF21 variant with PEG on the Ni-NTA resin as solid-phase.

2. Materials and methods

2.1 Materials

The PCR purification kit, gel extraction kit, bicinchoninic acid (BCA) kit, QuikChange site-directed mutagenesis kit, plasmid miniprep kit, *Pyrobest*® DNA Polymerase and restriction enzymes, *Nde* I and *Xho* I, were purchased from TaKaRa Company (Japan). In addition, 20 kDa PEG-maleimides (mPEG-MAL), isopropyl-1-thio-β-d-galactopyranoside (IPTG) were purchased from Sigmae Aldrich (St. Louis, MO, USA). The Ni-NTA resin column and Q-Sepharose FF column, and AKTA purifier were purchased from GE Healthcare (Piscataway, NJ, USA). Dulbecco's modified Eagle medium (DMEM) and small ubiquitin-like modifier (SUMO) protease were purchased from Invitrogen (Carlsbad, CA). All solvents were of analytical grade.

2.2 Expression and purification of SUMO-FGF21 variants

Recombinant human FGF21 (FGF21^{WT}) and its variant proteins were expressed in *Escherichia coli*. For the cysteine mutants, an FGF21^{WT} construct was used, and Ala59Cys (FGF21^{A59C}), Gly71Cys (FGF21^{G71C}), and Ala59Cys/Gly71Cys (FGF21^{A59C,G71C}) mutations were introduced into the expression vector using the QuikChange site-directed mutagenesis kit. Next, using a PCR fusion technique, the amplified PCR products (containing the fusion gene consisting of SUMO and mutant FGF21) was digested with *Nde* I and *Xho* I, and then ligated into the previously digested pET3c expression vectors to create pET3c-SUMO-FGF21 constructs, and transformed into BL21(DE3) competent cells. The recombinant plasmids encoding FGF21 variant proteins were cultured in a shaker at 37℃ and 200 rpm in 1 L Luriae Bertani (LB) medium containing 2% glucose and 100 μg/ml ampicillin until the cell density reached an OD_{600} of 0.6–0.8. The cells were induced with a final concentration of 1 mM isopropyl-L-thio-β-D-galactopyranoside (IPTG) and then incubated for an additional 4 h at 37℃ with shaking at 200 rpm. The expressed FGF21 variant proteins were confirmed using 12% sodium dodecyl sulfate polyacrylamide gel electrophoresis (SDS-PAGE) and western blotting analyses.

The bacteria were harvested by centrifugation at 5 000 rpm for 10 min at 4℃, and the cell pellets were resuspended in 20 mM PBS buffer. Next, the cells were dissolved by sonication in an ice bath. The suspensions were centrifuged at 12 000 rpm for 30 min at 4℃, and the cleared supernatant was collected (soluble fraction). The desired protein was purified using a DEAE-Sepharose FF column, followed by further purification with Ni-NTA resin. Finally, His-tagged SUMO-FGF21 variant proteins were collected from the column with elution buffer (20 mM PBS containing 300 mM imidazole and 150 mM NaCl, pH 8.0). The purity of SUMO-FGF21 was assessed using 12% SDS-PAGE and the concentration was evaluated using a bicinchoninic acid (BCA) kit (Perbio Science, Bonn, Germany).

2.3 Solid-phase PEGylation and purification of FGF21 variants

For the production of PEGylated FGF21 variants, we adopted solid-phase PEGylation for the site-specific modification of FGF21 variants. Three major procedures were performed: (1) 2 ml of 0.1 mM SUMO-FGF21 in HEPES buffer (20 mM HEPES, pH 7.5) was applied and bound on Ni-NTA affinity chromatography. Due to the high binding affinity, SUMO-FGF21 completely bound onto the column as evidenced by the fact that no protein was detected in the flow-through after application of the protein sample on the column. (2) A solution containing 4.8 ml of 0.5 mM mPEG-MAL was circulated in the column at low flow rate (0.01 ml/min) for specific reaction time at 4℃. Finally, 20 ml of equilibrium buffer (20 mM HEPES, 25 mM NaCl, pH 7.5) was used to wash the non-reacted mPEG-MAL. (3) The reaction complex was completely eluted by applying 200 mM imidazole in HEPES buffer (pH 7.5) at a rate of 1 ml/min. The eluate was collected and confirmed using 12% SDS-PAGE and stored at –20℃ for subsequent experiments.

The eluted fusion protein was concentrated and diluted to a concentration of 1 mg/ml. Ten units of SUMO protease were added to the dilution and the mixture was incubated in HEPES buffer (20 mM HEPES, pH 7.5) for 1 h at 4 ℃. Following incubation, the mixture was loaded onto the Q-Sepharose Fast Flow column, The column was further washed with 10 column volumes (CVs) of TriseHCl buffer (20 mM TriseHCl, pH 8.0), and then eluted with TriseHCl buffer containing different concentrations of NaCl. All elution fractions were collected and analyzed using 12% SDS-PAGE. The FGF21 variant proteins was further concentrated and desalted by ultrafiltration at 4 ℃.

2.4 Cell culture, adipocyte differentiation, glucose uptake experiments

3T3-L1 preadipocytes (American Type Culture Collection, Rockville, MD, USA) were seeded at 25×10^3 cells/well, and differentiation was induced 2 days later in DMEM supplemented with 10% fetal bovine serum (FBS), 1 μM dexamethasone, 0.25 mM 3-isobutyl-1-methylxanthine (IBMX), 2 μM insulin, 10 mM HEPES/MEM, nonessential amino acids, and penicillin/streptomycin, and differentiation medium without dexamethasone and IBMX for as additional 2 days [4]. Thereafter, the cells were incubated for an additional 9–20 days in DMEM/10% FBS (changed every other day). Accumulation of lipid droplets was observed in >95% of cells after 7 days, and the cells at day 7–10 were used for further experiments.

For glucose uptake, 3T3-L1 adipocytes were serum-starved overnight, and then stimulated with 100 nM of FGF21^{WT}, FGF21 variants (FGF21^{A59C}, FGF21^{G71C} and FGF21^{A59C,G71C}), and PEGylated FGF21 variant (PEG-FGF21^{G71C}) for 24 h, and then washed twice with KRP buffer (15 mM HEPES, pH 7.4, 118 mM NaCl, 4.8 mM KCl, 1.2 mM MgSO$_4$, 1.3 mM CaCl$_2$, 1.2 mM KH$_2$PO$_4$, and 0.1% BSA), and 100 μl of KRP buffer containing 2-deoxy-D-$^{[14C]}$glucose (2-DOG) (0.1 μCi, 100 μM) was added to each well. Furthermore, the control wells contained 100 μl of KRP buffer with 2-DOG (0.1 μCi, 100 μM) to monitor for nonspecificity. The uptake reaction was performed at 37 ℃ for 1 h, terminated by the addition of cytochalasin B (20 μM), and measured using the Wallac 1450 MicroBeta counter (Perkin Elmer, Waltham, MA, USA).

2.5 Mass spectrometry and circular dichroism spectroscopy analysis

Mass spectra were acquired using an Applied Biosystems Voyager System DE PRO MALDI-TOF mass spectrometer (Carlsbad, CA, USA) with a nitrogen laser. The matrix was a saturated solution of R-cyano-4-hydroxycinnamic acid in a 50:50 mixture of acetonitrile and water containing 0.1% trifluoroacetic acid. Purified solid-phase PEG-FGF21^{G71C} and matrix were mixed at a ratio of 1:1, and 1 μl was spotted onto a 100-well sample plate. All spectra were acquired in positive mode, and over the range of 600–2500 Da under reflectron conditions (20 kV accelerating voltage, 350 ns extraction delay time), and 2–100 kDa under linear conditions (25 kV accelerating voltage, 750 ns extraction delay time).

The secondary structure of the FGF21^{WT}, FGF21^{G71C} and solid-phase PEGylated FGF21 (PEG-FGF21^{G71C}) were determined using a circular dichroic (CD) spectropolarimeter (Jasco, Tokyo, Japan). Far-UV CD spectra were recorded at wave-lengths between 190 and 250 nm using a 0.1 cm path length cell at 25 ℃ with a protein concentration of 6 μM in 10 μM PBS, pH 7.5. Each spectrum was a representative of three scans and the CD spectra were corrected for buffer contributions.

2.6 Bio-stability and pharmacokinetic evaluation of solid-phase PEGylated FGF21^{G71C}

To determine the effect of site-directed mutation and solid-phase PEGylation on the biological stability of FGF21 at a physiologically relevant temperature, FGF21^{WT}, FGF21^{G71C} and PEG-FGF21^{G71C} were incubated at a concentration of 0.01 mM at 37 ℃ in mouse serum at specific time periods as described previously [28]. The samples were then subjected to the glucose uptake assay, and quantified using the human FGF21 immunoassay ELISA assay as reported previously [29]. To more specifically evaluate the thermal stability of proteins, the FGF21^{WT}, FGF21^{G71C} and PEG-FGF21^{G71C} were incubated at 37 ℃ for different time points in PBS buffer and the activity of proteins was examined using glucose uptake assay as described above.

The in vivo half-life of non-PEGylated and PEGylated proteins were analyzed by intravenously (i.v.) injecting a single dose of 0.5 mg/kg of FGF21^{WT}, FGF21^{A59C}, FGF21^{G71C}, FGF21^{A59C,G71C} or PEG-FGF21G71C in Male Sprague Dawley (SD) adult rats (220–250 g), and measurements of the dynamic levels of proteins in blood using the human FGF21 immunoassay ELISA kit (R&D, MN, USA). The pharmacokinetic parameters of the test proteins were determined using the Drug and Statistics Software (DAS, v2.0; Mathematical Pharmacology Professional Committee of China). The elimination half-life ($t_{1/2}$) was calculated using the formula, $t_{1/2} = 0.693/K_e$ (K_e stands for elimination rate constant). Furthermore, the test proteins of various tissues were also quantified using the human FGF21 immunoassay ELISA kit.

2.7　Functional evaluation of PEG-FGF21^{G71C} in ob/ob mice

2.7.1　Animal models

Adult (aged 11–12 weeks) obese $Lep^{ob/ob}$ C57BL/6 (*ob/ob*) mice and normal control C57BL/6 mice (aged 8–12 weeks) were purchased from the Model Animal Research Center of Nanjing University, China. All mice were housed in a temperature-controlled environment with a 12 h light/dark cycle, had free access to water, and were fed with a standard chow diet containing 60% carbohydrate, 13% fat and 27% protein on a caloric basis. The animal care and experiments were performed according to the Guide for the Care and Use of Laboratory Animals provided by U.S. National Institutes of Health and was approved by the Animal Care and Use Committee of Wenzhou Medical University, China. The *ob/ob* mice were randomly divided into four groups (*n* = 6): where three groups of mice were treated with 0.5 mg/kg FGF21^{WT}, FGF21^{G71C}, or PEG-FGF21^{G71C} and one group was treated with 0.9% physiological saline and served as the negative sham. In adition, normal control C57BL/6 mice treated with 0.9% physiological saline (*n*=6).

2.7.2　Anti-diabetic effects of PEG-FGF21^{G71C}

For chronic efficacy evaluation, the animals were subcutaneously dosed once daily for 7 days. The glucose, body weight, and food consumption were monitored as indicated after the commencement of treatment. On days 3 and 7 of treatment, the animals were tail bled (by tail snip) 1 h after injection. In addition, the long-lasting anti-diabetic effects of PEGylated FGF21 variant were compared by examining the plasma glucose and triglyceride levels in *ob/ob* mice at 3 and 7 days after cessation of the 7-day treatment with FGF21^{WT}, FGF21^{G71C}, or PEG-FGF21^{G71C}. The glucose and plasma triglyceride levels were measured using the Precision G Blood Glucose Testing System (Abbott Laboratories, Abbott Park, IL, USA) and the Hitachi 912 Clinical Chemistry Analyzer (Roche Diagnostics, Indianapolis, IN, USA), respectively.

The livers were fixed in 4% paraformaldehyde and embedded in paraffin. Paraffin sections (5 mm) were stained with hematoxylin and eosin (H&E). Liver tissue staining was performed as previously described [18]. To estimate the extent of damage, the specimen was observed under a light microscope (400× amplification; Nikon). For immunofluorescence, 5 mm liver sections were treated with 3% H_2O_2 for 10 min and with 1% BSA in PBS for 30 min. The slides were incubated overnight at 4℃ with anti-CD68 antibody (Santa Cruz, sc-9139, 1:100) then incubated with IgG-PE secondary antibody (Santa Cruz, sc-3745, 1:100) for 2 h at room temperature. Next, the cell nuclei were stained with Hoechst for 5 min, and the images were viewed using a fluorescence microscope (400× amplification; Nikon).

2.8　Western blotting analyses

To compare insulin signaling using phospho-AKT as a marker, 3T3-L1 adipocytes were starved for 12 h, stimulated with FGF21^{WT}, FGF21^{G71C} and PEG-FGF21^{G71C} (100 nM) for 15 min, and then lysed. Additionally, the liver tissue of male *ob/ob* mice was collected and lysed at 7 days after cessation of the 7-day treatment with FGF21^{WT}, FGF21^{G71C}, or PEG-FGF21^{G71C}. Ninety micrograms of lysates from 3T3-L1 adipocytes or liver tissue were separated using 10% SDS-PAGE and electrotransferred onto a nitrocellulose membrane. Each membrane was pre-incubated for 1 h at room temperature in Tris-buffered saline, pH 7.6, containing 0.05% Tween 20 and 5% non-fat milk. Each nitrocellulose membrane was incubated with phospho-Akt (Santa Cruz, sc-7985, 1:500) and GAPDH (Santa Cruz, 1:5 000). The immunoreactive bands were then detected by incubating with IgG-HRP secondary antibody (Santa Cruz, sc-2004, 1:300) conjugated with horseradish peroxidase and visualizing using enhanced chemiluminescence reagents (Bio-Rad, Hercules, CA, USA). The amount of the proteins were then analyzed using Image J analysis software version 1.38e (NIH, Bethesda, MD, USA) and normalized against their respective control.

2.9　Statistical analysis

The *in vitro* experiments were performed three times with triplicate samples for each individual experiment. Data obtained from the animal study were obtained from five mice or six rats All data were expresseal as the mean ± SD and subjected to statistical analysis by ANOVA and Student t-test using statistical software NASDAQ: SPSS from SPSS Inc. Furthermore, $P < 0.05$ and <0.01 was considered statistically significant.

3. Results and discussion

3.1 Preparation and determination of FGF21 variants

Recent attempts have focused on the engineering of human FGF21 analogs to address its shortcomings (*in vivo* stability, auto-proteolysis, aggregation, etc.) *via* mutations, Fc fusions, PEGylation and conjugation to other scaffolding proteins [30–36]. With relevance to our study, Kharitonenkov and his colleague described a FGF21 variant, LY2405319, which was generated by introducing an additional disulfide bond (Leu118CyseAla134Cys) based on distance and orientation constraints assessed *via* the structural modeling [33]. Although LY2405319 exhibited improved thermal stability, its serum half-life still remained short similar to wild-type FGF21 [19,33]. Xu and his colleague used an alternative strategy by introducing surface-exposed cysteines for site-specific PEGylation in solution. However, all the mutated FGF21 variants and their PEGylated products exhibited significant lower bioactivity than wild-type FGF21 [35].

To gain insight into the causes for the poor stability of FGF21, we compared the physical differences between FGF21 to that of FGF19, which exhibits good bio-stability *in vitro* and *in vivo* [37]. We first compared their amino acid sequences using alignment analysis, and found an intriguing difference between FGF19 and FGF21 (Fig. 1A), namely, four cysteine residues located at positions 58th, 70th, 102nd and 120th in FGF19. Two disulfide bonds were formed between Cys58 and 70, and between Cys102 and 120 in FGF19, while FGF21 demonstrated only one equivalent cysteine at the second disulfide position [6] (Fig. 1). In addition, time-of-flight mass spectrometry (TOF-MS) results showed that

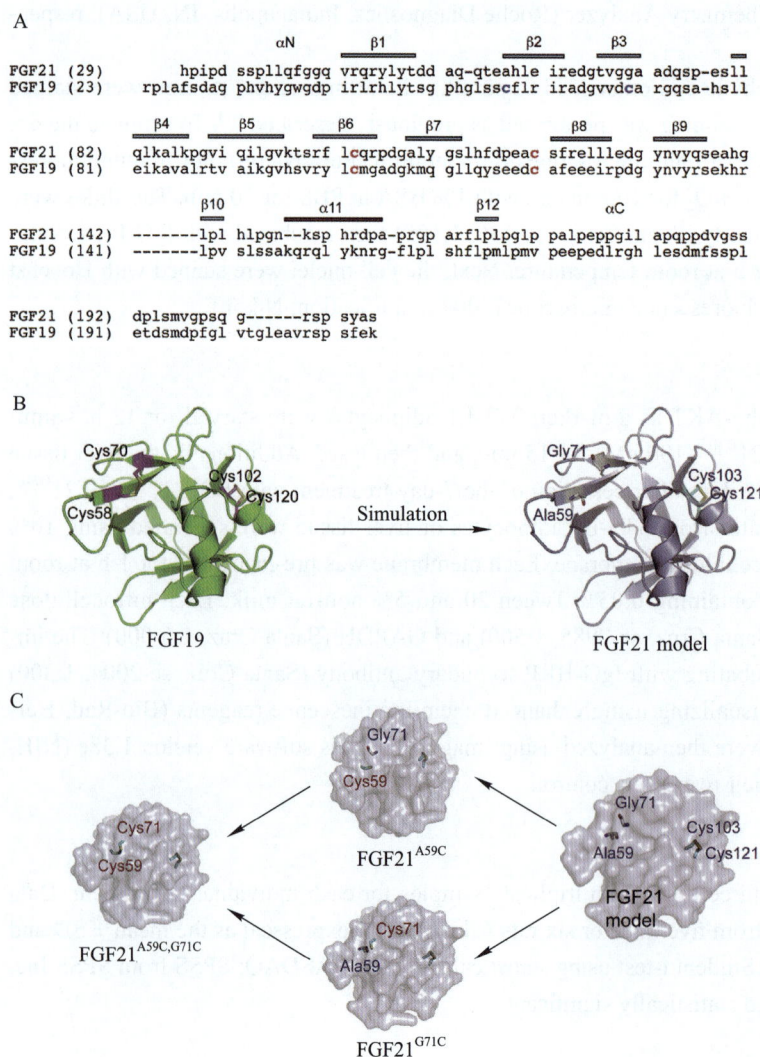

A

```
                           αN          β1            β2        β3
FGF21 (29)      hpipd  sspllqfggq  vrqrylytdd  aq-qteahle  iredgtvgga  adqsp-esll
FGF19 (23)      rplafsdag  phvhygwgdp  irlrhlytsg  phglsscflr  iradgvvdca  rgqsa-hsll

                β4        β5         β6        β7              β8          β9
FGF21 (82)      qlkalkpgvi  qilgvktsrf  lcqrpdgaly  gslhfdpeac  sfrellledg  ynvyqseahg
FGF19 (81)      eikavalrtv  aikgvhsvry  lcmgadgkmq  gllqyseedc  afeeeirpdg  ynvyrsekhr

                   β10         α11              β12       αC
FGF21 (142)     -------lpl  hlpgn--ksp  hrdpa-prgp  arflplpglp  palpeppgil  apqppdvgss
FGF19 (141)     -------lpv  slssakqrql  yknrg-flpl  shflpmlpmv  peepedlrgh  lesdmfsspl

FGF21 (192)     dplsmvgpsq  g------rsp  syas
FGF19 (191)     etdsmdpfgl  vtgleavrsp  sfek
```

B

Simulation

FGF19 → FGF21 model

C

FGF21^A59C

FGF21^A59C,G71C

FGF21 model

FGF21^G71C

Fig. 1. Design of FGF21 variants on the basis of the FGF19 structure and sequence. (A) Structure-based sequence alignment of wild-type FGF19 and FGF21. (B, C) FGF21 homology model. Based on the structural homology modeling and sequence analysis, cysteines were introduced into FGF21 variants at the 59th and/or 71st position, which are labeled in red.

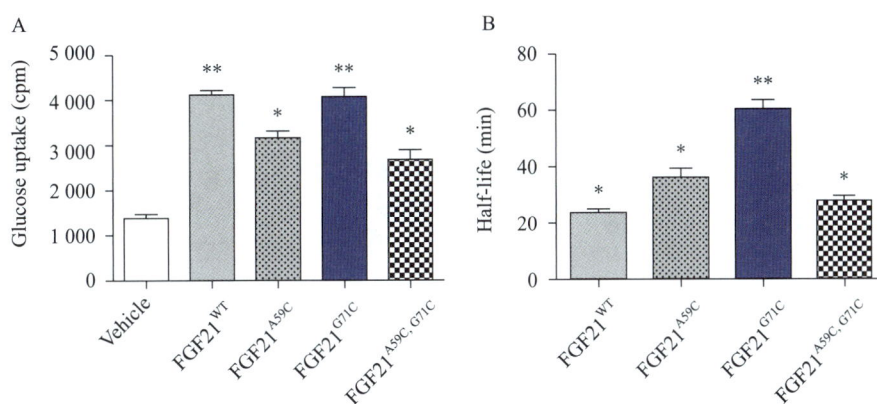

Fig. 2. Cell-based functional characterization and pharmacokinetics of FGF21 mutants. (A) Cellular glucose uptake stimulated by FGF21^{WT}, FGF21 mutants (FGF21^{A59C}, FGF21^{G71C} and FGF21^{A59C,G71C}) on 3T3-L1 adipocytes, as measured using a Wallac 1450 MicroBeta counter (Perkin Elmer). $^*P < 0.05$, and $^{**}P < 0.01$ vs. vehicle control; $n = 3$. (B) Comparison of the half-life of FGF21^{WT}, FGF21 mutants (FGF21^{A59C}, FGF21^{G71C} and FGF21^{A59C,G71C}) in SD rats. Normal male SD rats were injected intravenously with 0.5 mg/kg FGF21^{WT}, FGF21^{A59C}, FGF21^{G71C} and FGF21^{A59C,G71C}. Blood samples were collected at the indicated time points. The amount of FGF21 was measured using the human FGF21 immunoassay ELISA Kit. $^*P < 0.05$, $^{**}P < 0.01$ vs. the corresponding FGF21^{WT} group; $n = 3$.

the native amino acids (Ala59 and Gly71) were the primary degradation sites in FGF21. Thus, we hypothesized that residues at the 59th and/or 71st position might play an important role in stabilizing the structure of FGF21. On the basis of structural homology modeling and this sequence analysis, cysteines were introduced into FGF21 variants at the 59th and/or 71st position (Fig. 1B).

Three FGF21 variants (FGF21^{A59C}, FGF21^{G71C} and FGF21^{A59C,G71C}) were successfully expressed and purified for biological and physical characterization. In our previous study, we discovered that fusing small ubiquitin-like modifier (SUMO) to human FGF21 significantly enhanced the soluble expression level of human FGF21 in E. coli [38]. Thus, we designed FGF21 fusion proteins to facilitate the large-scale production and purification of our protein target.

To evaluate the effect of the mutation on the in vitro activity of FGF21, we tested the variants in glucose uptake assays in 3T3-L1 adipocytes. The in vitro activity of FGF21^{G71C} variant was more pronounced compared to the other two variants (FGF21^{A59C} and FGF21^{A59C,G71C}), and was similar to that of FGF21WT (Fig. 2A). Our in vivo study also showed that FGF21^{G71C} was more stable than FGF21^{WT} and the other two variants (FGF21^{A59C} and FGF21^{A59C,G71C}) (Fig. 2B, Supplemental Fig. 1A; Table 1). Thus, we selected the FGF21^{G71C} variant for subsequent experiments.

3.2 Solid-phase PEGylation and purification of FGF21 variants

Solid-phase synthesis techniques are routinely used to consume fewer reagents and to increase the desired product-to-side product ratio [39]. Taking advantage of our SUMO-tagged fusion proteins, we proposed to PEGylate FGF21 directly onto the Ni-NTA column, which we hypothesized would facilitate the purification and mono-PEGylation efficiency of the protein. The recombinant fusion protein (SUMO-FGF21) was first bound to a Ni-NTA affinity column, and mPEG-MAL was then passed through the Ni-NTA column at a low flow rate to ensure covalent attachment to the 71st cysteine residue of FGF21^{G71C} (Fig. 3A). To determine the optimal conditions for the site-specific PEGylation of the recombinant protein, the effects of different PEG/protein molar ratios (ranging from 5/1 to 30/1) and reaction times (ranging from 2 to 12 h) were examined. Our data showed that the optimized yield of mono-PEGylation was achieved when the reaction was performed at 4 ℃ for 12 h using a PEG/protein molar ratio of 12/1 (Fig. 3B). In fact, our SDS-PAGE and scanning densitometry analysis showed, under optimal conditions, 48.9% of the SUMO-FGF21^{G71C} was successfully PEGylated. Next, the pre-purified fusion protein (PEG-SUMO-FGF21^{G71C}) was diluted and cleaved by SUMO protease. As demonstrated in Fig. 3C, fractions containing PEG-FGF21^{G71C} were finally eluted off the Q Sepharose Fast Flow column using 20 mM TriseHCl (pH 8.0) containing 80 mM NaCl.

To confirm that FGF21^{G71C} was mono-PEGylated, MALDI-TOF mass spectrometry (MALDI-TOF-MS) was employed. Our data showed that the PEGylated FGF21^{G71C} had a molecular weight of 39.3 kDa (Fig. 3D), which indicated that a single 20 kDa PEG molecule was conjugated to non-PEGylated FGF21^{G71C} (19.3 kDa, Fig. 3E).

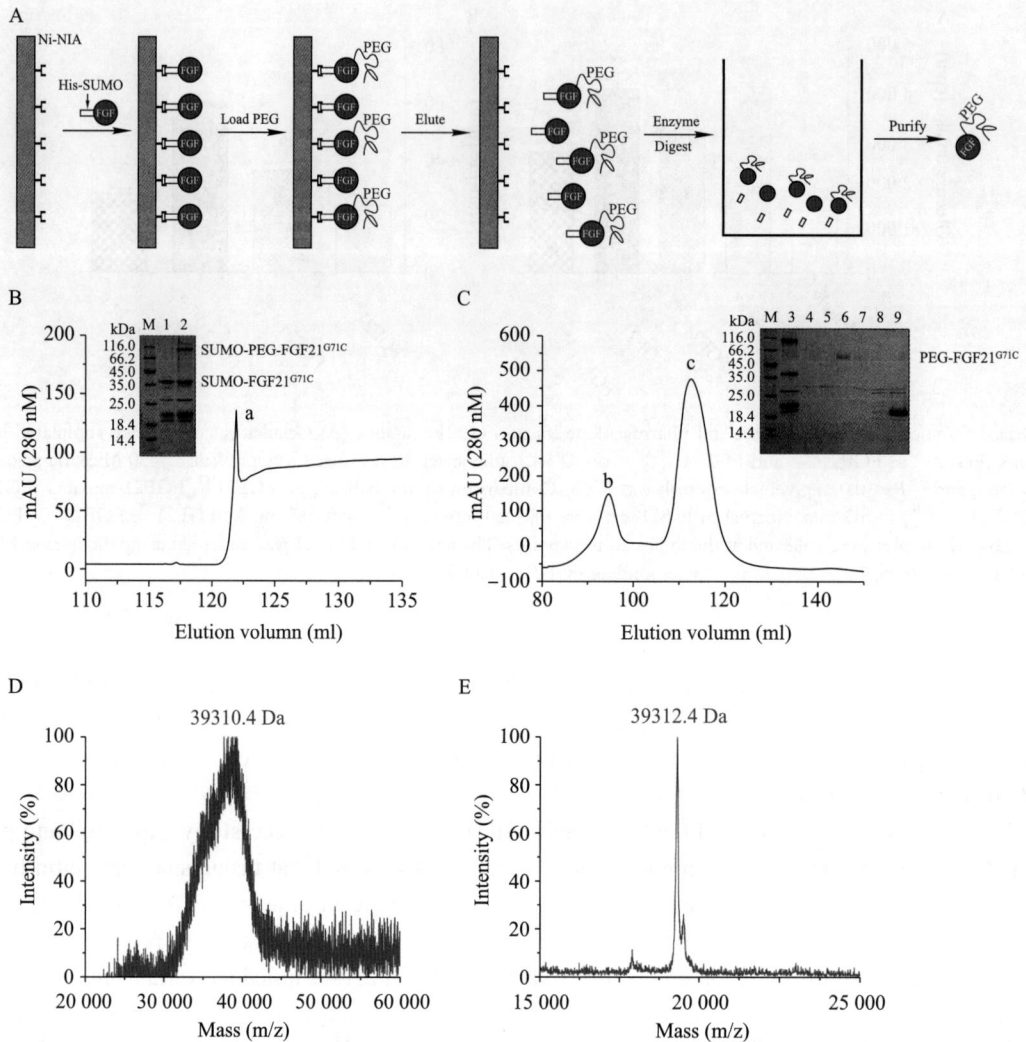

Fig. 3. SDS-PAGE analysis and identification of solid-phase PEGylated FGF21^{G71C}. (A) Schematic illustration of the solid-phase PEGylation strategies. (B) The elution profile of PEG-SUMO-FGF21^{G71C} from Ni-NTA affinity column following PEGylation. Inset Panel. SDS-PAGE analysis of the fractions collected from Ni-NTA affinity chromatography: lane M, molecular weight standards; lane 1, SUMO-FGF21^{G71C}; lane 2, eluted fraction of Peak a from Ni-NTA affinity column. (C) The elution chromatogram of PEG-FGF21^{G71C} from Q-Sepharose Fast Flow column after cleavage. Inset Panel. SDS-PAGE analysis of the fractions collected from Q-Sepharose Fast Flow column: lane M, molecular weight standards; lane 3, PEGylation mixture; lanes 4–9, eluted fraction were collected from different concentrations of NaCl (lane 6, the fraction of Peak b were eluted from Q-Sepharose Fast Flow column using 20 mM TriseHCl containing 80 mM NaCl). (D) MALDI-TOF mass spectrometry of PE-Gylated FGF21^{G71C} showing the molecular mass of PEGylated FGF21^{G71C} (39 310 Da). (E) MALDI-TOF mass spectrometry of non-PEGylated FGF21^{G71C} showing the molecular mass of non-PEGylated FGF21^{G71C} (19 312 Da).

3.3 Structural and biochemical evaluation of PEGylated FGF21^{G71C}

To rule out secondary structure changes, circular dichroism (CD) spectroscopy was performed on the protein samples. The approximate overlap in wavelength from 200 to 250 nm (Fig. 4A), indicated that the relative population of secondary structures calculated from the CD spectra showed minor difference among the variant and wild-type proteins, suggesting that site-specific mutation and solid-phase PEGylation didn't change the structure of FGF21^{WT}. Moreover, glucose uptake assays showed that the biological activity of FGF21^{G71C} and PEGylated FGF21^{G71C} were totally consistent with FGF21^{WT} (Fig. 4B). Analysis of the activation of cellular pathways also supported the fact that FGF21 signaling was preserved in the variants (Fig. 4C).

3.4 Bio-stability and pharmacokinetic evaluation of solid-phase PEGylated FGF21^{G71C}

The biological stabilities of FGF21^{WT}, FGF21^{G71C} and PEG-FGF21^{G71C} were compared by incubating proteins at 37 ℃ for different time points in mouse serum, which was applied to mimic the physiological environment in vivo. The

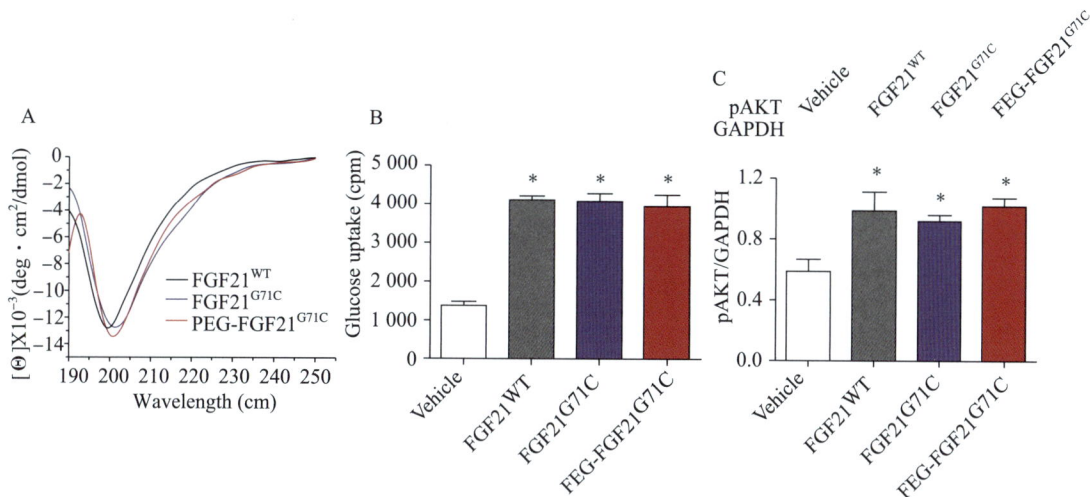

Fig. 4. Structural and biochemical evaluation of PEG-FGF21[G71C]. (A) Far-UV CD spectra of FGF21[WT] (black line), FGF21[G71C] (blue line), and solid-phase PEGylated FGF21[G71C] (red line). The ellipticities were reported as the mean residue ellipticity (MRE) (deg · cm²/dmol). (B) Cellular glucose uptake stimulated by FGF21[WT], FGF21[G71C] and PEG-FGF21G71C on 3T3-L1 adipocytes, as measured using the Wallac 1450 MicroBeta counter (Perkin Elmer). [*]$P < 0.05$ vs. vehicle control; $n = 3$. (C) The levels of phospho-AKT were examined using western blotting analyses with GAPDH as the loading control. [*]$P < 0.05$ vs. vehicle control; $n = 3$.

capacity of stimulating glucose uptake was reduced for all proteins after incubation with serum in a time-dependent manner. Interestingly, after 120 h of incubation, FGF21[WT] and FGF21[G71C] retained 34.3% and 45.1% of the original cellular bioactivity, respectively, while PEGylated FGF21[G71C] preserved 60.6% (Fig. 5A). The ELISA data also showed that the PEG-FGF21[G71C] was much slower degraded than FGF21[G71C] and FGF21[WT] (Supplemental Fig. 1B), which were totally consistent with the bioactivity analysis. To more specifically evaluate the thermal stability of proteins, we examined the bioactivity of proteins by incubating FGF21[WT], FGF21[G71C] and PEG-FGF21[G71C] at 37 ℃ for different time points in PBS. The result showed the same pattern of stability as obtained in serum incubation (Supplemental Fig. 1C). All these assays indicated that both mutation and solid-phase PEGylation can increase the biological and thermal stability of FGF21, albeit the effect of PEGylation was more profound compared to the Gly71Cys mutation alone.

In order to compare our FGF21 variant with the previously reported shortcomings of an FGF21 variant in the clinic [19], the in vivo half-life of PEG-FGF21[G71C] was analyzed by intravenously injecting a single dose of 0.5 mg/kg of FGF21[WT], FGF21[G71C] or PEG-FGF21[G71C] in male SD rats and then measuring the levels of three forms of FGF21 in blood using the human FGF21 immunoassay ELISA Kit. Compared with the half-life of FGF21[WT] (23.7 min), the mutation prolonged the half-life of FGF21[G71C] to 59.8 min (Fig. 5B, C; Table 1). More importantly, the solid-phase PEGylated FGF21[G71C] variant increased the half-life of FGF21 to 211.3 min, which is nearly 9-fold higher compared to FGF21[WT] (Fig. 5C; Table 1), and also 9-fold more compared to LY, a FGF21 variant currently in clinical trials [33]. The PEGylated form of FGF21 was also more prone to accumulate in target tissues such as the liver, pancreas, and subcutaneous fat, which are known to co-express the principal receptor (FGFR1c) and coreceptor (β-klotho) of FGF21 [7,40].

Table 1. Pharmacokinetic parameters of FGF21[WT] and its variants

	FGF21[WT]	FGF21[A59C]	FGF21[G71C]	FGF21[A59C,G71C]	PEG-FGF21[G71C]
$t_{1/2}\beta$ (min)	23.7	35.9	59.8	26.3	211.3
AUC (0–t) (µg/L*min)	28 457.961	47 689.059	84 441.784	31 081.463	323 675.793
AUC (0–∞) (µg/L*min)	34 998.212	55 909.936	95 756.481	39 145.125	489 833.626

3.5. Anti-diabetic effects of PEG-FGF21G71C in ob/ob mice

Accumulating pharmacological studies have shown that the activity of FGF21[WT] results in glucose-lowering activity [4,13]. These properties were investigated for PEG-FGF21[G71C] via subcutaneous injection of ob/ob mice once daily with FG-

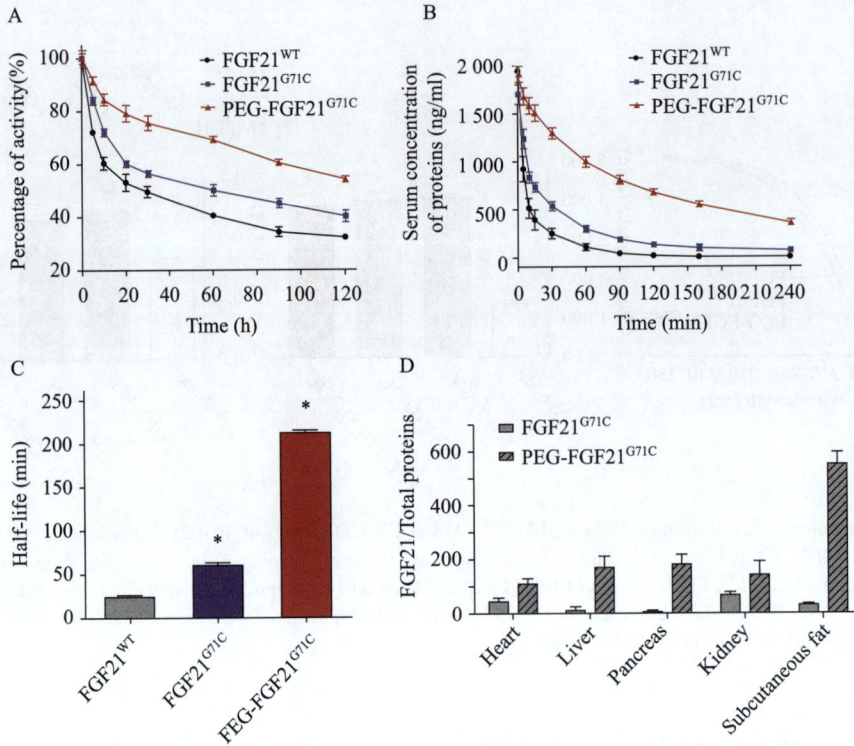

Fig. 5. The biological stability and pharmacokinetics study of solid-phase PEGylated FGF21^{G71C}. (A) The biological stability of FGF21^{WT}, FGF21^{G71C} and PEGylated FGF21^{G71C}. The protein samples were incubated in mouse serum at 37 ℃ for the indicated times, and then the serum-incubated proteins were added onto 3T3-L1 adipocytes for which the glucose uptake was measured to determine the functional integrity of each FGF21 variants. (B) Pharmacokinetic profiles of FGF21^{WT}, FGF21^{G71C} and PEG-FGF21^{G71C}. Normal male SD rats were injected intravenously with 0.5 mg/kg FGF21^{WT}, FGF21^{G71C} and PEG-FGF21^{G71C}. Blood samples were collected at the indicated time points. The amount of FGF21 was measured using the human FGF21 immunoassay ELISA kit. A standard curve was made for each FGF21, $n = 5$. Values were expressed as the mean ± SD. (C). Comparison of half-life of FGF21WT, FGF21^{G71C} and PEG-FGF21^{G71C}. $^*P < 0.05$, $^{**}P < 0.01$ $vs.$ the corresponding FGF21^{WT} group; $n = 3$. (D) After treatment, PEG-FGF21^{G71C} was distributed in various tissues.

F21^{WT}, FGF21^{G71C} and PEG-FGF21^{G71C} at a dose of 20 nmol/kg. Three days after treatment showed significantly lowered blood glucose and triglyceride levels for all variants (Fig. 6A, B).

After cessation of the 7-day treatment, the plasma glucose and triglyceride levels gradually returned to approximately vehicle treatment levels, although FGF21^{G71C} afforded a slightly better glucose-lowering effect compared to FGF21^{WT}. Importantly, the plasma glucose and triglyceride levels remained at significantly lower levels in ob/ob mice treated with PEGylated FGF21^{G71C}, even after 14 days post-treatment, indicating it's superior biological application in the T2D model. We also observed throughout the treatment period that ob/ob mice treated with the FGF21, FGF21^{G71C} and PEG-FGF21^{G71C} (0.5 mg/kg/d) demonstrated relatively reduced body weight (Fig. 6C).

In previous studies, systemic rhFGF21 was reported to significantly reverse hepatic steatosis and decrease tissue lipid contents in the type 2 diabetic animal model [18]. We examined liver tissues 7 days after the cessation of 7-day treatment with FGF21. Histological examination of liver sections obtained from vehicle-treated ob/ob mice showed the extensive existence of micro- and macrovesicular hepatocyte vacuolation (Fig. 6D). In contrast, hepatocellular vacuolation was significantly reduced in the liver sections of ob/ob mice treated with PEG-FGF21^{G71C}, even 7 days post-treatment cessation (Fig. 6D). To demonstrate that the metabolic effects of PEGylated FGF21^{G71C} occurred in an insulin-sensitive state, we profiled phosphorylated AKT levels in the liver, a major metabolic tissue [3,41]. As shown in Fig. 6E, AKT signaling was not only present, but was increased when treated with PEGylated FGF21^{G71C}.

3.6 PEG-FGF21^{G71C} reduces interstitial macrophage infiltration in the livers of ob/ob mice

Because T2D patients exhibit pro-inflammatory responses in a number of tissues (liver, kidney and adipose tissue) [42,43], we aimed to investigate the effect of PEG-FGF21^{G71C} on macrophage infiltration in the liver of ob/ob mice. Infiltration of CD68-positive (CD68$^+$) is used as a marker of decreasing insulin sensitivity and reflected the inflammato-

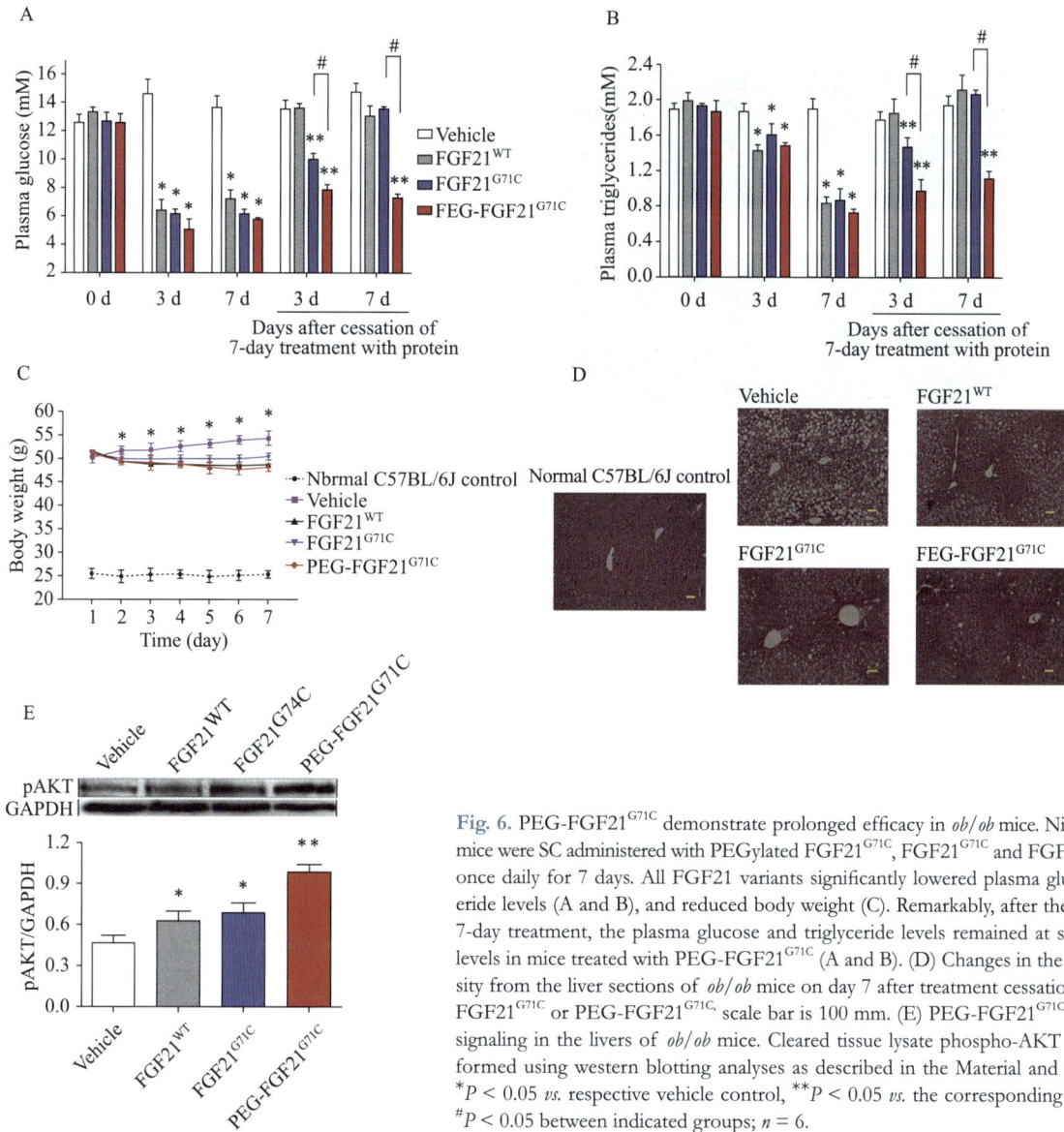

Fig. 6. PEG-FGF21^{G71C} demonstrate prolonged efficacy in *ob/ob* mice. Nine-week-old *ob/ob* mice were SC administered with PEGylated FGF21^{G71C}, FGF21^{G71C} and FGF21^{WT} (0.5 mg/kg) once daily for 7 days. All FGF21 variants significantly lowered plasma glucose and triglyceride levels (A and B), and reduced body weight (C). Remarkably, after the cessation of the 7-day treatment, the plasma glucose and triglyceride levels remained at significantly lower levels in mice treated with PEG-FGF21^{G71C} (A and B). (D) Changes in the fat droplet intensity from the liver sections of *ob/ob* mice on day 7 after treatment cessation with FGF21^{WT}, FGF21^{G71C} or PEG-FGF21^{G71C}, scale bar is 100 mm. (E) PEG-FGF21^{G71C} improves insulin signaling in the livers of *ob/ob* mice. Cleared tissue lysate phospho-AKT analysis was performed using western blotting analyses as described in the Material and methods section. $^*P < 0.05$ *vs.* respective vehicle control, $^{**}P < 0.05$ *vs.* the corresponding FGF21^{WT} group, $^#P < 0.05$ between indicated groups; $n = 6$.

ry state of the affected tissue [44]. *CD68* expression can be found in the resident macrophages of multiple tissues, such as microglia in the brain, Kupffer cells in the liver, and bone marrow macrophages (BMMs) [45]. Consistent with previous reports [46], *ob/ob* mice exhibited high levels of CD68-positive macrophage numbers *and CD68* gene expression (Fig. 7). When treated with FGF21^{WT} and variants, both hepatic CD68-positive macrophage infiltration and *CD68* expression showed a clear reduction in the liver, and compared with FGF21^{WT} and FGF21^{G71C}, PEG-FGF21^{G71C} showed a statistically significant higher reduction in hepatic CD68$^+$ macrophage infiltration and *CD68* expression. This effect was observed even after 7 days post-treatment (Fig. 7), confirming the longevity of the conjugated hormone *in vivo*.

4. Conclusion

In this study, we developed a recombinant human FGF21 variant by strategically introducing Gly71Cys using site-directed mutagenesis. For the first time, PEG was conjugated to this mutant *via* site-specific PEGylation with mPEG-MAL at Cys71 using Ni-NTA in a solid-phase reaction. Compared to non-PEGylated forms, the mono-PEGylated FGF21^{G71C} demonstrated improved biostability and increased *in vivo* half-life. Importantly, this solid-phase PEGylation of FGF21 is superior to previous reports on FGF21 modification as indicated by the increase in the yield of the mono-

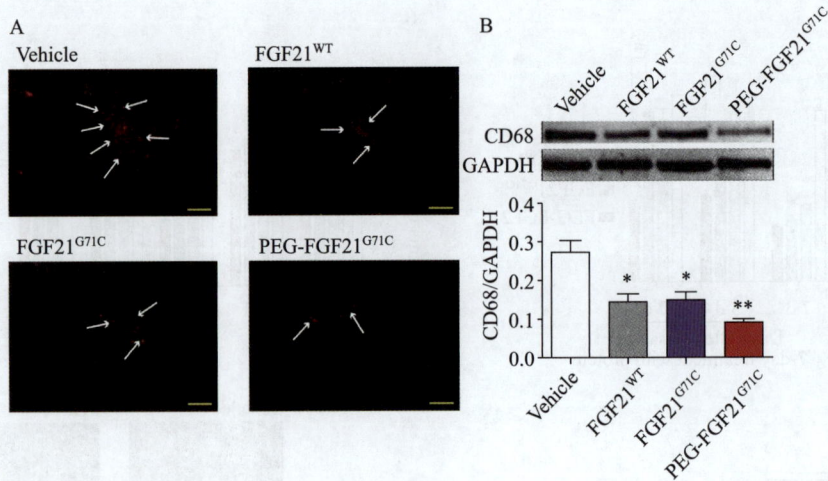

Fig. 7. PEG-FGF21^{G71C} inhibits hepatic macrophage infiltration in *ob/ob* mice. The mice were treated, and liver samples were prepared as described in the Material and Methods section. (A) Macrophage infiltration was evaluated using anti-CD68 antibodies. The arrows indicate stained interstitial inflammatory cells, scale bar 100 mm. (B) The mouse liver tissues obtained from the control group (vehicle), FGF21^{WT} group, FGF-21^{G71C} group and PEG-FGF21^{G71C} group were collected and homogenized. The protein levels of CD68 was detected using western blotting analyses. The column figures display the normalized optical density of CD68/GAPDH. $^*P < 0.05$ *vs.* vehicle control, $^{**}P < 0.05$ *vs.* the corresponding FGF21^{WT} group and FGF21^{G71C} group; $n = 6$.

PEGylated form and an improvement of downstream processing performance. Moreover, our study clearly demonstrated that Gly71Cys mutation together with solid-phase PEGylation could enhance FGF21 function *in vivo* by sustaining anti-diabetic effects in *ob/ob* mice for approximately 1 week without additional treatment. Thus, PEG-FGF21^{G71C} is a potent and efficacious long-acting FGF21 analog molecule with highly desirable anti-diabetic therapeutic effects.

Supplementary data

Supplementary data related to this article can be found online at http://dx.doi.org/10.1016/j.biomaterials.2014.03.023.

References

[1] Baird A, Klagsbrun M. The fibroblast growth-factor family[J]. Cancer Cells-a Monthly Review, 1991, 3(6): 239-243.

[2] McKeehan WL, Wang F, Kan M. The heparan sulfate fibroblast growth factor family: Diversity of structure and function[A]. In: *Progress In Nucleic Acid Research And Molecular Biology, Vol 59* (Moldave K, ed), Vol. 59, 1998: 135-176.

[3] Nishimura T, Nakatake Y, Konishi M, *et al.* Identification of a novel FGF, FGF-21, preferentially expressed in the liver[J]. Biochimica Et Biophysica Acta-Gene Structure And Expression, 2000, 1492(1): 203-206.

[4] Kharitonenkov A, Shiyanova TL, Koester A, *et al.* FGF-21 as a novel metabolic regulator[J]. Journal Of Clinical Investigation, 2005, 115(6): 1627-1635.

[5] Zhang X, Ibrahimi OA, Olsen SK, *et al.* Receptor specificity of the fibroblast growth factor family - The complete mammalian FGF family[J]. Journal Of Biological Chemistry, 2006, 281(23): 15694-15700.

[6] Goetz R, Beenken A, Ibrahimi OA, *et al.* Molecular insights into the klotho-dependent, endocrine mode of action of fibroblast growth factor 19 subfamily members[J]. Molecular And Cellular Biology, 2007, 27(9): 3417-3428.

[7] Kurosu H, Choi M, Ogawa Y, *et al.* Tissue-specific expression of beta Klotho and fibroblast growth factor (FGF) receptor Isoforms determines metabolic activity of FGF19 and FGF21[J]. Journal Of Biological Chemistry, 2007, 282(37): 26687-26695.

[8] Kharitonenkov A, Shanafelt AB. Fibroblast growth factor-21 as a therapeutic agent for metabolic diseases[J]. Biodrugs, 2008, 22(1): 37-44.

[9] Zimmet P, Alberti K, Shaw J. Global and societal implications of the diabetes epidemic[J]. Nature, 2001, 414(6865): 782-787.

[10] Lillioja S, Mott DM, Spraul M, *et al.* Insulin-resistance and insulin secretory dysfunction as precursors of non-insulin-dependent diabetes-melli TUS - prospective studies of pima-indians[J]. New England Journal Of Medicine, 1993, 329(27): 1988-1992.

[11] Weyer C, Funahashi T, Tanaka S, *et al.* Hypoadiponectinemia in obesity and type 2 diabetes: Close association with insulin resistance and hyperinsulinemia[J]. Journal Of Clinical Endocrinology & Metabolism, 2001, 86(5): 1930-1935.

[12] Kharitonenkov A. FGFs and metabolism[J]. Current Opinion In Pharmacology, 2009, 9(6): 805-810.

[13] Xu J, Lloyd DJ, Hale C, *et al.* Fibroblast growth factor 21 reverses hepatic steatosis, increases energy expenditure, and improves insu-

lin sensitivity in diet-induced obese mice[J]. Diabetes, 2009, 58(1): 250-259.

[14] Xu J, Stanislaus S, Chinookoswong N, et al. Acute glucose-lowering and insulin-sensitizing action of FGF21 in insulin-resistant mouse models-association with liver and adipose tissue effects[J]. American Journal Of Physiology-Endocrinology And Metabolism, 2009, 297(5): E1105-E1114.

[15] Kliewer SA, Mangelsdorf DJ. Fibroblast growth factor 21: from pharmacology to physiology[J]. American Journal Of Clinical Nutrition, 2010, 91(1): 254S-257S.

[16] Kharitonenkov A, Wroblewski VJ, Koester A, et al. The metabolic state of diabetic monkeys is regulated by fibroblast growth factor-21[J]. Endocrinology, 2007, 148(2): 774-781.

[17] Badman MK, Koester A, Flier JS, et al. Fibroblast growth factor 21-deficient mice demonstrate impaired adaptation to ketosis[J]. Endocrinology, 2009, 150(11): 4931-4940.

[18] Hotta Y, Nakamura H, Konishi M, et al. Fibroblast growth factor 21 regulates lipolysis in white adipose tissue but is not required for ketogenesis and triglyceride clearance in liver[J]. Endocrinology, 2009, 150(10): 4625-4633.

[19] Gaich G, Chien JY, Fu H, et al. The effects of LY2405319, an FGF21 analog, in obese human subjects with type 2 diabetes[J]. Cell Metabolism, 2013, 18(3): 333-340.

[20] Reitman ML. FGF21 Mimetic shows therapeutic promise[J]. Cell Metabolism, 2013, 18(3): 307-309.

[21] Harris JM, Martin NE, Modi M. Pegylation - a novel process for modifying pharmacokinetics[J]. Clinical Pharmacokinetics, 2001, 40(7): 539-551.

[22] Katre NV, Knauf MJ, Laird WJ. Chemical modification of recombinant interleukin-2 by polyethylene-glycol increases its potency in the murine meth-a sarcoma model[J]. Proceedings Of the National Academy Of Sciences Of the United States Of America, 1987, 84(6): 1487-1491.

[23] Kitamura K, Takahashi T, Takashina K, et al. Polyethylene-glycol modification of the monoclonal-antibody a7 enhances its tumor-localization[J]. Biochemical And Biophysical Research Communications, 1990, 171(3): 1387-1394.

[24] Lee BK, Kwon JS, Kim HJ, et al. Solid-phase PEGylation of recombinant interferon alpha-2a for site-specific modification: Process performance, characterization, and in vitro bioactivity[J]. Bioconjugate Chemistry, 2007, 18(6): 1728-1734.

[25] Filpula D, Yang K, Basu A, et al. Releasable PEGylation of mesothelin targeted immunotoxin SS1P achieves single dosage complete regression of a human carcinoma in mice[J]. Bioconjugate Chemistry, 2007, 18(3): 773-784.

[26] Hu J, Duppatla V, Harth S, et al. Site-specific PEGylation of bone morphogenetic protein-2 cysteine analogues[J]. Bioconjugate Chemistry, 2010, 21(10): 1762-1772.

[27] Jevsevar S, Kunstelj M, Porekar VG. PEGylation of therapeutic proteins[J]. Biotechnology Journal, 2010, 5(1): 113-128.

[28] Pan LQ, Wang HB, Lai J, et al. Site-specific PEGylation of a mutated-cysteine residue and its effect on tumor necrosis factor (TNF)-related apoptosis-inducing ligand (TRAIL)[J]. Biomaterials, 2013, 34(36): 9115-9123.

[29] Kaminskas LM, Ascher DB, McLeod VM, et al. PEGylation of interferon alpha 2 improves lymphatic exposure after subcutaneous and intravenous administration and improves antitumour efficacy against lymphatic breast cancer metastases[J]. Journal Of Controlled Release, 2013, 168(2): 200-208.

[30] Carter PJ. Introduction to current and future protein therapeutics: A protein engineering perspective[J]. Experimental Cell Research, 2011, 317(9): 1261-1269.

[31] Hecht R, Li YS, Sun J, et al. Rationale-based engineering of a potent long-acting FGF21 analog for the treatment of type 2 diabetes[J]. Plos One, 2012, 7(11).

[32] Adams AC, Halstead CA, Hansen BC, et al. LY2405319, an engineered FGF21 variant, improves the metabolic status of diabetic monkeys[J]. Plos One, 2013, 8(6).

[33] Kharitonenkov A, Beals JM, Micanovic R, et al. Rational design of a fibroblast growth factor 21-based clinical candidate, LY2405319[J]. Plos One, 2013, 8(3).

[34] Veniant MM, Komorowski R, Chen P, et al. Long-acting FGF21 has enhanced efficacy in diet-induced obese mice and in obese rhesus monkeys[J]. Endocrinology, 2012, 153(9): 4192-4203.

[35] Xu J, Bussiere J, Yie J, et al. Polyethylene glycol modified FGF21 engineered to maximize potency and minimize vacuole formation[J]. Bioconjugate Chemistry, 2013, 24(6): 915-925.

[36] Zhang J, Li Y. Fibroblast growth factor 21, the endocrine FGF pathway and novel treatments for metabolic syndrome[J]. Drug Discovery Today, 2014, 19(5): 579-589.

[37] Beenken A, Mohammadi M. The structural biology of the FGF19 subfamily[A]. In: Endocrine Fgfs And Klothos (KuroO M, ed), Vol. 728, 2012: 1-24.

[38] Wang H, Xiao Y, Fu L, et al. High-level expression and purification of soluble recombinant FGF21 protein by SUMO fusion in Escherichia coli[J]. Bmc Biotechnology, 2010, 10.

[39] Huang Z, Ye C, Liu Z, et al. Solid-phase N-terminus PEGylation of recombinant human fibroblast growth Factor 2 on heparin-sepharose column[J]. Bioconjugate Chemistry, 2012, 23(4): 740-750.

[40] Ito S, Kinoshita S, Shiraishi N, et al. Molecular cloning and expression analyses of mouse ss klotho, which encodes a novel Klotho family protein[J]. Mechanisms Of Development, 2000, 98(1-2): 115-119.

[41] Badman MK, Pissios P, Kennedy AR, et al. Hepatic fibroblast growth factor 21 is regulated by PPAR alpha and is a key mediator of hepatic lipid metabolism in ketotic states[J]. Cell Metabolism, 2007, 5(6): 426-437.

[42] Donath MY, Shoelson SE. Type 2 diabetes as an inflammatory disease[J]. Nature Reviews Immunology, 2011, 11(2): 98-107.

[43] Calle MC, Fernandez ML. Inflammation and type 2 diabetes[J]. Diabetes & Metabolism, 2012, 38(3): 183-191.

[44] Trevaskis JL, Gawronska-Kozak B, Sutton GM, et al. Role of adiponectin and inflammation in insulin resistance of Mc3r and Mc4r knockout mice[J]. Obesity, 2007, 15(11): 2664-2672.

[45] Holness CL, Dasilva RP, Fawcett J, et al. Macrosialin, a mouse macrophage-restricted glycoprotein, is a member of the lamp/lgp family[J]. Journal Of Biological Chemistry, 1993, 268(13): 9661-9666.

[46] Xu HY, Barnes GT, Yang Q, et al. Chronic inflammation in fat plays a crucial role in the development of obesity-related insulin resistance[J]. Journal Of Clinical Investigation, 2003, 112(12): 1821-1830.

One-step production of bioactive proteins through simultaneous PEGylation and refolding

Jianlou Niu, Xiaokun Li, Zhifeng Huang

1. Introduction

Overexpression of recombinant proteins in different host cells, particularly *Escherichia coli* (*E. coli*), often results in protein product accumulation in inactive and insoluble deposits inside host cells, termed inclusion bodies.[1] Inclusion body proteins must be refolded *in vitro* to gain solubility and bioactivity,[2] although theoretically, an unfolded protein can spontaneously recover its native structure following denaturant dilution. Intermolecular aggregates, as well as partially oxidized or misfolded species, compete against productive refolding, especially in cases of high protein concentration, resulting in low activity yields.[3] To improve *in vitro* protein refolding yield, a number of additives and compounds have been tested, and the molecular mechanisms by which they assist protein refolding have been reported.[4] Among these chemical additives, polyethylene glycol (PEG) has been reported to suppress aggregation by preventing the association of refolding intermediates or unfolded species through hydrophobic interaction.[5]

PEG can also be covalently conjugated to recombinant proteins, a process termed PEGylation,[6] which has been proposed as an effective approach to improve the stability and absorption, thereby reducing serious side-effects caused by acutely peaking drug concentrations, and also prolongs the half-life of drugs, therefore improving patient compliance by greatly reducing the frequency of drug injections.[8] However, the modification of proteins by PEG *via* nonselective groups often does not result in homogeneous products. To address this shortcoming, site-directed PEGylation techniques have been developed so that the definite numbers of PEGs could be coupled selectively to proteins. N-terminal residues of the peptide have been proposed as useful selective targets for PEGylation with an advantage of producing homogeneous products without changing the peptide structure.[6] For example, PEG aldehyde derivative such as PEG-butyraldehyde has highly specific affinity to the N-terminal α-amine of the peptide.[9,10]

In general, PEGylation has been performed with highly purified proteins harvested from inclusion bodies by *in vitro* refolding and purification, followed by multistep purification to attain the desired PEG–protein conjugates. We have provided several pieces of in-depth understanding to the molecular basis of polymer-assisted protein refolding and protein PEGylation.[11,13] Accordingly, we reasoned that the integration of site-specific PEGylation and protein refolding (IPPR) is a promising strategy for obtaining modified protein with preserved bioactivity and improved stability directly from inclusion bodies (Fig. 1).

In the present study, we investigated the feasibility of IPPR using lysozyme as a model protein. Several different complementary assays, including reverse phase HPLC (RP-HPLC), ion

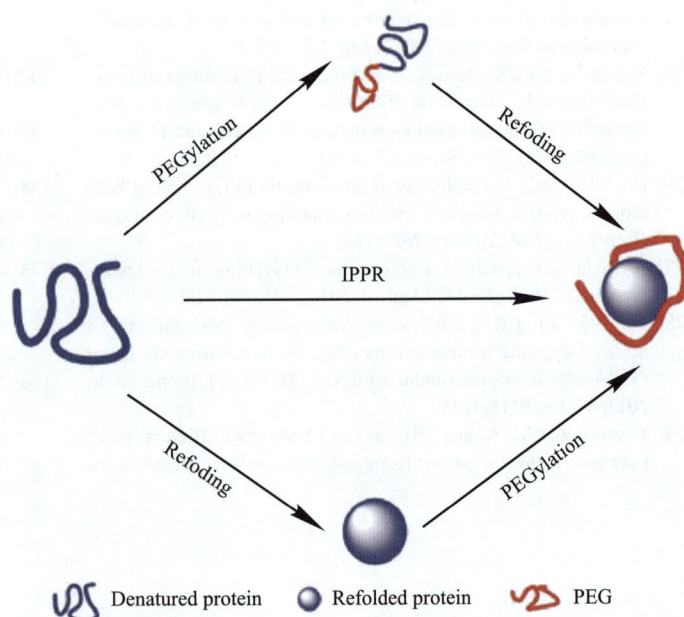

Fig. 1. Schematic illustration for the integration of PEGylation and refolding (IPPR) of denatured recombinant proteins. Using IPPR, highly purified, site-specific PEGylated proteins, which were successfully refolded, can be obtained directly from inclusion bodies.

exchange chromatography (IEC), and SDS-PAGE, were used to examine whether PEG-conjugated refolded lysozyme can be obtained by mixing mPEG20kD-butyraldehyde with denatured lysozyme in a protein refolding buffer. RP-HPLC and IEC were used to monitor the IPPR reaction at specific time-points and examined whether PEGylation and protein refolding were performed simultaneously. Subsequently, we used this novel IPPR approach to refold and modify the recombinant human FGF21 (rhFGF21) protein at its N-terminal residues, with mPEG20kD-butyraldehyde. The rhFGF21 protein is an important endocrine regulator of glucose and lipid metabolism[14] and is usually expressed in inclusion bodies in *E. coli*. Our bioactivity and circular dichroism (CD) analyses showed that IPPR-PEGylated rhFGF21 is comparable to the native rhFGF21 protein. In addition, we also applied *in vitro* and *in vivo* biostability analyses to examine whether IPPR-PEGylated rhFGF21 is more stable than non-PEGylated rhFGF21, which allowed for a significantly longer effect on lowering blood glucose and lipid levels in the ob/ob diabetic mouse model.

2. Experimental procedures

2.1 Reagents

Pyrobest DNA Polymerase and restriction enzymes, *Nde*I and *Hin*dIII, were purchased from TaKaRa Company (Japan). PCR purification, gel extraction, and plasmid miniprep kits were obtained from Promega Company (Madison, WI, USA). Isopropyl-1-thio-β-D-galactopyranoside (IPTG) was purchased from Gold BioTechnology (St. Louis, MO, USA). Hen egg white lysozyme, mPEG20 kDa- butyraldehyde (mPEG20K), reduced and oxidized glutathione (GSH and GSSG), dithiothreitol (DTT), urea, and *Micrococcus lysodeikticus* were purchased from Sigma-Aldrich (St. Louis, MO, USA). Anti-hFGF21 antibody was purchased from Santa Cruz Biotechnology Inc. (Santa Cruz, CA, USA). Bradford protein assay reagents used for quantitative protein analysis were purchased from Bio-Rad (Hercules, CA, USA). All chemicals were analytical grade.

2.2 Expression of insoluble rhFGF21

DNA coding for human FGF21 was PCR amplified. Following *Nco*I and *Hin*dIII digestion, PCR fragments were subcloned into a pET bacterial expression vector and the recombinant vector used to transform bacterial host BL21 (DE3) cells. Next, BL21 (DE3) cells were incubated at 37℃ in Luria-Bertani medium containing ampicillin (50 μg/ml) until the cell density reached an OD_{600} of 0.6. The cells were then incubated at 30℃ and 1.0 mM IPTG added to the medium to induce recombinant product expression. After incubation for 3−4 h, bacteria were collected by centrifugation and the cell pellet was resuspended in 25 mM Tris-HCl (pH 7.5), 1 mM EDTA, 0.6−0.9 M NaCl, and 1 mM phenylmethylsulfonyl fluoride. Cells were lysed by sonication and separated by centrifugation.

2.3 Protein denaturation−reduction

Lysozymes and rhFGF21 inclusion bodies were denatured by incubating 25 mg of proteins in 2.5 ml denaturing buffer (20 mM PB, 8 M urea, 100 mM dithiothreitol, pH 7.0) for 3 h at room temperature, forming a final denatured reduced protein concentration of 10 mg/ml. Complete denaturation of proteins was confirmed by RP-HPLC (Agilent Technologies, Palo Alto, CA).

2.4 IPPR of lysozyme and rhFGF21

Each denatured protein solution was applied to a PD-10 column (GE Healthcare Life Sciences, Piscataway, NJ, USA) for DTT removal. IPPR was initiated by rapid dilution of the denatured protein solution into refolding buffer (4 mM EDTA, 1 mM GSSG, 10 mM GSH, 1.5 M urea, 100 mM PB, pH 6.0) either in the absence or in the presence of increasing mPEG20K concentrations and 30 mM sodium cyanoborohydride (NaBH₃CN), to obtain final lysozyme and rhFGF21 concentrations of 1 mg/ml. Samples were incubated for different times (2, 4, 8, 12, or 24 h) at different temperatures (4, 16, or 25℃) and reactions were terminated by adding 2% (*w/v*) glycine. The progress of refolding and PEGylation over time was monitored and quantified using 12% SDS-PAGE and RP-HPLC, as described previously.[10]

Additionally, as controls, conventional PEGylation of native lysozyme and native rhFGF21 with mPEG20K were performed at 25 and 4℃ for 8 h in a phosphate buffer (100 mM PB, pH 6.0) in the presence of 10-fold molar ratios of mPEG20K and 30 mM NaBH$_3$CN, respectively.

2.5 RP-HPLC analysis

RP-HPLC was performed using Agilent 1 100 RP-HPLC (Agilent Technologies, Palo Alto, CA) equipped with an automatic injector and a 300SB-C18 column (Agilent Technologies, Palo Alto, CA). The mobile phase comprised two buffers: Buffer A (distilled H$_2$O, 0.1% TFA) and Buffer B (acetonitrile, 0.1% TFA). The RP column was first subjected to an isocratic 10% (*v/v*) acetonitrile–water gradient for 10 min, followed by a 10~70% (*v/v*) acetonitrile–water gradient over 60 min, at a total solvent flow rate of 1 ml/min. Absorbance was measured at 280 nm using a UV detector. RP-HPLC was used to analyze denatured protein, refolding protein, PEGylated mixture of native protein, and IPPR-PEGylated mixture. Yields of IPPR-PEGylated and overall IPPR-refolded proteins were quantified as the mass ratio of PEGylated proteins and final refolded protein to initial denatured protein. Protein mass eluted from the RP-HPLC column was measured by peak integration, based on standard curves obtained by calibration using known concentrations of native protein.

Moreover, RP-HPLC profiles obtained at different IPPR reaction times were used to quantitatively determine the refolding and PEGylated yield of proteins. Specifically, elution peaks of RP-HPLC of IPPR reaction at indicated time-points were identified by SDS-PAGE and quantified based on a standard curve obtained by calibration using known concentrations of native protein as described above.

2.6 IEC analysis and purification of IPPR-PEGylated proteins

Lysozyme reaction mixtures were applied to CM Sepharose fast flow column (1 ml bed volume; GE Healthcare Life Sciences), pre-equilibrated with 15 column volumes (CVs) of binding buffer (20 mM PB, pH 7.0) at a flow rate of 0.5 ml/min. Samples were washed with 10 CVs of binding buffer, and then eluted with elution buffer A (0.2 M NaCl, 20 mM SPB, pH 7.0) and buffer B (1.0 M NaCl, 20 mM SPB, pH 7.0) over 10 CVs.

RhFGF21 reaction mixtures were applied to HiTrap Q Sepharose fast flow column (1 ml bed volume; GE Healthcare Life Sciences), pre-equilibrated with 15 CVs of binding buffer (20 mM Tris-HCl, pH 8.0) at a flow rate of 0.5 ml/min. Samples were washed with 10 CVs of binding buffer, and then eluted with elution buffer A (80 mM NaCl, 20 mM Tris-HCl, pH 8.0) and buffer B (200 mM NaCl, 20 mM Tris-HCl, pH 8.0) over 10 CVs. All elution fractions were collected and analyzed by 12% SDS-PAGE.

2.7 Activity assays for IPPR-PEGylated proteins

2.71. Lysozyme activity assay

The activity of lysozyme and IPPR-PEGylated lysozyme was measured from their bioactivity on *Micrococcus lysodeikticus* (*M. lysodeikticus*), as described previously.[11]

2.7.2 Cell Culture and Glucose Uptake Experiments for IPPR- PEGylated rhFGF21

3T3-L1 preadipocytes (American Type Culture Collection, Rockville, MD, USA) were maintained in DMEM containing 10% fetal bovine serum (Invitrogen, Carlsbad, CA, USA). Adipocyte differentiation was induced by culturing the cells for 2 days in differentiation medium (DMEM with 10% FBS, 10 mM HEPES/MEM, nonessential amino acids (NEAA), penicillin/streptomycin (PC/SM), 2 μM insulin, 1 μM dexamethasone, 0.25 mM 3-isobutyl-1-methyl-xanthine (IBMX); all from Sigma-Aldrich, St. Louis, MO, USA), and then in differentiation medium without dexamethasone and IBMX for a further 2 days.[14] Thereafter, the medium was changed every 2 days with DMEM supplemented with 10% FBS, 10 mM HEPES, NEAA, and PC/SM. Lipid droplet accumulation was observed in >95% of cells after 7 days, and cells at days 7–10 were used for experiments.

For glucose uptake, cells cultured in multiwell plates were serum-starved overnight and then treated with different concentrations of either native or IPPR rhFGF21 (0.1, 1, 10, and 100 nmol/L) for 24 h. Plates were washed twice with KRP buffer [15 mM HEPES (pH 7.4), 118 mM NaCl, 4.8 mM KCl, 1.2 mM MgSO$_4$, 1.3 mM CaCl$_2$, 1.2 mM KH$_2$PO$_4$, 0.1% BSA], and then 100 μl of KRP buffer containing 2-deoxy-D- [^{14}C]glucose (2-DOG; 0.1 μCi, 100 μM) was added to each well. To eliminate nonspecificity, control wells contained 100 μl of KRP buffer with 2-DOG (0.1 μCi, 10 mM). Uptake reactions were performed at 37℃ for 1 h, terminated by addition of cytochalasin B (20 μM), and measured using a Wallac 1 450 MicroBeta counter (Perkin-Elmer, Waltham, MA, USA).

2.8 Mass spectrometry and N-terminal analysis of IPPR- PEGylated rhFGF21

Mass spectra were acquired using an Applied Biosystems Voyager System DE PRO MALDI-TOF mass spectrometer (Carlsbad, CA, USA) with a nitrogen laser. The matrix was a saturated solution of *R*-cyano-4-hydroxycin- namic acid in a 50:50 mixture of acetonitrile and water containing 0.1% trifluoroacetic acid. Purified IPPR-PEGylated rhFGF21 and matrix were mixed at a ratio of 1:1, and 1 µl spotted onto a 100-well sample plate. All spectra were acquired in positive mode, and over the range 600~2 500 Da under reflectron conditions (20 kV accelerating voltage, 350 ns extraction delay time), and 2~100 kDa under linear conditions (25 kV accelerating voltage, 750 ns extraction delay time). The N-terminal amino acid sequence of IPPR-PEGylated rhFGF21 was examined using the Edman degradation method,[15] followed by MALDI-TOF mass spectroscopy as described above.

2.9 Circular dichroism spectroscopy analysis

Secondary structures of native and IPPR-PEGylated rhFGF21 were determined using a CD spectropolarimeter (Model J-810; Jasco, Japan). Far-UV CD spectra were recorded at wavelengths between 190 and 250 nm using a 0.1 cm path length cell at 25 ℃ with a protein concentration of 6 µM in 10 mM PBS, pH 7.0. Each spectrum was obtained from an average of six scans, and CD spectra were corrected for buffer contributions. CD data were presented as a function of wavelength, in terms of the mean residue ellipticity. The thermodynamic stability of IPPR- PEGylated rhFGF21 was also determined by CD spectroscopy. In thermal stability experiments, the protein solution was heated with a temperature gradient of 20−60 ℃, and protein conformation changes monitored by CD spectroscopy as described above.

2.10 Functional evaluation of IPPR-PEGylated rhFGF21

2.10.1 Animal models

Adult (aged 11−12 weeks) obese *Lep*[ob/ob] C57BL/6 (ob/ob) mice and normal control C57BL/6 mice (aged 8−12 weeks) were purchased from the Model Animal Research Center of Nanjing University, China. All mice were housed in a temperature-controlled environment with a 12 h light/dark cycle, free access to water, and a standard chow diet containing 60% carbohydrate, 13% fat, and 27% protein on a caloric basis. Animal care and experiments were followed the Guide for the Care and Use of Laboratory Animals provided by National Institutes of Health and were approved by the Animal Care and Use Committee of Wenzhou Medical University, China. The ob/ob mice were randomly divided into three groups ($n = 9$): two groups of mice were treated either with 20 nmol/kg IPPR-rhFGF21 or with 20 nmol/kg native rhFGF21 and one group were treated with 0.9% physiological saline as positive sham. In addition, normal control C57BL/6 mice treated with 0.9% physiological saline ($n = 9$) were used as negative sham. IPPR-PEGylated and native rhFGF21 were given once a day for 1 week *via* subcutaneous injection.

2.10.2 Antidiabetic effects of IPPR-PEGylated rhFGF21

On days 4 and 7 after treatment, animals were tail bled (by tail snip) 1 h after the last injection of physiological saline, native, or IPPR-PEGylated rhFGF21. Glucose and plasma triglyceride levels were determined using the Precision G Blood Glucose Testing System (Abbott Laboratories, Abbott Park, IL, USA) and the Hitachi 912 Clinical Chemistry Analyzer (Roche Diagnostics, Indianapolis, IN, USA), respectively. In addition, the long-lasting antidiabetic effect of rhFGF21 was also compared by examining plasma glucose and triglyceride levels in ob/ob mice at 4 and 7 days after cessation of a 1-week treatment with native or IPPR-PEGylated rhFGF21. At the end of the study (day 7 after treatment cessation), all ob/ob mice were sacrificed and liver tissues were fixed in 10% zinc-formalin for processing, embedding with paraffin, sectioning at a thickness of 5 µm, and staining with hematoxylin-eosin (HE), as described previously.[16]

2.11 Protein concentration

Protein concentrations were measured using the Bradford method with BSA as the protein standard.[17]

2.12 Statistical analysis

For cell-based studies, data were collected from three independent experiments, and for *in vivo* studies, nine rats used per group. Results are expressed as mean ± standard deviation. One-way ANOVA followed by a *post hoc* Turkey's test was used for determining statistical differences between groups. Statistical tests were performed using Origin 7.5 laboratory data analysis and graphing software. *P* values <0.05 or 0.01 were considered statistically significant.

3. Results

3.1 Determining the feasibility of IPPR using lysozyme as a model protein

In order to determine if protein refolding and PEGylation can occur simultaneously in the chosen refolding buffer (described in Experimental Procedures), chemically denatured lysozyme (1 mg/ml) was refolded in the presence of mPEG20K (5 mg/ml) for designated reaction times. The reaction mixture was analyzed by RP-HPLC, with elution fractions identified by SDS-PAGE and then subsequently quantitated by RP-HPLC. As shown in Fig. 2A, when the reaction samples were incubated for 12 h at 25℃, IPPR-PEGylated lysozyme had the same retention time as PEGylated lysozyme, obtained from a conventional PEGylation approach with native lysozyme, and the retention time of non-PEGylated refolded lysozyme was identical to native lysozyme. SDS-PAGE analysis of IPPR fractions, eluted from RP-HPLC columns, showed refolded lysozyme was conjugated to a single mPEG20kD molecule (Fig. 2B). Additionally, RP-HPLC profiles obtained at different IPPR reaction times were used to quantitatively determine, based on protein mass quantification, the refolding yield, and PEGylated efficiency of lysozyme. The amount of IPPR and overall refolded lysozyme at specific reaction time-points during IPPR are shown in Fig. 2C, the yield of IPPR lysozyme increased accompanied by an enhancement of refolding yield, which was also confirmed by IEC (Fig. 2D). Table 1 summarizes the enzymatic activities of native, unfolded, refolded, and PEGylated lysozyme forms. Importantly, the enzymatic activity of IPPR-PEGylated lysozyme was exactly similar to PEGylated native lysozyme, indicating that IPPR had no detrimental effect on protein. Additionally, the PEGylated lysozyme showed significantly reduced enzymatic activity compared with the unmodified enzyme, because PEGylation had adverse effect on lysozyme bioactivity as previously documented.[9]

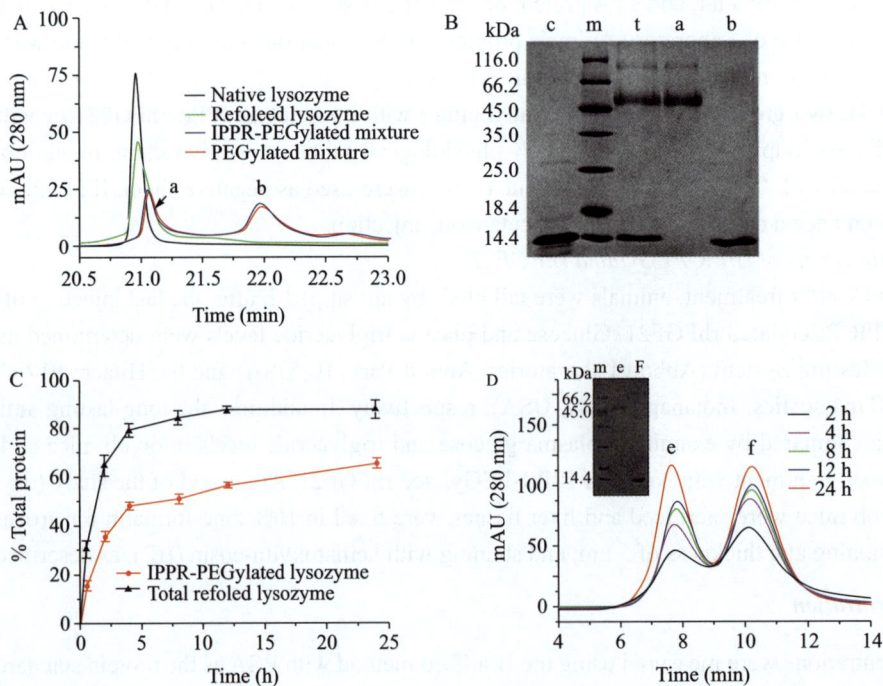

Fig. 2. Determining IPPR feasibility using lysozyme as a model protein. (A) RP-HPLC analysis of native, refolded, PEGylated native, and IPPR-PEGylated lysozyme. (B) SDS-PAGE analysis of RP-HPLC fractions. Lane c, native lysozyme; lane m, molecular weight standards; lane t, IPPR reaction mixture; lane a, eluted fraction (IPPR) of Peak A from RP-HPLC; lane b, eluted fraction (IPPR) of Peak B from RP-HPLC. (C) Yields of IPPR-PEGylated and overall IPPR refolded lysozyme at different time-points. Yields were calculated from RP-HPLC relative peak areas, based on the standard calibration curve. (D) Elution chromatogram, from CM Sepharose fast flow column, of the IPPR mixture which obtained at different reaction times. Insert panel. SDS-PAGE analysis of fractions collected from CM Sepharose fast flow column. Lane m, molecular weight standards; lane e, eluted fraction (IPPR) of Peak e from IEC; lane f, eluted fraction (IPPR) of Peak f from IEC.

Table 1. Enzymatic activity of different forms of lysozyme

	relative activity
native lysozyme	100%
unfolded lysozyme	0%
refolded lysozyme	89%
PEGylated native lysozyme	5%
IPPR-PEGylated lysozyme	5%

3.2 IPPR application for rhFGF21

To determine optimal conditions for IPPR of denatured rhFGF21, the effects of different PEG/protein molar ratios (ranging from 1/1 to 20/1), reaction times (2, 4, 8, 12, or 24 h) and temperatures (4, 16, or 25℃), on the yield and efficiency of site-specific mono-PEGylation were examined. We found the optimal yield of mono-PEGylated refolded rhFGF21 was achieved when the reaction was performed under the following conditions: denatured rhFGF21 was diluted 10 times into refolding buffer (4 mM EDTA, 1 mM GSSG, 10 mM GSH, 1.5 M urea, 100 mM PB, pH 6.0) to a final protein concentration of 1 mg/ml, in the presence of 10-fold molar ratios of mPEG20K and 30 mM NaBH3CN, at 4℃ for 8 h. Under optimal conditions, RP-HPLC and SDS-PAGE analysis showed 59.3% of total rhFGF21 was successfully mono-PEGylated (Fig. 3A, B). In parallel, we compared the modification efficiency of IPPR with conventional PEGylation, which was performed using native rhFGF21. Under the optimized IPPR conditions, the PEGylated yield of native rhFGF21 was 61.2%, similar to levels obtained by IPPR (Fig. 3A, B). Additionally, both RP-HPLC and IEC behaviors of IPPR-refolded and IPPR-PEGylated rhFGF21 were consistent with non-PEGylated and PEGylated native rhFGF21, respectively (Figs. 3A, 4A), indicating that denatured rhFGF21 was successfully refolded and PEGylated by IPPR.

3.3 Purification and validation of IPPR-PEGylated rhFGF21

To purify IPPR-PEGylated rhFGF21, IPPR reaction mixtures were subjected to salt gradient cation-exchange chromatography on a HiTrap Q Sepharose fast flow column. After cation-exchange chromatography, IPPR-PEGylated and non-PEGylated rhFGF21 were eluted in two separate peaks, as confirmed by SDS-PAGE (Fig. 4A, B). To verify that IPPR-PEGylated rhFGF21 was mono-PEGylated, MALDI-TOF mass spectrometry (MALDI-TOF-MS) was employed. Our MS data showed IPPR-PEGylated rhFGF21 had a molecular weight of 39.76 kDa (Fig. 4C), confirming that a single 20kD PEG molecule was conjugated to rhFGF21 (MW: 19.42 kDa).[12,18] The broad MS peak corresponding to IPPR-PEGylated rhFGF21 was most likely due to PEG polydispersity, as reported previously.[10] Next, we used automated N-terminal sequencing by Edman degradation to determine the IPPR-PEGylated site on refolded rhFGF21. Us-

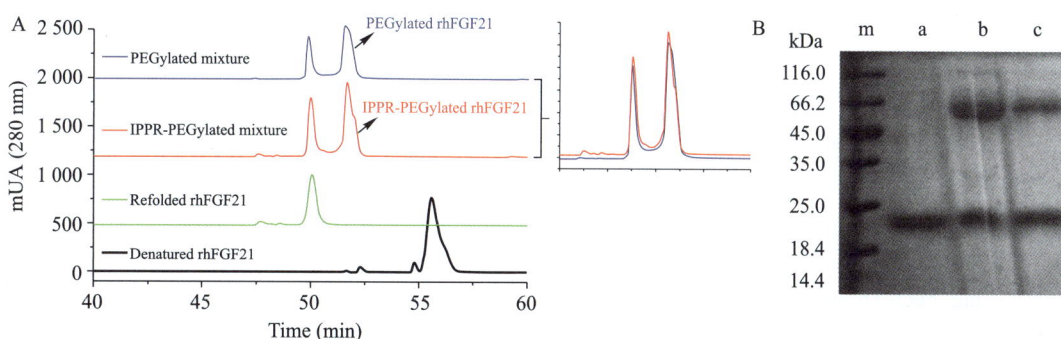

Fig. 3. IPPR of denatured rhFGF21. (A) RP-HPLC analysis of denatured rhFGF21, refolded rhFGF21, PEGylated products of native rhFGF21, and IPPR-PEGylated products of refolded rhFGF21 obtained at a PEG-to-protein ratio of 10:1, reaction time of 8 h, reaction temperature of 4℃, and pH of 6.0, respectively. Superimposition of RP-HPLC profiles of PEGylated products of native rhFGF21 and IPPR-PEGylated products of refolded rhFGF21 (insert panel). (B) SDS-PAGE analysis of IPPR-PEGylated and conventionally PEGylated products. Lane M, molecular weight standards; lane a, native rhFGF21; lanes b and c, IPPR-PEGylated and conventional PEGylated products.

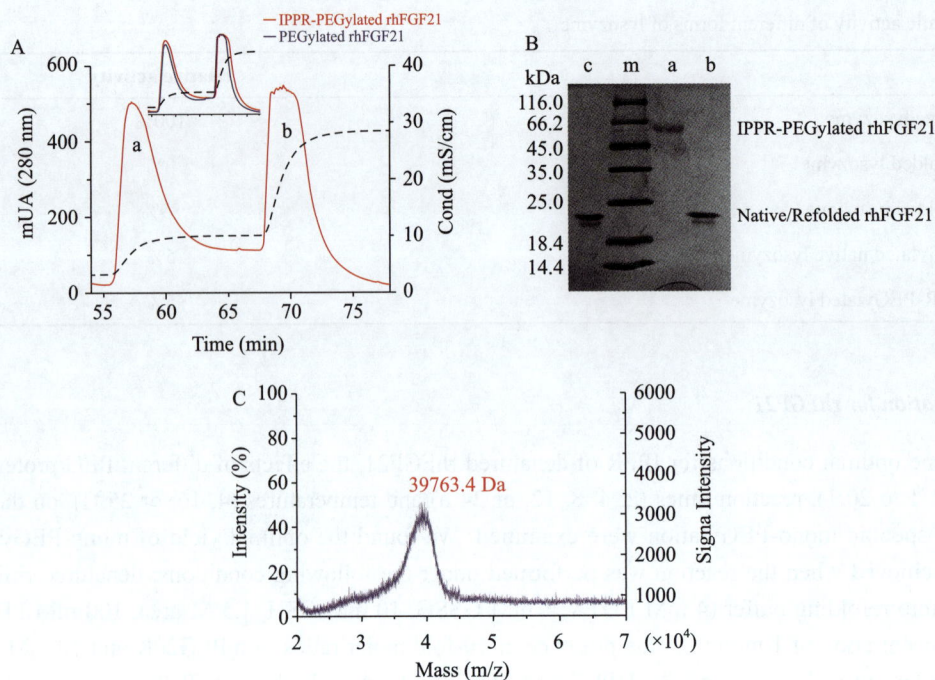

Fig. 4. Purification and validation of IPPR-PEGylated rhFGF21. (A) Elution profile of the IPPR mixture from HiTrap Q Sepharose fast flow column. Comparison of elution profiles of PEGylated native rhFGF21 and IPPR-PEGylated rhFGF21 (insert panel). (B) SDS-PAGE analysis of fractions collected from HiTrap Q Sepharose fast flow column. Lane c, native rhFGF21; lane m, molecular weight standards; lane a, eluted fraction (IPPR) of Peak a from IEC; lane b, eluted fraction (IPPR) of Peak b from IEC. (C) Molecular mass determination of IPPR-PEGylated rhFGF21 (39 763 Da) using MALDI-TOF mass spectrometry.

ing this method of sequencing, the five N-terminal amino acids (His-Pro-Ile-Pro-Asp) were detected in non-PEGylated rhFGF21 only (data not shown). The N-terminal residues of IPPR-PEGylated rhFGF21 were not detected, suggesting covalent attachment of PEG to the N-terminal α-amino group does not allow the N-terminal Ser residue to be modified by 1-fluoro-2,4-dinitrobenzene in the sequencing reaction, therefore making it unrecoverable.[15] Taken together, the MS and sequencing data unambiguously confirmed that a PEG molecule was site-directly attached to the N-terminus of rhFGF21 by IPPR-PEGylation.

3.4 Analysis of bioactivity of IPPR-PEGylated rhFGF21

To evaluate the bioactivity of IPPR-PEGylated rhFGF21, its effect on glucose uptake in differentiated mouse 3T3-L1 adipocytes[14] was compared with non-PEGylated native rhFGF21. As shown in Fig. 5A, IPPR-PEGylated rhFGF21 and native rhFGF21 induced a comparable response on enhancing glucose uptake in 3T3-L1 adipocytes, further demonstrating that denatured rhFGF21 was correctly refolded by IPPR and there was no adverse effect of IPPR on rhFGF21 bioactivity.

3.5 Effect of IPPR on the structural integrity and stability of rhFGF21

To investigate the effect of IPPR on rhFGF21 structure, the secondary structure of IPPR-PEGylated rhFGF21 was compared with native rhFGF21 using CD spectroscopy. Far-UV CD spectra recorded for IPPR-PEGylated rhFGF21 was comparable to non-PEGylated native rhFGF21 (Fig. 5B), demonstrating that IPPR aided protein refolding and did not alter the secondary structure of rhFGF21.

PEGylation has been shown to stabilize protein structures while also making their activities substantially more robust, with respect to temperature changes.[19] The thermal stability of native and IPPR-PEGylated rhFGF21 was compared by incubating the proteins in temperature gradients ranging from 20 to 60°C, and monitoring any protein conformation changes or heat effects by CD spectroscopy. Far UV-CD spectra showed native rhFGF21 had a disordered structure when the temperature was increased from 20 to 40°C (or higher), as determined from its large negative ellipticity around 200 nm and its low ellipticity at 190 nm (Fig. 5C). In contrast, the secondary structure of IPPR-PEGylated

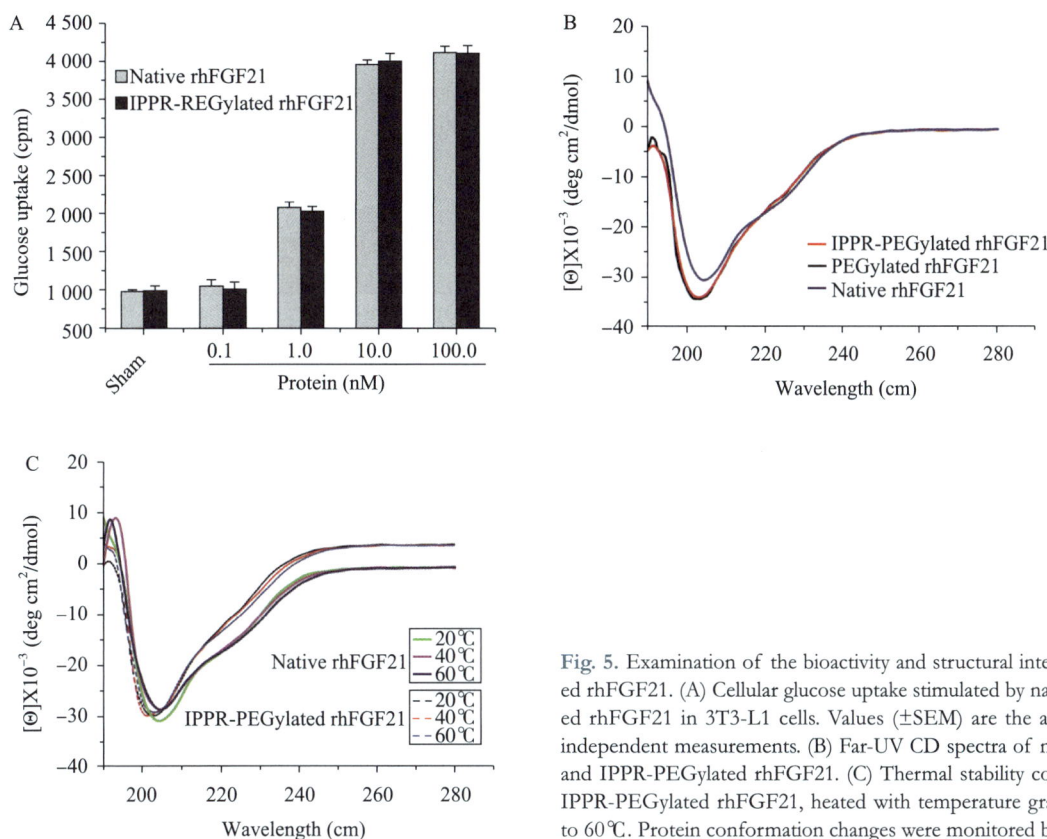

Fig. 5. Examination of the bioactivity and structural integrity of IPPR-PEGylated rhFGF21. (A) Cellular glucose uptake stimulated by native and IPPR-PEGylated rhFGF21 in 3T3-L1 cells. Values (±SEM) are the average of at least three independent measurements. (B) Far-UV CD spectra of native, PEGylated native, and IPPR-PEGylated rhFGF21. (C) Thermal stability comparison of native and IPPR-PEGylated rhFGF21, heated with temperature gradients ranging from 20 to 60 ℃. Protein conformation changes were monitored by CD spectroscopy.

rhFGF21 was minimally impacted in the thermostability assay.

3.6 Antidiabetic effects of IPPR-PEGylated rhFGF21 in ob/ob mice

The preserved function and increased thermostability of IPPR-PEGylated rhFGF21 promoted us to determine whether the modified protein could provide similar or even better therapeutic effect on diabetes *in vivo* as or than the native rhFGF21. We administered both rhFGF21 forms to ob/ob mice, a mouse model of hyperglycemia and insulin resistance.[20] Our results demonstrated that 4-day treatment with both native and IPPR-PEGylated rhFGF21 significantly lowered blood glucose, and this effect on 7-day treatment was even more pronounced (Fig. 6A). Similarly, the triglyceride-lowering effect was also evident for IPPR-PEGylated rhFGF21 treatment in ob/ob mice (Fig. 6B). Moreover, compared with the native rhFGF21 on days 7 of the treatment, IPPR-PEGylated rhFGF21 produced an observable improvement in the hypoglycemic effect (Fig. 6A). The improved hypoglycemic effect of IPPR-PEGylated rhFGF21 may be due to the increase in its *in vivo* biostability.

To test this above assumption, we examined plasma glucose and triglyceride levels at different times (immediately (0), 4 days, and 7 days) after cessation of 7-day treatment with native or IPPR-PEGylated rhFGF21. Plasma glucose and triglyceride levels gradually returned to approximately vehicle control levels in ob/ob mice treated with native rhFGF21, but remained at significantly low levels in mice treated with IPPR-PEGylated rhFGF21 (Fig. 6A,B).

In previous studies, systemic rhFGF21 was reported to significantly reverse hepatic steatosis and decrease tissue lipid contents in the type 2 diabetic animal model.[21] Therefore, we examined liver tissues on days 7 after cessation of 7-day treatment with either native or IPPR-PEGylated rhFGF21. Histological examination for the liver sections of ob/ob mice treated with native rhFGF21 (Fig. 6C) showed the extensive existence of micro- and macrovesicular hepatocyte vacuolation, reflecting intrahepatic fat accumulation. In contrast, hepatocellular vacuolation and lipid droplets were significantly reduced in the liver sections of ob/ob mice treated with IPPR-PEGylated rhFGF21, even on days 7 after treatment cessation (Fig. 6C), consistent with liver weight indexes (Fig. 6D). These results strongly support our hypothesis that (1) denatured rhFGF21 can be correctly refolded by IPPR; and (2) improved *in vivo* biostability of the IPPR-PEGylated rhFGF21 provides a significantly and long-lasting antidiabetic effect, compared with the native rhFGF21.

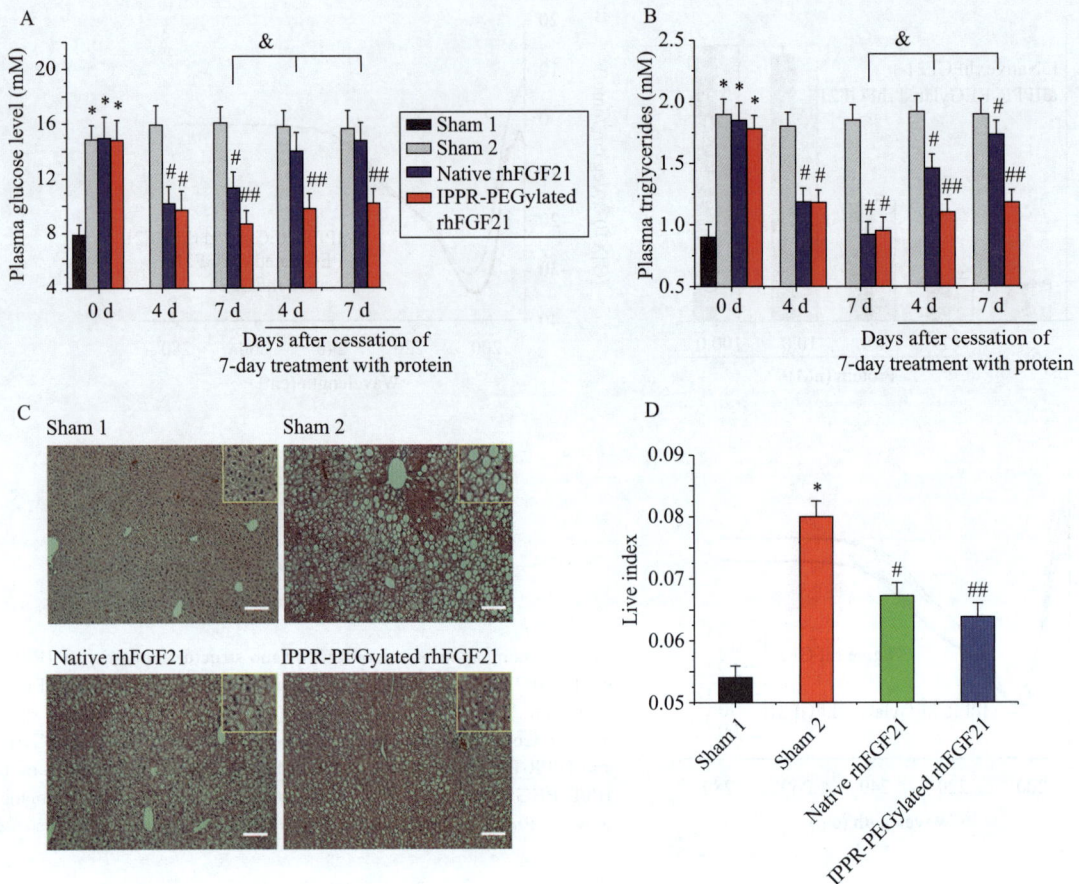

Fig. 6. Therapeutic effect of IPPR-PEGylated rhFGF21 in the *ob/ob* mouse model. (A,B) Effect of IPPR-PEGylated rhFGF21 on plasma glucose and triglyceride levels. Animals were treated (*via* subcutaneous injection) with IPPR-PEGylated and native rhFGF21 once a day for 1 week. On days 4 and 7, glucose (A) and plasma triglyceride (B) levels were determined. In addition, the long-lasting antidiabetic effects of the two rhFGF21 forms were compared by examining plasma glucose (A) and triglyceride (B) levels of days 4 and 7 after cessation of 7-day treatment with native or IPPR- PEGylated rhFGF21. $^{*}P < 0.01$ vs sham 1 (negative sham, normal C57BL/6 mice treated with vehicle); $^{#}P < 0.05$ vs sham 2 (positive sham, *ob/ob* mice treated with vehicle); $^{##}P < 0.05$ vs corresponding native rhFGF21; $^{&}P < 0.01$ vs corresponding 7-day treatment. (C,D) Changes in fat droplet intensity (C) and liver index (liver weight/total body weight) (D) from liver sections of ob/ob mice, on days 7 after treatment cessation with native or IPPR-PEGylated rhFGF21. $^{*}P < 0.01$ *vs.* sham 1; $^{#}P < 0.01$ *vs.* sham 2; $^{##}P < 0.05$ vs corresponding native rhFGF21.

4. Discussion

Recombinant proteins in bacteria, such as *E. coli* are often expressed in the form of inclusion bodies inside the cells.[1] To recover bioactive forms of expressed protein from *E. coli* inclusion bodies, a multistep, delicate refolding process is required. The process usually consists of *in vitro* refolding and purification steps,[22] although even after recovery of the refolded protein other common problems are encountered, for example, poor stability and relatively short half-life *in vivo*,[14,23,24] which have restricted their potential clinical applications. Surface modifications, such as PEGylation of therapeutic proteins, are widely studied as a means to improve in-serum circulation stability and reduce immunogenicity.[13,25,26] Combining PEGylation with a refolding process to obtain bioactive and PEGylated proteins directly from inclusion bodies (*i.e.*, IPPR) would significantly improve downstream processing performance. Additionally, the efficiency of this process may be drastically improved by simplifying the conventional steps of inclusion body refolding, purification of refolded protein, PEGylation, and purification of PEGylated protein.

In the present study, we sought to determine the feasibility of IPPR, first using denatured lysozyme as a model protein for PEGylation under specific refolding conditions. IPPR-refolded and IPPR-PEGylated lysozyme, representing non-PEGylated and conventionally PEGylated native protein, respectively, exhibit comparable hydrophobic and structural characteristics. It is encouraging that we have shown PEGylation and refolding can be performed simultaneously under the correct lysozyme refolding conditions, which is different from the previous study did by Minyoung Kim and his colleague.[27] In their study, lipase was used as a model protein for PEGylation under a reducing and denaturing condition and then *in vitro* refolding of PEGylated protein was performed by a traditional 'dilution' method.

We also extended our novel IPPR method to rhFGF21, which is an attractive candidate for the potential treatment of human type 2 diabetes and associated metabolic syndrome.[14,28] Until now, rhFGF21 was mostly produced in *E. coli*-expression systems within inclusion bodies. The *in vitro* stability and *in vivo* half-life of rhFGF21 are short, and the immunogenic activity is high,[14] all properties that have strongly restricted its clinical applications. Denatured rhFGF21 was successfully refolded and mono-PEGylated by IPPR under the determined optimal reaction conditions. Although it has already been reported that N-terminal α-amine of proteins is highly amenable for site- specific modifications,[29,30] our current study extends this knowledge to proteins which are insoluble, expanding the potential application to a vast number of protein therapeutics. Theoretically, as an alternative downstream processing technique, IPPR should not affect the folding or the intracellular action of proteins (Fig. 5A,B). The increased thermostability of PEGylated protein species further demonstrates its appealing application (Fig. 5C). Changes in CD spectroscopy observed at elevated temperatures (20 to 60℃) may be explained by reduced thermodynamic stability of the protein structure and increased hydrophobic interactions from exposed hydrophobic patches;[19,30] therefore, conjugated PEG may "swim around" the hydrophobic rhFGF21 patches to suppress hydrophobic interactions.[12]

More importantly, our physiological results suggested that IPPR-PEGylated rhFGF21 can sustainably lower blood glucose and triglyceride levels in the ob/ob mouse model. We found both plasma glucose and triglyceride levels in IPPR-PEGylated rhFGF21 treatment group were 40% lower than those in native rhFGF21-treated diabetic rats on days 7 after cessation of 7-day treatment (Fig. 6A,B). In addition, hepatocellular vacuolation and lipid droplets were significantly reduced in the liver sections from ob/ob mice, even on days 7 after treatment cessation (Fig. 6C,D). This clearly demonstrated that denatured rhFGF21 was successfully refolded and IPPR-PEGylation can enhance rhFGF21 function *in vivo* by sustaining antidiabetic effects in ob/ob mice for approximately 1 week without additional treatment. Thus, IPPR-PEGylated rhFGF21 shows favorable parameters for clinical application as it requires less frequent administration.

In conclusion, IPPR offers a one-step facile approach for high yield production of bioactive proteins. Importantly, IPPR is both time- and cost-effective compared to existing methodologies and hence will have a major impact on the drug development arena by facilitating the manufacturing of protein therapeutics for use in variety of human diseases.

References

[1] Baneyx F, Mujacic M. Recombinant protein folding and misfolding in Escherichia coli[J]. Nature Biotechnology, 2004, 22(11): 1399-1408.

[2] Gautam S, Dubey P, Singh P, *et al.* Smart polymer mediated purification and recovery of active proteins from inclusion bodies[J]. Journal Of Chromatography A, 2012, 1235: 10-25.

[3] Goldberg ME, Rudolph R, Jaenicke R. A kinetic-study of the competition between renaturation and aggregation during the refolding of denatured reduced egg-white lysozyme[J]. Biochemistry, 1991, 30(11): 2790-2797.

[4] Yamaguchi S, Yamamoto E, Mannen T, *et al.* Protein refolding using chemical refolding additives[J]. Biotechnology Journal, 2013, 8(1): 17-31.

[5] Cleland JL, Hedgepeth C, Wang DIC. Polyethylene-glycol enhanced refolding of bovine carbonic anhydrase-b - reaction stoichiometry and refolding model[J]. Journal Of Biological Chemistry, 1992, 267(19): 13327-13334.

[6] Roberts MJ, Bentley MD, Harris JM. Chemistry for peptide and protein PEGylation[J]. Advanced Drug Delivery Reviews, 2002, 54(4): 459-476.

[7] Caliceti P, Veronese FM. Pharmacokinetic and biodistribution properties of poly(ethylene glycol)-protein conjugates[J]. Advanced Drug Delivery Reviews, 2003, 55(10): 1261-1277.

[8] Fishburn CS. The pharmacology of PEGylation: Balancing PD with PK to generate novel therapeutics[J]. Journal Of Pharmaceutical Sciences, 2008, 97(10): 4167-4183.

[9] Shang X, Yu D, Ghosh R. Integrated Solid-Phase Synthesis and Purification of PEGylated Protein[J]. Biomacromolecules, 2011, 12(7): 2772-2779.

[10] Lee BK, Kwon JS, Kim HJ, *et al.* Solid-phase PEGylation of recombinant interferon alpha-2a for site-specific modification: Process performance, characterization, and *in vitro* bioactivity[J]. Bioconjugate Chemistry, 2007, 18(6): 1728-1734.

[11] Ye C, Ilghari D, Niu J, *et al.* A comprehensive structure-function analysis shed a new light on molecular mechanism by which a novel smart copolymer, NY-3-1, assists protein refolding[J]. Journal Of Biotechnology, 2012, 160(3-4): 169-175.

[12] Huang Z, Wang H, Lu M, *et al.* A better anti-diabetic recombinant human fibroblast growth factor 21 (rhFGF21) modified with polyethylene glycol[J]. Plos One, 2011, 6(6).

[13] Huang Z, Ye C, Liu Z, *et al.* Solid-Phase N-Terminus PEGylation of Recombinant Human Fibroblast Growth Factor 2 on Heparin-Sepharose Column[J]. Bioconjugate Chemistry, 2012, 23(4): 740-750.

[14] Kharitonenkov A, Shiyanova TL, Koester A, *et al.* FGF-21 as a novel metabolic regulator[J]. Journal Of Clinical Investigation, 2005, 115(6): 1627-1635.

[15] Guerra PI, Acklin C, Kosky AA, *et al.* PEGylation prevents the N-terminal degradation of megakaryocyte growth and development factor[J]. Pharmaceutical Research, 1998, 15(12): 1822-1827.

[16] Hotta Y, Nakamura H, Konishi M, *et al.* Fibroblast growth factor 21 regulates lipolysis in white adipose tissue but is not required for ketogenesis and triglyceride clearance in liver[J]. endocrinology, 2009, 150(10): 4625-4633.

[17] Bradford MM. Rapid and sensitive method for quantitation of microgram quantities of protein utilizing principle of protein-dye binding[J]. Analytical Biochemistry, 1976, 72(1-2): 248-254.

[18] Wang H, Xiao Y, Fu L, *et al.* High-level expression and purification of soluble recombinant FGF21 protein by SUMO fusion in Escherichia coli[J]. Bmc Biotechnology, 2010, 10.

[19] Manning MC, Chou DK, Murphy BM, *et al.* Stability of protein pharmaceuticals: an update[J]. Pharmaceutical Research, 2010, 27(4): 544-575.

[20] Kennedy AJ, Ellacott KLJ, King VL, *et al.* Mouse models of the metabolic syndrome[J]. Disease Models & Mechanisms, 2010, 3(3-4): 156-166.

[21] Xu J, Lloyd DJ, Hale C, *et al.* Fibroblast growth factor 21 reverses hepatic steatosis, increases energy expenditure, and improves insulin sensitivity in diet-induced obese mice[J]. Diabetes, 2009, 58(1): 250-259.

[22] Mollania N, Khajeh K, Ranjbar B, *et al.* An efficient *in vitro* refolding of recombinant bacterial laccase in Escherichia coli[J]. Enzyme And Microbial Technology, 2013, 52(6-7): 325-330.

[23] Chen BL, Arakawa T. Stabilization of recombinant human keratinocyte growth factor by osmolytes and salts[J]. Journal Of Pharmaceutical Sciences, 1996, 85(4): 419-422.

[24] Nguyen TH, Kim SH, Decker CG, *et al.* A heparin-mimicking polymer conjugate stabilizes basic fibroblast growth factor[J]. Nature Chemistry, 2013, 5(3): 221-227.

[25] Huang Z, Ni C, Chu Y, *et al.* Chemical modification of recombinant human keratinocyte growth factor 2 with polyethylene glycol improves biostability and reduces animal immunogenicity[J]. Journal Of Biotechnology, 2009, 142(3-4): 242-249.

[26] Gong N, Ma A-N, Zhang L-J, *et al.* Site-specific PEGylation of exenatide analogues markedly improved their glucoregulatory activity[J]. British Journal Of Pharmacology, 2011, 163(2): 399-412.

[27] Kim MY, Kwon JS, Kim HJ, *et al. In vitro* refolding of PEGylated lipase[J]. Journal Of Biotechnology, 2007, 131(2): 177-179.

[28] Seo JA, Kim NH. Fibroblast Growth Factor 21: A Novel Metabolic Regulator[J]. Diabetes & Metabolism Journal, 2012, 36(1): 26-28.

[29] Xiao J, Burn A, Tolbert TJ. Increasing solubility of proteins and peptides by site-specific modification with betaine[J]. Bioconjugate Chemistry, 2008, 19(6): 1113-1118.

[30] Manning MC, Patel K, Borchardt RT. Stability of protein pharmaceuticals[J]. Pharmaceutical Research, 1989, 6(11): 903-918.

Structural mimicry of A-loop tyrosine phosphorylation by a pathogenic FGF receptor 3 mutation

Zhifeng Huang, Xiaokun Li, Moosa Mohammadi

1. Introduction

Fibroblast growth factor receptor (FGFR) tyrosine kinases mediate the pleiotropic effects of FGFs in human biology and pathology. Gain-of-function mutations in the tyrosine kinase domains of FGFRs underlie a wide array of human develop- mental disorders and malignancies (Beenken and Mohammadi, 2009; Goriely et al., 2009; Webster and Donoghue, 1997b; Wilkie, 2005). FGFs act in concert with either heparin sulfate cofactors or Klotho coreceptors to bind and dimerize the ectodomains of FGFRs, bringing the cytoplasmic tyrosine kinase domains into proper proximity and orientation, which allows *trans*-phosphorylation on activation loop (A-loop) tyrosines to occur (Goetz and Moham- madi, 2013). This event triggers kinase activation and causes additional *trans*-phosphorylation reactions on tyrosines in the kinase C-terminal tail and juxtamembrane (JM) region to create specific recruitment sites for substrates, thereby increasing the proximity of substrate to the kinase and facilitating substrate phosphorylation (Bae et al., 2009; Chen et al., 2008; Goetz and Mohammadi, 2013; Moham madi et al., 1996a).

Crystallographic and nuclear magnetic resonance (NMR) studies of FGFR kinase domains in the unphosphorylated and A-loop phosphorylated states, as well as constitutively active FGFR kinases that harbor pathogenic gain-of-function mutations (Bae et al., 2009; Chen et al., 2007, 2013; Mohammadi et al., 1996a), show that the FGFR kinase is principally regulated at the protein dynamics level by an autoinhibitory network of hydrogen bonds in the kinase hinge/interlobe region (termed "molecular brake"), which restrains the kinase from transitioning into the active state (Chen et al., 2007, 2013). Upon A-loop tyrosine phosphorylation, the phosphate moiety of the phosphorylated A-loop tyrosine makes intramolecular hydrogen bonds with an RTK-invariant arginine at the N-terminal end of the A-loop, helping to restructure the A-loop into the active conformation. The change in the conformation of the A-loop is then allosterically communicated to the kinase hinge region, causing disengagement of the molecular brake, and hence maximal kinase activation (Chen et al., 2007, 2013). In FGFRs, the kinase hinge and A-loop are the two hotspots for pathogenic gain-of-function mutations (Bellus et al., 1995, 2000; Kan et al., 2002; Wilkie, 2005). Previously, we explored the mechanisms for FGFR activation by the pathogenic mutations at the kinase hinge, which led to the discovery of the autoinhibitory molecular brake (Chen et al., 2007). The K650E mutation in the A-loop of FGFR3 kinase is one of the most activating, and hence pathogenic mutations (Bellus et al., 2000; Naski et al., 1996; Webster et al., 1996; Webster and Donoghue, 1997a). When occurring in the germline, the K650E mutation causes Thanatophoric Dysplasia type II, a neonatal lethal dwarfism syndrome (Tavormina et al., 1995; Wilcox et al., 1998).If acquired somatically, it contributes to the progression of multiple myeloma, bladder cancer and benign skin tumors (Cappellen et al., 1999; Chesi et al., 1997; Logie´ et al., 2005).

There is a wealth of literature on the molecular mechanisms by which the hyperactive K650E mutant reduces proliferation of chondrocytes, causing them to prematurely enter into hypertrophic differentiation in the developing cartilage tissue. The effects of the K650E mutation on FGFR activation, maturation/ trafficking, and downstream signaling pathways have been extensively studied (Foldynova-Trantirkova et al., 2012; Guo et al., 2008). Webster and colleagues showed that the A-loop tyrosines are dispensable for the constitutive activity of the K650E FGFR3 mutant, implying that K650E mutation activates the kinase in an A-loop phosphorylation-independent fashion (Webster et al., 1996). Hence, it was proposed that this pathogenic mutation mimics the action of A-loop tyrosine phosphorylation to activate the kinase (Webster et al., 1996). The molecular mechanism by which this mutation imparts constitutive activation upon FGFR3 kinase is perplexing, however, because in accordance with the crystal structures of A-loop phosphorylated

FGFR1 and FGFR2 kinases, the corresponding lysine residues, namely, K656 and K659, make intramolecular hydrogen bonds with the phosphate moiety of the phosphorylated A-loop tyrosine and residues in the A-loop that actually help supporting the active A-loop conformation (Bae *et al.*, 2010; Chen *et al.*, 2007). Lievens and Liboi showed that the K650E mutation affects receptor maturation and that the constitutively active mutant accumulates as a mannose-rich and phosphorylated form in the endoplasmic reticulum, where it signals through activating STAT1 and Src (Lievens and Liboi, 2003). Using a neurite outgrowth differentiation assay in PC12 cells as readout, Nowroozi and colleagues suggested that activation of STAT1 and 3 may not be required for the K650E mutant to induce hypertrophic differentiation of the growth plate (Nowroozi *et al.*, 2005). Agazie and colleagues showed that the K650E mutant requires SHP2 to induce oncogenic transformation of cells (Agazie *et al.*, 2003).

The importance of elucidating the molecular mechanism by which the K650E mutation confers gain-of-function on FGFR3 kinase is 2-fold; first, it may provide new insight into the physiological mechanisms of FGFR kinase regulation, and second, it may facilitate the rational design of small molecule inhibitors that can specifically silence the hyperactivity of this pathogenic FGFR3 mutant. Here, we report the crystal structure of FGFR3 kinase that harbors the K650E mutation. The structure shows that the mutation functionally mimics the action of A-loop phosphorylation in activating the kinase by introducing a network of hydrogen bonds that stabilize the active-state conformation of the A-loop. Moreover, the structure provides a snapshot of two FGFR kinase molecules engaged in the act of *trans*-phosphorylation on the kinase insert tyrosine. Comparison of this *trans*-phosphorylation complex with a previously reported kinase *trans*-phosphorylation complex involving the C-terminal tail tyro-sine (Chen *et al.*, 2008) provides valuable insights into the molecular mechanism that controls *trans*-phosphorylation specificity. Based on our structural data, targeted inhibition of this pathogenic FGFR3 kinase can be achieved by small molecule kinase inhibitors that selectively bind the active-state conformation of FGFR3 kinase.

2. Results

To elucidate the molecular basis by which the pathogenic K650E mutation imparts constitutive activation upon FGFR3 kinase in human diseases, we solved the crystal structure of the FGFR3K^{K650E} mutant in complex with AMP-PCP, a nonhydrolyzable ATP analog, at 2.35 Å resolution (Fig. 1A). Data collection and structure refinement statistics

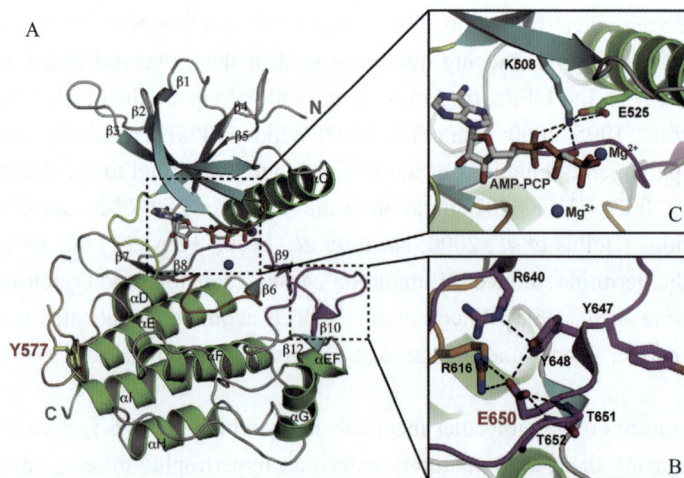

Fig. 1. The pathogenic K650E mutation drives the FGFR3 kinase into the active conformation. (A) Ribbon diagrams of the FGFR3K^{K650E} structure. b strands and a helices are colored cyan and green, respectively. The A-loop, catalytic loop, nucleotide-binding loop, kinase insert, and kinase hinge are colored magenta, orange, smudge, wheat, and yellow, respectively. In all of the figures, the ATP analog (AMP-PCP) and magnesium ions are rendered as sticks and blue spheres, respectively. (B) Close-up view of the catalytically critical salt bridge between K508 and E525 in the kinase N-lobe important for ATP coordination and hydrolysis. (C) The carboxylate group of E650 introduces a network of intramolecular hydrogen bonds that tether the flexible A-loop to the rigid core of the C-lobe, thereby stabilizing the activestate conformation of the A-loop. Side chains of selected residues are shown as sticks. Atom colorings in this figure and the following figures are as follows: oxygens in red, nitrogens in blue, and coloring for carbons follow the coloring scheme of the specific region of the kinase to which they belong. The mutant residue E650 and kinase insert tyrosine Y577 are labeled in red; other residues are labeled in black. The hydrogen bonds are shown as black dashed lines. See also Fig. S1–S3.

are given in Table 1. The refined model consists of residues L459 to T755, one AMP-PCP molecule, two Mg^{2+} ions, and 128 water molecules. FGFR3K^{K650E} exhibits the canonical two-lobe architecture of protein kinases with the smaller N-lobe comprising a twisted five-stranded β sheet and the α helix C, and the larger C-lobe consists mainly of a helices (Fig. 1). The ATP analog AMP-PCP is tucked snugly in the ATP-binding cleft between the two lobes, where it makes numerous hydrogen bonds and hydrophobic contacts with residues in both lobes as well as in the kinase hinge region (Fig. 1). The entire A-loop, bracketed between 635DFG and LPV^{658} motifs, is ordered, including the two tyrosine residues (Y647 and Y648), the phosphorylation of which is necessary for kinase activation. Most of the loop between the aD and aE helices, better known as the kinase insert region, is ordered as well (Fig. 1A). The ordering of this highly flexible loop is attributable to the fact that the autophosphorylation site Y577 from this loop inserts into the catalytic pocket of a neighboring kinase in the crystal, thereby forming an enzyme-substrate *trans*-phosphorylation complex.

Table 1. X-ray data collection and refinement statistics

Construct	FGFR3K^{K650E}
Data Collection	
Resolution (Å)	50–2.35 (2.39–2.35)[a]
Space group	P212121
Unit cell parameters (Å, °)	a = 54.226 α = 90.00
	b = 61.427 β = 90.00
	c = 100.666 γ = 90.00
Content of the asymmetric unit	1
No. of measured reflections	67 586
No. of unique reflections	14 385
Data redundancy	4.7
Data completeness (%)	97.0 (61.1)
R_{sym} (%)[b]	7.1 (24.3)
I/sig	32.4
Refinement	
R factor/R free	17.92/22.05
No. of protein atoms	2 322
No. of solvent atoms	128
No. of nonprotein/solvent atoms	33
Rmsd bond length (Å)	0.003
Rmsd bond angle (°)	0.776
PDB ID	4K33

[a]The numbers in parentheses refer to the highest resolution shell.

[b]Rsym = Σ|I − <I>|/Σ I, where I is the observed intensity of a reflection, and <I> is the average intensity of all of the symmetry-related reflections.

2.1 The K650E mutation confers gain-of-function by stabilizing the active conformation of the kinase A-loop

Superimposition of the FGFR3K^{K650E} structure onto the structures of unphosphorylated (low activity state) and A-loop phosphorylated (active state) FGFR1 (Bae *et al.*, 2009; Mohammadi *et al.*, 1996a) and FGFR2 (Chen *et al.*, 2007, 2008) kinases unambiguously shows that FGFR3K^{K650E} is in the active-state conformation (Fig. 1B; Fig. S1 available online). The A-loop of FGFR3K^{K650E} superimposes onto that of phosphorylated FGFR1 and FGFR2 kinases with root-mean-square deviations (rmsd) of 0.81 and 1.2 Å, respectively, and features the b strands 10 and 12 that are characteristics of the activated kinases (Fig. 1). A network of intramolecular hydrogen bonds introduced by the K650E mutation facilitates and stabilizes the active-state conformation of the A-loop in the FGFR3K^{K650E} structure (Fig. 1B). Specifically, the carboxylate group of E650 makes five hydrogen bonds: two with R616 in the catalytic loop, one each with the backbone amides of T651 and T652, and one with Y648 within the A-loop (Fig. 1B and S2). The latter hydrogen bond helps position the side chain of Y648 into a nearly identical location as that of the corresponding phosphorylated tyrosine residue in the A-loop phosphorylated wild-type (WT) FGFR1 and FGFR2 kinases (Fig. S1). The hydroxyl group of Y648 in FGFR3K^{K650E} makes an intramolecular hydrogen bond with R640 at the N-terminal end of the A-loop, which is reminiscent of the hydrogen bonds that the phosphate moiety of the phosphorylated A-loop tyrosine makes with the invariant A-loop arginine (Fig. 1B, S2). This hydrogen bond likely also contributes to the active-state conformation of the A-loop.

As in the crystal structures of A-loop phosphorylated, activated FGFR1 and FGFR2 kinases (Bae *et al.*, 2009; Chen *et al.*, 2007), the autoinhibitory molecular brake at the kinase hinge/ interlobe region of FGFR3K^{K650E} is disengaged, providing further evidence that the mutation drives the kinase into the active state (Fig. S3). The active-state conformation of FGFR3K^{K650E} is also apparent by the formation of a

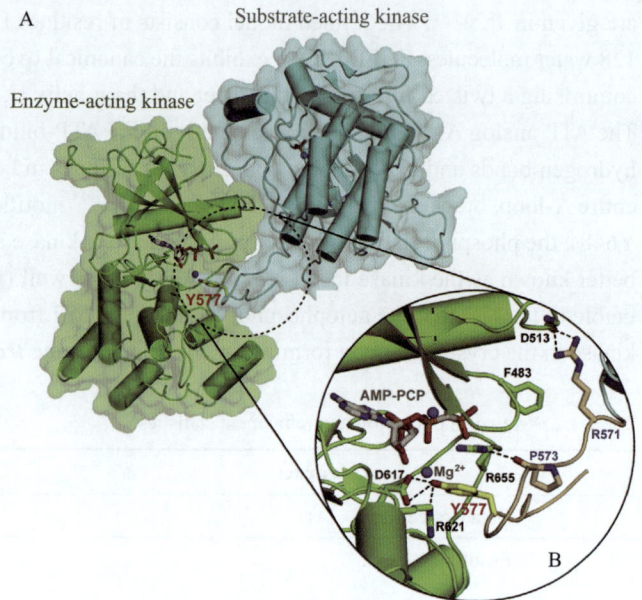

Fig. 2. Crystallographic snapshot of the kinase insert *trans*-phosphorylation reaction. (A) The substrate-acting kinase (in cyan) interacts with both N- and C-lobe of the enzyme-acting kinase (in green) during the *trans*-phosphorylation on Y577. (B) A detailed view of the interface formed between the enzyme-acting and substrate-acting kinases. The interacting residues are shown as sticks and labeled in black for the enzyme-acting kinase and in blue for the substrate-acting kinase. The kinase insert region is colored wheat, and the side chain of the Y577 residue is shown as yellow sticks and labeled in red. The hydrogen bonds are shown as black dashed lines. Atom coloring is as in Fig. 1. See also Fig. S1.

catalytically important salt bridge between the invariant E525 in the αC helix and K508 in the β3 strand of the kinase N-lobe (Fig. 1C). This salt bridge primes K508 for hydrogen bonding with the α and β phosphate groups of AMP-PCP (Fig. 1C). Analysis of crystal packing contacts provides additional strong evidence that the mutated FGFR3 kinase has adopted the active-state conformation. In the crystal, FGFR3K^{K650E} molecules are trapped in the act of *trans*-phosphorylation, whereby one kinase molecule acts as the enzyme, while the other serves as the substrate, offering a phosphorylatable tyrosine residue from the kinase insert region (Y577) (Fig. 2). The hydroxyl moiety Y577 of the substrate-acting kinase engages in two short-range hydrogen bonds with the catalytic base D617 of the enzyme-acting kinase and is about 5Å away from the g-phosphate of the ATP analog AMP-PCP, indicating that Y577 from the substrate-acting kinase is poised for deprotonation and phosphorylation by the enzyme-acting kinase (Fig. 2). Given the fact that substrate binding is strictly dependent on kinase activation (Hubbard and Till, 2000), this observation lends further support for the fact that the K650E mutation has forced the FGFR3 kinase into the active state. Taken together, these structural findings unambiguously demonstrate that the pathogenic K650E mutation confers gain-of-function by functionally mimicking the action of A-loop tyrosine phosphorylation in stabilizing the active-state conformation of the A-loop.

2.2 *The K650E mutation activates FGFR3 kinase independent of A-loop tyrosine phosphorylation*

To functionally validate our structural finding that the K650E mutation circumvents the requirement for A-loop tyrosine phosphorylation for FGFR3 kinase activation, we next compared the kinase activity of FGFR3K^{K650E} with that of FGFR3K^{K650E} harboring Y647F or Y648F single mutations or the Y647F/ Y648F double mutation *in vitro* (Fig. 3A–3E). As expected, FGFR3K^{K650E} exhibited greater activity than wild-type FGFR3K (FGFR3K^{WT}) at every time point examined, with the greatest difference (over 20-fold) seen at 20 s, the earliest measured time point (Fig. 3F). The difference in activity between FGFR3K^{K650E} and FGFR3K^{WT} tapered off at later time points, however. This is expected, as A-loop tyrosine phosphorylation takes place over time, amplifying the catalytic activity of FGFR3K^{WT}. The activity of the FGFR3K^{K650E} mutants in which one or both A-loop tyrosine residues has been replaced with phenylalanine remains

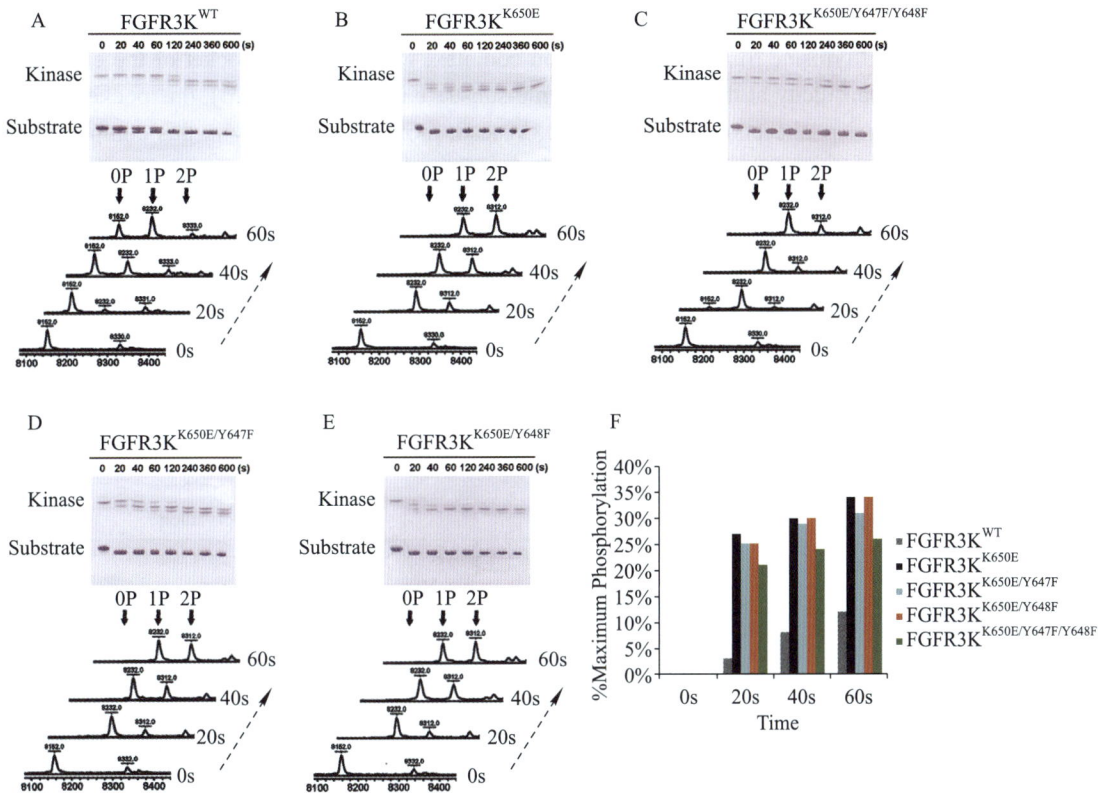

Fig. 3. The pathogenic K650E mutation circumvents the requirement for A-loop tyrosine phosphorylation for FGFR3 kinase activation (A–E) The substrate phosphorylation activities of FGFR3K^{WT}, FGFR3K^{K650E}, and its A-loop tyrosine mutant derivatives (FGFR3K$^{K650E/Y647F}$, FGFR3K$^{K650E/Y648F}$, and FGFR3K$^{K650E/Y647F/Y648F}$) were compared using native-PAGE (upper panel) coupled with time-resolved MALDI Q-TOF MS (lower panel). (F) The percentage of at least one site phosphorylation on the substrate was quantitated using the peak intensity data generated by mass spectrometry. For the sake of accuracy, only the MS data of the early time points (20, 40, and 60 s), which are in the linear phase of the kinase assay, were processed and presented.

comparable to that of the parent FGFR3K^{K650E} molecule (Fig. 3F), corroborating that kinase activation by the K650E mutation occurs independent of A-loop tyrosine phosphorylation. Our data are consistent with the previously published data by Webster and colleagues showed that the A-loop tyrosines are dispensable for the constitutive activity of the K650E FGFR3 mutant, implying that K650E mutation activates the kinase in an A-loop phosphorylation-independent fashion (Webster *et al.*, 1996). Notably, unlike FGFR3K^{WT}, the activity of FGFR3K^{K650E} did not increase significantly over time (Fig. 3F), further substantiating that the K650E mutation activates the kinase independent of A-loop tyro- sine phosphorylation. Taken together, these biochemical data support the structural finding that the K650E mutation confers constitutive activation by essentially mimicking the action of A-loop tyrosine phosphorylation in stabilizing the active-state conformation of the kinase.

2.3 Structural basis for specificity of tyrosine trans-phosphorylation in FGFR3 kinase

The crystal structure of FGFR3K^{K650E} depicts, as already mentioned, a snapshot of a *trans*-phosphorylation reaction on the kinase insert tyrosine residue Y577. We previously reported the crystal structure of FGFR2 kinases caught in the act of *trans*-phosphorylation on the FGFR-invariant C-terminal tail tyrosine (Chen *et al.*, 2008). Comparison of the two kinase *trans*-phosphorylation complexes provides important insights into the molecular determinants of specificity of kinase tyrosine *trans*-phosphorylation. Similar to the C-terminal tail tyrosine *trans*-phosphorylation complex, the kinase insert tyrosine *trans*-phosphorylation complex is also asymmetric, wherein the C-lobe of the substrate-acting kinase engages both the N- and C-lobe of the enzyme-acting kinase (Fig. 2). The enzyme-substrate interface can be roughly divided into a proximal and a distal site, with the former in the vicinity of the catalytic cleft of the enzyme-acting kinase and the latter remote from the catalytic cleft of the enzyme-acting kinase.

At the proximal interface, several contacts in the kinase insert tyrosine *trans*-phosphorylation complex (Fig. 4A) diverge from those observed in the C-terminal tail tyrosine *trans*-phosphorylation complex (Fig. 4B). Notably, in stark contrast to the C-terminal tail tyrosine *trans*-phosphorylation complex, where the P+1 pocket of the enzyme plays an important role in providing specificity at the proximal enzyme-substrate interface (Fig. 4B), this pocket is not utilized in the kinase insert tyrosine *trans*-phosphorylation complex. Instead, proximal specificity in this complex is primarily achieved by R655 from the A-loop of the enzyme-acting kinase. The guanidinium moiety of R655 stacks against the phenyl ring of Y577 *via* a π-cation interaction and also forms a hydrogen bond with the backbone carbonyl oxygen of P573 in the kinase insert of the substrate-acting kinase (Fig. 4A).

At the distal interface, the contacts in the kinase insert tyrosine *trans*-phosphorylation complex are completely different from those observed in the C-terminal tail tyrosine *trans*-phosphorylation complex. The main specific contacts in the distal site of the kinase insert tyrosine *trans*-phosphorylation complex are two hydrogen bonds between R571 (from the N-terminal end of the kinase insert of the substrate-acting kinase) and the backbone carbonyl oxygen atom of D513

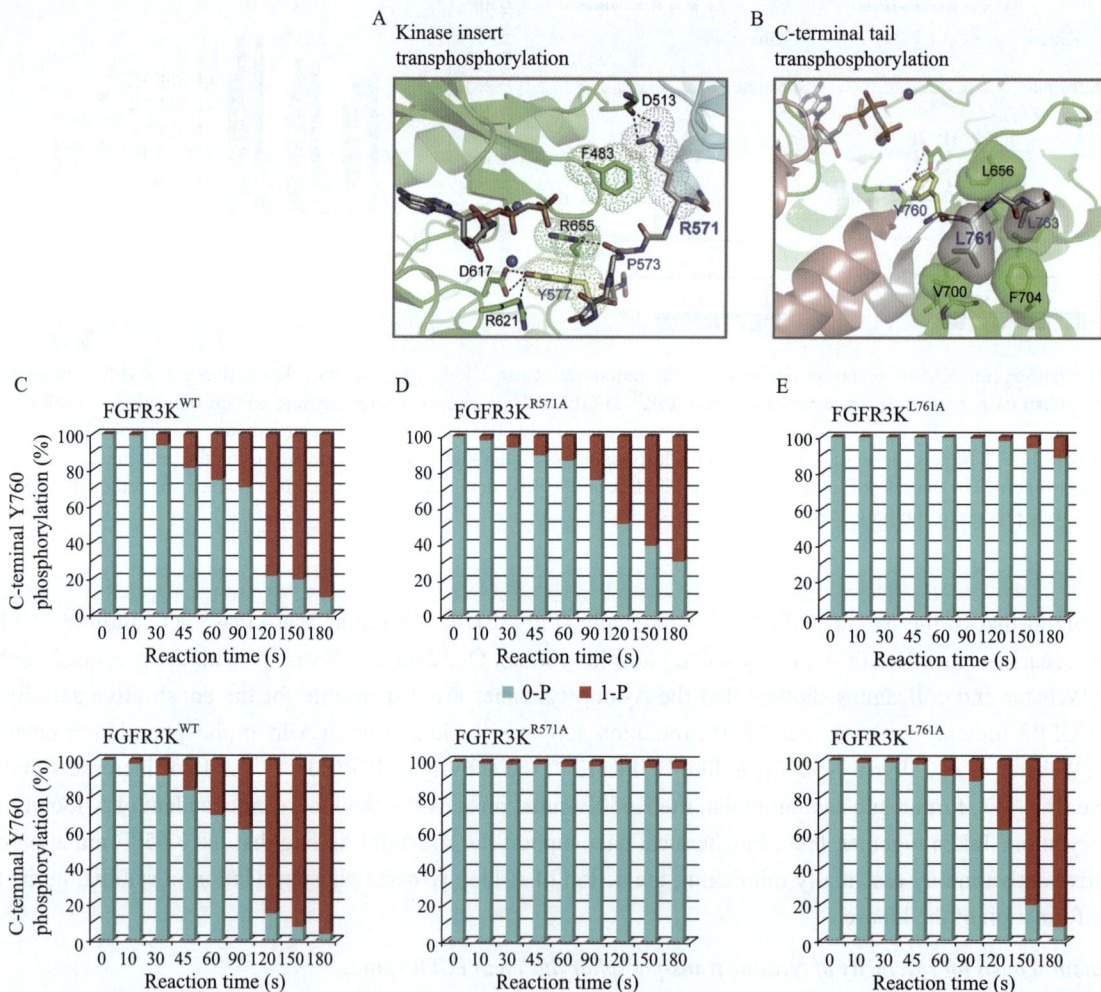

Fig. 4. Structural determinants of tyrosine *trans*-phosphorylation specificity in FGFR kinases. (A) Contacts between R571 of substrate and F483 of enzyme at the distal site mediate FGFR3 tyrosine *trans*-phosphorylation specificity on the kinase insert tyrosine Y577. Van der Waals surfaces of R571 and F483 are shown in mesh to emphasize their contacts. Likewise, meshed surfaces are used to indicate the π-cation interaction between the guanidinium moiety of R655 and the phenyl ring of Y577. (B) Based on the crystal structure of FGFR2 kinases trapped in the act of *trans*-phosphorylation on C-terminal tail tyrosine, the hydrophobic contacts between L761 of substrate and the P+1 pocket of the enzyme are critical for tyrosine *trans*-phosphorylation specificity on the C-terminal tail tyrosine Y760 in FGFR3. To highlight the hydrophobic contacts between the substrate and the enzyme at the P+1 pocket, the molecular surfaces of P+1 and P+3 residues (L761 and L763) of the substrate and residues in the P+1 pocket of the enzyme (L656, V700, and F704) are shown. Enzyme-acting kinases in both *trans*-phosphorylation complexes are colored green. Substrate-acting kinases are colored cyan and salmon in kinase insert and C-terminal tail tyrosine *trans*-phosphorylation complexes, respectively. (C–E) Analysis of autophosphorylation by mass spectrometry corroborates the importance of R571 and L761 in substrate recognition in the kinase insert and C-terminal tail tyrosine *trans*-phosphorylation. The R571A mutation diminishes *trans*-phosphorylation on the kinase insert tyrosine Y577 without a major impact on the C-terminal tail tyrosine phosphorylation (D). The L761A mutation (equivalent to L770A in FGFR2) impairs the *trans*-phosphorylation of the C-terminal tail tyrosine Y760 (E).

in the loop between β3 strand and αC helix of the enzyme-acting kinase (Fig. 4A). All of the remaining interactions at this distal contact site are of van der Waals nature with the most notable ones being the contacts between F483 from the nucleotide-binding loop of the enzyme-acting kinase and R571 of the substrate-acting kinase.

To functionally probe the observed mode of *trans*-phosphorylation specificity on the kinase insert tyrosine in the FGFR3K[K650E] crystal, we studied the impact of mutating R571 to alanine on phosphorylation of the kinase insert tyrosine Y577. Consistent with the structural data, the R571A mutation drastically impaired phosphorylation of the kinase insert tyrosine (Y577) but had only a minor effect on the phosphorylation of the C-terminal tail tyrosine (Y760) (Fig. 4D). As expected based on our previous crystal structure of the C-terminal tail tyrosine *trans*-phosphorylation complex (Chen *et al.*, 2008), substitution of L761, which engages the P+1 pocket of the enzyme, with alanine caused a major decrease in the kinase C-terminal tail tyrosine phosphorylation but had little impact on phosphorylation of the kinase insert tyrosine (Fig. 4E).

3. Discussion

In this study we elucidated the molecular mechanism by which the pathogenic K650E mutation in FGFR3, which underlies a lethal skeletal dysplasia in humans, confers gain-of-function on FGFR3. Our data unambiguously demonstrate that the K650E mutation mimics the action of A-loop tyrosine phosphorylation to cause ligand-independent activation of FGFR3. It should be noted that enzymes, in general, and tyrosine kinases, in particular, are intrinsically dynamic protein moieties, and in fact the catalytic turnover rate of enzymes is strongly correlated with magnitude and timescales of internal motions that enzymes undergo (Eisenmesser *et al.*, 2005; Villali and Kern, 2010). Using X-ray crystallography and NMR spectroscopy, we have recently shown that FGFR kinases swing between an inhibited state, which is conformationally rigid and stable, and an active state, which is conformationally dynamic and hence inhomogeneous (Chen *et al.*, 2013). The unphosphorylated wild-type FGFR kinase can sample the active state albeit with low frequency and hence predominately populates the inhibited state. Patho-genic mutations, such as the K650E mutation, introduce intra-molecular contacts that facilitate the ability of the kinase to adopt and remain longer in the active state, thereby increasing the population of kinase molecules in the active state (Chen *et al.*, 2013). In other words, the crystallographically fixed intramolecular hydrogen bonding contacts introduced by the mutation are dynamic in solution, and the FGFR3K[K650E] pathogenic kinase also oscillates between inhibited and active states with the equilibrium being skewed toward the active state.

Comparison of the kinase insert tyrosine *trans*-phosphorylation complex in the FGFR3K[K650E] crystal with the FGFR2 kinase C-terminal tail tyrosine *trans*-phosphorylation complex (Chen *et al.*, 2008) shows that kinase *trans*-phosphorylation entails a great degree of sequence specificity and structural complementarities. It remains to be determined whether Y577 of FGFR3 is phosphorylated in living cells. However, the equivalent tyrosine in FGFR1, Y583, is a bona fide *in vivo* phosphorylation site (Mohammadi *et al.*, 1996b) and is also a second major autophosphorylation site *in vitro* (Furdui *et al.*, 2006). Y577 is readily phosphorylated *in vitro*, both in the wild-type and in the K650E mutant FGFR3 kinases. Based on these observations, we surmise that Y577 undergoes phosphorylation *in vivo* as well. Future efforts should be directed toward elucidating the structural basis for *trans*-phosphorylation on the A-loop tyrosines, the earliest *trans*-phosphorylation event necessary for kinase activation. A full comprehension of the molecular details of FGFR *trans*-phosphorylation reactions will be essential to understanding FGFR signaling and devising novel strategies for targeted modulation of FGF signaling for therapeutic purposes.

4. Experimental procedures

Please refer to the Supplemental Experimental Procedures for full details.

4.1 Protein expression and purification

The human FGFR3 kinase domains FGFR3K[450-758] and FGFR3K[429-768], including their mutated forms, and the C-terminal tail peptide of FGFR2 kinase (FGFR2K[761-821]) were all expressed using pET bacterial expression vectors with an N-terminal 6XHis-tag to aid in protein purification.

4.2 Crystallization and structure determination

Crystals of the FGFR3K^{K650E} protein in complex with the ATP-analog (AMP- PCP) were grown by vapor diffusion at 20°C using crystallization buffer composed of 0.1 M HEPES (pH 7.5), 20% (*w/v*) PEG 4000, and 4% (*v/v*) (±)-1,3 Butanediol. Diffraction data were processed using the *HKL2000* suite (Otwinowski and Minor, 1997), and the structure was solved by the molecular replacement program *AMoRe* (Navaza, 1994), using the crystal structure of FGFR2 kinase that harbors the K659N mutation (Protein Data Bank [PDB] ID code 2PVY) (Chen *et al.*, 2007) as the search model. Model building was carried out using *O* (Jones *et al.*, 1991), and at later stages *Coot* (Emsley and Cowtan, 2004) was used, and refinement was completed using *PHENIX* (Adams *et al.*, 2002).

4.3 Dissection of the role of A-loop tyrosine phosphorylation in gain-of-function by the K650E mutation using peptide substrate phosphorylation

Peptide substrate phosphorylation activities of wild-type and mutated FGFR3 kinases (FGFR3K^{WT}, FGFR3K^{K650E}, FGFR3K$^{K650E/Y647F}$, FGFR3K$^{K650E/Y648F}$, and FGFR3K$^{K650E/Y647F/Y648F}$) were analyzed by MALDI-TOF MS (Bruker Autoflex MALDI-TOF, Bruker Daltonics) in positive ion linear mode.

4.4 Analysis of the specificity of tyrosine trans-phosphorylation

The *trans*-phosphorylation on kinase insert and C-terminal tail tyrosines in wild-type and mutated FGFR3 kinases (FGFR3K$^{440-778}$, FGFR3K$^{440-778/R571A}$, FGFR3K$^{440-778/R655A}$, and FGFR3K$^{440-778/L761A}$) were analyzed by LTQ Orbitrap (Thermo Electron) liquid chromatography-tandem mass spectrometry.

Supplemental information

Supplemental information to this article can be found online at http://dx.doi.org/10.1016/j.str.2013.07.017.

The coordinates and structure factors for the FGFR3K^{K650E} structure have been deposited in the Protein Data Bank under the accession number 4K33.

References

[1] Adams PD, Grosse-Kunstleve RW, Hung LW, *et al*. PHENIX: building new software for automated crystallographic structure determination[J]. Acta Crystallographica Section D-Biological Crystallography, 2002, 58: 1948-1954.

[2] Agazie YM, Movilla N, Ischenko I, *et al*. The phosphotyrosine phosphatase SHP2 is a critical mediator of transformation induced by the oncogenic fibroblast growth factor receptor 3[J]. Oncogene, 2003, 22(44): 6909-6918.

[3] Bae JH, Boggon TJ, Tome F, *et al*. Asymmetric receptor contact is required for tyrosine autophosphorylation of fibroblast growth factor receptor in living cells[J]. Proceedings Of the National Academy Of Sciences Of the United States Of America, 2010, 107(7): 2866-2871.

[4] Bae JH, Lew ED, Yuzawa S, *et al*. The selectivity of receptor tyrosine kinase signaling is controlled by a secondary SH2 domain binding site[J]. Cell, 2009, 138(3): 514-524.

[5] Beenken A, Mohammadi M. The FGF family: biology, pathophysiology and therapy[J]. Nature Reviews Drug Discovery, 2009, 8(3): 235-253.

[6] Bellus GA, McIntosh I, Smith EA, *et al*. A Recurrent mutation in the tyrosine kinase domain of fibroblast growth-factor receptor-3 causes hypochondroplasia[J]. Nature Genetics, 1995, 10(3): 357-359.

[7] Bellus GA, Spector EB, Speiser PW, *et al*. Distinct missense mutations of the FCFR3 Lys650 codon modulate receptor kinase activation and the severity of the skeletal dysplasia phenotype[J]. American Journal Of Human Genetics, 2000, 67(6): 1411-1421.

[8] Cappellen D, De Oliveira C, Ricol D, *et al*. Frequent activating mutations of FGFR3 in human bladder and cervix carcinomas[J]. Nature Genetics, 1999, 23(1): 18-20.

[9] Chen H, Huang Z, Dutta K, *et al*. Cracking the molecular origin of intrinsic tyrosine kinase activity through analysis of pathogenic gain-of-function mutations[J]. Cell Reports, 2013, 4(2): 376-384.

[10] Chen H, Ma J, Li W, *et al*. A molecular brake in the kinase hinge region regulates the activity of receptor tyrosine kinases[J]. Molecular Cell, 2007, 27(5): 717-730.

[11] Chen H, Xu C-F, Ma J, *et al*. A crystallographic snapshot of tyrosine trans-phosphorylation in action[J]. Proceedings Of the National Academy Of Sciences Of the United States Of America, 2008, 105(50): 19660-19665.

[12] Chesi M, Nardini E, Brents LA, *et al*. Frequent translocation t(4;14) (p16.3;q32.3) in multiple myeloma is associated with increased expression and activating mutations of fibroblast growth factor receptor 3[J]. Nature Genetics, 1997, 16(3): 260-264.

[13] Eisenmesser EZ, Millet O, Labeikovsky W, *et al*. Intrinsic dynamics of an enzyme underlies catalysis[J]. Nature, 2005, 438(7064): 117-121.

[14] Emsley P, Cowtan K. Coot: model-building tools for molecular

graphics[J]. Acta Crystallographica Section D-Biological Crystallography, 2004, 60: 2126-2132.

[15] Foldynova-Trantirkova S, Wilcox WR, Krejci P. Sixteen years and counting: the current understanding of fibroblast growth factor receptor 3 (FGFR3) signaling in skeletal dysplasias[J]. Human Mutation, 2012, 33(1): 29-41.

[16] Furdui CM, Lew ED, Schlessinger J, *et al.* Autophosphorylation of FGFR1 kinase is mediated by a sequential and precisely ordered reaction[J]. Molecular Cell, 2006, 21(5): 711-717.

[17] Goetz R, Mohammadi M. Exploring mechanisms of FGF signalling through the lens of structural biology[J]. Nature Reviews Molecular Cell Biology, 2013, 14(3): 166-180.

[18] Guo C, Degnin CR, Laederich MB, *et al.* Sprouty 2 disturbs FGFR3 degradation in thanatophoric dysplasia type II: A severe form of human achondroplasia[J]. Cellular Signalling, 2008, 20(8): 1471-1477.

[19] Hubbard SR, Till JH. Protein tyrosine kinase structure and function[J]. Annual Review Of Biochemistry, 2000, 69: 373-398.

[20] Jones TA, Zou JY, Cowan SW, *et al.* Improved methods for building protein models in electron-density maps and the location of errors in these models[J]. Acta Crystallographica Section A, 1991, 47: 110-119.

[21] Kan S, Elankko N, Johnson D, *et al.* Genomic screening of fibroblast growth-factor receptor 2 reveals a wide spectrum of mutations in patients with syndromic craniosynostosis[J]. American Journal Of Human Genetics, 2002, 70(2): 472-486.

[22] Lievens PMJ, Liboi E. The thanatophoric dysplasia type II mutation hampers complete maturation of fibroblast growth factor receptor 3 (FGFR3), which activates signal transducer and activator of transcription 1 (STAT1) from the endoplasmic reticulum[J]. Journal Of Biological Chemistry, 2003, 278(19): 17344-17349.

[23] Mohammadi M, Dikic I, Sorokin A, *et al.* Identification of six novel autophosphorylation sites on fibroblast growth factor receptor 1 and elucidation of their importance in receptor activation and signal transduction[J]. Molecular And Cellular Biology, 1996, 16(3): 977-989.

[24] Mohammadi M, Schlessinger J, Hubbard SR. Structure of the FGF receptor tyrosine kinase domain reveals a novel autoinhibitory mechanism[J]. Cell, 1996, 86(4): 577-587.

[25] Naski MC, Wang Q, Xu JS, *et al.* Graded activation of fibroblast growth factor receptor 3 by mutations causing achondroplasia and thanatophoric dysplasia[J]. Nature Genetics, 1996, 13(2): 233-237.

[26] Navaza J. Amore - an automated package for molecular replacement [J]. Acta Crystallographica Section A, 1994, 50: 157-163.

[27] Nowroozi N, Raffioni S, Wang T, *et al.* Sustained ERK1/2 but not STAT1 or 3 activation is required for thanatophoric dysplasia phenotypes in PC12 cells[J]. Human Molecular Genetics, 2005, 14(11): 1529-1538.

[28] Otwinowski Z, Minor W. Processing of X-ray diffraction data collected in oscillation mode[J]. Macromolecular Crystallography, Pt A, 1997, 276: 307-326.

[29] Tavormina PL, Shiang R, Thompson LM, *et al.* Thanatophoric dysplasia (type-i and type-II) caused by distinct mutations in fibroblast growth-factor receptor-3[J]. Nature Genetics, 1995, 9(3): 321-328.

[30] Villali J, Kern D. Choreographing an enzyme's dance[J]. Current Opinion In Chemical Biology, 2010, 14(5): 636-643.

[31] Webster MK, dAvis PY, Robertson SC, *et al.* Profound ligand-independent kinase activation of fibroblast growth factor receptor 3 by the activation loop mutation responsible for a lethal skeletal dysplasia, thanatophoric dysplasia type II[J]. Molecular And Cellular Biology, 1996, 16(8): 4081-4087.

[32] Webster MK, Donoghue DJ. Enhanced signaling and morphological transformation by a membrane-localized derivative of the fibroblast growth factor receptor 3 kinase domain[J]. Molecular And Cellular Biology, 1997, 17(10): 5739-5747.

[33] Webster MK, Donoghue DJ. FGFR activation in skeletal disorders: Too much of a good thing[J]. Trends In Genetics, 1997, 13(5): 178-182.

[34] Wilcox WR, Tavormina PL, Krakow D, *et al.* Molecular, radiologic, and histopathologic correlations in thanatophoric dysplasia[J]. American Journal Of Medical Genetics, 1998, 78(3): 274-281.

[35] Wilkie AOM. Bad bones, absent smell, selfish testes: The pleiotropic consequences of human FGF receptor mutations[J]. Cytokine & Growth Factor Reviews, 2005, 16(2): 187-203.

Dual delivery of bFGF- and NGF-binding coacervate confers neuroprotection by promoting neuronal proliferation

Yanqing Wu, Xiaokun Li, Jian Xiao

1. Introduction

Neurodegenerative diseases are a major socioeconomic burden and lead to unimaginable misery for millions of sufferers and their families around the world. With an increasing ageing population, the number of neurodegenerative diseases is expected to rise even further, prompting an urgent need for the development of rational and effective therapeutic strategies that can reverse or slow the degenerative process. Stem cell therapy, growth factors, and gene therapy are novel treatments that might prolong survival and delay progression of symptoms [1-4]. Growth factor treatment is one of the most promising therapies for neurodegenerative diseases, due to their great potential for neurorestoration and neuroprotection.

Within the family of neurotrophic factors, nerve growth factor (NGF) stimulates the survival and maturation of developing neurons in the peripheral nervous system and protects neurons in the degenerating mammalian brain [5-8]. It has been used as a therapeutic agent for the restoration and maintenance of neuronal function in both basic and clinical studies. Basic fibroblast growth factor (bFGF) is highly expressed in the nervous system and exerts multiple roles supporting the survival and growth of cultured neurons and neural stem cells [8-10]. Although bFGF and NGF have distinctive neuroprotective properties, their short half-life and rapid diffusion rate seriously hinders their clinical applicability. Thus, the development of a useful delivery system that not only protects the GFs from proteolytic degradation and controls their spatiotemporal release, but also avoids side effects from high concentrations of GFs for body would greatly improve their clinical efficacy.

[PEAD:heparin] coacervate is formed by a polycation, poly ethylene arginyl aspartate diglyceride (PEAD), and heparin [11]. PEAD is a biodegradable polycation with high biocompatibility and high charge density, which strongly binds to heparin and consequently is capable of incorporating growth factors with high efficiency [11]. Previous studies have demonstrated that [PEAD:heparin] coacervate controls the release of growth factors for over 30 days in a nearly linear fashion, can maintain the bioactivity of bFGF, and can increase the bioactivity of NGF [8], indicating that [PEAD:heparin] coacervate may be an optimal delivery system for growth factors for the treatment of neurodegenerative diseases.

Although the delivery of a single GF, bFGF or NGF, has shown promising therapeutic potency for neurodegenerative diseases, co-delivery of multiple GFs may be more successful in therapy. In this study, we co-delivered bFGF and NGF *via* [PEAD:heparin] coacervate and examined the effect of controlled co-release of bFGF and NGF on PC12 cells and SH-SY5Y cells. We hypothesized that co-delivery of bFGF and NGF would have a stronger and more robust neuroprotective effect than that of individual GF coacervates and the co-administration of free GFs.

2. Materials and methods

2.1 Reagents and antibodies

Recombinant human bFGF was purchased from Grost (Grost Biotechnology, Zhejiang, China). NGF and heparin were purchased from Sigma (Sigma-Aldrich, St. Louis, MO, USA). PEAD was a gift from the University of Pittsburgh. NGF and bFGF enzyme linked immunosorbent assay (ELISA) kits were purchased from Elabscience Biotechnology.

Dulbecco's modified Eagle's medium (DMEM) and fetal bovine serum (FBS) were purchased from Invitrogen (Carlsbad, CA, USA).

2.2　[PEAD:heparin] coacervate synthesis and maximal package loads of GFs

Poly ethylene argininylaspartate diglyceride (PEAD) was synthesized as previously described [11]. PEAD, heparin, NGF and bFGF were seriatim dissolved in 0.9% normal saline to obtain 10 mg/ml solutions and sterilized using 0.22 μm Millipore filter. We used a PEAD:heparin:GF with mass ratio of 500:100:1 to achieve maximal coacervation. The bFGF was loaded into the coacervate at doses of 50 ng, 100 ng and 10 μg respectively; the NGF was loaded at doses of 1 μg, 2 μg and 10 μg respectively. After 2 h, the solution was then centrifuged at 12 000 g for 10 min to pellet the coacervate at 4℃. The supernatant was aspirated and stored, and pellet was re-suspended using loading buffer to detect the maximal package loads of GFs in coacervate by Western blotting.

2.3　Western blotting

To detect the maximal package loads of GFs, protein concentrations were quantified using a BCA Protein Assay Kit (Thermo, Rockford, IL, USA). The equivalent of total protein was loaded onto SDS-PAGE, transferred to PVDF membrane (Bio-Rad), and blocked with 5% non-fat-milk in TBS with 0.05% Tween 20 (TBST) for 45 min. Primary antibodies were incubated overnight at 4℃. The membranes were washed with TBST for 3 times and incubated with horseradish peroxidase-conjugated secondary antibodies (1:10 000) for 4h at room temperature. Signals were visualized using the ChemiDocTM XRS + Imaging System (Bio-Rad).

2.4　Growth factors release assay

On day 1, 4, 7, 14, 21, 28 and 35, PEAD: heparin: GF coacervates with maximal package loads of bFGF and NGF were gently mixed and centrifuged at 12 000 g for 10 min. Then, the supernatant was collected to detect the amount of released GFs *via* ELISA kit. Standards containing 200 ng free-form GFs were used to determine the percent release. The samples and standards were reacted with assay buffer. The absorbance of the supernatant was recorded by a SynergyMX plate reader at 450/540 nm.

2.5　Cell viability measurements

MTT assay was used to determine cell viability and the optimal concentration of bFGF and NGF. Briefly, cells were plated at a density of 8 000 per well in a 96-well plate. After 6 h, the cells were washed with PBS and cultured in serum-free medium. Then, the cells were treated with bFGF and NGF at doses of 50 nM, 100 nM, 200 nM and 400 nM respectively. After 24 h incubation, 20 μl MTT buffer was added to each well. The absorbance was recorded by a SynergyMX plate reader at 490 nm.

2.6　Detection of cell growth status

PC12 cells and SH-SY5Y cells were plated at a density of 8000 per well in a 96-well plate. 6h after seeding, group-specific media was added and 8 groups were used with 5 wells per group: basal media, blank coacervate, free bFGF, free NGF, free bFGF+NGF, bFGF coacervate, NGF coacervate, and bFGF+NGF coacervate. Each GF was added at an optimal concentration according to MTT assay results. Cell growth status was observed and captured under an inverted microscope (Nikon ECLIPSE Ti-S). The area of cell number was quantitatively analyzed.

2.7　The proliferation of neuronal cells and live cell

Similar culture conditions were used for detecting the level of cell proliferation and performing live cell count assays. PC12 cells and SH-SY5Y cells were labeled with calcein AM for 2 h before seeding cells in 100 μl media per well in a 96-well plate. 6 h after seeding, group-specific media was added and 8 groups were used with 5 wells per group: basal media, blank coacervate, free bFGF, free NGF, free bFGF+NGF, bFGF coacervate, NGF coacervate, and bFGF+NGF coacervate. Each GF was added at an optimal concentration. For the BrdU cell proliferation assay, the plate was incubated at 37℃ for 16 h, then 20 μl of BrdU label was added to each well and incubated for 4 h. The proliferation assay protocol was then followed according to the kit's instruction manual. After the addition of stop solution, the absorbance at 450/540 nm was recorded by a SynergyMX plate reader and normalized to the basal media control. For the live cell count assay, the plate was incubated at 37℃ for 3 d, then cells were observed using a fluorescence microscope. The number of cells was determined by manually counting the cells in a 0.67 mm² field in the center of the well for 5 wells per group. Fluorescent images of cells were taken of 4 mm² fields.

2.8 Statistical analysis

Data is presented as the mean ± SD. Statistical differences were evaluated using One-way analysis of variance (ANOVA) followed by Tukey's test with GraphPad Prism 5 software. Differences were suggested to be statistically significant when $P < 0.05$.

3. Results

3.1 Loads and release efficiency of bFGF and NGF in [PEAD:heparin] coacervate

It had been demonstrated that maximal coacervation occurs at a mass ratio of 500:100:1 PEAD:heparin:GF [12]. In this study, we utilized PEAD:heparin:GF coacervate with this mass ratio and observed that the coacervate became turbid and precipitated immediately with bound GFs to the coacervate (Fig. 1A). After 24 h, the coavervate became pellucid and settled on the bottom of the tube (Fig. 1A). The maximal loads of bFGF and NGF in [PEAD:heparin] coacervate were detected by Western blotting. 100 ng, 200 ng and 10 µg of bFGF and 1 µg, 2 µg and 10 µg of NGF were bound to coacervate. The maximal loading capacity of each was found to be 10 µg (Fig. 1B). To further investigate the release efficiency of GFs that bound with coacervate, we measured the release amount of bFGF and NGF by ELISA on days 1, 4, 7, 14, 21, 28 and 35. NGF and bFGF were immediately released on day 1, and then sustained from day 1 to day 21. Afterwards, both were released slower and gradually trended to stabilize. By day 35, the total release of NGF and bFGF were approximately 60% and 30%, respectively. Taken together, this not only demonstrated that coavervate loading with GFs contributes to their slow release, but also indicated that the release efficiency of NGF was higher than that of bFGF in coacervate.

3.2 Determining the optimal protective concentration of bFGF and NGF on PC12 cells and SH-SY5Y cells

To test the optimal protective concentration of bFGF and NGF on PC12 cells and SH-SY5Y cells, we assessed the cell viability of PC12 cells and SH-SY5Y cells after treatment with different doses of each GF. We found 100 ng/ml to be the optimal protective concentration of bFGF on PC12 cells and SH-SY5Y cells (Fig. 2). Additionally, 100 ng/ml and 200 ng/ml of NGF were the optimal protective concentrations for

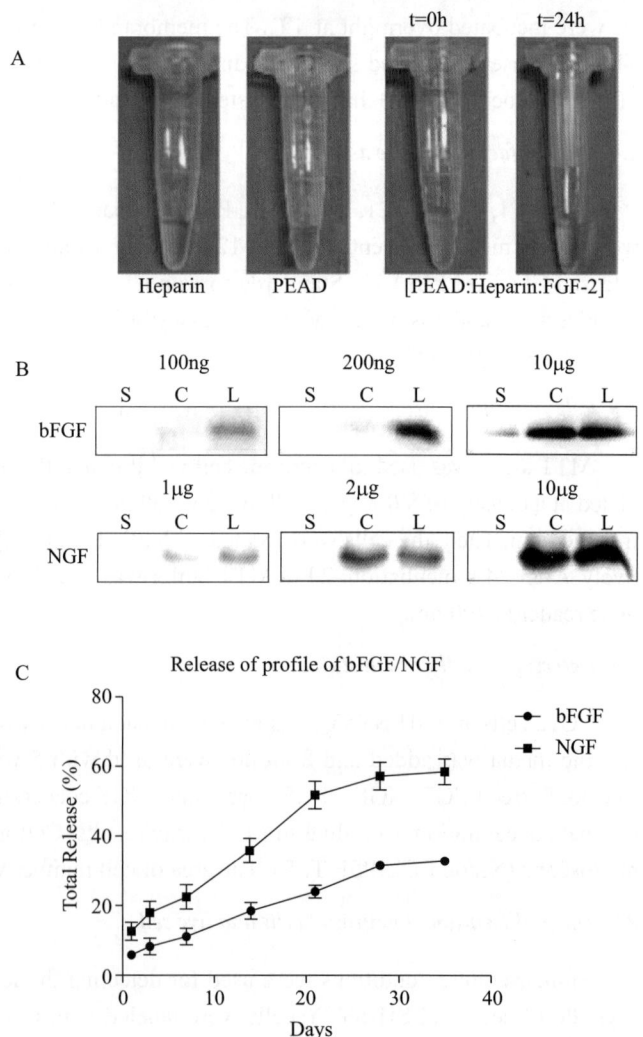

Fig. 1. Properties of [PEAD:heparin] coacervate binding with bFGF or NGF. (A) Preparation of [PEAD:heparin] coacervate. (B) Western blotting analysis of the loading efficiency of bFGF and NGF into coacervate. S: bFGF or NGF in supernatant after centrifugation. C: bFGF or NGF in settled coacervates. L: total amount of bFGF or NGF in loading solution. (C) Release efficiency of bFGF and NGF in [PEAD:heparin] coacervate. ($n=$ 3 per group).

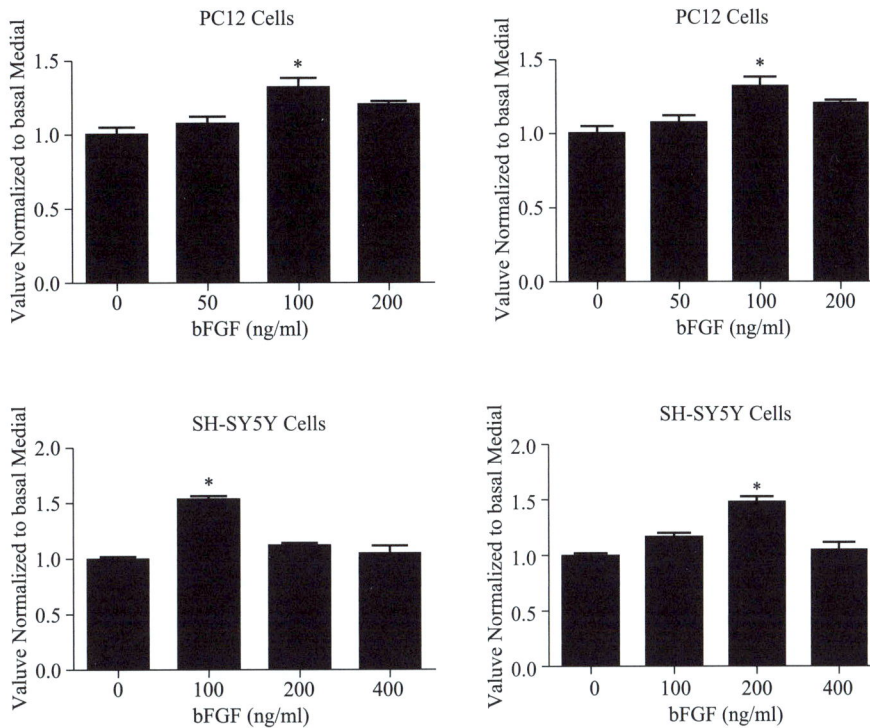

Fig. 2. The optimal protective concentration of bFGF and NGF on PC12 cells and SH-SY5Y cells. (A) The optimal protective concentration of bFGF and NGF on PC12 cells. (B) The optimal protective concentration of bFGF and NGF on SH-SY5Y cells. $^{*}P<0.05$ *vs.* the other groups.

PC12 cells and SH-SY5Y cells (Fig. 2).

3.3 bFGF+NGF coacervate promotes the growth of PC12 cells and SH-SY5Y cells

To assess how bFGF and NGF affect neuronal cell growth, PC12 cells were cultured in serum-free culture medium and each GF was applied separately or together in free-form or coacervate-bound. PC12 cells in serum-free culture medium had fewer cell number and abnormal morphology with karyopyknotic nuclei and shortened axons (Fig. 3A, B). Treatment with bFGF and NGF together in free-form recovered PC12 cell growth better than each GF alone. Moreover, each GF alone delivered by coacervate also significantly promoted PC12 cells growth when compared to free GF delivery. Importantly, compared to the other groups, dual delivery of bFGF and NGF in coavervate was the most beneficial to PC12 cells growth as evidenced by increased cell number and normal morphology (Fig. 3A, B). Consistent with our findings in PC12 cells, dual delivery of bFGF and NGF bound to coacervate also significantly promoted SH-SY5Y cells growth (Fig. 4A, B).

3.4 bFGF+NGF coacervate induces the proliferation of PC12 cells and SH- SY5Y cells

In this study, we further investigated the effect of bFGF and NGF on the proliferation of PC12 cells. PC12 cells were treated with each GF separately or together, in free-form or coacervate bound. 1 day after treatment, Free-form dual delivery of GFs and each GF alone delivered by coacervate significantly induced greater proliferation compared to each GF alone. Furthermore, dual delivery of bFGF and NGF with coacervate had a stronger effect compared to the other groups (Fig. 5A). Calcein staining was used to verify the cell proliferation beyond 1 day, and cells were still viable after 3 days culture. Consistent with these results, co-delivery of bFGF and NGF bound to coacervate exerted a stronger proliferative effect and induced more live cells compared to the other group (Fig. 5B, C). Additionally, the bFGF+NGF coacervate could significantly induce the proliferation of SH-SY5Y cells (Fig. 6A, B, C). Taken together, these results demonstrated that co-delivery of bFGF and NGF with coacervate had the greatest potential for promoting the proliferation of neuronal cells.

A.

B.

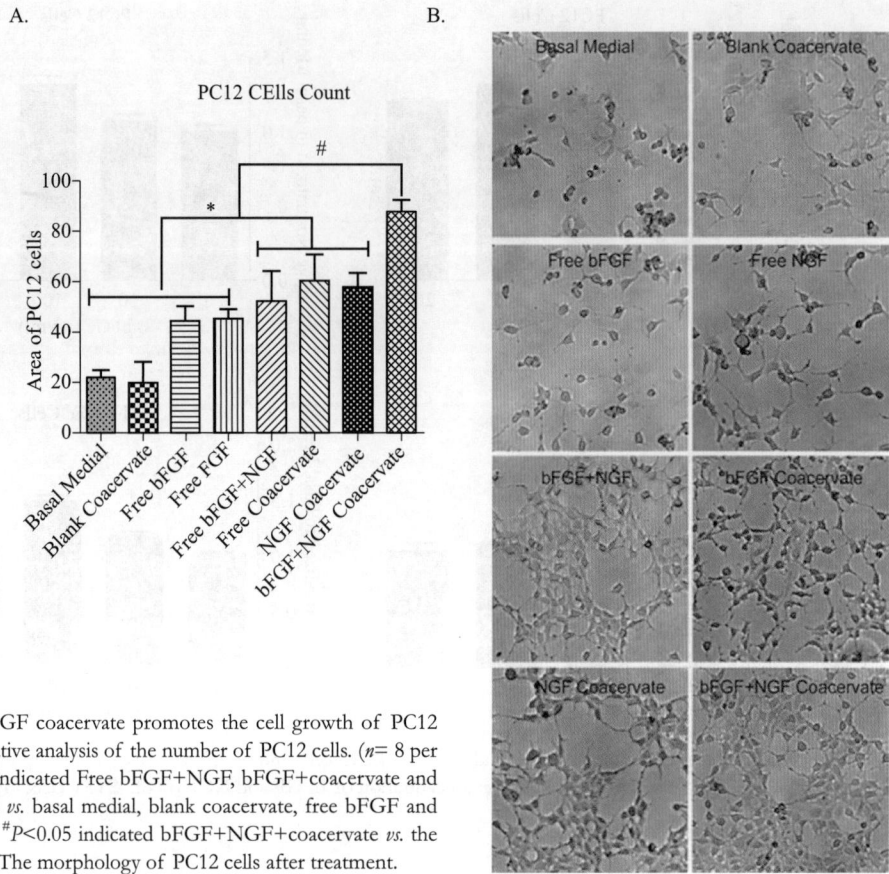

Fig. 3. bFGF+NGF coacervate promotes the cell growth of PC12 cells. (A) Quantitative analysis of the number of PC12 cells. ($n=$ 8 per group). *$P<0.05$ indicated Free bFGF+NGF, bFGF+coacervate and NGF+coacervate $vs.$ basal medial, blank coacervate, free bFGF and free NGF group; #$P<0.05$ indicated bFGF+NGF+coacervate $vs.$ the other groups. (B) The morphology of PC12 cells after treatment.

A

B

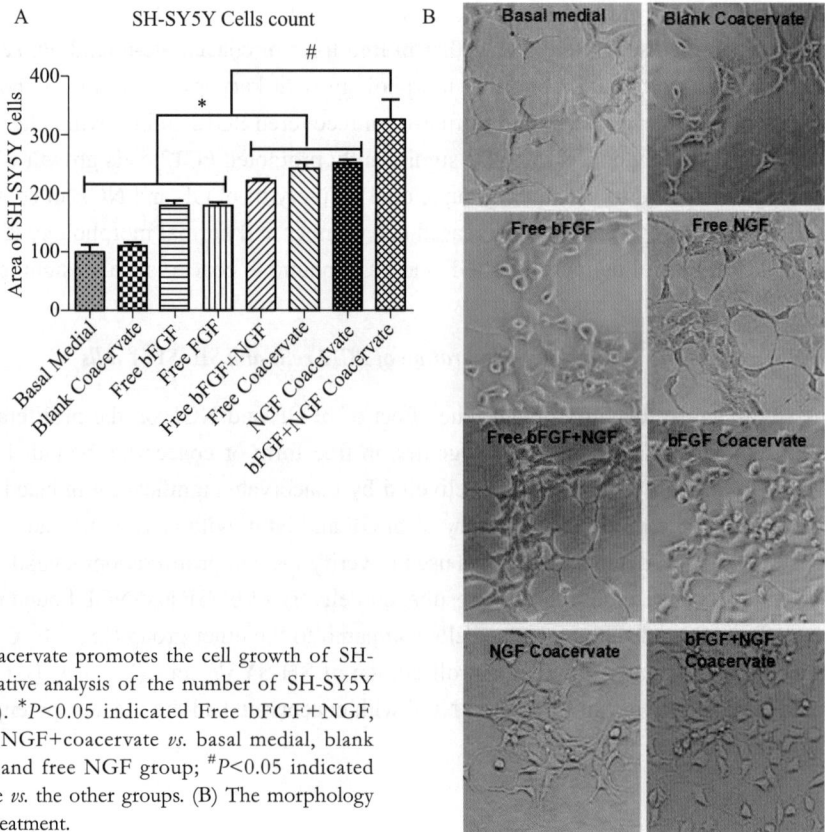

Fig. 4. bFGF+NGF coacervate promotes the cell growth of SH-SY5Y cells. (A) Quantitative analysis of the number of SH-SY5Y cells. ($n=$ 8 per group). *$P<0.05$ indicated Free bFGF+NGF, bFGF+coacervate and NGF+coacervate $vs.$ basal medial, blank coacervate, free bFGF and free NGF group; #$P<0.05$ indicated bFGF+NGF+coacervate $vs.$ the other groups. (B) The morphology of SH-SY5Y cells after treatment.

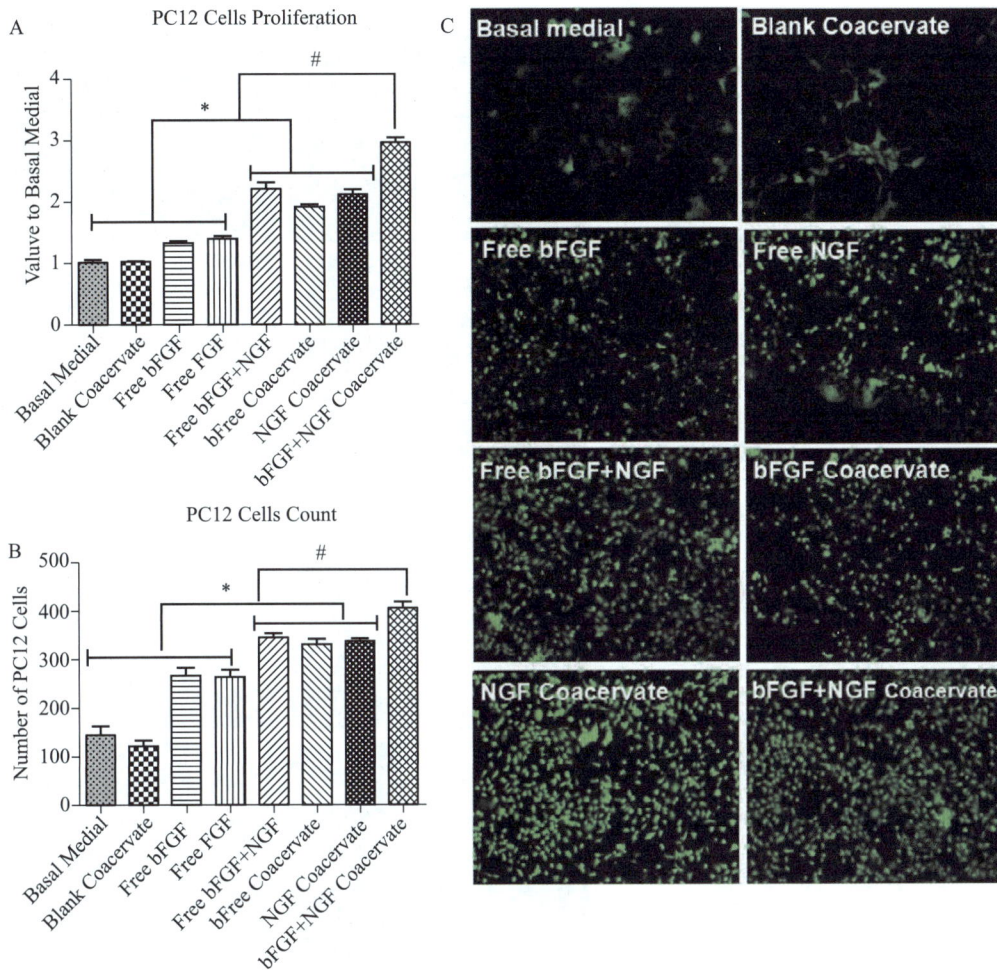

Fig. 5. bFGF+NGF coacervate induces the proliferation of PC12 cells. (A) The proliferation level of PC12 cells after treatment with free GFs or coacervate delivery of GFs. (B) Live PC12 cells number was quantified after 3 days incubation over 0.67 mm^2 fields in 3 wells per group. (C) Microscope images of calcein-stained PC12 cells. $^*P<0.05$ indicated Free bFGF+NGF, bFGF+coacervate and NGF+coacervate *vs.* basal medial, blank coacervate, free bFGF and free NGF group; $^\#P<0.05$ indicated bFGF+NGF+coacervate *vs.* the other groups.

4. Discussion

Neurodegenerative diseases are a more and more serious problem for the aging population in the world. They are characterized by progressive loss of neuronal function in defined regions of the nervous system. Elevated cellular stress, mitochondrial dysfunction, synapse loss, and neuronal apoptosis are the main physiological symptoms of neurodegenerative diseases [13]. No broadly effective strategies have been developed recently to reverse or halt the progression of these diseases in patients. bFGF and NGF have been extensively shown to promote the survival and maintainenance of neuronal function in neurological diseases [14, 15]. A deficiency of these two GFs may cause neuron susceptibility to injury and death [16, 17], suggesting that molecular therapy with exogenous bFGF and NGF may be a novel and challenging therapeutic strategy for neurodegenerative diseases.

However, the application of these GFs, including NGF and bFGF, in clinical therapy is greatly limited by their short half-life. Without efficient delivery systems, GFs degrade quickly and lose their bioactivities, which potentially lead to harmful effects when injected at high concentrations for effective therapy. Moreover, GFs diffuses broadly circulate throughout the body, which leads to adverse effects that can be intolerable. Previous studies reported that NGF led to pain and weight loss by stimulating nociceptive and hypothalamic neurons, respectively [18, 19]. Developing a controlled and useful delivery system that can preserve their processibility and biocompatibility is particularly attractive for their biomedical application. In this study, we utilized [PEAD:heparin] coacervate as a delivery system to deliver NGF and

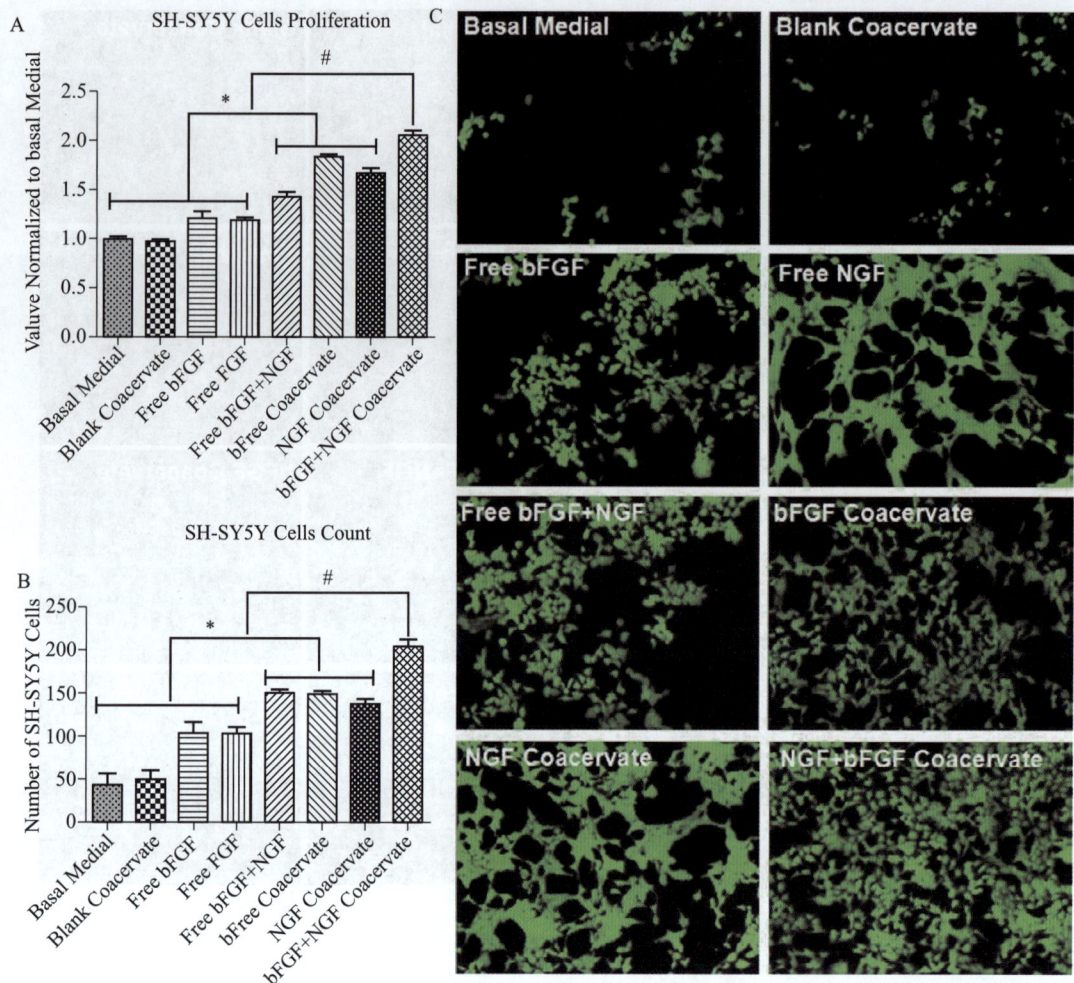

Fig. 6. bFGF+NGF coacervate induces the proliferation of SH-SY5Y cells. (A) The proliferation level of SH-SY5Y cells after treatment with free GFs or coacervate delivery of GFs. (B) Live SH-SY5Y cells number was quantified after 3 days incubation over 0.67 mm² fields in 3 wells per group. (C) Microscope images of calcein-stained SH-SY5Y cells. *P<0.05 indicated Free bFGF+NGF, bFGF+coacervate and NGF+coacervate vs. basal medial, blank coacervate, free bFGF and free NGF group; #P<0.05 indicated bFGF+NGF+coacervate vs. the other groups.

bFGF, and further confirmed the effects of bFGF and NGF on growth and proliferation of neuronal cells.

[PEAD:heparin] coacervate was formed by a polycation, poly(ethylene arginyl aspartate diglyceride) (PEAD) and heparin that can control the release of heparin-binding GFs [20]. The coacervate maintains the native properties and function of heparin through the direct, ionic interactions with PEAD [21], which not only improves GF loading efficiency and maintains their bioactivity, but also well controls the release of GFs to target tissues [20]. Thus, coacervate had been widely used to spatially and temporally control the release of GFs [22-25].

Wang et al. demonstrated that the molecular weight of PEAD and/or heparin, the charge density of PEAD, and the [PEAD:heparin] mass ratio affected the delivery function of [PEAD:heparin] coacervate. Moreover, a PEAD:heparin:GF mass ratio of 500:100:1 achieved maximal coacervation [21]. In this study, we developed [PEAD:heparin] coacervate with a PEAD: heparin: GF mass ratio of 500:100:1 to deliver bFGF and NGF. Maximal loading was reached with 10 μg of bFGF and NGF, and GFs-binding with coacervates sustained their release from day 1 to day 21 (Fig. 1B, C)., indicating that coacervate slows the release of GFs. Additionally, with the different dissociation constant (kd) of bFGF (2 nM) and NGF (600 nM), the release efficiency of NGF(60%) was higher than that of bFGF(30%) in coacervate(Fig. 1C), consistent with our previous study [8].

PC12 cells and SH-SY5Y cells are extensively used as neuronal cell models in vitro [26-28]. In this study, PC12 cells and SH-SY5Y cells were used as a model system to detect the neuroprotective effects of bFGF and NGF. Both bFGF and NGF are known to promotoe an appropriate environment for neurogenesis of stem cells as well as nerve regeneration [29, 30]. We found that bFGF and NGF together in free-form and each GF alone incorporated in coacervate significantly increased the growth and proliferation of PC12 cells and SH- SY5Y cells compared to each GF alone. This study in conjunction with previous studies have demonstrated that combined treatment with NGF and bFGF has a greater potential to promote the proliferation and differentiation of neural stem cells and nerve regeneration [8, 31] . Thus, dual delivery of bFGF and NGF using coacervate greatly increased the growth and proliferation of neuronal cells when compared to all the other groups, suggesting that controlled dual-delivery of bFGF and NGF using [PEAD:heparin] coacervate does not hinder the beneficial effects of bFGF and NGF, but rather improves it when compared to free application of both factors or coacervate delivery of each GF separately.

5. Conclusion

Our results further confirm the neuroprotective effects of NGF and bFGF on the growth and proliferation of neuronal cell types. Moreover, co-delivery of bFGF and NGF using coacervate displayed the most robust neuroprotective effect individual GF coacervates or co-administration of free GFs. These findings highlight that dual bFGF and NGF-incorporated coacervate may be more effective molecular therapeutics for neurodegenerative diseases.

References

[1] Pandya RS, Mao LLJ, Zhou EW, et al. Neuroprotection for amyotrophic lateral sclerosis: role of stem cells, growth factors, and gene therapy[J]. Central Nervous System Agents in Medicinal Chemistry, 2012, 12(1): 15-27.

[2] Kim SU, Lee HJ, Kim YB. Neural stem cell-based treatment for neurodegenerative diseases[J]. Neuropathology, 2013, 33(5): 491-504.

[3] Byrne JA. Developing neural stem cell-based treatments for neurodegenerative diseases[J]. Stem Cell Research & Therapy, 2014, 5.

[4] O'Connor DM, Boulis NM. Gene therapy for neurodegenerative diseases[J]. Trends In Molecular Medicine, 2015, 21(8): 504-512.

[5] Allen SJ, Watson JJ, Shoemark DK, et al. GDNF, NGF and BDNF as therapeutic options for neurodegeneration[J]. Pharmacology & Therapeutics, 2013, 138(2): 155-175.

[6] Tasset I, Sanchez-Lopez F, Agueera E, et al. NGF and nitrosative stress in patients with Huntington's disease[J]. Journal Of the Neurological Sciences, 2012, 315(1-2): 133-136.

[7] Cai J, Hua F, Yuan L, et al. Potential therapeutic effects of neurotrophins for acute and chronic neurological diseases[J]. Biomed Research International, 2014.

[8] Li R, Ma J, Wu Y, et al. Dual delivery of NGF and bFGF coacervater ameliorates diabetic peripheral neuropathy via inhibiting schwann cells apoptosis[J]. International Journal Of Biological Sciences, 2017, 13(5): 640-651.

[9] Cai P, Ye J, Zhu J, et al. Inhibition of endoplasmic reticulum stress is involved in the neuroprotective effect of bFGF in the 6-OHDA-induced parkinson's disease model[J]. Aging And Disease, 2016, 7(4): 336-349.

[10] Tooyama I. Fibroblast growth factors (FGFs) in neurodegenerative disorders[J]. Rinsho shinkeigaku = Clinical neurology, 1993, 33(12): 1270-1274.

[11] Chu H, Johnson NR, Mason NS, et al. A polycation:heparin complex releases growth factors with enhanced bioactivity[J]. Journal Of Controlled Release, 2011, 150(2): 157-163.

[12] Awada HK, Johnson NR, Wang Y. Dual delivery of vascular endothelial growth factor and hepatocyte growth factor coacervate displays strong angiogenic effects[J]. Macromolecular Bioscience, 2014, 14(5): 679-686.

[13] Winner B, Kohl Z, Gage FH. Neurodegenerative disease and adult neurogenesis[J]. European Journal Of Neuroscience, 2011, 33(6): 1139-1151.

[14] Andrades JA, Wu LT, Hall FL, et al. Engineering, expression, and renaturation of a collagen-targeted human bFGF fusion protein[J]. Growth Factors, 2001, 18(4): 261-275.

[15] Lane JT. The role of retinoids in the induction of nerve growth factor: a potential treatment for diabetic neuropathy[J]. Translational Research, 2014, 164(3): 193-195.

[16] Hellweg R, Hartung HD. Endogenous levels of nerve growth-factor (NGF) are altered in experimental diabetes-mellitus-a possible role for ngf in the pathogenesis of diabetic neuropathy[J]. Journal Of Neuroscience Research, 1990, 26(2): 258-267.

[17] Dobrowsky RT, Rouen S, Yu CJ. Altered neurotrophism in diabetic neuropathy: Spelunking the caves of peripheral nerve[J]. Journal Of Pharmacology And Experimental Therapeutics, 2005, 313(2): 485-491.

[18] Tuszynski MH, Yang JH, Barba D, et al. Nerve growth factor gene therapy activation of neuronal responses in alzheimer disease[J]. Jama Neurology, 2015, 72(10): 1139-1147.

[19] Bannwarth B, Kostine M. Targeting nerve growth factor (NGF) for pain management: what does the future hold for NGF antagonists? [J]. Drugs, 2014, 74(6): 619-626.

[20] Chu H, Johnson NR, Mason NS, et al. A polycation:heparin complex releases growth factors with enhanced bioactivity[J]. Journal Of Controlled Release, 2011, 150(2): 157-163.

[21] Awada HK, Johnson NR, Wang Y. Dual delivery of vascular endothelial growth factor and hepatocyte growth factor coacervate displays strong angiogenic effects[J]. Macromolecular Bioscience, 2014, 14(5): 679-686.

[22] Awada HK, Johnson NR, Wang Y. Dual delivery of vascular endothelial growth factor and hepatocyte growth factor coacervate displays strong angiogenic effects[J]. Macromolecular Bioscience, 2014, 14(5): 679-686.

[23] Chen WCW, Lee BG, Park DW, et al. Controlled dual delivery of fibroblast growth factor-2 and Interleukin-10 by heparin-based coacervate synergistically enhances ischemic heart repair[J]. Biomaterials, 2015, 72: 138-151.

[24] Chu H, Chen C-W, Huard J, et al. The effect of a heparin-based coacervate of fibroblast growth factor-2 on scarring in the infarcted

myocardium[J]. Biomaterials, 2013, 34(6): 1747-1756.

[25] Li H, Johnson NR, Usas A, *et al.* Sustained release of bone morphogenetic protein 2 *via* coacervate improves the osteogenic potential of muscle-derived stem cells[J]. Stem Cells Translational Medicine, 2013, 2(9): 667-677.

[26] Russo VC, Higgins S, Werther GA, *et al.* Effects of fluctuating glucose levels on neuronal cells *in vitro*[J]. Neurochemical Research, 2012, 37(8): 1768-1782.

[27] Zhou Y, Besner GE. Heparin-binding epidermal growth factor-like growth factor is a potent neurotrophic factor for PC12 cells[J]. Neurosignals, 2010, 18(3): 141-151.

[28] Agholme L, Lindstrom T, Kagedal K, *et al.* An *In Vitro* model for neuroscience: differentiation of SH-SY5Y cells into cells with morphological and biochemical characteristics of mature neurons[J]. Journal Of Alzheimers Disease, 2010, 20(4): 1069-1082.

[29] Mudo G, Bonomo A, Di Liberto V, *et al.* The FGF-2/FGFRs neurotrophic system promotes neurogenesis in the adult brain[J]. Journal Of Neural Transmission, 2009, 116(8): 995-1005.

[30] Otto D, Unsicker K, Grothe C. Pharmacological effects of nerve growth-factor and fibroblast growth-factor applied to the transected sciatic-nerve on neuron death in adult-rat dorsal-root ganglia[J]. Neuroscience Letters, 1987, 83(1-2): 156-160.

[31] Chen SQ, Cai Q, Shen YY, *et al.* Combined use of NGF/BDNF/bFGF promotes proliferation and differentiation of neural stem cells *in vitro*[J]. International Journal Of Developmental Neuroscience, 2014, 38: 74-78.

Design and evaluation of lyophilized fibroblast growth factor 21 and its protection against ischemia cerebral injury

Xuanxin Yang, Xiaokun Li, Xiaojie Wang

1. Introduction

FGF21 is an important member of the fibroblast growth factor family, which is preferentially secreted by the liver and involved in both glucose and lipid metabolism.[1-4] In combination with changes of FGF21 in the circadian rhythm, a recent study showed that FGF21 regulates the central nervous system and that intravenous injections of FGF21 can cross the blood-brain barrier, showing its potential as neuroprotective treatment.[5] However, in contrast to other proteins, long-term research and clinical practice have shown FGF21 to have poor stability and short shelf life, thus diminishing its therapeutic effect.[6]

Lyophilization is the most commonly used storage method for a therapeutic protein drug in the pharmaceutical industry to increase the long-term stability, and allow easy handling and storage of drug product.[7-9] This process may be used to maintain their quality, physicochemical characteristics, performance, and low residual moisture content, as well as distribution and good stability of the drug product.[10] Overall, the lyophilization process generally occurs in three sequential steps, freezing, primary drying, and secondary drying.[11] Specifically, it consists of freezing the samples, and removing the water by sublimation and desorption under vacuum. The exact mechanism for the freezing during the lyophilization is not clear. However, apparently during the freezing, ice crystals nucleate and grow, excluding the solutes in the formulation in lyophilization, such as cold shock, ice-water interfaces, pH changes, dehydration stress, easy aggregation, and chemical degradation during the process of lyophilization.[8,12-15] To stabilize the bioactivity of FGF21 during the process of preparation and storage, it is necessary to add protectants to the lyophilized formulation to protect them from freezing stresses.[16,17] The most common lyoprotectants have been considered, including sugars/polyols, polymers, surfactants, amino acids, metal ions, and inorganic substances,[15,18,19] which influence the glass transition temperature of formulation to with low residual moisture content, yielding better protein stability. Among these lyoprotectants, sugars (such as sucrose and trehalose) tend to produce an amorphous form, consequently enhancing protein stability during freeze-drying and storage.[9,20,21] Polyols, such as mannitol, can not only be used as bulking agents, but also as lyoprotectant in some formulations.[19,22,23] The purpose of this work was to understand how various physicochemical properties affect the stability of lyophilized FGF21 as a model therapeutic protein, and assess the effect of freezing on structural stability of FGF21. We examined the protecting effect of various excipients on the deterioration behavior of lyophilized FGF21 at elevated storage temperature. Furthermore, the effect of FGF21 was investigated against ischemia cerebral injury, using the middle cerebral artery occlusion (MCAO) model in rats.

2. Results and discussion

2.1 Glass transition temperature

T_g value is an important parameter of any lyophilized formulation. The T s of the five FGF21 formulations a to e were $51.36 \pm 0.75 \, ℃$, $50.96 \pm 0.90 \, ℃$, $51.56 \pm 0.09 \, ℃$, $47.35 \pm 0.12 \, ℃$, and $45.36 \pm 0.11 \, ℃$, respectively. T_g values were higher for mannitol-containing formulations (formulation a, b, and c) than of corresponding sorbitol-containing formulations (formulation d and e). The ingredients of five FGF21 formulations are shown in Table 1.

Table 1. Formulation excipients and their percent weight masses used for the preparation of FGF21 formulations

formulations	arginine	glycine	mannitol	trehalose	sorbitol	Poloxamer 188	buffer used	FGF21
a	0.6%	0.3%	4%			0.1%	2 mM sodium phosphate at pH 7.4	1 mg/ml
b	0.1%		4%	2%		0.1%		
c		0.05%	2%	2%		0.1%		
d		0.05%		3%	5%	0.1%		
e	0.6%			3%	5%	0.1%		
control	-	-	-	-	-	-		

2.2 Protein secondary structure of lyophilized FGF21 formulations

The secondary structure of lyophilized FGF21 in each formulation is shown in Fig. 1. The range of α-helix (11.02 ± 0.82%) > d (10.86 ± 1.18%) > b (10.38 ± 0.83%) > e (10.29 ± 1.10%) > control (9.97 ± 1.10%), while the differences between each formulation and the control group were not significant (Fig. 1G, $P > 0.05$, $n = 3$). Moreover, the contents of each of the formulations is c (11.18 ± 0.83%) > a range of β-pleated sheet contents resulted in the following order: control sample (45.98 ± 0.58%) > e (40.51 ± 0.42%) > d (40.50 ± 0.83%) > b (39.43 ± 1.67%) > a (39.39 ± 0.22%) > c (39.36 ± 0.61%). There was a significant difference between control group and the five lyophilized FGF21 formulations (Fig. 1H, $P < 0.05$ or $P < 0.01$, $n = 3$).

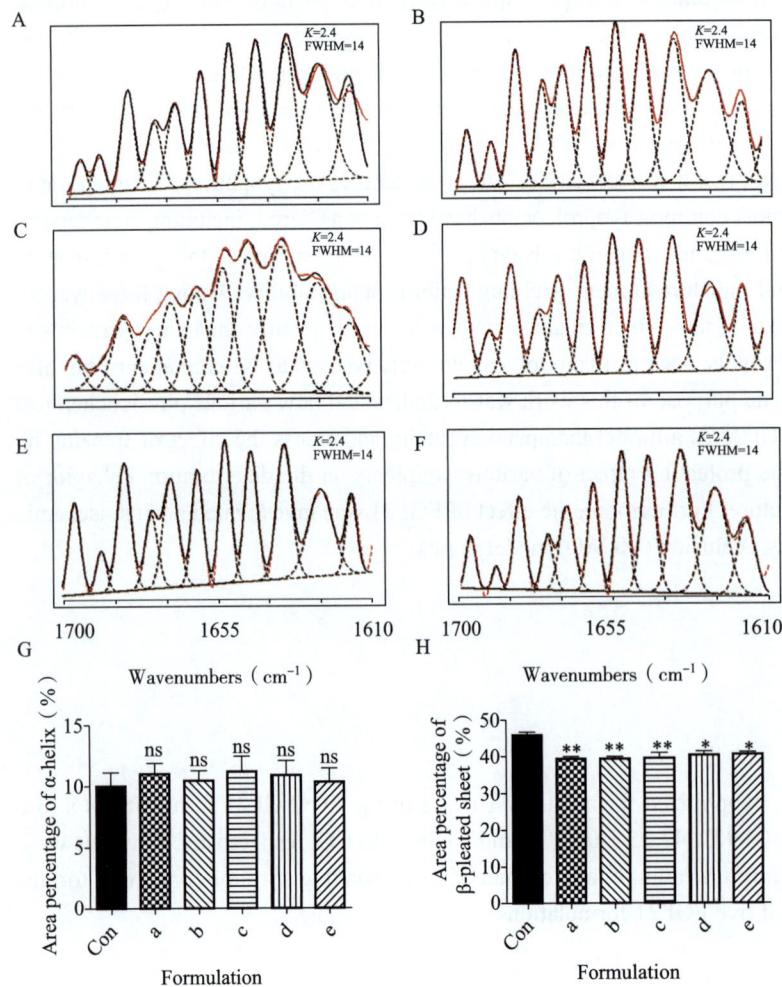

Fig. 1. FTIR spectra of lyophilized FGF21 Formulations. (A – E) shows the FTIR spectra of lyophilized FGF21 formulations a to e, respectively. (F) shows the FTIR spectra of lyophilized FGF21 formulations without any excipient. The solid lines represent the superimposed Fourier Self-Deconvolution (FSD) and the curve-fit, while the dashed curves represent individual Gaussian bands. (G) Area percentage of α-helix of five lyophilized FGF21 formulaions. (H) Area percentage of β-pleated sheet five lyophilized FGF21 formulaions. Con means lyophilized FGF21 without excipients. *, Significantly different from the control group ($P < 0.05$); **, Significantly different from the control group ($P < 0.01$) ($n = 3$).

2.3 Storage stability of lyophilized FGF21

As shown in Fig. 2F, the primary mode of deterioration under accelerated storage condition was aggregation. SDS-PAGE data showed that the aggregation of all five FGF21 formulations did not change significantly at 4℃ compared to right after lyophilization (Fig. 2A,B,C). However, SDS-PAGE data clearly showed visible polymerization in a band at 44 KDa at 37℃ in the five FGF21 formulations and control formulation (Fig. 2D,E,F). SE-HPLC data revealed a similar result. As shown in Fig. 2H, after three months of storage at 37℃, even though the aggregation content of each formulation increased, the aggregation content of all five FGF21 formulations were greatly reduced compared to that of the control formulation ($P < 0.001$). Furthermore, the aggregation rates in mannitol-containing formulations (formulation a, b, and c) were less than that of sorbitol-containing formulations (formulation d and e, Fig. 2H). Specifically, mannitol-containing formulation containing trehalose and glycine (formulation c) shows the least polymerization when stored at 37℃ (Fig. 2H, $P < 0.05$).

Furthermore, the bioactivity of FGF21 on the uptake of glucose in all formulations did not change significantly during three months storage at 4℃ (Fig. 3A, $P > 0.05$). However, it decreased significantly over time at 37℃ (Fig. 3B). This finding suggests that the FGF21 is unstable at higher temperature. Moreover, the bioactivity of FGF21 decreased sharply at 37℃ in the control formulation (Fig. 3B). Compared to control samples without excipients, all five formulations showed an apparent protective effect on FGF21 during lyophilization and storage processes (Fig. 3C, D, E, $P < 0.05$, 0.01, or 0.001). Particularly, the mannitol- containing formulation combined with trehalose and glycine (formulation c)

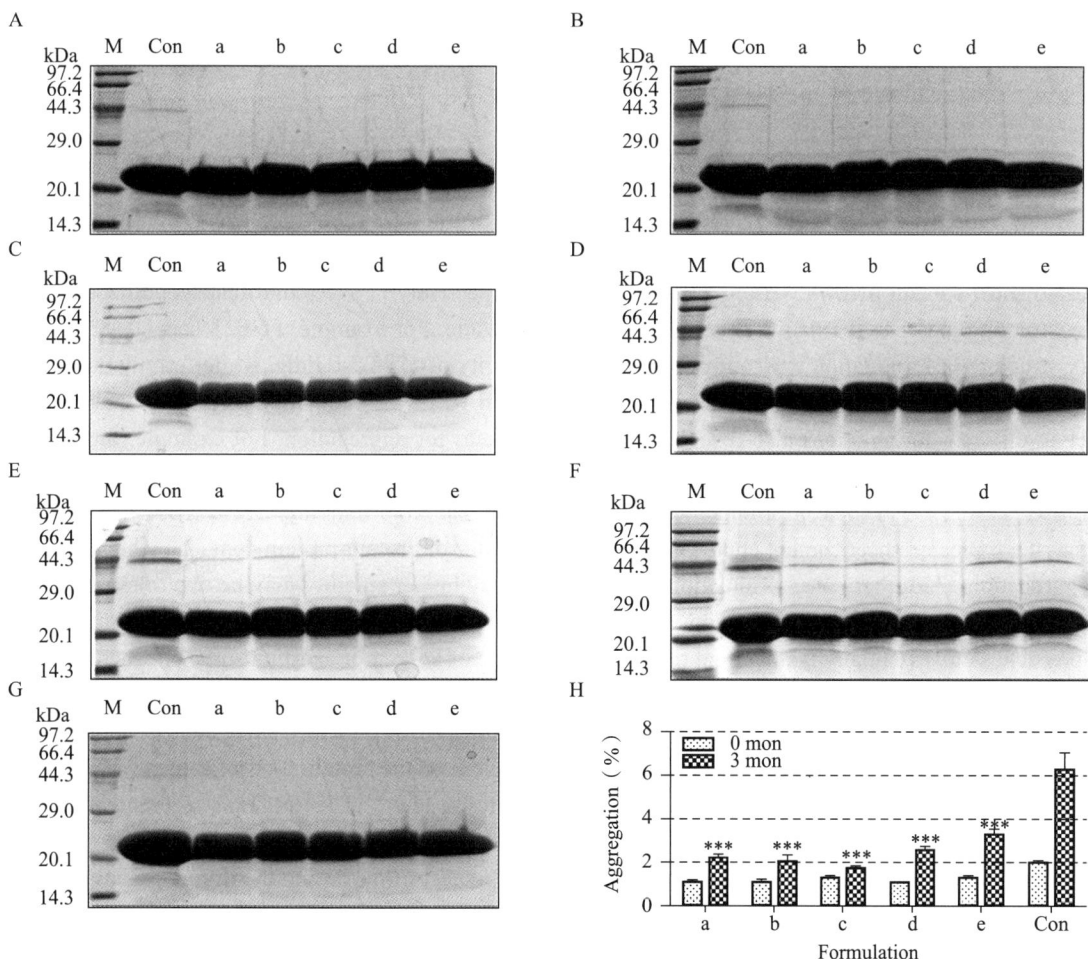

Fig. 2. Aggregation assay of lyophilized FGF21 formulations. (A – G) SDS-PAGE results of lyophilized FGF21 during a period of three months: (A, B, C) lyophilized FGF21 at 4℃ for one (A), two (B), and three (C) months; (D, E, F) lyophilized FGF21 at 37℃ for one (D), two (E), and three (F) months; (G) lyophilized FGF21 examined immediately after lyophilization. (H) Aggregation rate of lyophilized FGF21 for 0 and 3 months at 37℃ test *via* SE-HPLC. Compared to the control group, [*], Significantly different from the control group ($P < 0.05$); [**], Significantly different from the control group ($P < 0.01$); [***], Significantly different from the control group ($P < 0.001$) ($n = 3$).

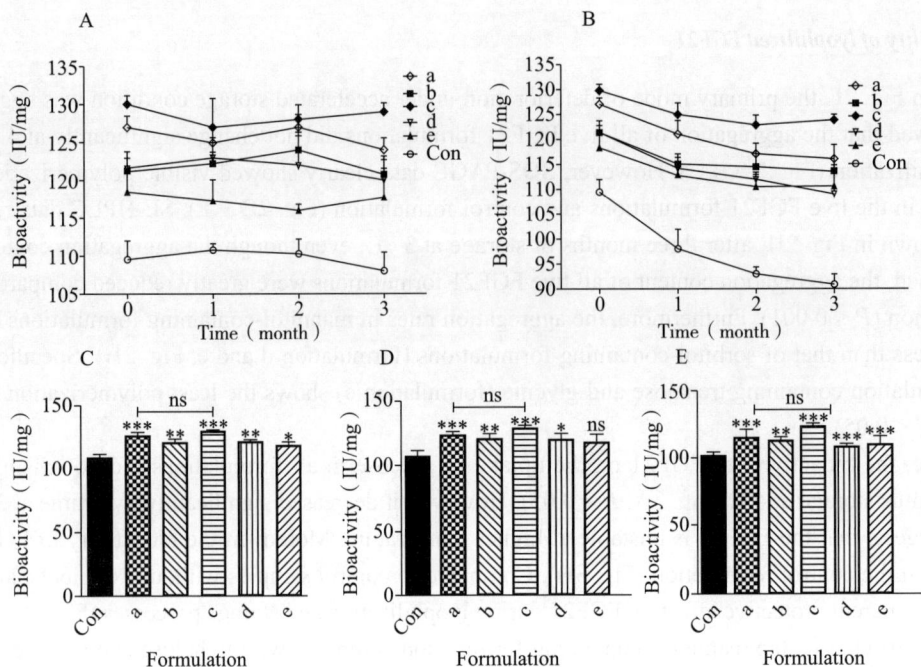

Fig. 3. Results of bioactivity assay of lyophilized FGF21 during three months. (A) Bioactivity of lyophilized FGF21 stored at 4℃. (B) Bioactivity of lyophilized FGF21 stored at 37℃. (C) Bioactivity of FGF21 immediately after lyophilization. (D) Bioactivity of lyophilized FGF21 stored at 4℃ after three months. (E) Bioactivity of lyophilized FGF21 stored at 37℃ after three months. Con: lyophilized FGF21 without excipients. Remaining groups stand for FGF21 formulation a to e. *, Significantly different from the control group ($P < 0.05$); **, Significantly different from the control group ($P < 0.01$); ***, Significantly different from the control group ($P < 0.001$) ($n = 3$).

showed the highest bioactivity for glucose uptake at 37℃ after three months storage (Fig. 3E, $P < 0.05$).

It was interesting to compare the relationship between the degree of structural conservation and the stability of lyophilized FGF21. Through predicting the secondary structure of FGF21 by the methods of SOPM, the α-helix and the β-pleated sheet content of FGF21 is 13.33% and 21.67% respectively.[24] We found that lyophilized FGF21 with a secondary structure closer to the native structure may be more stable. For example, FGF21 had 11.18% α-helix in the secondary structure in formulation c accompanied by the bioactivity of 127.25 IU/mg, while formulation e represented the lower α-helix content (10.29%) and a lower bioactivity of 116 IU/mg. Examination of the β-pleated sheet contents of FGF21 in different formulations also revealed similar tendencies for aggregation. For example, the total β-pleated sheet content of FGF21 in formulation c was 39.36%, while that of control formulation was 45.98%. The aggregation content of FGF21 at 37℃ in control formulation was more intense than in formulation c (Fig. 2D, E, F). This finding indicated that the β-pleated sheet content could be used as an indicator of protein-protein contacts, which likely influence protein aggregation.[25] Furthermore, formulation c with particularly higher stability may be due to more native α- helix and β-pleated sheet structures. Our results consequently suggest that the excipients of formulation c might offer a very suitable physical state, essentially maintaining the tertiary structure of FGF21 or exerting some effects on protein refolding after rehydration. Spectroscopic studies of FTIR, combined with simulations and predictions of protein structure, revealed that FGF21 was susceptible to loss of α-helix content and increase of β-pleated sheet content upon lyophilization. Moreover, previous study has shown that the drying process can increase the protein β-sheet content, while helix content substantially decreases due to the structure transition from helix to β-sheet.[26] This finding suggests that the protein aggregates or stronger intermolecular interaction occur during the drying process. Another independent report by Song L et al. based on the FGF19 model consistently suggests that more β-sheet forms during the drying process.[27] Our current study suggests that FGF21 protein can preserve more secondary structure with higher activity by comparing the protein structure and activity relationship, in good agreement with previous work.

2.4 Effect of FGF21 against cerebral ischemia

We next investigated the effect of FGF21 against ischemia cerebral injury using the MCAO model in SD rats. In contrast to the sham group, treatment with FGF21 significantly improved the behavioral ability of MCAO rats. Behav-

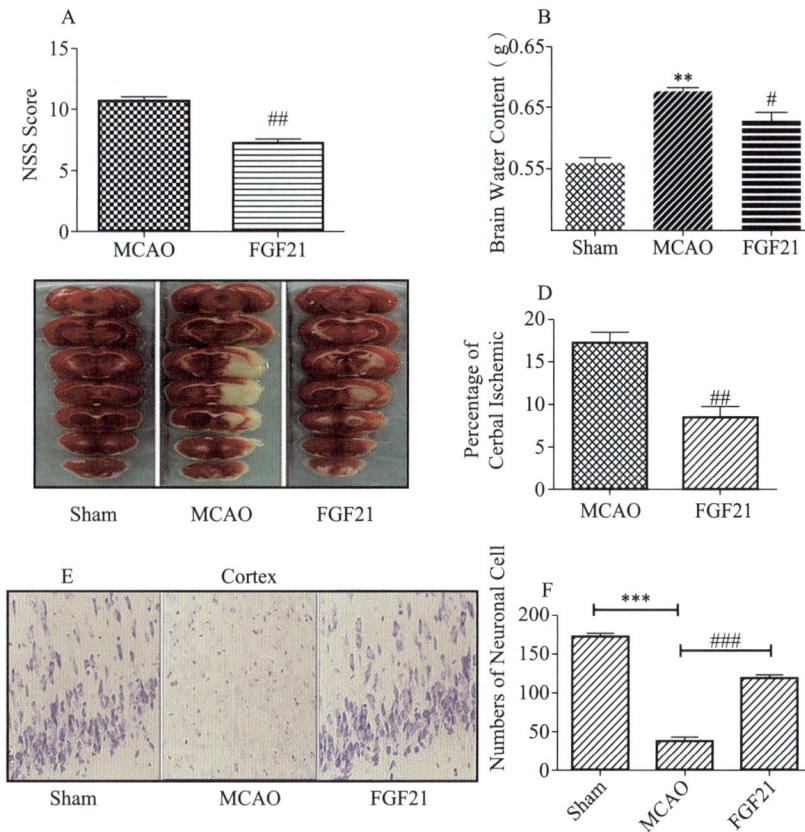

Fig. 4. Assay of cerebral ischemia of each group. (A) NSS score of MCAO rats ($n = 3$). (B) Water content of the brain foreach group ($n = 3$). (C) TTC staining of the right brain of each group. (D) Percentage of cerebral ischemia of MCAO rats ($n = 3$). (E) Nissl-staining of cortexes (400×). (F) Nissl-stained cell number in cortex; Compared to control group, [*]$P < 0.05$, [**]$P < 0.01$, [***]$P < 0.001$; Compared to MCAO group, [#]$P < 0.05$, [##]$P < 0.01$, [###]$P < 0.001$.

ioral score of the FGF21 administrated group was concentrated about 6 to 8. However, the score was nearly 10 to 12 in the MCAO group (Fig. 4A). The brain water content of MCAO group rats increased after ischemia-reperfusion for 24 h, while the water content in the FGF21 administered group was significantly lower than that of the MCAO group (Fig. 4B, $P < 0.01$). The cerebral ischemic area of MCAO rats was measured *via* TTC staining. Compared to the MCAO group, the ischemia infarct size of the FGF21- treated group was significantly reduced (Fig. 4C and D, $P < 0.01$). Nissl-staining is a very useful method to study the pathology of neurons. Histological observations of the cerebral cortex were performed *via* Nissl-staining (Fig. 4E, F). As shown in the Fig. 4E, the number of normal neurons in cortex area decreased in MCAO group, comparing to the sham group. Furthermore, the neuronal degeneration in MCAO group is more severe at reperfusion 24 h, comparing to the sham group. On the contrary, treatment with FGF21 significantly increased the numbers of neuron (Fig. 4G, $P < 0.01$). This finding implies that FGF21 can potentially act as a protective agent to against ischemia cerebral injury.

2.5 Expression of ER stress related proteins

Compared to the MCAO group after ischemia-reperfusion for 24 h, we found that the expression of XBP-1, Caspase-12, and ATF-6 proteins of the cortex in the MCAO group was significantly up-regulated (Fig. 5A, B, $P < 0.01$), indicating ER stress to be involved in ischemic injury. Compared to the MCAO group, it could also be observed that the decrement of the ER stress related proteins in the cortical region of the FGF21 treatment group (##, $P < 0.01$). In the brain hippocampus (Fig. 5C, D), expressions of ER stress related proteins were significantly increased compared to sham group (**, $P < 0.01$). The expression of these proteins in FGF21 treatment group was significantly decreased compared to the MCAO group (#, $P < 0.05$; ##, $P < 0.01$). Overall, these results show that the presence FGF21 in the formulations can decrease ER stress related proteins.

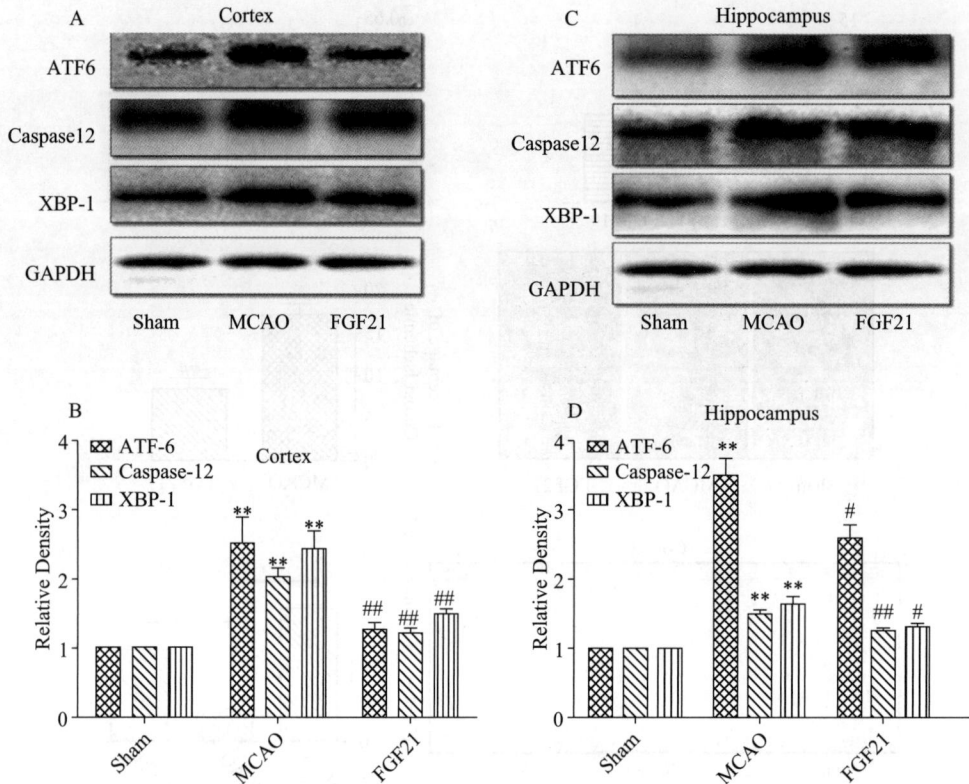

Fig. 5. Expression of ER stress related proteins in the cortexes of brain and hippocampus of the right hemisphere. (A) Expression of ATF-6, caspase-12, and XBP-1 in cortexes of brains for each group ($n = 3$); (B) Relative density of proteins in cortexes of brains ($n = 3$). (C) Expression of ATF-6, caspase-12, and XBP-1 in the hippocampus for each group. (D) Relative density of proteins in hippocampus. Compared to control group, $**P < 0.01$; compared to MCAO group, $#P < 0.05$, $##P < 0.01$.

2.6 The effect of FGF21 on the protection of neuron cell injury by hydrogen peroxide

Hydrogen peroxide (H_2O_2) induced oxidative stress in PC12 cell is the most common method of simulated endoplasmic reticulum stress (ERS) in recent years. To investigate the concentration of FGF21 on its effect of antiapoptosis induced by hydrogen peroxide on PC12, two dose-dependent MTT assays were designed (Fig. 6A, 6B). As a result, we finally confirmed that the concentration of H_2O_2 was 110 μM, at which the survival rate of PC12 cells was between 60% to 70% compared with control group. In addition, it was also determined that the concentration of FGF21 was 160 ng/ml, at which the survival rate of PC12 cells treated H_2O_2 was about 90%, showing good as an antioxidant (Fig. 6 B). The expression of GADD153, XBP-1, Caspase12, ATF6 and ATF4 in PC12 cells was detected by Western blot to evaluate the effect of FGF21 on endoplasmic reticulum stress. It was determined from results that the expression of intracellular endoplasmic reticulum stress-related protein in hydrogen peroxide induced PC12 cells were up-regulated (Fig. 6C, 6E), while treated with FGF21, the expression of these proteins was significantly decreased down ($P < 0.05$) in the molecular level. The results showed that FGF21 could inhibit the expression of ER stress-related proteins, which was consistent with the results obtained on animal experiments *in vivo*.

In order to determine whether FGF21 play the role in inhibition of ERS related proteins expression by activating ERK1/2, PI3K/Akt, JNK signaling pathway, thus protecting PC12 cells from oxidative stress injury, Western blot was used to detect the expression levels of p-ERK, p-Akt and p-JNK proteins, respectively. Furthermore, U0126, LY294002, SB203580, inhibitors of these signal pathways were made use of to confirm above surmise. The expression of p-ERk1/2 in H_2O_2 group was slightly decreased, while expression of p-Akt and p-JNK was significantly inhibited by H_2O_2 (*, $P < 0.05$). Otherwise, the phosphorylation levels of the ERK1/2, PI3K/ Akt, JNK signaling pathways were significantly up-regulated in the FGF21-administered group under stimulation of H_2O_2, including p-ERK1/2, p-Akt and p-JNK ($P < 0.05$) (Fig. 6F–H). When treated with three inhibitors of signal pathway, expression of these proteins was remarkably inhibited compared with FGF21-administered group (#, $P < 0.05$, ##, $P < 0.01$). From the results, it was indicated that FGF21

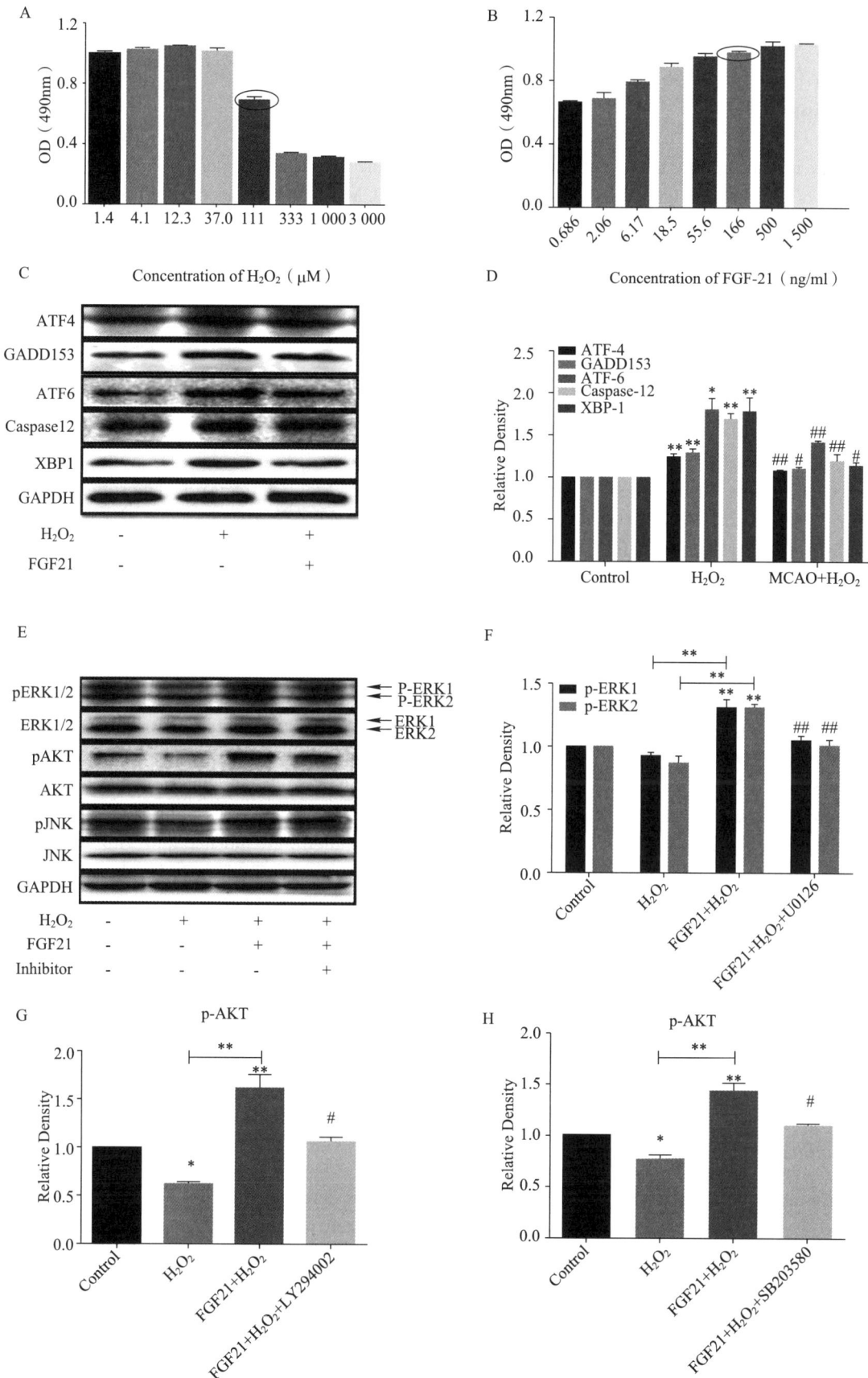

Fig. 6. Cytoprotective activity of FGF21 on H_2O_2-induced PC12 cell injury. (A) PC12 cells were treated with increasing concentrations of H_2O_2 for 10 h before cell viability was assessed by MTT assay ($n = 4$). (B) Relative number of PC12 cells after treatment with H_2O_2 in the presence of FGF21. (C, D) Expression of intracellular ERS-related protein in H_2O_2 induced PC12 cells after treatment with FGF21. (E) Phosphorylation levels of the ERK1/2, PI3K/Akt, JNK signaling pathways in PC12 cells after treatment with FGF21. (F) p-ERK 1/2 expression. (G) p-PI3K/Ak expression. (H) p-JNK expression.

was capable of activating ERK1/2, PI3K/Akt, JNK signaling pathways in ERS induced PC12 cells.

3. Conclusions

This study investigated various lyophilized formulations of the therapeutic protein FGF21. Aggregation was the primary mode of deterioration under accelerated storage conditions. Mannitol combined with trehalose and glycine formulations offers the most effective protein protection to prevent the protein from aggregation. Administration of FGF21 was found to protect the cerebral ischemia and decrease ER stress related proteins.

4. Materials and methods

4.1 Materials

FGF21was provided by the Key Laboratory Biotechnology Pharmaceutical Engineering at the Wenzhou Medical University, China. Poloxamer 188 was purchased from BASF SE Co., Ltd. (Germany). Trehalose was purchased from Linyuan Co., Ltd. (Japan). Arginine was purchased from Jinghai Amino Acid Co., Ltd. (Wuxi, China). Glycine was purchased from Tianyao Pharmaceuticals Co., Ltd. (Tianjin,China). Sorbitol and Mannitol were purchased from Sigma Chemical Co., Ltd. and the GOD-POD (Glucose Oxidase-Peroxidase) Kit was purchased from Huilin Co., Ltd. (Changchun, China).

4.2 Preparation and lyophilization of FGF21

FGF21 was dialyzed with 20 mM sodium phosphate buffer at pH 7.4 and subsequently concentrated at a concentration of 2 mg/ml in a high-speed refrigerated centrifuge at 4℃. Formulation excipients and their percent weight masses used for preparing formulations of FGF21 are all listed in Table 1. FGF21 without any excipients is used as control. The stock solutions of FGF21 and excipients were individually filtered using 0.22 μm Millipore sterile PVDF (polyvinylidene fluoride) hydrophobic filters. Finally, the protein solution and excipient stock solutions were mixed at a 1 to 1 ratio, arriving at a final protein concentration of 1 mg/ml. Aliquots of 1 ml solution were pipetted into 5 ml glass vials in a cold and clean environment at approximately 2 to 8℃. The vials were then sent to Tofllon- 20 lyophilizer (Tofflon, China) for the process of lyophilization. The vials were loaded at the shelf of the lyophilizer in a sterile environment, and then, ambient temperature and shelf temperature of lyophilizer were adjusted at −40℃ and maintained for 2 h. After that, the chamber was evacuated to 70 mTorr and the shelf temperature was increased from −40℃ to −20℃ at a speed of 2.5℃ per minute. Furthermore, the temperature of the lyophilizer was kept at −20℃ for 30 h during the process of primary drying. At the end of the primary drying, the shelf temperature was increased from −20 to 24℃ at a rate of 0.3℃ per minute. The temperature of the lyophilizer was held at 24℃ for 2 h during the process of secondary drying. When secondary drying was completed, the chamber was refilled with dry nitrogen and all vials were covered with rubber stoppers under nitrogen atmosphere. Finally, all vials were sealed with aluminum caps.

4.3 Glass transition temperature

The glass transition temperature (T_g) of lyophilized samples was determined *via* differential scanning calorimetry (DSC, Q-600, TA). A sample of approximately 5 to 10 mg was accurately weighed in an aluminum pan and hermetically sealed. An empty pan was used as reference. Pans were exposed to a liner heating ramp in a temperature range from −40 to 80℃ at a heating rate of 5℃ per minute.[28] When the DSC system started, the heat flow curve and data were recorded during heating. The T_g of samples was determined by analyzing heat flow curves with the software TA universal analysis 2000. For each formulation, three samples were analyzed ($n = 3$).

4.4 Analysis of FGF21 secondary structure

To obtain Fourier transform infrared (FTIR) spectra of FGF21 in the lyophilized formulations, lyophilized FGF21 (approximately 200 mg protein) was gently ground with 500 mg potassium bromide (KBr) using a mortar and pestle, and then transferred into a noncorrosive steel mold to form thickness pellets. Infrared spectra were recorded with a Nicolet Magna 560 ESP spectrometer (Nicolet Instrument, Madison, WI). Each spectrum had a resolution ratio of 4 cm^{-1} and a detection range of 4 000 cm^{-1} to 1 000 cm^{-1}. Water vapor spectra were subtracted, and all spectra were baseline corrected. The contents of α-helix and β-pleated sheet of the lyophilized FGF21 formulation were analyzed with OMNIC 8.0, methods of second derivatization, Fourier self-deconvolution (FSD), and Gaussian curve-fitting.[29-36].

4.5　Storage stability of FGF21

In this experiment, five lyophilized FGF21 formulations were incubated at 4 and 37℃ in temperature-controlled incubators. At various time points (0, 1, 2, and 3 months), samples were removed for analyses that are described below.

4.6　Aggregation analysis of lyophilized FGF21 via SDS-PAGE

The samples were prepared with 12% SDS-PAGE (sodium dodecyl sulfate polyacrylamide gel electrophoresis) nonreducing conditions of gel electrophoresis. Electrophoresis of the samples was done according to previously described protocol.[37]

4.7　Quantitation of lyophilized FGF21 aggregation via SE-HPLC

The polymerization of FGF21 was quantified *via* SE- HPLC (Size exclusion-High Performance Liquid Chromatography) (an Agilent 1100 HPLC system equipped with Chemstation software) at 0 and 3 months. Each sample was tested thrice. The conditions of high pressure liquid chromatography were as follows: The model number of the column was TSK gel G2000 SWxL. The mobile phase was a 20 mM PB buffer solution with 0.01 M sodium chloride with its pH value adjusted to 7.4. The flow rate was 0.8 ml per minute. The temperature of the column was 25℃. The loading amount of the FGF21 solution was 30 μl. The detection wavelength of the instrument was 280 nm. The method of elution was as follows: the column was first rinsed with distilled water for 1 h and then balanced with the mobile phase for more than 30 min. Finally, samples were eluted with mobile phase for 25 min.

4.8　Glucose uptake activity assay of lyophilized FGF21

HL-7702 cells were seeded into 96 well microplates at 1.6×10^5 cells/well, allowed to attach for 24 h, and then incubated in RPMI 1640 with 0.5% fetal bovine serum overnight at 37℃. Cells were supplemented with FGF21 (500 μg/ml) and incubated at 37℃ for 48 h. Each condition was performed in octuplicate and then the medium was changed at 48 h. The glucose uptake ability was measured *via* GOD-POD-assay kit according to the manufacturer's protocol.

4.9　Animal model of MCAO

Approximately 36 healthy male SD rats, each weighing around 200−250 g, were purchased from the Shanghai Slack experimental animals limited liability company. All animals were adaptively fed with free drinking water at a clean level in the Experimental Animal Center of Wenzhou Medical University, where the room temperature was around 23℃ and the relative humidity was about 60%. All animal experiments were approved by the Animal Institutional Ethics Committee of the Wenzhou Medical University (Wenzhou, China) and were performed following the guidelines for animal experimentation of the Wenzhou Medical University. Humane treatment of all research animals was assured. Animals were fasted for 12 h prior to surgery, then weighed, randomly numbered, and anesthetized with 10% chloral hydrate (0.40 mg/100 g). Animals were divided into sham surgeries, MCAO group, and FGF21-administrated group. The right middle cerebral artery ischemia-reperfusion animal model was established by using the modified Zea-Longa suture method with sterilized line-lock.[38-40] Exogenous Exogenous FGF21 at a dose of 100 μg/kg and normal saline were immediately intraperitoneally injected just after MCAO for the FGF21 treatment group and the MCAO model group, respectively. SD rats of sham group were performed with same surgery but without MCAO, which were immediately intra-peritoneally with same volume normal saline. For better evaluation of the neurological deficits in rats, neurological severity scores (NSS) were recorded for a period of 24 h after the operation.

4.10　Evaluation of the effects of FGF21 on ischemia cerebral injury and expression of ER stress related proteins

MCAO rats were anesthetized with 10% chloral hydrate (0.4 ml/100 g) and sacrificed after treatment of FGF21 for 24 h. TTC (2,3,5-triphenyltetrazolium chloride) staining, brain water content assay, Nissl staining, and Western blot were conducted as described below.

The brain of three rats in each group was then placed in a dish and placed in a refrigerator at −20℃ for 20 min. After freezing to a stiff form, the brain tissue was coronally sliced with a thickness of 2 mm, which started at the visual cross level with 7 slices. The brain slices were then placed in 0.5% TTC solution and incubated at 37℃ for approximately 20 min in the incubator in the dark. TTC solution was drawn out and 4% paraformaldehyde solution was added when the brain slices were turning from white to red (infarct brain tissue shows white, while normal brain tissue shows red). Each brain piece was labeled in accordance with the order from front to back, photographed with a camera, and analyzed *via* Image Pro Plus software.

The brain water content was tested with the dry-wet weight method to evaluate the hydrocephalus of the brain.[41] The brain of three rats in each group that removed olfactory bulb, cerebellum, and brain stem was weighted before and after drying, respectively until the difference of the weight was below 0.3 g (drying condition: oven at 80℃ and duration of 72 h). Fresh brains of three rats in each group were fixed with 4% paraformaldehyde, embedded in paraffin, then sliced, and finally used for Nissl staining to evaluate the histology of the cerebral cortex area. Both the cerebral cortex and the hippocampus of fresh brains of three rats in each group were separated and lysed at a ratio of 10 ml per gram. The expression of ER stress related proteins, such as caspase12 (1:1 000, Abcam), XBP-1 (1:1 000, Cell Signaling Technology) and ATF-6 (1:1 000, Cell Signaling Technology) were detected *via* Western blot.

4.11 Effect of FGF21 on the protection of neuron cell injury by hydrogen peroxide

Rat pheochromocytoma PC12 cells were obtained from the American Type Culture Collection (ATCC), Rockville, MD, USA). PC12 cells were grown in RPMI 1640 media containing 5% fetal bovine serum and 10% heat-inactivated horse serum (HIHS) and maintained at 37℃ in 5% CO_2 humidified incubator.

Cytoprotective activity of FGF21 on H_2O_2-induced PC12 cell injury was investigated by an MTT assay. The PC12 cells were seeded into 96 well plates at a density of 5×10^4 cells/well for 16 h and then pretreated with vehicle alone or different concentrations of FGF21 for 24 h before exposure to 110 mM H_2O_2 for 10 h. MTT test was done as described preriously.[42]

Expression of GADD153 (1:500, cell Signaling Technology), XBP-1 (1:1 000, cell Signaling Technology), Caspase12 (1:1 000, Abcam), ATF6 (1:1 000, Cell Signaling Technology), ATF4 (1:1 000, Cell Signaling Technology), and the phosphorylation levels of the ERK1/2, PI3K/Akt, JNK signaling pathways (Abcam) in PC12 cells after treatment with FGF21 was detected by Western blot. U0126, LY294002, SB203580 (Abcam), inhibitors of these signal pathways were made as control.

4.12 Statistic analysis

Statistical analysis of quantifiable results was performed by students, using ANOVA with GraphPad Prism 5.0. Statistical significance was set at a two-sided *P*-value of $P < 0.05$. All statistic data are written in the format of mean ± standard deviation.

References

[1] Itoh N, Ornitz DM. Evolution of the Fgf and Fgfr gene families[J]. Trends In Genetics, 2004, 20(11): 563-569.

[2] Izumiya Y, Bina HA, Ouchi N, *et al.* FGF21 is an Akt-regulated myokine[J]. Febs Letters, 2008, 582(27): 3805-3810.

[3] Micanovic R, Raches DW, Dunbar JD, *et al.* Different roles of N- and C-termini in the functional activity of FGF21[J]. Journal Of Cellular Physiology, 2009, 219(2): 227-234.

[4] Nishimura T, Nakatake Y, Konishi M, *et al.* Identification of a novel FGF, FGF-21, preferentially expressed in the liver[J]. Biochimica Et Biophysica Acta-Gene Structure And Expression, 2000, 1492(1): 203-206.

[5] Yu Y, Bai F, Wang W, *et al.* Fibroblast growth factor 21 protects mouse brain against D-galactose induced aging *via* suppression of oxidative stress response and advanced glycation end products

formation[J]. Pharmacology Biochemistry And Behavior, 2015, 133: 122-131.

[6] Yao W, Ren G, Han Y, *et al.* Expression and pharmacological evaluation of fusion protein FGF21-L-Fc[J]. Yaoxue Xuebao, 2011, 46(7): 787-792.

[7] Chang LQ, Shepherd D, Sun J, *et al.* Mechanism of protein stabilization by sugars during freeze-drying and storage: Native structure preservation, specific interaction, and/or immobilization in a glassy matrix?[J]. Journal Of Pharmaceutical Sciences, 2005, 94(7): 1427-1444.

[8] Devineni D, Gonschorek C, Cicerone MT, *et al.* Storage stability of keratinocyte growth factor-2 in lyophilized formulations: Effects of formulation physical properties and protein fraction at the solid-air interface[J]. European Journal Of Pharmaceutics And Biopharma-

ceutics, 2014, 88(2): 332-341.

[9] Park J, Nagapudi K, Vergara C, *et al.* Effect of pH and excipients on structure, dynamics, and long-term stability of a model IgG1 monoclonal antibody upon freeze-drying[J]. Pharmaceutical Research, 2013, 30(4): 968-984.

[10] Williams NA, Polli GP. The lyophilization of pharmaceuticals a literature review[J]. Journal of Parenteral Science and Technology, 1984, 38(2): 48-59.

[11] Franks F. Freeze-drying of bioproducts: putting principles into practice[J]. European Journal Of Pharmaceutics And Biopharmaceutics, 1998, 45(3): 221-229.

[12] Lipiainen T, Peltoniemi M, Sarkhel S, *et al.* Formulation and Stability of Cytokine Therapeutics[J]. Journal Of Pharmaceutical Sciences, 2015, 104(2): 307-326.

[13] Terakita A, Matsunaga H, Handa T. The Influence of water on the stability of lyophilized formulations with inositol and mannitol as excipients[J]. Chemical & Pharmaceutical Bulletin, 2009, 57(5): 459-463.

[14] Zeng XM, Martin GP, Marriott C. Effects of molecular weight of polyvinylpyrrolidone on the glass transition and crystallization of co-lyophilized sucrose[J]. International Journal Of Pharmaceutics, 2001, 218(1-2): 63-73.

[15] Wang W. Lyophilization and development of solid protein pharmaceuticals[J]. International Journal Of Pharmaceutics, 2000, 203(1-2): 1-60.

[16] Heller MC, Carpenter JF, Randolph TW. Protein formulation and lyophilization cycle design: Prevention of damage due to freeze-concentration induced phase separation[J]. Biotechnology And Bioengineering, 1999, 63(2): 166-174.

[17] Kadoya S, Fujii K, Izutsu K-i, *et al.* Freeze-drying of proteins with glass-forming oligosaccharide-derived sugar alcohols[J]. International Journal Of Pharmaceutics, 2010, 389(1-2): 107-113.

[18] Carpenter JF, Chang BS, Garzon-Rodriguez W, *et al.* Rational design of stable lyophilized protein formulations: theory and practice[J]. Pharmaceutical biotechnology, 2002, 13: 109-133.

[19] Remmele RL, Jr., Krishnan S, Callahan WJ. Development of Stable Lyophilized Protein Drug Products[J]. Current Pharmaceutical Biotechnology, 2012, 13(3): 471-496.

[20] Han Y, Jin B-S, Lee S-B, *et al.* Effects of sugar additives on protein stability of recombinant human serum albumin during lyophilization and storage[J]. Archives Of Pharmacal Research, 2007, 30(9): 1124-1131.

[21] Selva C, Malferrari M, Ballardini R, *et al.* Trehalose preserves the integrity of lyophilized phycoerythrin-antihuman CD8 antibody conjugates and enhances their thermal stability in flow cytometric assays[J]. Journal Of Pharmaceutical Sciences, 2013, 102(2): 649-659.

[22] Souillac PO, Middaugh CR, Rytting JH. Investigation of protein/carbohydrate interactions in the dried state. 2. Diffuse reflectance FTIR studies[J]. International Journal Of Pharmaceutics, 2002, 235(1-2): 207-218.

[23] Wu SL, Leung D, Tretyakov L, *et al.* The formation and mechanism of multimerization in a freeze-dried peptide[J]. International Journal Of Pharmaceutics, 2000, 200(1): 1-16.

[24] Geourjon C, Deleage G. SOPM - a self-optimized method for protein secondary structure prediction[J]. Protein Engineering, 1994, 7(2): 157-164.

[25] Costantino HR, Carrasquillo KG, Cordero RA, *et al.* Effect of excipients on the stability and structure of lyophilized recombinant

human growth hormone[J]. Journal Of Pharmaceutical Sciences, 1998, 87(11): 1412-1420.

[26] Costantino HR, Langer R, Klibanov AM. Aggregation of a lyophilized pharmaceutical protein, recombinant human albumin - effect of moisture and stabilization by excipients[J]. Bio-Technology, 1995, 13(5): 493-496.

[27] Song L, Zhu Y, Wang H, *et al.* A solid-phase PEGylation strategy for protein therapeutics using a potent FGF21 analog[J]. Biomaterials, 2014, 35(19): 5206-5215.

[28] Mosharraf M, Malmberg M, Fransson J. Formulation, lyophilization and solid-state properties of a pegylated protein[J]. International Journal Of Pharmaceutics, 2007, 336(2): 215-232.

[29] Byler DM, Susi H. Examination of the secondary structure of proteins by deconvolved ftir spectra[J]. Biopolymers, 1986, 25(3): 469-487.

[30] Griebenow K, Klibanov AM. On protein denaturation in aqueous-organic mixtures but not in pure organic solvents[J]. Journal Of the American Chemical Society, 1996, 118(47): 11695-11700.

[31] Griebenow K, Klibanov AM. Can conformational changes be responsible for solvent and excipient effects on the catalytic behavior of subtilisin Carlsberg in organic solvents?[J]. Biotechnology And Bioengineering, 1997, 53(4): 351-362.

[32] Kauppinen JK, Moffatt DJ, Mantsch HH, *et al.* Fourier self-deconvolution - a method for resolving intrinsically overlapped bands[J]. Applied Spectroscopy, 1981, 35(3): 271-276.

[33] Naumann D, Schultz C, Gornetschelnokow U, *et al.* Secondary structure and temperature behavior of the acetylcholine-receptor by fourier-transform infrared-spectroscopy[J]. Biochemistry, 1993, 32(12): 3162-3168.

[34] Susi H, Byler DM. Protein-structure by fourier-transform infrared-spectroscopy - 2nd derivative spectra[J]. Biochemical And Biophysical Research Communications, 1983, 115(1): 391-397.

[35] Susi H, Byler DM. Resolution-enhanced fourier-transform infrared-spectroscopy of enzymes[J]. Methods In Enzymology, 1986, 130: 290-311.

[36] Yang WJ, Griffiths PR, Byler DM, *et al.* Protein conformation by infrared-spectroscopy - resolution enhancement by fourier self-deconvolution[J]. Applied Spectroscopy, 1985, 39(2): 282-287.

[37] Zhang M, Jiang X, Su Z, *et al.* Large-scale expression, purification, and glucose uptake activity of recombinant human FGF21 in Escherichia coli[J]. Applied Microbiology And Biotechnology, 2012, 93(2): 613-621.

[38] Kokkinos J, Tang S, Rye K-A, *et al.* The role of fibroblast growth factor 21 in atherosclerosis[J]. Atherosclerosis, 2017, 257: 259-265.

[39] Ye X, Qi J, Yu D, *et al.* Pharmacological efficacy of FGF21 analogue, liraglutide and insulin glargine in treatment of type 2 diabetes[J]. Journal Of Diabetes And Its Complications, 2017, 31(4): 726-734.

[40] Longa EZ, Weinstein PR, Carlson S, *et al.* Reversible middle cerebral-artery occlusion without craniectomy in rats[J]. Stroke, 1989, 20(1): 84-91.

[41] Tamaki N, Yamashita H, Kimura M, *et al.* Changes in the components and content of biological water in the brain of experimental hydrocephalic rabbits[J]. Journal Of Neurosurgery, 1990, 73(2): 274-278.

[42] Cheong CU, Yeh CS, Hsieh YW, *et al.* Protective Effects of Costunolide against Hydrogen Peroxide-Induced Injury in PC12 Cells[J]. Molecules, 2016, 21(7).

Chapter 5
Signaling Pathway and Pharmacology

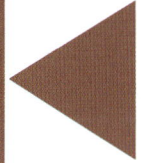

Fibroblast growth factor-1 released from a heparin coacervate improves cardiac function in a mouse myocardial infarction model

Zhouguang Wang, Xiaokun Li, Yadong Wang

1. Introduction

Despite decades of research, cardiovascular disease remains the largest cause of death as well as a major contributor to disability, affecting 5.8 million people in the United States with an estimated annual healthcare cost of $300 billion.[1] Within the myocardial infarction (MI) zone, insufficient blood supply to a region triggers both cell death and subsequent pathological remodeling, which eventually results in heart failure.[2] There has been a considerable amount of research interest in developing novel therapies, such as gene therapy, stem cell therapy, and direct administration of proangiogenic growth factors.[3] Although preclinical studies and initial clinical trials supported the beneficial effects of proangiogenic factors,[4,5] patients failed to show appreciable improvement in double-blinded clinical trials.[6-8] These negative findings may have resulted from a dearth of knowledge regarding how blood vessels form as well as the body's endogenous responses to ischemia as well as growth factor selection and/or the timing that growth factors reach the target zone. Moreover, the extent by directly administered growth factors are beneficial is restricted by their short half-lives after injection; enzymatic deactivation and proteolytic degradation occur within minutes of treatment. In this study, an injectable biocompatible and biodegradable coacervate is used to control the release of heparin-binding growth factors and offer an effective method of extending fibroblast growth factor 1 (FGF1) bioactivity.

We have developed a controlled delivery system that utilizes the charge interaction between a heparin, a natural polyanion, and poly(ethylene argininylaspartate diglyceride) (PEAD), a biodegradable polycation, which together form a complex coacervate. The coacervate is a phase separation of liquids where the polycation and polyanion forms a neutral complex and separates from the surrounding aqueous environment, encapsulating the heparin-binding proteins and protecting them from degradation. This heparin-based coacervate delivery platform functions to both protect and release heparin-binding growth factors, including nerve growth factor,[9] fibroblast growth factor-2 (FGF2),[9] heparin-binding epidermal growth factor-like growth factor,[10] and stromal cell-derived factor-1α.[11] Additionally, this system is retained within the heart for up to one month *in vivo* after injection.[12] In our previous study, we proved that Sonic Hedgehog (Shh) delivered by the coacervate combined with a degradable hydrogel is cardio-protective and promotes heart function and angiogenesis in rodents after MI.[13,14] We also utilized fibrin gel and the coacervate in order to sequentially deliver vascular endothelial growth factor (VEGF) and platelet-derived growth factor (PDGF) to rat ischemic hearts. Within 1 week, VEGF was released, and PDGF release was sustained a minimum of 3 weeks *in vitro*. Sequentially releasing VEGF and PDGF significantly enhanced heart function, which was assessed by measuring cardiac contractility through fractional area change (FAC), in an acute MI model in rats. We also demonstrated enhanced vascularization and survival of cardiomyocytes as well as reduced fibrosis, inflammation, left ventricle (LV) wall thinning, scar expansion, and fibrosis post-MI.[15]

FGF1 is a member of the FGF family and has many functions. FGF1 is synthesized by many different cell types, including cardiomyocytes, endothelial cells, and fibroblasts.[16] FGF1 has shown therapeutic potential in burns and wound healing.[17] Previous studies have reported that in acute ischemia and reperfusion, FGFs exert cardioprotective effects by inducing an ischemic preconditioning (IPC)-like state.[18-20] In the heart, FGF1 with its receptor FGFR1 is vital in the regulation of cardiac morphogenesis, arteriogenesis, and angiogenesis.[21] Furthermore, FGF1 greatly enhances cardiac remodeling after MI through the induction of cardiomyocyte proliferation.[22] By enhancing angiogenesis and reducing injury from ischemia-reperfusion, FGF1 would be expected to effectively treat cardiac ischemia. Indeed, constitutive over-expression of cardiac-specific FGF1 can delay myocardial infarct formation *in vivo*.[20] However, one major obstacle of growth factor therapies in the treatment of heart disease is their short half-lives *in vivo*.[23] Additionally, FGF1 in its free form possesses low levels of bioactivity but exhibits a much higher bioactivity when combined with heparin.[24] Because of the use of heparin in our delivery system, we therefore aim to extend the half-life and improve the bioactivity of FGF1, investigating its potential to reduce cardiac scar burden and improve heart function post-MI.

In this study, we formed the FGF1 coacervate and researched its bioactivity on endothelial and cardiac stem cells *in vitro*. Its therapeutic efficacy was evaluated in a murine MI model. Notably, the histological examination revealed that the FGF1 coacervate reduced inflammation and fibrosis post-MI, significantly increased the proliferation of endothelial and mural cells, and resulted in stable vasculature. Finally, we observed significantly improved cardiac function due to the controlled delivery of FGF1 to infarcted hearts.

2. Materials and methods

2.1 FGF1 coacervate characterization and release profile-PEAD and the complex coacervate were prepared as previously described[9,25]

PEAD and heparin were each dissolved separately in DI water at concentrations of 10 mg/ml. Heparin and FGF1 were first combined, then PEAD was added to form the coacervate. Following th addition of PEAD, the solution went from clear to turbid, indicating the coacervate had formed. The final mass ratios of PEAD:heparin:FGF1 were 500:100:1.

The release profile of the FGF1 coacervate was determined *in vitro* as previously described.[25] Briefly, 200 μl of FGF1 coacervate suspended in saline containing 500 ng of FGF1 was centrifuged at $12\,100 \times g$ for 10 min and the pellet stored at 37℃. On days 0, 1, 4, 7, 10, 14, 21, and 28, the supernatant was aspirated and stored at −80℃, and 200 μl of fresh saline was added to cover the pellet. The amount of released FGF1 in three separate fractions per time point was determined by ELISA (R&D Systems, Minneapolis, MN).

Coacervate size was determined by dynamic light scattering as previously described.[9] Heparin and PEAD were separately dissolved in DI water then combined at a 5:1 PEAD:heparin mass ratio in 1 ml total solution. Coacervate droplet size was then immediately measured using the Zetasizer Nano ZS (Malvern, Westborough, WA).

2.2 Measurement of cell proliferation and migration in vitro

Human umbilical vein endothelial cells (HUVEC) were purchased from ATCC (Manassas, VA) and cultured in EBM-2 media (Lonza, Basel, Switzerland) supplemented with 2.5% fetal bovine serum to simulate nutrient-deprived conditions. Human Sca-1+/ckit+ cardiac stem cells (hCSC) were purchased from Celprogen Inc. (Torrance, CA) and plated on extracellular expansion matrix-coated plates (Celprogen Inc.). To simulate nutrient deprivation in hCSCs, hCSC media with serum (Celprogen Inc.) was diluted 1:4 with basal DMEM media (25% hCSC-CM). HUVECs and hCSCs were each seeded at 2×10^3 cells per well in a 96-well plate for proliferation assays and incubated in 100 μl of nutrient-deprived media overnight to allow cells to attach. The following day, all cells were washed with DMEM, and 200 μl nutrient-deprived media containing no supplements, delivery vehicle, 50 ng/ml free FGF1, or 50 ng/ml FGF1 coacervate were added to each well to determine their effect on cell proliferation ($n = 4$ per group). This dose of FGF1 is based off previous *in vitro* studies utilizing FGF1.[26] The plates were then incubated for 72 h at 37℃. After washing all wells, CellTiter 96 AQueous One Solution Cell Proliferation Assay (MTS) reagent (Promega, Madison, WI, USA) in DMEM was added. The plate was incubated in 5% CO_2 at 37℃ for 3 h, at which point the absorbance at 490 nm (with reference at 650 nm) was read with the Infinite 200 PRO plate reader (Tecan, Switzerland).

The effect of FGF1 coacervate on the migration of hCSC and HUVEC was measured by transwell chemotaxis. Nutrient-deprived media containing no supplements, delivery vehicle, 50 ng/ml of free FGF1, or 50 ng/ml of FGF1 coacervate were loaded into bottom wells ($n = 4$ per group). hCSC and HUVEC were seeded in 24-well transwell inserts with 8 μm pore size (Millipore, Billerica, MA) at a density of 10 000 cells/cm². After incubation at 37℃ for 12 h, nonmigrated cells were removed with cotton swabs. Migrated cells were fixed in methanol for 10 min and stained with Quant-iT PicoGreen dsDNA reagent (P7581; Thermo Fisher Scientific, Waltham, MA, USA). Fluorescent images were captured by Nikon Eclipse Ti fluorescence microscope equipped with NIS-Elements AR imaging software (both from Nikon, Tokyo, Japan). The number of migrated cells was quantified and averaged from 3 independent images taken in 3 different areas per sample per group ($n = 4$). The cell number of each group was individually normalized to the average number of cells in the basal media control group.

2.3 Mouse acute MI model and intramyocardial injection

Male Balb/cJ mice (Jackson Laboratory, Bar Harbor, ME) at 9–12 weeks old were used and cared for in compliance with the Institutional Animal Care and Use Committee of the University of Pittsburgh. A total of 39 mice were used in this study, 13 for each of three treatments. At 2 weeks, 4–5 mice were chosen from each group at random and sacrificed for 2-week analysis. The remaining 8–9 in each group were sacrificed 6 weeks post-MI. MI and intramyocardial injections were performed as we previously reported.[12,27,28] Briefly, MI was induced by ligation of the left coronary artery. Five min after the induction of MI, a total volume of 35 μl saline, free FGF1 (500 ng of FGF1) or FGF1 coacervate (500 μg of PEAD, 100 μg of heparin and 500 ng of FGF1) was injected across three sites of the ischemic myocardium (one at the center and two at the border zone of the infarct). The FGF1 dose was chosen based on previous studies utilizing this coacervate system with other growth factors in a mouse MI model.[12,27] FGF1-free coacervate was not tested as it has shown to have no effect in cardiac repair in our previous studies.[15,27] The surgeon performing the surgical procedures and injections was blinded to the treatment received by each mouse.

2.4 Echocardiography

Echocardiography was repeatedly performed by a blinded investigator before surgery and at 2 and 6 weeks postinfarction to assess cardiac function. Briefly, the heart and respiratory rates were continuously monitored while the body temperature was maintained at 37℃ by a hot pad. Echocardiographic parameters were measured using a high-frequency linear probe (MS400, 30 MHz) connected to a high-resolution ultrasound imaging system (Vevo 2100; FUJIFILM VisualSonics, Toronto, Ontario, Canada). End-systolic area (ESA) and end-diastolic area (EDA) were measured from short-axis images of the LV by B-mode. FAC was calculated as [(EDA-ESA)/EDA]*100%. This has been validated as an accurate prediction of cardiac contractility.[29] LV ejection fraction (LVEF) was also calculated using echocardiography. The mice that were sacrificed for histological analysis prior to 6 weeks postinjection were not included in the echocardiographic study.

2.5 Histological analysis

At 2 and 6 weeks postinfarction, the mice were sacrificed and the hearts were harvested following the established methods.[30] The harvested hearts were frozen in OCT compound for staining. Specimens were serially sectioned at a thickness of 8 μm from apex to the ligation level (approximately 0.5 mm in length). For comparison of the ventricular wall thickness in the infarct zone, wall thickness was measured at the midinfarct point of each ventricle on H&E stained slides using NIH ImageJ software. Seven hearts for each treatment were used for this quantification. For observation of fibrosis, Masson's trichrome kit (IMEB, San Marcos, CA) was used to stain collagen fibers. Twelve sections from each treatment group were imaged to examine scar expansion through the ventricle wall. Inflammatory mast cells are known regulators of matrix metalloproteinase activity following MI.[31] To quantify their infiltration, we performed toluidine blue staining, and mast cell density was measured in two fields of view within the border zone of each heart. All wall thickness, fibrosis, and mast cell measurements were taken from mice sacrificed at the 6 week time point.

2.6. Immunofluorescent staining

For evaluation of inflammation, a rat antimouse CD68 (Abcam, Cambridge, MA) primary antibody was used, followed by an antirat IgG secondary antibody (Invitrogen, Carlsbad, CA). For detection of endothelial cells, a rat antimouse CD31 (BD Biosciences, San Jose, CA) and the same antirat IgG secondary antibody was used. For α-SMA staining, an FITC-conjugated anti-α-SMA monoclonal antibody (Sigma-Aldrich, St. Louis, MO) was utilized. To examine murine CSCs, we first incubated sections overnight at 4℃ with rat antimouse CD117/c-kit (Cedarlane Laboratories, Burlington, NC). For the detection of cardiomyocytes, sections were incubated overnight at 4℃ with mouse anticardiac troponin T (cTnT) primary antibody (Abcam), followed by goat antimouse Alexa 488 IgG at RT for 1 h. To detect proliferating cells, after the first staining for one of the cell lineage markers above, a second overnight incubation was performed at 4℃ with rabbit antimammalian Ki67 primary antibody (Abcam), followed by donkey antirabbit Alexa 488 IgG at RT for 1 h. The nuclei were stained with DAPI at RT for 10 min. Immunofluorescent images were taken using a Nikon Eclipse Ti fluorescence microscope equipped with NIS-Elements AR imaging software (both from Nikon). For quantification, four to six sections from different hearts were used for each group. Measures of inflammation, angiogenesis, and progenitor cell populations were taken as cells per mm^2 area; cTnT staining was measured by quantifying the fractional area of cTnT+ within the microscopic field.

2.7　Statistical analysis

All data are presented as the mean ± standard deviation (SD). Significant differences between groups were analyzed by Student's t test (two groups), one-way ANOVA (multiple groups), or two-way repeated ANOVA, and $P \leqslant 0.05$ was considered significantly different. Statistical analyses were performed with GraphPad Prism 5.0 (GraphPad Software, La Jolla, CA, USA).

3.　Results

3.1　Characterization of FGF1 coacervate

As shown in the chemical structure of PEAD, each repeating unit contains two functional groups with a positive charge: an ammonium and guanidinium group (Fig. 1A). The interactions between these positive charges on PEAD and the negative charges carried by the sulfates on heparin allow coacervate formation. FGF1 has a high-affinity binding site for heparin. Collectively, a ternary complex self-assembles: [PEAD:heparin:FGF1]. We fluorescently labeled FGF1 (DyLight 594, red), which showed that the coacervate droplets had an average size of 526.2 ± 106.4 nm (Fig. 1 B-D). To measure the controlled release of proteins *in vitro*, the amount of FGF1 released from the coacervate was measured by ELISA at 0, 1, 4, 7, 10, 14, 21, and 28 days. As shown in our result, less than 10% FGF1 was detectable in the supernatant after centrifugation (day 0 of release assay), and therefore, the loading efficiency was greater than 90%. After the initial release, FGF1 coacervate released approximately 15.1 ± 2.5% during the first 24 h. The total release of FGF1 was estimated to be 79.8 ± 6.3% over the 28-day duration (Fig. 1E). These results showed that FGF1 was released in a sustained manner without an initial burst at an approximately linear 2.31% day^{-1}.

3.2　FGF1 coacervate induces endothelial cell and cardiac stem cell chemotaxis and proliferation

The effect of FGF1 coacervate on HUVEC and hCSC proliferation was investigated *in vitro*. Cells were seeded on tissue culture treated polystyrene using nutrient-deprived media for the duration of the experiment in order to simulate nutrient starvation following coronary artery blockage. A fixed load of 50 ng/mL FGF1 was selected based on previous studies utilizing growth factors for *in vitro* assays.[26] DMEM basal medium served as the negative control. The treatment of HUVEC with 50 ng/ml of free FGF1 or FGF1 coacervate led to an increase in HUVEC proliferation, which was statistically significant ($P < 0.05$) (Fig. 2C). However, FGF1 coacervate could also significantly increase HUVEC proliferation in comparison to free FGF1 ($P < 0.05$) and saline ($P < 0.01$) (Fig. 2C). Consistent with these results, the hCSC proliferation test also showed that the FGF1 coacervate significantly increased hCSC proliferation compared to free FGF1 ($P < 0.05$) and saline ($P < 0.01$) (Fig. 2B). We did not observe any significant difference between the no-treatment control and the vehicle group in these two cell types ($P > 0.05$) (Fig. 2A–C).

We evaluated chemotaxis on HUVECs and hCSCs induced by FGF1 coacervate using a transwell assay. Fluorescent images of transwell insert membranes showed enhanced chemotaxis of HUVECs and hCSCs in both the free FGF1 (50 ng/ml) and FGF1 (50 ng/ml) coacervate groups relative to basal media ($P < 0.05$ for free FGF1, $P < 0.01$ for FGF1 coacervate) (Fig. 2A, D, E). However, an identical dose of FGF1 released by the coacervate exhibited greater chemotactic effects compared to the free FGF1 group in both HUVECs and hCSCs ($P < 0.05$) (panels D and E). The vehicle group demonstrated no effect on cell migration compared with the basal media group ($P > 0.05$). Thus, these results indicate that FGF1 released by the coacervate is highly bioactive and stimulates the proliferation and migration of HUVECs and hCSCs *in vitro*.

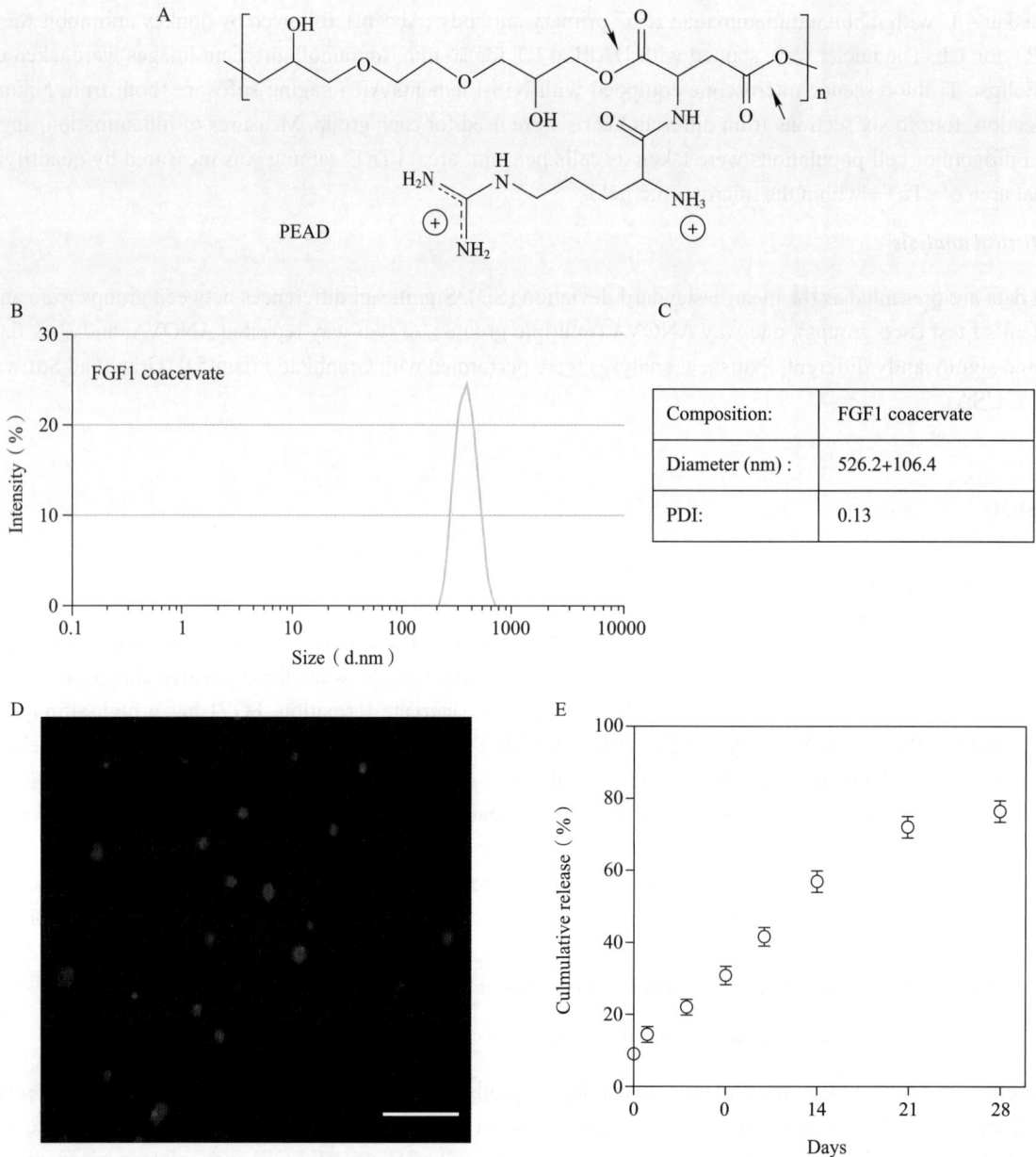

Fig. 1. Coacervate controls the release of FGF1 in a steady fashion. (A) Chemical structure of the PEAD polycation. (B, C) Analysis of coacervate droplet size with polydispersity index (PDI). (D) Confocal fluorescent imaging of fluorescein-labeled FGF1 shows spherical morphology with loading specifically within the coacervate droplet. Bar = 10 μm. (E) The release profile of FGF1 coacervate *in vitro* for 4 weeks as measured by ELISA. Data are presented as percent cumulative release (normalized to the original load). Error bars indicate means ± SD.

3.3 FGF1 coacervate protects cardiac structure and improves cell survival post-MI

To further elucidate how FGF1 coacervate affects the structure and function of the heart, we performed cTnT immunofluorescent staining in each group to examine the survival of cardiomyocytes (Fig. 3A). At 6 weeks post-MI, the saline and free FGF1 groups both showed significant reductions in cardiomyocyte (cTnT+) population in the infarct region. The FGF1 coacervate group, however, showed a significantly higher density of cTnT+ cells than the saline ($P <$ 0.01) and free FGF1 ($P <$ 0.05) groups, which suggests that FGF1 coacervate is more effective at preserving the cardomyocytes (Fig. 3B).

To evaluate the effect of FGF1 coacervate on cardiac structure, the infarct regions of the hearts were examined 6 weeks post-MI using H&E-stained sections (Fig. 3C). In the saline control, the ventricle wall where the infarct occurred was very thin. The ventricle was drastically dilated compared to a normal heart and healthy tissue was replaced by

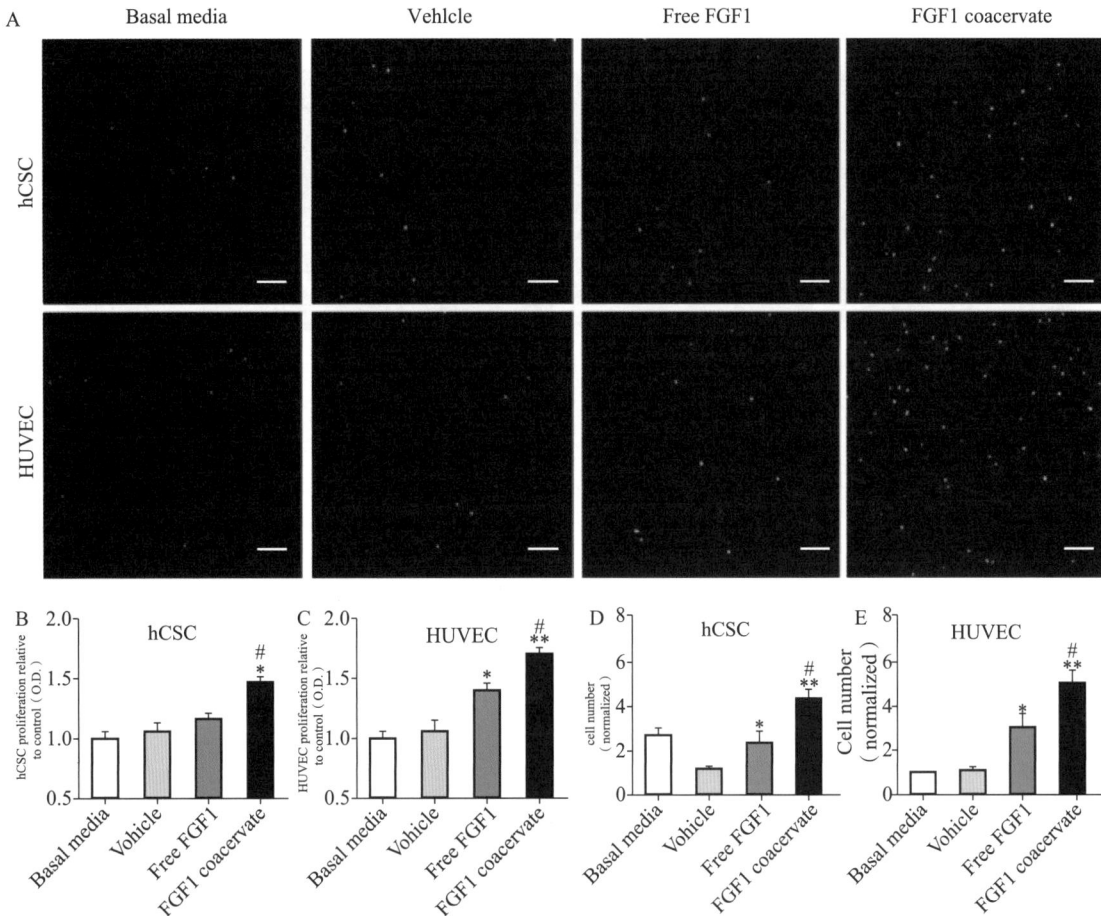

Fig. 2. Bioactivity of FGF1 coacervate on hCSC and HUVEC proliferation and migration. (A) Representative immunofluorescent images showing migration of hCSC and HUVEC in response to different treatments through a transwell chemotaxis assay. (B, C) Quantification of proliferation data showed that FGF1 coacervate significantly increased proliferation relative to both basal media and free FGF1 in both hCSC and HUVEC. Free FGF1 also increased proliferation of HUVEC relative to basal media but not hCSC. (D-E) Quantification of migration data showed enhanced chemotaxis of HUVEC and hCSC in both the free FGF1 and FGF1 coacervate groups. However, the same dose of FGF1 delivered by the coacervate had greater chemotactic effects compared to the both basal media and the free FGF1 group in both HUVEC and hCSC ($n = 4$ per group; data normalized to the respective basal media). $^*P < 0.05$, $^{**}P < 0.01$ compared to basal media; $^\#P < 0.05$ compared to free FGF1. All quantitative data represent means ± SD.

granulation and scar tissues. Free FGF1 could reduce the infarct area, but most fibers in this region were damaged, and the tissue architecture was not drastically different from the saline group. In contrast, FGF1 coacervate was capable of preventing these damaging effects on the infarcted tissue as well as preserving normal ventricular size. As a result (Fig. 3E), the FGF1 coacervate group showed significantly increased LV wall thickness in the infarct zone (274.8 ± 64.8 μm) compared to the saline (104.7 ± 31.8 μm, $P < 0.01$) and free FGF1 groups (153.4 ± 37.4 μm, $P < 0.05$). Overall, FGF1 coacervate reduced the infarct size (Fig. 3D), prevented ventricular dilation and preserved cardiac fiber morphology.

3.4 FGF1 coacervate reduces fibrosis and inhibits chronic infiltration of phagocytic cells in the infarcted myocardium

To examine the effect of FGF1 coacervate on cardiac fibrosis, we performed Masson's trichrome staining to observe collagen deposition in the infarcted myocardium 6 weeks post-MI. Consistent with the literature, there was significant deposition in the infarct zone post-MI (Fig. 4A). Fibrotic tissue was observed up to the border zone in the saline control group, as shown by dense collagen deposition along the border zone's ventricular wall (Fig. 4A). In the free FGF1 group, we observed similar fibrosis in this region. In contrast, images from the FGF1 coacervate group had reduced collagen deposition and scar formation in the infarct area in comparison to the saline and free FGF1 groups. FGF1 coacervate visibly reduced the amount of collagen in the border zone, indicating its efficacy at reducing fibrosis. Consequently, the tissue would be more compliant and should enhance cardiac contractility after MI, as shown below.

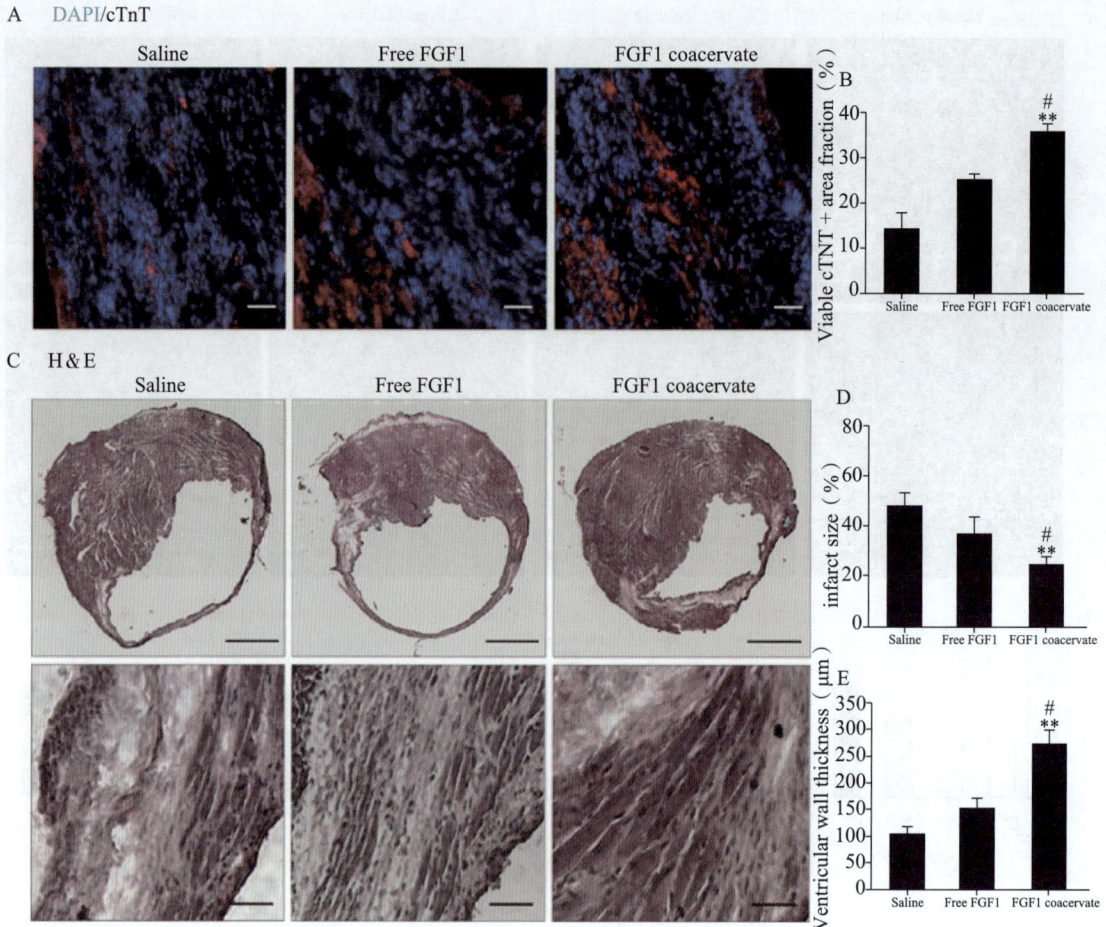

Fig. 3. FGF1 coacervate mitigates MI-associated injury. (A) cTnT staining (red) showed few viable cardiomyocytes in the saline and free FGF1 groups, while the FGF1 coacervate group showed a larger area of viable cardiac muscle in the infarct zone. Scale bars = 50 μm. (B) Quantitative analysis shows a significantly higher density of viable cardiomyocytes in hearts receiving FGF1 coacervate relative to saline or free FGF1. (C) H&E staining showed that MI caused wall thinning and ventricular dilation in the saline control group. The higher magnification micrographs revealed damaged cardiac myofibers surrounded by scar tissue. Similar morphology was observed in the free FGF1 groups. FGF1 coacervate reduced the infarct area and partially preserved the normal tissue structure in the infarct zone. Scale bars = 1 mm (top) and 50 μm (bottom). (D-E) Quantitative analysis showed significantly increased ventricular wall thickness and reduced infarct area in the FGF1 coacervate group compared with the saline and free FGF1 groups. $^{**}P < 0.01$, compared with saline, $^{#}P < 0.05$ compared with free FGF1. Data represent means ± SD.

In addition to cardiac fibrosis, MI could also trigger systemic and local inflammation in the infarcted zone. In our study, we detected phagocytic cells within the infarct area utilizing a pan-macrophage marker, CD68, at 2 weeks postinfarction. An earlier 2-week time point was selected for this analysis due to the large inflammatory response typically seen in the early acute phase of MI. Healthy myocardium has very few CD68+ cells; on the contrary, a significant number of CD68+ cells were present in the infarct area at 2 weeks postinfarction (Fig. 4B). Macrophage density was not affected by free FGF1 treatment, although significantly fewer CD68+ cells were observed in the FGF1 coacervate group (Fig. 4B). When analyzed, there was no significant difference in CD68+ cell density between the saline and free FGF1 groups ($P > 0.05$) (Fig. 4C). However, administration of FGF1 coacervate greatly decreased the number of CD68+ cells in the infarct area ($P < 0.01$ relative to saline, $P < 0.05$ relative to free FGF1) (Fig. 4C). In summary, these results showed that FGF1 coacervate could reduce macrophage infiltration post-MI in the infarcted tissue.

3.5 FGF1 coacervate promotes long-term revascularization

MI causes an ischemic environment, and vascularization to restore blood flow to the infarcted region is very important for both tissue regeneration and a functional recovery. To investigate mature and stable vasculature formation in the infarct zone, immunofluorescent staining was performed using the endothelial cell CD31 marker (mostly located in microvasculature/capillaries) and α-SMA marker for vascular smooth muscle cells, which surround large blood vessels,

A

B DAPI/CD68

C

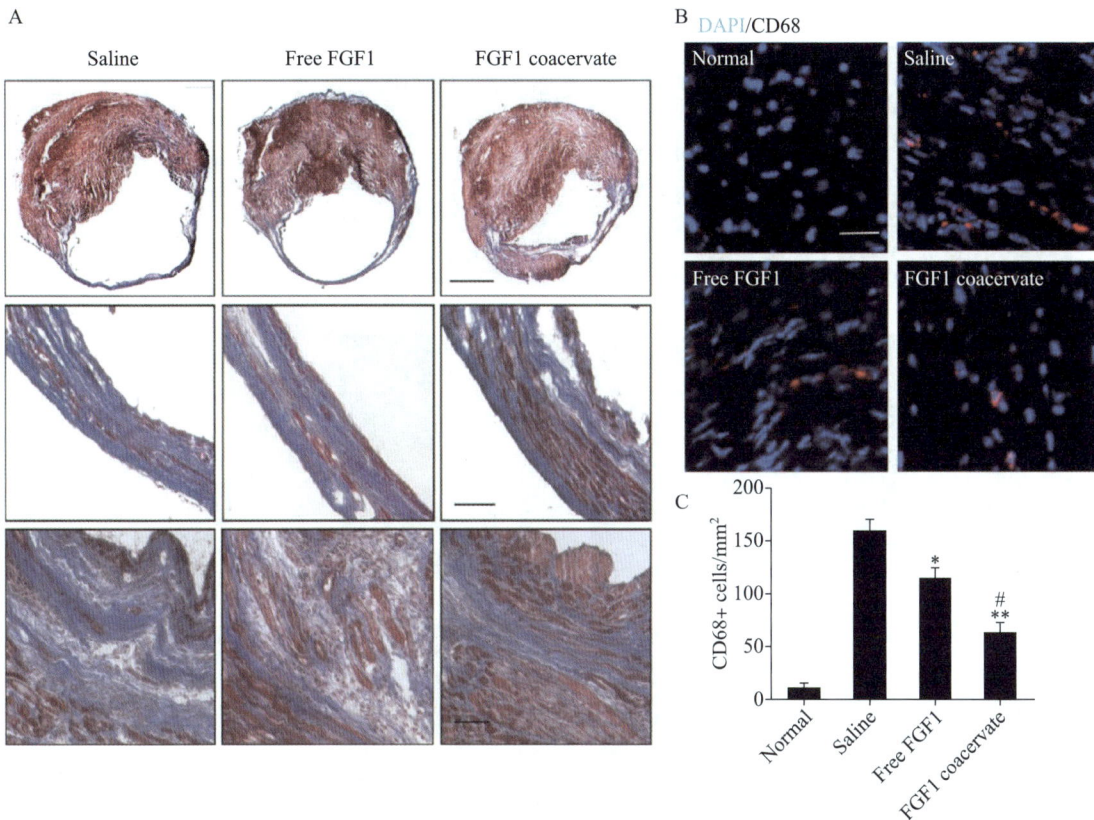

Fig. 4. FGF1 coacervate reduces inflammation and fibrosis post-MI. (A) Fibrosis in the border zone at 6 weeks as examined by Masson's tri-chrome staining. The saline control had many collagen fibers deposited along the inner wall. FGF1 coacervate effectively prevented propagation of fibrosis. Scale bars =1 mm for top row and 50 μm for bottom 2 rows. The second and third row are representative images showing collagen deposition in the infarct and border zones at higher magnification. (B) Distribution of macrophages in the infarct and border zone at 2 weeks as indicated by CD68 staining. Scale bars = 50 μm. (C) Quantitative analysis showed significantly reduced CD68+ cells in the FGF1 coacervate group compared with the saline and free FGF1 groups. $^*P < 0.05$, $^{**}P < 0.01$, compared with saline, $^\#P < 0.05$ compared with free FGF1. Data presented as means ± SD.

at 6 weeks post-MI. In the infarct region (Fig. 5A), there were very few CD31+ cells in the saline group, and the free FGF1 treatment group had higher CD31+ endothelial cell density compared to the saline control. However, the saline control was not different from the free FGF1 group after statistically analysis ($P > 0.05$). In contrast, the FGF1 coacervate treatment showed a much greater increase in CD31+ endothelial cell density than the saline ($P < 0.01$) and free FGF1 groups ($P > 0.05$) (Fig. 5B). To further detect endothelial cell proliferation 6 weeks postinfarction, the number of CD31+/Ki67+ cells in the ischemic myocardium were measured. Immunostaining showed that FGF1 coacervate-treated hearts had many more CD31+/Ki67+ proliferating endothelial cells than the free FGF1 ($P < 0.05$) and saline ($P < 0.01$) control groups at the infarct areas (Fig. 5C–D). This suggests that the FGF1 coacervate helped stimulate neovessel formation within the infarct and border zones.

    To further detect the stable vessel formation including arterioles, we costained CD31 and α-SMA to mark endothelial and mural cells together. As shown in our result, we could detect very few α-SMA+ cells after 6 weeks in the saline control (Fig. 5E). The saline control had 42.67 ± 12.01 α-SMA+ cells per mm^2 and had no significant difference from the free FGF1 group at 78.01 ± 15.87 per mm^2 ($P > 0.05$). However, the FGF1 coacervate treatment group had 163.1 ± 30.12 α-SMA+ cells per mm^2, which was much greater than the saline control ($P < 0.01$) and free FGF1 ($P < 0.01$) groups (Fig. 5F). In summary, free FGF1 had no significant effect in promoting angiogenesis compared with the saline group. Using coacervate delivery, the same dose of FGF1 formed substantially more blood vessels in the injured myocardium.

A DAPI/CD31

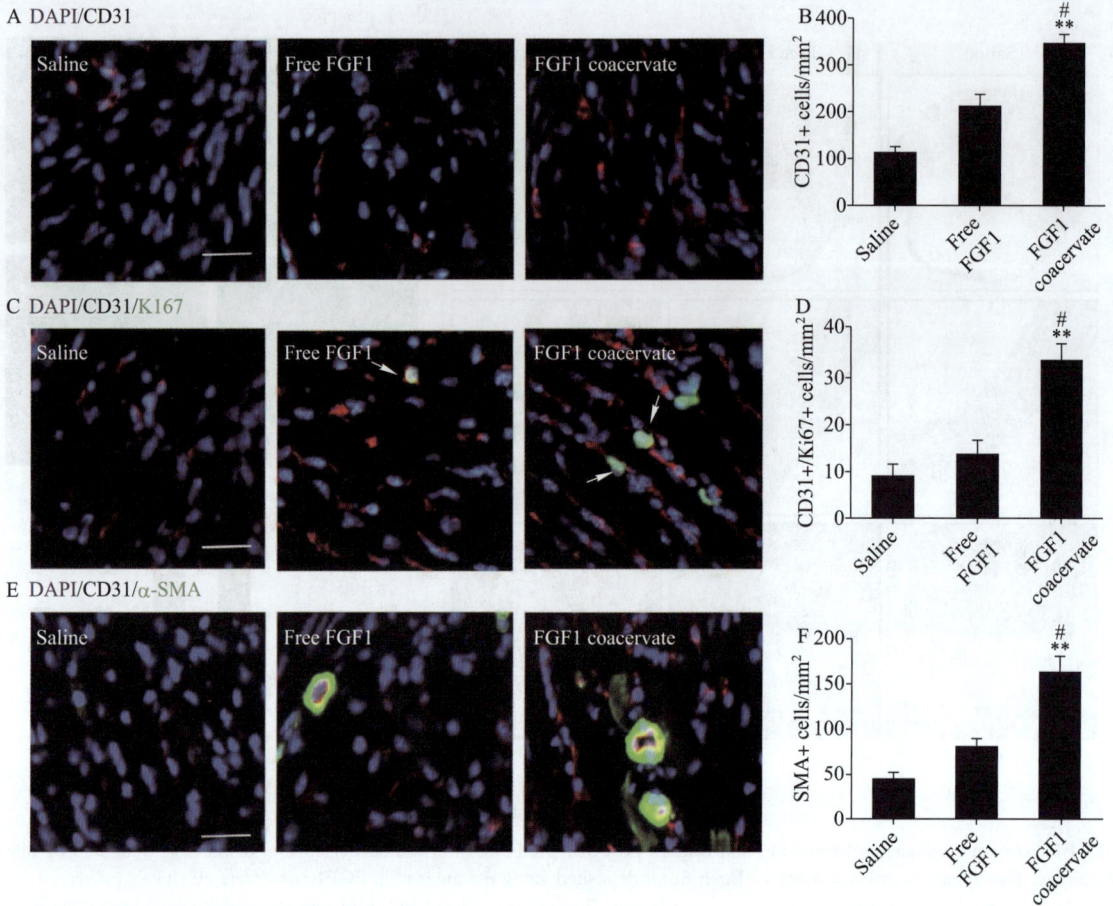

C DAPI/CD31/KI67

E DAPI/CD31/α-SMA

Fig. 5. FGF1 coacervate achieves stable vasculature in the infarcted myocardium. (A, B) CD31 staining for vascular endothelial cells in the infarct zone. At 6 weeks, significantly fewer CD31 positive cells were detected in the saline control group compared to the FGF1 coacervate group. FGF1 coacervate induced angiogenesis and achieved a significantly higher vessel density than saline and free FGF1. (C, D) CD31 & KI67 ww for proliferation of endothelial cells in the infarct zone. Analysis showed significantly higher numbers of proliferating CD31+ cells in the FGF1 coacervate group relative to both saline and free FGF1 groups. (E, F) CD31 & α-SMA costainingto mark endothelial and mural cells in the infarct zone, which could further detect the formation of stable vessels including arterioles. FGF1 coacervate exhibited significantly higher numbers of SMA+ cells relative to saline or free FGF1 groups. $^{**}P < 0.01$, compared to saline, $^{#}P < 0.05$, $^{##}P < 0.01$ compared to free FGF1. Data represent means ± SD.

3.6 FGF1 coacervate increases proliferation of cardiac precursor cell populations in vivo

To assess the effect of FGF1 coacervate on cardiac precursor cell density within the infarct area, we measured the number of c-kit+ cells in the myocardium. Quantitative analysis showed that while free FGF1 does not contain high numbers of c-kit+ cells relative to saline ($P > 0.05$), FGF1 coacervate shows a significantly higher density of c-kit+ cells as compared to saline ($P < 0.01$) and free FGF1 ($P < 0.05$) (Fig. 6B). We also investigated the effect of FGF1 coacervate on cardiac precursor cell proliferation by measuring the amount of c-kit+/Ki67+ cells in the ischemic myocardium. Immunohistochemistry conducted 6 weeks postinfarction showed that FGF1 coacervate-treated hearts had much higher numbers of c-kit +/Ki67+ proliferating CSCs than the free FGF1 ($P < 0.05$) and saline control ($P < 0.01$) groups at the infarct areas (c-kit: stem cell growth factor receptor or CD117; Ki67: a cellular proliferation marker) (Fig. 6A,C). Mast cells are also known to express this marker, so we performed toluidine blue staining to examine the effect of FGF1 on their infiltration. Staining at 6 weeks post-MI showed insignificant numbers of mast cells present in the infarct and border zone, regardless of treatment group (Fig. S1). Therefore, c-kit+ cells were predominantly progenitor cells rather than inflammatory mast cells. This result supports the postulation that FGF1 coacervate promotes cardiac precursor cell survival and proliferation in hearts after infarction that may in part be responsible for augmented cardiac function.

A DAPI/CD117/Ki67

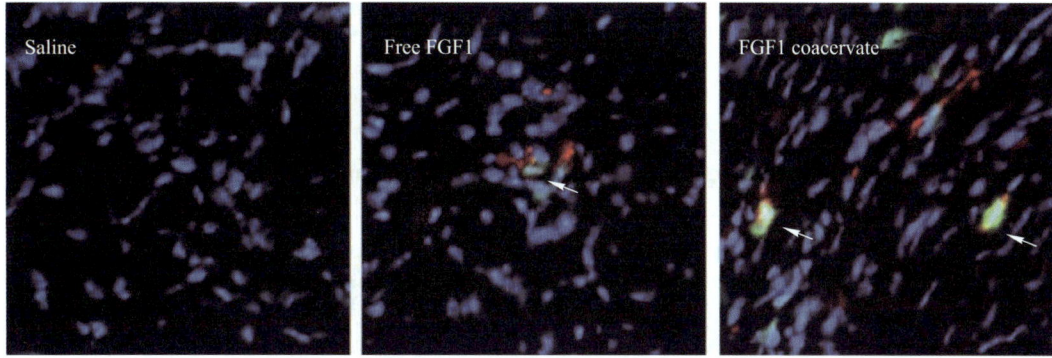

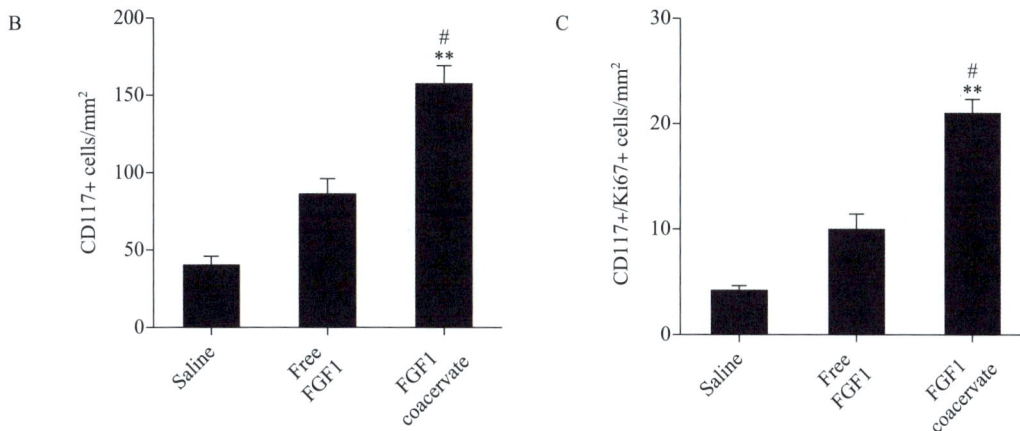

Fig. 6. FGF1 coacervate increases cardiac precursor cell proliferation. (A-C) Dual immunofluorescent detection and quantification of CD117+/ Ki67+ proliferating cardiac stem cells in infarct zone 6 weeks post-MI. $^{**}P < 0.01$ compared with saline, $^{#}P < 0.05$ compared with free FGF1. Data represent means ± SD.

3.7 Intramyocardial delivery of FGF1 coacervate improved post-MI cardiac function

To assess the therapeutic efficacy of FGF1 coacervate on cardiac function M-mode and B-mode 2-D echocardiography was used at 2 weeks and 6 weeks post-MI to monitor the changes in cardiac contractility (Fig. 7E, F). As shown in our results (Fig. 7A, B), EDA and ESA of the saline group increased to 18.99 ± 5.8 mm^2 and 13.45 ± 6.04 mm^2, respectively at 2 weeks post-MI. Both are significantly higher than healthy animals ($P < 0.05$), confirming that MI led to ventricular dilation. The ESA and EDA values were similar in the saline, free FGF1 and FGF1 coacervate groups, which suggests that the difference in ventricular dilation between the groups at 2 weeks post-MI is not significant ($P > 0.05$). FAC revealed that myocardial contractility in the saline control was lower than the normal value (from $52.82\% \pm 4.36\%$ to $29.29\% \pm 4.876\%$) (Fig. 7C). The free FGF1 groups ($36.36\% \pm 6.32\%$) showed no significant difference in comparison to the saline group ($P > 0.05$). The FAC of the FGF1 coacervate was higher than saline and free FGF1 at 2 weeks ($42.95\% \pm 4.06\%$), although this difference was not statistically significant ($P > 0.05$). A similar trend was seen in LVEF measurements (Fig. 7D).

At 6 weeks, the FAC declined slightly for the saline, free FGF1 and FGF1 coacervate groups, however the FGF1 coacervate group could maintain improved cardiac function with the highest FAC of all three groups ($P < 0.01$ *versus* saline, $P < 0.05$ *versus* free FGF1), which was consistent with the result at 2 weeks. The FAC values of the saline group were $21.25\% \pm 5.61\%$, $25.2\% \pm 3.8\%$ for the free FGF1 group, and $37.88\% \pm 4.27\%$ for the FGF1 coacervate group (Fig. 7C). Additionally, EDA and ESA values were significantly reduced in FGF1 coacervate group relative to saline (ESA $P < 0.01$, EDA $P < 0.05$) and free FGF1 (ESA and EDA $P < 0.05$). Consistent with FAC measurements, LVEF was greatly increased in the FGF1 coacervate group relative to saline(Fig. 7D).Taken together, these data demonstrate that the FGF1 coacervate can potently improve cardiac function 6 weeks post-MI by improving contractility and preventing ventricular dilation.

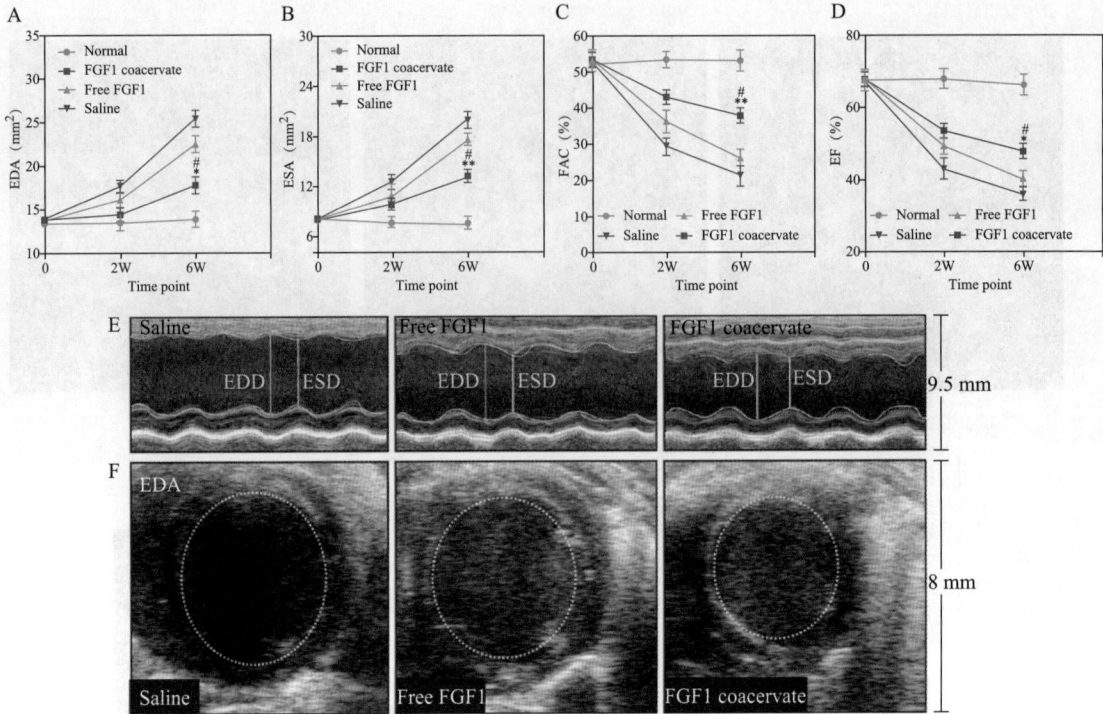

Fig. 7. Echocardiographic assessment suggests that FGF1 coacervate improves cardiac function. (A) Both at 2 and 6 weeks, the FGF1 coacervate group had the lowest EDA compared to the other groups, which was significant at 6 weeks. (B) Pairwise comparisons revealed that FGF1 coacervate treatment achieved a significantly lower ESA compared to saline and free FGF1 at 6 weeks. (C) FGF1 coacervate significantly increased FAC post-MI over saline or free FGF1 treatment at 6 weeks. (D) FGF1 coacervate significantly increased EF post-MI relatively to saline at 6 weeks. (E) Representative M-mode 2-D echocardiography at 6 weeks post-MI showed the changes of cardiac contractility in each group. (F) Representative B- mode 2-D echocardiography at 6 weeks post-MI showed the changes in cardiac contractility in each group. $^{*}P < 0.05$, $^{**}P < 0.01$ compared with saline, $^{#}P < 0.05$ compared with free FGF1. Data represent means $\pm$ SD.

4. Discussion

Protein therapy using proangiogenic factors that are capable of promoting cardiac repair as well as regeneration have been widely investigated.[32,33] To promote angiogenesis to revascularize ischemic myocardium, proangiogenic factors have been used with success in preclinical MI models.[34,35] However, in clinical trials, these methods of treatment have been ineffective with generally disappointing results. For example, FGF1, VEGF, granulocyte macrophage colony stimulating factor, FGF-2, hepatocyte growth factor, and neuregulin-1 therapies could not significantly improve revascularization and myocardial function in Phase I and II clinical trials on a consistent basis, despite being tolerable and reasonably safe at the different doses used.[3,33,36,37] One of the major obstacles of protein therapy utilizing exogenous growth factors or cytokines is the short half-life of the naked protein. In addition, systemically delivered growth factors have variable bioavailability in the target tissue largely due to the availability of local vasculature. These drawbacks have led to frequent administration of high growth factor doses in order to achieve therapeutic efficacy, but a systemic high quantity of the protein is potentially toxic. For example, a double-blind clinical trial showed that a high dose (50 ng/kg/min) of VEGF administered by intracoronary infusions in patients with myocardial ischemia can induce nitric oxide-mediated hypotension.[38] Thus, to better improve the local bioavailability and efficacy of exogenous growth factors and decrease the dosage required for ischemic injury, a suitable controlled release system for consistent, localized delivery is urgently needed.

Currently, there are many different types of vehicles for the controlled release of growth factors such as hydrogels, micro- and nanoparticles, and affinity-based delivery systems.[35,39] However, these systems suffer from different shortcomings including large initial burst release, low protein-loading efficiency, reduced bioactivity of cargo proteins due to the use of organic solvents, and high cost. Traditional hydrogels keep the protein within the aqueous phase where hydrolysis can rapidly degrade them. Unfortunately, these gels are characterized by a burst release of protein due to the swelling nature of hydrogels after implantation and incomplete loading of growth factor within the hydrogel matrix.[40,41] Thus, they are usually modified to better facilitate protein delivery. Micro- and nanoparticles are another commonly used vehicle; methods that fabricate micro- or nanoparticles require the use of organic solvents, which can denature the protein. The release of proteins from micro/nanoparticle-based systems follow first-order release kinetics, which is difficult to alter for various applications.[40,42] Thus, for efficient protein delivery, a vehicle that generates a high affinity between the vehicle and the delivered protein is warranted to increase the biological effect of growth factors.

In this study, we used a complex coacervate that composed of heparin and a polycation PEAD as the delivery vehicle. Heparin, the most negatively charged natural polymer in the body, can bind to more than 400 proteins and peptides such as extracellular matrix (ECM) proteins as well as growth factors and cytokines that are very important biologically. Contains basic amino acid residues such as lysine and arginine in the heparin-binding domain of many such proteins are vital to the intermolecular interactions and downstream signaling.[43] In our coacervate, electrostatic interactions in the complex immobilize heparin noncovalently, which can guarantee that its natural bioactivity will be preserved. Preservation of this bioactivity has been shown previously.[44] The polycation PEAD is designed specifically for protein delivery. Heparin facilitates the interaction between FGF1 and its receptor, and the coacervate phase separation isolates the protein from its aqueous environment, preventing its rapid degradation through hydrolysis or proteolysis.[25,44] It is a biodegradable polyester that exhibits minimal cytotoxicity regardless of its cationic charge.[25] With regard to cardiac repair, Shh delivery with our coacervate is both cardioprotective and capable of stimulating healthy vascularization and heart function in rodents post-MI. Additionally, FGF-2 coacervate was capable of stimulating vascular stromal cell recruitment and long-term angiogenesis in the infarct's border zone post-MI.[27] FGF2 coacervate could also reduce peri-infarct inflammation and fibrosis, most likely by replenishing a functional vasculature.

In our present study, we investigated whether FGF1 coacervate had potential cardioprotective effects. FGF1 was chosen due to its heparin-dependent bioactivity changes. Previous studies show that FGF1 activity is greatly increased when able to form a stable complex with heparin, which facilitates its interactions with receptors.[24]

There was an almost evenly homogeneous incorporation and distribution of FGF1 within coacervate droplets. Our delivery system not only had high loading efficiency for FGF1 (greater than 90%) but also exhibited low initial releases of approximately $15.1\% \pm 2.5\%$ during the first 24 h with a relatively linear trend of FGF1 release for the following 28 days (approximately linear at 10 ng day^{-1}). The in vitro assays indicated that FGF1 coacervate greatly improved the proliferation of HUVECs and hCSCs compared with free FGF1. The increase in cell proliferation in the presence of FGF1 is consistent with other studies,[45,46] and our results indicate a further increase in FGF1 activity when used in the coacervate. In addition to the proliferation assay, we performed transwell assays to evaluate the chemotaxis of HUVEC and hCSC induced by the FGF1 coacervate. We found that FGF1 coacervate had greater chemotactic effects compared to the free FGF1 group in both HUVEC and hCSC. These results are evidence that FGF1 released from the coacervate is highly bioactive and capable of stimulating both proliferation and migration of HUVECs and hCSCs in vitro.

In our animal study, we used a mouse MI model and demonstrated that the FGF1 coacervate system stimulated angiogenesis through the robust formation of mature and functional blood vessels in the infarct region. The number of CD31 and α-SMA positive vessels increased significantly, which indicated the formation of new stable and mature vasculature. Additionally, CD31+/Ki67+ staining showed that endothelial cells continued to proliferate in the FGF1 coacervate group at 6 weeks post-MI. Conversely, we observed a large increase in the proliferative capacity of cardiac precursor cells in the FGF1 coacervate group, consistent with our in vitro findings using HUVECs and hCSCs. We also saw reduced myocardial fibrosis, which helps to mitigate the loss in contractile function observed in the control groups.[47] Moreover, cardiomyocyte survival as a means of preserving contractile function, was greatly improved using our FGF1 coacervate delivery platform. In addition, FGF1 is capable of activating cardioprotective signaling pathways in cardiomyocytes.[48] Maintaining viable cardiac muscle is vital to better improve cardiac function post-MI, which has been shown in studies that attempt to stimulate the proliferation of cardiomyocytes, inhibit apoptosis, and stimulate the recruitment of cardiac progenitor cells to the heart.[49-52] Moreover, out study demonstrated that FGF1 coacervate was capable of reducing macrophage infiltration in the infarcted region 2 weeks after MI. This reduction could be linked to indirect FGF1 inhibition of pro-inflammatory cytokines. Another possibility is that the improved angiogenesis and better preservedcardiac muscle we observed could reduce tissue damage, which would in turn be able to reduce inflammation. Previous studies suggest similar trends using FGF1 in other applications, ultimately showing reduced presence of CD68+ and inflammatory M1 macrophages.[53] Thus, these benefits are manifested on a functional level through the improvements in cardiac contractility seen 6 weeks post-MI.

Overall, FGF1 coacervate exhibited higher therapeutic potential when compared with the saline and free FGF1 groups. Large preclinical animal models could help to validate this therapeutic approach and eventually pave the way for implementation of this controlled delivery approach in ischemic heart disease patients. Additional studies to optimize FGF1 dosing is necessary to maximize the efficacy of this therapy. In addition, future investigated is warranted to better delineate FGF1 coacervate could serve as a treatment of other ischemic conditions such as myocardial reperfusion injuries and peripheral artery disease. However, delivering a single growth factor still demonstrates limited therapeutic effect. In our delivery system, heparin had a high affinity to a wide range of proteins, so it is possible that multiple proteins could be delivered using the coacervate generating a synergistic effect for stronger MI therapy.

5. Conclusion

Taken together, our present findings demonstrated that controlled release of FGF1 with the coacervate triggered both formation and mature stabilization of neovasculature, and it could therefore better imrpove cardiac function post-MI in a mouse model. The improvement of cardiac function was observed at 2 weeks and reached a higher level at 6 weeks post-MI. This delivery system significantly improved myocardial function throughout the heart during post-MI remodeling by promoting angiogenesis, increased the formation of mature vasculature, promoting cardiomyocyte survival, inducing cardiac precursor cell proliferation, and decreasing collagen deposition and inflammation in the infarct zone. Large animal models could be used as a next step to validate the viability of the coacervate as a therapeutic approach in ischemic heart disease patients.

Supporting information

The supporting information is available on the ACS Publications website at DOI: 10.1021/acsbiomaterials.6b00509.

References

[1] Go AS, Mozaffarian D, Roger VL, et al. Executive Summary: Heart Disease and Stroke Statistics-2014 Update A Report From the American Heart Association[J]. Circulation, 2014, 129(3): 399-410.

[2] Orrego CM, Torre-Amione G. Is Myocardial Ischemia the Cause of the Progressive Decrease in Ejection Fraction during Acute Decompensated Heart Failure ?[J]. Journal Of Cardiac Failure, 2009, 15(6): S27-S27.

[3] Formiga FR, Tamayo E, Simon-Yarza T, et al. Angiogenic therapy for cardiac repair based on protein delivery systems[J]. Heart Failure Reviews, 2012, 17(3): 449-473.

[4] Tang Y, Hasan F, Giordano FJ, et al. Effects of recombinant human erythropoietin on platelet activation in acute myocardial infarction: Results of a double-blind, placebo-controlled, randomized trial[J]. American Heart Journal, 2009, 158(6): 941-947.

[5] Meier P, Gloekler S, de Marchi SF, et al. Myocardial Salvage Through Coronary Collateral Growth by Granulocyte Colony-Stimulating Factor in Chronic Coronary Artery Disease A Controlled Randomized Trial[J]. Circulation, 2009, 120(14): 1355-1363.

[6] Voors AA, Belonje AMS, Zijlstra F, et al. A single dose of erythropoietin in ST-elevation myocardial infarction[J]. European Heart Journal, 2010, 31(21): 2593-2600.

[7] Henry TD, Annex BH, McKendall GR, et al. Vascular endothelial growth factor in ischemia for vascular angiogenesis[J]. Circulation, 2003, 107(10): 1359-1365.

[8] Simons M, Annex BH, Laham RJ, et al. Pharmacological treatment of coronary artery disease with recombinant fibroblast growth fac-

tor-2-Double-blind, randomized, controlled clinical trial[J]. Circulation, 2002, 105(7): 788-793.

[9] Chu H, Johnson NR, Mason NS, et al. A polycation:heparin complex releases growth factors with enhanced bioactivity[J]. Journal Of Controlled Release, 2011, 150(2): 157-163.

[10] Johnson NR, Wang Y. Controlled delivery of heparin-binding EGF-like growth factor yields fast and comprehensive wound healing[J]. Journal Of Controlled Release, 2013, 166(2): 124-129.

[11] Lee K, Johnson NR, Gao J, et al. Human progenitor cell recruitment via SDF-1 alpha coacervate-laden PGS vascular grafts[J]. Biomaterials, 2013, 34(38): 9877-9885.

[12] Chen WCW, Lee BG, Park DW, et al. Controlled dual delivery of fibroblast growth factor-2 and Interleukin-10 by heparin-based coacervate synergistically enhances ischemic heart repair[J]. Biomaterials, 2015, 72: 138-151.

[13] Johnson NR, Kruger M, Goetsch KP, et al. Coacervate Delivery of Growth Factors Combined with a Degradable Hydrogel Preserves Heart Function after Myocardial Infarction[J]. Acs Biomaterials Science & Engineering, 2015, 1(9): 753-759.

[14] Johnson NR, Wang Y. Controlled Delivery of Sonic Hedgehog Morphogen and Its Potential for Cardiac Repair[J]. Plos One, 2013, 8(5).

[15] Awada HK, Johnson NR, Wang Y. Sequential delivery of angiogenic growth factors improves revascularization and heart function after myocardial infarction[J]. Journal Of Controlled Release, 2015, 207: 7-17.

[16] Battegay EJ. Angiogenesis: mechanistic insights, neovascular diseases, and therapeutic prospects[J]. Journal Of Molecular Medicine-Jmm, 1995, 73(7): 333-346.

[17] Ma B, Cheng D, Xia Z, et al. Randomized, multicenter, double-blind, and placebo-controlled trial using topical recombinant human acidic fibroblast growth factor for deep partial-thickness burns and skin graft donor site[J]. Wound Repair And Regeneration, 2007, 15(6): 795-799.

[18] Cuevas P, Reimers D, Carceller F, et al. Fibroblast growth factor-1 prevents myocardial apoptosis triggered by ischemia reperfusion injury[J]. Eur J Med Res, 1997, 2(11): 465-468.

[19] Htun P, Ito WD, Hoefer IE, et al. Intramyocardial infusion of FGF-1 mimics ischemic preconditioning in pig myocardium[J]. J Mol Cell Cardiol, 1998, 30(4): 867-877.

[20] Buehler A, Martire A, Strohm C, et al. Angiogenesis-independent cardioprotection in FGF-1 transgenic mice[J]. Cardiovasc Res, 2002, 55(4): 768-777.

[21] Fernandez B, Buehler A, Wolfram S, et al. Transgenic myocardial overexpression of fibroblast growth factor-1 increases coronary artery density and branching[J]. Circ Res, 2000, 87(3): 207-213.

[22] Palmen M, Daemen MJ, Bronsaer R, et al. Cardiac remodeling after myocardial infarction is impaired in IGF-1 deficient mice[J]. Cardiovasc Res, 2001, 50(3): 516-524.

[23] Silva AC, Rodrigues SC, Caldeira J, et al. Three-dimensional scaffolds of fetal decellularized hearts exhibit enhanced potential to support cardiac cells in comparison to the adult[J]. Biomaterials, 2016, 104: 52-64.

[24] Robinson CJ, Harmer NJ, Blundell TL, et al. Studying the role of heparin in the formation of FGF1-FGFR2 complexes using gel chromatography[J]. International Journal Of Experimental Pathology, 2004, 85(4): A72-A72.

[25] Chu H, Gao J, Wang Y. Design, synthesis, and biocompatibility of an arginine-based polyester[J]. Biotechnol Prog, 2012, 28(1): 257-264.

[26] Engel FB, Schebesta M, Duong MT, et al. p38 MAP kinase inhibition enables proliferation of adult mammalian cardiomyocytes[J]. Genes Dev, 2005, 19(10): 1175-1187.

[27] Chu H, Chen CW, Huard J, et al. The effect of a heparin-based coacervate of fibroblast growth factor-2 on scarring in the infarcted myocardium[J]. Biomaterials, 2013, 34(6): 1747-1756.

[28] Chen CW, Okada M, Proto JD, et al. Human pericytes for ischemic heart repair[J]. Stem Cells, 2013, 31(2): 305-316.

[29] Domanski MJ, Colleran JA, Cunnion RE, et al. Correlation of Echocardiographic Fractional Area Change with Radionuclide Left Ventricular Ejection Fraction[J]. Echocardiography-a Journal Of Cardiovascular Ultrasound And Allied Techniques, 1995, 12(3): 221-227.

[30] Okada M, Payne TR, Zheng B, et al. Myogenic endothelial cells purified from human skeletal muscle improve cardiac function after transplantation into infarcted myocardium[J]. J Am Coll Cardiol, 2008, 52(23): 1869-1880.

[31] Levick SP, Melendez GC, Plante E, et al. Cardiac mast cells: the centrepiece in adverse myocardial remodelling[J]. Cardiovasc Res, 2011, 89(1): 12-19.

[32] Nagai T, Komuro I. Gene and cytokine therapy for heart failure: molecular mechanisms in the improvement of cardiac function[J]. Am J Physiol Heart Circ Physiol, 2012, 303(5): H501-512.

[33] Hastings CL, Roche ET, Ruiz-Hernandez E, et al. Drug and cell delivery for cardiac regeneration[J]. Adv Drug Deliv Rev, 2015, 84: 85-106.

[34] Segers VF, Lee RT. Protein therapeutics for cardiac regeneration after myocardial infarction[J]. J Cardiovasc Transl Res, 2010, 3(5): 469-477.

[35] Chu H, Wang Y. Therapeutic angiogenesis: controlled delivery of angiogenic factors[J]. Ther Deliv, 2012, 3(6): 693-714.

[36] Srinivas G, Anversa P, Frishman WH. Cytokines and myocardial regeneration: a novel treatment option for acute myocardial infarction[J]. Cardiol Rev, 2009, 17(1): 1-9.

[37] Pascual-Gil S, Garbayo E, Diaz-Herraez P, et al. Heart regeneration after myocardial infarction using synthetic biomaterials[J]. J Control Release, 2015, 203: 23-38.

[38] Henry TD, Rocha-Singh K, Isner JM, et al. Intracoronary administration of recombinant human vascular endothelial growth factor to patients with coronary artery disease[J]. Am Heart J, 2001, 142(5): 872-880.

[39] Mohtaram NK, Montgomery A, Willerth SM. Biomaterial-based drug delivery systems for the controlled release of neurotrophic factors[J]. Biomed Mater, 2013, 8(2): 022001.

[40] Johnson NR, Wang Y. Drug delivery systems for wound healing[J]. Curr Pharm Biotechnol, 2015, 16(7): 621-629.

[41] Huang X, Brazel CS. On the importance and mechanisms of burst release in matrix-controlled drug delivery systems[J]. J Control Release, 2001, 73(2-3): 121-136.

[42] Soppimath KS, Aminabhavi TM, Kulkarni AR, et al. Biodegradable polymeric nanoparticles as drug delivery devices[J]. J Control Release, 2001, 70(1-2): 1-20.

[43] Ori A, Wilkinson MC, Fernig DG. A systems biology approach for the investigation of the heparin/heparan sulfate interactome[J]. J Biol Chem, 2011, 286(22): 19892-19904.

[44] Chu H, Gao J, Chen CW, et al. Injectable fibroblast growth factor-2 coacervate for persistent angiogenesis[J]. Proc Natl Acad Sci U S A, 2011, 108(33): 13444-13449.

[45] Reboucas JS, Santos-Magalhaes NS, Formiga FR. Cardiac Regeneration using Growth Factors: Advances and Challenges[J]. Arq Bras Cardiol, 2016, 107(3): 271-275.

[46] Yang GW, Jiang JS, Lu WQ. Ferulic Acid Exerts Anti-Angiogenic and Anti-Tumor Activity by Targeting Fibroblast Growth Factor Receptor 1-Mediated Angiogenesis[J]. Int J Mol Sci, 2015, 16(10): 24011-24031.

[47] Segura AM, Frazier OH, Buja LM. Fibrosis and heart failure[J]. Heart Fail Rev, 2014, 19(2): 173-185.

[48] Hsieh PC, Davis ME, Gannon J, et al. Controlled delivery of PDGF-BB for myocardial protection using injectable self-assembling peptide nanofibers[J]. J Clin Invest, 2006, 116(1): 237-248.

[49] Wang Z, Wang Y, Ye J, et al. bFGF attenuates endoplasmic reticulum stress and mitochondrial injury on myocardial ischaemia/reperfusion via activation of PI3K/Akt/ERK1/2 pathway[J]. J Cell Mol Med, 2015, 19(3): 595-607.

[50] Wang ZG, Wang Y, Huang Y, et al. bFGF regulates autophagy and ubiquitinated protein accumulation induced by myocardial ischemia/reperfusion via the activation of the PI3K/Akt/mTOR pathway[J]. Sci Rep, 2015, 5: 9287.

[51] Roberts WC, Burks KH, Ko JM, et al. Commonalities of cardiac rupture (left ventricular free wall or ventricular septum or papillary muscle) during acute myocardial infarction secondary to atherosclerotic coronary artery disease[J]. Am J Cardiol, 2015, 115(1): 125-140.

[52] Wang M, Zhang G, Wang Y, et al. Crosstalk of mesenchymal stem cells and macrophages promotes cardiac muscle repair[J]. Int J Biochem Cell Biol, 2015, 58: 53-61.

[53] Liu W, Struik D, Nies VJ, et al. Effective treatment of steatosis and steatohepatitis by fibroblast growth factor 1 in mouse models of nonalcoholic fatty liver disease[J]. Proc Natl Acad Sci U S A, 2016, 113(8): 2288-2293.

Basic fibroblast growth factor promotes melanocyte migration *via* activating PI3K/Akt-Rac1-FAK-JNK and ERK signaling pathways

Hongxue Shi, Xiaokun Li, Jian Xiao

1. Introduction

Vitiligo is an autoimmune disease characterized by the loss of pigment-producing melanocytes in the skin epidermis, leading to disfiguring white spots on the skin of affected individuals [1]. The prevalence of the disease ranges from less than 0.1% to greater than 8% worldwide [2] and is around 1% in the United States [3] and 0.56% in China [4]. The estimated direct health-care cost burden of vitiligo in the United States is $175 million each year, a cost that is particularly high due to the limited efficacy of available treatments [5]. Vitiligo also exerts devastating psychological effects. Vitiligo that occurs in exposed areas, such as the face and hands, has a major impact on self-esteem and perception of self, leading to depression, anxiety, feelings of discrimination, and even suicidal thoughts [2].

The factors that cause damage to melanocytes and con-tribute to their subsequent disappearance in vitiligo remain unknown. Autoimmune, neurohumoral, and autocytotoxic mechanisms, in addition to altered cellular environment, and impaired melanocyte migration and/or proliferation have been suggested to be implicated in the pathogenesis of vitiligo [6,7]. Recovery from vitiligo is initiated by the activation and proliferation of immature pigment cells, which then migrate either upward to the nearby epidermis to form perifollicular pigmentation islands or downward to the hair matrices to produce melanin. Normal melanocyte also migrates from the adjacent normal skin to the affected site [8,9].

Basic fibroblast growth factor (bFGF) is a member of the fibroblast growth factor (FGF) family, which is composed of 18 FGFs and 4 FGF receptors [10,11]. Our previous studies showed that bFGF promotes wound healing [12], reduces scar formation during wound healing process [13,14], and improves functional deficits in a spinal cord injury model [15,16] as a potent mitogen that stimulates the migration, proliferation, and differentiation of cells of mesenchymal and neuro-ectodermal origin [17,18]. Fibroblasts treated with bFGF showed increased activity of PI3K/Akt, Rho family proteins, and JNKs associated with cytoskeletal reorganization, leading to induction of fibroblast migration [17,19]. Moreover, bFGF stimulated melanocyte proliferation [20,21] and facilitated melanocyte migration [9].

Clinical studies have shown that levels of bFGF and stem cell factor are significantly lower in vitiligo skin than in control skin, whereas levels of tumor necrosis factor-alpha and inter-leukin 6 are much higher [22,23]; in contrast, an additional study showed that bFGF levels are increased in serum and blister fluid from patients with vitiligo [24], suggesting that this change in bFGF levels is correlated with vitiligo pathogenesis. Narrow-band ultraviolet (UVB), an effective therapy for vitiligo, increases bFGF release from keratinocyte, favoring melanocyte growth and enhancing melanocyte migration [25,26]. Based on these studies, a bFGF-based treatment for vitiligo disease is a promising potential therapeutic strategy that warrants further study. In this study, we used transwell assay to investigate the effects of bFGF on melanocyte migration, as well as its biochemical mechanism.

2. Materials and methods

2.1 Reagents

The Active Rac1 Pull-Down and Detection Kit was purchased from ThermoFisher Scientific (ThermoFisher, Shanghai, China). Fetal bovine serum (FBS), penicillin, and streptomycin were purchased from Life Technologies

(Shanghai, China). siRNA, second antibodies, and primary antibody p-Akt (Ser473), p-ERK (Thr202/Tyr204), Akt, ERK, and GAPDH were purchased from Santa Cruz Biotech (Santa Cruz, Shanghai, China), p-JNK (Thr183/Tyr185), p-FAK (Tyr397), JNK, and FAK were purchased from Cell Signaling Technology (Shanghai, China). Other reagents were purchased from Sigma-Aldrich (Shanghai, China).

2.2　Cell culture

Normal human epidermal melanocytes were purchased from Sciencell Research Laboratories (Carlsbad, CA). Melanocytes were cultured in special melanocyte medium (MelM), supplemented with a low percentage of FBS (0.5%), 100 U/ml penicillin, and 100 μg/ml streptomycin. The cells were grown in a humidified chamber containing 5% CO_2 at 37℃.

2.3　MTT assay

Melanocytes were seeded on 96-well plates (5×10^3 cells/well) and treated with different concentrations of bFGF (0, 5, 25, and 100 ng/ml) for 24 h after an overnight starvation. Then 20 μl of 3-(4,5-dimethylthiazol-2-yl)-2,5-diphenyltetrazolium bromide (MTT) (5 mg/ml in PBS) was added to each well and incubated for 4 h. Wells were washed with PBS (pH 7.4), after which dimethyl sulfoxide (DMSO) was added to each well to solubilize the formed formazan crystals. The absorbance was measured at 490 nm for each well on a Microplate Reader (Molecular Device, Beijing, China).

2.4　Transwell migration assay

The bottom chambers of the transwell were filled with 600 μl MelM supplemented with different concentrations of bFGF (0, 5, 25, and 100 ng/ml) and different selective inhibitors, while the top chambers were seeded with 5×10^4 inactivated cells per well in 100 μl MelM. After 24 h, the cells on the top surface of the membrane (nonmigrated cells) were scraped with a cotton swab and the cells spreading on the bottom side of the membrane (migrated cells) were fixed with cold 4% paraformaldehyde for 10 min. Migrated cells were stained with 0.1% hexamethylpararosaniline and imaged using a Nikon microscope after. Migrated cells were quantified by counting manually. All images shown were taken at high power (×100) magnification.

2.5　Rac1 pull-down assay

Rac1-GTP assays were performed using the Active Rac1 Pull-Down and Detection Kit according to the manufacturer's instruction. Briefly, the cells were scraped into 1× lysis buffer containing 25 mM Tris-HCl, pH 7.2, 5 mM $MgCl_2$, 1% NP-40, 5% glycerol, 150 mM NaCl, and a 1% protease inhibitor cock-tail and centrifuged for 15 min at 16 000 g at 4℃. The cleared cell lysates (which totaled 700 μl) were split into 20 μg aliquots. As negative and positive controls for the pull-down, two of the aliquots were added to 5 μl of 100 mM GDP or 10 mM GTPγS, respectively, and incubated for 1 h at 4℃ with gentle rocking. The beads were washed three times with lysis buffer and heated for 5 min at 100℃ in reducing SDS-PAGE sample buffer and then analyzed for active Rac1 by Western blotting with a monoclonal antibody (1:1 000 dilution) for Rac1. Total Rac1 levels were also determined for comparison with activated Rac1.

2.6　Western blot

Protein samples were collected, denatured, separated on 10% polyacrylamide gels, and transferred to a polyvinylidene difluoride membrane. The membranes were blocked in TBST containing 5% nonfat milk and 0.05% Tween-20 for 1 h at room temperature and blotted with primary antibodies (1:1 000 dilution) overnight at 4℃. The next day, membranes were washed with TBST, incubated for 1 h with secondary antibody (1:3 000 dilution), and washed once more with TBST. The labeled proteins were then detected using ECL substrate, and results were analyzed using Image J software (NIH).

2.7　Fluorescent labeling

The cells were plated in six-well tissue culture dishes in MelM for 24 h. After overnight starvation, cells were wounded with a linear scratch from a sterile pipette tip. Cells were washed with PBS to remove floating cells and cellular debris, then treated with 100 ng/ml bFGF for 24 h; control group were untreated. The cells were fixed with 4% paraformaldehyde in PBS for 20 min and permeabilized with 0.3% Triton X-100 in PBS for 15 min. Cells were then incubated with 5% bovine serum albumin (BSA) in PBS for 1 h at room temperature to block nonspecific antibody binding.

Cells were incubated with fluorescein isothiocyanate labeled phalloidin staining solution in PBS containing 1% BSA for 35 min and washed with PBS 3 times, for 5 min each wash. The nuclei were stained with 4,6-diamidino-2-phenylindole (DAPI) (1:1 000 dilution) for 10 min and washed with PBS at room temperature. Fluorescence images were taken using a Nikon fluorescence microscope. The images are shown at high power (× 400) magnification. Experiments were repeated three times.

2.8 Statistical analysis

Data are expressed as mean ± SEM. Statistical significance of differences between two experimental groups were determined using Student's t-test. To determine statistical difference of differences between more than two groups, data were evaluated using one-way ANOVA test, followed by Dunnett's *post hoc* test with a value of $P < 0.05$ considered significant.

3. Results

3.1 Effect of bFGF on melanocyte migration

bFGF is a keratinocyte-derived mitogen for melanocyte and promotes melanocytes migration [9,21,27]. We first investigated the effects of bFGF treatment on melanocyte proliferation using MTT assays. Incubation with different concentrations of bFGF (5, 25, and 100 ng/ml) for 24 h had negligible effects on melanocyte proliferation (Fig. 1A). We then examined the effects of bFGF on the melanocyte migration using transwell assay. As shown in Fig. 1B,C, incubation with bFGF for 24 h promoted melanocyte migration in a dose-dependent manner, compared to control group. This ef-

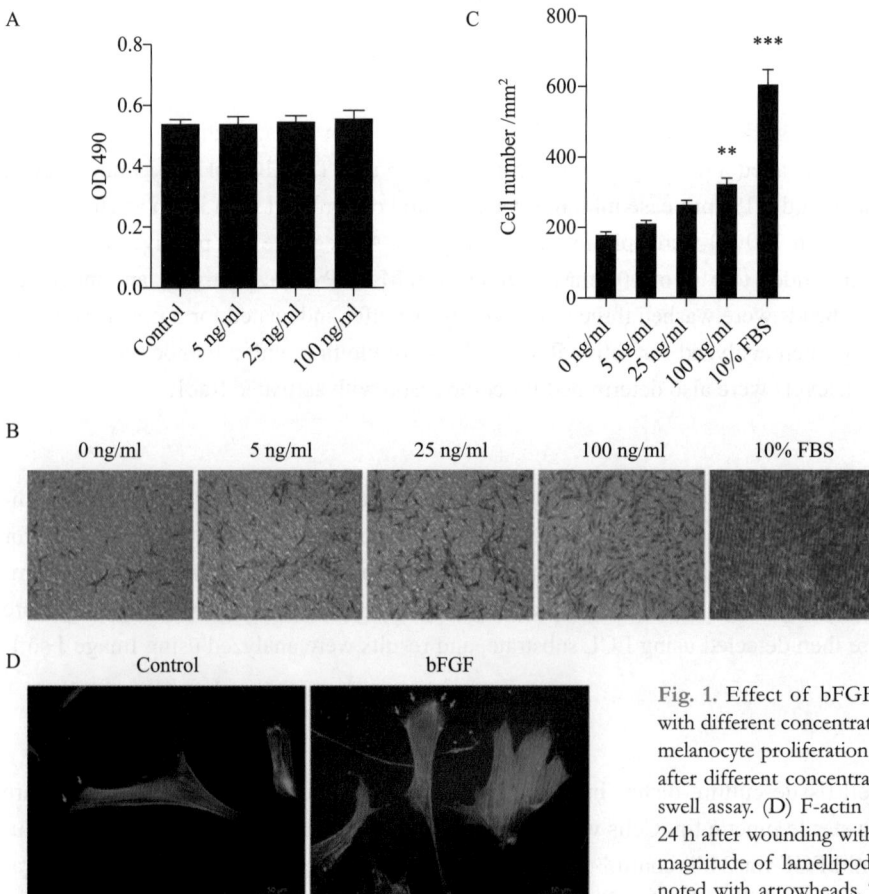

Fig. 1. Effect of bFGF on melanocyte migration. (A) Treatment with different concentrations of bFGF for 24 h showed no effect on melanocyte proliferation by MTT assay. (B, C) Melanocyte migration after different concentrations of bFGF treated within 24 h by transwell assay. (D) F-actin was labeled by FITC-conjugated phalloidin 24 h after wounding with or without bFGF treatment. The increased magnitude of lamellipodia formation in the migration cells were denoted with arrowheads. The experiments were repeated three times. Bar = 50 μm. Data were presented as mean ± SEM ($n = 3$). **$P < 0.01$ and ***$P < 0.001$ compared with control group.

fect was most obvious in melanocyte treated with 100 ng/ml of bFGF. Therefore, a dose of 100 ng/ml bFGF was used in subsequent experiments in this study.

Remodeling of the actin cytoskeleton is mediated by various actin-binding proteins and is necessary for migration of multiple cell types, including melanocytes [28,29]. We assessed the effects of bFGF on remodeling of the actin cytoskeleton by labeling the cells with rhodamine-conjugated phalloidin. As shown in Fig. 1D, activation of melanocytes with bFGF led to augmentation of cell migration and an increased magnitude of lamellipodia formation in the migrating cells. These data indicate that bFGF enhanced melanocyte migration, but not melanocyte proliferation by regulating remodeling of the actin cytoskeleton.

3.2 PI3K/Akt was involved in bFGF-promoted melanocyte migration

A wealth of studies have demonstrated that phosphatidylinositol 3-kinase (PI3K) is associated with cell polarization and is involved in cell migration [30]. PI3K and its downstream kinase effector Akt are also known to regulate cytoskeletal rearrangement, cell migration, survival, and apoptosis [31]. We found that incubation with bFGF for 5, 15, and 30 min increased Akt phosphorylation, Akt phosphorylation peaked at 5 min and 15 min, and returned to basal levels at 60 min (Fig. 2A,B). To test whether Akt is necessary for bFGF-promoted melanocyte migration, a selective inhibitor for PI3K, LY294002, was applied. Melanocyte was pretreated with 10 μM LY294002 for 30 min, the bFGF-induced increase in Akt phosphorylation was notably inhibited after treatment for 15 min (Fig. 2C,D). Furthermore, bFGF-induced melano-

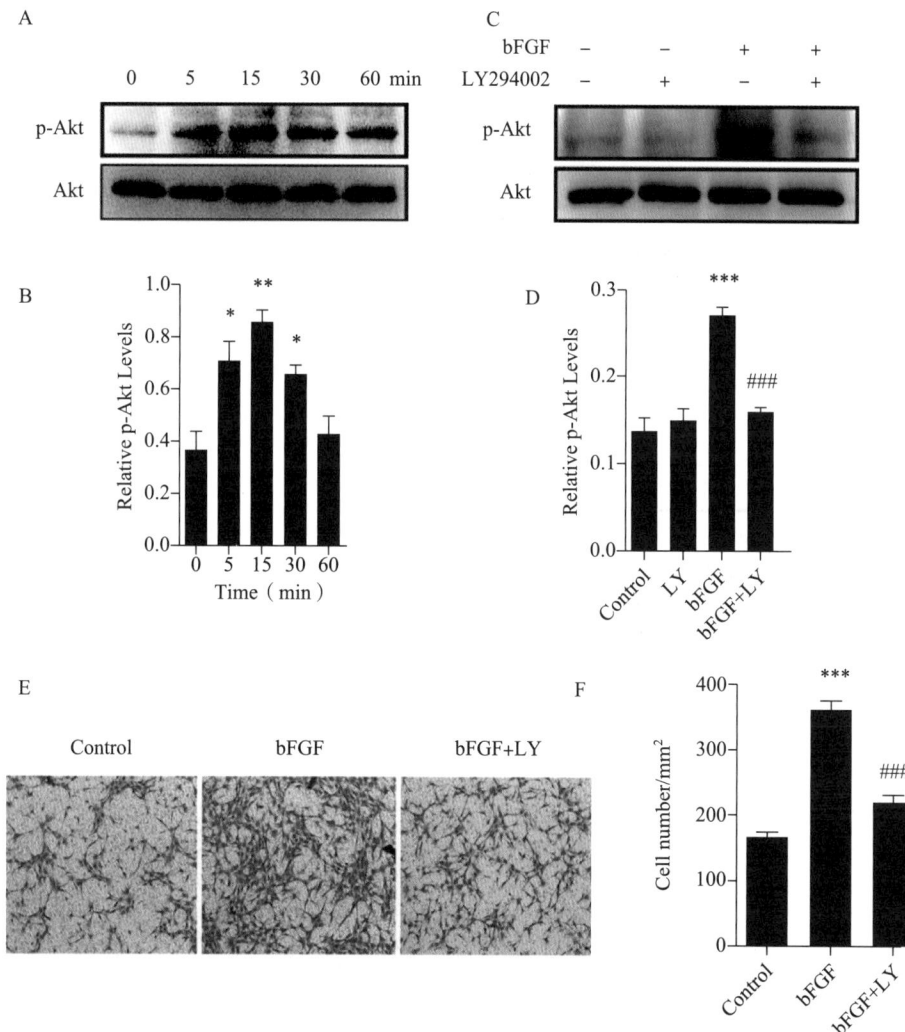

Fig. 2. PI3K/Akt was involved in bFGF-promoted melanocyte migration. (A, B) Induction of phosphorylation of Akt at indicated time after bFGF treated in melanocytes. (C, D) PI3K inhibitor LY294002 (10 μM) notably blocked Akt activity stimulated with bFGF at 15 min. (E, F) LY294002 significantly impeded bFGF-induced melanocytes migration by transwell assay. Data were presented as mean ± SEM ($n = 3$). $^*P < 0.05$, $^{**}P < 0.01$, and $^{***}P < 0.001$ compared with control group, $^{###}P < 0.001$ compared with bFGF group.

cyte migration remained significantly impaired after 24 h of incubation with LY294002 and bFGF (Fig. 2E,F).

3.3 Rac1 was implicated in bFGF-increased melanocyte migration

Activation of Rac1 induces the formation of lamellipodial protrusions *via* activation of the Wave complex. Lamellipodial protrusions provide the driving force for cell movements at the leading edge of migrating cells, thereby promoting cell migration [32]. We found that the level of active Rac1 was significantly increased at 15 and 30 min after bFGF treatment (Fig. 3A,B). Transfection of siRNA targeting Rac1 (siRac1) reduced Rac1 protein level (Fig. 3C) and was associated with suppression of melanocyte migration after bFGF treatment (Fig. 3D,E).

3.4 FAK was involved in bFGF-facilitated melanocyte migration

Focal adhesion kinase (FAK) plays important roles in cell adhesion, migration, and invasion by participating in signal transduction pathways initiated at sites of integrin-mediated cell adhesion to the extracellular matrix [33]. Treatment with bFGF increased the phosphorylation of FAK in a time-dependent manner. FAK phosphorylation peaked at 15 min and 30 min after bFGF administration and returned to basal levels at 60 min (Fig. 4A,B). Melanocytes pretreated with 10 μM FAK-selective inhibitor PF-562271 for 30 min, the bFGF dependent increase in FAK activity was completely eliminated (Fig. 4C,D). The bFGF-dependent increase in migration was blocked by PF-562271 (Fig. 4E,F).

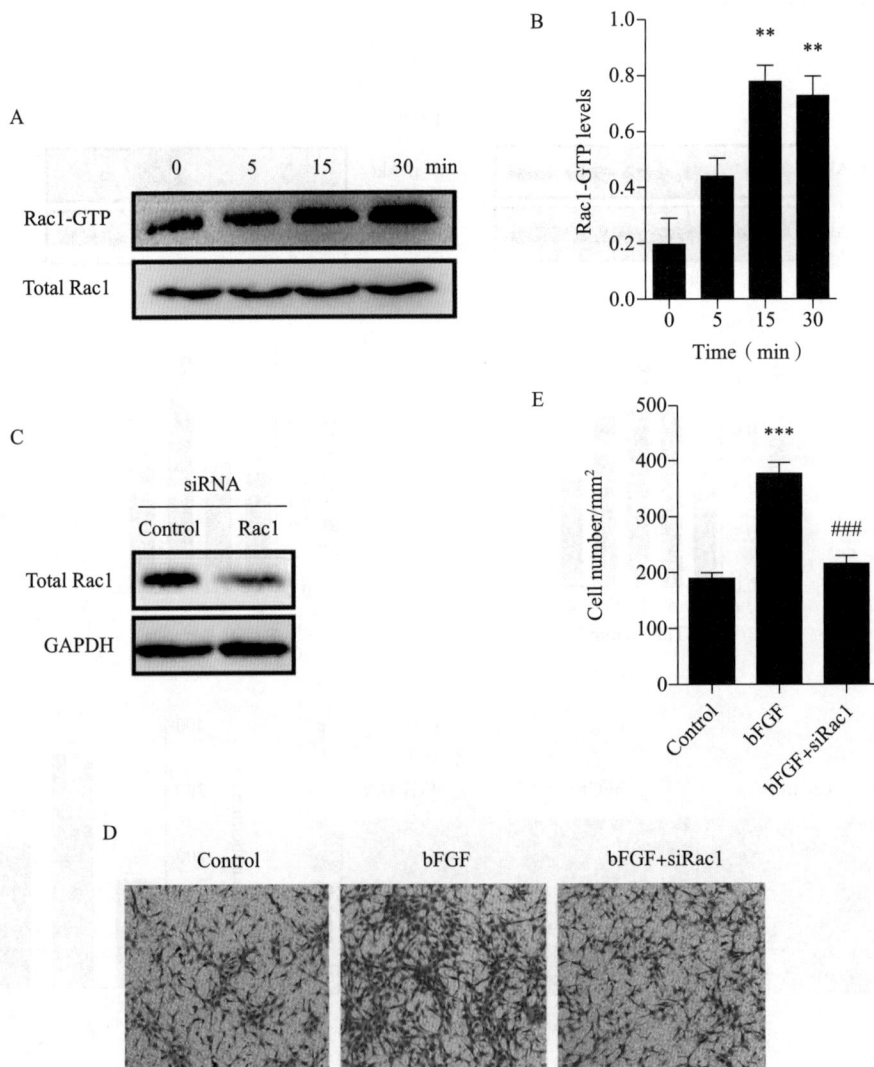

Fig. 3. Rac1 was implicated in bFGF-increased melanocyte migration. (A, B) Increased Rac1 activity at indicated time after bFGF treated in melanocytes. (C) siRNA Rac1 reduced total Rac1 protein level after 24 h. (D, E) siRNA Rac1 significantly prevented bFGF-induced melanocyte migration by transwell assay. Data were presented as mean ± SEM ($n = 3$). $^{**}P < 0.01$ and $^{***}P < 0.001$ compared with control group, $^{###}P < 0.001$ compared with bFGF group.

A

C

B

D

E

F

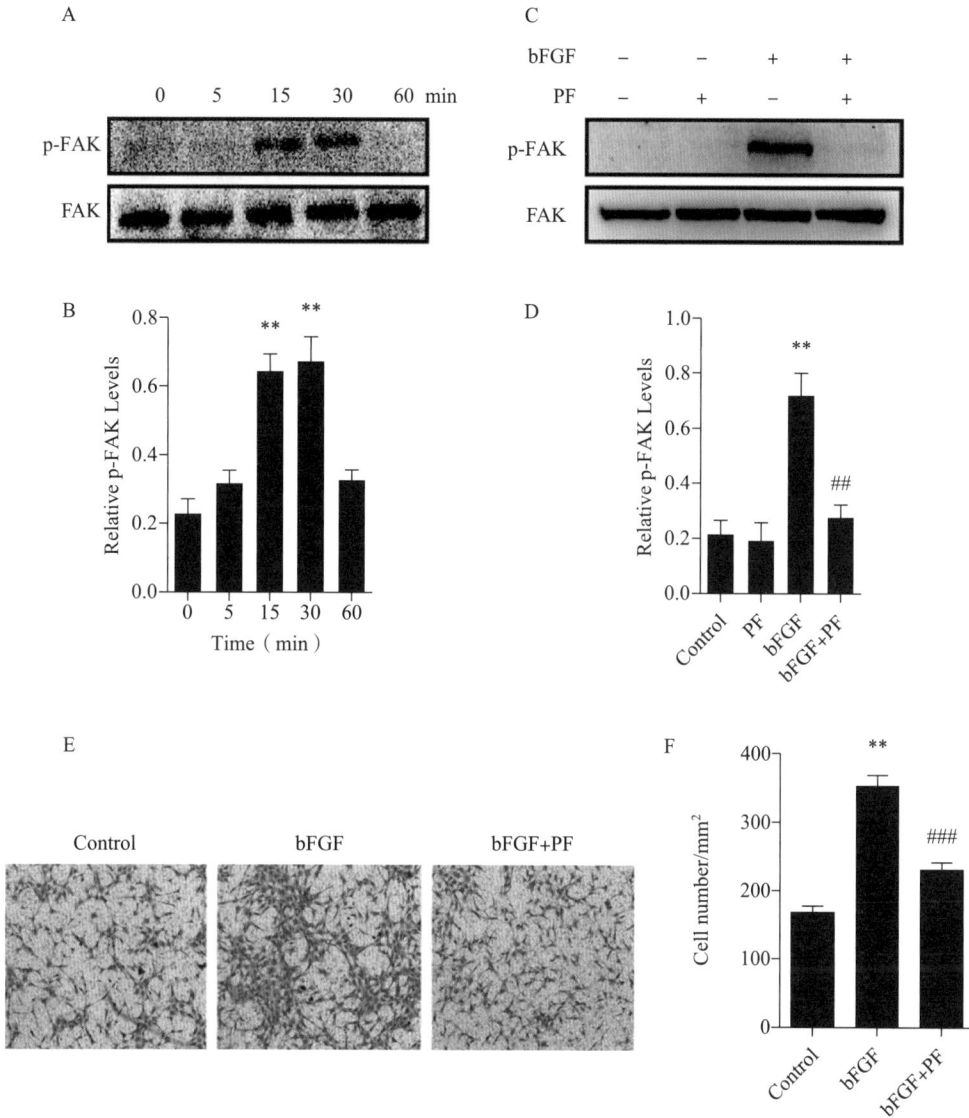

Fig. 4. FAK was involved in bFGF-facilitated melanocyte migration. (A, B) Induction of phosphorylation of FAK at indicated time after bFGF treated in melanocytes. (C, D) FAK inhibitor PF-562271 (10 μM) notably attenuated FAK activity stimulated with bFGF at 15 min. (E, F) PF-562271 significantly impaired bFGF-induced melanocytes migration by transwell assay. Data were presented as mean ± SEM ($n = 3$). ***$P < 0.01$ and ***$P < 0.001$ compared with control group, ##$P < 0.01$ and ###$P < 0.001$ compared with bFGF group.

3.5 bFGF-induced melanocyte migration in a JNK-dependent manner

Previous studies have demonstrated the importance of the c-Jun N-terminal kinase (JNK) pathway in the regulation of cell migration [34]. Based on these studies, we hypothesized that JNK is also involved in bFGF-induced melanocyte migration. As shown in Fig. 5A,B, phosphorylated JNK was upregulated at 5, 15, and 30 min after bFGF treatment. Levels of phosphorrylated JNK peaked at 5–30 min and returned to basal levels at 60 min. In melanocytes pretreated with 10 μM SP600125 for 30 min, bFGF-induced JNK activity was significantly reduced after treatment with bFGF for 15 min (Fig. 5C,D). Furthermore, bFGF-stimulated melanocyte migration was significantly reduced after incubation with SP600125 for 24 h (Fig. 5E,F).

3.6 ERK was involved in bFGF-promoted melanocyte migration

Extracellular signal-regulated protein kinase (ERK), one of the most characterized intracellular signaling pathways, plays a crucial role in regulating cell proliferation and migration in various cell types [35]. We found that treatment with bFGF for 5, 15, and 30 min significantly induced phosphorylation of ERK, ERK activity peaked at 5–30 min after bFGF treat-

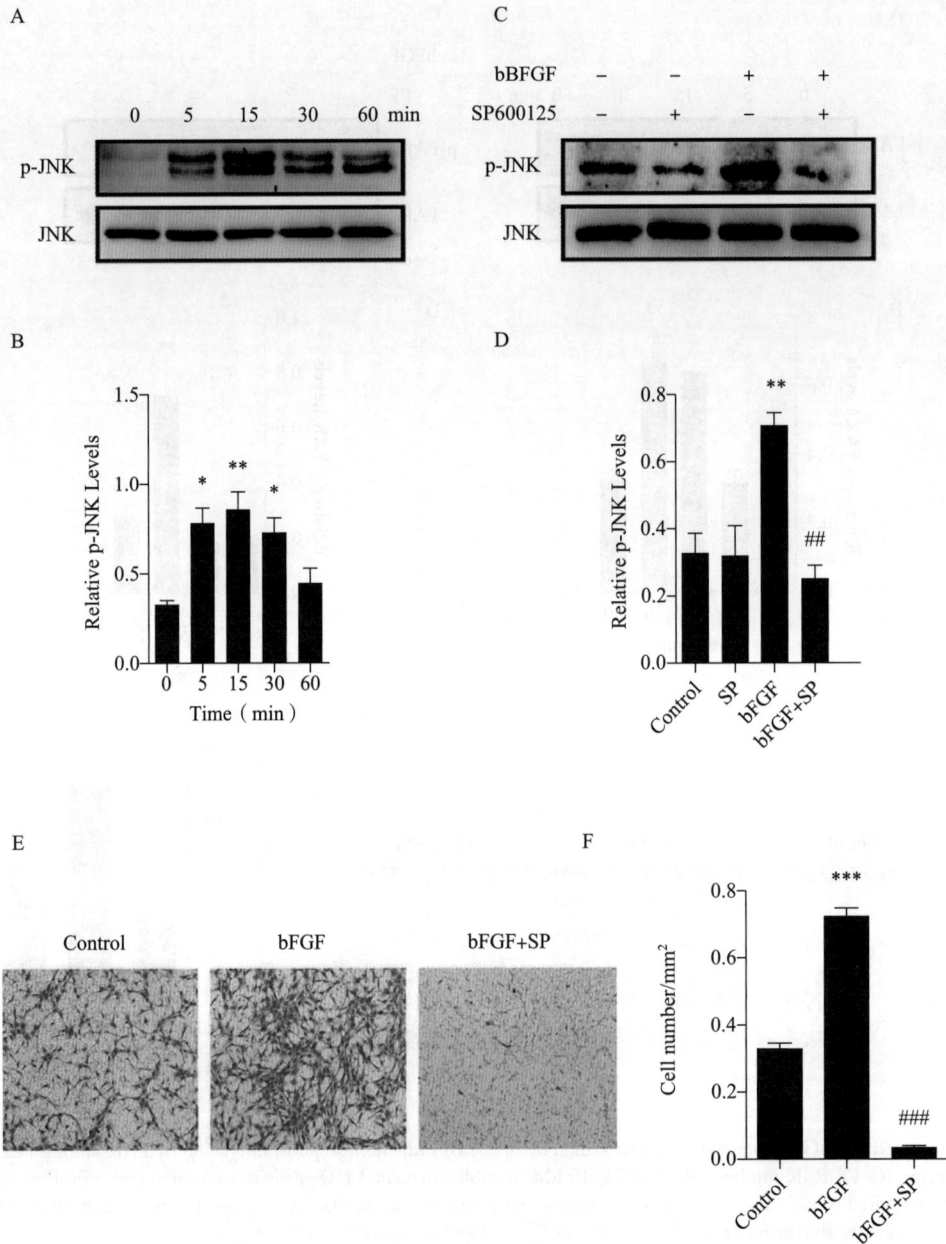

Fgi. 5. bFGF-induced melanocyte migration in JNK-dependent manner. (A, B) Induction of phosphorylation of JNK at indicated time after bFGF treated in melanocytes. (C, D) JNK inhibitor SP600125 (10 μM) notably inhibited JNK activity stimulated with bFGF at 15 min. (E, F) SP600125 significantly impaired bFGF-induced melanocyte migration by transwell assay. Data were presented as mean ± SEM (n = 3). $^*P < 0.05$, $^{**}P < 0.01$, and $^{***}P < 0.001$ compared with control group, $^{##}P< 0.01$ and $^{###}P< 0.001$ compared with bFGF group.

ment (Fig. 6A,B). In turn, melanocytes pretreated with 10 μM of U0126 for 30 min, bFGF-induced activity of ERK was significantly inhibited after 5 min of treatment with both bFGF and U0126 (Fig. 6C,D). Furthermore, bFGF-induced melanocyte migration was significantly hindered after 24 h treatment with U0126 (Fig. 6E,F).

3.7 PI3K/Akt contributed to bFGF-induced rac1 activation

Rac1 acts as a downstream effector of PI3K in several growth factor-stimulated pathways [17,19]. We measured the activation of Rac1 in melanocytes treated with LY294002 to determine whether PI3K/Akt is upstream of Rac1 in bFGF-promoted melanocyte migration. We found that in bFGF-treated melanocytes, activation of Rac1 was blocked by LY294002, but siRac1 did not block activation of Akt (Fig. 7A,B). In addition, the activation of FAK and JNK in bFGF-treated melanocytes was also blocked by LY294002 (Supporting Information Fig. 1A).

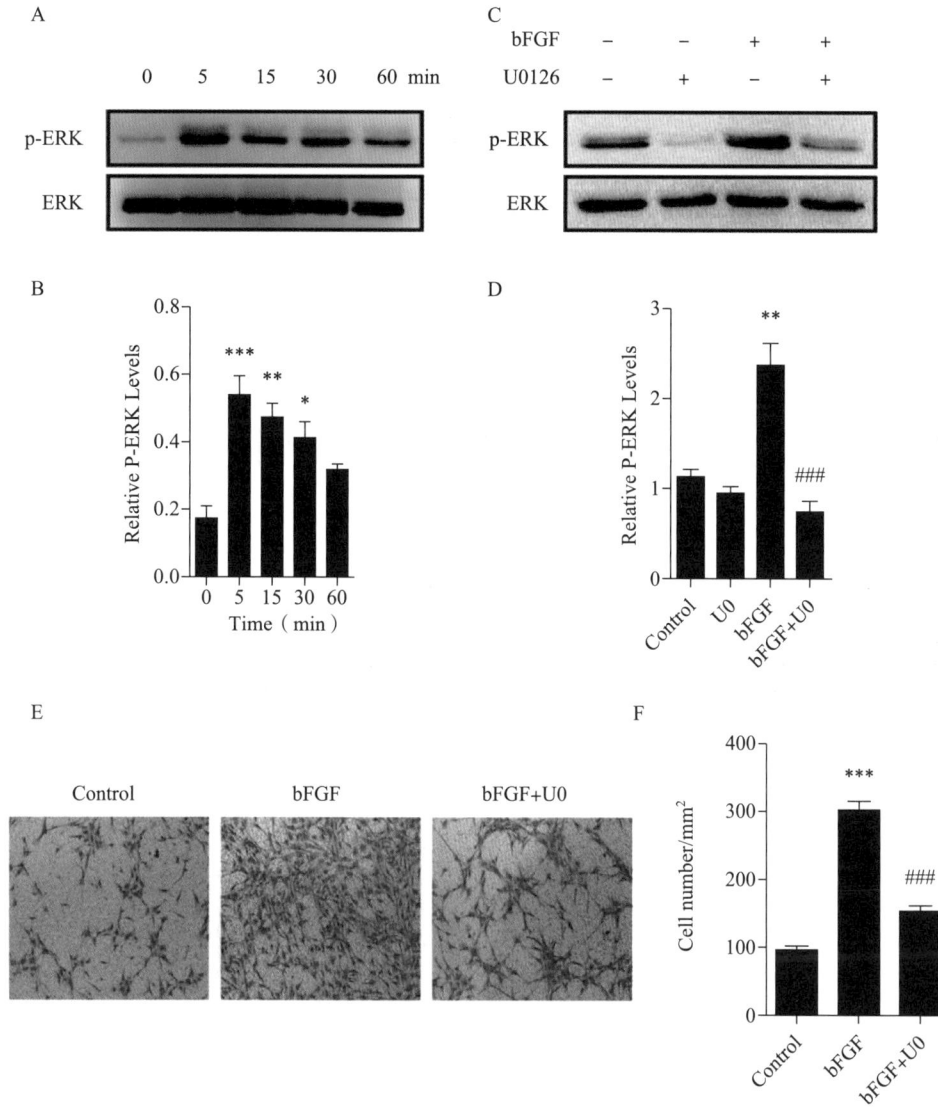

Fig. 6. ERK was involved in bFGF-promoted melanocyte migration. (A, B) Induction of phosphorylation of ERK at indicated time after bFGF treated in melanocytes. (C, D) ERK inhibitor U0126 (10 μM) notably inhibited ERK activity stimulated with bFGF at 5 min. (E, F) U0126 significantly blocked bFGF-induced melanocyte migration by transwell assay. Data were presented as mean ± SEM ($n = 3$). $^{*}P < 0.05$, $^{**}P < 0.01$, and $^{***}P < 0.001$ compared with control group, $^{###}P < 0.001$ compared with bFGF group.

3.8 bFGF-induced FAK activation depended on Rac1

The relationship between Rac1 and FAK in cell proliferation and migration is controversial [36,37]. We found that bFGF-induced FAK activation was blocked by siRac1, while bFGF-induced Rac1 activation was not blocked by PF-562271 (Fig. 7C,D). In addition, bFGF-induced Akt activation was also not blocked by PF-562271 (Supporting Information Fig. 1C).

3.9 JNK was downstream of FAK in bFGF signaling pathway

FAK is required for JNK phosphorylation and promotes cell migration [38]. We found that bFGF-induced JNK activation was completely blocked by PF-562271, while bFGF-induced FAK activation was not blocked by SP600125 (Fig. 7E,F). In addition, bFGF-induced JNK activation was blocked by siRac1, while bFGF-induced Akt and Rac1 activation was also not blocked by SP600125 (Supporting Information Fig. 1B, D).

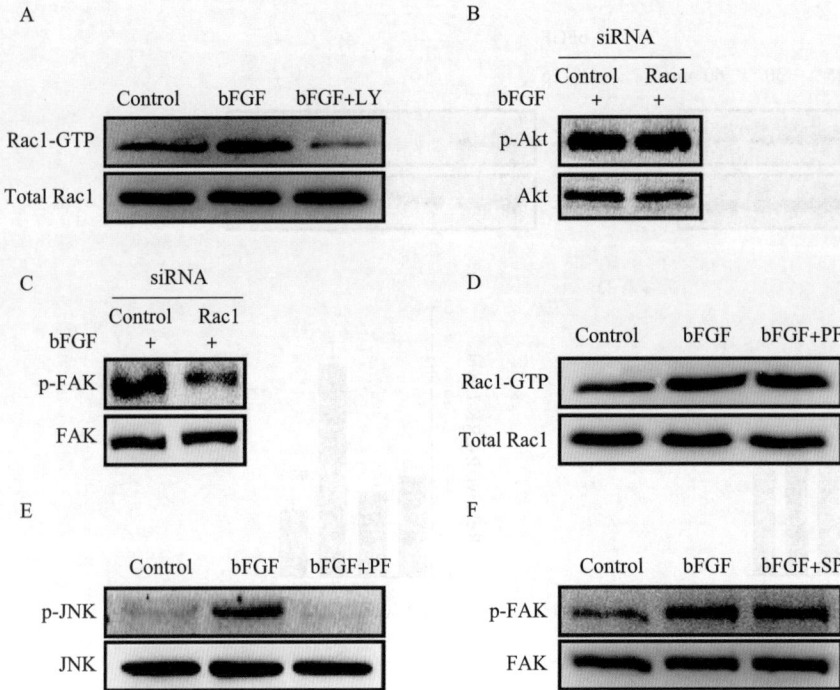

Fgi. 7. The role of PI3K/Akt, Rac1, FAK, and JNK in bFGF signaling pathway. (A, B) LY294002 inhibited the activity of Rac1, while siRNA Rac1 had negligible effect on Akt activity after bFGF treatment. (C, D) siRNA Rac1 blocked the FAK activity, while PF-562271 did not impair on Rac1 activity after bFGF administration. (E, F) PF-562271 impeded the JNK activity, while SP600125 showed no effect on FAK activity after bFGF stimulation.

4. Discussion

Previous studies have reported that bFGF induces melanocyte migration [9], and that the PI3K/Akt-Rac1-JNK signaling pathways are involved in bFGF-induced fibroblast migration [17,19]. However, it was not known whether PI3K/Akt-Rac1-JNK signaling pathway is involved in bFGF-induced melanocyte migration. The main aim of this study was to answer this question. In our study, we revealed that bFGF facilitated migration of primary human melanocytes. The mechanism of bFGF-promoted melanocyte migration was related to activation of PI3K/Akt-Rac1-FAK-JNK and ERK signaling pathways.

The PI3K/Akt signaling pathway plays important roles in regulating the cellular functions of various cell types, including cell proliferation, survival, and migration [39]. bFGF, via activating the PI3K/Akt signaling pathway, stimulates proliferation and migration of different cell types [17,19,40]. Our data showed that bFGF increased Akt phosphorylation and induced melanocyte migration (Fig. 2A,E). In addition, the Akt phosphorylation stimulated by bFGF was blocked by LY294002, which also the decreased melanocytes migration induced by bFGF (Fig. 2C,E). These findings suggest that PI3K/Akt signaling is necessary for bFGF-induced melanocyte migration.

Rho family proteins, including Rac1, Rho, and Cdc 42, are involved in cell migration via regulation of cytoskeletal rearrangement [41,42]. Zhang et al. demonstrated that hydrogen sulfide-promoted endothelial cell migration via actin cytoskeleton reorganization, an effect that was dependent on the activation of Rac1 [43]. Furthermore, bFGF induced activation of Rho family proteins and regulated cell growth and migration [44,45]. Our results showed that bFGF increased Rac1 activity and induced melanocytes migration (Fig. 3A,D). In addition, when Rac1 activity in melanocytes was decreased by transfection with Rac1 siRNA, bFGF-induced melanocyte migration was reduced. This suggests that Rac1 is involved in bFGF induced melanocyte migration.

FAK is necessary for integrin mediated cell migration and invasion [46], and lack of FAK impairs cell migration [47]. bFGF promotes melanocyte migration via increasing the expression of phosphorylated FAK, and herbimycin A, a potent FAK inhibitor, abolishes bFGF-induced melanocyte migration [9]. Consistent with these findings, we found that bFGF increased the phosphorylation of FAK, and that PF-562271 decreased FAK activity, reduced melanocyte migration stimulated by bFGF (Fig. 4A,C,E). These results suggest that FAK is also involved in bFGF-induced melanocyte migration.

The JNK pathway is involved in the regulation of inflammation, differentiation, and apoptosis [48]. Accumulating evidence also suggests that the JNK pathway is important for regulating cell migration stimulated by growth factors [49,50]. bFGF promotes fibroblast migration by upregulating JNK activity [17,51]. Melanocytes treated with bFGF showed significant induction of JNK phosphorylation, and melanocyte migration (Fig. 5A,E). In turn, reduction JNK phosphorylation by SP600125 was associated with a decrease in bFGF-induced melanocyte migration (Fig. 5C,E). This result suggests that JNK is also necessary for bFGF-induced melanocyte migration. The ERK signaling pathway also plays a role in the cell proliferation and migration of various cell types [52]. In endothelial progenitor cells, bFGF treatment contributed to cell proliferation and migration *via* upregulation of ERK [53]. In this study, bFGF induced phosphorylation of ERK and promoted melanocyte migration (Fig. 6A,E), but had no effect on their proliferation (Fig. 1A). In turn, ablation of ERK phosphorylation by U0126 was accompanied by a decrease in bFGF-induced melanocyte migration (Fig. 6C,E). This result indicates that ERK is also necessary for bFGF-induced melanocyte migration.

PI3K/Akt signaling contributes to Rac1 activation, and likewise, inhibition of PI3K/Akt signaling abolishes Rac1 activation [17,19,54]. In addition, a study has shown that Rac1 activation is often necessary for FAK activation and regulates cell adhesion [55]. However, different study revealed that FAK activity is required for Rac1 activation [56]. Knockdown of FAK decreases JNK phosphorylation and reduces cell invasion and metastasis [57]. In this study, melanocytes treated with LY294002 showed decreased bFGF-induced Rac1, FAK, and JNK activation, suggesting these proteins are downstream of PI3K/Akt in bFGF-induced melanocyte migration (Fig. 7A, Supporting Information Fig. S1A). Furthermore, in melanocyte treated with siRac1, FAK, and JNK activity was strongly down-regulated, but Akt activity was unaffected (Fig. 7B,C, Supporting Information Fig. S1B), suggesting Rac1 contributes to bFGF-induced FAK and JNK activation. In addition, melanocytes treated with PF-562271 showed a reduction in JNK activity, but not Akt activity and Rac1 activity (Fig. 7D,E, Supporting Information Fig. S1C), suggesting FAK is upstream of bFGF-induced JNK activation. Finally, melanocytes treated with SP600125 showed no effects on Akt, Rac1, or FAK activity after bFGF treatment (Fig. 7F, Supporting Information Fig. S1D). Accordingly, we concluded that a PI3K/Akt-Rac1-FAK-JNK signaling pathway is involved in bFGF-induced melanocyte migration.

Several additional questions about our findings remain to be addressed. ERK is a well-known signaling pathway that is critical for cell proliferation and migration [58]. Consistent with these findings, we found that the ERK signaling pathway was associated with bFGF-induced melanocyte migration (Fig. 6). Previous studies have also showed that bFGF produced by human keratinocytes is a natural mitogen for human melanocytes [20,21]. However, our data showed that treatment with bFGF for 24 h had no effect on melanocyte proliferation (Fig. 1A). Ruth *et al.* demonstrated that bFGF was mitogenic for melanocytes only in the presence of cAMP stimulators [20]. Furthermore, studies by Viki *et al.* showed that bFGF alone maintained the viability but did not induce the proliferation of melanocyte, and that bFGF promoted melanocyte proliferation in the presence of *a*-Melanotropin and Endothelin-1 [59]. Consistent with the Viki study, bFGF had no effect on proliferation of the melanocyte in this study, which were treated with bFGF alone in MTT assay and transwell assay after overnight starvation.

We did not explore the cross-talk between the ERK and PI3K/Akt-Rac1-FAK-JNK signaling pathways because FAK is also downstream of ERK in bFGF-mediated endothelial cell migration, which could confound interpretation of results [60]. However, since the classical signaling pathways with which the FGF family interacts are PI3K/Akt, MAPK/ERK, and PLCγ [11], we speculate that the ERK and PI3K/Akt-Rac1-FAK-JNK signaling pathways act in parallel but co-modulate FAK activity to facilitate melanocyte migration. Further studies using selective inhibitors or siRNA are needed to identify the relationship between these pathways.

It is well-known that melanocytes dysfunction contributes to the pathogenesis of vitiligo. Previous studies have demonstrated that adhesion and proliferation of melanocytes isolated from the lesioned skin of vitiligo patients is significantly impaired compared to melanocytes isolated from normal human skin [61,62]. In addition, clinical studies have shown that bFGF expression is decreased in skin tissue [22] but increased in serum and blister fluid from patients with vitiligo [24], implying that dysregulation of bFGF expression is involved in the pathogenesis of vitiligo through its regulation of melanocyte function. However, the exact role of bFGF in vitiligo development and progression is not known. A study found that narrow-band UVB, therapy used for treatment of vitiligo in the clinic, induced cultured keratinocytes to release bFGF and promoted melanocyte migration *in vitro* [26] and induced neonatal melanocytes to migrate to the epidermal basal layer [63]. These studies led us to speculate that bFGF has beneficial effects in treating the development and progression of vitiligo. Our current findings have provided a strong foundation for future *in vivo* studies.

In conclusion, bFGF promoted the migration of melanocytes by regulating PI3K/Akt, Rac1, FAK, JNK, and ERK activity. Inhibition of the activities of these proteins using selective inhibitors or siRNA reversed bFGF-induced melanocyte migration in transwell assays. Taken together, our data show that bFGF-induced activation of ERK and PI3K/Akt-Rac1-FAK-JNK signaling pathways leads to cytoskeleton reorganization, thereby contributing to melanocyte migration.

Supporting information

Additional supporting information may be found in the online version (doi:10.1002/iub.1531).

References

[1] Agarwal P, Rashighi M, Essien KI, et al. Simvastatin prevents and reverses depigmentation in a mouse model of vitiligo[J]. J Invest Dermatol, 2015, 135(4): 1080-1088.

[2] Alikhan A, Felsten LM, Daly M, et al. Vitiligo: a comprehensive overview Part I. Introduction, epidemiology, quality of life, diagnosis, differential diagnosis, associations, histopathology, etiology, and work-up[J]. J Am Acad Dermatol, 2011, 65(3): 473-491.

[3] Cooper GS, Stroehla BC. The epidemiology of autoimmune diseases[J]. Autoimmun Rev, 2003, 2(3): 119-125.

[4] Wang X, Du J, Wang T, et al. Prevalence and clinical profile of vitiligo in China: a community-based study in six cities[J]. Acta Derm Venereol, 2013, 93(1): 62-65.

[5] Bickers DR, Lim HW, Margolis D, et al. The burden of skin diseases: 2004 a joint project of the American Academy of Dermatology Association and the Society for Investigative Dermatology[J]. J Am Acad Dermatol, 2006, 55(3): 490-500.

[6] Miniati A, Weng Z, Zhang B, et al. Neuro-immuno-endocrine processes in vitiligo pathogenesis[J]. Int J Immunopathol Pharmacol, 2012, 25(1): 1-7.

[7] Qiu L, Song Z, Setaluri V. Oxidative stress and vitiligo: the Nrf2-ARE signaling connection[J]. J Invest Dermatol, 2014, 134(8): 2074-2076.

[8] Wu CS, Lan CC, Wang LF, et al. Effects of psoralen plus ultraviolet A irradiation on cultured epidermal cells in vitro and patients with vitiligo in vivo[J]. Br J Dermatol, 2007, 156(1): 122-129.

[9] Wu CS, Lan CC, Chiou MH, et al. Basic fibroblast growth factor promotes melanocyte migration via increased expression of p125(FAK) on melanocytes[J]. Acta Derm Venereol, 2006, 86(6): 498-502.

[10] Du X, Xie Y, Xian CJ, et al. Role of FGFs/FGFRs in skeletal development and bone regeneration[J]. J Cell Physiol, 2012, 227(12): 3731-3743.

[11] Beenken A, Mohammadi M. The FGF family: biology, pathophysiology and therapy[J]. Nat Rev Drug Discov, 2009, 8(3): 235-253.

[12] Xiang Q, Xiao J, Zhang H, et al. Preparation and characterisation of bFGF-encapsulated liposomes and evaluation of wound-healing activities in the rat[J]. Burns, 2011, 37(5): 886-895.

[13] Shi HX, Lin C, Lin BB, et al. The anti-scar effects of basic fibroblast growth factor on the wound repair in vitro and in vivo[J]. PLoS One, 2013, 8(4): e59966.

[14] Jia X, Tian H, Tang L, et al. High-efficiency expression of TAT-bFGF fusion protein in Escherichia coli and the effect on hypertrophic scar tissue[J]. PLoS One, 2015, 10(2): e0117448.

[15] Zhang HY, Wang ZG, Wu FZ, et al. Regulation of autophagy and ubiquitinated protein accumulation by bFGF promotes functional recovery and neural protection in a rat model of spinal cord injury[J]. Mol Neurobiol, 2013, 48(3): 452-464.

[16] Zhang HY, Zhang X, Wang ZG, et al. Exogenous basic fibroblast growth factor inhibits ER stress-induced apoptosis and improves recovery from spinal cord injury[J]. CNS Neurosci Ther, 2013, 19(1): 20-29.

[17] Shi H, Cheng Y, Ye J, et al. bFGF Promotes the Migration of Human Dermal Fibroblasts under Diabetic Conditions through Reactive Oxygen Species Production via the PI3K/Akt-Rac1- JNK Pathways[J]. Int J Biol Sci, 2015, 11(7): 845-859.

[18] Kottakis F, Polytarchou C, Foltopoulou P, et al. FGF-2 regulates cell proliferation, migration, and angiogenesis through an NDY1/KDM2B-miR-101-EZH2 pathway[J]. Mol Cell, 2011, 43(2): 285-298.

[19] Kanazawa S, Fujiwara T, Matsuzaki S, et al. bFGF regulates PI3-kinase-Rac1-JNK pathway and promotes fibroblast migration in wound healing[J]. PLoS One, 2010, 5(8): e12228.

[20] Halaban R, Ghosh S, Baird A. bFGF is the putative natural growth factor for human melanocytes[J]. In Vitro Cell Dev Biol, 1987, 23(1): 47-52.

[21] Halaban R, Langdon R, Birchall N, et al. Basic fibroblast growth factor from human keratinocytes is a natural mitogen for melanocytes[J]. J Cell Biol, 1988, 107(4): 1611-1619.

[22] Seif El Nasr H, Shaker OG, Fawzi MM, et al. Basic fibroblast growth factor and tumour necrosis factor alpha in vitiligo and other hypopigmented disorders: suggestive possible therapeutic targets[J]. J Eur Acad Dermatol Venereol, 2013, 27(1): 103-108.

[23] Moretti S, Spallanzani A, Amato L, et al. New insights into the pathogenesis of vitiligo: imbalance of epidermal cytokines at sites of lesions[J]. Pigment Cell Res, 2002, 15(2): 87-92.

[24] Ozdemir M, Yillar G, Wolf R, et al. Increased basic fibroblast growth factor levels in serum and blister fluid from patients with vitiligo[J]. Acta Derm Venereol, 2000, 80(6): 438-439.

[25] Samson Yashar S, Gielczyk R, Scherschun L, et al. Narrow-band ultraviolet B treatment for vitiligo, pruritus, and inflammatory dermatoses[J]. Photodermatol Photoimmunol Photomed, 2003, 19(4): 164-168.

[26] Wu CS, Yu CL, Wu CS, et al. Narrow-band ultraviolet-B stimulates proliferation and migration of cultured melanocytes[J]. Exp Dermatol, 2004, 13(12): 755-763.

[27] Hirobe T. How are proliferation and differentiation of melanocytes regulated?[J]. Pigment Cell Melanoma Res, 2011, 24(3): 462-478.

[28] Weidemann A, Breyer J, Rehm M, et al. HIF-1α activation results in actin cytoskeleton reorganization and modulation of Rac-1 signaling in endothelial cells[J]. Cell Commun Signal, 2013, 11: 80.

[29] Schnoor M. Endothelial actin-binding proteins and actin dynamics in leukocyte transendothelial migration[J]. J Immunol, 2015, 194(8): 3535-3541.

[30] Okada M, Oba Y, Yamawaki H. Endostatin stimulates proliferation and migration of adult rat cardiac fibroblasts through PI3K/Akt pathway[J]. Eur J Pharmacol, 2015, 750: 20-26.

[31] Dienstmann R, Rodon J, Serra V, et al. Picking the point of inhibition: a comparative review of PI3K/AKT/mTOR pathway inhibitors[J]. Mol Cancer Ther, 2014, 13(5): 1021-1031.

[32] Braun A, Dang K, Buslig F, *et al.* Rac1 and Aurora A regulate MCAK to polarize microtubule growth in migrating endothelial cells[J]. J Cell Biol, 2014, 206(1): 97-112.

[33] Deramaudt TB, Dujardin D, Noulet F, *et al.* Altering FAK-paxillin interactions reduces adhesion, migration and invasion processes[J]. PLoS One, 2014, 9(3): e92059.

[34] Cho HJ, Hwang YS, Mood K, *et al.* EphrinB1 interacts with CNK1 and promotes cell migration through c-Jun N-terminal kinase (JNK) activation[J]. J Biol Chem, 2014, 289(26): 18556-18568.

[35] Naci D, Aoudjit F. Alpha2beta1 integrin promotes T cell survival and migration through the concomitant activation of ERK/Mcl-1 and p38 MAPK pathways[J]. Cell Signal, 2014, 26(9): 2008-2015.

[36] Chang F, Lemmon CA, Park D, *et al.* FAK potentiates Rac1 activation and localization to matrix adhesion sites: a role for betaPIX[J]. Mol Biol Cell, 2007, 18(1): 253-264.

[37] Jung ID, Lee J, Yun SY, *et al.* Cdc42 and Rac1 are necessary for autotaxin-induced tumor cell motility in A2058 melanoma cells[J]. FEBS Lett, 2002, 532(3): 351-356.

[38] Zhong D, Ran JH, Tang WY, *et al.* Mda-9/syntenin promotes human brain glioma migration through focal adhesion kinase (FAK)-JNK and FAK-AKT signaling[J]. Asian Pac J Cancer Prev, 2012, 13(6): 2897-2901.

[39] Hemmings BA, Restuccia DF. PI3K-PKB/Akt pathway[J]. Cold Spring Harb Perspect Biol, 2012, 4(9): a011189.

[40] Pratsinis H, Kletsas D. PDGF, bFGF and IGF-I stimulate the proliferation of intervertebral disc cells *in vitro via* the activation of the ERK and Akt signaling pathways[J]. Eur Spine J, 2007, 16(11): 1858-1866.

[41] Tapon N, Hall A. Rho, Rac and Cdc42 GTPases regulate the organization of the actin cytoskeleton[J]. Curr Opin Cell Biol, 1997, 9(1): 86-92.

[42] Zhang Z, Yang M, Chen R, *et al.* IBP regulates epithelial-to-mesenchymal transition and the motility of breast cancer cells *via* Rac1, RhoA and Cdc42 signaling pathways[J]. Oncogene, 2014, 33(26): 3374-3382.

[43] Zhang LJ, Tao BB, Wang MJ, *et al.* PI3K p110alpha isoform-dependent Rho GTPase Rac1 activation mediates H2S-promoted endothelial cell migration *via* actin cytoskeleton reorganization[J]. PLoS One, 2012, 7(9): e44590.

[44] Kim EG, Shin EY. Nuclear Rac1 regulates the bFGF-induced neurite outgrowth in PC12 cells[J]. BMB Rep, 2013, 46(12): 617-622.

[45] Biname F, Sakry D, Dimou L, *et al.* NG2 regulates directional migration of oligodendrocyte precursor cells *via* Rho GTPases and polarity complex proteins[J]. J Neurosci, 2013, 33(26): 10858-10874.

[46] Hood JD, Cheresh DA. Role of integrins in cell invasion and migration[J]. Nat Rev Cancer, 2002, 2(2): 91-100.

[47] Sieg DJ, Hauck CR, Schlaepfer DD. Required role of focal adhesion kinase (FAK) for integrin-stimulated cell migration[J]. J Cell Sci, 1999, 112 (Pt 16): 2677-2691.

[48] Sabapathy K. Role of the JNK pathway in human diseases[J]. Prog Mol Biol Transl Sci, 2012, 106: 145-169.

[49] Kim EJ, Eom SJ, Hong JE, *et al.* Benzyl isothiocyanate inhibits basal and hepatocyte growth factor-stimulated migration of breast cancer cells[J]. Mol Cell Biochem, 2012, 359(1-2): 431-440.

[50] Chen JC, Lin BB, Hu HW, *et al.* NGF accelerates cutaneous wound healing by promoting the migration of dermal fibroblasts *via* the PI3K/Akt-Rac1-JNK and ERK pathways[J]. Biomed Res Int, 2014, 2014: 547187.

[51] Xuan YH, Huang BB, Tian HS, *et al.* High-glucose inhibits human fibroblast cell migration in wound healing *via* repression of bFGF-regulating JNK phosphorylation[J]. PLoS One, 2014, 9(9): e108182.

[52] Williams KA, Zhang M, Xiang S, *et al.* Extracellular signal-regulated kinase (ERK) phosphorylates histone deacetylase 6 (HDAC6) at serine 1035 to stimulate cell migration[J]. J Biol Chem, 2013, 288(46): 33156-33170.

[53] Guo S, Yu L, Cheng Y, *et al.* PDGFRbeta triggered by bFGF promotes the proliferation and migration of endothelial progenitor cells *via* p-ERK signalling[J]. Cell Biol Int, 2012, 36(10): 945-950.

[54] Ni B, Wen LB, Wang R, *et al.* The involvement of FAK-PI3K-AKT-Rac1 pathway in porcine reproductive and respiratory syndrome virus entry[J]. Biochem Biophys Res Commun, 2015, 458(2): 392-398.

[55] Havel LS, Kline ER, Salgueiro AM, *et al.* Vimentin regulates lung cancer cell adhesion through a VAV2-Rac1 pathway to control focal adhesion kinase activity[J]. Oncogene, 2015, 34(15): 1979-1990.

[56] Bae YH, Mui KL, Hsu BY, *et al.* A FAK-Cas-Rac-lamellipodin signaling module transduces extracellular matrix stiffness into mechanosensitive cell cycling[J]. Sci Signal, 2014, 7(330): ra57.

[57] Xiao W, Jiang M, Li H, *et al.* Knockdown of FAK inhibits the invasion and metastasis of Tca8113 cells *in vitro*[J]. Mol Med Rep, 2013, 8(2): 703-707.

[58] Albeck JG, Mills GB, Brugge JS. Abstract 4946: Control of cellular proliferation by ERK: A quantitative analysis in single cells[J]. Cancer Research, 2012, 72: 4946-4946.

[59] Swope VB, Medrano EE, Smalara D, *et al.* Long-term proliferation of human melanocytes is supported by the physiologic mitogens alpha-melanotropin, endothelin-1, and basic fibroblast growth factor[J]. Exp Cell Res, 1995, 217(2): 453-459.

[60] Shi C, Lu J, Wu W, *et al.* Endothelial cell-specific molecule 2 (ECSM2) localizes to cell-cell junctions and modulates bFGF-directed cell migration *via* the ERK-FAK pathway[J]. PLoS One, 2011, 6(6): e21482.

[61] Gauthier Y, Cario Andre M, Taieb A. A critical appraisal of vitiligo etiologic theories. Is melanocyte loss a melanocytorrhagy?[J]. Pigment Cell Res, 2003, 16(4): 322-332.

[62] Dell'anna ML, Cario-Andre M, Bellei B, *et al. In vitro* research on vitiligo: strategies, principles, methodological options and common pitfalls[J]. Exp Dermatol, 2012, 21(7): 490-496.

[63] Walker GJ, Kimlin MG, Hacker E, *et al.* Murine neonatal melanocytes exhibit a heightened proliferative response to ultraviolet radiation and migrate to the epidermal basal layer[J]. J Invest Dermatol, 2009, 129(1): 184-193.

Regulation of caveolin-1 and junction proteins by bFGF contributes to the integrity of blood–spinal cord barrier and functional recovery

Libing Ye, Xiaokun Li, Hongyu Zhang

1. Introduction

Traumatic spinal cord injury (SCI) is a devastating disease that results in permanent disability. Previous research focuses largely on improving neurological manifestations through the improvement of sensory function and locomotor function [1-4], but study of the blood–spinal cord barrier (BSCB) still lacks sufficient investigation. Similarly to the blood–brain barrier (BBB), BSCB plays a protective and regulatory role in spinal cord parenchyma. Endothelial cells, basement membranes, pericytes, and astrocytic end-feet processes constitute a specialized system for this functional barrier [5]. Early microvascular reactions and BSCB disruption are instrumental in the pathophysiology of SCI and repair [6, 7].

Caveolin-1 (Cav-1), a major structural protein of caveolae that is known to be involved in endocytosis, vesicular trafficking, and signal transduction [8, 9], regulates the permeability of the BBB. In several models of adult brain injuries, Cav-1 is increased in the endothelium for several days following cold cortical injury and brain ischemia [10, 11]. The knockdown of Cav-1 reduces matrix metalloproteinase (MMPs) activity in endothelial cells and their angiogenic response to vascular endothelial growth factor (VEGF) [12]. On the contrary, the loss of Cav-1 is crucial in the activation of MMPs and BBB breakdown in stroke animal models [13]. Cav-1 regulates expression of junction-associated proteins in brain microvascular endothelial cells, and attenuated Cav-1 levels are correlated with heightened permeability of endothelia [14]. In addition, Cav-1 knockout mice present higher vascular permeability, which has been found to aggravate disorders in rodent models [15, 16]. Although the exact role of Cav-1 in SCI remains unclear, it is plausible that Cav-1 is a critical mediator of BSCB integrity.

Basic fibroblast growth factor (bFGF) is a neurotrophic factor that functions as a neuroprotective agent and rescues neurons from various insults *in vitro* and *in vivo*. Administration of exogenous growth factors following SCI promotes functional recovery [17, 18]; intrathecal administration of bFGF also significantly enhances functional recovery after moderate and severe contusions in SCI rats [19, 20], but the precise mechanism underlying the observed therapeutic effects has not been elucidated. In our latest studies, bFGF was demonstrated to inhibit excessive autophagy and endoplasmic reticulum stress in SCI, which contributed to functional recovery [21, 22]. In addition, it has been reported that bFGF preserves BBB integrity after intracerebral hemorrhage in mice [23]. However, the effect of bFGF on BSCB has not been reported.

In this study, a contusive SCI rat model was constructed using an Infinite Horizon Impactor Device, to evaluate the effects of bFGF on BSCB integrity *in vivo*. Furthermore, an oxygen-glucose deprivation (OGD) cell model was established to clarify the role of Cav-1 in bFGF-mediated endothelial barrier function *in vitro*. Our data indicate, for the first time, that Cav-1 is essential for the function of bFGF in the recovery of the BSCB and correlates with fibroblast growth factor receptor 1 (FGFR1) regulation that contributes substantially to the repair of SCI.

2. Materials and methods

2.1 Experimental animals and surgical procedures

Eighty adult female Sprague–Dawley rats (weighing 220–250 g) were obtained from the Animal Center of Chinese Academy of Science. All experimental procedures were approved by the ethics committee of Wenzhou Medical University and performed in accordance with the Guide for the Care and Use of Laboratory Animals. Rats were anesthetized with 10% chloral hydrate (3.5 ml/kg) before a laminectomy. The vertebral column was stabilized by clamping the T8 and T10 vertebral bodies with forceps fixed to the base of an Infinite Horizon Impact Device. Rats were situated on the platform, and the 2.5-mm stainless steel impactor tip was positioned over the midpoint of T9 and impacted with 150 kdyn force with no dwell time. The force/ displacement graph was used to monitor impact consistency and any animals that exhibited an abnormal impact graph or > 10% deviation from 150 kdyn were immediately excluded from the study. The incision sites were then closed in layers and a topical antibiotic (cefazolin sodium salt, 50 mg/kg, i.p.) was applied to the incision site. For the sham-operated controls, the animals underwent a T9 laminectomy without contusion injury. Postoperative care involved manually emptying the urinary bladder twice a day (until the return of bladder function). The SCI rats were randomly divided into 2 groups, a bFGF-treated group (bFGF) and a vehicle group (SCI). Based on our previous study [22], recombinant human bFGF purchased from Sigma-Aldrich (St. Louis, MO, USA) was injected subcutaneously near the back wound at a dose of 80 μg/kg at 30 min post injury; after this, the recombinant human bFGF was administered every 2 days until the animals were euthanized. The death rate of our model was zero.

2.2 Tissue preparation

At specific time points after SCI, animals were anesthetized with 10% chloral hydrate (3.5 ml/kg) and perfused *via* cardiac puncture initially with 0.9% saline solution. For immunohistochemistry, animals were perfused with 4% paraformaldehyde in 0.1 M phosphate-buffered saline (PBS) after saline solution. A 0.5-cm section of the spinal cord, centered at the lesion site, was dissected out, postfixed by immersion in 4% paraformaldehyde for 24 h. and then placed in 30% sucrose in 0.1 M PBS for 2 days. The segments were embedded in optimal cutting temperature for frozen sections, and longitudinal or transverse sections were then cut at 10 or 20 μm on a cryostat (Leica Microsystems Wetzlar GmbH, Hesse-Darmstadt, Germany). For Western blot, a spinal cord segment (0.5 cm length) at the contusion epicenter was dissected and immediately stored at $-80\,^{\circ}\text{C}$.

2.3 Measurement of BSCB disruption

The integrity of BSCB was investigated with Evans Blue dye and fluorescein isothiocyanate (FITC)–dextran (MW 70 kDa; Sigma-Aldrich) extravasation, according to previous reports [24, 25]. At 1 day after SCI, animals were injected with 4 ml/kg 2% Evans Blue (Sigma-Aldrich) into the tail vein. Two hours later, animals were anesthetized and killed by intracardiac perfusion with saline. For qualitative examination of Evans Blue extravasation, the animals were perfused with PBS and subsequently with 4% formaldehyde, as described above. The spinal cords were separated into 20-μm thick sections with a cryostat. The fluorescence of Evans Blue in spinal tissues was observed with a fluorescence microscope and the relative fluorescence intensity was determined by Image Pro-Plus (Media Cybernetics, Rockville, MD, USA). In order to quantify leakage of larger molecular weight molecules, FITC–dextran (4 mg/kg) was injected into the tail vein and allowed to circulate for 2 h. The animals were killed and perfused with saline. The T8–T10 segment was removed, homogenized in PBS, and centrifuged. The supernatant fluorescence (excitation at 493 nm and emission at 517 nm) was then measured.

2.4 Locomotion recovery assessment

In order to examine the locomotor function after injury, the Basso, Beattie, and Bresnahan scale were scored by trained investigators who were blind to the experimental conditions [26]. It is performed in an open-field scale everyday postoperation. Briefly, the Basso, Beattie, and Bresnahan locomotion rating scale ranges from 0 points (complete paralysis) to 21 points (normal locomotion). The scale is based upon the natural progression of locomotion recovery in rats with thoracic SCIs.

2.5 Cell culture and treatment

Human brain microvascular endothelial cells (HBMEC) and endothelial cell medium were purchased from Scien-Cell Research Laboratories (ScienCell Research Laboratories, San Diego, CA, USA). HBMEC were grown as a monolayer in endothelial cell medium. All cells were incubated at $37\,^{\circ}\text{C}$ in a humidified atmosphere of 5% CO_2 and 95% air. The cells were subcultured into 60-mm or 35-mm dishes coated with fibronectin and confluent cells were exposed to a hypoxia chamber (1029; Thermo Fisher Scientific, Waltham, MA, USA) for 12 h after overnight starvation with 0.5%

fetal calf serum. Before OGD, the medium was then changed to sugarfree basic medium. The oxygen concentration was < 0.2%, as monitored by an oxygen analyzer. bFGF (50 ng/ml) was treated for 30 min before OGD. The bFGF powder was dissolved in PBS to make the stock solution (50 μg/μl). For the control group, PBS without drug was used. Primary astrocytes and the SHSY-5Y cell line were purchased from the Cell Storage Center of Wuhan University (Wuhan, Hubei, China). Both cell types were cultured with 10% F12/ DMEM medium (Gibco, Carlsbad, CA, USA) at 37℃ in a humidified atmosphere of 5% CO_2 and 95% air. The OGD conditions and procedure of these cells were same with HBMEC.

2.6 Primary hippocampal neuron culture

Primary hippocampal neurons were established from the brains of neonatal Sprague–Dawley rats (<4 h of age). Hippocampi were dissected from the brains and rinsed in ice-cold dissection buffer. Blood vessels and white matter were removed and tissues were treated with 0.125% trypsin in Hank's balanced salt solution for 20 min at 37℃. The whole solution was filtered through stainless steel (200 mesh; BD Biosciences, San Jose, CA, USA). Cell suspension was centrifuged twice at 198 g for 5 min and the cell pellets resuspended in DMEM/F-12 with 10% fetal bovine serum, 100 U/L penicillin, 100 mg/L streptomycin and 0.5 mM glutamine. Cells were seeded at a density of $1–5× 10^5$/ml in 6-well plates kept at 37℃ in a 5% CO_2 incubator. After 24 h, the culture medium was changed to Neurobasal Medium (Gibco) with 2% B27 and changed every 2–3 days. Arabinosylcytosin (10 mg/L; Sigma-Aldrich) was added at 72 h to prevent the growth of non-neuronal cells. All experiments were performed at 8–11 days after seeding. The procedure of OGD is same with other cells.

2.7 Small interfering RNA transfection

HBMEC at 70%–80% confluence were transfected with 100 pmol Cav-1 small interfering RNA (siRNA) or negative-control siRNA (Bioneer, Daejeon, Korea) using lipofectamine 2000 (Life Technologies, Carlsbad, CA, USA), according to the manufacturer's instructions. Twenty-four hours after transfection, cells were subjected to OGD treatment. Specific silencing was confirmed by Western blot.

2.8 HBMEC monolayer permeability assay

The effect of OGD on endothelial monolayer permeability to FITC–dextran was assessed using polyethylene terephthalate membrane 24-well cell culture inserts with a 0.4-μm pore size (Corning Life Sciences, Corning, NY, USA). Cells were placed on the upper side of the insert and allowed to grow to confluence. FITC–dextran at a concentration of 1 mg/ml was added to the endothelial monolayer after exposure to OGD [27]. Two hours later, relative fluorescence passed through the chamber was determined using a fluorescence plate reader at an excitation wavelength at 493 nm and an emission wavelength at 517 nm (SpectraMax M2e; Molecular Devices, Sunnyvale, CA, USA). Endothelial monolayer permeability was assessed by the intensity of FITC–dextran in the lower chamber. To test whether bFGF could protect the integrity of endothelial monolayer permeability, cells were pretreated with bFGF (40 ng/ml) for 1 h. In addition, cells were pretreated with Cav-1 siRNA for 24 h, to clarify the role of Cav-1 in endothelial cell.

2.9 Gelatin zymography

In vivo, the activity of MMP-2 and MMP-9 at 1 day after injury was examined by gelatin zymography. Briefly, the protein concentration of the homogenates was determined by the bicinchoninic acid method (BCA protein assay kit; Thermo Fisher Scientific, Rockford, IL, USA). After determination of protein concentration of the homogenates, equal amounts of protein (30 μg) were loaded on 10% sodium dodecyl sulfate polyacrylamide gel electrophoresis, co-polymerized with1 mg/ml gelatin (Sigma-Aldrich). Gels were washed in 2.5% Triton X-100 (Sigma-Aldrich) for 1 h and then incubated for 24 h in a developing buffer, including Tris 50 mM/(pH 7.6), CaCl 25 mM, NaCl 0.2 mM, and 0.02% (*w/v*) Brij-35 (Sigma-Aldrich) at 37℃, followed by staining with Coomassie blue (Sigma-Aldrich). Gels were destained to visualize gelatinolytic bands (MMP-2/MMP-9) on a dark blue background. *In vitro*, after OGD treatment, MMP-2/ MMP-9 in conditioned media was analyzed by gelatin zymography as described above.

2.10 Western blot

For *in vivo* protein analysis, a spinal cord segment (0.5 cm length) at the contusion epicenter was dissected at 6 h, and 1, 3 and 7 days and immediately stored at –80℃ for Western blotting. For protein extraction, the tissue was homogenized in modified buffer [50 mM Tris-HCl, 1% NP-40, 20 mM dithiothreitol, 150 mM NaCl (pH 7.4)] containing protease inhibitor cocktail (10 μl/ml; GE Healthcare Biosciences, Pittsburgh, PA, USA). The complex was then centrifuged at 13,362 g and the supernatant obtained for protein assay. *In vitro*, HBMEC were lysed in RIPA buffer (25 mM Tris-HCl, 150 mM NaCl, 1% Nonidet P-40, 1% sodium deoxycholate, and 0.1% sodium dodecyl sulfate) with protease and phosphatase inhibitors. The extracts above were quantified with BCA reagents. We separated proteins on a 10% or 12% gel and transferred them onto a polyvinylidene fluoride membrane (Bio-Rad, Hercules, CA, USA). The membrane was blocked with 5% milk (Bio-Rad) in TBS with 0.05% Tween 20 (TBST) for 1.5 h and incubated with the antibodies p120-catenin (1:1 000), β-catenin (1:1 000), occludin (1:300), claudin-5 (1:300), Cav-1 (1:300) in TBST for 2 h at room temperature or overnight at 4℃. The membranes were washed with TBST 3 times and treated with horseradish peroxidase-conjugated secondary antibodies (1:3000) for 1 h at room temperature. Signals were visualized by Chemi-DocXRS + Imaging System (Bio-Rad). β-Actin (1:300) was used as an internal control. Experiments were repeated 3 times and the densitometric values of the bands on Western blots obtained by Image J software (National Institutes of Health, Bethesda, MD, USA) were subjected to statistical analysis. Anti-p120-catenin and β-catenin were from Abcam (Cambridge, UK); all other antibodies were from Santa Cruz Biotechnology (Santa Cruz, CA, USA).

2.11　Real-time polymerase chain reaction

Total RNA was isolated using Trizol reagents according to manufacturer's protocol. RNA (0.5 μg) was used as a template for first-strand cDNA synthesis using the High-Capacity cDNA Reverse Transcription Kit (Applied Biosystems, Life Technologies, Carlsbad, CA, USA). Reverse transcription products were amplified with the 7900HT Fast Real-Time PCR System in a 10-μl final reaction volume using SYBR Green PCR Master Mix (Bio-Rad, Hercules, CA, USA) under the following conditions: 2 min at 50℃ and 10 min at 95℃, followed by a total of 40 cycles of 2 temperature cycles (15 s at 95℃ and 1 min at 60℃). Primers for MMP-2, MMP-9, and actin were designed against known rat sequences and human sequences as follows: rat, MMP-2 forward: 5'-GGACAGTG ACACCACGTGACA,-3', reverse: 5'-ACTCATTCCCTG CGAAGAACA-3'; MMP-9 forward: 5'-AACCCTGG TCACCGGACTTC-3', reverse: 5'-CACCCGGTTGTGGA AACTCAC-3'; β-actin forward: 5'-AAGATCCTGACCG AGCGTGGC-3', reverse: 5'-CAGCACTGTGTTGGCA TAGAGG-3'; Cav-1 forward: 5'-GCCCTCACAGGGACAT CTCTACA-3', reverse: 5'-CCGCAATCACATCTTC AAAGTCA-3'; human, MMP-2 forward: 5'-CCCAGACA GGTGATCTTGACC-3', reverse: 5'-CTTGCGAGGGA AGAAGTTGTAG-3'; MMP-9 forward: 5'-ATCCGGCACC TCTATGGTC-3', reverse: 5'-CTGAGGGGTGG ACAGTGG-3'; β-actin forward: 5'-CCTGGCACCCAG CACAAT-3', reverse: 5'-GCCGATCCA-CACGGAGTACT -3'. The fluorescence threshold value (Ct value) was calculated using the SDS Enterprise Database software. The relative value of mRNA expression was calculated by the comparative ΔΔCt method. In brief, mean Ct values were normalized to the internal control actin and the difference was defined as ΔCt. The difference between the mean ΔCt values of SCI group and bFGF treatment group was calculated and defined as ΔΔCt. The comparative mRNA expression level was expressed as $2^{-\Delta\Delta Ct}$. All agents mentioned were from Life Technologies.

2.12　Immunohistochemistry

Frozen sections were processed for double labeling with antibodies against claudin-5 (1:100; Santa Cruz), p120-catenin (1:200; Santa Cruz), NeuN (1:500; Abcam), glial fibrillary acidic protein (1:100; Santa Cruz), and CD31 (1:100, Santa Cruz). Alexa Fluor 488 (1:1 000; Abcam) or Texas Red-conjugated secondary antibodies (1:200; Santa Cruz) were used. Nuclei were labeled with Hoechst (Beyotime Institute of Biotechnology, Shanghai, China). The control study was performed by using PBS instead of primary antibody. For cell immunostaining, the HBMEC grown to confluence on fibronectin-coated coverslips were subjected to the indicated treatments. Cells were washed 3 times with PBS, fixed in 4% paraformaldehyde for 30 min, and blocked for 30 min at 37℃ with 5% bovine serum albumin. The cells were then incubated with anti-p120-catennin (1:200), anti-β-catenin (1:200), anticlaudin-5 (1:50), antioccludin (1:50), anti-Cav-1 (1:100), or anti-FGFR1 (1:100) overnight at 4℃. Alexa Fluor 488 (1:1 000) or TR-conjugated secondary antibodies were used. Anti-CD31, anti-FGFR1, and TR-conjugated secondary antibodies were from Santa Cruz, Alexa Fluor 488 was from Abcam, and others antibodies are same as used in the Western blot experiments.

2.13 Statistical analysis

All quantitative data are expressed as means ± SEM if normally distributed. Student's t test was used between 2 groups if data were normally distributed. Otherwise, we used the Wilcoxon rank sum test instead. For analyzing 3 or more groups, differences were assessed by 1-way ANOVA if data were normally distributed and variance homogeneous; otherwise, the Kruskal–Wallis test was performed, followed by post-hoc adjustment using Bonferroni's multiple comparisons test. Normality was checked using the Kolmogorov–Smirnov test and the homogeneity of variance was checked by the Levene test. A probability value $P < 0.05$ was considered to show statistical significance.

3. Results

3.1 bFGF attenuates BSCB disruption after SCI

To determine the effect of bFGF on BSCB integrity, we assessed the degree of BSCB disruption after SCI by Evans Blue and FITC–dextran assay. As is shown in Fig. 1A, we assessed the intensity of Evans Blue dye extravasation at 6 h, 1 d, 3 d, 7 d, and 14 d postinjury with or without bFGF. We found that the extravasation of Evans Blue significantly increased after injury, and showed maximal BSCB disruption at 1 d after injury. bFGF showed a remarkable reduction of the intensity of Evans Blue at 6 h, 1 d, 3 d, and 7 d postinjury. As 1 d is the peak of BSCB permeability and the effect of

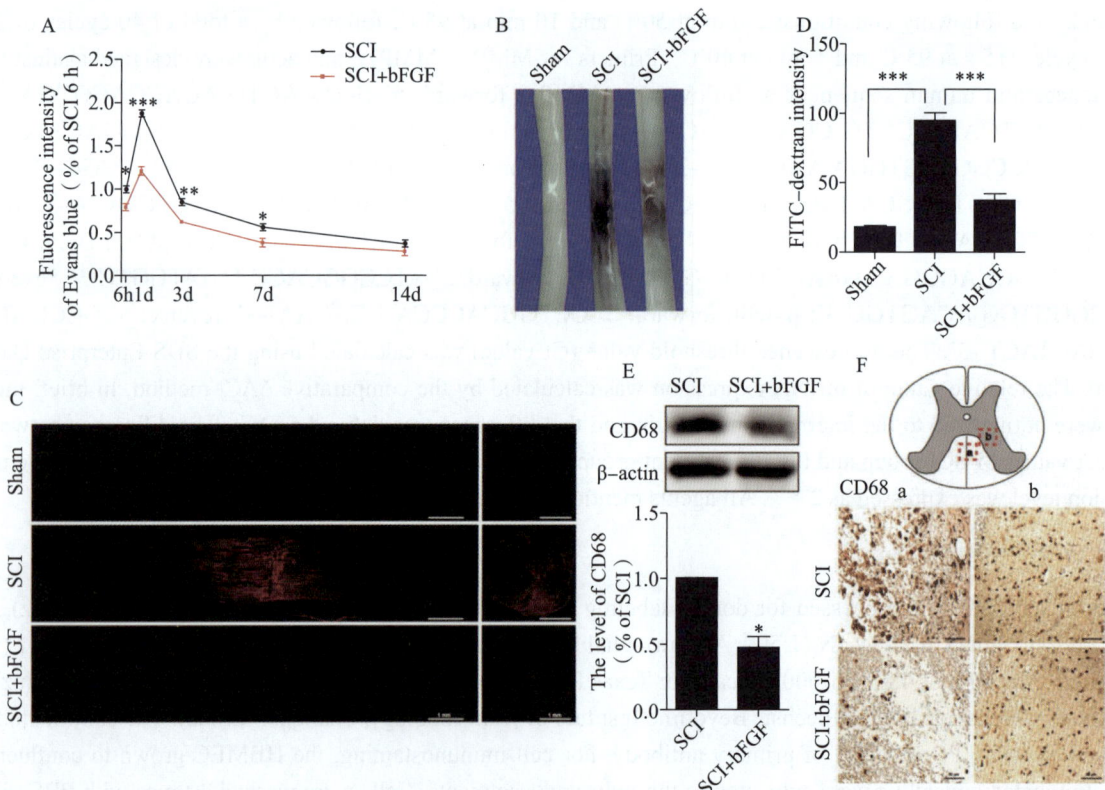

Fig. 1. Basic fibroblast growth factor (bFGF) reduces blood–spinal cord barrier (BSCB) permeability after contusive spinal cord injury (SCI). After SCI, rats were treated with bFGF and barrier permeability was measured at 1 d after injury, using Evans Blue dye and fluorescein isothiocyanate (FITC)–dextran. (A) Quantification of Evans Blue dye extracted from spinal cord at 6 h–14 d postinjury with or without bFGF. Data were analyzed by Student's t test (6 h: t = 4.444, P = 0.011; 1 d: t= 10.398, P < 0.001; 5 d: t = 5.013, P = 0.007; 7 d: t = 2.895, P = 0.044). (B) Representative whole spinal cords showing Evans Blue dye permeabilized into the spinal cord at 1 d. (C) Representative confocal images of sham, SCI, and bFGF-treatment groups. Scale bar = 1 mm. (D) Quantification of the FITC–dextran extravasation (excitation at 490 nm and emission at 520 nm). Data were analyzed by ANOVA ($F_{(2, 9)}$= 79.682, P < 0.001). Post-hoc analyses were done using Bonferroni's multiple comparison test (***P < 0.001). (E) Western blot and densitometric analysis of CD68 at 1 d with or without bFGF. Data were analyzed by Student's t test (t = 6.444, P = 0.023). (F) Immunochemical staining of CD68. Scale bar = 50 μm. *P < 0.05, **P < 0.01, ***P < 0.001.

bFGF at 1 d is most obvious, we suggest that there is a relatively large time window in which to exploit the disruption of the BSCB. From Fig. 1(B, C), it is easy to see that the fluorescence intensity of Evans Blue in spinal cord sections is much weaker in the bFGF treatment group than the SCI group, which suggests that bFGF increased the integrity of BSCB after SCI. To quantify the leakage of larger molecular weight molecules, FITC–dextran was injected into the tail vein. The intensity of FITC–dextran extravasation was obviously enhanced and bFGF reduced the fluorescence intensity compared with the SCI group (Fig. 1D). To further support the role of bFGF in increasing BSCB integrity, we analyzed immune cell infiltration. CD68, the marker of macrophages, was detected at 1 d postinjury with or without bFGF. As is shown in Fig. 1(E, F), bFGF reduced the expression of CD68.

Furthermore, to verify the protective effect of bFGF on functional recovery post-SCI, the functional recovery and pathologic morphology after bFGF treatment were evaluated (see Supplementary Fig. 1). The Basso, Beattie, and Bresnahan scores of SCI were assessed at 1, 3, 5, 7, and 14 d postinjury (Supplementary Fig. 1A). There was no obvious difference in the Basso, Beattie, and Bresnahan scores between the SCI model and the bFGF groups at 1 d after injury. However, the Basso, Beattie, and Bresnahan scores of the bFGF group were increased from d 3 to d 14 after injury, indicating that bFGF stimulated the recovery of locomotor activity. As shown in Supplementary Fig. 1B, footprint analyses for bFGF-treated rats at 14 d post-SCI disclosed fairly consistent hindlimb coordination and some toe dragging, while the SCI group showed inconsistent coordination and extensive drags, as revealed by ink streaks extending from both hindlimbs. From Supplementary Fig. 1(C, D), the results of hematoxylin and eosin stain, and NeuN stain, also demonstrated that bFGF ameliorated the pathological morphology of tissues and increased the number of neurons at 3 d postinjury (Supplementary Fig. 1E). All these data indicate that bFGF attenuates BSCB disruption in the early stages after SCI, which is beneficial for the functional recovery of SCI.

3.2 bFGF inhibits the expression and activation of MMP-9 after SCI

Although many factors are known to contribute to BBB/BSCB disruption, MMPs play a critical role [28]. Therefore, we measured the expression and activation of MMP-2 and MMP-9 after bFGF treatment. First, we examined the expression of MMP-2/MMP-9 mRNA at 6 h–7 d after injury by real-time polymerase chain reaction ($n = 5$/group). As shown in Fig. 2(A, B), the mRNA levels of MMP-9 markedly increased at 1 d after injury, whereas the level of MMP-2 exhibited no significant changes (Fig. 2B). In addition, bFGF treatment significantly inhibited MMP-9 mRNA expression at 1 d after injury compared with the vehicle controls (Fig. 2C). Next, the activities of MMP-2/MMP-9 were analyzed by gelatin zymography. Fig. 2E shows that MMP-9 activation was markedly enhanced at 1 d after injury, consistent with previous reports [29], with bands corresponding to the active form of MMP-9 and the inactive zymogen (pro-MMP-9). Although pro-MMP-2 appeared in the SCI group, there was no active MMP-2, which is consistent with the report of Lee *et al.* reports [25]. bFGF significantly decreased the level of active MMP-9 and pro-MMP-2 compared with the vehicle controls at 1 d after injury. In addition, we also performed double-labeling immunofluorescence between MMP-9 and other cell markers. As shown in Supplementary Fig. 2, the results of the Western blot suggest that the expression of MMP-9 was up-regulated after SCI, and bFGF significantly reduced its expression. Further staining indicated that MMP-9 was mainly expressed in endothelial cells and neurons (Supplementary Fig. 2B, C); however, in astrocytes, there is no co-localization with GFAP, but some positive points were found in the nuclear of astrocytes (Supplementary Fig. 2D). These data suggest that bFGF might prevent BSCB disruption by inhibiting the expression and activation of MMP-9 after SCI.

3.3 bFGF inhibits the disruption of tight and adherens junction after SCI

It was previously discovered the tight junction (TJ) proteins are critical structural proteins in the BSCB [21]. To determine whether SCI-induced hyperpermeability is caused by TJ alterations, the expression of claudin-5 and occludin, the major TJ proteins present in the BBB [30], were examined by Western blot in spinal cord lysates. After injury, the expression of occludin and claudin-5 decreased, and the decrease was especially prominent at 1 day after injury (Fig. 3A, C). However, the level of occludin returned nearly to the level of the sham group after 7 days. Furthermore, we examined the levels of adherens junctions (AJ) proteins. Catenins, a family of proteins found in complexes with adhesion molecules of animal cells, were degraded and were present in significant numbers at 1 d postinjury (Fig. 3A, B). However, bFGF-treated groups showed significantly higher levels of occludin, claudin-5, p120-catenin, and β-catenin at 1 d after injury (Fig. 3D, E, F). In addition, a double-labeling immunofluorescence was performed in blood vessels. The

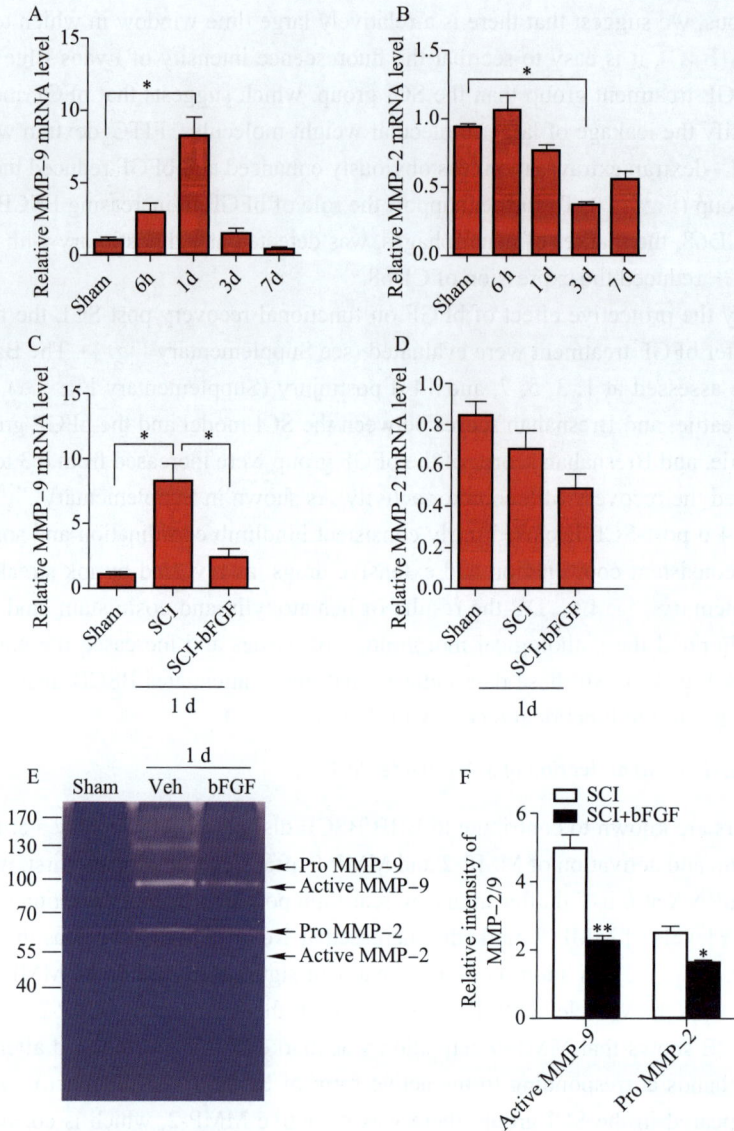

Fig. 2. Basic fibroblast growth factor (bFGF) inhibits the expression and activation of matrix metalloproteinase (MMP)-9 after spinal cord injury. Spinal cord tissues were isolated at 6 h–7 d after injury. Real-time polymerase chain reaction and gelatin zymography were processed as described in the ₚMaterials and Methods^ ($n = 5$/group). (A, B) mRNA level of MMP-2/MMP-9 at 6 h–7 d after injury. Data were analyzed by Kruskal–Wallis test (MMP-9: $P = 0.002$; MMP-2: $P = 0.002$). Post-hoc analyses were done using Bonferroni's multiple comparison test ($^*P < 0.05$). (C, D) mRNA level of MMP-2/MMP-9 at 1 d after injury with administration of bFGF. MMP-9 data were analyzed by Kruskal–Wallis test (MMP-9: $P = 0.005$). MMP-2 data were analyzed by ANOVA ($F[2, 9] = 3.828$, $P = 0.063$). Post-hoc analyses were done using Bonferroni's multiple comparison test ($^*P < 0.05$). (E) Gelatin zymography at 1 d after injury. (F) Densitometric analysis of zymography. Data were analyzed by Student's t test (active MMP-9: t = 6.819, $P = 0.002$; pro-MMP-2: t = 4.394, $P = 0.039$).

fluorescence intensity of claudin-5 and p120-catenin immunoreactivities were de-creased in endothelial cells (labeled by CD31) after injury compared with sham controls, and bFGF treatment attenuated the decrease in its intensity (Fig. 3G, H). These data indicate that bFGF prevents BSCB disruption by inhibiting the degradation of TJ and AJ molecules after SCI.

3.4 bFGF prevents loss of Cav-1 in endothelial cells after SCI

It is reported that reduced Cav-1 accompanied the diminished expression of TJ-associated proteins following stimulation of HBMECs with the chemokine CCL2, which contributes to BBB disruption [14]. However, the relationship of Cav-1 and BSCB disruption is still unclear. In our study, we found that in addition to the loss of TJ and AJ proteins following SCI, Cav-1 expression significantly decreased at 1 d after injury, shown by both mRNA and protein levels (Fig.

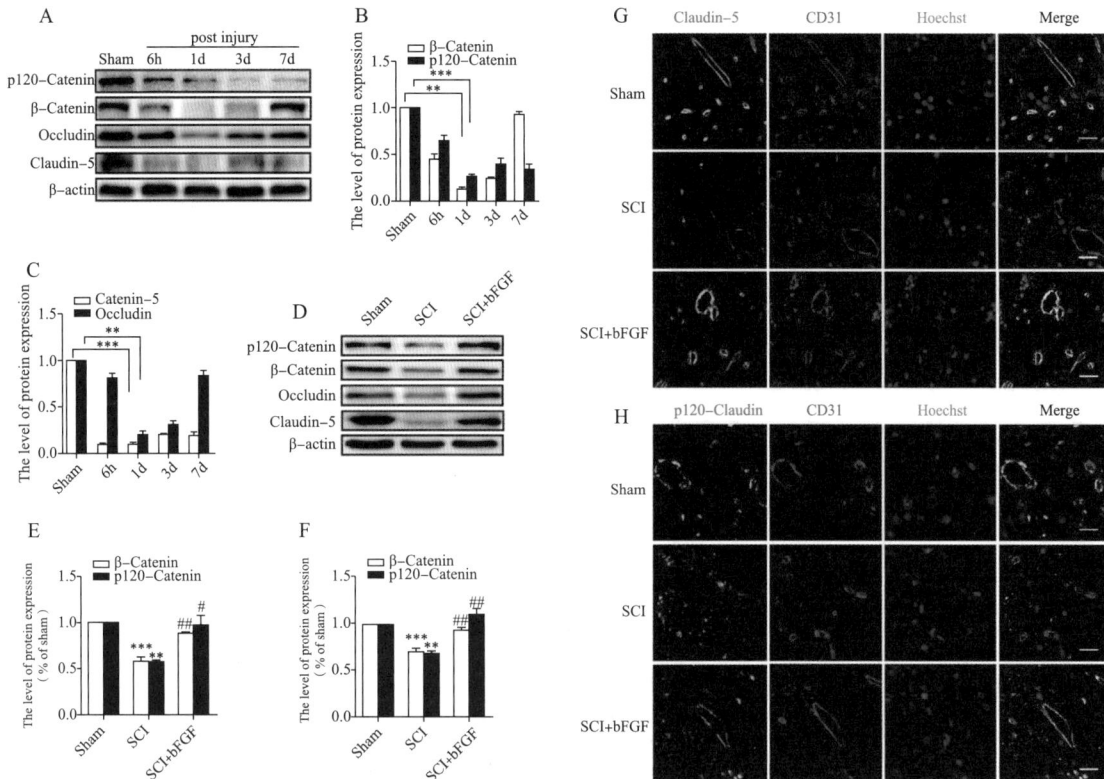

Fig. 3. Basic fibroblast growth factor (bFGF) prevents the loss of tight junction (TJ) and adherens junction (AJ) proteins after spinal cord injury (SCI). (A) The protein levels of p120-catenin, β-catenin, occludin, and claudin-5 at 6 h–7 d after injury. (B) Densitometric analyses of p120-catenin and β-catenin. Data were analyzed by ANOVA (β-catenin: $F_{(4, 10)} = 158.458$, $P < 0.001$; p120-catenin: $F_{(4, 10)} = 39.625$, $P < 0.001$). Post-hoc analyses were done using Bonferroni's multiple comparison test ($^{**}P < 0.01$, $^{***}P < 0.001$). (C) Densitometric analyses of occludin and claudin-5. Data were analyzed by ANOVA (claudin-5: $F_{(4, 10)} = 360.991$, $P < 0.001$; occludin: $F_{(4, 10)} = 70.827$, $P < 0.001$). Post-hoc analyses were done using Bonferroni's multiple comparison test ($^{**}P < 0.01$, $^{***}P < 0.001$). (D) Protein levels of TJ and AJ proteins 1 d after bFGF treatment. (E) Densitometric analyses of p120-catenin and β-catenin. Data were analyzed by ANOVA (β-catenin: $F_{(2, 6)} = 68.213$, $P < 0.001$; p120-catenin: $F_{(2, 6)} = 15.736$, $P = 0.004$). Post-hoc analyses were done using Bonferroni's multiple comparison test ($^{**}P < 0.01$, $^{***}P < 0.001$ vs Sham, $^{#}P < 0.05$, $^{##}P < 0.01$ vs SCI). (F) Densitometric analyses of occludin and claudin-5. Data were analyzed by ANOVA (claudin-5: $F_{(2, 6)} = 36.956$, $P < 0.001$; occludin: $F_{(2, 6)} = 32.484$, $P = 0.001$). Post-hoc analyses were done using Bonferroni's multiple comparison test ($^{**}P < 0.01$ vs sham, $^{##}P < 0.01$ vs SCI). (G) Double immunofluorescence shows that claudin-5 (green) co-localizes in endothelial cells (CD31, red). The background is staining of the blood cells. (H) Double immuno- fluorescence of p120-catenin (green) and CD31 (red). Scale bar = 25 μm.

4A, B, C). In addition, bFGF increased the expression of Cav-1 (Fig. 4D, E). Interestingly, as shown in Fig. 4F, Cav-1 was co-localized with CD31 (marker of endothelial cells) but not with NeuN (marker of neurons) or GFAP (marker of astrocytes), suggesting that Cav-1 was only located in endothelial cells in normal spinal cord. Therefore, we presume that bFGF exerts its beneficial role in BSCB integrity in relation to its regulation of Cav-1.

3.5 bFGF inhibits the levels of TJ and the activation of MMP-9 in HBMEC after OGD

Endothelial monolayer is the main component of the BBB or BSCB. Its partitioning, underlying tissue from blood components in the vessel wall, maintains the tissue fluid balance and host defense through dynamically opening intercellular junctions. To investigate the effect of bFGF on barrier integrity, we exposed HBMEC to OGD conditions. First, we examined whether bFGF affects the alteration of TJ and AJ proteins. The expression levels of p120-catenin, β-catenin, occludin, and claudin-5 decreased at 12 h after exposure to OGD conditions, and this effect was significantly reversed by bFGF (Fig. 5A, C, D). Moreover, expression and activation of MMP-9 were detected in HBMEC. We found that bFGF inhibited MMP-9 expression and activation, which was stimulated under OGD conditions, but MMP-2 presented no significant changes (Fig. 5F). As is known, astrocytes and neurons are important sources of MMP-2/MMP-9. Therefore, it would be interesting to deter-mine whether bFGF can affect MMP-2/MMP-9 activation in these 2 cell types. We found that the rapid activation of MMP-2/MMP-9 was inhibited by bFGF in astrocytes under OGD conditions (Fig. 5;

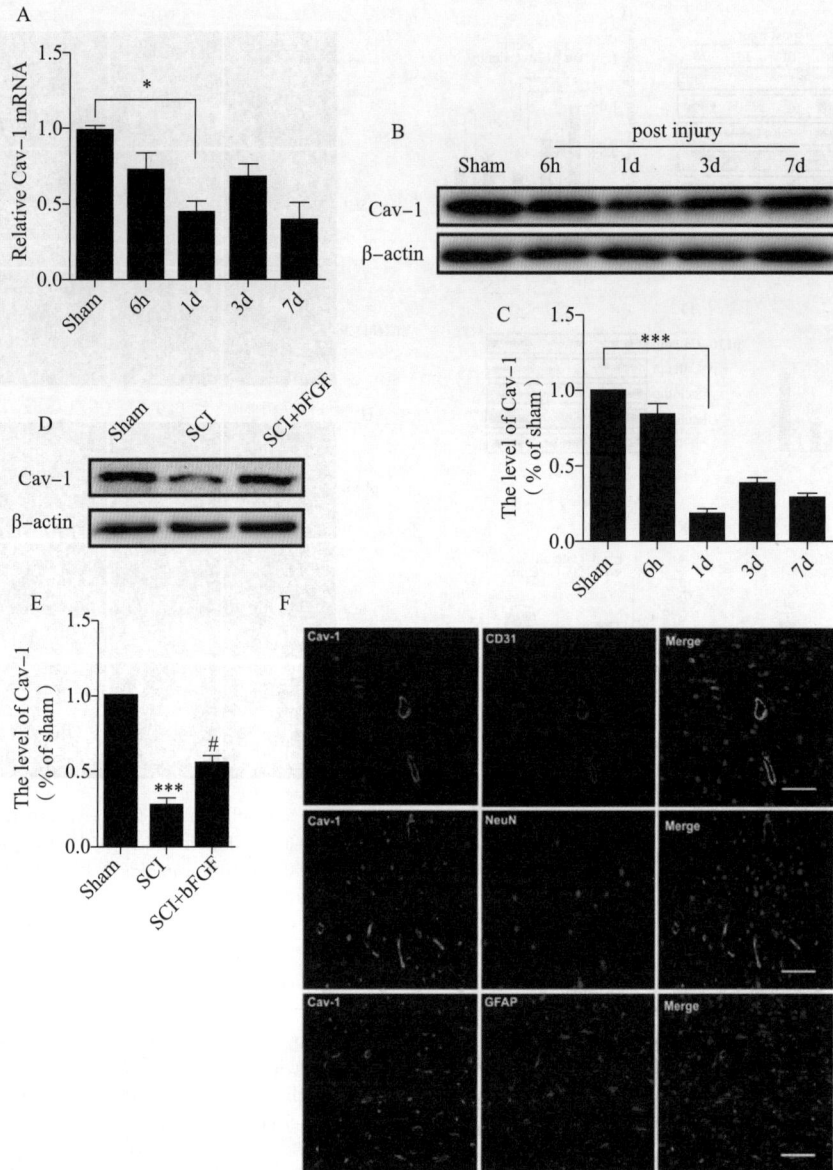

Fig. 4. Basic fibroblast growth factor (bFGF) increases the level of caveolin-1 (Cav-1) in endothelial cells after spinal cord injury. (A) mRNA levels of Cav-1 at 6 h–7 d after injury. Data were analyzed by ANOVA ($F_{[4, 19]} = 4.816$, $P = 0.007$). Post-hoc analyses were done using Bonferroni's multiple comparison test ($^{*}P < 0.05$). (B) Protein level of Cav-1 at 6 h–7 d after injury. (C) Densitometric analyses of Western blots. Data were analyzed by ANOVA ($F_{[4, 10]} = 71.280$, $P < 0.001$). Post-hoc analyses were done using Bonferroni's multiple comparison test ($^{*}P < 0.05$). (D) Protein level of Cav-1 at 1 d after bFGF treatment. (E) Densitometric analyses of Western blots. Data were analyzed by ANOVA ($F_{[2, 6]} = 74.499$, $P < 0.001$). Post-hoc analyses were done using Bonferroni's multiple comparison test ($^{***}P < 0.001$ vs Sham, $^{#}P < 0.05$ vs SCI). (F) Double immunofluorescence of Cav-1 (green) with CD31 (red, marker of endothelial cell), NeuN (red, marker of neuron), and glial fibrillary acidic protein (red, marker of astrocyte). Scale bar = 50 μm.

upper panel). However, there was no apparent MMP-9 activation in SH-SY5Y (middle panel; Fig. 5H). As our *in vivo* results have shown that MMP-9 was also expressed in neurons (Supplementary Fig. 2C), to clarify the inconsistent results, we performed the same experiments in cultured primary hippocampal neurons. As is shown in Fig. 5H (bottom panel), bFGF inhibited the activation of MMP-9 induced by OGD. These data imply that bFGF inhibits the loss of junction proteins, and reduces the expression and activation of MMP-9, but not MMP-2, in endothelial cells under OGD conditions.

3.6 The repair effect of bFGF on endothelial barrier is partly mediated by Cav-1

To support our hypothesis that the effect of bFGF is related to Cav-1 *in vitro*, Cav-1 siRNA was transfected to en-

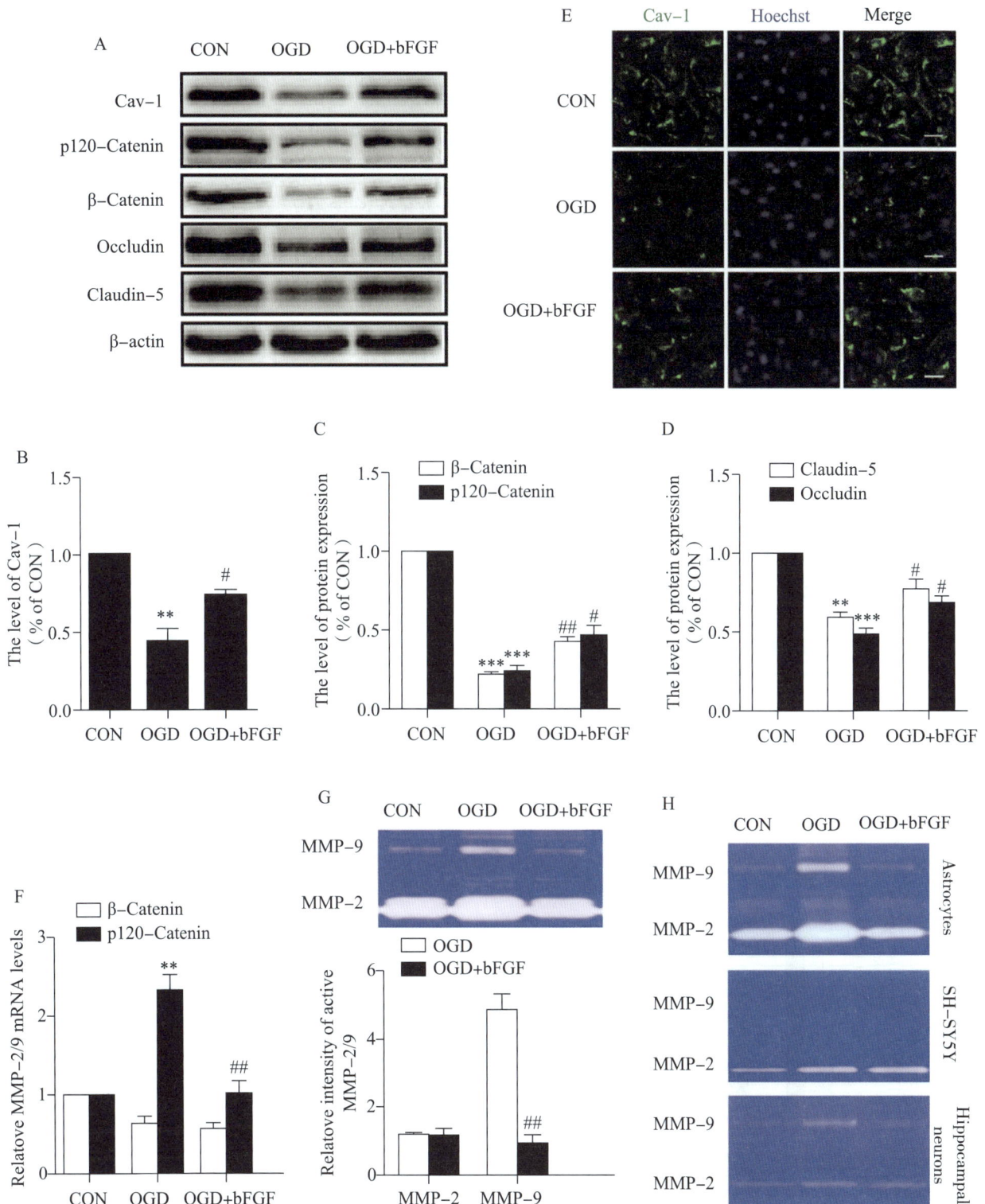

Fig. 5. Basic fibroblast growth factor (bFGF) inhibits the loss of caveolin-1 (Cav-1) and junction proteins, and attenuates the elevation of extracellular matrix metalloproteinase (MMP)-9 levels in endothelial cells after oxygen–glucose deprivation (OGD). (A) Protein levels of Cav-1, p120-catenin, β-catenin, occludin, and claudin-5 after 12 h of OGD. Densitometric analyses of (B) Cav-1, (C) adherens junction proteins, (D) and tight junction proteins. Data were analyzed by ANOVA (Cav-1: $F_{(2, 6)}$ = 26.702, P = 0.001; p120-catenin: $F_{(2, 6)}$ = 91.763, P < 0.001; β-catenin: $F_{(2, 6)}$ = 472.576, P < 0.001; occludin: $F_{(2, 6)}$ =53.484, P < 0.001; claudin-5: $F_{(2, 6)}$ = 27.251, P = 0.001). Post-hoc analyses were done using Bonferroni's multiple comparison test [**P < 0.01, ***P < 0.001 vs control (CON), #P < 0.05, ##P < 0.01 vs OGD]. (E) Immunocytochemistry of Cav-1 from fixed human brain microvascular endothelial cells after OGD for 12 h. Scale bar = 50 μm. (F) The mRNA levels of MMP-2/MMP-9 after 12 h of OGD in each group. Data were analyzed by ANOVA (MMP-9: $F_{(2, 6)}$ = 23.723, P = 0.001). Post-hoc analyses were done using Bonferroni's multiple comparison test (**P <0.01 vs. CON, ##P < 0.01 vs OGD). (G) Gelatin zymography and densitometric analyses for cell medium in endothelial cell after OGD. Data were analyzed by Student's t test (MMP-9: t = 7.623, P = 0.002, ##P <0.01 vs. OGD). (H) Gelatin zymography for cell medium in astrocytes (upper panel), neuronal cells line SH-SY5Y (middle panel), and primary hippocampal neuron (bottom panel). *P < 0.05, **P < 0.01 vs. CON, #P < 0.05 vs. OGD.

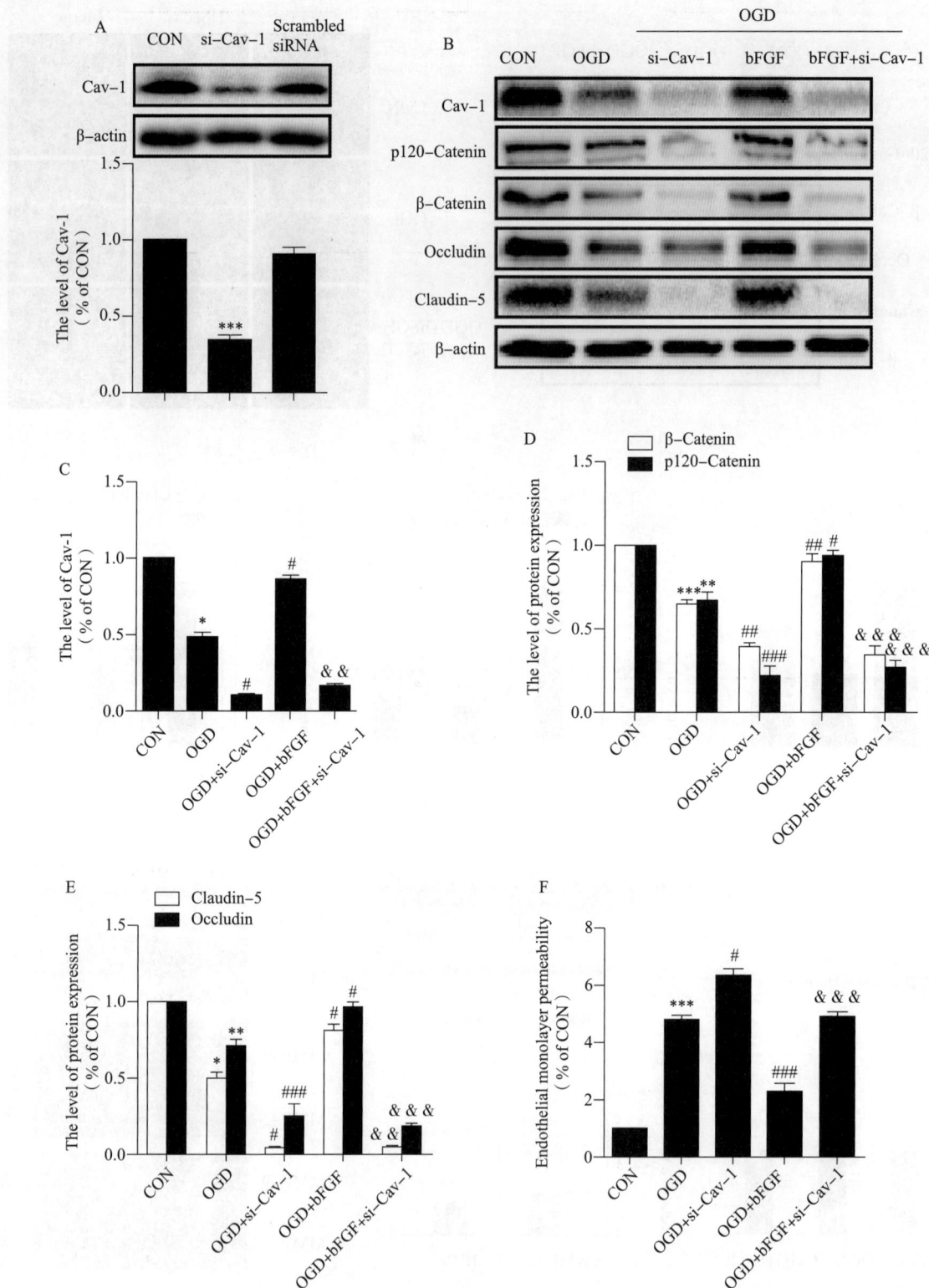

Fig. 6. Knockdown of caveolin-1 (Cav-1) reversed the protective effect of basic fibroblast growth factor (bFGF). (A) The effect of Cav-1 small interfering RNA (siRNA) under normal conditions. Data were analyzed by ANOVA ($F_{(2, 6)} = 122.751$, $P < 0.001$). Post-hoc analyses were done using Bonferroni's multiple comparison test ($^{***}P < 0.01$). (B) The protein levels of Cav-1, p120-catenin, β-catenin, occludin and claudin-5. Densitometric analyses of (C) Cav-1, (D) adherens junction proteins and tight junction proteins. Data were analyzed by ANOVA (Cav-1: $F_{(4, 10)} = 313.787$, $P < 0.001$; p120-catenin: $F_{(4, 10)} = 65.428$, $P < 0.001$; β-catenin: $F_{(4, 10)} = 70.302$, $P < 0.001$; occludin: $F_{(4, 10)} = 76.124$, $P < 0.001$; claudin5: $F_{(4, 10)} = 320.234$, $P < 0.001$). Post-hoc analyses were done using Bonferroni's multiple comparison test [$^*P < 0.05$, $^{**}P < 0.01$, $^{***}P < 0.001$ vs control (CON), $^#P < 0.05$, $^{##}P < 0.01$, $^{###}P < 0.001$ vs. OGD, $^{&&}P < 0.01$, $^{&&&}P < 0.001$ vs. OGD + bFGF]. (E) The permeability of FITC– dextran across endothelial cells monolayers in the endothelial cells transfected with Cav-1 siRNA under oxygen–glucose deprivation conditions. Data were analyzed by ANOVA ($F_{(4, 10)} = 100.817$, $P < 0.001$). Post-hoc analyses were done using Bonferroni's multiple comparison test ($^{***}P < 0.001$ vs. CON, $^#P < 0.05$, $^{###}P < 0.001$ vs. OGD, $^{&&&}P < 0.001$ vs. OGD + bFGF).

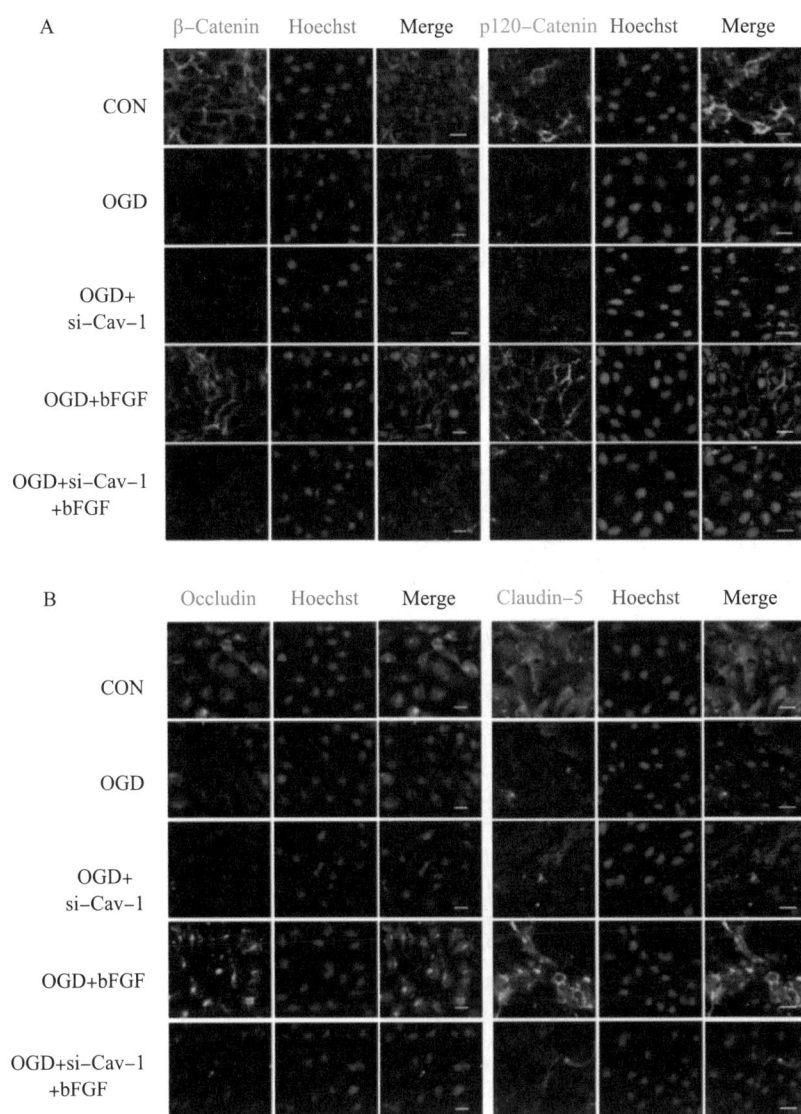

Fig. 7. Immunofluorescence of adherens junction and tight junction proteins. (A) Immunofluorescence of p120-catenin and β-catenin. (B) Immunofluorescence of occludin and claudin-5. Scale bar = 50 μm. All results represent 3 independent experiments.

dothelial cells. bFGF attenuated the reduction of Cav-1 expression by OGD in both Western blot and immunofluorescence analyses (Fig. 5A, B, E), which was consistent with our *in vivo* results . To assess the full level of knockdown, we checked the effects of Cav-1 siRNA on Cav-1 protein under control conditions. The results showed the rate of knockdown is about 65% and a scrambled siRNA control gives no significant difference compared with normal control. Fig. 6(B–E) shows that the effect of bFGF on junction proteins was significantly reversed by Cav-1 siRNA. The results of immunofluorescence further confirmed that bFGF mediating junction protein was partly through Cav-1 (Fig. 7A, B). To study the roles of bFGF and Cav-1 on endothelial barriers, cell monolayer permeability was examined by FITC–dextran permeating to the lower chamber. As illustrated in Fig. 6F, OGD remarkably elevated the quantity of FITC–dextran across the endothelial barrier, and the knockdown of Cav-1 enhanced this disruption, demonstrating the essential role of Cav-1 in the maintenance of barrier integrity. bFGF treatment alone significantly reduced the permeability of the OGD-treated cell monolayer to FITC–dextran, suggesting the protective role of bFGF in endothelial barrier integrity, which further confirmed our results *in vivo*. Moreover, Cav-1 siRNA strongly reversed the effect of bFGF. These data demonstrate that the repair function of bFGF on the endothelial barrier is partly mediated by Cav-1.

3.7 Interaction of Cav-1 and FGFR1 is essential for the function of bFGF in endothelial cells

To further investigate how Cav-1 exerts its role, we examined the expression of FGFR1, a major receptor of bFGF. As shown in Fig. 8(A, B), the expression of Cav-1 decreased under OGD conditions, while FGFR1 showed no obvi-

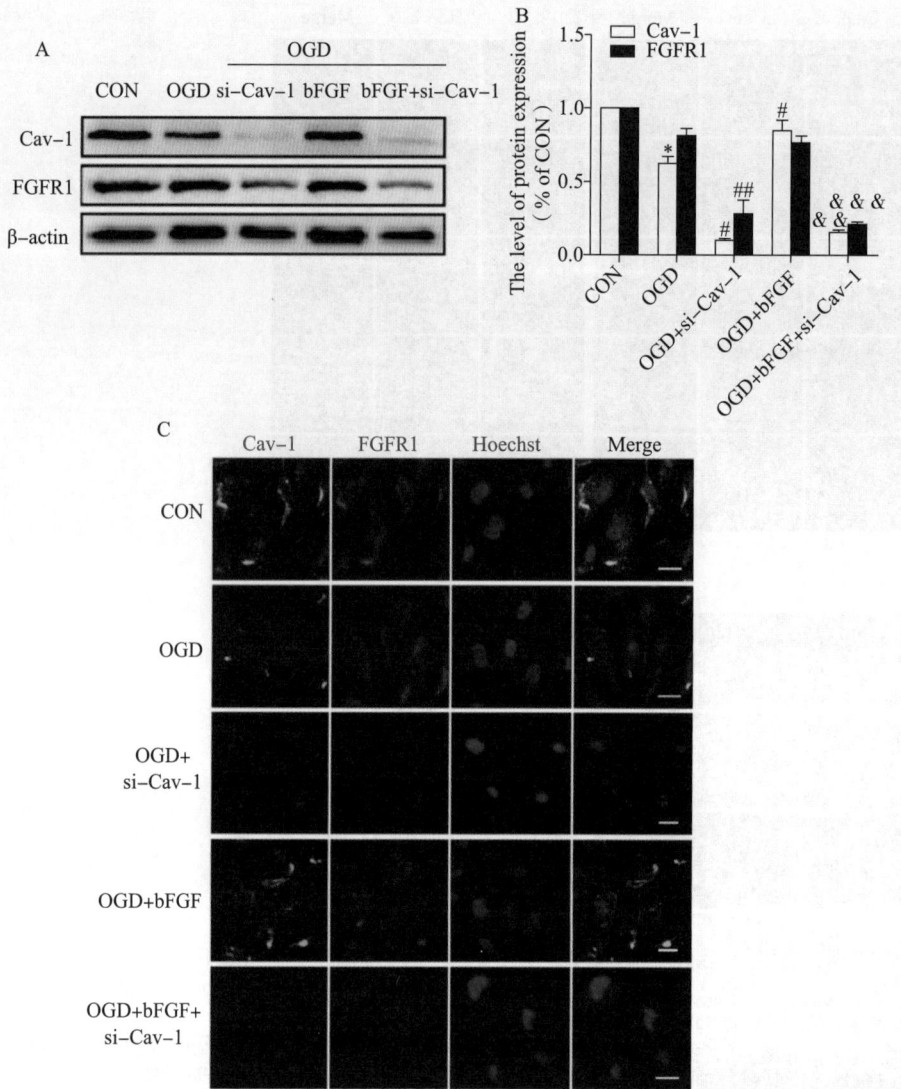

Fig. 8. Expression and co-localization of caveolin-1 (Cav-1) and fibroblast growth factor receptor 1 (FGFR1_ in the endothelial cells. (A) Protein levels of Cav-1 and FGFR1 in the endothelial cells transfected with Cav-1 small interfering RNA under oxygen–glucose deprivation (OGD) conditions for 12 h, treated by basic fibroblast growth factor (bFGF). (B) Densitometric analyses of Cav-1 and FGFR1. Data were analyzed by ANOVA (FGFR1: $F^{[4, 10]} = 37.415$, $P < 0.001$; Cav-1: $F^{[4, 10]} = 313.787$, $P < 0.001$). Post-hoc analyses were done using Bonferroni's multiple comparison test ([*]$P < 0.05$ *vs.* CON, [#]$P < 0.05$, [##]$P < 0.01$ *vs.* OGD, [&&]$P < 0.01$, [&&&]$P < 0.001$ *vs.* OGD + bFGF). (C) Co-localization detection by immunofluorescence staining of Cav-1 (green) and FGFR1 (red), and the nucleus is labeled by Hoechst (blue). Scale bar = 20 μm.

ous change. The transfection of Cav-1 siRNA reduced the level of Cav-1 significantly, and inhibited FGFR1 expression, which could not be reversed by bFGF treatment, suggesting that Cav-1 was closely related to the regulation of FGFR1. To elucidate the interaction of Cav-1 and FGFR1, immunofluorescence detection was applied. We found the co-localization of Cav-1 and FGFR1 on the membranes of endothelial cells in normal conditions, and the level of Cav-1 and FGFR1 decreased significantly in the siRNA transfected cells. bFGF treatment could not preserve FGFR1 compared with untransfected cells (Fig. 8C). Collectively, these data suggest that Cav-1 might be essential for the protective effect of bFGF, largely owing to its co-localization with FGFR1, which might relate to the activation of downstream FGF signal pathways.

4. Discussion

BSCB disruption occurs under various pathological conditions, such as SCI and amyotrophic lateral sclerosis. Traumatic SCI results in dramatic alteration of the spinal cord blood flow and causes systemic hypotension as a result of the interruption of descending sympathetic circuits [31]. SCI pathology resulted in rapid, permanent changes to the structure and function of the microvessels at the cellular level [32, 33]. In our study, the BSCB was significantly disrupted at 1 d after injury, *via* the evaluation of the extravasation of Evans Blue dye and FITC–dextran (Fig. 1), which is in agreement with previous reports [29, 34-36]. bFGF is demonstrated to preserve blood-brain barrier (BBB) integrity through RhoA inhibition after intracerebral hemorrhage in mice [23]. Moreover, in the *in vitro* BBB model, initial contact of glioblastoma cells with normal brain endothelial cells strengthens the barrier function *via* bFGF secretion, and a neutralization antibody for bFGF inhibits the recovery of BBB function [37]. Our previous reports show that bFGF treatment improves functional recovery after SCI, in part by inhibiting the apoptosis of neurons by inhibiting excessive autophagy and endoplasmic reticulum stress [21, 22]. However, whether bFGF has a beneficial role in BSCB recovery remains unclear. In this study, we found that bFGF treatment effectively prevented BSCB disruption both *in vivo* and *in vitro*. Changes in the expression and distribution of TJ and AJ proteins are closely related to the permeability of BSCB during SCI [38]. The levels of occludin, or zonula occludens 1 (ZO-1), are decreased at 1 or 3 d after SCI [25, 39]. It has been reported that occludin, claudin-5, and ZO-1 are lost or degraded at 48 h post injury, which aggravates the disruption of BSCB integrity [40]. Our data showed that the expression of occludin and claudin-5 apparently decreased at 1 d after injury, while bFGF significantly inhibited the reduction of these molecules *in vivo* and *in vitro* (Figs. 3, 5). Moreover, bFGF treatment enhanced the expression of AJ protein in endothelial cells. Consistent with our previous study, we concluded that bFGF had a therapeutic effect in the early stage of SCI *via* improving the BBB scores and pathological morphology at 3 d postinjury.

Upregulation of MMP-9 mediates BSCB disruption by degrading the basal components of TJ junctions and AJ junctions, thereby facilitating the infiltration of immune cells and initiating SCI-induced secondary damage [41]. Valproic acid inhibits ischemia-induced BBB disruption and brain edema by inhibiting MMP-9 induction and TJ breakdown. In our study, the expression and enzyme activity of MMP-9 were upregulated at 1 d after SCI, and inhibited by bFGF significantly (Fig. 2 and Supplementary Fig. 2). Moreover, the upregulation of MMP-2 also contributes to the initial opening of the BBB by degrading the basal lamina leading to neuronal injury [42]. Several studies have reported that active MMP-2 appeared at 5 d after SCI [25]. Interestingly, our results showed no obvious activation of MMP-2 at 1 d after injury (Fig. 2). In addition, the expression and activity of MMP-9 was markedly inhibited by bFGF treatment in OGD-induced endothelial cells. The mechanism of bFGF inhibiting MMP-9 activity in SCI has no related investigation, which needs to be further discussed in our next projects.

After ischemia-reperfusion in the brain, Cav-1 is remarkably downregulated in brain microvessels [43]. Cav-1 deficiency in mice led to higher MMPs activities and BBB permeability than in wild-type mice [44]. Cav-1 regulates the expression of junction-associated proteins in the brain micro-vascular endothelial cells; attenuated Cav-1 level is correlated with heightened permeability of endothelia [14]. In addition, Cav-1 knockout mice present higher microvascular permeability in the tumor barrier, and the loss of Cav-1 increases tumor permeability and growth, which may relate to enhanced VEGF signaling or decreased vascular endothelial cadherin [45]. The opening of AJs observed in Cav-1 knockout endothelium suggests that Cav-1 is necessary for AJ assembly or maintenance, which contributes to endothelial barrier function [15]. Our results showed that Cav-1 expression was reduced after SCI, as shown by both mRNA and protein levels (Fig. 4), similar to the progress of TJ and AJ protein expression in SCI. The expression of Cav-1 was highly decreased at 1 d after SCI, which was increased with bFGF administration (Fig. 4), suggesting that degradation of TJ and AJ proteins may be associated with the expression of Cav-1. Our data showed that the upregulation of TJ and AJ proteins by bFGF were reversed by Cav-1 siRNA. Furthermore, Cav-1 siRNA strongly increased the permeability, but with bFGF (Fig. 6). These results indicated that the repair effect of bFGF on the endothelial barrier was partially mediated by Cav-1. However, views of the role of Cav-1 in different pathologies are contradictory. In several models of adult brain injuries, Cav-1 is increased in the endothelium for several days following cold cortical injury and brain ischemia [10, 11]. In the cortical cold injury model in rats, an increased expression of Cav-1 precedes the decreased expression of occludin and claudin-5 at 2 d postinjury [11]. The Cav-1 protein in the membrane fraction of microvessels begins to upregulate at 5 min and reached a peak 10 min after treatment, which was associated with diminished expression of several TJ-associated proteins (ZO-1, occludin, and claudin-5), which led to in-creased BBB permeability [10]. This evidence suggests that the functions of Cav-1 are differential in different models or different organizations.

A recent study has illustrated that Cav-1 mediated growth factor-induced disassembly of adherens junctions to support tumor cell dissociation [46]. In the blood–tumor barrier, Cav-1 also participates in VEGF-mediated permeability [47].

Many studies have shown that Cav-1 is closely involved in the regulation of FGFR [48, 49]. Herein, we found the co-localization of Cav-1 and FGFR1 on the membranes of endothelial cells in normal conditions. However, the levels of Cav-1 decreased under OGD conditions, but FGFR1 did not change. Cav-1 siRNA dramatically reduced the expression of FGFR1, which could not be reversed by bFGF treatment (Fig. 8). A recent study has claimed that Cav-1 orchestrated bFGF downstream signaling control of angiogenesis in placental artery endothelial cells [50], but the interaction mechanism of Cav-1 and FGFR1 needs to be further investigated.

However, although abundant evidence suggests that bFGF has a therapeutic effect on SCI in rats [19, 22, 51], there has been no clinical trial investigating this. In acute stroke, a 24-h intravenous infusion of 5 mg bFGF has been confirmed as safe for patients and results in an improved outcome [52]. As the therapeutic potential of bFGF has been well recognized for decades, and the neuroprotection of FGF in SCI has already been translated to clinical trials [53, 54], it is reasonable to believe that bFGF will be applied to the clinic. In addition, the combination of a delivery system or special biomaterials to increase its stability and prolong the half-life might contribute to the utility of bFGF.

In conclusion, this study has demonstrated that bFGF improves the recovery of BSCB in an SCI model by increasing junction proteins and the key element Cav-1, inhibiting the expression and activation of MMP-9. In endothelial cells, bFGF treatment also increases the levels of junction proteins; Cav-1 siRNA abolished the effect of bFGF under OGD conditions, which might be related to the co-localization of Cav-1 and FGFR1. Taken together, our results suggest that bFGF may provide an effective therapeutic intervention by preventing BSCB disruption *via* the critical determinant Cav-1 after SCI, which involves interactions with FGFR1.

Supplementary material

Supplementary material to this article can be found in the online version (doi:10.1007/s13311-016-0437-3).

References

[1] Kaneko S, Iwanami A, Nakamura M, et al. A selective Sema3A inhibitor enhances regenerative responses and functional recovery of the injured spinal cord[J]. Nat Med, 2006, 12(12): 1380-1389.

[2] Mikami Y, Toda M, Watanabe M, et al. A simple and reliable behavioral analysis of locomotor function after spinal cord injury in mice. Technical note[J]. J Neurosurg, 2002, 97(1 Suppl): 142-147.

[3] Jeong SR, Kwon MJ, Lee HG, et al. Hepatocyte growth factor reduces astrocytic scar formation and promotes axonal growth beyond glial scars after spinal cord injury[J]. Exp Neurol, 2012, 233(1): 312-322.

[4] Giszter SF. Spinal cord injury: present and future therapeutic devices and prostheses[J]. Neurotherapeutics, 2008, 5(1): 147-162.

[5] Bartanusz V, Jezova D, Alajajian B, et al. The blood-spinal cord barrier: morphology and clinical implications[J]. Ann Neurol, 2011, 70(2): 194-206.

[6] Sharma HS. Early microvascular reactions and blood-spinal cord barrier disruption are instrumental in pathophysiology of spinal cord injury and repair: novel therapeutic strategies including nanowired drug delivery to enhance neuroprotection[J]. J Neural Transm (Vienna), 2011, 118(1): 155-176.

[7] Fassbender JM, Whittemore SR, Hagg T. Targeting microvasculature for neuroprotection after SCI[J]. Neurotherapeutics, 2011, 8(2): 240-251.

[8] Okamoto T, Schlegel A, Scherer PE, et al. Caveolins, a family of scaffolding proteins for organizing "preassembled signaling complexes" at the plasma membrane[J]. J Biol Chem, 1998, 273(10): 5419-5422.

[9] Lisanti MP, Scherer PE, Tang Z, et al. Caveolae, caveolin and caveolin-rich membrane domains: a signalling hypothesis[J]. Trends Cell Biol, 1994, 4(7): 231-235.

[10] Wang P, Liu Y, Shang X, et al. CRM197-induced blood-brain barrier permeability increase is mediated by upregulation of caveolin-1 protein[J]. J Mol Neurosci, 2011, 43(3): 485-492.

[11] Nag S, Venugopalan R, Stewart DJ. Increased caveolin-1 expression precedes decreased expression of occludin and claudin-5 during blood-brain barrier breakdown[J]. Acta Neuropathol, 2007, 114(5): 459-469.

[12] Madaro L, Antonangeli F, Favia A, et al. Knock down of caveolin-1 affects morphological and functional hallmarks of human endothelial cells[J]. J Cell Biochem, 2013, 114(8): 1843-1851.

[13] Shen J, Ma S, Chan P, et al. Nitric oxide down-regulates caveolin-1 expression in rat brains during focal cerebral ischemia and reperfusion injury[J]. J Neurochem, 2006, 96(4): 1078-1089.

[14] Song L, Ge S, Pachter JS. Caveolin-1 regulates expression of junction-associated proteins in brain microvascular endothelial cells[J]. Blood, 2007, 109(4): 1515-1523.

[15] Siddiqui MR, Komarova YA, Vogel SM, et al. Caveolin-1-eNOS signaling promotes p190RhoGAP-A nitration and endothelial permeability[J]. J Cell Biol, 2011, 193(5): 841-850.

[16] Gu Y, Dee CM, Shen J. Interaction of free radicals, matrix metalloproteinases and caveolin-1 impacts blood-brain barrier permeability[J]. Front Biosci (Schol Ed), 2011, 3: 1216-1231.

[17] Schnell L, Schneider R, Kolbeck R, et al. Neurotrophin-3 enhances sprouting of corticospinal tract during development and after adult spinal cord lesion[J]. Nature, 1994, 367(6459): 170-173.

[18] Cheng H, Cao Y, Olson L. Spinal cord repair in adult paraplegic rats: partial restoration of hind limb function[J]. Science, 1996, 273(5274): 510-513.

[19] Rabchevsky AG, Fugaccia I, Fletcher-Turner A, et al. Basic fibroblast growth factor (bFGF) enhances tissue sparing and functional

recovery following moderate spinal cord injury[J]. J Neurotrauma, 1999, 16(9): 817-830.

[20] Rabchevsky AG, Fugaccia I, Turner AF, *et al.* Basic fibroblast growth factor (bFGF) enhances functional recovery following severe spinal cord injury to the rat[J]. Exp Neurol, 2000, 164(2): 280-291.

[21] Zhang HY, Wang ZG, Wu FZ, *et al.* Regulation of autophagy and ubiquitinated protein accumulation by bFGF promotes functional recovery and neural protection in a rat model of spinal cord injury[J]. Mol Neurobiol, 2013, 48(3): 452-464.

[22] Zhang HY, Zhang X, Wang ZG, *et al.* Exogenous basic fibroblast growth factor inhibits ER stress-induced apoptosis and improves recovery from spinal cord injury[J]. CNS Neurosci Ther, 2013, 19(1): 20-29.

[23] Huang B, Krafft PR, Ma Q, *et al.* Fibroblast growth factors preserve blood-brain barrier integrity through RhoA inhibition after intracerebral hemorrhage in mice[J]. Neurobiol Dis, 2012, 46(1): 204-214.

[24] Figley SA, Khosravi R, Legasto JM, *et al.* Characterization of vascular disruption and blood-spinal cord barrier permeability following traumatic spinal cord injury[J]. J Neurotrauma, 2014, 31(6): 541-552.

[25] Lee JY, Kim HS, Choi HY, *et al.* Fluoxetine inhibits matrix metalloprotease activation and prevents disruption of blood-spinal cord barrier after spinal cord injury[J]. Brain, 2012, 135(Pt 8): 2375-2389.

[26] Basso DM, Beattie MS, Bresnahan JC. A sensitive and reliable locomotor rating scale for open field testing in rats[J]. J Neurotrauma, 1995, 12(1): 1-21.

[27] Ma X, Zhang H, Pan Q, *et al.* Hypoxia/Aglycemia-induced endothelial barrier dysfunction and tight junction protein downregulation can be ameliorated by citicoline[J]. PLoS One, 2013, 8(12): e82604.

[28] Zhang H, Chang M, Hansen CN, *et al.* Role of matrix metalloproteinases and therapeutic benefits of their inhibition in spinal cord injury[J]. Neurotherapeutics, 2011, 8(2): 206-220.

[29] Lee JY, Choi HY, Na WH, *et al.* Ghrelin inhibits BSCB disruption/hemorrhage by attenuating MMP-9 and SUR1/TrpM4 expression and activation after spinal cord injury[J]. Biochim Biophys Acta, 2014, 1842(12 Pt A): 2403-2412.

[30] Daneman R, Zhou L, Kebede AA, *et al.* Pericytes are required for blood-brain barrier integrity during embryogenesis[J]. Nature, 2010, 468(7323): 562-566.

[31] Hagen EM, Rekand T, Gronning M, *et al.* Cardiovascular complications of spinal cord injury[J]. Tidsskr Nor Laegeforen, 2012, 132(9): 1115-1120.

[32] Benton RL, Maddie MA, Minnillo DR, *et al.* Griffonia simplicifolia isolectin B4 identifies a specific subpopulation of angiogenic blood vessels following contusive spinal cord injury in the adult mouse[J]. J Comp Neurol, 2008, 507(1): 1031-1052.

[33] Utepbergenov DI, Mertsch K, Sporbert A, *et al.* Nitric oxide protects blood-brain barrier *in vitro* from hypoxia/reoxygenation-mediated injury[J]. FEBS Lett, 1998, 424(3): 197-201.

[34] Popovich PG, Horner PJ, Mullin BB, *et al.* A quantitative spatial analysis of the blood-spinal cord barrier. I. Permeability changes after experimental spinal contusion injury[J]. Exp Neurol, 1996, 142(2): 258-275.

[35] Noble LJ, Wrathall JR. Distribution and time course of protein extravasation in the rat spinal cord after contusive injury[J]. Brain Res, 1989, 482(1): 57-66.

[36] Lee JY, Choi HY, Ahn HJ, *et al.* Matrix metalloproteinase-3 promotes early blood-spinal cord barrier disruption and hemorrhage and impairs long-term neurological recovery after spinal cord injury[J]. Am J Pathol, 2014, 184(11): 2985-3000.

[37] Toyoda K, Tanaka K, Nakagawa S, *et al.* Initial contact of glioblastoma cells with existing normal brain endothelial cells strengthen the barrier function *via* fibroblast growth factor 2 secretion: a new *in vitro* blood-brain barrier model[J]. Cell Mol Neurobiol, 2013, 33(4): 489-501.

[38] Liebner S, Czupalla CJ, Wolburg H. Current concepts of blood-brain barrier development[J]. Int J Dev Biol, 2011, 55(4-5): 467-476.

[39] Lee JY, Kim HS, Choi HY, *et al.* Valproic acid attenuates blood-spinal cord barrier disruption by inhibiting matrix metalloprotease-9 activity and improves functional recovery after spinal cord injury[J]. J Neurochem, 2012, 121(5): 818-829.

[40] Wu Q, Jing Y, Yuan X, *et al.* Melatonin treatment protects against acute spinal cord injury-induced disruption of blood spinal cord barrier in mice[J]. J Mol Neurosci, 2014, 54(4): 714-722.

[41] Noble LJ, Donovan F, Igarashi T, *et al.* Matrix metalloproteinases limit functional recovery after spinal cord injury by modulation of early vascular events[J]. J Neurosci, 2002, 22(17): 7526-7535.

[42] Dang AB, Tay BK, Kim HT, *et al.* Inhibition of MMP2/MMP9 after spinal cord trauma reduces apoptosis[J]. Spine (Phila Pa 1976), 2008, 33(17): E576-E579.

[43] Fu S, Gu Y, Jiang JQ, *et al.* Calycosin-7-O-beta-D-glucoside regulates nitric oxide /caveolin-1/matrix metalloproteinases pathway and protects blood-brain barrier integrity in experimental cerebral ischemia-reperfusion injury[J]. J Ethnopharmacol, 2014, 155(1): 692-701.

[44] Gu Y, Zheng G, Xu M, *et al.* Caveolin-1 regulates nitric oxide-mediated matrix metalloproteinases activity and blood-brain barrier permeability in focal cerebral ischemia and reperfusion injury[J]. J Neurochem, 2012, 120(1): 147-156.

[45] Lin MI, Yu J, Murata T, *et al.* Caveolin-1-deficient mice have increased tumor microvascular permeability, angiogenesis, and growth[J]. Cancer Res, 2007, 67(6): 2849-2856.

[46] Orlichenko L, Weller SG, Cao H, *et al.* Caveolae mediate growth factor-induced disassembly of adherens junctions to support tumor cell dissociation[J]. Mol Biol Cell, 2009, 20(19): 4140-4152.

[47] Zhao LN, Yang ZH, Liu YH, *et al.* Vascular endothelial growth factor increases permeability of the blood-tumor barrier *via* caveolae-mediated transcellular pathway[J]. J Mol Neurosci, 2011, 44(2): 122-129.

[48] Citores L, Wesche J, Kolpakova E, *et al.* Uptake and intracellular transport of acidic fibroblast growth factor: evidence for free and cytoskeleton-anchored fibroblast growth factor receptors[J]. Mol Biol Cell, 1999, 10(11): 3835-3848.

[49] Citores L, Khnykin D, Sorensen V, *et al.* Modulation of intracellular transport of acidic fibroblast growth factor by mutations in the cytoplasmic receptor domain[J]. J Cell Sci, 2001, 114(Pt 9): 1677-1689.

[50] Feng L, Liao WX, Luo Q, *et al.* Caveolin-1 orchestrates fibroblast growth factor 2 signaling control of angiogenesis in placental artery endothelial cell caveolae[J]. J Cell Physiol, 2012, 227(6): 2480-2491.

[51] Liu WG, Wang ZY, Huang ZS. Bone marrow-derived mesenchymal stem cells expressing the bFGF transgene promote axon regeneration and functional recovery after spinal cord injury in rats[J]. Neurol Res, 2011, 33(7): 686-693.

[52] Bogousslavsky J, Victor SJ, Salinas EO, *et al.* Fiblast (trafermin) in acute stroke: results of the European-Australian phase II/III safety and efficacy trial[J]. Cerebrovascular diseases, 2002, 14(3-4): 239-251.

[53] Wu JC, Huang WC, Chen YC, *et al.* Acidic fibroblast growth factor for repair of human spinal cord injury: a clinical trial[J]. J Neurosurg Spine, 2011, 15(3): 216-227.

[54] Wu JC, Huang WC, Tsai YA, *et al.* Nerve repair using acidic fibroblast growth factor in human cervical spinal cord injury: a preliminary Phase I clinical study[J]. J Neurosurg Spine, 2008, 8(3): 208-214.

The role of bFGF in the excessive activation of astrocytes is related to the inhibition of TLR4/NFκB signals

Libing Ye, Xiaokun Li, Li Lin, Hongyu Zhang

1. Introduction

In healthy neural systems, astrocytes have a critical role in immune defense, homeostasis of ions and transmitters, energy metabolism, regulation of blood flow, synaptic remodeling, and regulation of synapse function [1,2]. Astrocytes respond to all forms of CNS insults through a process that is referred to as reactive astrogliosis (also known as astrocyte activation), which shows an abnormal increase in the number of astrocytes [3,4]. These activated astrocytes undergo hypertrophy and show high levels of intermediate filaments, such as GFAP, vimentin, and nestin [5-7].

Although reactive astrogliosis is considered to be a defense mechanism of astrocytes to injury, such as limiting the infiltration of peripheral leukocytes, reconstructing the damaged barrier and migrating to the damaged area and filling the insult center [8-10], excessive glial activation can produce a pro-inflammatory environment and promote neuronal death [11-13]. Interleukin-1β (IL-1β), TNF-α and IL-6 are secreted in reactive astrocytes, which may be a first step in the development of several neurodegenerative diseases [14,15]. Furthermore, pro-inflammatory cytokines are known to further activate astrocytes [16,17]. Therefore, limiting the inflammatory response of activated astrocytes can serve to prevent neuroinflammation and neurodegeneration. Nuclear factor κB (NFκB), a transcription factor, has been shown to control inflammatory responses in astrocytes. As we all know, the activation of NFκB begins with the phosphorylation and the subsequent degradation of inhibitor of κB (IκB), which subsequently causes the translocation of free NFκB to the nucleus, where it promotes the expression of pro-inflammatory genes [18]. Toll-like receptor 4 (TLR4) is a member of the TLR family, which has a fundamental role in pathogen recognition and activation of innate immunity [19]. It is well known that TLR4-mediated signaling pathways mainly stimulate the activation of NFκB and the subsequent induction of genes that encode pro-inflammatory cytokines [20].

The secretion of bFGF from astrocytes and peripheral nerve pericytes under many injury conditions contributes to the modification of the blood-brain barrier and blood-nerve barrier function [21,22]. In spinal cord injury, bFGF is also upregulated in the spinal cord, which is beneficial for functional recovery [23,24]. Moreover, bFGF expression is induced in injured brain regions (mainly in astrocytes) after trauma and in the pathology of diseases [25,26], such as Alzheimer's, where astrogliosis is highly activated [27]. Conversely, exogenous bFGF treatment has been shown to decrease gliosis after spinal cord hemisection in mice [28]. Additionally, bFGF decreases the expression of GFAP both in mRNA and protein levels in astrocytes; moreover, it also inhibits transforming growth factor-β-mediated increase in GFAP [29]. Nevertheless, one study suggests that the activation of astrocyte is inhibited in both normal and injured brain *via* activating the FGF signaling [30]. Therefore, the exact role of bFGF after injury still remains unclear. In this present study, we used lipopolysaccharide (LPS) to stimulate primary astrocytes to mimic reactive astrogliosis and investigated the effect of different concentrations of bFGF in primary cultured astrocytes. Our data showed that astrocytes were activated by a low concentration of bFGF, which was reversed by a high dose of bFGF; the potential mechanism is related to the inhibition of TLR4/NFκB signals and the downregulation of the expression of GFAP and vimentin.

2. Results

2.1. LPS stimulates the expression and release of endogenous bFGF in primary cultured astrocytes

It has been reported that bFGF has a persistently up-regulated response to injury following the activation of as-

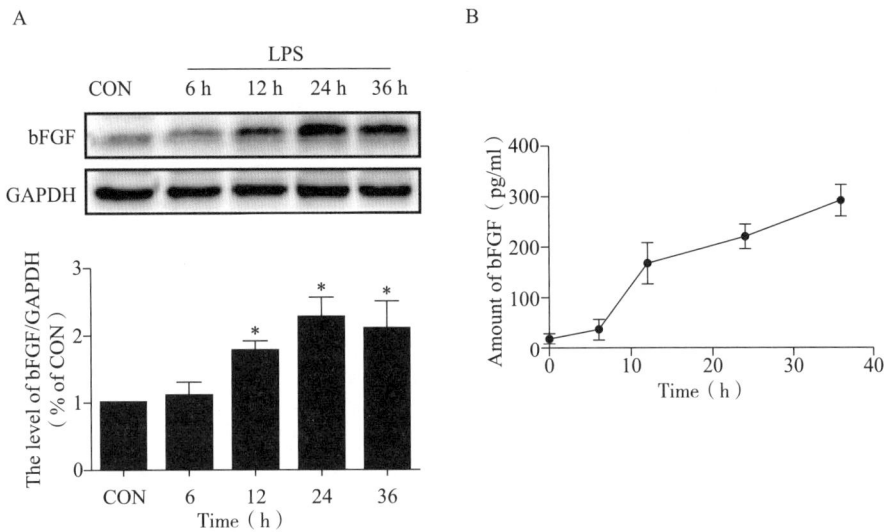

Fig. 1. Activation of astrocytes enhanced bFGF Release. LPS (2 μg/ml) was used to stimulate astrocytes for different times. (A) Western blot of bFGF and densitometric analyses; (B) ELISA of bFGF. *P < 0.05 *vs.* control (CON). All results represent at least three independent experiments.

trocytes [31]. Meanwhile, LPS is a classic activator of astrocytes *in vitro* [32,33]. To investigate the effect of LPS on the expression and release of endogenous bFGF in primary cultured astrocytes, we detected the protein level and release of bFGF at different times after LPS (2 μg/ml) treatment. bFGF was increased by LPS stimulation in a time-dependent manner (Fig. 1A) and significantly increased from 12 h after LPS administration (P < 0.01). Consistent with the results of protein blotting, the release of bFGF also showed a time-dependent increase in enzyme-linked immunosorbent assay (ELISA) analysis (Fig. 1B). The concentration of bFGF release was 16.7 ± 13.38 pg/ml under normal conditions, while it increased to 167.2 ± 70.63 pg/ml at 12 h after LPS stimulation (P < 0.01). These data suggest that the activation of astrocytes by LPS treatment enhances endogenous bFGF expression and release *in vitro*.

2.2 Exogenous bFGF attenuates the activation of astrocytes in a high concentration

The therapeutic potential of exogenous bFGF in CNS diseases has been well-recognized for decades [34,35], but the underlying mechanism in astrocyte activation is still under debate. It has been suggested that the observed increase of bFGF after neural injury would further activate astrocytes [36,37]. Interestingly, we found that bFGF with a low concentration, from 10 to 50 ng/ml, induced the activation of astrocytes, which was determined by GFAP immunofluorescence staining (Fig. 2A–E). Nevertheless, when the concentration increased to 100 or 200 ng/ml, there was less activation of GFAP in the primary cultured astrocytes (Fig. 2F,G). As is shown in Fig. 2H, the intensity of GFAP fluorescence is also enhanced after LPS treatment. These data indicate that bFGF might have dual roles in astrocyte activation.

2.3 Exogenous bFGF reduces the expression of GFAP and changes the morphology in LPS induced astrocytes

Currently, there are no relevant reports about whether bFGF can inhibit astrocytic activation in response to external stimulus, such as inflammation activators. To investigate the effect of bFGF on LPS-induced activation of astrocytes, we measured the expression of GFAP by western blot and immunofluorescence. As is shown in Fig. 3A, 25 ng/ml bFGF mentally decreased the protein level of GFAP after LPS stimulation (2 μg/ml). Furthermore, the expression of GFAP was significantly reduced at a dose of 100 ng/ml, which suggests that high doses of bFGF attenuated LPS-induced activation of astrocytes (Fig. 3A). Fig. 2B shows that following stimulation with LPS, most astrocytes displayed an extended cell body and enhanced fluorescence intensity, which indicates an activated reaction. However, treatment with bFGF at 100 ng/ml attenuated this morphological transformation. These data suggest that high doses of bFGF attenuate the activation of astrocytes which induced by LPS through reducing the expression of GFAP and blocking the changes in morphology.

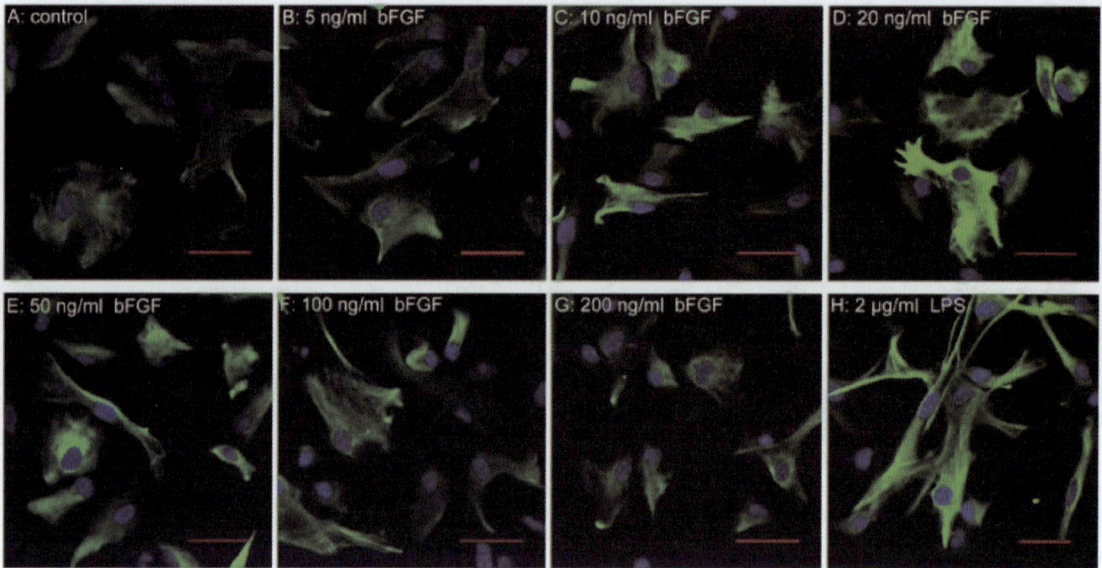

Fig. 2. Effect of bFGF on astrocyte activation. Immunofluorescence of GFAP (green) at different concentrations of bFGF and LPS (2 µg/ml). (A) Control; (B) 5 ng/ml; (C) 10 ng/ml; (D) 20 ng/ml; (E) 50 ng/ml; (F) 100 ng/ml; (G) 200 ng/ml; (H) LPS 2 µg/ml; Scale bar is 50 µm.

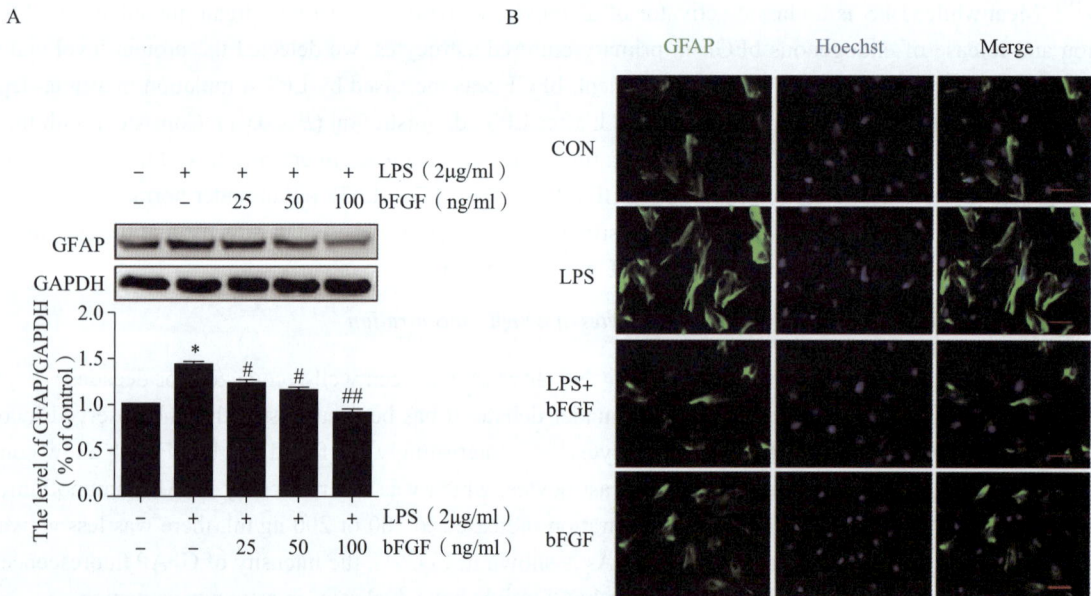

Fig. 3. Effect of bFGF on GFAP expression in astrocytes that were stimulated by LPS. LPS (2 µg/ml) was used to induce the activation of astrocytes for 24 h. Then, the effect of bFGF on astrocyte activation was investigated. (A) Western blot of GFAP at different concentrations of bFGF (25, 50, and 100 ng/ml); (B) Immunofluorescence of GFAP. $^*P < 0.05$ vs. CON, $^#P < 0.05$, $^{##}P < 0.01$ vs. LPS. All results represent at least three independent experiments; Scale bar is 50 µm.

2.4. Exogenous bFGF inhibits the expression of vimentin and neurocan in LPS-treated astrocytes

There are several markers in reactive astrocytes, such as GFAP, vimentin, nestin, and neurocan. To further verify the effect of bFGF in LPS-treated astrocytes, we detected the expression of vimentin and nestin. As is shown in Fig. 4A, LPS markedly increased the expression of vimentin, while exogenous bFGF (100 ng/ml) attenuated this increase. Notably, there was no significant change in nestin (Fig. 4A). At the same time, bFGF also decreased the upregulation of neurocan under LPS treatment (Fig. 4B). These data further confirm the role of bFGF in LPS-induced astrocytes, which also involves the activation of neurocan and vimentin.

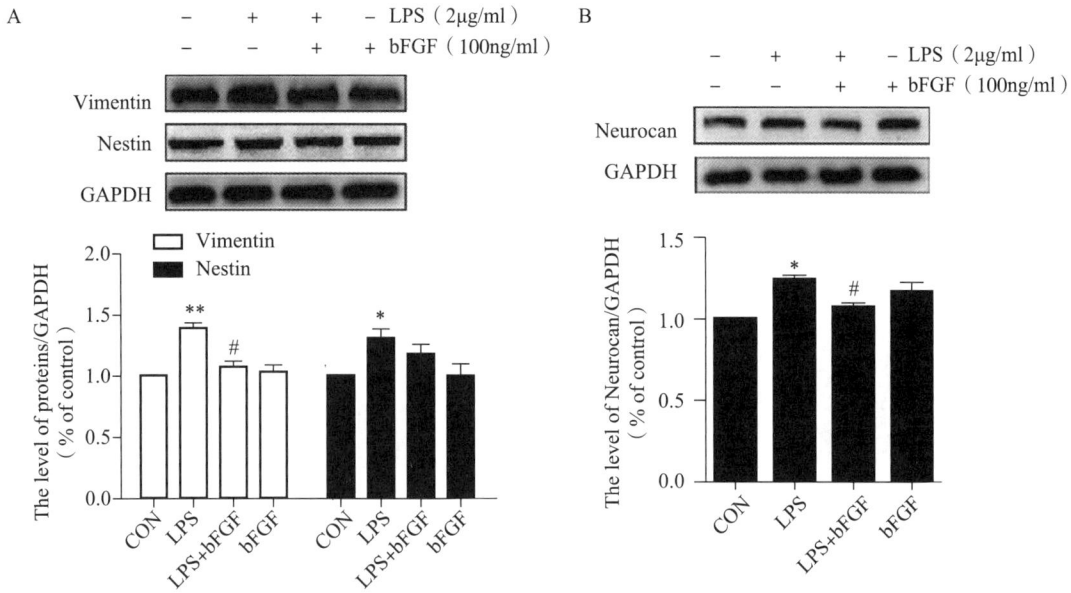

Fig. 4. Effect of bFGF on vimentin, nestin and neurocan in astrocytes stimulated by LPS. We measured additional markers of activated astrocytes. (A) Western blot of vimentin, nestin, and densitometric analyses; (B) Western blot of neurocan and densitometric analyses. $^{*}P < 0.05$, $^{**}P < 0.01$ vs. CON, $^{\#}P < 0.05$ vs. LPS. All results represent at least three independent experiments.

2.5　Exogenous bFGF inhibits the expression of pro-inflammatory cytokines in LPS-stimulated astrocytes

It is reported that astrocytes involve in normal and abnormal processes of the CNS via the release of cytokines [38]. Furthermore, the secretion of cytokines may further activate astrocytes [39]. We next evaluated the expression of pro-inflammatory cytokines following LPS stimulation with or without bFGF. We found that the expression of IL-6 and TNF-α were significantly increased when exposed astrocytes to LPS for 24 h (Fig. 5A,B), which was similar to the secretion level analysis (Fig. 5C,D). Nevertheless, bFGF at a high dose of 100 ng/ml reduced both the expression and secretion of IL-6 and TNF-α. These data indicate that bFGF might attenuate the activation of astrocytes induced by LPS via inhibiting inflammatory cytokines.

2.6　Exogenous bFGF reduces TLR4 expression induced by LPS

In CNS disorders, TLR4 is expressed in primary astrocytes, which relates to immune responses [40]. In our study, we measured the expression of TLR4 both in western blot and immunofluorescence stain. Our results suggest that the expression of TLR4 was markedly enhanced by LPS, and bFGF decreased the TLR4 level (Fig. 6A). The enhanced fluorescence intensity of TLR4 following LPS treatment was notably inhibited by exogenous bFGF addition (Fig. 6B). These results suggest that the role of bFGF in LPS-stimulated astrocytes was related to the inhibition of upstream TLR4 in inflammatory signals.

2.7　Exogenous bFGF inhibits the activation of NFκB in LPS-induced astrocytes

It is well known that TLR4-mediated signaling pathways mainly stimulate the activation of NFκB. Herein, we further detected the degradation of IκBα and the activation of NFκBp65. As Fig. 7A shows, LPS elevated the degradation of IκBα, which contributed to the phosphorylation of NFκBp65. Under normal conditions, NFκBp65 was mainly expressed in the cytoplasm, whereas it notably entered to the nucleus with LPS stimulation, and bFGF treatment significantly decreased its translocation (Fig. 7B). These results indicate that bFGF inhibited the activation of NFκBp65 in LPS-stimulated astrocytes. Collectively, all data suggest that in LPS-induced astrocytes, TLR4/NFκB might be the main pathway for bFGF to reduce the inflammation reaction, which attenuated the activation of astrocytes.

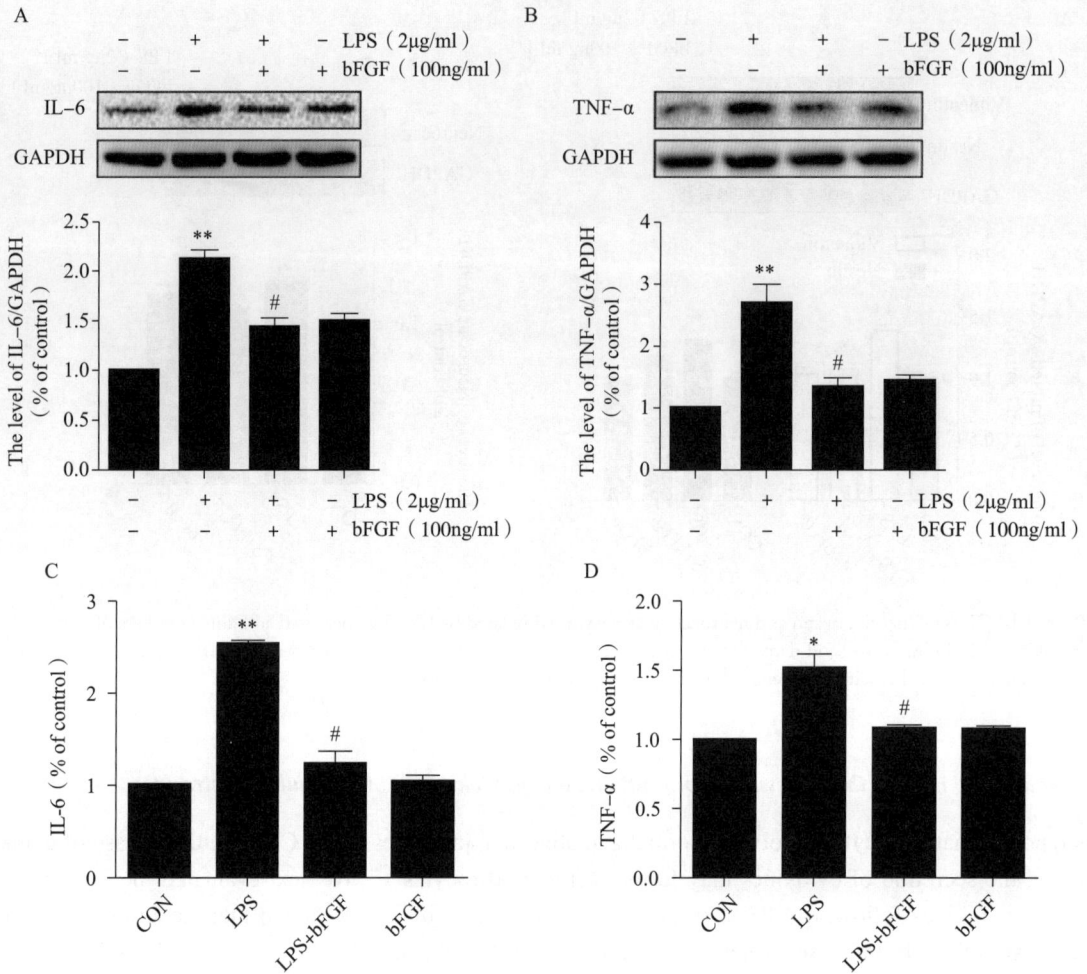

Fig. 5. Effect of bFGF on inflammatory cytokine expression and secretion in astrocytes that were induced by LPS. Cells were incubated in the presence of LPS (2 μg/ml) with or without bFGF (100 ng/ml) for 24 h. Cells and supernatants were collected for experiments. (A) Western blot of IL-6 and densitometric analyses; (B) Western blot of TNF-α and densitometric analyses; (C) ELISA of IL-6; (D) ELISA of TNF-α. $^{*}P < 0.05$, $^{**}P < 0.01$ vs. CON, $^{#}P < 0.05$ vs. LPS. All results represent at least three independent experiments.

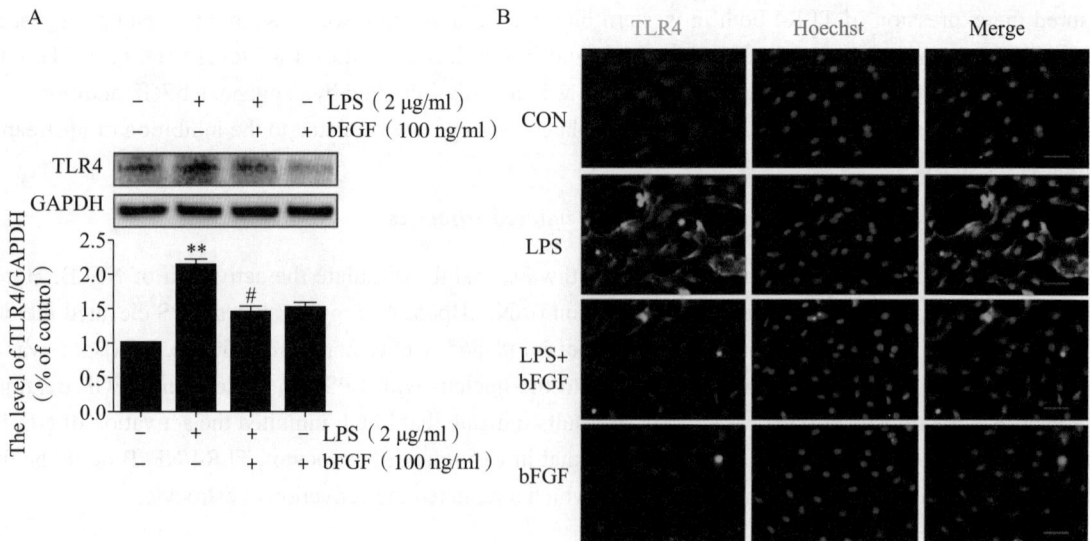

Fig. 6. Effect of bFGF on expression of TLR4 in LPS stimulated astrocytes. Cells were incubated in the presence of LPS (2 μg/ml) with or without bFGF (100 ng/ml) for 24 h. (A) Western blot of TLR4 and densitometric analyses; (B) Immunofluorescence of TLR4 (green), the nuclear is labeled by Hoechst (blue). $^{**}P < 0.01$ vs. CON, $^{#}P < 0.05$ vs. LPS. All results represent at least three independent experiments; Scale bar is 50 μm.

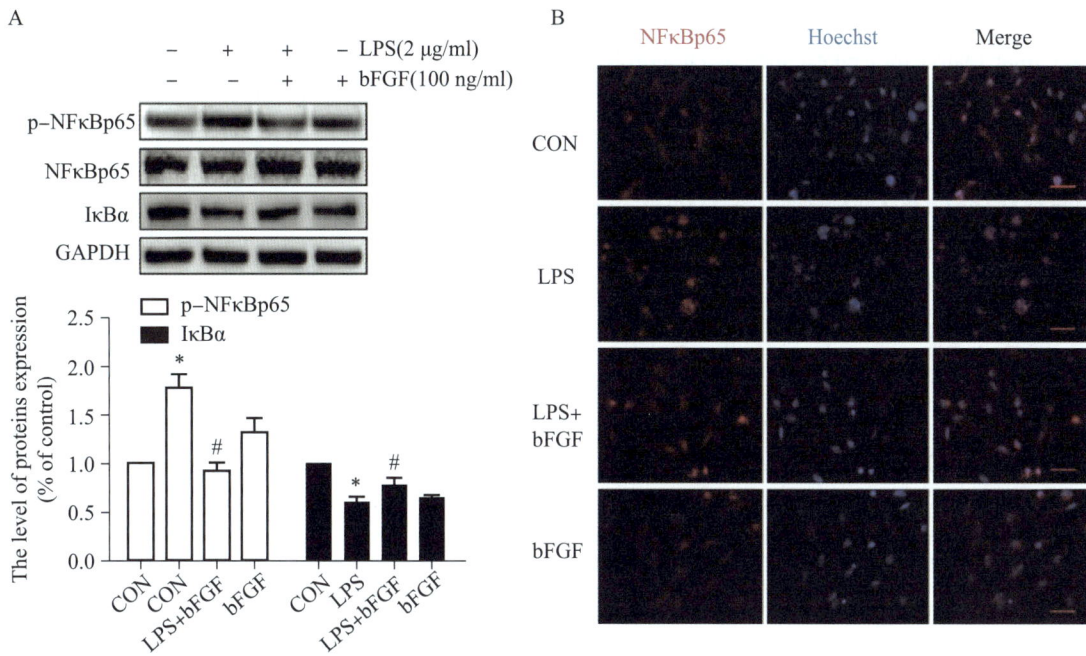

Fig. 7. Effect of bFGF on activation of NFκB in LPS-stimulated astrocytes. Cells were incubated in the presence of LPS (2 μg/ml) with or without bFGF (100 ng/ml) for 24 h. (A) Western blot of *P*-NFκBp65, NFκBp65 and IκB and densitometric analyses; (B) Immunofluorescence of NFκBp65 (red), the nuclear is labeled by Hoechst (blue). $^*P < 0.05$ *vs.* CON, $^#P < 0.05$ *vs.* LPS. All results represent at least three independent experiments. Scale bar is 50 μm.

3. Discussion

Astrogliosis is important in both physiological and pathological processes following brain injury, spinal cord injury, and other CNS diseases [30,41]. Astrogliosis, also called reactive astrocytes, has beneficial and detrimental effects on recovery from certain neuronal diseases. Reactive astrocytes enhance the dopaminergic differentiation of stem cells and promote brain repair through bFGF in brain injury [42]. Reactive astrocytes are also essential for minimizing the spread of damage and reducing leukocyte infiltration after spinal cord injury [43]. However, it is reported that reactive astrocytes inhibit the axonal regeneration in spinal cord injury [44]. Moreover, reactive astrocytes serve as a potential source of inflammatory cytokines. For example, the activation of astrocytes results in the production of diverse pro-inflammatory cytokines, such as IL-1β, TNF-α and IL-6, which may be a first step in the development of several neurodegenerative disease [14]. Therefore, the mechanism by which this activation of astrocytes is attenuated seems important and urgent. In this study, we investigated the effect of bFGF on reactive astrocytes that were stimulated by LPS in primary astrocytes culture. Our data showed that LPS stimulated the activation of astrocytes and was followed by the secretion of endogenous bFGF. Treatment with exogenous bFGF in a small dosage activated astrocytes, while this effect could not be detected in high concentrations of bFGF. Furthermore, high concentrations of bFGF inhibited LPS-induced activation of astrocytes by decreasing the expression of GFAP, vimentin, and pro-inflammatory cytokines. In addition, the TLR4/NFκB pathway was involved in this potential mechanism of bFGF activation of LPS-stimulated astrocytes.

As a maker of reactive astrocytes, the expression of GFAP always increased significantly. Studies have shown that LPS causes astrocytes activation, with the expression of high levels of GFAP or vimentin in primary astrocytes culture, while treatment with an activation inhibitor would reduce GFAP or vimentin expression [32,33]. In this study, we also found that GFAP is highly expressed after LPS stimulation and most astrocytes displayed an extended cell body and enhanced fluorescence intensity (Fig. 3 and 4); however, bFGF (100 ng/ml) markedly decreased the expression of GFAP and vimentin, and reversed the morphology of astrocytes. Nestin, a marker of reactive astrocytes, was reported to be highly expressed in astrocytes after focal cerebral ischemia injury [45]. Interestingly, our results suggest that there was no significant difference between the control group and LPS group in nestin expression, which implies that LPS might not influence all makers of reactive astrocytes, or it might be related to time points or dose points. This may be the reason why nestin is not widely used in such studies. It is known that excessive astrogliosis could produce growth inhibitory extracellular matrix molecules, such as chondroitin sulfate proteoglycans (CSPGs), after spinal cord injury [46]. In Jeong's study, hepatocyte growth factor was reported to prevent the expression of CSPGs, such as neurocan and phosphacan, which were secreted from reactive astrocytes during spinal cord injury [39]. Here, we measured the expression of neurocan and found that bFGF decreased neurocan levels in LPS-induced astrocytes (Fig. 4).

Evidence suggests that the pro-inflammatory cytokines TNF-α, IL-1β, and IL-6 are the initial triggers of reactive astrocytes in the acute phase of injury [47,48]. Interestingly, reactive astrocytes release a majority of these triggering molecules themselves, which result in a cyclic process of continuous activation [16,39]. In a latest study, IL-6, IL-1β, and TNF-α were inhibited by ulinastatin in LPS-stimulated astrocytes [33]. bFGF was found to down-regulate the expression of TNF-α and IL-1 following ischemia and reperfusion, which contributed to alleviating brain injury [35]. In the urinary tissue of the bladder, bFGF also reduced the production of TNF-α and IL-1β at early phases of radiation-induced injury [49]. Whether bFGF has an anti-inflammatory effect in LPS-stimulated astrocytes is unknown. Our results show that the production of TNF-α and IL-6 in astrocytes stimulated by LPS was significantly suppressed by exogenous bFGF (Fig. 5). The TLR4/NFκB pathway was reported to be activated in LPS-stimulated astrocytes [32,33]. TLR4 and phosphorylation of NFκBp65 were significantly up-regulated in LPS-induced astrocytes, which was reversed when astrocyte activation was inhibited by ketamine [32]. In this study, we also found that the exposure of astrocytes to LPS resulted in an increased expression of TLR4, degradation of IκBα, and phosphorylation of NFκBp65, followed by the translocation of active NFκBp65 from the cytoplasm to the nucleus, which was reversed by bFGF (Fig. 7). All of these data indicate that bFGF might inhibit the inflammation through the TLR4/NFκB pathway, which attenuated the activation of astrocytes. It is worth mentioning that other elements might also contribute to the effect of bFGF on astrocytes activation. Oxidative stress and endoplasmic reticulum stress are reported to be involved in astrogliosis after injury [50,51]. Extensive research suggests that bFGF is able to inhibit oxidative stress and endoplasmic reticulum stress post injury [34,52]. Therefore, it is reasonable to speculate that bFGF might, through other ways, weaken astrocytes activation, which should be further investigated.

Taken together, our study demonstrates that bFGF-attenuated astrocyte activation by reducing the expression of GFAP and other hallmark proteins, thereby inhibiting the production of pro-inflammation cytokines such as IL-6 and TNF-α, which might be regulated by the TLR4/NFκB pathway. Our study suggests the possibility that bFGF therapy may be suitable for excessive astrogliosis and glial scarring post-neuronal injury.

4. Materials and methods

4.1 Primary astrocyte cultures

Adult Sprague-Dawley (SD) rats were obtained from the Animal Center of the Chinese Academy of Science (Shanghai, China). All experimental procedures were approved by the Laboratory Animal Ethics Committee of Wenzhou Medical University (wydw2015-0048, 24-2-2014) and were performed in accordance with the Guide for the Care and Use of Laboratory Animals. Primary astrocytes were prepared from neonatal SD rats. Briefly, SD rats were anesthetized with ether and then dipped into 75% alcohol to sterilize. The cerebral cortex was separated from skulls, and the meningeal tissue was removed. Then, tissue was cut into small pieces and washed with phosphate buffer solution (PBS) three times. The tissue was chemically dissociated with 0.125% trypsin for 25 min (Invitrogen, Carlsbad, CA, USA). After centrifugation at 1 000 rpm for 5 min, the cells were suspended in DMEM/F12 with 10% fetal bovine serum and 100 U/ml penicillin (Invitrogen, Carlsbad, CA, USA) and plated in a flask coated with poly-L-lysine (Sigma–Aldrich, St. Louis, MO, USA). Cells were maintained in a humidified atmosphere, and culture medium was changed every 3–4 days. When the culture was reaching confluency, flasks were shaken at 200 rpm for 12 h to remove oligodendrocytes and microglial cells. Cells were passaged for at least three times for further purification. The purities of the cultured astrocytes were confirmed by immunofluorescence staining for glial fibrillary acidic protein (GFAP, Santa Cruz Biotechnology, Santa Cruz, CA, USA).

4.2 Cell treatment

Cell culture medium was switched to serum-free DMEM/F12 culture medium. Astrocytes were synchronized for 12 h in the absence of serum, and then incubated in the presence of LPS (2 μg/ml) with or without bFGF for 24 h. Cells were then harvested for analysis.

4.3 Western blot analysis

Astrocytes cells were lysed in RIPA buffer (25 mM Tris-HCl, 150 mM NaCl, 1% Nonidet P-40, 1% sodium deoxycholate, and 0.1% sodium dodecyl sulfate) with protease and phosphatase inhibitors (GE Healthcare Biosciences, Piscataway, NJ, USA). After centrifugation, the extracts above were quantified with bicinchoninic acid (BCA) reagents (Thermo, Rockford, IL, USA). The complex was then centrifuged at 12 000 rpm and the supernatant obtained for protein assay. Total proteins (20 μg) were loaded on 8% or 10% gel and transferred onto PVDF membrane (Bio-Rad, Hercules, CA, USA). The membrane was blocked with 5% milk (Bio-Rad) in TBST (TBS with 0.05% tween 20) for 1.5 h and incubated with the antibodies GFAP (1:300, Santa Cruz Biotechnology), vimentin (1:1 000, Abcam, Cambridge, UK), bFGF (1:300, Santa Cruz Biotechnology), neurcon (1:1 000, Merck Millipore, Billerica, MA, USA), IκBα (1:300, Santa Cruz Biotechnology), NFκBp65 (1:300, Santa Cruz Biotechnology), p-NFκBp65 (1:1 000, Cell Signaling, Boston, MA, USA), IL-6 (1:300, Santa Cruz Biotechnology), TNF-α (1:300, Santa Cruz Biotechnology) in TBST for 2 h at room temperature or overnight at 4 ℃. The membranes were washed with TBST for three times and treated with horseradish peroxidase-conjugated secondary antibodies (1:3 000) for 1 h at room temperature. Signals were visualized by ChemiDoc XRS+ Imaging System (Bio-Rad). GAPDH (1:300, Santa Cruz Biotechnology) was used as an internal control. Experiments were performed at least three times and the densitometric values of the bands on western blots obtained by Image J software were subjected to statistical analysis.

4.4 Immunofluorescence staining

Astrocytes were fixed with 4% paraformaldehyde (PFA) and rinsed three times with PBS. Next, the cells were incubated with 0.5% Triton X-100 for 15 min at room temperature, washed three times with 0.01 M PBS and incubated with 5% bovine serum albumin (BSA) for 30 min. Then, samples were incubated with anti-GFAP antibody (1:1 000, Abcam), anti-TLR4 antibody (1:200, Abcam), anti-inhibitor of κBα (IκBα) antibody (1:300, Santa Cruz Biotechnology), anti-toll-like receptor TLR4 antibody (1:100, Abcam) and anti-MD2 antibody (1:100, Abcam) overnight at 4 ℃ in 1% BSA. Alexa Fluor 488 (1:1 000, Abcam) or TR-conjugated secondary antibodies (1:200, Santa Cruz Biotechnology) were used. The nucleus was stained with Hoechst. All images were captured on Nikon ECLIPSE Ti microscope (Nikon, Tokyo, Japan).

4.5 Enzyme-linked immunosorbent assay (ELISA)

bFGF, IL-6 and TGFβ1 levels were measured using an enzyme-linked immunosorbent assay (ELISA). Cells were plated onto 6-well plates, 24 h after treatment with drugs. Cultured supernatants were then centrifuged at 12,000 rpm for 10 min and were assessed using ELISA kits (eBioscience, Vienna, Austria) according to manufacturer's instructions. Optional densities were measured at 405 nm using a microplate reader.

4.6 Statistical analysis

Data were expressed as the mean ± SEM. Statistical significance was determined using Student's t-test when there were two experimental groups. For more than two groups, statistical evaluation of the data was performed using a one-way analysis-of-variance (ANOVA) test, followed by Tukey's *post hoc* test. Statistical significance was accepted at $P < 0.05$.

5. Conclusions

This study demonstrates that bFGF-attenuated astrocyte activation by reducing the expression of GFAP and other hallmark proteins, thereby inhibiting the production of pro-inflammation cytokines such as IL-6 and TNF-α, which might be regulated by the TLR4/NFκB pathway. Our study suggests the possibility that bFGF therapy may be suitable for excessive astrogliosis and glial scarring post neuronal injury.

References

[1] Sofroniew MV, Vinters HV. Astrocytes: biology and pathology - eScholarship[J]. Acta Neuropathologica, 2010, 119(1): 7-35.

[2] Gordon GRJ, Mulligan SJ, Macvicar BA. Astrocyte control of the cerebrovasculature[J]. Glia, 2010, 55(12): 1214-1221.

[3] Kawano H, Kimura-Kuroda J, Komuta Y, et al. Role of the lesion scar in the response to damage and repair of the central nervous system[J]. Cell & Tissue Research, 2012, 349(1): 169-180.

[4] Hawthorne AL, Hu H, Kundu B, et al. The unusual response of serotonergic neurons after CNS Injury: lack of axonal dieback and enhanced sprouting within the inhibitory environment of the glial scar[J]. J Neurosci, 2011, 31(15): 5605-5616.

[5] Dharmarajan S, Gurel Z, Wang S, et al. Bone morphogenetic protein 7 regulates reactive gliosis in retinal astrocytes and Muller glia[J]. Mol Vis, 2014, 20: 1085-1108.

[6] Kelso ML, Liput DJ, Eaves DW, et al. Upregulated vimentin suggests new areas of neurodegeneration in a model of an alcohol use disorder[J]. Neuroscience, 2011, 197: 381-393.

[7] Lee HS, Lee SH, Cha JH, et al. Meteorin is upregulated in reactive astrocytes and functions as a negative feedback effector in reactive gliosis[J]. Mol Med Rep, 2015, 12(2): 1817-1823.

[8] Seo TB, Chang IA, Lee JH, et al. Beneficial function of cell division cycle 2 activity in astrocytes on axonal regeneration after spinal cord injury[J]. J Neurotrauma, 2013, 30(12): 1053-1061.

[9] Renault-Mihara F, Okada S, Shibata S, et al. Spinal cord injury: emerging beneficial role of reactive astrocytes' migration[J]. Int J Biochem Cell Biol, 2008, 40(9): 1649-1653.

[10] Herrmann JE, Imura T, Song B, et al. STAT3 is a critical regulator of astrogliosis and scar formation after spinal cord injury[J]. J Neurosci, 2008, 28(28): 7231-7243.

[11] Pekny M, Wilhelmsson U, Pekna M. The dual role of astrocyte activation and reactive gliosis[J]. Neurosci Lett, 2014, 565: 30-38.

[12] Zhu Z, Zhang Q, Yu Z, et al. Inhibiting cell cycle progression reduces reactive astrogliosis initiated by scratch injury in vitro and by cerebral ischemia in vivo[J]. Glia, 2007, 55(5): 546-558.

[13] Liu R, Wang Z, Gou L, et al. A cortical astrocyte subpopulation inhibits axon growth in vitro and in vivo[J]. Mol Med Rep, 2015, 12(2): 2598-2606.

[14] Barcia C, Ros CM, Annese V, et al. IFN-gamma signaling, with the synergistic contribution of TNF-alpha, mediates cell specific microglial and astroglial activation in experimental models of Parkinson's disease[J]. Cell Death Dis, 2011, 2: e142.

[15] Daginakatte GC, Gadzinski A, Emnett RJ, et al. Expression profiling identifies a molecular signature of reactive astrocytes stimulated by cyclic AMP or proinflammatory cytokines[J]. Exp Neurol, 2008, 210(1): 261-267.

[16] Cui M, Huang Y, Tian C, et al. FOXO3a inhibits TNF-alpha- and IL-1beta-induced astrocyte proliferation:Implication for reactive astrogliosis[J]. Glia, 2011, 59(4): 641-654.

[17] Sticozzi C, Belmonte G, Meini A, et al. IL-1beta induces GFAP expression in vitro and in vivo and protects neurons from traumatic injury-associated apoptosis in rat brain striatum via NFkappaB/Ca(2)(+)-calmodulin/ERK mitogen-activated protein kinase signaling pathway[J]. Neuroscience, 2013, 252: 367-383.

[18] Olajide OA, Bhatia HS, de Oliveira AC, et al. Inhibition of Neuroinflammation in LPS-Activated Microglia by Cryptolepine[J]. Evid Based Complement Alternat Med, 2013, 2013: 459723.

[19] Medzhitov R, Preston-Hurlburt P, Janeway CA, Jr. A human homologue of the Drosophila Toll protein signals activation of adaptive immunity[J]. Nature, 1997, 388(6640): 394-397.

[20] Wang Y, Li C, Cheng K, et al. Activation of liver X receptor improves viability of adipose-derived mesenchymal stem cells to attenuate myocardial ischemia injury through TLR4/NF-kappaB and Keap-1/Nrf-2 signaling pathways[J]. Antioxid Redox Signal, 2014, 21(18): 2543-2557.

[21] Proia P, Schiera G, Mineo M, et al. Astrocytes shed extracellular vesicles that contain fibroblast growth factor-2 and vascular endothelial growth factor[J]. Int J Mol Med, 2008, 21(1): 63-67.

[22] Shimizu F, Sano Y, Abe MA, et al. Peripheral nerve pericytes modify the blood-nerve barrier function and tight junctional molecules through the secretion of various soluble factors[J]. J Cell Physiol, 2011, 226(1): 255-266.

[23] Jia Y, Wu D, Zhang R, et al. Bone marrow-derived mesenchymal stem cells expressing the Shh transgene promotes functional recovery after spinal cord injury in rats[J]. Neurosci Lett, 2014, 573: 46-51.

[24] DeLeo JA, Colburn RW, Rickman AJ. Cytokine and growth factor immunohistochemical spinal profiles in two animal models of mononeuropathy[J]. Brain Res, 1997, 759(1): 50-57.

[25] Xiang Y, Liu H, Yan T, et al. Functional electrical stimulation-facilitated proliferation and regeneration of neural precursor cells in the brains of rats with cerebral infarction[J]. Neural Regen Res, 2014, 9(3): 243-251.

[26] Rotschafer JH, Hu S, Little M, et al. Modulation of neural stem/progenitor cell proliferation during experimental Herpes Simplex encephalitis is mediated by differential FGF-2 expression in the adult brain[J]. Neurobiol Dis, 2013, 58: 144-155.

[27] Gomez-Pinilla F, Cummings BJ, Cotman CW. Induction of basic fibroblast growth factor in Alzheimer's disease pathology[J]. Neuroreport, 1990, 1(3-4): 211-214.

[28] Goldshmit Y, Frisca F, Pinto AR, et al. FGF2 improves functional recovery-decreasing gliosis and increasing radial glia and neural progenitor cells after spinal cord injury[J]. Brain Behav, 2014, 4(2): 187-200.

[29] Reilly JF, Maher PA, Kumari VG. Regulation of astrocyte GFAP expression by TGF-beta1 and FGF-2[J]. Glia, 1998, 22(2): 202-210.

[30] Kang W, Balordi F, Su N, et al. Astrocyte activation is suppressed in both normal and injured brain by FGF signaling[J]. Proc Natl Acad Sci U S A, 2014, 111(29): E2987-E2995.

[31] Fahmy GH, Moftah MZ. FGF-2 in astroglial cells during vertebrate spinal cord recovery. Front Cell Neurosci, 2010, 4.

[32] Wu Y, Li W, Zhou C, et al. Ketamine inhibits lipopolysaccharide-induced astrocytes activation by suppressing TLR4/NF-kB pathway[J]. Cell Physiol Biochem, 2012, 30(3): 609-617.

[33] Li Y, Zhao L, Fu H, et al. Ulinastatin suppresses lipopolysaccharide induced neuro-inflammation through the downregulation of nuclear factor-kappaB in SD rat hippocampal astrocyte[J]. Biochem Biophys Res Commun, 2015, 458(4): 763-770.

[34] Zhang HY, Zhang X, Wang ZG, et al. Exogenous basic fibroblast growth factor inhibits ER stress-induced apoptosis and improves recovery from spinal cord injury[J]. CNS Neurosci Ther, 2013, 19(1): 20-29.

[35] Zhang M, Ma YF, Gan JX, et al. Basic fibroblast growth factor alleviates brain injury following global ischemia reperfusion in rabbits[J]. J Zhejiang Univ Sci B, 2005, 6(7): 637-643.

[36] Gomez-Pinilla F, Vu L, Cotman CW. Regulation of astrocyte proliferation by FGF-2 and heparan sulfate in vivo[J]. J Neurosci, 1995, 15(3 Pt 1): 2021-2029.

[37] Neary JT, Shi YF, Kang Y, *et al.* Opposing effects of P2X(7) and P2Y purine/pyrimidine-preferring receptors on proliferation of astrocytes induced by fibroblast growth factor-2: implications for CNS development, injury, and repair[J]. J Neurosci Res, 2008, 86(14): 3096-3105.

[38] Lau LT, Yu AC. Astrocytes produce and release interleukin-1, interleukin-6, tumor necrosis factor alpha and interferon-gamma following traumatic and metabolic injury[J]. J Neurotrauma, 2001, 18(3): 351-359.

[39] Jeong SR, Kwon MJ, Lee HG, *et al.* Hepatocyte growth factor reduces astrocytic scar formation and promotes axonal growth beyond glial scars after spinal cord injury[J]. Exp Neurol, 2012, 233(1): 312-322.

[40] Fellner L, Irschick R, Schanda K, *et al.* Toll-like receptor 4 is required for α-synuclein dependent activation of microglia and astroglia[J]. Glia, 2013, 61(3): 349-360.

[41] Li Z-W, Li J-J, Wang L, *et al.* Epidermal growth factor receptor inhibitor ameliorates excessive astrogliosis and improves the regeneration microenvironment and functional recovery in adult rats following spinal cord injury[J]. Journal of neuroinflammation, 2014, 11: 71-71.

[42] Yang F, Liu Y, Tu J, *et al.* Activated astrocytes enhance the dopaminergic differentiation of stem cells and promote brain repair through bFGF[J]. Nature communications, 2014, 5: 5627-5627.

[43] Faulkner JR, Herrmann JE, Woo MJ, *et al.* Reactive astrocytes protect tissue and preserve function after spinal cord injury[J]. J Neurosci, 2004, 24(9): 2143-2155.

[44] Liu Y, Ye H, Satkunendrarajah K, *et al.* A self-assembling peptide reduces glial scarring, attenuates post-traumatic inflammation and promotes neurological recovery following spinal cord injury[J]. Acta Biomater, 2013, 9(9): 8075-8088.

[45] Na JI, Na JY, Choi WY, *et al.* The HIF-1 inhibitor YC-1 decreases reactive astrocyte formation in a rodent ischemia model[J]. Am J Transl Res, 2015, 7(4): 751-760.

[46] Tang X, Davies JE, Davies SJ. Changes in distribution, cell associations, and protein expression levels of NG2, neurocan, phosphacan, brevican, versican V2, and tenascin-C during acute to chronic maturation of spinal cord scar tissue[J]. J Neurosci Res, 2003, 71(3): 427-444.

[47] Lin HW, Basu A, Druckman C, *et al.* Astrogliosis is delayed in type 1 interleukin-1 receptor-null mice following a penetrating brain injury[J]. J Neuroinflammation, 2006, 3: 15.

[48] Aranguez I, Torres C, Rubio N. The receptor for tumor necrosis factor on murine astrocytes: characterization, intracellular degradation, and regulation by cytokines and Theiler's murine encephalomyelitis virus[J]. Glia, 1995, 13(3): 185-194.

[49] Zhang S, Qiu X, Zhang Y, *et al.* Basic Fibroblast Growth Factor Ameliorates Endothelial Dysfunction in Radiation-Induced Bladder Injury[J]. Biomed Res Int, 2015, 2015: 967680.

[50] Yan BC, Park JH, Ahn JH, *et al.* Effects of high-fat diet on neuronal damage, gliosis, inflammatory process and oxidative stress in the hippocampus induced by transient cerebral ischemia[J]. Neurochem Res, 2014, 39(12): 2465-2478.

[51] Alberdi E, Wyssenbach A, Alberdi M, *et al.* Ca(2+) -dependent endoplasmic reticulum stress correlates with astrogliosis in oligomeric amyloid beta-treated astrocytes and in a model of Alzheimer's disease[J]. Aging Cell, 2013, 12(2): 292-302.

[52] Kocer G, Naziroglu M, Celik O, *et al.* Basic fibroblast growth factor attenuates bisphosphonate-induced oxidative injury but decreases zinc and copper levels in oral epithelium of rat[J]. Biol Trace Elem Res, 2013, 153(1-3): 251-256.

bFGF promotes the migration of human dermal fibroblasts under diabetic conditions through reactive oxygen species production *via* the PI3K/Akt-Rac1-JNK pathways

Hongxue Shi, Xiaokun Li, Jian Xiao

1. Introduction

Impaired wound healing is an emerging global public concern with considerable social, health, and economic consequences. One of the most common diseases associated with impaired tissue repair is diabetes mellitus, and foot ulcerations are the most frequent cause of hospitalization in patients with diabetes [1]. The healing of cutaneous wounds is a complex and highly orchestrated process that includes four main integrated and overlapping phases: hemostasis, inflammation, proliferation and tissue remodeling [2]. However, this orderly progression of the healing process is impaired in diabetic patients [3].

Cutaneous wounds require a well-orchestrated interaction of cell migration and proliferation from numerous different tissues and cell lineages. Among these cell types, fibroblasts play a pivotal role in all four phases of wound healing. After wounding, fibroblasts are attracted from the edge of the wound or from the bone marrow [4]. At the inflammation stage, fibroblasts produce a variety of chemokines [5]. At the stage of new tissue formation, fibroblasts are stimulated by macrophages, and some differentiate into myofibroblasts. Fibroblasts interact with myofibroblasts to produce extracellular matrix, mainly in the form of collagen [5]. At the tissue remodeling stage, most of the myofibroblasts, macrophages and endothelial cells undergo apoptosis or exit from the wound, leaving a mass that contains few cells and consists mostly of collagen and other extracellular matrix proteins [6]. However, diabetes has an adverse effect on the proliferation of fibroblasts [7, 8]. Accumulating evidence also suggests that the fibroblasts from diabetic mice and rats exhibit a marked reduction in migratory ability compared with those from normal control mice [9, 10].

Growth factors have been shown to play multiple and critical roles in the process of wound healing, and their decreased expression in diabetes mellitus may disrupt the normal healing process [11]. Among growth factors, basic fibroblast growth factor (bFGF) is a potent mitogen that stimulates the migration, proliferation, and differentiation of cells of mesenchymal and neuroectodermal origin, such as keratinocytes, fibroblasts, melanocytes and endothelial cells [12]. Animal studies have shown that recombinant human bFGF can promote wound healing in genetically diabetic mice and streptozotocin-induced diabetic rats [13, 14]. It has been suggested that recombinant bFGF promotes granulation and epithelialization and shortens the time required for healing in patients with diabetic ulcers as well as in patients with other types of skin ulcers [15, 16]. However, the mechanisms underlying the therapeutic effect of bFGF on skin wounds under diabetic conditions are not completely understood.

The migration of various cells mediated by bFGF and the underlying signal transduction pathways have been studied extensively [17]. However, the effect of bFGF on human dermal fibroblast migration under diabetic conditions remains unknown. In this study, we investigated the effect of bFGF on the migration of human dermal fibroblasts under diabetic conditions and further examined its molecular mechanism.

2. Materials and methods

2.1 Cell culture

Human foreskins were obtained from the First Affiliated Hospital of Wenzhou Medical University with approval by the Ethic Committee of First Affiliated Hospital of Wenzhou Medical University, Wenzhou, China. All of the experiments were performed in accordance with the relevant approved guidelines and regulations. The isolation and primary culture of human dermal fibroblasts were performed as described previously [16]. Briefly, the foreskins were washed three times in phosphate-buffered saline (PBS) solution containing 1% penicillin and streptomycin sulfate. Subsequently, the excised tissues were digested with 0.5% dispase II at 4℃ overnight. The epidermis and subcutaneous tissue were then re-moved from the excised tissues, cut into pieces with a size of approximately 1×1×0.5 cm and placed into T25 tissue culture flasks as explants. Dulbecco's modified eagle medium (DMEM) containing 5.5 mM D-glucose, 20% fetal bovine serum (FBS), 1% penicillin, streptomycin sulfate and 2 mM L-glutamine was used as the growth medium. The medium was replaced every three days. The primary fibroblasts were grown at 37℃ in an atmosphere of 5% CO_2 and were passaged every other day by trypsinization. Cells that had undergone three to six passages were used for all of our experiments.

2.2 Cell proliferation assay

Human dermal fibroblasts were plated in 35-mm tissue culture dishes at a density of $2.4×10^4$ cells/ml and cultured overnight. The culture medium was modified according to the experimental groups to include the following constituents: 5.5 mM D-glucose for the normal-glucose group, 30 mM D-glucose for the high glucose group and 5.5 mM D-glucose and 24.5 mM mannitol for the osmotic control group. Twenty-four hours later, the cells were treated with 100 ng/ml bFGF for 24 h in the presence or absence of 5 μg/ml mitomycin-C. The cells were then washed three times with PBS and harvested using 0.1% trypsin. The number of cells was counted in a microscopic counting chamber.

2.3 Wound-healing assay

Human dermal fibroblasts were plated overnight in six-well tissue culture dishes under standard culture conditions. The culture medium was modified as described previously for a period of 24 h. After another 24 h of serum starvation, the cells were wounded with a linear scratch using a sterile pipette tip and treated with 100 ng/ml bFGF in the presence of 5 μg/ml mitomycin-C. Twelve and 24 hours after wounding, the cells were washed with PBS to remove any floating cells and cellular debris. Images of the wound closure or cell migration were immediately photographed using an inverted microscope equipped with a digital camera. To observe the role of PI3K/Akt, JNK, ROS, and NADPH oxidases in the migration of human dermal fibroblasts, the cells were pretreated with 10 μM LY294002, 10 μM SP600125, 10 mM NAC or 10 μM diphenyleneiodonium chloride (DPI), respectively, for 1 h before wounding. The distances between the front edges of the selected cells and the wound edge 12 or 24 h after wounding were measured using the ImageJ software. The migration rate was expressed as the migration distance/time (μm/h). All of the wound-healing assays were performed in the presence of 5 μg/ml mitomycin-C to inhibit cell proliferation.

2.4 Analysis of cell polarity index

To migrate, cells must possess a defined front and rear to move in one direction. Without this front-rear polarity, the cells will be unable to coordinate a directed migration. To assess the effect of bFGF on cell polarity, the polarity index was calculated as the length of the major migration axis (parallel to the direction of movement) divided by the length of the perpendicular axis that intersects the center of the cell nucleus after treatment with 100 ng/ml bFGF for 1 h in the presence of 5 μg/ml mitomycin-C [10, 18].

2.5 Rac1 pull-down assay

The Rac1 pull-down assay was performed using the manufacturer's protocol. In brief, the cells were scraped into ice-cold lysis buffer and centrifuged for 10 min at 12,000 rpm. The cleared lysates (containing at least 500 μg) were incubated with 20 μg of Pak1-PBD agarose (Thermo scientific, Hangzhou, China) for 1 h at 4℃ with gentle rocking. The beads were washed three times with wash buffer, heated for 5 min at 100℃ in reducing SDS-PAGE sample buffer, and then centrifuged for 2 min at 6,000 rpm. Rac1-GTP expression was analyzed by western blot using anti-Rac1 antibody.

2.6 siRNA knockdown of Rac1

Scrambled control siRNA (sc-37007) and Rac1 siRNA (sc-36351) were purchased from Santa Cruz. Primary human fibroblasts were transfected with Rac1 siRNA (10 nM) using Lipofectamine 2000 reagent (Invitrogen, Shanghai,

China) with the manufacturer's protocol. Twenty-four hours after transfection, the cells were subjected to bFGF treatment. Specific silencing was confirmed by western blot.

2.7 Measurement of intracellular ROS production

The membrane-permeable indicator H2DCF-DA was used to detect intracellular ROS production. The cells were cultured in DMEM containing 5.5 mM glucose overnight. The cells were then cultured in DMEM containing 30 mM glucose for 24 h. After another 24 h of serum starvation, the cells were treated with 100 ng/ml bFGF for 24 h in the presence or absence of DPI or NAC. The cells were loaded with 10 µmol/l H2DCF-DA in serum-free DMEM at 37 ℃ for 30 min and washed three times with PBS. Fluorescent images were obtained using an upright fluorescence microscope.

2.8 Western blot analysis

The cells were lysed in RIPA buffer (50 mM Tris–HCl, pH 7.4, 150 mM NaCl, 0.25% Na deoxycholate, 1% NP-40, 1 mM EDTA, 1 mM PMSF, 1 mM Na_3VO_4, 1 mM NaF, and complete protease inhibitor cocktail), incubated for 10 min on ice and centrifuged at 12,000 rpm for 10 min at 4 ℃. The protein samples were denatured by incubating at 100 ℃ for 10 min in 5× loading buffer, separated on 10.6% polyacrylamide gels, and transferred to a polyvinylidene difluoride membrane. The membranes were incubated in TBS containing 5% nonfat milk and 0.05% Tween-20 for 1 h and blotted with primary antibodies at 4 ℃ overnight (p-Akt/Akt, Santa cruz, Shanghai, China. 1:500 dilution; p-JNK/JNK, p-FAK/FAK and p-Paxillin/Paxillin, Cell signaling technology, Shanghai, China. 1:1 000 dilution; NOX4, Abcam, Shanghai, China. 1:1 000 dilution). The membranes were washed with TBST for 15 min (three times for 5 min each) the next day. Subsequently, the membranes were incubated with second antibody (Santa cruz, Shanghai, China. 1:3 000 dilution) for 1 h at room temperature and washed with TBST for 21 min (three times for 7 min each). The membranes were then detected using ECL ECL (Bio-Rad, Hangzhou, China). The western blot results were further analyzed using the Quantity One software 4.1.1 (Bio-Rad, Hangzhou, China).

2.9 Immunofluorescence

The cells were plated in six-well tissue culture dishes. The cells were maintained in a high-glucose medium containing 10% FBS for 24 h and cultured in serum-free DMEM for 24 h. The cells were then treated with or without 100 ng/ml bFGF for 6 and 12 h after wounding in the presence of 5 µg/ml mitomycin C. The cells were fixed with 4% paraformaldehyde in PBS for 20 min, permeabilized with 0.3% Triton X-100 in PBS for 15 min and incubated with 5% bovine serum albumin (BSA) in PBS for 45 min to block nonspecific antibody binding at room temperature. The cells were incubated with fluorescein isothiocyanate-labeled phalloidin staining solution in PBS containing 1% BSA for 35 min and washed with PBS for 15 min. The nuclei were stained with DAPI. Fluorescence images were obtained using an upright fluorescence microscope. All of the illustrations were assembled and processed digitally.

2.10 Statistical analysis

Data are expressed as the mean ± SEM. Statistical significance was determined using Student's *t*-test for two experimental groups. For more than two groups, the statistical evaluation of data was performed using one-way analysis of variance (ANOVA) followed by Dunnett's *post hoc* test. For all tests, $P < 0.05$ was considered significant.

3. Results

3.1 bFGF promoted the migration of human dermal fibroblasts under diabetic conditions

High glucose mediated oxidative stress and impaired cell migration. To investigate the effect of high glucose on human dermal fibroblast migration, a wound-healing assay was performed. The migratory ability of dermal fibroblasts was markedly impaired in the presence of a high concentration of glucose for 12 and 24 h, and the migration rates of dermal fibroblasts incubated with mannitol showed no significant decrease (Supplementary Material: Fig. 1A, B). These results suggest that the high-glucose-impaired migration of dermal fibroblasts does not result from changes in osmotic pressure.

bFGF is a well-known potent mitogen for most cell types. In this study, we focused on investigating the effect of

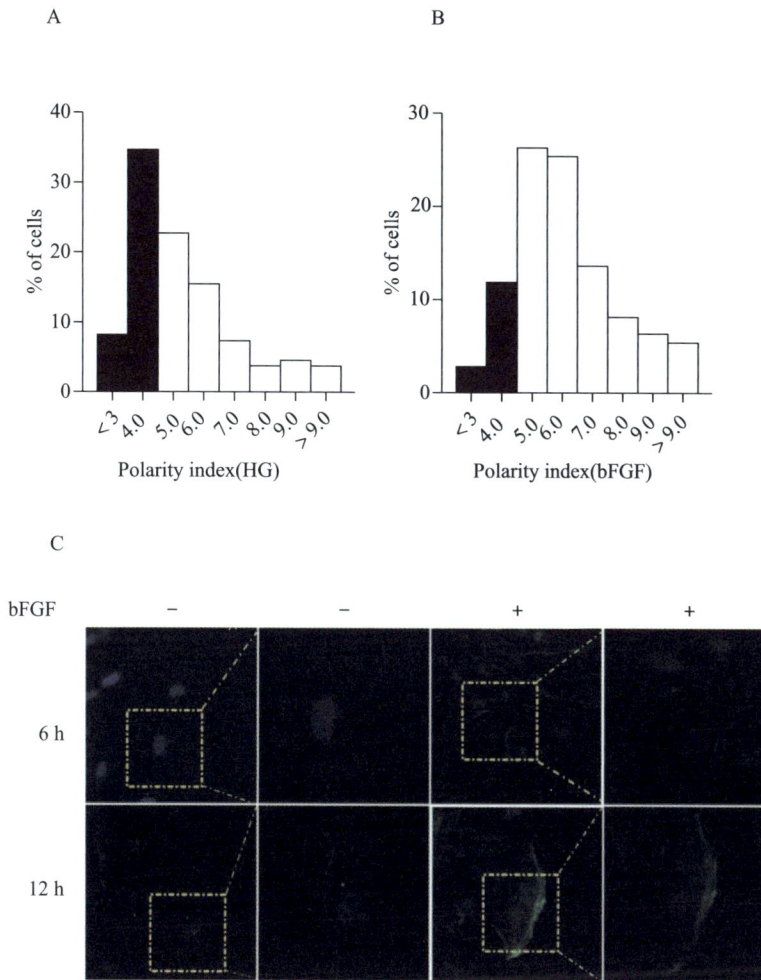

Fig. 1. bFGF altered human dermal fibroblast polarity impaired by high glucose. (A, B) The front-rear polarity index of dermal fibroblasts treated without or with 100 ng/ml bFGF under high-glucose conditions was calculated in single cell in scratch wound edge. (C) F-actin was labeled by FITC-conjugated phalloidin 6 h or 12 h after wounding with or without bFGF treatment.

bFGF on the migration of human dermal fibroblasts under high-glucose conditions. Therefore, to eliminate the impact of cell proliferation on the process of evaluating bFGF-induced dermal fibroblast migration, mitomycin C at a final concentration of 5 μg/ml was selected and used in all of our subsequent experimental procedures. Under such concentrations, mitomycin C completely blocked the proliferation of dermal fibroblasts while exhibiting no visible damage on cell viability (Supplementary Material: Fig. 1C). To migrate, a cell must normally establish morphological polarity and continuously protrude a single lamellipodium polarized in the direction of migration. To explore the impact of bFGF on cell polarity, the polarity index of dermal fibroblasts with or without bFGF treatment was determined. The results indicate that bFGF treatment significantly increased the cell number with elongated morphology. The fraction of those dermal fibroblasts under high-glucose conditions with a polarity index greater than 5 was 57.28%. When treated with bFGF for only 1 h, the percentage of cells with a polarity index greater than 5 sharply increased to 85.44% (Fig. 1A, B). To migrate, cells also require reorganization of the cytoskeleton, such as F-actin. bFGF promotes the remodeling of F-actin in dermal fibroblasts under high-glucose conditions and thus further boosts the formation of lamellipodia (Fig. 1C). These results suggest that the migratory ability of dermal fibroblasts is significantly impaired under high-glucose conditions and that bFGF promotes the migration of dermal fibroblasts impaired by high glucose by increasing the number of cells with a high polarity index and boosts cytoskeletal rearrangement, including F-actin.

3.2 PI3K/Akt is involved in bFGF-promoted der-mal fibroblast migration under high-glucose conditions

It has been widely reported that phosphatidylinositol 3-kinase (PI3K) is associated with cell polarization and migration in certain cell types [19]. However, it remains unclear whether PI3K is involved in bFGF-induced human dermal fibroblast migration under high-glucose conditions. The addition of bFGF at a final concentration of 100 ng/ml sharply increased the activity of Akt after 15 min of treatment. The level of phosphorylated Akt enhanced by bFGF in cultured human dermal fibroblasts was completely inhibited by LY294002, which is an Akt-specific inhibitor (Fig. 2D, E). Through a wound-healing assay, we found that bFGF treatment notably promoted the migration of dermal fibroblasts under high-glucose conditions with migratory rates of 20.200 ± 0.428 and 13.680 ± 0.333 μm/h 12 h or 24 h after wounding compared with 10.901 ± 0.200 and 7.812 ± 0.253 μm/h for the untreated control, respectively. However, when pretreated with LY294002, bFGF-induced fibroblast migration was completely blocked. The migratory rates were determined to be 8.343 ± 0.282 and 6.294 ± 0.252 μm/h at 12 h or 24 h after wounding, respectively (Fig. 2A–C). These results demonstrate that PI3K is involved in bFGF-promoted dermal fibroblast migration under high-glucose conditions.

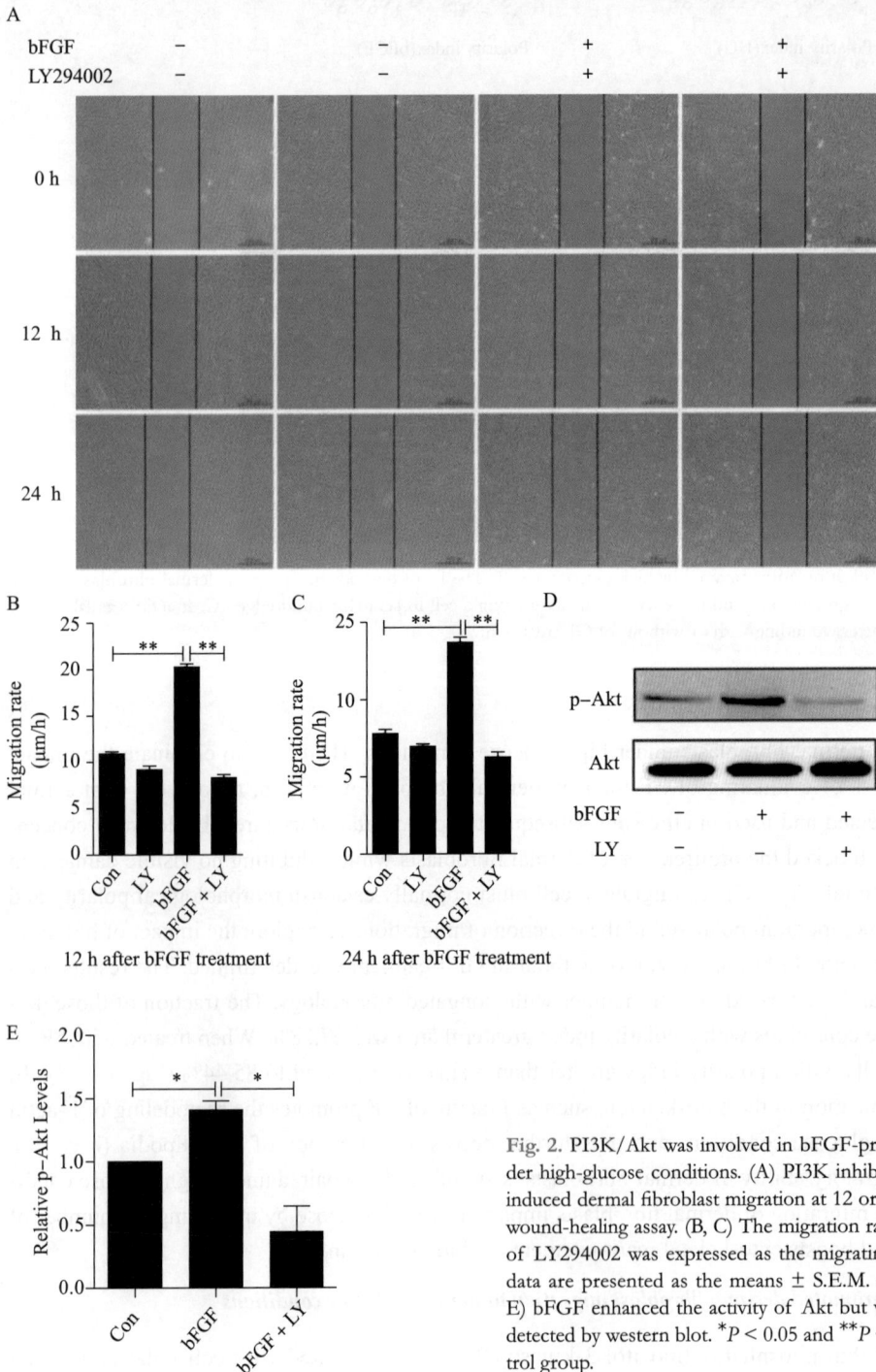

Fig. 2. PI3K/Akt was involved in bFGF-promoted dermal fibroblast migration under high-glucose conditions. (A) PI3K inhibitor LY294002 (10 μM) blocked bFGF-induced dermal fibroblast migration at 12 or 24 h after wounding as detected using a wound-healing assay. (B, C) The migration rate of dermal fibroblasts in the presence of LY294002 was expressed as the migrating distance per hour and analyzed. The data are presented as the means ± S.E.M. from six independent experiments. (D, E) bFGF enhanced the activity of Akt but was markedly inhibited by LY294002, as detected by western blot. $^*P < 0.05$ and $^{**}P < 0.01$ compared with the indicated control group.

3.3 Rac1 is involved in bFGF-promoted dermal fibroblast migration under high-glucose conditions

Rac1 is a member of the small GTPases of the Rho family and regulates cell cytoskeletal dynamics and cell migration [20]. To investigate the involvement of Rac1 in bFGF-induced fibroblast migration, we measured the activities of Rac1 in fibroblasts after treatment with bFGF. Rac1 activity was increased two-fold 10 min after bFGF stimulation and remained high for 30 min (Fig. 3D, F). The activity of Rac1 enhanced by bFGF in cultured human dermal fibroblasts

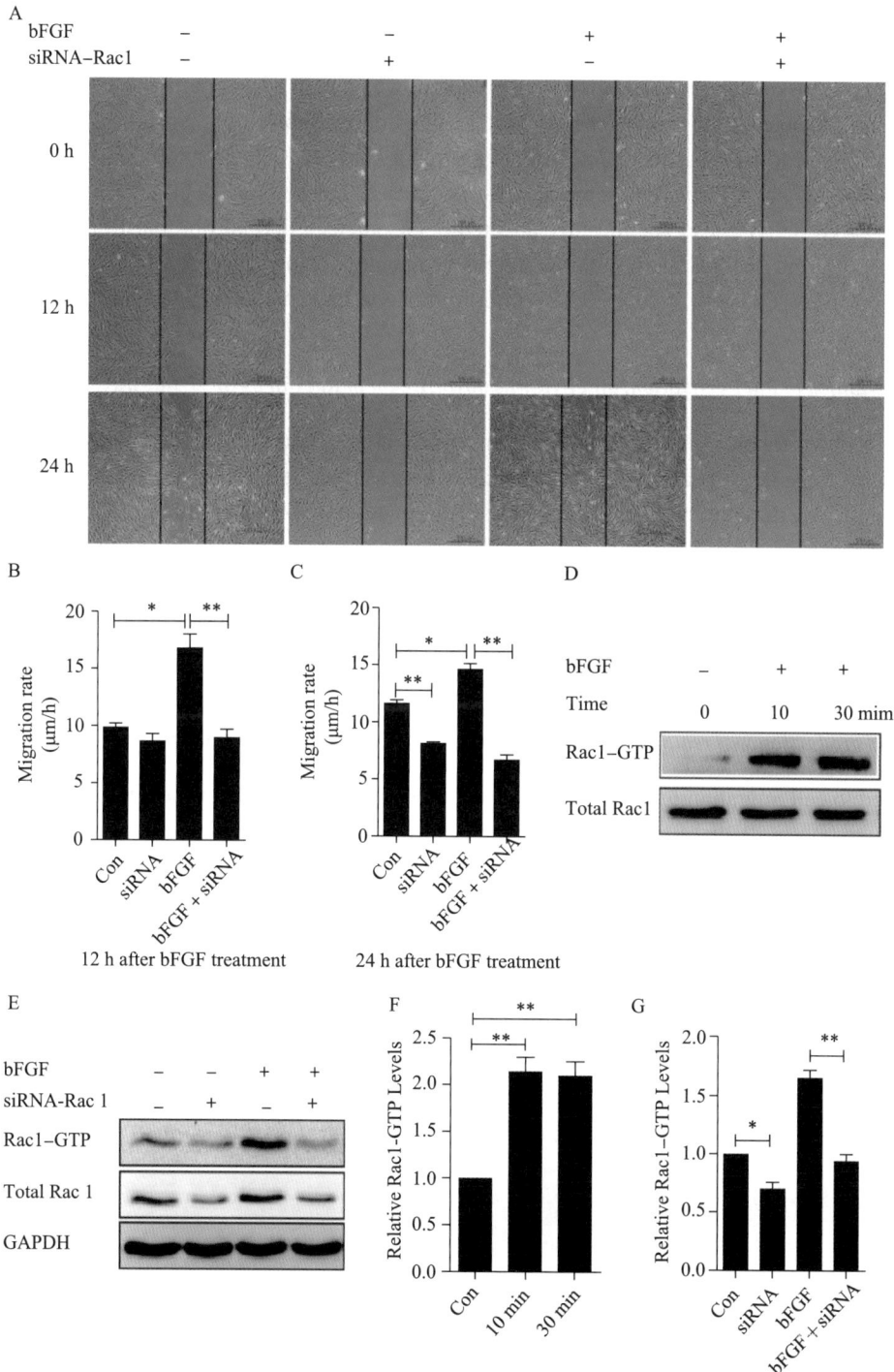

Fig. 3. Rac1 was involved in bFGF-promoted dermal fibroblast migration under high glucose conditions. (A) Rac1-siRNA (10 nM) blocked bFGF-induced dermal fibroblast migration at 12 or 24 h after wounding, as detected through a wound-healing assay. (B, C) The migration rate of dermal fibroblast in the presence of Rac1 siRNA is expressed as the migrating distance per hour and analyzed. The data are presented as the means ± S.E.M. from six independent experiments. (D, F) bFGF enhanced the activity of Rac1, as detected by western blot. (E, G) Rac1-siRNA reduced the total Rac1 protein and the activity of Rac1 after bFGF treatment. *P < 0.05 and **P < 0.01 compared with the indicated group.

was partially inhibited by Rac1 interference (Fig. 3E, G). The transfection of Rac1 siRNA led to a significant reduction in the Rac1 protein levels and Rac1-GTP levels in response to bFGF stimulation. The inhibition of Rac1 activity also significantly affected bFGF-induced dermal fibroblast migration under high-glucose conditions in a wound-healing assay, with the migratory rate decreasing to 8.995 ± 0.742 and 6.733 ± 0.485 μm/h compared with 16.741 ± 1.259 and 14.660 ± 0.513 μm/h for the non-treated control at 12 h or 24 h after wounding (Fig. 3A–C).

3.4 JNK is involved in bFGF-promoted dermal fibroblast migration under high-glucose conditions

JNK was initially identified and purified as a p54 microtubule-associated protein kinase and is activated by a wide range of stresses. JNK has also been reported to be involved in a wide variety of cellular processes, such as cell proliferation, migration and cytoskeleton reorganization [21]. To explore whether JNK also participates in the process of dermal fibroblast migration promoted by bFGF under high-glucose conditions, SP600125, a specific JNK inhibitor, was added into the culture medium for the subsequent detection of phosphorylated JNK levels and the migratory rate. bFGF treatment increased the activity of JNK, and its activation was completely blocked by SP600125 (Fig. 4D, E). The inhibition of phosphorylated JNK activity also significantly affected bFGF-induced dermal fibroblast migration under high-glucose conditions in a wound-healing assay, with the migratory rate decreasing to 6.679 ± 0.319 and 7.197 ± 0.214 μm/h compared with 16.310 ± 0.669 and 14.100 ± 0.228 μm/h for the non-treated control at 12 h or 24 h after wounding, respectively (Fig. 4A–C).

3.5 PI3k/Akt contributed to Rac1 activation, and JNK was downstream of Rac1 in bFGF signal-ing

Rac1 acts as a downstream effector of PI3-kinase in several growth factor-stimulated pathways, and the activity of JNK is regulated by the small GTPases [22]. Consequently, we measured the activation of Rac1 treated with LY294002 and the activation of JNK through treatment with Rac1 siRNA in dermal fibro-blasts after bFGF stimulation to examine whether PI3-kinase is upstream of Rac1, and JNK was found to be downstream of Rac1 in bFGF-induced dermal fibro-blast migration. The level of Rac1-GTP showed a 30% reduction in the presence of LY294002 (Fig. 5A, C), and the activity level of JNK showed a 50% reduction in the presence of Rac1 siRNA after bFGF stimulation (Fig. 5B, D). These data indicate that PI3K/Akt contributes to bFGF-induced Rac1 activation and that JNK is downstream of Rac1 in bFGF signaling.

3.6 Increased ROS production was required for bFGF-promoted dermal fibroblast migration under diabetic conditions

ROS is linked to cell migration in certain cell types. To identify whether ROS production was also involved in the bFGF-induced migration of dermal fibroblasts under high-glucose conditions, the intracellular ROS generation follow-

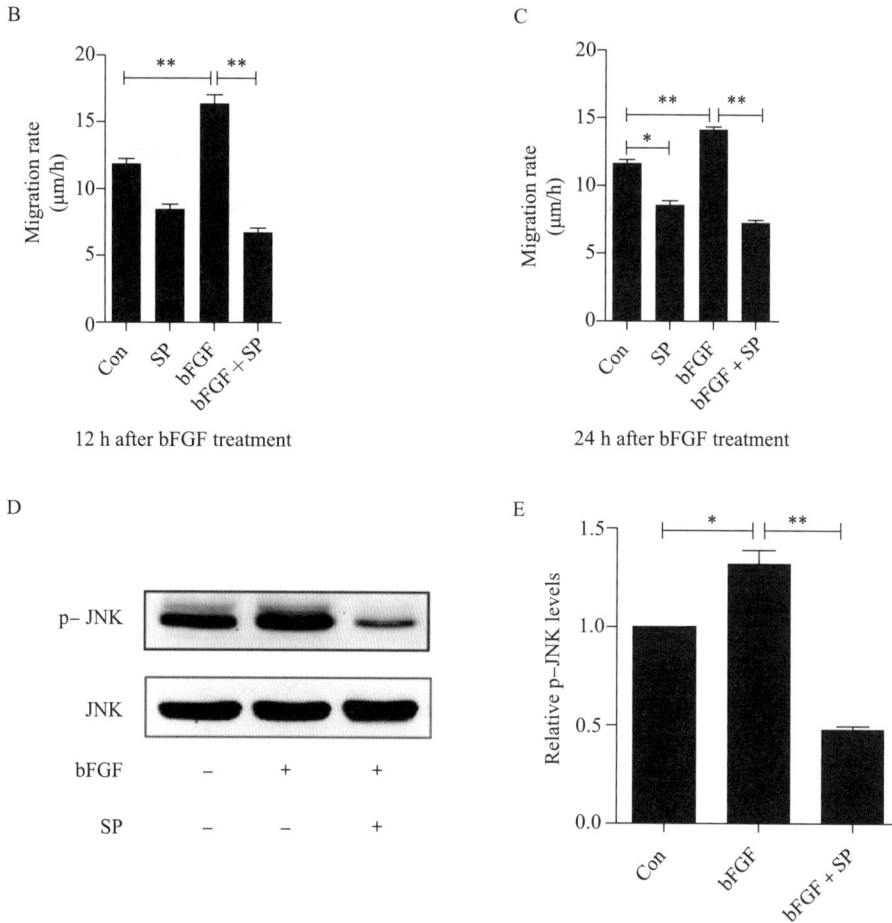

Fig. 4. JNK mediated bFGF-induced dermal fibroblast migration under diabetic conditions. (A) JNK inhibitor SP600125 (10 μM) suppressed bFGF-stimulated dermal fibroblast migration at 12 or 24 h after wounding, as detected through a wound-healing assay. (B, C) The migration rate of dermal fibroblast in the presence of SP600125 is expressed as the migrating distance per hour and analyzed. The data are represented as the means ± S.E.M. from six independent experiments. (D, E) bFGF increased the activity of JNK but was markedly inhibited by SP600125, as detected by western blot. $^{*}P < 0.05$ and $^{**}P < 0.01$ compared with the indicated control group.

ing bFGF treatment was detected using the fluorescent probe H2DCFDA. bFGF can significantly induce the generation of intracellular ROS after 24 h of incubation. Treatment with 10 μM N-acetyl-l-cysteine (NAC), a potent ROS scavenger, strongly suppressed the increased ROS levels induced by bFGF in dermal fibroblasts (Fig. 6A). In the wound-healing assay, the inhibition of bFGF-induced ROS generation by NAC apparently attenuated the migration of dermal fibroblasts promoted by bFGF with their migratory rate decreasing to 6.952 ± 0.6419 μm/h compared with a migratory rate of 11.27 ± 0.6327 μm/h in the control group at 24 h after wounding (Fig. 6B, D).

NADPH oxidase (NOX) is considered a major source of ROS in several physiological and pathological processes. Thus, we determined whether bFGF-upregulated ROS production was dependent on NADPH oxidase [23]. Pretreatment with DPI, a potent inhibitor of NADPH oxidase, completely blocked bFGF-induced ROS production (Fig. 6A). DPI also significantly suppressed bFGF-boosted dermal fibro blast migration, with the migratory rate decreasing to 6.069 ± 0.3205 μm/h at 24 h after wounding in the wound-healing assay (Fig. 6C, D). In addition, the NOX4 mRNA and protein levels were significantly up-regulated after bFGF treatment compared with the control group (Fig. 6E, F). These results suggest that bFGF induces ROS production in a NADPH oxidase-depending manner to promote the migration of dermal fibroblast under high-glucose conditions.

3.7　bFGF induced intracellular ROS production via the PI3K/Akt and JNK pathways

To evaluate whether ROS is involved in the bFGF-induced migration of human dermal fibroblasts, we investigated the potential interaction be-tween ROS production and the phosphorylation of PI3K/Akt and JNK. The pretreatment of

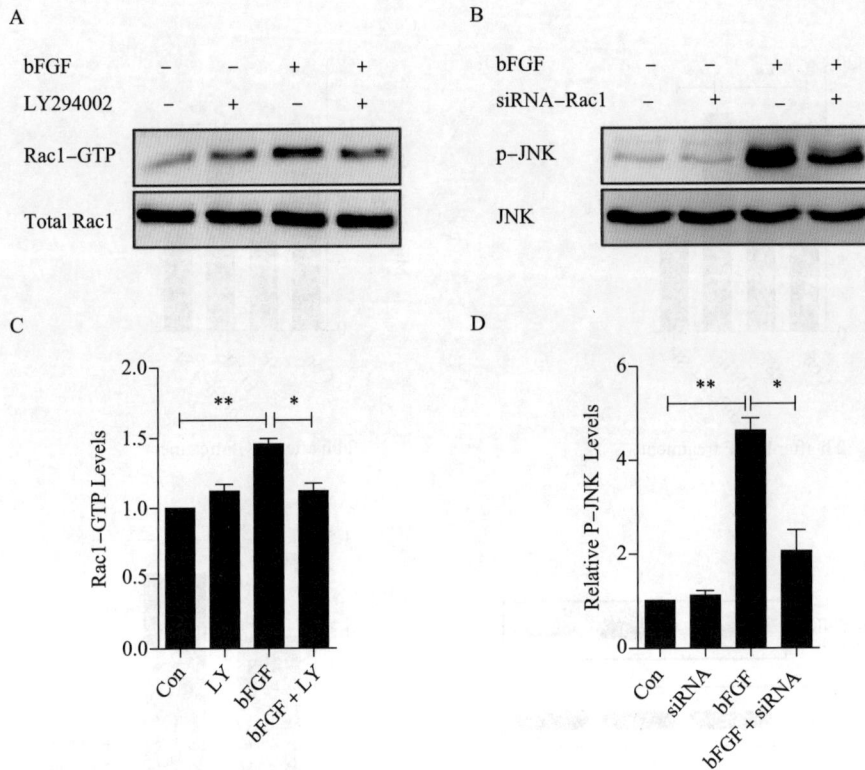

Fig. 5. PI3k/Akt contributed to Rac1 activation, and JNK was downstream of Rac1 in bFGF signaling. (A, C) The activities of Rac1 after treatment with or without 10 μM LY294002 were analyzed 15 min after stimulation with 100 ng/ml bFGF. (B, D) The activities of JNK after treatment with or without 10 nM Rac1-siRNA were analyzed 15 min after stimulation with 100 ng/ml bFGF.

dermal fibroblasts with NAC or DPI did not block the phosphorylation of either Akt or JNK induced by bFGF (Fig. 7A-D), suggesting that NADPH oxidase-derived ROS are not necessary for the bFGF-induced activation of both Akt and JNK. However, the addition of LY294002 or SP600125 sharply suppressed bFGF-induced ROS production (Fig. 7E). These results indicate that bFGF induces the generation of ROS *via* the Akt and JNK pathways to promote the migration of human dermal fibroblasts under high-glucose conditions.

3.8 *Increased ROS production is indispensible for the activation of FAK and paxillin induced by bFGF*

Focal adhesion kinase (FAK) has been widely reported to be involved in the control of several bio-logical processes, including cell proliferation and migration. Paxillin is phosphorylated by FAK and thus provides a docking site for the recruitment of other signaling molecules to focal adhesions to promote cell migration [23, 24]. Therefore, we further investigated whether these molecules mediate the bFGF-induced migration of dermal fibroblasts in the presence of a high concentration of glucose. The level of phosphorylated FAK was significantly up-regulated after 15 min of treatment with bFGF compared with the level of total FAK (Fig. 8A). Nevertheless, both the ROS scavenger NAC and the NADPH oxidase inhibitor DPI nearly completely blocked the phosphorylation of FAK induced by bFGF, but these had no effect on the level of total FAK (Fig. 8B, C). Paxillin began to be phosphorylated after incubation with bFGF for 5 min and reached a maximum level 15 min after bFGF addition (Fig. 8D). Similarly, the phosphorylation of paxillin following treatment with bFGF was also significantly inhibited by NAC and DPI, suggesting that increased ROS production by bFGF was indispensable for the activation of FAK and paxillin (Fig. 8E, F). These data suggested that the activation of FAK and paxillin is involved in the process of bFGF-induced fibroblast migration under high-glucose conditions. Furthermore, bFGF-induced ROS production is required for the activation of FAK and paxillin to promote the migration of dermal fibroblasts under high-glucose conditions.

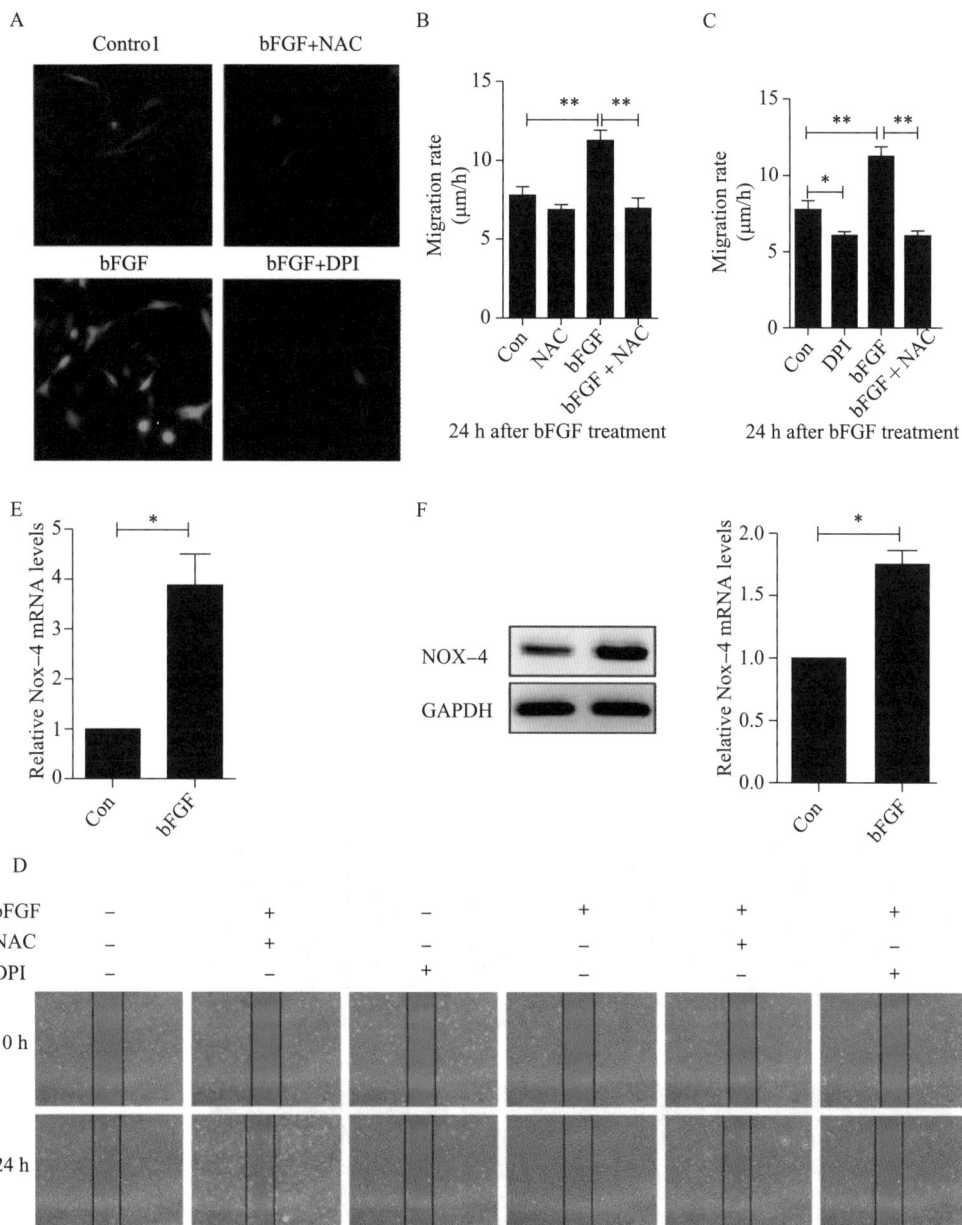

Fig. 6. Increased reactive oxygen species (ROS) production was required for bFGF-promoted dermal fibroblast migration under high-glucose conditions. (A) bFGF induced the generation of intracellular ROS in dermal fibroblasts but was suppressed by the ROS scavenger N-acetyl-l-cysteine (NAC) or the NADPH oxidase inhibitor DPI, as detected using the fluorescent probe H2DCFDA. (B, C, D) The suppression of bFGF-induced intracellular ROS production by NAC or DPI blocked bFGF-promoted dermal fibroblast migration. $^*P < 0.05$ and $^{**}P < 0.01$ compared with the indicated control group. (E, F) The NOX4 mRNA and protein levels in dermal fibroblasts after treatment with bFGF were determined by RT-PCR and western blot. $^*P < 0.05$ compared with the indicated control group.

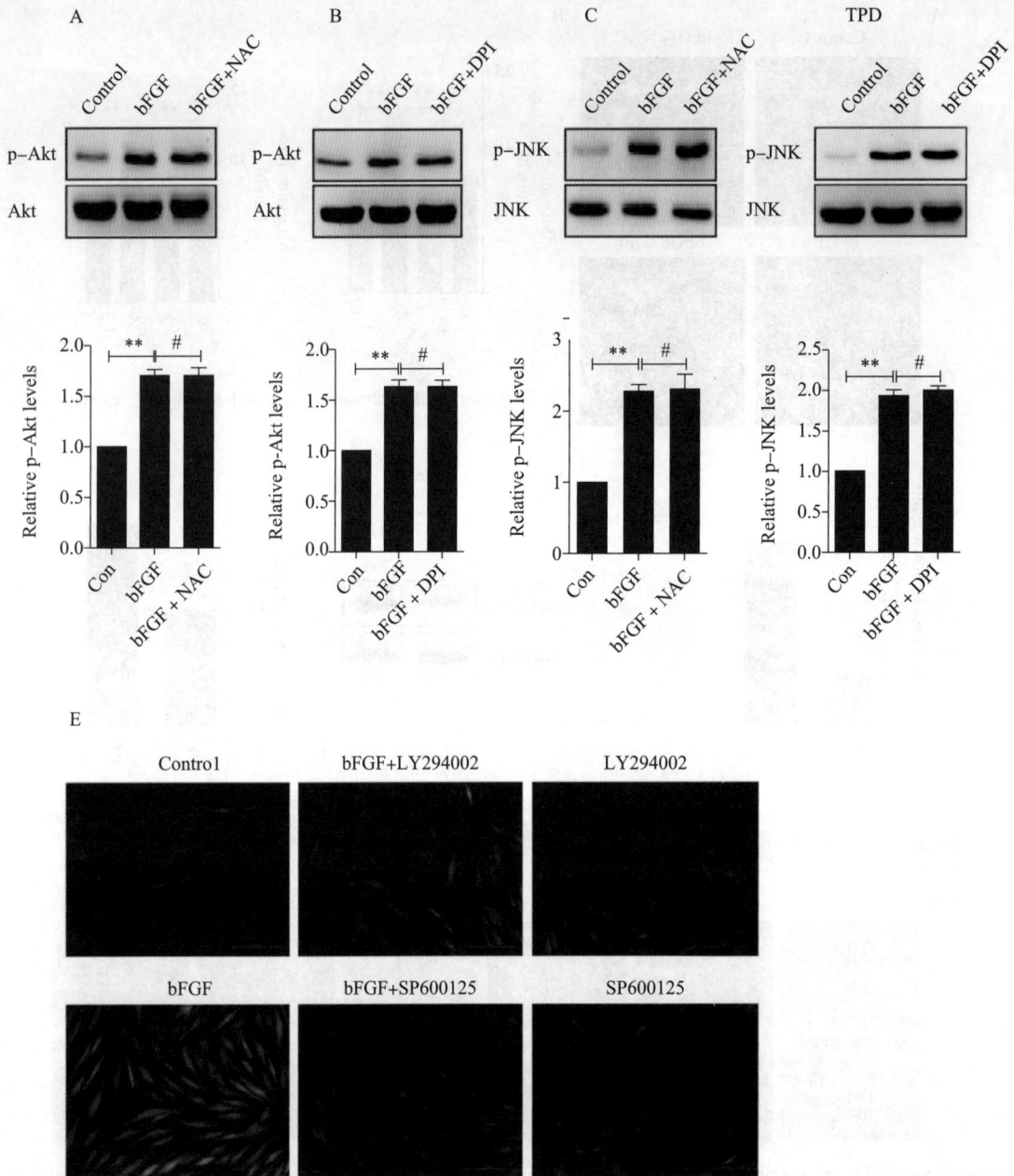

Fig. 7. bFGF induced intracellular ROS production *via* the PI3K/Akt and JNK pathways. (A–D) The ROS scavenger N-acetyl-l-cysteine (NAC) or NADPH oxidase inhibitor DPI did not block the phosphorylation of either Akt or JNK induced by bFGF, as detected by western blot. The optical density of p-Akt or p-JNK was normalized to Akt or JNK using the Quantity One software. The results are presented as fold changes compared with the control. (E) The PI3K inhibitor LY294002 or JNK inhibitor SP600125 suppressed bFGF-increased reactive oxygen species production, as detected using the fluorescent probe H2DCFDA. $^*P < 0.05$ and $^{**}P < 0.01$ compared with the indicated control group.

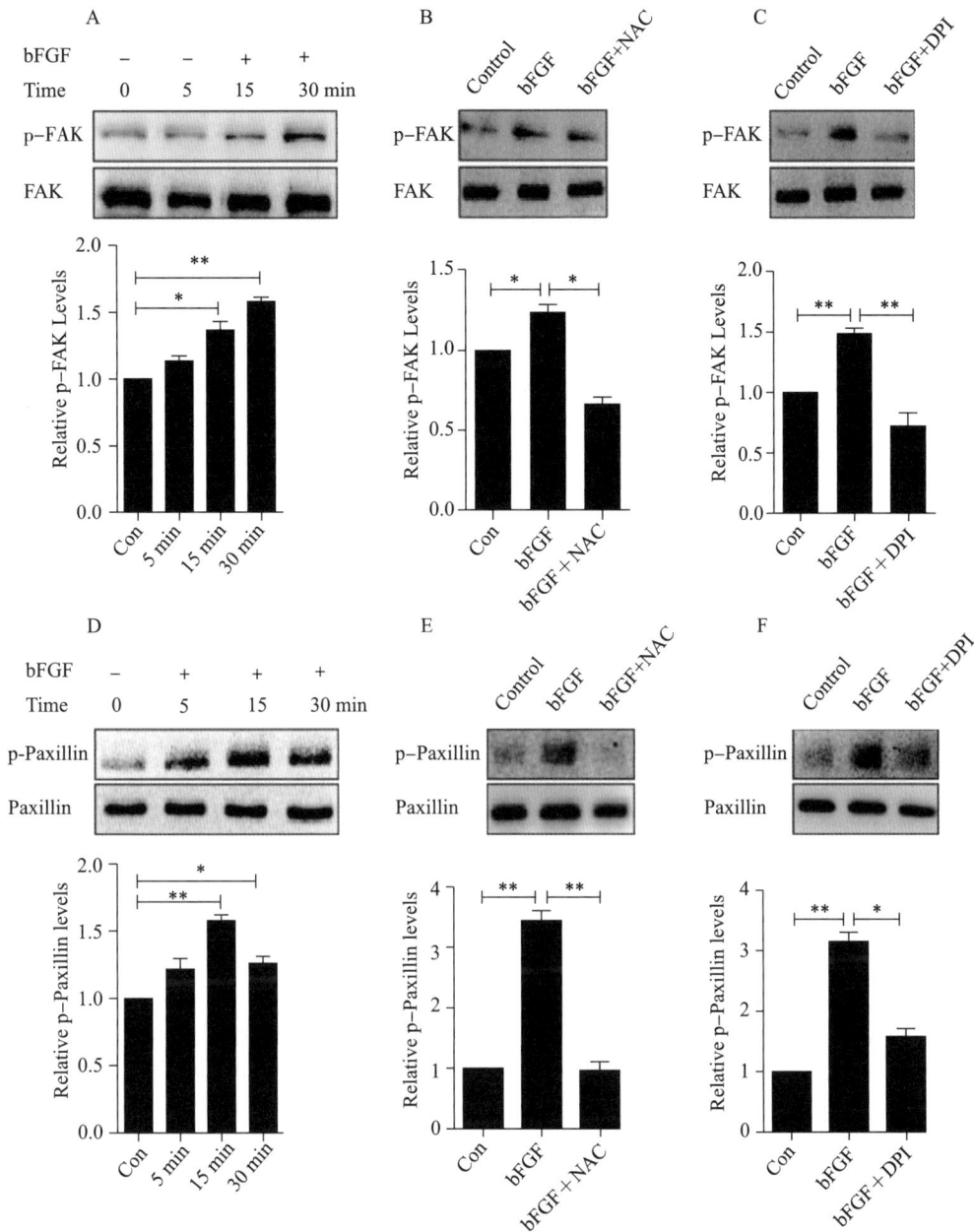

Fig. 8. Increased ROS production was necessary for the activation of FAK and paxillin induced by bFGF. (A, D) The activity of focal adhesion kinase (FAK) or paxillin was significantly up-regulated following bFGF treatment at the indicated time point, as detected by western blot. The optical density of p-FAK or p-paxillin was measured using the Quantity One software and normalized to that of FAK or paxillin. The results are presented as fold changes compared with the non-treated control. (B, E) The ROS scavenger N-acetyl-L-cysteine (NAC) blocked the activity of FAK or paxillin induced by bFGF, as detected by western blot. (C, F) The NADPH oxidase inhibitor DPI suppressed the phosphorylation of FAK or paxillin stimulated by bFGF. $^*P < 0.05$ and $^{**}P < 0.01$ compared with the indicated control group.

4. Discussion

The proliferation and migration of dermal fibroblasts are essential for cutaneous wound repair be-cause dermal fibroblasts migrate to damaged sites, repopulate the wound, and remodel fibrin and collagen deposits [25]. Cutaneous wound healing is severely impaired in diabetic patients, and high glucose is thought to be main reason for delaying wound healing in diabetes, we investigated the effect of a high concentration of glucose on the migration of human dermal fibroblasts. In this study, we showed that the migratory ability of dermal fibroblasts from human dermal skin was markedly impaired in a high-glucose environment and that bFGF activated the PI3K/Akt-Rac1-JNK signal pathway and significantly promoted the migration of human dermal fibroblasts by increasing the number of cells with a high polarity index and boosting cytoskeletal rearrangement under diabetic conditions. In addition, we demonstrated that bFGF induces dermal fibroblast migration by upregulating the NOX4 level to mediate ROS production in the presence of a high concentration of glucose.

Akt is a major transducer of the phosphoinositide 3-kinase pathway and plays a crucial role in the regulation of cellular processes, including growth, metabolism, survival, proliferation and migration [19]. The activation of the PI3K/Akt pathway plays a central role in establishing cell polarity and migration speed and is therefore required for the migration of various cell types, including fibroblasts [26]. Rac1 is required at the front of the cell to regulate actin polymerization and membrane protrusion [20], and c-Jun N-terminal kinase (JNK) is involved in the regulation of inflammation, differentiation and apoptosis [21]. Accumulating evidence also suggests that the JNK pathway is important for regulating cell migration [27]. bFGF has been shown to stimulate the directed migration of periodontal ligament cells *via* PI3K/Akt [28]. Epidermal growth factor stimulates Rac1 activation through Src and PI3K to promote colonic epithelial cell migration [29] and induces the ERK/Rac1 signaling pathway to promote cell migration in human hepatoma HepG2 cells [30]. In our study, the cultured human dermal fibroblasts showed significant increases in Akt, Rac1 and JNK activity following bFGF treatment. The inhibition of their activities by a chemical inhibitor or siRNA interference significantly inhibited the migration of dermal fibroblasts induced by bFGF under diabetic conditions, implying that PI3K/Akt, Rac1 and JNK are involved in the regulation of bFGF-promoted dermal fibroblast migration. Several studies showed that Rac1 activation was dependent on PI3K activity and that inhibitors of PI3K/Akt blocked Rac1 activation [22, 31]. Moreover, inhibition of the activity of Rac1 reduced JNK activity [32, 33]. In our study, the activity of Rac1 was abolished by the PI3-kinase/Akt inhibitor LY294002, suggesting that PI3-kinase/Akt contributes to bFGF-induced Rac1 activation. Furthermore, the inhibitory activity of Rac1 achieved with Rac1 siRNA down-regulated JNK activation after treatment with bFGF. Thus, we concluded that bFGF promotes dermal fibroblast migration through the PI3K/Akt-Rac1-JNK pathway under diabetic conditions. Shigeyuki Kanazawa *et al.* also showed that bFGF regulates the PI3K/Akt-Rac1-JNK pathway and promotes dermal fibroblast migration in rodents [34]. However, the difference between our studies is the culture medium conditions. Primary rat dermal fibroblasts were cultured in normal DMEM medium in their experiments, whereas human dermal fibroblasts were cultured in high-glucose medium in our study to mimic the diabetic conditions in diabetes patients. The data demonstrated that the PI3K/Akt-Rac1-JNK signal pathway is a cell-dependent pathway in bFGF that promotes dermal fibroblast migration.

ROS are a family of molecules that have historically been viewed as purely harmful metabolites resulting in oxidative stress and damage in aging and diseases, such as diabetes mellitus [35, 36]. Diabetes mellitus is a group of metabolic disorders that cause chronic hyperglycemia, and hyperglycemia has been linked to impaired wound healing, particularly altered angiogenesis and extracellular matrix remodeling [10, 37]. It has been shown that alterations in cell function associated with diabetic conditions and oxidative stress are the result of diabetes that damage the cell [38, 39]. High glucose modulates ROS formation and induces inflammation and cell apoptosis [40, 41], and a high-glucose environment enhances oxidative stress, increased interleukin-8 secretion and impaired keratinocyte migration. Fibroblasts from diabetic mice migrate 75% less than those from normoglycemic mice, and Lamers *et al.* showed that high glucose mediates oxidative stress, causes cell polarity loss and impairs cell migration [10]. In addition, advanced glycation end-products (AGEs) mediate the activation of ROS and blocks wound healing through impairing dermal fibroblast proliferation and migration [42]. Anti-AGE agents appear to facilitate wound healing by reducing AGE-associated inflammation and promoting the recovery process [43, 44]. However, there is no difference in ROS production between normal glucose and high glucose group in our study. Unexpectedly, we found that bFGF increased ROS generation in high glucose, the reasons for this maybe the different kinds of cell, the glucose concentration and cell culture time in high glucose condition. Wealth of evidence shows that ROS produced in certain situations may also function as important physiological regulators of intracellular signaling pathways [45]. Furthermore, studies have shown that ROS play a pivotal role in mediating the migration of certain cell types. It has been reported that ROS are involved in vascular endothelial growth factor (VEGF)-mediated endothelial migration [46], platelet-derived growth factor-induced smooth muscle cell migration [47], vascular cell adhesion molecule-1 (VCAM-1)-regulated leukocyte migration [48], and insulin-like growth factor-I (IGF-I)-stimulated vascular smooth muscle cell migration [49]. In accordance with the literature, our data suggest that increased ROS production is required for bFGF-induced human dermal fibroblast migration and that NAC significantly inhibits bFGF-promoted human dermal fibroblast migration under diabetic conditions. There are numerous potential sources of

ROS within the cell, and NADPH oxidases are one of the major enzymatic sources of ROS in different tissues [50]. Our data show that DPI significantly inhibits bFGF-promoted dermal fibroblast migration, suggesting that bFGF-induced ROS production in human dermal fibroblasts under high-glucose conditions is dependent on NDAPH oxidases. Classic NADPH oxidase consist of the two membrane bound subunits Nox2 and p22phox and the cytosolic components p47phox, p67phox, p40phox, and Rac-1, and several isoforms of the NADPH oxidase, such as NOX1, NOX3, and NOX4, have been reported [51]. Sampson *et al.* showed that NADPH oxidase 4 (NOX4)-derived ROS mediate fibroblast-to-myofibroblast transdifferentiation [52] and that NOX4 expression is increased in pulmonary fibroblasts and mediates TGF-beta1-induced fibroblast differentiation into myofibroblasts [53]. Thus, we tested whether NOX4 is up-regulated and mediates ROS production after bFGF treatment in dermal fibroblasts under diabetic conditions. Our data showed that the NOX4 mRNA and protein levels were up-regulated in the presence of bFGF, indicating that bFGF induces ROS production and mediates dermal fibroblast migration by up-regulating the NOX4 mRNA and protein levels. In adherent cells, ROS production participates in actin cytoskeletal reorganization by increasing FAK activity during cell spreading and participates in further control of gene expression and cell proliferation and migration [54]. In our study, bFGF was found to promote the migration of dermal fibroblasts through the activation of FAK and paxillin, and NAC and DPI inhibited the bFGF-induced activation of FAK and paxillin, suggesting that intracellular ROS are necessary for the activation of FAK and paxillin and participate in actin cytoskeletal reorganization in the presence of bFGF. The data demonstrated that the NOX-ROS signal pathway is another cell-dependent pathway in bFGF-induced dermal fibroblast migration under high-glucose conditions.

Endogenously generated ROS following treatment with peptide growth factors leads to the activation of the PI3K/Akt/JNK pathway [55, 56]. For example, the bFGF-induced migration of rodent vascular smooth muscle cells depends on the ROS-mediated activation of JNK [57]. The data indicated that ROS is upstream of PI3K/Akt and JNK activation and regulates cell proliferation, migration and apoptosis. The ROS-mediated activation of Akt induces apoptosis in prostate cancer cells [58], and cathepsin S plays an important role in the regulation of autophagy and apoptosis *via* ROS and serves upstream of the PI3K/AKT/mTOR/p70S6K and JNK signaling pathways in human glioblastoma cells [21]. However, in our study, we found that the blockade of intracellular ROS production with NAC or DPI did not affect the bFGF-induced activation of Akt or JNK. On the contrary, inhibition of the PI3K/Akt or JNK pathway significantly suppressed bFGF-induced ROS formation, suggesting that bFGF induces the generation of ROS in human dermal fibroblasts through the PI3K/Akt-Rac1-JNk pathway. All of the above findings indicated that ROS formation and the activation of PI3K/Akt and JNK are involved in cell proliferation, survival and migration. In addition, most of these results showed the ROS is upstream of the activation of PI3K/Akt and JNK and modulates cell physiological activity. However, our data are contrary to the specificity of the cells, and the cell culture microenvironment differences may be taken into consideration, but the PI3K/Akt and JNK mechanisms that regulate ROS formation in dermal fibroblasts under diabetic environment remain to be elucidated.

A duality in the roles of ROS with respect to wound healing. Injury to the skin initiates a series of events, such as inflammation, tissue regeneration, and matrix remodeling. During the early inflammatory phase, leukocytes and macrophages infiltrate the wounded tissue and produce large amounts of reactive oxygen species (ROS) as part of their defense mechanism once activated [59]. ROS are essential during various stages of the healing process, ranging from the initial signal that instigates the immune response, to the triggering of intracellular redox-dependent signaling pathways and the defence against invading bacteria [60]. For example, galectin-1 induced myofibroblast activation, migration, and proliferation by upregulating NOX4, triggered intracellular ROS production and accelerated the healing of general and pathological wounds and decreased the mortality of diabetic mice with skin wounds [61]. Further, study showed that ROS were essential mediators in epidermal growth factor (EGF)-stimulated corneal epithelial cell proliferation, adhesion, migration, and wound healing [55]. Although this process is beneficial, increased levels of ROS can inhibit cell migration and proliferation and even cause severe tissue damage, such as diabetes and diabetic complications [62, 63]. Based on above, increased appropriate ROS are helpful in promoting wound healing, excessive ROS cause cell dysfunction and impair wound healing. In our study, bFGF increased ROS formation which were essential for promoting dermal fibroblasts migration, indicating that the beneficiary of increased ROS in the wound healing may be wound stage or context dependent. Therefore, we are going to observe the synergistic effect during cutaneous wound repair by combining use low level of hydrogen peroxide (H_2O_2) and bFGF in future study, which could be helpful for clinical use of bFGF.

It should be noted that the detailed interaction of bFGF with ROS and PI3K/Akt-Rac1-JNK has not been fully es-

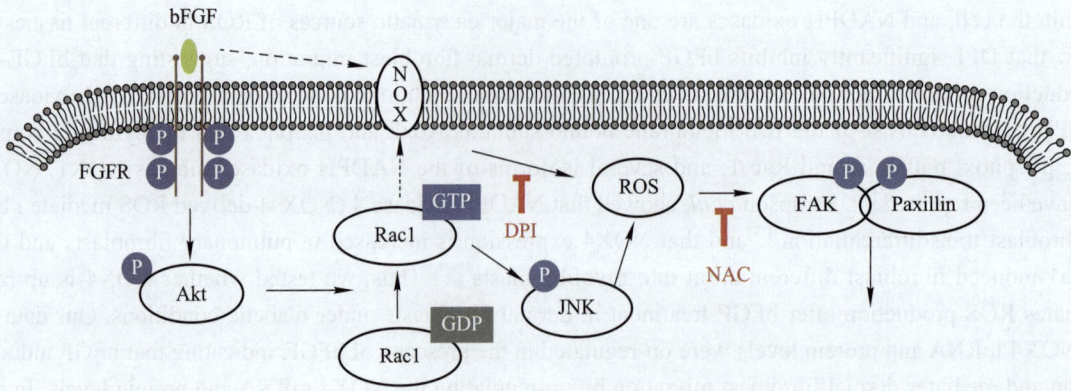

Fig. 9. The proposed mechanism of bFGF promotes the migration of human dermal fibroblasts under diabetic conditions. Schematic representation of the mechanism through which bFGF promotes human dermal fibroblast migration under diabetic conditions.

tablished in the present study. In addition, why AKT and JNK activation lead to ROS production *via* NADPH oxidase activation are also unclear. A further clarification of these issues utilizing knock down of Akt, JNK and NOX4 will provide novel insights into these questions and provide more evidence to support our conclusions. In addition, whether NOX4 is the source of ROS responsible for bFGF-induced dermal fibroblast migration and whether the Rac1, p47phox, and p67phox cytosolic subunits have to assemble with the membrane-bound subunits to induce ROS formation after bFGF treatment in dermal fibroblasts under high glucose. The knock down of NOX4 protein should be performed to confirm whether NOX4 is the specific NADPH oxidase that induces ROS formation. Meanwhile, co-immunoprecipitation assays should also be performed to verify whether Rac1, p47phox, and p67phox transfer from the cytoplasm to the membrane, assemble with the membrane-bound subunits, allow the transfer of electrons from NADPH to molecular oxygen and induce ROS formation in the presence of bFGF.

In conclusion, our results indicate that bFGF induces ROS formation and promotes the migration of dermal fibroblasts, leading to the activation of FAK and paxillin in human dermal fibroblasts under high-glucose conditions (Fig. 9). In addition, we have shown that inhibition of the activation of PI3K/Akt, Rac1, JNK and ROS using special inhibitors or siRNA interference can block the bFGF-induced migratory properties of human dermal fibroblasts under diabetic conditions. Taken together, our results suggest that bFGF promotes the migration of dermal fibroblasts by NOX4 and mediates ROS production *via* the PI3K/Akt-Rac1-JNK pathways in a diabetic environment.

Supplementary material

Supplementary material to this article can be found online at http://www.ijbs.com/v11p0845s1.pdf.

References

[1] Boulton AJ, Vileikyte L, Ragnarson-Tennvall G, et al. The global burden of diabetic foot disease[J]. Lancet, 2005, 366(9498): 1719-1724.

[2] Sun DP, Yeh CH, So E, et al. Interleukin (IL)-19 promoted skin wound healing by increasing fibroblast keratinocyte growth factor expression[J]. Cytokine, 2013, 62(3): 360-368.

[3] Falanga V. Wound healing and its impairment in the diabetic foot[J]. Lancet, 2005, 366(9498): 1736-1743.

[4] Opalenik SR, Davidson JM. Fibroblast differentiation of bone marrow-derived cells during wound repair[J]. Faseb j, 2005, 19(11): 1561-1563.

[5] Werner S, Krieg T, Smola H. Keratinocyte-fibroblast interactions in wound healing[J]. J Invest Dermatol, 2007, 127(5): 998-1008.

[6] Wang T, Feng Y, Sun H, et al. miR-21 regulates skin wound healing by targeting multiple aspects of the healing process[J]. Am J Pathol, 2012, 181(6): 1911-1920.

[7] Hehenberger K, Hansson A. High glucose-induced growth factor resistance in human fibroblasts can be reversed by antioxidants and protein kinase C-inhibitors[J]. Cell Biochem Funct, 1997, 15(3): 197-201.

[8] Hehenberger K, Heilborn JD, Brismar K, et al. Inhibited proliferation of fibroblasts derived from chronic diabetic wounds and normal dermal fibroblasts treated with high glucose is associated with increased formation of l-lactate[J]. Wound Repair Regen, 1998, 6(2): 135-141.

[9] Lerman OZ, Galiano RD, Armour M, et al. Cellular dysfunction in

the diabetic fibroblast: impairment in migration, vascular endothelial growth factor production, and response to hypoxia[J]. Am J Pathol, 2003, 162(1): 303-312.

[10] Lerman OZ, Galiano RD, Armour M, et al. Cellular dysfunction in the diabetic fibroblast: impairment in migration, vascular endothelial growth factor production, and response to hypoxia[J]. Am J Pathol, 2003, 162(1): 303-312.

[11] Blakytny R, Jude E. The molecular biology of chronic wounds and delayed healing in diabetes[J]. Diabet Med, 2006, 23(6): 594-608.

[12] Bennett SP, Griffiths GD, Schor AM, et al. Growth factors in the treatment of diabetic foot ulcers[J]. Br J Surg, 2003, 90(2): 133-146.

[13] Liu Y, Cai S, Shu XZ, et al. Release of basic fibroblast growth factor from a crosslinked glycosaminoglycan hydrogel promotes wound healing[J]. Wound Repair Regen, 2007, 15(2): 245-251.

[14] Mizuno K, Yamamura K, Yano K, et al. Effect of chitosan film containing basic fibroblast growth factor on wound healing in genetically diabetic mice[J]. J Biomed Mater Res A, 2003, 64(1): 177-181.

[15] Marti-Carvajal AJ, Gluud C, Nicola S, et al. Growth factors for treating diabetic foot ulcers[J]. Cochrane Database Syst Rev, 2015, (10): Cd008548.

[16] Shi HX, Lin C, Lin BB, et al. The anti-scar effects of basic fibroblast growth factor on the wound repair in vitro and in vivo[J]. PLoS One, 2013, 8(4): e59966.

[17] Boosani CS, Nalabothula N, Sheibani N, et al. Inhibitory effects of arresten on bFGF-induced proliferation, migration, and matrix metalloproteinase-2 activation in mouse retinal endothelial cells[J]. Curr Eye Res, 2010, 35(1): 45-55.

[18] Vicente-Manzanares M, Koach MA, Whitmore L, et al. Segregation and activation of myosin IIB creates a rear in migrating cells[J]. J Cell Biol, 2008, 183(3): 543-554.

[19] Lu JW, Liao CY, Yang WY, et al. Overexpression of endothelin 1 triggers hepatocarcinogenesis in zebrafish and promotes cell proliferation and migration through the AKT pathway[J]. PLoS One, 2014, 9(1): e85318.

[20] Magi S, Takemoto Y, Kobayashi H, et al. 5-Lipoxygenase and cysteinyl leukotriene receptor 1 regulate epidermal growth factor-induced cell migration through Tiam1 upregulation and Rac1 activation[J]. Cancer Sci, 2014, 105(3): 290-296.

[21] Zhang L, Wang H, Xu J, et al. Inhibition of cathepsin S induces autophagy and apoptosis in human glioblastoma cell lines through ROS-mediated PI3K/AKT/mTOR/p70S6K and JNK signaling pathways[J]. Toxicol Lett, 2014, 228(3): 248-259.

[22] Murga C, Zohar M, Teramoto H, et al. Rac1 and RhoG promote cell survival by the activation of PI3K and Akt, independently of their ability to stimulate JNK and NF-kappaB[J]. Oncogene, 2002, 21(2): 207-216.

[23] Wang H, Yang Z, Jiang Y, et al. Endothelial NADPH oxidase 4 mediates vascular endothelial growth factor receptor 2-induced intravitreal neovascularization in a rat model of retinopathy of prematurity[J]. Mol Vis, 2014, 20: 231-241.

[24] Ben Mahdi MH, Andrieu V, Pasquier C. Focal adhesion kinase regulation by oxidative stress in different cell types[J]. IUBMB Life, 2000, 50(4-5): 291-299.

[25] Hata S, Okamura K, Hatta M, et al. Proteolytic and non-proteolytic activation of keratinocyte-derived latent TGF-beta1 induces fibroblast differentiation in a wound-healing model using rat skin[J]. J Pharmacol Sci, 2014, 124(2): 230-243.

[26] Yu J, Wang Q, Wang H, et al. Activation of liver X receptor enhances the proliferation and migration of endothelial progenitor cells and promotes vascular repair through PI3K/Akt/eNOS signaling pathway activation[J]. Vascular pharmacology, 2014, 62(3): 150-161.

[27] Mendes KN, Wang GK, Fuller GN, et al. JNK mediates insulin-like growth factor binding protein 2/integrin alpha5-dependent glioma

cell migration[J]. Int J Oncol, 2010, 37(1): 143-153.

[28] Shimabukuro Y, Terashima H, Takedachi M, et al. Fibroblast growth factor-2 stimulates directed migration of periodontal ligament cells via PI3K/AKT signaling and CD44/hyaluronan interaction[J]. J Cell Physiol, 2011, 226(3): 809-821.

[29] Dise RS, Frey MR, Whitehead RH, et al. Epidermal growth factor stimulates Rac activation through Src and phosphatidylinositol 3-kinase to promote colonic epithelial cell migration[J]. Am J Physiol Gastrointest Liver Physiol, 2008, 294(1): G276-G285.

[30] Hu Z, Du J, Yang L, et al. GEP100/Arf6 is required for epidermal growth factor-induced ERK/Rac1 signaling and cell migration in human hepatoma HepG2 cells[J]. PLoS One, 2012, 7(6): e38777.

[31] Huang JS, Cho CY, Hong CC, et al. Oxidative stress enhances Axl-mediated cell migration through an Akt1/Rac1-dependent mechanism[J]. Free Radic Biol Med, 2013, 65: 1246-1256.

[32] Yamauchi J, Miyamoto Y, Kokubu H, et al. Endothelin suppresses cell migration via the JNK signaling pathway in a manner dependent upon Src kinase, Rac1, and Cdc42[J]. FEBS Lett, 2002, 527(1-3): 284-288.

[33] Chen JC, Lin BB, Hu HW, et al. NGF accelerates cutaneous wound healing by promoting the migration of dermal fibroblasts via the PI3K/Akt-Rac1-JNK and ERK pathways[J]. Biomed Res Int, 2014, 2014: 547187.

[34] Kanazawa S, Fujiwara T, Matsuzaki S, et al. bFGF regulates PI3-kinase-Rac1-JNK pathway and promotes fibroblast migration in wound healing[J]. PLoS One, 2010, 5(8): e12228.

[35] Rojas A, Mercadal E, Figueroa H, et al. Advanced Glycation and ROS: a link between diabetes and heart failure[J]. Curr Vasc Pharmacol, 2008, 6(1): 44-51.

[36] Rovira-Llopis S, Rocha M, Falcon R, et al. Is myeloperoxidase a key component in the ROS-induced vascular damage related to nephropathy in type 2 diabetes?[J]. Antioxid Redox Signal, 2013, 19(13): 1452-1458.

[37] Browning AC, Alibhai A, McIntosh RS, et al. Effect of diabetes mellitus and hyperglycemia on the proliferation of human Tenon's capsule fibroblasts: implications for wound healing after glaucoma drainage surgery[J]. Wound Repair Regen, 2005, 13(3): 295-302.

[38] Takahashi A, Aoshiba K, Nagai A. Apoptosis of wound fibroblasts induced by oxidative stress[J]. Exp Lung Res, 2002, 28(4): 275-284.

[39] Lan CC, Wu CS, Huang SM, et al. High-glucose environment enhanced oxidative stress and increased interleukin-8 secretion from keratinocytes: new insights into impaired diabetic wound healing[J]. Diabetes, 2013, 62(7): 2530-2538.

[40] Liu D, Zhang H, Gu W, et al. Effects of exposure to high glucose on primary cultured hippocampal neurons: involvement of intracellular ROS accumulation[J]. Neurol Sci, 2014, 35(6): 831-837.

[41] Jayakumar T, Chang CC, Lin SL, et al. Brazilin ameliorates high glucose-induced vascular inflammation via inhibiting ROS and CAMs production in human umbilical vein endothelial cells[J]. Biomed Res Int, 2014, 2014: 403703.

[42] Loughlin DT, Artlett CM. Precursor of advanced glycation end products mediates ER-stress-induced caspase-3 activation of human dermal fibroblasts through NAD(P)H oxidase 4[J]. PLoS One, 2010, 5(6): e11093.

[43] Chang PC, Tsai SC, Jheng YH, et al. Soft-tissue wound healing by anti-advanced glycation end-products agents[J]. J Dent Res, 2014, 93(4): 388-393.

[44] Goova MT, Li J, Kislinger T, et al. Blockade of receptor for advanced glycation end-products restores effective wound healing in diabetic mice[J]. Am J Pathol, 2001, 159(2): 513-525.

[45] Finkel T. Signal transduction by reactive oxygen species[J]. J Cell Biol, 2011, 194(1): 7-15.

[46] Yamaoka-Tojo M, Ushio-Fukai M, Hilenski L, et al. IQGAP1, a novel vascular endothelial growth factor receptor binding protein, is involved in reactive oxygen species--dependent endothelial migration and proliferation[J]. Circ Res, 2004, 95(3): 276-283.

[47] Weber DS, Taniyama Y, Rocic P, *et al*. Phosphoinositide-dependent kinase 1 and p21-activated protein kinase mediate reactive oxygen species-dependent regulation of platelet-derived growth factor-induced smooth muscle cell migration[J]. Circ Res, 2004, 94(9): 1219-1226.

[48] Weber DS, Taniyama Y, Rocic P, *et al*. Phosphoinositide-dependent kinase 1 and p21-activated protein kinase mediate reactive oxygen species-dependent regulation of platelet-derived growth factor-induced smooth muscle cell migration[J]. Circ Res, 2004, 94(9): 1219-1226.

[49] Meng D, Lv DD, Fang J. Insulin-like growth factor-I induces reactive oxygen species production and cell migration through Nox4 and Rac1 in vascular smooth muscle cells[J]. Cardiovasc Res, 2008, 80(2): 299-308.

[50] Dickinson BC, Chang CJ. Chemistry and biology of reactive oxygen species in signaling or stress responses[J]. Nat Chem Biol, 2011, 7(8): 504-511.

[51] Nam HJ, Park YY, Yoon G, *et al*. Co-treatment with hepatocyte growth factor and TGF-beta1 enhances migration of HaCaT cells through NADPH oxidase-dependent ROS generation[J]. Exp Mol Med, 2010, 42(4): 270-279.

[52] Sampson N, Plas E, Berger P. NADPH oxidase 4 (NOX4) derived ROS mediate fibroblast to myofibroblast transdifferentiation in the diseased prostatic stroma. In: Federation of American Societies for Experimental Biology, 2009.

[53] Rocic P, Lucchesi PA. NAD(P)H oxidases and TGF-beta-induced cardiac fibroblast differentiation: Nox-4 gets Smad[J]. Circ Res, 2005, 97(9): 850-852.

[54] Gregg D, de Carvalho DD, Kovacic H. Integrins and coagulation: a role for ROS/redox signaling?[J]. Antioxid Redox Signal, 2004, 6(4): 757-764.

[55] Huo Y, Qiu WY, Pan Q, *et al*. Reactive oxygen species (ROS) are essential mediators in epidermal growth factor (EGF)-stimulated corneal epithelial cell proliferation, adhesion, migration, and wound healing[J]. Exp Eye Res, 2009, 89(6): 876-886.

[56] Yang Y, Du J, Hu Z, *et al*. Activation of Rac1-PI3K/Akt is required for epidermal growth factor-induced PAK1 activation and cell migration in MDA-MB-231 breast cancer cells[J]. J Biomed Res, 2011, 25(4): 237-245.

[57] Schroder K, Helmcke I, Palfi K, *et al*. Nox1 mediates basic fibroblast growth factor-induced migration of vascular smooth muscle cells[J]. Arterioscler Thromb Vasc Biol, 2007, 27(8): 1736-1743.

[58] Chetram MA, Bethea DA, Odero-Marah VA, *et al*. ROS-mediated activation of AKT induces apoptosis *via* pVHL in prostate cancer cells[J]. Mol Cell Biochem, 2013, 376(1-2): 63-71.

[59] Steiling H, Munz B, Werner S, *et al*. Different types of ROS-scavenging enzymes are expressed during cutaneous wound repair[J]. Exp Cell Res, 1999, 247(2): 484-494.

[60] Vermeij WP, Backendorf C. Skin cornification proteins provide global link between ROS detoxification and cell migration during wound healing[J]. PLoS One, 2010, 5(8): e11957.

[61] Lin YT, Chen JS, Wu MH, *et al*. Galectin-1 accelerates wound healing by regulating the neuropilin-1/Smad3/NOX4 pathway and ROS production in myofibroblasts[J]. J Invest Dermatol, 2015, 135(1): 258-268.

[62] Li JM, Shah AM. ROS generation by nonphagocytic NADPH oxidase: potential relevance in diabetic nephropathy[J]. J Am Soc Nephrol, 2003, 14(8 Suppl 3): S221-226.

[63] Bitar MS, Al-Mulla F. ROS constitute a convergence nexus in the development of IGF1 resistance and impaired wound healing in a rat model of type 2 diabetes[J]. Dis Model Mech, 2012, 5(3): 375-388.

Fibroblast growth factor 21 protects the heart from apoptosis in a diabetic mouse model *via* extracellular signal-regulated kinase 1/2-dependent signalling pathway

Chi Zhang, Yi Tan, Xiaokun Li

1. Introduction

Diabetic cardiomyopathy is attributed to multiple pathogenic factors, including hyperglycaemia, hyperlipidaemia, hypertension and inflammation [1–3]. Cardiomyopathy is the late consequence of diabetes-induced early cardiac responses. One of the key early cardiac responses is apoptosis [2, 4, 5]. Inhibition of the early cardiac apoptosis can prevent subsequent diabetic cardiomyopathy [4, 6]. Thus, reducing cardiac apoptosis may be beneficial to prevent diabetic cardiomyopathy.

Fibroblast growth factor 21 (FGF21) has been identified as a potent metabolic regulator with specific effects on glucose and lipid metabolism [7–9]. It has been predominantly investigated in the liver and adipose tissue [10]. However, FGF21 is also expressed in other tissues such as the myocardium [11]. FGF21 was found to be an acute response protein to protect tissues from acute toxicity [12, 13]. Additionally, the anti-apoptotic effects of FGF21 on islet beta cells and endothelial cells were also reported [14, 15]. However, the effect of FGF21 on the heart remains largely unknown. FGF21 functions through binding to fibroblast growth factor receptor FGFR 1 and the co-factor β-klotho [16]. The existence of FGFR1, β-klotho [17] and FGF21 [11] in the myocardium implies that FGF21 may play certain physiological roles in the heart. Recently, several studies have demonstrated FGF21-mediated protection against myocardial ischaemia/ reperfusion injury [18, 19] and isoprenaline-induced cardiac hypertrophy [20]. However, the effect of FGF21 on diabetic heart remains elusive.

In the present study, we examined whether FGF21 protects the heart from NEFA-or diabetes-induced cardiac apoptosis and dysfunction *in vitro* and *in vivo*.

2. Methods

2.1 Animal experiments

Five sets of animal studies were performed: (1) measuring cardiac *Fgf21* mRNA expression; (2) assessing cardiac FGF21-mediated protection from lipotoxicity induced by NEFA infusion; (3) evaluating acute FGF21-mediated protection from diabetes-induced cardiac apoptosis; (4) testing whether *Fgf21*-knockout (*Fgf21*-KO) mice are susceptible to diabetic cardiac apoptosis; and (5) testing whether FGF21 prevents diabetic cardiomyopathy in a model of chronic diabetes. All animal experiments were conducted in accordance with the guideline of the Institutional Animal Care and Use committees of Wenzhou Medical University and University of Louisville. See electronic supplementary material (ESM) Methods for details.

2.2 Cardiac function and BP assay

Cardiac function and BP were measured by echocardiography and tail-cuff manometry, respectively [21, 22]. See ESM Methods for details.

2.3 Biochemical and histochemical assay

Plasma triacylglycerol was measured using a triacylglycerol assay kit. Cardiac apoptosis was detected by TUNEL or DNA fragmentation [23]. Cardiac fibrosis was examined using Sirius Red staining. The expression and/or phosphorylation of target genes was detected by western blot or real-time quantitative (q)PCR. See ESM Methods for details.

2.4 Primary cardiomyocyte isolation, cell culture, palmitate and FGF21 treatments and small interfering RNA transfection

Adult mouse cardiomyocytes were isolated as described previously [24]. H9c2 cells and/or cardiomyocytes were pre-treated with pharmaceutical inhibitors or specific small interfering (si)RNAs against *Erk1* (also known as *Mapk3*)/*Erk2* (also known as *Mapk1*), *p38Mapk* (also known as *Mapk14*) and *Ampk* with or without FGF21 (50 ng/ml), followed by palmitate treatment for 15 h. A pilot time-course study has been performed to optimise the transfection efficiency with *p38Mapk* siRNA in adult mouse cardiomyocytes (ESM Fig. 1). See ESM Methods for details.

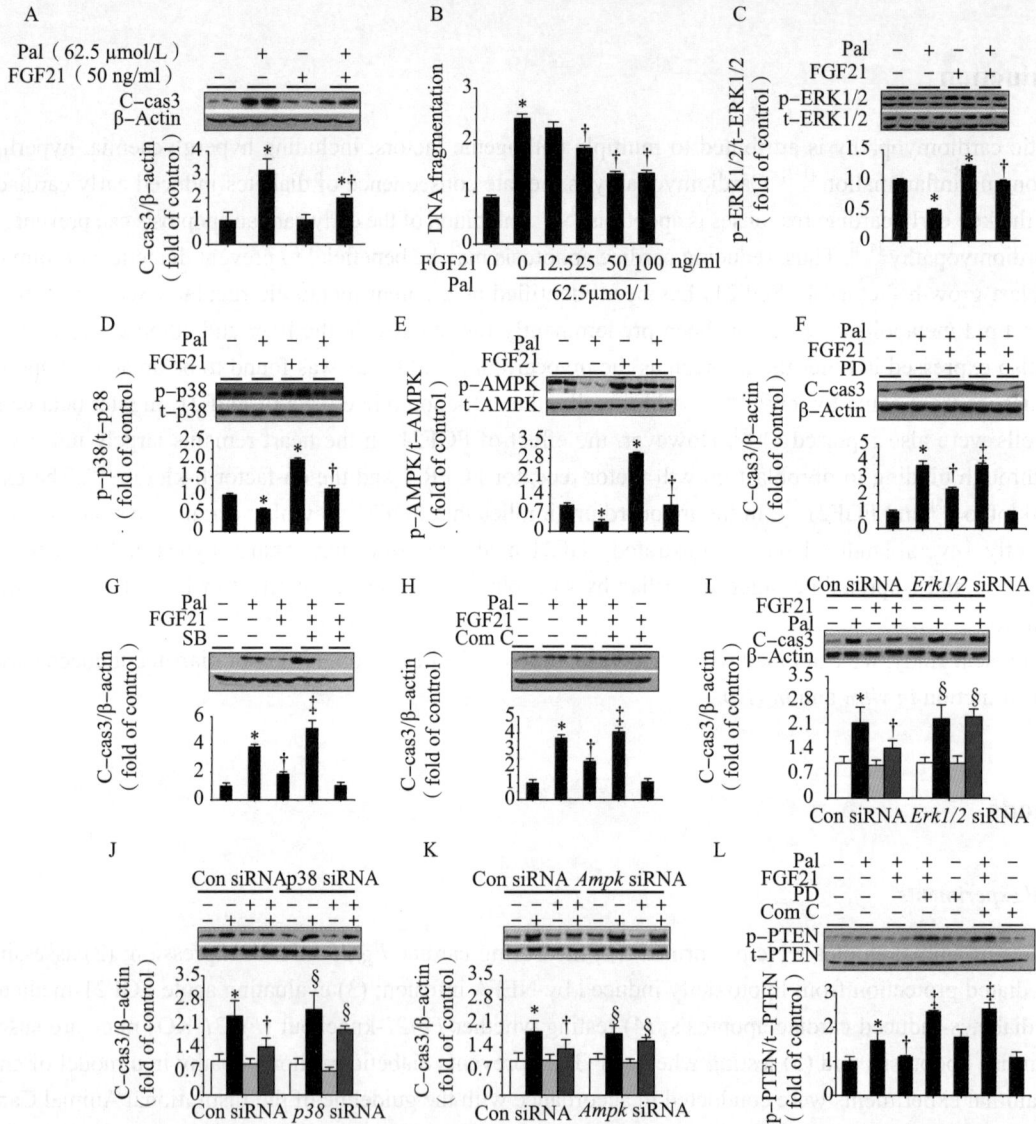

Fig. 1. FGF21 prevents palmitate-induced cardiac apoptosis and inactivation of ERKg1/2, p38 MAPK and AMPK. Pre-treatment of H9c2 cells with FGF21 (50 ng/ml) for 1 h was followed by co-treatment with palmitate (62.5 μmol/L) for 15 h. Caspase-3 cleavage (A) and DNA fragmentation (B) were detected as markers of apoptosis, and phosphorylation levels of ERK1/2 (C), p38 MAPK (D) and AMPK (E) were examined as markers of FGF21-mediated protection. Some H9c2 cells were treated with both FGF21 (50 ng/ml) and PD98059 (20 μmol/L), SB203580 (20 μmol/L) or compound C (10 μmol/L) 1 h before and during 15 h palmitate treatment, and then caspase-3 cleavage (F–H) and PTEN phosphorylation (L) were examined by western blot. Primary cardiomyocytes were pre-treated with FGF21 (50 ng/ml, light grey bar) or PBS (white bar) for 1 h followed by co-treatment with palmitate (62.5 μmol/L; black bar, PBS+palmitate; dark grey bar, FGF21+palmitate) in the presence of either siRNA against *Erk1/2*, *p38Mapk* or *Ampk* or control siRNA. Caspase-3 cleavage (I–K) was examined as above. Data were collected from at least three independent experiments and presented as mean ± SD. $^*P < 0.05$ vs control; $^\dagger P < 0.05$ vs. palmitate; $^\ddagger P < 0.05$ vs. palmitate/FGF21; $^\S P<0.05$ vs. control in *Erk1/2*, *p38Mapk* or *Ampk* siRNA treatment. C-cas3, caspase-3 cleavage; Com C, compound C; Con, control; p38, p38 MAPK; Pal, palmitate; PD, PD98059; SB, SB203580

2.5 *Statistical analysis*

Data were collected from three replicates of cell-culture experiments, or from $n \geq 5$ mice per group for *in vivo* studies and presented as mean ± SD. One-way ANOVA was used to determine general differences, followed by a *post hoc* Tukey's test for the difference between groups, using Origin 7.5 software (Northampton, MA, USA). Statistical significance was considered as $p < 0.05$.

3. Results

3.1 *Fgf21 mRNA expression is increased in the heart of mice with diabetes*

We found that fasting for 24 h increased *Fgf21* mRNA expression about nine fold in the heart (ESM Fig. 2A) and 26-fold in the liver (ESM Fig. 2B). The endoplasmic reticulum stress inducer thapsigargin [25, 26] also significantly increased *Fgf21* mRNA in the heart (ten fold) (ESM Fig. 2C) and liver (14-fold) (ESM Fig. 2D). In streptozotocin (STZ)-induced diabetic mice, the hepatic *Fgf21* mRNA expression was significantly decreased at 2, 4 and 6 months after diabetes onset (ESM Fig. 2F), while cardiac *Fgf21* mRNA was unexpectedly increased 40-fold at 2 months and 1.5–2.5-fold at 4–6 months (ESM Fig. 2E).

3.2 *FGF21 prevents palmitate-induced cardiac apoptosis via ERK1/2-mediated pathways*

To define the remarkable induction of cardiac *Fgf21* expression at the early stage of diabetes as a protective response to diabetic lipotoxicity, H9c2 cells were treated with palmitate to mimic diabetic hyperlipidaemia [27]. Exposure of H9c2 cells to palmitate at 62.5 μmol/L for 15 h induced a significant increase of apoptosis, detected by caspase-3 cleavage and DNA fragmentation (Fig. 1A, B), which was prevented by FGF21 in a dose range of 25–100 ng/ml. The mechanistic study revealed that palmitate inhibited the phosphorylation of extracellular signal-regulated kinase (ERK)1/2 (Fig. 1C), mitogen-activated protein kinase 14 (p38 MAPK) (Fig. 1D) and AMP-activated protein kinase (AMPK) (Fig. 1E), and this effect was reduced by FGF21 treatment (Fig. 1C–E).

To establish whether the upregulation of these kinases is required for FGF21-mediated protection, H9c2 cells were treated with both FGF21 (50 ng/ml) and an inhibitor of ERK1/2 (PD98059, 20 μmol/L), p38 MAPK (SB203580, 20 μmol/L) or AMPK (compound C, 10 μmol/L) for 1 h before and during palmitate treatment for 15 h (Fig. 1F–H). The FGF21-mediated protection from palmitate-induced apoptosis was attenuated by each kinase inhibitor (Fig. 1F–H). To exclude a non-specific effect of an inhibitor, we further evaluated the role of these kinases in FGF21-mediated protection by using specific siRNAs against *Erk1/2* (ESM Fig. 3A–C), *p38Mapk* (ESM Fig. 3D–F) and *Ampk* (ESM Fig. 3G–I). We found that the specific siRNA, but not the control, efficiently silenced the expression and phosphorylation of each kinase (ESM Fig. 3A–I), and also abolished FGF21-mediated protection from palmitate-induced apoptosis in adult cardiomyocytes (Fig. 1I–K). Inhibition of ERK1/2 or AMPK also increased phosphatase and tensin homologue (PTEN) phosphorylation (Fig. 1L).

Time-course studies showed that FGF21 treatment for 1–15 h increased ERK1/2 phosphorylation at 1–3 h and 9–12 h, peaking at 1 h and 9 h (ESM Fig. 4A), p38 MAPK phosphorylation at 3–9 h, peaking at 6 h (ESM Fig. 4B), and AMPK phosphorylation at 6–15 h, peaking at 12 h (ESM Fig. 4C). To dissect whether these kinases are in the same signaling pathway, H9c2 cells were treated with FGF21 and each inhibitor for 15 h (ESM Fig. 4D–L). PD98059 inhibited not only ERK1/2 (ESM Fig. 4D), but also p38 MAPK (ESM Fig. 4E) and AMPK (ESM Fig. 4F). SB203580 did not affect ERK1/2 (ESM Fig. 4G), but significantly inhibited p38 MAPK (ESM Fig. 4H) and AMPK phosphorylation (ESM Fig. 4I). Com-pound C inhibited only AMPK (ESM Fig. 4J–L). These results suggest that FGF21 activates an ERK1/2-mediated p38 MAPK–AMPK signaling pathway.

To rule out inhibitor non-specificity, the direct role of ERK1/2 in the top position of the signaling pathway was confirmed with *Erk1/2* siRNA that almost completely abolished ERK1/2 phosphorylation (Fig. 2A, B) and expression (Fig. 2A, C) and the subsequent *Fgf21*-increased phosphorylation of p38 MAPK (Fig. 2A, D) and AMPK (Fig. 2A, E), which also abolished FGF21-mediated protection against palmitate-induced apoptosis (Fig. 2A, F). To further validate the role of ERK1/2–p38 MAPK–AMPK signaling in FGF21-mediated cardiac protection in a more physiological context, the

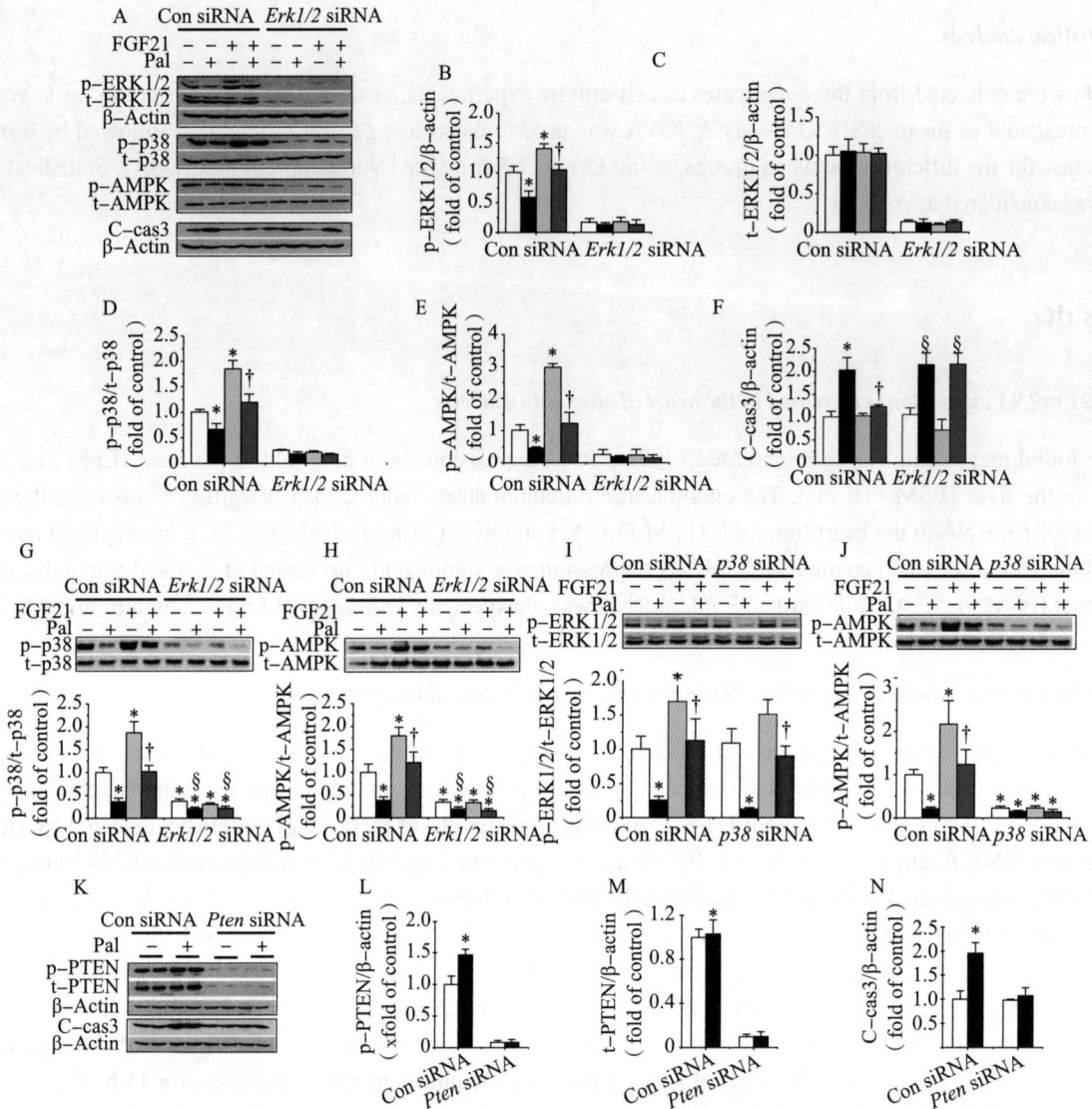

Fig. 2. Inhibition of ERK1/2 or PTEN with siRNA attenuates FGF21- mediated anti-apoptotic function against palmitate. H9c2 cells were treated with FGF21 (50 ng/ml, light grey bar) or PBS (white bar) for 1 h followed by co-treatment with palmitate (62.5 μmol/L; black bar, PBS+ palmitate; dark grey bar, FGF21+palmitate) in the presence of either control or *Erk1/2*-specific siRNA and then western blotting was used to detect the phosphorylation levels of ERK1/2 (A–C), p38 MAPK (A, D) and AMPK (A, E), and caspase-3 cleavage (A, F). Primary cardiomyocytes were pre-treated with FGF21 (50 ng/ml, light grey bar) or PBS (white bar) for 1 h followed by co-treatment with palmitate (62.5 μmol/L; black bar, PBS+palmitate; dark grey bar, FGF21+palmitate) in the presence of either siRNA against *Erk1/2* (G, H) or *p38Mapk* (I, J) or control siRNA. p38 MAPK, AMPK and ERK1/2 phosphorylation was examined by western blot. Some H9c2 cells were treated with PBS (white bar) or palmitate (black bar) in the presence of control or *Pten* siRNA, and the phosphorylation (K, L) and levels of PTEN (K, M) and caspase-3 cleavage (K, N) were examined by western blot. Data collection and presentation are the same as in Fig. 1. *$P<0.05$ *vs.* control in the control siRNA group; †$P<0.05$ *vs.* palmitate in the control siRNA group; §$P<0.05$ *vs.* control in *Erk1/2* siRNA group. Con, control; p38, p38 MAPK; Pal, palmitate.

specific siRNAs against *Erk1/2* (ESM Fig. 3A–C) and *p38Mapk* (ESM Fig. 3D–F) were also used to knockdown these kinases in adult cardiomyocytes. We found that *Erk1/2* siRNA, but not control, almost completely abolished the FGF21-mediated increase in p38 MAPK and AMPK phosphorylation (Fig. 2G, H), and *p38Mapk* siRNA had no significant effects on FGF21-mediated increase in ERK1/2 phosphorylation (Fig. 2I), but significantly abolished the FGF21-mediated increase in AMPK phosphorylation (Fig. 2J).

In addition, *Pten* siRNA almost completely abolished the phosphorylation (Fig. 2K, L) and abundance of PTEN (Fig. 2K, M), which also prevented palmitate-induced apoptosis (Fig. 2K, N), confirming the pivotal role of PTEN in the palmitate-induced apoptotic signalling pathway.

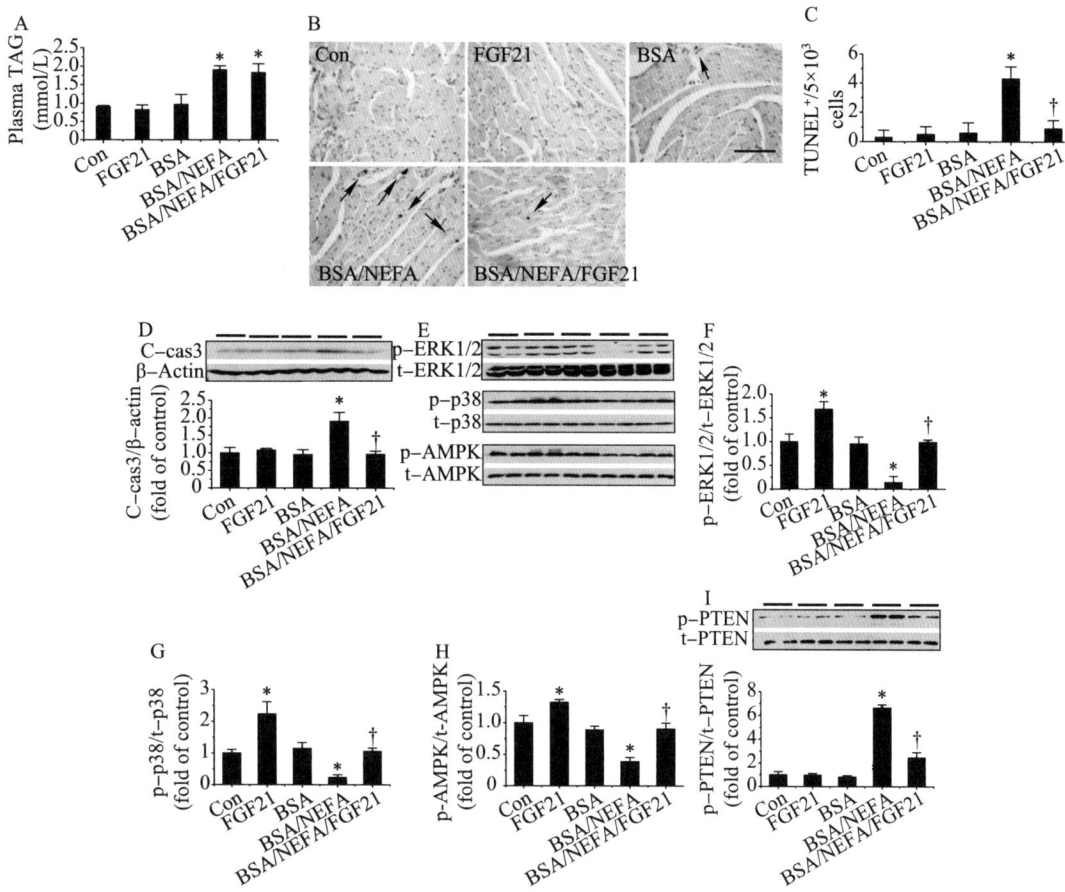

Fig. 3. FGF21 prevents NEFA-infusion-induced cardiac apoptosis. Mice were infused with NEFA (0.1 g/10 g body weight) with or without FGF21 (100 μg/kg/day) for 10 days. Plasma triacylglycerol was measured using an assay kit (A). Cardiac apoptosis was detected by TUNEL (B, C) and caspase-3 cleavage (D); arrows in micrographs indicate apoptotic nuclei. Phosphorylation of ERK1/2 (E, F), p38 MAPK (E, G), AMPK (E,H) and PTEN (E, I) was examined by western blot. Data are presented as mean ± SD. $n \geq 5$ for each group. *$P<0.05$ *vs.* control; †$P<0.05$ *vs.* NEFA treatment. Scale bar, 100 μm. Con, control; p38, p38 MAPK; TAG, triacylglycerol.

3.3 FGF21 prevents acute NEFA-infusion-induced cardiac apoptosis in mice

To see whether FGF21 can also protect the heart from lipotoxicity *in vivo*, mice were intraperitoneally given NEFA (0.1 g/10 g) with and without FGF21 (100 μg/kg/day) for 10 days.

NEFA significantly increased serum triacylglycerol levels, and this was not affected by FGF21 (Fig. 3A). Significant cardiac apoptosis was observed in NEFA-infused mice, but not in mice with BSA or mice treated with FGF21 (Fig. 3B–D). FGF21 also significantly prevented the NEFA-mediated decrease in ERK1/2 (Fig. 3E, F), p38 MAPK (Fig. 3E, G) and AMPK phosphorylation (Fig. 3E, H) and increase in PTEN phosphorylation (Fig. 3I).

3.4 FGF21 prevents diabetes-induced cardiac apoptosis through ERK1/2 activation

To confirm whether the anti-apoptotic effect of FGF21 observed in the above studies can be replicated in type 1 diabetes, FGF21 (100 μg/kg/day) or vehicle was administered to diabetic and control mice for 10 days. FGF21 slightly decreased the blood glucose in diabetes, but had no effect on controls (Fig. 4A). Additionally, FGF21 did not affect the plasma triacylglycerol level in either control or diabetic mice (Fig. 4B).

TUNEL staining (Fig. 4C, D) and caspase-3 cleavage (Fig. 4E) showed that FGF21 prevented diabetes-induced cardiac apoptosis. Diabetes also significantly decreased cardiac ERK1/2 (Fig. 4F), p38 MAPK (Fig. 4G) and AMPK (Fig. 4H) phosphorylation and increased PTEN phosphorylation (Fig. 4I), all of which were completely prevented by FGF21. These results suggest that FGF21 prevents diabetes-induced cardiac apoptosis *via* increasing ERK1/2, p38 MAPK and AMPK phosphorylation and inhibiting PTEN phosphorylation, as found in the *in vitro* study.

Inhibition of ERK1/2 by PD98059 (10 mg/kg daily, Fig. 4J, L) completely abolished FGF21-mediated prevention

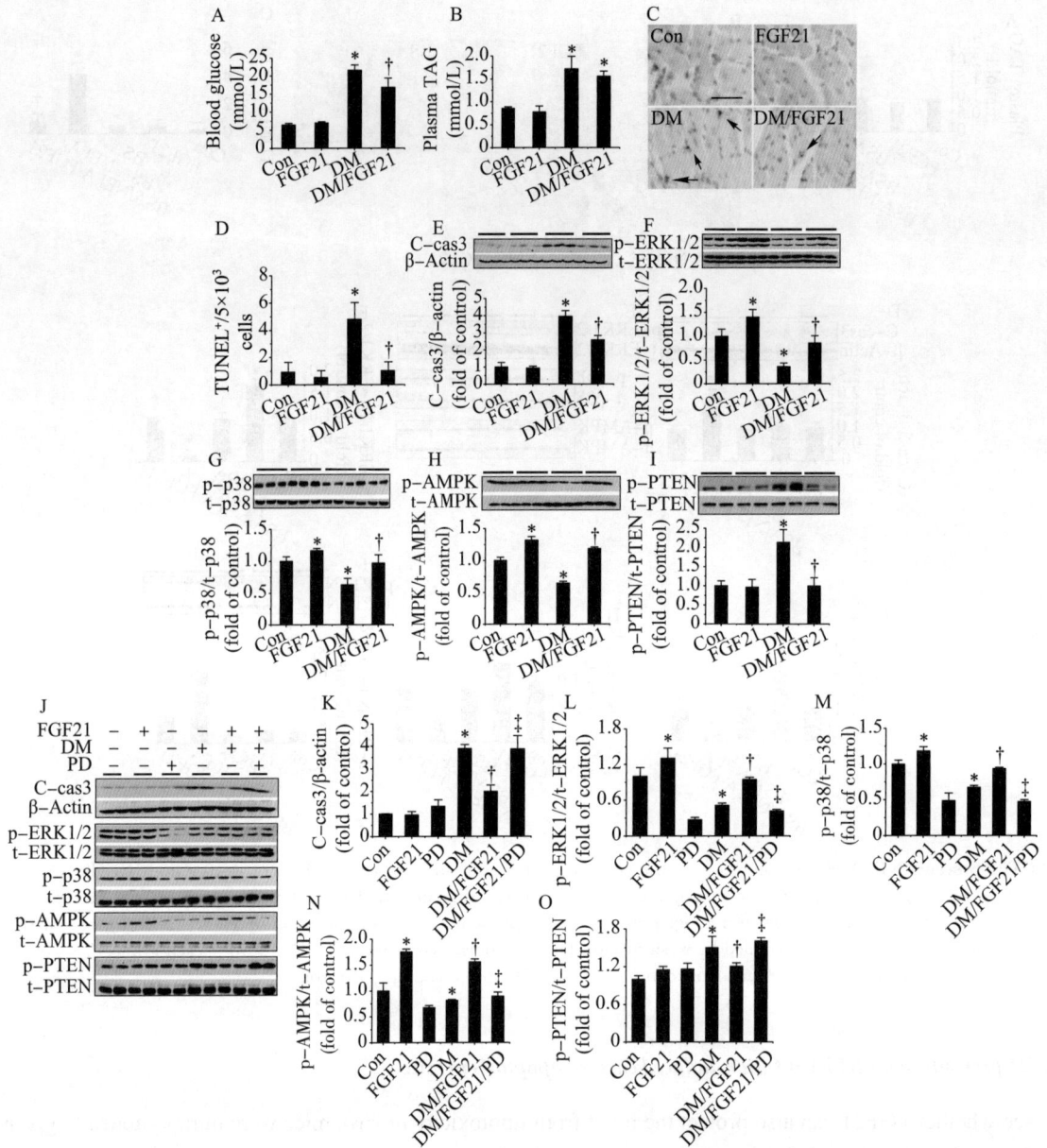

Fig. 4. FGF21 prevention of diabetes-induced cardiac apoptosis is mediated by ERK1/2 activation. Diabetic and control mice were given FGF21 (100 μg/kg/day) or PBS daily for 10 days. Blood glucose (A) and plasma triacylglycerol (B) levels were examined using a blood glucose monitor or a triacylglycerol assay kit. Cardiac apoptosis was assessed by TUNEL (C, D) and caspase-3 cleavage (E); arrows in micrographs indicate the apoptotic nuclei. Phosphorylation of ERK1/2 (F), p38 MAPK (G), AMPK (H) and PTEN (I) was examined by western blot. Some mice were treated with both FGF21 and the ERK1/2 inhibitor PD98059 for 10 days. Caspase-3 cleavage (J, K) and ERK1/2 (J, L), p38 MAPK (J, M), AMPK (J, N) and PTEN (J, O) phosphorylation were detected by western blot. Data are presented as mean ± SD. $n=8$ for each group. *$P<0.05$ vs. control; †$P<0.05$ vs. diabetes; ‡$P<0.05$ vs. diabetes/FGF21. Scale bar, 100 μm. C- cas3, caspase-3 cleavage; Con, control; DM, diabetes; p38, p38 MAPK; PD, PD98059; TAG, triacylglycerol.

of diabetes-induced cardiac apoptosis (Fig. 4J, K), and FGF21-maintained cardiac p38 MAPK (Fig. 4J, M) and AMPK phosphorylation (Fig. 4J, N). Furthermore, inactivation of ERK1/2 also abolished FGF21-mediated prevention of diabetes-induced PTEN phosphorylation (Fig. 4J, O). These results demonstrated that FGF21 prevented diabetes-related inhibition of ERK1/2, resulting in a reduction of diabetes-induced PTEN-activation-mediated apoptosis.

Fgf21-KO mice are more susceptible to diabetes-induced cardiac apoptosis To further define the protective role of endogenous FGF21, diabetes was induced in both Fgf21-KO and wild-type (WT) control mice. Compared with WT mice with diabetes, Fgf21-KO mice with diabetes showed a further elevation of blood glucose (Fig. 5A) and plasma triacylglycerol (Fig. 5B). Treatment of Fgf21-KO diabetic mice with FGF21 (100 μg/kg/day for 10 days) significantly

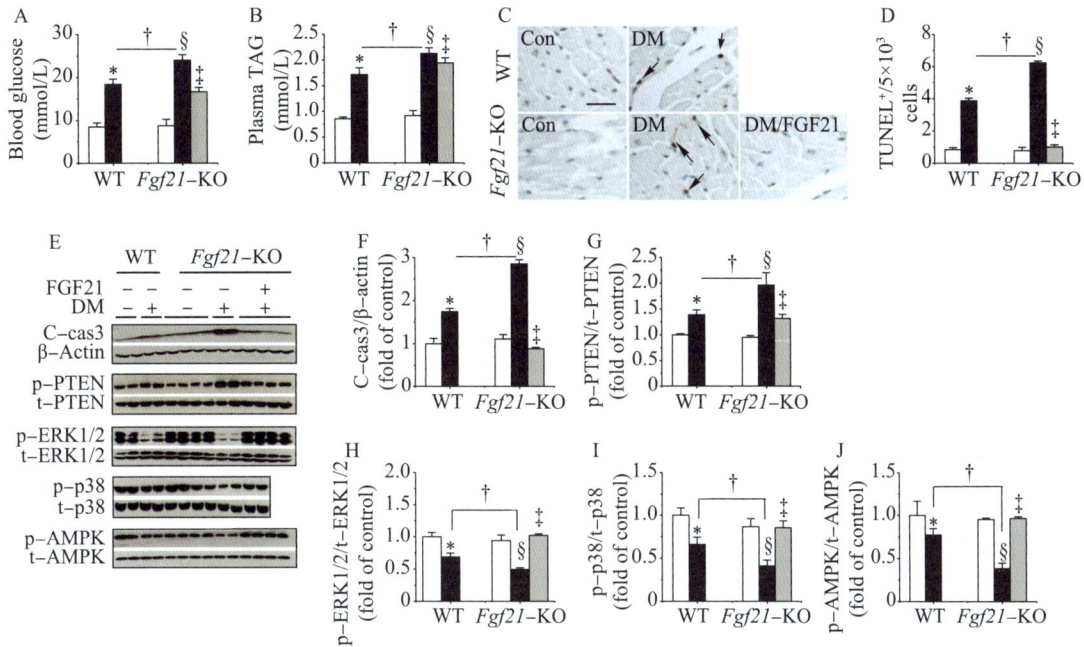

Fig. 5. *Fgf21*-KO mice are more sensitive to diabetes-induced cardiac apoptosis. *Fgf21*-KO and WT mice were induced to develop diabetes (black bar) with STZ and treated with FGF21 (100 μg/kg/day, light grey bar) or PBS (white bar) for 10 days. Blood glucose (A) and plasma triacylglycerol (B) levels were examined as above. Cardiac apoptosis was assessed by TUNEL (C, D) and caspase-3 cleavage (E, F); arrows in micrographs indicate the apoptotic nuclei. Phosphorylation of PTEN (E, G), ERK1/2 (E, H), p38 MAPK (E, I) and AMPK (E, J) was examined by western blot. $n=8$ for each group. *$P<0.05$ *vs.* WT control; †$P<0.05$ *vs.* WT diabetes; ‡$P<0.05$ *vs.* diabetes; *Fgf21*. Scale bar, 100 μm. C-cas3, caspase-3 cleavage; Con, control; DM, diabetes; TAG, triacylglycerol.

decreased blood glucose compared with non-treated *Fgf21*-KO diabetic mice (Fig. 5A).

Apoptosis was significantly more abundant in the heart of *Fgf21*-KO mice with diabetes than in WT mice with diabetes (Fig. 5C–F), which was same as the PTEN phosphorylation profile (Fig. 5E, G). The inhibition of ERK1/2 (Fig. 5E, H), p38 MAPK (Fig. 5E, I) and AMPK (Fig. 5E, J) was also more evident in heart from *Fgf21*-KO mice with diabetes than in heart from WT mice with diabetes. FGF21 treatment of *Fgf21*-KO mice with diabetes completely reversed diabetes-increased apoptosis and PTEN phosphorylation and diabetes-decreased ERK1/2, p38 MAPK and AMPK phosphorylation (Fig. 5C–J).

3.5 FGF21 prevents diabetes-induced cardiac remodelling and dysfunction through ERK1/2

activation The next study examined whether FGF21 prevention of cardiac apoptosis can result in prevention of cardiac remodelling and dysfunction. WT and *Fgf21*-KO mice with diabetes chronically treated with FGF21 (100 μg/kg/day) for 2 months showed a significant reduction in blood glucose, which was abolished by ERK1/2 inhibition in WT diabetes (Fig. 6A). However, FGF21 treatment did not affect plasma triacylglycerol, which was significantly higher in *Fgf21*-KO diabetic mice compared with WT diabetic mice; the presence or absence of ERK1/2 inhibition did not affect plasma triacylglycerol in either the WT or the *Fgf21*-KO diabetic mice (Fig. 6B).

Cardiac apoptosis was detected by TUNEL staining (Fig. 6C, ESM Fig. 5) and caspase-3 cleavage (Fig. 6D, E). There was significant cardiac apoptosis in diabetes, particularly in *Fgf21*-KO mice. Consistent with an apoptotic effect, PTEN phosphor-ylation was increased in diabetes (Fig. 6D, F), and ERK1/2 (Fig. 6D, E), p38 MAPK (Fig. 6D, H) and AMPK inhibition (Fig. 6D, I) were also more evident in *Fgf21*-KO diabetic mice than in WT diabetic mice. These diabetes-induced apoptosis and associated signalling changes were prevented by FGF21 treatment (Fig. 6A–I), but FGF21-mediated protection was significantly abolished by PD98059 treatment (Fig. 6A–I). Diabetes also induced cardiac remodelling, shown by an increase in connective tissue growth factor (CTGF) expression (Fig. 6D, J) and collagen accumulation (Fig. 6K, L), which was significantly different in *Fgf21*-KO diabetic mice than in WT diabetic mice.

Diabetes-induced hypertension was significantly prevented by FGF21 treatment in both WT and *Fgf21*-KO diabetic

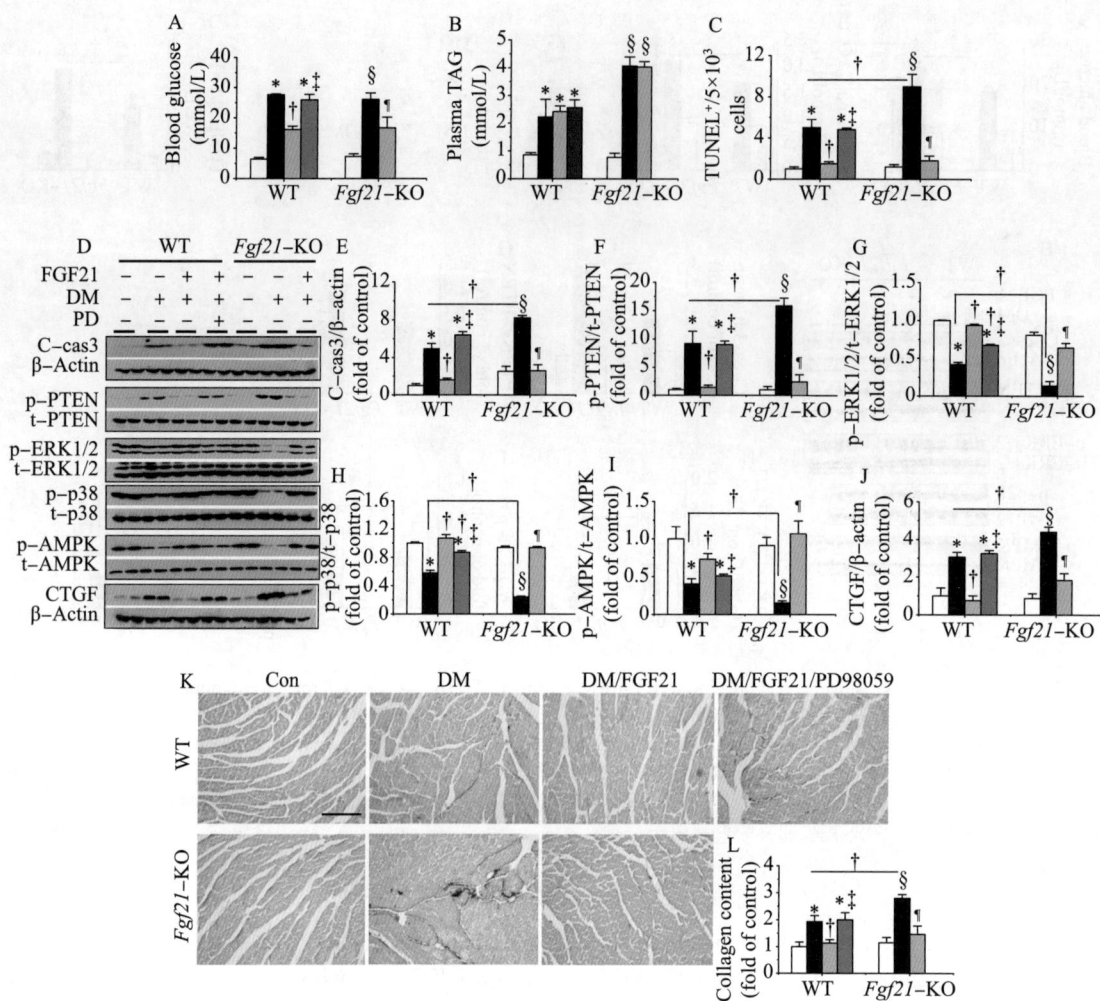

Fig. 6. FGF21 prevents diabetes-induced cardiac remodelling and dysfunction through ERK1/2 activation. *Fgf21*-KO and WT mice were induced as diabetic (black bar) with STZ, and treated with PBS (white bar) or FGF21 (100 µg/kg/day, light grey bar) for 2 months. One set of WT diabetic mice were treated with FGF21 + ERK1/2 inhibitor (PD98059, dark grey bar). Blood glucose (A) and plasma triacylglycerol (B) were examined as above. Cardiac apoptosis was assessed by TUNEL (C) and caspase-3 cleavage (D, E). Phosphorylation of PTEN (D, F), ERK1/2 (D, G), p38 MAPK (D, H) and AMPK (D, I) was examined by western blot. Cardiac remodelling was examined by CTGF expression (D, J) and Sirius Red staining (K, L). Data are presented as mean ± SD. $n=8$ for each group. *$P<0.05$ *vs.* control; †$P<0.05$ *vs.* WT diabetic mice; ‡$P<0.05$ *vs.* diabetic mice receiving FGF21; §$P <0.05$ *vs.* *Fgf21*-KO control; ¶$P<0.05$ *vs.* *Fgf21*-KO diabetic mice. Scale bar, 100 µm. Con, control; DM, diabetes; p38, p38 MAPK; TAG, triacylglycerol.

mice (Table 1). The preventive effects of FGF21 were abolished by ERK1/2 inhibition (Table 1). Diabetes significantly reduced cardiac function, indicated by decreased ejection fraction (EF) and fractional shortening (FS) in both WT and *Fgf21*-KO mouse hearts (Table 1). At the same time, diabetes also induced alterations in several structural indices (Table 1), including decreased left ventricular (LV) postal wall thickness, increased end systolic LV inner diameter and volume, together with a small decrease in LV mass, but a significant increase in LV mass index, which reflects a greater body weight loss, in both WT and *Fgf21*-KO diabetes (Table 1). All these cardiac functional and structural changes were mildly but significantly improved by FGF21 treatment in both WT and *Fgf21*-KO diabetic mice, an effect that was abolished by ERK1/2 inhibition (Table 1). *Fgf21* deletion had no significant effects on cardiac structural and functional variables under basal conditions.

Table 1.   Biometric and echocardiographic characteristics of diabetic mice at 2 months

Characteristic	Wild type				Fgf21-KO		
	Control	DM	DM/FGF21	DM/FGF21/PD98059	Control	DM	DM/FGF21
Body weight (g)	33.12±3.42	24.14±1.57*	34.12±4.16[†]	25.12±3.72[‡]	35.42±4.33	22.43±2.56[§]	31.92±3.09[¶]
Diastolic BP (mmHg)	68.11±4.43	86.40±4.10*	73.29±3.02[†]	91.55±7.48[‡]	67.28±8.92	97.92±9.11[§]	70.70±5.50[¶]
Systolic BP (mmHg)	101.40±2.73	115.80±4.60*	102.24±4.25[†]	116.70±2.81[‡]	101.17±6.22	123.32±18.43[§]	100.45±4.98[¶]
Mean BP (mmHg)	78.90±3.65	101.2±1.86*	83.41±4.86[†]	103.01±7.58[‡]	78.22±7.73	109.02±13.63[§]	81.34±5.94[¶]
cHR (bpm)	647±32	641±15	641±17	627±11	637±16	631±14	634±10
aHR (bpm)	435±12.97	446±15.33	426±12.11	451±20.54	441±20.34	425±25.63	432±25.74
IVSd (mm)	0.62±0.05	0.61±0.01	0.614±0.01	0.63±0.02	0.64±0.01	0.63±0.02	0.64±0.01
LVIDd (mm)	3.75±0.12	3.78±0.1	3.78±0.04	3.74±0.1	3.89±0.17	3.76±0.22	3.83±0.05
LVPWd (mm)	0.79±0.07	0.65±0.05*	0.68±0.06	0.67±0.07	0.75±0.03	0.67±0.05[§]	0.67±0.04
IVSs (mm)	1.09±0.16	1.0±0.03	1.01±0.02	1.02±0.05	1.11±0.16	1.02±0.05[§]	1.04±0.03
LVIDs (mm)	1.69±0.16	2.42±0.02*	2.22±0.06	2.37±0.1	2.0±0.22	2.42±0.18[§]	2.26±0.07
LVPWs (mm)	1.59±0.11	1.07±0.13*	1.15±0.19	1.04±0.07	1.39±0.07	1.05±0.05[§]	1.13±0.05
LVVold (μl)	60.19±4.29	61.47±3.83	61.04±1.67	59.74±3.84	65.81±6.8	60.74±8.71	63.21±2.1
LVVols (μl)	8.43±2.04	20.61±0.49*	16.66±1.1[†]	19.71±1.91	13.04±3.84	20.82±3.8[§]	17.44±1.34[¶]
EF, %	86.14±2.77	66.43±1.96*	72.81±1.61[†]	67.05±2.71[‡]	82.35±1.18	65.89±2.55[§]	71.9±1.62[¶]
FS, %	55.07±3.41	35.96±1.46*	40.64±2.52[†]	36.24±2.74[‡]	47.82±3.52	35.68±1.89[§]	40.97±1.48[¶]
LV mass (mg)	89.37±7.46	77.82±4.03*	82.63±1.07[†]	79.75±9.99	93.39±5.24	80.94±13.18	83.48±2.73
LV mass/body weight (mg/g)	2.70±0.23	3.21±0.16*	2.41±0.13[†]	3.17±0.18[‡]	2.63±0.35	3.61±0.15[§]	2.62±0.11[¶]

Values are mean ± SD; n=8 for each group

*P<0.05 vs. WT control; [†]P<0.05 vs. WT with diabetes; [‡]P<0.05 vs. diabetes/FGF21; [§]P<0.05 vs. Fgf21-KO control; [¶] P<0.05 vs. Fgf21-KO diabetes

aHR; heart rate under anaesthetised conditions; cHR, hear rate under conscious conditions; DM, diabetes; IVSd, end diastolic interventricular septum; IVSs, end systolic interventricular septum; LVIDd, LVend diastolic diameter; LVIDs, LVend systolic diameter; LVPWd, LVend diastolic posterior wall; LVPWs, LV end systolic posterior wall; LVVold, end diastolic LV volume; LVVols, end systolic LV volume.

4. Discussion

The early upregulation of cardiac *Fgf21* mRNA expression was found to gradually decrease with the progression of diabetes (ESM Fig. 2E). We hypothesised that, besides induction of lipolysis to meet cardiac energy requirements, the early upregulation of cardiac FGF21 expression may be a compensatory effect to protect from the acute toxic effect of the accumulated intermediates of lipid metabolism in the heart. Here, we provide direct evidence for the anti-apoptotic effect of FGF21 in cardiac tissue, with protection against palmitate in the cultured cardiac cell line and primary cardio-myocytes and STZ-induced diabetes or NEFA infusion in mice. We have also demonstrated that FGF21 supplementation prevents the progression of diabetes-induced cardiomyopathy in both WT and *Fgf21*-KO mice, a finding that is supportive of previous studies showing FGF21 protects against myocardial ischaemia/reperfusion injury [18, 19] and isoprenaline induced cardiac hypertrophy [20].

Mice with *Fgf21* deletion were more susceptible to diabetes-induced cardiac apoptosis, but cardiac structural and functional derangements were not exacerbated in these mice (Fig. 6A–L and Table 1). This could be attributed to the relative time span of the diabetic model, as we have established that diabetes-induced cardiac apoptosis at an early stage

(7–21 days) leads to the development of diabetic cardio-myopathy in later life (4–6 months) [28]. Therefore, we could see increased apoptosis in *Fgf21*-KO diabetic mice at the early stage (2 months), but could not yet see any exacerbation of diabetes-induced cardiac structural and functional changes.

The insulin-sensitising and lipid-manipulating effects of FGF21 [29, 30] may not be the predominant contributor to cardiac protection by FGF21 in mice with STZ-induced type 1 diabetes, as these mice have severe insulin deficiency. We also only observed a slight glucose-lowing effect (Figs. 4A, 5A, 6A), but without global lipid-lowering potency (Figs. 4B, 5B, 6B) at a lower FGF21 dose level (100 μg/kg/day), which is consistent with previous reports [30, 31]. Based on our *in vitro* studies showing that FGF21 protects against palmitate-induced cardiac apoptosis in H9c2 cells and primary cardiomyocytes, and also previous reports indicating that liver-and adipose-tissue-secreted FGF21 protects the heart from ischaemia/reperfusion injury [18] and exogenous FGF21 protects the heart from isoprenaline-induced cardiac hypertrophy [20], we presume that cardiac protection from diabetes by FGF21 may predominantly be attributed to its direct actions on the heart.

The present study elucidated the intracellular mechanisms by which FGF21 prevents palmitate-mediated apoptosis *in vitro* and NEFA-infusion-or diabetes-mediated apoptosis *in vivo*. The activation of ERK1/2 by FGF21 in cardiac cells and heart plays a pivotal role in FGF21-mediated anti-apoptotic effects by activation of downstream p38 MAPK and AMPK (Figs. 1F–K, 2, 4 and 6). These findings corroborate previous studies that provided indirect evidence for this mechanism. Chau *et al* demonstrated that FGF21 regulates mitochondrial activity and enhances oxidative capacity through an AMPK-dependent mechanism in adipocytes [32]. Ge *et al.* reported that FGF21 increases glucose uptake through sequential activation of ERK1/2 and serum response factor (SRF)/ELK1, member of ETS oncogene family (ELK-1) in adipocytes [33]. Wente *et al* also documented the important role of ERK1/2 in the anti-apoptosis effects of FGF21 [14]. Here, we found that inhibition of ERK1/2, p38 MAPK or AMPK abolishes FGF21-mediated cardiac protection from palmitate-induced apoptosis *in vitro* (Figs. 1F–K and 2A, F, K, M), and that inhibition of ERK1/2 abolished the protection by FGF21 against diabetes-induced cardiac apoptosis and cardio-myopathy (Figs. 4J–O, 6C–L and Table 1). Although FGF21 activation of ERK1/2 has not been documented in cardiac cells and tissues, it has been widely studied in adipocyte, hepatocyte and beta cells, in which FGF21 induces heparin-independent tyrosine phosphorylation of FGFR substrate-2, a docking protein linking FGFRs to the Ras–MAPK pathway, and transient activation of MAPK, including ERK1/2 [14, 31, 34]. Whether FGF21 activation of ERK1/2 occurs in a similar manner in cardiac cells needs to be verified.

Clinical studies have demonstrated that elevated serum FGF21 is closely associated with hypertension [35–37]. Zhu *et al* revealed that FGF21 ameliorates BP in a fructose-induced hypertension model [38]. In the present study hyper-tension observed in a mouse model of type 1 diabetes was also prevented by FGF21 supplementation (Table 1). Therefore, FGF21-mediated anti-hypertension effects might provide an additional beneficial effect on the diabetic heart in addition to FGF21-mediated direct protection from diabetes. This important issue will be further defined in future studies.

We found that the FGF21-activated AMPK following inhibition of PTEN function provided the anti-apoptotic effect, as either inhibition or knockdown of ERK1/2 or AMPK could completely abolish the inactivation of PTEN by FGF21 (Figs. 1L, 4J, O and 6D, F). PTEN is a lipid phosphatase that inhibits the phosphatidylinositol 3-kinase (PI3K) pathway, in which PI3K phosphorylates Akt to promote cell survival. The present study implies that the prevention of palmitate-induced cardiac apoptosis by FGF21 may partially depend on Akt. Our findings not only support previous studies showing that FGF21-mediated cardiac protection against ischaemia/ reperfusion injury is mediated by PI3K/Akt cell survival signalling under both *in vitro* and *in vivo* conditions [18, 19], but also further establish FGF21-mediated cardiac protection against diabetic pathogenic changes *via* upregulation of ERK1/2-p38 MAPK-AMPK-mediated cell survival pathways.

It should be mentioned that the preventive effects of FGF21 on diabetic cardiac dysfunction were incomplete (84.5% for EF and 89.3% for LV mass index). This partial prevention may be related to the multiple pathogenic factors of diabetic cardiomyopathy [1–3]. Also, the prevention of diabetic cardiac apoptosis using FGF21 at 100 μg kg body/weight/day for 2 months may not be enough to completely prevent diabetes-induced cardiac dysfunction, and the dose will be optimised in future studies.

5. Conclusions

In summary, our study reveals the following new findings: (1) FGF21 is expressed in the heart, and increases in cardiac FGF21 expression in type 1 diabetes is a protective mechanism for lipotoxicity-induced cardiac apoptosis *in vitro* and *in vivo*; (2) the cardioprotective effect of FGF21 against diabetic damage is mediated by ERK1/2–p38 MAPK–AMPK cell survival pathways. This study lays the groundwork for the potential clinical use of FGF21 to treat heart disease, particularly in diabetes.

Supplementary material

Electronic supplementary material to this article can be found in the online version (doi:10.1007/s00125-015-3630-8).

References

[1] Bugger H, Abel ED. Molecular mechanisms of diabetic cardiomyopathy[J]. Diabetologia, 2014, 57(4): 660-671.

[2] Boudina S, Abel ED. Diabetic cardiomyopathy, causes and effects[J]. Rev Endocr Metab Disord, 2010, 11(1): 31-39.

[3] Cai L, Kang YJ. Oxidative stress and diabetic cardiomyopathy: a brief review[J]. Cardiovasc Toxicol, 2001, 1(3): 181-193.

[4] Cai L, Kang YJ. Cell death and diabetic cardiomyopathy[J]. Cardiovasc Toxicol, 2003, 3(3): 219-228.

[5] Boudina S, Abel ED. Diabetic cardiomyopathy revisited[J]. Circulation, 2007, 115(25): 3213-3223.

[6] Cai L, Wang J, Li Y, et al. Inhibition of superoxide generation and associated nitrosative damage is involved in metallothionein prevention of diabetic cardiomyopathy[J]. Diabetes, 2005, 54(6): 1829-1837.

[7] Adams AC, Kharitonenkov A. FGF21: The center of a transcriptional nexus in metabolic regulation[J]. Curr Diabetes Rev, 2012, 8(4): 285-293.

[8] Cuevas-Ramos D, Almeda-Valdes P, Aguilar-Salinas CA, et al. The role of fibroblast growth factor 21 (FGF21) on energy balance, glucose and lipid metabolism[J]. Curr Diabetes Rev, 2009, 5(4): 216-220.

[9] Laeger T, Henagan TM, Albarado DC, et al. FGF21 is an endocrine signal of protein restriction[J]. J Clin Invest, 2014, 124(9): 3913-3922.

[10] Mraz M, Bartlova M, Lacinova Z, et al. Serum concentrations and tissue expression of a novel endocrine regulator fibroblast growth factor-21 in patients with type 2 diabetes and obesity[J]. Clin Endocrinol (Oxf), 2009, 71(3): 369-375.

[11] Fon Tacer K, Bookout AL, Ding X, et al. Research resource: Comprehensive expression atlas of the fibroblast growth factor system in adult mouse[J]. Mol Endocrinol, 2010, 24(10): 2050-2064.

[12] Feingold KR, Grunfeld C, Heuer JG, et al. FGF21 is increased by inflammatory stimuli and protects leptin-deficient ob/ob mice from the toxicity of sepsis[J]. Endocrinology, 2012, 153(6): 2689-2700.

[13] Ye D, Wang Y, Li H, et al. Fibroblast growth factor 21 protects against acetaminophen-induced hepatotoxicity by potentiating peroxisome proliferator-activated receptor coactivator protein-1α-mediated antioxidant capacity in mice[J]. Hepatology, 2014, 60(3): 977-989.

[14] Wente W, Efanov AM, Brenner M, et al. Fibroblast growth factor-21 improves pancreatic beta-cell function and survival by activation of extracellular signal-regulated kinase 1/2 and Akt signaling pathways[J]. Diabetes, 2006, 55(9): 2470-2478.

[15] Lu Y, Liu JH, Zhang LK, et al. Fibroblast growth factor 21 as a possible endogenous factor inhibits apoptosis in cardiac endothelial cells[J]. Chin Med J (Engl), 2010, 123(23): 3417-3421.

[16] Suzuki M, Uehara Y, Motomura-Matsuzaka K, et al. betaKlotho is required for fibroblast growth factor (FGF) 21 signaling through FGF receptor (FGFR) 1c and FGFR3c[J]. Mol Endocrinol, 2008, 22(4): 1006-1014.

[17] Kurosu H, Choi M, Ogawa Y, et al. Tissue-specific expression of betaKlotho and fibroblast growth factor (FGF) receptor isoforms determines metabolic activity of FGF19 and FGF21[J]. J Biol Chem, 2007, 282(37): 26687-26695.

[18] Liu SQ, Roberts D, Kharitonenkov A, et al. Endocrine protection of ischemic myocardium by FGF21 from the liver and adipose tissue[J]. Sci Rep, 2013, 3: 2767.

[19] Cong WT, Ling J, Tian HS, et al. Proteomic study on the protective mechanism of fibroblast growth factor 21 to ischemia-reperfusion injury[J]. Can J Physiol Pharmacol, 2013, 91(11): 973-984.

[20] Planavila A, Redondo I, Hondares E, et al. Fibroblast growth factor 21 protects against cardiac hypertrophy in mice[J]. Nat Commun, 2013, 4: 2019.

[21] Zhou G, Li X, Hein DW, et al. Metallothionein suppresses angiotensin II-induced nicotinamide adenine dinucleotide phosphate oxidase activation, nitrosative stress, apoptosis, and pathological remodeling in the diabetic heart[J]. J Am Coll Cardiol, 2008, 52(8): 655-666.

[22] Tan Y, Li X, Prabhu SD, et al. Angiotensin II plays a critical role in alcohol-induced cardiac nitrative damage, cell death, remodeling, and cardiomyopathy in a protein kinase C/nicotinamide adenine dinucleotide phosphate oxidase-dependent manner[J]. J Am Coll Cardiol, 2012, 59(16): 1477-1486.

[23] Zhao Y, Tan Y, Xi S, et al. A novel mechanism by which SDF-1beta protects cardiac cells from palmitate-induced endoplasmic reticulum stress and apoptosis *via* CXCR7 and AMPK/p38 MAPK-mediated interleukin-6 generation[J]. Diabetes, 2013, 62(7): 2545-2558.

[24] Luo J, Hill BG, Gu Y, et al. Mechanisms of acrolein-induced myocardial dysfunction: implications for environmental and endogenous aldehyde exposure[J]. Am J Physiol Heart Circ Physiol, 2007, 293(6): H3673-H3684.

[25] Cameron TL, Bell KM, Tatarczuch L, et al. Transcriptional profiling of chondrodysplasia growth plate cartilage reveals adaptive ER-stress networks that allow survival but disrupt hypertrophy[J]. PLoS One, 2011, 6(9): e24600.

[26] Schaap FG, Kremer AE, Lamers WH, et al. Fibroblast growth factor 21 is induced by endoplasmic reticulum stress[J]. Biochimie, 2013, 95(4): 692-699.

[27] Wang J, Song Y, Elsherif L, et al. Cardiac metallothionein induction plays the major role in the prevention of diabetic cardiomyopathy by zinc supplementation[J]. Circulation, 2006, 113(4): 544-554.

[28] Cai L, Wang Y, Zhou G, et al. Attenuation by metallothionein of early cardiac cell death *via* suppression of mitochondrial oxidative stress results in a prevention of diabetic cardiomyopathy[J]. J Am Coll Cardiol, 2006, 48(8): 1688-1697.

[29] Potthoff MJ, Inagaki T, Satapati S, et al. FGF21 induces PGC-

1alpha and regulates carbohydrate and fatty acid metabolism during the adaptive starvation response[J]. Proc Natl Acad Sci U S A, 2009, 106(26): 10853-10858.

[30] Xu J, Lloyd DJ, Hale C, et al. Fibroblast growth factor 21 reverses hepatic steatosis, increases energy expenditure, and improves insulin sensitivity in diet-induced obese mice[J]. Diabetes, 2009, 58(1): 250-259.

[31] Kharitonenkov A, Shiyanova TL, Koester A, et al. FGF-21 as a novel metabolic regulator[J]. J Clin Invest, 2005, 115(6): 1627-1635.

[32] Chau MD, Gao J, Yang Q, et al. Fibroblast growth factor 21 regulates energy metabolism by activating the AMPK-SIRT1-PGC-1alpha pathway[J]. Proc Natl Acad Sci U S A, 2010, 107(28): 12553-12558.

[33] Ge X, Chen C, Hui X, et al. Fibroblast growth factor 21 induces glucose transporter-1 expression through activation of the serum response factor/Ets-like protein-1 in adipocytes[J]. J Biol Chem, 2011, 286(40): 34533-34541.

[34] Kouhara H, Hadari YR, Spivak-Kroizman T, et al. A lipid-anchored Grb2-binding protein that links FGF-receptor activation to the Ras/MAPK signaling pathway[J]. Cell, 1997, 89(5): 693-702.

[35] Semba RD, Crasto C, Strait J, et al. Elevated serum fibroblast growth factor 21 is associated with hypertension in community-dwelling adults[J]. J Hum Hypertens, 2013, 27(6): 397-399.

[36] Lin Z, Wu Z, Yin X, et al. Serum levels of FGF-21 are increased in coronary heart disease patients and are independently associated with adverse lipid profile[J]. PLoS One, 2010, 5(12): e15534.

[37] Chow WS, Xu A, Woo YC, et al. Serum fibroblast growth factor-21 levels are associated with carotid atherosclerosis independent of established cardiovascular risk factors[J]. Arterioscler Thromb Vasc Biol, 2013, 33(10): 2454-2459.

[38] Zhu SL, Ren GP, Zhang ZY, et al. [Therapeutic effect of fibroblast growth factor 21 on hypertension induced by insulin resistance][J]. Yao Xue Xue Bao, 2013, 48(9): 1409-1414.

Pharmacokinetics of topically applied recombinant human keratinocyte growth factor-2 in alkali-burned and intact rabbit eye

Jianqiu Cai, Xiaokun Li , Xiaojie Wang

1. Introduction

Keratinocyte growth factor-2 (KGF-2), also called fibroblast growth factor-10 (FGF-10), is a soluble 170-amino-acid polypeptide secreted by fibroblasts and endothelial cells that acts primarily on epithelial cells (Saksena et al., 2013). Its diverse effects are mainly mediated by FGF-2 IIIb receptor, a transmembrane receptor, expressed exclusively by epithelial cells (Wang et al., 2009). KGF-2 promotes the growth, proliferation, and differentiation of epithelial cells (Kruse and Tseng, 1993; Marchese et al., 2001). It has been extensively investigated for its promising effects in treating epithelial damage (Han et al., 2000; Jimenez and Rampy, 1999; Miceli et al., 1999; She et al., 2012; Smith et al., 2000; Xia et al., 1999).

The surface of the cornea consists of a stratified squamous epithelium that must be continuously renewed (Pajoohesh-Ganji and Stepp, 2005). The corneal epithelium plays important roles in the maintenance of corneal function and integrity. Corneal surface injuries are among the most frequent traumas of the eye, however, no commercial eye drops have been approved for clinical treatment (Martin et al., 2013). Corneal epithelium is very vulnerable to chemical, thermal, and mechanic injury. Chemical and thermal injuries are often used in animal model study. Chemical injury accounts for up to one-fifth of ocular traumas. Alkali injury happens more frequently than acid injury as alkali materials are more commonly used in building materials and cleaning agents (Wagoner, 1997). Since it can promote corneal epithelial cell growth and inhibit injury-induced neovascularization, KGF-2 may be a therapeutic option to treat corneal diseases with corneal epithelial defects. Topical application of KGF-2 enhanced corneal wound healing in a rabbit model of carbon dioxide laser-induced corneal Injury (Wang et al., 2010). In consistent with our report, topical administration of KGF-2 has been shown to significantly enhance corneal wound healing in rabbit alkali-burned corneas (Liu et al., 2007). The promising wound healing effect of KGF-2 on injured corneas encourages us to perform pharmacokinetic study, a critical component in drug development (Chen et al., 2012). Tissue distribution and pharmacokinetics of KGF-2 upon topical application have not been explored for in eye and are paramount in the characterization of both physiological and pathological conditions, particularly those of the cornea.

We have successfully developed a rapid and efficient expression and purification system for large-scale production of biologically active KGF-2 (Wu et al., 2009), which has been modified to improve biostability and reduce immunogenicity (Huang et al., 2009). KGF-2 produced by this system significantly promoted the proliferation of conjunctival epithelial cells in vitro and stimulated the expression and synthesis of mucins (Ma et al., 2011). By topical application of this recombinant KGF-2, we studied tissue distribution of rhKGF-2 in alkali-burned and control rabbit eyes and determined pharmacokinetic parameters of rhKGF-2 in cornea, iris, aqueous humor, and lens. Our results showed that KGF-2 predominantly distributes in corneas and alkali injury leads to further accumulation of KGF-2 in the corneas.

2. Materials and methods

2.1 Preparation and biological activity assay of ^{125}I-rhKGF-2

RhKGF-2 protein was produced as previously described (Wang et al., 2010). 1 mg iodogen was dissolved in 0.5 ml chloroform. Iodogen solution was aliquoted into the tubes (50 ml, each) and dried with nitrogen gas. 6 mg rhKGF-2 and

4 mCi Na ^{125}I (PerkinElmer™) were pipetted into the tube, mixed, and kept at 15℃ for 30 min for iodination reaction. The reaction mixture was chromatographed on Sephacryl S-300 HR (1 50 cm, GE Health, Connecticut, USA). The purity of ^{125}I-rhKGF-2 was confirmed by high-performance liquid chromatography (HPLC).

The biological activity of ^{125}I-rhKGF-2 was determined by 3-(4,5-dimethylthiazol-2-yl)-2,5-diphenyltetrazolium bromide (MTT) proliferation assay of NIH3T3 cells. Briefly, NIH3T3 cells at 7×10^3 cells per well were seeded in 96-well plates for 24 h in DMEM with 10% fetal bovine serum and then starved for overnight in DMEM with 0.5% fetal bovine serum. ^{125}I-rhKGF-2 or rhKGF-2 was diluted in DMEM supplemented with 0.5% fetal bovine serum to prepare samples of different concentrations. Starved NIH3T3 cells were incubated for 48 h with 0, 1.56, 3.12, 6.25, 12.5, 25, 50 and 100 mg/ml of ^{125}I-rhKGF-2 or rhKGF-2 (final volume, 100 ml/well) in 6 replicates and 4 replicates respectively in each concentration. 0.5% fetal bovine serum was used as blank control. At the end of the incubation, the medium was replaced with 50 ml of MTT solution (0.5 mg/ml in PBS buffer; Sigmae–Aldrich Corp., St. Louis, MO, USA) and the plates were incubated at 37℃ for 4 h followed by the addition of 200 ml of dimethyl sulfoxide to each well and incubation with shaking at 37℃ for 20 min to ensure complete dissolution of the formazan crystals. The plates were read at 570 nm with SpectraMax M2 microplate reader (Molecular Devices, USA). Cell proliferation rates were presented as percentage of control.

2.2 Animals protocols

Japanese white rabbits, obtained from Laboratory Animal Center of Academy of Military Medical Science, Beijing, China, were handled in compliance with the ARVO Statement for the Use of Animals in Ophthalmic and Vision Research. All animal protocols in this study (license No. SYXK (jing) 2013-0007) were approved by the Institutional Animal Care and Use Committee (IACUC) of the Academy of Military Medical Science. All procedures were performed under deep anesthesia using 30 mg/kg of ketamine and proparacaine hydrochloride (0.5%) was used for topical anesthesia. A round filter paper with 6 mm diameter was soaked for 3 s in 0.5 N NaOH and then applied to the cornea of one eye for 30 s. The eyes were then washed with 10 ml of 0.9% NaCl. Three animals were sacrificed by air embolism at the end of each time point after topical application of ^{125}I-rhKGF-2.

2.3 Analysis of ^{125}I-rhKGF-2 with TCA-RA method

Trichloroacetic acid precipitation-radiometric assay (TCA-RA) method was used to determine the concentration of iodinated rhKGF-2 in eye tissue samples. The rabbit eye tissue samples were isolated and weighed. Approximately 0.5 g of the each tissue sample was individually mixed with 5 volumes (w/w) of deionized water in a clean tube and homogenized. Equal amount of each tissue homogenate was mixed with various amount of ^{125}I-rhKGF-2 to prepare a serial calibration standard of ^{125}I-rhKGF-2 at concentrations of 0.51 ng/ml, 1.49 ng/ml, 19.6 ng/ml, 463.1 ng/ml. Proteins were precipitated by addition of equal volume of 20% TCA and centrifuged at 2 000 g at 4 C for 5 min. The radioactivity in the pellets was counted with a scintillation counter. The standard recovery curves of ^{125}I-rhKGF-2 from different rabbit eye tissues were generated by graphing experimental data against added concentrations of ^{125}I-rhKGF-2. The limit of quantitation (LoQ), linearity and accuracy of the method were determined and validated.

2.4 Tissue distribution and pharmacokinetics of ^{125}I-rhKGF-2 in rabbit eye tissues

Twenty-four Japanese white rabbits, approximately 2.5–3.0 kg each, were randomly assigned into two groups, 12 animals each. In treated group, rabbit eyes were burned with NaOH. Rabbit eyes in control group received a vehicle treatment. Three animals in each group were sacrificed at 1, 2, 4, and 24 h after topical application of 50 μg/ml ^{125}I-rhKGF-2. Cornea, iris, ciliary body, sclera, lens, aqueous humor, vitreous body, and serum samples were isolated and weighed. Another 33 Japanese white rabbits were given topical application of ^{125}I-rhKGF-2 50 ml (2032.27 Bq, 25 μg/ml). Three animals were sacrificed by air embolism at time points 0, 0.5, 1, 2, 3, 4, 6, 8, 12, 24, and 48 h after topical application of ^{125}I-rhKGF-2. Cornea, aqueous humor, iris and lens tissue samples were isolated and weighed. Each aliquot of tissue homogenate was vortex-mixed with the same volume of 20% TCA to precipitate proteins, and then was centrifuged at 2000 g at 4 C for 5 min. The total radioactivity assay and the radioactivity assay after precipitation with trichloroacetic acid (TCA-RA method) were both used to determine the tissue distribution and pharmacokinetics of ^{125}I-rhKGF-2.

2.5 Data and statistical analysis

Pharmacokinetic parameters were calculated using the software package DAS (version 3.0, Bontz Inc., Beijing, China). The terminal elimination half-life ($t_{1/2}$) was obtained by non-compartmental analysis of ^{125}I-rhKGF-2 concentrations in the eye tissues. Maximum concentration (C_{max}) and the time to reach the maximum concentration (T_{max}) were obtained directly from the experimental data. Area under the concentrationetime curve (AUC) was calculated using the trapezoidal rule. All values were expressed as the mean ± SD. Statistical analysis was performed with the Statistical Package for Social Science program (SPSS). $P < 0.05$ was considered significant for all experiments.

3. Results

3.1 The purity determination of 125I-rhKGF-2

After separation on Sephacryl S-300 HR, purity of the ^{125}I-rhKGF-2 was evaluated with HPLC. The calculated purities of three independent experiments were 99.35%, 99.44%, and 99.84%, respectively. The mean value was 99.54% ± 0.26% (Fig. 1), demonstrating that free ^{125}I is almost completely removed from ^{125}I-rhKGF-2 preparation. The lower radioactivity in the experiment 2 might be due to incomplete sample loading, yet the purity analysis will not be affected as the result is presented as percentage. The concentration of ^{125}I-rhKGF-2 was 0.996 mg/ml. The radioactivity of ^{125}I-KGF-2 was 4 258.8 Bq/μl.

3.2. The biological activity of ^{125}I-rhKGF-2

NIH3T3 cell proliferation assay was carried out to address whether iodination alters biological activity of rhKGF-2. Starved NIH3T3 cells were treated with various concentrations of rhKGF-2 and ^{125}I-rhKGF-2, respectively for 48 h, cell numbers were determin ed. As shown in Fig. 2, no difference in the proliferation rate of NIH3T3 cell was detected between rhKGF-2-and ^{125}I-rhKGF-2-stimulated groups at all concentrations tested. This data reveals that iodination does not change biological activity of rhKGF-2.

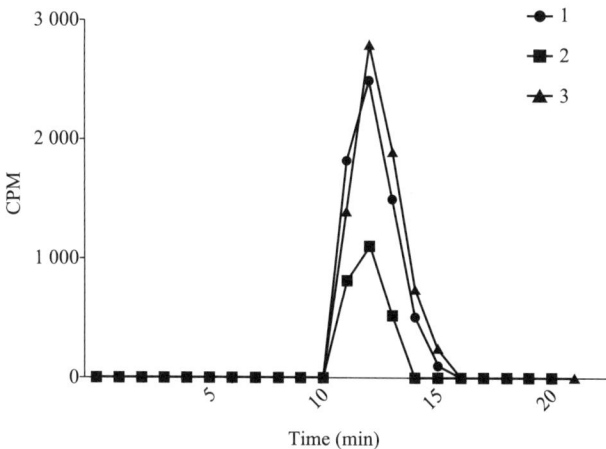

Fig. 1. Purity analysis of ^{125}I-rhKGF-2. After separation on Sephacryl S-300 HR, purity of ^{125}I-rhKGF-2 was analyzed with TSK-GEL G300 HPLC column (300 mm × 7.8 mm). The TSK-GEL column was eluted with 0.1 M PBS in the presence of 0.1 M NaCl and 0.05% sodium azide. The absorbance was measured continuously at 280 nm. Data shown were radioactivity of three independent experiments. Area under the radio activityetime curve was calculated using the trapezoidal. HPLC: high-performance liquid chromatography; rhKGF-2: recombinant human Keratinocyte growth factor-2.

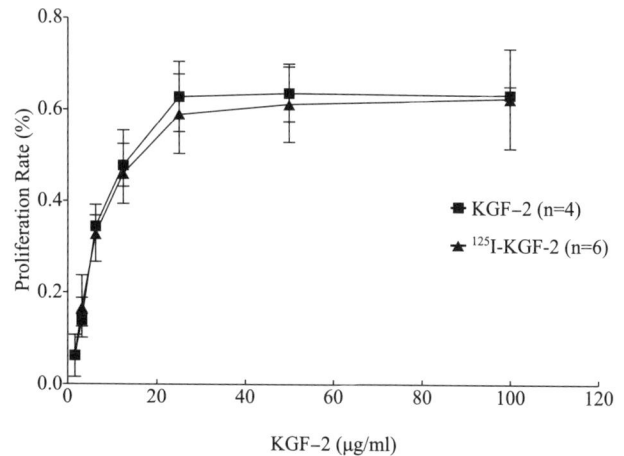

Fig. 2. No effect of iodination on biological activity of rhKGF-2. NIH3T3 cells were seeded into 96-well microplates at 7 000 cells/well. After 4–6 h attachment, cells were then starved in DMEM with 0.5% fetal bovine serum for overnight at 37 ℃. The starved cells were stimulated with various concentrations of rhKGF-2 and ^{125}I-rhKGF-2, respectively at 37 ℃ for 48 h. Cell proliferation was determined as described in Materials and methods. No statistical difference between cell proliferation responses to rHKGF-2 and 125I-rhKGF-2 ($P > 0.05$). rhKGF-2: recombinant human keratinocyte growth factor-2; ^{125}I-rhKGF-2: iodinated rhKGF-2.

3.3. Validation of the TCA-RA method for ^{125}I-rhKGF-2 quantification

Trichloroacetic acid precipitation coupled with radiometric assay (TCA-RA) was applied for determination of io-dinated rhKGF2. A series of concentrations of ^{125}I-rhKGF-2 were added into the blank tissues and the radioactivity was measured before and after TCA precipitation. The calibration curves for different rabbit eye tissues were generated by graphing experimental data against added concentrations of ^{125}I-rhKGF-2. The accuracy and precision were determined at three levels: linearity, coefficient of variance (CV), and lower limit of quantification (LoQ). Excellent linearity ($r^2 >$ 0.996) was obtained between 0.5 and 463 ng/ml, with a LoQ of 2 Bq/g or Bq/ml (equivalent to 0.5 ng/g or/ml) for ^{125}I-rhKGF-2 (Fig. 3). The precision (CV) was <20% for all matrices. More than 80% of the added ^{125}I-rhKGF-2 in all sam-ples was recovered by TCA precipitation (Fig. 3). These results demonstrated that the TCA-RA method was accurate,

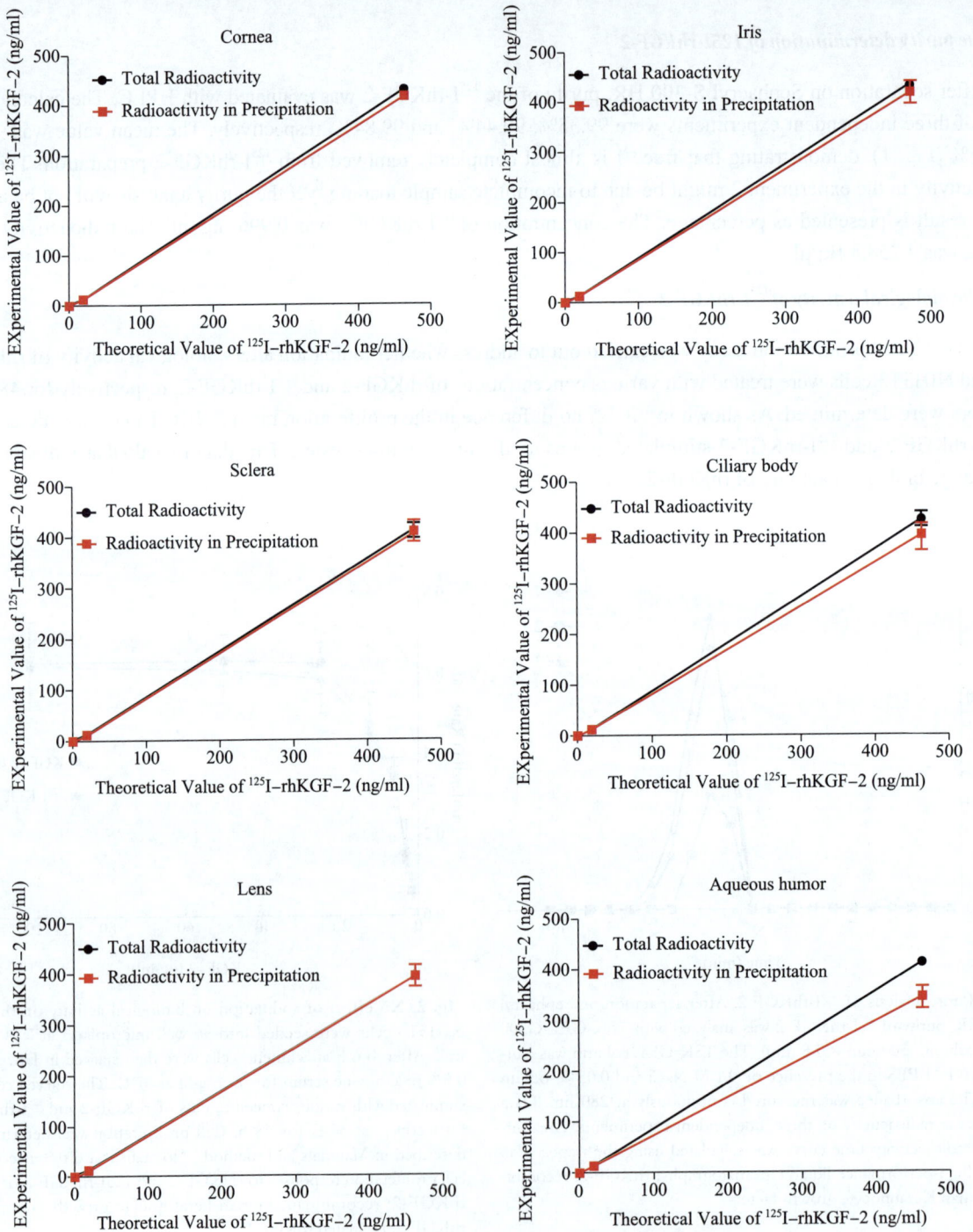

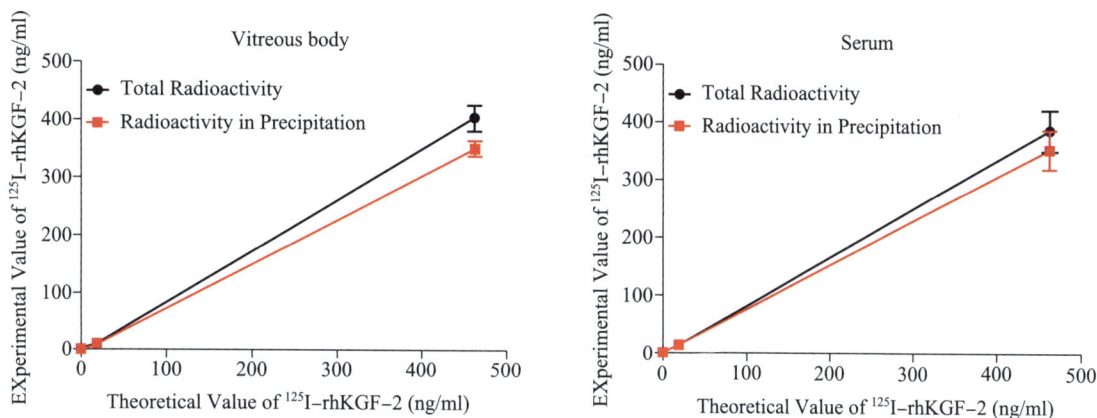

Fig. 3. rhKGF-2 recovery by the TCA precipitation. The rabbit eye tissue samples were isolated and weighed. Approximately 0.5 g of the each tissue sample was individually mixed with 5 volumes (w/w) of deionized water in a clean tube and homogenized. The standard recovery curves of ^{125}I-rhKGF-2 from different rabbit eye tissues were generated by adding a series of concentrations of ^{125}I-rhKGF-2 into the blank tissues. Data shown were mean values ± SD of three independent experiments. No statistical difference between total radioactivity and TCA-precipitated radioactivity ($P > 0.05$). TCA: trichloroacetic acid.

reliable, and reproducible. This method would be applicable for studies of the tissue distribution and pharmacokinetics of ^{125}I-rhKGF-2.

3.4 Tissue distribution of ^{125}I-rhKGF-2

Tissue distribution of ^{125}I-rhKGF-2 was evaluated by measuring radioactivity in eye tissues at 1, 2, 4, and 24 h post topical application of 50 mg/ml ^{125}I-rhKGF-2. ^{125}I-rhKGF-2 was detected in all eye tissues obtained from control group (Fig. 4A) and alkali-burned group (Fig. 4B). The highest radioactivity level was found in the cornea, followed by iris, sclera, ciliary body, lens, aqueous humor, vitreous body, and serum in a greatest to least order. A longer time is required for rhKGF-2 to reach peak concentration in control eye tissues than in alkali-burned eye tissues. This is more likely due to barrier effect of epithelial layer that is destroyed after alkali injury.

AUC calculation revealed that the radioactivity levels of ^{125}IrhKGF2 in alkali-burned corneas were higher than those in control corneas (Fig. 5).

3.5 Pharmacokinetics of ^{125}I-rhKGF-2 in rabbit eye tissues

Our previous studies showed that wound healing effect of rhKGF-2 is better at 25 μg/ml than at 50 μg/ml in laser-

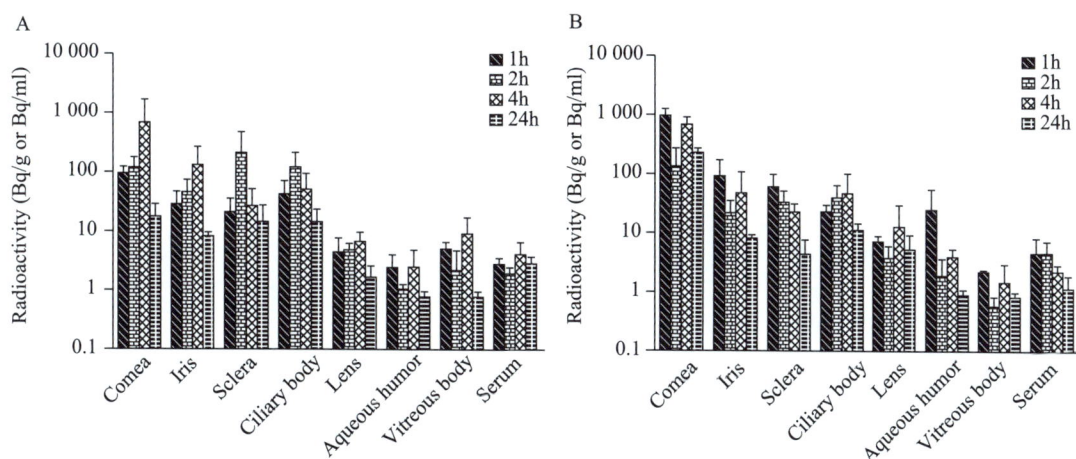

Fig. 4. Tissue distribution of ^{125}I-rhKGF-2. After topically application of 50 μg/ml ^{125}I- rhKGF-2 on rabbit eyes, three rabbits were sacrificed at 1, 2, 4, and 24 h and eye tissues were collected. Radioactivity of ^{125}I-rhKGF-2 was measured by TCA-RA method. Data shown were mean values ± SD of control group (A) and alkali-burned group (B). TCA- RA: radioactivity assay after TCA precipitation.

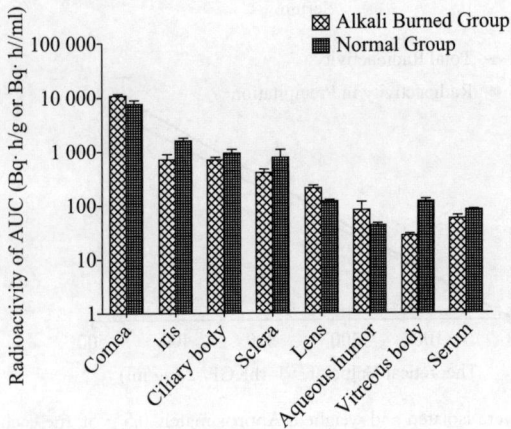

Fig. 5. The comparison of AUC radioactivity between alkali-burned group and control group. After topical application of ^{125}I-rhKGF-2, three rabbits were sacrificed at 1, 2, 4, and 24 h and eye tissues were collected. Radioactivity of ^{125}I-rhKGF-2 was measured by TCA-RA method. Area under the radioactiv/time curve was calculated using the trapezoidal from 0 to 24 h. Data shown were mean values ± SD of three rabbits. No statistical difference of rhKGF-2 concentrations between alkali-injured group and control group ($P > 0.05$). AUC: area under the curve.

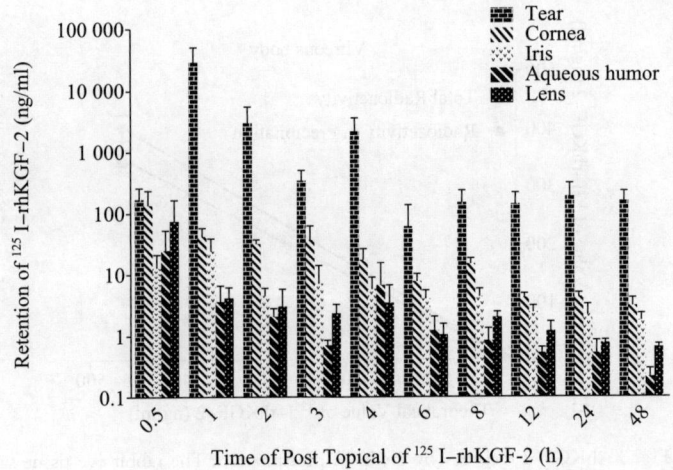

Fig. 6. Retention of ^{125}I-rhKGF-2 in eye tissues. After topical application of 25 μg/ml ^{125}I-rhKGF-2, radioactivity in the cornea, iris, aqueous humor, lens and tear was measured at time points of 0.5, 1, 2, 3, 4, 6, 8, 12, 24, and 48 h. Data shown were mean values ± SD of three rabbits.

injured rabbit model (Wang *et al.*, 2010). 25 μg/ml of rhKGF-2 was chosen for pharmacokinetic study and tissue samples were collected at 10 time points for accuracy of calculated pharmacokinetic parameters. Alkali injury appears not to significantly alter tissue distribution of rhKGF-2, thus, pharmacokinetic study was only carried out in normal rabbit eyes.

Concentration-time profiles in four rabbit eye tissues and tear for ^{125}I-rhKGF-2 were shown in Fig. 6. Radioactivity reached maximal values in the cornea, aqueous humor, and lens at 0.5 h after topically application of ^{125}I-rhKGF-2. However, a maximal value was reached at 1 h in iris tissue and declined gradually over time. Except in corneas and tear, radioactivity levels declined to background by 24 h after topical application in the other three eye tissues. The calculated pharmacokinetic parameters of $t_{1/2}$, T_{max}, and C_{max} were 3.4, 6.2, 6.5, 5.2, 2.5 h; 0.5, 1.0, 0.5, 0.5, 1.0 h; and 135.2, 23.2, 4.5, 24.1, 29,498.9 ng/ml, respectively in cornea, iris, lens, aqueous humor, and tear (Table 1).

Table 1. Pharmacokinetics data of 125I-rhKGF-2 in rabbit eye tissues

	Cornea	Iris	Aqueous humor	Lens	Tear
$t_{1/2}$[a] (h)	3.4	6.2	5.2	6.5	2.5
T_{max}[b] (h)	0.5	1.0	0.5	0.5	1.0
C_{max}[c] (ng/ml)	135.15	23.2	24.08	4.48	29 498.94

[a] $t_{1/2}$, the terminal elimination half-time.

[b] T_{max}, time to peak value.

[c] C_{max}, peak drug concentration.

4. Discussion

KGF-2, a potent epithelial cell mitogen, plays an important role in organ morphogenesis and epithelial differentiation (Fang *et al.*, 2010). The ability to promote re-epithelialization and wound healing in multiple models of tissue injury makes it a promising therapeutic for tissue repair (Plichta and Radek, 2012). Most importantly, KGF-2 has been in phase I/II clinical trials for evaluation of safety and efficacy in ulcerative colitis and in mucositis after chemotherapy with bone marrow transplantation (Freytes *et al.*, 2004). Although pharmacokinetic profile of KGF-2 has been evaluated in cynomolgus monkeys and healthy humans during a phase I trial (Sung *et al.*, 2002), the tissue distribution and pharmacokinetics of KGF-2 in alkali-burned and control rabbit eyes was first time reported, to our knowledge.

RhKGF-2 effectively penetrated the cornea epithelium and distributed to eye tissues such as cornea, iris, ciliary body, lens, aqueous humor and vitreous body in control rabbit eyes (Fig. 4). Small molecular mass of KGF-2 (19.3 kDa) may make it penetrate the corneal epithelium easier than high molecular mass drugs that do not generally cross the corneal epithelium (Koevary, 2003; Lambiase *et al.*, 2005). However, the underlining mechanisms are unclear at present. The fact that rhKGF-2 reached high levels in the corneas 1 h after topical application, strongly suggested that the eye drops of rhKGF-2 was an efficient route of administration for cornea. Moreover, very limited amount of rhKGF-2, about 1% of that in the cornea was detected in the serum, indicating that little rhKGF-2 enters into the systemic circulation. This characteristic of KGF-2 will minimize possible systemic side effects when clinically used.

Under physiological condition, the corneal epithelium annular tight junctions surround and effectively seal the superficial epithelial cells (Sasaki *et al.*, 1999), thus limiting its permeability. RhKGF-2 can penetrate into cornea, therefore, rhKGF-2 should penetrate into cornea easily under pathological condition where annular tight junctions are broken. As expected, concentration of rhKGF-2 increased more quickly in injured corneas (Fig. 4B) than in control corneas (Fig. 4A). More intriguing, the concentration of ^{125}I-rhKGF-2 was higher in the corneas of alkali-burned rabbit group (pathological condition) than in those of control group (physiological condition). In contrast, the concentration of ^{125}I-rhKGF-2 was lower in all other eye tissues of alkali-burned group when compared with control group, though not statistically significant (Fig. 5). These findings suggest that predominant and preferred accumulation of rhKGF-2 in injured corneas could promote repair process under pathological conditions causing corneal injuries.

Pharmacokinetic studies of rhKGF-2 were carried out in cornea, iris, aqueous humor, lens and tear. In corneas, concentration of rhKGF-2 reached peak at 135.2 ng/ml 30 min upon topical application and declined to 4.3 ng/ml 24 h later (Fig. 6). A rapid turnover was observed in lens and aqueous humor. The initial amount of rhKGF-2 detected in the lens and aqueous humor was 74.3 ng/ml and 24.1 ng/ml, respectively, which promptly decreased to 4.0 ng/ ml and 3.67 ng/ml just 0.5 h later (Fig. 6). Only 1%–2% of the initial amount of rhKGF-2 was left in the lens and aqueous humor 24 h after topical delivery. These results implied that there was almost no accumulation of rhKGF-2 in the lens and aqueous humor after topical administration of it 24 h later, which may be a safe factor for the application of rhKGF-2.

$t_{1/2}$, C_{max}, and T_{max} are important pharmacokinetic parameters. Our study showed that the $t_{1/2}$, C_{max}, and T_{max} of rhKGF-2 in the rabbit corneas were 3.4 h, 135.2 ng/ml, and 0.5 h (Table 1). RhKGF-2 concentration in corneas diminished from an initial 135.2 ng/ml to ng/ml from 0.5 to 24 h after topical administration. KGF has been showed to enhance proliferation of human corneal epithelial cells as low as 1 ng/ml (Zhong and Gong, 1998). We have also demonstrated that KGF-2 ranging from 1 to 200 ng/ml significantly stimulated the proliferation of rat conjunctival epithelial cells (Ma *et al.*, 2011). Our current pharmacokinetic data suggest that KGF-2 may provide the proliferative effect on corneal epithelial cells for at least 24 h upon a single dose topical application.

It appears increasingly likely that the events occurring within the earliest stages of corneal wound healing alter prognosis (Jester *et al.*, 1997; Møller-Pedersen *et al.*, 1998). Early application of treatment will be essential to minimize adverse healing and optimize repair for corneal wound healing (Carrington *et al.*, 2006). It is worth to note that T_{max} of rhKGF-2 was just 0.5 h in the corneas after topical delivery. Rapid increase in rhKGF-2 in corneas could effectively promote wound healing process and limit damage at the earliest stages, which would be beneficial for corneal wound recovery.

In conclusion, rhKGF-2 distributed predominantly into corneas among eye tissues examined upon topical delivery. Chemical injury led to more accumulation of rhKGF-2 in the injured corneas, potentially facilitating wound healing processes. The pharmacokinetic profile of rhKGF-2 showed 3.4 h half-life in rabbit corneas and maintained biologically active level in rabbit corneas upon single dose topical application, suggesting that topical application of rhKGF-2 is an efficient route of administration for corneal wound healing. Our findings provide additional support for the ongoing development of rhKGF-2 for eye diseases involving epithclial injury.

References

[1] Carrington LM, Albon J, Anderson I, *et al.* Differential regulation of key stages in early corneal wound healing by TGF-beta Isoforms and their inhibitors[J]. Investigative Ophthalmology & Visual Science, 2006, 47(5): 1886-1894.

[2] Chen X, Zaro JL, Shen W-C. Pharmacokinetics of recombinant bifunctional fusion proteins[J]. Expert Opinion on Drug Metabolism & Toxicology, 2012, 8(5): 581-595.

[3] Fang X, Bai C, Wang X. Potential clinical application of KGF-2 (FGF-10) for acute lung injury/acute respiratory distress syndrome[J]. Expert Review Of Clinical Pharmacology, 2010, 3(6): 797-805.

[4] Freytes CO, Ratanatharathorn V, Taylor C, *et al.* Phase I/II randomized trial evaluating the safety and clinical effects of repifermin administered to reduce mucositis in patients undergoing autologous hematopoietic stem cell transplantation[J]. Clinical Cancer Research, 2004, 10(24): 8318-8324.

[5] Han DS, Li FL, Holt L, *et al.* Keratinocyte growth factor-2 (FGF-10) promotes healing of experimental small intestinal ulceration in rats[J]. American Journal Of Physiology-Gastrointestinal And Liver Physiology, 2000, 279(5): G1011-G1022.

[6] Huang Z, Ni C, Chu Y, *et al.* Chemical modification of recombinant human keratinocyte growth factor 2 with polyethylene glycol improves biostability and reduces animal immunogenicity[J]. Journal Of Biotechnology, 2009, 142(3-4): 242-249.

[7] Jester JV, BarryLane PA, Petroll WM, *et al.* Inhibition of corneal fibrosis by topical application of blocking antibodies to TGF(beta) in the rabbit[J]. Cornea, 1997, 16(2): 177-187.

[8] Jimenez PA, Rampy MA. Keratinocyte growth factor-2 accelerates wound healing in incisional wounds[J]. Journal Of Surgical Research, 1999, 81(2): 238-242.

[9] Koevary SB. Pharmacokinetics of topical ocular drug delivery: Potential uses for the treatment of diseases of the posterior segment and beyond[J]. Current Drug Metabolism, 2003, 4(3): 213-222.

[10] Kruse FE, Tseng SCG. Growth-factors modulate clonal growth and differentiation of cultured rabbit limbal and corneal epithelium[J]. Investigative Ophthalmology & Visual Science, 1993, 34(6): 1963-1976.

[11] Lambiase A, Tirassa P, Micera A, *et al.* Pharmacokinetics of conjunctivally applied nerve growth factor in the retina and optic nerve of adult[J]. Investigative Ophthalmology &Visual Science, 2005, 46(10): 3800-3806.

[12] Liu L, Li Y, Huang S, *et al.* Keratinocyte growth factor-2 on the proliferation of corneal epithelial stem cells in rabbit alkali burned cornea[J]. Yan ke xue bao = Eye science, 2007, 23(2): 107-116.

[13] Christman KL, Singelyn JM, Salvatore M, *et al.* Catheter-deliverable hydrogel derived from decellularized ventricular extracellular matrix increases cardiomyocyte survival and preserves cardiac function post-myocardial infarction[J]. Journal Of the American College Of Cardiology, 2011, 57(14): E2017-E2017.

[14] Marchese C, Felici A, Visco V, *et al.* Fibroblast growth factor 10 induces proliferation and differentiation of human primary cultured keratinocytes[J]. Journal Of Investigative Dermatology, 2001, 116(4): 623-628.

[15] Miceli R, Hubert M, Santiago G, *et al.* Efficacy of keratinocyte

growth factor-2 in dextran sulfate sodium-induced murine colitis[J]. Journal Of Pharmacology And Experimental Therapeutics, 1999, 290(1): 464-471.

[16] Pajoohesh-Ganji A, Stepp MA. In search of markers for the stem cells of the corneal epithelium[J]. Biology Of the Cell, 2005, 97(4): 265-276.

[17] Plichta JK, Radek KA. Sugar-Coating Wound Repair: A Review of FGF-10 and Dermatan Sulfate in Wound Healing and Their Potential Application in Burn Wounds[J]. Journal Of Burn Care & Research, 2012, 33(3): 299-310.

[18] Saksena S, Priyamvada S, Kumar A, *et al.* Keratinocyte growth factor-2 stimulates P-glycoprotein expression and function in intestinal epithelial cells[J]. American Journal Of Physiology-Gastrointestinal And Liver Physiology, 2013, 304(6): G615-G622.

[19] Sasaki H, Yamamura K, Mukai T, *et al.* Enhancement of ocular drug penetration[J]. Critical Reviews In Therapeutic Drug Carrier Systems, 1999, 16(1): 85-146.

[20] She J, Goolaerts A, Shen J, *et al.* KGF-2 targets alveolar epithelia and capillary endothelia to reduce high altitude pulmonary oedema in rats[J]. Journal Of Cellular And Molecular Medicine, 2012, 16(12): 3074-3084.

[21] Smith PD, Polo M, Soler PM, *et al.* Efficacy of growth factors in the accelerated closure of interstices in explanted meshed human skin grafts[J]. Journal Of Burn Care & Rehabilitation, 2000, 21(1): 5-9.

[22] Sung C, Pary TJ, Riccobene TA, *et al.* Pharmacologic and pharmacokinetic profile of repifermin (KGF-2) in monkeys and comparative pharmacokinetics in humans[J]. Aaps Pharmsci, 2002, 4(2).

[23] Taranta Martin LF, Rocha EM, Garcia SB, *et al.* Topical Brazilian propolis improves corneal wound healing and inflammation in rats following alkali burns[J]. Bmc Complementary And Alternative Medicine, 2013, 13.

[24] Wagoner MD. Chemical injuries of the eye: Current concepts in pathophysiology and therapy[J]. Survey Of Ophthalmology, 1997, 41(4): 275-313.

[25] Wang J, Cai X, Zou M, *et al.* Construction and characterization of a high activity mutant of human keratinocyte growth factor-2[J]. Biotechnology Letters, 2009, 31(6): 797-802.

[26] Wang X, Zhou X, Ma J, *et al.* Effects of Keratinocyte Growth Factor-2 on Corneal Epithelial Wound Healing in a Rabbit Model of Carbon Dioxide Laser Injury[J]. Biological & Pharmaceutical Bulletin, 2010, 33(6): 971-976.

[27] Wu X, Tian H, Huang Y, *et al.* Large-scale production of biologically active human keratinocyte growth factor-2[J]. Applied Microbiology And Biotechnology, 2009, 82(3): 439-444.

[28] Xia YP, Zhao YN, Marcus J, *et al.* Effects of keratinocyte growth factor-2 (KGF-2) on wound healing in an ischaemia-impaired rabbit ear model and on scar formation[J]. Journal Of Pathology, 1999, 188(4): 431-438.

[29] Zhong X, Gong X. Effect of keratinocyte growth factor on corneal epithelial wound healing[J]. [Zhonghua yan ke za zhi] Chinese journal of ophthalmology, 1998, 34(1): 15-18.

Fibroblast growth factors stimulate hair growth through β-catenin and shh expression in C57BL/6 mice

Weihong Lin, Xiaokun Li, Xiaojie Wang, Jian Xiao

1. Introduction

Hair is considered accessory structure of the integument along with sebaceous glands, sweat glands, and nails. Hair follicle morphogenesis requires the intricately controlled regulation of apoptosis, proliferation, and differentiation. Hair follicles are miniorgans that, during postnatal life, cycle through periods of anagen (growth phase), catagen (regression phase), and telogen (resting phase) [1, 2]. Hair loss is generally not a life-threatening event, but the number of patients suffering from it has increased dramatically. Meanwhile, hair loss takes impact on social interactions and patients' psychological well beings. To date, there are only two anti-hair loss drugs, finasteride and minoxidil, which have been used in clinical, but the effect of these drugs is limited, transient, and somewhat unpredictable [3]. Therefore, it is urgent to develop novel pharmacological treatments.

Various cytokines and growth factors are involved in the regulation of hair morphogenesis and cycle hair growth. The fibroblast growth factor (FGF) family is composed of 22 members with a wide range of biological functions involved in angiogenesis, embryonic development, cell growth, and tissue repair [4, 5]. The early literature reported that acidic fibroblast growth factor (aFGF or FGF-1) and basic fibroblast growth factor (bFGF or FGF-2) may affect the growth of hair follicles, but people have different conclusion. D.C DL demonstrated that exogenous FGF-1 and FGF-2 interfere with follicle morphogenesis and ultimately suppress the hair cycle [6, 7]. On the other hand, Katsuoka *et al.*, reported that FGF-2 promotes papilla cell proliferation and the increase in the size of hair follicle in mice [8, 9]. The controlled release study also showed that gelatin hydrogel enables FGF-2 to positively act on the hair growth cycle of mice [10,11]. Recent evidence explored another FGF, named keratinocyte growth factor 2 (KGF-2 or FGF-10), which also significantly stimulated human hair-follicle cell proliferation in organ culture [12]. Moreover, FGF-1 has been identified as a crucial endogenous mediator of normal hair follicle growth, development, and differentiation [13], but KGF is not required for wound healing [14]. Therefore, it is necessary for enhanced *in vivo* efficacy to contrive the administration form of FGF.

It should be noted that FGF-1, FGF-2, and FGF-10 have been approved by SFDA for wound healing, and China is the only country in the world for clinical application of these drugs. Thus, the commercial growth factors were used in this study, the hair growth promoting activity was scientifically proven, and the mechanism of action was investigated.

2. Materials and methods

2.1 Materials

The DAB chromogen kit (ZSGB-BIO, Beijing, China) was purchased. Anti-β-catenin (rabbit polyclonal antibody, Abcam, UK), anti-FGF9 (rabbit polyclonal antibody, Abcam, UK), and anti-Shh (rabbit polyclonal antibody, Santa Cruz Biotech, Santa Cruz, CA, USA) antibodies were purchased. Hematoxylin (Beyotime Institute of Biotechnology, China) and eosin (Beyotime Institute of Biotechnology, China) were purchased. FGF-1 (Shanghai Wanxing Co.), FGF-2 (Zhuhai Essexbio Co.), and FGF-10 (Anhui Xin-huakun Co.) were applied to the experimental group. The concentration of FGFs was diluted at 500 μg/ml.

2.2 Experimental animals

Healthy C57BL6/N mice (6-week-old, 15 mice per group) were obtained from Laboratory Animals Center of Wenzhou Medical University. All animals were from the Laboratory Animals Center of Wenzhou Medical University and were treated strictly in accordance with international ethical guidelines and the National Institutes of Health Guide concerning the Care and Use of Laboratory Animals. The experiments were carried out with the approval of the Animal Experimentation Ethics Committee of Wenzhou Medical University. Temperature ($23 \pm 2°C$), humidity (35%–60%), and photoperiod (12 h light and 12 h darkness cycle) were kept constant.

2.3 Experimental studies with FGFs

60 animals in 4 randomized groups ($n = 15$) were used for the study of hair promoting activity. All animals were shaved using depilatory cream (Veet, USA) at 6 weeks of age, at which all hair follicles were synchronized in the telogen stage. FGF-10, FGF-1, FGF-2 (all500 µg/ml dissolved in 10 µl normal saline, 5 µg/12 cm^2 per mouse), or vehicle (100 µl normal saline) was applied topically on dorsal skin of C57BL/6N mice with subcutaneous injection for 14 d. At every 1,7,14, and 28 d, three mice of each group were sacrificed to obtain skin specimen. Visible hair growth was recorded at every 1, 7, 14, and 28 d.

2.4 Histological studies

Dorsal skin was excised after topical application with FGFs at the indicated time points. Dorsal skin was maintained in 4% paraformaldehyde at 4°C and embedded in paraffin blocks to obtain longitudinal and transverse section. 5 mm sections were stained with hematoxylin and eosin (H&E). The other skin was stored at –80°C for protein extraction. Digital photomicrographs were taken from representative areas at a fixed magnification of 100 ×.

2.5 Hair follicle count

The H&E stained slides were photographed using a digital photomicrograph and all of the images were cropped in a fixed area of 300 pixels width. We counted hair follicles manually in a fixed area (0.09 mm^2). Digital photomicrographs were taken from representative areas at a fixed magnification of 100 ×.

2.6 Hair length determination

Hairs were plucked randomly from shaved dorsal area at 1,7,14,21, and 28 days. After plucking 20 hairs per mouse, we measured the average hair length manually.

2.7 Immunohistochemistry

Dorsal skins were stained with anti-β-catenin and Sonic hedgehog (Shh) antibodies. Sections were dewaxed and hydrated. To quench endogenous peroxidase activity, deparaffinized sections were pretreated with 3% peroxidase for 10 min. After washing with PBS, the sections were incubated with serum to block nonspecific binding of biotinylated secondary antibody for 30 min and then incubated with anti-β-catenin (1:200) and Shh (1:500) antibodies overnight at 4°C. Slides were incubated with biotinylated secondary antibody for 30 min. After incubating with HRP-streptavidin complex to detect secondary antibody for 30 min, slides were developed until light brown staining was visible with DAB chromogen kit. The immunopositivity in fields was counted for per sections using Image-Pro Plus software (Nikon, Tokyo, Japan).

2.8 Statistical analysis

Results are expressed as mean ± SD. Statistical significance was determined with Student's t-test when there were two experimental groups. For more than two groups, statistical evaluation of the data was performed using One-way Analysis-of-variance (ANOVA) test, followed by Dunnett's *post hoc* test with the values $P < 0.05$ considered significant.

3. Results

3.1 The effect of FGFs on hair growth

The black pigmentation was taken as evidence for transition of hair follicles from telogen to anagen phase. To evaluate the hair growth activity of FGFs, we topically applied FGF-1, FGF-2, and FGF-10 on the shaved dorsal skin of telogenic C57BL/6 mice for 14 d. Each week, we evaluated the degree of hair growth by observing the skin color. At 2 weeks, three FGFs induced black coloration in the shaved skin of C57BL/6 mice significantly; FGF-10 group showed the most black coloration, while very less visible hair growth and black coloration were observed in control group (Fig. 1A). At 3 weeks, the FGFs group showed markedly hair growth, and FGF-10 stimulated hair growth over 1/2 area on the shaved dorsal skin. At 4 weeks, we observed that hair growth from FGF-1 and FGF-2 was confined to the proximal parts of epidermis; FGF-10 treated group showed overall hair growth which was not confined to the proximal parts. However, the control group only showed less hair growth (Fig. 1A). To confirm whether FGFs promoted hair growth, we measured the length of 10 hairs plucked from the dorsal skin of each mouse at 2, 3, and 4 weeks. Since visible hair shaft was observed after 2 weeks, we measured length of 2-, 3-, and 4-week-old hairs. As shown in Fig. 1B, the length of hairs in FGF-10, FGF-1, and FGF-2 treated group was remarkably longer than that of control group, and FGF-10 exists with the strongest activity of hair growth. Taken together, these results indicated commercialized drugs, FGF-10, FGF-1, and FGF-2, promote hair growth and FGF-10 appears with the highest efficiency in the three protein drugs.

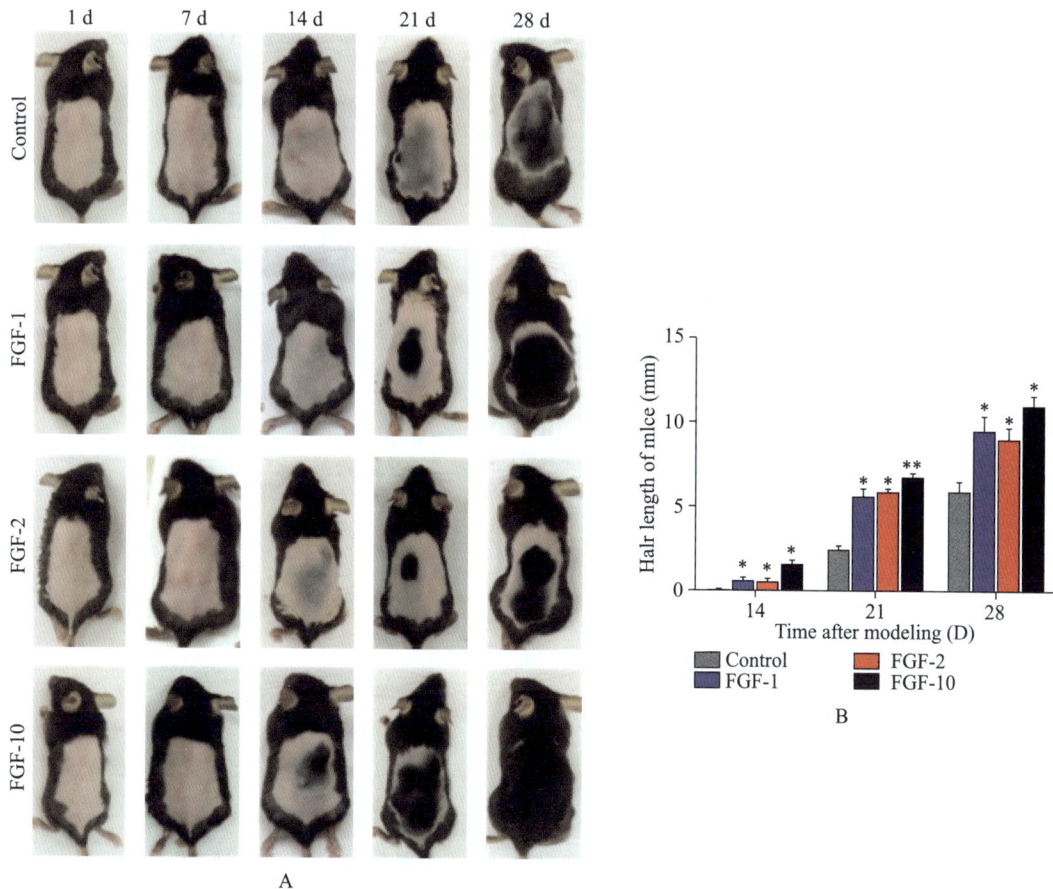

Fig. 1. Hair growth promoting effect of FGFs. (A) 6-week-old C57BL6/N mice were shaved and topically applied with vehicle, FGF-1, FGF-2, and FGF-10. Photographs were taken every week after applying FGFs or vehicle on the shaved dorsal skin. (B) Hair length was measured after topical application ofFGFs. The hair length of randomly plucked hairs ($n = 10$) was measured at 14, 21, and 28 days after topical application of FGFs. Data shown represent means ± S.D, [*]$P < 0.05$, < 0.01 vs. control group.

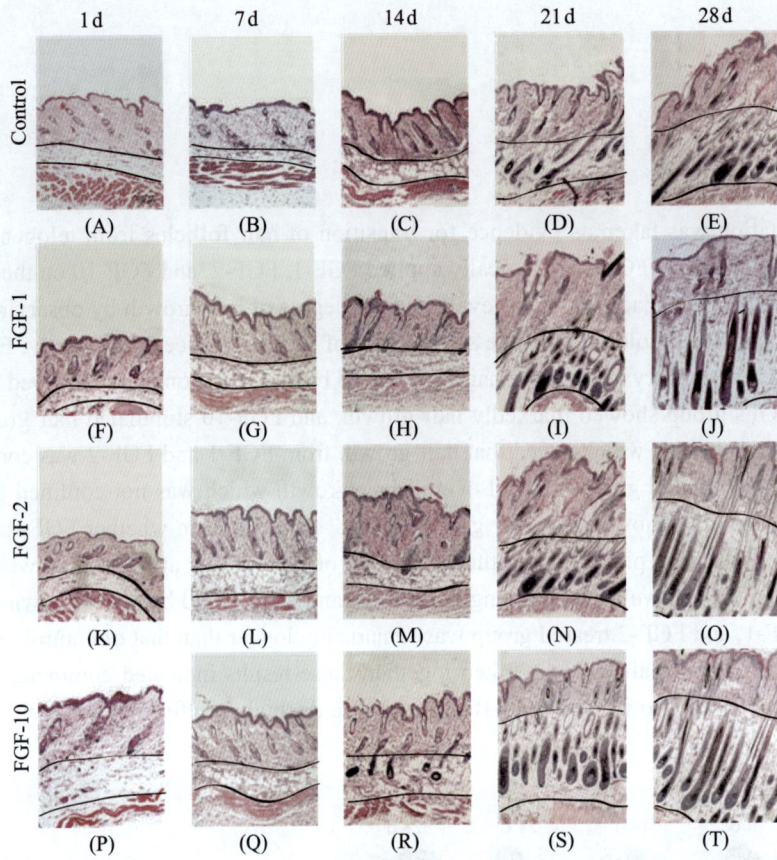

A

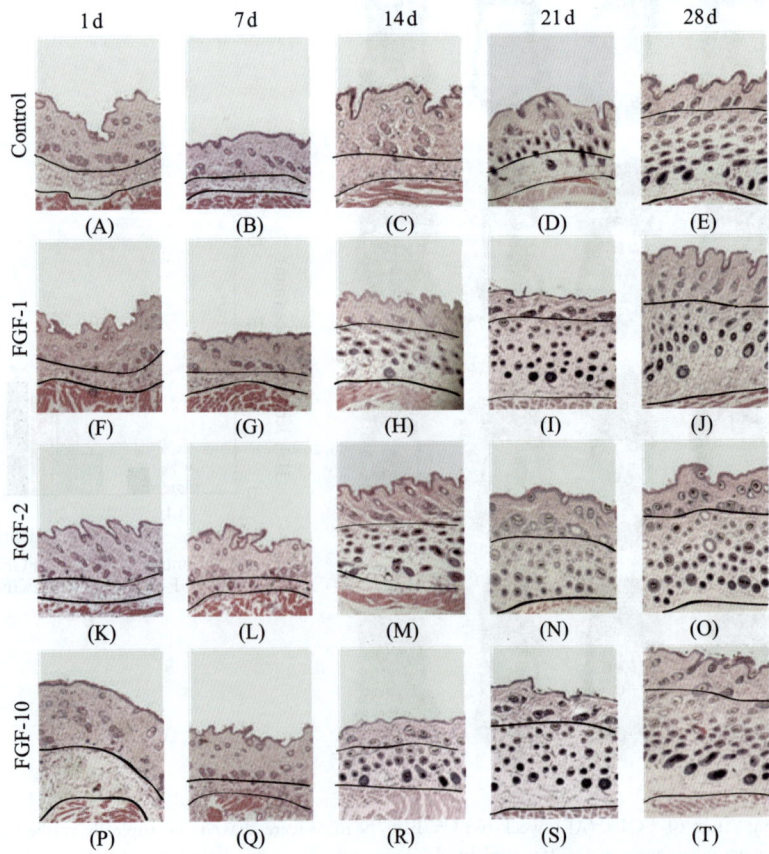

B

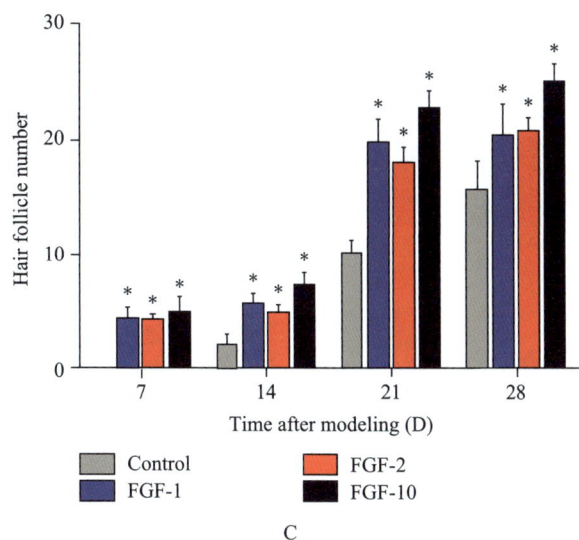

C

Fig. 2. The effect ofFGFs on the hair follicles was analyzed by H&E staining. (A) Longitudinal sections of the dorsal skins. (B) Transverse sections ofthe dorsal skins. (C) The number ofhair follicles in deep subcutis. Data shown represent means ± S.D, $^{*}P < 0.05$, $^{**}P < 0.01$ *vs.* control group.

3.2. Effect of FGFs on hair follicle number

It has reported increasing in the number and the size of hair follicles during anagen phase induction [15]. An increase in the density of hair follicles is an indicator for the transition of hair growth from the telogen to anagen phases [16,17]. To investigate the progression of hair follicles in the hair cycle, HE staining was performed. In the representative longitudinal and transverse sections, the hair follicles in FGF-10, FGF-1, and FGF-2 treated group appeared earlier than those in the control group (Fig. 2A, 2B). Meanwhile, the number of hair follicles of the relative area in FGFs treated group was higher than in the control group, consistent with the above results, and topical application of FGF-10 showed the maximum amount of hair follicles as compared to FGF-1 and FGF-2 group (Fig. 2C). These data suggested that FGFs including FGF-10, FGF-1, and FGF-2 stimulate hair growth by inducing anagen phase of hair follicles.

3.3 FGFs induced the expression of β-catenin and sonic hedgehog (Shh)

Evidence showed that β-catenin induced the transition of the hair growth cycle from the telogen to anagen phases [18, 19]. To elucidate the mechanism of the early events of anagen induction by FGFs, immunohisto chemistry analysis was performed to detect the expression of β-catenin. We observed that β-catenin protein expression appears in FGF-10, FGF-1, and FGF-2 at 1 week, and the levels of β-catenin were higher in FGFs group than in control group at 2 weeks (Fig. 3). It should be noted that, at 3 weeks, the expression of β-catenin was remarkable in control group, while it is decreased in FGF-10 group compared to the appearance at 2 weeks. At 4 weeks, only the control group showed significant expression of β-catenin.

The secreted signaling molecule Sonic hedgehog (Shh) plays an important role in both embryonic and adult hair development. In adult mice, Shh expression is upregulated in early anagen, and ectopic application of Shh can prematurely induce anagen in resting telogen follicles [20]. Immunohistochemical analysis result showed that Shh expression was upregulated in FGF-10, FGF-1, and FGF-2 treated group compared to that in control group at 2 weeks (Fig. 4). Taking together, these data indicated that the three FGFs drugs promote hair growth partly through upregulating β-catenin and Shh.

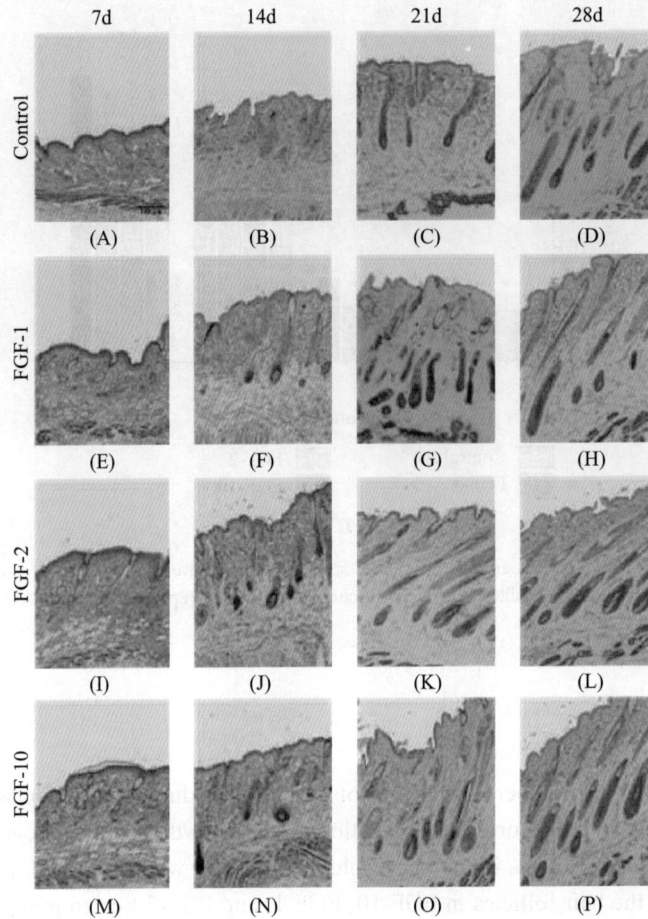

Fig. 3. The expression of β-catenin after topical application of FGFs. Longitudinal sections of the dorsal skins from each group were stained for β-catenin by immunohistochemistry (brown staining). Digital photomicrographs were taken from representative areas at a fixed magnification of 100 ×.

4. Discussion

Hair loss disorders are not life-threatening, but it may make afflicte the people vulnerable and lower their quality of life [21]. The estimated annual market value for hair growth promoting agents is multibillion dollars in the all world. Minoxidil is a widely used hair growth promoting drug for androgenic alopecia patients by inducing hair follicles in the telogen stage to undergo transition into the anagen stages [22]; however, it would also cause adverse dermatological effects, such as dryness, scaling, local irritation, and dermatitis [23, 24]. Finasteride has been reported to be efficacious for androgenic alopecia patients, but it is not recommended for female patients [25]. Therefore, developing new drugs for promoting hair growth is urgently.

Several growth factors (e.g., FGF-1, FGF-2, FGF-7, FGF-10, IGF-1, IGF-2, and EGF) can promote cell cycle and proliferation and have the potential to rescue hair loss and facilitate hair cell regeneration in vivo and in vitro. It has been shown that EGF and transforming growth factor-α (TGF-α) are contributed to hair cell proliferation and regeneration in avian utricles [26]. Regeneration of lost hair cells has also been found in rat utricular after treatment with FGF-2 and IGF-1 [27]. KGF protects hair follicles from cell death induced by UV irradiation, chemotherapeutic, or cytotoxic agents [28]. EGF, FGF-1, or FGF-2 maintains high proliferation and multipotent potential of human hair follicle-derived mesenchymal stem cells [29]. All of this literature demonstrated that growth factors may be potential for treating hair loss. Therefore, we searched all of the growth factors which proved by SFDA (China) and we found that FGF-1, FGF-2, and KGF have been applicated in clinical for wound healing, so we purchased these three drugs and investigated the hair growth promoting activity in vivo.

C57BL/6 mice are useful models for screening hair growth promoting agents, as their truncal pigmentation is de-

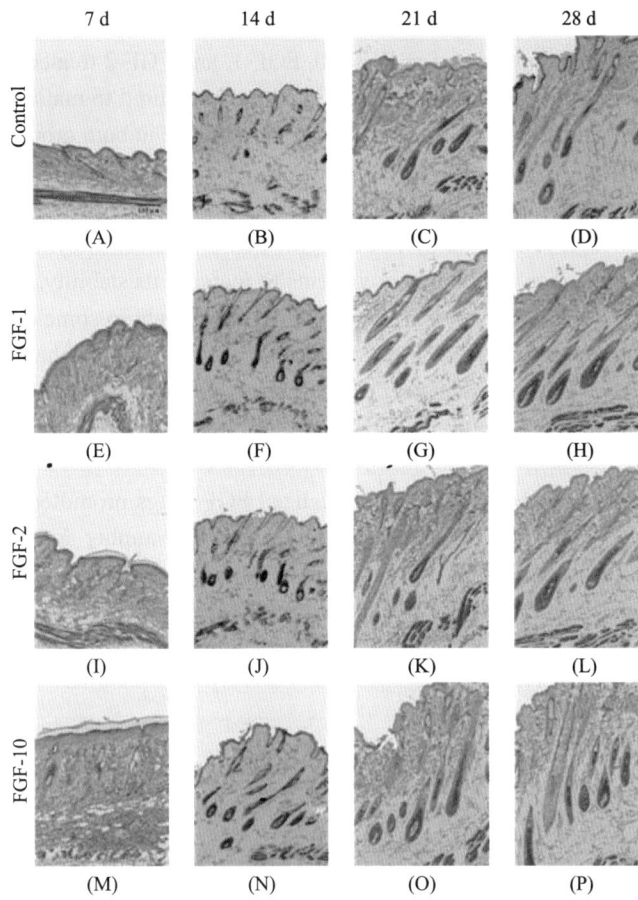

Fig. 4. The expression of Shh after topical application of FGFs. Longitudinal sections of the dorsal skins from each group were stained for Shh by immunohistochemistry (brown staining). Digital photomicrographs were taken from representative areas at a fixed magnification of 100 ×.

pendent on their follicular melanocytes, producing pigment only during anagen [30]. The shaved back skins of C57BL6/N were treated with topical application of FGFs for 1, 2, 3, and 4 weeks. At 2 weeks, FGF-1, FGF-2, and FGF-10 induced hair growth in the telogenic C57BL/6 mice, while no less visible hair growth was observed in the control group. To further investigate the hair growth promoting effect, we plucked 10 hairs per mouse randomly from the treated area and measured the hair length. The hair length of FGFs treated mice was significantly longer than that of control group. Although FGF-2 is one of the most well-known mitogenic cytokine, interestingly, FGF-2 is not the strongest mitogenic cytokine for hair growth and FGF-10 exerts more potential hair growth promoting effect than FGF-1 and FGF-2. As we know, hair-follicle morphogenesis is governed by epithelial-mesenchymal interactions, between hair placode keratinocytes and fibroblasts of underlying mesenchymal condensations [31]. FGF-10 is found in the dermal papilla fibroblasts and its receptor FGFR2IIIb is found in the neighboring outer root sheath of the keratinocytes [32], suggesting that FGF-10 is a mesenchymally derived stimulator of hair-follicle cells, which contribute to the hair promoting activity.

The Wnt/β-catenin pathway plays an important role in the initiation, development, and growth of hair follicles. The transient activation of β-catenin results in hair regrowth in mice, while ablation of β-catenin results in dramatic hair shortening and abnormal regeneration of hair in the dermal papilla of mouse hair follicles [19, 33]. The levels of β-catenin in the dermal papilla are high in the anagen phase but low in the catagen and the telogen phases [18, 34]. Furthermore, the interaction between β-catenin, androgen receptors, and keratinocyte growth inhibition through modification of Wnt signaling contributes to androgenic alopecia, a common form of hair loss [35, 36]. Like β-catenin, Sonic hedgehog (Shh) also plays a vital role in the morphogenesis of hair follicles and acts as anagen-inducing signaling molecules. Mice lacking Shh activity exhibits follicles arrested at the hair germ stage of development [37, 38]. In the adult, Shh serves as a key regulator to induce the transition from the resting (telogen) to the growth stage (anagen) of the hair follicle cycle [20, 39]. Conversely, antibodies that block the activity of Shh are able to prevent hair growth in adult mice [40]. To elucidate the molecular mechanism underlying the ability of FGFs to induce anagen hair follicles, we examined the protein levels of β-catenin and Shh and in the shaved dorsal skin. Our immunohistochemical analysis results showed that the expression levels of β-catenin and Shh were upregulated in FGF-10, FGF-1, and FGF-2 treated group compared to that in the control group at 14 days. Its reported continuous β-catenin signaling is required to maintain hair follicle tumors [41]; we observed that Shh and β-catenin expression levels gradually began to reduce in both groups at 3 and 4 weeks, indicating that anagen phase of hair follicles was ceased.

However, there is no doubt that the limitations of this study still need further investigations and improvements. For example, FGFs are not stable enough which is easy to be degradated by various enzymes *in vitro,* resulting in the loss of biological activity. So the combination with delivery systems to increase its stability may contribute to the functions of promoting hair growth. Moreover, mixtures of several growth factors might to some extent promote cooperation between growth factors and their receptors and contribute together for the protection of hair cells in a sequencing manner or at multiple steps. Further study also should consider the hair growth effect and the mechanism of these FGFs during wound healing. Nevertheless, the effect of FGF-1, FGF-2, and FGF-10 in the therapy ofhair loss is confirmative and feasible.

Collectively, our study demonstrated that the commercialized FGF drugs promoted hair growth by inducing anagen in telogenic C57BL6/N mice. FGFs showed significant increase in the number and the size of hair follicles that is considered evidence for anagen phase induction. Immunohistochemical analysis revealed that β-catenin and Shh were expressed earlier in FGFs treated group than that in controlgroup. Taken together, these results strongly suggest that FGF-1, FGF-2, and FGF-10 promote hair growth by inducing anagen phase of hair follicles, which is beneficial for the clinical therapy.

References

[1] Wosicka H, Cal K. Targeting to the hair follicles: current status and potential[J]. J Dermatol Sci, 2010, 57(2): 83-89.

[2] Cotsarelis G. Epithelial stem cells: a folliculocentric view[J]. J Invest Dermatol, 2006, 126(7): 1459-1468.

[3] Jain R, De-Eknamkul W. Potential targets in the discovery of new hair growth promoters for androgenic alopecia[J]. Expert Opin Ther Targets, 2014, 18(7): 787-806.

[4] Shi HX, Lin C, Lin BB, et al. The anti-scar effects of basic fibroblast growth factor on the wound repair *in vitro* and *in vivo*[J]. PLoS One, 2013, 8(4): e59966.

[5] Coutu DL, Galipeau J. Roles of FGF signaling in stem cell self-renewal, senescence and aging[J]. Aging (Albany NY), 2011, 3(10): 920-933.

[6] du Cros DL. Fibroblast growth factor and epidermal growth factor in hair development[J]. J Invest Dermatol, 1993, 101(1 Suppl): 106s-113s.

[7] du Cros DL. Fibroblast growth factor influences the development and cycling of murine hair follicles[J]. Dev Biol, 1993, 156(2): 444-453.

[8] Katsuoka K, Schell H, Wessel B, et al. Effects of epidermal growth factor, fibroblast growth factor, minoxidil and hydrocortisone on growth kinetics in human hair bulb papilla cells and root sheath fibroblasts cultured *in vitro*[J]. Arch Dermatol Res, 1987, 279(4): 247-250.

[9] Katsuoka K, Schell H, Hornstein OP, et al. Epidermal growth factor and fibroblast growth factor accelerate proliferation of human hair bulb papilla cells and root sheath fibroblasts cultured *in vitro*[J]. Br J Dermatol, 1987, 116(3): 464-465.

[10] Ozeki M, Tabata Y. Promoted growth of murine hair follicles through controlled release of basic fibroblast growth factor[J]. Tissue Eng, 2002, 8(3): 359-366.

[11] Ozeki M, Tabata Y. *In vivo* promoted growth of mice hair follicles by the controlled release of growth factors[J]. Biomaterials, 2003, 24(13): 2387-2394.

[12] Jang JH. Stimulation of human hair growth by the recombinant human keratinocyte growth factor-2 (KGF-2)[J]. Biotechnol Lett, 2005, 27(11): 749-752.

[13] Danilenko DM, Ring BD, Yanagihara D, et al. Keratinocyte growth factor is an important endogenous mediator of hair follicle growth, development, and differentiation. Normalization of the nu/nu follicular differentiation defect and amelioration of chemotherapy-induced alopecia[J]. Am J Pathol, 1995, 147(1): 145-154.

[14] Guo L, Degenstein L, Fuchs E. Keratinocyte growth factor is required for hair development but not for wound healing[J]. Genes Dev, 1996, 10(2): 165-175.

[15] Nakamura M, Schneider MR, Schmidt-Ullrich R, et al. Mutant laboratory mice with abnormalities in hair follicle morphogenesis, cycling, and/or structure: an update[J]. J Dermatol Sci, 2013, 69(1): 6-29.

[16] Shin HS, Lee JM, Park SY, et al. Hair growth activity of Crataegus pinnatifida on C57BL/6 mouse model[J]. Phytother Res, 2013, 27(9): 1352-1357.

[17] Park HJ, Zhang N, Park DK. Topical application of Polygonum multiflorum extract induces hair growth of resting hair follicles through upregulating Shh and beta-catenin expression in C57BL/6 mice[J]. J Ethnopharmacol, 2011, 135(2): 369-375.

[18] Bierie B, Nozawa M, Renou JP, et al. Activation of beta-catenin in prostate epithelium induces hyperplasias and squamous transdifferentiation[J]. Oncogene, 2003, 22(25): 3875-3887.

[19] Van Mater D, Kolligs FT, Dlugosz AA, et al. Transient activation of beta -catenin signaling in cutaneous keratinocytes is sufficient to trigger the active growth phase of the hair cycle in mice[J]. Genes Dev, 2003, 17(10): 1219-1224.

[20] Sato N, Leopold PL, Crystal RG. Induction of the hair growth phase in postnatal mice by localized transient expression of Sonic hedgehog[J]. J Clin Invest, 1999, 104(7): 855-864.

[21] Patel M, Harrison S, Sinclair R. Drugs and hair loss[J]. Dermatol Clin, 2013, 31(1): 67-73.

[22] Gregoriou S, Papafragkaki D, Kontochristopoulos G, et al. Cytokines and other mediators in alopecia areata[J]. Mediators Inflamm,

2010, 2010: 928030.

[23] Gelfuso GM, Gratieri T, Delgado-Charro MB, *et al.* Iontophoresis-targeted, follicular delivery of minoxidil sulfate for the treatment of alopecia[J]. J Pharm Sci, 2013, 102(5): 1488-1494.

[24] Tarlow JK, Clay FE, Cork MJ, *et al.* Severity of alopecia areata is associated with a polymorphism in the interleukin-1 receptor antagonist gene[J]. J Invest Dermatol, 1994, 103(3): 387-390.

[25] D'Amico AV, Roehrborn CG. Effect of 1 mg/day finasteride on concentrations of serum prostate-specific antigen in men with androgenic alopecia: a randomised controlled trial[J]. Lancet Oncol, 2007, 8(1): 21-25.

[26] Zine A, de Ribaupierre F. Replacement of mammalian auditory hair cells[J]. Neuroreport, 1998, 9(2): 263-268.

[27] Zheng JL, Helbig C, Gao WQ. Induction of cell proliferation by fibroblast and insulin-like growth factors in pure rat inner ear epithelial cell cultures[J]. J Neurosci, 1997, 17(1): 216-226.

[28] Braun S, Krampert M, Bodo E, *et al.* Keratinocyte growth factor protects epidermis and hair follicles from cell death induced by UV irradiation, chemotherapeutic or cytotoxic agents[J]. J Cell Sci, 2006, 119(Pt 23): 4841-4849.

[29] Zhang X, Wang Y, Gao Y, *et al.* Maintenance of high proliferation and multipotent potential of human hair follicle-derived mesenchymal stem cells by growth factors[J]. Int J Mol Med, 2013, 31(4): 913-921.

[30] Plonka PM, Michalczyk D, Popik M, *et al.* Splenic eumelanin differs from hair eumelanin in C57BL/6 mice[J]. Acta Biochim Pol, 2005, 52(2): 433-441.

[31] Osada A, Kobayashi K. Appearance of hair follicle-inducible mesenchymal cells in the rat embryo[J]. Dev Growth Differ, 2000, 42(1): 19-27.

[32] Saksena S, Priyamvada S, Kumar A, *et al.* Keratinocyte growth factor-2 stimulates P-glycoprotein expression and function in intestinal epithelial cells[J]. Am J Physiol Gastrointest Liver Physiol, 2013, 304(6): G615-G622.

[33] Enshell-Seijffers D, Lindon C, Kashiwagi M, *et al.* beta-catenin activity in the dermal papilla regulates morphogenesis and regeneration of hair[J]. Dev Cell, 2010, 18(4): 633-642.

[34] Ouji Y, Yoshikawa M, Shiroi A, *et al.* Wnt-10b promotes differentiation of skin epithelial cells *in vitro*[J]. Biochem Biophys Res Commun, 2006, 342(1): 28-35.

[35] Singh R, Artaza JN, Taylor WE, *et al.* Testosterone inhibits adipogenic differentiation in 3T3-L1 cells: nuclear translocation of androgen receptor complex with beta-catenin and T-cell factor 4 may bypass canonical Wnt signaling to down-regulate adipogenic transcription factors[J]. Endocrinology, 2006, 147(1): 141-154.

[36] Ito M, Yang Z, Andl T, *et al.* Wnt-dependent *de novo* hair follicle regeneration in adult mouse skin after wounding[J]. Nature, 2007, 447(7142): 316-320.

[37] Chiang C, Swan RZ, Grachtchouk M, *et al.* Essential role for Sonic hedgehog during hair follicle morphogenesis[J]. Dev Biol, 1999, 205(1): 1-9.

[38] St-Jacques B, Dassule HR, Karavanova I, *et al.* Sonic hedgehog signaling is essential for hair development[J]. Curr Biol, 1998, 8(19): 1058-1068.

[39] Stenn KS, Paus R. Controls of hair follicle cycling[J]. Physiol Rev, 2001, 81(1): 449-494.

[40] Wang LC, Liu ZY, Gambardella L, *et al.* Regular articles: conditional disruption of hedgehog signaling pathway defines its critical role in hair development and regeneration[J]. J Invest Dermatol, 2000, 114(5): 901-908.

[41] Lo Celso C, Prowse DM, Watt FM. Transient activation of beta-catenin signalling in adult mouse epidermis is sufficient to induce new hair follicles but continuous activation is required to maintain hair follicle tumours[J]. Development, 2004, 131(8): 1787-1799.

High-efficiency expression of TAT-bFGF fusion protein in *Escherichia coli* and the effect on hypertrophic scar tissue

Xuechao Jia, Xiaokun Li, Xiaojie Wang

1. Introduction

Basic fibroblast growth factor (bFGF) is a member of the fibroblast growth factor family, which is widely distributed throughout various human and animal cells. bFGF was first abstracted and purified by Gospodarowicz in 1974[1]. In 1986, Abraham cloned the cDNA sequence of human bFGF[2]. Since then, human bFGF has been under extensive experimentation for improvement, and in these works, bFGF has been expressed in various species, such as E. coli[3], Picher pastoris[4] and silkworms[5]. Eventually, a recombinant human fibroblast growth factor (rhbFGF) was made for clinic treatment. bFGF is well known for its role in the process of wound healing[6], neuro-protection[7], cell proliferation and apoptosis[8]. Specifically, bFGF has been shown to play a significant role in wound healing in which bFGF promotes faster healing and fewer scars[9].

Hypertrophic scars are a common clinical skin disorder. The development of hypertrophic scars usually occurs in darker skinned patients and is associated with the proliferation of fibroblasts and the excessive deposition of extracellular matrix (ECM)[10,11]. In the wound, the invasive proliferation of fibroblasts leads to excessive expression of collagen proteins and keloids. bFGFs are believed to alleviate scar formation in a rabbit ear model by decreasing the collagen expression[12]. Because bFGF is a high molecular weight protein, it is difficult to deliver bFGF to the dermal tissue except through direct injection. In this work, we utilized cell-penetrating peptides (CPPs) to help the protein penetrate the scar.

CPPs are vehicles for the intracellular and transdermal delivery of macromolecules, and several transporters of CPPs have been previously described[13,14]. The HIV trans-activator of transcription (TAT) peptide has 9 basic amino acids and is a type of high-efficiency CPP. The TAT fusion protein has been investigated and was confirmed to be efficient in transdermal administration[15,16]. Because the recombinant protein solution was difficult to adhere to the skin surface, we utilized carbomer gel to maintain the protein on the skin for an extended period of time. Carbomer is a high-molecular weight, water-soluble polymeric resin. Carbomer is widely used for auxiliary substances in drug development[17]. Therefore, we fused the TAT peptide with rhbFGF and manufactured the carbomer gel to evaluate its potential effect on hypertrophic scars.

2. Materials and methods

2.1 Reagents

Restriction enzymes NdeI, EcoRI, T4 DNA Ligase, DNA polymerase, plasmid purification kit and agarose gel DNA extraction kit were purchased from Dalian Takara (Dalian, China). DH5α and BL21 (DE₃) pLsS were obtained from the Key Laboratory of Zhejiang Province Biotechnology and Pharmaceutical Engineering. The bFGF antibody was purchased from Santa Cruz Biotechnology (Santa Cruz, CA, USA). Hematoxylin, eosin and the One Step TUNEL Apoptosis Assay Kit were purchased from Beyotime (Shanghai, China).

2.2 Animals

BALB/c mice ($n = 15$, 20 g) and Japanese big-ear white rabbits ($n = 6$, 2–2.5 kg), were obtained from the Laboratory Animal Center of Wenzhou Medical University and were treated strictly in accordance with international ethical guidelines and the National Institutes of Health Guide Concerning the Care and Use of Laboratory Animals. The experiments were carried out with the approval of the Animal Experimentation Ethics Committee of Wenzhou Medical University.

2.3 Expression and purification of TAT-rhbFGF

2.3.1 Construction of TAT-rhbFGF expression vector

The coding sequence of rhbFGF was obtained from a pET3c vector containing the sequence of recombinant human basic fibroblast growth factor (rhbFGF). Two forward primers containing the coding sequence of the transactivator of transcription protein transduction domain were used to fuse the TAT_{49-57} coding sequence with rhbFGF. The primers used to recombine and amplify the TAT_{49-57}-rhbFGF were the following: forward primers: F1-5'-CGC CAT ATG CGC AAA AAA CGT CGT CAGC-3', F2-5'-ACGTCGTCAGCGTCGCCGTCCAGCTTTGC-3'; reverse primer: R-5'-CCGGAATTCTTAGCTCTTAGCAGACATTGG-3'. The forward primer F1 and the reverse primer contained NdeI and EcoRI, respectively. To fuse the TAT_{49-57} coding sequence to rhbFGF, we first amplified a partial TAT sequence and a complete rhbFGF sequence with primers F2 and R. Primers F1 and R were then used to amplify the product obtained from the previous step to acquire the TAT-rhbFGF coding sequence. PCR was conducted with a 50 μl reaction mixture containing 0.5 μl PrimeSTAR HS DNA Polymerase (2.5 U/μl), 10 μl 5x PS buffer (Mg^{2+} plus), 4 μl dNTPs (2.5 mM each), 1 μl of both the forward and the reverse primers (10 μM each), 0.0625 μl pET3c-rhbFGF, and 33.5 μl ultra-pure water. The thermo-cycling parameters used for the PCR were the following: 10 s at 98℃ for denaturation, 15 s at 61℃ for annealing, and 1 min at 72℃ for extension. After 28 cycles, the final product generated by primers F1 and R was digested with NdeI and EcoRI and was then ligated into the previously digested pET3c expression vector to create the pET3c-TAT-rhbFGF construct. The construct was transformed into E. coli DH5α. The accurate insertion of the gene into the plasmid was confirmed by automated DNA sequencing. After being amplified in E. coli DH5α, the expression vector was extracted and transformed into competent cells of E. coli strain BL21 (DE3) PlysS.

2.3.2 Production and screening of TAT-rhbFGF

To obtain the best expression strains of TAT-rhbFGF, the recombinant E. coli BL21 (DE3) PlysS with the correct TAT-rhbFGF sequence was shaken and cultured at 37℃ and 200 rpm in 5 ml Luria-Bertani (LB) medium containing 100 μg/ml ampicillin. When the cell density reached an OD_{600} of 0.6, the cells were diluted with a final concentration of 1 mM IPTG as an inducer. After adding the inducer, we continued to incubate the cells at 37℃ for 4 h with shaking at 200 rpm. The expression of each culture was analyzed using Coomassie brilliant blue staining of 15%(v/v) sodium dodecyl sulfate polyacrylamide gel electrophoresis (SDS-PAGE), and the expression level of the TATrhbFGF fusion protein was determined by densitometry. The greatest expression of the fusion protein transformant was reserved and used for subsequent experiments.

We then investigated the relationship of the IPTG concentration, the temperature, and the time after introduction with the expression of the fusion protein. After the best parameters were confirmed, we amplified and incubated the transformant in 500 ml LB medium. The bacteria were harvested by centrifugation at 8 000 rpm for 10 min at 4℃. The cells were then resuspended in 20 mM Tris-HCl (pH 8.0) buffer containing 0.1 M NaCl and 10 mM ethylene diamine tetraacetic acid (EDTA). Subsequently, the cells were lysed by sonication for 20 min in an ice bath. The lysates were the centrifuged at 20000 rpm and 4℃ for 30 min. Finally, the supernatant was transferred to a fresh tube and used for subsequent purification.

2.3.3 Purification and identification of TAT-rhbFGF

Considering the isoelectric point of the target protein, CM Sepharose Fast Flow was chosen for the purification of TAT-rhbFGF. Because the target protein had an affinity with heparin, we selected a heparin sepharose column for further purification The CM column was equilibrated with 200 ml equilibrium liquid (20 mM PB, 0.1 M NaCl, pH 7.0) at a rate of 2 ml/min. Subsequently, the supernatant was applied to the column at a rate of 1.5 ml/min. After the target protein was bound to the column, we washed the column with 50 ml equilibrium liquid at a flow rate of 2 ml/min and then washed with elution buffer (20 mM PB, 0.6 M NaCl, pH 7.0). The elution liquid was subsequently bound to the heparin sepharose column that was previous equilibrated using equilibrium buffer (20 mM PB, 0.6 M NaCl, pH 7.0). After binding to the column, we re-equilibrated the column and eluted with elution buffer (20 mM PB, 1.2 M NaCl, pH 7.0). The purity of the fusion protein was assessed using SDS-PAGE, and the concentration was determined using the Bradford method. The immune reactivity of the target protein was verified by western blotting, and the purified protein was sub-packaged and reserved at −70℃.

2.3.4 Analysis of the mitogenic activity of TAT-rhbFGF

The biological activity of the TAT-rhbFGF was assessed by its ability to accelerate proliferation in the NIH 3T3 cell line (American Type Culture Collection, Rockville, MD). The cells were transferred into a 96-well plate ($7×10^3$ cells per well) and were incubated in DMEM supplemented with 10% fetal bovine serum (FBS), 100 U/ml ampicillin, and 100 U/ml streptomycin for 12 h at 37℃ with 5% CO_2. The medium was then replaced by DMEM containing 0.5% FBS. The cells were starved for 24 h. Subsequently, the cells were treated with different concentrations of TAT-rhbFGF and rhbFGF for 48 h. The cell density was measured by adding 20 μl MTT (5 mg/ml) per well for 4 h. Finally, the medium was replaced with 100 μl DMSO, and the absorbance was detected at 570 nm after shaking for 10 min.

2.4 The effect of TAT-rhbFGF on hypertrophic scars

2.4.1 The preparation of TAT-rhbFGF gel

First, 0.25 g carbomer was combined with 500 μl mannitol solution and allowed to swell in 45 ml deionized water for 24 hours. Then, we added 1 ml 1 mol/L PB to the Carbomer gel. Additionally, 0.015 g methylparaben and 0.005 g ethylparaben were used as antiseptic substances. We utilized triethanolamine to adjust the pH of the Carbomer gel to 7.0. The viscosity of the Carbomer gel increased with increased basicity. The Carbomer gel was then sterilized *via* standard autoclaving. Finally, we mixed the recombined protein with the Carbomer gel to the required concentration after sterilization and stored it in the freezer.

2.4.2 The ability of TAT-rhbFGF to penetrate cells

Human foreskin fibroblasts (HFFs) were used for the penetration trials. The cells ($10×10^4$ per well) were seeded into a 6-well plate containing a sterilized microslide and DMEM. The microslide was dipped in 75% ethyl alcohol for 8 h on a clean bench and was washed with PBS before use. The DMEM contained 10% FBS, 100 U/ml ampicillin, 100 U/ml streptomycin, and 1.5 g/L glucose. After 12 hours, the cells had adhered to the microslide. We then treated the cells with TAT-rhbFGF and rhbFGF for 15 min with a final concentration of 15 ng/ml. Then, the microslides were washed 3 times in PBS and fixed for 15 min by previously frozen 4% paraformaldehyde at 4℃. Next, the cells were exposed to 0.3% Triton X-100 for 10 min. The proteins penetrating into the cells were detected using rabbit anti-human FGF-2 polyclonal antibodies followed by goat anti-rabbit fluorescent secondary antibodies.

2.4.3 The ability of TAT-rhbFGF to penetrate the skin of a mouse

BALB/c male mice (20–25 g, $n = 15$) were anesthetized with chloral hydrate (300 mg/kg, Sigma, Germany), and their dorsal hair was carefully shaved (3 cm×3 cm segment). The animals were divided into three groups ($n = 5$): a normal group, a control group and a treatment group. The treatment group was daubed with 200 μl TAT-rhbFGF gel containing 40 μg TAT-rhbFGF, and the control group was treated the same except the rhbFGF protein was utilized. The normal group was treated with a blank Carbomer gel. After 30 minutes, the mice were euthanasia by cervical dislocation. The skin segments were fixed and embedded in paraffin. Then, the skin samples were cut into 5 μm thick sections using standard procedures. Finally, the sections were subjected to immunohistochemical analysis.

2.4.4 The effect of TAT-rhbFGF gel on hypertrophic scars in a rabbit ear model

The rabbit ear model of hypertrophic scars was established as described previously with a minor modification[18]. Six Japanese big-ear white rabbits were anesthetized with sodium pentobarbital (30 mg/kg, Sigma, Germany) by intraperitoneal injection. Four identical, full-thickness, circular wounds with a 1 cm diameter were created down to the cartilage on the ventral surface of each ear using a surgical blade. The wounds were exposed to air and cleaned every day. Four weeks later, the hypertrophic scar model was established with a prominence in the central scar. Then, the hypertrophic scars were randomly divided into three groups ($n = 8$): control, TAT-rhbFGF, and rhbFGF and were treated with blank Carbomer gel, TAT-rhbFGF gel (6 μg), and rhbFGF gel (6 μg), respectively, for 30 days. Every ten days, two rabbits were sacrificed by air embolism. The scar tissue in every group was harvested and embedded in paraffin after being fixed in 4% paraformaldehyde. The hypertrophic scar was assessed in terms of thickness, fibroblast density, the content of collagen and cell apoptosis. The thickness of hypertrophic scars is the ratio of the central thickness of the model group to the normal group. All measurements were performed within the confines of the scar using 40 × magnification of the H&E stained tissue sections. The fibroblast density was measured by 6 random microscopic inspections of the H&E stained slices at 400×. To determine of the number of fibroblasts in a unit area and the average fibroblast densities for the entire group, the ratios between the cell numbers of the model group and those of the normal group were computed. The transition of collagen content in the scars was detected by Masson staining. The stained slices were randomly selected for microscopic examination at 200×. The One Step TUNEL Apoptosis Assay Kit was used to detect cell apoptosis and was implemented in accordance with the manufacturer's protocol.

3. Results

3.1 Construction of TAT-rhbFGF expression vector

To acquire the TAT-rhbFGF coding sequence, we amplified the gene as described in the methods section. The first and second PCR products are shown in Fig. 1(A, B). Then, we digested the second PCR product and connected it to the pet3c expression vector. We abstracted and digested the plasmid, which formed the DH5α E. coli containing target sequence. Additionally, we detected the gene sequence by bacterium polymerase chain reaction (Fig. 1C). The lengths of all the products were in accordance with their theoretical value. The TAT-rhbFGF sequence was confirmed by automated DNA sequencing.

Fig. 1. Agarose gel electrophoresis results from the identified recombinant gene. In section A, lane 1 is the product of the first PCR step; in section B, lane 1 is the final recombinant gene; in section C, lane 1 is the pET3c plasmid vector, lane 2 is the PCR product of the transformant, and lane 3 is the digested recombinant vector product.

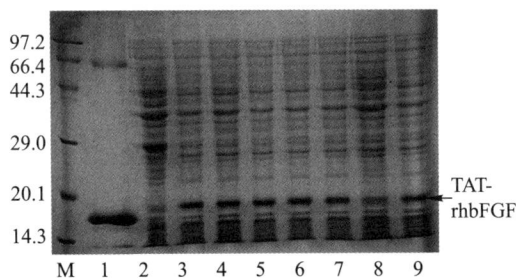

3.2 Production and screening of TAT-rhbFGF

To obtain the TAT-rhbFGF protein, we utilized BL21 (DE3) pLsS bacteria for an expression screening and performed several small-scale experiments. The main protein was highly produced in the BL21 (DE3) pLsS cells, as verified by SDS-PAGE and shown in Fig. 2. For this work, we harvested the highly expressed cells and stored them in a freezer at −70 ℃.

3.3 Purification and identification of TAT-rhbFGF

The purification of TAT-rhbFGF was conducted as described in the "materials and methods" section. The supernatant of the cell lysate was applied to CM sepharose, and quantities of the mixed proteins were discarded. Then, the protein was purified by a heparin sepharose column, and the protein purity was confirmed to be greater than 95%. As shown in the Fig. 3A, the final purified product was almost a single band tested by SDS-PAGE. We identified

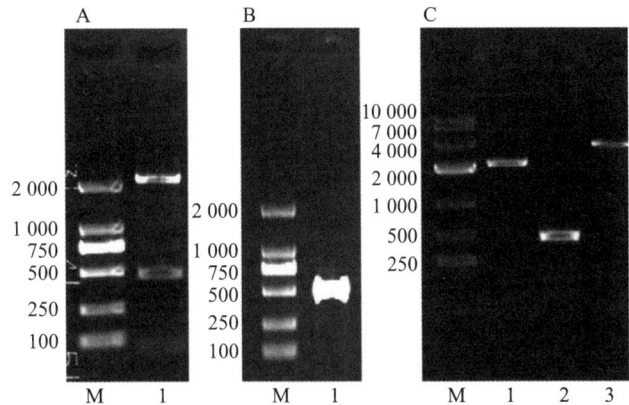

Fig. 2. The analysis of TAT-rhbFGF expression using SDS-PAGE. Lane M is a MW marker (low), lane 1 is the rhbFGF control, lane 2 is the expression of the BL21 (DE3)pLsS cells without the inducer, and lanes 3 through 6 are the expression of BL21 (DE3)pLsS cells after being induced for 1 to 4 hours.

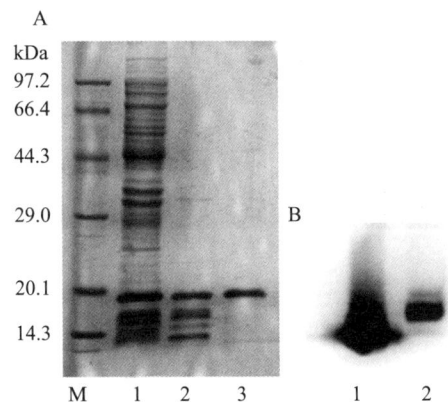

Fig. 3. The purification and identification of TAT-rhbFGF. In section a, lane 1 is the supernatant of the cell lysate, lane 2 is the purified product from the CM Sepharose, and lane 3 is the final product of the heparin sepharose chromatography. In section b, lane 1 and lane 2 are the western blot results for rhbFGF and TAT- rhbFGF, respectively.

TAT-rhbFGF *via* western blot (Fig. 3B), in which the protein was transformed to a nitrocellulose membrane and detected using the bFGF antibody.

3.4 Analysis of the mitogenic activity of TAT-rhbFGF

In the MTT assay, the bioactivity of TAT-rhbFGF was similar to the mitogenic activity of rhbFGF. The bioactivity of TAT-rhbFGF was slightly greater than that of rhbFGF at very low concentrations; however, the bioactivity was slightly less than that of rhbFGF when the protein concentration was greater, as shown in Fig. 4.

3.5 The ability of TAT-rhbFGF to penetrate cells

To determine whether TAT-rhbFGF has the ability to penetrate fibroblasts, we utilized the human foreskin fibroblasts. The detailed processing was conducted in accordance with the "materials and methods" section. The proteins were detected using cell immunofluorescence, and the result is shown in Fig. 5. In the figure, we can see that both TAT-rhbFGF and rhbFGF could penetrate into cells. However, the amount of TAT-rhbFGF penetrating into the cells was much greater than that of rhbFGF.

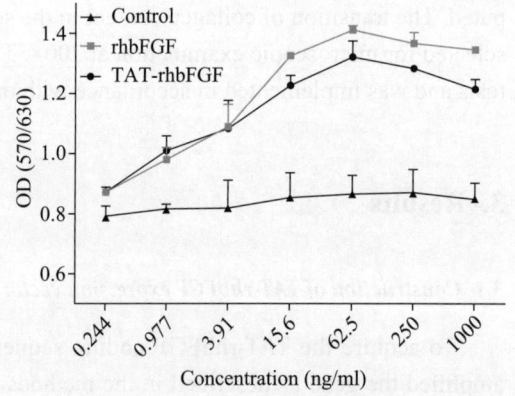

Fig. 4. The proliferation activity of TAT-rhbFGF was tested using NIH 3T3 Cells. NIH3T3 cells, which were seeded into 96-well microplates at 7000 cells/well, were allowed to attach (4–6 hours) and were then incubated in DMEM with 0.5% fetal bovine serum overnight at 37 ℃. Cells were supplemented with rhbFGF and TAT-rhbFGF and were incubated at 37 ℃ for 48 hours. PBS was used as a control.

3.6 The ability of TAT-rhbFGF to penetrate the skin of a mouse

In this trial, the skins were embedded in paraffin and detected *via* immunohistochemistry. As shown in Fig. 6, rhbFGF primarily aggregated in the hair follicle and in the surface of the mouse skin. However, TAT-rhbFGF could not only aggregate in the subcutaneous hair follicle but could also directly penetrate into the dermal tissue through the skin barrier. In this study, we can conclude that the subcutaneous penetration of TAT-rhbFGF was readily available and was

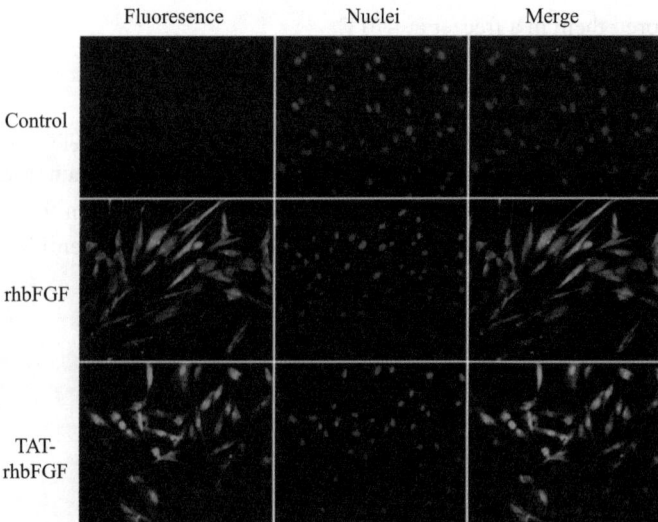

Fig. 5. The ability of TAT-rhbFGF to penetrate cells. These images were produced using immunofluorescence. The target protein was identified by green fluorescence.

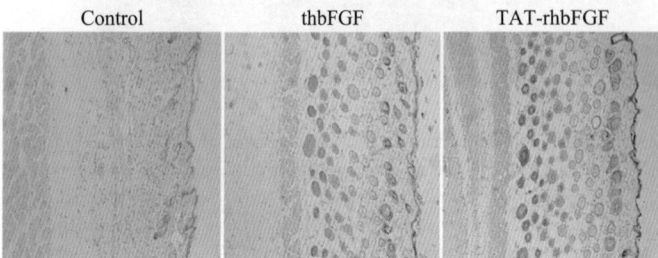

Fig. 6. TAT-rhbFGF and rhbFGF penetrated into the skin of a mouse. The nuclei stained blue, and the positive proteins stained brown.

absorbed faster than rhbFGF.

3.7 Analysis of the effect of TAT-rhbFGF gel on hypertrophic scars in the rabbit ear model

The physical appearance of the hypertrophic scars gradually turned to a pale red after treatment for 30 days. Compared with the control group, the protuberant scars became flat in the TAT-rhbFGF groups. The thickness of the scar tissue is shown in Table 1. From the data, we concluded that TAT-rhbFGF improved the hypertrophic scars by reducing the thickness and the overall appearance.

The cell density of the TAT-rhbFGF treatment group was much lower than that of the rhbFGF group and the control group, and there was a similar cell density compared with the normal group (Fig. 7A). In the scar tissue, there was greater collagen accumulation, and the distribution of collagen was uneven compared with the normal group (Fig. 7B). After topical application of TAT-rhbFGF for 30 days, type I and III collagen in the scar tissue were reduced and evenly distributed. From the results of the TUNEL staining, we found that the number of apoptotic cells in the TAT-rhbFGF group was greater compared with the control and rhbFGF groups. Apoptotic cells were absent in the control group (showed in Fig. 7E).

Table 1.   Effect of TAT-rhbFGF on the index of hypertrophic scar thickness

group	n	10 days after therapy	20 days after therapy	30 days after therapy
control	8	2.79±0.10	2.75±0.11	2.58±0.13
rhbFGF	8	2.80±0.11	2.54±0.12*	2.46±0.13*
TAT-rhbFGF	8	2.77±0.12*	2.05±0.17*	1.61±0.10*

Note: Data are presented as the mean±SD.

* Compared with the control, $P<0.05$.

4. Discussion

rhbFGF has been shown to be a powerful wound healing factor, and its effect on mature scars has yet to be researched extensively[12]. To improve rhbFGF's penetration ability, we utilized the TAT peptide as a transport vessel in this study. Expression of the exogenous protein in *Escherichia coli* is a technique that has being used more in recent years due to its success rate and cost effectiveness[19–21]. The pET3c vector is a frequently used vector that adopts the T7 RNA polymerase to selectively activate the T7 phage promoter in *E. coli*. The T7 RNA polymerase that is inserted into the pET3c vector is transient and inducible during the expression of exogenous proteins[22]. Considering that the bioactivity of rhbFGF may be inhibited when a fusion protein attaches to its C terminal[23], we fused the TAT sequence to rhbFGF's N terminal. Therefore, we acquired a pET3c vector containing the TAT-rhbFGF encoding sequence.

The recombinant TAT-rhbFGF protein was purified *via* three purification columns, which included CM Sepharose FF, heparin sepharose column and Sephadex G-25. These columns have been broadly and successfully used for the purification of rhbFGF and TAT-rhbFGF[24]. The purity of this recombinant protein was greater than 95%, as detected by SDS-PAGE, and was identified by western blot. The bioactivity of TAT-rhbFGF was verified by stimulating the proliferation of NIH-3T3 cells, which demonstrated that the TAT peptide may assist rhbFGF penetration into the cell and deposition to the receptor location. Furthermore, our cell penetration trial combined with the bioactivity trial demonstrated that the TAT peptide may cause nuclear localization of the fusion protein[25,26]. Previous studies showed that some biological activities of bFGF may be mediated by the direct binding of bFGF to DNA, which supports the effect of the TAT peptide in its role to assist in cell penetration[27]. In the transdermal trial, the fusion protein could penetrate into the skin as described in previous studies[28,29].

Hypertrophic scars are formed through a complicated and multifactorial participation process[30]. Many scientists have attempted to resolve the intractable symptom through the development of pressure therapy, corticosteroids, laser therapy, cryotherapy and even surgery for the treatment of exuberant scars[31–33]. Recently, rhbFGF was confirmed to prevent and alleviate hypertrophic scar formation in a rabbit hypertrophic scar model[34]. The aberrant proliferation of fibro-

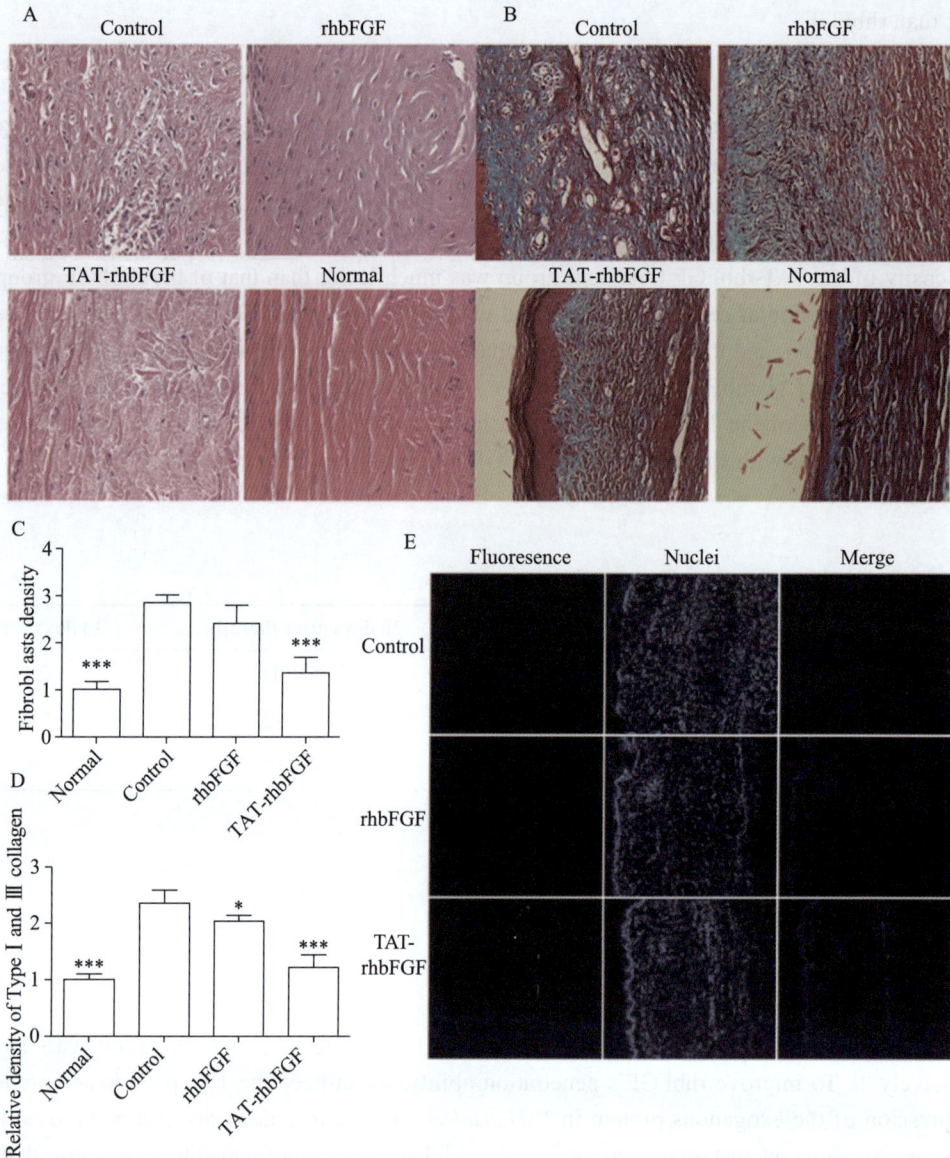

Fig. 7. The effect of rhbFGF and TAT-rhbFGF gel on the hypertrophic scar model. (A, C): the tissue slices of the hypertrophic scar stained using H&E, (A) observed at 400×, (C) the relative density of fibroblasts; all the data are compared with the mean density of the normal derma. *Compared with the control, $P<0.05$; (B, D): the content of type I and III collagen in the scars, (B) the collagen stained using a Masson kit, observed at 200×, (D) the relative content of type I and III collagen; all the data are compared with the mean content of the normal derma. *$P<0.05$ and ***$P<0.01$ compared with the control; (E) the apoptosis cells in HTS after treatment observed at 200×.

blasts is seen as an important inducing factor of hypertrophic scars not only in inducing the scar to become hypertrophic but also in the excessive deposition of ECM. The ECM products primarily consist of type I and III collagen. Although type I and III collagen are indispensable components for wound healing, they can lead to scarring with excessive expression[35,36]. TAT-rhbFGF was able to reduce the incidence of type I and III collagen, which may lead to an increase in scar formation. To have a further understand of how the scar was improved after the application of TAT-rhbFGF, we detected the proliferation of fibroblasts in the scar. The TUNEL trial indicated that the effect of the TAT-rhbFGF on improving the scar was linked to the apoptosis of fibroblasts.

In summary, we have successfully expressed and purified a TAT-rhbFGF fusion protein in this study. Our results demonstrated that the fusion protein had better penetration to the dermal areas of the skin. Additionally, TAT-rhbFGF improved the physical appearance of the hypertrophic scars. TAT-rhbFGF may be a potential fusion protein for the treatment of dermal disorders including hypertrophic scars.

References

[1] Gospodarowicz D. Localisation of a fibroblast growth factor and its effect alone and with hydrocortisone on 3T3 cell growth[J]. Nature, 1974, 249(453): 123-127.

[2] Abraham JA, Whang JL, Tumolo A, et al. Human basic fibroblast growth factor: nucleotide sequence and genomic organization[J]. Embo j, 1986, 5(10): 2523-2528.

[3] Gasparian ME, Elistratov PA, Drize NI, et al. Overexpression in Escherichia coli and purification of human fibroblast growth factor (FGF-2)[J]. Biochemistry (Mosc), 2009, 74(2): 221-225.

[4] Mu X, Kong N, Chen W, et al. High-level expression, purification, and characterization of recombinant human basic fibroblast growth factor in Pichia pastoris[J]. Protein Expr Purif, 2008, 59(2): 282-288.

[5] Wu X, Kamei K, Sato H, et al. High-level expression of human acidic fibroblast growth factor and basic fibroblast growth factor in silkworm (Bombyx mori L.) using recombinant baculovirus[J]. Protein Expr Purif, 2001, 21(1): 192-200.

[6] Andres C, Hasenauer J, Ahn HS, et al. Wound-healing growth factor, basic FGF, induces Erk1/2-dependent mechanical hyperalgesia[J]. Pain, 2013, 154(10): 2216-2226.

[7] Abe K, Saito H. Effects of basic fibroblast growth factor on central nervous system functions[J]. Pharmacol Res, 2001, 43(4): 307-312.

[8] Sgadari C, Barillari G, Palladino C, et al. Fibroblast Growth Factor-2 and the HIV-1 Tat Protein Synergize in Promoting Bcl-2 Expression and Preventing Endothelial Cell Apoptosis: Implications for the Pathogenesis of AIDS-Associated Kaposi's Sarcoma[J]. Int J Vasc Med, 2011, 2011: 452729.

[9] Ono I, Akasaka Y, Kikuchi R, et al. Basic fibroblast growth factor reduces scar formation in acute incisional wounds[J]. Wound Repair Regen, 2007, 15(5): 617-623.

[10] Burd A, Huang L. Hypertrophic response and keloid diathesis: two very different forms of scar[J]. Plast Reconstr Surg, 2005, 116(7): 150e-157e.

[11] Miller MC, Nanchahal J. Advances in the modulation of cutaneous wound healing and scarring[J]. BioDrugs, 2005, 19(6): 363-381.

[12] Xie J, Qi S, Xu Y, et al. Effects of basic fibroblast growth factors on hypertrophic scarring in a rabbit ear model[J]. J Cutan Med Surg, 2008, 12(4): 155-162.

[13] Koren E, Torchilin VP. Cell-penetrating peptides: breaking through to the other side[J]. Trends Mol Med, 2012, 18(7): 385-393.

[14] Nasrollahi SA, Taghibiglou C, Azizi E, et al. Cell-penetrating peptides as a novel transdermal drug delivery system[J]. Chem Biol Drug Des, 2012, 80(5): 639-646.

[15] Kim DW, Eum WS, Jang SH, et al. Ginsenosides enhance the transduction of tat-superoxide dismutase into mammalian cells and skin[J]. Mol Cells, 2003, 16(3): 402-406.

[16] Lim JM, Chang MY, Park SG, et al. Penetration enhancement in mouse skin and lipolysis in adipocytes by TAT-GKH, a new cosmetic ingredient[J]. J Cosmet Sci, 2003, 54(5): 483-491.

[17] Rabiskova M, Sedlakova M, Vitkova M, et al. [Carbomers and their use in pharmaceutical technology][J]. Ceska Slov Farm, 2004, 53(6): 300-303.

[18] Morris DE, Wu L, Zhao LL, et al. Acute and chronic animal models for excessive dermal scarring: quantitative studies[J]. Plast Reconstr Surg, 1997, 100(3): 674-681.

[19] Kwong KW, Wong WK. A revolutionary approach facilitating co-expression of authentic human epidermal growth factor and basic fibroblast growth factor in both cytoplasm and culture medium of Escherichia coli[J]. Appl Microbiol Biotechnol, 2013, 97(20): 9071-9080.

[20] Nuc P, Nuc K. [Recombinant protein production in Escherichia coli][J]. Postepy Biochem, 2006, 52(4): 448-456.

[21] Song L, Huang Z, Chen Y, et al. High-efficiency production of bioactive recombinant human fibroblast growth factor 18 in Escherichia coli and its effects on hair follicle growth[J]. Appl Microbiol Biotechnol, 2014, 98(2): 695-704.

[22] Mohamed MR, Niles EG. Transient and inducible expression of vaccinia/T7 recombinant viruses[J]. Methods Mol Biol, 2004, 269: 41-50.

[23] Sakiyama H, Kaji K, Nakagawa K, et al. Inhibition of bFGF activity by complement C1s: covalent binding of C1s with bFGF[J]. Cell Biochem Funct, 1998, 16(3): 159-163.

[24] Chen XJ, Sun FY, Xie QL, et al. Cloning and high level nonfusion expression of recombinant human basic fibroblast growth factor in Escherichia coli[J]. Acta Pharmacol Sin, 2002, 23(9): 782-786.

[25] Efthymiadis A, Briggs LJ, Jans DA. The HIV-1 Tat nuclear localization sequence confers novel nuclear import properties[J]. J Biol Chem, 1998, 273(3): 1623-1628.

[26] Vaysse L, Gregory LG, Harbottle RP, et al. Nuclear-targeted minicircle to enhance gene transfer with non-viral vectors in vitro and in vivo[J]. J Gene Med, 2006, 8(6): 754-763.

[27] Tessler S, Neufeld G. Basic fibroblast growth factor accumulates in the nuclei of various bFGF-producing cell types[J]. J Cell Physiol, 1990, 145(2): 310-317.

[28] Manosroi J, Lohcharoenkal W, Gotz F, et al. Transdermal absorption enhancement of N-terminal Tat-GFP fusion protein (TG) loaded in novel low-toxic elastic anionic niosomes[J]. J Pharm Sci, 2011, 100(4): 1525-1534.

[29] Wang Y, Su W, Li Q, et al. Preparation and evaluation of lidocaine hydrochloride-loaded TAT-conjugated polymeric liposomes for transdermal delivery[J]. Int J Pharm, 2013, 441(1-2): 748-756.

[30] Bloemen MC, van der Veer WM, Ulrich MM, et al. Prevention and curative management of hypertrophic scar formation[J]. Burns, 2009, 35(4): 463-475.

[31] Jin R, Huang X, Li H, et al. Laser therapy for prevention and treatment of pathologic excessive scars[J]. Plast Reconstr Surg, 2013, 132(6): 1747-1758.

[32] van der Veer WM, Ferreira JA, de Jong EH, et al. Perioperative conditions affect long-term hypertrophic scar formation[J]. Ann Plast Surg, 2010, 65(3): 321-325.

[33] Ward RS. Pressure therapy for the control of hypertrophic scar formation after burn injury. A history and review[J]. J Burn Care Rehabil, 1991, 12(3): 257-262.

[34] Shi HX, Lin C, Lin BB, et al. The anti-scar effects of basic fibroblast growth factor on the wound repair in vitro and in vivo[J]. PLoS One, 2013, 8(4): e59966.

[35] Verhaegen PD, Marle JV, Kuehne A, et al. Collagen bundle morphometry in skin and scar tissue: a novel distance mapping method provides superior measurements compared to Fourier analysis[J]. J Microsc, 2012, 245(1): 82-89.

[36] Verhaegen PD, Schouten HJ, Tigchelaar-Gutter W, et al. Adaptation of the dermal collagen structure of human skin and scar tissue in response to stretch: an experimental study[J]. Wound Repair Regen, 2012, 20(5): 658-666.

bFGF protects against blood-brain barrier damage through junction protein regulation *via* PI3K-Akt-Rac1 pathway following traumatic brain injury

Zhouguang Wang, Xiaokun Li, Hongyu Zhang, Jian Xiao

1. Introduction

Traumatic brain injury (TBI) is a leading cause of death and disability in the Western World [1]. More than 1.7 million new cases of TBI occur in the USA each year, causing 60% of all trauma-related deaths [2]. TBI damage is highly heterogeneous and can also trigger other neurological complications including epilepsy, depression, and dementia. The initial injury often leads to the development of secondary sequelae including neurovascular dysfunction, inflammation, oxidative stress, and apoptosis [3–6]. Among all these pathological events, blood-brain barrier (BBB) breakdown is one key mechanism that leads to progression of brain injury and long-term neurological deficits. The BBB integrity is compromised soon after TBI due to mechanical breach or functional breakdown of endothelial cells and other essential BBB components. BBB disruption results in uncontrolled efflux of ions and proteins from the intravascular space to the interstitial brain compartments with water accumulation, vasogenic brain edema, elevated intracerebral pressure, and secondary ischemic injuries [5]. Therefore, targeting the molecular mechanisms that regulate BBB permeability may lead to more efficacious therapeutic strategies for TBI [7, 8]. In the previous study, bFGF treatment shows the efficacy to reduce cerebral edema and neurological deficits after ischemia/reperfusion injury in stroke models [9]. In our study, we first reported that the protective role of bFGF on TBI-induced BBB breakdown is related to the upregulation of tight junction proteins and inhibition of RhoA *via* Rac-1.

Tight junctions (TJs) are the hallmark of BBB integrity that essentially contributes to its structural inviolacy. The paracellular flux of hydrophilic molecules across the BBB is thereby limited which is essential for the functional integrity of the CNS [10]. TJs are composed of transmembrane proteins such as occludin, claudins, and junctional adhesion molecules. All of these proteins are anchored to endothelial cells by cytoplasmic protein complexes comprising zonula occludens-1 [ZO-1], zonula occludens-2 [ZO-2], and cingulin [11, 12]. The TJs limit the flux of hydrophilic molecules across the BBB while smaller lipophilic substances such as O_2 and CO_2 diffuse freely across plasma membranes along their concentration gradient [13]. The development of vasogenic brain edema after TBI is caused by BBB rupture and consists of protein-rich fluid [11]. The alteration of TJ assemblies may contribute to the loss of BBB integrity and BBB breakdown [14]. A wide array of growth factors, cytokines, and drugs influence TJs and their barrier function. For example, steroids [15] or unsaturated fatty acids [16] enhance TJ tightness by increasing the expression of occludin. Cytokines, VEGF [17], and tumor necrosis factor-[18] perturb TJ integrity by decreasing occludin and ZO-1 expression and causing cl5 and ZO-1 protein disruption. It is safe to suggest that any pathologic stimulus affecting the expression and localization of TJ proteins will profoundly affect the integrity of the BBB.

Basic fibroblast growth factor (bFGF or FGF-2) is a member of the fibroblast growth factor family which regulates a variety of biological functions including proliferation, morphogenesis, and suppression of apoptosis during development *via* a complex signal transduction system [19–21]. bFGF is highly expressed in the nervous system where it has multiple roles including the regulation of vascular integrity. Inhibition of fibroblast growth factors receptor (FGFR) signaling resulted in a decrease in cell-cell adhesions through disintegration of the p120-catenin/VE-cadherin complex [22]. Furthermore, previous studies demonstrated that bFGF inhibited RhoA by activating Ras-related C3 botulinum toxin substrate 1 (Rac1) through the phosphatidylinositol 3-kinase (PI3K)-Akt signaling pathway in human endothelial cells of the cornea [23], as well as in bone marrow stromal cells [24]. Activated Rac1 inhibits RhoA [25] which may preserve BBB integrity and reduce the development of vasogenic brain edema after TBI.

The goal of the present study was to explore the mechanisms by which exogenous bFGF treatment preserves BBB integrity, specifically by upregulating TJs proteins, attenuating neurofunctional deficits in TBI mice. We demonstrate that bFGF activation of the PI3K-Akt-Rac1 signaling pathway and consequent inhibition of RhoA results in preservation of tight junction proteins. Collectively, our results suggest that the bFGF may be an effective and feasible target for drug development of TBI both *in vivo* and *in vitro*.

2. Material and methods

2.1 Reagents and antibodies

Recombinant human basic fibroblast growth factor (bFGF) was purchased from Sigma (Sigma-Aldrich, St. Louis, MO), and PI3K inhibitor LY294002 (Sigma-Aldrich, St Louis, MO) was dissolved in 25% dimethylsulfoxide solution (DMSO). FITC-dextran and Evans Blue were purchased from Sigma-Aldrich, St. Louis, MO. Anti-β-catenin, anti-p120-catenin, and anti-CD31 were purchased from Abcam, Cambridge, MA. GTP-Rac1, total-Rac1, GTP-RhoA, and total-RhoA were detected using Rac1/Cdc42 and Rho Activation Assay Kits (Millipore, Temecula, CA). Anti-Akt and anti-p-Akt (Ser473), anti-claudin-5, anti-occludin, and anti-zonula occludens-1 were from Proteintech. Human brain microvascular endothelial cells (HBMECs) and endothelial cell medium (ECM) were purchased from Sciencell (Carlsbad, CA, USA). The appropriate secondary antibodies were obtained from Santa Cruz Biotechnology.

2.2 Animals and surgical procedures

C57BL/6N male mice (20–25 g) were purchased from the Animal Center of the Chinese Academy of Sciences. The animal use and care protocol conformed to the Guide for the Care and Use of Laboratory Animals from the National Institutes of Health and was approved by the Animal Care and Use Committee of Wenzhou Medical University. The animals were housed under standard conditions, including adequate temperature and humidity (60%) control with a 12-h light/12-h dark cycle, and free access to water and food. All procedures used in this study were approved by the ethics committee for the use of experimental animals at Wenzhou Medical University. All animals remained in the animal care facility for a minimum of 7 days prior to the experiments. The TBI model was used as previously described [26]. The C57BL/6N mice were anesthetized with 4% choral hydrate (10 ml/kg IP), and surgery was performed under aseptic conditions and mounted in a stereotaxic system (David Kopf Instruments, Tujunga, California). The following steps were all performed using aseptic techniques. A midline incision on the scalp exposed the skull, without requiring muscle retraction. Craniotomy was performed by hand-held trephine. For the trephine method, a 3-mm-diameter manual trephine (Roboz Surgical Instrument Co., Gaithersburg, MD) was carefully used to penetrate the skull for removal of the bone flap. Mice were subjected to TBI on the right part of the brain between the lambda and the bregma about 1 mm from the midline. The stereotaxic frame was inclined so as to make the plane of the cortex perpendicular to the impactor tip. The impact velocity was set at 4 m/s with the penetration depth at 1.5 mm and the impactor dwell time was 600 ms, as described previously [27]. The craniotomy which did not significantly affect physiological parameters (arterial pressure, heart rate, or body weight) was closed immediately after TBI. For the sham operation group, only the surgical procedure was performed on the animals without cortical impact. Inhibitor LY294002 (50 nmol/kg) was injected into the left striatum at a rate of 2 μl/min. After completed injection, the needle was left in place for an additional 10 min to prevent backflow of collagenase along the needle tract, before being withdrawn at a rate of 1 mm/min. To explore the effect of bFGF in the TBI mouse, a dose of 0.5 μg/g bFGF was intranasally administrated 1 h before induction of the TBI model. Vehicle animals received same volume of PBS. After the surgical incisions were closed, the mice were allowed to recover for 24 h. Animals were housed under a 12-h light/dark cycle in a pathogen-free area with free access to water and food. All efforts were made to minimize the number of animals used and their suffering.

2.3 Evans Blue extravasation assay

Evans Blue [13] extravasation assays were conducted 24 h after surgery. Briefly, mice received an intraperitoneal injection of 0.25 ml EB dye (2%) 22 h after TBI. Two hours after EB dye injection (24 h after TBI), the anesthetized animals were perfused with saline to wash away any remaining dye in the blood vessels prior to sample collection. The right hemisphere was weighed. The EB dye was extracted by formamide, and the supernatant was allowed to incubate for 3 days at 72℃ and was then re-centrifuged. The quantity of extravasated Evans Blue dye was detected by spectro-photometer at an excitation wavelength of 610 nm and an emission wavelength of 680 nm and quantified according to a standard curve.

2.4 Determination of BBB vascular permeability

TBI or sham procedure was performed (n = 6 per group). Twenty-two hours later, the mice were injected with 0.2 ml 70 kDa FITC-dextran (100 μg/ml). Two hours later, the animals were subjected to systemic intracardiac perfusion with 1 USP U/ml of heparin in saline to flush the intravascular FITC-dextran out of the vasculature. The perfused brains were then harvested. Thereafter, relative fluorescence passing through the tissues was determined using an EnSpire Manager (PerkinElmer Company, USA) multimode plate reader at an excitation wavelength of 485 nm and an emission wave-length of 535 nm.

2.5 Behavior assessments

The sensorimotor Garcia Test [28] was conducted in a blinded fashion and was used to assess neurofunctional defi-cits in mice at 24 after surgery. The Garcia Test has been modified and consisted of 7 individual tests, examining spon-taneous activity (1), axial sensation (2), vibrissae proprioception (3), limb symmetry (4), as well as the animal's ability of lateral turning (5), forelimb outstretching (6), and climbing (7). A score of 0 (worst performance) to 3 (best perfor-mance) was given for each sub-test, and a total Garcia score was calculated as the sum of all sub-tests (maximum score of 21).

2.6 Immunofluorescence staining

Brain tissues were embedded in OCT and cut into 10-mm sections. The sections were then stained with specific antibodies for analysis. To determine claudin-5, ZO-1, CD31, and occluding activities, sections were incubated with 3% H_2O_2 in methanol for 10 min, followed by blocking with 5% bovine albumin in PBS for 30 min incubated 37℃. Next, sections were incubated at 4℃ overnight with a primary antibody against claudin-5 (1:100), ZO-1 (1:100), oc-cludin (1:100), or CD31 (1:500), followed by incubation with Alexa-Fluor594/647 donkey anti-mouse/rabbit, Alexa-Fluor488/594 donkey anti-rabbit/mouse, or Alexa-Fluor 488/594 donkey anti-goat secondary antibody (1:500; Invit-rogen Corporation, Carlsbad, CA, USA) for 1 h at 37℃. Cellular nuclei were counterstained with Hoechst 33258. The saline injection group was considered to be the negative control. The results were imaged at ×400 magnifications using a Nikon ECLPSE 80i.

2.7 Cell culture and in vitro oxygen glucose deprivation/reoxygenation model

HBMECs were incubated at 37℃ in a humidified atmosphere of 5% CO_2 and 95% air and cultured in endothelial cell medium (ECM). Normal growth medium was then replaced with ECM without FBS, and the cells were incubated in an anaerobic chamber for 24 h. This ensured that the oxygen level remained below 0.5%. After oxygen glucose depri-vation (OGD), the cells were incubated under normal culture conditions for 12 h. Basic fibroblast growth factor (bFGF) (50 ng/ml) was added 1 h before of OGD and maintained during the reoxygenation process. To further evaluate the ef-fect of PI3K/Akt activation on OGD. Cells were pre-treated for 1 h with specific inhibitor LY294002 (20 μM). After 12 h, cells were detached and collected for further study. All experiments were performed in triplicate.

2.8 Paracellular permeability assay

Flux of 70 kDa FITC-dextran across HBMECs was analyzed. Briefly, HBMECs was seeded at a density of 2×10^4 cells/well in 100 μl medium onto polycarbonate 24-well transwell chambers with a 0.4-mm mean pore size and a 0.3-cm^2 surface area (Millicell Hanging Cell Culture Inserts, USA). Cells were incubated with FITC-dextran (1 mg/ml) in me-dium for 4 h. Thereafter, relative fluorescence passing through the chamber (in the lower chambers) was determined by using an EnSpire Manager (PerkinElmer Company, USA) multimode plate reader at an excitation wavelength of 485 nm and an emission wavelength of 520 nm.

2.9 siRNA preparation and transfections

Transient transfection of siRNA was carried out using Lipofectamine 2000 (Invitrogen). One day before transfection, cells were trypsinized and plated on a 6-well plate at 2×10^5 cells/well in 1 ml of DMEM 10% serum without antibiotics. In all, 100 pmol of siRNA diluted in 250 µl of serum-free DMEM and 3.5 µl of Oligofectamine diluted in 250 µl of serum-free DMEM was pre-incubated for 5 min. The two mixtures were combined and incubated for 20 min at room temperature for complex formation. After the addition of 500 µl of serum-free DMEM, the entire mixture (1 ml) was added to each well. Cells were assayed 1 day after transfection.

2.10 Western blot analysis

Total proteins were purified using protein extraction reagents for the right brain cortical region and HBMEC. The equivalent of 60 µg of protein was separated by 12% gel and then transferred onto a PVDF membrane. After blocking with 5% fat-free milk, the membranes were incubated with the following antibodies: claudin-5 (1:500), ZO-1 (1:200), occluding (1:500), p-Akt (1:500), p120-catenin (1:1 000), β-catenin (1:1 000), CD31 (1:1 000), GTP-Rac1 (1:1 000), total-Rac1 (1:1 000), GTP-RhoA (1:1 000), and total-RhoA (1:1 000) overnight. The membranes were washed with TBS and treated with horseradish peroxidase-conjugated secondary antibodies for 2 h at room temperature. The signals were visualized with the ChemiDicTM XRS+ Imaging System (Bio-Rad Laboratories, Hercules, CA, USA), and the band densities were quantified with Multi Gauge Software of Science Lab 2006 (FUJIFILM Corporation, Tokyo, Japan).

2.11 Statistical analysis

The data were expressed as the mean ± SEM. Statistical significance was determined with Student's t test when there were two experimental groups. For more than two groups, statistical evaluation of the data was performed using the one-way analysis of variance (ANOVA) test, followed by Dunnett's *post hoc* test with values of $P < 0.05$ being considered significant.

3. Results

3.1 bFGF treatment reduces neurofunctional deficits after TBI in mice

In order to evaluate the role of bFGF in TBI, neurofunctional deficits and BBB disruption were evaluated at 24 h after TBI. As evaluated by the Garcia Test, the Garcia neuroscore of mice subjected to TBI significantly decreased compared to sham-operated animals at 24 h after surgery. bFGF (15 µg) treatments significantly ameliorated neurofunctional deficits compared with the TBI control group (Fig. 1A). BBB breakdown results in cerebral edema and secondary neuronal injury after brain ischemia or trauma [29]. In our previous study, bFGF treatment demonstrated efficacy at reducing cerebral edema and neurological deficits after ischemia/reperfusion injury in stroke models; we were therefore motivated to investigate the effects of bFGF on BBB integrity after TBI. EB leakage, an indicator of BBB injury, was also prominent in brain specimens at 24 h after TBI (Fig. 1B). Compared to vehicle-treated animals, bFGF-treated animals had significantly reduced EB content following TBI, as demonstrated by fluorescence intensity quantification (Fig. 1C). Consistent with the EB content test, the level of FITC-dextran that leaked through the BBB was also statistically significantly increased after TBI, but reduced by treatment with bFGF (Fig. 1D). Taken together, our results suggest that bFGF treatment reduces neurological deficits by ameliorating BBB disruption following TBI.

3.2 The protective role of bFGF on TBI-induced BBB breakdown is mediated by the activation of TJs, adherens junction proteins, and PI3K/Akt pathways in mice

To determine whether bFGF protects the BBB from disruption by regulating TJ proteins, Western blot analysis of the ipsilateral brain cortex was conducted. We analyzed the effect of bFGF on the activity of TJ proteins claudin-5, occluding, and zonula occludens-1, and adherens junction (AJ) proteins p120-catenin and β-catenin, 24 h after TBI. As shown in Fig. 2, bFGF significantly increased the expression of these TJ and AJ proteins compared to the TBI control group. Consistent with the Western blot results, dual-label immuno-fluorescence shows that the co-localization of ZO-1,

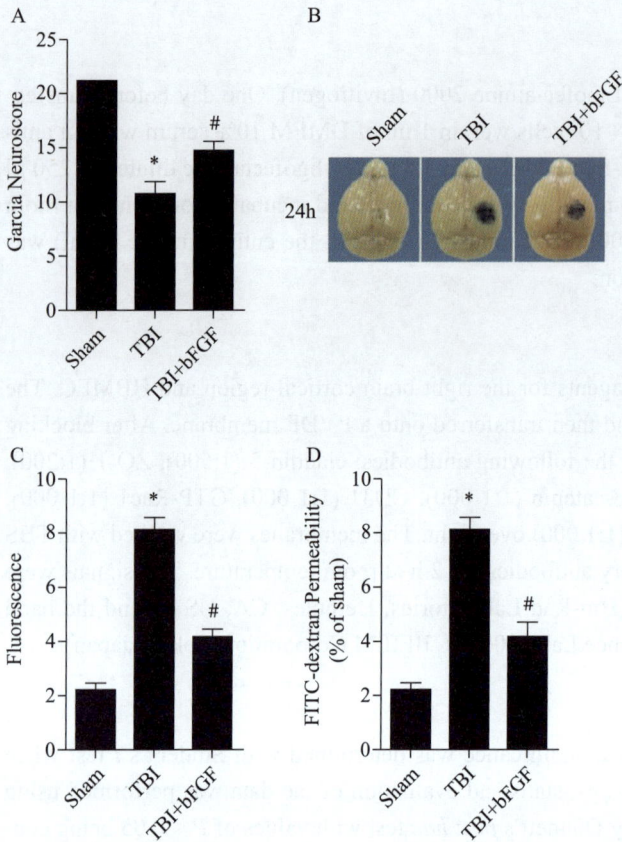

Fig. 1. Effects of exogenous bFGF (15 μg) or PBS on Garcia scores (A) at 24 h after TBI. Effects of bFGF on Evans Blue fluorescence (B, C) and FITC-dextran permeability (D) at 24 h after TBI. $*P < 0.05$ vs. the sham group. $#P < 0.05$ vs. the TBI group. Data are the mean values± SEM, $n = 6$.

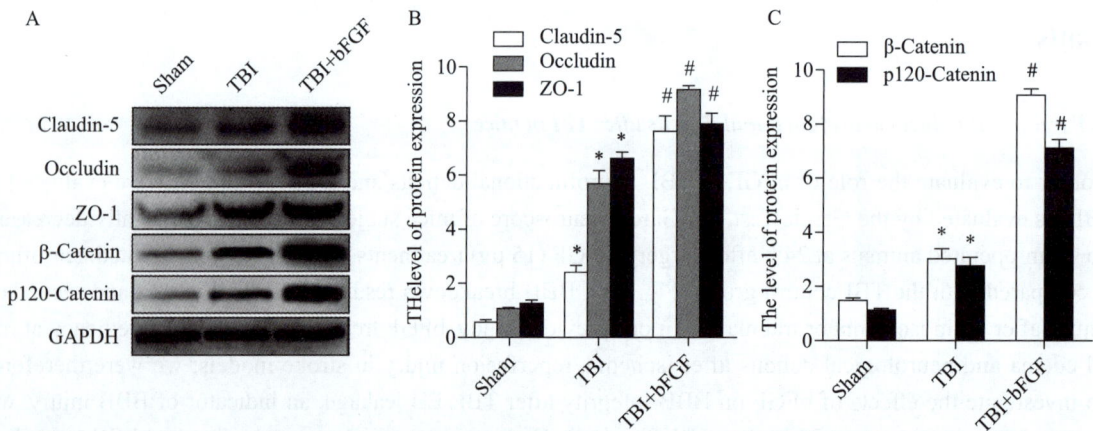

Fig. 2. Protein expression of claudin-5, occludin, zonula occludens-1, p120-catenin, and β-catenin for the sham, TBI, and bFGF treatment groups. GAPDH was used as the loading control and for band density normalization (A). The optical density analysis of claudin-5, occludin, zonula occludens-1, p120-catenin and β-catenin protein (B, C). $*P < 0.05$ vs. the sham group. $#P < 0.05$ vs. the TBI group. Data are the mean values ± SEM, $n = 6$

claudin-5, occludin, and the microvessel marker CD31 were markedly increased after bFGF treatment compared to vehicle-treated TBI animals (Fig. 3). These results suggest that bFGF treatment preserves BBB integrity after TBI, at least in part by increasing these TJ proteins. To further evaluate whether the PI3K/Akt pathway is involved in the neuroprotective effect of bFGF, the PI3K/Akt inhibitor LY294002 was injected into the left striatum. Neurofunctional deficits, EB fluorescence, and FITC-dextran fluorescence were analyzed at 24 h after TBI. LY294002 co-administration reversed the neuroprotection of bFGF as shown by the Garcia Test results. As expected, bFGF + LY294002 treated animals showed significant lower neuroscores than bFGF-treated animals and the bFGF + DMSO group (Fig. 4A). Furthermore, mice

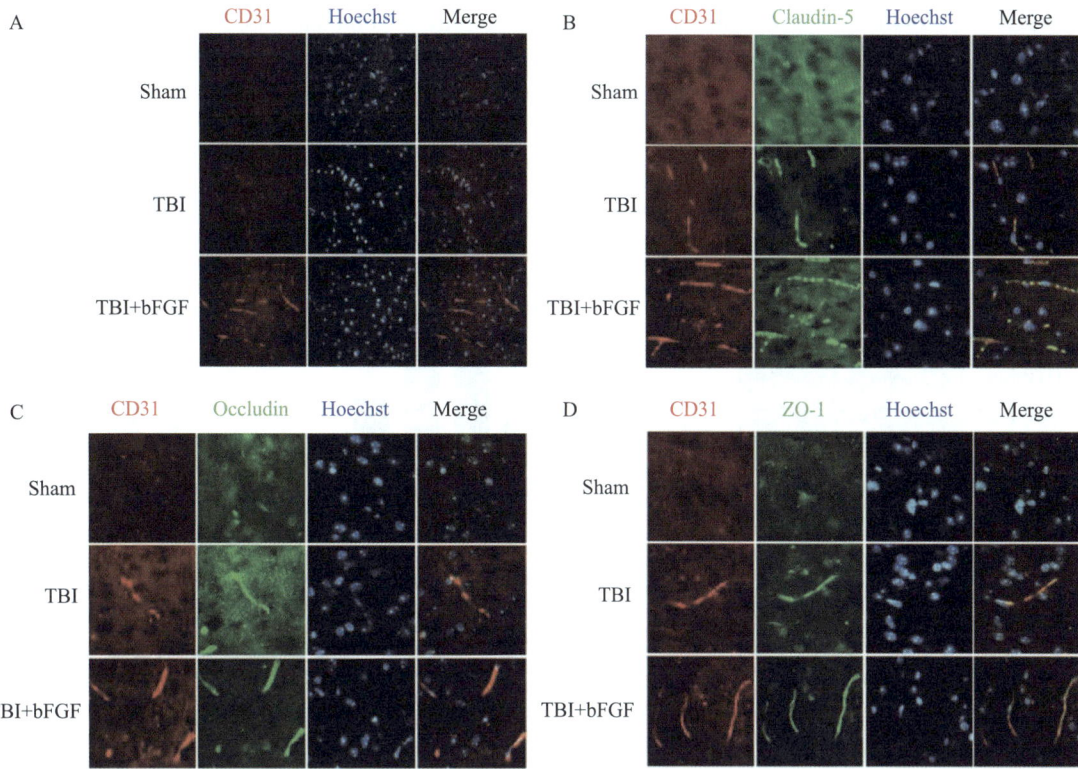

Fig. 3. Dual-label immunofluorescence staining results of endothelial cell marker (A) CD31 (*red*) and different tight junction proteins (B) Claudin-5 (C) Occludin, and (D) ZO-1 in the mouse brain 1 day after TBI. The nuclei are labeled by Hoechst. Scale bar = 10 μm. The proteins with obvious bright signals are labeled. Magnification was ×40.

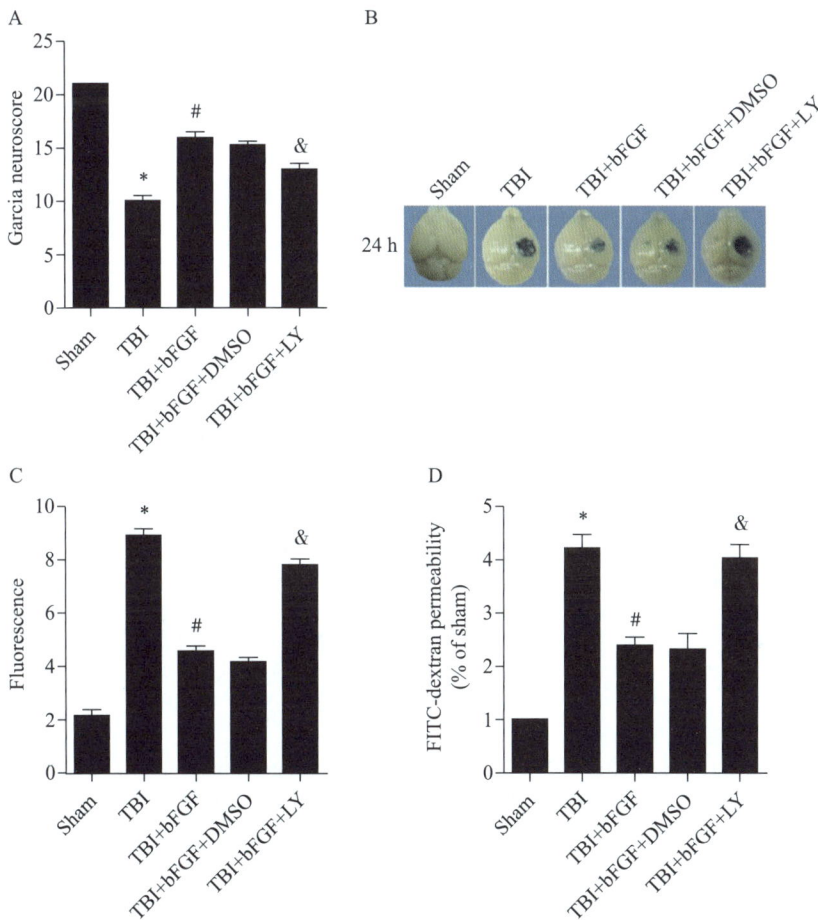

Fig. 4. Effects of the PI3K/Akt inhibitor LY294002 (50 nmol/kg) on bFGF induced attenuation of brain injury at 24 h after TBI. Evaluation of Garcia test (A) and Evans Blue fluorescence (B, C) and FITC-dextran permeability (D) in mice subjected to TBI. *$P < 0.05$ *vs.* the sham group. #$P < 0.05$ *vs.* the TBI group. &$P < 0.05$ *vs.* the TBI + bFGF group. Data are the mean values ± SEM, n =6.

receiving bFGF + LY294002 showed significantly more EB dye extravasation than bFGF treated animals (Fig. 4B–D). The protein expression of TJ and AJ proteins claudin-5, occludin, zonula occludens-1, p120-catenin, and β-catenin were also tested by Western blot. As shown in Fig. 5D–F, LY294002 treatment inhibited the activation by bFGF of the levels

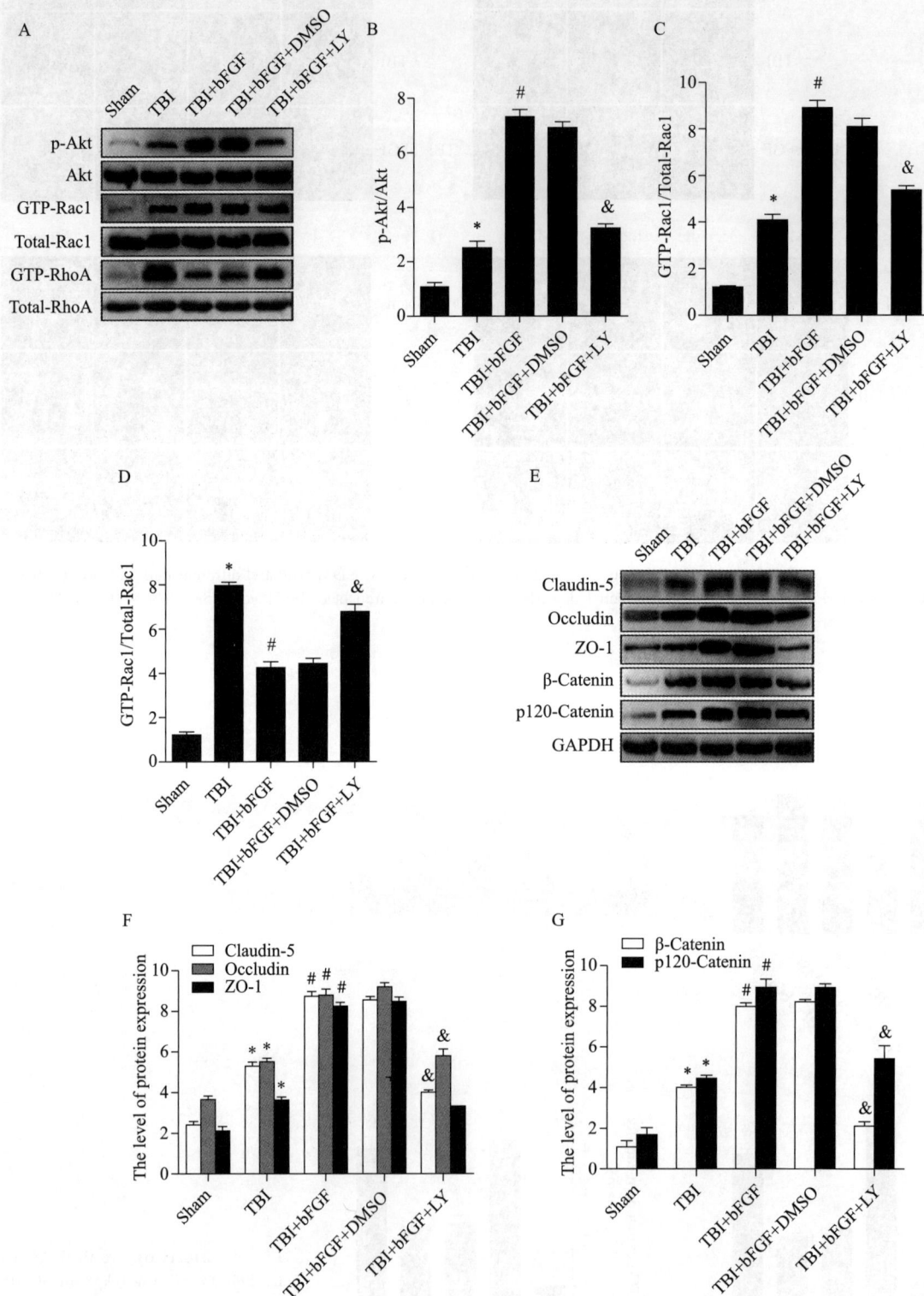

Fig. 5. The protein expression of p-Akt, GTP-Rac1, and GTP-RhoA after TBI-induced BBB destruction treated with bFGF and LY294002. GAPDH was used as the loading control and for band density normalization (A). The optical density analysis of p-Akt, GTP-Rac1, and GTP-RhoA protein (B, C). The protein expression of claudin-5, occluding, ZO-1, p120-catenin, and β-catenin after TBI-induced BBB destruction treated with bFGF and LY294002. GAPDH was used as the loading control and for band density normalization (D). The optical density analysis of pclaudin-5, occluding, ZO-1, p120-catenin, and β-catenin protein (E, F). $^*P < 0.05$ vs. the sham group. $^\#P < 0.05$ vs. the TBI group. $^\&P < 0.05$ vs. the TBI + bFGF group. Data are the mean values ± SEM, $n = 6$.

of these junction proteins. The DMSO control group showed no significant difference compared to the bFGF group ($P >$ 0.05). Taken together, all of these results suggested that bFGF treatment protects against BBB breakdown after TBI, at least in part by regulating the PI3K/Akt pathway.

3.3 bFGF treatment inhibits RhoA activity via the PI3K-Akt-Rac1 signaling pathway in mice

RhoA and Rac1 are members of the Rho subfamily of small GTPases which play crucial roles in the regulation of cytoskeletal organization in many cell types. It has been reported that Rac1 maintains and stabilizes the barrier function of microvascular endothelial cells, whereas RhoA antagonistically impairs endothelial barrier properties. To evaluate the role of RhoA and Rac1 in the protective effect of bFGF on BBB integrity, Western blot analysis was performed using the ipsilateral hemispheres of animals 24 h after TBI and subsequent co-administration of bFGF and LY294002. The results of the quantification of all target proteins were compared to groups treated with vehicle, bFGF, and bFGF + DMSO. As shown in Fig. 5A, LY294002 treatment reversed the activation by bFGF of the protein level of p-Akt as well as the GTP-Rac-1/Total-Rac-1 ratio. The ratio of GTP-RhoA/Total-RhoA was significantly increased in the bFGF + LY group compared to the bFGF alone group. Taken together, these results demonstrate that the protective role of bFGF on BBB integrity is related to the inhibition of RhoA through activation of the PI3K/Akt/Rac-1 signaling pathway in TBI mice.

3.4 bFGF ameliorates OGD-induced BBB injury and inhibition of the PI3K/Akt pathway partially reverses the protective effect of bFGF in vitro

To further confirm the hypothesis that bFGF can ameliorate OGD-induced BBB injury in a cellular model, HBMECs were subjected to OGD conditions, followed by treatment with bFGF or bFGF combined with LY294002. As shown in Fig. 6A, paracellular permeability of HBMECs increased dramatically after OGD; however, bFGF adminis-

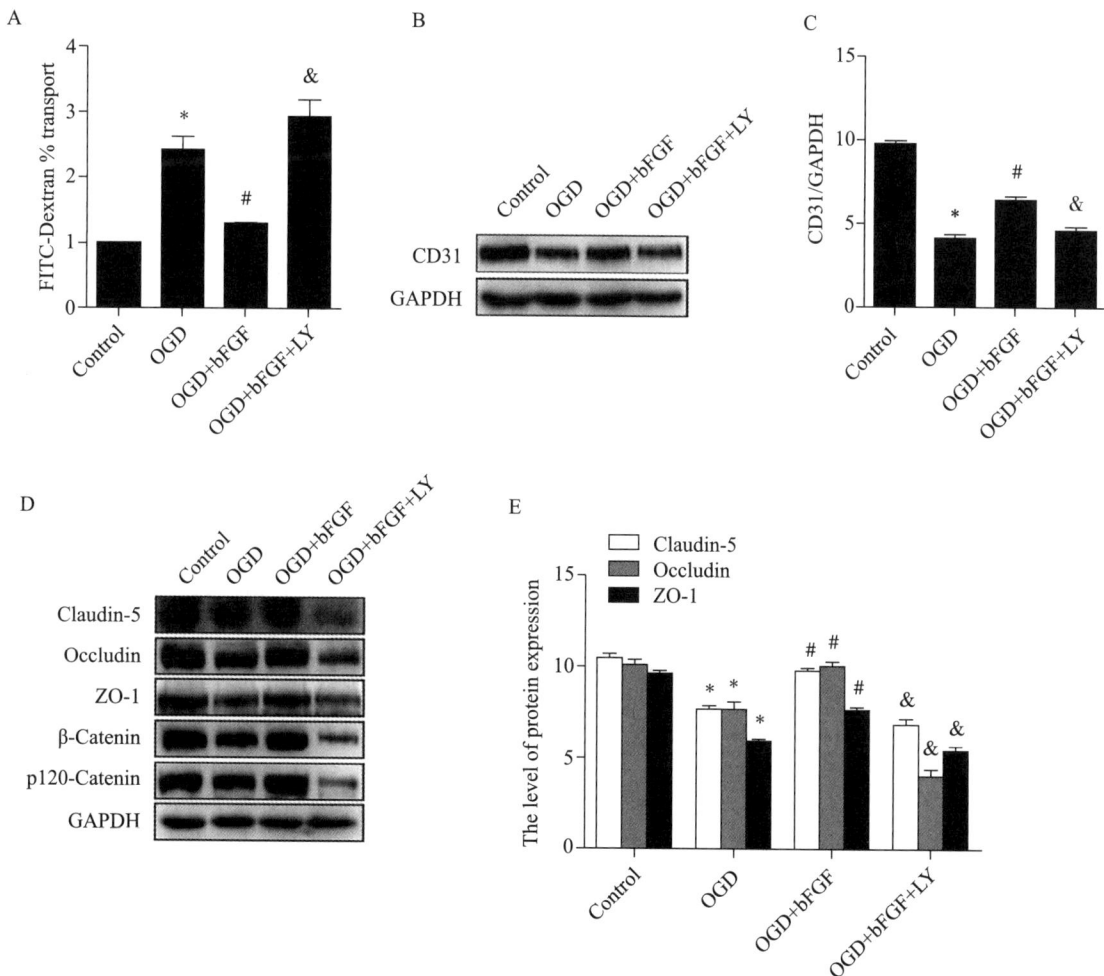

F

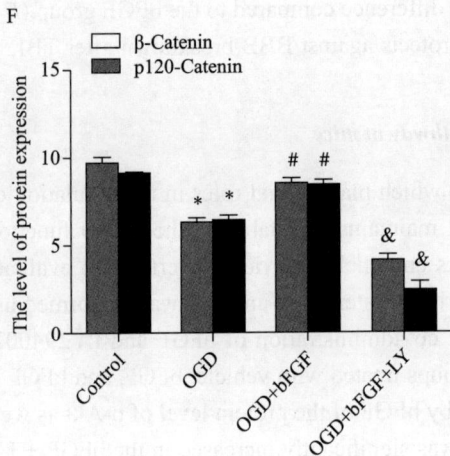

Fig. 6. HBMECs were pre-treated with 50 ng/ml bFGF with or without inhibitor LY294002 (20 μM) for 1 h, and then OGD conditions for 24 h and reperfusion for 12 h. The cells were analyzed for FITC-dextran transport (A). The cell lysates were analyzed by western blotting for the expression of CD31, claudin-5, occluding, ZO-1, p120-catenin, and β-catenin, and GAPDH was used as the loading control and for band density normalization (B, C). The optical density analysis of CD31, claudin-5, occluding, ZO-1, p120-catenin and β-catenin protein (C, E, F). $^*P<0.05$ vs. the control group. $^\#P<0.05$ vs. the OGD group. $^\&P<0.05$ vs. the OGD+bFGF group. Data are the mean values±SEM, $n=6$

tration significantly decreased the FITC-dextran permeability. On the other hand, the Akt inhibitor LY294002 partially reversed the protective effect of bFGF. In our previous study, BBB integrity was shown to be mainly dependent on the presence of TJs.

Therefore, we hypothesized that OGD-induced alterations in TJs and AJs may be responsible for the increased BBB permeability. We measured the protein levels of CD31, claudin-5, occludin, zonula occludens-1, p120-catenin, and β-catenin after OGD and their expression was significantly decreased when compared with the control group. bFGF treatment significantly increased the expression of these proteins while Akt inhibitor LY294002 reversed their activation by bFGF (Fig. 6B–F). Consistent with the Western blot results, immunostaining of claudin-5, ZO-1, β-catenin, and p120-catenin proteins also showed that OGD treatment decreased expression of these TJ and AJ proteins while bFGF administration significantly increased their expression. As shown in Fig. 7, LY294002 incubation partially reversed the activation effect of bFGF on TJ and AJ proteins. All of these findings illustrate that bFGF ameliorates OGD-induced BBB destruction by regulating TJ and AJ proteins *via* the PI3K/Akt pathway *in vitro*.

3.5 bFGF treatment preserves BBB integrity by inhibiting RhoA activity via the PI3K-Akt-Rac1 signaling pathway

In order to evaluate whether the PI3K/Akt pathways is involved in the preservation of BBB *in vitro*, HBMECs under OGD conditions were treated with bFGF. Our data shows that bFGF improved the expression of p-Akt and GTP-Rac1 and decreased the expression of GTP-RhoA under OGD conditions. Co-treatment with Akt inhibitor LY294002 and bFGF significantly reversed the activation effect of bFGF on protein levels of p-Akt, GTP-Rac1, and GTP-RhoA (Fig. 8). These data suggest that the PI3K-Akt-Rac1 pathway is involved in the protective effect of bFGF and is dependent on the inhibition of RhoA.

To further confirm the role of Rac1 in the protective effect of bFGF on TBI-induced BBB breakdown, RNA interference by transfection with Lipofectamine 2000 was used in HBMECs. The results showed that after treatment with Rac1 siRNA, the expression of TJs (claudin-5, occludin, zonula occludens-1), AJs (p120-catenin and β-catenin), and GTP-Rac1 were decreased significantly when compared with the control group while the expression of GTP-RhoA was significantly increased (Fig. 9A–D). As expected, silencingRac1 markedly reduced the stimulatory effect on these TJ and AJ protein levels by bFGF and fully abolished the inhibitory effect by bFGF on GTP-RhoA (Fig. 9A, E). All of these results further confirmed that the protective effect of bFGF on BBB integrity is mediated by inhibiting RhoA signaling through the PI3K-Akt-Rac1 pathway *in vitro*.

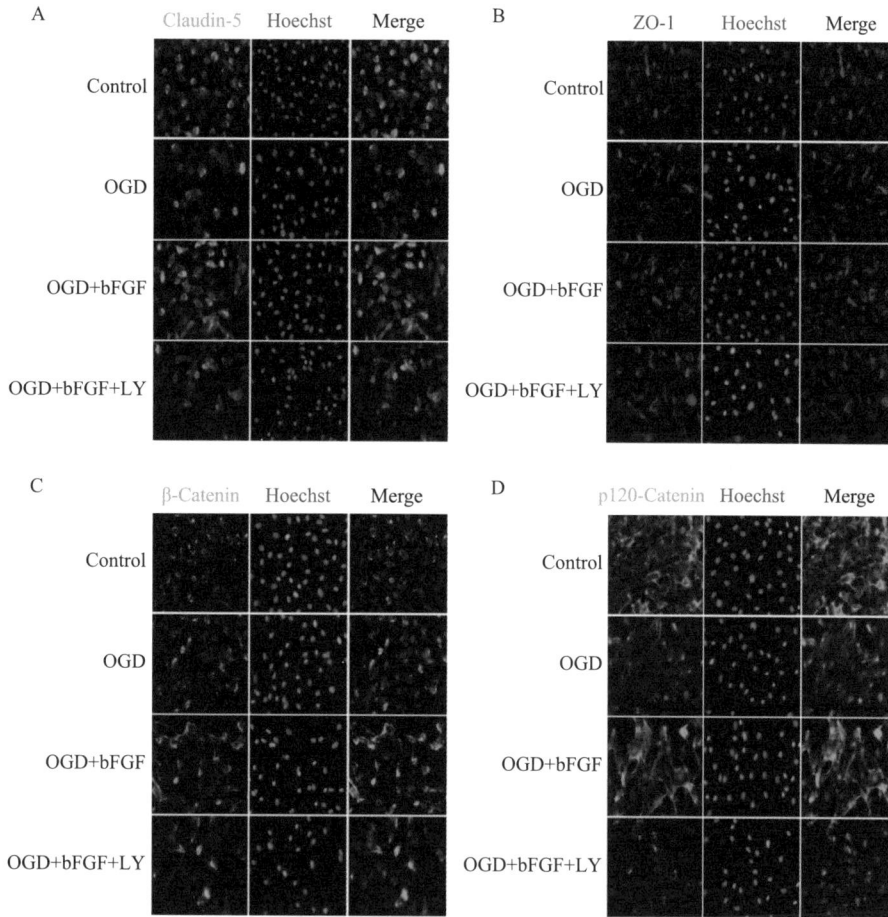

Fig. 7. HBMECs were pre-treated with bFGF for 1 h, and then OGD conditions for 24 h, and reperfusion for 12 h. Immunofluorescence staining of confluent HBMECs monolayers for (A) claudin-5, (B) occluding, (C) p120-catenin, and (D) β-catenin. Nuclei were labeled by Hoechst. The proteins with obvious bright signals are labeled. Magnification was ×40.

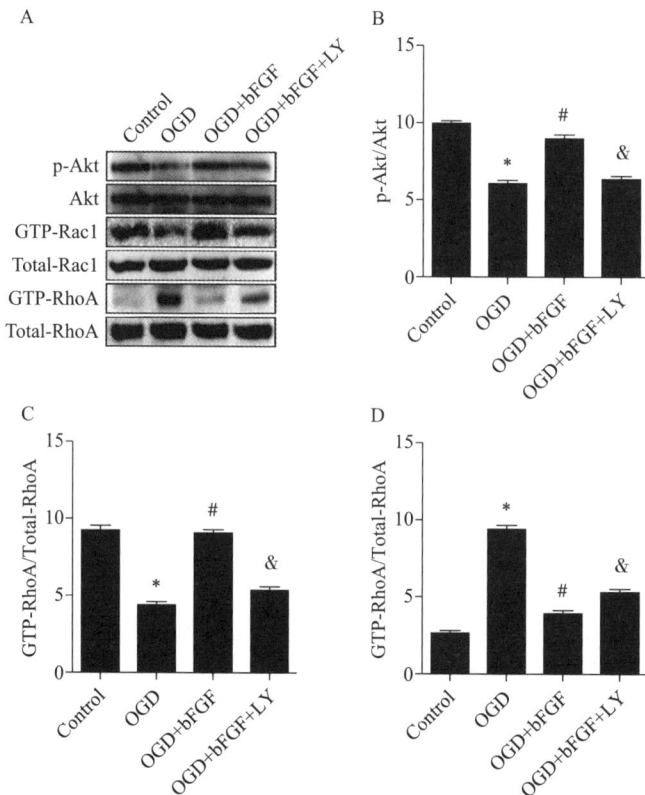

Fig. 8. The protein expression of p-Akt, GTP-Rac1 and GTP-RhoA in OGD-induced HBMECs treated with bFGF and LY294002 inhibitor. GAPDH was used as the loading control and for band density normalization (A). The optical density analysis of p-Akt, GTP-Rac1 and GTP-RhoA protein (B, C, D). *$P < 0.05$ vs. the control group. #$P < 0.05$ vs. the OGD group. &$P < 0.05$ vs. the OGD + bFGF group. Data are the mean values ± SEM, $n =6$.

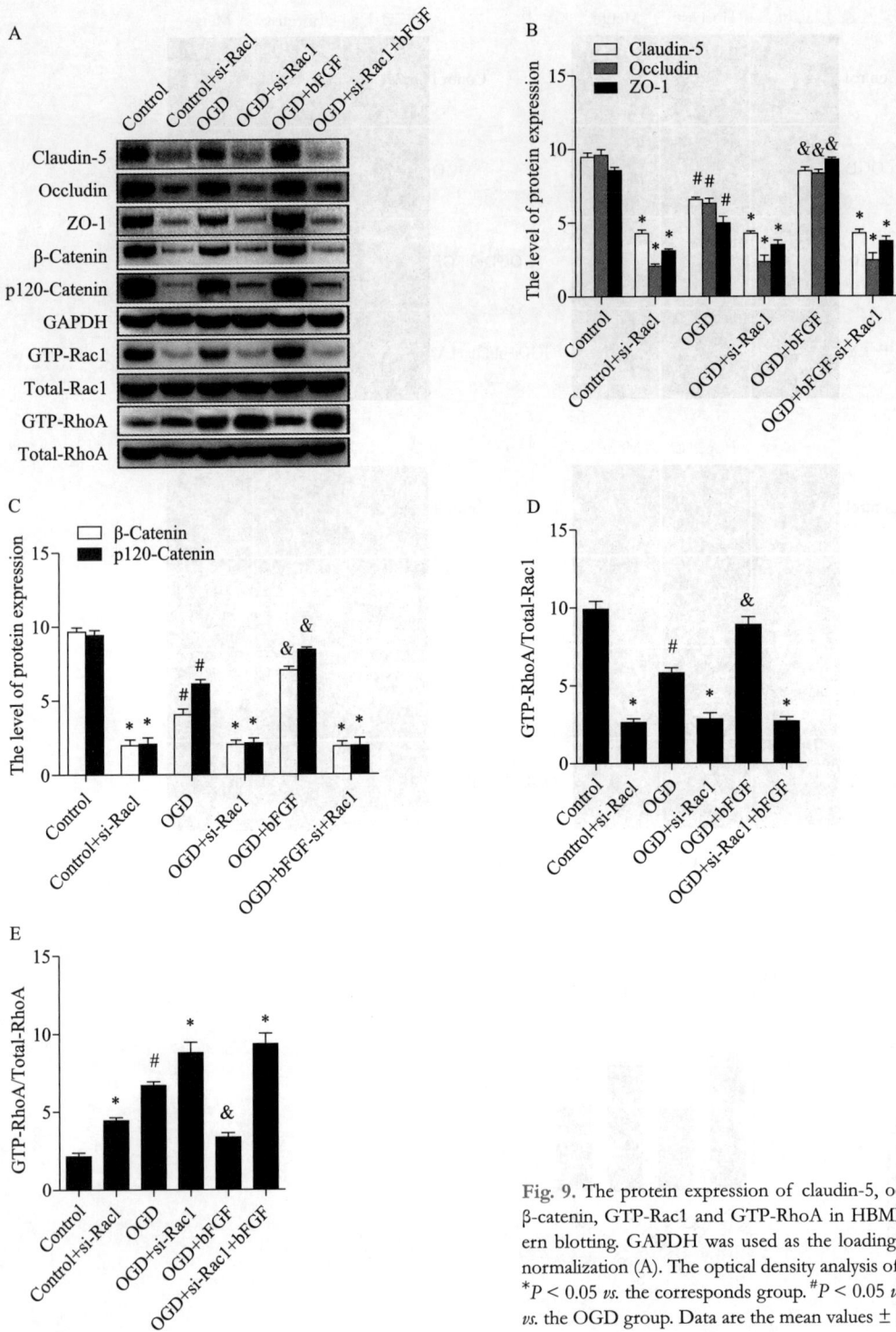

Fig. 9. The protein expression of claudin-5, occluding, ZO-1, p120-catenin, β-catenin, GTP-Rac1 and GTP-RhoA in HBMECs was determined by Western blotting. GAPDH was used as the loading control and for band density normalization (A). The optical density analysis of all these proteins (B, C, D, E). *$P < 0.05$ vs. the corresponds group. #$P < 0.05$ vs. the control group. &$P < 0.05$ vs. the OGD group. Data are the mean values ± SEM, $n = 6$.

4. Discussion

Patients experience TBI as a result of traffic accidents, sports injuries, or other types of trauma, which can lead to lifelong disability and significant economic costs [30]. After TBI, the initial traumatic injury to brain tissue is followed by a long period of secondary damage including neurovascular dysfunction, inflammation, oxidative stress, and cell apoptosis [31]. The breakdown of BBB is one of the main contributors interfering brain recovery from secondary damage. The BBB normally restricts free transcellular water movement from the vascular compartment to the brain interstitium and thereby supports the restricted and closely controlled environment necessary for normal brain function [32]. Although improved emergency medicine has led to decreases in TBI mortality in recent years, many survivors suffer sustained physical disability and cognitive impairments due to the lack of defined therapies to reduce TBI-associated long-term brain damage and neurological dysfunction. In the present study, we showed that post-injury bFGF treatment robustly reduced brain damage and improved neurological functions evaluated in the mouse model of TBI. Moreover, the results presented here suggest that preserved BBB integrity is a key underlying mechanism of bFGF-afforded neuroprotection against TBI. Understanding this mechanism will be crucial for translating these results to human clinical trials, in which most subjects have chronic neurological impairments.

In line with our findings, Huang *et al.* demonstrated that bFGF treatment can effectively preserve BBB integrity through RhoA inhibition after intracerebral hemorrhage in mice [9]. We therefore investigated the effects of bFGF on BBB integrity after TBI in the current study. Our results support the notion that BBB breakdown plays a key role in the pathogenesis of TBI and may be a potential therapeutic target [3]. The present study reveals that bFGF treatment can improve BBB integrity and attenuate neurological deficits following TBI. Although the exact mechanism of bFGF-conferred BBB protection is unclear, our results suggest that it is likely associated with the upregulation of TJ proteins. There is compelling evidence that the upregulation of TJ proteins mediates BBB disruption after TBI [33, 34]. The present study revealed that TBI animals have increased EB leakage (Fig. 1B), neurofunctional deficits (Fig. 1A), and EB fluorescence intensities (Fig. 1C). However, bFGF treatment significantly attenuated neurofunctional deficits and reduced EB extravasation following TBI (Fig. 1A–C). Western blot results showed that bFGF also upregulates TJ proteins (claudin-5, occludin, and zonula occludens-1) and AJ proteins (p120-catenin and β-catenin) at 24 h after TBI (Fig. 2). Consistent with the Western blot results, dual-label immunofluorescence showed that co-localization between ZO-1, claudin-5, occludin, and the microvessel marker CD31 was markedly increased after bFGF treatment compared to vehicle-treated TBI animals (Fig. 3). Notably, bFGF also upregulated these TJ and AJ proteins after OGD conditions in HBMECs (Figs. 6 and 7). To the best of our knowledge, this is the first study demonstrating that bFGF treatment preserves BBB integrity after TBI, at least in part by increasing these TJ proteins.

As a main downstream signal activated by bFGF, PI3K/Akt has essential neruoprotective effects [35]. The PI3K/Akt pathway is particularly important for mediating neuronal survival under a wide variety of circumstances and plays an important role in cellular angiogenesis, protein synthesis, metabolism, and proliferation [36, 37]. Activation of the PI3K/Akt pathway is also essential for growth factor-mediated cell survival. In this study, we focused on the role of the PI3K/Akt pathway in order to understand the signaling mechanisms involved in TBI-induced BBB breakdown. We demonstrated that the role of bFGF in TBI-induced BBB breakdown recovery is related to the activation of the PI3K/Akt pathway *in vivo*. We used the pathway inhibitor LY294002 combined with bFGF in the TBI mouse model, and the results showed significantly more dye extravasation than animals receiving bFGF treatment only; LY294002 also reversed the neuroprotective effect of bFGF (Fig. 4). To further confirm that the PI3K/Akt pathway is essential for the protective effect of bFGF on the BBB, we used HBMECs under OGD conditions (and additionally with the PI3K/Akt inhibitor LY294002) to show that the BBB breakdown induced by OGD was inhibited by bFGF treatment and further abolished by the inhibitor (Fig. 6A). In order to investigate how the PI3K/Akt signal pathway preserves BBB integrity, TJ proteins (claudin-5, occludin, and zonula occludens-1) and AJ proteins (p120-catenin and β-catenin) were detected after treatment with bFGF combined with LY294002. Western blot revealed that LY294002 treatment reversed the TJ and AJ protein upregulation effect by bFGF (Fig. 6D). Finally, our immunostaining results reinforced those shown by Western blot (Fig. 7). Taken together, all of these results suggest that bFGF ameliorates TBI or OGD-induced BBB destruction by regulating TJ and AJ proteins *via* the PI3K/Akt pathway.

Members of the Rho subfamily of small GTPases, including Rho, Rac, and Cdc42, play crucial roles in the regulation of cytoskeletal organization in many cell types. It has been previously reported that Rac1 maintains and stabilizes the barrier function of microvascular endothelial cells whereas RhoA antagonistically impairs endothelial barrier properties [38]. There is accumulating evidence that Rho regulates endothelial permeability, which depends on the integrity of intercellular junctions and actomyosin contractility [39]. One report showed that inhibition of Rho-kinase activity, following cerebral ischemia, may represent a viable therapeutic option to neutralize a variety of phenomena, including BBB dysfunction [40]. RhoA can disintegrate AJs through ROCK phosphorylation and has further been identified to increase actomyosin contractility which also results in breakdown of intercellular junctions. In our present study, we found that administration of bFGF increased the protein level of the GTP-Rac-1/Total-Rac-1 ratio. Additionally, the ratio of GTP-

RhoA/Total-RhoA was significantly decreased after bFGF treatment (Fig. 5A). In order to figure out how bFGF regulated these Rho-kinase proteins, the inhibitor LY was co-administered with bFGF and our results showed that the protein regulation effects of bFGF were reversed by LY (Fig. 5A). The results of our *in vitro* study (Fig. 8) were also consistent with the results showed *in vivo*. To further validate the role of Rac-1 in the protective effect of bFGF, siRNA-Rac-1 was used in HBMECs. As demonstrated in Fig. 9, silencing Rac-1 partially inhibited the ability of bFGF to upregulate these TJ proteins and reversed the RhoA inhibition effect by bFGF. These results indicate that the protective function of bFGF on the BBB may be involved in the inhibition of RhoA protein and upregulation of TJ proteins *via* the Rac-1 pathway.

There are certainly limitations of bFGF as a therapy for TBI-induced BBB breakdown and still require further study and investigation. For example, a single dose of bFGF was administered immediately after injury; however, post-injury treatment with an optimized dose and extended treatment time would provide a better evaluation of its therapeutic value. In this study, we looked at the 1-day outcome but the long-term neurological outcomes, such as 2–4 weeks or longer, also need to be evaluated in the future. Moreover, HBMECs used *in vitro* are informative, yet future transwell assays of the effect of bFGF on astrocytes combined with HBMECs in co-culture would be more persuasive. Nevertheless, the neuroprotective effect of bFGF on TBI-induced BBB breakdown is confirmed and it is feasible to elucidate the pharmacodynamic properties and underlying mechanisms in future studies.

In conclusion, bFGF significantly reduced the extent of damage and preserved the BBB integrity after TBI. We first reported that the protective role of bFGF on BBB is related to the upregulation of TJ proteins and the inhibition of RhoA *via* Rac-1. Furthermore, activation of the downstream signaling pathway PI3K/Akt/Rac-1 is essential for the protective effect of bFGF on BBB integrity both *in vivo* and *in vitro*. Our study demonstrates that therapeutic strategies using bFGF may be suitable for recovery from TBI.

References

[1] Maas AIR, Stocchetti N, Bullock R. Moderate and severe traumatic brain injury in adults[J]. Lancet Neurology, 2008, 7(8): 728-741.

[2] Coronado VG, Xu L, Basavaraju SV, *et al.* Surveillance for Traumatic Brain Injury-Related Deaths-United States, 1997-2007[J]. Morbidity and Mortality Weekly Report, 2011, 60(SS5, Suppl. S): 1-32.

[3] Shlosberg D, Benifla M, Kaufer D, *et al.* Blood-brain barrier breakdown as a therapeutic target in traumatic brain injury[J]. Nature Reviews Neurology, 2010, 6(7): 393-403.

[4] Nag S, Kapadia A, Stewart DJ. Molecular pathogenesis of blood-brain barrier breakdown in acute brain injury[J]. Neuropathology And Applied Neurobiology, 2011, 37(1): 3-23.

[5] Werner C, Engelhard K. Pathophysiology of traumatic brain injury[J]. British Journal Of Anaesthesia, 2007, 99(1): 4-9.

[6] Potts MB, Koh SE, Whetstone WD, *et al.* Traumatic injury to the immature brain: inflammation, oxidative injury, and iron-mediated damage as potential therapeutic targets[J]. NeuroRx : the journal of the American Society for Experimental NeuroTherapeutics, 2006, 3(2): 143-153.

[7] Lin Y, Pan Y, Wang M, *et al.* Blood-brain barrier permeability is positively correlated with cerebral microvascular perfusion in the early fluid percussion-injured brain of the rat[J]. Laboratory Investigation, 2012, 92(11): 1623-1634.

[8] Loane DJ, Faden AI. Neuroprotection for traumatic brain injury: translational challenges and emerging therapeutic strategies[J]. Trends In Pharmacological Sciences, 2010, 31(12): 596-604.

[9] Huang B, Krafft PR, Ma Q, *et al.* Fibroblast growth factors preserve blood-brain barrier integrity through RhoA inhibition after intracerebral hemorrhage in mice[J]. Neurobiology Of Disease, 2012, 46(1): 204-214.

[10] Abbott NJ, Patabendige AAK, Dolman DEM, *et al.* Structure and function of the blood-brain barrier[J]. Neurobiology Of Disease, 2010, 37(1): 13-25.

[11] Huber JD, Egleton RD, Davis TP. Molecular physiology and pathophysiology of tight junctions in the blood-brain barrier[J]. Trends In Neurosciences, 2001, 24(12): 719-725.

[12] Engelhardt B, Sorokin L. The blood-brain and the blood-cerebrospinal fluid barriers: function and dysfunction[J]. Seminars In Immunopathology, 2009, 31(4): 497-511.

[13] Grieb P, Forster RE, Strome D, *et al.* O-2 exchange between blood and brain-tissues studies with o-18(2) indicator-dilution technique[J]. Journal Of Applied Physiology, 1985, 58(6): 1929-1941.

[14] Luh C, Kuhlmann CR, Ackermann B, *et al.* Inhibition of myosin light chain kinase reduces brain edema formation after traumatic brain injury[J]. Journal Of Neurochemistry, 2010, 112(4): 1015-1025.

[15] Antonetti DA, Wolpert EB, DeMaio L, *et al.* Hydrocortisone decreases retinal endothelial cell water and solute flux coincident with increased content and decreased phosphorylation of occludin[J]. Journal Of Neurochemistry, 2002, 80(4): 667-677.

[16] Jiang WG, Bryce RP, Horrobin DF, *et al.* Regulation of tight junction permeability and occludin expression by polyunsaturated fatty acids[J]. Biochemical And Biophysical Research Communications, 1998, 244(2): 414-420.

[17] Harhaj NS, Antonetti DA. Regulation of tight junctions and loss of barrier function in pathophysiology[J]. International Journal Of Biochemistry & Cell Biology, 2004, 36(7): 1206-1237.

[18] Wachtel M, Bolliger MF, Ishihara H, *et al.* Down-regulation of occludin expression in astrocytes by tumour necrosis factor (TNF) is mediated *via* TNF type-1 receptor and nuclear factor-kappa B activation[J]. Journal Of Neurochemistry, 2001, 78(1): 155-162.

[19] Wang Z, Zhang H, Xu X, *et al.* bFGF inhibits ER stress induced by ischemic oxidative injury *via* activation of the PI3K/Akt and ERK1/2 pathways[J]. Toxicology Letters, 2012, 212(2): 137-146.

[20] Wang ZG, Wang Y, Huang Y, *et al.* bFGF regulates autophagy and ubiquitinated protein accumulation induced by myocardial ischemia/reperfusion *via* the activation of the PI3K/Akt/mTOR

pathway[J]. Scientific Reports, 2015, 5.

[21] Zhang HY, Wang ZG, Wu FZ, et al. Regulation of Autophagy and Ubiquitinated Protein Accumulation by bFGF Promotes Functional Recovery and Neural Protection in a Rat Model of Spinal Cord Injury[J]. Molecular Neurobiology, 2013, 48(3): 452-464.

[22] Murakami M, Nguyen LT, Zhang ZW, et al. The FGF system has a key role in regulating vascular integrity[J]. Journal Of Clinical Investigation, 2008, 118(10): 3355-3366.

[23] Lee JG, Kay EP. PI 3-Kinase/Rac1 and ERK1/2 Regulate FGF-2-Mediated Cell Proliferation through Phosphorylation of p27 at Ser10 by KIS and at Thr187 by Cdc25A/Cdk2[J]. Investigative Ophthalmology & Visual Science, 2011, 52(1): 417-426.

[24] Kamura S, Matsumoto Y, Fukushi Ji, et al. Basic fibroblast growth factor in the bone microenvironment enhances cell motility and invasion of Ewing's sarcoma family of tumours by activating the FGFR1-PI3K-Rac1 pathway[J]. British Journal Of Cancer, 2010, 103(3): 370-381.

[25] Wojciak-Stothard B, Ridley AJ. Shear stress-induced endothelial cell polarization is mediated by Rho and Rac but not Cdc42 or PI 3-kinases[J]. Journal Of Cell Biology, 2003, 161(2): 429-439.

[26] Zhang M, Shan H, Wang T, et al. Dynamic Change of Hydrogen Sulfide After Traumatic Brain Injury and its Effect in Mice[J]. Neurochemical Research, 2013, 38(4): 714-725.

[27] Luo CL, Chen XP, Yang R, et al. Cathepsin B Contributes to Traumatic Brain Injury-Induced Cell Death Through a Mitochondria-Mediated Apoptotic Pathway[J]. Journal Of Neuroscience Research, 2010, 88(13): 2847-2858.

[28] Garcia JH, Wagner S, Liu KF, et al. Neurological deficit and extent of neuronal necrosis attributable to middle cerebral-artery occlusion in rats - statistical validation[J]. Stroke, 1995, 26(4): 627-634.

[29] Lo EH, Dalkara T, Moskowitz MA. Mechanisms, challenges and opportunities in stroke[J]. Nature Reviews Neuroscience, 2003, 4(5): 399-415.

[30] Zlokovic BV. The blood-brain barrier in health and chronic neurodegenerative disorders[J]. Neuron, 2008, 57(2): 178-201.

[31] Roth TL, Nayak D, Atanasijevic T, et al. Transcranial amelioration of inflammation and cell death after brain injury[J]. Nature, 2014, 505(7482): 223-228.

[32] Chodobski A, Zink BJ, Szmydynger-Chodobska J. Blood-Brain Barrier Pathophysiology in Traumatic Brain Injury[J]. Translational Stroke Research, 2011, 2(4): 492-516.

[33] Vajtr D, Benada O, Kukacka J, et al. Correlation of Ultrastructural Changes of Endothelial Cells and Astrocytes Occurring during Blood Brain Barrier Damage after Traumatic Brain Injury with Biochemical Markers of Blood Brain Barrier Leakage and Inflammatory Response[J]. Physiological Research, 2009, 58(2): 263-268.

[34] Higashida T, Kreipke CW, Rafols JA, et al. The role of hypoxia-inducible factor-1a, aquaporin-4, and matrix metalloproteinase-9 in blood-brain barrier disruption and brain edema after traumatic brain injury Laboratory investigation[J]. Journal Of Neurosurgery, 2011, 114(1): 92-101.

[35] Zhang H-Y, Zhang X, Wang Z-G, et al. Exogenous Basic Fibroblast Growth Factor Inhibits ER Stress-Induced Apoptosis and Improves Recovery from Spinal Cord Injury[J]. Cns Neuroscience & Therapeutics, 2013, 19(1): 20-29.

[36] Hossain MS, Ifuku M, Take S, et al. Plasmalogens Rescue Neuronal Cell Death through an Activation of AKT and ERK Survival Signaling[J]. Plos One, 2013, 8(12).

[37] Zhao J, Cheng Y-Y, Fan W, et al. Botanical Drug Puerarin Coordinates with Nerve Growth Factor in the Regulation of Neuronal Survival and Neuritogenesis via Activating ERK1/2 and PI3K/Akt Signaling Pathways in the Neurite Extension Process[J]. Cns Neuroscience & Therapeutics, 2015, 21(1): 61-70.

[38] Gerhard R, John H, Aktories K, et al. Thiol-modifying phenylarsine oxide inhibits guanine nucleotide binding of Rho but not of Rac GTPases[J]. Molecular Pharmacology, 2003, 63(6): 1349-1355.

[39] Zandy NL, Playford M, Pendergast AM. Abl tyrosine kinases regulate cell-cell adhesion through Rho GTPases[J]. Proceedings Of the National Academy Of Sciences Of the United States Of America, 2007, 104(45): 17686-17691.

[40] Gibson CL, Srivastava K, Sprigg N, et al. inhibition of rho kinase protects cerebral barrier from ischaemia-evoked injury through modulations of endothelial cell oxidtive stress and tight junctions[J]. Journal Of Neurochemistry, 2014, 129(5): 816-826.

bFGF attenuates endoplasmic reticulum stress and mitochondrial injury on myocardial ischaemia/reperfusion *via* activation of PI3K/Akt/ERK1/2 pathway

Zhouguang Wang , Jian Xiao,Xiaokun Li

1. Introduction

Despite current optimal treatment, ischaemic heart disease is still the leading cause of death throughout the world [1]. Because of the lack of effective therapies, myocardial ischaemia/reperfusion (I/R) injury remains a major medical problem today [2]. The current standard treatment for myocardial ischaemia is rapid reperfusion, which can attenuate myocardial infarction, reduce cardiomyocyte apoptosis and restore contractile dysfunction. Reduction in infarct size by reperfusion in patients with acute myocardial infarction was also quickly translated to clinical practise [3]; however, reperfusion also has the potential for additional injury, the overproduction of reactive oxygen species (ROS), mitochondrial dysfunction and overloading of calcium in the early reperfusion period. Unbalanced and high steady-state levels of reactive oxygen and nitrogen species (ROS/RNS) are responsible for cytotoxicity, which in turn leads to contractile dysfunction and cell death [4]. Oxidative stress resulting from the overload of toxic ROS, such as hydroperoxide, also leads to various modifications of proteins, DNA, and lipids that induce cell proliferation, growth arrest, apoptosis or necrosis [5, 6]. Therefore, therapeutic strategies focusing on delaying or inhibiting apoptosis induced by oxidative stress may facilitate the treatment of myocardial I/R injury.

Basic fibroblast growth factor (bFGF or FGF-2) regulate a variety of biological functions including proliferation, morphogenesis and the suppression of apoptosis [7]; it is an important angiogenic factor produced by hearts subjected to ischaemia. It acts on cells through transmembrane receptors with tyrosine kinase activity. Activation of FGFR induces a variety of intracellular signaling cascades, including the MAPK/ERK and PI3K/Akt pathways [8]. In the heart, bFGF expression was shown to be up-regulated after cardiac injury, such as ischaemia/reperfusion, or in the process of cardiac remodeling [9]. Moreover, the overexpression of bFGF increases cardiac myocyte viability after injury in isolated mouse hearts [10]. bFGF delivered during reperfusion protects the heart against ischaemia-reperfusion injury through increased relative levels of PKC subtypes alpha, epsilon and zeta [11]. In our previous study, we also proved that bFGF protects the heart against I/R-induced oxidative damage and cell death; however, the molecular mechanism by which bFGF treatment reduces myocardial I/R injury is unknown.

The increased generation of free radicals without a concomitant increase in antioxidant protection has been shown to induce apoptosis during I/R [12]. The resulting oxidative stress leads to the peroxidation of phospholipid cardiolipin in the inner mitochondrial membrane, which contributes to the induction of mitochondrial fragmentation and dysfunction and triggers apoptosis [13, 14]. Mitochondrial processes have been demonstrated to be major events during apoptosis, and the Bcl-2 family, including Bax and Bak, is involved in the alteration of mitochondrial membrane potential as well as the release of mitochondrial apoptotic factors [15]. Mitochondria are crucial signaling elements and potential effectors. The mitochondrial respiratory chain accepts electrons from NADH/H and flavine adenine dinucleotide (FADH)/H and transports them over four complexes ultimately onto oxygen generates, creating a proton gradient that then drives adenosine triphosphate (ATP) production [16]. A previous study showed that exogenous taurine provides cardioprotection against myocardial ischaemic reperfusion by regulating the mitochondrial dysfunction induced by ROS generation [17]. In addition, myocardial I/R injury is exacerbated by the promotion of myocardial mitochondrial dysfunction. The role and clinical impact of apoptosis needs to be further assessed to enable the development of more effective therapies to prevent myocardial damage during I/R. Such therapies must prevent mitochondrial dysfunction to preserve myocardial physiology. Although many reports have identified mitochondrial apoptosis as critical for myocardial I/R, whether bFGF may reduce myocardial mitochondrial dysfunction remains unclear.

Concurrently, endoplasmic reticulum (ER) stress is often accompanied by increased ROS generation in the myocardium [18, 19]. Excessive ROS production, which initiates the perturbation of the cellular redox balance, causes cell apoptosis [20, 21]. ROS generation appears to be one of the important stimuli that triggers ER stress [22], a paradigm called 'ROS-dependent ER stress'. ER stress plays an important role in cell growth, differentiation and apoptosis. A previous study provided evidence for the involvement of ER stress in the cardiac apoptosis in the myocardial I/R model [23]. These experimental data suggested that ER stress was initiated in myocardial I/R hearts, and the ER stress-induced apoptosis took part in the pathogenesis and development of myocardial I/R injury. Investigations have also demonstrated that ER stress induces cell apoptosis independently from mitochondria and death receptor-dependent pathways [24]. New research also suggests that the ROS-stimulated activation of the PERK signaling pathway, rather than the IRE1 or activating transcription factor 6 (ATF-6) signaling pathways, is primarily responsible for ROS-mediated ER stress-induced myocyte apoptosis [18]. Although many reports have identified that ER stress-induced apoptosis is critical for myocardial I/R, whether bFGF ameliorates myocardial ER stress is not clear.

In this study, we demonstrated that ER stress and mitochondrial dysfunction-induced apoptosis under oxidative stress *in vitro* and *in vivo*. bFGF inhibits ER stress and mitochondrial dysfunction-related protein expression *via* activation of the PI3K/Akt and ERK1/2 pathways. Our results reveal a potential drug target for treating myocardial I/R injuries.

2. Materials and methods

2.1 Reagents and antibodies

DMEM and foetal bovine serum (FBS) were purchased from Invitrogen (Carlsbad, CA, USA). Recombinant human bFGF was purchased from Sigma-Aldrich (St. Louis, MO, USA). Anti-Akt, p-Akt (Ser473), anti-ERK1/2, p-ERK1/2 (Thr202/Tyr204), anti-cleaved-caspase-3, cleaved-caspase-9, Bax, Bcl-2, cleaved-PARP, cytochrome *c*, anti-CHOP, cleaved-caspase-12, glucose-regulated protein (GRP-78), ATF-6 and GAPDH antibodies were purchased from Santa Cruz Biotechnology (Santa Cruz, CA, USA). Goat antirabbit and antimouse IgG-HRP were purchased from Cell Signaling Technology, Inc. (Danvers, MA, USA). An enhanced chemiluminescence (ECL) kit was purchased from Bio-Rad (Hercules, CA, USA). TBHP, PI3K/Akt inhibitor LY294002, ERK1/2 inhibitor PD98059 and all other reagents were purchased from Sigma-Aldrich unless otherwise specified.

2.2 Cell culture and viability assay

Rat cardiomyocyte H9C2 cells were purchased from the American Type Culture Collection and maintained in DMEM containing 10% foetal bovine serum under 5% CO_2. H9C2 cells were seeded on 96-well plates and treated with different doses of the TBHP for 8 h. To determine the effective concentration for cytoprotection, cells were also pre-treated with various concentrations of recombinant bFGF. Cell viability was assessed using the methyl thiazolyl tetrazolium assay. To further evaluate the effect of PI3K/Akt and ERK1/2 activation on oxidative injury, cells were pre-treated for 2 h with specific inhibitors, namely LY294002 (20 μM) and PD98059 (20 μM), before the addition of TBHP, as previously described. All experiments were performed in triplicate.

2.3 Myocardial I/R model in mice and bFGF treatment

Adult male C57/B6 mice (8–12 weeks of age) were supplied by the Animal Center of the Chinese Academy of Sciences. The animal use and care protocol conformed to the Guide for the Care and Use of Laboratory Animals from the National Institutes of Health and was approved by the Animal Care and Use Committee of Jilin University. Experimental MI/R was induced by transient myocardial ischaemia for 30 min. and was followed by reperfusion for 4 h, as described previously. Mice were anaesthetized with 4% chloral hydrate (100 mg/kg, i.p) and placed on a ventilator (Harvard Rodent Ventilator, Harvard Apparatus, Holliston, MA, USA) in the right lateral decubitus position, and core temperature was maintained at 37 ℃ with a heating pad. After a left lateral thoracotomy and pericardiectomy, the left anterior descending coronary artery was occluded for 30 min. with an 8-0 nylon suture and polyethylene tubing to prevent arterial injury and then re-perfused for 4 h. The mice that survived surgery were assigned randomly to the different treatment groups ($n = 6$–15 per group). Control group operations were performed in which animals underwent the same surgical procedure without coronary artery ligation ($n = 4$–8 per group). The I/R mice were administered 2 µg bFGF/mouse through intramyocardial injection at 30 min after ischaemia.

2.4 TUNEL assay

DNA fragmentation *in vivo* was detected using a one-step TUNEL Apoptosis Assay KIT (Roche, Mannheim, Germany). The images were captured with a Nikon ECLIPSE Ti microscope (Nikon, Melville, NY, USA). The apoptotic rates of the H9C2 cells treated with TBHP and bFGF were measured using a PI/Annexin V-FITC kit (Invitrogen) and then analysed by a FACScan flow cytometer (Becton Dickinson, Franklin Lakes, NJ, USA) according to the kit's manual.

2.5 Fluorescence activated cell sorting (FACS) analysis

The cells were cultured at a density of 2×10^5 cells per well in growth medium for 24 h in 6-well plates. The cells were then pre-incubated with 50 nM bFGF which was followed 2 h later by exposure to 100 µM TBHP for 8 h. Meanwhile, inhibitors of PI3K and ERK phosphorylation were added to the cells 2 h prior to TBHP at a final concentration of 20 µM. Annexin V assays were performed with the Annexin V-FITC Apoptosis Detection Kit (Becton Dickinson, San Jose, CA, USA). Cells were washed twice with cold PBS and re-suspended in binding buffer before the addition of Annexin V-FITC and propidium iodide (PI). Cells were vortexed and incubated for 15 min. in the dark at room temperature before analysis using a FACSCalibur flow cytometer (BD Biosciences, San Jose, CA, USA) and FlowJo software (Tree Star, San Carlos, CA, USA).

2.6 Immunofluorescence staining

To determine CHOP, GRP-78, cleaved-PARP and cleaved caspase-12 activities, sections were incubated with 0.3% H_2O_2 in methanol for 30 min, followed by blocking with 1% bovine albumin in PBS for 1 h at room temperature. Next, the sections were incubated at 4 ℃ over-night with a primary antibody against CHOP (1:200), GRP-78 (1:200), cleaved-PARP (1:200) or cleaved caspase-12 (1:1 000). After primary antibody incubation, the sections were washed for 4 × 10 min at room temperature and then incubated with donkey antimouse/rabbit, donkey antirabbit/mouse or donkey antigoat secondary antibody (1:500; Invitrogen) for 1 h at room temperature. The saline injection group was considered the negative control. The images were captured using a Nikon ECLPSE 80i.

2.7 Western blot

Total proteins were purified using protein extraction reagents for the heart tissue and H9C2 cells. The equivalent of 50 µg of protein was separated by 12% gel and then transferred onto a PVDF membrane. After blocking with 5% fat-free milk, the membranes were incubated with the relevant protein antibodies overnight. The membranes were washed with TBS and treated with secondary antibodies for 2 h at room temperature. The signals were visualized with the ChemiDicTM XRS + Imaging System (Bio-Rad Laboratories), and the band densities were quantified with Multi Gauge Software of Science Lab 2006 (FUJIFILM Corporation, Tokyo, Japan).

2.8 Statistical analysis

Data are expressed as the mean ± SEM. Statistical significance was determined using Student's *t*-test when there were two experimental groups. When more than two groups were compared, statistical evaluation of the data was performed with one-way ANOVA and Dunnett's *post hoc* test. $P < 0.05$ was considered statistically significant.

3. Results

3.1 bFGF decreases myocardial apoptosis in myocardial I/R mouse

To determine the role of bFGF in cardiac protection, bFGF was delivered into the mouse myocardium at 30 min after ischaemia. The myocardial apoptosis in the myocardial I/R group was detected using TUNEL staining. As shown in Fig. 1A, there were no apoptosis-positive cells in the control group. The numbers of TUNEL-positive cells increased

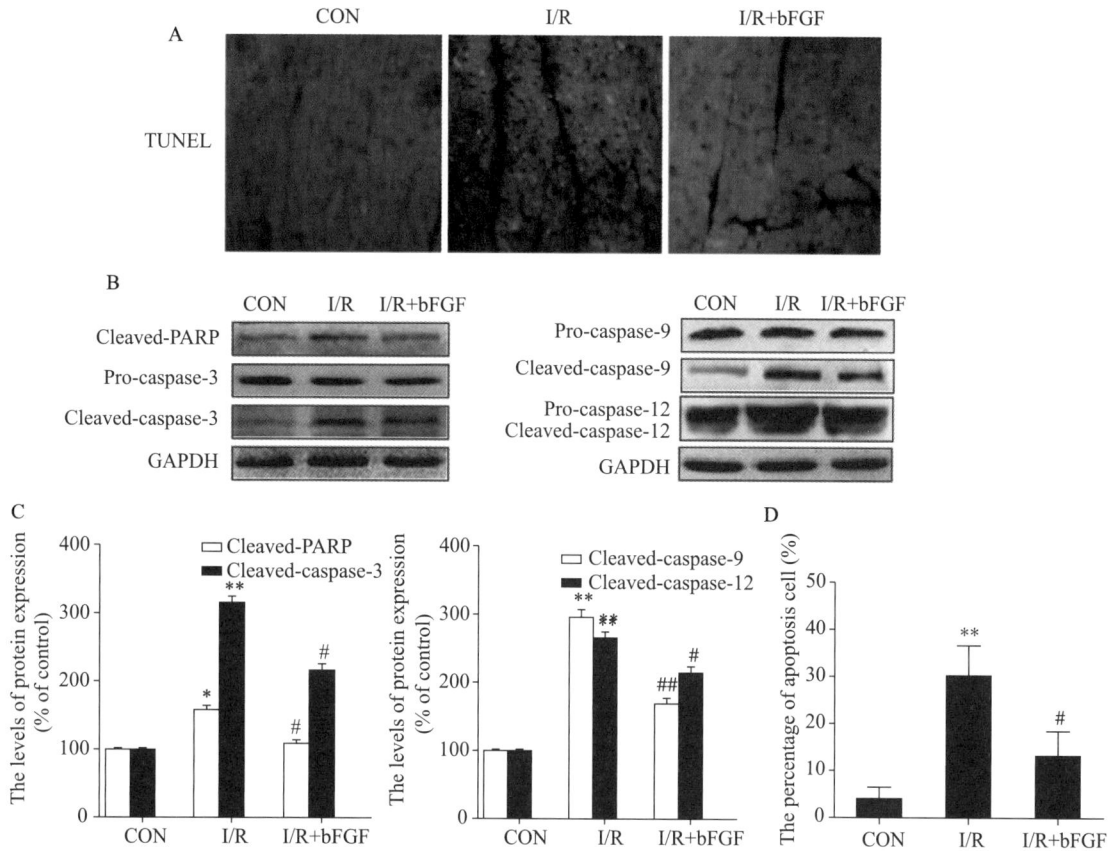

Fig. 1. Basic fibroblast growth factor (bFGF) reduces myocardial apoptosis and the caspase cascade pathway in the hearts of mice after myocardial ischaemia/reperfusion. (A) Representative terminal deoxynucleotidyl transferase-mediated dUTP nick end labelling (TUNEL) immunofluorescence of sections from the ischaemic area in the hearts of mice that received bFGF or vehicle. (B) The detection of endoplasmic reticulum (ER) stress-related and mitochondrial dysfunction-related apoptosis proteins was performed by western blotting. The protein expression levels of cleaved-PARP, caspase-3, caspase-9 and caspase-12 in the hearts of control, ischaemia/reperfusion (I/R) mice and I/R mice treated with bFGF. (C) The optical density analysis of cleaved-PARP, caspase-3, caspase-9 and caspase-12 in the heart. (D) The percentage of apoptosis was counted from three random 1 mm2 areas. $^*P < 0.05$, $^{**}P < 0.01$, $vs.$ the Control group, $^#P < 0.05$, $^{##}P < 0.01$ $vs.$ the I/R group; $n = 6$.

significantly after 4 h of ischaemia reperfusion, and the bFGF treatment group showed significant protective effects.

To further confirm the protective effect of bFGF, the protein expression levels of the caspase cascade pathway in the heart after myocardial ischaemia reperfusion were detected by western blot. We found that the levels of the cleaved-PARP, cleaved-caspase-3, cleaved-caspase-9 and cleaved-caspase-12 proteins decreased significantly after bFGF treatment compared with the I/R group 4 h after injury (Fig. 1B, C). Our data indicated that bFGF administration has a cardioprotective effect and significantly reduces caspase cascade pathway activation.

3.2 bFGF inhibits ER stress and mitochondrial dysfunction in myocardial I/R mouse

To determine whether the cardioprotective effect of bFGF is related to ER stress and mitochondrial dysfunction, we measured the expression of ER stress and mitochondrial dysfunction proteins. Our western blot results indicated that the protein levels of C/EBP homologous protein (CHOP), 78 kD GRP-78, ATF-6 and cleaved caspase-12 were significantly up-regulated in the hearts of I/R mice when compared with the sham group. Moreover, bFGF treatment inhibited the activation of ER stress-related proteins in the hearts of I/R mice (Fig. 2A). We also determined via CHOP, GRP-78 and cleaved caspase-12 immunofluorescent analysis that there are few ER stress protein-positive cells in the control group. The numbers of ER stress protein-positive cells increased significantly after 4 h of ischaemia reperfusion, and the bFGF treatment group showed significant protective effects (Fig. 3A). In addition, western blot and immunofluorescent results all suggested that bFGF inhibits the up-regulation of mitochondrial dysfunction-related proteins cytochrome c (Cyt c), Bax and Bcl-2, which were induced by I/R injury (Figs. 2B, 3A). To further understand the mechanism underlying behind the effect of bFGF on I/R injury, the activation of PI3K/Akt and ERK1/2 downstream signals were also analysed by western blot. As expected, bFGF treatment increased the phosphorylation of Akt and ERK1/2 in the hearts of I/R mice when compared with controls (Fig. 2C, D). Taken together, these results suggest that the protective role of bFGF in I/R injury is related to the inhibition of ER stress and mitochondrial dysfunction through the activation of the PI3K/Akt and ERK1/2 signaling pathways.

3.3 bFGF reduces oxidative stress-induced cell death in H9C2 cells

To establish a suitable concentration of TBHP and bFGF in H9C2 cells, we conducted dose-response experiments (Fig. 4A) and determined that TBHP incubation resulted in dose-dependent cell death after 8 h exposure. In addition, bFGF increased cell viability at concentrations under 75 ng/ml (Fig. 4B). Based on these data, 100 μM TBHP and 50 ng/ml bFGF were chosen for subsequent experiments. To further confirm the effect of bFGF on TBHP-induced apoptosis, cells were subjected to PI and Annexin V-FITC staining, and the apoptotic cells were then quantified by FACS. As

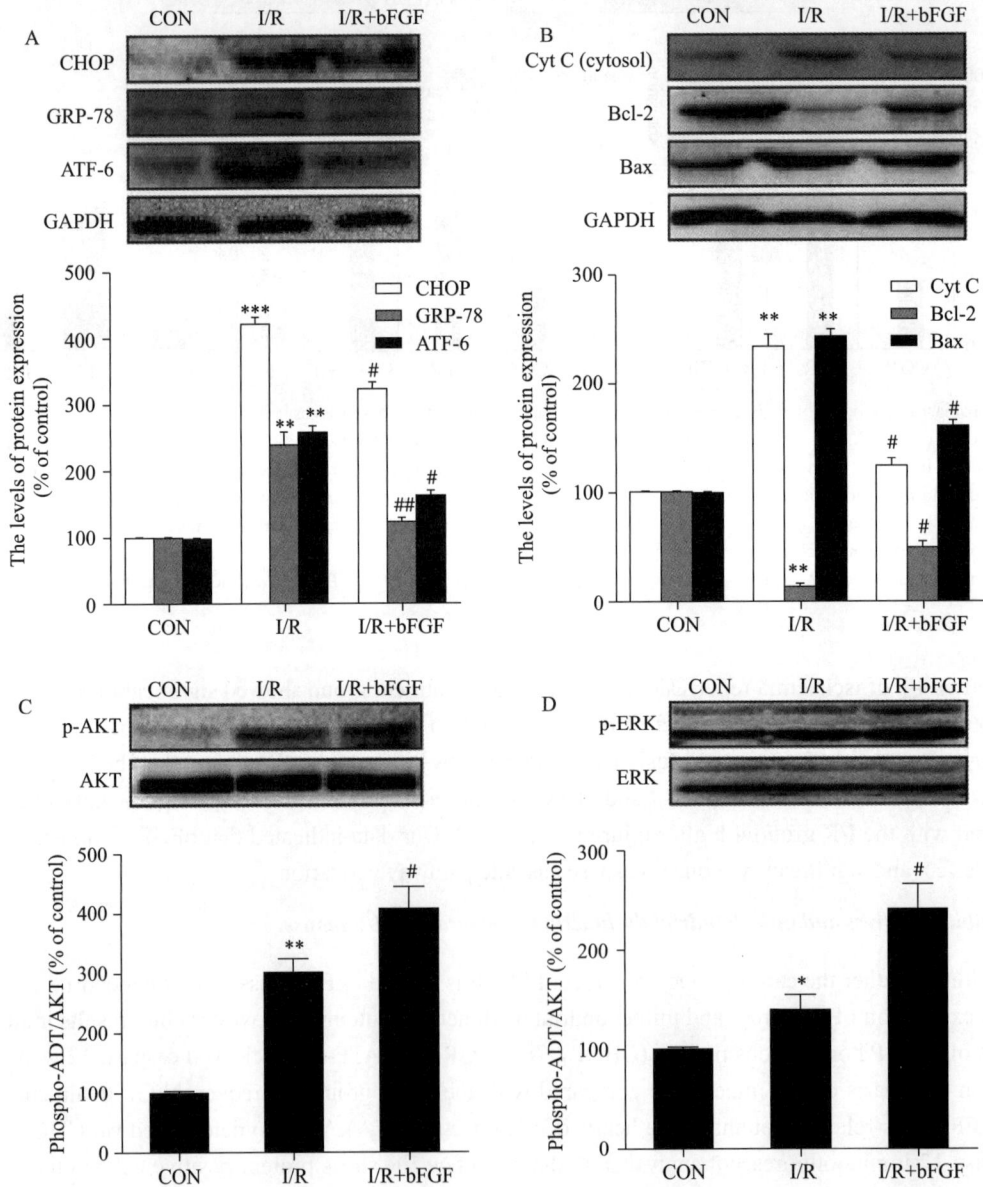

Fig. 2. The effect of basic fibroblast growth factor (bFGF) on endoplasmic reticulum (ER) stress and mitochondrial dysfunction-related proteins in the hearts of mice after myocardial ischaemia/reperfusion (I/R). (A) The protein expression levels and optical density analysis of CHOP, GRP-78 and ATF-6 in the hearts of control, I/R mice and I/R mice treated with bFGF. (B) The protein expression levels and optical density analysis of Cyt c, Bcl-2 and Bax in the hearts of control, I/R mice and I/R mice treated with bFGF. (C) The protein expression levels and optical density analysis of p-AKT and AKT in the heart. (D) The protein expression levels and optical density analysis of p-ERK and ERK in the heart. $^{*}P < 0.05$, $^{**}P < 0.01$, vs. the control group, $^{#}P < 0.05$, $^{##}P < 0.01$ vs. the I/R group; $n = 6$.

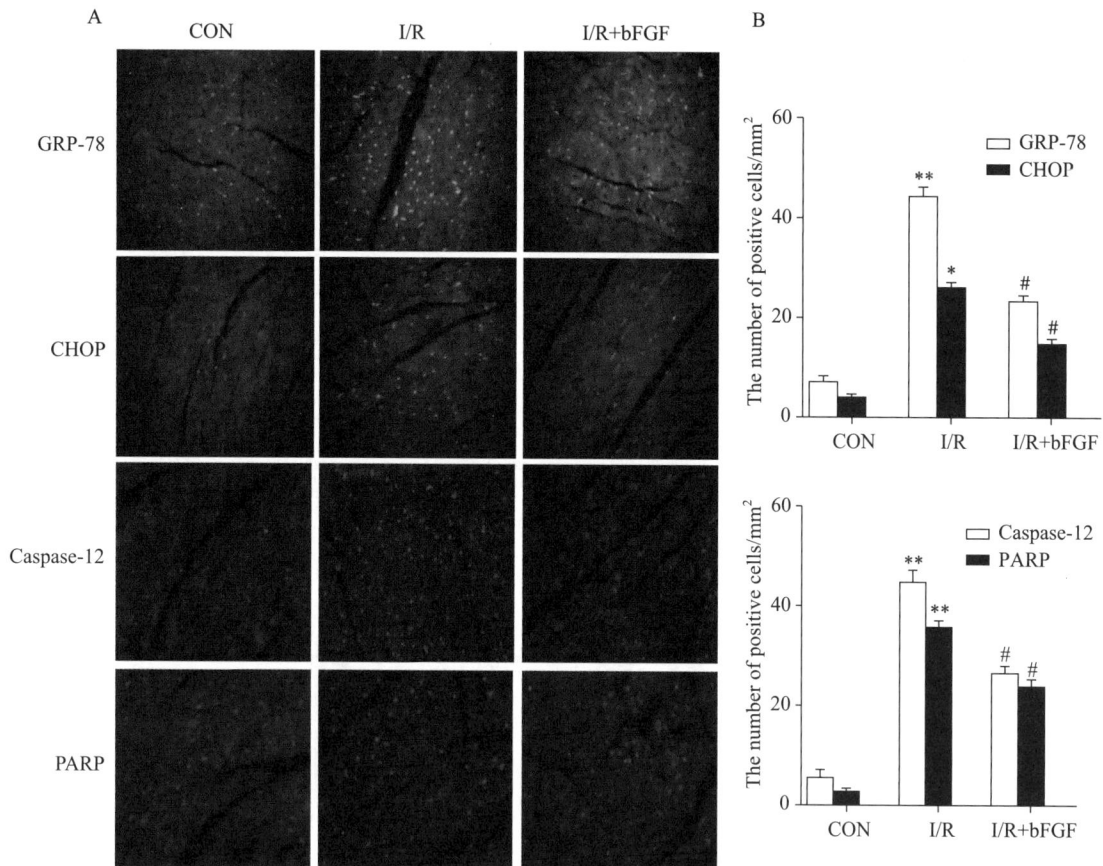

Fig. 3. Immunofluorescent staining of endoplasmic reticulum (ER) stress and mitochondrial dysfunction-related proteins in the hearts of mice. (A) Immunofluorescent staining for GRP-78, CHOP, cleaved caspase-12 and cleaved-PARP in the hearts of control, ischaemia/reperfusion (I/R) mice and I/R mice treated with basic fibroblast growth factor (bFGF). (B) Analysis of the positive cells of the immunofluorescent results. $^{*}P < 0.05$, $^{**}P < 0.01$, *vs.* the control group, $P < 0.05$, *vs.* the I/R group; $n = 5$.

shown in Fig. 4C and D, TBHP-induced apoptosis was decreased after treatment with bFGF. The apoptotic cells were also detected by TUNEL assay, producing results consistent with the flow cytometry results indicating that apoptosis was suppressed by bFGF treatment. Our results suggested that bFGF inhibits TBHP-induced apoptosis and may play a protective role in oxidative stress injury in H9C2 cells.

3.4　bFGF decreases ER stress and mitochondrial dysfunction-induced apoptosis in H9C2 cells

To investigate whether the apoptosis induced by TBHP and the effect of bFGF were related to chronic ER stress and mitochondrial dysfunction in H9C2 cells, the levels of the ER stress and mitochondrial dysfunction-related proteins were measured by western blot or immunofluorescent analysis. As shown in Fig. 5, the expression of CHOP, cleaved caspase-12, GRP-78 and ATF-6 were higher in the TBHP-treated group than in the control group. bFGF treatment significantly inhibited the ER stress-related proteins that had been induced by TBHP. On the other hand (Fig. 6A and B), the mitochondrial dysfunction-related proteins Bax, Bcl-2, cleaved-PARP, cleaved-caspase-9 and cytochrome *c* were also significantly increased in the TBHP-treated group, whereas these proteins attenuated significantly after bFGF treatment. Taken together, our data suggest that the protective role of bFGF may involve the inhibition of ER stress-related and mitochondrial dysfunction-related proteins.

3.5　bFGF activate the PI3K/Akt and ERK1/2 pathways

Based on our previous experiments, we hypothesized that the PI3K/Akt and ERK1/2 pathways may be involved in the bFGF-mediated inhibition of ER stress and mitochondrial dysfunction in an oxidative stress injury model. As shown in Fig. 7A and B, an increase in p-Akt and p-ERK1/2 was observed in the cells exposed to TBHP compared with the

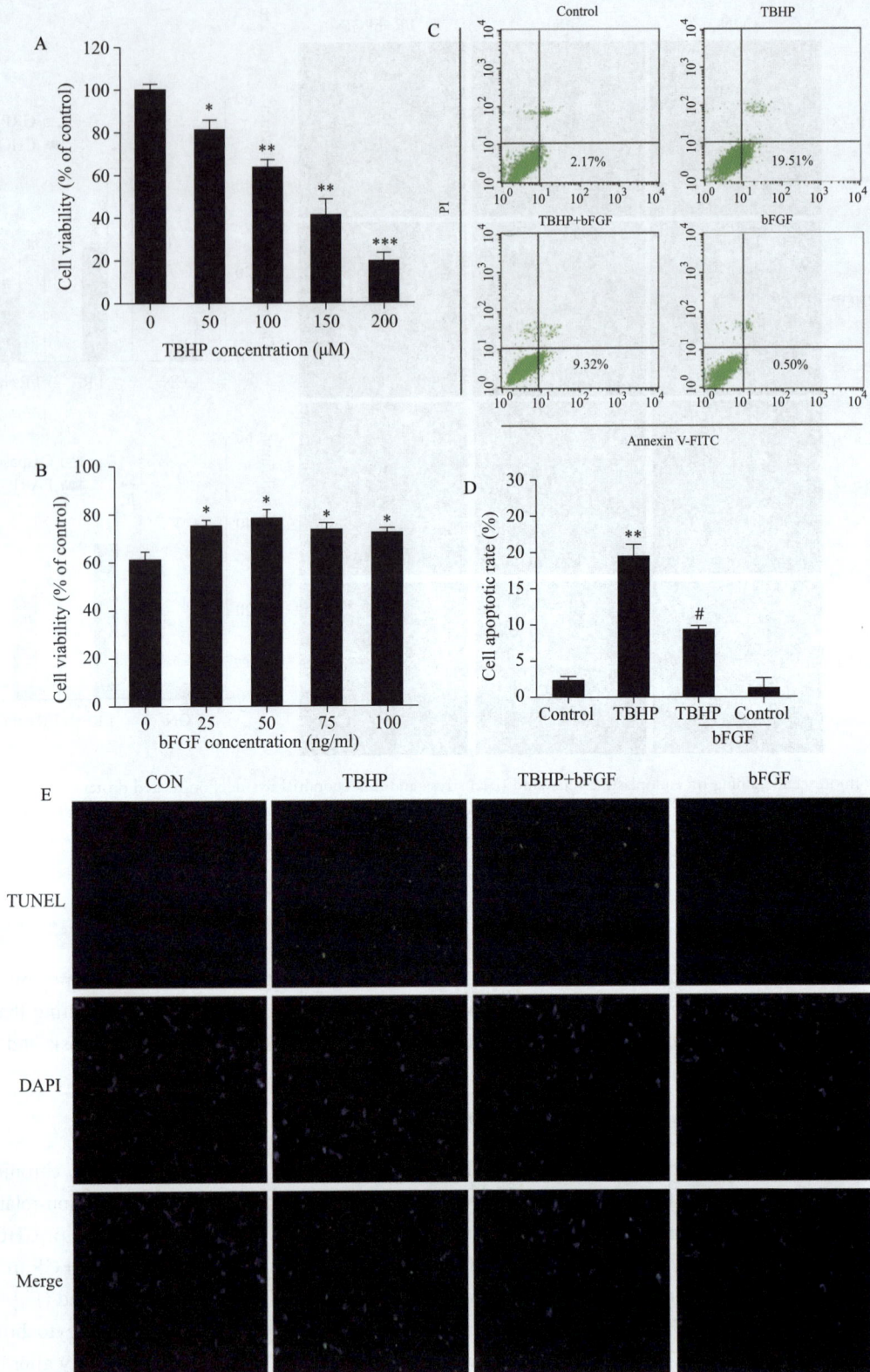

Fig. 4. Basic fibroblast growth factor (bFGF) inhibits apoptosis induced by hydroperoxide (TBHP) in H9C2 cells. (A) PC12 cells were treated with different concentrations of TBHP (0, 50, 100, 150, 200 μM) for 8 h, and then cell viability was assessed by the 3-(4,5-Dimethylthiazol-2-yl)-2,5-diphenyltetrazolium bromide (MTT) assay. (B) H9C2 cells were pre-treated with bFGF (0, 25, 50, 75, 100 ng/ml) for 2 h, 100 μM TBHP was added for an additional 8 h, and then cell viability was assessed by the MTT assay. (C) H9C2 cells were pre-treated with 50 ng/ml bFGF for 2 h, and then 100 μM TBHP was added for an additional 8 h. Cells were then stained with Annexin V-FITC/propidium iodide and detected by flow cytometry; the lower right panel indicates the apoptotic cells. (D) Bar diagram of apoptotic cell rates from three separate experiments. (E) Detection of apoptotic cells by TUNEL (green) and DAPI (blue) staining assay. $^*P < 0.05$, $^{**}P < 0.01$, vs. the control group, $^#P < 0.05$, $^{##}P < 0.01$ vs. the TBHP group.

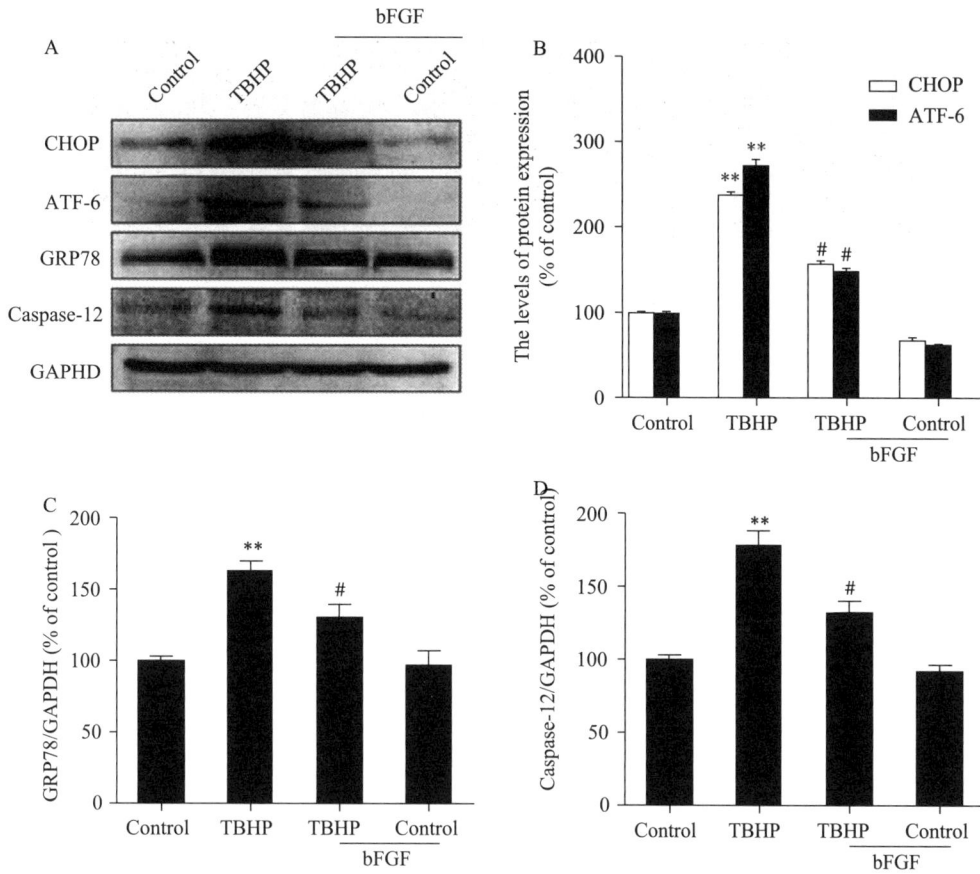

Fig. 5. Basic fibroblast growth factor (bFGF) attenuates endoplasmic reticulum (ER) stress-related proteins induced by hydroperoxide (TBHP) in H9C2 cells. (A) H9C2 cells were pre-treated with 50 ng/ml bFGF for 2 h, and then 100 μM TBHP was added for an additional 8 h. The cell lysates were analysed for the expression of CHOP, GRP-78, ATF-6 and caspase-12 by western blotting. Bar diagram of (B) CHOP, ATF-6, (C) GRP-78 and (D) caspase-12 expression from three Western blot analyses. $^*P < 0.05$, $^{**}P < 0.01$, *vs.* the control group, $^#P < 0.05$, $^{##}P < 0.01$ *vs.* the TBHP group.

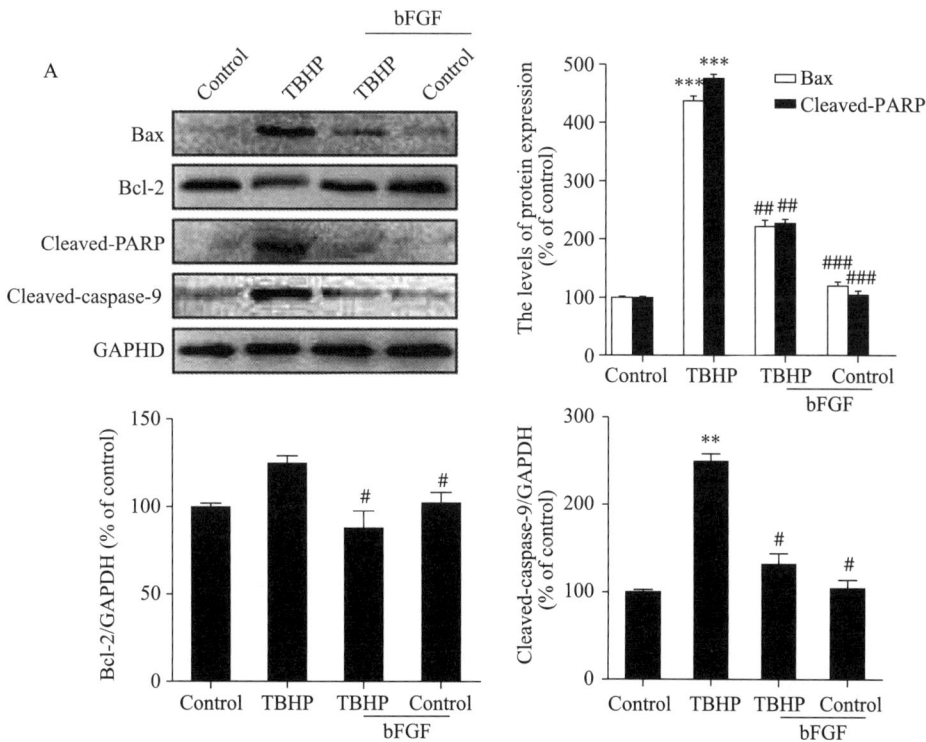

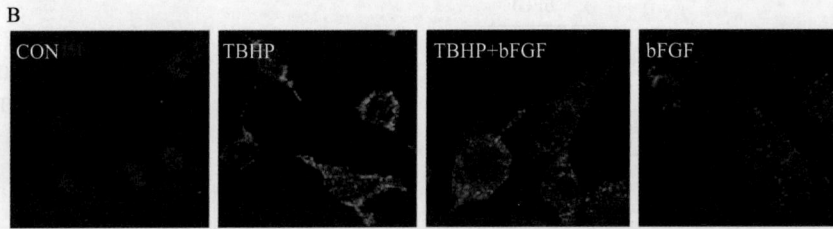

Fig. 6. The effect of basic fibroblast growth factor (bFGF) on mitochondrial dysfunction-related proteins induced by hydroperoxide (TBHP) in H9C2 cells. (A) H9C2 cells were pre-treated with 50 ng/ml bFGF for 2 h, and then 100 μM TBHP was added for an additional 8 h. The cell lysates were analysed for the expression of Bax, Bcl-2, cleaved-PARP and cleaved-caspase-9 by western blotting. Bar diagram of Bax, Bcl-2, cleaved-PARP and cleaved-caspase-9 expression from three Western blot analyses. (B) Immunofluorescence results of the mitochondrial apoptotic marker cytochrome c in H9C2 cells. $^{*}P < 0.05$, $^{**}P < 0.01$, $vs.$ the control group, $^{#}P < 0.05$, $^{##}P < 0.01$ $vs.$ the TBHP group.

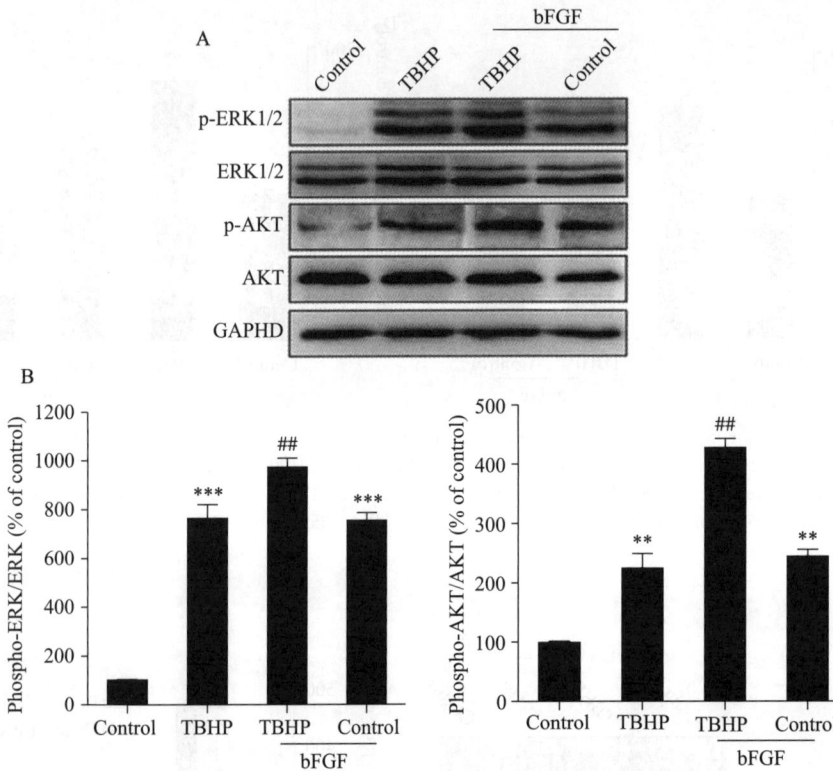

Fig. 7. Basic fibroblast growth factor (bFGF) activates PI3K/Akt and ERK1/2 in H9C2 cells. (A) H9C2 cells were pre-treated with 50 ng/ml bFGF for 2 h, and then 100 μM hydroperoxide (TBHP) was added for an additional 8 h. The cell lysates were analysed by western blotting for the expression of phospho-Akt, Akt, phospho-ERK and ERK. (B) Bar diagram of phospho-Akt/Akt and phosphorylated-ERK/ERK levels from three Western blot analyses. GAPDH was used as a protein loading control and for band density normalization. $^{*}P < 0.05$, $^{**}P < 0.01$, $vs.$ the control group, $^{#}P < 0.05$, $^{##}P < 0.01$ $vs.$ the TBHP group.

control group. The pre-treatment of bFGF significantly increased the activation of the PI3K/Akt and ERK1/2 pathways in the H9C2 cells exposed to TBHP. These data suggest that both the PI3K/ Akt and ERK1/2 pathways are involved in the protective effect of bFGF.

3.6 Inhibition of the PI3K/Akt and ERK1/2 pathway partially reverses the protective effect of bFGF

To further confirm the important role of PI3K/Akt and ERK1/2 activation by bFGF, the PI3K inhibitor LY294002 and the ERK1/2 inhibitor PD98059 were added to the media. LY294002 and PD98059 inhibited the activation of Akt and ERK1/2, respectively, when compared with the bFGF group (Fig. 8A, B). Moreover, the expression of CHOP, GRP-78, cleaved caspase-12 and ATF-6 increased after the combined exposure to LY294002 and PD98059 when compared with the bFGF treatment group (Fig. 7A, C). In addition, LY294002 and PD98059 can also reverse the inhibitory effect

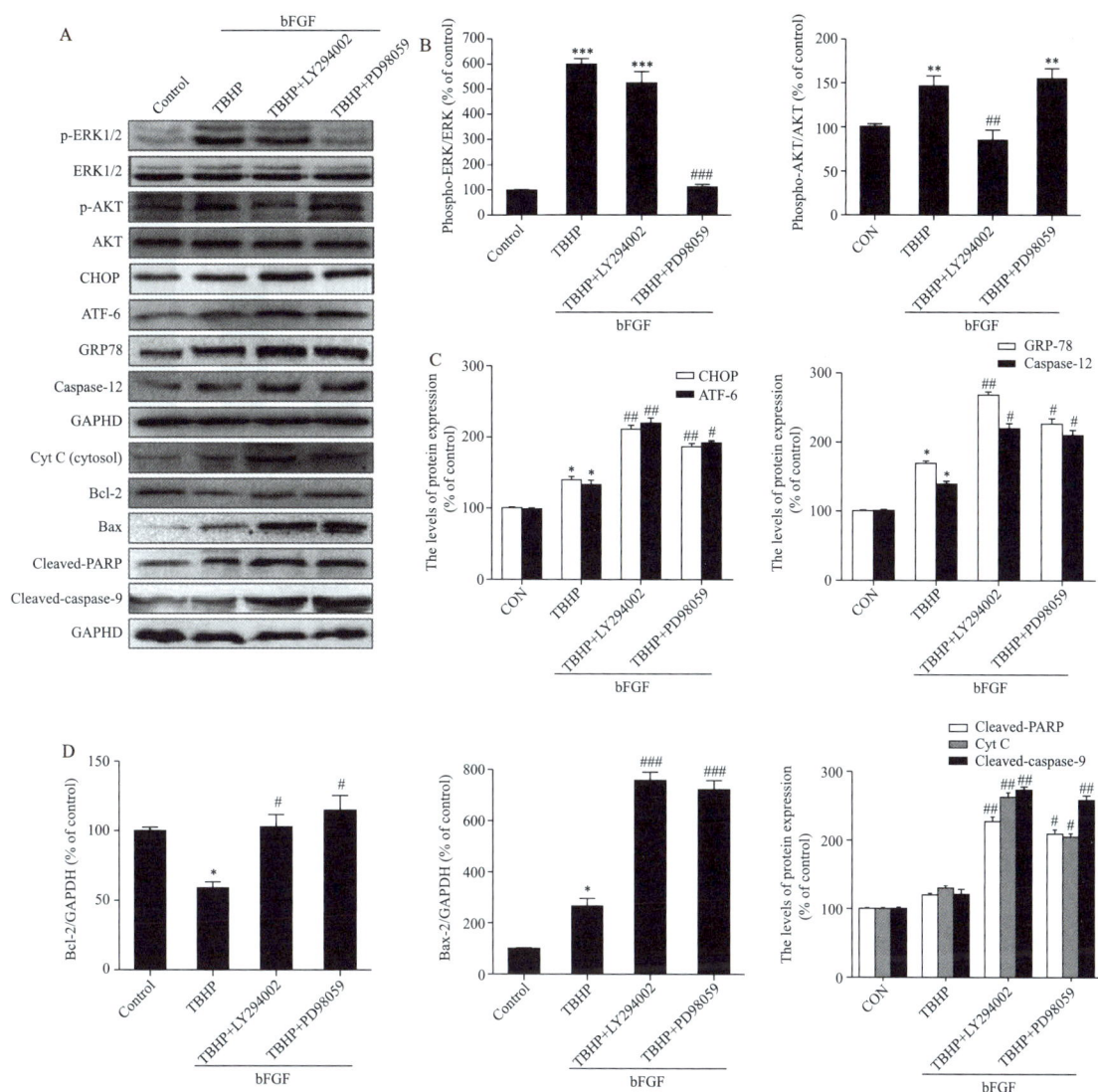

Fig. 8. Inhibition of the PI3K/Akt and ERK1/2 pathways partially attenuates the basic fibroblast growth factor (bFGF)-mediated reduction in the endoplasmic reticulum (ER) stress and mitochondrial dysfunction effects in H9C2 cells. H9C2 cells were pre-treated with 50 ng/ml bFGF with or without the specific inhibitors LY294002 (20 μM) and PD98059 (20 μM) for 2 h, and then 100 μM hydroperoxide (TBHP) was added for an additional 8 h. The cell lysates were analysed by western blotting to detect the expression of phospho-Akt, phospho-ERK and ERK, CHOP, GRP-78, ATF-6, caspase-12, Bax, Bcl-2, Cyt c, cleaved-PARP and cleaved-caspase-9. Bar diagram of the (B) phospho-Akt/Akt ratio, phospho-ERK/ERK ratio, (C) CHOP, GRP-78, ATF-6 and caspase-12, (D) Bax, Bcl-2, Cyt c, cleaved-PARP and cleaved-caspase-9 expression from three Western blot analyses. GAPDH was used as a protein loading control and for band density normalization. $^*P < 0.05$, $^{**}P < 0.01$ and $^{***}P < 0.001$ vs. the control group, $^#P < 0.05$, $^{##}P < 0.01$ vs. the TBHP group.

of bFGF on the expression of Bax, Bcl-2, cleaved-PARP, cleaved-caspase-9 and Cyt c. These results suggest that the mitochondrial dysfunction and ER stress-induced apoptosis were aggravated by the addition of Akt or ERK inhibitors. The apoptotic cell rate was determined by FACS. As shown in Fig. 9A and B, the addition of LY294002 or PD98059 significantly increased cell apoptosis when compared with the bFGF group. All of these results suggest that the protective effect of bFGF is mediated by both the PI3K/Akt and ERK1/2 signaling pathways.

4. Discussion

Ischaemic heart disease secondary to acute myocardial infarction, is among the most prevalent health problems in the world and is a major cause of morbidity and mortality. After ischaemia, myocardial reperfusion is followed by a long period of secondary myocardial injury that may include oxidative stress, inflammation, necrosis and

from ischaemia/reperfusion heart disease.

References

[1] Forouzanfar MH, Moran AE, Flaxman AD, et al. Assessing the Global Burden of Ischemic Heart Disease Part 2: Analytic Methods and Estimates of the Global Epidemiology of Ischemic Heart Disease in 2010[J]. Global Heart, 2012, 7(4): 331-342.

[2] Penna C, Perrelli MG, Tullio F, et al. Diazoxide postconditioning induces mitochondrial protein S-Nitrosylation and a redox-sensitive mitochondrial phosphorylation/translocation of RISK elements: no role for SAFE[J]. Basic Research In Cardiology, 2013, 108: 371.

[3] Heusch G. Cardioprotection: chances and challenges of its translation to the clinic[J]. Lancet, 2013, 381(9861): 166-175.

[4] Tullio F, Angotti C, Perrelli M-G, et al. Redox balance and cardioprotection[J]. Basic Research In Cardiology, 2013, 108: 392.

[5] Wang YP, Schmeichel AM, Iida H, et al. Ischemia-reperfusion injury causes oxidative stress and apoptosis of Schwann cell in acute and chronic experimental diabetic neuropathy[J]. Antioxidants & Redox Signaling, 2005, 7(11-12): 1513-1520.

[6] Wang Z, Zhang H, Xu X, et al. bFGF inhibits ER stress induced by ischemic oxidative injury via activation of the PI3K/Akt and ERK1/2 pathways[J]. Toxicology Letters, 2012, 212(2): 137-146.

[7] Xiao J, Lv Y, Lin S, et al. Cardiac Protection by Basic Fibroblast Growth Factor from Ischemia/Reperfusion-Induced Injury in Diabetic Rats[J]. Biological & Pharmaceutical Bulletin, 2010, 33(3): 444-449.

[8] Wang X, Lin G, Martins-Taylor K, et al. Inhibition of Caspase-mediated Anoikis Is Critical for Basic Fibroblast Growth Factor-sustained Culture of Human Pluripotent Stem Cells[J]. Journal Of Biological Chemistry, 2009, 284(49): 34054-34064.

[9] Detillieux KA, Sheikh F, Kardami E, et al. Biological activities of fibroblast growth factor-2 in the adult myocardium[J]. Cardiovascular Research, 2003, 57(1): 8-19.

[10] Sheikh F, Sontag DP, Fandrich RR, et al. Overexpression of FGF-2 increases cardiac myocyte viability after injury in isolated mouse hearts[J]. American Journal Of Physiology-Heart And Circulatory Physiology, 2001, 280(3): H1039-H1050.

[11] Jiang ZS, Padua RR, Ju HS, et al. Acute protection of ischemic heart by FGF-2: involvement of FGF-2 receptors and protein kinase C[J]. American Journal Of Physiology-Heart And Circulatory Physiology, 2002, 282(3): H1071-H1080.

[12] Machado NG, Alves MG, Carvalho RA, et al. Mitochondrial Involvement in Cardiac Apoptosis During Ischemia and Reperfusion: Can We Close the Box?[J]. Cardiovascular Toxicology, 2009, 9(4): 211-227.

[13] Lee CF, Liu CY, Chen SM, et al. Attenuation of UV-induced apoptosis by coenzyme Q10 in human cells harboring large-scale deletion of mitochondrial DNA[J]. Ann N Y Acad Sci., 2005, 1042: 429-438.

[14] Apostolova N, Gomez-Sucerquia LJ, Moran A, et al. Enhanced oxidative stress and increased mitochondrial mass during Efavirenz-induced apoptosis in human hepatic cells[J]. British Journal Of Pharmacology, 2010, 160(8): 2069-2084.

[15] Buja LM, Entman ML. Modes of myocardial cell injury and cell death in ischemic heart disease[J]. Circulation, 1998, 98(14): 1355-1357.

[16] Heusch G, Boengler K, Schulz R. Cardioprotection Nitric Oxide, Protein Kinases, and Mitochondria[J]. Circulation, 2008, 118(19): 1915-1919.

[17] Takahashi K, Takatani T, Uozumi Y, et al. Molecular mechanisms of cardioprotection by taurine on ischemia-induced apoptosis in cultured cardiomyocytes[J]. Adv Exp Med Biol., 2006, 583: 257-263.

[18] Liu ZW, Zhu HT, Chen KL, et al. Protein kinase RNA-like endoplasmic reticulum kinase (PERK) signaling pathway plays a major role in reactive oxygen species (ROS)-mediated endoplasmic reticulum stress-induced apoptosis in diabetic cardiomyopathy[J]. Cardiovascular Diabetology, 2013, 12: 158.

[19] Malhotra JD, Kaufman RJ. Endoplasmic reticulum stress and oxidative stress: A vicious cycle or a double-edged sword?[J]. Antioxidants & Redox Signaling, 2007, 9(12): 2277-2293.

[20] Sun X, Chen RC, Yang ZH, et al. Taxifolin prevents diabetic cardiomyopathy in vivo and in vitro by inhibition of oxidative stress and cell apoptosis[J]. Food And Chemical Toxicology, 2014, 63: 221-232.

[21] Qi XF, Zheng L, Lee KJ, et al. HMG-CoA reductase inhibitors induce apoptosis of lymphoma cells by promoting ROS generation and regulating Akt, Erk and p38 signals via suppression of mevalonate pathway[J]. Cell Death & Disease, 2013, 4: e518.

[22] Ding W, Yang L, Zhang M, et al. Reactive oxygen species-mediated endoplasmic reticulum stress contributes to aldosterone-induced apoptosis in tubular epithelial cells[J]. Biochemical And Biophysical Research Communications, 2012, 418(3): 451-456.

[23] Li Z, Zhang T, Dai H, et al. Involvement of endoplasmic reticulum stress in myocardial apoptosis of streptozocin-induced diabetic rats[J]. Journal Of Clinical Biochemistry And Nutrition, 2007, 41(1): 58-67.

[24] Nakagawa T, Zhu H, Morishima N, et al. Caspase-12 mediates endoplasmic-reticulum-specific apoptosis and cytotoxicity by amyloid-beta[J]. Nature, 2000, 403(6765): 98-103.

[25] Manning JR, Perkins SO, Sinclair EA, et al. Low molecular weight fibroblast growth factor-2 signals via protein kinase C and myofibrillar proteins to protect against postischemic cardiac dysfunction[J]. American Journal Of Physiology-Heart And Circulatory Physiology, 2013, 304(10): H1382-H1396.

[26] Sontag DP, Wang J, Kardami E, et al. FGF-2 and FGF-16 Protect Isolated Perfused Mouse Hearts from Acute Doxorubicin-Induced Contractile Dysfunction[J]. Cardiovascular Toxicology, 2013, 13(3): 244-253.

[27] Starkov AA, Polster BM, Fiskum G. Regulation of hydrogen peroxide production by brain mitochondria by calcium and Bax[J]. Journal Of Neurochemistry, 2002, 83(1): 220-228.

[28] Iwawaki T, Hosoda A, Okuda T, et al. Translational control by the ER transmembrane kinase/ribonuclease IRE1 under ER stress[J]. Nature Cell Biology, 2001, 3(2): 158-164.

[29] Brocheriou V, Hagege AA, Oubenaissa A, et al. Cardiac functional improvement by a human Bcl-2 transgene in a mouse model of ischemia/reperfusion injury[J]. Journal Of Gene Medicine, 2000, 2(5): 326-333.

[30] Chen ZY, Chua CC, Ho YS, et al. Overexpression of Bcl-2 attenuates apoptosis and protects against myocardial I/R injury in transgenic mice[J]. American Journal Of Physiology-Heart And Circulatory Physiology, 2001, 280(5): H2313-H2320.

[31] Hochhauser E, Kivity S, Offen D, et al. Bax ablation protects against myocardial ischemia-reperfusion injury in transgenic mice[J]. American Journal Of Physiology-Heart And Circulatory Physiology, 2003, 284(6): H2351-H2359.

[32] Hammadi M, Oulidi A, Gackiere F, et al. Modulation of ER stress and apoptosis by endoplasmic reticulum calcium leak via translocon during unfolded protein response: involvement of GRP78[J]. Faseb Journal, 2013, 27(4): 1600-1609.

[33] Wu T, Dong Z, Geng J, et al. Valsartan protects against ER stress-

induced myocardial apoptosis *via* CHOP/Puma signaling pathway in streptozotocin-induced diabetic rats[J]. European Journal Of Pharmaceutical Sciences, 2011, 42(5): 496-502.

[34] Zhang Z, Tong N, Gong Y, *et al.* Valproate protects the retina from endoplasmic reticulum stress-induced apoptosis after ischemia-reperfusion injury[J]. Neuroscience Letters, 2011, 504(2): 88-92.

[35] Belaidi E, Decorps J, Augeul L, *et al.* Endoplasmic reticulum stress contributes to heart protection induced by cyclophilin D inhibition[J]. Basic Research In Cardiology, 2013, 108(4).

[36] Yang C, Wang Y, Liu H, *et al.* Ghrelin Protects H9C2 Cardiomyocytes From Angiotensin II-induced Apoptosis Through the Endoplasmic Reticulum Stress Pathway[J]. Journal Of Cardiovascular Pharmacology, 2012, 59(5): 465-471.

[37] Kim DS, Ha KC, Kwon DY, *et al.* Kaempferol protects ischemia/reperfusion-induced cardiac damage through the regulation of endoplasmic reticulum stress[J]. Immunopharmacology And Immunotoxicology, 2008, 30(2): 257-270.

[38] Beenken A, Mohammadi M. The FGF family: biology, pathophysiology and therapy[J]. Nature Reviews Drug Discovery, 2009, 8(3): 235-253.

[39] Boyce M, Yuan J. Cellular response to endoplasmic reticulum stress: a matter of life or death[J]. Cell Death And Differentiation, 2006, 13(3): 363-373.

[40] Brunet A, Bonni A, Zigmond MJ, *et al.* Akt promotes cell survival by phosphorylating and inhibiting a forkhead transcription factor[J]. Cell, 1999, 96(6): 857-868.

[41] Yuan Y, Xue X, Guo RB, *et al.* Resveratrol Enhances the Antitumor Effects of Temozolomide in Glioblastoma *via* ROS-dependent AMPK-TSC-mTOR Signaling Pathway[J]. CNS Neuroscience & Therapeutics, 2012, 18(7): 536-546.

[42] Zhang H, Kong X, Kang J, *et al.* Oxidative Stress Induces Parallel Autophagy and Mitochondria Dysfunction in Human Glioma U251 Cells[J]. Toxicological Sciences, 2009, 110(2): 376-388.

[43] Datta SR, Dudek H, Tao X, *et al.* Akt phosphorylation of BAD couples survival signals to the cell-intrinsic death machinery[J]. Cell, 1997, 91(2): 231-241.

[44] Yin Y, Guan Y, Duan J, *et al.* Cardioprotective effect of Danshensu against myocardial ischemia/reperfusion injury and inhibits apoptosis of H9C2 cardiomyocytes *via* Akt and ERK1/2 phosphorylation[J]. European Journal Of Pharmacology, 2013, 699(1-3): 219-226.

[45] Zhang HY, Zhang X, Wang ZG, *et al.* Exogenous Basic Fibroblast Growth Factor Inhibits ER Stress-Induced Apoptosis and Improves Recovery from Spinal Cord Injury[J]. CNS Neuroscience & Therapeutics, 2013, 19(1): 20-29.

Selection of a novel FGF23-binding peptide antagonizing the inhibitory effect of FGF23 on phosphate uptake

Tao Huang, Xiaokun Li, Xiaoping Wu

1. Introduction

Hypophosphatemia is a common clinical condition and mainly originates from the renal phosphate wasting in which the renal tubular reabsorption of phosphate is impaired (Imel and Econs, 2005; Negri, 2007). Replacement therapy including oral administration or intravenous injection (i.v.) of inorganic phosphate salts is the primary means for current clinical treatment of hypophosphatemia. However, the occurrence of diverse complications including diarrhea, gastric irritation (Shiber and Mattu, 2002), and metastatic calcification (Gaasbeek and Meinders, 2005) are currently observed in patients subjected to the replacement therapy. Moreover, renal phosphate wasting is still significant with the replacement therapy, which only remiss hypophosphatemia by temporarily supplementing the inorganic phosphate. Therefore, understanding the precise mechanisms of renal phosphate wasting will greatly contribute to the development of novel strategies with high efficacy and low side effect for hypophosphatemia therapy.

Fibroblast growth factor 23 (FGF23) belongs to the FGF19 subfamily consisting of FGF19, FGF21, and FGF23 (Yamashita *et al.*, 2000). Compared with other FGF subfamilies which regulate cell proliferation, differentiation, and migration, the FGF19 subfamily members appear to serve as metabolic regulators and hormones (Benet-Pages *et al.* 2005; Inagaki *et al.*, 2005; Kharitonenkov *et al.*, 2005; Kobayashi *et al.*, 2006a, b; Larsson *et al.*, 2004; Shimada *et al.*, 2004; Strewler, 2001; Yu and White, 2005). Accumulating evidences showed that FGF23 is an essential regulator of phosphate homeostasis by inhibiting phosphate uptake by renal proximal tubule epithelium. Increased plasma levels of FGF23 are found in hypophosphatemia patients. As FGF23 is the pathogenic factor in phosphate wasting disorders including autosomal dominant hypophosphatemic rickets (ADHR), tumor-induced osteomalacia (TIO), X-linked hypophosphatemic rickets (XLH), and fibrous dysplasia (FD), targeting FGF23 may provide the causative pharmacotherapy for hypophosphatemia.

The phage display technology is a useful tool for identifying peptides with desirable biological properties. In previous studies, we have used phage display technology to isolate a high-affinity bFGF-binding peptide (named P7) with strong inhibitory activity against bFGF-induced cell proliferation and angiogenesis (Wang *et al.*, 2010; Wu *et al.*, 2010, 2011). Results suggest that P7 peptide blocks the biological activities of bFGF by interrupting its interactions with its receptors. Herein, we attempt to isolate a high-affinity FGF23-binding peptide from a phage display library and evaluate its effects on the phosphaturic actions of FGF23.

2. Materials and methods

2.1 Materials

Ph.D.-7™ Phage Display Peptide Library Kit (complexity ~2.8×10^9 transformants) including *Escherichia coli* ER2738 host strain and −96 gIII sequencing primer (5′-CCCTCA TAGTTAGCGTAACG-3′) was purchased from New England Biolabs (Beverly, MA, USA). The recombinant human FGF23, FGF21, and bFGF were obtained from Pepro-Tech (Rocky Hill, NJ, USA). The FGF23$_{180-205}$ fragment was synthesized by SBS Genetech (Beijing, China). The opossum kidney cells (OK cells) were from the American Type Culture Collection (Manassas, VA, USA). RPMI 1640 and fetal bovine serum (FBS) were purchased from Invitrogen (Carlsbad, CA, USA). Phosphate Colorimetric Assay Kit was from BioVision (San Francisco, CA, USA). Anti-phospho-Erk1/2, anti-Erk1/2, anti-phospho-P38, anti-P38, anti-phospho-Akt, anti-Akt antibodies, and goat anti-rabbit IgG conjugated with horseradish peroxidase (HRP) antibody were from Cell Signaling Technology (Danvers, MA, USA). TRIZOL reagent and First-Strand cDNA Synthesis Kit were purchased from Bio-Rad (Hercules, CA, USA). DreamTaq Green PCR Master Mix (2×) was from Thermo Scientific (Waltham, MA, USA).

2.2 Phage biopanning

A sterile polystyrene petri dish (35×10 mm^2) was coated with 1 000 μg of the synthetic FGF23$_{180–205}$ at 4℃ in 0.1 M NaHCO$_3$ (pH 8.6). After coated overnight, the dish was further blocked with bovine serum albumin (BSA) at 5 mg/ml in 0.1 M NaHCO$_3$ for 2 h at room temperature, and washed six times (1 min each) with PBS containing 0.05% Tween-20 (0.05% PBST). The diluted original Ph.D.-7 library was added to the dish and incubated for 3 h with shaking at room temperature. After washing ten times (1 min each) with 0.05% PBST to remove the unbound phages, the attached phages were eluted with continuous shaking in 1 ml of 0.1 M glycine-HCl (pH 2.2) for 10 min at room temperature and neutralized with 100 μl of 1 M Tris-HCl (pH 9.1). Amplification, purification, and titration of the eluate were successively performed as described in the standard protocol (NEB) prior to the next round of screening. Three more rounds of selection were carried out under more stringent conditions. Briefly, dishes were blocked with different agents (non-fat milk, gelatin, and BSA in the second, third, and fourth rounds, respectively), incubated with the eluate for a shorter time (2, 1.5, and 1 h in the second, third, and fourth rounds, respectively), and washed with higher concentration of PBST (0.1, 0.2, and 0.3% for the second, third, and fourth rounds, respectively) for a longer time (10×2, 10×3, and 10×5 min for the second, third, and fourth rounds, respectively). The phage clones obtained from the fourth round selection were further subjected to the enzyme-linked immunosorbent assay (ELISA).

2.3 Selection of the positive phage clones by ELISA

The maxi-sorp 96-well microtiter plates (Nunc) were coated with 2.5 μg/ml FGF23 and an equal amount of control proteins including bFGF and FGF21 overnight at 4℃. The plates were blocked with the blocking buffer (PBSM, PBS with 2% dry milk) at room temperature for 1 h and washed with 0.05% PBST three times. The phage clones (10^{10} pfu/well) and control phage vcsM13 were then added and incubated at room temperature for 1 h. After washing three times with 0.05% PBST, 200 μl of horseradish peroxidase (HRP)–anti-M13 (1:5 000) was added and incubated for 1 h at room temperature. The plates were washed with 0.05% PBST three times prior to addition of the substrate 3,3′,5,5′-tetramethylbenzidine (TMB). After 20 min, 50 μl per well of 2 M H$_2$SO$_4$ was added to terminate the reaction. The absorbance was measured at 450 nm with a reference wave-length of 655 nm.

2.4 DNA sequencing and peptide synthesis

ssDNA was prepared as described by the standard protocol (NEB). Briefly, the positive phage clones selected by ELISA were precipitated with polyethylene glycol (PEG)/NaCl for 10 min at room temperature followed by centrifugation at 12 000 rpm for 10 min. The pellet was resuspended in 100 μl iodide buffer, and DNA was precipitated with 250 μl ethanol for 10 min at room temperature, washed with 70% ethanol, and resuspended in 30 μl TE buffer [10 mM Tris-HCl (pH 8.0), 1 mM EDTA]. DNA sequencing was performed with −96 gIII primer by Shanghai Sangon Company (Shanghai, China). The BioEdit Sequence Alignment Editor software and the ProtParam programs were used to analyze the DNA sequence.

The phages display random heptapeptides fused to the N terminus of the M13 phage coat protein pIII by a short spacer (Gly-Gly-Gly-Ser), resulting in the displaying peptide with free N terminus and C terminus fused to the phage, having no free negatively charged carboxylate. Therefore, when synthesizing the selected peptide, a spacer sequence (Gly-Gly-Gly-Ser) was added to the C terminus and the C-terminal carboxylate was amidated to avoid introducing a negative charge which may influence binding. The selected peptide was synthesized by SBS Genetech (Beijing, China).

2.5 Phosphate uptake assay

OK cells were seeded in six-well plates (1×10^5 cells/well) in RPMI 1640 containing 10% FBS and allowed to attach overnight. Cells were grown in RPMI 1640 with 0.4% FBS for 24 h and then pretreated with peptides for 5 min before stimulation with FGF23 (200 ng/ml) alone or FGF23 plus peptides for 3 h (Goetz *et al.*, 2010). A previously isolated bFGF-binding peptide (named as P7) (Wu *et al.*, 2010) was used as the control. Cells were washed with the medium (137 mM NaCl, 5.4 mM KCl, 1 mM CaCl$_2$, 1.2 mM MgSO$_4$, and 15 mM HEPES, pH 7.4) before incubation with the above medium supplemented with 2 mM KH$_2$PO$_4$ at 37℃ for 5 min. The medium was collected and subjected to phosphate assay by the Phosphate Colorimetric Assay Kit according to the manufacturer's instructions.

2.6 Analysis of mitogen-activated protein kinase (MAPK) and AKT activation

OK cells were seeded in 12-well plates (1×10^5 cells/ well) in RPMI 1640 containing 10% FBS and allowed to attach overnight. Starved cells were treated with peptides for 5 min prior to stimulation with FGF23 for 10 min (Goetz *et al.*, 2010). After being washed with cold PBS, cells were lysed in 1× SDS-PAGE loading buffer. The lysate was clarified by centrifugation at 12 000 rpm for 10 min at 4℃, and the supernatant was subjected to separate by 10% SDS-PAGE and transferred to a PVDF membrane (350 mA, 70 min). The membrane was incubated with the primary antibodies at 4℃ overnight, followed by goat anti-rabbit IgG, HRP-linked antibody at room temperature for 1 h. The blots were visualized with an ECL detection kit and analyzed by Quantity One 4.6 software.

2.7 Semi-quantitative RT-PCR analysis of NaPi-2a and NaPi-2c expression

OK cells were seeded in six-well plates with 1×10^5 cells per well in RPMI 1640 containing 10% FBS and allowed to attach overnight. Starved cells were treated with peptides for 5 min prior to stimulation with 200 ng/ml FGF23 for 1 h. Total RNA was extracted using the TRIZOL reagent and reverse-transcribed to cDNA by the First-Strand cDNA Synthesis Kit according to the manufacturer's instructions. The resulting cDNA was used as a template for PCR amplification. Opossum type IIa sodium-phosphate cotransporter (NaPi-2a) was amplified with the primers 5′-TATTGCC-GCTCTTAGGTCACC-3′ (forward) and 5′-GTGCCGATATTAGAACCCAGG-3′ (reverse). Type IIc sodium-phosphate cotransporter (NaPi-2c) was amplified with the primers 5′-CAAGGACAATGTGGTGCTGTC-3′ (forward) and 5′-ACT-GTGGAGCCAGTTGAAGTT-3′ (reverse). Glyceraldehyde-3-phosphate dehydrogenase (GAPDH) was amplified as an internal control with the primers 5′-CTGCACCACCAACTGCTTAGC-3′ (forward) and 5′-GCCTGCTTCAC-CACCTCTTG-3′ (reverse) (Ito *et al.*, 2010). PCR reaction system containing 10 μl of DreamTaq Green PCR Master Mix (2×), 1 μl of forward primer (2 μM), 1 μl of reverse primer (2 μM), 2 μl of cDNA, and 6 μl of nuclease-free water was established and subjected to PCR running (95℃ for 5 min followed by 40 cycles of 95℃ for 30 s, 54℃ for 30 s, and 72℃ for 30 s). After PCR, the same volume of reaction products is electrophoresed on an agarose gel. Images of stained DNA are then obtained and the intensities of the PCR product bands were analyzed by Quantity One 4.6 software. The relative NaPi-2a and NaPi-2c mRNA levels were calculated by comparison of the intensities of NaPi-2a and NaPi-2c PCR product bands against the intensities of the corresponding GAPDH control bands, respectively.

2.8 Statistical analysis

Data were presented as mean ± standard deviations (SD) from at least three independent experiments. Statistical differences between the groups were determined with one-way ANOVA (GraphPad Prism 5.0), followed by Tukey's multiple comparison test. Statistical significance for all tests was set at $P < 0.05$.

3. Results

3.1 Selection of specific FGF23-binding phage clones

Ph.D.-7™ Phage Display Peptide Library was subjected to four cycles of biopanning with gradually increased stringency of selection. As shown in Table 1, P/N value gradually increased to 2.5, and the phage recovery increased from 3.0×10^{-3} to 5.0×10^{-3}%, indicating that the phages specifically bound to FGF23$_{180-205}$ were enriched. After four rounds of selection, high-affinity FGF23-binding clones were further identified from the recovered phage clones by ELISA. In order to determine binding specificities, we also detected the ability of phage clones binding to the other two members of the FGF family, bFGF and FGF21, respectively. Phage clones were considered to possess high affinity and specificity for FGF23 if their O.D. values were two times greater than those of the control phage vcsM13, bFGF, and FGF21 (Wu *et al.*, 2010). As shown in Fig. 1, after four rounds of panning, three positive clones with higher affinity and specificity

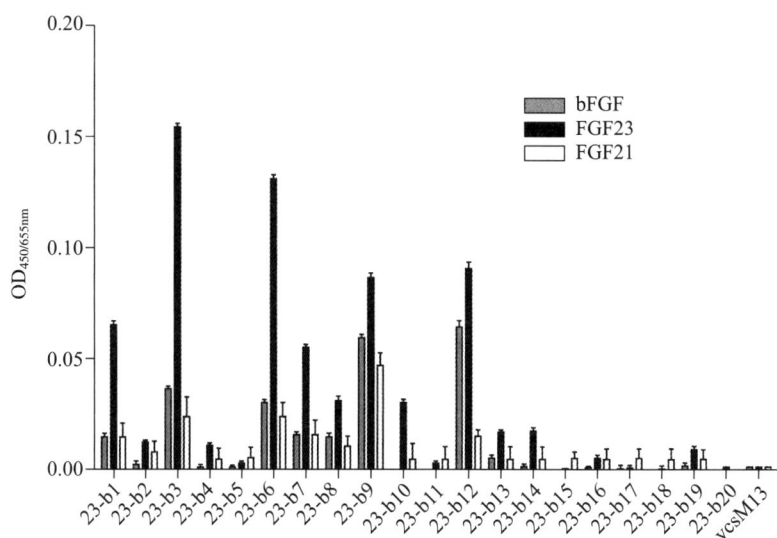

Fig. 1. Selection of the positive phage clones specifically binding to FGF23. The binding affinity of the 20 phage clones and the control vcsM13 to FGF23, bFGF, and FGF21 was determined by ELISA assay. Data displayed are the mean O.D. values (±SD) of triplicate samples.

for FGF23 (clones b1, b3, and b6) were selected from 20 clones detected and further subjected to sequencing.

Table 1.　Selective enrichment for FGF23$_{180-205}$-binding phages

Round	FGF23 (μg)	Input phage (pfu)	Output phage (pfu) P	Output phage (pfu) of negative control N	Recovery (%)	P/N
1	1 000	1.0×10^{11}	3.0×10^{6}	1.8×10^{7}	3.0×10^{-3}	0.17
2	500	2.2×10^{10}	3.7×10^{5}	1.6×10^{6}	1.7×10^{-3}	0.23
3	500	2.2×10^{11}	7.0×10^{6}	5.0×10^{6}	3.2×10^{-3}	1.4
4	500	2.0×10^{11}	1.0×10^{7}	4.0×10^{6}	5.0×10^{-3}	2.5

3.2　Sequence analysis and property prediction of FGF23-binding phage clones

The amino acid sequences of the peptides displayed on the selected phages were obtained from the DNA sequences and analyzed by the BioEdit and ProtParam programs (Table 2). The amino acid sequences of the selected peptides were compared with that of FGFR1 (GenBank AAH15035.1) using BioEdit Sequence Alignment Editor. Phage clone no. 6 (23-b6) shows the highest sequence similarity to FGFR1 (0.0012165, PAM250 Matrix) and contains seven amino acids in D3 domain of FGFR1 (S271, S281, P283, P285, K291, S298, P302). Moreover, in the physiological condition, the panning target FGF23$_{180-205}$ carries negative charges (pI 4.86) and displays hydrophilicity with a grand average of hydropathicity (GRAVY) of −1.038. Among the three selected phage clones, only 23-b6 peptide carries positive charges (pI 8.47) and also is hydrophilic with the GRAVY value of −1.586. It is likely that 23-b6 peptide with the sequence similarity to FGFR1 may bind to FGF23 via electrostatic and hydrophilic interactions and therefore may have a greater potential to interrupt FGF23 binding to its receptor than other identified heptapeptides.

Table 2.　Properties of peptides displayed by specific FGF23-binding phages

Peptides	Sequences	Similarities with FGFR	Similarities with Klotho	Theoretical pI	Gravy
23-b1	LPLGPHT	0	0.006917	6.74	0.014
23-b3	TDHSMPP	0	0.006917	5.05	−1.357
23-b6	SSPPKSP	0.0012165	0.006917	8.47	−1.586

A

B

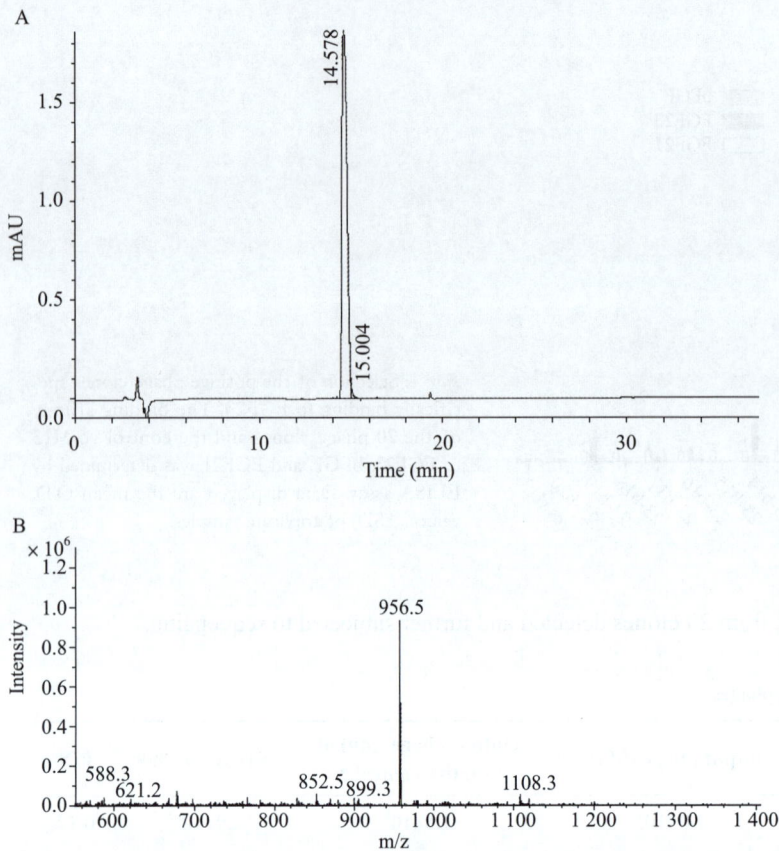

Fig. 2. Analysis of the synthetic 23-b6 peptide. (A) HPLC chromatogram at 214 nm. (B) Electrospray ionization mass spectrum of the synthetic peptide.

The selected 23-b6 peptide was subsequently synthesized on solid phase using a Fmoc strategy. As shown in Fig. 2, the synthetic 23-b6 peptide with 98% purity was obtained after purification by reverse-phase HPLC and characterized for its identity by mass spectrometry analysis.

3.3 Heptapeptide-library-derived peptide 23-b6 counteracts the regulatory effect of FGF23 on phosphate uptake

FGF23 inhibits phosphate uptake in renal proximal tubule epithelium. To determine the ability of 23-b6 peptide to block the actions of FGF23, we tested the effects of the peptide on the phosphate uptake in OK cells, an *in vitro* model for kidney proximal tubule cells, using a Phosphate Colorimetric Assay Kit. As shown in Fig. 3, 23-b6 peptide exhibited a significant antagonistic effect on the inhibition of phosphate uptake by FGF23, increasing the phosphate uptake to the

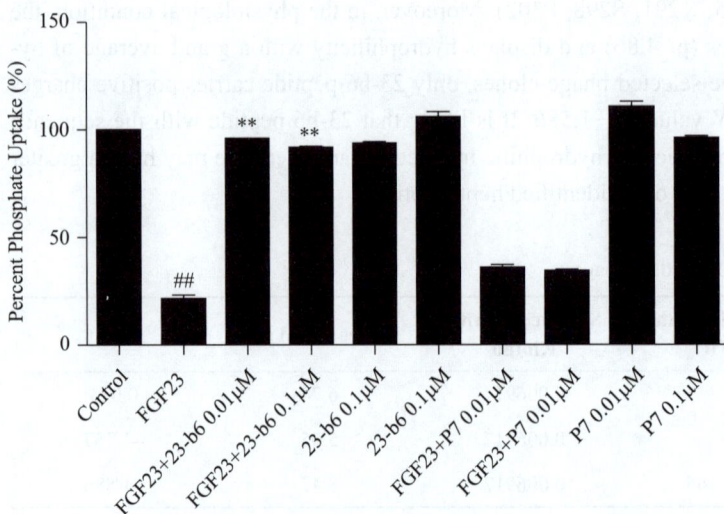

Fig. 3. Synthetic 23-b6 peptide counteracts the phosphate uptake inhibition by FGF23. OK cells were treated with 200 ng/ml FGF23 alone, 200 ng/ml FGF23 plus 23-b6 or control peptide P7, 23-b6, or P7 peptides alone. Effects of the synthetic peptides on phosphate uptake were measured with Phosphate Colorimetric Assay Kit. Data are presented as the mean±SD of three independent experiments performed in triplicate. $^{\#\#}P<0.01$ *vs.* control group; $^{**}P<0.01$ *vs.* FGF23 group.

control level even at a low concentration of 0.01 μM. When 23-b6 peptide was applied alone, little effect was observed on the alteration of phosphate uptake in OK cells. Moreover, the control peptide P7 targeting bFGF has no effect on the phosphate uptake in cells treated with or without FGF23. The results indicated that the isolated peptide 23-b6 has specifically antagonistic potentials targeting FGF23.

3.4 Effects of 23-b6 on MAPK and Akt activation in FGF23-stimulated OK cells

It is known that FGFs modulate their cellular activities through MAPK and Akt signal pathways. In order to examine whether 23-b6 peptide counteract the phosphate uptake inhibition by FGF23 *via* influencing the intracellular signaling pathway of FGFs, we examined the effects of 23-b6 peptide on phosphorylation of Erk1/2, P38, and Akt in FGF23-stimulated OK cells by Western blotting analysis. As shown in Fig. 4, exogenous FGF-23 significantly induced phosphorylation of Erk1/2, but not that of P38 and Akt. Pretreatment with 23-b6 peptide for 5 min before stimulation with FGF23 resulted in significant blockage of the activation of Erk1/2. Little effect was found on the activation of signal molecules when applied 23-b6 peptide alone in OK cells.

3.5 Effects of 23-b6 on NaPi-2a and NaPi-2c expression in FGF23-induced OK cells

The sodium-dependent phosphate (Na/Pi) transporters NaPi-2a and NaPi-2c expressed primarily in the proximal tubule contribute to the renal phosphate reabsorption (Sorribas *et al.*, 1994). FGF23 inhibits phosphate uptake by decreasing NaPi-2a and NaPi-2c expression in the renal proximal tubule (Gattineni *et al.*, 2009). To assess whether 23-b6 peptide antagonized the phosphate uptake inhibition by up-regulating the expression of NaPi-2a and NaPi-2c, semi-quantitative RT-PCR was applied to analyze the effects of 23-b6 peptide on mRNA levels of NaPi-2a and NaPi-2c in

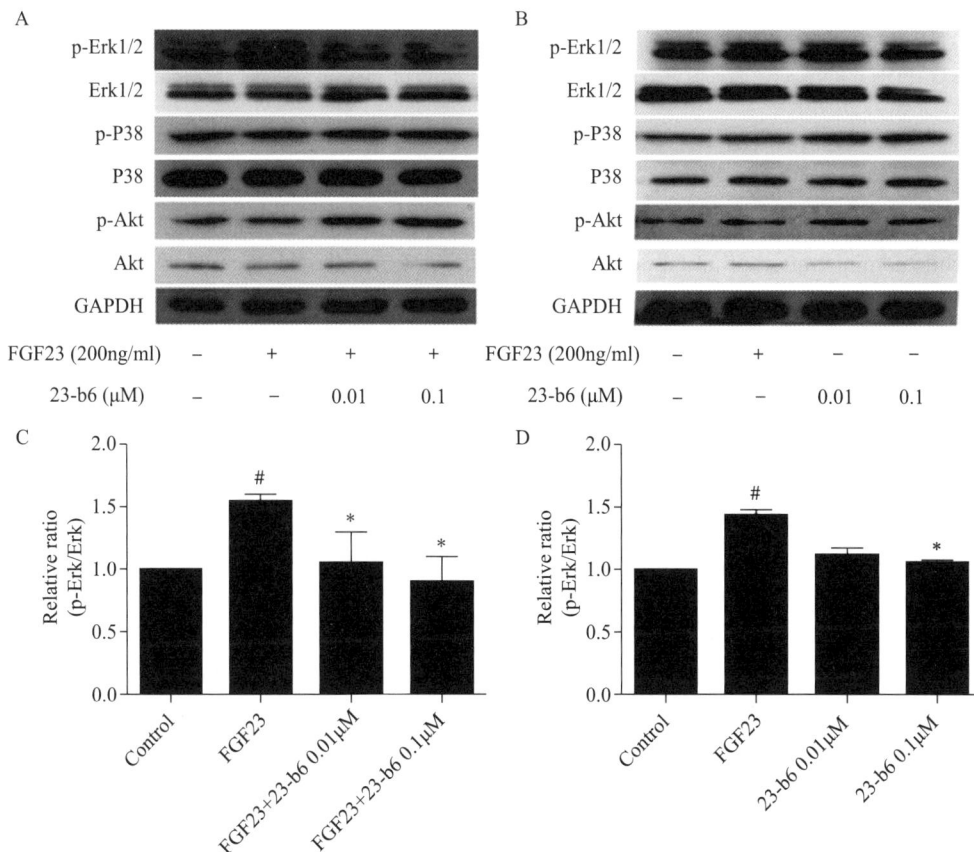

Fig. 4. Effects of synthetic 23-b6 peptide on MAPK and Akt activation in FGF23-stimulated OK cells. OK cells were pretreated with 23-b6 at the indicated concentrations for 5 min before stimulation with 200 ng/ml FGF23 for 10 min (A) or treated with 23-b6 alone (B). After treatment, phosphorylated Erk1/2 (p-Erk1/2), phosphorylated P38 (p-P38), and phosphorylated Akt (p-Akt) were detected by Western blotting analysis with the corresponding antibodies. (C, D) Density ratios of phosphorylated proteins to total proteins are presented as the mean±SD of three independent experiments. [#]P<0.05 vs. control group; [*]P<0.05 vs. FGF23 group.

A

NaPi-2a

NaPi-2c

GAPDH

FGF23 (200ng/ml)　　−　　+　　+　　+

23-b6 (μM)　　−　　−　　0.01　　0.1

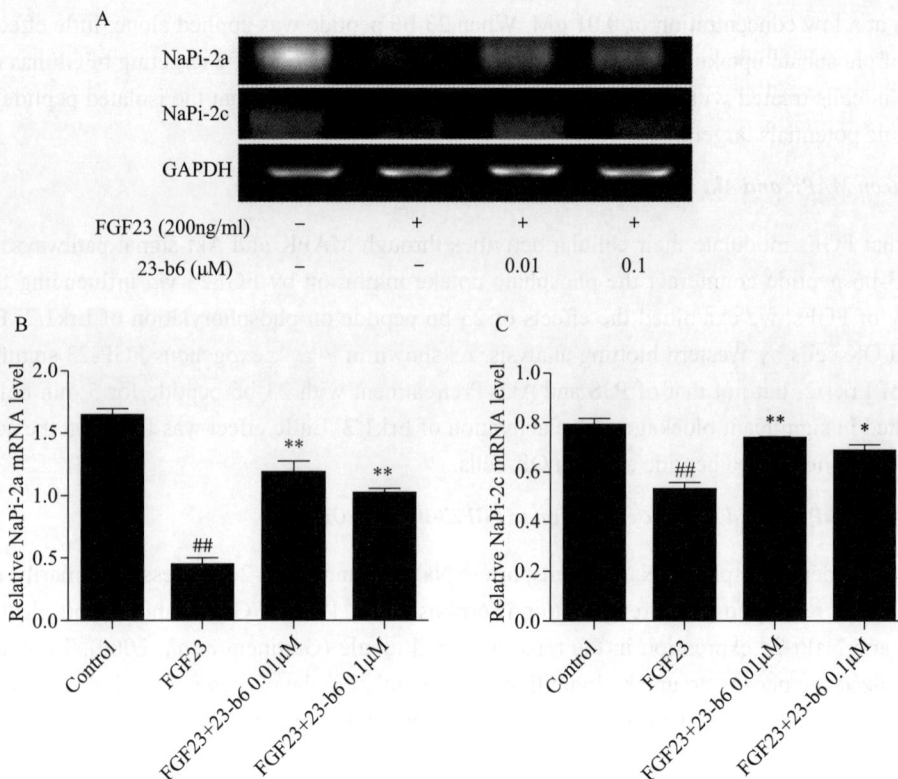

Fig. 5. Effects of synthetic 23-b6 peptide on NaPi-2a and NaPi-2c mRNA expression in FGF23-stimulated OK cells. (A) Starved cells were treated with peptides for 5 min prior to stimulation with 200 ng/ml FGF23 for 1 h. Total RNA was extracted and subjected to analysis of the expression levels of NaPi-2a and NaPi-2c mRNA by semi-quantitative RT-PCR. (B, C) The relative mRNA levels of NaPi-2a and NaPi-2c were calculated as ratios to GAPDH mRNA level. Results are presented as the mean±SD of three independent experiments. $^{\#\#}P<0.01$ vs. control group; $^{*}P<0.05$, $^{**}P<0.01$ vs. FGF23 group.

OK cells stimulated by FGF23. As expected, exogenous FGF23 significantly decreased mRNA expression of NaPi-2a and NaPi-2c, while administration of 23-b6 peptide significantly reversed the down-regulation of NaPi-2a and NaPi-2c expression by FGF23 in OK cells (Fig. 5). The results suggested that the synthetic 23-b6 peptide counteracts the phosphaturic actions of FGF23 through increasing the expression of NaPi-2a and NaPi-2c.

4. Discussion

FGF23 is predominantly expressed in the bone and regulates phosphate reabsorption in the kidney. FGF23 knockout mice showed hyperphosphatemia with increased renal phosphate reabsorption. Elevated plasma levels of FGF23 are found in patients with phosphate wasting disorders. Therefore, antagonists targeting FGF23 have been considered a potential therapeutic strategy for renal phosphate wasting.

FGF23 initials the phosphaturic actions by binding to the FGFR-Klotho complex. Goetz et al. have narrowed down the minimal binding epitope for the FGFR-Klotho complex to FGF23 residues S180 to T205 (Goetz et al., 2010). Garringer and colleagues also showed that residues P189 to P203 are required for FGF23 signaling (Garringer et al., 2008). The ability of the FGF23$_{180-205}$ fragment to specifically recognize the binary receptor complex makes it the desirable target to isolate FGF23 antagonists. Therefore, when we applied the phage displaying technology to identify FGF23 antagonists, the FGF23$_{180-205}$ fragment was chosen as the panning target for obtaining peptides specifically binding to the active epitope on FGF23 and interrupting the interaction between FGF23 and the FGFR-Klotho complex. It is known that depending on the target, directly coating the target on a plastic surface can cause an inaccessible ligand binding site either due to steric blocking or partial denaturation of the target along the surface. Considering that the target used composed of only 26 amino acid residues may induce less steric blocking or denaturation than the full-length protein when coated on the surface, we tried the surface panning method by directly coating a plastic surface with the target.

After four rounds of panning, the phages specifically bound to $FGF23_{180\text{-}205}$ were enriched, and three positive clones with higher affinity and specificity for FGF23 were selected. It has been reported that FGF23 exerts the hypophosphatemic actions by activating the predominant receptor (FGFR1c) in a Klotho-dependent manner. The extracellular domain of FGFR1 consists of three immunoglobulin-like domains (D1 to D3). Given that the FGFR1c-Klotho complex comprises the high-affinity receptor for FGF23 (Kurosu et al., 2006), and the D3 domain (270–359 aa) is involved in FGFR1 binding to both the ligand and the Klotho coreceptor (Goetz et al., 2012), alignment of the selected peptide sequences with FGFR1, which is the predominant receptor for the hypophosphatemic action of FGF23, showed high sequence homology between 23-b6 and FGFR1. Moreover, analysis of the properties of 23-b6 and $FGF23_{180\text{-}205}$ predicted that 23-b6 may have the capability to bind FGF23 via electrostatic and hydrophilic interactions, resulting in suppression of the biological activity of FGF23. Further functional analysis demonstrates that the synthetic 23-b6 peptide counteracts the phosphate uptake inhibition by FGF23 in OK cells, which is consistent with the speculation. Different from the 72-residue-long C-terminal tail of FGF23, $FGF_{180\text{-}251}$, which was identified as an FGF23 antagonist by competing with FGF23 for binding to a de novo site generated at the composite FGFR1c-Klotho interface (Goetz et al., 2010), the isolated 23-b6 peptide may antagonize the phosphaturic actions of FGF23 through occupying the binding site on FGF23 for the binary FGFR-klotho complex by targeting the FGFR-Klotho complex binding epitope $FGF_{180\text{-}205}$.

FGF23 has been found to inhibit renal phosphate reabsorption via a mitogen-activated protein kinase (MAPK) pathway (Yamashita et al., 2002). In order to determine which MAPK pathway is involved in mediating the inhibitory effect of 23-b6 on phosphaturic actions of FGF23, phosphorylation levels of Erk1/2 and P38 were detected by Western blotting, respectively. Our results demonstrating that FGF23 triggered activation of Erk1/2 but not P38 are consistent with several groups (Andrukhova et al., 2012; Kurosu et al., 2006; Urakawa et al., 2006), who revealed that FGF23 induced phosphaturic actions through activation of the Erk1/2 signaling pathway, but in contrast to another report suggesting that FGF23 significantly induces phosphorylation of both Erk and P38 MAPK (Yamashita et al., 2002). Moreover, little effect of FGF23 was found on the phosphorylation of PI3K/Akt in OK cells. Administration of 23-b6 peptide suppressed FGF23-induced Erk1/2 phosphorylation, suggesting that the Erk cascade may be involved in mediating the inhibitory effects of 23-b6 on FGF23-triggered phosphaturic actions.

It has been demonstrated that the type II sodium-coupled phosphate (Na/Pi) transporters are the molecules responsible for the renal reabsorption of Pi (Biber et al., 2009). FGF23 decreases the expression of an electrogenic phosphate transporter (NaPi-2a) and an electroneutral phosphate transporter (NaPi-2c) primarily expressed in the kidney proximal tubule, resulting in several hypophosphatemic disorders (Gattineni et al., 2009). Alteration of the expression levels of NaPi-2a and NaPi-2c by 23-b6 peptide may contribute to counteracting the phosphate uptake inhibition by FGF23. Consistent with the speculation, semi-quantitative RT-PCR analysis indicated that 23-b6 peptide significantly reversed the down-regulation of NaPi-2a and NaPi-2c expression by FGF23 in OK cells. As FGF23 directly down-regulates the expression of the sodium-phosphate transporters through Erk1/2 signaling, combined with the results of our present studies, we propose that the mechanisms by which 23-b6 peptide antagonized the inhibition of phosphate uptake by FGF23 may be in part blocking the activation of Erk1/2 pathway, leading to up-regulation of the expression of NaPi-2a and NaPi-2c.

In summary, we successfully isolated an FGF23-binding peptide 23-b6 by screening a phage display heptapeptide library with $FGF23_{180\text{-}205}$, which provides an effective FGF23 antagonist, and may have potentials for counteracting the phosphaturic actions of FGF23 in hypophosphatemic disorders. Moreover, we also provided a successful strategy for identifying the desirable peptides antagonizing the actions of the target protein from the phage display library by using a minimal active epitope on the target protein as the panning target.

References

[1] Andrukhova O, Zeitz U, Goetz R, et al. FGF23 acts directly on renal proximal tubules to induce phosphaturia through activation of the ERK1/2-SGK1 signaling pathway[J]. Bone, 2012, 51(3): 621-628.

[2] Benet-Pages A, Orlik P, Strom TM, et al. An FGF23 missense mutation causes familial tumoral calcinosis with hyperphosphatemia[J]. Human Molecular Genetics, 2005, 14(3): 385-390.

[3] Biber J, Hernando N, Forster I, et al. Regulation of phosphate transport in proximal tubules[J]. Pflugers Archiv-European Journal Of Physiology, 2009, 458(1): 39-52.

[4] Gaasbeek A, Meinders AE. Hypophosphatemia: An update on its

etiology and treatment[J]. American Journal Of Medicine, 2005, 118(10): 1094-1101.

[5] Garringer HJ, Malekpour M, Esteghamat F, *et al.* Molecular genetic and biochemical analyses of FGF23 mutations in familial tumoral calcinosis[J]. American Journal Of Physiology-Endocrinology And Metabolism, 2008, 295(4): E929-E937.

[6] Gattineni J, Bates C, Twombley K, *et al.* FGF23 decreases renal NaPi-2a and NaPi-2c expression and induces hypophosphatemia *in vivo* predominantly *via* FGF receptor 1[J]. American Journal Of Physiology-Renal Physiology, 2009, 297(2): F282-F291.

[7] Goetz R, Nakada Y, Hu MC, *et al.* Isolated C-terminal tail of FGF23 alleviates hypophosphatemia by inhibiting FGF23-FGFR-Klotho complex formation[J]. Proceedings Of the National Academy Of Sciences Of the United States Of America, 2010, 107(1): 407-412.

[8] Goetz R, Ohnishi M, Ding X, *et al.* Klotho Coreceptors Inhibit Signaling by Paracrine Fibroblast Growth Factor 8 Subfamily Ligands[J]. Molecular And Cellular Biology, 2012, 32(10): 1944-1954.

[9] Imel EA, Econs MJ. Fibroblast growth factor 23: Roles in health and disease[J]. Journal Of the American Society Of Nephrology, 2005, 16(9): 2565-2575.

[10] Inagaki T, Choi M, Moschetta A, *et al.* Fibroblast growth factor 15 functions as an enterohepatic signal to regulate bile acid homeostasis[J]. Cell Metabolism, 2005, 2(4): 217-225.

[11] Ito M, Sakurai A, Hayashi K, *et al.* An apical expression signal of the renal type IIc Na$^+$-dependent phosphate cotransporter in renal epithelial cells[J]. American Journal Of Physiology-Renal Physiology, 2010, 299(1): F243-F254.

[12] Kharitonenkov A, Shiyanova TL, Koester A, *et al.* FGF-21 as a novel metabolic regulator[J]. Journal Of Clinical Investigation, 2005, 115(6): 1627-1635.

[13] Kobayashi K, Imanishi Y, Koshiyama H, *et al.* Expression of FGF23 is correlated with serum phosphate level in isolated fibrous dysplasia[J]. Life Sciences, 2006, 78(20): 2295-2301.

[14] Kobayashi K, Imanishi Y, Miyauchi A, *et al.* Regulation of plasma fibroblast growth factor 23 by calcium in primary hyperparathyroidism[J]. European Journal Of Endocrinology, 2006, 154(1): 93-99.

[15] Kurosu H, Ogawa Y, Miyoshi M, *et al.* Regulation of fibroblast growth factor-23 signaling by Klotho[J]. Journal Of Biological Chemistry, 2006, 281(10): 6120-6123.

[16] Larsson T, Marsell R, Schipani E, *et al.* Transgenic mice express-ing fibroblast growth factor 23 under the control of the alpha 1(I) collagen promoter exhibit growth retardation, osteomalacia, and disturbed phosphate homeostasis[J]. Endocrinology, 2004, 145(7): 3087-3094.

[17] Negri AL. Hereditary hypophosphatemias: New genes in the bone-kidney axis[J]. Nephrology, 2007, 12(4): 317-320.

[18] Shiber JR, Mattu A. Serum phosphate abnormalities in the emer-gency department[J]. Journal Of Emergency Medicine, 2002, 23(4): 395-400.

[19] Shimada T, Hasegawa H, Yamazaki Y, *et al.* FGF-23 is a potent regulator of vitamin D metabolism and phosphate homeostasis[J]. Journal Of Bone And Mineral Research, 2004, 19(3): 429-435.

[20] Sorribas V, Markovich D, Hayes G, *et al.* Cloning of a Na/Pi co-transporter from opossum kidney-cells[J]. Journal Of Biological Chemistry, 1994, 269(9): 6615-6621.

[21] Strewler GJ. FGF23, hypophosphatemia, and rickets: Has phos-phatonin been found?[J]. Proceedings Of the National Academy Of Sciences Of the United States Of America, 2001, 98(11): 5945-5946.

[22] Urakawa I, Yamazaki Y, Shimada T, *et al.* Klotho converts canoni-cal FGF receptor into a specific receptor for FGF23[J]. Nature, 2006, 444(7120): 770-774.

[23] Wang C, Lin S, Nie Y, *et al.* Mechanism of antitumor effect of a novel bFGF binding peptide on human colon cancer cells[J]. Can-cer Science, 2010, 101(5): 1212-1218.

[24] Wu X, Jia X, Ji Y, *et al.* Effects of a Synthetic bFGF Antagonist Peptide on the Proteome of 3T3 Cells Stimulated with bFGF[J]. International Journal Of Peptide Research And Therapeutics, 2011, 17(1): 53-59.

[25] Wu X, Yan Q, Huang Y, *et al.* Isolation of a novel basic FGF-binding peptide with potent antiangiogenetic activity[J]. Journal Of Cellular And Molecular Medicine, 2010, 14(1-2): 351-356.

[26] Yamashita T, Konishi M, Miyake A, *et al.* Fibroblast growth factor (FGF)-23 inhibits renal phosphate reabsorption by activation of the mitogen-activated protein kinase pathway[J]. Journal Of Biological Chemistry, 2002, 277(31): 28265-28270.

[27] Yamashita T, Yoshioka M, Itoh N. Identification of a novel fibro-blast growth factor, FGF-23, preferentially expressed in the ventro-lateral thalamic nucleus of the brain[J]. Biochemical And Biophysi-cal Research Communications, 2000, 277(2): 494-498.

[28] Yu XJ, White KE. FGF23 and disorders of phosphate homeostasis[J]. Cytokine & Growth Factor Reviews, 2005, 16(2): 221-232.

Effects of fibroblast growth factor 21 on cell damage *in vitro* and atherosclerosis *in vivo*

Wenhe Zhu, Xiaokun Li, Huiyan Wang

1. Introduction

Atherosclerosis (AS) is a chronic and degenerative disease of the large artery walls. It is the single most important cause of cardiovascular disease (CVD), which is a predominant health problem worldwide and a leading cause of mortality (Tan *et al.*, 2013). AS has a long asymptomatic phase, and the first manifestation of the disease may lead to sudden cardiac death (Mizuguchi *et al.*, 2008). Hypercholesterolemia, particularly of low-density lipoprotein cholesterol (LDL-C), is a well-established risk factor for the development of atherosclerosis and its pathologic complications (Mizuguchi *et al.*, 2008). At present, drugs used to reduce LDL-C in the treatment of AS have the potential for serious adverse reactions. Thus, the development of new effective therapeutic agents with minimal side effects is highly warranted.

The fibroblast growth factor family plays multiple roles in de fining and regulating functions of some endocrine-relevant tissues and organs. Of the 23 known members of the family, FGF-21 is a novel member (Nishimura *et al.*, 2000; Izumiya *et al.*, 2008; Muise *et al.*, 2008). FGF-21 is a key regulator in glucose and lipid metabolism, and its plasma levels are increased in different situations, such as type 2 diabetes, obesity, and nonalcoholic fatty liver disease (Shu *et al.*, 2002). FGF-21 directly protects pancreatic a and β cells from glucolipotoxicity and cytokine-induced cell apoptosis (Kharitonenkov *et al.*, 2007). Systemic administration of FGF-21 has been shown to reduce plasma glucose and triglycerides to near normal levels in genetically compromised diabetic rodents (Coskun *et al.*, 2008). Importantly, these effects were durable and did not come at the expense of weight gain or hypoglycemia, and also led to significant improvements in lipoprotein profiles, including lowering levels of LDL-C and raising levels of high-density lipoprotein cholesterol (Kharitonenkov *et al.*, 2007). Transgenic mice overexpressing FGF-21 in liver are resistant to diet-induced obesity (Badman *et al.*, 2007). Knockdown of hepatic FGF-21 transcript leads to hyperlipidemia and fatty liver in mice fed a ketogenic diet, whereas overexpression of FGF-21 in liver leads to the production of ketone bodies (Badman *et al.*, 2007). FGF-21 increases energy expenditure and improves insulin sensitivity in diet-induced obese mice (Inagaki *et al.*, 2007). These data support the development of FGF-21 as a potential treatment for diabetes and other metabolic diseases, including AS.

Previous studies have demonstrated that FGF-21 can be expressed and purified using a commercial vector containing a small ubiquitin-like modifier (SUMO) tag to promote the soluble expression of FGF-21 in *Escherichia coli* (Wang *et al.*, 2010). In this study, the *FGF21* gene was cloned to vector pET22b (+) and expressed in *E. coli*. We describe the purification of the recombinant protein and the role of this recombinant FGF-21 in improving resistance to cell damage *in vitro* and atherosclerosis *in vivo*.

2. Materials and methods

2.1 Reagents and cell culture

Restriction enzymes and Pyrobest DNA polymerase were purchased from the TaKaRa Company. The PCR purification kit, gel extraction kit, and plasmid miniprep kit were obtained from the Omega Company. Antibodies against Bax (sc20067), Bcl-2 (sc509), caspase-3 (sc22171R), P38 (sc81621), p-P38 (sc7973), p-JNK (sc6254), JNK (sc7345), and β-actin (sc8432) were purchased from Santa Cruz Biotechnology (Santa Cruz, California, USA). These were used at a concentration of 1:1 000 except for β-actin (conc. 1:5 000). Primers were synthesized by Sangon Biotech (Shanghai, China). Q-Sepharose Fast F and Sephadex G-25 Fine were obtained from Amersham Pharmacia (Piscataway, New Jersey, USA). Wistar rats were purchased from the Experimental Animal Holding of Jilin University (Changchun City, Jilin, China). For the experimental animals, approval was obtained from the Institutional Review Committee of Ji Lin Medical College. All experimental procedures involving the rats were performed in accordance with the Regulations for the Administration of Affairs Concerning Experimental Animals approved by the State Council of People's Republic of China. Test kits for glucose, total cholesterol (TC), LDL-C, high-density lipoprotein cholesterol (HDL-C), and triglycerides (TG) were obtained from the Beijing BHKT Clinical Reagent Company (Beijing, China).

Human umbilical vein endothelial cells (HUVECs; Invitrogen Life Technology, Carlsbad, Calif.) were maintained in M199 medium and supplemented with 10% fetal bovine serum, 1% penicillin and streptomycin, 10 ng/ml human fibroblast growth factor, and 18 mU/ml heparin. The cells were incubated at 37℃ under 5% CO_2. HUVECs were grown to approximately 80% confluence, maintained with fresh medium as described above, and subcultured every 2 to 3 days. The cells were used within passages 4 to 9 during these experiments.

2.2 Expression and purification of FGF-21

The expression vector pET22b-rFGF-21 was provided by the Engineering Research Center of Bioreactor and Pharmaceutical Development, Ministry of Education, Jilin Agricultural University. The *FGF21* DNA fragments of human *FGF21* that were 543 bp long (GenBank database accession number NM_019113; the mRNA was 940 bp long. The gene that extended from 235 to 777 codes for a mature peptide of FGF-21 was cloned.) were ligated into corresponding sites of the expression vector pET22b (+) digested with *Nco* I and *Xho* I. The recombinant plasmids were transformed into *E. coli* BL21 (DE3). Expression of FGF-21 was induced with 0.5 mM isopropyl β-D-1-thiogalactopyranoside (IPTG) at 37℃ for 4 h. The induced bacteria were then pelleted by centrifugation at 4℃. The culture pellet was obtained by centrifugation at 10 000 *g* at 4℃ for 10 min, exposed to osmotic shock by suspension in ice-cold 40% sucrose in 50 mM Tris-HCl, pH 7.2, and then lysozyme (600 μg/g cells) was added. Following 20 min incubation on ice, the suspension was pelleted at 10 000 *g* at 4℃ for 15 min and then resuspended in the same volume of ice-cold 50 mM Tris-HCl and 2.0 mM $MgSO_4$, at pH 7.2. After centrifugation as described above, the supernatant was stored at 4℃ for subsequent purification. The supernatant was loaded to a 2.6 cm × 15 cm Q-Sepharose Fast Flow column pre-equilibrated with buffer A [20 mM phosphate-buffered saline (PBS), pH 7.2]. The column was washed with buffer A and the protein was eluted with a linear gradient from 0 to 1.0 M NaCl in 20 mM PBS, pH 7.2. The fractions containing *FGF21* were loaded onto a 1.6 cm × 90 cm Sepharose G-25 column to harvest the FGF-21 protein. The concentration of purified protein was determined using a Thermo ND2000 Spectrophotometer and a bicinchoninic acid (BCA) assay. The expression of FGF-21 was analyzed using SDS-polyacrylamide gel electrophoresis (PAGE), and the expression level of FGF-21 was detected by densitometer scanning. For Western blotting, the protein in the gel was transferred to a PVDF membrane using a semidry electro-blotting apparatus at 15 V for 30 min in the buffer with 25 mM Tris and 192 mM glycine. The membrane was blocked with 5% nonfat milk for 1 h at room temperature. The membrane was incubated with rabbit anti-FGF-21 antibody. After being washed, the membrane was incubated with the goat anti-rabbit IgG conjugated to horseradish peroxidase (HRP; Sangon Biotech). The bound antibody was detected using an enhanced chemiluminescence (ECL) Western blotting analysis system (Beckton Dickinson).

2.3 Cell viability and apoptosis assay

The HUVECs were treated with FGF-21 (12.5, 25.0, 50.0, or 100.0 ng/ml) for 12 h before testing for the presence of H_2O_2 for another 1 h. Cell viability was detected using the MTT assay according to the method of Singh (2008).

Apoptosis was detected by staining with Hoechst 33258. HUVECs were collected, washed with PBS, and fixed with 2% paraformaldehyde at room temperature for 15 min, and then the cells were washed with PBS again and stained with Hoechst 33258 (25 μg/ml) for 30 min at room temperature. The stained nuclei were observed using a fluorescence photomicroscope (Olympus, Shinjuku Monolith, Tokyo, Japan).

2.4 Western blot analysis

After treatment for 24 h, 5×10^5 cells from each group were harvested and sonicated in radioimmunoprecipitation assay (RIPA) buffer [1% Nonidet P-40, 50 mM Tris-HCl (pH 7.5), 150 mM NaCl, 1 mM NaF, 1 mM phenylmethylsulfonyl fluoride, 4 mg/ml leupeptin, and 1 mg/ml aprotinin]. After centrifugation at 12 000 g for 10 min at 4℃, the protein content was estimated according to the Bio-Rad protein assay, and 50 μg protein per lane were loaded on to 12% poly-acrylamide SDS gel. The separated proteins were then transferred electrophoretically to nitrocellulose paper and soaked in transfer buffer (25 mM Tris, 192 mM glycine) and 20% methanol v/v. Non-specific binding was blocked by incubation of the blots in 5% nonfat dry milk in TBS–0.1% Tween (25 mM Tris, 150 mM NaCl, 0.1% Tween v/v) for 60 min. After washing, the blots were incubated overnight at 4℃ with the different primary antibodies. After a 30 min wash, the membranes were incubated with secondary antibody conjugated to horseradish peroxide for 1 h at room temperature. The membranes were then washed for 30 min and exposed to ECL reagents for 1 min and developed on film. The Bio Rad Laboratories Quantity One software was used to quantify the blots.

2.5 Animal model

All procedures involving animals were first approved by the Institutional Animal Care and Use Committee at Ji Lin Medical College. Sixty adult male Wistar rats (180–220 g) were purchased from the Experimental Animal Holding of Ji-lin University. The animals were housed in standard polypropylene cages and maintained under conditions of controlled room temperature and humidity with 12 h (light) – 12 h (dark) cycle. The rats were randomly distributed in 2 groups: (*i*) the control group ($n = 10$), which was fed a normal diet (NC), and (*ii*) the high-fat group ($n = 50$), which was fed a high-fat diet for 12 weeks, then further divided into 4 groups. The blood concentrations of TC, TG, HDL-C, and LDL-C were measured using kits according to the manufacturer's directions. Twelve weeks later, 3 rats from the high-fat diet group were randomly selected. After euthanasia of the animals by intravenous injection of pentobarbital, the aortas of each animal were obtained to assess the success of the atherosclerotic model construction.

When the atherosclerotic model had been successfully constructed, the group containing rats fed the high fat diet was further divided into 4 different groups: model group 1 (AS1), model group 2 (AS2), model group 3 (AS3), and model group 4 (AS4). NC and AS1 rats received an intraperitoneal (i.p.) injection of physiological saline. Rats in the AS2 group were given simvastatin (10 mg/kg body mass). Rats in the AS3 and AS4 groups were given FGF-21 at doses of 1.2 and 0.6 mg/kg, respectively. Body mass and food intake were recorded every week. After receiving once-daily injections for 8 weeks, the fasted rats were sacrificed under general anesthesia induced with pentobarbital, and the blood was collected. Blood samples were drawn from the ophthalmic venous plexus.

2.6 Measurement of TG, TC, HDL-C, and LDL-C

After centrifugation (1 000 g, 10 min, 4℃), the serum samples were collected and stored at –20℃. The liver and kidneys were excised, rinsed in ice-cold physiological saline, weighed, and then stored at –20℃. Serum levels of TC, TG, HDL-C, and LDL-C were measured using commercially available enzyme kits.

2.7 Determination of serum SOD activity and GSH and MDA levels

The activity of superoxide dismutase (SOD) and the levels of reduced glutathione (GSH) and malondialdehyde (MDA) in the collected serum of rats were evaluated, respectively, using a colorimetric method with kits for xanthine oxidase and thiobarbituric acid (Nanjing jian cheng Bioengineering Institute, Nanjing, China). The absorbance was measured, according to the manufacturer's instructions (kits), with a UV–VIS spectrophotometer at the wave-lengths of 550 nm and 532 nm, respectively.

2.8 Morphological measurements

Immediately after opening the chest, the aorta was excised. For oil red O staining, the aorta was stained with oil red O for 30 min, then transferred to 70% alcohol for differentiation. After 15 min, samples were washed and images were taken with a digital camera. For staining with hematoxylin and eosin (H&E), the aortas were stored in 10% (w/v) neutral formalin for at least one day, as was previously described (Kharitonenkov *et al.*, 2007). In brief, the roots of the aortas were cut off and then the samples were washed, dehydrated, cleared, embedded in wax, sliced, coated, and stained with H&E. Finally, the thickness of the intima and media were examined and photographed with an image operation system under a 1/10 mm lens and with ×400 amplification.

2.9 Statistics

Values are the mean ± SD. Statistical analyses of the data were performed using one-way analysis of variance (ANOVA) followed by a Tukey *post hoc* test. In all cases, values for $P < 0.05$ were considered statistically significant.

3. Results

To obtain recombinant FGF-21 proteins, we constructed the plasmid pET22b-rFGF-21 to promote the soluble expression of FGF-21 in *E. coli* BL21 (DE3) cells. After culture and induction with IPTG, more than 55.2% of the recombinant FGF-21 protein was secreted to the periplasmic space by the *pelB* signal sequence in the vector. The expressed protein in the cell lysate had an apparent molecular mass of 21 kDa, which corresponds to the predicted size for FGF-21 (Figs. 1A, 1C). The periplasmic protein was purified with Q-Sepharose FF and Sepharose G-25 columns. The results showed that FGF-21 was highly purified by SDS–PAGE (Fig. 1E). HPLC analysis of the target protein showed a major peak for FGF-21, with a purity of 96.5%.

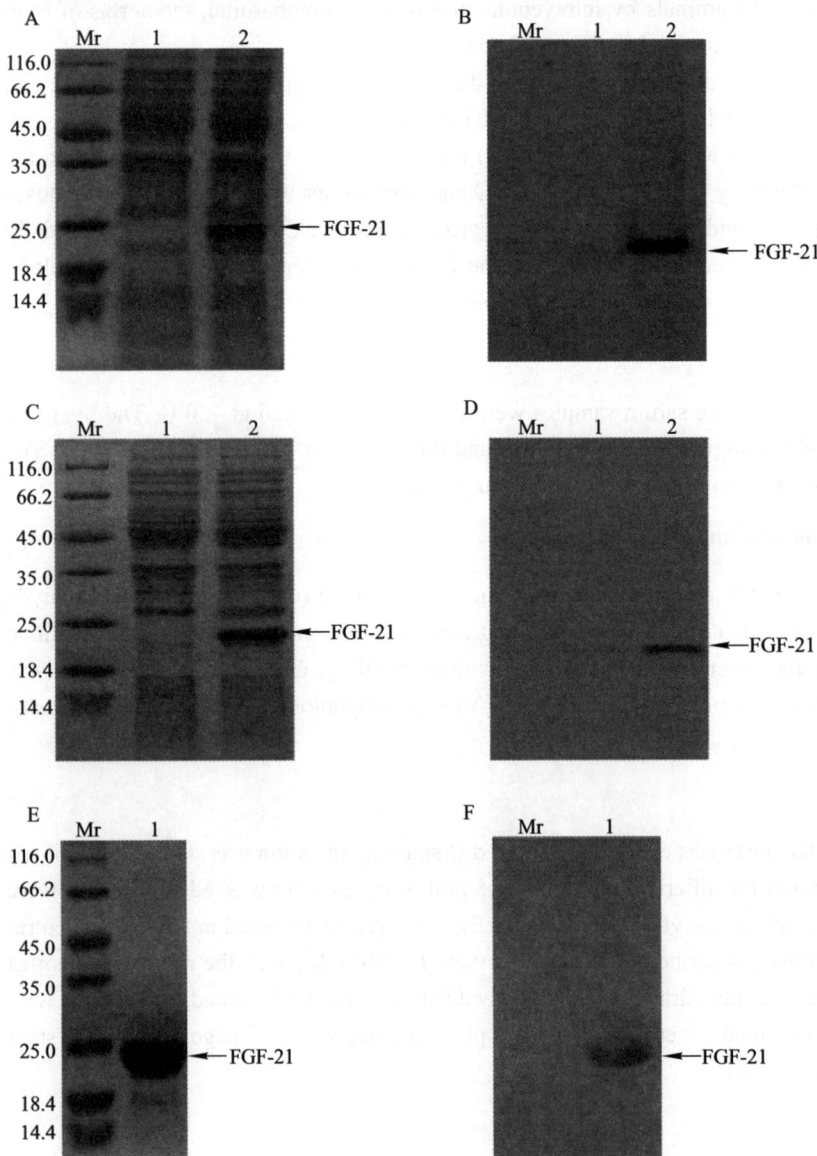

Fig. 1. Expression and purification of recombinant fibroblast growth factor 21 (FGF-21). (A) SDS–PAGE analysis of the expression of FGF-21. Lane 1 shows the results for whole bacteria (*E. coli*) with FGF-21, which were not induced with isopropyl β-D-1-thiogalactopyranoside (IPTG). Lane 2, shows the results for *E. coli* where the expression of *FGF21* was induced with IPTG. (B) Western blot analysis showing the expression of FGF-21. (C) SDS–PAGE analysis of recombinant the FGF-21 in *E. coli*. Lane 1 shows the extraction precipitation of periplasmic protein. Lane 2 shows the extraction supernatant of the periplasmic protein. (D) Western blot analysis of recombinant FGF-21 in *E. coli*. (E) SDS–PAGE results for the purification of FGF-21. Lane 1 shows the results for the purified FGF-21. (F) Western blot analysis of the expressed protein with anti-FGF-21, Mr, low range protein marker.

To further verify the authenticity of the purified FGF-21, we examined it by Western blotting analysis with anti-FGF-21 antibody. The result showed that the protein was recognized specifically by anti-FGF-21, indicating that the heterogeneous product was recombinant FGF-21 protein (Fig. 1B, D, F).

3.1 FGF-21 attenuated H_2O_2-induced cell damage

Studies have suggested that cardiac endothelial dysfunction induced by various pathological factors is the initiating factor that promotes the formation of atherosclerotic plaque (Singh, 2008). Therefore, exploration of active endogenous factors against endothelial dysfunction to antagonize the development of AS have become important strategies for treatment.

To evaluate the cyto-protective effect of FGF-21, HUVECs were pretreated with increasing concentrations of FGF-21 for 12 h before testing for the presence of H_2O_2 for another 1 h. After H_2O_2 treatment, cell viability of each condition was measured by MTT assay. H_2O_2 significantly depressed the viability of control cells without FGF-21 treatment (Fig. 2, columns 1 and 2). Compared with the control group (Fig. 2, column 1), 1 h incubation with of H_2O_2 led to a 55% decrease in cell viability (Fig. 2, column 2). However, pretreatment of cells with FGF-21 partially negated the effects from H_2O_2-induced cytotoxicity, in a dose-dependent manner (Fig. 2). The cell viability increased 35% (treated, 80.72% and untreated, 45.96%) at the concentration of 100 ng/ml FGF-21 compared with the untreated cells (Fig. 2, column 6), suggesting that FGF-21 protected the HUVECs from oxidative-stress-induced cell injuries.

3.2 FGF-21 prevented H_2O_2-induced apoptosis

To investigate the effects of FGF-21 on cell apoptosis, we stained some of the HUVECs with Hoechst 33258. Hoechst 33258 is a marker for apoptosis that detects apoptotic nuclei with condensed and (or) fragmented DNA. The uniform morphology of the nuclei is revealed through Hoechst 33258 staining (well-distributed deep-blue fluorescence). As shown in Fig. 3, without H_2O_2 induction, chromatin in the cell nuclei stained uniform blue and displayed an organized structure [Fig. 3(I)]. After incubation with 100 μM H_2O_2 for 1 h, HUVECs showed the typical features of apoptosis [Fig. 3(II)]. Pretreatment with FGF-21 reduced the level of H_2O_2-induced apoptosis in a dose-dependent manner [Fig. 3(III)–3(V)]. Interestingly, very few apoptotic nuclei were observed in the HUVECs pre-treated with 100 ng/ml FGF-21 [Fig. 3(V)], which were similar to the control group [Fig. 3(I)]. The data show that the apoptotic index increased dramatically in cells stimulated with H_2O_2, but FGF-21 improved the morphology of HUVECs that had been undergoing apoptosis-related changes.

3.3 Effect of FGF-21 on the expression of H_2O_2-induced apoptotic-related proteins

Members of the Bcl-2 family of proteins such as Bcl-2 and Bax are critical regulators of the apoptotic pathway. Bcl-2 proteins protect against multiple signals that lead to cell apoptosis, whereas Bax proteins induce apoptosis. Our study found that the expression of Bcl-2 was decreased, whereas Bax was increased, i.e., the ratio of Bax/Bcl-2 increased upon treatment with H_2O_2 in the HUVECs, but pretreatment with FGF-21 decreased the ratio (Fig. 4). We further investigated the protein expression of caspase-3. Caspase-3 is one of the primary executioner caspases activated during apoptosis (Inoue *et al.*, 2009). Our data showed that incubating HUVECs with H_2O_2 also led to increased cleaved caspase-3,

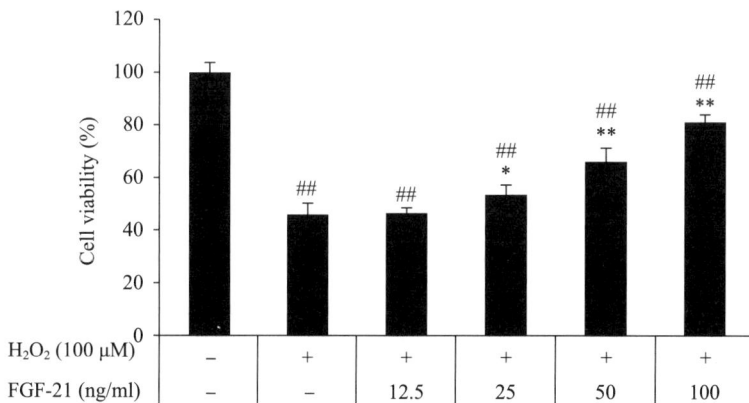

Fig. 2. Fibroblast growth factor 21 (FGF-21) attenuated H_2O_2-induced cytotoxicity in human umbilical vein endothelial cells (HUVECs). The HUVECs were pretreated with FGF-21 for 12 h and then exposed to 100 μM H_2O_2 for 1 h. Values are the mean ± SD, $n = 5$. $^{\#\#}P < 0.01$ compared with the untreated group (control); $^{*}P < 0.05$ compared with the HUVECs treated with H_2O_2 only; $^{**}P < 0.01$ compared with the HUVECs treated with H_2O_2 only.

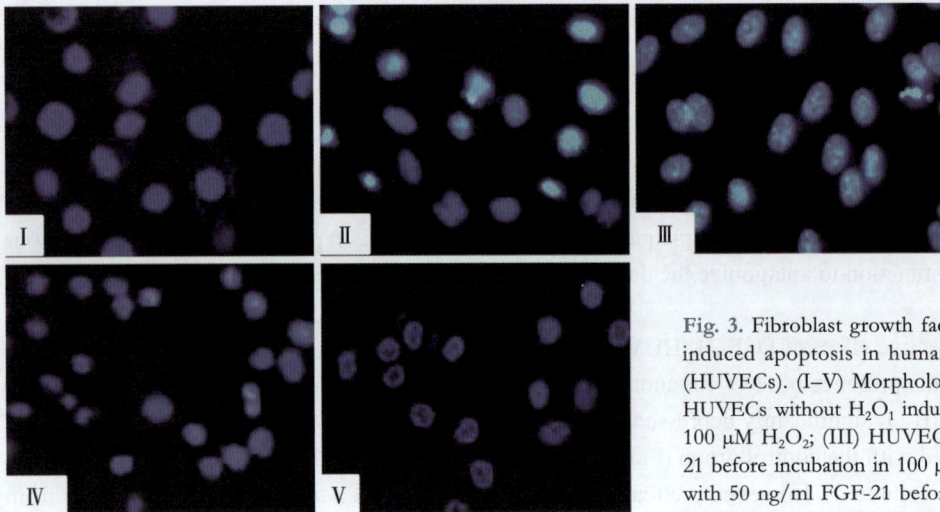

Fig. 3. Fibroblast growth factor 21 (FGF-21) prevented H_2O_2-induced apoptosis in human umbilical vein endothelial cells (HUVECs). (I–V) Morphological analysis of the HUVECs. (I) HUVECs without H_2O_1 induction; (II) HUVECs incubated with 100 μM H_2O_2; (III) HUVECs pretreated with 25 ng/ml FGF-21 before incubation in 100 μM H_2O_2; (IV) HUVECs pretreated with 50 ng/ml FGF-21 before incubation in 100 μM H_2O_2; (V) HUVECs pretreated with 100 ng/ml FGF-21 before incubation in 100 μM H_2O_2. Cell nuclei were stained with Hoechst 33258 (fluorescence microscope, 200×).

whereas pretreatment with FGF-21 inhibited the H_2O_2-induced cleavage of caspase-3 (Fig. 4).

3.4 FGF-21 regulates the MAPK signaling pathway in H_2O_2-treated HUVECs

The mitogen-activated protein kinase (MAPK) family, especially p-38 and JNK, are reportedly involved in oxidative stress and cell apoptosis (Sun *et al.*, 2006). We attempted to determine whether FGF-21 inhibits apoptosis in cells exposed to H_2O_2 through blocking MAPK signaling cascades. H_2O_2 induction increased p-P38 and p-JNK expression, whereas treatment with FGF-21 exerted antagonistic effects on p-P38 and p-JNK expression (Fig. 5), suggesting that FGF-21 prevents H_2O_2-induced cell apoptosis by decreasing activation of p-38.

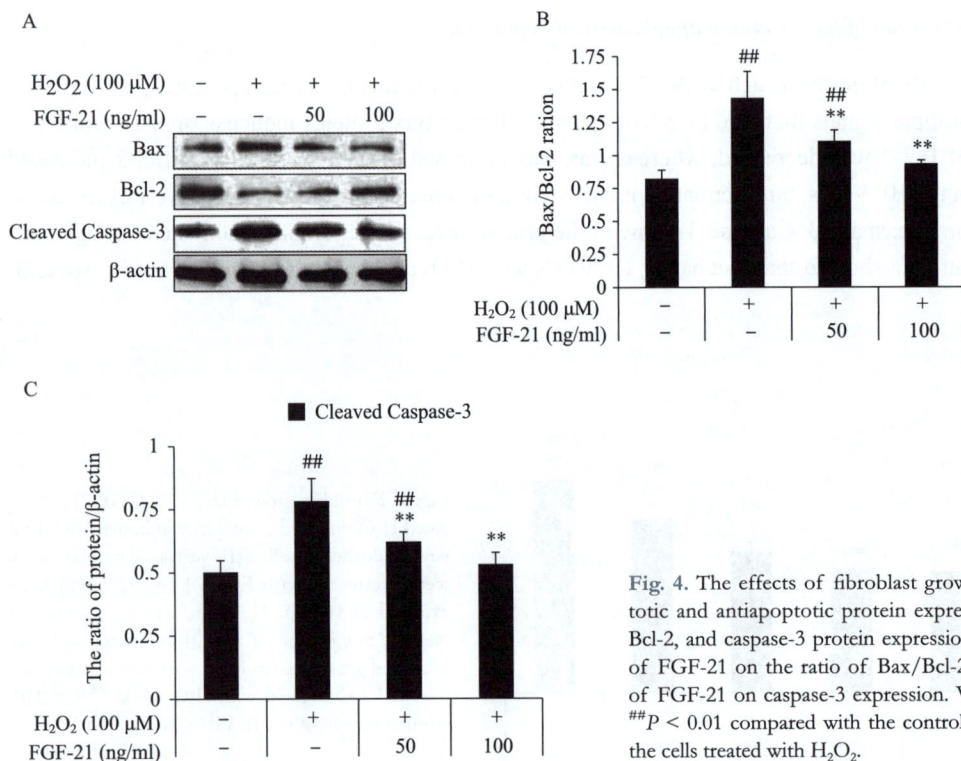

Fig. 4. The effects of fibroblast growth factor 21 (FGF-21) on apoptotic and antiapoptotic protein expression. (A) Western blot for Bax, Bcl-2, and caspase-3 protein expression. (B) Quantitation of the effects of FGF-21 on the ratio of Bax/Bcl-2. (C) Quantitation of the effects of FGF-21 on caspase-3 expression. Values are the mean ± SD, $n = 5$. ##$P < 0.01$ compared with the control cells; **$P < 0.01$ compared with the cells treated with H_2O_2.

A

H$_2$O$_2$ (100 μM)   –   +   +   +
FGF-21 (ng/ml)   –   –   50   100

Phospho-p38

p38

Phospho-JNK

JNK

B

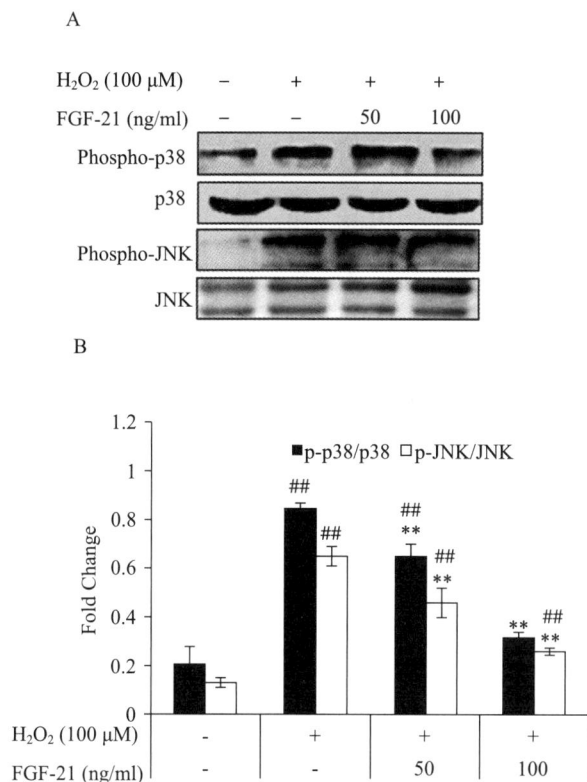

Fig. 5. Representative blots showing the effects of fibroblast growth factor 21 (FGF-21) on phosphorylated and total p38 and JNK expression. (A) Western blot for phosphorylated and total p38 and JNK protein expression. (B) Quantitation of effect of FGF-21 on phosphorylated and total p38 and JNK protein expression. Values are the mean ± SD, $n = 5$. [##]$P < 0.01$ compared with the control cells; [**]$P < 0.01$ compared with the cells treated with H$_2$O$_2$.

3.5 FGF-21 improved atherosclerosis in vivo

To establish an animal model with atherosclerosis, rats were fed with either regular food or a high-fat diet. As shown in Fig. 6A, using oil red O stain, there were no signs of atherosclerosis in the normal control group, and the morphologies of the aortas were normal with smooth intima. However, there were obvious signs of atherosclerosis in the rats fed the high-fat diet (Fig. 6B). These symptoms included serious lesions in the intima of the aortas and fused plaque areas that were spreading into the intima (Fig. 6B).

To test the effects of FGF-21 on atherosclerosis, rats on the high-fat diets were treated with or without FGF-21 protein, or with simvastatin as a control. Levels of TC, TG, HDL-C, and LDL-C were examined in the sera from each group of rats. Compared with the NC group, serum levels of TC and LDL-C in the rats with atherosclerosis (SA1) were significantly increased, and the HDL-C content was significantly reduced ($P < 0.05$) (Fig. 6C). Meanwhile, the content of TG from the atherosclerosis-model group was significantly increased compared with that of the normal group. This finding suggested that atherosclerotic rats have a lipid metabolism disorder. Simvastatin plays a regulatory role in lipid metabolism, and this was used for the "intervention group" of rats (SA2): for these rats the serum levels of TC, LDL-C, and TG were lower, whereas the HDL-C content was significantly increased by comparison with the AS1 group (Fig. 6C). Levels of TC, LDL-C, and TG in the rats from the AS3 and AS4 groups were significantly lower than those from the AS2 group ($P < 0.05$), whereas the HDL-C content was significantly increased compared with the AS2 group (Fig. 6C), indicating that treatment with FGF-21 dramatically improved lipid metabolism in the atherosclerotic rats. There were no statistically significant differences in the serum levels of TC, HDL-C, LDL-C, and TG among the NC, AS2, AS3, and SA4 groups (Fig. 6C).

To evaluate the antioxidant effects of FGF-21 on the vascular parameters of the rats used in our experiment, we measured the serum levels of SOD, MDA, and GSH, which are commonly used standards for assessing antioxidant properties. The results are shown in Fig. 6D. From the results, we can surmise that, compared with the NC group, serum levels of SOD and GSH in the AS1 group dropped greatly ($P < 0.01$), whereas serum levels of MDA increased remarkably in rats fed the high-fat diet. After treatment with simvastatin or FGF-21, levels of SOD and GSH increased and levels of MDA were significantly reduced, compared with the NC group. The results also indicated that FGF-21 had a

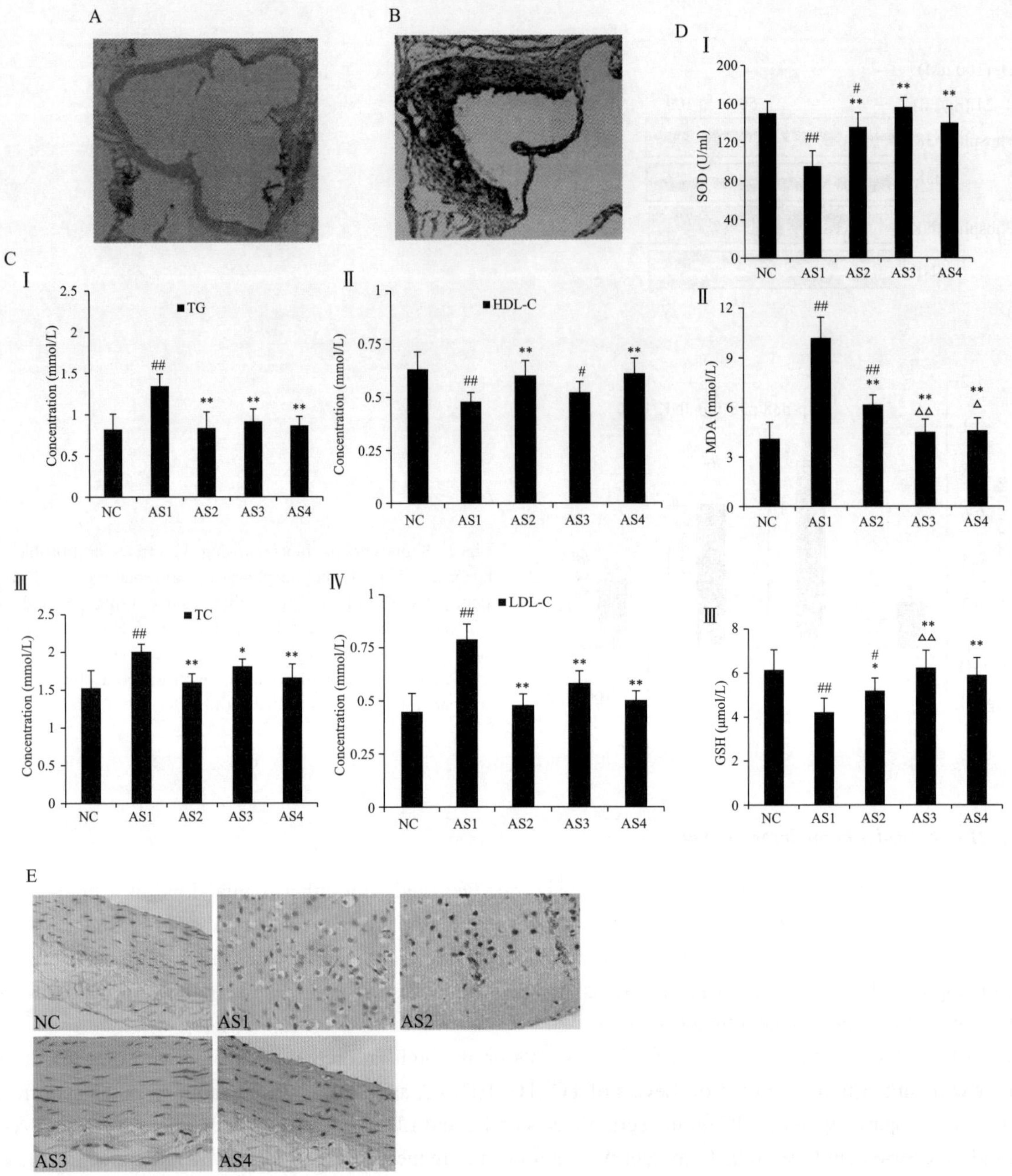

Fig. 6. Effect of fibroblast growth factor 21 (FGF-21) treatment on atherosclerosis *in vivo*. (A) Oil red O staining of aorta from normal rats (the control group rats fed with normal diet). (B) Oil red O staining of aorta from atherosclerotic rats (rats fed a high-fat diet for 12 weeks). (C) Variation in blood fat levels among the various experimental groups. The serum levels of triglycerides (TG), total cholesterol (TC), and low-density lipoprotein cholesterol (LDL-C) in groups AS2, AS3, and AS4 were significantly lower than that in the group AS1 ($P < 0.05$). There were no statistically significant differences between groups AS2 and AS3 or AS2 and AS4. The serum levels of HDL-C in groups AS2, AS3, and AS4 were significantly higher than that in group AS1 ($P < 0.05$). There were no statistically significant differences between groups AS2 and AS3, and AS4. Values are the mean ± SD, $n = 10$. $^{\#}P < 0.05$ and $^{\#\#}P < 0.01$ compared with the NC group; $^{*}P < 0.05$ and $^{**}P < 0.01$ compared with the AS1 group. (D) The effects of FGF-21 on the oxidative stress parameters for superoxide dismutase (SOD), reduced glutathione (GSH), and malondialdehyde (MDA) enzyme activity. (I) Serum SOD activity. (II) Serum MDA content. (III) Serum GSH activity. Values are the mean ± SD. $^{\#}P < 0.05$ and $^{\#\#}P < 0.01$ compared with the NC group; $^{*}P < 0.05$ and $^{**}P < 0.01$ compared with the AS1 group; $^{\triangle}P < 0.05$ and $^{\triangle\triangle}P < 0.01$ compared with the AS2 group. (E) Hematoxylin and eosin stained sections of rat aorta (magnification, 400×). The vessel walls are thin and smooth with an even thickness in the control group (NC). Foam cells, atheronecrotic substances, and calcification are present in the intima in group AS1, compared with the NC group. In group AS2, the vessel walls are rough, but no foam cells are present. The vessels in groups AS3 and AS4 were rougher and thicker than in AS1, and foam and inflammatory cells were detected.

stronger antioxidant effect than simvastatin.

We analyzed the pathology of the rat tissues using tissue stained with H&E. The vessel walls in the NC group were round and even in thickness, and the inner and outer elastic plates were clear and complete. The endotheliocyte cores were stained blue and evenly arranged. Also, no smooth muscle cells were observed underneath the endoderm (Fig. 6E; NC).

In contrast, the vessel walls in AS1 group were rough and uneven in thickness. The intima exhibited signs of hyperplasia. Numerous foam cells and atheronecrotic substances were observed under the fiber caps. Cholesterol crystals and inflammatory cells were also observed (Fig. 6E; AS1). The vessel walls in groups AS2, AS3, and AS4 were not as smooth as in NC group, and a few foam cells and inflammatory cells were observed (Fig. 6E; AS2, AS3, and AS4).

4. Discussion

FGF-21 is a potent metabolic regulator, and pharmacological evaluation of mammals treated with FGF-21 shows lowered levels of glucose and lipids (Kharitonenkov *et al.*, 2013). Pharmacologically speaking, FGF-21 has become recognized as a modulator of glucose and lipid homeostasis *in vivo*. Recombinant FGF-21 therapy has corrected many metabolic perturbations in diseased rodent models and nonhuman primates. Systemic administration of FGF-21 reduces plasma glucose, triglycerides, insulin, and glucagon in diabetic rhesus monkeys (Qiang and Accili, 2012). FGF-21 administration led to significant improvements in lipoprotein profiles, by lowering LDL-C and by raising HDL-C, as well as causing weight loss in the animals (Veniant *et al.*, 2012). However, the precise therapeutic mechanism for FGF-21 in AS is still elusive.

In this study, the effects of FGF-21 on H_2O_2-induced apoptosis of HUVECs *in vitro*, and on the rat model of AS *in vivo* were investigated. FGF-21 has recently been described as a potential new drug for combating metabolic diseases (Kharitonenkov *et al.*, 2007). However, it is difficult to highly express and purify recombinant FGF-21 because recombinant FGF-21 forms inclusion bodies in *E. coli*, making it difficult to purify and obtain high concentrations of bioactive FGF-21 (Liu *et al.*, 2012; Zhang *et al.*, 2012). For this study we expressed FGF-21 with vector pET22b (+) to express FGF-21 in *E. coli*. After IPTG induction, more than 55.2% of FGF-21 protein was secreted to the periplasmic space using the *pelB* signal sequence of the pET22b (+) vector. The harvested protein purity of FGF-21 was higher than 96% when using Q-Sepharose FF and Sepharose G-25 columns. The results indicated that expressing *FGF21* with the pET22b (+) vector made it easier to obtain high concentrations of bioactive protein.

Animal and clinical research have revealed that FGF-21 is associated with the morbidity of many metabolic syndromes caused by various kinds of obesity, and more importantly, overexpression or treatment with recombinant *FGF21* protects mice from developing obesity and fatty liver and improves insulin sensitivity, thus treatment with *FGF21* significantly deceases the level of risk for cardiovascular diseases *in vitro* (Kharitonenkov *et al.*, 2005). However, no data have been found that define the relation-ship between *FGF21* and AS in animal or clinical research. AS is a slowly progressing and multifactorial disease, in which abnormalities in endothelial cell (EC) structure and function play an initial role in its development (Crosby *et al.*, 2000). Healthy endothelial cells maintain vascular homeostasis through tight control of permeability, inflammation, vascular tone, and injury repair. Many risk factors for AS can lead to endothelial damage, proceeding to the accumulation of atheroma in the lumen of blood vessels (Ozcan, 2012). Apoptosis also plays an essential role in different pathological processes, including AS, in which it affects all cell types in the atherosclerotic lesion, including endothelial cells, vascular smooth muscle cells, and macrophages (Guevara *et al.*, 2001). We examined the effects of FGF-21 on H_2O_2-induced HUVEC apoptosis *in vitro*. Caspase-3 is one of the primary executioner caspases activated during apoptosis. It is activated during programmed cell death and leads to apoptosis (Lee *et al.*, 2012). MAPK signal transduction pathways differentially relay numerous extra-cellular signals within cells, and are involved in diverse cellular functions including stress responses and apoptosis (Kiel and Serrano, 2012). Western blot analysis revealed that caspase-3 cleavage was blocked, and the rapid phosphorylation of p38 MAPK and phosphorylation of JNK in H_2O_2-exposed HUVEC was substantially down-regulated by FGF-21. Our data indicated that FGF-21 protects HUVECs from oxidative-stress-induced cell injury and from the apoptosis induced by H_2O_2.

Since its discovery as a member of FGF super family, FGF-21 has been thought to be mainly expressed in the liver (Suzuki *et al.* 2008). However, FGF-21 has also been detected in skeletal muscles, implying that it might be secreted by cells of various origins, and its expression profile is likely broader than initially thought (Christodoulides *et al.*, 2009).

FGF-21 has recently been identified as a novel adipokine, which enhances insulin sensitivity and regulates lipid metabolism (Kharitonenkov and Larsen, 2011). Serum FGF-21 levels are significantly higher in obese populations with increased cardiovascular risk, as characterized by the symptoms of metabolic syndrome in obese subjects (Berglund et al., 2009; Hotta et al., 2009). It has been speculated that the paradoxical increase of this protein in populations with risk of cardiovascular disease such as AS, is a compensatory mechanism to counteract metabolic stress (Amira et al., 2012). This gives us a speculative clue that the mechanism of increased FGF-21 levels in cardiovascular disease is similar to obesity-associated resistance to insulin. However, whether using a disease-associated animal model can prove that the systemic administration of FGF-21 can regulate blood lipid metabolism for the treatment of AS has not been reported. Numerous animal species have been used to study the pathogenesis of and the potential treatment for atherosclerotic lesions (Olson et al., 2012). In this study, we examined the therapeutic effects of FGF-21 on AS in an animal model and found that FGF-21 reduced TC, LDL-C, and TG levels, and significantly increased HDL-C content in the atherosclerotic rat. The vessel walls of the FGF-21 treatment group were smooth and few foam or inflammatory cells were detected. These data demonstrated that FGF-21 had obvious therapeutic effects on AS in an atherosclerotic animal model. Besides, our results suggested that FGF-21 has antioxidant effects in the atherosclerotic rat, for which increased SOD, GSH and reduced MDA were observed. It is known that free radicals are strongly associated with cardiovascular disease, and thus the antioxidant properties of FGF-21 could protect against the development of CVD.

In conclusion, we have successfully expressed FGF-21 fused with pET22b (+) vector, and obtained a high purity of FGF-21. The recombinant FGF-21 can significantly resist oxidative stress induced cell apoptosis by preventing the cleavage of caspase-3 and blocking MAPK signaling cascades in vitro. In vivo, treatment with FGF-21 dramatically improved lipid metabolism and antioxidant effects in the atherosclerotic rat. Therefore, the possible mechanisms of FGF-21 on atherosclerosis may be mediated by its antioxidant capacity, in vitro and in vivo.

Our study suggests that FGF21 is a potential candidate for therapeutic application against AS, but the precise mechanism of FGF-21 action still needs further study.

References

[1] Amira OC, Naicker S, Manga P, et al. Adiponectin and atherosclerosis risk factors in African hemodialysis patients: A population at low risk for atherosclerotic cardiovascular disease[J]. Hemodialysis International, 2012, 16(1): 59-68.

[2] Badman MK, Pissios P, Kennedy AR, et al. Hepatic fibroblast growth factor 21 is regulated by PPAR alpha and is a key mediator of hepatic lipid metabolism in ketotic states[J]. Cell Metabolism, 2007, 5(6): 426-437.

[3] Berglund ED, Li CY, Bina HA, et al. Fibroblast Growth Factor 21 Controls Glycemia via Regulation of Hepatic Glucose Flux and Insulin Sensitivity[J]. Endocrinology, 2009, 150(9): 4084-4093.

[4] Christodoulides C, Lagathu C, Sethi JK, et al. Adipogenesis and WNT signalling[J]. Trends In Endocrinology And Metabolism, 2009, 20(1): 16-24.

[5] Coskun T, Bina HA, Schneider MA, et al. Fibroblast Growth Factor 21 Corrects Obesity in Mice[J]. Endocrinology, 2008, 149(12): 6018-6027.

[6] Crosby JR, Kaminski WE, Schatteman G, et al. Endothelial cells of hematopoietic origin make a significant contribution to adult blood vessel formation[J]. Circulation Research, 2000, 87(9): 728-730.

[7] Guevara NV, Chen KH, Chan L. Apoptosis in atherosclerosis: Pathological and pharmacological implications[J]. Pharmacological Research, 2001, 44(2): 59-71.

[8] Hotta Y, Nakamura H, Konishi M, et al. Fibroblast Growth Factor 21 Regulates Lipolysis in White Adipose Tissue But Is Not Required for Ketogenesis and Triglyceride Clearance in Liver[J]. Endocrinology, 2009, 150(10): 4625-4633.

[9] Inagaki T, Dutchak P, Zhao G, et al. Endocrine regulation of the fasting response by PPAR alpha-mediated induction of fibroblast growth factor 21[J]. Cell Metabolism, 2007, 5(6): 415-425.

[10] Inoue S, Browne G, Melino G, et al. Ordering of caspases in cells undergoing apoptosis by the intrinsic pathway[J]. Cell Death And Differentiation, 2009, 16(7): 1053-1061.

[11] Izumiya Y, Bina HA, Ouchi N, et al. FGF21 is an Akt-regulated myokine[J]. Febs Letters, 2008, 582(27): 3805-3810.

[12] Kharitonenkov A, Beals JM, Micanovic R, et al. Rational Design of a Fibroblast Growth Factor 21-Based Clinical Candidate, LY2405319[J]. Plos One, 2013, 8(3).

[13] Kharitonenkov A, Larsen P. FGF21 reloaded: challenges of a rapidly growing field[J]. Trends In Endocrinology And Metabolism, 2011, 22(3): 81-86.

[14] Kharitonenkov A, Shiyanova TL, Koester A, et al. FGF-21 as a novel metabolic regulator[J]. Journal Of Clinical Investigation, 2005, 115(6): 1627-1635.

[15] Kharitonenkov A, Wroblewski VJ, Koester A, et al. The metabolic state of diabetic monkeys is regulated by fibroblast growth factor-21[J]. Endocrinology, 2007, 148(2): 774-781.

[16] Kiel C, Serrano L. Challenges ahead in signal transduction: MAPK as an example[J]. Current Opinion In Biotechnology, 2012, 23(3): 305-314.

[17] Lee JS, Jung WK, Jeong MH, et al. Sanguinarine Induces Apoptosis of HT-29 Human Colon Cancer Cells via the Regulation of Bax/Bcl-2 Ratio and Caspase-9-Dependent Pathway[J]. International Journal Of Toxicology, 2012, 31(1): 70-77.

[18] Liu X, Chen Y, Wu X, et al. SUMO fusion system facilitates soluble expression and high production of bioactive human fibroblast growth factor 23 (FGF23)[J]. Applied Microbiology And Biotechnology, 2012, 96(1): 103-111.

[19] Mizuguchi Y, Oish Y, Miyoshi H, et al. Impact of statin therapy on left ventricular function and carotid arterial stiffness in patients

with hypercholesterolemia[J]. Circulation Journal, 2008, 72(4): 538-544.

[20] Muise ES, Azzolina B, Kuo DW, *et al.* Adipose fibroblast growth factor 21 is up-regulated by peroxisome proliferator-activated receptor gamma and altered metabolic states[J]. Molecular Pharmacology, 2008, 74(2): 403-412.

[21] Nishimura T, Nakatake Y, Konishi M, *et al.* Identification of a novel FGF, FGF-21, preferentially expressed in the liver[J]. Biochimica Et Biophysica Acta-Gene Structure And Expression, 2000, 1492(1): 203-206.

[22] Olson ES, Whitney MA, Friedman B, *et al. In vivo* fluorescence imaging of atherosclerotic plaques with activatable cell-penetrating peptides targeting thrombin activity[J]. Integrative Biology, 2012, 4(6): 595-605.

[23] Ozcan L. Endoplasmic Reticulum Stress in Cardiometabolic Disorders[J]. Current Atherosclerosis Reports, 2012, 14(5): 469-475.

[24] Qiang L, Accili D. FGF21 and the Second Coming of PPAR gamma[J]. Cell, 2012, 148(3): 397-398.

[25] Shu XD, Wu WC, Mosteller RD, *et al.* Sphingosine kinase mediates vascular endothelial growth factor-induced activation of Ras and mitogen-activated protein kinases[J]. Molecular And Cellular Biology, 2002, 22(22): 7758-7768.

[26] Singh S. Scaling up anti-mycobacterial drug susceptibility testing services in India: it is high time[J]. Indian Journal Of Medical Microbiology, 2008, 26(3): 209-211.

[27] Sun HY, Wang NP, Halkos M, *et al.* Postconditioning attenuates cardiomyocyte apoptosis *via* inhibition of JNK and p38 mitogen-activated protein kinase signaling pathways[J]. Apoptosis, 2006, 11(9): 1583-1593.

[28] Suzuki M, Uehara Y, Motomura-Matsuzaka K, *et al.* beta Klotho is required for fibroblast growth factor (FGF) 21 signaling through FGF receptor (FGFR) 1c and FGFR3c[J]. Molecular Endocrinology, 2008, 22(4): 1006-1014.

[29] Tan SM, Sharma A, Yuen DYC, *et al.* The Modified Selenenyl Amide, M-hydroxy Ebselen, Attenuates Diabetic Nephropathy and Diabetes-Associated Atherosclerosis in ApoE/GPx1 Double Knockout Mice[J]. Plos One, 2013, 8(7): e69193.

[30] Veniant MM, Komorowski R, Chen P, *et al.* Long-Acting FGF21 Has Enhanced Efficacy in Diet-Induced Obese Mice and in Obese Rhesus Monkeys[J]. Endocrinology, 2012, 153(9): 4192-4203.

[31] Wang H, Xiao Y, Fu L, *et al.* High-level expression and purification of soluble recombinant FGF21 protein by SUMO fusion in *Escherichia coli*[J]. BMC Biotechnology, 2010, 10.

[32] Zhang M, Jiang X, Su Z, *et al.* Large-scale expression, purification, and glucose uptake activity of recombinant human FGF21 in *Escherichia coli*[J]. Applied Microbiology And Biotechnology, 2012, 93(2): 613-621.

ATF4- and CHOP-dependent induction of FGF21 through endoplasmic reticulum stress

Xiaoshan Wan, Jian Xiao, Xiaokun Li

1. Introduction

The fibroblast growth factor family contains 22 members with a wide range of biological functions relevant to regulating cell growth, differentiation, wound healing, development, and angiogenesis [1-3]. Fibroblast growth factor 21 (FGF21) is a unique member of the FGF family and has broad metabolic functions, including stimulating glucose uptake insulin-independently and improving hyperglycemia and dyslipidemia [4-7]. FGF21 has a protective effect on the preservation of pancreatic β-cell function and promotes hepatic and peripheral insulin sensitivity *via* the prevention of lipolysis, which improves insulin resistance [8-10]. In addition, FGF21 can resist the diet-induced obesity and induce fatty acid oxidation [8, 11, 12]. At present, FGF21 is considered as a novel metabolism regulator and has become a focus of metabolic disease research.

FGF21 is expressed predominantly in liver and, to a lower extent, in white adipose tissue, thymus, skeletal muscle, and pancreatic β-cells [4, 9,13]. Substantial clinical research has focused on detecting FGF21 expression levels in various pathological states. It has been reported that serum FGF21 and hepatic mRNA expression levels in patients with NAFLD are significantly higher than levels in control subjects, which correlates with a substantial increase in liver triglyceride levels [14-16]. Plasma FGF21 was also found to elevate in type 2 diabetic or impaired glucose tolerance patients [17-19]. Circulating FGF21 levels were significantly higher in overweight subjects than those in lean individuals [20, 21]. Animal studies have reported similar results, showing increased FGF21 mRNA levels and serum FGF21 concentrations in the hepatic and adipose tissue of high fat diet-induced and genetically obese mice compared with wild-type mice [6, 8, 22]. An increase in FGF21 mRNA levels is similarly induced by fasting [23-25]. It seems likely that FGF21 levels are unchanged in different physiological states but increased with stress in individuals who are either overweight or have type 2 diabetes, or NAFLD. Based on these findings, we propose that the mechanism of increased FGF21 levels in metabolism disease may be due to feedback regulation, but the mechanism responsible for the effect is still unclear.

Numerous studies indicated that ER stress was closely related to metabolic diseases and it contributed to triggering insulin resistance, obesity, and type 2 diabetes [26-29]. ER is the site of synthesis, folding, and routing of proteins and it plays a prominent role in maintaining Ca^{2+} homeostasis in the cytosol. ER stress is a compensatory process that aims to preserve cellular functions and survival and induce by hypoxia, toxicity, infection, unfold protein accumulation, and perturbation of Ca^{2+} homeostasis [30]. ER stress transducers, including PKR-like ER kinase (PERK), activating transcription factor 6 (ATF6), and inositol-requiring enzyme 1 (IRE1), can be activated [31]. Phosphorylation of eukaryotic initiation factor α (eIF2α), *via* activation by PERK, leads to translational induction of ATF4. BiPfree pATF6(p) is transported to the Golgi apparatus where it is processed to a transcriptionally active nuclear form pATF6(N). Activated IRE1 site-specifically cleaves X-box-binding protein 1 (XBP1) mRNA precursor to create the mature XBP1 mRNA (XBP1-sp). ATF4, pATF6(N), and XBP1-sp then activate transcription of CCAAT enhancer binding protein homologous protein (CHOP) by binding to the appropriate promoter region, and CHOP plays a crucial role in ER stress-mediated apoptosis and in diseases including diabetes, brain ischemia, and neurodegenerative disease [32].

Several studies have shown that upregulation of FGF21 is mediated by ATF4 under conditions causing cellular stress, such as amino acid deprivation, autophagy, and mitochondrial dysfunction [33-36]. ATF4 directly increases FGF21 expression in cells with ER stress by binding to both amino acid-responsive element 1 (AARE1) and amino acid-responsive element 2 (AARE2) sequence on FGF21 [35, 37]. ATF4 activates the CHOP gene downstream, but not much is known on the relationship between CHOP and FGF21. To investigate whether FGF21 is regulated by ER stress *via* effects on AFT4 and CHOP, we establish an ER stress cell model using TG (thapsigargin) in which we detect FGF21 and ER stress-specific gene expression levels. We then demonstrated that TG-induced ER stress upregulates the expression and secretion of FGF21 by influencing ATF4 and CHOP providing insights on the mechanisms that link FGF21 and metabolic diseases.

2. Materials and methods

2.1 Materials

Dulbecco's modified Eagle's medium (DMEM), penicillin-streptomycin (p-s), newborn calf serum (NCS), and fetal bovine serum (FBS) were obtained from Gibco BRL (Grand Island, NY, USA). TRIzol reagent was obtained from Invitrogen (Carlsbad, CA, USA). High-Capacity cDNA Reverse Transcription Kits were obtained from Applied Biosystems (Foster City, CA, USA). QIAprep spin miniprep kits were obtained from Qiagen. Restriction endonucleases *Hin*d III and *Xho* I were purchased from NEB (Ipswich, MA, USA). Vector pGL4.17-Luc, Fugene HD reagents, and Luciferase Assay System were obtained from Promega (Sunnyvale, CA, USA). Mouse FGF21 ELISA Kits were obtained from R&D Systems (Minneapolis, MN, USA). Isobutyl-1-methylxanthine (IBMX), Dexamethasone (DEX), Insulin, Thapsigargin (TG), Actnomycin D, and all other chemical reagents were obtained from Sigma-Aldrich (St. Louis, MO).

2.2 Cell culture and differentiation

3T3-L1 murine preadipocytes were obtained from the American Type Culture Collection (Manassas, VA, USA). Cells were cultured in DMEM containing 10% NCS and 1% p-s; cells were induced to differentiate with DMEM plus 10% FBS, 1% p-s, 0.5 mM IBMX, 1 μM of DEX, and 1.7 μM Insulin for two days. Then the induction medium was replaced by DMEM with 10% FBS, 1% p-s, and 1.7 μM Insulin for another two days, followed by 10% FBS/DMEM medium, which was changed every two days. After 5-6 additional days, more than 85% cells differentiated to mature adipocytes, which can be used for the experiments.

2.3 Isolation and culture of mouse primary hepatocytes

Primary hepatocytes were isolated from C57BL/6J wild type (WT) and CHOP knockout (CHOP−/−)mice(male, 8 weeks) and cultured as described previously [38]. Cells were maintained in serum-free William'E medium containing 0.1 μM Dex, 1% penicillin, and 1 μM thyroxine. Before treatment, cells were incubated at 37℃, in 5% CO_2 for approximately 16 h or until they had attached.

2.4 RNA isolation and real-time reverse transcription-polymerase chain reaction (RT-PCR)

Total RNA was extracted from 3T3-L1 adipocytes using the TRIzol reagent according to the manufacturer's instructions. Total RNA (2 μg) was used as a template for first-strand cDNA synthesis using the High-Capacity cDNA Reverse Transcription Kit. The mRNA levels of ATF4, splicing of XBP1 (XBP1-sp), CHOP, and FGF21 were quantified using the following primers. ATF4 forward primer 5′-CCT AGG TCT CTT AGA TGA CTA TCT GGA GG-3′, ATF4 reverse primer 5′-CCA GGT CAT CCA TTC GAA ACA GAG CAT CG-3′; XBP1-sp forward primer 5′-TGA GTC CGC AGC AGG TG-3′, XBP1-sp reverse primer 5′-GAC AGG GTC CAA CTT GT-3′; CHOP forward primer 5′-GCT CCT GCC TTT CAC CTT GG-3′, CHOP reverse primer 5′-GGT TTT TGA TTC TTC CTC TTC-3′; FGF21 forward primer 5′-GCA GTC CAG AAA GTC TCC-3′, FGF21 reverse primer 5′-TGT AAC CGT CCT CCA GCA G-3′; iQ SYBR Green Supermix was used as a fluorescent dye to detect the presence of double-stranded DNA. The mRNA levels of each target gene were normalized to an endogenous control Glyceraldehyde-3-phosphate dehydrogenase (GAPDH). GAPDH forward primer 5′-GTC GTG GAT CTG ACG TGC C-3′, GAPDH reverse primer 5′-GAT GCC TGC TTC ACC ACC TT-3′. The ratio of normalized mean value for each treatment group to vehicle control group (DMSO) was calculated.

2.5 Enzyme-linked immunosorbent assay (ELISA) of FGF21

3T3-L1 adipocytes were treated with TG (0,12.5, 25, 50, and 100 nM) for 24 h, or TG (100 nM) for 0, 2, 4, 8, 16, and 24 h. The accumulated FGF21 in the culture medium was determined using ELISA Kit according to the manufacturer's instructions. The total protein concentrations of viable cells were determined using the Bio-Rad Protein Assay reagent. The total amounts of the FGF21 in medium were normalized to the total protein amounts and reported as pg/mg protein.

2.6 Plasmids construction and luciferase assay

The mouse FGF21 promoter constructs −1497/+5 were generously provided by Dr. Wenke Feng (The University of Louisville, Louisville, USA) and subcloned into pGL4.17-Luc luciferase report vector using *Hind* III and *Xho* I sites. The expression vector containing the coding sequence of ATF4 or CHOP was preserved in our laboratory. All plasmids were propagated in *Escherichia coli* DH5α and isolated using QIAprep spin miniprep kit (Qiagen). 293T cells were plated in 6-well plates 24 h before transfection. Cells were transfected with 2 μg of pGL4.17 promoter FGF21 (−1497/+5), 2 μg of ATF4, or CHOP expression vector using Fugene HD (Promega). 48 h after transfection, the cells were harvested and lysed, and the luciferase activity was measured using the Luciferase Assay System (Promega). The transfection efficiency was normalized to cotransfection of 1 μg of GFP vector.

2.7 Assessment of FGF21 mRNA stability

3T3-L1 mature adipocytes were treated with TG (100 nM)/DTT or vehicle control for 4 h; then Actinomycin D (5.0 μg/ml) was added to the medium (time 0 h). The mRNA of the cells was isolated after added Actinomycin D for 0.5, 1, 2, 4, and 6 h. FGF21, ATF4, XBP1-sp, and CHOP mRNA levels were detected using real-time RT-PCR as described in the previous section; the results are expressed as the fold of the mRNA value at the time of Actinomycin D addition.

2.8 Statistical analysis

All of the experiments were repeated at least three times; results were stated as the mean ± standard error. One-way ANOVA was employed to analyze the differences between sets of data. Statistics were performed using GraphPad Pro. A value of $P < 0.05$ was considered significant.

3. Results

3.1 ER stress increases FGF21 expression

To investigate the effect of ER stress on FGF21 mRNA levels, we treated 3T3-L1 adipocytes with TG, a potent ER stress activator, by disturbing ER calcium homeostasis. The mRNA levels of ER stress-specific genes (ATF4, XBP1-sp, and CHOP) and FGF21 were detected using real-time RT-PCR. We observed that TG increased FGF21 mRNA expression in a time-dependent manner (Fig. 1A). However, the expression levels at 24 h were lower than those at 16 h, perhaps due to cell toxicity. As shown in Fig. 1B, after the 3T3-L1 adipocytes were incubated with 12.5, 25, and 100 nM TG for 16 h, the levels of FGF21 mRNA were significantly increased in a concentration-dependent manner compared with the vehicle control group.

3.2 ER stress induces FGF21 secretion

Based on the above findings, a model of TG-induced stress in 3T3-L1 adipocytes was established, and we used this model to examine whether ER stress increases FGF21 secretion. Differentiated 3T3-L1 cells were treated with TG; the FGF21 protein levels in the medium were measured using ELISA. As shown in Fig. 2A and 2B, TG-induced ER stress led to increase in secreted FGF21 in a time- and dose-dependent manner. TG induced FGF21 protein level to a 40-fold rise at concentration of 100 nM for 24 h.

3.3 Knockout of CHOP decreases FGF21 expression

CHOP is a major transcription factor involved in ER stress. To determine whether CHOP expression contributes to ER stress-induced upregulation of FGF21, we isolated MPH from WT and CHOP-/-mice and treated the cells with TG for 24 h. In WT MPH, TG promoted the mRNA levels of CHOP and FGF21. However, in CHOP-/-MPH, TG failed to induce FGF21 expression, because ATF4 is upstream gene of CHOP and there is no effect of CHOP knockout on the ac-

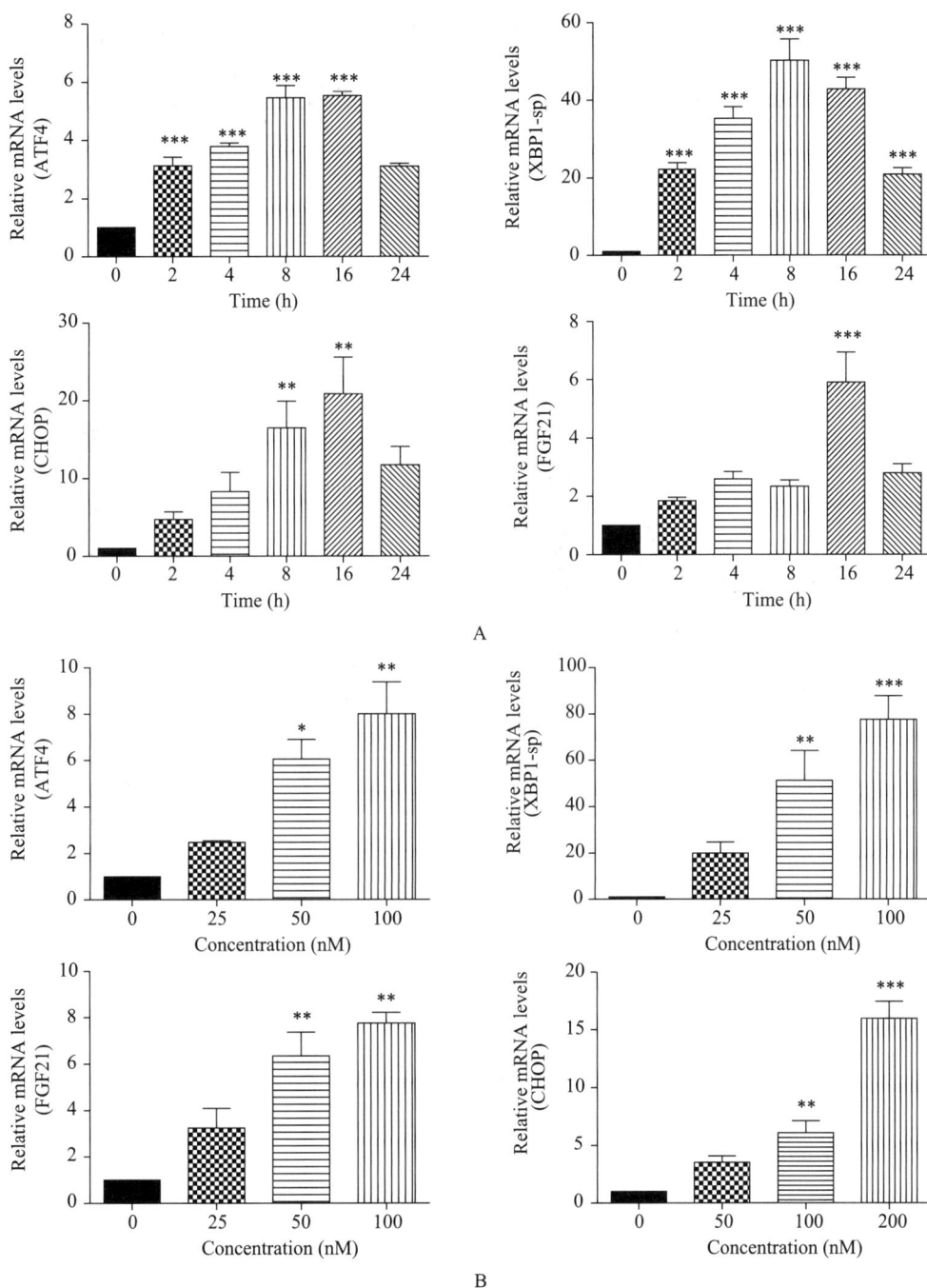

Fig. 1. ER stress increases FGF21 mRNA levels. (A) 3T3-L1 adipocytes were treated with TG (100 nM) for 0, 2,4, 8,16, and 24 h; (B) 3T3-L1 adipocytes were treated with TG (25, 50, and 100 nM) for 16 h. Total cellular RNA was isolated. The mRNA levels of ATF4, XBP1-sp, CHOP, and FGF21 were measured by real-time RT-PCR. Values are mean ± S.E. of three independent experiments. Statistical significance relative to vehicle control: $^{*}P < 0.05$; $^{**}P < 0.01$; $^{***}P < 0.001$.

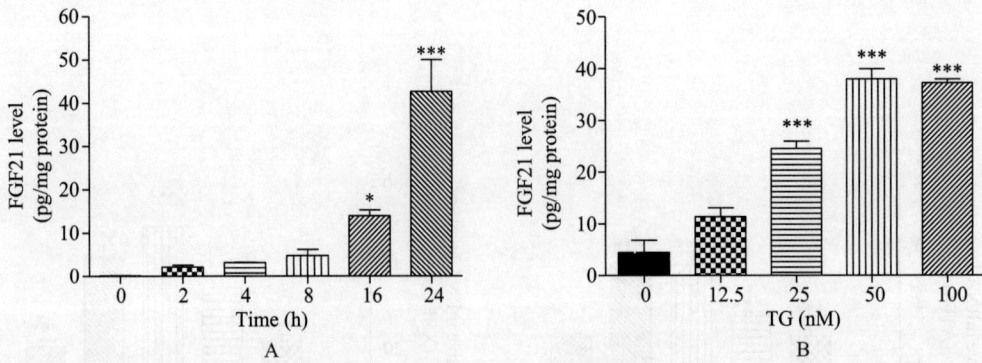

Fig. 2. ER stress induces FGF21 secretion. Differentiated 3T3-L1 cells were treated with 100 nM TG for 0,2,4,8,16, and 24 h(A); or different concentrations of TG for 24 h (B), at the end of treatment, cell culture medium was collected. The protein level ofFGF21 was determined by ELISA. Values are mean ± S.E. of three independent experiments. Statistical significance relative to vehicle control: *P < 0.05; ***P < 0.001.

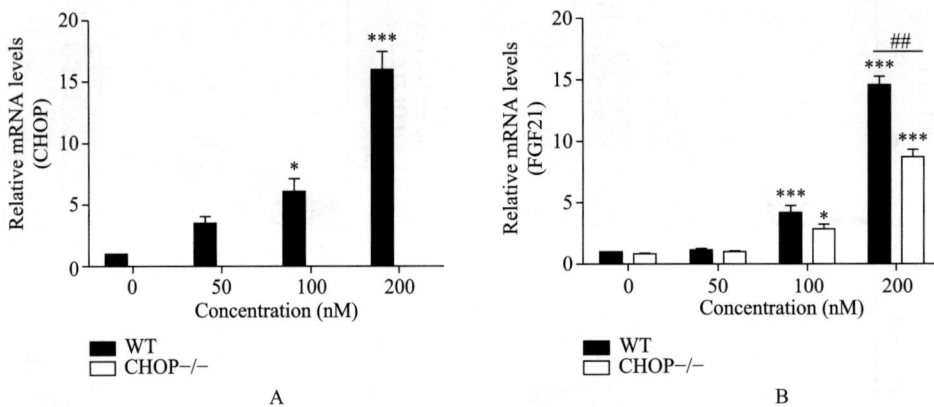

Fig. 3. Knockout of CHOP decreases FGF21 expression. WT and CHOP−/− mouse primary hepatocytes were treated for 24 h with increasing concentration of TG. Total cellular RNA was isolated and the mRNA levels of CHOP and FGF21 were measured by real-time RT-PCR. Values are mean ± S.E. of three independent experiments. Statistical significance relative to WT vehicle control: * P < 0.05; ***P < 0.001; statistical significance relative of the same TG concentration between WT group and CHOP−/− group: ##P< 0.01.

tivation of ATF4. Moreover, much research indicated that ATF4 can induce FGF21 expression under stress [33-37]. As depicted in Fig. 3, an absence of CHOP expression significantly increased FGF21 gene expression by 30%. These results indicate that CHOP may be a key player in the mechanism by which TG-induces increased FGF21 expression in MPH.

3.4 ATF4 and CHOP increase FGF21 promoter-driven transcription

To address the mechanism of TG-induced stress regulating FGF21 expression, we subcloned the FGF21 promoter (−1497/+5) into the pGL4.17-Luc luciferase report vector and measured the ability of ATF4 or CHOP to regulate the activation of the FGF21 promoter using a cotransfection assay. A previous study has reported that FGF21 expression could be mimicked by overexpression of ATF4 [37]. Unlike 3T3-L1 cell line, 293T cells can be transfected with high efficiency. 293T cells were cotransfected with pGL4.17-Luc luciferase report vector, which was inserted the mouse FGF21 promoter and expression vector for ATF4 or CHOP. Luciferase activity was determined at 48 h after transfection. Fig. 4A demonstrates that, compared with the control group, ATF4 overexpression enhanced FGF21 promoter activity more than 3-fold. This is consistent with the result of a previous study [37] that reported that there are two conserved ATF4-binding sites in the promoter region of the FGF21 gene and that FGF21 expression can be mimicked by overexpression of ATF4. CHOP is one of the genes that is downstream of ATF4. We hypothesized that CHOP would induce FGF21 expression similar to ATF4. We transfected HEK293 cells with the FGF21 reporter construct and CHOP. As shown in Fig. 4B, similar to ATF4, CHOP overexpression significantly increased the transcription of an FGF21 promoter-driven reporter. These findings indicate that ATF4 and CHOP upregulate FGF21 expression by activating the promoter in an environment of TG-induced ER stress.

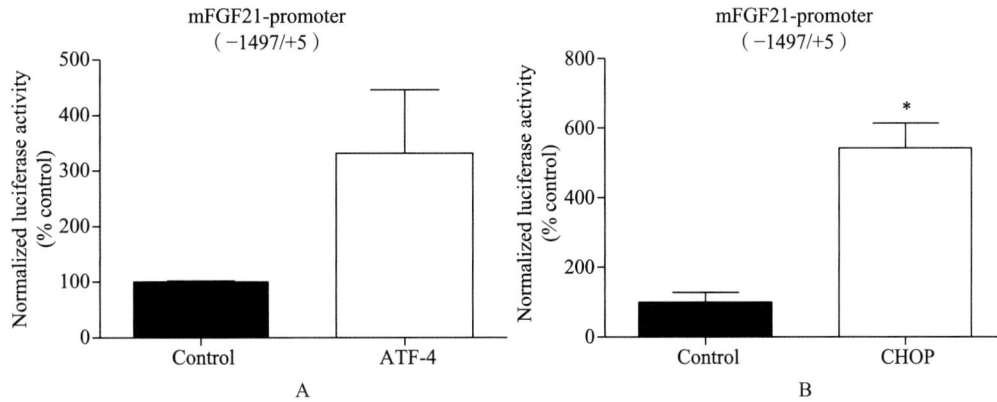

mFGF21-promoter
(−1497/+5)

mFGF21-promoter
(−1497/+5)

A

B

Fig. 4. ATF4 and CHOP increase FGF21 promoter-driven transcription. 293T cells were transfected with FGF21 promoter reporter construct along with the expression plasmid ATF4 or CHOP. Values are mean ± S.E. of three independent experiments. Statistical significance relative to control vector: * $P < 0.05$.

3.5 ER stress increases FGF21 mRNA stability

Posttranscriptional regulation is a major mechanism for the expression of cytokines. To determine whether TG- or DTT-(dithiothreitol-) induced ER stress increases FGF21 expression by regulating mRNA stability, we examined the effects of TG/DTT on the mRNA stability of FGF21 in 3T3-L1 adipocytes. The results indicated that TG and DTT increased the half-life of mRNA of FGF21 significantly but had no effect on ER stress-specific genes (Fig. 5). This result suggested TG- and DTT-induced ER stress activate FGF21 expression by increasing mRNA stability specifically.

4. Discussion

FGF21 acts as a hormone-like cytokine on multiple tissues to coordinate carbohydrate and lipid metabolism [4]. Clinical research has shown that serum FGF21 levels are higher in subjects who are overweight, have NAFLD, or are type 2 diabetic [14-18, 20]. Similarly, circulating FGF21 concentrations in *db/db* mice were much higher than normal, as were the FGF21 mRNA levels in both the liver and white adipose tissue [6, 8, 22]. Previous studies have reported that FGF21 expression is mediated by several transcriptional activators and their DNA response elements. Gene expression of FGF21 is induced directly by PPARα in response to starvation and ketotic states and PPARα agonists in liver [23, 25] as well as in cultured adipocytes and adipose tissue by PPARγ [39-41]. Activation of the farnesoid X receptor (FXR) in-

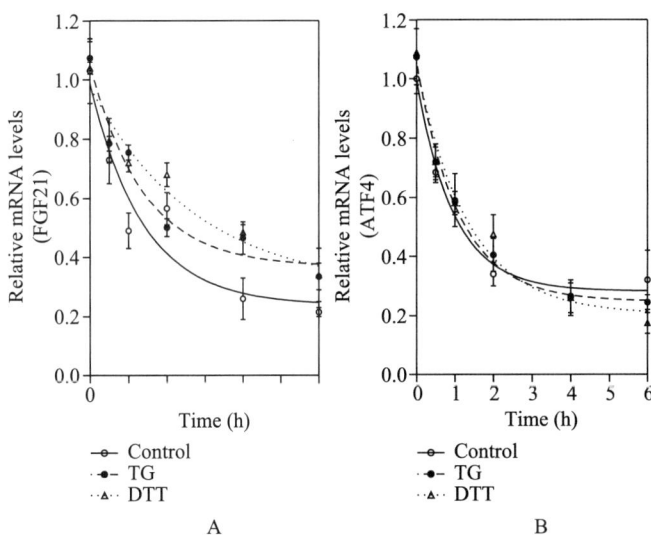

A

B

Fig. 5. ER stress increases FGF21 mRNA stability. 3T3-L1 adipocytes were pretreated with 100 nM TG/DTT or vehicle control (DMSO) for 4 h and then treated with 5.0 μg/ml actinomycin D (time 0). Total cellular RNA was extracted at 0, 0.5,1,2, 4, and 6 h after actinomycin D addition. FGF21 mRNA levels were determined by real-time RT-PCR. Values are mean ± S.E. of three independent experiments.

creased FGF21 gene expression and secretion was mediated by FXR/retinoid X receptor binding site in 5′-flanking region of the FGF21 gene [42]. A study demonstrated that glucose activation of carbohydrate response element binding protein (ChREBP) is involved in the upregulation of FGF21 mRNA expression in liver [43]. Retinoic acid receptor-related receptor α (RORα) also induces expression and secretion of FGF21, and there is a canonical ROR response element in the proximal promoter of FGF21 gene that exhibits functional activity [44]. PGC-1α-mediated reduction of FGF21 expression is dependent on the expression of its ligand, ALAS-1, and Rev-Erbα [45].

In addition, studies by Schaap *et al.* suggest that FGF21 expression is regulated by ER stress [37]. The authors reported that FGF21 mRNA is increased by TG-induced ER stress in rat H4IIE cells and rat primary hepatocytes. Moreover, intraperitoneal injection of the ER stressor tunicamycin induced hepatic FGF21 expression in mice and resulted in marked elevation of serum FGF21 levels [37]. Consistent with these new findings, we observed that TG-induced ER stress elevated FGF21 expression and secretion in murine 3T3-L1 adipocytes along with increasing ATF4 expression.

PERK (PKR-like ER kinase) is one of the major ER stress pathways. PERK can induce CHOP *via* activating ATF4. However, there was no information regarding the regulation of FGF21 by CHOP. We show for the first time that CHOP can increase FGF21 expression by activating transcription *via* promoter elements and enhancing mRNA stability in ER stress. We analyzed mouse FGF21 (−1497/+5) promoter and confirmed the absence of the conserved CHOP binding site 5′-(A/G) (A/G) TGCAAT (A/C) CCC-3′. Thus, FGF21 was not directly responsive to CHOP directly. To the contrary, our data demonstrates that CHOP can induce the transcription of a FGF21 promoter-driven reporter (Fig. 4B). CHOP may also regulate the expression of FGF21 indirectly by activating other cytokines and intracellular stress signaling pathways, though this remains to be determined conclusively.

Gene expression can be regulated by posttranscriptional control of mRNA stability [46]. The presence of AU-rich elements (AREs) in the 3′-untranslated region (3′-UTR) is essential for stabilization or degradation of mRNA of inflammatory factor [47]. The RNA-binding proteins (RBPs), such as HuR, AUF1, and CUG-BP1, positively regulate stability of many target mRNA *via* binding AREs present in the 3′-UTR [48, 49]. In this study, we identified for the first time that increased FGF21 mRNA stability, through the binding of RBPs to its target mRNAs, is responsible for elevated FGF21 levels by TG- or DTT-induced ER stress in differentiated 3T3-L1 cells.

In conclusion, these findings suggest that FGF21 is the target gene for ATF4 and CHOP, and transcription and mRNA stabilization are responsible for ATF4 and CHOP mediated induction of FGF21 expression in ER stress. Thus, we indicate ER stress is the key mechanism for regulating FGF21 in several metabolic diseases. Moreover, our studies provide important information about the FGF21 signaling pathway and the clinical significance of FGF21 in the development of metabolic diseases. Compared with WT MPH, FGF21 mRNA levels are reduced in CHOP−/− MPH treated with TG; however, the effects of CHOP overexpression on FGF21 levels are not understood. And it remains to be detected that the synergistic effect of ATF4 and CHOP on FGF21 expression. Moreover, further prospective studies are needed to determine the specific RBPs and their binding sites in FGF21 3′-UTR as well as the signaling pathway of CHOP-dependent activation of FGF21 in ER stress.

References

[1] Beenken A, Mohammadi M. The FGF family: biology, pathophysiology and therapy[J]. Nature Reviews Drug Discovery, 2009, 8(3): 235-253.

[2] Olsen SK, Garbi M, Zampieri N, *et al*. Fibroblast growth factor (FGF) homologous factors share structural but not functional homology with FGFs[J]. Journal Of Biological Chemistry, 2003, 278(36): 34226-34236.

[3] Smallwood PM, MunozSanjuan I, Tong P, *et al*. Fibroblast growth factor (FGF) homologous factors: New members of the FGF family implicated in nervous system development[J]. Proceedings Of the National Academy Of Sciences Of the United States Of America, 1996, 93(18): 9850-9857.

[4] Kharitonenkov A, Shiyanova TL, Koester A, *et al*. FGF-21 as a novel metabolic regulator[J]. J Clin Invest, 2005, 115(6): 1627-1635.

[5] Kharitonenkov A, Wroblewski VJ, Koester A, *et al*. The metabolic state of diabetic monkeys is regulated by fibroblast growth factor-

21[J]. Endocrinology, 2007, 148(2): 774-781.

[6] Coskun T, Bina HA, Schneider MA, *et al*. Fibroblast Growth Factor 21 Corrects Obesity in Mice[J]. Endocrinology, 2008, 149(12): 6018-6027.

[7] Seo JA, Kim NH. Fibroblast Growth Factor 21: A Novel Metabolic Regulator[J]. Diabetes & Metabolism Journal, 2012, 36(1): 26-28.

[8] Xu J, Lloyd DJ, Hale C, *et al*. Fibroblast Growth Factor 21 Reverses Hepatic Steatosis, Increases Energy Expenditure, and Improves Insulin Sensitivity in Diet-Induced Obese Mice[J]. Diabetes, 2009, 58(1): 250-259.

[9] Wente W, Efanov AM, Brenner M, *et al*. Fibroblast growth factor-21 improves pancreatic beta-cell function and survival by activation of extracellular signal-regulated kinase 1/2 and Akt signaling pathways[J]. Diabetes, 2006, 55(9): 2470-2478.

[10] Arner P, Pettersson A, Mitchell PJ, *et al*. FGF21 attenuates lipolysis in human adipocytes-A possible link to improved insulin

sensitivity[J]. Febs Letters, 2008, 582(12): 1725-1730.

[11] Mai K, Andres J, Biedasek K, et al. Free fatty acids link metabolism and regulation of the insulin-sensitizing fibroblast growth factor-21. Diabetes, 2009, 58(7): 1532-1538.

[12] Hotta Y, Nakamura H, Konishi M, et al. Fibroblast Growth Factor 21 Regulates Lipolysis in White Adipose Tissue But Is Not Required for Ketogenesis and Triglyceride Clearance in Liver[J]. Endocrinology, 2009, 150(10): 4625-4633.

[13] Mashili FL, Austin RL, Deshmukh AS, et al. Direct effects of FGF21 on glucose uptake in human skeletal muscle: implications for type 2 diabetes and obesity[J]. Diabetes-Metabolism Research And Reviews, 2011, 27(3): 286-297.

[14] Li H, Fang Q, Gao F, et al. Fibroblast growth factor 21 levels are increased in nonalcoholic fatty liver disease patients and are correlated with hepatic triglyceride[J]. Journal Of Hepatology, 2010, 53(5): 934-940.

[15] Dushay J, Chui PC, Gopalakrishnan GS, et al. Increased Fibroblast Growth Factor 21 in Obesity and Nonalcoholic Fatty Liver Disease[J]. Gastroenterology, 2010, 139(2): 456-463.

[16] Yilmaz Y, Eren F, Yonal O, et al. Increased serum FGF21 levels in patients with nonalcoholic fatty liver disease[J]. European Journal Of Clinical Investigation, 2010, 40(10): 887-892.

[17] Chen WW, Li L, Yang GY, et al. Circulating FGF-21 levels in normal subjects and in newly diagnose patients with type 2 diabetes Mellitus[J]. Experimental And Clinical Endocrinology & Diabetes, 2008, 116(1): 65-68.

[18] Li L, Yang G, Ning H, et al. Plasma FGF-21 levels in type 2 diabetic patients with ketosis[J]. Diabetes Research And Clinical Practice, 2008, 82(2): 209-213.

[19] Chavez AO, Molina-Carrion M, Abdul-Ghani MA, et al. Circulating Fibroblast Growth Factor-21 Is Elevated in Impaired Glucose Tolerance and Type 2 Diabetes and Correlates With Muscle and Hepatic Insulin Resistance[J]. Diabetes Care, 2009, 32(8): 1542-1546.

[20] Zhang X, Yeung DCY, Karpisek M, et al. Serum FGF21 levels are increased in obesity and are independently associated with the metabolic syndrome in humans[J]. Diabetes, 2008, 57(5): 1246-1253.

[21] Mraz M, Bartlova M, Lacinova Z, et al. Serum concentrations and tissue expression of a novel endocrine regulator fibroblast growth factor-21 in patients with type 2 diabetes and obesity[J]. Clinical Endocrinology, 2009, 71(3): 369-375.

[22] Fisher FM, Estall JL, Adams AC, et al. Integrated Regulation of Hepatic Metabolism by Fibroblast Growth Factor 21 (FGF21) in Vivo[J]. Endocrinology, 2011, 152(8): 2996-3004.

[23] Badman MK, Pissios P, Kennedy AR, et al. Hepatic fibroblast growth factor 21 is regulated by PPAR alpha and is a key mediator of hepatic lipid metabolism in ketotic states[J]. Cell Metabolism, 2007, 5(6): 426-437.

[24] Inagaki T, Dutchak P, Zhao G, et al. Endocrine regulation of the fasting response by PPAR alpha-mediated induction of fibroblast growth factor 21[J]. Cell Metabolism, 2007, 5(6): 415-425.

[25] Lundasen T, Hunt MC, Nilsson L-M, et al. PPAR alpha is a key regulator of hepatic FGF21[J]. Biochemical And Biophysical Research Communications, 2007, 360(2): 437-440.

[26] Ozcan U, Cao Q, Yilmaz E, et al. Endoplasmic reticulum stress links obesity, insulin action, and type 2 diabetes[J]. Science, 2004, 306(5695): 457-461.

[27] Hotamisligil GS. Endoplasmic Reticulum Stress and the Inflammatory Basis of Metabolic Disease[J]. Cell, 2010, 140(6): 900-917.

[28] Ozcan L, Tabas I. Role of Endoplasmic Reticulum Stress in Metabolic Disease and Other Disorders[J]. Annual Review Of Medicine, 2012, 63: 317-328.

[29] Cao SS, Kaufman RJ. Targeting endoplasmic reticulum stress in metabolic disease[J]. Expert Opinion on Therapeutic Targets, 2013, 17(4): 437-448.

[30] Kaufman RJ. Stress signaling from the lumen of the endoplasmic reticulum: coordination of gene transcriptional and translational controls[J]. Genes & Development, 1999, 13(10): 1211-1233.

[31] Oyadomari S, Mori M. Roles of CHOP/GADD153 in endoplasmic reticulum stress[J]. Cell Death And Differentiation, 2004, 11(4): 381-389.

[32] Zinszner H, Kuroda M, Wang XZ, et al. CHOP is implicated in programmed cell death in response to impaired function of the endoplasmic reticulum[J]. Genes & Development, 1998, 12(7): 982-995.

[33] Luisa De Sousa-Coelho A, Marrero PF, Haro D. Activating transcription factor 4-dependent induction of FGF21 during amino acid deprivation[J]. Biochemical Journal, 2012, 443: 165-171.

[34] Kim KH, Jeong YT, Oh H, et al. Autophagy deficiency leads to protection from obesity and insulin resistance by inducing Fgf21 as a mitokine[J]. Nature Medicine, 2013, 19(1): 83-92.

[35] Jiang X, Zhang C, Xin Y, et al. Protective effect of FGF21 on type 1 diabetes-induced testicular apoptotic cell death probably via both mitochondrial- and endoplasmic reticulum stress-dependent pathways in the mouse model[J]. Toxicology Letters, 2013, 219(1): 65-76.

[36] Luo Y, McKeehan WL. Stressed Liver and Muscle Call on Adipocytes with FGF21[J]. Frontiers in endocrinology, 2013, 4: 194-194.

[37] Schaap FG, Kremer AE, Lamers WH, et al. Fibroblast growth factor 21 is induced by endoplasmic reticulum stress[J]. Biochimie, 2013, 95(4): 692-699.

[38] Zhou H, Gurley EC, Jarujaron S, et al. HIV protease inhibitors activate the unfolded protein response and disrupt lipid metabolism in primary hepatocytes[J]. American Journal Of Physiology-Gastrointestinal And Liver Physiology, 2006, 291(6): G1071-G1080.

[39] Muise ES, Azzolina B, Kuo DW, et al. Adipose fibroblast growth factor 21 is up-regulated by peroxisome proliferator-activated receptor gamma and altered metabolic states[J]. Molecular Pharmacology, 2008, 74(2): 403-412.

[40] Moyers JS, Shiyanova TL, Mehrbod F, et al. Molecular determinants of FGF-21 activity-synergy and cross-talk with PPAR gamma signaling[J]. Journal Of Cellular Physiology, 2007, 210(1): 1-6.

[41] Wang H, Qiang L, Farmer SR. Identification of a domain within peroxisome proliferator-activated receptor gamma regulating expression of a group of genes containing fibroblast growth factor 21 that are selectively repressed by SIRT1 in adipocytes[J]. Molecular And Cellular Biology, 2008, 28(1): 188-200.

[42] Cyphert HA, Ge X, Kohan AB, et al. Activation of the Farnesoid X Receptor Induces Hepatic Expression and Secretion of Fibroblast Growth Factor 21[J]. Journal Of Biological Chemistry, 2012, 287(30): 25123-25138.

[43] Iizuka K, Takeda J, Horikawa Y. Glucose induces FGF21 mRNA expression through ChREBP activation in rat hepatocytes[J]. Febs Letters, 2009, 583(17): 2882-2886.

[44] Wang Y, Solt LA, Burris TP. Regulation of FGF21 Expression and Secretion by Retinoic Acid Receptor-related Orphan Receptor alpha[J]. Journal Of Biological Chemistry, 2010, 285(21): 15668-15673.

[45] Estall JL, Ruas JL, Choi CS, et al. PGC-1 alpha negatively regulates hepatic FGF21 expression by modulating the heme/Rev-Erb alpha axis[J]. Proceedings Of the National Academy Of Sciences Of the United States Of America, 2009, 106(52): 22510-22515.

[46] Schwanhaeusser B, Busse D, Li N, et al. Global quantification of mammalian gene expression control[J]. Nature, 2011, 473(7347): 337-342.

[47] Brennan CM, Steitz JA. HuR and mRNA stability[J]. Cellular And Molecular Life Sciences, 2001, 58(2): 266-277.

[48] Raineri I, Wegmueller D, Gross B, et al. Roles of AUF1 isoforms, HuR and BRF1 in ARE-dependent mRNA turnover studied by RNA interference[J]. Nucleic Acids Research, 2004, 32(4): 1279-1288.

[49] Lu JY, Schneider RJ. Tissue distribution of AU-rich mRNA-binding proteins involved in regulation of mRNA decay[J]. Journal Of Biological Chemistry, 2004, 279(13): 12974-12979.

Protective effect of FGF21 on type 1 diabetes-induced testicular apoptotic cell death probably *via* both mitochondrial- and endoplasmic reticulum stress-dependent pathways in the mouse model

Xin Jiang, Xiaokun Li, Lu Cai

1. Introduction

The fibroblast growth factor (FGF) family plays multiple roles in determining and regulating functions of some endocrine-relevant tissues or organs (Angelin *et al.*, 2012; Kharitonenkov, 2009). Of the 23 known members of the family, FGF21 is a novel member identified by Nishimura *et al.* (2000). Accumulating evidence indicates the role of FGF21 as a critical regulator of long-term energy balance and metabolism. Mice lacking FGF21 cannot respond appropriately to a ketogenic diet, resulting in an impaired ability to mobilize and utilize lipids (Badman *et al.*, 2009). The FGF21 expresses pre-dominantly in pancreas, liver and adipose tissues, and relatively less in other organs, including the testis (Fon Tacer *et al.*, 2010). Numerous studies have focused on the role of FGF21 in metabolic regulation in the liver, fat, and even skeletal muscle (Angelin *et al.*, 2012; Cuevas-Ramos *et al.*, 2012; Kharitonenkov, 2009). However, the role of FGF21 in other organs has not been well addressed.

The expression of FGF21 mRNA was found in the testis (Fon Tacer *et al.*, 2010), but what is the biological function of FGF21 in the testis remains unclear. In fact, it has been appreciated that the other FGF family members such as FGF1, 2, 4, 8, and 9 are also expressed in the male reproductive tract and are intimately involved in testicular maturation, Sertoli cell proliferation and differentiation (El Ramy *et al.*, 2005; Elo *et al.*, 2012; Hiramatsu *et al.*, 2010; Lahr *et al.*, 1992); some members of FGF family such as FGF4 play important anti-apoptotic role in the protection of the testicular cells against the toxic effect (Hirai *et al.*, 2004; Yamamoto *et al.*, 2002).

Testicular apoptotic cell death occurs in many conditions, including the normal spermatogenesis and also chronic diseases such as diabetes (Cai *et al.*, 2000; Guneli *et al.*, 2008; Mohasseb *et al.*, 2011; Zhao *et al.*, 2011). We have demonstrated that diabetes induces testicular apoptotic cell death predominantly through mitochondrial and endoplasmic reticulum (ER) stress associated cell death pathways, which may be metabolic abnormality induced oxidative damage (Cai *et al.*, 2000; Zhao *et al.*, 2010, 2011). Whether FGF21 as an important metabolic mediator is also involved in the maintenance of the spermatogenesis and whether FGF21 protects the germ cells from diabetes-induced apoptotic cell death have never been investigated.

Reportedly FGF21 improves the survival of pancreatic β-cells (Wente *et al.*, 2006). Islets and INS-1E cells isolated from FGF21-treated diabetic rats were partially protected from glucose-, lipid-, and cytokine-induced apoptosis (Wente *et al.*, 2006). In addition, the protection of FGF21 from oxidized-low density lipoprotein (ox-LDL)-induced apoptotic cell death was also observed in cardiac microvascular endothelial cells (Lu *et al.*, 2010).

Therefore, the present study aimed to test our hypothesis that the testicular FGF21 expression is required for the normal spermatogenesis and able to protect the germ cells from diabetes-induced apoptotic cell death. To these ends, we have examined the mRNA expression of FGF21 in the testis of fasting and non-fasting mice or mice with type 1 diabetes. The type 1 diabetes mouse model was induced with streptozotocin (STZ). We also examined the effect of *Fgf21* gene deletion on the testicular apoptotic cell death spontaneously or induced by type 1 diabetes with *Fgf21* gene knockout (FGF21-KO) mice and their age-matched wild-type (WT) mice. In addition, we also supplemented exogenous FGF21 to FGF21-KO diabetic mice to directly define the anti-apoptotic effect of FGF21 on diabetes-induced testicular cell death.

2. Materials and methods

2.1 Animals

FGF21-KO mice with C57BL/6J background were given as a gift from Dr. Steve Kliewer, University of Texas Southwestern Medical Center. Age-matched WT (C57BL/6J) controls were obtained from Jackson Laboratory. Total 26 male WT mice and 34 male FGF21-KO mice, 10 weeks of age, were assigned to this study. There were two sets of experiments. The first experiment used 10 WT and 10 FGF21-KO mice for examining testicular and hepatic expression of FGF21 mRNA under fasting and non-fasting conditions ($n = 5$). The liver was included as a positive tissue control for FGF21 mRNA expression under fasting condition (Badman $et~al.$, 2007; Chavez $et~al.$, 2008). The rest 16 WT and 24 FGF21-KO mice were used for the second experiment as diabetic model (see Section 2.2).

All animal procedures were approved by Institutional Animal Care and Use Committee, which is certified by the American Association for Accreditation of Laboratory Animal Care. All mice were housed in the University of Louisville Research Resources Center at $22\,^{\circ}\mathrm{C}$ with a 12:12-h light–dark cycle and provided with free access to rodent chow and tap water. All mice were kept under these conditions for 1 week.

2.2 Diabetes model

Sixteen WT and 24 FGF21-KO mice were randomly allocated into five groups ($n = 8$), including WT control (WT-CON), WT diabetes (WT-DM), FGF21-KO control (KO-CON), FGF21-KO diabetes (KO-DM), and KO-DM with treatment of exogenous FGF21 (KO-DM-FGF21). To make type 1 diabetes, STZ (Sigma–Aldrich, St. Louis, MO) was dissolved in 0.1 M sodium citrate (pH 4.5) and was given intraperitoneally to the mice of WT-DM, KO-DM, and KO-DM-FGF21 groups at single dose of 200 mg/kg body weight. Corresponding control mice were given the same volume of sodium citrate buffer as control. Whole blood glucose obtained from the mouse tail vein was detected using a SureStep complete blood glucose monitor (LifeScan, Milpitas, CA) at the third day after STZ injection. Mice with blood glucose level $\geqslant 250$ mg/dl were considered as diabetic (Cai $et~al.$, 2002). The mice in the KO-DM-FGF21 group were intraperitoneally injected with FGF21 at 100 μg/kg body weight daily for 10 days while mice in other groups were given the same volume of phosphate buffer. When these mice were sacrificed at 6 h after the last injection of FGF21 on the 10th day after the onset of diabetes bilateral testes were harvested. One side testis of each mouse was fixed in 10% buffered formalin for histopathological studies, while the other was stored at $-80\,^{\circ}\mathrm{C}$ for biochemical studies.

2.3 Terminal deoxynucleotidyl transferase-mediated dUTP nick end labeling (TUNEL) assay

Every testis was fixed in 10% formalin for 24 h, embedded in paraffin, and sectioned at 5 μm. Four sections were selected from each testis at each interval 30 pieces along with horizontal axis and stained for TUNEL with the ApopTag Peroxidase $In~Situ$ Apoptosis Detection Kit (Chemicon, CA, USA), as described in previous studies (Cai $et~al.$, 2000; Zhao $et~al.$, 2011). Briefly, each slide was deparaffinized and rehydrated, and treated with proteinase K (20 mg/L) for 15 min at room temperature. Slides were treated with 3% hydrogen peroxide to quench endogenous peroxidases for 5 min, and then were incubated with TUNEL reaction mixture containing terminal deoxynucleotidyl transferase (TdT) and digoxigenin-11-dUTP at $37\,^{\circ}\mathrm{C}$ for 1 h. Then 3,3-diaminobenzidine chromogen was applied. Hematoxylin was used as counterstaining. For negative control, TdT was omitted from the reaction mixture.

Under microscope apoptotic cells would exhibit a brown nuclear stain as the TUNEL positive and were quantitatively counted manually. From each of the three sections at least from each testis (mouse) we randomly selected 30 seminiferous tubule's cross-sections that were selected in a same pattern to move each slide without repetitive counting in a blinded fashion, i.e., the examiner was unaware of the grouping information of slides. At least 3 sections were counted from each testis, and at least 5 animals were counted in each group. The apoptotic cells were counted from spermatogonia, primary spermatocytes, and secondary spermatocytes, but not spermatid and spermatozoa because total cells of the former can be easily identified for the quantification. Results were presented as TUNEL positive cells per 10^{3} cells.

We also calculated the apoptotic index (AI) that was the percentage of essentially round seminiferous tubules with more than three TUNEL-positive cells. Thirty fields from each of the three sections at least were counted for each of the five testes (mice) in each group.

2.4 Western blotting

Western blots were performed as described in our previous studies (Cai *et al.*, 2000; Zhao *et al.*, 2011). Briefly, testicular tissues were homogenized in RIPA lysis buffer (Santa Cruz Biotechnology, CA) for collecting the protein by centrifuging at 12000 rpm at 4 ℃ for 15 min. The testicular protein concentration was measured. The protein sample was diluted in loading buffer and heated at 95 ℃ for 5 min, separated by electrophoresis on 10% sodium dodecyl sulfate polyacrylamide gel electrophoresis (SDS-PAGE) at 120 V, and then transferred to a nitrocellulose membrane. Membranes were rinsed briefly in Tris-buffered saline (pH 7.2) containing 0.1% Tween 20 and blocked with blocking buffer (5% milk and 0.5% BSA) for 1 h, and incubated overnight at 4 ℃ with the following antibodies: anti-cleaved-caspase-8, anti-Bax, anti-Bcl-2, anti-cleaved-caspase-3, anti-apoptosis-inducing factor (AIF), and anti-glucose-regulated protein 78 (GRP78) (all at 1:1 000 and purchased from Cell Signaling, MA); anti-cleaved-caspase-12 (1:1000; Exalpha Biologicals, MA), anti-activating transcription factor 4 (ATF4, 1:1000; Abcam, MA), and anti-C/EBP homologous protein (CHOP) and anti-β-actin (1:1 000; Santa Cruz Biotechnology, CA). After the unbound antibodies were removed, the membranes were incubated with the horseradish peroxidase-conjugated secondary antibody for 1 h at room temperature. Blots were visualized using an enhanced chemiluminescence detection kit (ECL; Thermo Scientific, IL). All experiments were performed in triplicate and repeated at least three times. Quantitative densitometry was performed on the identified bands by using a computer-based measurement system, as employed in previous studies (Cai *et al.*, 2002; Zhao *et al.*, 2011).

2.5 RNA isolation and real-time RT-PCR

Total RNA was extracted from testicular tissues using Trizol reagent (RNA STAT 60 Tel-Test; Ambion, Austin, TX). RNA concentration and purity were quantified using a Nanodrop ND-1000 spectrophotometer (Thermo Scientific, Wilmington, DE) and the A260/A280 ratio of all RNA samples was >1.8. One microgram of total RNA was reversely transcribed using an avian myeloblastosis virus reverse transcriptase kit (Promega, Madison, WI) following the manufacturer's protocol. For real-time PCR, primers (mouse FGF21: Mm00840165_g1; mouse β-actin: Mm00607939_s1) were purchased from Applied Biosystems (Carlsbad, CA). The amplification reactions were carried out in triplicate of a 20 μl reaction system that was composed of TaqMan Universal PCR Master Mix (Applied Biosystems) 10 μl, Primers 1 μl, cDNA 2 μl, and DD H_2O 7 μl, in the ABI 7300 Real-Time PCR system (Life Technologies Corporation, Carlsbad, CA) with initial hold steps (50 ℃ for 2 min), followed by 95 ℃ for 10 min, for 60 cycles of a two-step PCR (92 ℃ for 15 s and 60 ℃ for 1 min). The comparative cycle time (Ct) method was used to determine fold differences between samples and determined the amount of tar-get, normalized to an endogenous reference (β-actin) and relative to a calibrator ($2^{-\Delta\Delta Ct}$).

2.6 Immunohistochemical and immunofluorescence staining

Testicular tissues fixed in 10% neutral-buffered formalin were embedded in paraffin and sectioned at 5 μm. Four sections for each animal were selected as described for TUNEL staining. The sections were deparaffinized in xylene and rehydrated in graded alcohol solutions. After sections were incubated with retrieval solution (Dako, Carpinteria, CA) for 15 min at 98 ℃ and then treated with 3% hydrogen peroxide for 15 min at room temperature, followed by blocking with 5% BSA for 30 min.

For immunohistochemical staining sections were incubated with primary antibodies including anti-proliferating cell nuclear antigen (PCNA, 1:4000; Cell Signaling), anti-tumor necrosis factor-α (TNF-α, 1:200 dilution; Abcam), anti-plasminogen activator inhibitor-1 (PAI-1, 1:100; BD Biosciences, CA), anti-AIF (1:50 dilution; Cell Signaling), anti-3-nitrotyrosine (3-NT, 1:200; Millipore, MA), and anti-4-hydroxy-2-nonenal (4-HNE, 1:200; Alpha Diagnostic International, TX) at 4 ℃ overnight. After washing with PBS, these sections were incubated with horseradish peroxidase conjugated secondary antibody for 1 h at room temperature. For the development of color, sections were treated with peroxidase substrate 3,3-Dsity relative to WT control. AIF positive cells were counted and presented as the positive cells per 1000 cells in the manner same as described above for TUNEL studies.

For immunofluorescence staining sections were incubated with the primary antibodies including anti-AIF (1:100; Cell Signaling) and anti-β-actin (1:500; Santa Cruz Biotechnology). The secondary antibodies CY3-conjugated IgG (1:200; Cell Signaling) and FITC-conjugated IgG (1:100; Abcam) were applied for 1 h at room temperature. Slides were counterstained with DAPI (Sigma–Aldrich), covered with aqueous mounting medium (Sigma–Aldrich) and analyzed under fluorescent micro-scope (Nikon, Tokyo, Japan).

2.7 Quantitative analysis of lipid peroxides

The lipid peroxide concentration was detected by measuring thiobarbituric acid (TBA) reactivity reflected by the amount of malondialdehyde (MDA) formed during acid hydrolysis of the lipid peroxide compound. The reaction mixtures contained 50 μl protein sample, 20 μl 8.1% sodium dodecyl sulfate, 150 μl 20% acetic acid solution (pH 3.5), and 210 μl 0.571% TBA. Each sample was duplicated. The mixtures were incubated at 90℃ for 1 h, cooled on ice, added 100 μl distilled water, and centrifuged at 4000 rpm for 15 min. After centrifugation, 150 μl supernatant of each samples was take out to measure the absorbance at 540 nm. The lipid peroxide (MDA) level was expressed in nmol MDA per milligram tissue.

2.8 Statistical analysis

Data were presented as mean ± S.D. (n = 5–8). One-way ANOVA was used to determine whether differences exist and if so, a *post hoc* Tukey's test was used for analysis for the difference between groups, with Origin 7.5 laboratory data analysis and graphing software. Statistical significance was considered as $P < 0.05$.

3. Results

3.1 General feature of FGF21-KO animal model

Reportedly there was relative high expression of FGF21 mRNA in the testis of mice (Fon Tacer *et al.*, 2010). We examined the testicular FGF21 mRNA expression in FGF21-KO and WT mice by real-time RT-PCR and found that FGF21 mRNA expression in both the testis and the liver was detectable and also comparable between two tissues in WT mice, but not FGF21-KO mice, under non-fasting condition (Fig. 1A). Functionally testicular and hepatic expression of FGF21 mRNA was examined in mice under 24 h fasting, a condition that is well-defined for the stimulation of hepatic FGF21 mRNA expression (Archer *et al.*, 2012; Hsuchou *et al.*, 2007; Palou *et al.*, 2008). As shown in Fig. 1A, the testicular expression of FGF21 mRNA was not significantly changed under 24 h fasting condition, but the hepatic expression of FGF21 mRNA was elevated about 30-fold at the same condition, implying that FGF21 expression in the testis does not predominantly involve in energy metabolism.

Fig. 1B shows that testicular mRNA expression was significantly increased in diabetic mice compared to the WT mice. The testicular expression of FGF21 mRNA was not affected by supplementation of exogenous FGF21 in FGF21-KO mice.

By examination of testicular weights and the tibia length, no significant difference among groups was seen for the testicular weight to body weight ratio although there was a slight decreasing trend of the testicular weight in the diabetic FGF21-KO mice (Fig. 1C).

3.2 FGF21-KO shows high incidence of spontaneous and diabetes-induced testicular apoptotic cell death, which could be prevented by exogenous FGF21

Compared to the WT control, FGF21-KO mice showed a significant elevation of spontaneous testicular apoptotic cell death, examined by TUNEL staining (Fig. 2A).

Consistent with our previous studies (Cai *et al.*, 2000; Zhao *et al.*, 2011), diabetes induced a significant increase in testicular apoptosis, examined by TUNEL staining (Fig. 2A). Apoptotic cells occur predominantly in spermatogonia and primary spermatocytes and less secondary spermatocytes. Semi-quantitative analysis by both total TUNEL positive cells/1000 germ cells including spermatogonia, primary and secondary spermatocytes (Fig. 2B) and apoptotic index (Fig. 2C) showed that FGF21-KO diabetic mice showed a significantly higher incidence of testicular apoptotic cell death than WT diabetic mice, which could be almost completely attenuated by supplementation of exogenous FGF21 (Fig. 2B, C).

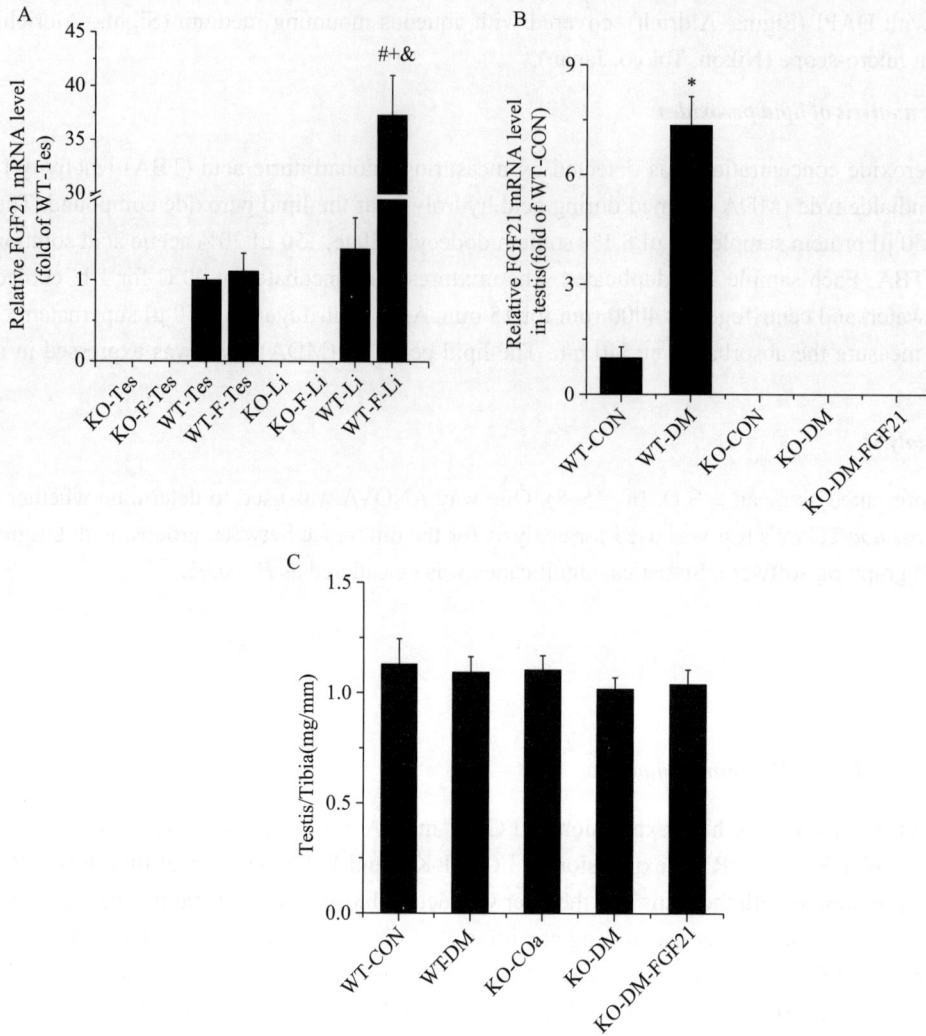

Fig. 1. General features of FGF21-KO animal model. (A) Relative FGF21 mRNA levels in testicular tissues and livers under fasting or no fasting condition. (B) The relative FGF21 mRNA expression in the testicular tissues. Type 1 diabetes was induced with STZ (200 mg/kg) in WT and FGF21-KO mice. Some of FGF21-KO diabetic mice were administered daily intraperitoneal injections of FGF21 (100 μg/kg) and others were administered PBS for 10 days. (C) The ratio of testicular weight to tibia length. All data are presented as mean S.D. (n = 5 at least in each group). KO: FGF21-KO mice; DM: diabetes; F: fasting; Tes: testis; Li: liver. *P < 0.05 $vs.$ WT-CON; #P < 0.05 $vs.$ WT-Tes; +P < 0.05 $vs.$ WT-F-Tes; &P < 0.05 $vs.$ WT-Li.

3.3 Deletion of Fgf21 gene increases diabetes-induced mitochondrial and ER stress-associated cell death pathway

Our previous studies have demonstrated the involvement of both mitochondrial and ER stress-associated cell death pathways in diabetes-induced testicular cell death (Zhao et $al.$, 2011). In the present study we did not see any significant change of caspase-8 cleavage among groups, examined by Western blot (Fig. 3A). Therefore, we have focused on examining mitochondrial and ER stress cell death pathways in the following studies. Western blotting revealed a significant increase in the Bax to Bcl2 expression ratio (Fig. 3B), but no change of caspase-3 cleavage level among groups (Fig. 3C). This may suggest the involvement of caspase-3 independent mitochondrial cell death pathway in the diabetes-induced cells death. Since mitochondrial release of AIF can activate apoptotic cell death via caspase-3 dependent and independent pathways, we next examined the AIF expression with a finding of the significantly elevated expression of AIF in the testis of diabetic mice (Fig. 3D). AIF expression was further examined with immunohistochemical staining that ensured the localization of the positive staining predominantly in spermatogonia or primary spermatocytes (indicated by arrows, Fig. 4A). Immunofluorescent staining confirmed the nuclear localization of AIF (Fig. 4B), as observed by immunohistochemical staining. Compared to WT diabetic mice, these changes were significantly increased in FGF-KO diabetic mice, which was significantly prevented by supplementation of exogenous FGF21 (Figs. 3 and 4).

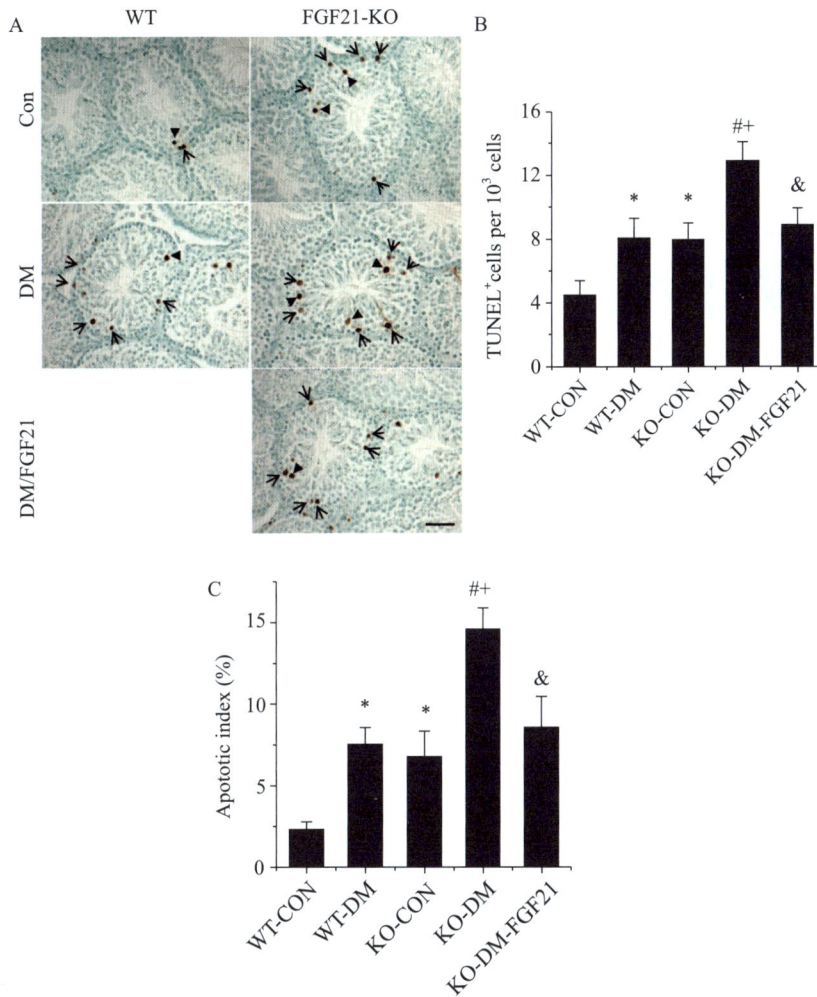

Fig. 2. FGF21 prevents diabetes-induced testicular apoptosis. (A) Testicular apoptosis cell death was examined by TUNEL staining. Bar = 50 μm. (B) TUNEL-positive cells were quantitatively analyzed by total positive cells/1000 germ cells (spermatogonia, primary and secondary spermatocytes). (C) Apoptotic index (AI) for the percentage of testicular tubules with more than 3 TUNEL positive cells. Data are presented as mean S.D. (n = 5 at least in each group). [*]$P < 0.05$ *vs.* WT-CON; [#]$P < 0.05$ *vs.* WT-DM; [+]$P < 0.05$ *vs.* KO-CON; [&]$P < 0.05$ *vs.* KO-DM.

Diabetes induced testicular ER stress, shown by the increased expression of GRP78 (Fig. 5A), ATF4 (Fig. 5B), CHOP (Fig. 5C), and cleaved caspase-12 (Fig. 5D), as reported in our previous studies (Zhao *et al.*, 2011). Deletion of *Fgf21* gene does not significantly increase the spontaneously testicular expression of ER stress proteins GRP78 and ATF4, and cell death mediators CHOP and caspase-12, compared to the WT control. However, deletion of *Fgf21* gene significantly increased the expression of diabetes-induced these ER stress proteins and cell death mediators in FGF21-KO diabetic mice, compared to the WT diabetic mice (Fig. 5).

3.4 Deletion of FGF21 gene does not affect spontaneous and diabetes-induced testicular cell proliferation and inflammation

Since several other members of FGF family play important role in the spermatogenesis, Sertoli cell proliferation and differentiation (El Ramy *et al.*, 2005; Elo *et al.*, 2012; Hiramatsu *et al.*, 2010; Lahr *et al.*, 1992), whether FGF21 has any stimulating effect on testicular cell proliferation was also examined here with immunohistochemical staining for PCNA, a marker of cell proliferation in various tissues. There was no significant change of the immunohistochemical staining for PCNA among groups (Fig. 6A and B), suggesting no effect of *Fgf21* gene deletion or exogenous FGF21 supplementation on the testicular cell proliferation in non-diabetic and diabetic conditions.

Next we performed immunohistochemical staining for of TNF-α (Fig. 6C) and PAI-1 (Fig. 6D) to reflect the status of testicular inflammation, which also showed no any significant change among groups no matter in control, diabetes or with and without FGF21.

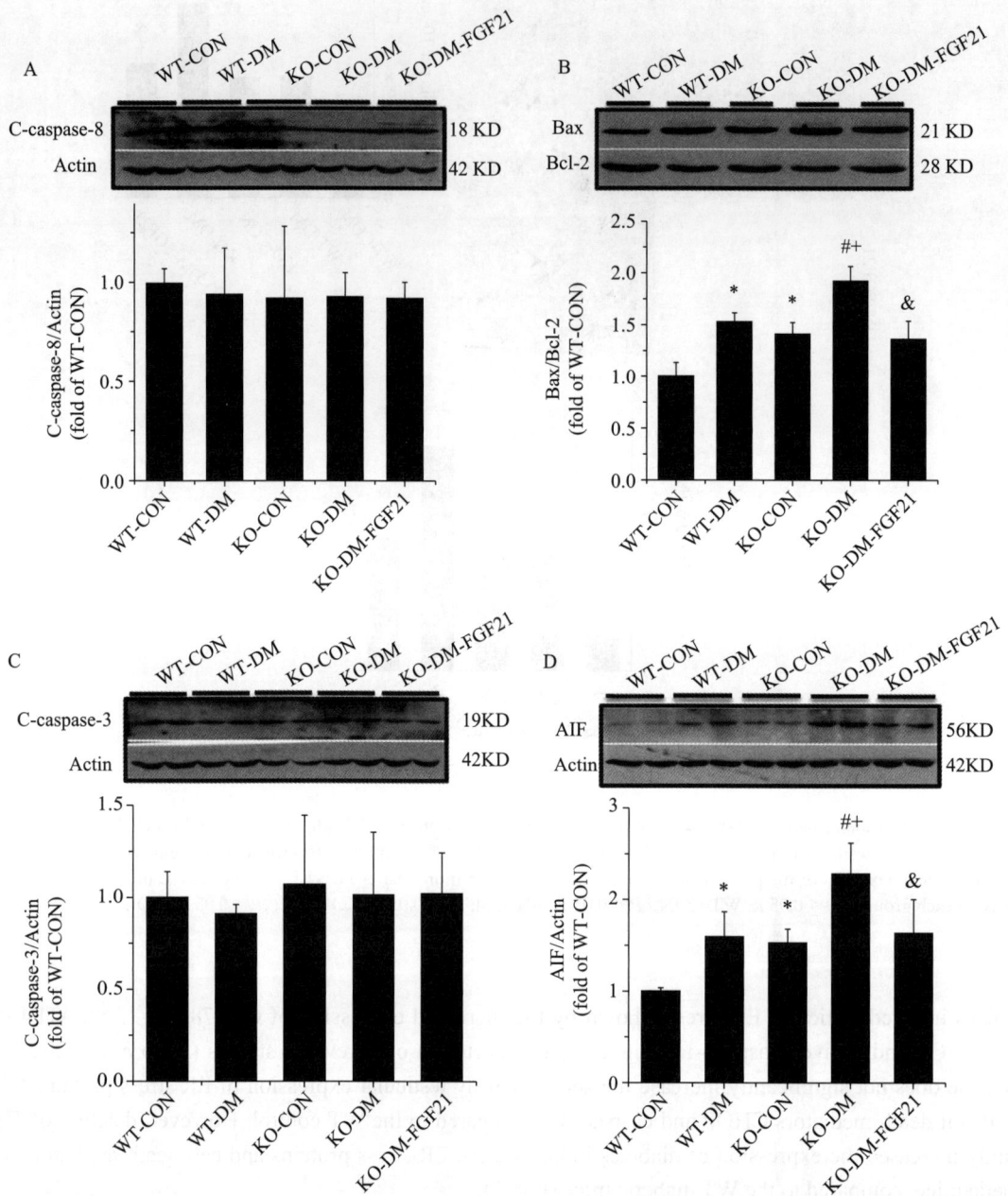

Fig. 3. Deletion of Fgf gene induces testicular apoptotic cell death *via* activation the mitochondrial cell death pathway. (A) The expression of cleaved-caspase-8 in testis was detected by Western blotting assay and the ratio of cleaved-caspase-8 to actin was presented. (B) The expression of Bax and Bcl-2 in testis was detected by Western blotting assay and the expression ratio of Bax to Bcl-2 was presented. (C) The expression of cleaved-caspase-3 in testis was examined by Western blotting assay and the ratio of cleaved-caspase-3 to actin was presented. (D) The expression of AIF in testis was examined by Western blotting assay and the ratio of AIF to actin was presented (D). Data are presented as mean ± S.D. ($n = 5$ at least in each group). *$P < 0.05$ *vs.* WT-CON; #$P < 0.05$ *vs.* WT-DM; +$P < 0.05$ *vs.* KO-CON; &$P < 0.05$ *vs.* KO-DM.

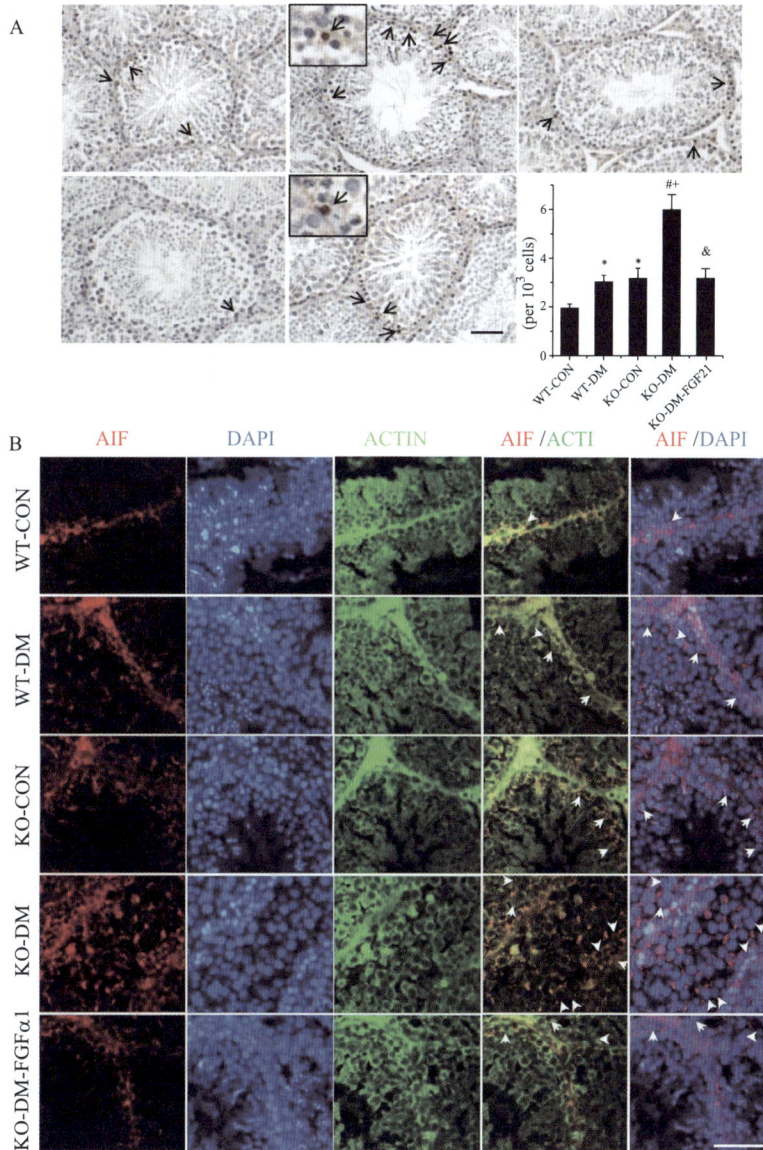

Fig. 4. Immunohistochemical and immunofluorescent staining for AIF. (A) AIF expression was examined by immunohistochemical staining, followed by semi-quantitative analysis, as described in Section 2. AIF positive cells were found predominantly in spermatogonia (indicated by arrows). (B) AIF nuclear localization was further defined by immunofluorescent staining, by which AIF and β-action were probed by CY3-conjugated IgG (red) and FITC-conjugated IgG (green), respectively. White arrow indicated the nuclear accumulation of AIF (×400). Bar = 50 μm. Data are presented as mean ± S.D. (n = 5 at least in each group). *$P < 0.05$ vs. WT-CON; #$P < 0.05$ vs. WT-DM; +$P < 0.05$ vs. KO-CON; $P < 0.05$ vs. KO-DM.

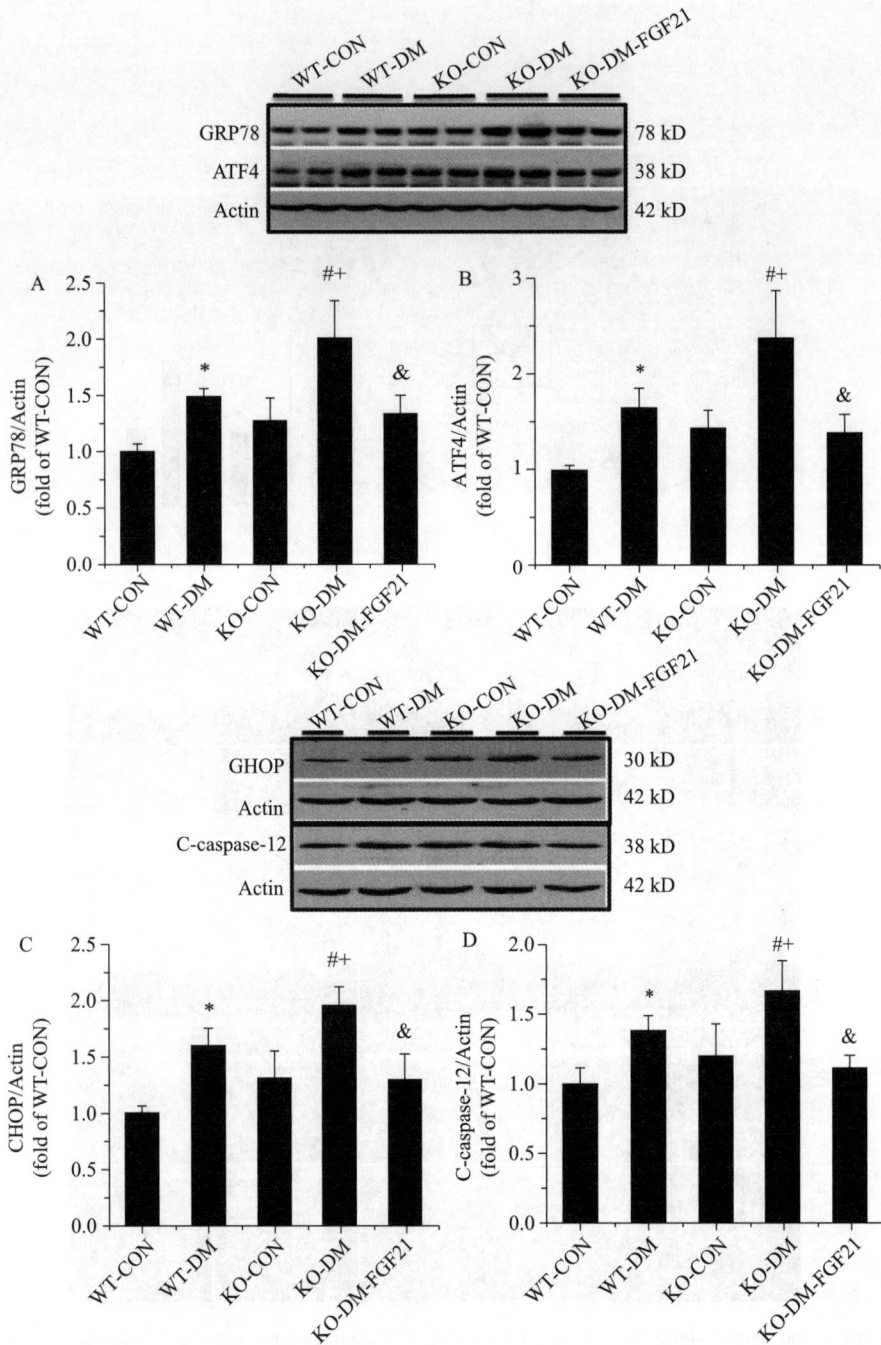

Fig. 5. FGF21 and diabetes-induced testicular ER stress. ER stress-associated cell death was examined by Western blotting assay for the expression of GRP78, ATF4, CHOP and cleaved caspase-12. (A–D) Quantitative analysis of GRP78 ATF4, CHOP and cleaved caspase-12. Data are presented as mean S.D. (n = 5 at least in each group). $^{*}P$ < 0.05 vs. WT-CON; $^{\#}P$ < 0.05 vs. WT-DM; ^{+}P < 0.05 vs. KO-CON; $^{\&}P$ < 0.05 vs. KO-DM.

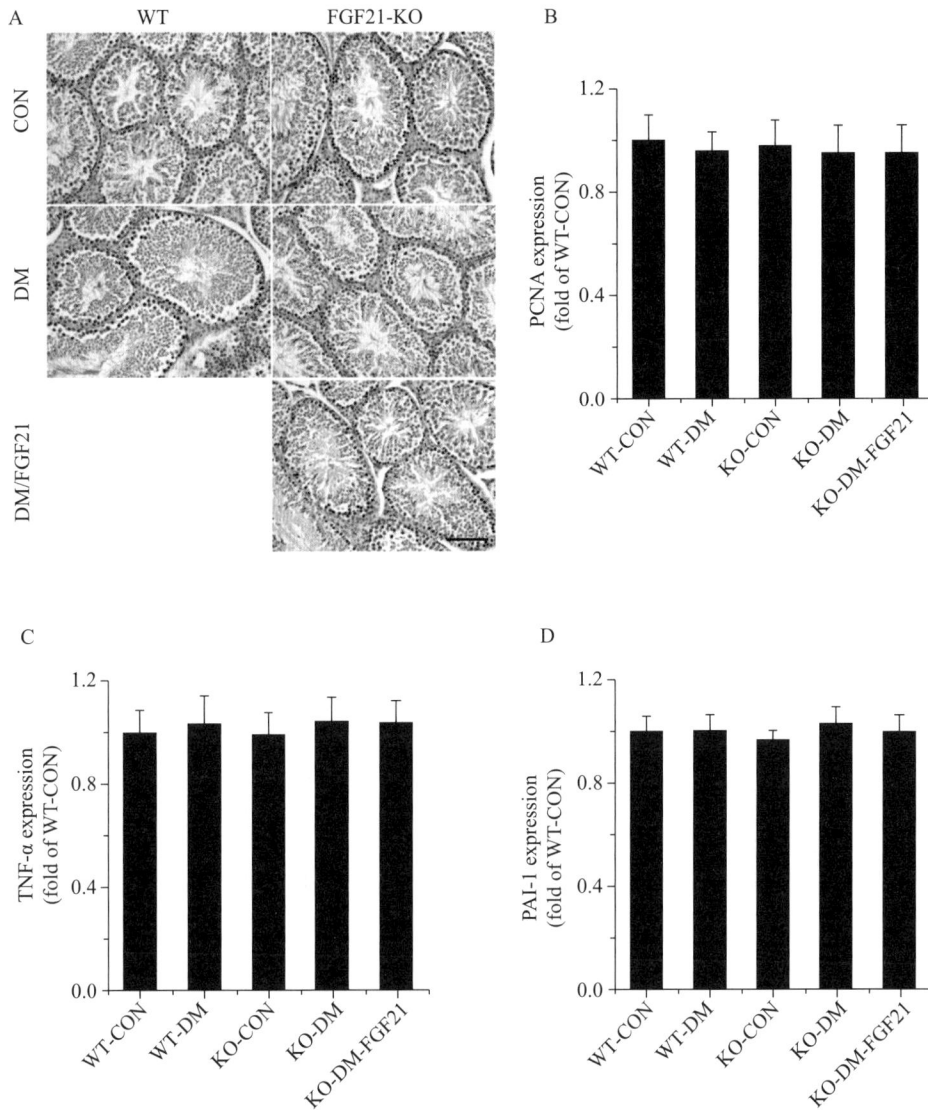

Fig. 6. Effects of FGF21 on diabetes-induced testicular cell proliferation and inflammation. (A) Immunohistochemistry staining of PCNA. Bar = 100 μm. (B) Quantitative analysis of PCNA expression. (C) Quantitative analysis of TNF-α expression by immunohistochemistry staining. (D) Quantitative analysis of PAI-1 expression by immunohistochemistry staining. Data are presented as mean ± S.D. ($n = 5$ at least in each group).

3.5 Deletion of Fgf21 gene does not affect spontaneous, but significantly increases diabetes-induced, testicular oxidative damage

Immunohistochemical staining for 3-NT, as the marker of protein nitration (Fig. 7A), and 4-HNE, as the marker of lipid peroxidation (Fig. 7B), showed that deletion of *Fgf21* gene did not significantly elevated testicular accumulation of 3-NT and 4-HNE, but diabetes significantly increased the contents of these two markers as nitrosative and oxidative damage. The diabetes-induced accumulation of 3-NT and 4-HNE was significantly enhanced by *Fgf21* gene deletion in FGF21-KO diabetic mice and significantly prevented by supplementation of exogenous FGF21, respectively. These findings were further confirmed by biochemical measurement of MDA (Fig. 7C).

4. Discussion

The present study was the first one to explore the expression of FGF21 mRNA in the testis under physiological and pathological conditions. We demonstrated that there was no significant response of testicular FGF21 mRNA expression to fasting condition that is a well-defined condition to stimulate the hepatic expression of FGF21 mRNA and protein

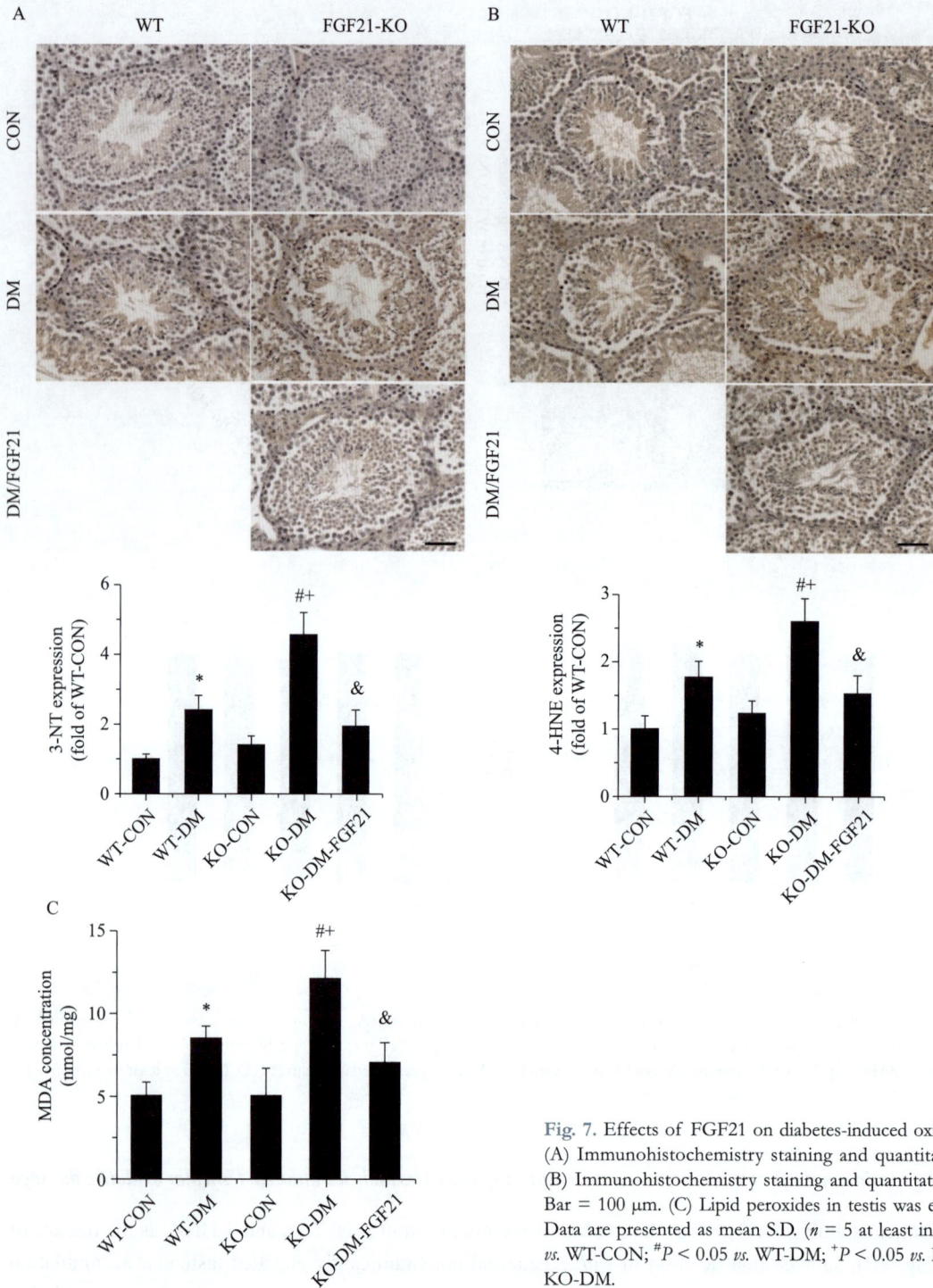

Fig. 7. Effects of FGF21 on diabetes-induced oxidative damage in testis. (A) Immunohistochemistry staining and quantitative analysis of 3-NT. (B) Immunohistochemistry staining and quantitative analysis of 4-HNE. Bar = 100 μm. (C) Lipid peroxides in testis was evaluated by TBA assay. Data are presented as mean S.D. ($n = 5$ at least in each group). [*]$P < 0.05$ vs. WT-CON; [#]$P < 0.05$ vs. WT-DM; [+]$P < 0.05$ vs. KO-CON; [&]$P < 0.05$ vs. KO-DM.

(Archer et al., 2012; Hsuchou et al., 2007; Inagaki et al., 2007; Palou et al., 2008).

Numerous studies have shown the increase of FGF21 protein in serum and tissues (liver and adipose) in diabetic patients and animals (Bobbert et al., 2013; Dostalova et al., 2009; Kamimura et al., 2011; Lundasen et al., 2007; Schaap et al., 2013; Xu et al., 2009). However, there was no information regarding the condition that stimulates or depresses the expression of FGF21 in the testis. Here we showed for the first time that testicular FGF21 mRNA expression was significantly increased at the 10th day after diabetes was onset. We do not know whether this elevation of testicular expression of FGF21 mRNA in response to diabetes can be sustained during the chronic pathogenesis of diabetes based on this acute study.

The mechanism by which diabetes increased testicular FGF21 mRNA expression may be related to diabetic induction of ER stress, particularly ATF4, since a recent study demonstrated the induction of hepatic expression of FGF21 by ER stress *in vitro* and *in vivo*; (Schaap *et al.*, 2013). In that study, ER stress stimuli were found to induce the expression of FGF21 mRNA in H4IIE hepatoma cells and in isolated rat hepatocytes. Moreover, intraperitoneal injection of the ER stressor tunicamycin to normal mice also induced hepatic FGF21 expression with a marked elevation of serum FGF21 levels. The effect of ER stress on FGF21 expression could be mimicked by overexpression of ATF4 as one component of ER stress pathways. There was also a study reporting that mitochondrial dysfunction or damage could increase FGF21 expression in an ATF4 dependent manner (Kim *et al.*, 2013). Both studies suggest the important role of ATF4 in up-regulating FGF21. This notion was further appreciated by the finding that there are two conserved ATF4-binding sequences in the 5′ regulatory region of the human *Fgf21* gene, which are responsible for the ATF4-dependent transcriptional activation of this *Fgf21* gene (De Sousa-Coelho *et al.*, 2012). Consistent with these new findings, we showed here that diabetes induced a significant increase in FGF21 mRNA expression in the testis along with the increased ATF4 expression and ER stress.

Generally there are three major pathways of ER stress: (1) PERK [PKR (double-stranded RNA-activated protein kinase)-like ER kinase], (2) ATF6, and (3) inositol requiring enzyme-1 (IRE-1). Both PERK, *via* activation of ATF4, and ATF6 can induce CHOP (also known as growth arrest-and DNA damage-inducible gene 153, GADD153) to conduct the apoptosis induction through the suppression of Bcl2 family, the activation of JNK or calcium/calmodulin-dependent protein kinase II, and cross-reaction with the mitochondrial apoptotic pathways while IRE-1 itself can induce the apoptotic cell death through an ASK-1/JNK or TRAF2/caspase-12-related pathway (Badiola *et al.*, 2011). Chaperone GRP78 binds the N-termini of PERK, ATF6, and IRE-1, preventing their activation. Unfolded proteins in the ER cause GRP78 to release PERK, ATF, and IRE-1, leading to their oligomerization and activation in ER membranes. Therefore, during ER stress, GRP78 overexpression maintains protein folding (Hammadi *et al.*, 2013). In the present study, we demonstrated significant increases in the expression of ER stress marker, GRP78, suggesting the existence of ER stress in the diabetic testis, and the expression of CHOP that may explain the down-regulation of Bcl2 expression, suggesting the induction of ER stress associated mitochondrial cell death pathway.

Our previous study showed the involvement of both ER stress-associated and mitochondrial apoptotic cell death pathways in diabetes-induced testicular apoptotic cell death (Zhao *et al.*, 2011). In line with the previous study, here diabetes was found to induce a significant increase in apoptotic cell death (TUNEL positive cells), associated with both ER-stress, shown by increased expression of CHOP and cleaved caspase-12, and mitochondrial cell death pathway, shown by increased expression ratio of Bax to Bcl2 expression with the increased AIF expression and nuclear localization. However, we did not find any significant change of caspase-3 cleavage (Fig. 3C). Therefore, the diabetes-induced apoptotic cell death is caspase-3 independent. Several studies have demonstrated the possible induction of caspase-3 independent cell death *in vitro* and *in vivo* (Asmis and Begley, 2003; Puertollano *et al.*, 2003; Zhang *et al.*, 2009). More interestingly, a recent study has compared the apoptotic effect of three stimuli, high glucose, NOC-18 and hydrogen peroxide in retinal endothelial cells (Leal *et al.*, 2009). They found that caspase-3 activation did not increase in high glucose-or NOC-18-treated cells, but it increased in cells exposed to hydrogen peroxide. However, the protein levels of AIF increased in nuclear fractions, in all conditions (Leal *et al.*, 2009). Combined these previous studies with our fining, it seems whether kinds of apoptotic stimuli determines whether the apoptotic mechanism is caspase-3-dependent or independent; therefore, our *in vivo* study is supportive of this *in vitro* effect of high glucose on caspase-3 independent cell death since hyperglycemia is the predominant feature of the type 1 diabetes, particularly at the early stage.

Another one of the novel findings in the present study is the increase of spontaneous incidence of testicular apoptotic cell death in FGF21-KO mice compared to the age-matched WT mice; however, deletion of *Fgf21* gene did not significantly enhance the spontaneous level of testicular ER stress-related apoptotic cell death signaling (only marginally, Fig. 5), but indeed significantly enhanced the spontaneous level of mitochondrial apoptotic cell death pathway (Fig. 3 and 4), suggesting that there may be another mechanism by which FGF21 inhibits the spontaneously caspase-3 independent mitochondrial apoptosis. Under diabetic conditions, however, deletion of *Fgf21* gene significantly exacerbated diabetcs-induced ER stress and mitochondrial cell death (Fig. 2–5).

Although FGF21 have been recognized predominantly as an important endogenous regulator for systemic glucose and lipid metabolism (Angelin *et al.*, 2012; Cuevas-Ramos *et al.*, 2012; Woo *et al.*, 2012), its cytoprotective effect was also reported in certain conditions (Feingold *et al.*, 2012; Lu *et al.*, 2010; Wente *et al.*, 2006; Zhang *et al.*, 2010). For instance, islets and INS-1E cells treated with FGF21 were partially protected from glucolipotoxicity and cytokine-induced apoptosis (Wente *et al.*, 2006). Syrian hamster islet (HIT-T15) cells treated with palmitic acid have significantly higher apoptotic rates than controls, which could be significantly prevented by FGF21 (Zhang *et al.*, 2010). In the cultured cardiac microvascular endothelial cells, bezafibrate-increased FGF21 expression could reduce, but inhibition of FGF21 expression by shRNA could significantly increase, the apoptotic cell death induced by oxidized-low density lipoprotein (Lu *et al.*, 2010). However, these studies were done *in vitro*, here we presented for the first time that deletion of *Fgf21* gene enhanced, and supplementation of exogenous FGF21 significantly reduced, the testicular apoptotic cell death induced by diabetes *in vivo*, suggesting the anti-apoptotic role in the testis of diabetic mice.

Based on the present study it remains unclear for the mechanism by which deletion of FGF21 increases both mitochondrial apoptotic and/or ER stress cell death in diabetic condition. This anti-apoptotic effect of FGF21 in the testis of diabetic mice was not related to testicular cell proliferation since there was no change for the testicular PCNA positive cells. Our finding is in line with a previous study that showed no effect of FGF-21 on islet cell proliferation (Wente *et al.*, 2006). Although FGF21 is able to be induced by inflammation and also protects inflammation-induced toxicity (Feingold *et al.*, 2012), its anti-inflammation effect was not the case in the present study since there was not significant change for testicular inflammation, shown by no change of TNF-α and PAI-1 as the two typical markers of inflammation, among groups (Fig. 6C and D). However, the protective role of FGF21 on testicular apoptotic cell death in normal and diabetic condition was found to be significantly associated with its prevention of oxidative damage that was reflected by increased immunohistochemical staining for the accumulation of 3-NT and 4-HNE and biochemical levels of MDA (Fig. 7). Although several studies have demonstrated the anti-oxidative function of other FGF family members such as FGF1 and FGF2 (Li *et al.*, 2007; Mark *et al.*, 1997; Xiao *et al.*, 2010), there was no evidence to indicate the anti-oxidative capacity of FGF21 up to date. Therefore, how FGF21 decreases oxidative stress remains further exploration.

References

[1] Angelin B, Larsson TE, Rudling M. Circulating Fibroblast Growth Factors as Metabolic Regulators-A Critical Appraisal[J]. Cell Metabolism, 2012, 16(6): 693-705.

[2] Archer A, Venteclef N, Mode A, *et al.* Fasting-Induced FGF21 Is Repressed by LXR Activation *via* Recruitment of an HDAC3 Corepressor Complex in Mice[J]. Molecular Endocrinology, 2012, 26(12): 1980-1990.

[3] Asmis R, Begley JG. Oxidized LDL promotes peroxide-mediated mitochondrial dysfunction and cell death in human macrophages - A caspase-3-independent pathway[J]. Circulation Research, 2003, 92(1): E20-E29.

[4] Badiola N, Penas C, Minano-Molina A, *et al.* Induction of ER stress in response to oxygen-glucose deprivation of cortical cultures involves the activation of the PERK and IRE-1 pathways and of caspase-12[J]. Cell Death & Disease, 2011, 2.

[5] Badman MK, Koester A, Flier JS, *et al.* Fibroblast Growth Factor 21-Deficient Mice Demonstrate Impaired Adaptation to Ketosis[J]. Endocrinology, 2009, 150(11): 4931-4940.

[6] Badman MK, Pissios P, Kennedy AR, *et al.* Hepatic fibroblast growth factor 21 is regulated by PPAR alpha and is a key mediator of hepatic lipid metabolism in ketotic states[J]. Cell Metabolism, 2007, 5(6): 426-437.

[7] Bobbert T, Schwarz F, Fischer-Rosinsky A, *et al.* Fibroblast Growth Factor 21 Predicts the Metabolic Syndrome and Type 2 Diabetes in Caucasians[J]. Diabetes Care, 2013, 36(1): 145-149.

[8] Cai L, Chen SL, Evans T, *et al.* Apoptotic germ-cell death and testicular damage in experimental diabetes: prevention by endothelin antagonism[J]. Urological Research, 2000, 28(5): 342-347.

[9] Cai L, Li W, Wang GW, *et al.* Hyperglycemia-induced apoptosis in mouse myocardium - Mitochondrial cytochrome c-mediated caspase-3 activation pathway[J]. Diabetes, 2002, 51(6): 1938-1948.

[10] Chavez AO, Molina-Carrion M, Abdul-Ghani M, *et al.* Fibroblast growth factor-21 (FGF-21), a novel peptide, is associated with whole body and hepatic insulin resistance[J]. Diabetes, 2008, 57: A33-A34.

[11] Cuevas-Ramos D, Aguilar-Salinas CA, Gomez-Perez FJ. Metabolic actions of fibroblast growth factor 21[J]. Current Opinion In Pediatrics, 2012, 24(4): 523-529.

[12] Dostalova I, Haluzikova D, Haluzik M. Fibroblast Growth Factor 21: A Novel Metabolic Regulator With Potential Therapeutic Properties in Obesity/Type 2 Diabetes Mellitus[J]. Physiological Research, 2009, 58(1): 1-7.

[13] El Ramy R, Verot A, Mazaud S, *et al.* Fibroblast growth factor (FGF) 2 and FGF9 mediate mesenchymal-epithelial interactions of peritubular and Sertoli cells in the rat testis[J]. Journal Of Endocrinology, 2005, 187(1): 135-147.

[14] Feingold KR, Grunfeld C, Heuer JG, *et al.* FGF21 Is Increased by Inflammatory Stimuli and Protects Leptin-Deficient ob/ob Mice from the Toxicity of Sepsis[J]. Endocrinology, 2012, 153(6): 2689-2700.

[15] Guneli E, Tugyan K, Ozturk H, *et al.* Effect of melatonin on testicular damage in streptozotocin-induced diabetes rats[J]. European Surgical Research, 2008, 40(4): 354-360.

[16] Hirai K, Sasaki H, Yamamoto H, *et al.* HST-1/FGF-4 protects male germ cells from apoptosis under heat-stress condition[J]. Experimental Cell Research, 2004, 294(1): 77-85.

[17] Hiramatsu R, Harikae K, Tsunekawa N, *et al.* FGF signaling directs a center-to-pole expansion of tubulogenesis in mouse testis differentiation[J]. Development, 2010, 137(2): 303-312.

[18] Hsuchou H, Pan W, Kastin AJ. The fasting polypeptide FGF21 can enter brain from blood[J]. Peptides, 2007, 28(12): 2382-2386.

[19] Inagaki T, Dutchak P, Zhao G, *et al.* Endocrine regulation of the

fasting response by PPAR alpha-mediated induction of fibroblast growth factor 21[J]. Cell Metabolism, 2007, 5(6): 415-425.

[20] Kamimura N, Nishimaki K, Ohsawa I, *et al.* Molecular Hydrogen Improves Obesity and Diabetes by Inducing Hepatic FGF21 and Stimulating Energy Metabolism in db/db Mice[J]. Obesity, 2011, 19(7): 1396-1403.

[21] Kharitonenkov A. FGFs and metabolism[J]. Current Opinion In Pharmacology, 2009, 9(6): 805-810.

[22] Kim KH, Jeong YT, Oh H, *et al.* Autophagy deficiency leads to protection from obesity and insulin resistance by inducing Fgf21 as a mitokine[J]. Nature Medicine, 2013, 19(1): 83-92.

[23] Lahr G, Mayerhofer A, Seidl K, *et al.* Basic fibroblast growth-factor (BFGF) in rodent testis-presence of bfgf messenger-rna and of a 30-KDa bFGF protein in pachytene spermatocytes[J]. Febs Letters, 1992, 302(1): 43-46.

[24] Leal EC, Aveleira CA, Castilho AF, *et al.* High glucose and oxidative/nitrosative stress conditions induce apoptosis in retinal endothelial cells by a caspase-independent pathway[J]. Experimental Eye Research, 2009, 88(5): 983-991.

[25] Li XK, Lin ZF, Li Y, *et al.* Cardiovascular protection of nonmitogenic human acidic fibroblast growth factor from oxidative damage *in vitro* and *in vivo*[J]. Cardiovascular Pathology, 2007, 16(2): 85-91.

[26] Lu Y, Liu JH, Zhang LK, *et al.* Fibroblast growth factor 21 as a possible endogenous factor inhibits apoptosis in cardiac endothelial cells[J]. Chinese Medical Journal, 2010, 123(23): 3417-3421.

[27] Luisa De Sousa-Coelho A, Marrero PF, Haro D. Activating transcription factor 4-dependent induction of FGF21 during amino acid deprivation[J]. Biochemical Journal, 2012, 443: 165-171.

[28] Lundasen T, Hunt MC, Nilsson L-M, *et al.* PPAR alpha is a key regulator of hepatic FGF21[J]. Biochemical And Biophysical Research Communications, 2007, 360(2): 437-440.

[29] Mark RJ, Keller JN, Kruman I, *et al.* Basic FGF attenuates amyloid beta-peptide-induced oxidative stress, mitochondrial dysfunction, and impairment of Na$^+$/K$^+$-ATPase activity in hippocampal neurons[J]. Brain Research, 1997, 756(1-2): 205-214.

[30] Mohasseb M, Ebied S, Yehia MAH, *et al.* Testicular oxidative damage and role of combined antioxidant supplementation in experimental diabetic rats[J]. Journal Of Physiology And Biochemistry, 2011, 67(2): 185-194.

[31] Nishimura T, Nakatake Y, Konishi M, *et al.* Identification of a novel FGF, FGF-21, preferentially expressed in the liver[J]. Biochimica Et Biophysica Acta-Gene Structure And Expression, 2000, 1492(1): 203-206.

[32] Palou M, Priego T, Sanchez J, *et al.* Sequential changes in the expression of genes involved in lipid metabolism in adipose tissue and liver in response to fasting[J]. Pflugers Archiv-European Journal Of Physiology, 2008, 456(5): 825-836.

[33] Puertollano MA, De Pablo MA, De Cienfuegos GA. Polyunsaturated fatty acids induce cell death in YAC-1 lymphoma by a caspase-3-independent mechanism[J]. Anticancer Research, 2003, 23(5A): 3905-3910.

[34] Schaap FG, Kremer AE, Lamers WH, *et al.* Fibroblast growth factor 21 is induced by endoplasmic reticulum stress[J]. Biochimie, 2013, 95(4): 692-699.

[35] Elo T, Sipila P, Valve E, *et al.* Fibroblast growth factor 8b causes progressive stromal and epithelial changes in the epididymis and degeneration of the seminiferous epithelium in the testis of transgenic mice[J]. Biology of Reproduction, 2012, 86(157): 112-151.

[36] Wente W, Efanov AM, Brenner M, *et al.* Fibroblast growth factor-21 improves pancreatic beta-cell function and survival by activation of extracellular signal-regulated kinase 1/2 and Akt signaling pathways[J]. Diabetes, 2006, 55(9): 2470-2478.

[37] Xiao J, Lv Y, Lin S, *et al.* Cardiac Protection by Basic Fibroblast Growth Factor from Ischemia/Reperfusion-Induced Injury in Diabetic Rats[J]. Biological & Pharmaceutical Bulletin, 2010, 33(3): 444-449.

[38] Xu J, Lloyd DJ, Hale C, *et al.* Fibroblast Growth Factor 21 Reverses Hepatic Steatosis, Increases Energy Expenditure, and Improves Insulin Sensitivity in Diet-Induced Obese Mice[J]. Diabetes, 2009, 58(1): 250-259.

[39] Yamamoto H, Ochiya T, Tamamushi S, *et al.* HST-1/FGF-4 gene activation induces spermatogenesis and prevents adriamycin-induced testicular toxicity[J]. Oncogene, 2002, 21(6): 899-908.

[40] Zhang L, Zhang M, Wang C, *et al.* Protective effect of fibroblast growth factors-21 and rosiglitazone sodium on palmitic acid-induced apoptosis in HIT-T15 cells[J]. Journal of Sichuan University. Medical science edition, 2010, 41(2): 218-221.

[41] Zhang X, Chen F, Huang Z. Apoptosis induced by acrylamide is suppressed in a 21.5% fat diet through caspase-3-independent pathway in mice testis[J]. Toxicology Mechanisms And Methods, 2009, 19(3): 219-224.

[42] Zhao H, Xu S, Wang Z, *et al.* Repetitive exposures to low-dose X-rays attenuate testicular apoptotic cell death in streptozotocin-induced diabetes rats[J]. Toxicology Letters, 2010, 192(3): 356-364.

[43] Zhao Y, Tan Y, Dai J, *et al.* Exacerbation of diabetes-induced testicular apoptosis by zinc deficiency is most likely associated with oxidative stress, p38 MAPK activation, and p53 activation in mice[J]. Toxicology Letters, 2011, 200(1-2): 100-106.

Fibroblast growth factor 2 protects against renal ischaemia/reperfusion injury by attenuating mitochondrial damage and proinflammatory signalling

Xiaohua Tan , Xiaokun Li, Jinsan Zhang

1. Introduction

AKI, previously known as 'acute renal failure', is a common clinical syndrome characterized by sudden loss of the ability of the kidneys to excrete wastes, concentrate urine, conserve electrolytes, and maintain fluid balance [1]. The principal cause of AKI is hypoxia induced by I/RI, which can be caused by numerotions, such as surgical interventions, organ transplantation, circulatory shock, toxic insults like haemorrhagic shock or sepsis and diseases such as myocardial infarction [2–4]. Despite advances in preventive strategies and support measures, AKI continues to be associated with high morbidity and mortality, particularly in those admitted to the Intensive Care Unit, where in-hospital mortality rates may exceed 50% [5]. Extensive research has been carried out about the mechanism and intervention method of renal I/RI in the past decades, but the complex pathophysiology of AKI is yet to be fully understood and there remains a lack of definitively effective treatment for AKI. Current treatment is focused on maintaining renal perfusion and avoiding volume overload [6].

The destructive role of reactive oxygen species (ROS) in I/RI is well recognized. ROS are generated from several different sources, including NADPH oxidase, xanthine oxidase-hypoxanthine, inflammatory cells, and mitochondria of parenchymal cells, as the result of ischaemia-provoked derangement of the electron transport chain [7, 8]. Overproduction of ROS by mitochondria plays a critical role in the pathogenesis of I/RI *via* loss of mitochondrial membrane potential (MMP), destabilizing the electron transport chain [9, 10], triggering mitochondrial DNA (mtDNA) injury [11], and direct damage to cellular components that can result in necrosis and apoptosis [12–16]. Mitochondria are the main source of cellular ROS and contain a number of enzymes that convert molecular oxygen to superoxide or its derivative hydrogen peroxide (H_2O_2) [17]. Mitochondrial processes have been demonstrated to be major events during apoptosis, and the Bcl-2 family is involved in the alteration of MMP as well as the release of mitochondrial apoptotic factors. In addition, agents that open the mitochondrial ATP-dependent potassium (K_{ATP}) channel have been found to be effective in preventing renal injury *via* inhibition of mitochondrial DNA damage [11, 18–22]. Therefore, therapeutic strategies aiming at inhibiting ROS production and protection of mitochondrial from oxidative damage may ameliorate renal I/R injury.

Inflammatory response is another key and integral process of I/R–induced pathogenesis. The initial non-immune injury to the renal parenchyma, such as ROS-induced renal tubular cell apoptosis/necrosis, inevitably triggers an innate immune response leading to activation of inflammatory cells and cytokine secretion. The inflammation then imposes further damage to the renal parenchyma cells [23, 24]. Accumulating evidence suggests that High-Mobility Group Box-1 (HMGB1) serves as a crucial link between the initial I/RI-induced cell damage and the activation of inflammatory signaling cascade. Although previously known as a DNA-binding transcription factor, HMGB1 has recently been recognized as a potent proinflammatory cytokine released from I/R injured cells. Circulating HMBG1 is capable of activating multiple cell surface receptors, including toll-like receptors (TLRs), which act as a central mediator of inflammation through activation of NF-jB and expression of proinflammatory cytokines [25]. Targeting HMGB1/TLRs has been proposed and investigated as a therapeutic approach to protect renal tissue in various animal renal and other I/RI models with some promising results [26–29].

Basic FGF2 is a member of a large family of growth factors consisting of 22 evolutionarily and structurally related proteins that signal through FGF receptors (FGFRs). FGF2 was first identified as a 146-amino acid protein isolated from the pituitary [30]. Extensive research has documented FGF2 as a pleiotropic cytokine, which exerts its effects *via* all four high affinity receptors (FGFR-1 to 4) through a paracrine/autocrine mechanism. Exogenous FGF2 stimulates migration and proliferation of endothelial cells *in vivo* [31], has anti-apoptotic activity and promotes mitogenesis of smooth muscle cells and fibroblasts, which induces the development of large collateral vessels with adventitia [32, 33]. In certain disorders of the central nervous system (CNS), including ischaemic injury, FGF2 has also been examined for its therapeutic effects on the maintenance of Na^+/K^+-ATPase activity against oxidative injury [34]. The protective role of FGF2 against I/RI is best documented for myocardial infarction. FGF2 has been reported to reduce the size of the ischaemic region and ameliorates the associated symptoms in ischaemic myocardium [35–37]. Using cardiac-specific FGF-2 overexpression transgenic mouse model, House *et al.* elegantly demonstrate the myocardial protection effect of FGF2 against I/RI, which involves its activation of both MAPK and PKC pathways [38–40]. The role of endogenous FGF2 in renal I/ RI and repair has also been recognized. Villanueva *et al.* first reported that FGF2 is expressed early during kidney development, re-expressed in the regeneration phase after I/RI, and that FGF2 participates in the recovery process of I/RI by inducing an altered expression of morphogens through FGFR2 [41–43]. Despite the prominent role of FGF2 in I/RI pathogenesis and repair processes, the molecular mechanism underlying FGF2 signaling-mediated protection against I/RI remains incompletely understood, and whether exogenous FGF2 can deliver therapeutic benefit towards renal I/RI is unknown. In studies of the brain and heart, some evidence indicates that FGF2 can modulate oxidative stress caused by the formation of ROS [37, 44]. Our previous studies have demonstrated that excessive mitochondrial ROS production plays an important role in renal I/RI [6, 11]. Herein, we show that either pre-or post-I/R administration of FGF2 protects against renal I/RI by attenuating multiple mitochondrial damage parameters, as well as HMGB1/TLR2-mediated proinflammatory response.

2. Materials and methods

2.1 Reagents and antibodies

Bovine serum albumin (BSA), recombinant human FGF2, sodium pentobarbital, 5-hydroxydecanoate (5-HD) and mitochondria isolation kits were purchased from Sigma-Aldrich (St Louis, MO, USA). 5,5′,6,6′-*Tetrachloro-1,1′,3,3′*-tetraethylbenzimidazolylcarbocyanine iodide (JC-1) and 40, 6-diamidino-2-phenylindole (DAPI) were pur chased from Invitrogen (Carlsbad, CA, USA). Rat HMGB1 ELISA Kit was purchased from CUSABIO (Hubei, China). Antibodies against 8-hydroxy-2-deoxyguanosine (8-OHdG), phospho-FGFR, TNFα and caspase-9 were purchased from Abcam (Cambridge, MA, USA). Anti-3-Nitrotyrosine (3-NIT) antibody was purchased from Invitrogen. Anti-Kir6.2 antibody was purchased from Santa Cruz Biotechnology (Santa Cruz, CA, USA). Antibodies against the voltage-dependent anion channel (VDAC), cleaved caspase-3, HMGB1 and GAPDH were purchased from Cell Signaling Technology (Beverly, MA, USA). The secondary antibodies were purchased from Abcam or Santa Cruz Biotechnology.

2.2 Animals and renal I/RI model

Male Sprague-Dawley rats (SD rats, 8–10 weeks old) were purchased from Shanghai SLAC Laboratory Animal Co., Ltd. and were housed in our SPF facility under standard conditions of temperature and 12 h light/dark cycle with *ad libitum* feeding. The Institutional Animal Ethical Committee and Use Committee of Wenzhou Medical University approved the animal research protocol. Rats were positioned on a homoeothermic surgical platform after being anaesthetized with an intra-peritoneal (i.p) injection of 25 mg/kg sodium pentobarbital and underwent right nephrectomy. Renal ischaemic condition was achieved by renal artery clamping for 45 min (50 min for survival studies) and then renal blood flow was re-established. Kidneys were harvested 2 days after artery ischaemia and stored at -80℃ until further analysis. Serum creatinine (Cr) and Blood Urea Nitrogen (BUN) were measured 2 days following renal ischaemia by the hospital laboratory. Rats were divided into four groups: (*i*) Sham-operated animals with an unrestricted renal artery; (*ii*) I/R animals: kidneys were subjected to 45 min. of ischaemia followed by reperfusion; (*iii*) I/R+FGF2 Group, rats were treated with single dose of 0.5 mg/kg FGF2 (i.p) 1 hr before ischaemia and then subjected to 45 min. of ischaemia followed by reperfusion; (*iv*) I/R+FGF2 + 5-HD Group, animals were treated with 0.5 mg/kg FGF2 (i.p) 1 hr before ischaemia and then treated with 5 mg/kg 5-HD (i.m) 15 min. before ischaemia. The lyophilized recombinant FGF2 was freshly dissolved in sterile saline before use. 5-HD was dissolved in saline. For post-I/R treatment, rats were treated with one dose of 0.5 mg/kg FGF2 (i.p) at 1, 3, or 12 h after reperfusion as indicated. Twenty rats from each group were used for survival assessments.

2.3 Histology and pathological scoring of the renal tubules

Kidney tissues were fixed in 10% formaldehyde, embedded in paraffin, and sectioned for haematoxylin and eosin (H&E) staining. Renal pathological changes were observed using light microscopy. To measure the pathological score of the renal tubules, 12 visual fields from each section were selected randomly under the microscope using previously reported methods [45, 46]. Based on the assessment of tubular expansion, cast formation, brush border loss, and epithelial cell necrosis, the following 5-point scoring system was used to assess renal pathology: 0 point (normal kidney morphology without damage); 1 point (necrosis of the renal tubules $\leq 10\%$); 2 points (necrosis of the renal tubules $11\% - 25\%$); 3 points (necrosis of the renal tubules $26\% - 45\%$); 4 points (necrosis of the renal tubules $46\% - 75\%$); 5 points (necrosis of the renal tubules $\geq 76\%$). The pathologists were blinded to rat allocation group.

2.4 Immunohistochemistry staining (IHC)

Kidneys were excised and harvested 2 days following 45 min. of ischaemic condition. Paraffin-embedded sections (5 μm) were stained with H&E. Slides were incubated with anti-FGFR antibody (1 : 200) at 4℃ overnight and stained with diaminobenzidine tetrahydrochloride (DAB) and counterstained with haematoxylin. Oxidative damage was detected using anti-8-OHdG antibody (1 : 100) and antibody against nitrotyrosine (1 : 200). For caspase-3 and caspase-9 staining, slides were incubated with anti-cleaved caspase-3 antibody (1 : 200) and anti-cleaved caspase-9 antibody (1 : 200), respectively. Apoptosis was detected using a one-step TUNEL Apoptosis Assay KIT (Roche, Mannheim, Germany) according to the manufacturer's instructions. Slides were also counterstained with DAPI at 37℃ for 5 min. to identify nuclei. The images were captured with a Nikon ECLIPSE Ti microscope (Nikon, Melville, NY, USA). The percentage of positive cells with dual TUNEL and DAPI staining at five randomly selected 4009 fields served as the index of apoptosis. For Kir6.2 and VDAC double staining, sections were incubated with goat anti-Kir6.2 antibody (1 : 200) and mouse anti-VDAC antibody (1 : 200) at 4℃ overnight and then with fluorescein isothiocyanate-labelled donkey anti-goat IgG (1 : 200) and phycoerythrin-labelled donkey antimouse IgG (1 : 200) for 60 min. Cell nuclei were counterstained blue with DAPI at 37℃ for 5 min. Sections were analysed by fluorescence microscopy.

2.5 Western blot analysis

For protein analysis of *in vivo* samples, renal tissues were dissected, snap frozen and stored at -80℃. Protein extracts from renal tissues were prepared by centrifuging the complex mixed 0.1 g kidney with protein extraction reagents and subjected to Western blot. Protein concentrations were measured with a BCA Protein Assay Kit. Equal amounts of protein were loaded into lanes and separated on SDSPAGE, followed by transfer to a polyvinylidene fluoride membrane. After blocking in 5% skim milk in Tris-buffered saline/0.1% Tween-20 (TBST), the membrane was incubated with following antibodies against Kir6.2, Bcl-2, Bax, 3-Nit, cytochrome C, caspase-3, VDAC and GAPDH, respectively. After washing with TBST three times, membranes were incubated with secondary antibodies for 1 hr at room temperature. The signals were visualized with the ChemiDoc XRS+Imaging System (Bio-Rad Laboratories, Hercules, CA, USA). The band densities were quantified with Multi Gauge Software of Science Lab 2006 (FUJIFILM Corporation, Tokyo, Japan).

2.6 Determination of MMP

We measured MMP with freshly isolated mitochondria and paraffin-embedded sections (5 μm). Kidney tissue was homogenized in 50 mM Tris-HCl buffer (pH7.4) and centrifuged at $2000\times g$ in 4℃ for 5 min to precipitate the nuclear fraction. The supernatant was then centrifuged at $11,000\times g$ in 4℃ for 10 min. to yield the mitochondrial fraction. The mitochondrial pellet was suspended in 40 ll of storage buffer. Mitochondria protein and paraffin sections were incubated with 1 μg/ml JC-1 for 10 min. at 37℃ according to the manufacturer's instructions. The electrical potential across the inner mitochondrial membrane ($\Delta\Psi$) was detected using the laser confocal at an excitation wavelength of 485 nm and an emission wavelength of 590 nm.

2.7 ELISA

Serum HMGB1 was measured using ELISA kit (CUSABIO) according to the manufacturer's instructions. The result was expressed as pg/ml. The lower detection limit was 62.5 pg/ml.

2.8　Real-time quantitative RT-PCR

Total RNA was isolated from kidney using RNeasy column (QIAGEN, Germantown, MD, USA), reverse transcribed using PrimeScript™ RT reagent Kit (TaKaRa, Berkeley, CA, USA) according to the manufacturer's instructions. Real-time PCR was performed using the SYBR Green gene expression assays (TaKaRa) for detection of mRNA expression levels. The PCR primers used for mRNA expression analysis for GAPDH, KIM1, TLR2, TLR4, IL-Iα, IL-6 and TNF-α are shown in Table 1. The target values were normalized to GAPDH.

Table 1.　Primers used to amplify rat cDNAs

Gene	GenBank	Primer sequences
GAPDH	NM_012675	5′-GACATGCCGCCTGGAGAAAC-3′ 5′-AGCCCAGGATGCCCTTTAGT-3′
IL-1β	NM_031512	5′-TGCAGGCTTCGAGATGAAC-3′ 5′-GGGATTTTGTCGTTGCTTGTC-3′
IL-6	NM_012589	5′-AAGCCAGAGTCATTCAGAGC-3′ 5′-GTCCTTAGCCACTCCTTCTG-3′
KIM-1	NM_173149	5′-CTCTGTTGATAGTGATAGTGGTCTG-3′ 5′-TGTGGGTCTTGTAGTTGTGG-3′
TLR2	NM_198769	5′-ATGAACACTAAGACATACCTGGAG-3′ 5′-CAAGACAGAAACAGGGTGGAG-3′
TLR4	NM_019178	5′-CATGACATCCCTTATTCAACCAAG-3′ 5′-GCCATGCCTTGTCTTCAATTG-3′
TNF-α	NM_012675	5′-CTTCTCATTCCTGCTCGTGG-3′ 5′-TGATCTGAGTGTGAGGGTCTG-3′

IL-1β: interleukin-1β; IL-6: interleukin-6; TLR2: Toll-like receptor-2; TLR-4: Toll-like receptor-4; KIM1: Kidney Injury Molecule-1; TNF-α: tumour necrosis factor-α; GAPDH: Glyceraldehyde 3-phosphate dehydrogenase.

2.9　Statistical analysis

SPSS 19.0 statistical software (Cary, NC, USA) was used for data analysis. The Kaplan–Meier method was used to compare the survival rates. Data are expressed as the mean ± S.E.M. of n independent experiments. When more than two groups were compared, statistical evaluation of the data was performed using one-way analysis of variance (ANOVA). Tukey multiple comparison was used as a *post hoc* analysis. A value of $P < 0.05$ was considered statistically significant.

3.　Results

3.1　FGF2 pre-treatment attenuates I/RI-induced renal dysfunction and pathologic damage

To assess the histology of AKI and protective effect of FGF2 on renal function, we employed a rat model of I/R-induced AKI (Fig. 1A). Two days following I/R, the serum levels of Cr and BUN were significantly higher in I/R rats compared with sham-operated rats (Fig. 1B and C). Strikingly, serum levels of both Cr and BUN in I/R+FGF2 rats were much lower compared to I/R rats ($P < 0.001$) and revealed no significant difference to the sham-operated rats, whereas 5-HD treatment partially reversed the action of FGF2. We next evaluated the histopathological changes in the kidney tissuc 2 days after reperfusion. Representative H&E stained kidney sections from each group are shown in Fig. 2A. No significant damage was observed in the kidney sections from rats of the sham group (Fig. 2A-a, e). In contrast, the I/R group displayed typical features of AKI characterized by cellular swelling, intraluminal necrotic cellular debris, vacuolar degeneration, luminal narrowing, interstitial congestion and oedema, and formation of proteinaceous casts (Fig. 2A-b, f). Quantification analysis of renal damages indicated that a near 15-fold increase in tubular injury score in I/R group

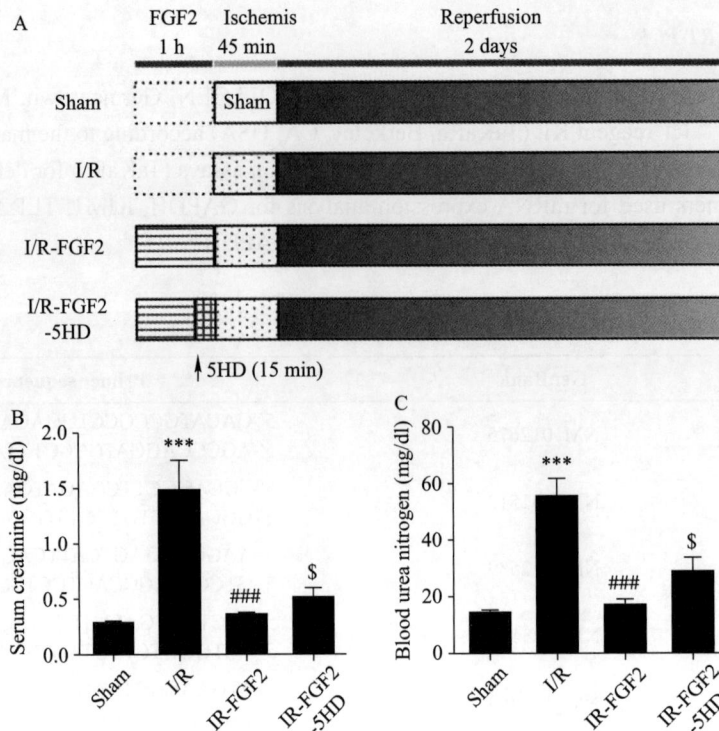

Fig. 1. FGF2 sustains renal function after I/ R injury. (A) Protocol for renal ischaemia/ reperfusion injury model in rat. (B) Determination of serum Cr levels in indicated animal groups at 48 h after reperfusion (mean ± S.E.; $n = 8$). ***$P < 0.001$ vs. Sham group, ###$P < 0.001$ vs. I/R group; $^{\$}P < 0.05$ vs. FGF2 + I/R group. (C) Determination of blood urea nitrogen (BUN) levels in indicated animal groups at 48 h after reperfusion (mean ± S.E.; $n = 8$). ***$P < 0.001$ vs. sham group; ###$P < 0.001$ vs. I/R group; $^{\$}P < 0.05$ versus FGF2 + I/R group.

as compared to sham control ($P < 0.001$), whereas FGF2 pre-treatment significantly lowered the score compared to, an effect largely blunted by 5-HD co-treatment (Fig. 2C). Consistent with the reduced levels of serum Cr and BUN, FGF2 administration markedly reduced kidney tissue damage compared to the I/R group (Fig. 2A-c, g), whereas 5-HD significantly antagonized the protection activity of FGF2 (Fig. 2A-d, h).

3.2 FGF2 treatment enhances I/RI-induced activation of endogenous FGFR

To investigate the relationship between FGF2/FGFR pathway and renal I/RI, we determined the activation status of FGFR by IHC staining of kidney tissue sections with anti-p-FGFR antibody. Very few p-FGFR and weak positive renal tubular epithelial cells were present in kidneys of sham rats (Fig. 2B-a, e), while this number is perceptibly increased 2 days after reperfusion (Fig. 2B-b, f). However, both the number of p-FGFR positive cells and the staining intensity were markedly increased in renal tubules of I/R kidney with FGF2 alone or combined with 5-HD (Fig. 2B-c, d, g, h) compared to sham group and I/R alone. Quantification analysis shown in Fig. 2D indicated that the number of p-FGFR positive cells was already significantly increased by I/RI ($P < 0.05$), whereas FGF2 treatment led to more robust increase ($P < 0.001$).

3.3 FGF2 pre-treatment protects the renal tubular cells from I/R-induced apoptosis

TUNEL staining of kidney tissue sections revealed a small number of TUNEL-positive tubular epithelial cells were present in the sham rats (Fig. 3A-a). Consistent with I/RI-induced apoptotic phenotype, the number of TUNEL-positive cells was dramatically increased after 2 days of reperfusion (Fig. 3A-b). Importantly, FGF2 pre-treatment largely prevented the I/RI-induced apoptotic cell death (Fig. 3A-c), whereas co-treatment with 5-HD significantly reduced the FGF2 protection effect (Fig. 3A-d). To determine the possible pathway of I/ R injury, we performed IHC staining of activated caspase-3 and observed that its expression was significantly increased in kidneys of I/R group and I/R+FGF2+5-HD group, but was dramatically lower in I/R+FGF2 group (Fig. 3B). This result was confirmed by Western blot, which indicated that the expression of cleaved caspase-3 was significantly decreased in I/R+FGF2 kidney tissues compared

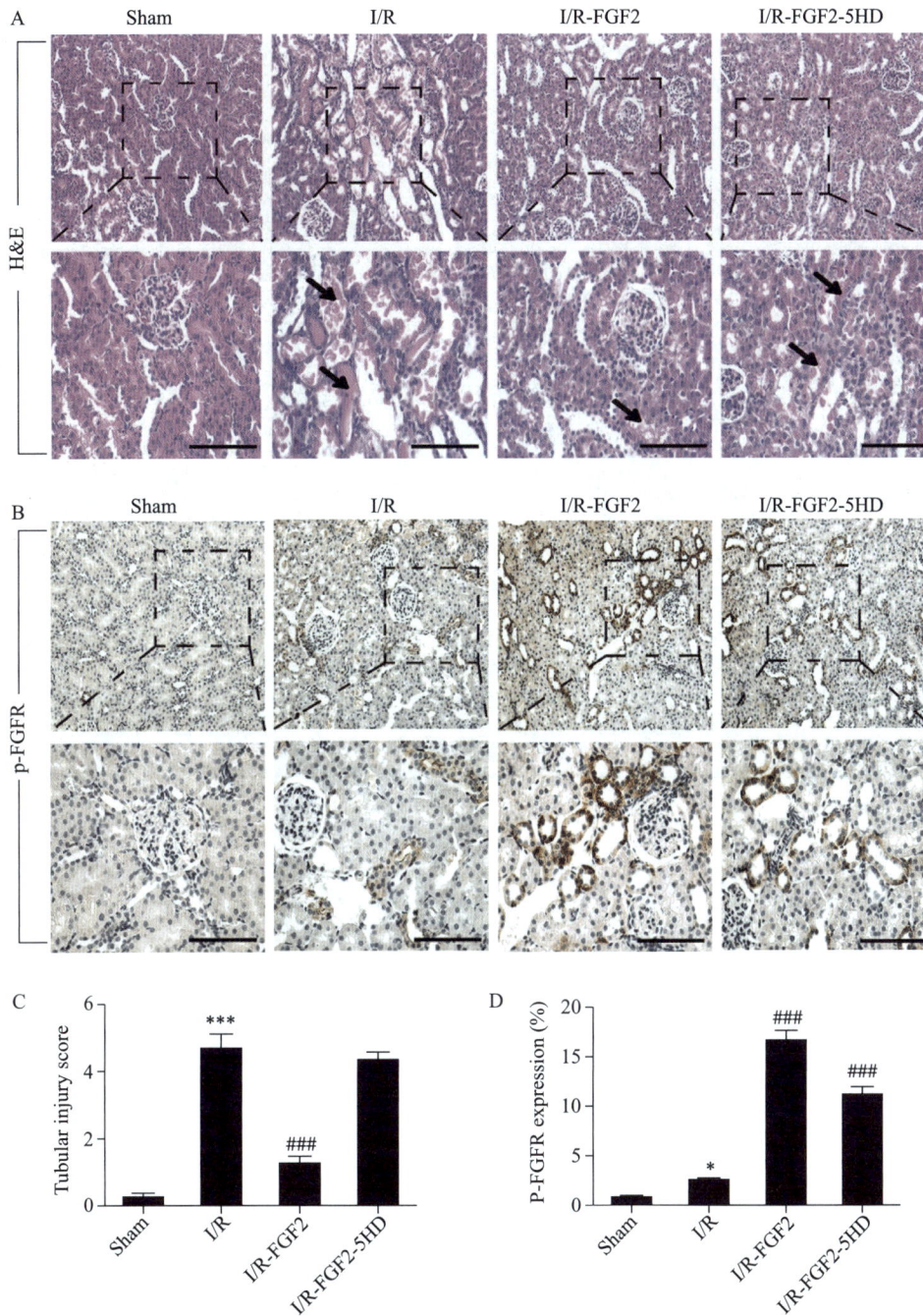

Fig. 2. FGF2 protects renal histological integrity and robustly activates FGFR. (A) Histological evaluations of renal tissue with H&E after 2 days of reperfusion (original magnification ×20 and ×40, respectively). Arrows show intraluminal necrotic cellular debris, interstitial congestion and oedema, and formation of proteinaceous casts. Scale bars represent 50 μm. (B) Immunohistochemical staining for phospho-FGFR (p-FGFR, original magnification ×20 and ×40, respectively). Scale bars represent 50 μm. (C) Renal tubular injury scores were calculated based on H&E staining using the criteria and procedure described in the material and methods. Results are representative of eight animals in each group. ***$P < 0.001$ vs. sham group), ###$P < 0.001$ vs. I/R group. Results are representative of eight animals in each group. (D) Quantification and statistical analysis of p-FGFR positive cells in the kidney. Data are representative of five animals in each group. *$P < 0.05$ vs. sham group.

with I/R or I/R+FGF2+5-HD groups (Fig. 3C–E). The results indicated that FGF2 administration exerted potent renal protective effects against I/R-induced apoptosis by reducing the caspase activation.

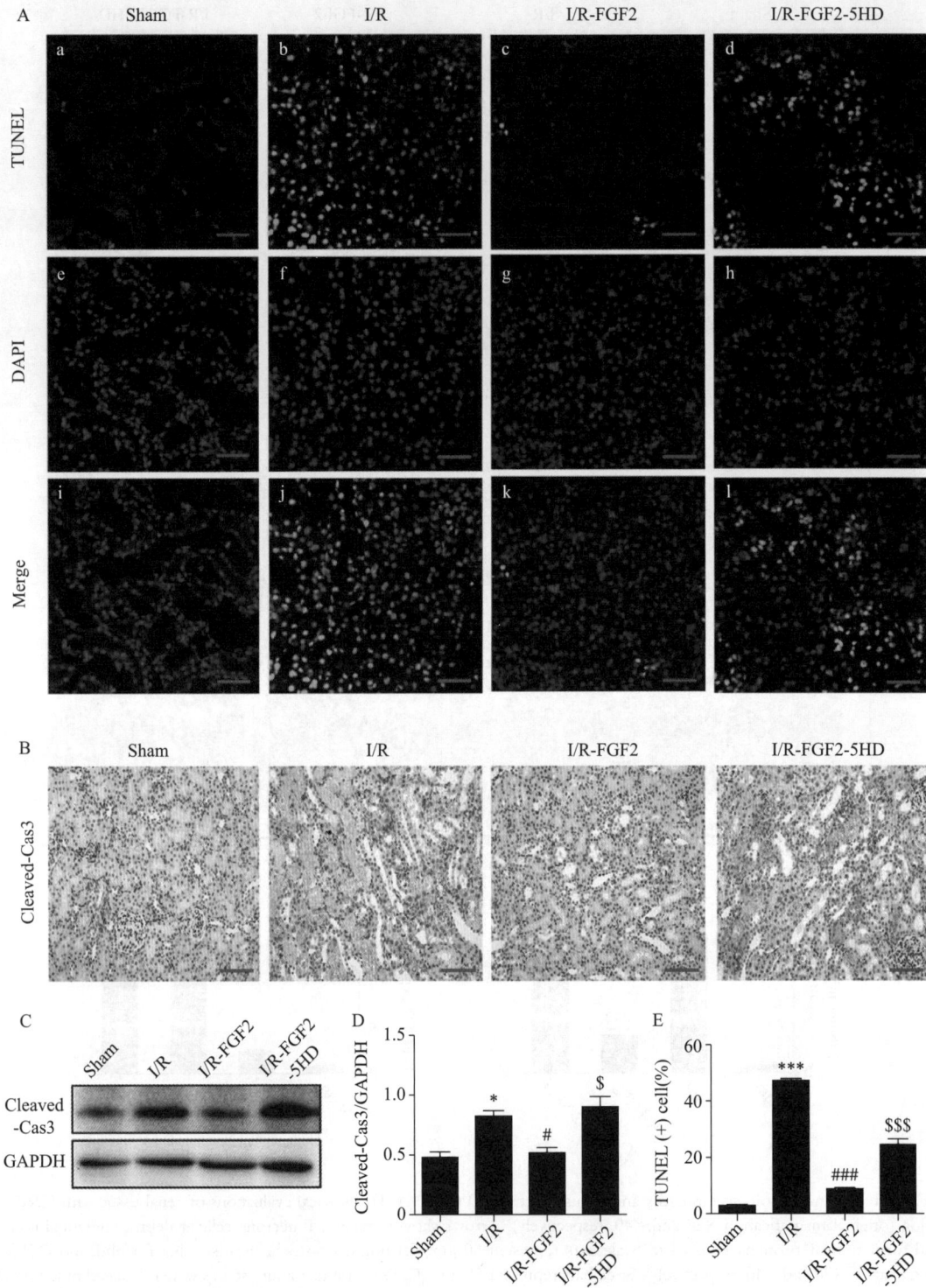

Fig. 3. FGF2 protects renal tubular cells from I/R-induced apoptosis. (A) Representative sections of nuclear DNA fragmentation after 2 days of reperfusion. Staining was achieved by TdT-mediated dUTP nick-end labelling (TUNEL) immunofluorescence. Original magnification ×40, scale bars represent 50 μm. Results are representative of five animals in each group. (B) IHC staining for Cleaved caspase-3 (Original magnification ×40, scale bars represent 50 μm). Data are representative of five animals in each group. (C) Western blot analyses of Cleaved caspase-3 expression. GAPDH was used as a loading control. Representative data of three individual samples per group. (D) The optical density analysis of Cleaved caspase-3 in the kidney. $^*P < 0.05$ $vs.$ sham group, $^#P < 0.05$ $vs.$ I/R group; $^$P < 0.05$ $vs.$ I/R+FGF2 group. (E) The percentage of TUNEL-positive cells was counted from five random 1 mm^2 areas. Data are presented as the mean S.D. $^{***}P < 0.001$ $vs.$ sham group; $^{###}P < 0.001$ $vs.$ I/R group; $^{$$$}P < 0.001$ $vs.$ I/R+FGF2 group.

3.4 FGF2 pre-treatment alters the expression of key mitochondrial apoptosis-regulatory proteins

To determine whether the renal protective effect of FGF2 is related to its ability to maintain mitochondrial integrity following I/RI, we measured the expression of several key mitochondrial proteins involved in apoptosis by immunoblot. Observation revealed that the level of Bax expression was significantly up-regulated in renal tissues of I/R rats compared with sham control (Fig. 4A, B). However, increased Bax expression was partially inhibited by FGF2 pre-treatment. In contrast, the protein levels of Bcl-2 and cytochrome c in mitochondria (Cyto-c) were significantly down-regulated in the kidneys of I/R rats compared with sham rats. Importantly, FGF2 treated animals did not show a significant loss of either Bcl-2 or Cyto-c compared with sham group (Fig. 4A, C, D). IHC analysis indicated that FGF2 inhibited the up-regulation of cleaved caspase-9 that was induced by I/RI (Fig. 4E).

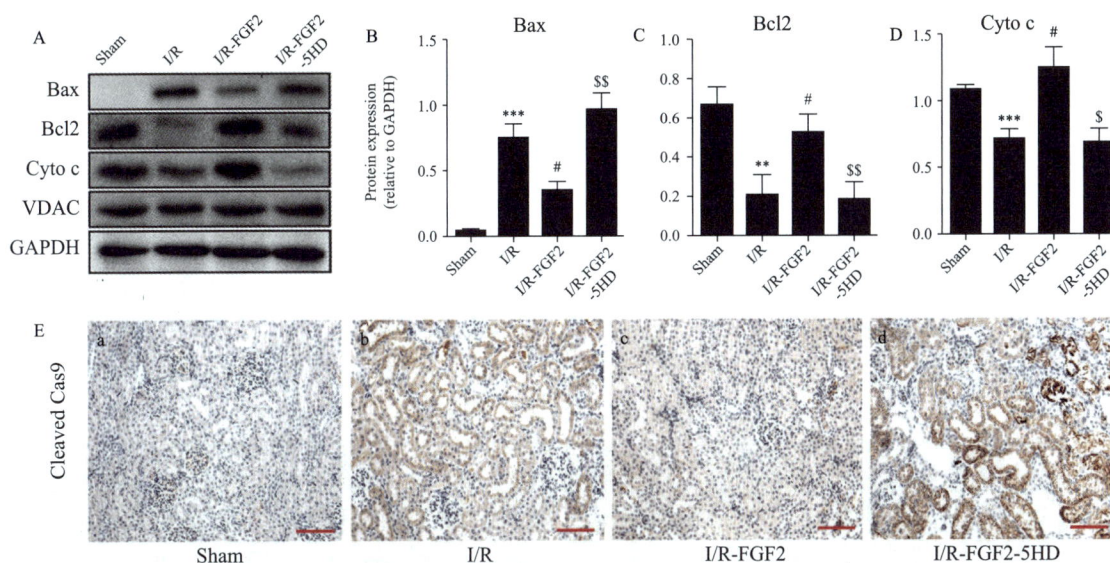

Fig. 4. FGF2 ameliorates pro-apoptotic mitochondrial protein expression. (A) Immunoblot analysis of mitochondrial damage-related proteins in the kidneys 2 days after reperfusion. (B-D). Optical density analysis to quantify protein expression levels for Cytochrome c (Cyto-c), Bax and Bcl2 in kidneys of sham rats, I/R rats, I/R+FGF2 rats and I/R+FGF2 + 5-HD rats (mean ± S.E.; $n = 5$). $^{**}P < 0.01$ and $^{***}P < 0.001$ $vs.$ sham group, $^{#}P < 0.01$ $vs.$ I/R group, $^{\$}P < 0.05$ and $^{\$\$}P < 0.01$ $vs.$ FGF2 + I/R group. (E) IHC staining of Cleaved caspase-9 (original magnification ×20, scale bars represent 100 μm). Data are representative of five animals in each group.

3.5 FGF2 pre-treatment greatly alleviates I/RI-induced mitochondrial oxidative damage

Nitrotyrosine immunohistochemistry staining was performed to reveal peroxynitrite formation caused by mitochondrial oxidative damage. I/RI increased nitrotyrosine production after reperfusion, as demonstrated by strong tubular epithelial cell staining of kidney tissue sections (Fig. 5A-b). The production of nitrotyrosine was significantly lower in I/R+FGF2 kidneys when compared with I/R kidneys (Fig. 5A-c). Immunoblot analysis of nitrotyrosine is consistent with IHC staining as I/R-induced nitrotyrosine accumulation is largely abolished by FGF2 (Fig. 5B and C). It is well accepted that mtDNA is more susceptible than nuclear DNA to increase oxidative stress due to the lack of histone protection [47]. MtDNA damage caused by oxidative stress can be assessed staining with 8-OHdG staining. Indeed, we detected increased production of 8-OHdG in the cytoplasm of tubular cells in ischaemic kidneys by IHC (Fig. 5A-f), while FGF2 treatment inhibited the production of 8-OHdG (Fig. 5A-g). Of note, staining of 8-OHdG was primarily localized in the cytoplasm, indicating that this oxidative adduct was mainly present in the mitochondria.

3.6 FGF2 pre-treatment mitigates the loss of MMP following I/RI

Mitochondria isolation kit (Sigma-Aldrich) was used to prepare the mitochondria containing intact inner and outer membranes [11, 48]. MMP was detected in paraffin-embedded sections 2 days after reperfusion by use of the fluorescent probe JC-1 (Invitrogen). We observed that relative fluorescence intensity of red to green was lower in I/R kidneys

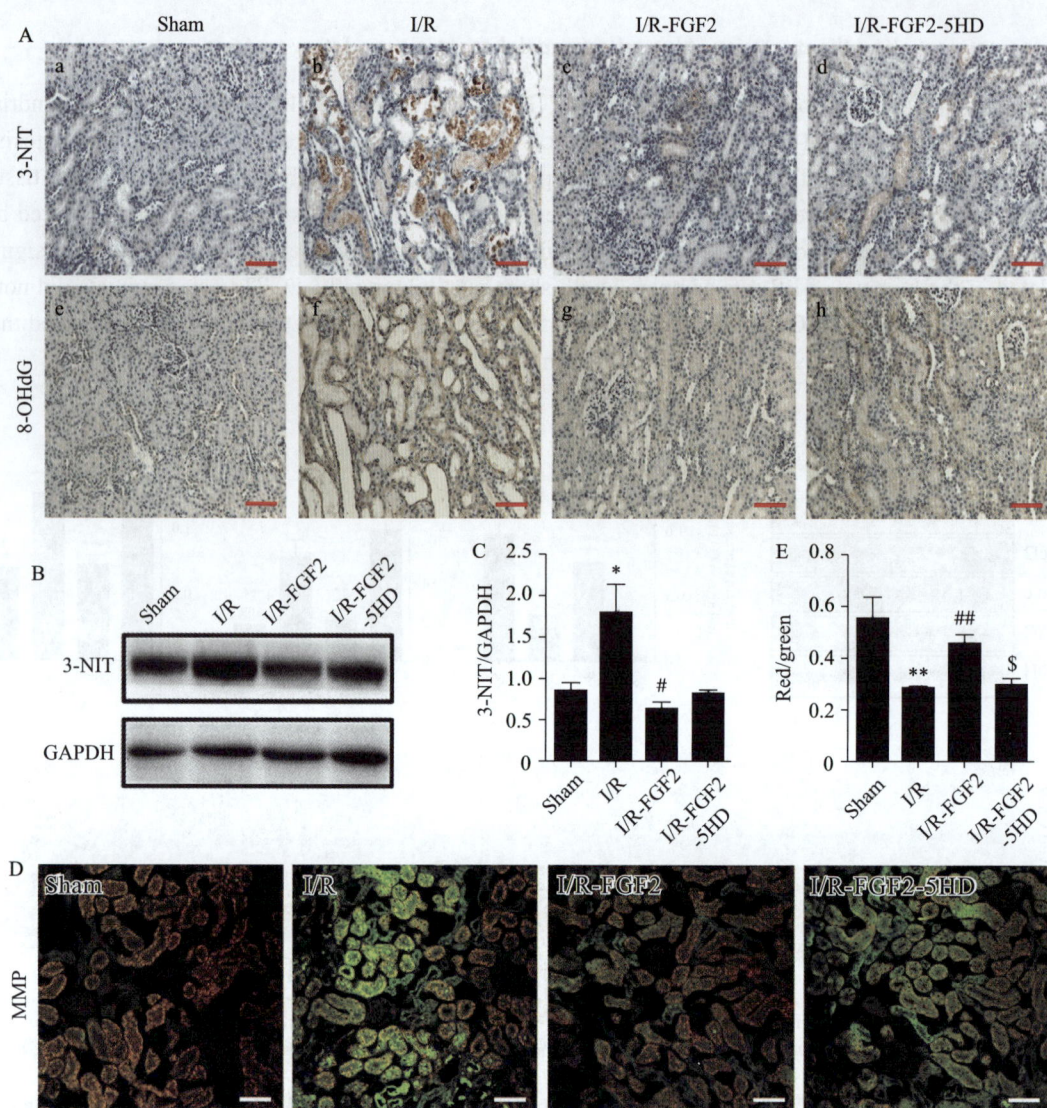

Fig. 5. FGF2 alleviates I/R-induced mitochondrial oxidative damage. (A) Immunohistochemistry staining for 3-nitrotyrosine and 8-OHdG 2 days after reperfusion. Results show positive staining of 3-nitrotyrosine and 8-OHdG primarily localized in tubular epithelial cells. FGF2 treatment reduced 3-nitrotyrosine and 8-OHdG to levels similar to sham rats. Original magnification ×20, scale bars represent 100 μm. Renal tissue sections from 1 of 4 animals in each group are shown. (B) Western blot analysis of 3-nitrotyrosine expression in the kidney. GAPDH was used as a loading control. (C) Optical density analysis to quantify protein expression for 3-nitrotyrosine in the kidney (mean ± S.E.; $n = 4$). $^{*}P < 0.05$ vs. sham group, $^{#}P < 0.05$ vs. I/R group. (D) Detection of mitochondrial membrane potential (MMP) in kidney using the JC-1 MMP detection Kit and confocal microscope imaging analysis. MMP declined in I/R kidney after 2 days of reperfusion as indicated by JC-1 fluorescence shift from red towards green, a phenomenon reversed by FGF2 treatment. Original magnification ×20, scale bars represent 100 μm. Data are representative of five animals in each group. (E) MMP in freshly isolated kidney mitochondria was also measured by the JC-1 MMP detection Kit. $^{**}P < 0.01$ vs. sham group, $^{##}P < 0.01$ vs. I/R group, $^{$}P < 0.05$ vs. I/R+FGF2 group.

compared with the sham control, whereas relative fluorescence intensity of red to green was contrastively higher in I/R+FGF2 kidneys compared to I/R kidneys (5D). We also measured the MMP using JC-1 in freshly isolated mitochondria 2 days after reperfusion. Consistent with results of measurements in tissue sections, the intensity of red fluorescence was reduced almost half in I/R kidneys compared with sham control. The lack of significant difference in MMP between I/R+FGF2 and sham control (Fig. 5E) suggests that FGF2 could contribute in maintaining a near homoeostatic MMP; which may be essential for the functional integrity of mitochondria and cell survival [49].

3.7 FGF2 pre-treatment contributes to sustain mitochondrial KATP channel upon I/RI

Previous studies have shown that Kir6.2, a subunit of the mitochondrial K_{ATP} channel, is localized to the mitochondria of renal tubular epithelial cells, smooth muscle cells and cardiomyocytes [50, 51]. To determine whether FGF2 treat-

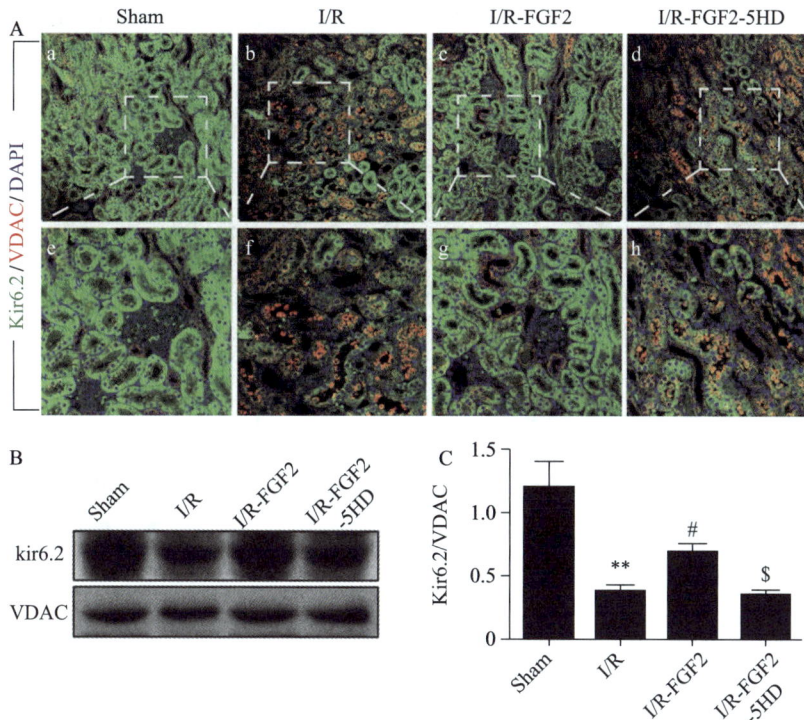

Fig. 6. FGF2 contributes to maintain mitochondrial $K_&$ channel expression and functional integrity. (A) Expression of mitochondrial ATP-dependent potassium (K_{ATP}) channel subunit Kir6.2 was determined by immunofluorescence staining 2 days after reperfusion. Kir6.2 (in green) was widely distributed in renal tubular epithelial cells and was more abundant than VDAC (in red) in sham-operated kidney, but Kir6.2 expression declined dramatically in I/R animals, which was largely reversed by FGF2 treatment. The effect of FGF2 in reversing the decrease of Kir6.2 expression is counteracted by 5-HD co-treatment. Results are representative of four animals from each group. (B) Western blot analysis of Kir6.2 protein expression. VDAC was used as an internal control. FGF2 treatment sustained Kir6.2 expression, but this effect was reversed by 5-HD (mean ± S.E.; $n = 4$). $^{**}P < 0.01$ vs. sham group, $^{#}P < 0.05$ vs. I/R group, $^{$}P < 0.05$ vs. FGF2 + I/R group. (C) The optical density analysis of Kir6.2 in the kidney tissue sections.

ment influenced mitochondrial KATP channels, subunit Kir6.2 was examined by immunofluorescence staining, using VDAC as an internal control. Immunofluorescence staining showed that Kir6.2 expression (green fluorescence) was decreased in ischaemic kidneys after 2 days of reperfusion. However, FGF2 treatment sustained Kir6.2 expression and this effect was reversed in the 5-HD treatment (Fig. 6A). Western blot analysis confirmed that the decrease of Kir6.2 expression relative to VDAC (Kir6.2/VDAC) was largely prevented upon FGF2 treatment of I/R kidneys, whereas 5-HD treatment abolished this protection effect (Fig. 6B, C).

3.8 Delayed FGF2 treatment exerts equal protection against renal I/RI

To explore the potential of FGF2 for therapy, we further investigated the effect of delayed FGF2 administration on renal I/RI and repair. Animals were treated with FGF2 at 1, 3 and 12 hrs, respectively, post renal ischaemic exposure besides the pre-I/R treatment as above. We assessed and compared the degree of renal dysfunction in each group by measuring their serum creatinine levels. Serum Cr measurement indicated that post-I/R FGF2 treatment at all three time-points displayed similar and marked alleviation of renal functional impairment to the pre-I/R treatment compare to sham-treated group (Fig. 7A). H&E staining of renal tissue sections and quantification analysis of tubular injury score indicated that post-I/R FGF2 was equally effective in preserving the renal histology as pre-I/R administration (Fig. 7B, C). The potent effect of exogenous FGF2 against I/R-induced functional impairment and histology damage prompt us to determine whether FGF2 would bring any survival benefit to the injured animals. Kaplan–Meier analysis revealed that no mortality was observed in the rats from the sham-operated group, whereas shamtreated I/R animals exhibited a survival rate of 60% with most of fatalities occurring within 3 days of reperfusion. Importantly, both the pre-I/R and 12 h post-I/R FGF2 treatment significantly improved the animal survival of I/R rats (Fig. 7D). Consistent with the protection against ROS damage and apoptosis, post-I/R FGF2 also induced Bcl2 expression, while markedly decreased the levels of both Bax and 3-NIT expression. Overall these results indicate that post-I/R administration of FGF2 equally protects

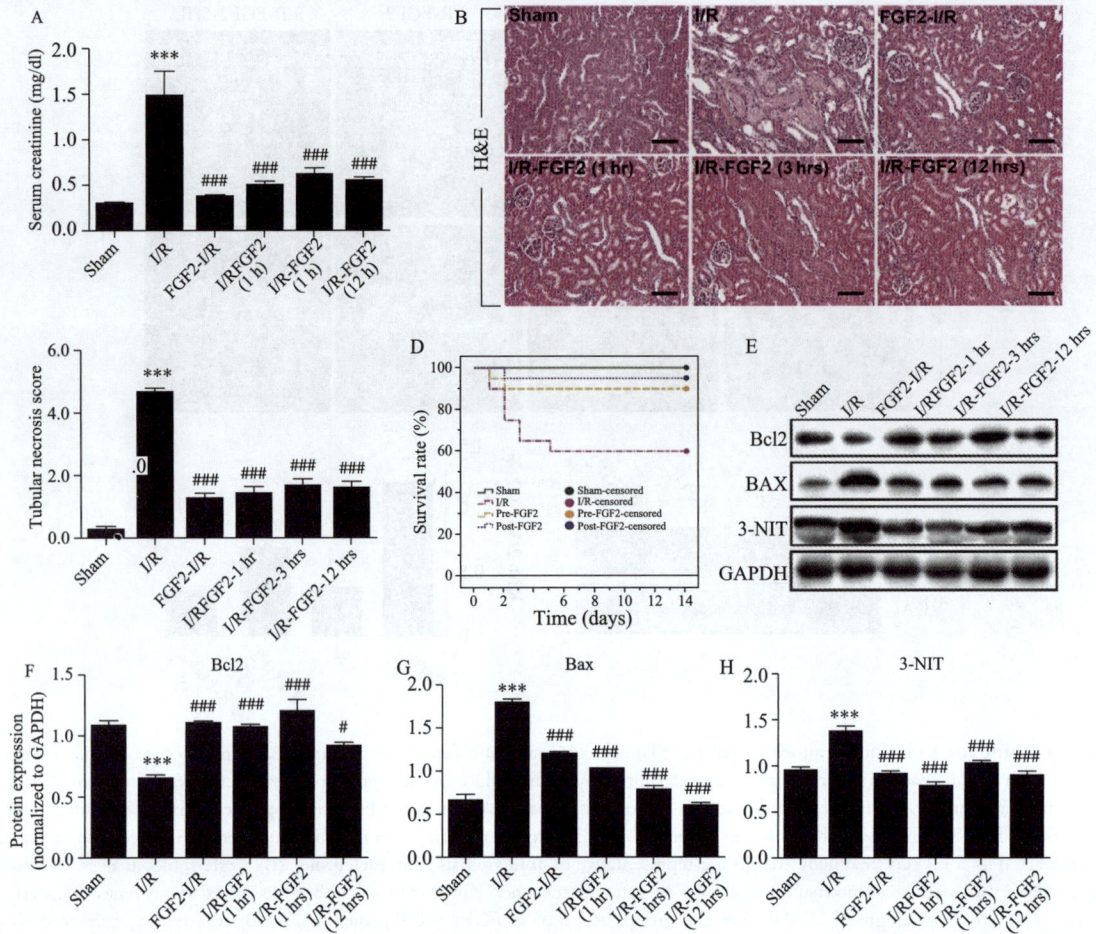

Fig. 7. Delayed FGF2 treatment exhibits potent protection against I/RI. Animals were divided into six groups, including sham-operated control, I/RI group, and I/RI rat with FGF2 pre-treatment or post-I/R treatment at 1, 3 and 12 h, respectively, after reperfusion as indicated. Except for the animal survival analysis, which was carried out for 2 weeks, all other experiments were performed at 48 h after reperfusion. (A) The serum creatinine (Cr) levels of animals receiving indicated treatment, including sham-operated (sham), ischaemia-reperfusion (I/R), I/R pre-treated with FGF2 (FGF2-I/R), or I/R with delayed FGF2 treatment at 1, 3, or 12 h, respectively, after reperfusion as indicated. ***$P < 0.001$ vs. sham group, ###$P < 0.001$ vs. I/R group. (B) Representative H&E stained renal tissue sections. Original magnification ×20, scale bars represent 100 μm. (C) Histological evaluation and pathological scoring based on H&E staining. Renal tubular necrosis scores were calculated using the criteria and procedure described in the material and methods. Results are representative of eight animals in each group. ***$P < 0.001$ vs. sham group), ###$P < 0.001$ vs. I/R group. (D) Effect of FGF2 treatment on the survival of I/R rats. Twenty rats were assigned to each group as indicated and animal survival curves (Kaplan–Meier analysis) were constructed at 14 days after reperfusion. Upon 50 min. of ischaemic exposure, the survival rate of I/RI rats was 60% compared to 100% in sham-operated control. Notably, FGF2 pre-treatment (Pre-FGF2) or delayed treatment (Post-FGF2, 12 h after reperfusion) resulted in significantly increased animal survival rates (90% and 95%, respectively). $P < 0.05$ vs. I/R alone group). There was no significant difference between pre- and post-FGF2 group. (E) Renal protein extracts were subjected to Western blot analysis with indicated antibodies to determine the expression of Bcl2, Bax, 3-NIT with GAPDH as loading control. (F–H) Optical density analysis to quantify the expression levels of Bax, Bcl-2 and 3-NIT, respectively, with indicated treatments. The data were shown as mean S.E. ($n = 5$). ***$P < 0.001$ vs. sham group, ###$P < 0.001$ and #$P < 0.05$ vs. I/R group.

kidney from I/R-induced mitochondrial damage and improves animal survival.

3.9 FGF2 inhibits I/RI-induced HMGB1 release and inflammatory cytokine gene expression

HMGB1 is a major damage-associated molecular pattern (DAMP) molecule released by damaged cells upon I/RI, which contributes to proinflammatory signaling to inflict broader tissue damage. To determine whether FGF2 could affect the nuclear–cytoplasmic trafficking and extracellular release of HMGB1 in I/R kidneys, we first assessed the expression of HMGB1 by immunoblot analysis. HMGB1 is readily detected in protein extract of sham-operated kidney (Fig. 8A), but was markedly decreased upon I/RI. Significantly, either pre-or post-I/R exposure to exogenous FGF2 blunted the I/R-induced decrease of HMGB1. TNF-α, a key downstream inflammatory cytokine, was significantly induced in

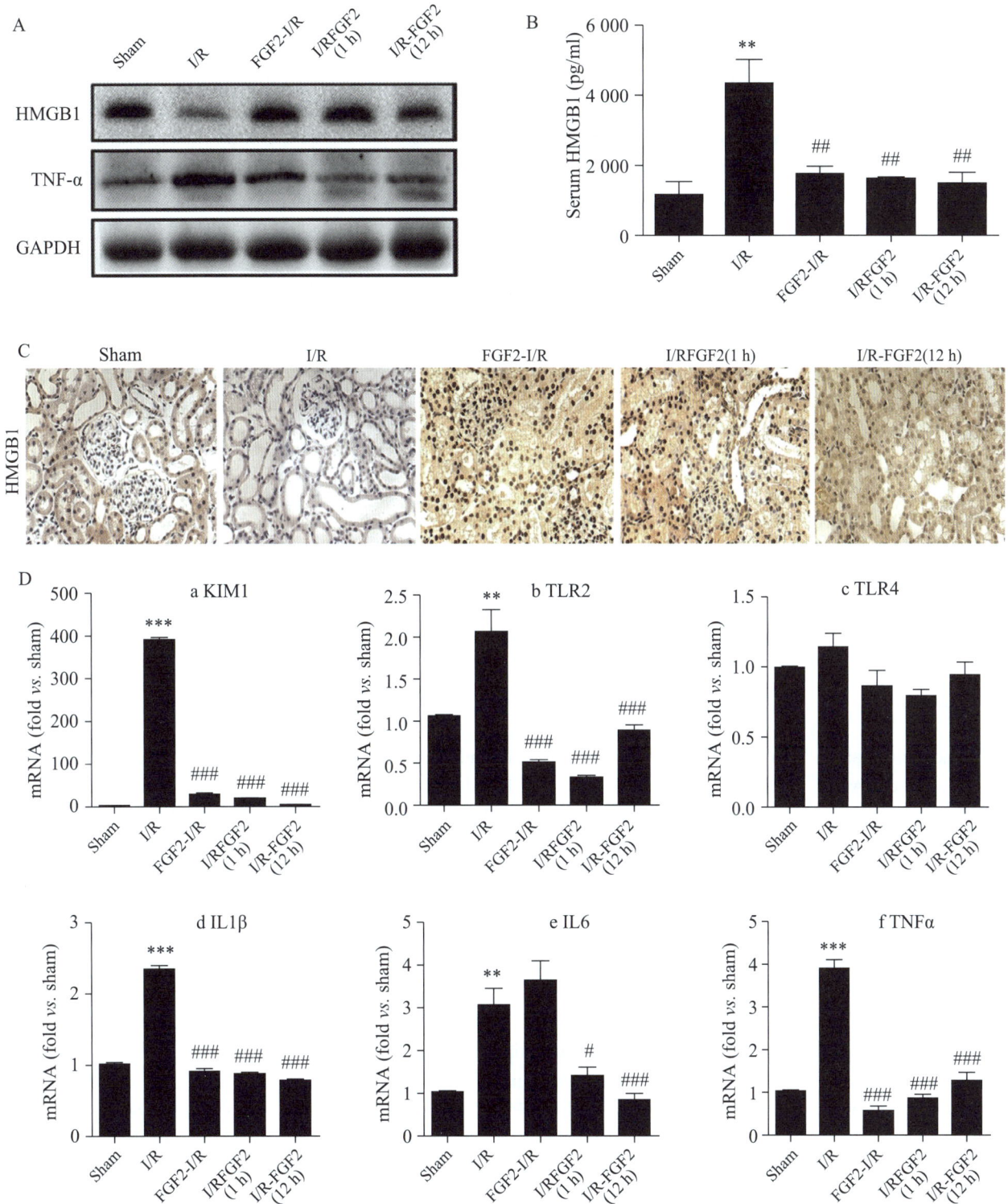

Fig. 8. FGF2 inhibits I/RI-induced HMGB1 serum release and inflammatory response. Animals were divided into 5 groups ($n = 4$), including sham-operated control, I/RI group, and I/RI with FGF2 pre-treatment or delayed treatment at 1 and 12 h, respectively, after reperfusion as indicated. The samples were collected at 48 h following reperfusion for Western blot, ELISA, Immunohistochemistry staining (IHC) and qRT-PCR analysis as detailed below. (A) Western blot analysis to determine the expression of HMGB1 and TNF-α in renal tissues with GAPDH as loading control. (B) ELISA assay was used to determine the levels of HMGB1 in the serum of animals receiving indicated treatments. $^{**}P < 0.01$ vs. sham group, $^{##}P < 0.01$ vs. I/R group. (C) IHC of kidney tissue sections for expression of HMGB1. Original magnification ×20. One representative area of renal tissue staining from 1 of 4 animals in each group is shown. (D) Real-time PCR quantification of mRNA levels for KIM1, TLR2, TLR4, IL-1α, IL-6 and TNF-α in the kidney, respectively. The result is normalized to GAPDH. The data are presented as mean ± S.E. ($n = 4$). $^{***}P < 0.001$, $^{**}P < 0.001$ vs. sham group; $^{###}P < 0.001$, $^{#}P < 0.05$ vs. I/R group.

I/R kidney, and conversely largely prevented by FGF2 treatment (Fig. 8A). Contrary to the decrease in kidney tissue, serum HMGB1 level, as measured by ELISA, was increased to nearly fourfold in the I/R group. Notably, either 1 or 12 h post-I/R given FGF2 achieved similar levels of inhibition towards HMGB1 release to the serum (Fig. 8B). IHC staining further confirmed the HMGB1 release following ischaemia (Fig. 8C). Compared to the sham control (Fig. 8C-a), HMGB1 staining intensity was greatly reduced in I/R kidney (Fig. 8C-b), with minimal nuclear HMGB1 left in the tubular cells. Strikingly, either pre-or post-I/R FGF2 treatment effectively pre-served the intracellular level of HMGB1, particularly its nuclear localization (Fig. 8C-c, d, e). These results together indicate that either pre-or post-IR FGF2 prevented I/RI-induced HMGB1 nucleus to cytoplasm translocation and extracellular release.

Extracellular HMGB1 activates proinflammatory response mainly *via* activation of cell surface receptors including TLRs. TLR2 and TLR4, in particular, are essential in mediating renal I/R-induced damage and inflammatory cytokine gene expression, such as IL1β, IL-6 and TNF-α. We next measured the mRNA expression of these inflammatory factors *via* real-time PCR. As expected, the expression of Kidney Injury Molecule-1 (KIM-1), a biomarker for renal proximal tubule injury, was dramatically increased upon I/RI with up to a nearly 400-fold induction over the sham-operated control (Fig. 8D-a). Consistent with its protective effect, FGF2 treatment dramatically reduced I/RI-induced KIM1 expression (Fig. 8D-a). In the same cDNA samples, TLR2 expression was increased twofold in the I/R group, which was completely prevented by either Pre-or post-ischaemic FGF2 treatment (Fig. 8D-b). We did not observe significant change with TLR4 expression in any of the I/R groups regardless of FGF2 treatment (Fig. 8D-c). The expression for IL-1β, IL-6 and TNF-α all showed significant increases in I/RI kidney relative to sham control (Fig. 8D-d, e, f). Importantly, FGF2 treatment effectively blunted the I/R-induced expression of these five pro-inflammatory genes. The only exception is IL-6, for which the I/R-induced expression was not inhibited by pre-ischaemic FGF2 (Fig. 8D-e). The data together strongly indicate that FGF2 exerts potent inhibitory activity towards I/R-induced HMGB1 release and the expression of key proinflammatory genes, such as IL-1β, IL-6, TLR2 and TNF-α.

4. Discussion

The molecular mechanism of I/RI remains incompletely understood and there are no definitive treatment measures for I/RI-induced AKI [52]. Current work demonstrates that I/R-induced renal tubular cell apoptosis is associated with pro-apoptotic alteration of key mitochondria protein (Bcl2 and Bax) expression, decreased MMP and caspase activation. The accumulation of oxidative mtDNA damage in this I/R-induced AKI model is also evident and likely contributes to the mitochondria dysfunction and apoptosis. Strikingly, FGF2 treatment dramatically alleviated the various damaging parameters of I/RI, including oxidative mtDNA damage and decrease in MMP. Furthermore, the reduced expression of the mitochondrial KATP channel subunit Kir6.2 following I/R was largely rescued in FGF2 treated animals. Nonetheless, blocking of KATP channels with the classic mKATP inhibitor 5-HD reduced the protective effect of FGF2. Therefore, FGF2 appears to act upon several key aspects of mitochondrial function to mediate its protection effect.

A number of previous studies including those from our own group have reported the protective effect of FGF2 against I/RI in myocardial, retinal, Intestinal and neural tissues in various experimental models [34–37, 41]. However, the protective mechanism of FGF2 on renal I/R model remains unclear. In this study, we found that both renal functional and morphological integrity were largely preserved in I/R kidney group receiving pre-or post-ischaemic FGF2 treatment. Interestingly FGF2 has previous been identified as an I/R-induced nephrogenic protein with the inhibition of FGFR2 by antisense oligonucleotides enhancing ischaemic AKI damage, thus suggesting that endogenous FGF2/FGFR2 signaling is involved in the renal I/RI repair process. To determine how effectively FGF2 activated the FGFRs in this model, we further analysed the expression of activated FGFR using a phospho-FGFR antibody. Consistent with the reported increase of FGF2 following I/RI, we observed mild and localized activation of FGFR in proximal renal tubular cells, whereas FGF2 administration robustly enhanced the level of phospho-FGFR compared with control I/R animals. Therefore our experimental data combined with the published work strongly suggest that the protective effect of FGF2 towards renal I/RI is mediated through its activation of FGFRs.

It is well-established that apoptosis plays an important role in renal I/R pathogenesis [53]. The Bcl-2 family of anti-apoptotic proteins has a major role in maintaining the integrity of the external mitochondrial membrane and preventing the release of cytochrome C from the mitochondria. Conversely, several pro-apoptotic proteins such as Bax promote mitochondrial injury and cytochrome C release into cytoplasm from cell mitochondria. Released cytochrome C combined with apoptotic protease activating factor-1 (Apaf-1) and caspase-9 produce the Cytc-Apaf-1-Caspase-9 complex. This leads to the activation of pro-caspase-9 and subsequent downstream activation of caspase-3, which initiates the apoptotic cascade leading to cells death *via* either apoptosis or necrosis [54, 55]. To address if FGF2 has an impact on AKI-induced apoptotic process and how it may affect the apoptotic regulatory proteins, we first demonstrated that exogenous FGF2 dramatically reduced the number of TUNEL-positive tubular cells and decreased the activation of caspase-3, as well as caspase-9 in renal tubular cells compared with I/R alone (Fig. 3B). Western blot analysis revealed that the levels of mitochondrial cytochrome C and cytoplasmic Bcl-2 were increased. On the contrary, cytoplasmic Bax expression induced by I/RI was significantly decreased by FGF2 treatment (Fig. 4A). Together our results suggest that FGF2 prevents I/RI-induced apoptosis in a mitochondrial dependent mechanism *via* regulation of Bcl2 family of proteins.

Generation of ROS by mitochondria also contributes to damage of cellular components and initiation of cell death. MtDNA is more susceptible than nuclear DNA to increased oxidative stress because of the lack of histone protection and limited capacity of DNA repair capability [47, 56]. 8-OHdG is a biomarker of oxidative DNA damage, which stains nuclear DNA as well as mtDNA. Nitrotyrosine, a marker of nitrosative stress, was increased in renal tubular epithelial cells after I/R. ROS reacts with nitric oxide generating peroxynitrite, which may bind to protein residues such as tyrosine and yield highly cytotoxic nitrotyrosine [57, 58]. In our previous study, we demonstrate that ROS, the major initiator of lethal effects of I/R injury, were rapidly produced in the mitochondria of renal tubular cells following reperfusion. Agents that open the mitochondrial K_{ATP} channel reduced the generation of ROS by the mitochondria in as early as 1 hr post reperfusion [11]. However, whether FGF2 can protect damage to mtDNA had not been previously investigated. In the current study, protection of mtDNA by FGF2 was reflected by lowering the amounts of 3-NIT generation and less mtDNA oxidative damage when compared with those in I/R rats (Fig. 5A, B). We have previously proposed that mtDNA damage may be the cause of renal injury and could occur even before cell death [11]. To determine whether mtDNA damage indeed influenced mitochondrial function, we further measured MMP with an immunofluorescence-based assay. MMP was significantly decreased 2 days after reperfusion; however, FGF2 treatment largely sustained MMP level in the treated animals (Fig. 5D, E).

K_{ATP} channels have a critical role in maintaining cellular energetic homoeostasis under physiological conditions, highlighted by the fact they sustain MMP during oxidative stress [59]. Opening of the K_{ATP} channel has been proposed to be associated with an uptake of potassium in the mitochondrial matrix, which could constitute a parallel potassium influx and attenuate Ca^{2+} overload. The reduction in mitochondrial Ca^{2+} uptake would prevent mitochondrial swelling and inhibit opening of the mitochondrial permeability transition pore during reperfusion [60]. Additionally, mitochondrial K_{ATP} channel activity effectively inhibits the development and release of ROS [61], which are the reactive molecules and possible initiators of all deleterious effects seeing following reperfusion. A number of studies have concluded that activation of mitochondrial K_{ATP} channels confer protection against I/RI, which has been shown not only by pharmacological means using mitochondrial K_{ATP} channel activators and inhibitors, but also by direct evidence of Kir6.2 gene overexpression [62–64].

We speculated that the protective mechanisms of FGF2 were related to its effect on mitochondrial K_{ATP} channels. To test this hypothesis, 5-HD, an ischaemia-selective mitochondrial K_{ATP} antagonist [65], was administered before ischaemia. 5-HD was chosen, due to its acceptance as a more specific blocker of mitochondrial K_{ATP} channel than glibenclamide [66]. In our present study, Kir6.2 expression was significantly decreased in renal tubular epithelial cells 2 days after reperfusion, while FGF2 treatment resulted in significant up-regulation of Kir6.2 expression, which was completely antagonized by 5-HD (Fig. 6). We speculate that opening of mitochondrial K_{ATP} channels may be a protective mechanism of FGF2; therefore, blocking of mitochondrial K_{ATP} channels blunted its protection effect.

The innate immune response is another key pathogenic aspect of I/RI. The initial hypoxic damage to parenchymal cells, particularly the highly susceptible proximal tubular cells, inevitably triggers sterile inflammatory response contributing to the infliction of broad tissue damage. HMGB1 has been identified as a major DAMP protein capable of imposing potent proinflammatory response once released by damaged cells. Thus far, we are unaware of any published research on I/RI linking FGF2 to regulation of inflammatory response. By combining analysis of immunoblot, ELISA and IHC of the same samples, we obtained convincing evidence that I/R-associated cytoplasmic translocation and extracellular release of HMGB1 can be completely inhibited by either pre-I/R or delayed FGF2 treatment. As circulating HMGB1 is known to activate proinflammatory signaling pathways through its interaction with pattern recognition receptors such as TLR2 and TLR4; both of which are crucial pro-inflammatory factors in exacerbating I/RI as demonstrated using their respective knockout mouse models [45, 67]. We therefore further measured the mRNA expression of TLR2 and TLR4 in the kidneys, and confirmed that I/RI significantly induced TLR2 expression, which is completely obliterated upon FGF2 treatment. Contrary to the earlier report on I/RI-induced TLR4 expression, we found TLR4 to be only marginally induced in the same samples measured at 48 h post-I/R exposure. This result was confirmed by testing two independent sets of primers with the same result (Fig. 8D-c, and data not shown). Consistent with the potent inhibitory effect of FGF2 treatment on I/R-induced HMGB1 release and TLR2 expression, we affirmed complete obliteration, by FGF2 treatment, of I/R-induced IL-1α, IL-6 and TNFα expression, which are three key inflammatory cytokines downstream of HMGB1/ TLRs signaling pathway. Therefore, current work provides the first experimental evidence that FGF2-mediated protection against I/RI involves its ability to mitigate subsequent inflammatory responses. Whether this potent anti-inflammatory effect of FGF2 is due to its protection of renal parenchymal cells from initial hypoxic damage, alleviating the extracellular release of HMGB1 and subsequent proinflammatory response, or additional mechanism involving direct interaction FGF2/FGFR signaling with the immune cells will be an interesting topic for future study.

From the clinical translational point of view, FGF2 has been successfully used as a repair/regeneration factor in a variety of conditions such as burns, chronic wounds, oral ulcers, vascular ulcers, diabetic ulcers, pressure ulcers and surgical incisions. To date all of these indications have been limited to topical application [68].

However, a number of recent studies including those from our group have reported the protective effect of FGF2 against I/R injuries in various disease models; particularly in cardiac infarction [36-40]. The current work investigated the effect of both pre-I/R and delayed FGF2 administration and demonstrated its potent protection against I/R-induced mitochondrial damage and anti-inflammatory response. Given that delayed FGF2 treatment at 12 h post-IR still showed significant protective activity and improved animal survival, our findings further highlight the potential of FGF2 in the prevention and treatment of I/R-induced AKI. As the prototype member of the FGF family, FGF2 is known to engage all four FGFRs and activate signaling pathways including Ras-MAPK and PI3K/AKT pathways, which contribute to cell proliferation and survival. Indeed, in several ischaemic disease models such as the cardiac infarction, activation of MAPK, PI3K/AKT, or PKC signaling pathway by FGF2 is essential to mediate its protection [38-40]. The fact that FGF2 administered at 12 h post-I/R still delivered significant protection strongly suggests a role of FGF2 in the repair process of AKI in addition to its aid in the protection from initial damage. It has been reported that exogenous FGF2 promotes cardiac stem cell-mediated myocardial regeneration and enhance the viability of cord blood-derived mesenchymal stem cells transplanted to ischaemic limbs [69, 70]. Further study is required to delineate the role as well as the molecular mechanism of FGF2 on renal tissue repair and regeneration through stem cell differentiation and/or mobilization.

In summary, current study provides the first experimental evidence that exogenously administered FGF2 exhibits robust protection against renal I/RI and significantly improves animal survival. The remarkable protective effect pertains to its ability to attenuate several I/RI-induced mitochondrial-damaging parameters including pro-apoptotic alteration of Bcl2/Bax expression and caspase-3 activation. FGF2 also contributes to maintain the expression of mitochondrial K_{ATP} channels under hypoxic condition, which may help to alleviate oxidative stress and I/R-induced mtDNA damage. Beside the above protection on renal parenchyma, FGF2 treatment is also capable of obliterating I/R-triggered HMGB1 release and activation of TLRs-mediated signaling and inflammatory cytokine gene expression. These new mechanistic insights into FGF2-mediated protection against renal I/RI may also shed light to understand I/RI-related disorders in other tissues. Given that either pre-ischaemic or post-I/R FGF2 treatment delivers similar potency of protection, our work suggests that FGF2 has the potential to be used for the prevention as well as treatment of I/RI-related AKI.

References

[1] Schrier RW, Wang W, Poole B, et al. Acute renal failure: definitions, diagnosis, pathogenesis, and therapy[J]. Journal Of Clinical Investigation, 2004, 114(1): 5-14.

[2] Chertow GM, Burdick E, Honour M, et al. Acute kidney injury, mortality, length of stay, and costs in hospitalized patients[J]. Journal Of the American Society Of Nephrology, 2005, 16(11): 3365-3370.

[3] Ishani A, Xue JL, Himmelfarb J, et al. Acute Kidney Injury In-creases Risk of ESRD among Elderly[J]. Journal Of the American Society Of Nephrology, 2009, 20(1): 223-228.

[4] Mehta RL. Outcomes research in acute renal failure[J]. Seminars In Nephrology, 2003, 23(3): 283-294.

[5] Bonventre JV, Yang L. Cellular pathophysiology of ischemic acute kidney injury[J]. Journal Of Clinical Investigation, 2011, 121(11): 4210-4221.

[6] Tan X, Yin R, Chen Y, et al. Postconditioning attenuates renal isch-

emia-reperfusion injury by mobilization of stem cells[J]. Journal Of Nephrology, 2015, 28(3): 289-298.

[7] Akki A, Zhang M, Murdoch C, *et al.* NADPH oxidase signaling and cardiac myocyte function[J]. Journal Of Molecular And Cellular Cardiology, 2009, 47(1): 15-22.

[8] Lambeth JD. Nox enzymes and the biology of reactive oxygen[J]. Nature Reviews Immunology, 2004, 4(3): 181-189.

[9] Meneshian A, Bulkley GB. The physiology of endothelial xanthine oxidase: From urate catabolism to reperfusion injury to inflammatory signal transduction[J]. Microcirculation, 2002, 9(3): 161-175.

[10] Rauen U, de Groot H. New insights into the cellular and molecular mechanisms of cold storage injury[J]. Journal Of Investigative Medicine, 2004, 52(5): 299-309.

[11] Tan X, Zhang L, Jiang Y, *et al.* Postconditioning ameliorates mitochondrial DNA damage and deletion after renal ischemic injury[J]. Nephrology Dialysis Transplantation, 2013, 28(11): 2754-2765.

[12] Kalogeris T, Bao Y, Korthuis RJ. Mitochondrial reactive oxygen species: A double edged sword in ischemia/reperfusion vs preconditioning[J]. Redox Biology, 2014, 2: 702-714.

[13] Wang YP, Schmeichel AM, Iida H, *et al.* Ischemia-reperfusion injury causes oxidative stress and apoptosis of Schwann cell in acute and chronic experimental diabetic neuropathy[J]. Antioxidants & Redox Signaling, 2005, 7(11-12): 1513-1520.

[14] Zhang H, Kong X, Kang J, *et al.* Oxidative Stress Induces Parallel Autophagy and Mitochondria Dysfunction in Human Glioma U251 Cells[J]. Toxicological Sciences, 2009, 110(2): 376-388.

[15] Thadhani R, Pascual M, Bonventre JV. Medical progress-Acute renal failure[J]. New England Journal Of Medicine, 1996, 334(22): 1448-1460.

[16] Sun Z, Zhang X, Ito K, *et al.* Amelioration of oxidative mitochondrial DNA damage and deletion after renal ischemic injury by the K-ATP channel opener diazoxide[J]. American Journal Of Physiology-Renal Physiology, 2008, 294(3): F491-F498.

[17] Lee HL, Chen CL, Yeh ST, *et al.* Biphasic modulation of the mitochondrial electron transport chain in myocardial ischemia and reperfusion[J]. American Journal Of Physiology-Heart And Circulatory Physiology, 2012, 302(7): H1410-H1422.

[18] Domoki F, Bari F, Nagy K, *et al.* Diazoxide prevents mitochondrial swelling and Ca^{2+} accumulation in CA1 pyramidal cells after cerebral ischemia in newborn pigs[J]. Brain Research, 2004, 1019(1-2): 97-104.

[19] Miura T, Miki T. ATP-sensitive K^+ channel openers: Old drugs with new clinical benefits for the heart[J]. Current Vascular Pharmacology, 2003, 1(3): 251-258.

[20] Ren R, Zhang Y, Li B, *et al.* Effect of beta-Amyloid (25-35) on Mitochondrial Function and Expression of Mitochondrial Permeability Transition Pore Proteins in Rat Hippocampal Neurons[J]. Journal Of Cellular Biochemistry, 2011, 112(5): 1450-1457.

[21] Robin E, Simerabet M, Hassoun SM, *et al.* Postconditioning in focal cerebral ischemia: Role of the mitochondrial ATP-dependent potassium channel[J]. Brain Research, 2011, 1375: 137-146.

[22] Zhang H, Song LC, Jia CH, *et al.* Effects of ATP sensitive potassium channel opener on the mRNA and protein expressions of caspase-12 after cerebral ischemia-reperfusion in rats[J]. Neuroscience Bulletin, 2008, 24(1): 7-12.

[23] Kaczorowski DJ, Tsung A, Billiar TR. Innate immune mechanisms in ischemia/reperfusion[J]. Frontiers in Bioscience (Elite edition), 2009, 1: 91-98.

[24] Jang HR, Rabb H. The innate immune response in ischemic acute kidney injury[J]. Clinical Immunology, 2009, 130(1): 41-50.

[25] Arslan F, Keogh B, McGuirk P, *et al.* TLR2 and TLR4 in Ischemia Reperfusion Injury[J]. Mediators Of Inflammation, 2010.

[26] Musumeci D, Roviello GN, Montesarchio D. An overview on HMGB1 inhibitors as potential therapeutic agents in HMGB1-related pathologies[J]. Pharmacology & Therapeutics, 2014, 141(3): 347-357.

[27] Li J, Gong Q, Zhong S, *et al.* Neutralization of the extracellular HMGB1 released by ischaemic-damaged renal cells protects against renal ischaemia-reperfusion injury[J]. Nephrology Dialysis Transplantation, 2011, 26(2): 469-478.

[28] Chen Q, Guan X, Zuo X, *et al.* The role of high mobility group box 1 (HMGB1) in the pathogenesis of kidney diseases[J]. Acta Pharmaceutica Sinica B, 2016, 6(3): 183-188.

[29] Kim HJ, Park SJ, Koo S, *et al.* Inhibition of kidney ischemia-reperfusion injury through local infusion of a TLR2 blocker[J]. Journal Of Immunological Methods, 2014, 407: 146-150.

[30] Bohlen P, Baird A, Esch F, *et al.* Isolation and partial molecular characterization of pituitary fibroblast growth-factor[J]. Proceedings Of the National Academy Of Sciences Of the United States Of America-Biological Sciences, 1984, 81(17): 5364-5368.

[31] Ware JA, Simons M. Angiogenesis in ischemic heart disease[J]. Nature Medicine, 1997, 3(2): 158-164.

[32] Yanagisawamiwa A, Uchida Y, Nakamura F, *et al.* Salvage of infarcted myocardium by angiogenic action of basic fibroblast growth-factor[J]. Science, 1992, 257(5075): 1401-1403.

[33] Scholz D, Cai W-J, Schaper W. Arteriogenesis, a new concept of vascular adaptation in occlusive disease[J]. Angiogenesis, 2001, 4(4): 247-257.

[34] Mark RJ, Keller JN, Kruman I, *et al.* Basic FGF attenuates amyloid beta-peptide-induced oxidative stress, mitochondrial dysfunction, and impairment of Na^+/K^+-ATPase activity in hippocampal neurons[J]. Brain Research, 1997, 756(1-2): 205-214.

[35] Ruel M, Laham RJ, Parker JA, *et al.* Long-term effects of surgical angiogenic therapy with fibroblast growth factor 2 protein[J]. Journal Of Thoracic And Cardiovascular Surgery, 2002, 124(1): 28-34.

[36] Manning JR, Perkins SO, Sinclair EA, *et al.* Low molecular weight fibroblast growth factor-2 signals *via* protein kinase C and myofibrillar proteins to protect against postischemic cardiac dysfunction[J]. American Journal Of Physiology-Heart And Circulatory Physiology, 2013, 304(10): H1382-H1396.

[37] Wang Z, Zhang H, Xu X, *et al.* bFGF inhibits ER stress induced by ischemic oxidative injury *via* activation of the PI3K/Akt and ERK1/2 pathways[J]. Toxicology Letters, 2012, 212(2): 137-146.

[38] House SL, Bolte C, Zhou M, *et al.* Cardiac-specific overexpression of fibroblast growth factor-2 protects against myocardial dysfunction and infarction in a murine model of low-flow ischemia[J]. Circulation, 2003, 108(25): 3140-3148.

[39] House SL, Branch K, Newman G, *et al.* Cardioprotection induced by cardiac-specific overexpression of fibroblast growth factor-2 is mediated by the MAPK cascade[J]. American Journal Of Physiology-Heart And Circulatory Physiology, 2005, 289(5): H2167-H2175.

[40] House SL, Melhorn SJ, Newman G, *et al.* The protein kinase C pathway mediates cardioprotection induced by cardiac-specific overexpression of fibroblast growth factor-2[J]. American Journal Of Physiology-Heart And Circulatory Physiology, 2007, 293(1): H354-H365.

[41] Villanueva S, Cespedes C, Gonzalez A, *et al.* bFGF induces an earlier expression of nephrogenic proteins after ischemic acute renal failure[J]. American Journal Of Physiology-Regulatory Integrative And Comparative Physiology, 2006, 291(6): R1677-R1687.

[42] Villanueva S, Cespedes C, Vio CP. Ischemic acute renal failure induces the expression of a wide range of nephrogenic proteins[J]. American Journal Of Physiology-Regulatory Integrative And Comparative Physiology, 2006, 290(4): R861-R870.

[43] Villanueva S, Cespedes C, Gonzalez AA, *et al.* Inhibition of bFGF-receptor type 2 increases kidney damage and suppresses nephrogenic protein expression after ischemic acute renal failure[J]. American Journal Of Physiology-Regulatory Integrative And Comparative Physiology, 2008, 294(3): R819-R828.

[44] Wang Z, Wang Y, Ye J, *et al.* bFGF attenuates endoplasmic reticulum stress and mitochondrial injury on myocardial ischaemia/reperfusion *via* activation of PI3K/Akt/ERK1/2 pathway[J]. Journal Of

Cellular And Molecular Medicine, 2015, 19(3): 595-607.

[45] Wu H, Chen G, Wyburn KR, et al. TLR4 activation mediates kidney ischemia/reperfusion injury[J]. Journal Of Clinical Investigation, 2007, 117(10): 2847-2859.

[46] Yamada K, Miwa T, Liu JN, et al. Critical protection from renal ischemia reperfusion injury by CD55 and CD59[J]. Journal Of Immunology, 2004, 172(6): 3869-3875.

[47] Lum H, Roebuck KA. Oxidant stress and endothelial cell dysfunction[J]. American Journal Of Physiology-Cell Physiology, 2001, 280(4): C719-C741.

[48] Zhang X, Tachibana S, Wang H, et al. Interleukin-6 Is an Important Mediator for Mitochondrial DNA Repair After Alcoholic Liver Injury in Mice[J]. Hepatology, 2010, 52(6): 2137-2147.

[49] Kulkarni GV, Lee W, Seth A, et al. Role of mitochondrial membrane potential in concanavalin A-induced apoptosis in human fibroblasts[J]. Experimental Cell Research, 1998, 245(1): 170-178.

[50] Flagg TP, Enkvetchakul D, Koster JC, et al. Muscle K-ATP Channels: Recent Insights to Energy Sensing and Myoprotection[J]. Physiological Reviews, 2010, 90(3): 799-829.

[51] Zhou M, He HJ, Suzuki R, et al. Expression of ATP sensitive K^+ channel subunit Kir6.1 in rat kidney[J]. European Journal Of Histochemistry, 2007, 51(1): 43-51.

[52] Wang W, Tang T, Zhang P, et al. Postconditioning Attenuates Renal Ischemia-Reperfusion Injury by Preventing DAF Down-Regulation[J]. Journal Of Urology, 2010, 183(6): 2424-2431.

[53] Oberbauer R, Schwarz C, Regele HM, et al. Regulation of renal tubular cell apoptosis and proliferation after ischemic injury to a solitary kidney[J]. Journal Of Laboratory And Clinical Medicine, 2001, 138(5): 343-351.

[54] Sun K, Liu ZS, Sun Q. Role of mitochondria in cell apoptosis during hepatic ischemia-reperfusion injury and protective effect of ischemic postconditioning[J]. World Journal Of Gastroenterology, 2004, 10(13): 1934-1938.

[55] Buja LM, Entman ML. Modes of myocardial cell injury and cell death in ischemic heart disease[J]. Circulation, 1998, 98(14): 1355-1357.

[56] Stadtman ER, Levine RL. Free radical-mediated oxidation of free amino acids and amino acid residues in proteins[J]. Amino Acids, 2003, 25(3-4): 207-218.

[57] Vinas JL, Hotter G, Pi F, et al. Role of peroxynitrite on cytoskeleton alterations and apoptosis in renal ischemia-reperfusion[J]. American Journal Of Physiology-Renal Physiology, 2007, 292(6): F1673-F1680.

[58] Vinas JL, Sola A, Hotter G. Mitochondrial NOS upregulation during renal I/R causes apoptosis in a peroxynitrite-dependent manner[J]. Kidney International, 2006, 69(8): 1403-1409.

[59] Storey NM, Stratton RC, Rainbow RD, et al. Kir6.2 limits Ca^{2+} overload and mitochondrial oscillations of ventricular myocytes in response to metabolic stress[J]. American Journal Of Physiology-Heart And Circulatory Physiology, 2013, 305(10): H1508-H1518.

[60] Wu L, Shen F, Lin L, et al. The neuroprotection conferred by activating the mitochondrial ATP-sensitive K+ channel is mediated by inhibiting the mitochondrial permeability transition pore[J]. Neuroscience Letters, 2006, 402(1-2): 184-189.

[61] Facundo HTF, de Paula JG, Kowaltowski AJ. Mitochondrial ATP-sensitive K^+ channels are redox-sensitive pathways that control reactive oxygen species production[J]. Free Radical Biology And Medicine, 2007, 42(7): 1039-1048.

[62] Garlid KD, Paucek P, YarovYarovoy V, et al. Cardioprotective effect of diazoxide and its interaction with mitochondrial ATP-Sensitive K^+ channels - Possible mechanism of cardioprotection[J]. Circulation Research, 1997, 81(6): 1072-1082.

[63] Garlid KD, Dos Santos P, Xie ZJ, et al. Mitochondrial potassium transport: the role of the mitochondrial ATP-sensitive K^+ channel in cardiac function and cardioprotection[J]. Biochimica Et Biophysica Acta-Bioenergetics, 2003, 1606(1-3): 1-21.

[64] Ljubkovic M, Marinovic J, Fuchs A, et al. Targeted expression of Kir6.2 in mitochondria confers protection against hypoxic stress[J]. Journal Of Physiology-London, 2006, 577(1): 17-29.

[65] Auchampach JA, Grover GJ, Gross GJ. Blockade of ischemic preconditioning in dogs by the novel ATP dependent potassium channel antagonist sodium 5-hydroxydecanoate[J]. Cardiovascular Research, 1992, 26(11): 1054-1062.

[66] Liu YG, Sato T, Seharaseyon J, et al. Mitochondrial ATP-dependent potassium channels: Viable candidate effectors of ischemic preconditioning[J]. Ann N Y Acad Sci., 1999,874: 27-37.

[67] Trentin-Sonoda M, da Silva RC, Kmit FV, et al. Knockout of Toll-Like Receptors 2 and 4 Prevents Renal Ischemia-Reperfusion-Induced Cardiac Hypertrophy in Mice[J]. Plos One, 2015, 10(10).

[68] Nunes QM, Li Y, Sun C, et al. Fibroblast growth factors as tissue repair and regeneration therapeutics[J]. Peer J, 2016, 4.

[69] Zhang YH, Zhang GW, Gu TX, et al. Exogenous basic fibroblast growth factor promotes cardiac stem cell-mediated myocardial regeneration after miniswine acute myocardial infarction[J]. Coronary Artery Disease, 2011, 22(4): 279-285.

[70] Bhang SH, Lee T-J, La W-G, et al. Delivery of fibroblast growth factor 2 enhances the viability of cord blood-derived mesenchymal stem cells transplanted to ischemic limbs[J]. Journal Of Bioscience And Bioengineering, 2011, 111(5): 584-589.

Hedgehog signaling contributes to basic fibroblast growth factor-regulated fibroblast migration

Zhongxin Zhu, Xiaokun Li, Litai Jin

1. Introduction

Skin plays an important role in life sustenance by protecting the internal organs and tissues from external injury [1]. Skin wounds are readily caused by tears, cuts, and contusions [2], making their existence a common occurrence of daily life. Given that injury to the skin can culminate in death due to disruption of its barrier function with accompanying infection, fluid loss, and so on, it becomes essential that any wound sustained by the skin be healed to restore homeostasis [1].

Wound healing is a complex orchestration of molecular and biological events, involving cell migration, cell proliferation, and extracellular matrix (ECM) synthesis and remodeling. It also requires the coordinated actions of multiple cell types, including fibroblasts [3,4], which produce ECM molecules and remodel the matrix to direct re-epithelialization and control contraction. Moreover, fibroblast proliferation and migration are essential for the formation of granulation tissue and wound closure [5].

Numerous cytokines and growth factors regulate assorted processes in wound repair. For example, basic fibroblast growth factor (bFGF, also known as fibroblast growth factor 2), a well-known member of the fibroblast growth factor family, participates in cell migration, cell and tissue differentiation, and cell proliferation [6,7]. Previously, we showed that bFGF activates the phosphoinositide 3-kinase (PI3K)-Rac1 signaling pathway to induce c-Jun N-terminal kinase (JNK) phosphorylation, which results in the promotion of fibroblast migration [5,6]. Furthermore, the results of our recent RNA-sequencing analysis showed that bFGF stimulation modulates many other signaling cascades, including the Wnt and Hedgehog (Hh) pathways.

Hh signaling is crucial during the development of vertebrate and invertebrate organisms, and exerts a wide variety of regulatory functions [8]. Hh was initially identified as a secreted signaling protein required for specification of positional identity in the *Drosophila melanogaster* embryonic segment [9]. The three mammalian *hh* genes, *Sonic hedgehog*, *Indian hedgehog*, and *Desert hedgehog* (*Shh*, *Ihh*, and *Dhh*, respectively), are important in the patterning of many tissues and biological structures [9]. Accordingly, loss or reduction of Hh signaling is associated with severe developmental deficits, including holoprosencephaly, polydactyly, and various craniofacial defects and skeletal malformations. Moreover, inappropriate activation of Hh signaling is responsible for nearly all basal cell carcinomas, some medulloblastomas, and rhabdomyosarcomas; excessive Hh signaling is also implicated in other tumors [8,10–12]. Under normal unstimulated conditions, the transmembrane protein Patched1 (Ptch1) binds to a second transmembrane protein, Smoothened (Smo), to maintain the Hh pathway in an inactive or "off" state. In contrast, when the secreted protein, Shh, binds to and inactivates Ptch1, allowing activation of Smo [11,13], Smo may then triggers target gene transcription through the Gli-Kruppel family of transcription factors, leading to the control of cell survival, proliferation, and differentiation [13].

A recent investigation identified a novel aspect of Gli-Kruppel family member 1 (Gli1) function in modulating E-cadherin/β-catenin-regulated cancer cell properties. Gli1 interfered with the membrane localization of E-cadherin by up-regulating a gel-forming mucin, MUC5AC, which in turn weakened E-cadherin-dependent cell-cell adhesions and enhanced pancreatic ductal adenocarcinoma cell migration and invasiveness [14]. Another study found that Shh can stimulate bone marrow-derived endothelial progenitor cell proliferation, migration, and production of vascular endothelial growth factor (VEGF), which may then promote neovascularization of ischemic tissucs [15]. In addition, the Shh pathway also induces cell migration and invasion in liver cancer *via* focal adhesion kinase/AKT signaling-mediated production and activation of matrix metalloproteinases 2 and 9 [16]. All of these studies advance our understanding of the role of Hh pathway proteins (Smo/Gli1) in fibroblast migration and skin wound healing. However, the molecular basis of the relationship between Hh signaling and bFGF-stimulated fibroblast migration is not clear.

Here, we showed that bFGF induces Smo/Gli1 expression to facilitate fibroblast migration. Smo acts upstream of PI3K-JNK signaling, which in turn increases levels of glycogen synthase kinase 3 beta phosphorylated at Ser 9 (pGSK3β-Ser9) and the nuclear accumulation of β-catenin. Furthermore, experiments with β-*catenin*-knock-down cells demonstrated that β-catenin contributes to a feedback mechanism to modulate the transcription of Hh pathway genes. In conclusion, the results of this study identify a new mechanism of bFGF-Hh-mediated regulation of fibroblast migration.

2. Materials and methods

2.1 Ethics statement

Human foreskin samples were collected from the volunteers at the Second Affiliated Hospital of Wenzhou Medical University (Wenzhou, China). All volunteers were informed of the purpose and procedures of this study, and agreed to offer their tissue specimens with written consent. All protocols were approved by the Ethics Committee of the Second Affiliated Hospital of Wenzhou Medical University.

2.2 Human foreskin fibroblast cell culture

All fat was removed from the human foreskin samples obtained from the volunteers, and the tissue was cut into 3 mm strips and incubated with 0.05% dispase neutral protease (Sigma-Aldrich) in Dulbecco's Modified Eagle's Medium (DMEM, Gibco) supplemented with 10% fetal bovine serum (FBS, Gibco) and 1% penicillin-streptomycin (Gibco) at 4 °C overnight. Next, the epidermis was removed from the dermis, and the dermis was finely minced and placed into 25 cm^2 tissue culture flasks coated with FBS. The flasks were placed horizontally for 1 h and then vertically for 3 h in an atmosphere of 5% CO_2 at 37 °C. The tissues were transferred into DMEM supplemented with 5.5 mM glucose, 10% FBS, and 1% penicillin-streptomycin, with subsequent changes of the medium every 3 days. Cultured cells were passaged by using 0.25% trypsin (Gibco) when cell confluency reached ~80%. Primary human fibroblasts at passage 5–6 were used in experiments described below.

2.3 MTT assay

The cells in suspension were digested using trypsin, the cell concentration adjusted to 5,000/mL, and 200 µL of this cell suspension was placed in 96-well plates. The medium containing low FBS (0.5%), 5 mg/mL mitomycin-C and SAG (0.5 µM) or SAG (0.5 µM) plus LY294002 (1.0 µM) was added until the cell adherence. Each group was used in three parallel control wells. Before adding MTT reagents, images of the cells were taken under a Model IX70 Microscope (Olympus, Tokyo, Japan) at 24 h. After addition of MTT reagent, the cells were incubated for 4 h at 37 °C and the plates were shaken for an additional 10 min and the absorbance values were read at 490 nm using a Microplate Reader (Bio-Rad Co., USA).

2.4 Creation of skin wounds on rats and treatment with SAG, Cyc, Shh or GANT61

Male SD rats, weighting 220~300 g, were anesthetized with pentobarbital (45 mg/ml). The dorsal area of rats was totally depilated using Na_2S (8.0%, *w/v*) and two full-thickness circular wounds (about 250 mm^2 each) were created on the lower back of each rat using a pair of sharp scissors and a scalpel. The rat skin wounds were treated by applying SAG (0.5 µM), Cyc (0.5 µM), Shh (0.1 µg/ml), GANT61 (0.5 µM), or SAG (0.5 µM) plus GANT61 (0.5 µM) to the wound area.

2.5 Microscopic evaluation of wound healing area in rats

The wound areas in rat skins were examined after treatment for 0, 4, 8, 12 or 16 days. The skin wounds of five rats were photographed, and the healed wound areas were measured based on the analysis of images using Image-ProPlus 6.0 software (Media Cybernetics, UK) [17].

2.6 Cell migration assay

Cell migration was measured by using a scratch wound-healing assay. Cells (primary human fibroblasts, the mouse NIH 3T3 fibroblast cell line, and target gene knock-down NIH 3T3 cells, including β-*catenin*, *Smo*, *Gli1* knock-down cells (see below)) were plated into six-well plates at a plating density sufficient to create a confluent monolayer after 12 h of culture at 37℃ in an incubator with 5% CO_2. Cells were cultured in medium containing low FBS (0.5%) and 5 mg/ml mitomycin-C for 24 h to inhibit cell proliferation. The monolayer was then scraped in a straight line with a P200 pipette tip to create a "scratch wound". Images of the wounded cell monolayers were taken under a Model IX70 Microscope (Olympus, Tokyo, Japan) at 0, 12, and 24 h after wounding. Cell migration into the wounded area was recorded by using the same microscope equipped with a CoolSNAP HQ CCD Camera (Nippon Roper, Chiba, Japan) and MetaMorph Software (Universal Imaging Co., Ltd., Buckinghamshire, UK). The healing rate was quantified using measurements of gap size after culture. Ten different areas in each assay were chosen to measure the distance of migrating cells to the origin of the wound edge. The distance and the wound edge were measured using the "measurement length" function in Image J Software (National Institutes of Health, Bethesda, MD, USA).

2.7 3D spheroid cell invasion assay

The invasive activity of fibroblasts after SAG, Cyc, Shh or GANT61 treatment was measured using 96 well 3D spheroid cell invasion assay (Trevigen, Cat. 3500-096-K). Cells of 80% confluence were harvested and re-suspended in 1× Spheroid Formation ECM, and then which was added into this plate 50 μL per well, centrifuged at 200 *g* for 3 min at room temperature, and incubated at 37℃ in a tissue culture incubator for 72 h to promote spheroid formation. Working on ice, 50 μL of Invasion Matrix was added into per well and centrifuged plates at 300 *g* for 5 min at 4℃, and then plate was transferred to the incubator at 37℃ for 1 h to promote gel formation. After 1 h, 100 μl of cell culture mediums containing 0.5 μM SAG, 0.5 μM Cyc, 0.1 μg/ml Shh, or 0.5 μM GANT61, respectively were added, and incubated at 37℃ in the incubator for 4 days. The spheroid in each well every 24 h was photographed using the 4× objective and the invasion area was measured by Image-ProPlus 6.0 software (Media Cybernetics, UK).

2.8 Western blot analysis

For nuclear β-catenin accumulation assays, primary human fibroblasts were harvested and lysed to obtain cytoplasmic and nuclear lysates using the Keygen Nuclear-Cytosol Protein Extraction Kit from Nanjing KeyGen Biotech. Co., Ltd. (China). For immunoblotting of total and phosphorylated JNK and AKT, and phosphorylated GSK3β-Ser9, total GSK3β, Gli1, and Smo, whole cell lysates were employed. Skin tissues around healing wound were sampled, grinded into powder, and homogenized in an ice-cold lysis solution (AR0101-100, Boster, Wuhan, China). Cytoplasmic protein extracts were obtained by centrifugation at 15 000 rpm at 4℃ in a Biofuge Stratos centrifuge (Thermo Fisher Scientific, Bremen, Germany) for 15 min. Lysates (equal amounts of protein) were separated in sodium dodecyl sulfate polyacrylamide gels and transferred onto polyvinylidene difluoride membranes. The membranes were blocked at room temperature for 2 h and incubated at 4℃ overnight with the following primary antibodies: anti-glyceraldehyde 3-phosphate dehydrogenase (GAPDH; Abcam), anti-Lamin B1 (Cell Signaling Technology), anti-β-catenin (Abcam), anti-pGSK3β-Ser9 (Cell Signaling Technology), anti-GSK3β (Cell Signaling Technology), anti-Gli1 (Santa Cruz Biotechnology), anti-pAKT-Ser473 (Cell Signaling Technology), anti-AKT (Cell Signaling Technology), anti-pJNK (stress activated protein kinase/ JNK-Thr183/Tyr185; Cell Signaling Technology), anti-JNK1+JNK2+JNK3 (Abcam), and anti-Smo (Abcam). The membranes were then incubated for 1 h with an anti-mouse or anti-rabbit horseradish peroxidase-conjugated secondary antibody (Cell Signaling Technology), and immunoreactive signals were visualized *via* enhanced chemiluminescence. Quantitation of relative band intensities were performed by scanning densitometry using ImageJ software.

2.9 RNA interference

SiRNA for *Smo* (ON-TARGETplus SMART pool, J-047917-17), *Gli1* (ON-TARGET plus SMART pool, J-041026-05), β-*catenin* (ON-TARGET plus SMART pool, L-004018) and negative control siRNA (ON-TARGET plus si CONTROL non-targeting pool, D-001810) were purchased from Dharmacon RNA Technologies (Chicago, IL, USA). The NIH 3T3 cells were seeded 12 h before transfection. After reaching 30%–50% confluence (day 0), 30 nM of the siRNA duplex was transfected using Lipofectamine 2000 (Invitrogen) and Opti-MEM®I Reduced Serum Medium (Gibco) according to the instructions of the manufacturers. On reaching confluence on day 1 (24 h after transfection), siRNA solution was exchanged against full growth medium. The transfected cells were then used in two analyses: the cell migration assay using cells at 60%–80% confluence on day 2 (48 h after transfection) and Western blot analysis or qRT-PCR using cells at 80%–90% confluence at the time of harvesting for RNA or protein preparation on day 3 (72 h after transfection).

2.10 Knock-down of endogenous β-catenin by lentivirus-mediated siRNA

Lentivirus-mediated siRNA transfection was performed as previously described [18,19] by using NIH 3T3 cells. Stably transduced cells were selected after 2 weeks of puromycin (2 μg/mL) stress. Silencing efficiency was confirmed by Western blotting.

2.11 RNA isolation and quantitative real-time polymerase chain reaction (qRT-PCR)

Total RNA was extracted from cells by using TRIzol Reagent (Invitrogen). Next, total RNA (2 μg) was reverse transcribed into cDNA by using GoScript Reverse Transcription Kit (Promega). The cDNA was then subjected to qRT-PCR analysis, and gene expression was quantified as previously described [20]. The mRNA levels of target genes were normalized against that of *GAPDH*. Gene-specific primer sequences used for qRT-PCR are listed in Table S1.

2.12 RNA sequencing

Total RNA extracted from NIH 3T3 cells and *β-catenin* knock-down NIH 3T3 cells were used in RNA-Seq experiments. RNA-Seq experiments were performed according to the manufacturer's protocol and data analyses were performed by Lc. Bio tech Co., Ltd. (Hangzhou, China, http://www.lc-bio.com/).

2.13 Statistical analysis

Statistical analysis was performed with GraphPad Prism 5 (GraphPad, San Diego, CA). All data were expressed as mean ± SE and analyzed by ANOVA with post-and Student's *t*-test. Comparison between two groups was performed by the *t*-test. And one-way or two-way analysis of variance (ANOVA) with post-Bonferroni corrections was used to compare the effect of different treatments or compare the effect of treatment along time. A value of $^*P < 0.05$ denotes statistical significance, $^{**}P < 0.01$ denotes, high level of significance and $^{***}P < 0.001$ denotes, very high level of statistical significance.

3. Results

3.1 Hh signaling positively regulates fibroblast migration, invasion, and skin wound healing

The capacity of bFGF to promote fibroblast migration is well known, but the regulatory mechanism behind bFGF pro-migratory action is still poorly understood. To gain insight into this mechanism, we previously performed RNA-sequencing analysis using bFGF-stimulated fibroblasts. The results showed that Hh signaling genes (*e.g.*, *Smo*) are regulated by bFGF signaling (Table S2). Thereby, in this study, we employed a specific small-molecule agonist of Smo (SAG and Shh) and a Smo inhibitor (Cyc) to assess whether the Hh pathway participates in the control of fibroblast migration. As shown in Fig. 1A, SAG (0.5 μM) expedited primary human fibroblast migration at 24 h after wounding in a scratch wound healing assay. Moreover, 0.5 μM SAG was verified to facilitate activation of the Hh cascade by qRT-PCR (Fig. S1A). Thus, 0.5 μM SAG was selected as the optimal concentration for use in subsequent experiments. By contrast, fibroblast migration was delayed by the addition of 0.5 μM Cyc, a cell-permeable drug that inhibits Hh signaling *via* direct inhibition of Smo (Fig. S1B), and the expression levels of Hh-related genes were also evaluated by qRT-PCR (Fig. S1C). Moreover, recombinant human Shh significantly increased fibroblast migration at a concentration of 0.1 μg/ml (Fig. S1D), and 0.1 μg/ml Shh was also demonstrated to activate the Hh pathway (Fig. S1E). To confirm the impact of the Hh pathway on fibroblast migration, *Smo*-specific small interfering RNA (siRNA) was transformed into NIH 3T3 cells and the protein expression level of Smo was monitored (Fig. S1F). The migratory ability of NIH 3T3 cells was markedly impaired upon *Smo* silencing (Fig. S1G).

Wound healing is a multistep process including cell invasion, proliferation, and stabilization [21], and involves cell-

cell as well as cell-ECM interaction in tissues. Therefore, fibroblasts were subjected to a 3D spheroid cell invasion assay where the cells were grown as spheroids surrounded by ECM prior to inducing cell invasion with SAG, Cyc, or Shh treatment [22]. Similar to the effects seen in the cell migration, SAG and Shh markedly enhanced invasion of fibroblasts into the ECM, while the invasion was reduced by Cyc compared with the control group (Fig. 1B).

To verify the effects of Hh signaling *in vivo*, we established a Sprague-Dawley (SD) rat wound healing model composed of rats with two full-thickness circular wounds on their waists and monitored the wound repair rate. The results indicated that SAG and Shh treatment accelerated wound closure (Fig. 1C and S1I), while it was delayed by Cyc treatment (Fig. S1H). These findings suggest that activation of the Hh pathway promotes fibroblast migration, similar to bFGF stimulation.

3.2　Activation of Hh signaling by bFGF

Our previous data revealed that bFGF alters Hh pathway-related gene expression in fibroblasts at the transcriptional level and accelerates fibroblast migration [6]. To determine the relationship between the Hh pathway and bFGF-regulated fibroblast migration, a pharmacologic activator (SAG) and an inhibitor (Cyc) of Smo were employed. The migration rate of fibroblasts incubated with bFGF plus SAG was much higher than that of fibroblasts incubated with bFGF alone, however, the pro-migratory effect induced by bFGF was largely abolished by Cyc treatment (Fig. 2A, B).

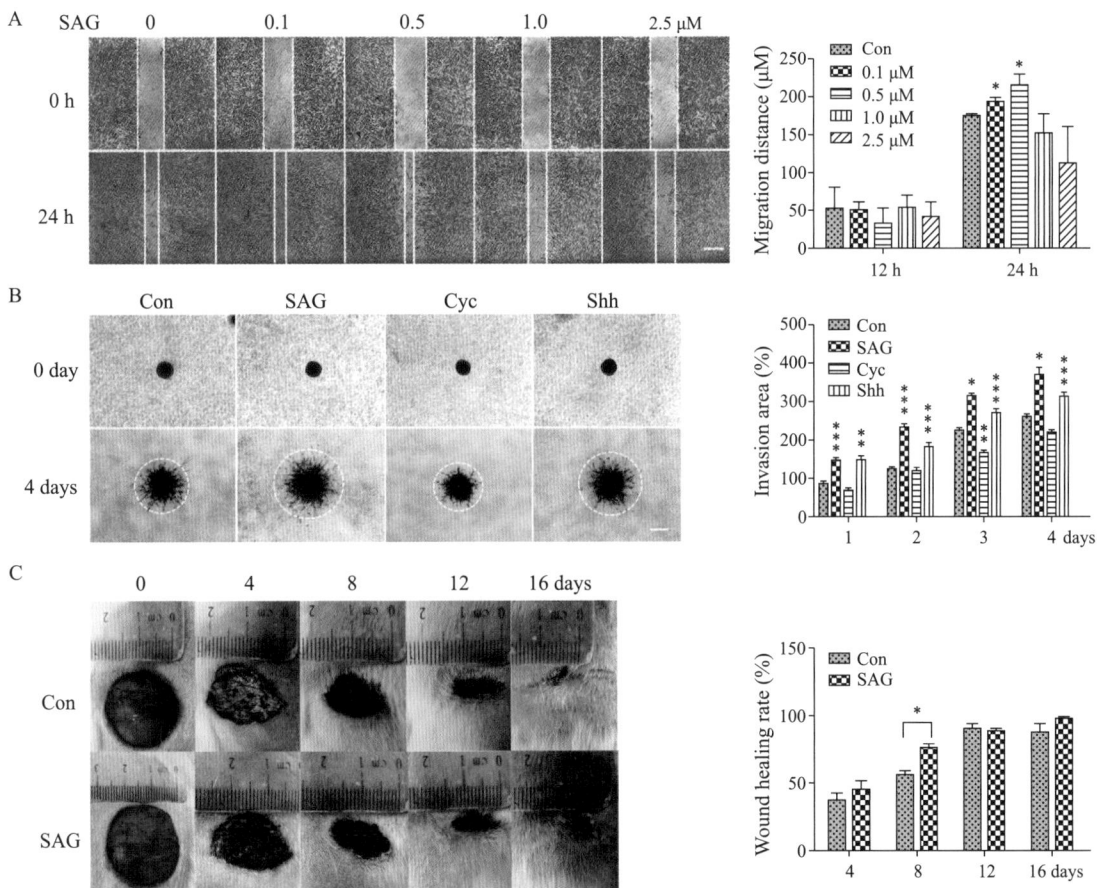

Fig. 1. Hh signaling directs primary human fibroblast migration, invasion, and wound healing. (A) A scratch wound healing assay was performed in the presence of SAG (0, 0.1, 0.5, 1.0, and 2.5 μM). Cell monolayers were imaged at 0, 12, and 24 h after wounding. White vertical lines indicate the wound area borders. Scale bar=500 μm. Cell migration distances were measured based on the data. Data represent mean values ± SE of five replicates ($^*P$ < 0.05 compared with the untreated group). (B) A 3D spheroid cell invasion assay was performed with SAG (0.5 μM), Cyc (0.5 μM), or Shh (0.1 μg/mL) treatment for 4 days. Cells invading into the surrounding matrix were photographed after 0, 1, 2, 3, and 4 days. White dashed circles indicate the borders of cell invasion areas. Bar=500 μm. The cell invasion area was measured according to the data. Data represent mean values ± SE of five replicates ($^*P$ < 0.05, $^{**}P$ < 0.01, $^{***}P$ < 0.001 compared with the control group). (C) Representative images of skin wounds from normal rats treated with or without SAG (0.5 μM). SAG (0.5 μM) was supplied every day. Data represent mean values ± SE of five independent experiments ($^*P$ < 0.05 compared with the control). Wound healing was monitored until 16 days after wounding (n=5 per group). Each rat had two wound sites (the one on the left was the control and the one on the right was treated with SAG).

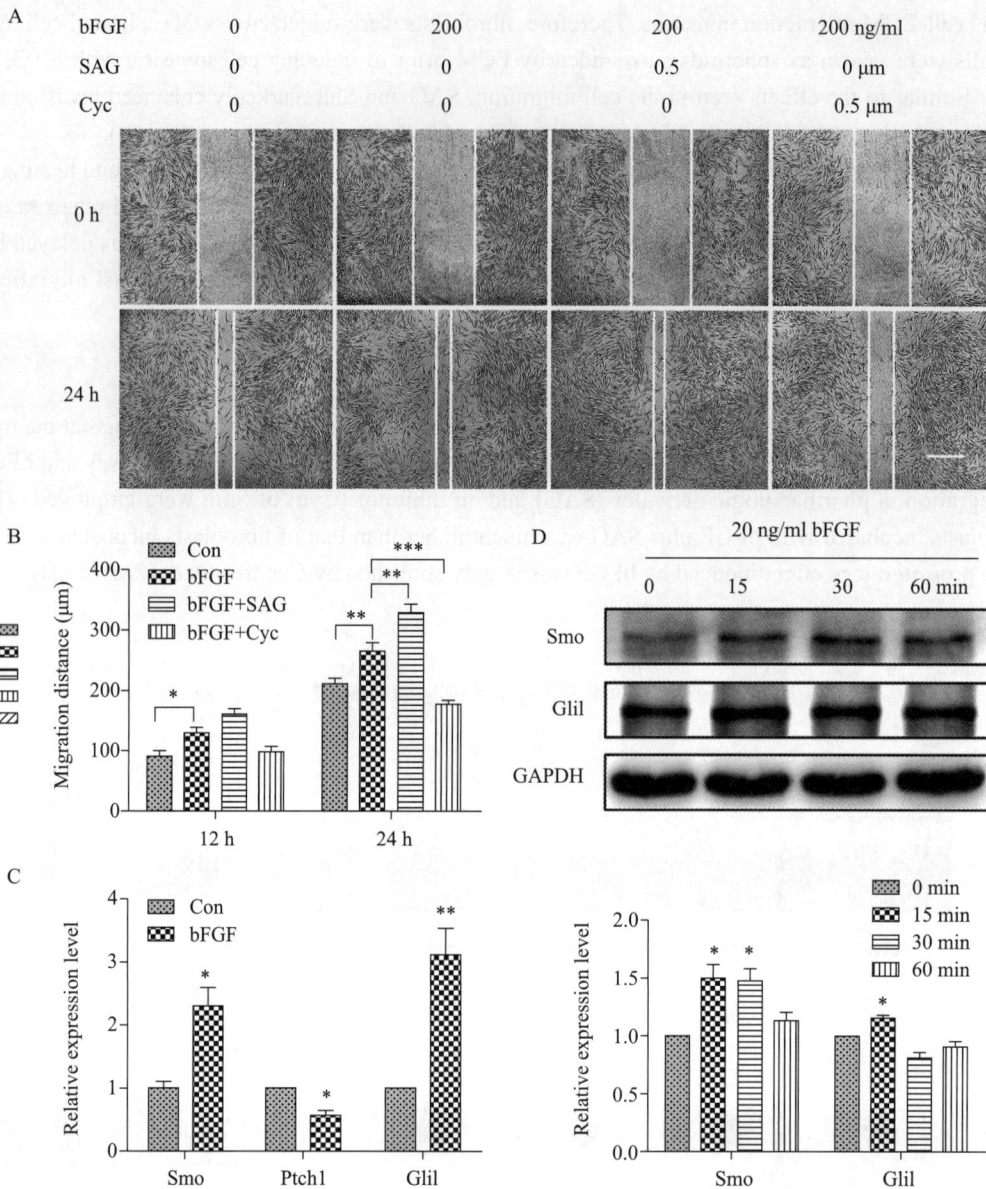

Fig. 2. Activation of Hh signaling by bFGF. (A) A scratch wound healing assay was performed in the presence of bFGF (200 ng/ml), bFGF (200 ng/ml) plus SAG (0.5 μM), and bFGF (200 ng/ml) plus Cyc (0.5 μM). Cell monolayers were imaged at 0, 12, and 24 h after wounding. White vertical lines indicate the wound area borders. Scale bar=500 μm. (B) Cell migration distances shown in (A) were measured. Data represent mean values ± SE of five replicates ($^{*}P < 0.05$, $^{**}P < 0.01$, $^{***}P < 0.001$). (C) qRT-PCR analysis was performed to monitor the mRNA levels of *Smo*, *Ptch1*, and *Gli1*. *GAPDH* was used as an internal control. All data represent mean values ± SE of five replicates ($^{*}P < 0.05$, $^{**}P < 0.01$ compared with the untreated group). (D) Protein levels of Smo and Gli1 were assessed by Western blot analysis after the fibroblasts treated with bFGF (200 ng/mL) for the indicated durations. GAPDH was used as a loading control. Densitometry data for Smo and Gli1 from the blots shown were normalized to the level of GAPDH. Data represent mean values ± SE of five replicates ($^{*}P< 0.05$ *vs.* untreated group).

To ascertain the impact of bFGF on activation of the Hh pathway, the expression of Hh signaling marker genes and proteins were evaluated. bFGF treatment altered the expression of Hh signaling genes, including *Smo*, *Gli1*, and *Ptch1* (Fig. 2C). In addition, the protein levels of Smo and Gli1 in primary human fibroblasts were also altered by bFGF (Fig. 2D). These results indicate that bFGF activates Hh signaling, and that Hh signaling mediates the pro-migratory effects of this growth factor, at least partly.

3.3 Relationship between Hh signaling and bFGF-stimulated PI3K-JNK signaling

Our previous results have showed that bFGF regulates fibroblast migration *via* the PI3K-Rac1-JNK pathway [5,6], and the Hh pathway is involved in fibroblast migration (Figs. 1 and S1). Thus, further experiments were performed to analyze the relationship between the Hh pathway and PI3K-JNK signaling cascades. PI3K facilitates AKT phosphorylation at Ser 473 [23]; therefore, the AKT phosphorylation level was used to measure the activation of PI3K. SAG (0.5 μM) treatment significantly increased the phosphorylation levels of both AKT and JNK, without affecting their protein levels (Fig. 3A). To confirm this result, cells were treated with Shh (a Hh pathway activator) and Cyc, and increased phosphorylation levels of AKT and JNK were detected by Shh treatment (Fig. 3B), but decreased by Cyc (0.5 μM) (Fig. 3C).

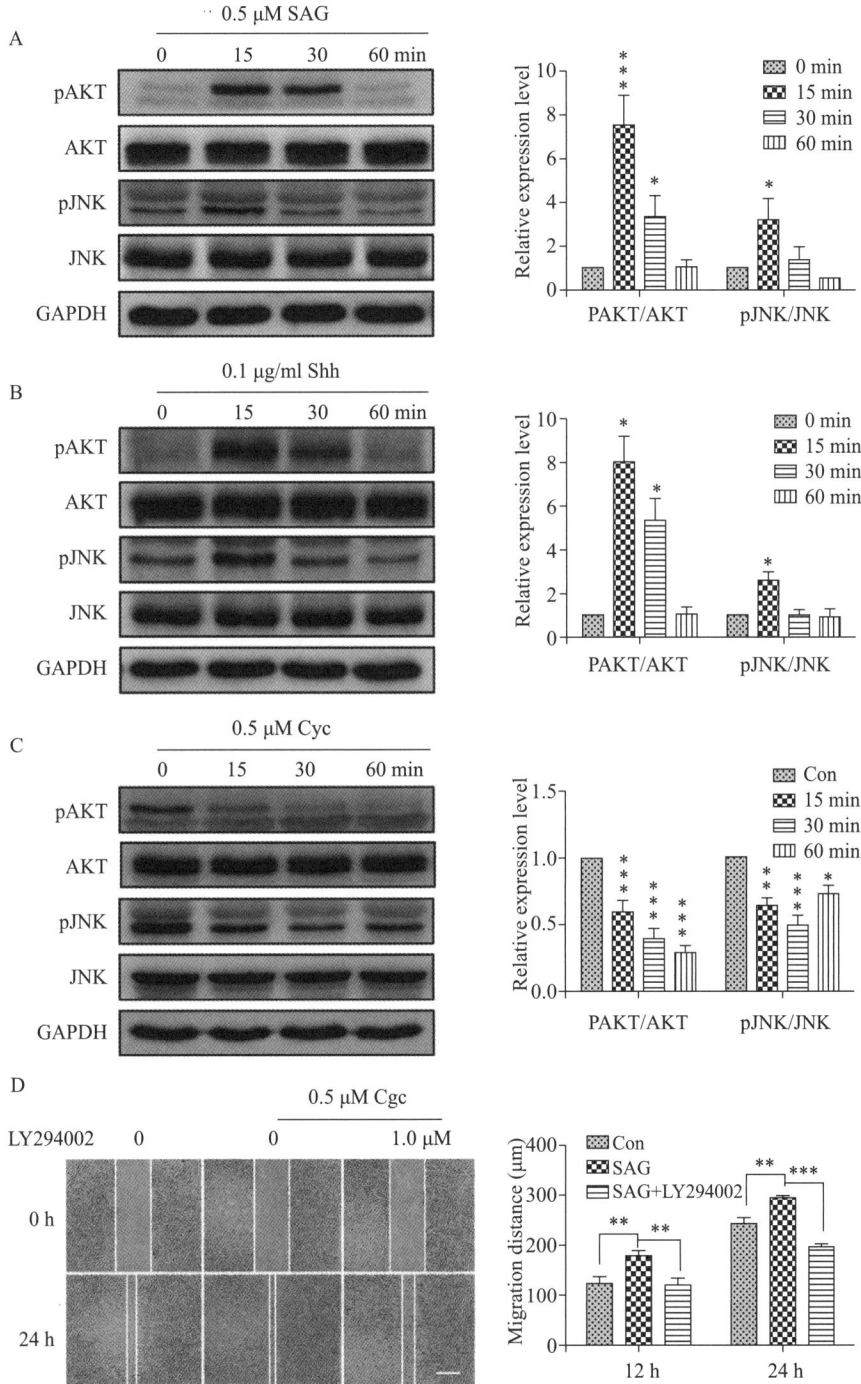

Fig. 3. The Hh pathway acts upstream of the bFGF-stimulated PI3K-JNK pathway. Primary human fibroblasts were stimulated with vehicle and (A) 0.5 μM SAG, (B) 0.1 μg/ml Shh or (C) 0.5 μM Cyc for the indicated durations, and the protein levels of pAKT, AKT, pJNK, and JNK were determined by Western blot analysis. GAPDH was used as a loading control. Densitometry data for pAKT and pJNK from the blots shown were normalized to data of AKT and JNK, respectively. The Data are given as means ± SE (n=5 replicates; $^{*}P < 0.05$, $^{**}P < 0.01$, $^{***}P < 0.001$ vs. untreated group). (D) A scratch wound healing assay was performed for fibroblasts treated with SAG (0.5 μM) or SAG plus LY294002 (1.0 μM), and cell migration distances were measured at 0, 12, and 24 h after wounding. White vertical lines indicate the borders of the wound areas. Scale bar=500 μm. The Data are given as means ± SE (n=5 replicates; $^{**}P < 0.01$, $^{***}P < 0.001$).

On the other hand, fibroblast migration in the scratch wound healing assay was blocked by LY294002, a PI3K inhibitor, even with continued SAG treatment (Fig. 3D). Also, no significant effect on fibroblast viability was observed with either LY294002 or LY294002 plus SAG treatment (Fig. S2A). And the Cyc-inhibited cell migration was aggravated by LY294002 treatment (Fig. S2B). To further confirm the effect of Smo on PI3K-JNK pathway in fibroblast migration, a JNK inhibitor (SP600125) was employed. We found that increased fibroblast migration rate induced by SAG was decreased under the condition of SP600125 (Fig. S2C).

Moreover, to verify that PI3K-JNK pathway is responsible for the SAG-promotion of fibroblast migration *in vivo*, the SD rat wound healing experiment was used to confirm the viewpoint. Wound treatment with SAG or Shh increased PI3K-JNK pathway activity relative to that of the control (Fig. S2D and S2E), while Cyc reversed this effect (Fig. S2F), indicating that Smo functions at upstream of the PI3K-JNK signaling pathway to promote fibroblast migration during wound healing.

3.4 Effects of PI3K-JNK and Smo on the GSK3β/β-catenin pathway

PI3K modulates GSK3β phosphorylation at Ser 9 [23,24], which allows β-catenin translocation into the nucleus to initiate the transcription of target genes, with subsequent regulation of a wide array of biological processes [25–29]. Therefore, we directly evaluated whether the PI3K-JNK pathway affects β-catenin translocation by treating primary human fibroblasts with SP600125. According to the result, SP600125 suppressed the accumulation of nuclear β-catenin and induced the increase of cytoplasmic β-catenin (Fig. 4A), implying that the movement of β-catenin from the cytosol into the nucleus is modulated by PI3K-JNK signaling.

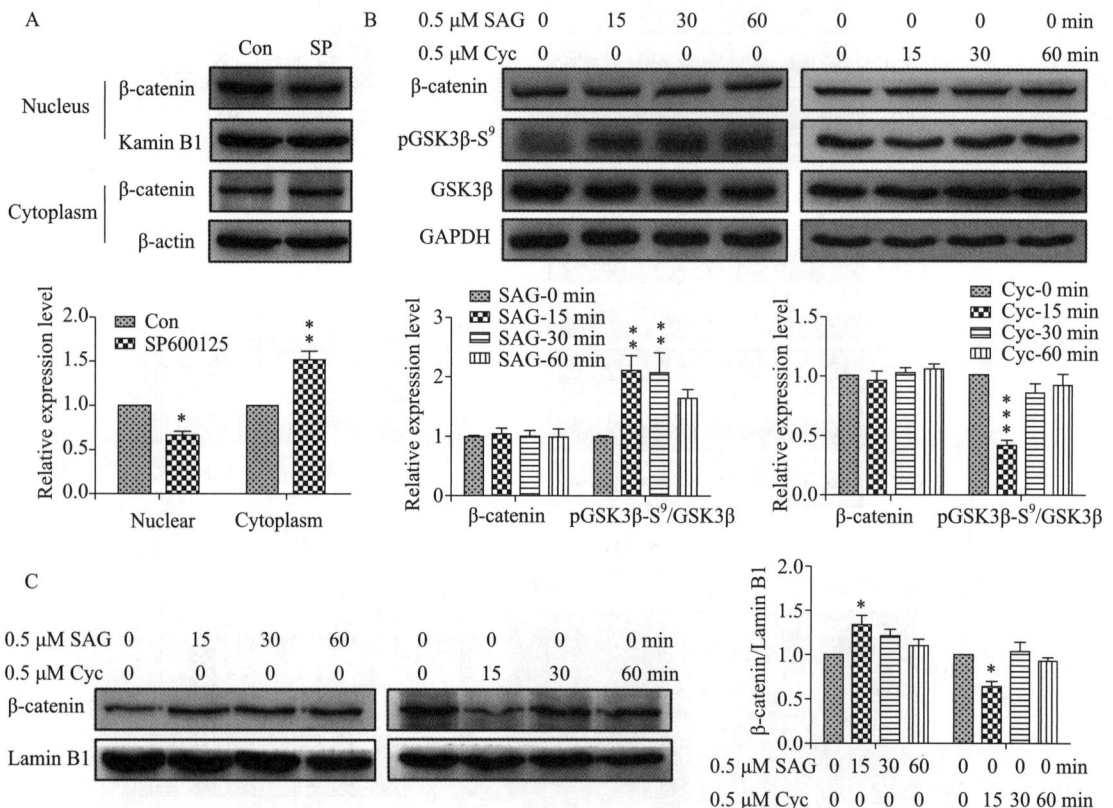

Fig. 4. Hh signaling affects the GSK3β/β-catenin pathway. (A) Nuclear and cytoplasmic β-catenin levels were measured in primary human fibroblasts treated with the JNK inhibitor SP600125 (SP). β-catenin densitometry data were normalized using Lamin B1 (Nucleus) or β-actin (Cytoplasm) densitometry data. (B) The levels of phosphorylated GSK3β at Ser 9, total GSK3β, and total (cytoplasmic plus nuclear) β-catenin were detected under SAG (0.5 μM) or Cyc (0.5 μM) treatment for 0, 15, 30, or 60 min pGSK3β-Ser9 (pGSK3β-S⁹) and β-catenin densitometry data were obtained from the blots shown and were normalized using GSK3β or GAPDH densitometry data, respectively. (C) Nuclear β-catenin levels were monitored after treatment with SAG (0.5 μM) or Cyc (0.5 μM) for 0, 15, 30 or 60 min β-catenin densitometry data were obtained from the blots shown and were normalized using Lamin B1 densitometry data. Data in (A-C) are given as fold changes and represent mean values ± SE of five independent experiments (*P < 0.05, **P < 0.01, ***P < 0.001 vs. untreated control group).

In light of these results and growing evidence indicating that Hh signaling modulates β-catenin translocation in various cell types and organs to elicit opposing or synergistic cellular effects [30], we next examined the effect of Smo stimulation or blockade on the GSK3β/β-catenin pathway. This was done by assessing whether SAG, Cyc or Shh treatment of primary human fibroblasts alters GSK3β-Ser9 phosphorylation levels and β-catenin nuclear translocation. As shown in Fig. 4B and C, pGSK3β-Ser9 and nuclear β-catenin levels were significantly higher in SAG-treated cells, while the total β-catenin level remained unchanged. Conversely, Cyc significantly decreased pGSK3β-Ser9 and nuclear β-catenin levels when total β-catenin was stable. Consistent with the effect of SAG, pGSK3β-Ser9 levels and nuclear β-catenin accumulation were also higher in fibroblasts after Shh treatment approximately 15 min, whereas total β-catenin was invariable (Fig. S3), which further confirmed that Smo positively regulates the GSK3β/ β-catenin pathway.

3.5 Role of β-catenin in fibroblast migration

Stabilization of nuclear β-catenin is a key step in the transduction of Wnt signaling, which may activate the transcription of downstream Wnt target genes [31]. We previously found that bFGF stimulation of fibroblasts modulates the expression levels of several canonical Wnt pathway genes. To further investigate whether β-catenin similarly influences the transcription of Hh pathway genes, *β-catenin*-specific siRNA was introduced to suppress *β-catenin* expression. As human primary fibroblasts remain active for a maximum of six generations, they are not suitable for the lentivirus-mediated transfection experiments described here.

Thus, RNA-sequencing analysis was performed using NIH 3T3 cells with and without siRNA-mediated *β-catenin*-specific suppression. The RNA-sequencing results showed that 127 genes were differentially expressed (at least 2.0-fold change; $P < 0.03$) in *β-catenin*-silencing NIH 3T3 cells (Table S3), namely, 54 down-regulated and 73 up-regulated genes involved in diverse biological pathways under the control of β-catenin (Fig. 5A). And the differentially expressed genesets were classified into the known signal pathway according to KEGG (Kyoto Encyclopedia of Genes and Genomes). The results revealed that six up-regulated and six down-regulated clusters (including Hh pathway) were significantly enriched by silencing of *β-catenin* (Fig. 5A). qRT-PCR analysis verified that the expression levels of Hh pathway genes (*e.g.*, *Smo*, *Gli1*, *Gli2*, *Gli3*, and *Ptch1*) were altered when *β-catenin* was suppressed (Fig. 5B). Moreover, Western blot analysis confirmed that Gli1 and Smo were significantly down-regulated in *β-catenin*-knock-down NIH 3T3 cells relative to control siRNA-transfected cells (Fig. 5C). Likewise, migration rates were also markedly decreased in β-*catenin*-knock-down cells and were partly restored by SAG treatment (Fig. 5D).

In addition, modulation of the transcription of Hh pathway genes by β-catenin was further confirmed by performing plasmid-mediated transfection experiments using Lipofectamine 2000. Notably, siRNA-mediated knock-down of *β-catenin* resulted in important alterations in the activation of well-characterized targets of the Hh pathway, including *Smo*, *Gli1*, *Gli2*, *Gli3*, and *Ptch1* (Fig. S4A), and Hh symbolic proteins, such as Smo and Gli1 (Fig. S4B). Consistently, migratory ability was attenuated by *β-catenin* silencing in NTH 3T3 cells, but was slightly restored by SAG treatment (Fig. S4C).

3.6 The function of β-catenin-regulated Gli1 expression in fibroblast migration and skin wound healing

For the expression level of Gli1 was suppressed by *β-catenin* silencing (Figs. 5B, C, S4A and S4B), Gli1 function was further analyzed by examining cell migration in the scratch wound healing assay. Firstly, GANT61, a selective antagonist of Gli1/Gli2 [32], notably delayed fibroblast migration (Fig. 6A) and inhibited Hh pathway activity (Fig. S5A), indicating that attenuation of Gli1 expression inhibits fibroblast migration. Secondly, *Gli1*-specific siRNA was transformed into NIH 3T3 cells and exhibited a dramatic reduction in migration compared with control cells (Figs. S5B and 6B). Moreover, GANT61 blocked SAG-stimulated cell migration (Fig. 6C). Lastly, to confirm whether Gli1 is a determining factor for skin wound healing and cell invasion ability, the skin closure rate in SD rats and the invasion activity in fibroblasts under GANT61 treatment were determined. The results shown in Fig. 6D and E indicate that wound closure and invasion activity were delayed by GANT61 treatment. However, GANT61 only had a negligible effect on skin closure in SD rats when it was used in combination with SAG (Fig. 6F).

In addition, to understand whether Gli1 participates in bFGF-facilitated fibroblast migration, the scratch wound healing assay was performed in the presence of both bFGF and GANT61. According to the results, fibroblast migration was delayed by GANT61, which was partly restored by bFGF (Fig. 6G).

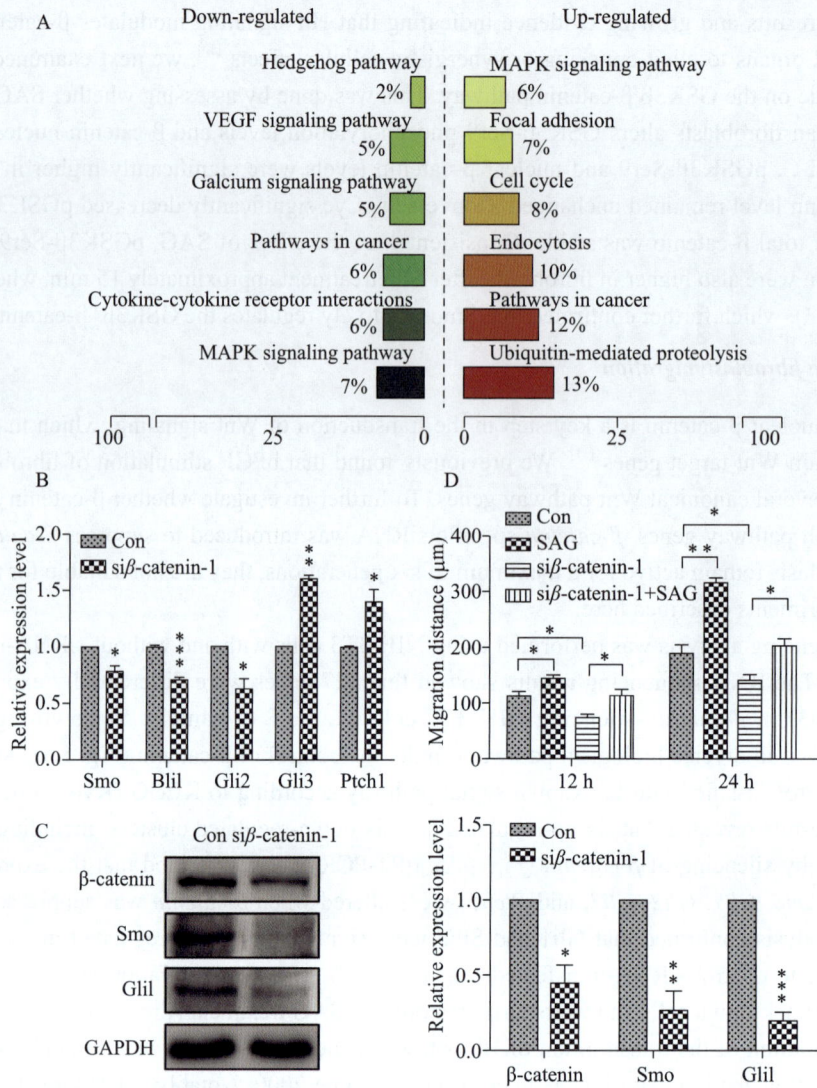

Fig. 5. β-catenin affects Hh signaling-mediated fibroblast migration. (A) RNA-sequencing analysis was performed of RNA from *β-catenin*-specific siRNA (lentivirus-mediated *β-catenin* siRNA, si*β-catenin*-1)- and control (scrambled) siRNA-transfected NIH 3T3 cells. The differentially expressed gene sets were classified into the known pathway according to KEGG (Kyoto Encyclopedia of Genes and Genomes), which revealed that six up-regulated and six down-regulated clusters were significantly enriched by silencing of *β-catenin*. (B) qRT-PCR analysis was performed to monitor the mRNA levels of *Smo*, *Gli1*, *Gli2*, *Gli3*, and *Ptch1* in lentivirus-mediated *β-catenin*-specific siRNA (si*β-catenin*-1)-transfected NIH 3T3 cells. *GAPDH* was used as an internal control. (C) Western blot analysis was performed to examine the protein levels of β-catenin, Smo, and Gli1 in control (scrambled) siRNA- and *β-catenin*- specific siRNA (si*β-catenin*-1)-transfected cells. Densitometry data for β-catenin, Smo, and Gli1 from the blots shown were normalized to data for GAPDH. (D) A scratch wound healing assay was performed with control siRNA- and *β-catenin*-specific siRNA (si*β-catenin*-1)-transfected cells with or without SAG (0.5 μM). The cell monolayers were photographed at 0, 12, and 24 h after wounding. Cell migration distances were measured. All data are given as means ± SE (n=5 replicates; $^*P < 0.05$, $^{**}P < 0.01$, $^{***}P < 0.0001$).

4. Discussion

The pro-migratory growth factor bFGF is important for skin wound repair and is employed in various experimental and clinical models of skin wound healing. However, its underlying mechanism remains unclear. Our previous work showed that bFGF stimulation modifies the expression levels of Hh signaling genes in fibroblasts. Markedly, the Hh pathway exerts mitogenic and morphogenic functions during development [33], modulates adult tissue homeostasis and repair, and facilitates cancer cell migration [33,34]. Recently, Yan *et al.* showed that human gastric cancer cells require active Hh signaling for survival, proliferation, and migration [34]. Similarly, we found that treatment of primary human fibroblasts with a Smo agonist (SAG and Shh) and antagonist (Cyc) promoted and inhibited, respectively, cell migration, invasion, and skin wound healing (Fig. 1, S1A–S1E, and S1H–S1I). Also, the migratory ability of *Smo*-silenced

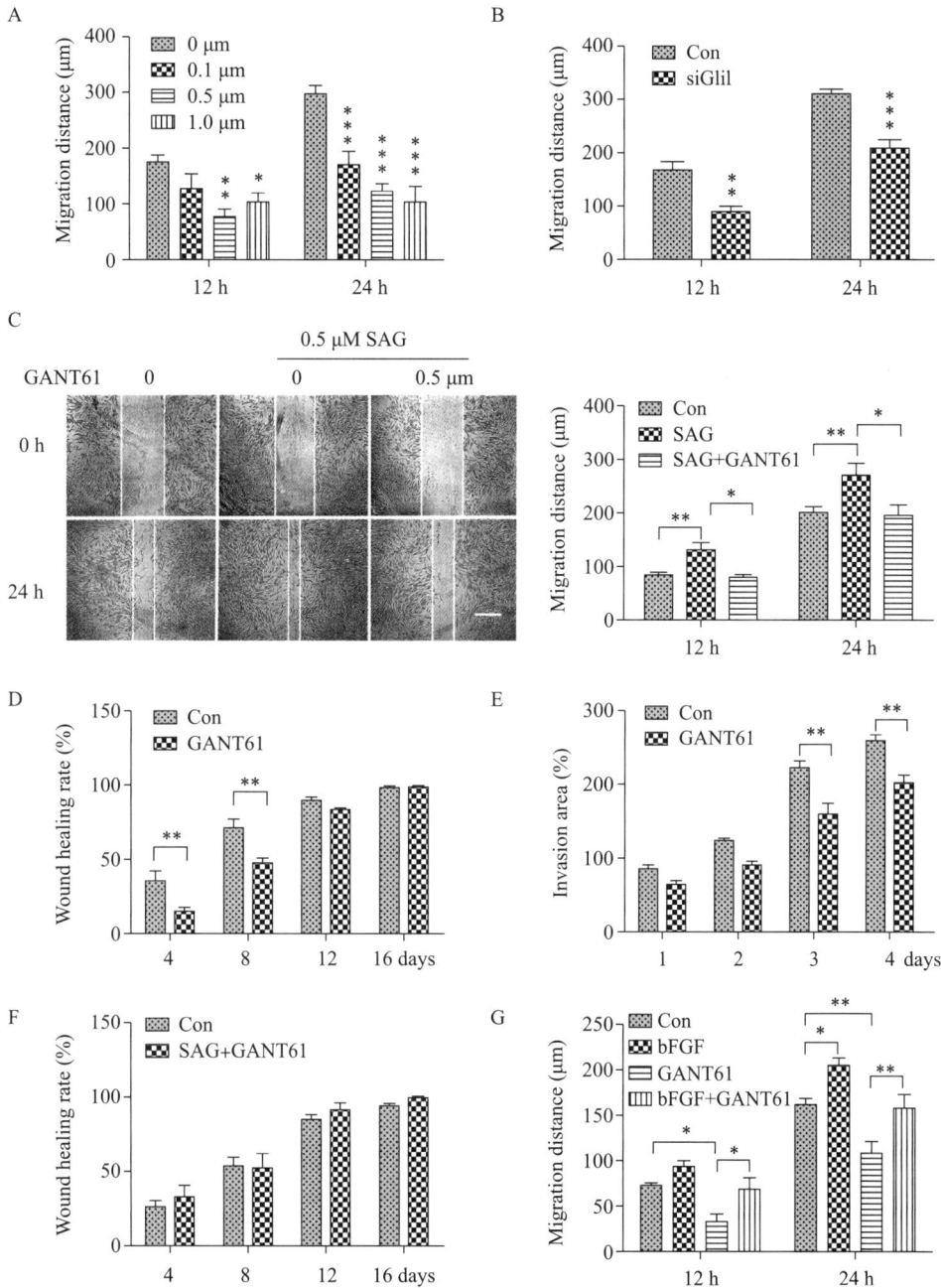

Fig. 6. Gli1 modulates bFGF-stimulated ftbroblast migration, invasion, and wound healing. (A, C, G) A scratch wound healing assay was per-formed with primary human fibroblasts in the presence of (A) GANT61 (0, 0.1, 0.5, and 1.0 μM), (C) SAG (0.5 μM) or SAG plus GANT61 (0.5 μM), or (G) bFGF (200 ng/mL), GANT61 (0.5 μM), or bFGF plus GANT61. The cell monolayers were photographed at 0, 12, and 24 h after wounding. Cell migration distances were measured. The data are given as means ± SE (*n*=5 replicates; $^*P< 0.05$, $^{**}P < 0.01$, $^{***}P < 0.001$). (B) A scratch wound healing assay was performed with control siRNA- and *Gli1*-specific siRNA-transfected cells. The cell monolayers were pho-tographed at 0, 12, and 24 h after wounding. All data are given as means ± SE (*n*=5 replicates; $^{**}P < 0.01$, $^{***}P < 0.001$ *vs.* the control). (D, F) The skin wounds of normal rats treated with or without (D) GANT61 (0.5 μM) or (F) GANT61 (0.5 μM) plus SAG (0.5 μM). Wound healing was monitored up to 16 days after wounding. Wound areas of each rat were measured using Prism 5 software (GraphPad, San Diego, CA). Data represent mean values ± SE of five independent experiments (3-month-old male rats; *n*=5 animals/group; $^{**}P < 0.01$ *vs.* the control). (E) A 3D spheroid cell invasion assay was performed with GANT61 (0.5 μM) treatment for 4 days. Cells invading into the surrounding matrix were photo-graphed after 0, 1, 2, 3, and 4 days. White dashed circles indicate the borders of cell invasion areas. Bar=500 μm. Cell invasion area was measured according to the data. Data represent mean values ± SE of five replicates ($^{**}P <0.01$ compared with the control group).

NIH 3T3 cells was impaired (Fig. S1F–G), indicating the involvement of Hh signaling. Furthermore, SAG and Shh increased the levels of phosphorylated AKT and JNK both *in vitro* and *in vivo*, but contrary to those of Cyc. And the PI3K inhibitor, LY294002, reversed SAG-promoted fibroblast migration, as well as JNK inhibitor, SP600125 (Figs. 3 and S2). Thus, Smo functions at upstream of the bFGF-regulated PI3K-JNK pathway to expedite fibroblast migration.

Interestingly, the data herein established that SP600125 suppressed the translocation of cytoplasmic β-catenin into nucleus in fibroblasts relative to those untreated controls (Fig. 4A). Moreover, SAG-and Shh-facilitated agonism of Smo increased GSK3β phosphorylation at Ser 9 and β-catenin translocation into the nucleus, while Cyc-facilitated antagonism of Smo had the opposite effect on GSK3β (Ser9) phosphorylation and β-catenin nuclear accumulation (Figs. 4B, C and S3). Additionally, migration rates were significantly lower in SAG-treated, *β-catenin*-specific siRNA-transfected NIH 3T3 cells than in SAG-treated cells (Figs. 5D and S4C). In conclusion, these results suggest that Smo contributes to nuclear β-catenin accumulation *via* PI3K-JNK signaling and then promotes cell migration.

It should be noted that, besides its potential anti-migratory role in the fibroblasts with a pathogenesis based on such "Hh signaling" herein reported (Fig. 1), Cyc also delayed cell migration in the presence of bFGF (Fig. 2A, B), indicating that bFGF acts upstream of Smo to accelerate cell migration. Consistently, bFGF significantly increased the levels of Hh target genes both at the transcriptional and protein levels (Fig. 2C, D). However, the expression levels of these genes were reduced when the endogenous β-catenin level was suppressed (Figs. 5B, C and S4A, B). Correspondingly, the inhibition of β-*catenin*-mediated Gli1 expression with the selective Gli1/Gli2 inhibitor GANT61 or by *Gli1*-specific siRNA had an inhibitory effect on fibroblast migration, invasion activity, as well as wound healing (Fig. 6A, B, D, E). These findings suggest that Gli1 functions downstream of bFGF/β-catenin and that β-catenin is a key regulator of fibroblast migration.

With regard to β-catenin as a transcription factor, we performed RNA-sequencing analysis of *β-catenin*-knock-down NIH 3T3 cells to determine whether Hh signaling genes are under the control of β-catenin (Fig. 5A). When β-catenin expression was down-regulated, *Smo*, *Gli1*, and *Gli2* levels were all decreased, while *Gli3* and *Ptch1* levels were increased (Figs. 5B and S4A). These observations are consistent with those of an earlier report showing that Smo, Gli1, and Gli2 are positive regulators of Hh pathway gene transcription, while Gli3 and Ptch1 are negative regulators [34]. Furthermore, exposure of fibroblasts to SAG increased the nuclear accumulation of β-catenin (Fig. 4B, C), but, as noted above, a reduction in the level of endogenous β-catenin down-regulated the expression of both Smo and Gli1 (Figs. 5C and S4B). Moreover, Cyc and GANT61, inhibitors of Smo and Gli1, respectively, retarded cell migration, and bFGF rescued the delayed cell migration induced by the inhibition of Gli1 (Figs. S1B and 6G). Moreover, SAG-induced fibroblast migration and -accelerated wound healing were abolished by treatment with GANT61 (Fig. 6C and F). Therefore, a regulatory loop involving Smo, β-catenin, and Gli1 may, when activated, facilitate fibroblast migration.

Lastly, we identified several up-and down-regulated pathways under the control of β-catenin in NIH 3T3 cells, including VEGF signaling and mitogen-activated protein kinase (MAPK) pathways (Fig. 5A). Ample evidence demonstrates that MAPK regulates mesangial cell proliferation and migration [35], while VEGF signaling directs endothelial cell migration [36–38], probably through AKT-mediated phosphorylation of endothelial nitric oxide synthase [38]. Thus, β-catenin may direct fibroblast migration *via* modulation of diverse signaling events encompassing the MAPK, VEGF, Wnt, and Hh pathways. Therefore, further studies will be required to unravel the mechanisms underlying the interactions between these different pathways. Besides, it should be noted that the promotion effect of Hh pathway on tissue regeneration and skin wound healing was not only attribute to the pro-migratory aspects, but also to the proliferation function [39]. Thus, the relationship between cell proliferation and wound healing bridged by Hh pathway is still needed to thoroughly investigate.

Based on the present results and previous work, our experimental findings support the following conclusions: (1) the Hh pathway participates in bFGF-mediated fibroblast migration; (2) Smo facilitates β-catenin translocation into the nucleus to increase migration rates; (3) Gli1 positively regulates fibroblast migration; and (4) β-catenin, acting downstream of bFGF signaling, plays a feedback role in fibroblast migration by modulating the expression of *Smo* and *Gli1*. Taken together, our observations provide evidence for a new regulatory mechanism for bFGF-mediated cell migration (Fig. 7), and may contribute to the identification of novel therapeutic targets for wound repair.

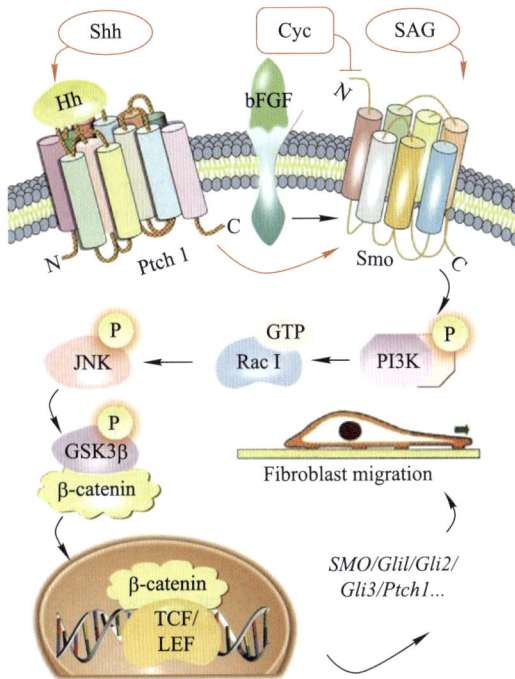

Fig. 7. A working model illustrating the role of the Hh pathway in bFGF-regulated fibroblast migration. A working model depicting how the Hh pathway participates in bFGF pro-migratory action is shown. The Hh ligand binds to Ptch1, helping to stimulate Smo. Activation of the Hh pathway is symbolized by Smo stimulation. Shh, SAG, and Cyc are pharmacological molecules targeting Hh or Smo to activate or inhibit the Hh pathway. Smo stimulated by bFGF activates the PI3K-Rac1-JNK pathway and then facilitates β-catenin translocation into the nucleus. Accumulation of nuclear β-catenin accelerates fibroblast migration by modulating the expression of Hh pathway-related genes, including *Smo*, *Gli1*, *Gli2*, *Gli3*, and *Ptch1*.

5. Conclusion

Our findings provide evidence that Hh signaling contributes to fibroblast migration *via* bFGF and that β-catenin, downstream of bFGF signaling, plays a feedback role in fibroblast migration by modulating the expression of *Smo* and *Gli1*.

Supporting information

Supplementary data associated this article can be found in the online version at doi:10.1016/j.yexcr.2017.03.054.

References

[1] McMahon AP, Ingham PW, Tabin CJ. Developmental roles and clinical significance of hedgehog signaling[A]. In: *Current Topics In Developmental Biology, Vol 53* (Schatten GP, ed), Vol. 53, 2003: 1-114.

[2] Pazyar N, Yaghoobi R, Rafiee E, *et al.* Skin Wound Healing and Phytomedicine: A Review[J]. Skin Pharmacology And Physiology, 2014, 27(6): 303-310.

[3] Wagner W, Wehrmann M. Differential cytokine activity and morphology during wound healing in the neonatal and adult rat skin[J]. Journal Of Cellular And Molecular Medicine, 2007, 11(6): 1342-1351.

[4] Broughton IG, Janis JE. Wound healing: an overview, Plast. econstr. [J]. Surg., 2006, 117: 1e-S-32e-S.

[5] Kanazawa S, Fujiwara T, Matsuzaki S, *et al.* bFGF Regulates PI3-Kinase-Rac1-JNK Pathway and Promotes Fibroblast Migration in Wound Healing[J]. Plos One, 2010, 5(8).

[6] Xuan YH, Bin Huang B, Tian HS, *et al.* High-Glucose Inhibits Human Fibroblast Cell Migration in Wound Healing *via* Repression of bFGF-Regulating JNK Phosphorylation[J]. Plos One, 2014, 9(9).

[7] Dvorak P, Hampl A. Basic fibroblast growth factor and its receptors in human embryonic stem cells[J]. Folia Histochemica Et Cytobiologica, 2005, 43(4): 203-208.

[8] Bushman W. *Hedgehog signaling in development and cancer*, 2007.

[9] Taipale J, Beachy PA. The Hedgehog and Wnt signaling pathways in cancer[J]. Nature, 2001, 411(6835): 349-354.

[10] Beauchamp EM, Ringer L, Bulut G, *et al.* Arsenic trioxide inhibits human cancer cell growth and tumor development in mice by blocking Hedgehog/GLI pathway[J]. Journal Of Clinical Investigation, 2011, 121(1): 148-160.

[11] Wang K, Pan L, Che X, *et al.* Sonic Hedgehog/GLI1 signaling pathway inhibition restricts cell migration and invasion in human gliomas[J]. Neurological Research, 2010, 32(9): 975-980.

[12] Huangfu D, Anderson KV. Signaling from Smo to Ci/Gli: conservation and divergence of Hedgehog pathways from Drosophila to vertebrates[J]. Development, 2006, 133(1): 3-14.

[13] Rohatgi R, Milenkovic L, Scott MP. Patched1 regulates Hedgehog signaling at the primary cilium[J]. Science, 2007, 317(5836): 372-376.

[14] Inaguma S, Kasai K, Ikeda H. GLI1 facilitates the migration and invasion of pancreatic cancer cells through MUC5AC-mediated attenuation of E-cadherin[J]. Oncogene, 2011, 30(6): 714-723.

[15] Fu J-R, Liu W-L, Zhou J-F, et al. Sonic hedgehog protein promotes bone marrow-derived endothelial progenitor cell proliferation, migration and VEGF production via PI 3-kinase/Akt signaling pathways[J]. Acta Pharmacologica Sinica, 2006, 27(6): 685-693.

[16] Chen J-S, Huang X-h, Wang Q, et al. Sonic hedgehog signaling pathway induces cell migration and invasion through focal adhesion kinase/AKT signaling-mediated activation of matrix metalloproteinase (MMP)-2 and MMP-9 in liver cancer[J]. Carcinogenesis, 2013, 34(1): 10-19.

[17] Yang Y, Xia T, Zhi W, et al. Promotion of skin regeneration in diabetic rats by electrospun core-sheath fibers loaded with basic fibroblast growth factor[J]. Biomaterials, 2011, 32(18): 4243-4254.

[18] Ma J, Cheng J, Gong Y, et al. Downregulation of Wnt signaling by sonic hedgehog activation promotes repopulation of human tumor cell lines[J]. Disease Models & Mechanisms, 2015, 8(4): 385-391.

[19] Singh R, Bhasin S, Braga M, et al. Regulation of Myogenic Differentiation by Androgens: Cross Talk between Androgen Receptor/beta-Catenin and Follistatin/Transforming Growth Factor-beta Signaling Pathways[J]. Endocrinology, 2009, 150(3): 1259-1268.

[20] Zittermann SI, Issekutz AC. Basic fibroblast growth factor (bFGF, FGF-2) potentiates leukocyte recruitment to inflammation by enhancing endothelial adhesion molecule expression[J]. American Journal Of Pathology, 2006, 168(3): 835-846.

[21] Diegelmann RF, Evans MC. Wound healing: An overview of acute, fibrotic and delayed healing[J]. Frontiers In Bioscience-Landmark, 2004, 9: 283-289.

[22] Miron-Mendoza M, Seemann J, Grinnell F. Collagen fibril flow and tissue translocation coupled to fibroblast migration in 3D collagen matrices[J]. Molecular Biology Of the Cell, 2008, 19(5): 2051-2058.

[23] Engelman JA, Luo J, Cantley LC. The evolution of phosphatidylinositol 3-kinases as regulators of growth and metabolism[J]. Nature Reviews Genetics, 2006, 7(8): 606-619.

[24] Cohen P, Frame S. The renaissance of GSK3[J]. Nature Reviews Molecular Cell Biology, 2001, 2(10): 769-776.

[25] Moon RT, Kohn AD, De Ferrari GV, et al. WNT and beta-catenin signalling: Diseases and therapies[J]. Nature Reviews Genetics, 2004, 5(9): 689-699.

[26] Clevers H. Wnt/β-catenin signaling in development and disease[J]. Cell, 2006, 127(3): 469-480.

[27] Brack AS, Conboy MJ, Roy S, et al. Increased Wnt signaling during aging alters muscle stem cell fate and increases fibrosis[J]. Science, 2007, 317(5839): 807-810.

[28] Aberle H, Bauer A, Stappert J, et al. beta-catenin is a target for the ubiquitin-proteasome pathway[J]. Embo Journal, 1997, 16(13): 3797-3804.

[29] Gordon MD, Nusse R. Wnt signaling: Multiple pathways, multiple receptors, and multiple transcription factors[J]. Journal Of Biological Chemistry, 2006, 281(32): 22429-22433.

[30] Zinke J, Schneider FT, Harter PN, et al. beta-Catenin-Gli1 interaction regulates proliferation and tumor growth in medulloblastoma[J]. Molecular Cancer, 2015, 14.

[31] Salic A, Lee E, Mayer L, et al. Control of beta-catenin stability: Reconstitution of the cytoplasmic steps of the wnt pathway in Xenopus egg extracts[J]. Molecular Cell, 2000, 5(3): 523-532.

[32] Kern D, Regl G, Hofbauer SW, et al. Hedgehog/GLI and PI3K signaling in the initiation and maintenance of chronic lymphocytic leukemia[J]. Oncogene, 2015, 34(42): 5341-5351.

[33] Petrova R, Joyner AL. Roles for Hedgehog signaling in adult organ homeostasis and repair[J]. Development, 2014, 141(18): 3445-3457.

[34] Yan R, Peng X, Yuan X, et al. Suppression of growth and migration by blocking the hedgehog signaling pathway in gastric cancer cells[J]. Cellular Oncology, 2013, 36(5): 421-435.

[35] Choudhury GG, Karamitsos C, Hernandez J, et al. PI-3-kinase and MAPK regulate mesangial cell proliferation and migration in response to PDGF[J]. American Journal Of Physiology-Renal Physiology, 1997, 273(6): F931-F938.

[36] Barleon B, Sozzani S, Zhou D, et al. Migration of human monocytes in response to vascular endothelial growth factor (VEGF) is mediated via the VEGF receptor flt-1[J]. Blood, 1996, 87(8): 3336-3343.

[37] Cleaver O, Krieg PA. VEGF mediates angioblast migration during development of the dorsal aorta in Xenopus[J]. Development, 1998, 125(19): 3905-3914.

[38] Dimmeler S, Dernbach E, Zeiher AM. Phosphorylation of the endothelial nitric oxide synthase at Ser-1177 is required for VEGF-induced endothelial cell migration[J]. Febs Letters, 2000, 477(3): 258-262.

[39] Wang Y, Lu P, Zhao D, et al. Targeting the hedgehog signaling pathway for cardiac repair and regeneration[J]. Herz, 2016, 42(7): 662-668.

Fibroblast growth factor 18 promotes proliferation and migration of H460 cells *via* the ERK and p38 signaling pathways

Taotao Chen, Xiaokun Li, Chao Jiang

1. Introduction

Lung cancer is the leading cause of cancer-associated mortality in the United States, with 157,000 cases of lung cancer-associated mortality in 2010 and 160,000 people in 2013, accounting for 26% and 28% of all female and male cancer-associated deaths, respectively [1,2]. Lung cancer is classified into two main histological types: Non-small cell lung cancer (NSCLC) and small cell lung cancer (SCLC), accounting for 87% and 13% of all lung cancer cases, respectively [3]. The predominant histological subtypes of NSCLC are adenocarcinoma (50%–60%), squamous cell carcinoma (30%–35%) and large-cell carcinoma (5%–10%) [4]. At present despite improvements in the diagnosis and treatment of lung cancer, factors such as postoperative recurrence and metastatic infiltration mean the prognosis of patients with lung cancer is still poor. However, the precise mechanisms of cancer recurrence and metastasis remain unclear.

The family of fibroblastic growth factors (FGF) has 23 identified members, which bind with 4 FGF receptor (FGFR) ligands, consisting of an extracellular portion, a transmembrane region and an intracellular domain. FGF family members are involved in cell growth, differentiation, morphogenesis, tissue repair, inflammation, angiogenesis, tumor growth and numerous developmental processes including embryonic and skeletal development [5-9]. As such, the role of the FGF family has been widely studied during tumor growth and metastasis and has been shown to increase the proliferation, motility and invasiveness of a range of cell types [10,11]. FGF18 has been demonstrated to serve an important role in skeletal growth and limb development, potentially through the modulation of osteoblasts, chondrocytes, and osteoclasts [12,13]. Furthermore, FGF18 expression was upregulated in colon cancer and ovarian cancer, and increased expression of FGF18 mRNA and protein is associated with tumor progression and poor overall survival in patients [14-16].

Mitogen activated protein kinase (MAPK) is an intra-cellular signaling pathway, with physiological functions including cell proliferation, apoptosis and differentiation. The extracellular signal-regulated kinase (ERK) signaling pathway, which is one of the MAPKs, plays the role of prolifration, migration, differentiation [17]. FGF activated FGFRs then activate a number of downstream signaling pathways, including ERK and p38, phospholipase Cγ, protein kinase C and phosphatidylinositol 3-kinase [11,17,18]. The majority of these signaling pathways are involved in the growth and metastasis of cancer cells. In the present study, we aimed to investigate the effect of FGF18 and short interfering RNA (siRNA)-FGF18 on the proliferation and migration of NSCLC cells, in addition to the underlying mechanisms.

2. Materials and methods

2.1 Cell culture

The H460 human NSCLC line was obtained from Chemical Biology Research Center (Wenzhou Medical University, Wenzhou, China). The cells were cultured in Roswell Park Memorial Institute (RPMI)-1640 medium (Gibco; Thermo Fisher Scientific, Inc., Waltham, MA, USA) containing 10% fetal bovine serum (Gibco; Thermo Fisher Scientific, Inc.), and 1% antibiotic-antimycotic (Gibco) at 37℃ and 10% CO_2.

2.2 Cell proliferation assay

A 3-(4,5-dimethylthiazol-2-yl)-2, 5-diphenyltetrazolium bromide (MTT) assay (Beyotime Institute of Biotechnology, Haimen, China) was used to determine the proliferation of H460 cells. The cells (4,000 cells/well) were seeded and cultured for 24 h in 96-well plates, and serum-free medium was added for 4 h, following which cells were stimulated with (0, 5, 10, 50, 100 and 200 ng/ml rhFGF18 (Bioreactor, Wenzhou, China) (19), 5 μmol ERK inhibitor (FR180204, Sigma-Aldrich), 5 μmol p38 inhibitor (SB203580, Sigma-Aldrich) and further incubated for 0, 24, 48 and 72 h. Subsequently, 20 μl of 5 mg/ml MTT (BioSharp, Hefei, China) was added to each well, the plate was incubated for 4 h and the absorbance at 490 nm (SpectraMax M2, Molecular Devices, Sunnyvale, CA, USA) was subsequently detected. In each group, three wells were measured for cell proliferation; the data are shown as the mean ± standard deviation (SD).

2.3 Cell cycle analysis

Cell cycle distribution was analyzed by propidium iodide (PI; BD Bioscience, San jose, CA, USA) staining and flow cytometry. The H460 cells (20,000 cells/well) were seeded in 6-well plates and exposed to (0, 5, 10 and 50 ng/ml) FGF18 for 48 h. The cells were then harvested, fixed with 70% ice-cold ethanol, and stored at -20℃ until analysis. After fixation, the cells were washed twice with cold phosphate-buffered saline (PBS) and centrifuged, following which the supernatants were removed. The pellet was resuspended and stained with PBS containing 50 mg/ml PI and 100 mg/ml RNaseA for 20 min in the dark. The DNA content was analyzed by flow cytometry using a FACSCalibur instrument and CellQuest software (BD Bioscience). The cell cycle data were analyzed using FlowJo 7.6 software, version (FlowJo, LLC, Ashland, OR, USA) and the data are shown as the mean ± SD.

2.4 Would healing assay

H460 cells were seeded into 6-well plates and were cultured at 37℃ until they reached 100% confluence. The monolayers were scratched with a pipette tip and cultured under normal conditions or (0, 5, 10 and 50 ng/ml) FGF18 after the cell fragments were removed by washing with PBS. Images (Olympus IX51, magnification: ×40, Olympus Corporation, Tokyo, Japan) were captured at 0, 24, 48 and 72 h, and the data are shown as the migration distance between the two edges. The migration distance was assessed using ToupView software. The data are shown as the mean ± SD.

2.5 Cell transfection

Chemically synthesized FGF18 siRNA (Guangzhou Ribobio Co., Ltd., Guangzhou, China) were used for transfection. To make the transfection mixture, riboFECT™ CP buffer and siRNA were first prepared in 1.5 ml micro-centrifuge tubes. Subsequently, they were mixed with riboFECT CP reagent and allowed to incubate at room temperature for 15 min. Cells in 6-well plates were washed with PBS twice and the transfection mixture was added to the cells. The plates were gently rocked following which the medium was added to the cells. Subsequently, the H460 cells were transfected with FGF18 siRNA for 48 h.

2.6 Reverse transcription-quantitative polymerase chain reaction (RT-qPCR)

Total RNA was isolated from the cells using a TRIzol plus kit (Takara Bio, Inc., Otsu, Japan) according to the manufacturer's protocol. RNA was reverse transcribed using PrimeScript™ RT Master Mix (Takara Bio, Inc.) according to the manufacturer's instructions. The PCR amplifications were performed for 40 cycles of 94℃ for 30 sec, 60℃ for 30 sec, and 72℃ for 30 sec, using a Applied CFX96™ Real-Time PCR (Bio-Rad Laboratories, Inc., Hercules, CA, USA) with 1.0 μl of cDNA and SYBR Green Real-time PCR Master Mix (Takara Bio, Inc.). Data were collected and analyzed by Bio-Rad CFX Manager software. The expression level of each sample was internally normalized against that of the glyceraldehyde 3-phosphate dehydrogenase (GAPDH). The relative quantitative value was calculated using the $2^{-\Delta\Delta Ct}$ method [20]. Each experiment was performed in triplicate. The primers used in real-time PCR were as follow: Matrix metalloproteinase 26 (MMP26), forward 5′-GGCCAGGTGGTAT CTTAGGC-3′ and reverse 5′-AGCT-GACCAGTGTTCATT CTTG-3′; FGF18 forward sequence 5′-GGACATGTGCAG GCTGGGCTA-3′ and reverse 5′-GTAGAATTCCGTCTC CTTG CCCTT-3′; and GAPDH forward 5′-ACAACAGCCT CAAGATCATCAG-3′ and reverse 5′-GGTCCACCACTGACACGTTG-3′. The primers were designed and chemically synthesized in Genewiz, Inc. (South Plainfield, NJ, USA).

2.7 Western blotting

Cell samples were digested in lysis buffer (Beyotime Institute of Biotechnology), and the protein concentrations were measured using the bicinchoninic acid protein assay kit (Beyotime Institute of Biotechnology). Total protein (40 μg) was resolved by 12% odium dodecyl sulfate-polyacrylamide gel electrophoresis and transferred onto 0.22 μm polyvi- nylidene fluoride membranes and probed with the following primary antibodies, overnight at −4℃: Anti-human FGF18 and anti-MMP26 (Abcam, Cambridge, MA, USA), anti-phosphorylated (p)-ERK1/2, anti-ERK1/2, anti-p-p38, anti-p38 and anti-β-actin (Cell Signaling Technology, Inc., Danvers, MA, USA). Following three washes, the membranes were incubated with horseradish peroxidase conjugated anti-rabbit IgG secondary antibodies (Santa Cruz Biotechnology, Inc., Dallas, TX, USA) for 1 h at room temperature. The detection of specific proteins was carried out using an enhanced chemiluminscence western blotting kit (Santa Cruz Biotechnology, Inc.).

2.8　Statistical analysis

For each experiment, three independent replicates were performed. All data are expressed as the mean ± SD. Statis- tical evaluation was conducted using Student's test. The intergroup differences were compared using one-way analysis of variance followed by Dunnett's test.

$P<0.05$ was considered to indicate a statistically significant difference. $^*P<0.05$, $^{**}P<0.01$, and $^{***}P<0.001$ vs. control.

3.　Results

3.1　FGF18 promotes the proliferation of H460 cells

A cell proliferation assay was used to investigate the effect of FGF18 on H460 cells. Cells were treated with 0, 5, 10, 50, 100 and 200 ng/ml of FGF18 for 0, 24, 48 or 72 h. As shown in Fig. 1, stimulation with FGF18 significantly in- creased H460 cell proliferation in a time and concentration-dependent manner. At concentrations of 5, 10 and 50 ng/ml, FGF18 had a remarkable effect on H460 cell proliferation. When time reached 72 h, however, FGF18 was unable to affect the growth as a consequence of the too long culture. The results suggest that FGF18 has a role in promoting the proliferation of lung cancer cells.

3.2　FGF18 promotes cell cycle progression

Different concentrations of FGF18 promoted proliferation of H460 cells, indicating that FGF18 may alter cell cy- cle-related events in H460 cells. Therefore, the effects of FGF18 on cell cycle kinetics were investigated to understand how FGF18 may regulate the cell cycle. As shown in Fig. 2A–E, stimulation with FGF18 increased the proportion of cells in the G0/G1 phase and reduced the proportion of cells in the S or G2/M phases compared with untreated H460 cells. These results suggest that the FGF18-mediated increase in H460 cell proliferation occurred via increasing the pro- portion of cells in G0/G1 phase and S phase.

3.3　FGF18 promotes the migration of H460 cells and modulates the migration-related factor

A wound healing assay was used to investigate the effects of FGF18 on cell migration. Following treatment with 5, 10 and 50 ng/ml FGF18 for 24, 48 or 72 h, the migration distance was increased in H460 cells compared with the

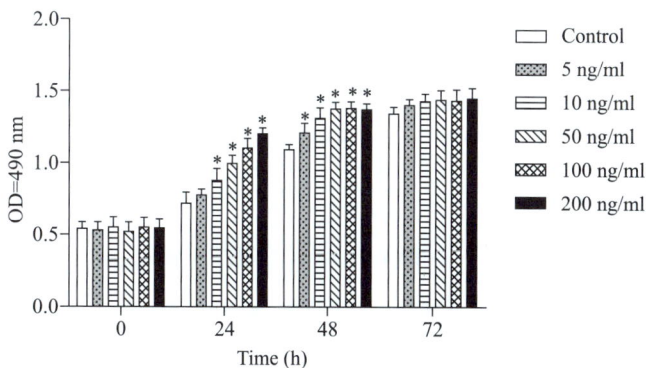

Fig. 1. Effect of FGF18 on the proliferation of H460 cells. H460 cells were cultured in 96-well plates for 24 h and treated with dif- ferent concentrations (0, 5, 10, 50, 100 and 200 ng/ml) of FGF18 for 0, 24, 48 or 72 h. Subsequently, cell proliferation was assessed by the 3-(4,5-dimethylthiazol-2-yl)-2,5-di- phenyltetrazolium bromide assay. Values are presented as the mean ± SD. ($n=3$). $^*P<0.05$ vs. control group. FGF18, fibroblast growth factor 18; OD, optical density.

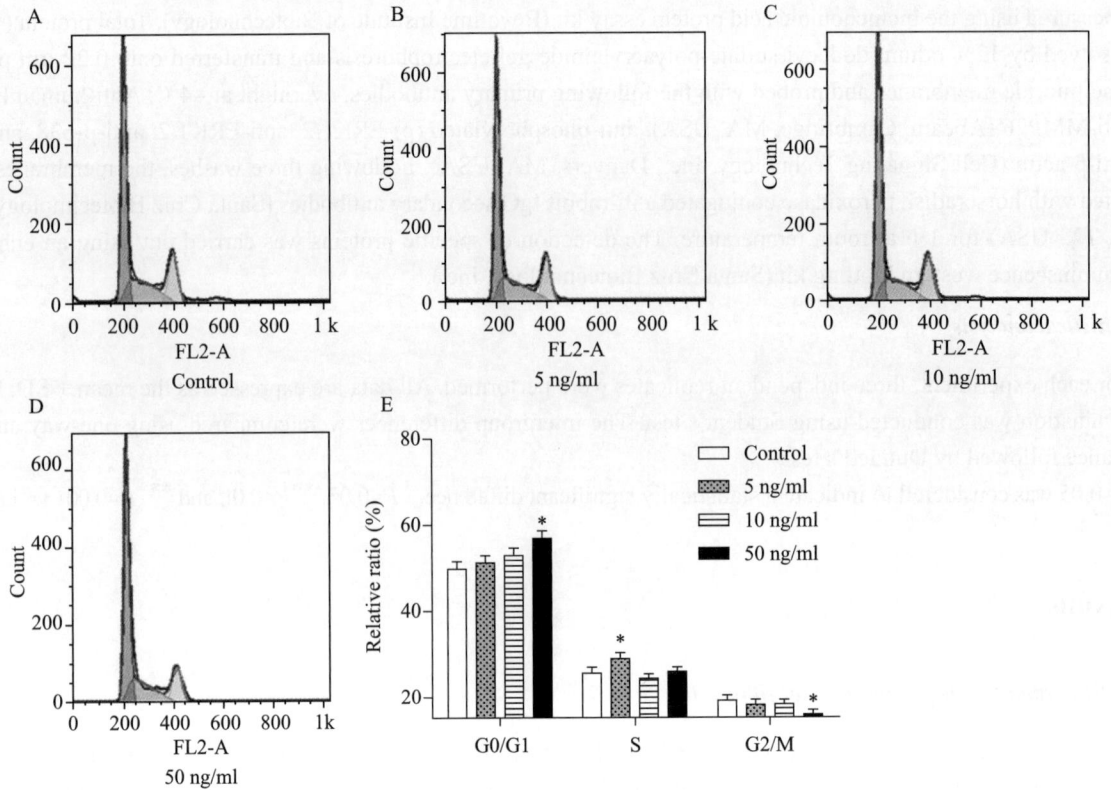

Fig. 2. Effect of FGF18 on the cell cycle of H460 cells. (A–D) H460 cells were cultured in 6-well plates and treated with different concentrations (0, 5, 10, 50 ng/ml) of FGF18 for 48 h. (E) Cell cycle kinetics were analyzed by flow cytometry using propidium iodide staining. Values are presented as the mean ± SD (n=3). *$P<0.05$ vs. control group. FGF18, fibroblast growth factor 18.

control untreated cells (Fig. 3A, B). Additionally, the effect of FGF18 on the expression of the migration-related factor MMP26, was investigated in H460 cells. As shown in the results of the western blot and RT-qPCR assays in Fig. 3C and E, FGF18 increased the mRNA and protein expression levels of MMP26 in a dose-dependent manner, particularly at 10 and 50 ng/ml concentrations. These results suggest that FGF18 promotes the migration of H460 cells and affects the migration-related factor MMP26.

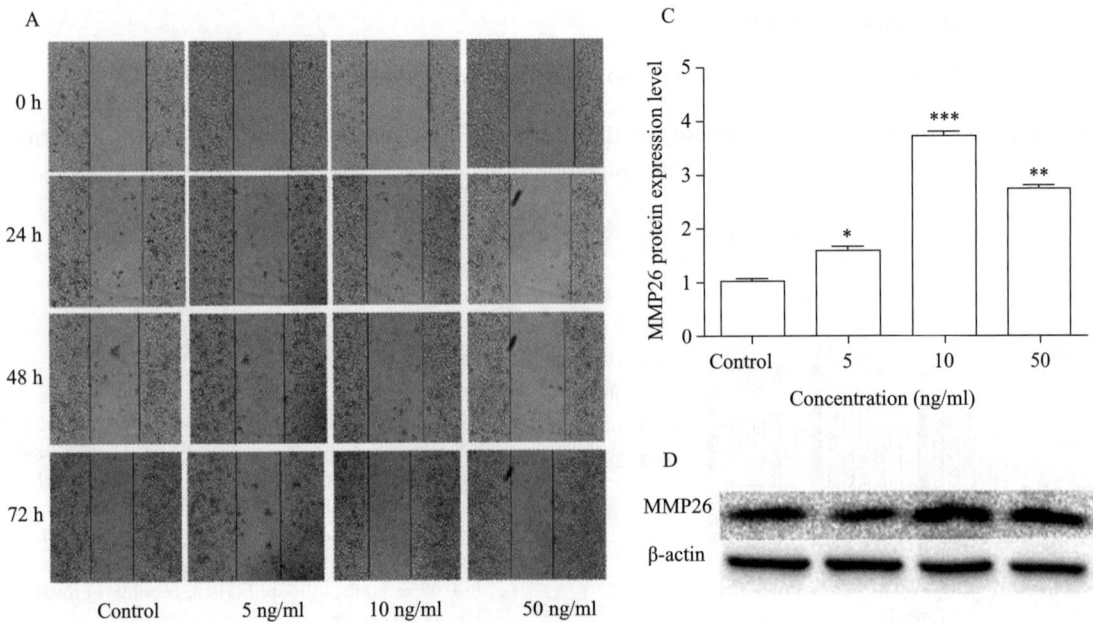

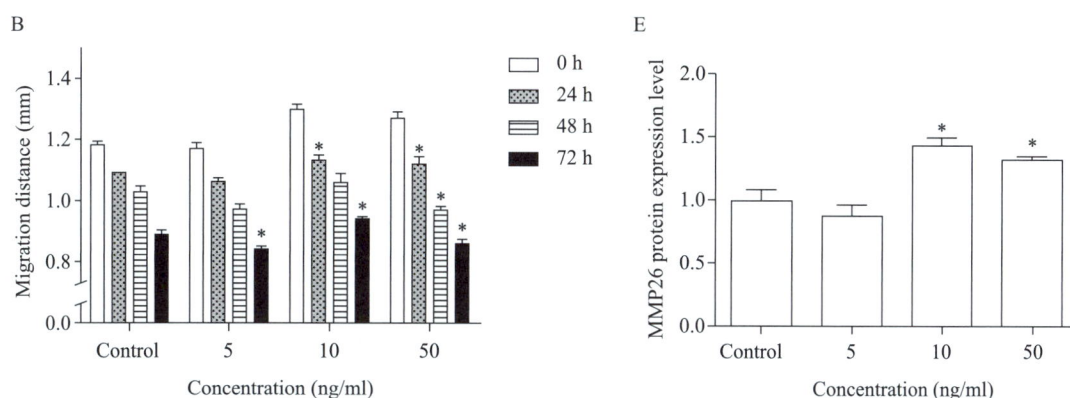

Fig. 3. Effects of FGF18 on the migration of H460 cells. (A and B) H460 cells were cultured in 6-well plates and grown to 100% confluence. Cells were scratched with a sterile pipette tip and then treated with FGF18 (0, 5, 10 or 50 ng/ml) for 24, 48 or 72 h. The cell migration activity was expressed as the distance of cells migrating into the wound. (C and D) MMP-26 was assayed by reverse transcription-quantitative polymerase chain reaction and western blotting. (E) Quantification of the protein levels. Values are presented as the mean ± SD ($n=3$). $^*P<0.05$, $^{**}P<0.0l$ and $^{***}P<0.001$ *vs.* control. FGF18, fibroblast growth factor 18; MMP, matrix metalloproteinase.

3.4　ERK and p38 signaling are involved in FGF18 mediated promotion of proliferation and migration in H460 cells

The above findings indicate that FGF18 significantly promotes the proliferation and migration of H460 cells. Moreover, the expression of MMP26 was promoted by FGF18 in H460 cells. However, the underlying mechanisms responsible for the effect of FGF18 are unclear. Hence, the effect of FGF18 on the signal transduction of MAPKs was further assessed by western blot analysis. H460 cells were treated with 5, 10 and 50 ng/ml FGF18 for 48 h, and the total protein lysates collected and subjected to western blotting with p-ERK1/2, ERK1/2, p38 MAPK and p-p38 MAPK antibodies. As shown in Fig. 4A and B, FGF18 increased the levels of p-ERK1/2 and p-p38. To address which of these pathways are regulating these effects, we used the specific inhibitors, FR180204 FERK inhibitor) and SB203580 (p38 inhibitor). Results showed that the effect of FGF18 stimulation on proliferation and migration was inhibited by application of 5 µmol/L FR180204 and 5 µmol/l SB203580 (Fig. 4C–E). However, MMP26 protein did not change by the inhibitors (Fig. 4F, G). These data suggest that the effects of FGF18 in proliferation and migration of H460 cells is potentially mediated *via* modulations of the ERK1/2 pathway and p38 MAPK pathways.

3.5　FGF18 expression in H460 cells is downregulated by FGF18-siRNA

The RT-qPCR results indicated that the mRNA expression of FGF18 in H460 cells transfected with siFGF18 was reduced compared with control group (Fig. 5A).

Additionally, FGF18 protein expression was examined using western blot analyses (Fig. 5B, C), with the results consistent with the mRNA data. These results demonstrate the successful knockdown of FGF18 using siRNA.

3.6　FGF18 siRNA inhibits cell proliferation and migration in the ERK and p38 signaling pathways in H460 cells

The proliferation and migration of cancer cells are key steps in the progression of cancer. Following cell transfection, the effect of FGF18 siRNA on cell proliferation was evaluated in H460. The OD values were significantly reduced in the siFGF18 group compared with the control group (Fig. 6A), indicating that FGF18 siRNA inhibited cell proliferation in H460 cells.

However, as shown in Fig. 6B and C, the siFGF18 group did not exhibit alterations in the cell cycle of H460 cells. In addition, the migration distance of siFGF18-transfected H460 cells was reduced compared with the control groups (Fig. 6D, E). Expression of MMP26 gene and protein was addition-ally significantly reduced following siFGF18, with a 57% gene inhibition rate and 62% protein inhibition rate, respectively (Fig. 6F–H). The levels of p-ERK and p-p38 protein were significantly lower in the siFGF18 group compared with the cells in the control group (Fig. 6I, J). Taken together, these results suggest that FGF18 siRNA is able to repress cell proliferation and migration, and this effect is potentially mediated through the ERK and pP38 signaling pathways in H460 cells.

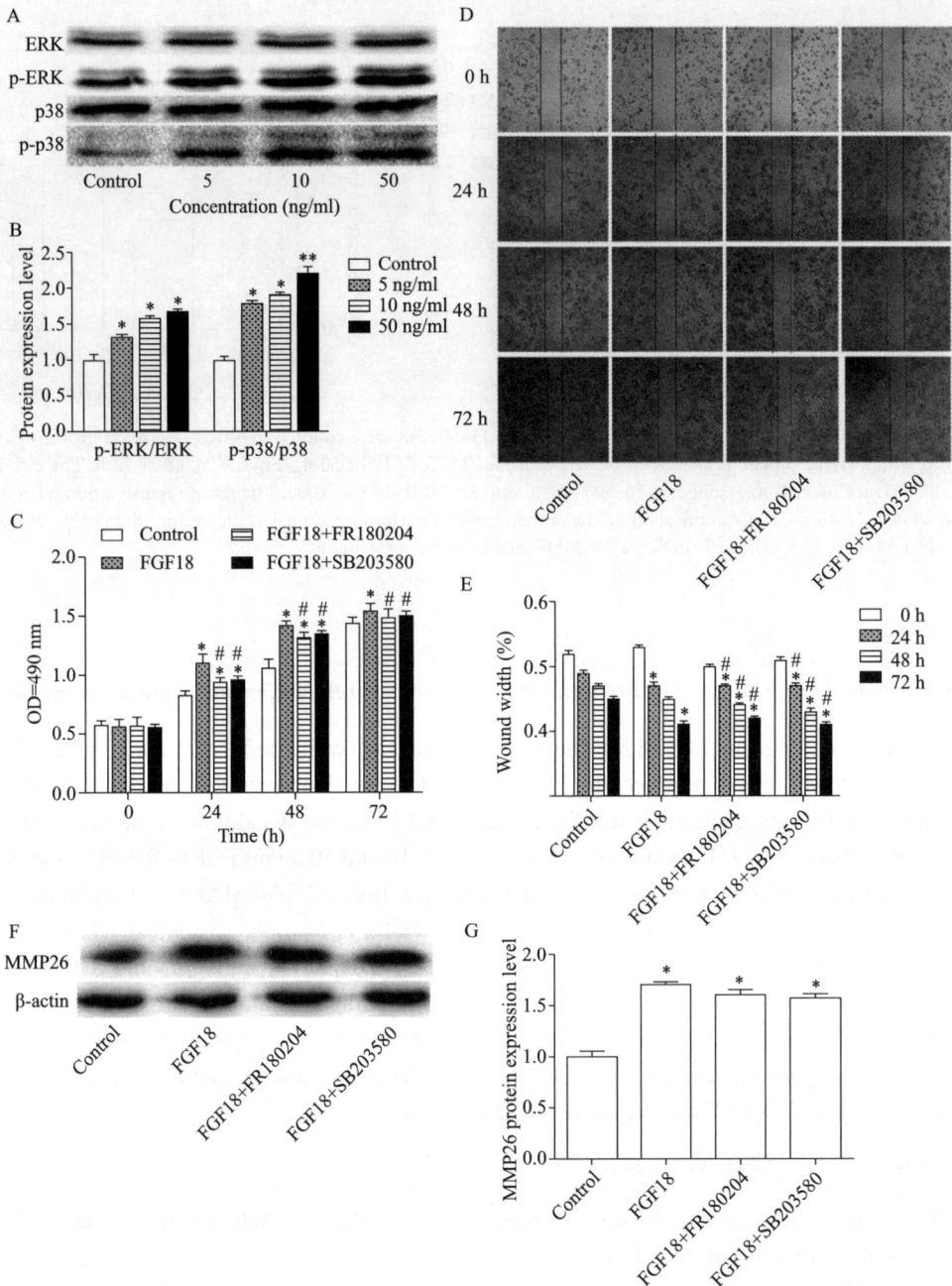

Fig. 4. Effect of FGF18 on ERK, p-ERK, p38 and p-p38 expression levels in H460 cells. (A) H460 cells were treated with various concentrations of FGF18 (0, 5, 10 or 50 ng/ml) for 48 h, then cells were collected and subjected to western blot analysis. (B) Quantification of the protein expression levels. (C) H460 cells were cultured on 96-well plates for 24 h and treated with FGF18 (50 ng/ml), FGF18+FR180204 (ERK inhibitor, 5 μmol), FGF18+SB203580 (p38 inhibitor, 5 μmol) for 0, 24, 48 or 72 h. Subsequently, cell proliferation was assessed by 3-(4,5-dimethylthiazol-2-yl)-2, 5-diphenyltetrazolium bromide assay. (D and E) Effects of FGF18, FGF18+FR180204, and FGF18+SB203580 on the migration of H460 cells. (F and G) Effect of FGF18, FGF18+FR180204, and FGF18+SB203580 on MMP26 expression levels in H460 cells. Values are presented as the mean ± SD (n=3). $^{*}P<0.05$, $^{**}P<0.01$ $vs.$ control. $^{\#}P<0.05$ $vs.$ FGF18. FGF18, fibroblast growth factor 18; ERK, extracellular signal-regulated kinase; p-ERK, phosphorylated ERK; MMP, matrix metalloproteinase.

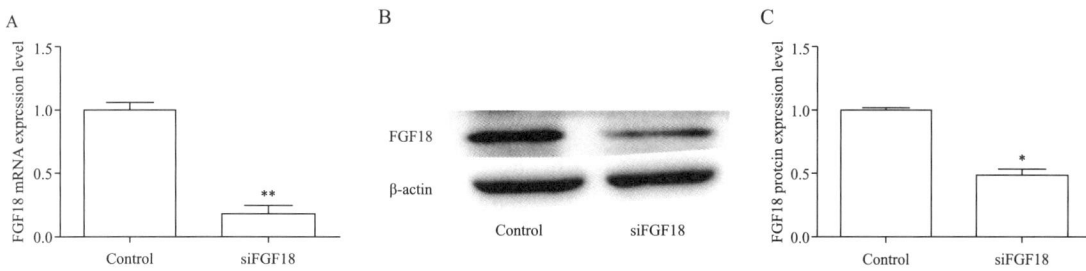

Fig. 5. siRNA against FGF18 specifically inhibit its expression. H460 cells were cultured in 6-well plates and were transfected with FGF18 siRNA. (A) Reverse transcription-quantitative polymerase chain reaction analysis of FGF18 mRNA expression and (B and C) western blot analysis of FGF18 protein expression were performed 48 h following transfection. *$P<0.05$, **$P<0.01$ vs. control. siRNA, short interfering RNA; FGF18, fibroblast growth factor 18.

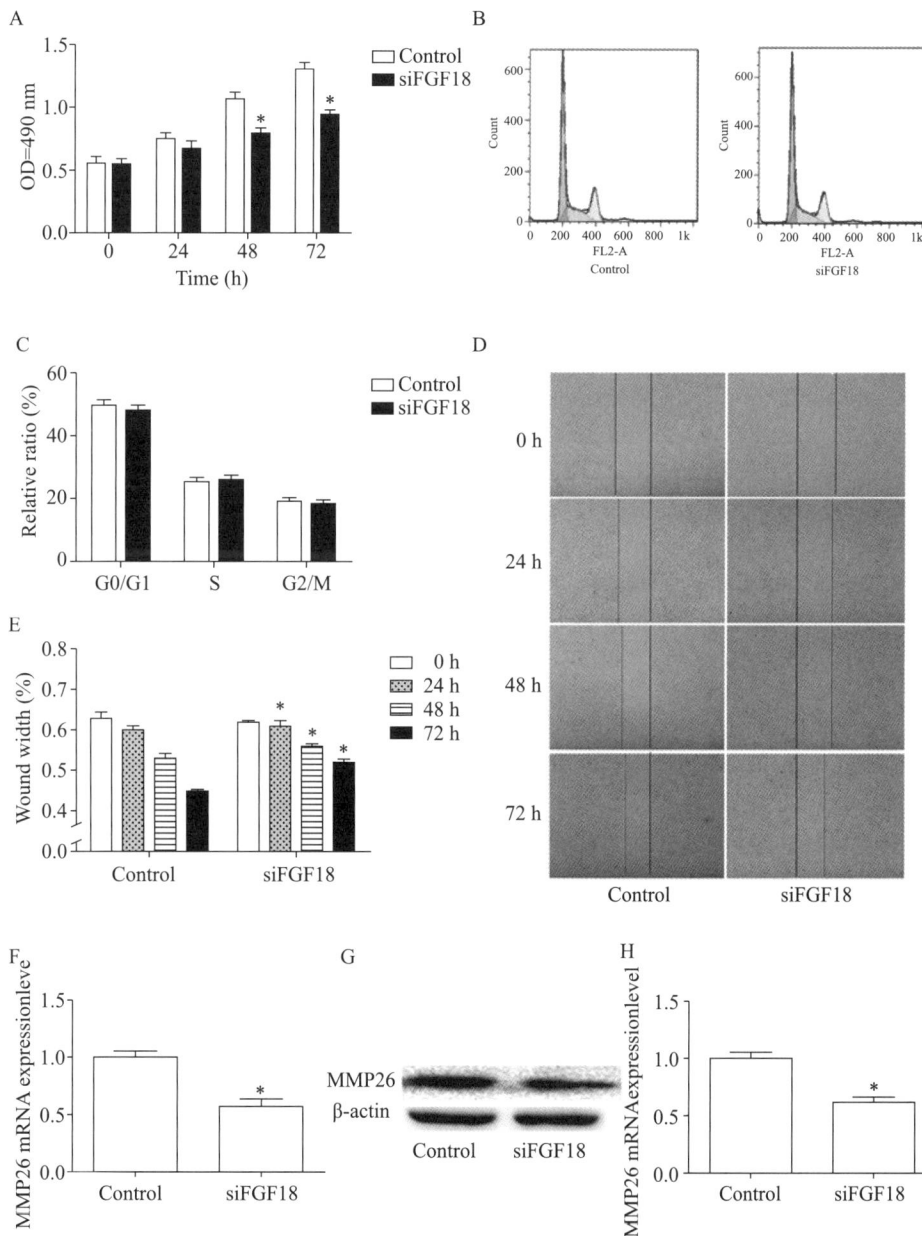

Fig. 6. Effect of siFGF18 on H460 cells. (A) H460 cells were cultured on 96-well plates for 24 h and treated with siFGF18 for 0, 24, 48 or 72 h. Subsequently, cell proliferation was assessed by 3-(4,5-dimethylthiazol-2-yl)-2, 5-diphenyltetrazolium bromide assay. (B and C) Effect of siFGF18 on the cell cycle of H460 cells. (D and E) Effects of siFGF18 on the migration of H460 cells. (F–H) RNA and protein levels of MMP26 in H460 cell. MMP, matrix metalloproteinase; OD, optical density. *$P<0.05$ vs. control.

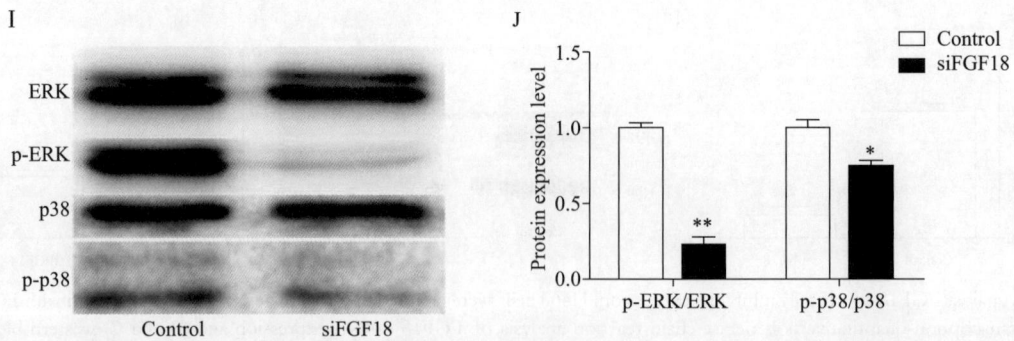

Fig. 6. Continued. Effect of siFGF18 on H460 cells. (I) Effect of siFGF18 on ERK, p-ERK, p38 and p-p38 expression levels in H460 cells. (J) Quantification of protein expression levels. Values are presented as the mean ± SD (n=3). *P<0.05, **P<0.01 *vs.* control. siFGF18, short interfering RNA against fibroblast growth factor 18; ERK, extracellular signal-regulated kinase; p-ERK, phosphorylated ERK.

4. Discussion

In NSCLC, the FGF and FGFR family has been demonstrated to be associated with its progression. FGF1 expression has been identified in the cytoplasm, or both cytoplasm and nucleus of NSCLC cells, and high expression levels of FGF1 in cancer cells were significantly correlated with larger primary tumor size and vascular invasion [21]. FGF9-FGFR3 signaling has a complex role in the initiation, growth and propagation of lung cancer [22]. Nevertheless, the role of FGF18 has not been previously studied in the context of lung cancer. Previous studies have indicated that elevated expression of FGF18 promotes the growth of colon cancer cells in culture [23], and demonstrated the pronounced oncogenic effect of FGF18 on ovarian tumor growth and metastasis [16]. These observations are in agreement with our conclusion that FGF18 promoted the proliferation and migration of H460 cells. The present study, to the best of our knowledge, is the first report of the effects of FGF18 on NSCLC cells.

A number of studies have shown that MAPKs (JNK1/2, ERK1/2, and p38) are involved in the growth, migration, and alterations in MMPs activity [24,25] in various cancers including lung, prostate, colorectal and ovarian cancer [26-30]. Furthermore, the ERK signaling pathway in addition to the p38 signaling pathway may regulate numerous factors that are associated with cancer progression and poor prognosis in NSCLC [31-33]. The MMP family comprises 24 zinc-dependent endopeptidases, and serves important roles in tumor metastasis and MMP26 is associated with the invasion and metastasis of non-small cell lung cancer [34-36]. It has been reported that the expression of MMPs is regulated by MAPK pathways [37,38]. To confirm whether ERK and p38 signaling pathway is involved in this situation, we applied specific inhibitors for ERK and p38, respectively, to the FGF18-stimulated H460 cells. We found that the inhibition of ERK and p38 decreased the proliferation and migration in response to FGF18 stimulation, while the activation of MMP26 did not change, suggesting that the activation of ERK and p38 signaling may cause an increase in proliferation and migration of H460 cells without MMP26 protein. However, using either ERK inhibitor or p38 inhibitor could not completely inhibit the H460 proliferation and migration, which may be due to the presence and activation of another signal transduction cascade. The present study suggests that the stimulation with FGF18 in NSCLC cells activated the ERK and p38 signaling pathways, and additionally upregulated the level of MMP26. This suggests that the underlying molecular mechanism may involve activated ERK and p38 signaling pathways in NSCLC cells inducing proliferative and migratory signals.

The present study additionally demonstrated that the transfection of cancer cells with siRNA targeted against the FGF18 gene can effectively reduce FGF18 gene expression and suppress the effects on proliferation, and migration in H460 cells. However, the effect of siFGF18 on proliferation was not accompanied by alterations in the cell cycle. Therefore further studies are required to explore the mechanisms of FGF18 on proliferation. Western blot analysis was used to investigate the expression of ERK, p38 and MMP26 in human H460 cells following siRNA-FGF18 treatment for 48 h, which demonstrated marked inhibition of the ERK and p38 signaling pathways. These results imply that the use of siRNA holds potential in treating lung cancer cells, and that the FGF18 gene may be a potential therapeutic target in NSCLC.

In conclusion, the present study suggests that FGF18 serves a key role in the proliferation and migration of NSCLC cells by regulating the ERK, p38 signaling pathways and MMP26 protein expression levels, indicating that FGF18 may represent a potential molecular drug target in NSCLC. Nevertheless, further studies using NSCLC cell lines and investigating the *in vivo* physiological role of FGF18 are required.

References

[1] Jemal A, Siegel R, Xu J, *et al.* Cancer Statistics, 2010[J]. Ca-a Cancer Journal for Clinicians, 2010, 60(5): 277-300.

[2] Siegel R, Naishadham D, Jemal A. Cancer statistics, 2013[J]. Ca-a Cancer Journal for Clinicians, 2013, 63(1): 11-30.

[3] Travis WD, Brambilla E, Nicholson AG, *et al.* The 2015 World Health Organization Classification of Lung Tumors Impact of Genetic, Clinical and Radiologic Advances Since the 2004 Classification[J]. Journal Of Thoracic Oncology, 2015, 10(9): 1243-1260.

[4] Ettinger DS, Akerley W, Bepler G, *et al.* Non Small Cell Lung Cancer[J]. Journal Of the National Comprehensive Cancer Network, 2010, 8(7): 740-801.

[5] Antoine M, Wirz W, Tag CG, *et al.* Expression pattern of fibroblast growth factors (FGFs), their receptors and antagonists in primary endothelial cells and vascular smooth muscle cells[J]. Growth Factors, 2005, 23(2): 87-95.

[6] Hu MCT, Qiu WR, Wang YP, *et al.* FGF-18, a novel member of the fibroblast growth factor family, stimulates hepatic and intestinal proliferation[J]. Molecular And Cellular Biology, 1998, 18(10): 6063-6074.

[7] Canalis E, McCarthy TL, Centrella M. GROWTH-FACTORS AND CYTOKINES IN BONE CELL-METABOLISM[J]. Annual Review Of Medicine, 1991, 42: 17-24.

[8] Liu ZH, Xu JS, Colvin JS, *et al.* Coordination of chondrogenesis and osteogenesis by fibroblast growth factor 18[J]. Genes & Development, 2002, 16(7): 859-869.

[9] Dailey L, Ambrosetti D, Mansukhani A, *et al.* Mechanisms underlying differential responses to FGF signaling[J]. Cytokine & Growth Factor Reviews, 2005, 16(2): 233-247.

[10] Turner N, Grose R. Fibroblast growth factor signalling: from development to cancer[J]. Nature Reviews Cancer, 2010, 10(2): 116-129.

[11] Beenken A, Mohammadi M. The FGF family: biology, pathophysiology and therapy[J]. Nature Reviews Drug Discovery, 2009, 8(3): 235-253.

[12] Marie PJ. Fibroblast growth factor signaling controlling osteoblast differentiation[J]. Gene, 2003, 316: 23-32.

[13] Moore EE, Bendele AM, Thompson DL, *et al.* Fibroblast growth factor-18 stimulates chondrogenesis and cartilage repair in a rat model of injury-induced osteoarthritis[J]. Osteoarthritis And Cartilage, 2005, 13(7): 623-631.

[14] Sonvilla G, Allerstorfer S, Staettner S, *et al.* FGF18 in colorectal tumour cells: autocrine and paracrine effects[J]. Carcinogenesis, 2008, 29(1): 15-24.

[15] Koneczny I, Schulenburg A, Hudec X, *et al.* Autocrine Fibroblast Growth Factor 18 Signaling Mediates Wnt-Dependent Stimulation of CD44-Positive Human Colorectal Adenoma Cells[J]. Molecular Carcinogenesis, 2015, 54(9): 789-799.

[16] Wei W, Mok SC, Oliva E, *et al.* FGF18 as a prognostic and therapeutic biomarker in ovarian cancer[J]. Journal Of Clinical Investigation, 2013, 123(10): 4435-4448.

[17] Rubinfeld H, Seger R. The ERK cascade - A prototype of MAPK signaling[J]. Molecular Biotechnology, 2005, 31(2): 151-174.

[18] Krejci P, Prochazkova J, Bryja V, *et al.* Molecular Pathology of the Fibroblast Growth Factor Family[J]. Human Mutation, 2009, 30(9): 1245-1255.

[19] Song L, Huang Z, Chen Y, *et al.* High-efficiency production of bioactive recombinant human fibroblast growth factor 18 in Escherichia coli and its effects on hair follicle growth[J]. Applied Microbiology And Biotechnology, 2014, 98(2): 695-704.

[20] Livak KJ, Schmittgen TD. Analysis of relative gene expression data using real-time quantitative PCR and the 2(T)(-Delta Delta C) method[J]. Methods, 2001, 25(4): 402-408.

[21] Li J, Wei Z, Li H, *et al.* Clinicopathological significance of fibroblast growth factor 1 in non-small cell lung cancer.[J]. Hum Pathol, 2015, 46: 1821-1828.

[22] Arai D, Hegab AE, Soejima K, *et al.* Characterization of the cell of origin and propagation potential of the fibroblast growth factor 9-induced mouse model of lung adenocarcinoma[J]. Journal Of Pathology, 2015, 235(4): 593-605.

[23] Shimokawa T, Furukawa Y, Sakai M, *et al.* Involvement of the FGF18 gene in colorectal carcinogenesis, as a novel downstream target of the beta-catenin/T-cell factor complex[J]. Cancer Research, 2003, 63(19): 6116-6120.

[24] Tang S-W, Yang T-C, Lin W-C, *et al.* Nicotinamide N-methyltransferase induces cellular invasion through activating matrix metalloproteinase-2 expression in clear cell renal cell carcinoma cells[J]. Carcinogenesis, 2011, 32(2): 138-145.

[25] McCubrey JA, Steelman LS, Chappell WH, *et al.* Roles of the Raf/MEK/ERK pathway in cell growth, malignant transformation and drug resistance[J]. Biochimica Et Biophysica Acta-Molecular Cell Research, 2007, 1773(8): 1263-1284.

[26] Sun L, Zhang Q, Li Y, *et al.* CCL21/CCR7 up-regulate vascular endothelial growth factor-D expression *via* ERK pathway in human non-small cell lung cancer cells[J]. International Journal Of Clinical And Experimental Pathology, 2015, 8(12): 15729-15738.

[27] Han Y, Luo Y, Wang Y, *et al.* Hepatocyte growth factor increases the invasive potential of PC-3 human prostate cancer cells *via* an ERK/MAPK and Zeb-1 signaling pathway[J]. Oncology Letters, 2016, 11(1): 753-759.

[28] Li L, Duan T, Wang X, *et al.* KCTD12 Regulates Colorectal Cancer Cell Stemness through the ERK Pathway[J]. Scientific Reports, 2016, 6.

[29] Xia ZX, Li ZX, Zhang M, *et al.* CARMA3 regulates the invasion, migration, and apoptosis of non-small cell lung cancer cells by activating NF-kappa B and suppressing the P38 MAPK signaling pathway[J]. Experimental And Molecular Pathology, 2016, 100(2): 353-360.

[30] Bai RX, Wang WP, Zhao PW, *et al.* Ghrelin attenuates the growth of HO-8910 ovarian cancer cells through the ERK pathway[J]. Brazilian Journal Of Medical And Biological Research, 2016, 49(3).

[31] Kim JH, Cho EB, Lee J, *et al.* Corrigendum to "Emetine inhibits migration and invasion of human non-small-cell lung cancer cells *via* regulation of ERK and p38 signaling pathways" [J]. Chemico-Biological Interactions, 243: 150.

[32] Zhang Y, Zhao J, Qiu L, *et al.* Co-expression of ILT4/HLA-G in human non-small cell lung cancer correlates with poor prognosis and ILT4-HLA-G interaction activates ERK signaling[J]. Tumor Biology, 2016, 37(8): 11187-11198.

[33] Zhang C, Shi J, Mao S, *et al.* Role of p38 MAPK in enhanced human cancer cells killing by the combination of aspirin and ABT-737[J]. Journal Of Cellular And Molecular Medicine, 2015, 19(2): 408-417.

[34] Zhang Y, Zhao H, Wang Y, *et al.* Non-small cell lung cancer invasion and metastasis promoted by MMP-26[J]. Molecular Medicine Reports, 2011, 4(6): 1201-1209.

[35] Ming SH, Sun TY, Xiao W, *et al.* Matrix metalloproteinases-2,-9 and tissue inhibitor of metalloproteinase-1 in lung cancer invasion and metastasis[J]. Chinese Medical Journal, 2005, 118(1): 69-72.

[36] Zhao D, Lu Y, Yang C, *et al.* Activation of FGF receptor signaling promotes invasion of non-small-cell lung cancer[J]. Tumor Biol-ogy, 2015, 36(5): 3637-3642.

[37] Wu X, Yang L, Zheng Z, *et al.* Src promotes cutaneous wound healing by regulating MMP-2 through the ERK pathway[J]. International Journal Of Molecular Medicine, 2016, 37(3): 639-648.

[38] Xia Y, Lian S, Khoi PN, *et al.* Chrysin Inhibits Tumor Promoter-Induced MMP-9 Expression by Blocking AP-1 *via* Suppression of ERK and JNK Pathways in Gastric Cancer Cells[J]. Plos One, 2015, 10(4).

Chapter 6
Pharmaceutics and New Material

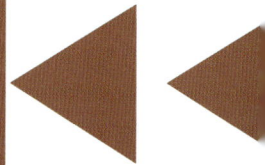

Prevent diabetic cardiomyopathy in diabetic rats by combined therapy of aFGF-loaded nanoparticles and ultrasound-targeted microbubble destruction technique

Yingzheng Zhao, Xiaokun Li

1. Introduction

Diabetic cardiomyopathy (DCM) is described as the structural and functional changes in the myocardium that are associated with diabetes (DM) in the absence of ischemic heart diseases, hypertension, or other cardiac pathologies [1,2]. The structural changes include fibrosis, apoptosis, angiopathy of myocytes and the functional changes include endothelium-myocytes uncoupling, impairment for contractility of cardiomyocytes, decrease in survival and differentiation of cardiac stem cells as well as diastolic and systolic dysfunction [3,4]. DCM has been identified as the leading cause of morbidity and mortality in DM patients. However, up to date there is no effective treatment for this common yet lethal pathological condition.

Acidic fibroblast growth factor (aFGF, also known as FGF-1) is a 15.8 kDa peptide and is also referred to as heparin-binding growth factor 1 because of its affinity for heparin. aFGF induces endothelial and smooth muscle cell proliferation and angiogenesis *in vivo* [5]. In addition, aFGF has shown to be an important pro-survival anti-apoptotic factor in a variety of cell types [6]. Zhang *et al.* showed that the non-mitogenic aFGF has the therapeutic effects on DCM by the suppression of oxidative stress and damage in diabetes rats [7]. aFGF is thus a potentially valuable therapeutic agent for DCM treatment. However, there is a strong need to optimize the mode of aFGF delivery aiming at minimizing the impact on systemic tissues (*e.g.* liver, spleen, lung and kidney), while retaining the aFGF bioactivity on the myocardial tissues. The current strategies for delivery of exogenous aFGF or aFGF gene to the damaged myocardial tissue include direct cardiac injection of bolus dose and delivery by drug carrier. The use of carriers such as nanoparticles (NP) is less risky, and may also improve the stability of aFGF both during storage and in blood circulation. But without additional strategy to increase the selectivity for cardiac tissue, aFGF encapsulated nanoparticles still may not be able to improve the aFGF delivery to the heart without causing unnecessary impact on the other body tissues.

Recently, low-intensity ultrasound (US) in combination with microbubbles has been shown to improve the efficiency and tissue/organ specificity of *in vivo* uptake for nanoparticles [8]. When exposed to the low intensity ultrasound, microbubbles would lead to a stable cavitation (the oscillations of microbubbles) [9]. Such stable oscillations created a liquid flow around the microbubbles, the so-called microstreaming [10]. When these oscillating microbubbles were in close vicinity of cells, these cells would experience shear stress. Consequently, these US induced elevated shear stress levels can enhance cellular uptake of macromolecular drugs [11–13]. Therefore, this ultrasound-targeted microbubble destruction (UTMD) technique, which has been conventionally used as a clinical diagnosis, holds considerable promise as an effective strategy to achieve targeted delivery of aFGF from nanoparticle formulation to the heart.

The present study aimed at determining whether the combination therapy of UTMD technique with novel aFGF-loaded nanoparticles (aFGF-NP) is effective to prevent DCM in a diabetes animal model. In a previous study, we developed Poloxamer 188-grafted heparin copolymer which demonstrated high affinity for aFGF as a result of interaction with its heparin content [14]. This copolymer was therefore chosen for preparation of aFGF-NP in this study. To achieve an in-depth understanding of the therapeutic impact of the aFGF-NP/UTMD technique, a broad range of commonly used pathophysiological indicators of the heart conditions were measured in a DCM rat model induced by streptozotocin (STZ). These measurements allowed thorough preclinical evaluation of the *in vivo* effects of 12 weeks aFGF-NP + UTMD treatment on the cardiac functions and related structural damages. Overall, this study has generated comprehensive data that are critical for the translation of this promising combination therapy of DCM, a frequently occurred and deadly disease.

2. Methods

2.1 Preparation and characterization of aFGF-NP

2.1.1 Preparation of phospholipid-based aFGF-NP

aFGF (20 mg/ml) (Sigma-Aldrich, USA) was dissolved in 1 ml of 20% *w/v* Poloxamer 188-grafted heparin co-polymer solution. The resulting solution was added into 2 ml of 2.0% *w/v* gelatin solution to produce a homogeneous mixture. Under sonication (110 w, 15℃) using a probe sonicator, D, L-glyceraldehyde was injected into the mixture until its final concentration reached 0.1% *w/v*. The mixture solution was kept at 5℃ and aFGF-NP was formed by the cross-linking reaction under magnetic stirring at 2,500 rpm for 5 h. Empty nanoparticles (blank nanoparticles, using Poloxamer 188-grafted heparin solution instead of aFGF Poloxamer 188-grafted heparin solution in preparation) and free aFGF solution (aFGF dissolved in 0.9% NaCl solution) were also prepared for comparison. Final aFGF concentration in the aFGF-containing solutions (aFGF-NP or aFGF solution) was 2 mg/ml.

2.1.2 Preparation phospholipid-based microbubbles

Lyophilized phospholipid-based microbubbles (PMB) were prepared by sonication-lyophilization method which was reported in our previous study [15]. The PMB concentration in the solution formed was about 2×10^9 bubble/ml with an average diameter of 3.4 μm as measured by coulter counter (Coulter Corporation, Hialeah, FL).

2.1.3 Characterization of aFGF-NP

The morphologies of aFGF-NP and blank NP were observed by scanning electron microscopy (SEM). Size and zeta potential values of aFGF-NP and blank NP were measured by dynamic light scattering using a Zeta Potential/Particle Sizer Nicomp™ 380 ZLS (PSS. Nicomp, Santa Barbara, CA, USA).

To determine the aFGF encapsulation efficiency of aFGF-NP, aFGF-NP dispersion was centrifuged at 10,000 *g* for 40 min. The supernatant was then collected and diluted for aFGF determination using an ELISA kit [16]. The drug encapsulation efficiency was calculated as indicated below. The analyses were performed in triplicate.

Encapsulation efficiency (%) = (total amount of drugs − amount of drugs in supernatant)/total amount of drugs added initially ×100%.

To evaluate the aFGF bioactivity after encapsulation in aFGF-NP, NIH-3T3 cells were grown in RPMI-1640 medium supplemented with 10% fetal bovine serum (FBS) in a 96-well plate (7,000 cells per well). The cells were incubated in 0.1% FBS 1640 medium for 24 h and treated with aFGF-NP suspension for 72 h. The number of viable cells was determined by MTT cell proliferation kit in accordance with the manufacture protocol.

To evaluate the stability of aFGF-NP in sonoportation, aFGF-NP encapsulation values before and after sonoportation were compared. 100 μl PMB and 100 μl aFGF-NP were mixed for 5 min in a sealed container and then added into 12-well plates. 200 μl 10% FBS was added into the mixture which was rotated at approximately 30 rpm for 60 s before ultrasound exposure. Sonoportation experiments were performed in a device described in a previous study [17]. A linear array transducer (15LSw.S probe, 12 – 14 MHz, Acuson Sequoia 512C system, Siemens) was used to generate the sonoportation. The ultrasound transducer was inserted in a 37℃ water tank and directly faced the bottom of the cell plate. A spongy rubber ultrasound shield was used to focus ultrasound on experimented cells. Each sample received designed ultrasound exposure in the water bath. The 12-well plate was held 4 cm from the submersed transducer (US exposure duration per time: 5 s, 10 s and 15 s respectively; repeat three times with off intervals of 1 s). After ultrasound exposure, the aFGF encapsulation efficiency of aFGF-NP was determined by the ELISA kit mentioned above.

2.2 Animal studies

2.2.1 Type 1 DM animal model

DM was induced in male Sprague Dawley (SD) rats (42–49 days, 180–220 g) by intraperitoneal single injection of streptozotocin (STZ, Sigma Corporation, USA) at 70 mg/kg after 12 h of fasting. On the 3rd day, 7th day, and 2nd week after STZ administration, the fasting blood glucose was measured from the tail tip using an autoanalyzer (Surestep, Roche, Germany). Only the rats with fasting blood glucose levels exceeding 16.7 mM and stabilized in the next two weeks were selected as diabetic rats. The normal control rats were injected with STZ-free citrate buffer instead. All animal experiments were performed under the approval and guidance of the Institutional Animal Care and Use Committee of Wenzhou Medical University.

2.2.2 Groups and treatments of animals

After the model of diabetic rats was induced, the experimental rats were randomized into seven groups (n = 8 per group): (1) DM group: DM rats were administered 1 ml normal saline. (2) Control: non-diabetic rats were administered 1 ml normal saline; (3) aFGF group: DM rats were treated with free aFGF (15 μg/kg) in 1 ml normal saline without PMB and US; (4) aFGF-NP group: DM rats were treated with aFGF-NP (15 μg/kg) in 1 ml normal saline without PMB and US; (5) UTMD group: DM rats were treated with 1 ml PMB solution only combined with US; (6) aFGF + UTMD group: DM rats were treated with a mixture of free aFGF (15 μg/kg) and PMB in 1 ml normal saline combined with US; (7) aFGF-NP + UTMD group: DM rats were treated with a mixture of aFGF-NP (15 μg/kg) and PMB in 1 ml normal saline combined with US. For all animals, aFGF and PMB were administered *via* tail vein injection twice weekly for 12 consecutive weeks.

2.2.3 Drug and microbubble administration method

Animals were treated with therapeutic agents and ultrasound-targeted microbubble destruction (UTMD) as shown in supplemental Fig. S1A. Each rat was anesthetized with an intraperitoneal injection of 30 mg/kg sodium pentobarbital. The thoracic region was shaved, and the rats were placed in the supine position. A 20-gauge cannula was inserted into the tail vein and experimental solution was infused. A linear array transducer (15LSw.S probe, 12–14 MHz, Acuson Sequoia 512C system, Siemens) was used to generate the UTMD effect. In the groups with UTMD, the linear array transducer was placed over the heart (short axis view; depth = 3.0–4.0 cm) to view papillary muscles of the left ventricle. There was no microbubbe signal before the filling of microbubbes and aFGF-containing treatment (supplemental Fig. S1B). When a large number of PMB were seen filling the heart (supplemental Fig. S1C), the microbubble destruction (MBD) function key (the key for controlling the bursting of microbubbles) attached to the machine was employed to disrupt PMB for UTMD (US exposure duration per time = 10 s, repeat three times with off intervals of 1 s to allow refill of the tissue with more MBs) (supplemental Fig. S1D). After the bursting, the microbubbles completely disappeared in heart (supplemental Fig. S1E).

2.3 Measurement of cardiac dimensions and function

2.3.1 Transthoracic echocardiography

All subjects underwent an echocardiographic study (Siemens Sequoia 512) in the 2nd week after modeling (before treatment) and the 12th week after diabetes (*i.e.* the week after treatment). The data was analyzed offline in Siemens Sygno US Workplace 3.01 (Sygno VVI, Siemens). In this study, the LV wall at mid-level from the short-axis view was divided into six segments according to the standard 16-segment model of the American Society of Echocardiography. The segments of the LV wall were plotted, the endocardial and epicardial borders were manually identified in a single frame of a cine-loop, and the borders in other frames were automatically generated, allowing operators to alter any of those contours. Next, segmental mean peak systolic radial velocity (Vs), systolic circumferential strain (Sc), and systolic circumferential strain rate (SRc) were obtained from the velocity, strain, and strain rate curves provided by Sygno VVI.

2.3.2 Hemodynamic evaluation

A terminal surgical procedure was performed to all rats to evaluate LV hemodynamics as described previously [18]. The LV end-systolic pressure (LVESP), end-diastolic pressure (LVEDP), and the maximum rising and dropping rates of LV pressure (±dp/dt) were measured by using a commercially available analog-to-digital converter and analyzed by Chart 5 for Windows Analysis Software.

2.4 Histological and molecular analyses

After all the experiments were completed and the animals euthanized, the body weight (BW), heart weight (HW), blood glucose, and HW/BW were measured. Left ventricular tissue samples were obtained and stored in 2.5% glutaraldehyde for electron microscope studies. Samples were fixed in 10% formalin for paraffin sectioning. The remaining tissues were stored at −80 ℃ for western blot and other molecular analyses.

2.4.1 Masson staining

Briefly, 4 μm thick paraffin-embedded cardiac tissue sections were stained according to standard Masson trichrome staining. Digital pictures were taken with identical exposure settings for all sections. Cardiac collagen volume fraction (CVF) was quantified by use of computer-assisted image analysis software (Image-Pro plus 6.0 imaging software, NIH).

2.4.2 Transmission electron microscopy

A portion of the left ventricle was cut into 1 mm fragments and fixed in 2.5% glutaraldehyde for 4 h for electron microscopic examination. Then myocardial tissues were fixed in 1% osmic acid. After dehydration by acetone and embedded by epoxy resins, the myocardial tissue was sectioned at 1 μm and stained with toluidine blue. Ultrathin sections were cut in from this block and studied under a JEM-1230 (Jeol Limited, Japan) transmission electron microscope.

2.4.3 TUNEL staining

The apoptotic cells of myocardiums were detected by TUNEL staining. An *in situ* detection kit from Roche Biochemicals was used according to the manufacturer's instructions. Briefly, the sections of each group were treated with H_2O_2 and incubated with the reaction mixture containing terminal deoxynucleotidyl transferase (TdT) and digoxigenin-conjugated dUTP for 1 h at 37℃. Labeled DNA was visualized with peroxidase-conjugated anti-digoxigenin antibody using 3,3-diaminobenzidine (DAB) as the chromogen. The group which TdT was omitted from the reaction mixture served as the negative control.

2.4.4 Immunohistochemical staining

4 μm thick paraffin sections of LV were stained with polyclonal rabbit anti-rat caspase-3 and Ser473-phospho-Akt (Ser473-phospho-Protein Kinase B) antibodies (1 ∶ 200) (Santa Cruz biotechnology, USA). The staining was visualized by reaction with 3,3-diaminobenzidine (1 ∶ 20) (DAB; Sigma Chemical Co, USA). The sections were then lightly counterstained with Mayer's hematoxylin, dehydrated, and xylene-based mounted under glass cover slips. Negative controls were treated as above except that the primary antibody was replaced with PBS. Brown colored sites were quantified at final magnification of 200 × and 400× with an optical microscope connected to a video camera.

2.4.5 Myocardial capillary density

Myocardial capillary density (MCD) was measured by counting the number of brown-stained capillaries in 20 visual fields using high power (400×), and presented as the number of blood vessels per high power field (n/hpf). CD31 immunohistochemical staining was used to identify capillaries to measure MCD.

2.4.6 Western blot assay

Proteins were isolated from homogenized tissues with Trizol reagent (Invitrogen, Carlsbad, CA) using standard Invitrogen protocols. The protein concentration was measured by Braford protein assay. Equal amounts of protein (20 μg) were electrophoresed through a 10% SDS-PAGE gel and transferred to PVDF membranes (Millipore Company, USA). The membrane was blocked with 5% skim milk powder in PBS overnight. Then the membrane was incubated with primary antibody including aFGF, Akt, Ser473-phospho-Akt (pAkt), BCL-2, Bax and β-actin primary antibody (all antibodies purchased from Santa Cruz Biotechnology, USA). Proteins were then treated with goat anti-rabbit IgG-horseradish peroxidase as the secondary antibody (1 ∶ 5,000) (Santa Cruz Biotechnology, USA) and visualized with a chemiluminescence system. The signals were quantified by Quantity One software.

3 Results

3.1 Characterization of aFGF-NP

Characteristics of the blank NP and aFGF-NP are summarized in supplement Table S1. Dynamic light scattering results demonstrated that the average particle size of blank and aFGF-NP were 106 ± 1.84 nm and 128 ± 1.65 nm, respectively. Polydispersity index (PI) represents the distribution of particle size. Low PI values (≈0.1) were observed in both blank NP and aFGF-NP, which indicated that blank NP and aFGF-NP approached a monodisperse stable system. Moderately negative zeta potential values (≤ 15 mV) were observed in both nanoparticles. As indicated by the low PI values, the electrostatic repulsive forces between nanoparticles surfaces in combination with the steric forces provided by the poloxamer were likely sufficient to maintain the dispersion stability of the nanosystems.

The encapsulation efficiency of aFGF-NP reached 84.3 ± 2.8%. The bioactivity of aFGF-NP was about 7.20×10^5 IU/ml (supplement Table S1). There was no significant difference comparing the bioactivity between the aFGF-NP with the close quantity of free aFGF (about 7.80×10^5 IU/ml) ($P > 0.05$). These results indicate that the preparation of aFGF-NP did not diminish the original aFGF bioactivity.

From the comparison of aFGF-NP encapsulation before and after UTMD treatment (supplemental Fig. S2), only very small amount of encapsulated aFGF could be released from aFGF-NP after UTMD treatment. Therefore, aFGF-NP was the major form during UTMD treatment, corresponding to a previous study [17].

3.2 Improvement on heart-to-body weight ratio

Blood glucose, body weight (BW) and heart-to-body weight ratio (HW/BW) of the animals (Fig. 1A) was measured to evaluate the general effects of UTMD/aFGF-NP therapy on glucose metabolism and cardiomyopathy. As expected, all 6 groups using diabetic animals had similarly higher blood glucose levels and lower body weights when compared with the non-diabetic control. The differences were all significant ($P < 0.05$) regardless of the treatments, indicating that the aFGF and UTMD treatment both did not significantly modify the metabolic abnormalities of the diabetic animals.

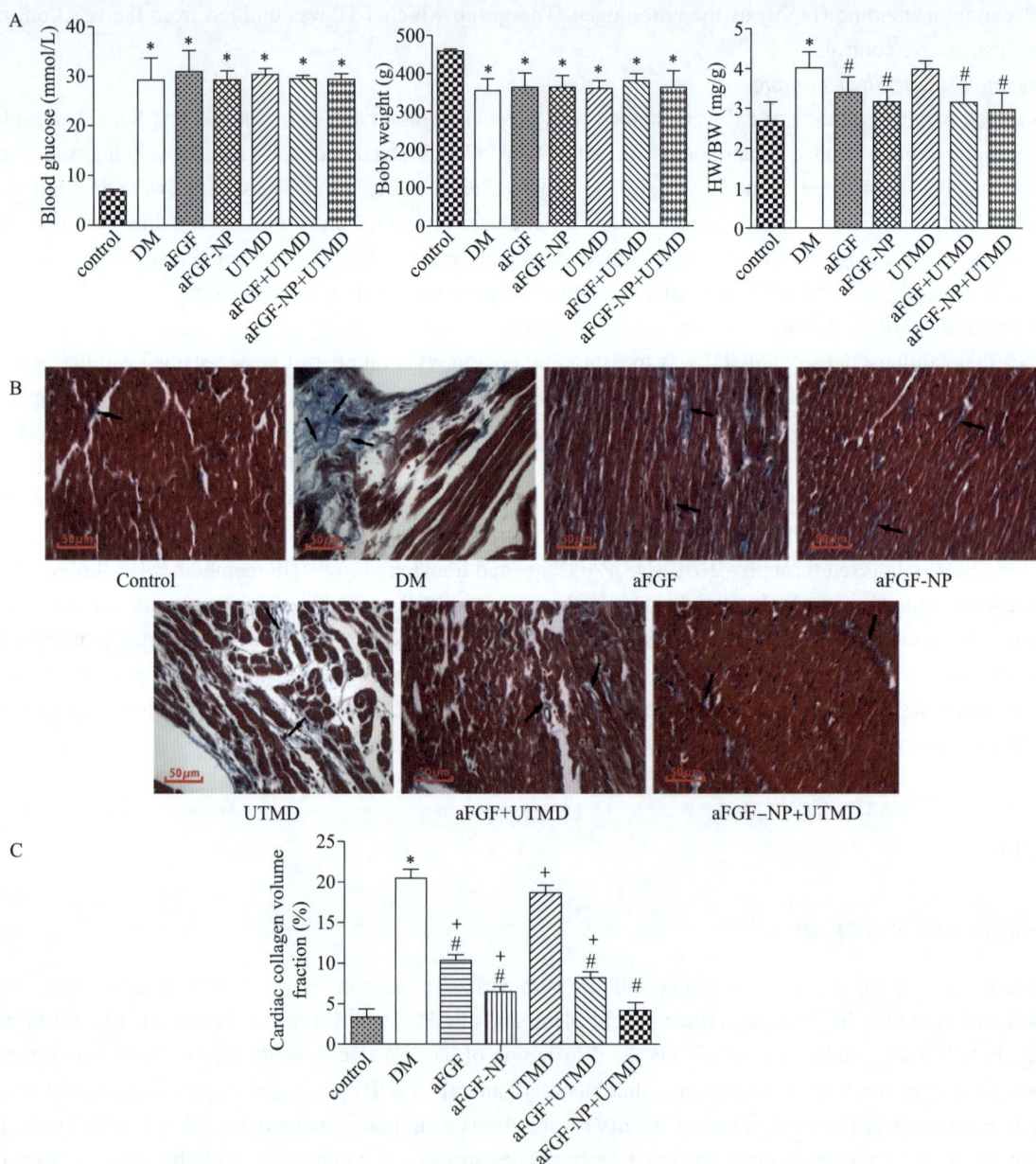

Fig. 1. aFGF-NP prevented DM-induced metabolism abnormalities and cardiomyocyte interstitial fibrosis. (A): quantitative analysis of the blood glucose of rats (left), the body weight of rats (middle) and the heart-to-body ratio (HW/BW) of rats (right). $n = 8$ per group. (B) representative pictures of myocardial tissue sections stained with Masson trichrome (400×). $n = 8$ per group. Arrow indicates myocardial fibrosis stained in blue. (C) quantitative analysis of cardiac collagen volume fraction. $n = 8$ per group. Date are expressed as Mean ± SD. *$P < 0.05$ vs. control group; #$P < 0.05$ vs. DM group; +$P < 0.05$ vs. aFGF-NP + UTMD group.

However, Fig. 1A shows that all 4 groups with aFGF or aFGF-NP possessed lower HW/BW than the untreated diabetic animals (DM group, $P < 0.05$) and UTMD only. The results indicate all aFGF treatment modified cardiomyopathy without altering the blood glucose levels.

3.3 Prevention of left ventricle dysfunction in diabetic rats

Myocardial velocity, strain and strain rate data by VVI are shown in Table 1. Right after induction of DM with STZ, there was no statistically significant difference among control and all the study groups in Vs, Sc and SRc (*i.e.* left column under each parameter). After 12 weeks (right column) the absolute values of all three parameters were noticeably decreased to various extents in all diabetic animals indicating deterioration of ventricular function caused by DM. In comparison, after treatment with a combination of aFGF-NP + UTMD (Group 7) minimal differences comparing with the non-diabetic control (Group 2) were observed, and all three parameters were significantly smaller than other groups including the remaining three aFGF treated groups (Group 3, 4, 6). In brief, aFGF-NP + UTMD led to the least ventricular dysfunction in diabetic animals.

Table 1.　Results of peak velocity, strain, and strain rate in control and study groups (mean ± SD, $n = 8$)

Group	Vs (cm/s)		Sc (%)		SRc (1/s)	
	0th after DM	12th after DM	0th after DM	12th after DM	0th after DM	12th after DM
1. DM	0.843 ± 0.051	0.526 ± 0.078*	−14.4 ± 2.0	−10.3 ± 1.5*	−3.69 ± 0.46	−2.46 ± 0.41*
2. Control	0.855 ± 0.059	0.870 ± 0.061	−14.6 ± 1.8	−14.8 ± 1.7	−3.76 ± 0.44	−3.82 ± 0.27
3. aFGF	0.848 ± 0.071	0.667 ± 0.061[#,+]	−14.3 ± 2.2	−12.0 ± 1.6[#,+]	−3.66 ± 0.46	−2.89 ± 0.45[#,+]
4. aFGF-NP	0.831 ± 0.074	0.671 ± 0.062[#,+]	−14.5 ± 1.9	−12.5 ± 1.6[#,+]	−3.69 ± 0.20	−3.01 ± 0.37[#,+]
5. UTMD	0.851 ± 0.081	0.519 ± 0.084*	−14.3 ± 1.8	−10.3 ± 1.3*	−3.72 ± 0.36	−2.49 ± 0.39*
6. aFGF + UTMD	0.835 ± 0.082	0.675 ± 0.097[#,+]	−14.4 ± 1.7	−12.5 ± 1.1[#,+]	−3.48 ± 0.49	−2.99 ± 0.35[#,+]
7. aFGF-NP + UTMD	0.839 ± 0.096	0.829 ± 0.080[#]	−14.6 ± 1.6	−14.4 ± 1.5[#]	−3.73 ± 0.32	−3.71 ± 0.44[#]

Note: Vs = peak systolic velocity; Sc = peak circumferential strain; SRc = peak circumferential strain rate. Data are Mean ± SD.

*$P < 0.05$ *vs.* control.

[#]$P < 0.05$ *vs.* DM group.

[+]$P < 0.05$ *vs.* aFGF-NP + UTMD.

The invasive hemodynamic data by intracardiac catheters were shown in Table 2. All aFGF formulations did not significantly affect the blood pressure and heart rate. During the study, no morality of the animals was observed. Compared with control animals, the DM group showed significantly lower LVSP, LV + dp/dtmax, and LV −dp/dtmax but a higher LVEDP ($P < 0.05$). In contrast to the DM group, the animals with aFGF treatment (Group 3, 4, 6 and 7) exhibited significantly improvement in LVSP, LVEDP, and LV + dp/dtmax and −dp/dtmax ($P < 0.05$). Moreover, the LVSP, LV + dp/dtmax and −dp/dtmax in the animals treated with aFGF-NP + UTMD group were significantly higher and LVEDP lower than the other aFGF treatment groups without nanoparticles or UTMD, and no difference in LVSP, LVEDP, and LV + dp/ dtmax and −dp/dtmax between this group (Group 7) and the control group.

3.4 Attenuation of DM-induced cardiomyocyte interstitial fibrosis

Fig. 1B–C presented the results of Mason staining (collagen in blue). CVF significantly increased in DM group (20.5%) with altered and disorganized collagen network structure in the interstitial and perivascular areas compared with control and other animals. In comparison with DM group, CVF was significantly reduced (*i.e.* reduced% blue staining) in the groups treated with aFGF (10.32%) or aFGF-NP (6.47%). Furthermore, CVF was significantly lower in the aFGF-NP + UTMD group (4.15%) than other aFGF groups without NP or UTMD. In fact, there was no significant difference in CVF between this group and the non-diabetic control (3.37%). It should be noted that UTMD alone did not reduce CVF.

Table 2. The hemodynamic data in experiment *in vivo* (mean ± SD, $n = 6$)

Group	LVESP (mmHg)	LVEDP (mmHg)	LV + dp/dtmax (mmHg)	LV −dp/dtmax (mmHg)	HR (bpm)
1. DM	$72.3 \pm 7.1^*$	$3.92 \pm 0.45^*$	$3.11 \times 10^3 \pm 212^*$	$2.80 \times 10^3 \pm 188^*$	$291.17 \pm 37.30^*$
2. Control	95.3 ± 7.5	2.83 ± 0.43	$4.79 \times 10^3 \pm 198$	$4.02 \times 10^3.65 \pm 289$	410.52 ± 46.81
3. aFGF	$83.5 \pm 7.7^{\#,+}$	$3.44 \pm 0.31^{\#,+}$	$4.04 \times 10^3 \pm 297^{\#,+}$	$3.50 \times 10^3 \pm 206^{\#,+}$	$342.49 \pm 48.72^{\#,+}$
4. aFGF-NP	$83.9 \pm 7.1^{\#,+}$	$3.42 \pm 0.29^{\#,+}$	$4.11 \times 10^3 \pm 340^{\#,+}$	$3.57 \times 10^3 \pm 314^{\#,+}$	$350.68 \pm 47.87^{\#,+}$
5. UTMD	$73.7 \pm 6.9^+$	$3.87 \pm 0.38^+$	$3.17 \times 10^3 \pm 307^+$	$2.84 \times 10^3 \pm 248^+$	$293.03 \pm 35.70^+$
6. aFGF + UTMD	$83.5 \pm 6.1^{\#,+}$	$3.45 \pm 0.31^{\#,+}$	$3.96 \times 10^3 \pm 335^{\#,+}$	$3.58 \times 10^3 \pm 235^{\#,+}$	$362.86 \pm 46.33^{\#,+}$
7. aFGF-NP + UTMD	$93.0 \pm 7.3^{\#}$	$2.91 \pm 0.33^{\#}$	$4.66 \times 10^3 \pm 248^{\#}$	$3.99 \times 10^3 \pm 211^{\#}$	$401.45 \pm 44.76^{\#}$

Notes: LVESP = left ventricular systolic pressure; LVEDP = left ventricular end diastolic pressure; ±dp/dtmax − maximum rate of the rise and fall of left ventricular pressure.

$^*P < 0.05$ *vs.* control.

$^{\#}P < 0.05$ *vs.* DM group.

$^+P < 0.05$ *vs.* aFGF-NP + UTMD.

3.5 Effects of aFGF-NP/UTMD combined treatment on electron microscopic findings

As shown in Fig. 2A, alterations in myofilaments, Z-line myofibers (Z in Fig. 2A), and degeneration and destruction in myofibril were seen in the myocardial samples by electron microscopy in study animals compared with control ones. In addition, the mitochondria (M in Fig. 2A) of the cardiomyocytes in the DM group showed swelling, and loss of cristae and granular matrix with vacuolization. In comparison, few alterations in myocardial ultrastructures were observed in the aFGF treatment groups. Furthermore, there were well organized and symmetric myofibrils in the Z lines and sarcomeres as well as relatively well-integrated ultra-structures in the mitochondria in aFGF-NP + UTMD group as compared with other treatment and DM groups. Again, the myocardial samples after UTMD treatment alone were structurally similar to untreated DM group.

3.6 Effects of UTMD treatment with aFGF-NP on expression of Caspase-3, BCL-2, Bax and aFGF levels

As shown in Fig. 2B-D, increased expression of pro-apoptotic proteins Caspase-3 and Bax but reduced expression of anti-apoptotic protein Bcl-2 were detected in DM group when compared with the control group ($P < 0.05$). Remark-

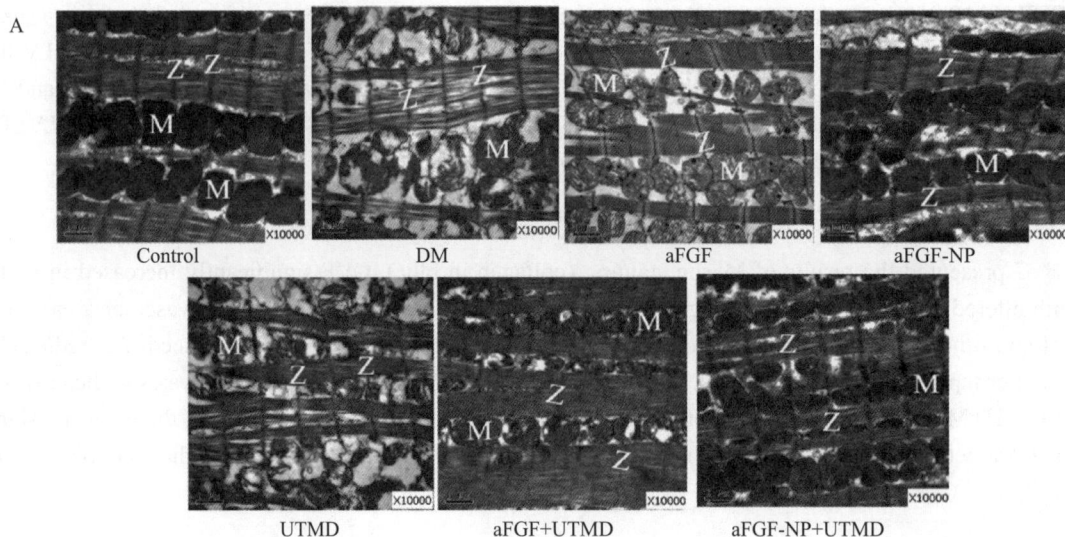

A   Control   DM   aFGF   aFGF-NP
UTMD   aFGF+UTMD   aFGF-NP+UTMD

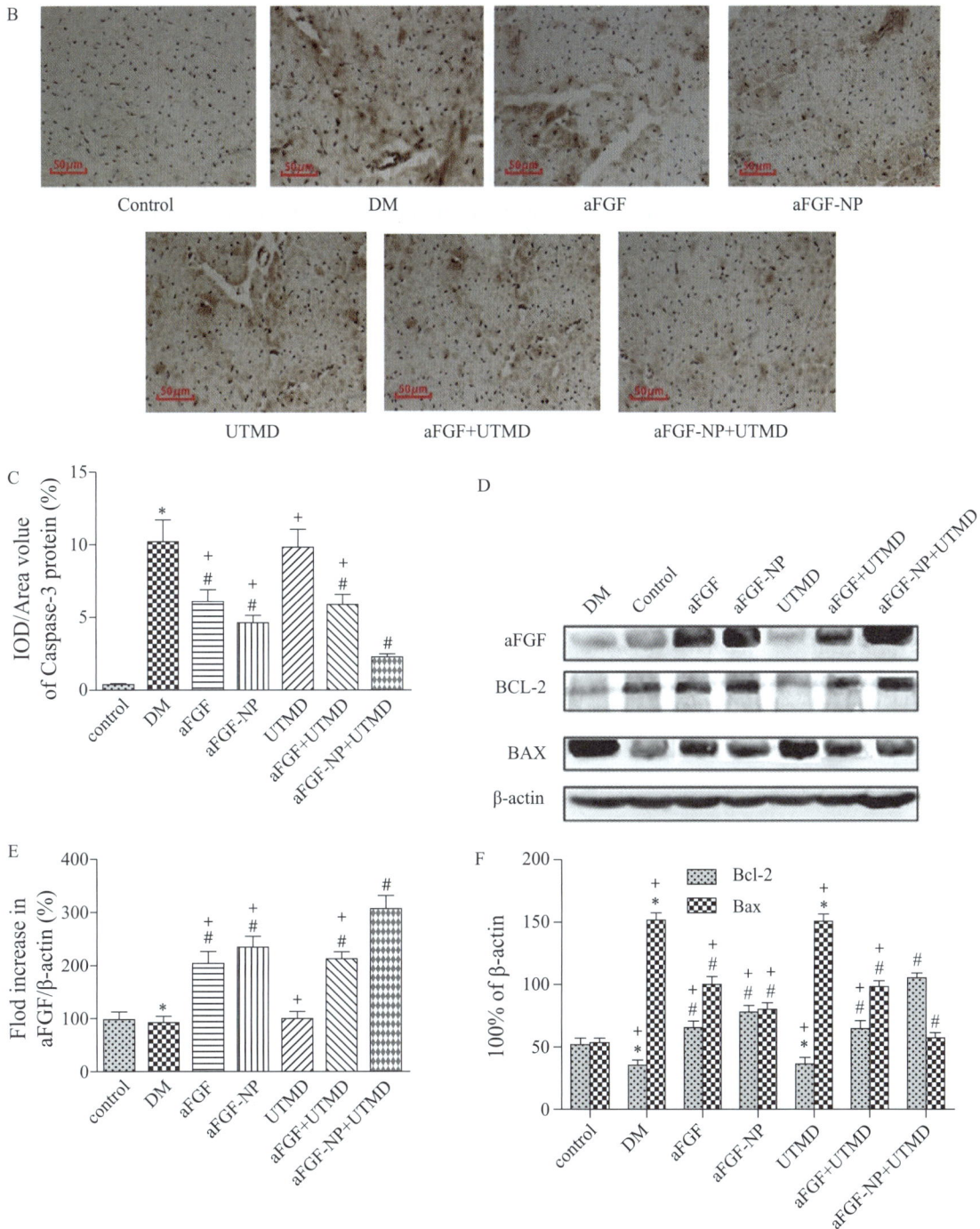

Fig. 2. aFGF-NP prevents cardiomyocyte from DM-induced injury and attenuated the expression of Caspase-3, BCL-2, Bax and aFGF in the hearts of DM rats. (A) representative pictures of electron micrographs (magnification 10,000×) of left ventricular heart muscle sections from the rats of each group. $n = 8$ per group. Z represented the Z-line in myofiber and M represented the mitochondria. (B) representative immunohisto-chemical staining of Caspase-3 expression (400×). (C) Quantitative analyses of the expression of Caspase-3; (D) Western blot analysis of aFGF, Bcl-2 and Bax expression; (E, F) Quantitative analyses of the expression of aFGF (panel E), Bcl-2 and Bax (panel F), respectively. $n = 8$ per group. Data are presented as Mean ± SD. $^*P < 0.05$ vs. control group; $^#P < 0.05$ vs. DM group; $^+P < 0.05$ vs. aFGF-NP + UTMD group.

ably, the groups treated with aFGF had significantly lower level expression of Caspase-3 and Bax as well as higher level expression of Bcl-2 than DM group. Quantitative analysis also confirmed that the aFGF-NP + UTMD group could significantly up-regulate Bcl-2 and down regulate expression of Bax and Caspase-3 when compared with other treatment groups ($P < 0.05$).

Furthermore, the aFGF levels in the hearts of aFGF treated groups were all significantly higher than DM and control groups as detected by Western blot (Fig. 2D). Comparing among the various aFGF treated groups, the aFGF-NP + UTMD group demonstrated higher level of aFGF than the other aFGF treated groups ($P < 0.05$), which was confirmed by quantitative analyses (Fig. 2 E–F).

3.7 Effects of UTMD treatment with aFGF-NP on cardiomyocyte apoptosis

As shown in Fig. 3, the apoptotic indexes were significantly increased in the DM group (10.5%) compared with the control animals (0.92%) ($P < 0.01$). However, aFGF treatment groups significantly attenuated DM-induced myocyte apoptosis in study groups ($P < 0.01$). Among the four aFGF treated groups, the aFGF-NP + UTMD group (2.31%) had a significantly lower apoptotic index than the other treatment groups. Quantitative analysis also demonstrated that the TU-NEL-positive cardiomyocytes were significantly less in the group combined aFGF-NP with UTMD than the other treatment groups ($P < 0.05$).

3.8 Effects of UTMD treatment with aFGF-NP on expression of pAkt and pAkt/Akt

As shown in Fig. 4A–B, immunohistochemical staining confirmed that the expression of phosphorylated Akt (pAkt, stained in brown) was significantly reduced in the DM group compared with control group. In general, all four aFGF treated groups all pAkt expression levels were elevated when compared with DM group ($P < 0.05$) as well as the non-diabetic control. Among these aFGF treated groups, the aFGF-NP + UTMD group had higher pAkt level than the other groups ($P < 0.05$). Western blot analysis (Fig. 4C) has confirmed this trend. The ratio of pAkt/Akt in the aFGF-NP + UTMD group was significantly higher (Fig. 4D) than other aFGF treated groups ($P < 0.05$).

3.9 Effects of UTMD treatment with aFGF-NP on myocardial capillary density

It was known that diabetes caused microvascular rarefaction in myocardium and reduced cardiac perfusion [19]. As

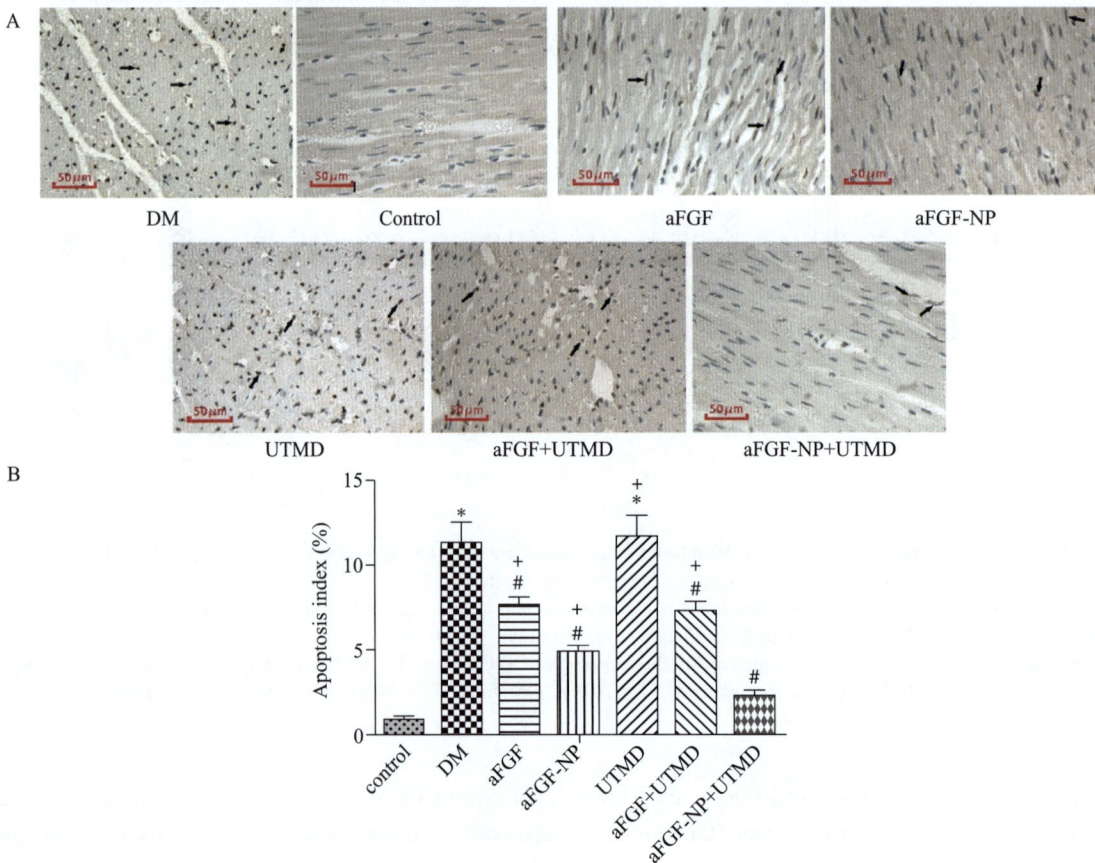

Fig. 3. aFGF-NP prevented DM-induced cardiomyocytes apoptosis. (A) representative pictures of TUNEL assay (400×, Arrow indicates TU-NEL-positive cardiomyocytes stained in brown); (B) Quantitative analysis of cardiomyocyte apoptosis index. $n = 8$ per group. Date are presented as Mean ± SD. *$P < 0.01$ vs. control group; #$P < 0.01$ vs. DM group; +$P < 0.05$ vs. aFGF-NP + UTMD group.

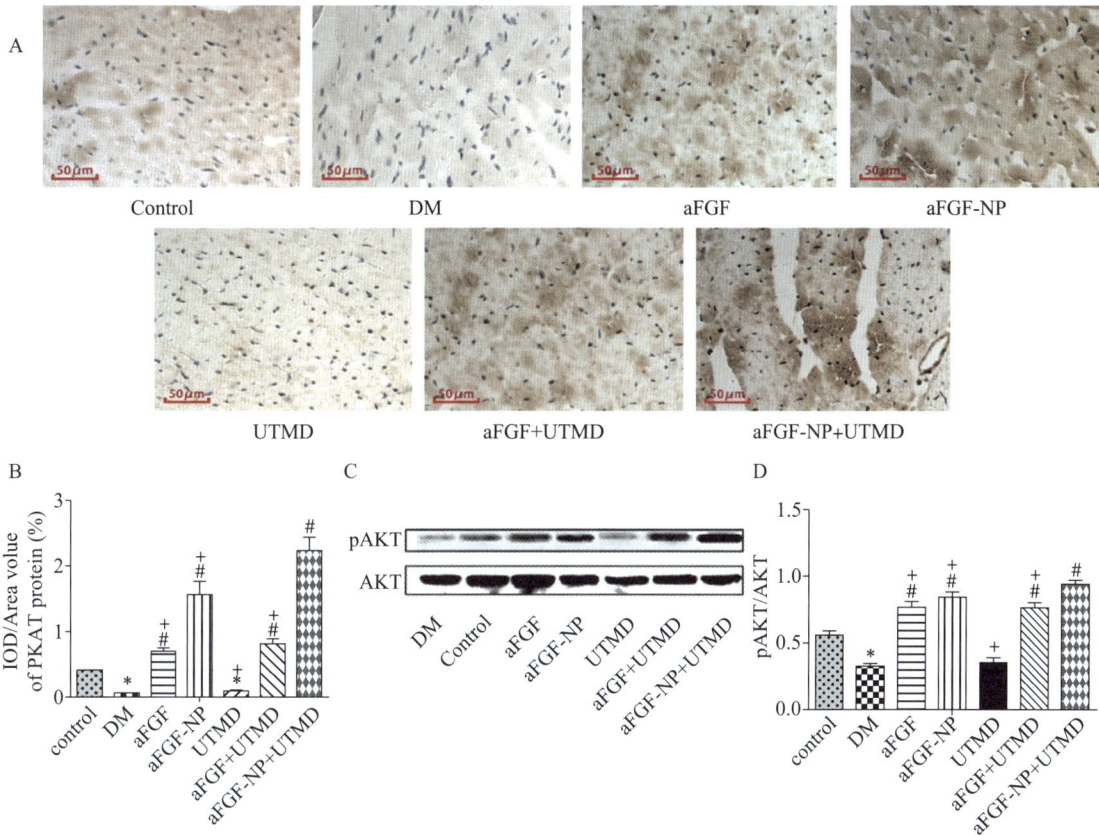

Fig. 4. aFGF-NP increased the expression of pAkt and up-regulated the ratio of pAkt/Akt in diabetic rats. (A) representative immunohistochemical staining of PAkt expression (400×); (B) Quantitative analyses of the expression of Caspase-3; (C) western blot analysis of the expression of PAkt and Akt; (D) Quantitative analyses of the ratio of PAkt/Akt. $n = 8$ per group. Data are presented as Mean ± SD. [*]$P < 0.05$ *vs.* control group; [#]$P < 0.05$ *vs.* DM group; [+]$P < 0.05$ *vs.* aFGF-NP + UTMD group.

shown in Fig. 5A–B, myocardial microvascular density (MCD, vascular cells in brown) was significantly lower in DM group (14 n/hpf) than the control group (40 n/hpf) ($P < 0.01$). The aFGF treated groups had significantly higher MCD than the DM group ($P < 0.05$). Additionally, the group treated with both aFGF-NP and UTMD had higher MCD (35 n/hpf) than the other aFGF groups ($P < 0.05$).

4. Discussion

Recently, clinical studies suggested that the increased risk of cardiac infraction and cardiac failure in diabetic patients could be caused by significantly reduced serum levels of bFGF [20,21]. As an analog of bFGF, aFGF induce similar beneficial effects in the diabetic heart [7]. Due to the surface charge, aFGF has a better biocompatibility, higher affinity with heart cells when compared with bFGF [22]. Researchers therefore studied aFGF as a therapeutic agent for DCM prevention. However, it remains difficult to apply aFGF clinically due to current inefficient delivery methods.

Before proceeding to extensive evaluation of the *in vivo* therapeutic and pharmacodynamic effects, the obvious concerns about the biological stability and encapsulation efficiency of aFGF in our new nanoparticle system needed to be addressed. These are common issues associated with any protein drugs carried by delivery systems. From the characterization studies (Supplement Table S1), aFGF-NP was shown to have high encapsulation efficiency and good bioactivity *in vitro*. Our novel Poloxamer 188-grafted heparin copolymer apparently helped to bind aFGF as this protein has a natural affinity for heparin, and the good binding and encapsulation likely have preserved the aFGF stability as indicated by the bioactivity data. In addition, the encapsulation of aFGF-NP showed little changes after UTMD treatment (supplemental Fig. S2), supporting the high stability of NP for aFGF transportation.

Although the mechanisms of UTMD-facilitated drug delivery have not yet been fully understood, a direct physi-

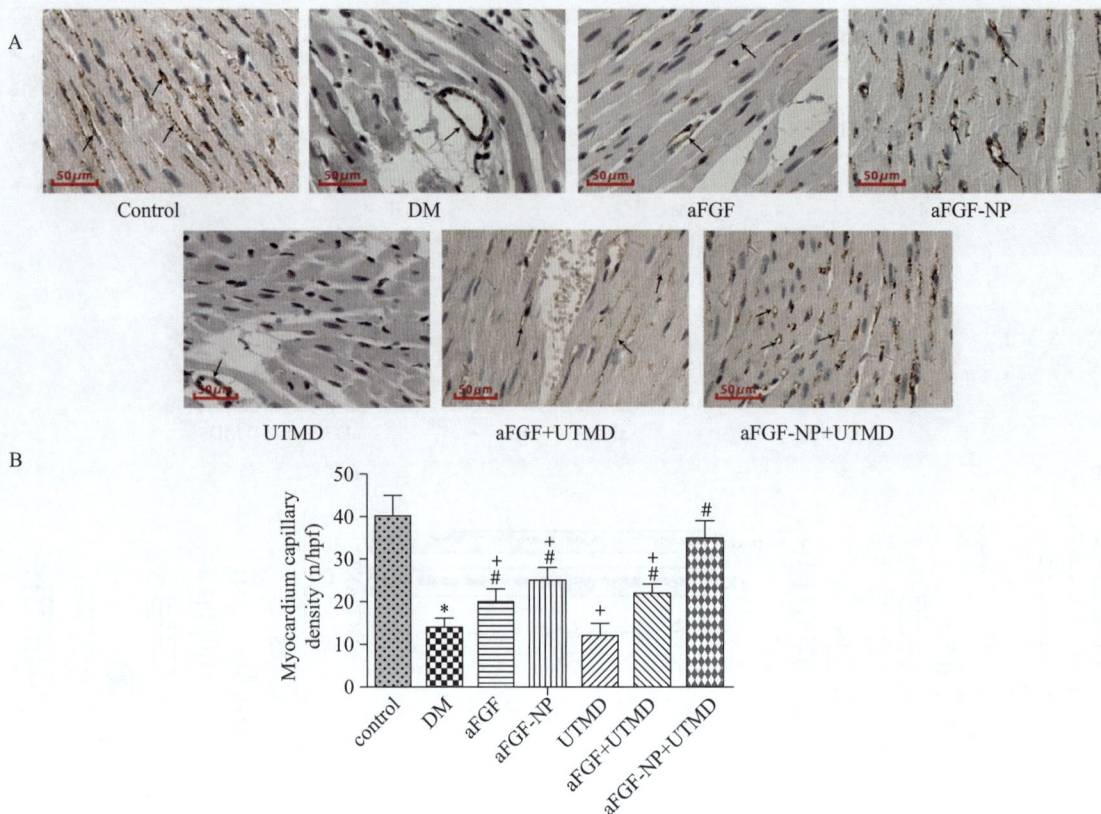

Fig. 5. aFGF-NP increased myocardial microvascular density of the diabetic heart and improves myocardial perfusion. (A) representative immunohistochemical staining of CD31 expression. (200×, arrow indicates CD31-positive cardiomyocytes stained in brown); (B) Quantitative analyses of the value of MCD. $n = 8$ per group. Data are presented as Mean ± SD. $^*P < 0.05$ vs. control group; $^\#P < 0.05$ vs. DM group; $^+P < 0.05$ vs. aFGF-NP + UTMD group.

cal route of transport often termed sonoporation is most likely involved [23,24]. Sonoporation is the use of ultrasound for modifying the permeability of the cell plasma membrane. Sonoporation is transient and dynamic, involving complex processes of bubble physics, bubble–cell interactions, and subsequent cellular effects that all affect the ultimate delivery outcome. As the basis of sonoporation, ultrasound cavitation depends highly on the amplitude and frequency of the ultrasound wave, as well as the size and material properties of the compressible objects [25]. Unlike gas-filled microbubbles used for ultrasound imaging, normal nanoparticles present a thick shell and a weakly compressible core, which can hardly produce effective volumetric oscillations in ultrasound field. [26]. But volumetric oscillations are the mechanism for facilitating drug release, increasing drug penetration and producing backscattered echoes that can be used for imaging [25]. Under the PMB sonoportion, the microjet formation from intertially collapsing microbubbles can create pores mechanically in the cytomembrane which is composed of a phospholipid bilayer [27]. Endocytosis and subsequent transcytosis can be stimulated through this localized sonoportion on adjacent cells, which can increase the membrane permeability for aFGF-NP [24]. In addition, sonoporation on cell membranes resulted from PMB's cavitation can last for a period of time because the enlarged membrane pores needed time to restore back to normal size [28,29]. Therefore, the mechanism of aFGF-NP combined with UTMD technique is mainly based on the synergistic effects of NP's transportation and PMB's cavitation.

No doubt, nanoparticles have many other advantages facilitating UTMD-mediated targeted delivery for aFGF. For example, the long circulation time of nanoparticles in vivo can improve the heart accumulation of aFGF-NP, because the lasting sonoporation effects after UTMD treatment will remain beneficial for the absorption of residual aFGF-NP in the blood circulation by the myocardial cells [30].

Notably, some researchers reported that the application of ultrasound to solid polymeric nanoparticles appears to be effective in reducing cavitation threshold in water, even in the absence of preformed gas bubbles. But other investigators did not report whether these particles lowered thresholds or enhanced ultrasound activity [31,32]. Considering the physical mechanism of ultrasound cavitation, different conditions (especially the setting of ultrasound wave and physiochemical properties of the objects) may result in large variation of delivery outcome which should be further investigated in detailed study.

Another issue needing clarification is the efficiency of aFGF delivery to diabetic hearts. Without knowing if aFGF-NP + UTMD therapy had led to sufficient aFGF accumulation in the damaged heart tissues, it would not be possible to attribute the various *in vivo* effects to this combined therapy. Western blot analysis of heart tissues at 12 weeks has confirmed that the aFGF-NP + UTMD group demonstrated the highest aFGF level among all groups (Fig. 2E). The results indicated the effectiveness of *in vivo* aFGF delivery to heart.

It may be questioned that the duration of UTMD treatment was too limited (US exposure duration per time = 10 s, repeat three times with off intervals of 1 s) to achieve the observed long-term aFGF build-up. But the sonoporation on a cell membrane resulting from UTMD would continue for a period of time because the enlarged membrane pores needed time to restore to normal size [28]. Even though the microbubbles completely disappeared in the heart, the lasting sonoporation in the heart remained beneficial for the absorption of residual aFGF-NP or aFGF in the blood circulation. The finding suggests that the duration of the UTMD treatment to enhance aFGF-NP delivery does not have to be unduly long and frequent, which makes this treatment more clinically feasible. Though some reports mentioned the potential security problems of aFGF in intravenous injection [7], little pathological change was observed in both adjacent and remote tissues (brain, kidney, liver) in our study.

In this study, western blot was used to detect the content of aFGF in cardiomyocytes *in vivo* after treatment. From the result, aFGF-NP + UTMD group showed the highest concentration of aFGF among the experimental groups. Under the dynamic process of pore formation on the targeted cells during the PMB's sonoporation [12], we can assume that aFGF-NP's accumulation in myocardial cells plays a main role in the following DCM prevention after UTMD-facilitated delivery. In a recent study on using gold NP and sonoporation strategy for the treatment of heart failure [33], similar conclusion has also been observed which supports our assumption.

The focus of this study is on the impact of the aFGF-NP/UTMD combined therapy on various pathophysiological aspects related to DCM progression. Consistent with previous reports [34], our data of transthoracic echocardiography (*i.e.* reduced absolute values of Vs, Sc and SRc) in Table 1 and hemodynamic evaluation in Table 2 showed that the diabetic rats left untreated for 12 weeks were characterized by declined diastolic and systolic myocardial performance when compared with the non-diabetic control.

These functional changes were associated with corresponding morphological damages such as excess collagen accumulation and cardiac damage (Figs. 1B and 2A) as well as molecular changes. Data in Fig. 2B–D show increasing expression of pro-apoptotic proteins Caspase-3 and Bax coupled with decreasing expression of anti-apoptotic protein BCL-2 and inactivating pro-survival pathways of PI3K/Akt in diabetic animals (*e.g.* DM group). These changes finally caused cell apoptosis (Fig. 3), which led to cardiac fibrosis and reduction of myocardial microvascular density in the untreated diabetic heart. In contrast, in all of these studies we have demonstrated that long-term aFGF-NP + UTMD combined treatment (twice weekly treatments for 12 consecutive weeks) can effectively prevent the development of such characteristic alterations of DCM. In fact, all of the parameters of cardiac functions and morphology (Tables 1 and 2, Fig. 1B and 3A) in aFGF-NP + UTMD group were comparable to the non-diabetic control. Our data indicate that 12 consecutive weeks of aFGF-NP + UTMD combined therapy nearly reversed the progress of DCM in diabetic animals.

We also noted that the amount of aFGF delivered by intravenous injection over the course of 12 weeks could increase the aFGF levels by upward of 300% in the best case. As reported in a previous study [21], diabetes was found to impair the expression of endogenous FGFs. Until now, no evidence has been reported to support the up-regulation of aFGF expression after aFGF treatment for diabetics. From the results in this study, the high efficiency of PMB's sonoporation and NP's transportation may contribute to the high aFGF level in heart.

The observed efficacy of aFGF-NP to prevent DCM in the diabetic rats can be attributed to two mechanisms. First of all, aFGF activated the important PI3K/Akt signaling pathway by phosphorylation. Phosphorylated Akt has been shown to reduce myocardial apoptosis in response to ischemia-reperfusion injury [35,36]. After Akt activation by aFGF, the activated Akt can modulate the activities of many downstream targets such as inhibition of Caspaes-3 activity and induction of anti-apoptotic effects by phosphorylation and translocation of Bax to the mitochondria to suppress the release of cytochrome [37]. It should be noted that to trigger all these potentially pro-survival molecular events in the diabetic hearts, the aFGF molecules first need to get access to individual cells of myocardium. This is a challenging task considering the large molecular weight of a protein drug like aFGF and its susceptibility to degradation especially in blood circulation when systemically administered. Our results confirmed that the aFGF-NP combined with UTMD had the best effects to deliver aFGF into the myocardial cells. aFGF-NP likely protected the aFGF and UTMD enhanced the local uptake by the myocardial tissues using the sonoportation effect as previously mentioned. The result was reduction in the apoptosis and fibrosis of cardiomyocytes, and these effects were not mediated *via* blood glucose level regulation (Fig. 1A) like most of the current standard drug treatment options.

aFGF can also improve cardiac perfusion by increasing microvascular density. "Microangiopathy" has been demonstrated in the myocardium of diabetic rats and becomes one of the marked characteristics of DCM [38]. As the diabetes disease progresses, the microangiopathy exerts changes in the morphology and density of microvasculature. Morphology changes include thickening of the capillary basement membrane, medial thickening of the arterial and perivascular fibrosis [39,40]. The density of the microvessel of diabetics is also significantly decreased due to the apoptosis of endothelial cells. Consequently, the perfusion to the diabetic heart tissue is compromised. The aFGF therapy can reduce apoptosis of endothelial cells, increases the density of the microvessel and reduces pervascular fibrosis. In our study, the CD31 immunohisto-chemical staining in Fig. 5 also confirmed comparable therapeutic effect against the DCM-related microangiopathy. Among various aFGF treated groups, the aFGF-NP + UTMD combined treatment again demonstrated the highest effectiveness in increasing density of microvasulature, and this was achieved without the need for the risky local injection procedure.

Taken together, our study has provided extensive *in vivo* evidence to strongly suggest that NPs combining with UTMD technique have great translational potential in delivery of aFGF for the prevention of DCM. Moreover, our novel drug delivery system has the potential for the diabetic heart targeted delivery for other biological macromoleculars with the similar physiological activities to aFGF. Once the optimal dose of drug is determined and the delivery system is fully standardized, this technique plus the current commonly-used glucose control treatment will provide diabetic patients with an effective and feasible strategy for DCM prevention efficient prevention of DCM, avoiding this dangerous medical condition.

Supplementary data

Supplementary data to this article can be found online at http://dx. doi.org/10.1016/j.jconrel.2015.12.030.

References

[1] Goyal BR, Mehta AA. Diabetic cardiomyopathy: pathophysiological mechanisms and cardiac dysfuntion[J]. Human & experimental toxicology, 2013, 32(6): 571-590.

[2] Miki T, Yuda S, Kouzu H, *et al.* Diabetic cardiomyopathy: pathophysiology and clinical features[J]. Heart failure reviews, 2013, 18(2): 149-166.

[3] Fowlkes V, Clark J, Fix C, *et al.* Type II diabetes promotes a myofibroblast phenotype in cardiac fibroblasts[J]. Life sciences, 2013, 92(11): 669-676.

[4] Papa G, Degano C, Iurato MP, *et al.* Macrovascular complication phenotypes in type 2 diabetic patients[J]. Cardiovascular diabetology, 2013, 12(1): 20.

[5] Fischer C, Schneider M, Carmeliet P. Principles and therapeutic implications of angiogenesis, vasculogenesis and arteriogenesis[J]. Handbook of experimental pharmacology, 2006, 176(2): 157-212.

[6] Chen W, Fu XB, Ge SL, *et al.* Intravenous acid fibroblast growth factor protects intestinal mucosal cells against ischemia-reperfusion injury *via* regulating Bcl-2/Bax expression[J]. World journal of gastroenterology, 2005, 11(22): 3419-3425.

[7] Zhang C, Zhang L, Chen S, *et al.* The prevention of diabetic cardiomyopathy by non-mitogenic acidic fibroblast growth factor is probably mediated by the suppression of oxidative stress and damage[J].

PloS one, 2013, 8(12): e82287.

[8] Chappell JC, Song J, Burke CW, *et al.* Targeted delivery of nanoparticles bearing fibroblast growth factor-2 by ultrasonic microbubble destruction for therapeutic arteriogenesis[J]. Small (Weinheim an der Bergstrasse, Germany), 2008, 4(10): 1769-1777.

[9] Lentacker I, de Cock I, Deckers R, *et al.* Understanding ultrasound induced sonoporation: definitions and underlying mechanisms[J]. Advanced drug delivery reviews, 2014, 72: 49-64.

[10] VanBavel E. Effects of shear stress on endothelial cells: possible relevance for ultrasound applications[J]. Progress in biophysics and molecular biology, 2007, 93(1-3): 374-383.

[11] Forbes MM, Steinberg RL, O'Brien WD. Examination of inertial cavitation of Optison in producing sonoporation of chinese hamster ovary cells[J]. Ultrasound in medicine & biology, 2008, 34(12): 2009-2018.

[12] Forbes MM, Steinberg RL, O'Brien WD. Frequency-dependent evaluation of the role of definity in producing sonoporation of Chinese hamster ovary cells[J]. Journal of ultrasound in medicine : official journal of the American Institute of Ultrasound in Medicine, 2011, 30(1): 61-69.

[13] Du J, Shi QS, Sun Y, *et al.* Enhanced delivery of monomethoxy-poly (ethylene glycol)-poly(lactic-co-glycolic acid)-poly l-lysine

nanoparticles loading platelet-derived growth factor BB small interfering RNA by ultrasound and/or microbubbles to rat retinal pigment epithelium cells[J]. The journal of gene medicine, 2011, 13(6): 312-323.

[14] Tian JL, Zhao YZ, Jin Z, et al. Synthesis and characterization of Poloxamer 188-grafted heparin copolymer[J]. Drug development and industrial pharmacy, 2010, 36(7): 832-838.

[15] Lu CT, Zhao YZ, Wu Y, et al. Experiment on enhancing antitumor effect of intravenous epirubicin hydrochloride by acoustic cavitation in situ combined with phospholipid-based microbubbles[J]. Cancer chemotherapy and pharmacology, 2011, 68(2): 343-348.

[16] Jiang Y, Wei N, Lu T, et al. Intranasal brain-derived neurotrophic factor protects brain from ischemic insult via modulating local inflammation in rats[J]. Neuroscience, 2011, 172: 398-405.

[17] Lu CT, Zhao YZ, Gao HS, et al. Comparing encapsulation efficiency and ultrasound-triggered release for protein between phospholipid-based microbubbles and liposomes[J]. Journal of microencapsulation, 2010, 27(2): 115-121.

[18] Kang NN, Fu L, Xu J, et al. Testosterone improves cardiac function and alters angiotensin II receptors in isoproterenol-induced heart failure[J]. Archives of cardiovascular diseases, 2012, 105(2): 68-76.

[19] Katare R, Caporali A, Zentilin L, et al. Intravenous Gene Therapy With PIM-1 Via a Cardiotropic Viral Vector Halts the Progression of Diabetic Cardiomyopathy Through Promotion of Prosurvival Signaling[J]. Circulation Research, 2011, 108(10): 1238-1251.

[20] Song Y, Song Z, Zhang L, et al. Diabetes enhances lipopolysaccharide-induced cardiac toxicity in the mouse model[J]. Cardiovascular toxicology, 2003, 3(4): 363-372.

[21] Yeboah J, Sane DC, Crouse JR, et al. Low plasma levels of FGF-2 and PDGF-BB are associated with cardiovascular events in type II diabetes mellitus (diabetes heart study)[J]. Disease markers, 2007, 23(3): 173-178.

[22] Beenken A, Mohammadi M. The FGF family: biology, pathophysiology and therapy[J]. Nature reviews. Drug discovery, 2009, 8(3): 235-253.

[23] Schlicher RK, Radhakrishna H, Tolentino TP, et al. Mechanism of intracellular delivery by acoustic cavitation[J]. Ultrasound in medicine & biology, 2006, 32(6): 915-924.

[24] Fan Z, Kumon RE, Park J, et al. Intracellular delivery and calcium transients generated in sonoporation facilitated by microbubbles[J]. Journal of controlled release : official journal of the Controlled Release Society, 2010, 142(1): 31-39.

[25] Sirsi SR, Borden MA. State-of-the-art materials for ultrasound-triggered drug delivery[J]. Advanced drug delivery reviews, 2014, 72: 3-14.

[26] Guédra M, Valier-Brasier T, Conoir JM, et al. Influence of shell compressibility on the ultrasonic properties of polydispersed suspensions of nanometric encapsulated droplets[J]. The Journal of the Acoustical Society of America, 2014, 135(3): 1044-1055.

[27] Ohl CD, Arora M, Ikink R, et al. Sonoporation from jetting cavitation bubbles[J]. Biophysical journal, 2006, 91(11): 4285-4295.

[28] Zhao YZ, Luo YK, Lu CT, et al. Phospholipids-based microbubbles sonoporation pore size and reseal of cell membrane cultured in vitro[J]. Journal of drug targeting, 2008, 16(1): 18-25.

[29] Fu H, Comer J, Cai W, et al. Sonoporation at Small and Large Length Scales: Effect of Cavitation Bubble Collapse on Membranes[J]. The journal of physical chemistry letters, 2015, 6(3): 413-418.

[30] Miller DL, Dou C, Lu X, et al. Use of Theranostic Strategies in Myocardial Cavitation-Enabled Therapy[J]. Ultrasound in medicine & biology, 2015, 41(7): 1865-1875.

[31] Larina IV, Evers BM, Ashitkov TV, et al. Enhancement of drug delivery in tumors by using interaction of nanoparticles with ultrasound radiation[J]. Technology in cancer research & treatment, 2005, 4(2): 217-226.

[32] Figueiredo M, Esenaliev R. PLGA Nanoparticles for Ultrasound-Mediated Gene Delivery to Solid Tumors[J]. Journal of Drug Delivery, 2012(2012): 767839.

[33] Spivak MY, Bubnov RV, Yemets IM, et al. Development and testing of gold nanoparticles for drug delivery and treatment of heart failure: a theranostic potential for PPP cardiology[J]. The EPMA journal, 2013, 4(1): 20.

[34] Meloni M, Descamps B, Caporali A, et al. Nerve growth factor gene therapy using adeno-associated viral vectors prevents cardiomyopathy in type 1 diabetic mice. Diabetes, 2012, 61(1): 229-240.

[35] Armstrong. Protein kinase activation and myocardial ischemia/reperfusion injury[J]. Cardiovascular Research, 2004, 61(3): 427-436.

[36] Bae S, Zhang L. Gender differences in cardioprotection against ischemia/reperfusion injury in adult rat hearts: focus on Akt and protein kinase C signaling[J]. The Journal of pharmacology and experimental therapeutics, 2005, 315(3): 1125-1135.

[37] Linseman DA, Butts BD, Precht TA, et al. Glycogen synthase kinase-3beta phosphorylates Bax and promotes its mitochondrial localization during neuronal apoptosis[J]. The Journal of neuroscience : the official journal of the Society for Neuroscience, 2004, 24(44): 9993-10002.

[38] Factor SM, Minase T, Sonnenblick EH. Clinical and morphological features of human hypertensive-diabetic cardiomyopathy[J]. American Heart Journal, 1980, 99(4): 446-458.

[39] Kawaguchi M, Techigawara M, Ishihata T, et al. A comparison of ultrastructural changes on endomyocardial biopsy specimens obtained from patients with diabetes mellitus with and without hypertension[J]. Heart and vessels, 1997, 12(6): 267-274.

[40] Yarom R, Zirkin H, Stämmler G, et al. Human coronary microvessels in diabetes and ischaemia. Morphometric study of autopsy material[J]. The Journal of pathology, 1992, 166(3): 265-270.

Functional and pathological improvements of the hearts in diabetes model by the combined therapy of bFGF-loaded nanoparticles with ultrasound-targeted microbubble destruction

Yingzheng Zhao, Xiaokun Li

1. Introduction

With the modern lifestyle, diabetes mellitus (DM) has become a serious threat to human health [1]. Among the complications of DM, diabetic cardiomyopathy (DCM) is a leading cause of morbidity and mortality [2].

Basic fibroblast growth factor (bFGF or FGF-2) is a member of the FGF family which consists of at least 22 homologous peptides. bFGF can stimulate proliferation of fibroblasts and capillary endothelial cells, thus promoting angiogenesis and wound healing [3,4]. Previous studies have shown that intramuscular injection of plasmids coding bFGF alone could improve ischemic hind limb blood flow and increase angiogenesis [5]. Animal experiments showed that bFGF and FGF receptor expressions are increased in the infarcted heart at an early stage following myocardial infarction, which is spatially and temporally coincident with angiogenesis. This indicates that bFGF is involved in the regulation of cardiac angiogenesis and repair [6]. All of these findings suggest that bFGF has good therapeutic potential for the DCM patients. This notion is further supported by our finding that bFGF protected the heart from ischemia/reperfusion-induced oxidative damage and infarction in diabetic rats [7].

An effective approach to increase exogenous bFGF concentration in the damaged heart tissue of DCM patients is currently unavailable. Although direct injection of bFGF into the heart has been intensively investigated, intramyocardial delivery poses many risks that prevent its clinical application. In addition, the cellular uptake of bFGF following this approach is also inefficient, resulting in a low level of gene expression [8]. Besides direct injection, the most prevalent method of bFGF therapy in the literature is via viral-mediated bFGF gene delivery. This approach has many drawbacks; for example, several human clinical trials with viral vectors have led to severe inflammatory responses with high fever [9] and hepatotoxicity [10]. These viral systems are also limited for bFGF gene transfer, and not for supplying an exogeneous source of therapeutic bFGF that can be readily utilized by the cardiac cells for damage recovery.

Comparing with the viral delivery approach, non-viral carrier systems are potentially safer and more convenient, and can be used not only for bFGF gene, but also for direct delivery of exogenous bFGF protein. Micro-or nano-carriers have been widely explored as the delivery systems of other protein drugs. These include nanoparticles (NP), liposomes, microspheres, microemulsion, and micelles. Emerging evidence indicates that NP are particularly advantageous for the delivery of bioactive drugs because NP are able to improve drug penetration capacity, protect the encapsulated drugs from biological and chemical degradation and be efficiently transported by active endocytosis or transcytosis mechanisms [11,12]. It should be noted that up to date, although nonviral approaches for delivery of bFGF-based therapeutics (bFGF or its gene) have been explored [13–15], their use for bFGF delivery to the heart especially the DCM areas has not been studied. The key of success to this application relies on efficient and specific delivery of the bFGF nanotherapeutics to the heart and demonstration of strong bFGF-mediated healing activities in the damaged cardiac tissues.

Ultrasound imaging has been used as an effective, noninvasive diagnostic method for cardiovascular diseases. When combined with the ultrasonic microbubble contrast agents, the resulting ultrasound-targeted microbubble destruction (UTMD) technique has been developed as a promising method for targeted delivery of bioactive agents to cardiac tissue [16]. The contrast agents enable visual imaging control and microbubble destruction can provide cavitation-facilitated drug absorption promoting effect. UTMD technique may therefore serve as a valuable tool to further improve the heart specificity and efficacy of bFGF nanotherapeutics for patients with DCM.

The overall goal of this study was to establish an efficient bFGF delivery approach for DCM treatment by combining the power of NP carriers and UTMD technique. In our previous study, we reported a novel copolymerknown as Poloxamer 188-grafted heparin copolymer. This copolymer has demonstrated a high affinity for bFGF and excellent physical strength and biocompatibility [17]. In this study, novel bFGF-loaded NP (bFGF-NP) composed of Poloxamer 188-grafted heparin copolymer was prepared by water-in-water emulsion technique, and this bFGF-NP was integrated with an UTMD system made of phospholipid-based microbubbles (PMBs). We hypothesized that the UTMD technique would significantly improve the performance of bFGF-NP nanotherapy in DCM-induced subjects. Specifically, two aims were studied: (1) to evaluate the various characteristics of bFGF-NP including their morphology, encapsulation efficiency and *in vitro* biological activities, and (2) to study the *in vivo* therapeutic effects of the bFGF-NP/UTMD combined treatment in a rat model with type 1 DM and DCM induced. The findings are significant for validating a less invasive, more efficient form of growth factor therapy to repair the damaged heart tissues of diabetes patients.

2.　Materials and methods

2.1　Chemicals

Hydrogenated phosphatidylcholine (HPC, HPC content > 99%) was purchased from Doosan Corporation Biotech BU, Kyonggi Do, Korea, polyethylene glycol 1,500 from Qingming Chemical Plant, Zhejiang, China, Poloxamer 188 from Shenyang Chemical Plant, Liaoning, China, streptozotocin (STZ) from Sigma Inc, St Louis, MO, USA. Butanol was analytical grade and purchased from Beijing Chemical Plant, Beijing, China, and perfluoropropane was electronic grade purchased from Institute of Special Gas, Tianjing, China. Basic fibroblast growth factor (bFGF) was ordered from Gelusite Biology Technology Company, Zhejiang, China. Poloxamer 188-grafted heparin copolymer was synthesized by our laboratory as previously reported [17].

2.2　Preparation of phospholipid-based microbubbles (PMBs)

PMBs were prepared by sonication-lyophilization method. Briefly, HPC, polyethylene glycol 1500, and Poloxamer 188 were dissolved in butanol and sonicated at 30℃ using JY 92-II ultrasonic processor (KunShan US Instrument Inc., China) at a frequency of 40 kHz and power of 160 W for 3 min. The solution was stored at 0℃ for 30 min and at −20℃ for 1 h. The coagulated solution was then lyophilized at 5×10^{-4} Pa pressure for 20 h (primary drying at −48℃ for 15 h and then the temperature was gradually raised to 10℃ < 5 h). PMB lyophilized powder was put in 10 ml vials (200 mg/vial) and saturated with perfluoropropane. PMB solution for animal experiments was obtained by adding 2 ml sterile 0.9% *w/v* NaCl solution in lyophilized PMB. As measured by a coulter counter (Coulter Corporation, Hialeah, FL), PMB concentration was about 2×10^{9} bubbles/ml with an average diameter of 3.4 μm.

2.3　Preparation and characterization of bFGF-NP

2.3.1　Preparation of bFGF-NP

Preparation of bFGF-NP was carried out using water-in-water emulsion technique. High concentration bFGF (10 mg/ml) was dissolved in 1 ml of 20% (*w/v*) Poloxamer 188-grafted heparin copolymer solution. The solution was added into 2 ml of 2.0% (*w/v*) gelatin solution to produce a homogeneous mixture. Under sonication (110 W, 15℃) using a probe sonicator, D, L-glyceraldehyde was injected into the mixture until its final concentration reached 0.1% *w/v* to initiate the cross-linking reaction. The mixture solution was bathed at 5℃ under magnetic stirring at 2,500 rpm for 5 h to form the bFGF-NP suspension. The final bFGF concentration in stock bFGF-NP solution was adjusted to 1 mg/ml.

Empty nanoparticles (blank NP, using gelatin solution instead of bFGF gelatin solution in preparation) and bFGF solution (bFGF dissolved in 0.9% NaCl solution) were also prepared for the following experiments. The final bFGF concentration in bFGF solution was adjusted to 1 mg/ml.

2.3.2　Characteristics of bFGF-NP

The morphology of bFGF-NP and blank NP was determined using scanning electron microscopy (SEM) (X-650, Hitachi Co., Ltd., Tokyo, Japan). Size and zeta potential values of bFGF-NP and blank NP were determined by dynamic light scattering using a Zeta Potential/Particle Sizer Nicomp™ 380 ZLS (PSS. Nicomp, Santa Barbara, CA, USA). The pH of bFGF-NP suspension used for zeta potential analysis is 7.0.

To determine the encapsulation efficiency of bFGF-NP, approximately 1.5 ml of the bFGF-NP dispersion was placed in microtubes and centrifuged at 10,000 g for 40 min. The supernatant was then collected and diluted for content determination of bFGF using an ELISA kit [18]. The drug encapsulation efficiency was calculated as indicated below. The experiments were performed in triplicate.

Encapsulation efficiency (%)=(total amount of drugs−amount of drugs in the supernatant)/total amount of drugs added initially × 100%

Bioactivity of bFGF in bFGF-NP was assayed using NIH-3 T3 cells. The cells were grown in RPMI-1640 medium supplemented with 10% fetal bovine serum (FBS) in a 96-well plate (7,000 cells per well). The cells were incubated for 24 h and placed in 0.1% FBS supplemented medium for 24 h, and incubated with bFGF-NP for another 72 h. The number of viable cells was determined by adding 20 μl of methylthiazoletetrazolium (MTT; 5 mg/ml) to each well and incubating for 5 h. After removal of the medium, 100 μl dimethyl sulfoxide (DMSO) was added to each well and the plate was kept at room temperature for 30 min. The absorbance of the solution in the plate was measured at 490/690 nm.

2.4 Fluorescent labeling of bFGF with fluorescein isothiocyanate

In order to trace the bFGF distribution in various *in vitro* experiments, bFGF used in the bFGF-NP and bFGF solution was labeled with fluorescein isothiocyanate (FITC) as follows. One ml of FITC solution (100 μg/ml in dimethylsulfoxide) was added slowly into 1 ml bFGF solution (10 mg/ml in bicarbonate buffer, pH = 8.8, 0.1 M). The mixture was incubated for 3 h at room temperature in darkness with gentle stirring. Unconjugated FITC was eliminated from the labeled bFGF (FITC-bFGF) by dialysis (cut-off 10 000 Da, Snake skin Dialysis Tubing, Permolecular BioScience, Erembodegem-Aalst, Belgium) and then gel chromatography (Sephadex G-25 M column, Sigma, St. Louis, MO, USA). The FITC-bFGF solution was desalted by dialysis against ultrapure water and lyophilized to obtain FITC-bFGF powder. Sodium dodecyl sulfate polyacrylamide gel electrophoresis (SDS-PAGE) of FITC-bFGF indicated that the bFGF molecules remained intact after the labeling procedure.

2.5 Fluorescence imaging in vitro

LV cardiomyocytes from 1-to 2-day-old Sprague–Dawley (SD) rats were cultured in 96-well plates. After 48 h, the cells received different treatments. PMB (3.4 μm in diameter, final volume concentration = 5%) and bFGF-containing treatment (bFGF-NP or bFGF solution, final concentration = 50 μg bFGF/ml) were added in fresh growth media containing 10% FBS. UTMD was generated by a linear array transducer (14 MHz, Acuson Sequoia 512C system, Siemens). Cultured LV cardiomyocytes were exposed to ultrasound radiation in a device as reported in our previous paper [19]. The ultrasound transducer was inserted into a 37℃ water tank and directly faced the bottom of the cell plate. A spongy rubber ultrasound shield was used to focus ultrasound on the cells. MBD function key attached to the machine was used to blast the microbubbles (MI = 1.9, exposure time = 10 s). After insonation, the cells were incubated for 4 h to settle and then imaged with a Nikon fluorescence microscope (Nikon ECLIPSE 80i, Ruikezhongyi Company, Beijing, China). MTT-based assay was performed to evaluate the percentage of cell viability on 24 h after the insonation.

2.6 Flow cytometry

Flow cytometry (FACS Calibur FCM, Becton Dickinson, San Jose, CA) was conducted to detect the effect of using NP or UTMD on FITC-bFGF uptake by H9c2 heart myoblast cells. The cells were cultured in 6-well plates overnight at standard cell culture conditions and subjected to treatments including UTMD only, bFGF only, bFGF-NP only, bFGF + UTMD or bFGF-NP + UTMD, respectively. Untreated H9c2 cells served as the blank control. 24 h after treatment, duplicate cell samples from each group were trypsinized, washed with ice cold PBS three times and resuspended for flow cytometry. Live cells were gated by forward/ side scattering from a total of 10,000 events. bFGF or bFGF-NP was detected in the fluorescence level (FL2) channel of the flow cytometer. The efficiency of bFGF cellular uptake was analyzed by Cell Quest software (B. D. Co., USA) using a Power Macintosh 7600 Computer (Becton–Dickinson, San Jose, CA). MTT-based assay was performed to evaluate the percentage of cell viability at 24 h after the insonation.

2.7 DCM rat model and treatment

Diabetes was induced in SD rats by intraperitoneal injection of STZ at 70 mg/kg after 12 h of fasting. STZ was prepared as 1% solution in 0.1 M citrate buffer (pH 4.0–4.5). On the 3rd day, 7th day, and 8th week after final STZ administration, the fasting blood glucose was measured from the tail tip using an autoanalyzer (Surestep, Roche, Germany). Only the rats with fasting blood glucose levels exceeding 16.7 mM and cardiac dysfunction 8 weeks after STZ treatment (confirmed by echocardiograph) were selected as diabetic rats with DCM (*i.e.* DCM rats). All animal experiments were performed under the approval and guidance of the Institutional Animal Care and Use Committee of Wenzhou Medical Universtiy.

DCM rats were randomized into six groups: (1) Control: DCM rats without any treatment; (2) bFGF alone; (3) bFGF-NP alone; (4) UTMD (*i.e.* PMB only); (5) bFGF + UTMD (*i.e.* bFGF/PMB mixture); and (6) bFGF-NP + UTMD (*i.e.* bFGF-NP/PMB mixture). The treatments in groups (2) to (6) were administered prior to ultrasound treatment on the 1 st, the 3rd, and the 5th day. The dose of bFGF in bFGF-NP or bFGF solution was 3 μg/kg weight.

The drug and ultrasound treatments were administered as follows. DCM rats were anesthetized with intraperitoneal injection of chloral hydrate (350 mg/kg body weight) 5 min before the experiment. The thoracic region was shaved, and the rats were placed in the supine position. A 20-gauge cannula was inserted into the tail vein and treatment solution was infused. Similar to the experiment *in vitro*, a linear array transducer (14 MHz, Acuson Sequoia 512C system, Siemens) was used to generate the UTMD effect. In the groups with UTMD, the linear array transducer was placed over the heart (short axis view; depth = 3.0–4.0 cm) to view papillary muscles of the left ventricle. When a large number of microbubbles were seen filling the heart, the MBD function key attached to the machine was used to blast the microbubbles (MI = 1.9, exposure time = 10 s).

2.8 Evaluation of the effects of bFGF treatment on cardiac function of DCM rats

Cardiac function was evaluated with two methods. Transthoracic echocardiography was performed on all rats during the 8th week (*i.e.* before treatment) and the 12th week (*i.e.* the 4th week after treatment) after diabetes induction. Rats were weighed and anesthetized by 10% chloral hydrate (3 ml/kg, peritoneal injection). The 2-D sequences of three consecutive cardiac beats were recorded with the highest possible frame rate at rest from the short axis views at the papillary muscle level. Imaging depth was adjusted to 35–40 mm, resulting in a temporal resolution at 70–90 Hz.

All images were stored as standard Digital Imaging and Communication in Medicine (DICOM) format images on MO and analyzed offline in Siemens Sygno US Workplace 3.01 (Sygno VVI, Siemens). In this study, the LV wall at mid-level from the short-axis view was divided into six segments according to the standard 16-segment model of the American Society of Echocardiography. The segments of the LV wall were plotted, the endocardial and epicardial borders were manually identified in a single frame of a cine-loop, and the borders in other frames were automatically generated, allowing operators to alter any of those contours. Next, segmental mean peak systolic radial velocity (Vs), systolic circumferential strain (Sc), and systolic circumferential strain rate (SRc) were obtained from velocity, strain, and strain rate curves provided by Sygno VVI. The system automatically set the end diastole as the baseline and Sc and SRc as negative values (Fig. 1).

Hemodynamic evaluation was also performed 4 weeks after treatment. A terminal surgical procedure was performed to evaluate LV hemodynamics as described previously [20]. Rats were anesthetized with 10% chloral hydrate (3 ml/kg, peritoneal injection), the trachea was exposed, and the animal ventilator (HX-300, TME Technology Co., Ltd, China) was connected. The pericardial cavity was opened and a 1.4 Fr miniature cardiac catheter was inserted into the LV from the apex. The LV end-systolic pressure (LVESP), end-diastolic pressure (LVEDP), and the maximum rising and dropping rates of LV pressure (± dp/dt) were measured by using a commercially available analog-to-digital converter and analyzed by Chart 5 for Windows Analysis Software.

2.9 CD31 immunohistochemical staining and cardiac capillary density measurement

After hemodynamic measurements were performed, the heart was arrested in diastole by intraventricular injection of potassium chloride solution (10% *w/v*). Hearts were excised, washed quickly in PBS, and cut into six short-axis slices from the apex to the base. Each slice was embedded in paraffin and cut into four-micron serial paraffin sections for CD31 immunohistochemistry staining with anti-rat CD31 antibody (1 ∶ 150, Sangon Biotech Co., Ltd. China) to determine the capillary density. A capillary was defined as a vessel with a diameter less than 20 μm. Myocardial capillary density (MCD) was measured by counting the number of brown-stained capillaries under 20 visual high power fields (400 ×), and presented as the mean numbers of blood vessels per high power field (n/hpf).

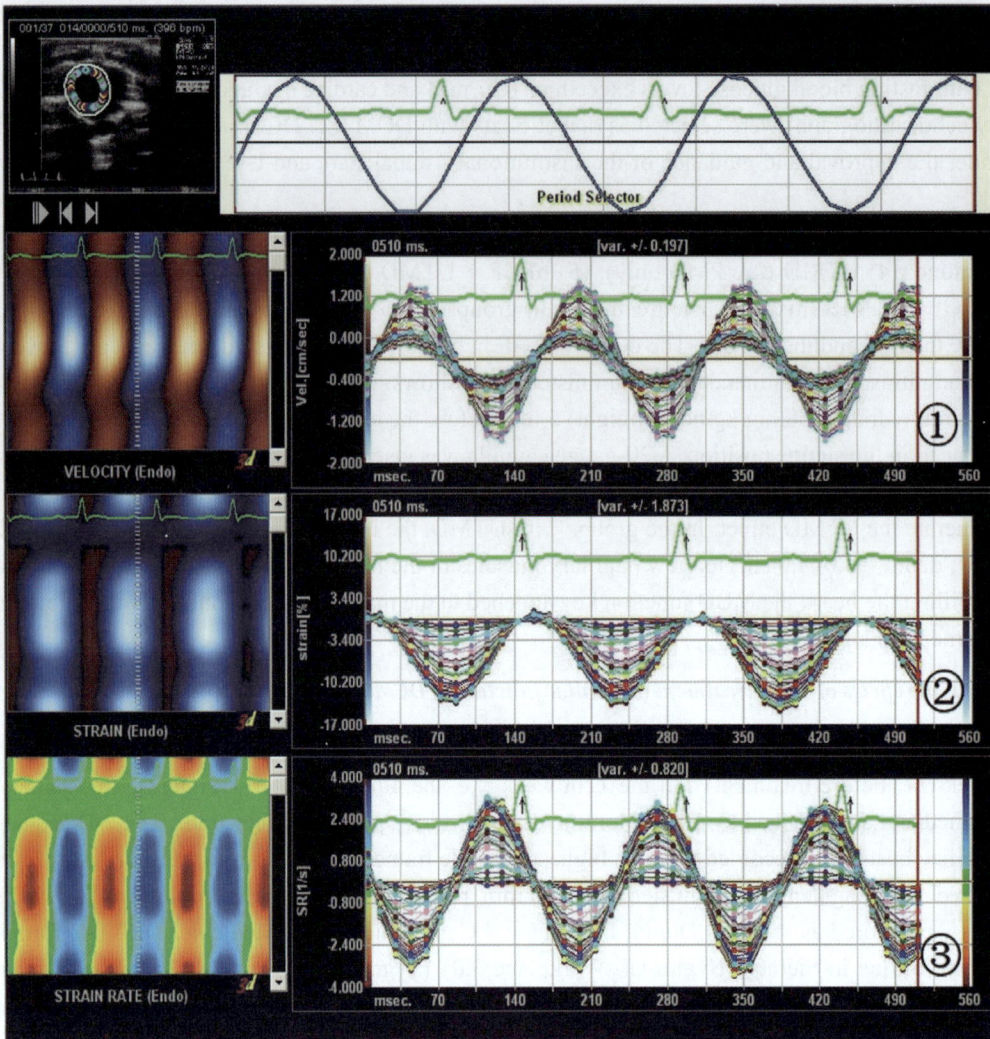

Fig. 1. Representative picture of the myocardial velocity, strain, and strain rate curve provided by Sygno VVI (1: the speed curve; 2: the strain curve; and 3: the strain rate).

2.10 Masson staining for cardiac collagen accumulation

Cardiac collagen was detected using Masson staining as described before [21]. Briefly, cardiac tissue sections were processed at 4 μm for dewaxing and rehydration and stained with Masson's trichrome staining solution. With this staining, the collagen was stained blue with a red background. Twenty fields were randomly selected per group and measured by a computer-assisted image analysis software (Image-Pro plus 6.0 imaging software, NIH). Cardiac collagen volume fraction (CVF) was obtained by calculating the mean ratio of connective tissue to the total tissue area of all the measurements of the section.

2.11 Statistical analysis

One-way ANOVA and Student's t-test or Kruskal–Wallis test were adopted for statistical comparison using the SAS 8.01 (1999–2000, SAS Institute Inc., Cary, NC, USA). The difference was considered to be statistically significant when the P-value was equal or less than 0.05.

3. Results

3.1 Characterization of bFGF-NP

Fig. 2 showed the representative SEM micrographs of the NP and bFGF-NP. Both bFGF-NP and blank NP showed good elliptical morphology. Characteristics of the NP and bFGF-NP are summarized in Table 1. Dynamic light scattering results demonstrated that the average particle size of blank NP and bFGF-NP were 106 ± 1.8 nm and 128 ± 1.7 nm, respectively. Polydispersity index (PI) is a measure of the particle size distribution. Low PI values (< 0.2) were observed in both blank NP and bFGF-NP, which indicated that blank NP and bFGF-NP approached a monodispersed system.

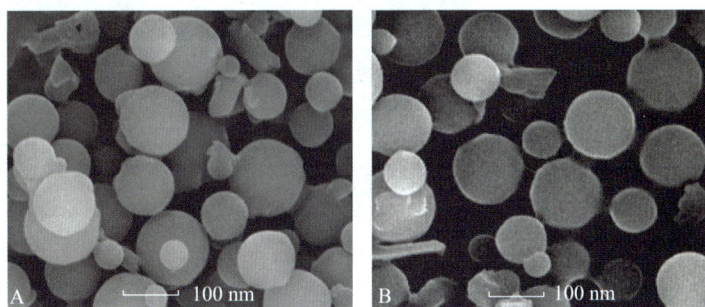

Fig. 2. Scanning electron micrographs of (A) blank NP and (B) bFGF-NP. Nanoparticles generally show uniformity with round shape.

Moderately negative zeta potential values (< -15 mV) were observed in both NP and bFGF-NP. The electrostatic repulsive forces in combination with the steric forces from the Pluronic portions would likely provide adequate dispersion stability of the nanosystems as supported by the low PI values. NP with negative charges are also less susceptible to elimination by the reticuloendothelial system than those with positive charges.

The encapsulation efficiency of bFGF-NP reached $(84.3 \pm 2.8)\%$. The bioactivity of bFGF-NP was about 7.4×10^5 IU/ml (Table 1), higher than that of bFGF-encapsulated liposomes (about 6.2×10^5 IU/ml) as reported in our previous study [4]. There was no significant difference comparing the bioactivity between the bFGF-NP and free bFGF at the same quantity (about 7.8×10^5 IU/ml) ($P > 0.05$). These results indicated that the preparation of bFGF-NP did not diminish the original bioactivity of bFGF.

Table 1. Characterization of blank NP and bFGF-NP ($n = 5$)

Formulation	Particle size (nm)	PI	Zeta potential (mV)	Encapsulation efficiency (%)	Bioactivity ($\times 10^5$ IU/ml)
Blank NP	106 ± 1.84	0.108	-16.1 ± 1.5	/	/
bFGF-NP	128 ± 1.65	0.089	-15.3 ± 1.6	84.3 ± 2.8	7.4 ± 0.546

3.2 Cellular uptake and cytotoxicity of bFGF in vitro

The cellular uptake of bFGF by primary cardiomyocytes *in vitro* is shown by green fluorescence (Fig. 3A), which is quantified and the data are presented in Fig. 3D. There was no fluorescent signal detected in the UTMD group, ruling out the presence of strong auto-fluorescence from the microbubbles and tested cells. Only weak bFGF signals were noted in the cells treated with bFGF alone. This confirms the poor cell permeability of bFGF without NP as the carrier. In comparison, the signals were significantly increased in the bFGF-NP alone group ($P < 0.05$). Combining with UTMD further significantly increased the bFGF uptake in bFGF-NP group comparing with bFGF-NP alone (Fig. 3D, $^\#P < 0.05$).

Flow cytometry showed that the H9c2 cells treated with only UTMD produced no shifts (right-shift and up-shift indicating increased fluorescence from cells) compared with control group (Fig. 3B and C). Meanwhile, only moderate shifts were observed in the cells treated with bFGF alone. Significantly stronger shifts were detected in the cells treated with bFGF-NP instead of bFGF. Similar to the fluorescence spectrophotometric studies, the flow cytometry analysis also showed that the use of UTMD could further increase the bFGF uptake in both the bFGF group (panel e *versus* b) and the bFGF-NP group (panel f *versus* c).

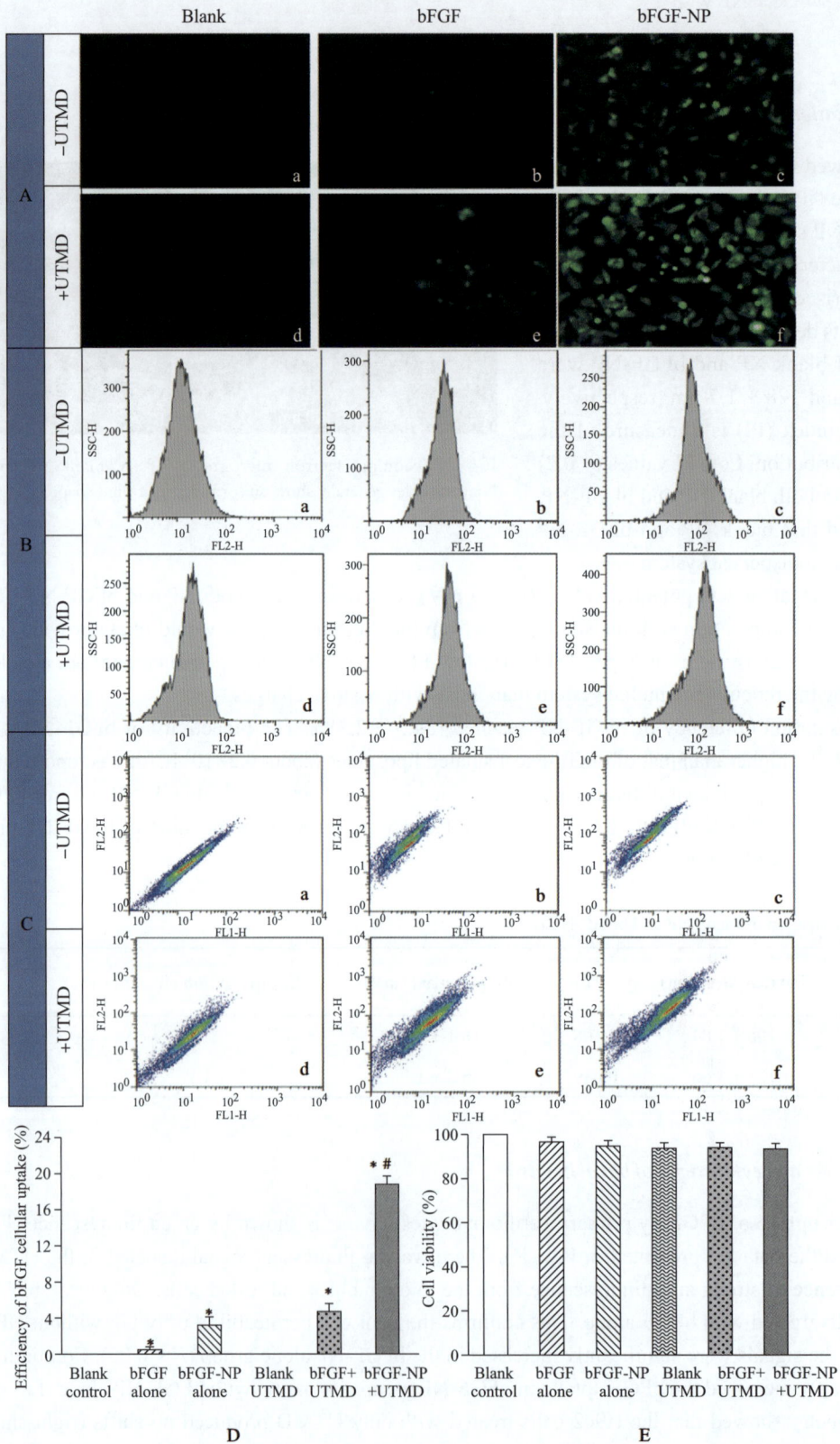

Fig. 3. Experiment of bFGF cellular uptake *in vitro*. (A) Fluroescence microscopy showing bFGF cellular uptake *in vitro*. (a: control group; b: bFGF group; c: bFGF-NP group; d: UTMD group; e: bFGF + UTMD group; f: bFGF-NP + UTMD group); (B and C) Flow cytometry results of H9c2 cells treated with FITC-bFGF; (D) quantitative analysis of efficiency of bFGF cellular uptake; (E) cell viability of various groups. Data are presented as Mean ± SD ($n = 5$). $^*P < 0.05$ *vs.* control; $^\#P < 0.05$ *vs.* other groups.

To rule out if the observed improved uptakes were caused by the cytotoxic effects of bFGF-NP or UTMD, the effects of bFGF and bFGF-NP with and without UTMD on cell viability were evaluated with MTT assay (Fig. 3E). Compared with a control, there was no toxic effect on the cell viability in any treatment groups (*i.e.* viability not significantly different from 100%).

3.3 *The application of UTMD technique with bFGF-NP in vivo*

The linear array transducer was applied over the area of the heart of DCM rats and the images at different stages of the UTMD process are shown in Fig. 4. Images were captured before the filling of microbubbles and bFGF-containing treatment (Fig. 4A), during infilling of microbubble agent to the heart (Fig. 4B), during MBD blasting of microbubbles (Fig. 4C) and after the blasting (Fig. 4D). It can be seen that the microbubbles began to accumulate in the ventricle of the heart (Fig. 4B) and were intensely burst during the MBD stage (Fig. 4C). According to a previous report, sonoporation on cell membranes resulting from UTMD would continue for a period of time because the enlarged membrane

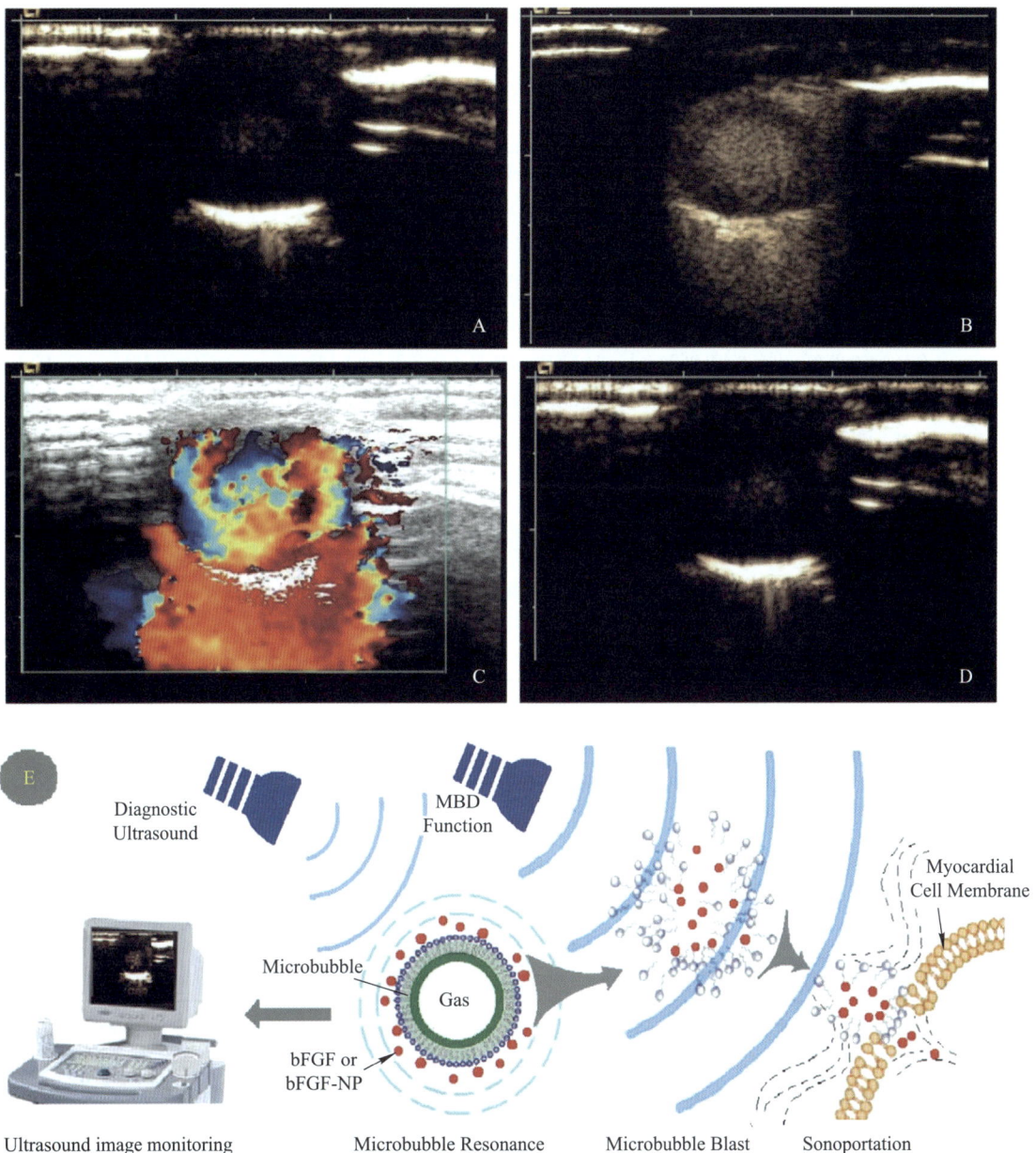

Fig. 4. Outline of UTMD technique for bFGF delivery in myocardium. (A) Ultrasound images before the filling of microbubble agent; following injection; (B) Left ventricular myocardium was gradually filled with microbubble agent; (C) Targeted bursting of microbubbles by MBD function; (D) Ultrasound images after UTMD treatment; (E) Schematic illustration of using UTMD technique in bFGF targeted delivery.

pores needed time to restore back to normal size [22] (please see Fig. 4E for the schematic illustration). Even though the microbubbles completely disappeared in the heart (Fig. 4D), the lasting sonoporation effect in the heart should remain beneficial for the absorption of residual bFGF in the blood circulation by the myocardial cells.

3.4 Echocardiography evaluation

Table 2 summarizes the echocardiographic indexes (Vs, Sc and SRc) before and after various treatments. Before treatments, all indexes in the DCM rats were significantly lower than those in the non-DCM control which confirmed the pathological conditions. These conditions deteriorated when the DCM rats did not receive any treatment (*i.e.* DCM control). All of the three indexes decreased in this group. Four-week intervention resulted in various degrees of changes in these indexes. UTMD alone did not demonstrate any therapeutic effects ($P > 0.05$ vs. DCM control), indicating that it only served to enhance the bFGF efficacy. Although moderate improvements on echocardiographic indexes were observed in the bFGF-NP alone group and the bFGF + UTMD group when compared with the DCM control, their differences were not statistically significant ($P > 0.05$). It was observed that only the indexes in bFGF-NP + UTMD group showed significant improvements ($P < 0.05$) over the DCM control. bFGF-NP + UTMD was also significantly better than all other treatment groups ($P < 0.05$).

Table 2. Results of velocity, strain, and strain rate in experiment *in vivo* (mean ± SD, $n = 10$)

Group	Vs(cm/s)		Sc (%)		SRc (1/s)	
	Before intervention	After intervention	Before intervention	After intervention	Before intervention	After intervention
Normal control	0.719 ± 0.093	0.721 ± 0.068	−13.961 ± 2.264	−14.369 ± 2.047	−3.773 ± 0.293	−3.848 ± 0.309
DCM control	0.564 ± 0.076	0.406 ± 0.078	−11.736 ± 0.727	−10.033 ± 1.020	−2.886 ± 0.358	−2.060 ± 0.295
bFGF alone	0.557 ± 0.087	0.412 ± 0.089	−11.695 ± 1.554	−10.054 ± 0.978	−2.862 ± 0.340	−2.045 ± 0.263
bFGF-NP alone	0.562 ± 0.080	0.478 ± 0.067	−11.674 ± 1.467	−12.083 ± 1.143	−2.876 ± 0.386	−2.402 ± 0.343
Blank UTMD	0.561 ± 0.092	0.432 ± 0.078	−11.687 ± 1.565	−10.043 ± 0.998	−2.798 ± 0.335	−2.144 ± 0.289
bFGF + UTMD	0.554 ± 0.067	0.503 ± 0.088	−11.732 ± 1.341	−12.244 ± 1.131	−2.844 ± 0.289	−2.527 ± 0.356
bFGF-NP + UTMD	0.568 ± 0.076	0.652 ± 0.075*	−11.804 ± 1.475	−13.265 ± 1.122*	−2.825 ± 0.363	−3.443 ± 0.354*

Note: Vs = peak systolic velocity; Sc = peak circumferential strain; SRc = peak circumferential strain rate.

*$P < 0.05$ vs. DCM control, bFGF alone, bFGF-NP alone, blank UTMD and bFGF + UTMD.

Table 3. The hemodynamic data in experiment *in vivo* (mean ± SD, $n = 10$)

Group	LVESP (mmHg)	LVEDP (mmHg)	LV + dp/dt$_{max}$ (mmHg)	LV − dp/dt$_{max}$ (mmHg)
Normal control	97.568 ± 6.222	2.824 ± 0.430	4 717.011 ± 204.734	4 059.807 ± 259.757
DCM control	69.546 ± 6.317	3.797 ± 0.354	3 247.850 ± 230.544	2 752.232 ± 160.066
bFGF alone	70.653 ± 6.537	3.923 ± 0.346	3 252.435 ± 262.655	2 743.808 ± 248.887
bFGF-NP alone	76.032 ± 4.768	3.575 ± 0.325	3 542.643 ± 234.342	2 956.464 ± 324.638
Blank UTMD	70.272 ± 6.161	3.763 ± 0.226	3 332.173 ± 217.235	2 843.808 ± 248.887
bFGF + UTMD	77.104 ± 5.104	3.513 ± 0.363	3 547.347 ± 224.624	3 032.643 ± 334.767
bFGF-NP + UTMD	83.424 ± 5.243*	3.102 ± 0.244*	4 345.344 ± 276.328*	3 624.537 ± 296.546*

Note: LVESP = left ventricular systolic pressure; LVEDP = left ventricular end diastolic pressure; ±dp/dtmax − maximum rate of the rise and fall of left ventricular pressure.

*$P < 0.05$ vs. DCM control, bFGF alone, bFGF-NP alone, blank UTMD and bFGF + UTMD.

3.5 Hemodynamic evaluation

As shown in Table 3, LVESP, LVEDP, and LV + dp/dt and −dp/dt were measured to evaluate hemodynamic characteristics. Compared with the control rats, DCM control rats showed lower values in LVESP, LV + dp/dt, and LV −dp/dt, but a higher value in LVEDP (P <0.05). DCM rats treated with bFGF alone did not exhibit any improvement in the hemodynamic characteristics ($P > 0.05$) compared with the DCM control. The hemodynamic characteristics in bFGF-NP + UTMD group, bFGF-NP alone group, and bFGF-NP + UTMD group were all improved (*i.e.* values closer to the normal control than DCM control); however, only the bFGF-NP + UTMD group demonstrated significant improvements ($P < 0.05$). In fact, bFGF-NP + UTMD was also significantly better than all other treatment groups except bFGF + UTMD group ($P < 0.05$). This finding is consistent with the data of *in vitro* bFGF cellular uptake and echocardiography evaluation.

3.6 Myocardial collagen volume fraction and capillary density

Cardiac dysfunction induced by diabetes and its recovery are predominantly attributed to cardiac remodeling. Masson staining of collagen (representative image in Fig. 5A, data of quantitative analysis in Fig. 5C) and CD31 immunohistochemical staining of newly formed blood capillaries (Fig. 5B and D) were performed to measure the myocardial collagen volume fraction (MCVF) and myocardial capillary density (MCD), respectively. As shown in Fig. 5C, MCVF was significantly increased ($P < 0.01$) in the heart of DCM rats (group b) as compared to the normal control rats (group a), revealing the pathological hypertrophic changes in these rats. Treatment with bFGF alone (group c) did not significantly reduce the MCVF in DCM rats ($P > 0.05$). Only when the DCM rats were subjected to the combination treatment of bFGF-NP/UTMD, the MCVF value was moderately but significantly reduced ($P < 0.05$).

One of the major functions of bFGF for DCM treatment is angiogenesis. Higher MCD value reflects the formation of new blood supplies and occurrence of the recovery process. The MCD values indicating angiogenesis are shown in Fig. 5D. When compared with the normal control rats (group a), hearts of DCM rats (group b) showed low values of MCD ($P < 0.01$), which was not improved by treatment with bFGF alone. In contrast, treatment with bFGF-NP/UTMD once again led to a moderate but significant improvement in MCD ($P < 0.05$) when compared with the untreated DCM group.

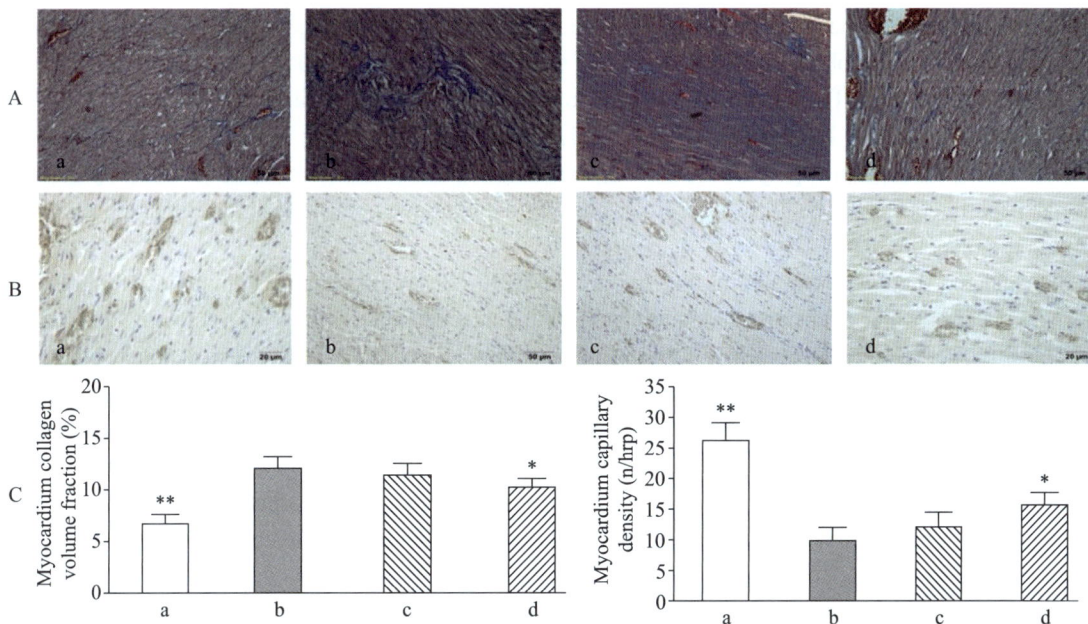

Fig. 5. Histological changes and improvement by bFGF-NP + UTMD treatment. (A) Representatives pictures of trichrome stained myocardium for collagen accumulation and the semi-quantitative analysis for all groups; (B) Representatives of CD31 immunohistochemical staining of MCD and the semi-quantitative analysis for all groups. (C) Myocardium collagen volume fraction of all groups; (D) Myocardium capillary density of all groups. a: Normal control; b: DCM control; c: bFGF-NP alone; d: bFGF-NP + UTMD. *$P < 0.05$ or **$P < 0.01$ *vs.* the DCM control.

4 Discussions

Current pharmacological therapy for DCM suffers from multiple limitations. Although several medications have been used to lower blood pressure, enhance insulin sensitivity, and reduce lipid levels in circulation, these conventional drug treatments only prevent further pathological damages to the heart. They do not directly reverse the established pathological changes of the heart. Molecular therapeutics offer an attractive alternative to the current pharmacologic therapies. By specifically manipulating the expression of genes and their downstream molecular pathways in cardiac tissues, it is possible to reverse the established pathologies. For example, gene therapy for ischemic heart disease has been reported to protect the heart from damages and stimulate its recovery [23].

FGFs bind to tyrosine kinase receptors and mediate mitogenic activities which stimulate tissue growth and cellular proliferation and migration [24,25]. As a member of FGFs, bFGF promotes endothelial cell proliferation and the physical organization of endothelial cells into tube-like structures. It was found that activation of bFGF-dependent signaling pathway following delivery of PR39 gene could also activate VEGF-dependent pathways to improve myocardial blood flow and functioning [26]. bFGF-based therapy thus offers a promising alternative for DCM patients, not only for prevention, but also for treatment of this practically incurable condition as well. Indeed, in the previous animal studies, bFGF gene therapy has been shown to improve arteriogenesis and echocardiographic parameters of LV function [27,28]. However, although these bFGF-based therapies certainly have potential for DCM treatment, their clinical application remains difficult due to the lack of an efficient and safe delivery strategy and device.

Non-viral carriers such as polymeric nanoparticles have drawn an increasing level of interest as the delivery systems for molecular therapeutics. They are often customizable to the desirable physicochemical properties for efficient delivery, can preserve the bioactivity of the easily degradable biomolecules, and generally have low inherent toxicity [29]. In a previous report [30], heparin conjugated PLGA NPs were developed to enhance tumor imaging and therapy. In our study, NPs containing Poloxamer 188-grafted heparin copolymer to improve bFGF encapsulation were used. In comparison to PLGA, Poloxamer 188 has many advantages, especially in terms of safety, amphiphilic properties and biocompatibility. As a non-ionic amphiphilic copolymer with low toxicity, Poloxamer 188 is an FDA-approved pharmaceutical excipient and can be used in cell culture to protect cells in suspension against possible damage during transfer, freeze-thawing and stirring. Poloxamer 188-grafted heparin copolymer maintains the high affinity of heparin with bFGF. Theoretically, Poloxamer 188-heparin copolymer cored NPs can load bFGF in the matrix of NP structure (not only on the NP surface as heparin-coated PLGA NPs). Therefore, our NPs should have good loading ability and protection for the loaded protein drug like bFGF.

These advantages were demonstrated in this study. The bFGF-NP prepared using Poloxamer 188-grafted heparin copolymer and water-in-water emulsion technique demonstrated adequate size (size ≈ 100 nm with PI < 0.2, Table 1), moderately negative zeta potential (≈−15 mV, Table 1) and round morphology (Fig. 2). These parameters are all comparable to the nanoformulations marketed for systemic use, e.g. Doxil (size averages 108 nm, zeta potential −13.3 mV and round shape) [31]. bFGF-NP also had a high bFGF encapsulation efficiency (> 80%, Table 1) and was able to preserve the bioactivity of bFGF in vitro (Table 1). Moreover, the inherent cellular toxicity of the delivery system was low as supported by the cytotoxicity assay results (Fig. 3E), which showed no significant reduction in cell viability after treatment with blank NP or bFGF-NP. All in all, these properties are all favorable for efficient and safe systemic delivery of a growth factor drug like bFGF.

The next concern was whether the NP system could deliver sufficient quantity of bFGF to the cardiac cells/tissues. We performed a fluorescence microscope study and flow cytometry study on two different cardiac cell types (LV primary cardiomyocytes and H9c2 heart myoblast cell line) to more accurately assess this issue (Fig. 3). Although in relative term, the NP noticeably improved the uptake of the labeled bFGF into the cardiac cells as compared to free bFGF (panel c versus panel b in Fig. 3A and B), in quantitative term the uptake efficiency using bFGF-NP was modest only (< 4%, Fig. 3D). It was clear that an additional mechanism would be essential to further increase the efficiency of bFGF-NP delivery to a more optimal rate.

UTMD was therefore studied for this purpose as this non-invasive, physical technique has previously shown some success in improving protein drug delivery to the heart. Bekeredjian et al. [32] used luciferase-loaded microbubbles to evaluate UTMD for heart-targeted delivery for proteins. In their study, luciferase proteins were loaded directly on microbubbles. This study proved that UTMD can non-invasively augment heart-specific delivery of proteins. However, the drug loading space in the gas-core microbubbles is limited, and the loaded drugs on the microbubble surface can also influence the effects of acoustic resonance and reduce ultrasonic image resolution. Therefore, protein loaded NP was introduced in UTMD technique to reduce the protein loading burden on the microbubbles. Vancraeynest et al. [33] used UTMD technique to enhance delivery of colloid nanoparticles to the rat myocardium. They demonstrated the positive correlation between the delivery efficacy of UTMD and various ultrasound parameters. However, this report only used normal animals to study the feasibility of UTMD technique to improve targeted drug delivery, without applying any disease models to explore the feasibility of clinical treatment. In our study, the efficiency and therapeutic effects of the bFGF-NP/UTMD combined therapy was extensively evaluated not only in vitro, but also in DCM animals. Our study is thus the much needed expanded study on the basis of previous UTMD related research from a therapeutic/clinical perspective.

The in vitro data confirmed that this approach was potentially effective and harmless. Fig. 3D quantitatively showed that the uptake efficiency of the labeled bFGF delivered by bFGF-NP was increased from less than 4% (bFGF-NP alone) to nearly 20% (bFGF-NP + UTMD), approximately a 5-fold improvement. It may be argued that the increased uptake could be caused by cell damage inflicted by UTMD. In a previous report, cytotoxicity was observed after 8 h in ultrasound-mediated transfection in vitro [34]. In another report, transient regional dysfunction was detected after repeated UTMD treatment on rat myocardium [33]. From its conclusion, the contractile dysfunction or tissue alteration in myocardium caused by UTMD are time-and pressure-dependent. Based on our preliminary studies, side effects can be reduced or even avoided by optimization of the insonation treatment conditions. In our study, we used only 10 s exposure treatment to produce the recoverable opening of myocardium. No significant cytotoxicity was observed during our study as shown by the viability assay data (Fig. 5E).

We proceeded to evaluate if the improved cellular bFGF uptake could translate into enhanced in vivo efficacy for DCM treatment. As shown in Table 2 and Table 3, all of the echocardiography evaluation criteria and hemodynamic evaluation indicated that UTMD together with NP delivery approach could significantly enhance the bFGF effects in restoring the cardiac functions in DCM animals. The histochemical staining data presented in Fig. 5 showed signs of moderate but significant structural recovery (reducing collagen and increasing new blood supplies), further suggesting that the improved functions were the result of structural remodeling of the cardiac tissues and thus may bring longer lasting therapeutic benefits. Overall, the bFGF-NP/UTMD combination therapy was able to reverse the DCM conditions both in functional and structural terms. This is a very appealing effect as compared to the current pharmacologic therapy, which primarily aims at preventing or slowing down the pathological progress instead of reversing it.

Given the exciting results obtained in the present study, there are limitations that need to be addressed. First, the low number of samples limited the optimization of experimental parameters for UTMD. We also noticed that the improved functional and reversed pathological changes in bFGF-NP + UTMD group still did not reach the levels of the control rats, which may be related to the short intervention (only 4 weeks after treatment). In addition, the complex mechanism of angiogenesis in DCM model remains to be explored before UTMD technique can be brought from bench to bedside [35]. Therefore, increasing dosing regimens and intervention time for bFGF-NP administration should be considered in the future studies. Molecular mechanisms and signaling pathways of bFGF in DCM therapy and other potential adverse effects of bFGF needs further investigation. While the goal of this study was to demonstrate safety, pathophysiology and short-term efficacy of this treatment, further studies for the long-term effect of single versus repeated treatments using this approach are warranted. Furthermore, alternative approaches, such as to deliver bFGF genes to the myocardium to achieve long term expression of bFGF, are also promising strategies.

In conclusion, while using non-viral vectors combined with UTMD technique for gene or protein therapy is still in its early stages, its future seems very promising. We demonstrated that bFGF delivery by this method can significantly improve or even reverse cardiac dysfunction and pathological abnormalities. Therefore, this pre-clinical study provides us with great hope for the future of treating DCM patients. We predict that once the optimal dose of bFGF is determined and the delivery system is optimized, this technique plus the current commonly-used systemic control for diabetic patients will provide DCM patients an efficient adjuvant therapy to cure their pathologically damaged and dysfunctional hearts.

References

[1] Pessin JE, Kwon H. How does high-fat diet induce adipose tissue fibrosis?[J]. Journal of investigative medicine : the official publication of the American Federation for Clinical Research, 2012, 60(8): 1147-1150.

[2] Rubler S. New type of cardiomyopathy associated with diabetic glomerulosclerosis[J]. American Journal of Cardiology, 1972, 30(6): 595-602.

[3] Barrientos S, Stojadinovic O, Golinko MS, et al. Growth factors and cytokines in wound healing[J]. Wound Repair And Regeneration, 2008, 16(5): 585-601.

[4] Xiang Q, Xiao J, Zhang H, et al. Preparation and characterisation of bFGF-encapsulated liposomes and evaluation of wound-healing activities in the rat[J]. Burns : journal of the International Society for Burn Injuries, 2011, 37(5): 886-895.

[5] Fujii T, Yonemitsu Y, Onimaru M, et al. VEGF function for up-regulation of endogenous PlGF expression during FGF-2-mediated therapeutic angiogenesis[J]. Atherosclerosis, 2008, 200(1): 51-57.

[6] Zhao T, Zhao W, Chen Y, et al. Acidic and basic fibroblast growth factors involved in cardiac angiogenesis following infarction[J]. International journal of cardiology, 2011, 152(3): 307-313.

[7] Xiao J, Lv YX, Lin SQ, et al. Cardiac Protection by Basic Fibroblast Growth Factor from Ischemia/Reperfusion-Induced Injury in Diabetic Rats[J]. Biological & Pharmaceutical Bulletin, 2009, 33(3): 444-449.

[8] Zhao W, Zhao T, Chen Y, et al. Reactive oxygen species promote angiogenesis in the infarcted rat heart[J]. International journal of experimental pathology, 2009, 90(6): 621-629.

[9] Ylä-Herttuala S, Alitalo K. Gene transfer as a tool to induce therapeutic vascular growth[J]. Nature medicine, 2003, 9(6): 694-701.

[10] Muruve DA, Barnes MJ, Stillman IE, et al. Adenoviral gene therapy leads to rapid induction of multiple chemokines and acute neutrophil-dependent hepatic injury in vivo[J]. Human gene therapy, 1999, 10(6): 965-976.

[11] Ischakov R, Adler-Abramovich L, Buzhansky L, et al. Peptide-based hydrogel nanoparticles as effective drug delivery agents[J]. Bioorganic & medicinal chemistry, 2013, 21(12): 3517-3522.

[12] Agnihotri SA, Mallikarjuna NN, Aminabhavi TM. Recent advances on chitosan-based micro- and nanoparticles in drug delivery[J]. Journal of controlled release : official journal of the Controlled Release Society, 2004, 100(1): 5-28.

[13] Rose LC, Kucharski C, Uluda H. Protein expression following non-viral delivery of plasmid DNA coding for basic FGF and BMP-2 in a rat ectopic model[J]. Biomaterials, 2012, 33(11): 3363-3374.

[14] Jean M, Smaoui F, Lavertu M, et al. Chitosan-plasmid nanoparticle formulations for IM and SC delivery of recombinant FGF-2 and PDGF-BB or generation of antibodies[J]. Gene therapy, 2009, 16(9): 1097-1110.

[15] Shah PB, Losordo DW. Non-viral vectors for gene therapy: clinical trials in cardiovascular disease[J]. Advances in genetics, 2005, 54: 339-361.

[16] Fujii H, Li SH, Wu J, et al. Repeated and targeted transfer of angiogenic plasmids into the infarcted rat heart via ultrasound targeted microbubble destruction enhances cardiac repair[J]. European heart journal, 2011, 32(16): 2075-2084.

[17] Tian JL, Zhao YZ, Jin Z, et al. Synthesis and characterization of Poloxamer 188-grafted heparin copolymer[J]. Drug development and industrial pharmacy, 2010, 36(7): 832-838.

[18] Jiang Y, Wei N, Lu T, et al. Intranasal brain-derived neurotrophic factor protects brain from ischemic insult via modulating local inflammation in rats[J]. Neuroscience, 2011, 172(1): 398-405.

[19] Luo YK, Zhao YZ, Lu CT, et al. Application of ultrasonic gas-filled liposomes in enhancing transfer for breast cancer-related antisense oligonucleotides: an experimental study[J]. Journal of liposome research, 2008, 18(4): 341-351.

[20] Wang J, Song Y, Elsherif L, et al. Cardiac metallothionein induction plays the major role in the prevention of diabetic cardiomyopathy by zinc supplementation[J]. Circulation, 2006, 113(4): 544-554.

[21] Song Y, Li C, Cai L. Fluvastatin prevents nephropathy likely through suppression of connective tissue growth factor-mediated extracellular matrix accumulation[J]. Experimental and molecular pathology, 2004, 76(1): 66-75.

[22] Zhao YZ, Luo YK, Lu CT, et al. Phospholipids-based microbubbles sonoporation pore size and reseal of cell membrane cultured in vitro[J]. Journal of drug targeting, 2008, 16(1): 18-25.

[23] Lavu M, Gundewar S, Lefer DJ. Gene therapy for ischemic heart disease[J]. Journal of Molecular & Cellular Cardiology, 2011, 50(5): 742-750.

[24] Ornitz DM, Itoh N. Fibroblast Growth Factors[J]. Genome biology, 2001, 2(3).

[25] Khurana R, Simons M. Insights from angiogenesis trials using fibroblast growth factor for advanced arteriosclerotic disease[J]. Trends in cardiovascular medicine, 2003, 13(3): 116-122.

[26] Post MJ, Sato K, Murakami M, et al. Adenoviral PR39 improves blood flow and myocardial function in a pig model of chronic myocardial ischemia by enhancing collateral formation[J]. American Journal of Physiology Regulatory Integrative & Comparative Physiology, 2006, 290(3): R494.

[27] Horvath KA, Doukas J, Lu CY, et al. Myocardial functional recovery after fibroblast growth factor 2 gene therapy as assessed by echocardiography and magnetic resonance imaging[J]. The Annals of thoracic surgery, 2002, 74(2): 481-486; discussion 487.

[28] Heilmann C, von Samson P, Schlegel K, et al. Comparison of protein with DNA therapy for chronic myocardial ischemia using fibroblast growth factor-2[J]. European journal of cardio-thoracic surgery : official journal of the European Association for Cardio-thoracic Surgery, 2002, 22(6): 957-964.

[29] Elsabahy M, Wooley KL. Design of polymeric nanoparticles for biomedical delivery applications[J]. Chemical Society Reviews, 2012, 41(7): 2545-2561.

[30] Xiao J, Lv YX, Lin SQ, et al. Cardiac Protection by Basic Fibroblast Growth Factor from Ischemia/Reperfusion-Induced Injury in Diabetic Rats[J]. Biological & Pharmaceutical Bulletin, 2010, 33(3): 444-449.

[31] Szebeni J, Bedocs P, Rozsnyay Z, et al. Liposome-induced complement activation and related cardiopulmonary distress in pigs: factors promoting reactogenicity of Doxil and AmBisome[J]. Nanomedicine : nanotechnology, biology, and medicine, 2012, 8(2): 176-184.

[32] Bekeredjian R, Chen S, Grayburn PA, et al. Augmentation of cardiac protein delivery using ultrasound targeted microbubble destruction[J]. Ultrasound in medicine & biology, 2005, 31(5): 687-691.

[33] Vancraeynest D, Havaux X, Pouleur AC, et al. Myocardial delivery of colloid nanoparticles using ultrasound-targeted microbubble destruction[J]. European heart journal, 2006, 27(2): 237-245.

[34] Kim HJ, Greenleaf JF, Kinnick RR, et al. Ultrasound-mediated transfection of mammalian cells[J]. Human gene therapy, 1996, 7(11): 1339-1346.

[35] Royen NV, Piek JJ, Buschmann I, et al. Stimulation of arteriogenesis; a new concept for the treatment of arterial occlusive disease[J]. Cardiovascular research, 2001, 49(3): 543-553.

Gelatin nanostructured lipid carriers-mediated intranasal delivery of basic fibroblast growth factor enhances functional recovery in hemiparkinsonian rats

Yingzheng Zhao, Xiaokun Li

Intranasal delivery of large molecular weight biologics such as proteins, gene vectors, and stem cells is a noninvasive strategy to treat a variety of diseases/disorders of the central nervous system (CNS).[1] The major disadvantages of the route, aside from the challenge of reproducibility, are the limited absorption across the nasal epithelium and short resident time in nasal cavity that restrict its application for particularly potent substances.[2,3] Vesicular systems have shown promising results in intranasal drug delivery of both small and large molecules to the CNS by overcoming limitations of nasal administration.[4] Intranasal mucoadhesive liposomes can enhance penetration of drug and provide better absorption into the brain compared to intranasal administration of drugs alone or oral administration.[5,6] However, drugs encapsulated in liposomes are not stable and are prone to leak. Nanoparticles may improve nose-to-brain drug delivery since they are able to protect the encapsulated drug from biological and/or chemical degradation, and promote extracellular transport by P-gp efflux proteins.[7] Recently, lipid nanoparticles with a solid matrix, including solid lipid nanoparticles (SLNs) and nanostructured lipid carriers (NLCs), received major attention as novel colloidal drug carriers for intranasal delivery because they combine the advantages of polymeric nanoparticles, fat emulsions, and liposomes, and avoid some of their disadvantages.[8]

Parkinson's disease (PD) is a chronic CNS disorder caused primarily by the progressive loss of dopaminergic cells in the substantia nigra pars compacta (SNc). In PD patients, expressions of brain-derived neurotrophic factor (BDNF) and bFGF were reduced in the remaining dopaminergic neurons of SNc.[9-12] BDNF depletion from the midbrain-hindbrain selectively leads to reduced tyrosine hydroxylase (TH) expression.[13] In neurotoxin-induced degeneration models of midbrain DA neurons, higher levels of DA neuron death occurred in bFGF null mutant mice whereas more DA neurons were preserved in bFGF overexpressing mice,[14] suggesting that bFGF protects DA neurons from the neurotoxicity. Neurotrophic factor (NTF) therapy has recently gained attention in the treatment of PD.[15] The intact BDNF can be made to cross the BBB by a high-capacity, saturable transport system,[16] but bFGF is unstable in solution and has very short half-life[17]; thus, it does not cross the blood–brain barrier (BBB) in pharmacologically significant amounts,[18,19] which limits its therapeutic value in the CNS.

The aim of the present study was to determine whether gelatin nanostructured lipid carriers (GNLs) encapsulated bFGF (bFGF-GNLs) could be efficiently delivered to the brain striata with effective bioactivity *via* nasal epithelium. Physicochemical characterizations of GNLs and its bFGF preparation, including micromorphology, particle size, polydispersity index and Zeta potential, were investigated. The neuroprotective effect of bFGF-GNLs was evaluated in hemiparkinsonian rats following intranasal administration.

1. Methods

1.1 Materials and animals

All reagents and animals used in this study were commercially available. The animals were handled according to protocols approved by the ethical committee of Wenzhou Medical University and all the experiments were performed according to the National Institutes of Health Guide for the Care and Use of Laboratory Animals (Supplemental Experimental Procedures).

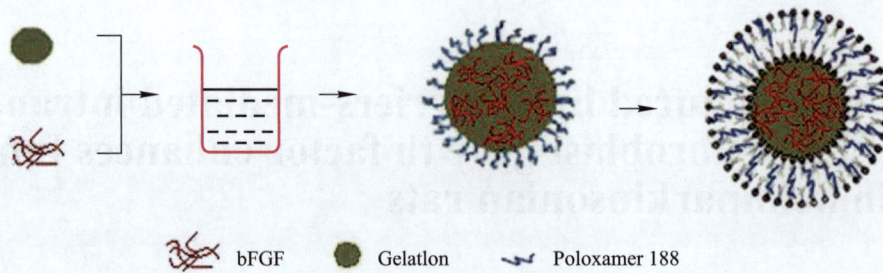

Fig. 1. Schematic diagram of the bFGF-GNLs preparation. The bFGF-GNLs were prepared using water-in-water emulsion and freeze-drying technique.

1.2 Preparation of gelatin nanostructured lipid carriers

The schematic diagram of the preparation for bFGF-loaded nanoparticles is shown in Fig. 1. The GNLs and its bFGF preparation were prepared using water-in-water emulsion and freeze-drying technique,[20-22] as described in Supplemental Experimental Procedures. The final bFGF concentrations in bFGF-GNs and bFGF-GNLs suspensions were 2 mg/ml, respectively.

1.3 Characterization of GNs and GNLs

The microscopic appearance of loaded or unloaded GNs and GNLs were examined by scanning electron microscopy (SEM). Zeta potential of the loaded or unloaded GNs and GNLs was determined by dynamic light scattering using a Zeta Potential/ Particle Sizer Nicomp™ 380 ZLS (PSS. Nicomp, Santa Barbara, CA, USA). The encapsulating efficiency, loading capacity, and bioactivity of bFGF in GNs and GNLs were measured as previous reports.[23,24] The details were described in Supplemental Experimental Procedures.

1.4 6-OHDA induced hemiparkinsonian rat model

The hemiparkinsonian rats were generated by injecting 10.0 μl 6-OHDA solution in the right-side striatum (or vehicle for sham animals) by use of the stereotaxic apparatus,[25,26] as described in Supplemental Experimental Procedures.

1.5 Behavioral evaluation of apomorphine-induced rotations in hemiparkinsonian rats

The post-operative rats received a subcutaneous injection of DA agonist apomorphine (0.5 mg/kg), and were transferred into an opaque cylinder with 30 cm diameter which was placed 45 cm below the recording camera. After a 5 min habituation period, movements were recorded over a 5 min timeframe. Both contra-and ipsi-lateral full-body rotations were measured and compared with the sham control rats. Animals scoring over 7 rpm (displaying at least 7 full-body contralateral rotations per minute) were considered as successfully lesioned (Supplemental Experimental Procedures).

1.6 bFGF intranasal administration, its distribution in the rat brain, and potential toxicity to the nasal mucosa

Deeply anesthetized rats (60 mg/kg pentobarbital sodium) were maintained in a supine position, with head and neck maintained horizontal using a small roll of gauze under the dorsal neck. Nanoparticles loaded with bFGF (5 μl) were administered to alternating nostrils using a pipette, with the untreated nostril occluded to maximize drug absorption over the 3 min of exposure, which allowed the rat to inhale all the preparation,[27] until about 30 μl of the nanoparticle solution was delivered (dosage of bFGF in each loaded GNs or GNLs suspension =0.2 mg/kg body weight). To determine if GN-and GNL-encapsulated bFGF administrations enhance the brain delivery *via* nasal mucosa, the tissues from olfactory bulb (OB), pallium, striatum, and hippocampus were dissected and collected 90 min after administration for Western blot analysis. To evaluate potential toxicity to the nasal mucosa, nasal mucosae were harvested for immunohistochemistry to test for pathological changes after two-weeks of daily treatments.

1.7 Western blot for bFGF assessment

Sprague–Dawley rats (N = 15) were randomized into the following five groups (Table 1, Group 1, Groups 3–6) to evaluate the bFGF level in different brain areas including olfactory bulb (OB), pallium, striatum, and hippocampus.

Rats were sacrificed 90 min after administration. The target tissues were quickly separated and homogenized in cold lysis buffer. Protein samples were extracted at 4 ℃ and immunoprecipitated with rabbit anti-bFGF (Abcam, Cambs, UK) using standard biochemical procedures (Supplemental Experimental Procedures). The band densities were quantified by densitometry (Quantity One software, Bio-Rad, Hercules, CA, USA).

1.8 Mucosal toxicity and tolerability — a histopathological study

Following two weeks of daily drug administration, rats were sacrificed and their nasal septum with the epithelial cell membrane was taken and embedded in paraffin and sectioned, stained with hematoxylin and eosin, and examined under a light microscope.

1.9 Pharmacodynamics of intranasal delivery of bFGF-GNLs in hemiparkinsonian rats

Rats were randomly divided into six groups (8/each group) and were examined one day before surgery to make sure there was no rotation behavior in animals. After the surgery, two-week daily treatment was applied in each animal. As shown in Table 1, Groups 1 and 2 were sham and PD rats, which received nasally administered PBS and unloaded GNLs. Groups 3 to 5 were all hemiparkinsonian rats that received intranasal bFGF, bFGF-GNs and bFGF-GNLs for therapeutic evaluation (bFGF/IN, bFGF-GNs/IN, and bFGF-GNLs/IN). Group 6 (bFGF-GNLs/IV) was administered bFGF-GNLs intravenously (0.2 mg/kg body weight) as a therapeutic control. Striata were dissected from rat brains carefully after two-week consecutive treatment for HPLC analysis of dopamine (DA), dihydroxyphenylacetic acid (DOPAC), and homovanillic acid (HVA). The amount of DA, DOPAC and HVA was quantified using a standard curve generated by determining the ratio between the known amounts of monoamine and a constant amount of an internal standard (DHBA), and represented as ng/g tissue weight (Supplemental Experimental Procedures).

Table 1. Designed groups for different pharmacodynamics study in rats

Experimental	Group Rat Model	Preparation	Route of Administration
1	Sham	PBS	Intranasal (IN)
2	PD	unload-GNLs	Intranasal (IN)
3	PD	bFGF	Intranasal (IN)
4	PD	bFGF-GNs	Intranasal (IN)
5	PD	bFGF-GNLs	Intranasal (IN)
6	PD	bFGF-GNLs	Intravenous (IV)

PD, hemiparkinsonian rats; PBS, phosphate buffered saline; bFGF-GNs and bFGF-GNLs stand for bFGF-loaded gelatin nanoparticles and bFGF-loaded gelatin nanostructured lipid carriers (2 mg/ml), respectively.

1.10 TH immunohistochemical staining

Following behavioral assessment on the 28th day post-surgery, rat brains of Groups 1 to 6 were collected for coronal sectioning across the SN region. The immunohistochemical staining with anti-TH antibody was performed to examine the extent of dopaminergic neuronal loss (Supplemental Experimental Procedures). The ratio of TH staining (grayscale) in the corresponding lesioned to unlesioned SN regions was calculated.

1.11 Statistical analysis

Statistically significant difference for multiple groups was determined using a one way ANOVA with a Newman–Keuls post-hoc test. Statistical significance between individual groups was determined using a Student's t test. All testing was done using the SAS 8.01 (1999-2000, SAS Institute Inc, Cary, NC, USA). Difference was considered statistically significant when the P value was less than 0.05.

2. Results

2.1 Physicochemical properties and bioactivity of GNs, GNLs, and the particles loaded with bFGF

Polymeric nanoparticles are defined as particulate dispersions or solid particles ranging in sizes between 10 and 1 000 nm. The representative SEM micrographs of the unloaded or loaded GN and GNL shapes revealed that GNLs (Fig. 2, A_3) and bFGF-GNLs (Fig. 2, A_4) were more uniform in size than GNs (Fig. 2, A_1) and bFGF-GNs (Fig. 2, A_2). Characterization of GNs and GNLs loaded with or without bFGF was shown in Table 2. The dynamic light scattering results demonstrated that the average particle size of GNs and GNLs was 91 nm ± 1.02 nm, 143 nm± 1.14 nm, respectively. The polydispersibility index (PDI) represents the distribution of particle size; lower PDI values were observed in both of GNLs and bFGF-GNLs, which indicated that GNLs and bFGF-GNLs approached a monodisperse stable system. After bFGF loading, mean nanoparticle diameters increased, but were still below 200 nm (Table 2). The zeta potential is an

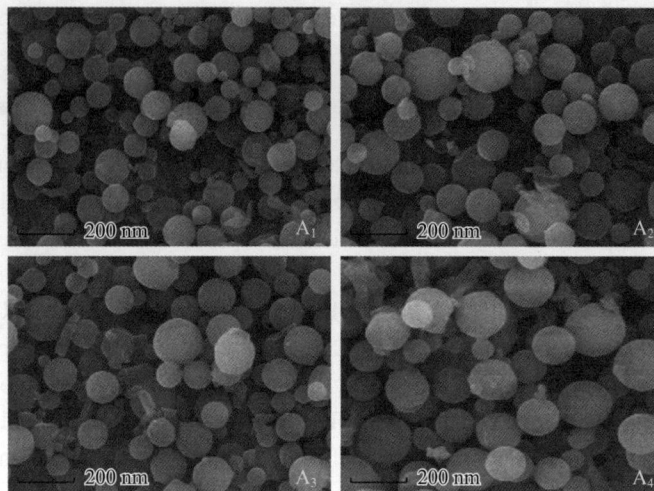

Fig. 2. Representative scanning electron micrographs of GNs (A_1), bFGF-GN (A_2), GNLs (A_3) and bFGF-GNLs (A_4). The GNLs (A_3) and bFGF-GNLs (A_4) possessed more uniform morphology than GNs (A_1) and bFGF-GNs (A_2). Bar = 200 nm.

important index evaluating the physical stability of nanoparticles. Nanoparticles with high absolute value of zeta potential are electrically stable while those with low absolute value of zeta potential tend to fluctuate. As shown in Table 2, the bFGF-GNLs and GNLs both possessed stronger negative charge on the surface with the potential value below −25 mV than bFGF-GNs and GNs, indicating that the GNL dispersion was more stable. The encapsulation efficiency and loading capacity of bFGF-GNs or bFGF-GNLs were 25.3% ± 1.4% and 1.1% ± 0.03% or 86.7% ± 1.1% and 4.6% ± 0.01%, respectively (Table 2). The bioactivity of bFGF-GNs and bFGF-GNLs was $(6.147 \pm 0.469) \times 10^5$ IU/ml and $(5.894 \pm 0.394) \times 10^5$ IU/ml, respectively ($P > 0.05$). The bioactivity was similar to that of liposome-encapsulated bFGF reported previously, [24]which indicated that the preparations of bFGF-GNs and bFGF-GNLs did not significantly reduce bFGF bioactivity.

Table 2. Characterization of GNs and GNLs loaded with or without bFGF ($n = 3$)

Formulation	Particle Size (nm)	PDI	Zeta Potential (mV)	Encapsulation Efficiency (%)	Loading Capacity (%)	Bioactivity ($\times 10^5$ IU/ml)
GNs	91 ± 1.02	0.252 ± 0.042	− 19.1 ± 0.6	–	–	–
GNLs	143 ± 1.14*	0.127 ± 0.038*	− 38.2 ± 1.2*	–	–	–
bFGF-GNs	123 ± 1.75	0.215 ± 0.034	− 17.2 ± 0.4	25.3 ± 1.4	1.10 ± 0.03	6.147 ± 0.469
bFGF-GNLs	172 ± 1.31#	0.105 ± 0.011#	− 27.6 ± 1.1#	86.7 ± 1.1#	4.60 ± 0.01#	5.894 ± 0.394

PDI, Polydispersity Index. *$P < 0.05$ (GNLs vs. GNs); #$P < 0.05$ (bFGF-GNLs vs. bFGF-GNs).

2.2 Regional distribution of exogenous bFGF in rat brains

It has been reported that intranasal administration of bFGF in adult rat brain promotes neurogenesis following cerebral ischemia.[28] However, no direct evidence has been provided that bFGF enters the brain nasally. To determine whether intranasal bFGF gains access to the brain, we examined the protein level of bFGF in different brain regions

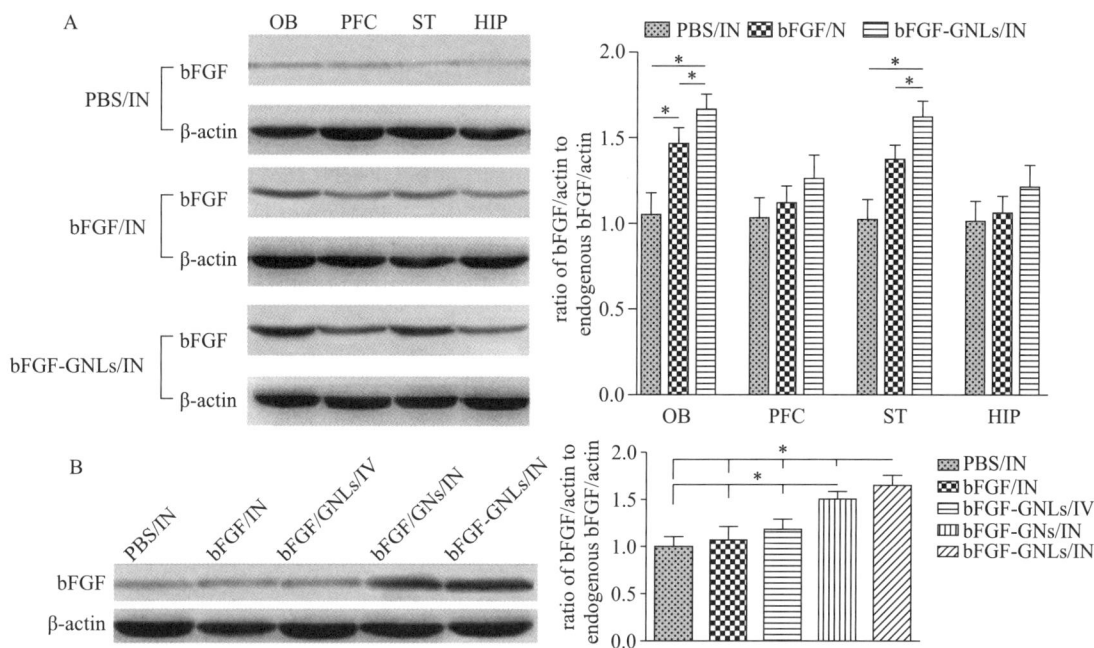

Fig. 3. Protein level of bFGF in different regions of rat brain after the administration with exogenous bFGF. (A) The presence of bFGF in olfactory bulb, prefrontal cortex, striatum and hippocampus after intranasal administration with PBS, bFGF, or bFGF-GNLs by Western blot analysis. Endogenous bFGF was rarely detected in all areas. In contrast, bFGF was significantly increased in olfactory bulb and striatum with intranasal administration of bFGF and bFGF-GNLs but not in prefrontal cortex or hippocampus. (B) The presence of bFGF in striatum after the administration with PBS/IN, bFGF/IN, bFGF-GNs/IN, bFGF-GNLs/ IN or bFGF-GNLs/IV. More bFGF-GNLs were detected in striatum than bFGF-GNs in the same area with intranasal administration. OB: olfactory bulb; PFC: prefrontal cortex; ST: striatum; HIP: hippocampus; GNs: gelatin nanoparticles; GNLs: gelatin nanostructured lipid carriers; IN: intranasal; IV: intravenous. Error bar: standard deviation. *P < 0.05 (n = 3).

after intranasal administration. In control vehicle rats, endogenous bFGF was rarely detected in olfactory bulb, cortex, striatum and hippocampus. In contrast, bFGF was significantly increased in olfactory bulb and striatum with intranasal administration of bFGF and bFGF-GNLs but not in prefrontal cortex or hippocampus (Fig. 3A). More bFGF-GNLs were detected in striatum than bFGF-GNs in the same area with intranasal administration (Fig. 3B).

2.3 Levels of monoamine neurotransmitters in striatum

Selective neurotoxic disruption of dopaminergic pathways can be reproduced by injection of 6-OHDA. As the most widely used parkinsonian rat model, 6-OHDA lesion model leads to massive irreversible neuronal loss and functional deficits. In unilaterally lesioned rats, an imbalance of DA activity between the two striata causes the rotational behavior. Because of dopaminergic neuron damage, D_2 receptors in postsynaptic neurons of the lesioned striatum are up-regulated. When rats are injected with the D_2 receptor agonist apomorphine, its effect is stronger on the lesioned side, inducing a rotating locomotor pattern in animals which have lost approximately 90% of SNc dopaminergic neurons. In our study, no rotational behavior was observed in any rats prior to surgery. Compared to the sham group (0 rpm), the apomorphine-induced rotation was clearly present in 6-OHDA lesioned rats after seven days (4.1 ± 0.6 rpm) and reached its maximum after 4 weeks (7 ± 1.3 rpm), indicating successful establishment of the hemiparkinsonian model (Table 3).

Table 3. Rotations per minute in apomorphine-induced behavior tests after 6-OHDA lesion surgery

Group	Number	1 st wk	2nd wk	3rd wk	4th wk	5th wk
PD	8	4.1 ± 0.6	5.0 ± 1.1	6.0 ± 1.4	7.0 ± 1.3	7.0 ± 1.2
Sham	8	0	0	0	0	0

PD, hemiparkinsonian rats; wk, week.

Consistent with behavioral changes in the hemiparkinsonian rats, DA levels in the lesioned striatum (right side) fell dramatically (Fig. 4A, $P < 0.05$). Administration with bFGF-GNs/IN (Group 4) and bFGF-GNLs/IN or IV (Group 5 and 6) but not bFGF/IN (Group 3) significantly increased DA levels in lesioned striata relative to unloaded-GNLs/IN controls (Group 2). Although, the DA amount in bFGF-GNLs/IN group (3 000.38 ± 331.03 ng/g tissue weight) was higher than that in bFGF-GNs/IN group (1 020 ± 141.3 ng/g tissue weight) or bFGF-GNLs/IV group (900 ± 121.3 ng/g tissue weight), it only reached approximately 37% of DA level in sham-PBS/IN group (Group 1). In the unlesioned stratum (left side) of the unloaded-GNLs/IN group, the DA level was about 93% of sham-PBS/IN group ($P < 0.05$). The intranasal administration with GNs-and GNLs-encapsulated bFGF2 (Group 4 and 5) significantly elevated the striatal DA level in the unlesioned striatum ($P < 0.05$). Notably, DA levels on the lesioned side were lower than those of the unlesioned side in sham-PBS/IN rats ($P < 0.05$).

DA can be metabolized into 3,4-Dihydroxyphenylacetic acid (DOPAC) and 3-methoxytyramine (3-MT). Both of these substances are eventually degraded to form homovanillic acid (HVA). As with DA levels in lesioned striata, more DOPAC and HVA were detected in bFGF-GNs/IN and bFGF-GNLs/IN or IV treated hemiparkinsonian rats compared

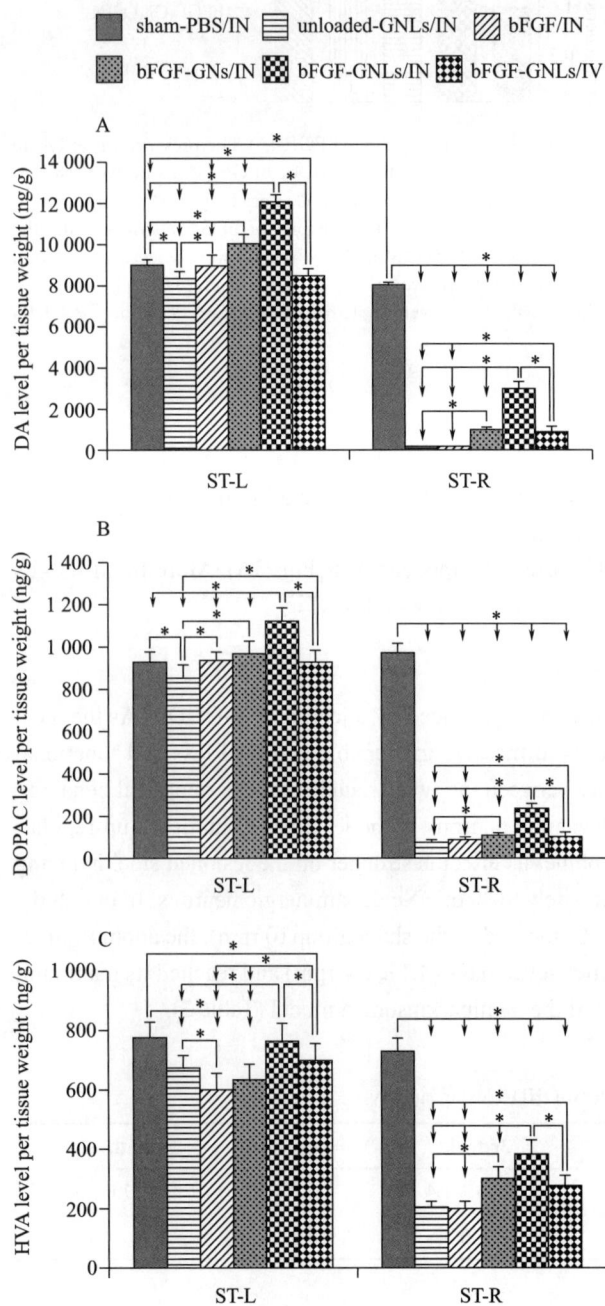

Fig. 4. Levels of DA (A), DOPAC (B), and HVA (C) in the striatum of 6-OHDA lesioned side (right side, ST-R) and unlesioned side (left side, ST-L) measured at the 14th day after intranasal administration of bFGF preparations. DA: dopamine; DOPAC: dihydroxyphenylacetic acid; HVA: homovanillic acid; GNs: gelatin nanoparticles; GNLs: gelatin nanostructured lipid carriers; IN: intranasal; IV: intravenous. Error bar: standard deviation. *$P < 0.05$ ($n = 7$).

to bFGF/IN and unloaded-GNLs/IN rats (Fig. 4B, C, $P < 0.05$). The lesioned striata of bFGF-GNLs/IN rats showed the highest levels of DOPAC (230.1 ± 21.7 ng/g tissue weight) and HVA (387.6 ± 43.2 ng/g tissue weight) among those three groups, but still significantly lower than sham-PBS/IN rats ($P < 0.05$). In unlesioned striata, DOPAC significantly rose in all bFGF-treated groups (Groups 3 to 6, $P < 0.05$) compared to unloaded GNLs/IN group (Group 2). Surprisingly, only intranasal bFGF-GNLs promoted the HVA level, which significantly declined after intranasal bFGF administration (Fig. 4B, C, $P < 0.05$).

2.4　bFGF-GNLs improves the retention of nigral dopaminergic neurons and attenuates rotational behavior in hemiparkinsonian rats

Tyrosine hydroxylase (TH) is the rate-limiting enzyme to catalyze the hydroxylation of L-tyrosine to L-3,4-dihydroxyphe-nylalanine (L-DOPA), the precursor to dopamine, norepinephrine and epinephrine. TH is considered a marker for catecholaminergic/dopaminergic neurons. TH immunohistochemistry in substantia nigra revealed severe loss of dopaminergic cells in the unload-GNLs/IN group (Fig. 5 B_R) compared with sham-PBS/IN group (Fig. 5 A_R). Enhanced cell retention was observed in the bFGF-GNs/IN, bFGF-GNLs/ IN and bFGF-GNLs/IV groups (Fig. 5 D_R, E_R and F_R), but not in the bFGF/IN group (Fig. 5 C_R). As semi-quantitative analysis of the result of immunohistochemistry with anti-TH antibody, bFGF-GNLs/IN group showed more TH-positive staining than bFGF-GNs/IN and bFGF-GNLs/IV groups (Fig. 5G, $P < 0.05$).

To further evaluate the therapeutic effect of bFGF by different delivery approaches, apomorphine-induced rotations were examined (Table 4). The hemiparkinsonian rats that received intranasal unloaded GNLs showed little difference from the untreated hemiparkinsonian rats (Table 3), indicating that blank GNLs had no therapeutic effect. Among the bFGF administration groups, only hemiparkinsonian rats treated with bFGF-GNLs/IN exhibited a significant decrease on apoorphine-induced rotation ($P < 0.05$), while the rats treated with bFGF-GNs/IN and bFGF-GNLs/IV showed a trend of improvement without statistical significance ($P > 0.05$).

Table 4.　Apomorphine-induced behavioral change at the 28th day after two-week daily treatment responding to different approaches of drug delivery

Experimental Group ($n = 8$)	1	2	3	4	5	6
Rotation (r/min)	0	7.3 ± 0.6	7.2 ± 1.1	6.3 ± 1.4	$5.1 \pm 0.8^*$	6.2 ± 1.2

$^*P < 0.05$ (Group 5 vs. Group 2 or 3).

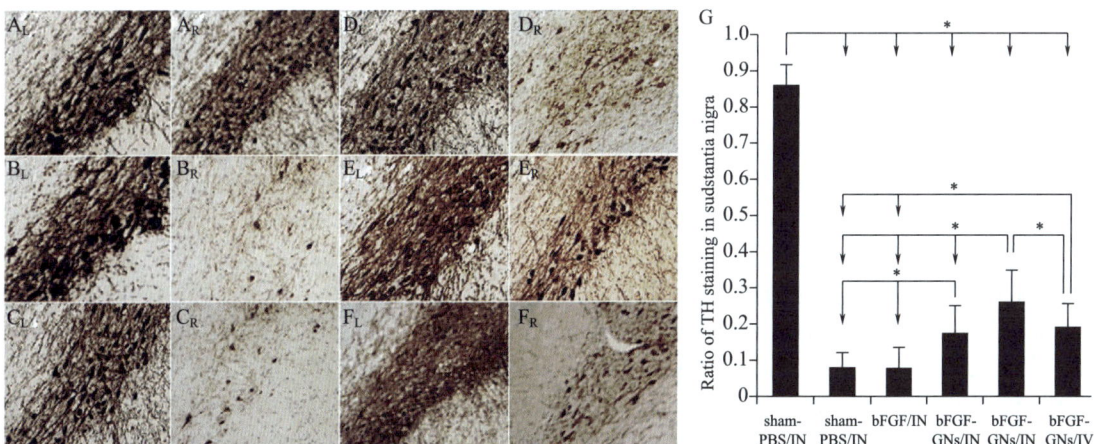

Fig. 5. TH immunohistochemical staining in the rat substantia nigra of lesioned (right, A_R-F_R) and unlesioned (left, A_L-F_L) sides on the 28th days after the surgery. Photomicrographs of immunostaining sections of rat substantia nigra from sham-PBS/IN (A_L, A_R), unload-GNLs/IN (B_L, B_R), bFGF/IN (C_L, C_R), bFGF-GNs/IN (D_L, D_R), bFGF-GNLs/IN (E_L, E_R) and bFGF-GNLs/IV (F_L, F_R) were shown. The ratio of TH staining (grayscale) in the corresponding lesioned to unlesioned SN regions was calculated in G. TH: tyrosine hydroxylase; GNs: gelatin nanoparticles; GNLs: gelatin nanostructured lipid carriers; IN: intranasal; IV: intravenous. Error bar: standard deviation. $^*P < 0.05$ ($n = 8$).

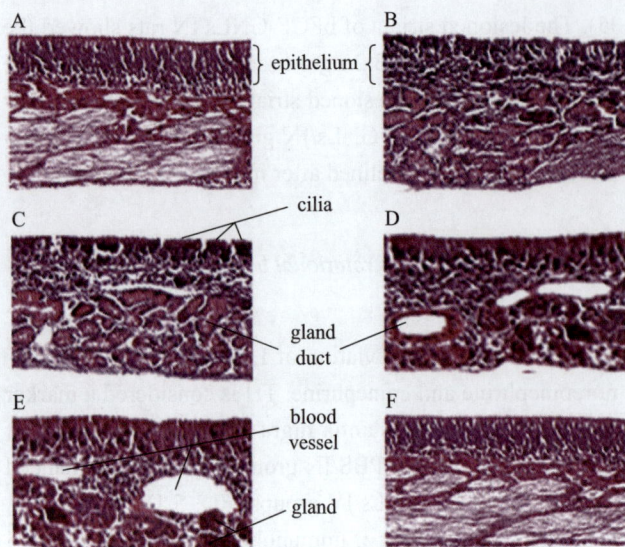

Fig. 6. Photomicrographs of the rat nasal mucosa after the administration with PBS/IN (A), unload-GNLs/IN (B), bFGF/IN (C), bFGF-GNs/IN (D), bFGF-GNLs/IN (E) and bFGF-GNLs/IV (F). All rats showed intact nasal epithelium with cilia. No adverse reactions (calcification, tumorigenesis, necrosis, sloughing of epithelium, hemorrhage, and infection etc.) were observed. GNs: gelatin nanoparticles; GNLs: gelatin nanostructured lipid carriers; IN: intranasal; IV: intravenous.

2.5 GNLs and its bFGF preparation do not elicit local epithelial damage of nasal mucosa

The potential of vesicular systems for use as an intranasal drug delivery system requires that this treatment be well-tolerated. Since the nanocubic vesicles are typically composed of phospholipids and surfactants, it is particularly important to consider potential nasal mucosal irritation induced by these vesicular formulations. In the sham-PBS/IN group, the nasal mucosa exhibited the orderly arrangement of the cilia on the surface (Fig. 6A). Similar observations were also evident in rats administered with unloaded GNLs (Fig. 6B) and bFGF preparations (Fig. 6C–F), respectively. No adverse reactions (calcification, tumorigenesis, necrosis, sloughing of epithelium, hemorrhage, and infection etc.) were observed at the administration site in any of the rats.

3. Discussion

Many brain diseases cannot receive effective treatment due to the presence of protective barriers (*e.g.* BBB) that inhibit free diffusion of circulating molecules from the blood into the brain. Recently, nanoparticles have emerged as a promising approach for delivering therapeutic agents across the BBB.[29] In this study, novel gelatin nanostructured lipid carriers (GNLs) with the nonionic copolymer-poloxamer 188 and solid lipids were developed, which effectively enhanced the brain delivery of bFGF *via* the noninvasive intranasal route and showed a significant neuroprotective improvement in hemiparkinsonian rats.

3.1 High stability, encapsulating efficiency, and loading capacity of GNLs

Lipid nanoparticles with solid matrix possess some advantages over other colloidal systems such as liposomes, emulsion, micro/nanoparticles, which include possibility of controlled release, drug targeting, increased stability, high payload, incorporation of both hydrophilic and hydrophobic drugs, and little biotoxicity.[30-32] Of the natural polymers, gelatin was selected for nanoparticle preparation due to its biocompatibility, biodegradability, low immunogenicity and surface modification. Being nonionic triblock copolymers with amphiphilic nature, the poloxamers have surfactant properties that make them widely used as both solubilizers and stabilizers for poorly soluble drugs in pharmaceutical applications.[33,34] It has been reported that modified gelatin mixed with Poloxamer 188 (Pluronic® F-68, PF-68) can generate nanoparticles that may be used in drug delivery.[35,36] Here, we adopted water-in-water emulsion followed by freeze-drying process to prepare the GNs and GNLs (Fig. 1). Negative charge was attributed to the lipid and surfactant in the system.[32] Generally, particle aggregation is less likely to occur for charged particles with higher absolute zeta potentials due to electric repulsion. As for the GNLs, high absolute zeta potentials and the presence of a steric stabilizer provided physical stability. The GNs had a statistically lower potential value than GNLs, possibly because the GNs without a phospholipid film were unstable. Smaller particles can easily penetrate into the cell and go through cell-to-cell junctions.

However, it is equally important to maintain a balance between size and properties such as distribution, polydispersity, stability, encapsulating efficiency, loading capacity and uptake capacity for drugs/bioactive materials. Although the GNLs had a larger particle size than the GNs, the GNLs and bFGF-loaded GNLs showed a better monodispersity (lower PDI), encapsulating efficiency and drug payload (Table 2).

3.2 GNLs improve the uptake of bFGF by nasal epithelium in the rat brain

It has been reported that nonionic surfactants, like poloxamer 188, might increase transcellular transport of olanzapine by reduction of the barrier function of the mucous layer due to their ability to reduce the mucous viscosity and elasticity, or to modulate the tight junction.[37,38] Poloxamer 188 interacted with the lipid bilayer may also induce a transition to the cubic phase,[34] act as a penetration enhancer,[39] and affect the lipid bilayer by perturbation.[40] Mucociliary clearance mechanisms rapidly remove drugs from the delivery site,[3] thus negatively charged drugs which increase the residence time at the delivery site have been shown to possess greater CNS bioavailability after intranasal administration compared to a neutral drug of similar size and lipophilicity.[41] The surface of bFGF-GNLs had strong negative charge with the potential value of -27.6 ± 1.1 mV, suggesting that GNL-mediated intranasal administration may be a promising approach to reduce clearance and enhance targeted delivery to the CNS. Compared to the level of bFGF in sham rats and wild-type rats administrated with bFGF alone *via* nasal cavity, more bFGF protein was detected in the olfactory bulbs of rats that received intranasally administered bFGF-GNLs, indicating a higher capacity of bFGF uptake by GNLs (Fig. 3A). It is believed that drugs can gain access to the CNS *via* the following pathways after intranasal administration: the systemic circulation in which the drug has to cross the BBB; the olfactory pathway in which the drug is taken up by the olfactory epithelium and enters the olfactory bulb; and the trigeminal pathway in which the drug is transported *via* the trigeminal nerve system.[42,43] Drug molecules can be delivered *via* axonal transport and transport through perineuronal channels[44] to the cerebrospinal fluid (CSF) and different brain parenchymal regions. The bFGF was significantly aggregated in striatum after intranasal administration with both bFGF-loaded GNs and GNLs, indicating that intranasal bFGF is able to be transported to specific brain areas. Moreover, the GNLs carried more bFGF to striatum than GNs (Fig. 3B). Intranasal bFGF alone significantly elevated bFGF level in olfactory bulb but not in striatum, suggesting that the intranasal uptake of bFGF was not efficient enough to result in its accumulation in striatal areas, perhaps also because of degradation that may occur due to its instability in solution.

3.3 Biological activity of GN-or GNL-mediated intranasal delivery of bFGF

As a neurotrophic factor, bFGF may block dopaminergic neuron death, retain striatal DA fibers, enhance dopaminergic graft survival, and thus induce functional recovery in parkinsonian rats.[45-47] However, its rapid denaturation in physiological conditions has been a major obstacle for its clinical application.[17] It was also reported that the bioactivity of bFGF is partially or totally lost when synthetic delivery vehicles such as poly(lactide-co-glycolide) and ethylene-vinyl acetate (EVAc) were used, since the protein is denatured during polymer processing conditions.[20,22,48,49] In our study, the GNLs had four times the loading capacity of bFGF than GNs (Table 2) but their bioactivities *in vitro* were almost the same, probably due to their different particle size. Compared to the bFGF-GNLs, the smaller bFGF-GNs had larger surface in a given volume and more opportunities to contact the cellular surface *in vitro*. Additionally, the bioactivity of bFGF-GNLs might be partially lost by double sonications during the two-step nanoparticle preparation.

Although bFGF-GNLs and bFGF-GNs had a similar bioactivity, more bFGF-GNLs were absorbed by nasal epithelium and delivered to the striatum (Fig. 3B). The bioactive effectiveness of the intranasal administration with the bFGF preparations was further assessed by monitoring the levels of DA and its metabolites DOPAC and HVA (Fig. 4). In sham rats, DA level in the striatum of surgery side was reduced around 10.5% ($P < 0.05$), indicating that the surgery procedure itself had an adverse impact on dopaminergic neurons or their DA synthesis. In the striata of both lesioned and unlesioned sides, DA and DOPAC were dramatically increased *via* intranasal administration with bFGF-GNLs when compared to any of the other preparations. Since not enough bFGF was able to be delivered to the striatal areas in bFGF/IN rats (Fig. 3), DA and DOPAC levels of lesioned side were not changed compared to those in sham-PBS/IN rats ($P > 0.05$). Surprisingly, HVA levels on the unlesioned side significantly declined in bFGF/IN rats, suggesting exogenous bFGF in striatum might activate an unidentified signaling pathway to inhibit the HVA formation. This inhibition was overcome when a sufficiently high level of exogenous bFGF accumulated in striatum to stimulate DA synthesis. Consistent with higher DA levels in the lesioned striatum, the hemiparkinsonian rats intranasally treated with bFGF-GNLs showed a significant improvement in their rotational behavior (Table 4). Of note, although there is no statistical difference of bFGF level among PBS/IN, bFGF/IN, and bFGF-GNLs/IV groups, more bFGF protein was detected in the bFGF-GNLs/IV group (Fig. 3B). Since bFGF elicits the biological effects under very low amounts, limited bFGF delivered by GNLs *via* intravenous administration may still increase the syntheses of DA, DA metabolites, and TH (Figs. 4 and 5G) in the striatum of 6-OHDA lesioned side. In general, intranasal bFGF-GNLs administration efficiently delivered exogenous bFGF in striatal areas where it exerted therapeutic effects on the PD rats.

3.4 Little toxicity of GNLs preparation to the nasal epithelium and dopaminergic neurons

Drug preparation and/or repeated administration may have harmful effects on the nasal epithelium including irritation (vascular congestion and subeptithelial edema), morphologic/functional changes of goblet cells, and chronic inflammatory response. GNLs and its bFGF preparations did not changethe integrity of nasal mucosa and mucosal cilia, indicating the safety of the developed GNLs for nasal administration (Fig. 6). However, GNLs may have a mild adverse effect on dopaminergic neurons and/or their DA synthesis since the levels of DA, DOPAC and HVA in unlesioned striata of unload-GNLs/IN rats were statistically lower than those of sham-PBS/IN rats (Fig. 4).

3.5 Therapeutic role of bFGF in 6-OHDA induced hemiparkinsonian rats

It is possible that the behavioral improvement of hemiparkinsonian rats that received bFGF-GNLs could be a physiologic rather than neuroprotective effect of treatment, i.e. boosting dopaminergic function in surviving synapses rather than boosting perikaryal survival. The ratio of DA metabolite to DA could identify such differences of DA metabolism in DA turnover.[50] In the 6-OHDA induced lesioned rats, the ratio of DOPAC to DA was not changed in the normal hemisphere of all groups even though higher DA levels were shown in bFGF-GNs/ IN and bFGF-GNLs/IN groups. However, the ratio was increased three-to four-fold in the injured hemisphere of unloaded GNLs/IN and bFGF/ IN groups but turned over in other groups, especially for bFGF-GNLs/IN group. Since the bFGF treatment was initiated just after the surgery and lasted for two weeks, DA turnover suggested that bFGF may not only stimulate the dopaminergic function in surviving synapses but also play a neuroprotective role. Consistent with this conjecture, an obvious retention of TH synthesis in substantia nigra was observed in the bFGF-GNLs/IN group compared with others (Fig. 5). In our study, bFGF alone was not striking enough to convert DA neuron loss and apomorphine-induced rotations; thus a therapeutic approach involving delivery of a cocktail of diverse NTFs should be considered for improving the survival rates of degenerating dopamine neurons and promoting regeneration of the nigrostriatal dopamine system.[15]

Overall, GNLs prepared by water-in-water emulsion and freeze-drying technique possessed better profile than GNs. GNLs efficiently enriched exogenous bFGF in olfactory bulb and striatum *via* nasal epithelium without damage to the mucous membrane. The bFGF not only stimulated dopaminergic function in surviving synapses but may play a neuroprotective role as well. However, bFGF alone is not able to completely reverse DA neuron loss and apomorphine-induced rotations in hemiparkinsonian rats. GNLs could be developed as carriers for nose-to-brain drug delivery, especially for the unstable macromolecular drugs such as bFGF.

Supplementary data

Supplementary data to this article can be found online at http://dx.doi.org/10.1016/j.nano.2013.10.009.

References

[1] Lochhead JJ, Thorne RG. Intranasal delivery of biologics to the central nervous system[J]. Advanced drug delivery reviews, 2012, 64(7): 614-628.

[2] Costantino HR, Illum L, Brandt G, *et al.* Intranasal delivery: physicochemical and therapeutic aspects[J]. International journal of pharmaceutics, 2007, 337(1-2): 1-24.

[3] Vyas TK, Shahiwala A, Marathe S, *et al.* Intranasal drug delivery for brain targeting[J]. Current drug delivery, 2005, 2(2): 165-175.

[4] Alsarra IA, Hamed AY, Mahrous GM, *et al.* Mucoadhesive polymeric hydrogels for nasal delivery of acyclovir[J]. Drug development and industrial pharmacy, 2009, 35(3): 352-362.

[5] Alsarra IA, Hamed AY, Alanazi FK. Acyclovir liposomes for intranasal systemic delivery: development and pharmacokinetics evaluation[J]. Drug delivery, 2008, 15(5): 313-321.

[6] Arumugam K, Subramanian GS, Mallayasamy SR, et al. A study of rivastigmine liposomes for delivery into the brain through intranasal route[J]. Acta pharmaceutica (Zagreb, Croatia), 2008, 58(3): 287-297.

[7] Mistry A, Stolnik S, Illum L. Nanoparticles for direct nose-to-brain delivery of drugs[J]. International journal of pharmaceutics, 2009, 379(1): 146-157.

[8] Doijad RC, Manvi FV, Godhwani DM, et al. Formulation and targeting efficiency of Cisplatin engineered solid lipid nanoparticles[J]. Indian journal of pharmaceutical sciences, 2008, 70(2): 203-207.

[9] Howells DW, Porritt MJ, Wong JY, et al. Reduced BDNF mRNA expression in the Parkinson's disease substantia nigra[J]. Experimental neurology, 2000, 166(1): 127-135.

[10] Parain K, Murer MG, Yan Q, et al. Reduced expression of brain-derived neurotrophic factor protein in Parkinson's disease substantia nigra[J]. Neuroreport, 1999, 10(3): 557-561.

[11] Tooyama I, Kawamata T, Walker D, et al. Loss of basic fibroblast growth factor in substantia nigra neurons in Parkinson's disease[J]. Neurology, 1993, 43(2): 372-376.

[12] Tooyama I, McGeer EG, Kawamata T, et al. Retention of basic fibroblast growth factor immunoreactivity in dopaminergic neurons of the substantia nigra during normal aging in humans contrasts with loss in Parkinson's disease[J]. Brain research, 1994, 656(1): 165-168.

[13] Baquet ZC, Bickford PC, Jones KR. Brain-derived neurotrophic factor is required for the establishment of the proper number of dopaminergic neurons in the substantia nigra pars compacta[J]. The Journal of neuroscience : the official journal of the Society for Neuroscience, 2005, 25(26): 6251-6259.

[14] Timmer M, Cesnulevicius K, Winkler C, et al. Fibroblast growth factor (FGF)-2 and FGF receptor 3 are required for the development of the substantia nigra, and FGF-2 plays a crucial role for the rescue of dopaminergic neurons after 6-hydroxydopamine lesion[J]. The Journal of neuroscience : the official journal of the Society for Neuroscience, 2007, 27(3): 459-471.

[15] Rangasamy SB, Soderstrom K, Bakay RA, et al. Neurotrophic factor therapy for Parkinson's disease[J]. Progress in brain research, 2010, 184: 237-264.

[16] Pan W, Banks WA, Fasold MB, et al. Transport of brain-derived neurotrophic factor across the blood-brain barrier[J]. Neuropharmacology, 1998, 37(12): 1553-1561.

[17] Edelman ER, Nugent MA, Karnovsky MJ. Perivascular and intravenous administration of basic fibroblast growth factor: vascular and solid organ deposition[J]. Proceedings of the National Academy of Sciences of the United States of America, 1993, 90(4): 1513-1517.

[18] Deguchi Y, Naito T, Yuge T, et al. Blood-brain barrier transport of 125I-labeled basic fibroblast growth factor[J]. Pharmaceutical research, 2000, 17(1): 63-69.

[19] Whalen GF, Shing Y, Folkman J. The fate of intravenously administered bFGF and the effect of heparin[J]. Growth factors (Chur, Switzerland), 1989, 1(2): 157-164.

[20] Tobío M, Gref R, Sánchez A, et al. Stealth PLA-PEG nanoparticles as protein carriers for nasal administration[J]. Pharmaceutical research, 1998, 15(2): 270-275.

[21] Varshosaz J, Eskandari S, Tabakhian M. Production and optimization of valproic acid nanostructured lipid carriers by the Taguchi design[J]. Pharmaceutical development and technology, 2010, 15(1): 89-96.

[22] Varshosaz J, Tabbakhian M, Mohammadi MY. Formulation and optimization of solid lipid nanoparticles of buspirone HCl for enhancement of its oral bioavailability[J]. Journal of liposome research, 2010, 20(4): 286-296.

[23] Jiang Y, Wei N, Lu T, et al. Intranasal brain-derived neurotrophic factor protects brain from ischemic insult via modulating local inflammation in rats[J]. Neuroscience, 2011, 172: 398-405.

[24] Xiang Q, Xiao J, Zhang H, et al. Preparation and characterisation of bFGF-encapsulated liposomes and evaluation of wound-healing activities in the rat[J]. Burns : journal of the International Society for Burn Injuries, 2011, 37(5): 886-895.

[25] Decressac M, Ulusoy A, Mattsson B, et al. GDNF fails to exert neuroprotection in a rat α-synuclein model of Parkinson's disease [J]. Brain, 2011, 134(8): 2302-2311.

[26] Kemeny S, Dery D, Loboda Y, et al. Parkin promotes degradation of the mitochondrial pro-apoptotic ARTS protein[J]. PloS one, 2012, 7(7): e38837.

[27] Berg MPVD, Verhoef JC, Romeijn SG, et al. Uptake of estradiol or progesterone into the CSF following intranasal and intravenous delivery in rats[J]. European journal of pharmaceutics and biopharmaceutics : official journal of Arbeitsgemeinschaft fur Pharmazeutische Verfahrenstechnik e.V, 2004, 58(1): 131-135.

[28] Wang ZL, Cheng SM, Ma MM, et al. Intranasally delivered bFGF enhances neurogenesis in adult rats following cerebral ischemia[J]. Neuroscience letters, 2008, 446(1): 30-35.

[29] Modi G, Pillay V, Choonara YE, et al. Nanotechnological applications for the treatment of neurodegenerative disorders[J]. Progress in neurobiology, 2009, 88(4): 272-285.

[30] Bondì ML, Fontana G, Carlisi B, et al. Preparation and characterization of solid lipid nanoparticles containing cloricromene[J]. Drug delivery, 2003, 10(4): 245-250.

[31] Das S, Chaudhury A. Recent advances in lipid nanoparticle formulations with solid matrix for oral drug delivery[J]. AAPS PharmSciTech, 2011, 12(1): 62-76.

[32] Patel S, Chavhan S, Soni H, et al. Brain targeting of risperidone-loaded solid lipid nanoparticles by intranasal route[J]. Journal of drug targeting, 2011, 19(6): 468-474.

[33] Katakam M, Bell LN, Banga AK. Effect of surfactants on the physical stability of recombinant human growth hormone[J]. Journal of pharmaceutical sciences, 1995, 84(6): 713-716.

[34] Salama HA, Mahmoud AA, Kamel AO, et al. Phospholipid based colloidal poloxamer-nanocubic vesicles for brain targeting via the nasal route[J]. Colloids and surfaces. B, Biointerfaces, 2012, 100: 146-154.

[35] Vandelli MA, Rivasi F, Guerra P, et al. Gelatin microspheres crosslinked with D,L-glyceraldhyde as a potential drug delivery system: preparation, characterisation, in vitro and in vivo studies[J]. International journal of pharmaceutics, 2001, 215(1): 175-184.

[36] Zhao YZ, Li X, Lu CT, et al. Experiment on the feasibility of using modified gelatin nanoparticles as insulin pulmonary administration system for diabetes therapy[J]. Acta diabetologica, 2012, 49(4): 315-325.

[37] Di Colo G, Zambito Y, Zaino C. Polymeric enhancers of mucosal epithelia permeability: synthesis, transepithelial penetration-enhancing properties, mechanism of action, safety issues[J]. Journal of pharmaceutical sciences, 2008, 97(5): 1652-1680.

[38] Zaki NM, Awad GA, Mortada ND, et al. Enhanced bioavailability of metoclopramide HCl by intranasal administration of a mucoadhesive in situ gel with modulated rheological and mucociliary transport properties[J]. European Journal of Pharmaceutical Sciences, 2007, 32(4): 296-307.

[39] Gizurarson S. Animal models for intranasal drug delivery studies. A review article[J]. Acta pharmaceutica Nordica, 1990, 2(2): 105-122.

[40] Lin HX, Gebhardt M, Bian SJ, et al. Enhancing effect of surfactants on fexofenadine·HCl transport across the human nasal epithelial cell monolayer[J]. International Journal of Pharmaceutics, 2007, 330(1): 23-31.

[41] Charlton ST, Whetstone J, Fayinka ST, et al. Evaluation of direct transport pathways of glycine receptor antagonists and an angiotensin antagonist from the nasal cavity to the central nervous system in the rat model[J]. Pharmaceutical research, 2008, 25(7): 1531-1543.

[42] Illum L. Transport of drugs from the nasal cavity to the central

nervous system[J]. European Journal of Pharmaceutical Sciences Official Journal of the European Federation for Pharmaceutical Sciences, 2000, 11(1): 1-18.

[43] Thorne RG, Frey WH. Delivery of neurotrophic factors to the central nervous system: pharmacokinetic considerations[J]. Clinical pharmacokinetics, 2001, 40(12): 907-946.

[44] Thorne RG, Emory CR, Ala TA, *et al.* Quantitative analysis of the olfactory pathway for drug delivery to the brain[J]. Brain Research, 1995, 692(1–2): 278-282.

[45] Date I, Yoshimoto Y, Imaoka T, *et al.* Enhanced recovery of the nigrostriatal dopaminergic system in MPTP-treated mice following intrastriatal injection of basic fibroblast growth factor in relation to aging[J]. Brain Research, 1993, 621(1): 150-154.

[46] Hsuan SL, Klintworth HM, Xia Z. Basic fibroblast growth factor protects against rotenone-induced dopaminergic cell death through activation of extracellular signal-regulated kinases 1/2 and phosphatidylinositol-3 kinase pathways[J]. The Journal of neuroscience:

the official journal of the Society for Neuroscience, 2006, 26(17): 4481-4491.

[47] Takayama H, Ray J, Raymon HK, *et al.* Basic fibroblast growth factor increases dopaminergic graft survival and function in a rat model of Parkinson's disease[J]. Nature medicine, 1995, 1(1): 53-58.

[48] Laham RJ, Chronos NA, Pike M, *et al.* Intracoronary basic fibroblast growth factor (FGF-2) in patients with severe ischemic heart disease: results of a phase I open-label dose escalation study[J]. Journal of the American College of Cardiology, 2000, 36(7): 2132-2139.

[49] Zhang L, Lu CT, Li WF, *et al.* Physical characterization and cellular uptake of propylene glycol liposomes *in vitro*[J]. Drug development and industrial pharmacy, 2012, 38(3): 365-371.

[50] Altar CA, Marien MR, Marshall JF. Time course of adaptations in dopamine biosynthesis, metabolism, and release following nigrostriatal lesions: implications for behavioral recovery from brain injury[J]. Journal of neurochemistry, 1987, 48(2): 390-399.

Heparin-based coacervate of FGF2 improves dermal regeneration by asserting a synergistic role with cell proliferation and endogenous facilitated VEGF for cutaneous wound healing

Jiang Wu, Xiaokun Li, Jian Xiao

1. Introduction

Human skin—the largest living organ in humans—not only serves as a the first physical barrier to protect the underneath organs from damage, but also possesses many biological functions including immunological surveillance and self-healing.[1] Any serious damage of skin integrity (*e.g.*, burns, lacerations, and diabetic wounds) will cause severe adverse effects on bacterial infection, the loss of blood and electrolytes, and tissue failure.[2] Skin wound healing is a highly complicated and coordinated process involving several distinct but overlapping stages. In general, it begins with hemostasis, followed by the prevalent inflammation, then leads to another stage for cell migration and proliferation, extracellular matrix deposition, angiogenesis, and tissue formation and remodeling.[3] Most severe skin wounds (i.e., non-healing wounds) are very difficult to heal spontaneously due to the lack of scaffold to guide cell growth and promote the angiogenesis of endogenous growth factors.[4-7]

Emerging evidence reveals that a number of growth factors play important but different roles in skin wound healing, including fibroblast growth factor (FGFs), epidermal growth factor (EGF), vascular endothelial growth factor (VEGF) and platelet derived growth factor (PDGF) families.[8,9] Among different endogenous growth factors, a number of *in vivo* studies of fibroblast growth factor-2 (FGF2;16−18.5 kDa) have shown that FGF2 is able to stimulate the proliferation and migration of a wide variety of cells (fibroblasts, endothelial cells, and kerotinocytes) at the wound area, accelerate acute wound closure, and promote tissue regeneration and angiogenesis in the process of wound healing.[6,8,10] Moreover, FGF2 can cross-talk with different neurotrophins and growth factors to promote wound healing. For instance, FGF2 interacts with α-smooth muscle actin (α-SMA) and increased its expression to form the connective tissue with the treatment of surgical periodontal defects in diabetic rats.[11] FGF2 also regulates the release of transforming growth factor β1 (TGF-β1) to promote re-epithelialization at the early stage.[12] Co-application of FGF2 and VEGF synergistically improves extracellular matrix deposition and neovascularization at wound sites in the diabetic mouse model.[13] In line with these studies, our previous work[14] also showed that regularly administered FGF2 every the other day (1 ml to each wound, 1 μg/ml, dissolved in 0.9% *w/v* saline) can accelerate the preformed healing wounds in the rat cutaneous wound model. The FGF2-improved wound healing is attributed to combinatorial effects by regulating inflammation response, stimulating fibroblast growth, and enhancing collagen deposition. All these studies above have demonstrated that FGF2 regulates many aspects of wound healing.[15,16]

On the hand other, like most of growth factors in clinical trials, FGF2 often requires high-dosages and frequent treatments (every the other day, even every day) to retain positive wound healing effects due to its short half-life caused by diffusion and susceptibility to enzymatic degradation.[17-19] Moreover, FGF2 is highly vulnerable to temperature and pH, and it degrades rapidly if surrounding temperature is above 40℃ or pH is less than 5.[20] Despite biological importance of FGF2, it is also equally important to design a suitable delivery system that protects and releases FGF2 in a sustained and controlled manner.[21-23] A number of particle-based delivery systems (hydrogels, nanogels, nano/microparticles) have been developed for encapsulation and controlled release of FGF2, but these delivery systems often suffer from low loading efficiency, high denaturation rate, and poor controlled-release.[24] To overcome these limits above, herein we developed a coacervate delivery system, which integrates poly(ethylene argininylaspartate digylceride) (PEAD) matrix (Fig. 1) with heparin and FGF2 together. In this delivery system, heparin is used to specifically bind to FGF2 to stabilize and prolong FGF2 half-life,[25] meanwhile PEAD matrix is designed to conjugate the heparin *via* non-

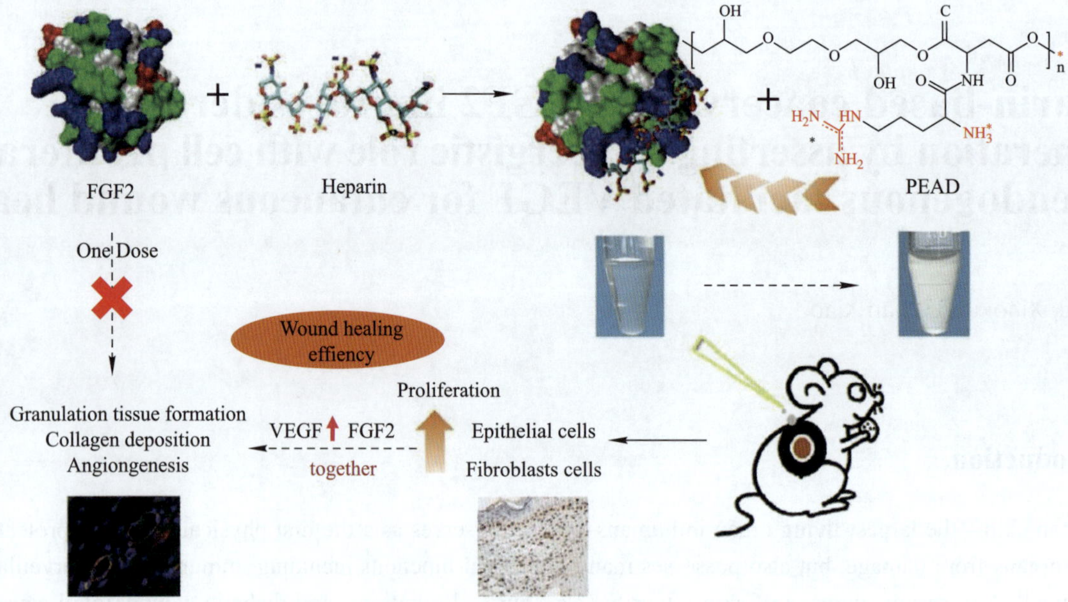

Fig. 1. Illustration of Heparin-FGF2@PEAD from preparation to wound healing process. Heparin-FGF2@PEAD enhances the cutaneous skin wound by promoting keratinocyte and fibroblast proliferation, stimulating the secretion of vascular endothelial growth factor (VEGF), and enhancing re-epithelization, granulation tissue formation, collagen deposition, and angiogenesis.

specific electrostatic interactions between the negatively charged heparins and the positively charged PEAD matrix.[26-28] The specific heparin-FGF2 binding also helps to prevent large burst release while providing tunable release profiles by attenuating diffusional release through transient interactions with the delivery PEAD matrix. The release of FGF2 from the heparin-FGF2@PEAD delivery system and its wound healing effect was examined in C57BL/6 mice. Additionally, we examined the biological roles of FGF2 in wound healing in mice models.

2. Experimental section

2.1 Preparation of FGF2 coacevate delivery system

The synthesis of PEAD was in two steps as previous described.[26] In brief, PEAD and heparin was each dissolved in 0.9% saline at 10 mg/ml and used a 0.22 μm filter membrane to sterilize. To prepare the delivery vehicle, FGF2 (the Key Laboratory of Biotechnology and Pharmaceutical Engineering, Wenzhou Medical University, China) was first mixed with 10 μl heparin, and then 50 μl PEAD was added (the heparin and PEAD mass ratio was 1:5) under constant stirring at room temperature. The mixed solution immediately turned cloudy to form the delivery vehicle.

2.2 FGF2 loading efficiency by Western blotting

To prepare FGF2-coacervates, 5 μg or 10 μg of FGF2 was mixed with 100 μg of heparin and 500 μg of PEAD at room temperature, separately. Upon mixing, 5 μg or 10 μg FGF2 was loaded into the coacervates, then the resulting FGF2-loaded coacervates were centrifuged at 12 100 g for 10 min. Both supernatant and the precipitate of FGF2-coacervates after centrifugation and FGF2-coacervate without centrifugation were mixed with the 5× loading buffer and denatured at 100 ℃ for 10 min, separated on 12% polyacrylamide gels, and transferred to a polyvinylidene difluoride (PVDF) membrane. The membranes were incubated in Tris-buffered saline (TBS) containing 5% skim milk for 90 min and incubated with primary antibodies at 4 ℃ overnight. The membranes were washed for 7 min three times with TBS containing 0.05% Tween-20. Then, the membranes were incubated with second antibody for 1 h at room temperature and washed with TBST as usual. FGF2 loading efficiency was detected with rabbit antihuman FGF-2 antibody (sc-79, 1:300, Santa Cruz Biotech, CA, USA) and then visualized using goat antirabbit horseradish peroxidase-conjugated antibody (AB22151, 1:10 000, Bioworld, Shanghai, China). The signals were then detected using Western blotting detection reagent, and the results were further analyzed by Image Lab (Bio-Rad, Hangzhou, China).

2.3 Heparin@PEAD complex by scanning electron microscopy

The scanning electron microscopy (SEM) samples were prepared by mixing 500 μg PEAD with 100 μg heparin to form the complex. The samples were rapidly frozen by liquid nitrogen, lyophilized, fixed on the aluminum stub, and sputtered with gold. Use of the liquid nitrogen to rapidly freeze the sample can greatly minimize the phase separation effect on the morphology of the sample. The surface of solid was then viewed by a scanning electron microscope (10 kV) (Hitachi, Tokyo, Japan).

2.4 Release of FGF2 from FGF2-coacervate

The controlled delivery system was formed by 500 ng of recombinant human FGF2 to 10 μl heparin and 50 μl PEAD. The solution was mixed and centrifuged for 10 min at 12 100 g. The supernatant was removed, and 500 μl 0.9% saline was added to the FGF2-coacervate. At days 0, 4, 7,10, 17, the supernatant was collected for analysis and added to fresh saline. The samples were stored at −80 ℃. The released FGF2 was analyzed by FGF2 enzyme-linked immunosorbent assay Kit (ELISA, Westang system, Shanghai, China). The amount of released FGF2 was calculated between the former and final concentrations. The FGF2 release system was carried out at 37 ℃. This trend of the release profile was maintained up to the end of the experiment.

2.5 Mice model

6−7 week-old male C57BL/6 mice were obtained from the Laboratory Animals Center of Wenzhou Medical University. The experiments on animals were conducted with adherence to the National Institutes of Health Guide Concerning the Care and Use of Laboratory Animals. All animal experiments were carried out with the guidelines approved by the Animal Experimentation Ethics Committee of Wenzhou Medical University, Wenzhou, China. Mice were maintained on a standard diet and water was freely available. Temperature (23 ± 2 ℃), humidity (35%−60%), and photoperiod (12 h light and 12 h darkness cycle) were kept constant.

2.6 Preparation of mice cutaneous wound healing model and analysis

Healthy C57BL/6 mice were randomly divided into four groups ($n = 7$). Group 1 was given saline as control. Group 2 was given heparin@PEAD as the vehicle. Group 3 was given free FGF2. Group 4 was given heparin-FGF2@PEAD. The treatment groups containing FGF2 were applied to the wound as a 10 μl solution.

In brief, animals were anaesthetized with intraperitoneal injection of 4% chloral hydrate (0.01 ml/g) and prepared for wounding under aseptic conditions. Mice were positioned on a form panel and the hair on the dorsum was shaved with an electric clipper. Depilatory creams was used to clear up the residual hair. Two silicone-splinted rings (external diameter of 16 mm, internal diameter of 8 mm, and 0.5 mm-thickness) were fixed on the wounds using 6-0 nylon sutures (Lingqiao, Ningbo, China). The use of silicone rings is of importance to reduce skin contraction upon wounding.[29] A 6 mm round skin biopsy punch (Acuderm inc., Ft Lauderdale, FL, USA) was used to create two full-thickness cutaneous wounds on either side of the dorsal midline. To prevent cross-contamination, the two wounds on each mouse received the same treatment. The experiment was single-dose topical administration on the healing of induced mice skin wounds. The appropriate dressing material was placed on the wounds. Mice were applied a Tegaderm transparent dressing (3 M Health Care, Brookings, USA) to prevent infection and wrapped in a thin layer of self-adhesive bandages (MDS, Shanghai, China) to deter chewing of the splints. In order to calculate the wound closure rate based on wound areas, photographs of wounds were taken immediately after surgery at different time points. These bandages only gently held the mice and did not limit the motion of the mice. Each mouse was fed separately with food and water. The bandage was removed and the size of the wounds was photographed from 7 to 17 days through the transparent dressing. Wound area was measured by Image-Pro plus to trace the wound margin, and all of the measured data were compared with postwounding. Since the fixed splints and wraps sometimes will be destroyed by mice, new splints and wraps should be provided to replace the damaged ones as soon as possible to keep the wounds in a consistent way.

Their wounds were harvested for histological analyses on the seventh day, four wounds per group, and the remaining animals were sacrificed at the day of terminal biopsy (on the 17th day). Wounds and surrounding tissue were excised for histological evaluation. The wound closure rate was calculated as follows:[30]

$$\text{Wound closure (\%)} = \frac{\text{area of original wound-area of actual wound}}{\text{area of original wound}} \times 100\%$$

2.7 Histological analysis

after anesthesia, wound tissue from the surrounding area was excised, maintained in cold 4% paraformaldehyde in 0.01 M phosphate buffered saline (PBS, pH = 7.4) overnight, and embedded in paraffin. Sections of 5-μm thickness were cut with a microtome (LEICA RM2235, Germany) and mounted in poly-L-lysine coating , stored at room temperature. Four wounds were analyzed at each time point, and only the sections from the wounded center were used for analysis. Skin sections were stained with Hematoxylin and Eosin (H&E) (Beyotime Institute of Biotechnology, China) for morphological evaluation and with Masson's trichrome staining (Beyotime) for assessment of collagen content following the manufacturer's protocols. The rest of skin was stored at −80°C for other tests.

2.8 Immunohistochemical staining

Sections were dewaxed and hydrated, and were pretreated with 3% H_2O_2 and 80% carbinol for 15 min to quench endogenous peroxidase activity. After washing by PBS, the sections were heated to antigen recovery, permeabilized with 0.5% Triton X-100 and blocked nonspecific antibody binding in 5% bovine serum albumin (BSA) (Beyotime) in PBS for 45 min at room temperature. Subsequently, primary antibodies diluted in PBS containing 1% BSA were used including rabbit polyclonal antiwide spectrum cytokeratin (ab9377, 1:75, Abcam), mouse monoclonal anti-PCNA (sc25280, 1:200, Santa Cruz Biotech, CA, USA), rabbit polyclonal anti-VEGF (sc-152, 1:200, Santa Cruz Biotech, CA, USA), rabbit polyclonal anticollagen III (ab7778, 1:1000, Abcam), rabbit polyclonal anti-TGF-β1 (ab92486, 1:500, Abcam) incubated at 4°C overnight. Followed by goat antimouse or goat antirabbit HRP-conjugated secondary antibodies, incubating for 2 h at room temperature and the reaction was stopped with DAB chromogen kit (ZSGB-BIO, Beijing, China) then counterstained with hematoxylin. The result images were acquired using Nikon positive position microscope (Nikon, 80i, Tokyo, Japan). The positive numbers of PCNA, VEGF were counted and quantified by optical density through Image-Pro plus. Immunohistochemistry for these markers were performed simultaneously in all wound samples as well as negative controls with 1% BSA.

2.9 Immunofluorescent staining

17-day skin sections were stained with rabbit polyclonal anti-CD31 (ab28364, 1:200, Abcam) and mouse monlclonal antialpha smooth muscle actin (α-SMA) (ab7817, 1:100, Abcam) followed by goat antirabbit IgG Alexa Fluor 647 (ab150083, 1:1 500, Abcam) and goat antimouse IgG Alexa Fluor 488 (ab150113, 1:1500, Abcam), respectively, and stained with 4',6-diamidino-2-phenylindole (DAPI; Beyotime). The fluorescent images were taken by Nikon confocal laser microscope (Nikon, A1 PLUS, Tokyo, Japan). The number of CD31 (endothelia cell) or α-SMA (mural cell) in the tissue was counted and confirmed by DAPI-positive nuclei. The diameter of blood vessels were measured and averaged by several randomly selected vessels using Image-Pro plus software. The value was divided by the area of the field and measured by NIS Elements Version 3.2 software (Nikon, Tokyo, Japan). All of the illustrations were assembled and processed digitally.

2.10 Statistical analysis

All data were expressed as mean ± standard deviations (SD). Statistical differences were performed using one-way analysis of variance (ANOVA) followed by Tukey's test with GraphPad Prism 5 software (GraphPad Software Inc., La Jolla, CA, USA). For all tests, $^*P$ value < 0.05, $^{**}P$ value < 0.01, $^{***}P$ value < 0.001.

3. Results and discussion

3.1 The characterizations, loading efficiency, and release kinetics of FGF2-coacervate

In Fig. 1, cationic PEAD contains two positively charged functional groups of amino and guanidine groups under physiological conditions, enabling PEAD to interact with heparin strongly. Fig. 2A shows the preparation process of

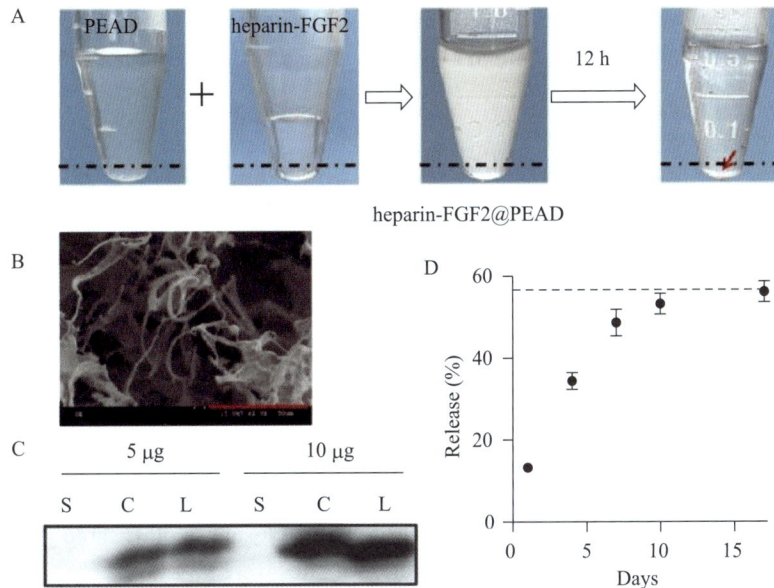

Fig. 2. The characterization, loading efficiency, and release kinetics of heparin-FGF2@PEAD. (A) The preparation process of FGF2-coacervate. The red arrow points to the precipitation particles. (B) Scanning electron micrograph of the interior morphology of heparin@ PEAD complex at 1000×. Heparin@PEAD complex was largely composed of ribbon-like structures. Scale bars: 500 μm. (C) The loading efficiency of FGF2 into the FGF2-coacervate. (D) The cumulative release profile of FGF2 from heparin-FGF2@PEAD during 17 days.

FGF2-coacervate (*i.e.*, heparin-FGF2@PEAD). It can be seen that both PEAD and heparin-FGF2 had excellent solubility in aqueous solution, as shown as transparent solutions. Upon mixing PEAD solution with heparin-FGF2 solution, the transparent solution became a milky suspension solution, and after 12 h, the heparin-FGF2@ PEAD complex precipitated down to the bottom (as indicated by a red arrow in Fig. 2A). These data indicate the formation of the heparin-FGF2@PEAD complex. To confirm the formation of heparin@PEAD *via* electrostatic interactions, cross-sectional images of heparin@PEAD samples were investigated using SEM. As shown in Fig. 2B, the cross-section area of heparin@ PEAD reflects their interior morphologies, which mainly consist of ribbon-like structures in globular domains. These ribbon-like domains further confirmed that this coacervate would provide superb accommodation for the loaded FGF2.

In Fig. 2C, the loading efficiency of FGF2 into the FGF2-coacervate was measured by Western blot. The amounts of FGF2 in the supernatant and in the settled coacervate after centrifugation were compared to the total amount of FGF2 in the loading solution. For the higher amount of growth factors (10 μg), the loading amounts of FGF2 in the settled coacervate and in the loading solution were almost same, and the loss of FGF2 was negligible after the incubation with PEAD matrix, indicating ~ 93% loading efficiency because of the large excess of heparin relative to FGF2. Then we utilized the FGF2-coacervate to evaluate the release of FGF2 from heparin-FGF2@PEAD. Fig. 2D shows the cumulative release profile of FGF2 from the FGF2-coacervate into saline over 17 days, and the FGF2 release was determined using ELISA. The FGF2 release behavior exhibited a typical two-phase release profile: an initial burst release during the first 24 h and a slow sustained release during the rest of the time course (day 2–day 17). The burst release percentage of FGF2 from supernatant was 13.2% ± 0.7% during the initial 24 h. After 24 h, the release percentage of FGF2 was slowly and gradually increased to a steady plateau of 56.1% ± 3.4% at day 17. The competency of the FGF2 release from heparin-FGF2@PEAD indicates a diffusion-controlled release at the initial phase (24 h) and a combined release behavior from the degradation, dissolution, and/or erosion of coacervates in the second phase (2–17 days). It has been reported that a sustained release of FGF2 for at least over 5 days is required to achieve regenerative in rat spinal cord injury model.[31] However, due to both positively charged nature of PEAD and FGF, there is no direct interactions between PEAD and FGF. Instead, the negatively charged heparin was used as a bridge to associate both positively charged PEAD and FGF2 together through its heparin domain in FGF2 and its negative-positive charge interactions between heparin and PEAD. Strong binding of FGF2 to heparin-PEAD may modulate its release from the heparin containing polymeric matrix, resulting in ~40% unreleased FGF2. All these results above only support that our designed FGF2-coacervate is workable *in vitro*, but do not necessarily mimic *in vivo* scenario, where enzymatic degradation of FGF2-

coacervate is anticipated. Next, we systematically performed a series of *in vivo* tests on the FGF2-coacervate to obtain different aspects of the wound healing capacity of the FGF2-coacervate in C57BL/6 mice model.

3.2 FGF2-coacervate enhances wound closure in mice

To evaluate the role of FGF2-coacervate in the skin wound healing process, we created full-thickness cutaneous wounds in C57BL/6 mice, followed by the examination of the wound healing process when treating the wounds with saline as control, heparin@PEAD as delivery vehicle, free FGF2, and FGF2-coacervate, respectively. Fig. 3A shows sequential photographs of the four types of treated wounds on day 7, 10, 14, and 17, respectively. It can be seen that the saline-treated and heparin@PEAD-treated wounds displayed similar wound closure rates of 14.5% ± 4.1% and 14.2% ± 7.0%. The wounds treated with both free FGF2 and FGF2-coacervate accelerated wound closure at day 7 and 14, but the wounds treated with the FGF2-coacervate recovered much faster with better skin appearance than other groups. In particularly, after day 17 the heparin-FGF2@PEAD-treated wounds were completely healed and almost scar-less, while FGF2-treated wounds still retained large residual wound areas. Quantitatively, Fig. 3B compares the wound closure rates for the four treated wounds. Consistent with visual inspection of wound healing in Fig. 3A, the rate of wound closure in heparin-FGF2@PEAD-treated mice was higher than that of wound closure in other three group mice at all treatment times (days 7, 10, 14, and 17). At day 17, the final wound closure rates were 98.2% ± 2.6% for heparin-FGF2@PEAD-treated group, 78.2% ± 6.7% for FGF2-treated group, 76.4% ± 10.8% for heparin@PEAD treated group, and 72.9% ± 4.6% for control group, respectively. The wounds were still covered with eschar. The FGF2-treated wounds showed comparable wound closure rates to the two control groups, but 20% lower than heparin-FGF2@PEAD-treated wounds, indicating that sustained release of FGF2 from the FGF2-coacervate has a positive effect on re-epithelialization.

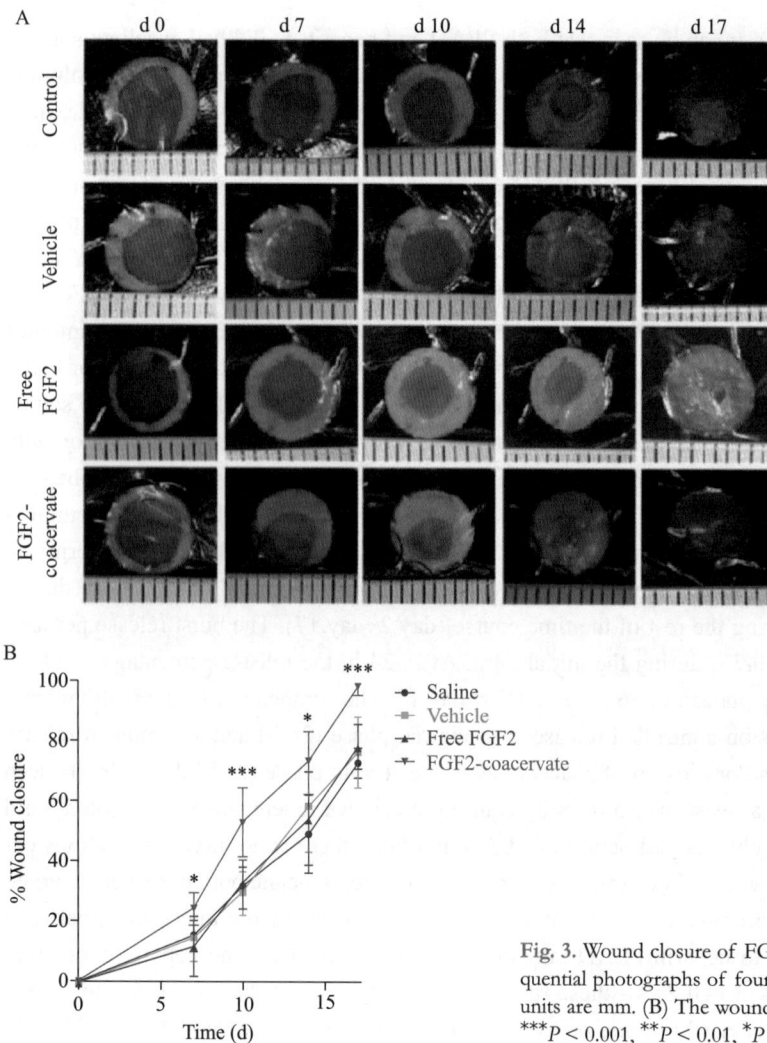

Fig. 3. Wound closure of FGF2-coacervate-treated wound closure in mouse. (A) Sequential photographs of four types of treated wounds on day 7, 10, 14, and 17. The units are mm. (B) The wound closure rates for the four types of the treated wounds. ***$P < 0.001$, **$P < 0.01$, *$P < 0.05$, compared to the control group, $n = 7$.

3.3　FGF2-coacervate induces more granulation tissue formation

Mice from each group were euthanized on days 7 and 17 post-treatment for clinical observation and histological analysis. Fig. 4 shows representative images of HE-stained (Hematoxylin and Eosin-stained) histological wound sites for four groups. In the control and vehicle groups, even at day 17, the wounds were still not fully closed. In the heparin-FGF2@PEAD-treated group, the regenerated skin was translucent and thin. The peripheral region was well integrated into the surrounding native skin tissue and there was complete appendage regeneration, as indicated by the formation of many hair follicles and blood vessels. In the other three groups, however, no obvious skin appendage regeneration was observed.

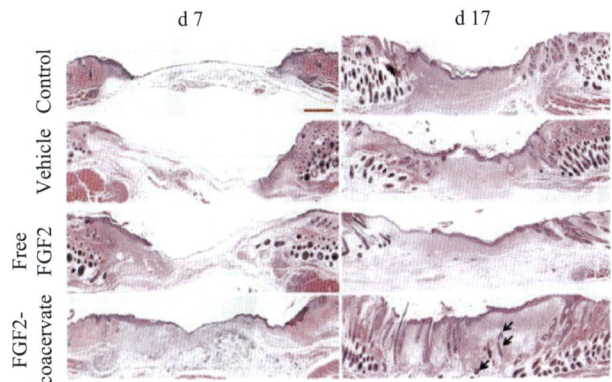

Fig. 4. Representative images of HE-stained histological wound sites for the four groups. The black arrows point to the skin appendages. Scale bars = 500 μm.

In parallel, Fig. 5 shows the histological collagen deposition in the dermis of regenerated skin in four groups at day 7 and 17 using masson trichrome staining (MTS). At day 7, MTS-stained sections of wounds treated with the heparin-FGF2@PEAD revealed the abundant granulation tissues formation with increased cellularity. This observation was similar to the HE-stained results in Fig. 4. However, for the control, vehicle, and free FGF2 groups, the gross appearance of granulation tissues were almost indistinguishable, suggesting that the delivery vehicle and free FGF2 had no apparently positive effect on wound sites (Fig. 5A–D). At day 17 postwounding, when more than 90% of wound closure was reached in the heparin-FGF2@PEAD group, the accelerated granulation tissue formation effect became even more pronounced. When compared to the untreated defects (Fig. 5E), extensive collagen deposition and thick wavy collagen fibers were observed in the wounds (Fig. 5H). Moreover, the underlying collagen fibers of heparin-FGF2@PEAD treated group (Fig. 5H, S1A, S1B) were well organized and morphologically similar to normal dermal skin (Fig. S1C). Consequently, both Fig. 4 and Fig. 5 show the expression of the newly formed blood vessels and skin appendage, indicating that the heparin-FGF2@PEAD group has a significantly higher blood vessel area and blood vessel numbers in the

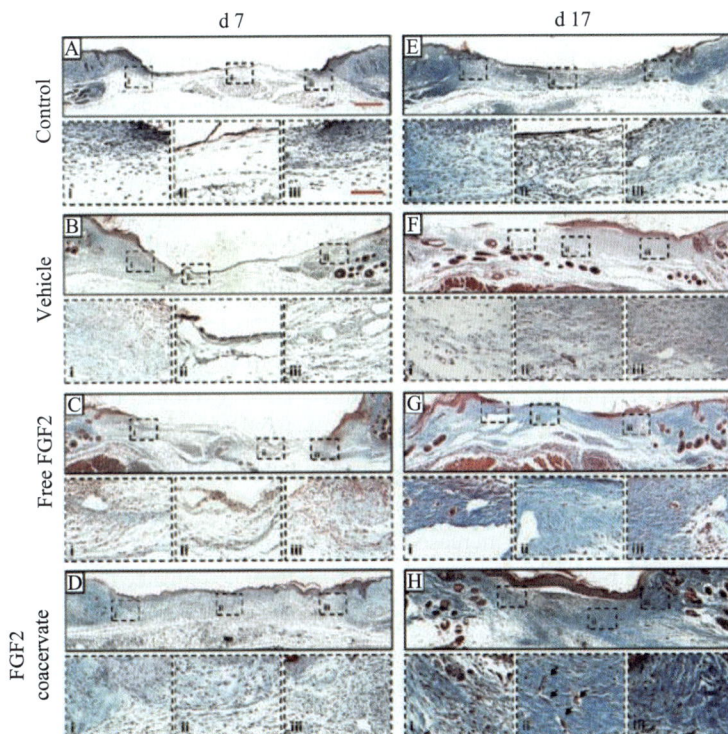

Fig. 5. The histological collagen deposition of MTS. (A) Representative images of MTS histological wound sites for the four groups. The black arrows point to the skin appendages. Scale bars (A–H) = 500 μm; scale bars (i, ii, iii) = 200 μm.

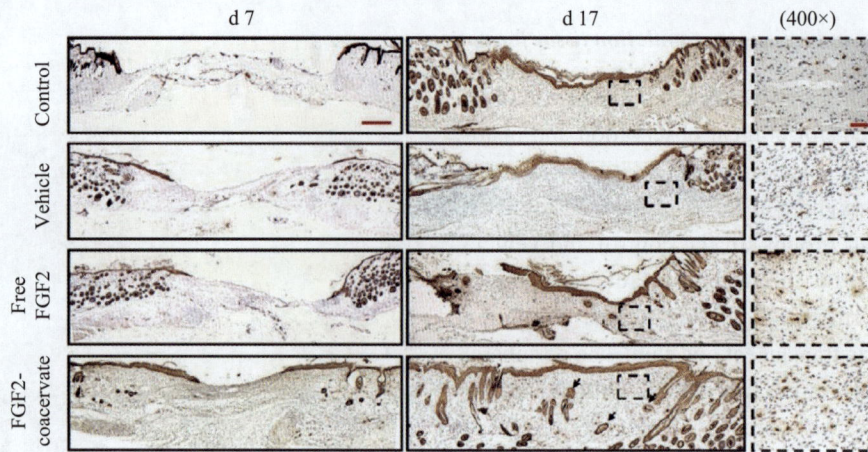

Fig. 6. Immunohistochemical results with the cytokeratin in wounds for the four groups. Representative light microscopy images indicates appendage regeneration in the presence of hair follicles within the granulation tissue after treated. Scale bars (low magnification) = 500 μm; scale bars (high magnification) = 50 μm.

healing wound area than the other three groups, suggesting that the FGF2-coacervate enables recruitment and proliferation of cells to form blood vessels in the wounded area.

In Fig. 6, the wounds were stained with wide-spectrum cytokeratin to evaluate re-epithelialization. Consistent with the HE and Masson results, the appendage regeneration of skin wounds were not observed in both control and the vehicle groups at 17 day postsurgery. Although the number of skin appendages increased from day 7 to day 17 postsurgery for both FGF2 and FGF2-coacervate groups, the FGF2-coacervate-treated wounds showed a much higher number of skin appendages and the thicker epithelial layers than the FGF2-treated wounds. Additionally, a close-up visualization (Fig. 6, 400×) also revealed the regeneration of hair follicles in the wounds treated with the FGF2-coacervate, demonstrating the accelerating effect of FGF2-coacervate on the wound re-epithelization *in vivo*. These *in vivo* data also had a good match to the results of wound closure rates.

Taken together, the FGF2-coacervate was demonstrated to exhibit the improved healing effect on re-epithelialization, granulation tissue formation, and collagen deposition, due to its sustaining release of FGF2.

3.4 FGF2-coacervate promotes keratinocytes and fibroblasts proliferation

Proliferating cell nuclear antigen (PCNA) was further used as a stained marker to evaluate cell proliferation as shown in Fig. 7. When treating with the FGF2-coacervate, cells around the wounds, such as keratinocytes, fibroblasts and others, proliferated very obviously, as compared to cells treated with no or vehicle and FGF2. Specifically, at day 7, the proliferation of cells in the epithelium and in the dermal with the treated of FGF2-coacervate were ~2.0 and 4.6 times higher than that of cells in the other three groups where most cells were inactive (Fig. 7B–C), indicating that the FGF2-coacervate possesses more active ability to stimulate cell proliferation at the wound sites. We performed further quantification of specific florescence staining of α-SMA to detect the density changes of activated fibroblast (the presence of myofibroblast) between different treated groups.[32,33] Using anti-α-SMA antibody to represent the formation of myofibroblast revealed that α-SMA-positive cells in FGF2-Heparin@PEAD group arranged more compactly and orderly than those in other groups (Fig. 8A). Quantitatively, FGF2-Heparin@PEAD group (7.8% ± 1.2%) exhibited the highest density of α-SMA-positive cells as compared to other three groups (3.6% ± 2.0% to 4.2% ± 2.6%,) (Fig. 8B), indicating more myofibroblast were also promoted by FGF2 coacervate leading to the quicker wound healing. Moreover, TGF-β1 is another important growth factor driving angiogenesis and myofibroblast differentiation during granulation tissue formation[12,34] At day 7 postwounding, the wounds in all groups revealed increased expression amounts of TGF-β1 (Fig. S2A), and the FGF2-coacervate-treated wounds showed the highest TGF-β1 level (Fig. S2B). The enhanced temporal expression of TGF-β1 concentration was driven by FGF2 stimulation from FGF2-coacervate groups and consequently accelerated the granulation tissue formation. However, at day 17, the TGF-β1 concentration was decreased in the FGF2-coacervate treated group (Fig. S2C and Fig. S2D), as compared to the other groups, indicating that the FGF2-coacervate group improved wound healing by releasing FGF2 to induce the higher TGF-β1, stimulating expression of cytokine at

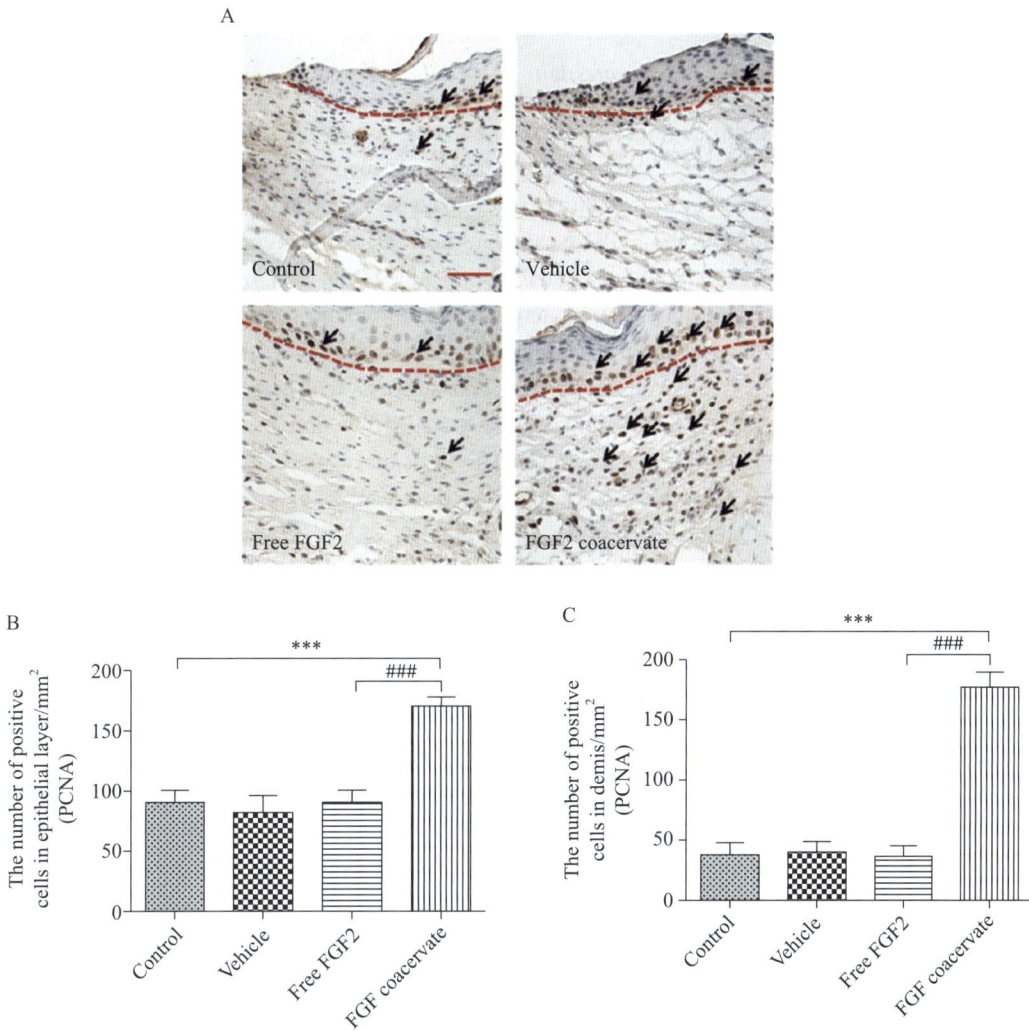

Fig. 7. Immunohistochemical results with the PCNA in wounds for the four groups. The histogram represents the positive cells and optical density of the immunohistochemistry results. The red dotted line is used to separate the epidermis and the dermis. Scale bars = 50 μm. ***$P < 0.001$ *vs.* control, ###$P < 0.001$ *vs.* free FGF2.

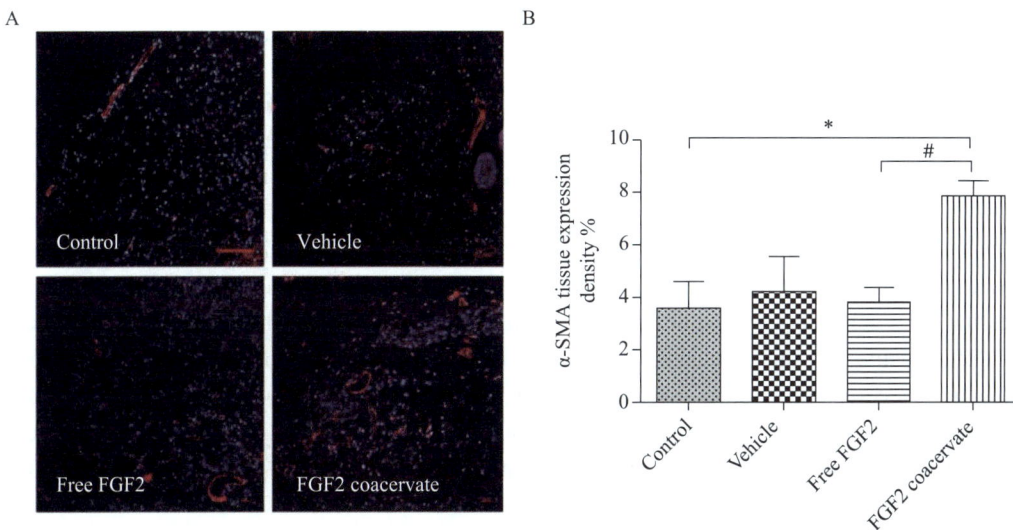

Fig. 8. (A) The presence of α-SMA expression myfibroblast upon post wounding for control, vehicle, free FGF2, and FGF2-coacervate group. (B) The histogram represents the quantitation of myofibroblasts through α-SMA expressions. Scale bars = 50 μm. *$P < 0.05$ *vs.* control, #$P < 0.05$, *vs.* free FGF2.

first, followed by reducing scar formation by decreasing the TGF-β1.

3.5 FGF2-coacervate facilitates endogenous VEGF expression

In addition to FGF2, a number of proangiogenic factors regulating cell division and cell survival, including VEGF, PDGF, and tumor necrosis factor (TNF-α),[35-37] not only are important for neovascularization,[38,39] but also stimulate with each other to assert a synergistic role in promoting angiogenesis.[40,41] At day 7, immunohistochemical staining showed significant expression of VEGF in the FGF2-coacervate-treated group as compared to the other three groups. The high expression of VEGF was observed not only in the wound edges (Fig. 9A), but also in the wound centers (Fig. 9B). This indicates that VEGF and FGF2 play a key synergistic role in wound healing by stimulating endothelial cell proliferation, migration into the wound area, and inducing angiogenesis. However, at day 17, there was no significant difference in VEGF expression between all groups (Fig. 9C). This suggests that FGF2-induced expression of VEGF to promote angiogenesis only occur at the first 7 days, not at the later stage of wound healing. A number of studies reported similar observation that FGF2 stimulated the expression of VEGF at the wound sites, and counterplay of FGF2 and VEGF resulted in a synergistic impact on skin wound healing.[42] Moreover, Nogami et al. demonstrated the fluctuation of the expression of VEGF in the wound healing process, revealing that VEGF was activated in the early stage of tissue repair process to induce vascularization.[43]

3.6 FGF2-coacervate increases vascularization in wound

The proper wound healing requires angiogenesis of the newly generated dermis, a process involving the proliferation and migration of endothelial and mural cells.[44,45] To evaluate neovascularization of the wounds, we quantified the expression of CD31 and α-SMA the biomarker of endothelial cells and mural cells in blood vessels in skin tissue sections stained with immunofluorescence. In Fig. 10, immunofluorescence detection of CD31 and α-SMA together after 17 days confirmed the number of newly formed and mature blood vessels in the wounds treated with FGF2-coacervate, but there was only a very small amount of vascular vessels and smooth muscle cells found in wounds treated with free FGF2 or saline. In Fig. 10C, blood vessel density as shown was significantly higher in wounds treated with FGF2-coacervate (13.2% ± 3.1%) vs wounds treated with vehicle (8.2% ± 1.7%) or saline only (6.6% ± 1.6%) or FGF2 only (7.4% ± 1.8%). Moreover, vessel diameter as shown in Fig. 10D was larger in the healing wounds of the FGF2-coacervate group (31.8 μm ± 8.7 μm), compared with the other groups (13.5 μm ± 7.7 μm, 9.4 μm ± 5.0 μm, and 5.3 μm ± 9.0 μm, respectively). It was also observed the colocation of both mural cells and endothelial cells around the wound treated with FGF2-coacervate, but the wounds from other three groups did not show the detectable cell proliferation. This is also consistent with the previous observation that there were approximately 3-fold more cells in the wounds of FGF2-coacervate-treated mice. These data indicate that the control release of FGF2 promotes the recruitment of endothelial cells to the wound area and enhances the vessel growth in healing wounds.

4. Conclusions

This work develops a heparin-FGF2@PEAD coacervate to efficiently and safely deliver FGF2 to full-thickness dermal wounds in mice, followed by an investigation of the mechanism of action of the controlled release of FGF2 for accelerating wound healing. The coacervate is demonstrated to play a synergistic role in increasing the proliferation and migration of the wound area related cells, improving granulation tissue formation and angiogenesis, up-modulating VEGF expression, thus enhancing wound healing. Additionally, we provide valuable data for better understanding the role of the FGF2 in healing full-thickness skin wounds, i.e., the controlled release of FGF2 is important for accelerating skin wound healing as compared to other cytokines. Hence, the FGF2-coacervate delivery system is highly promising for the future treatment of chronic wounds. On the other hand, we should also mention that for this coacervate system, the negatively charged heparin is used as a bridge to associate charged PEAD first, then binds to FGF2 through heparin domain, forming the coacervate. Both ionic and pH environments are very crucial for this coacervate system, especially for different growth factors (GFs) with different isoelectric points. Thus, different GF delivery systems should be carefully designed using heparin cross-linked hydrogels or modified heparin polymers especially for codelivery of varied GFs toward chronic wounds.

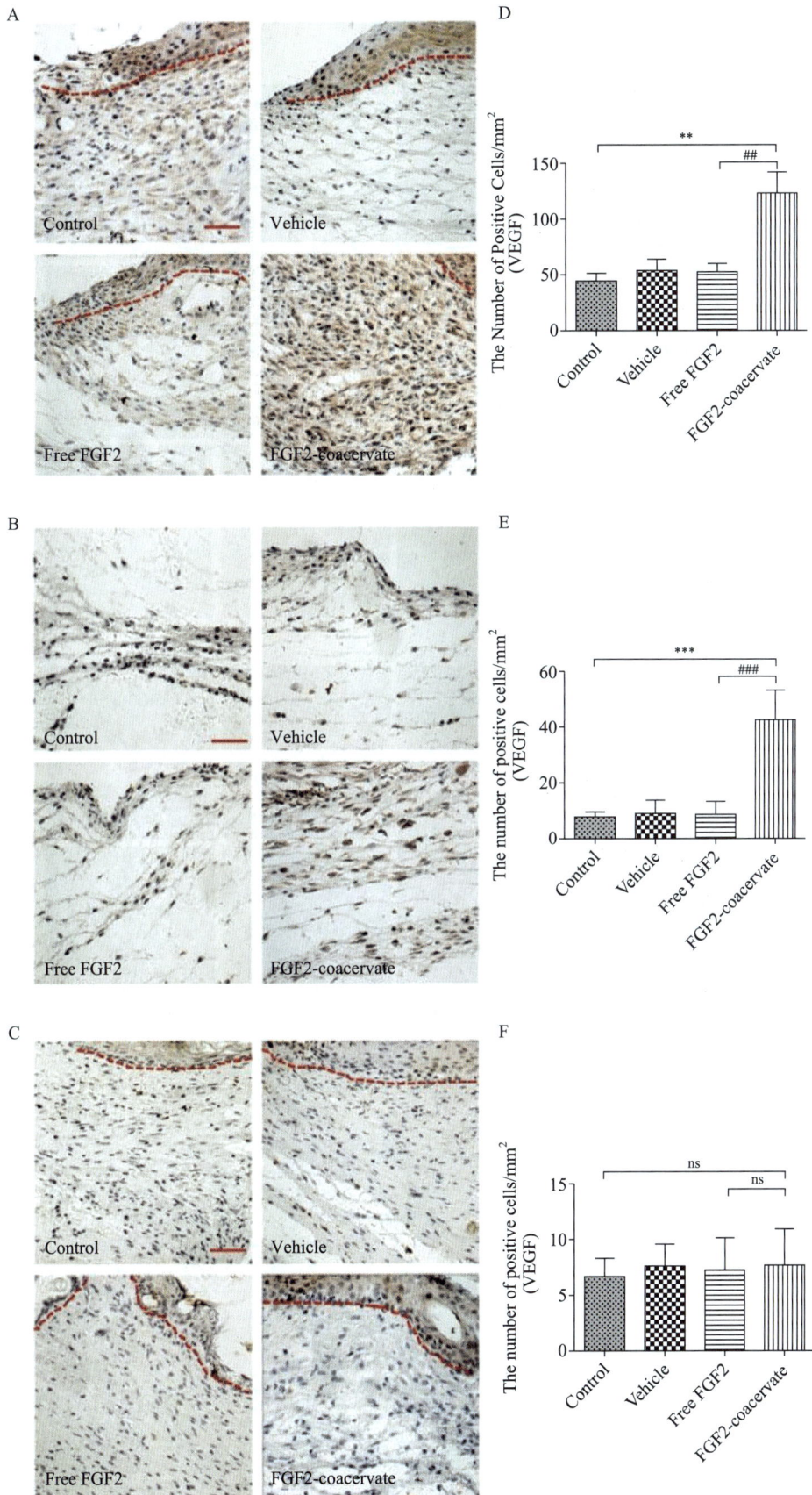

Fig. 9. Immunohistochemistry of the expression of VEGF. (A) at the wound edge at the day 7, (B) at the center of wound at the day 7, and (C) at the healing area at the day 17. The histogram represents the positive cells and optical density of the immunohistochemistry results (D,E,F). The red dotted line is used to separate the epidermis and the dermis. Scale bars = 50 μm. [***]$P < 0.001$ *vs.* control, [##]$P < 0.01$ *vs.* free FGF2, [###]$P < 0.001$ *vs.* free FGF2, NS means no significant difference between them.

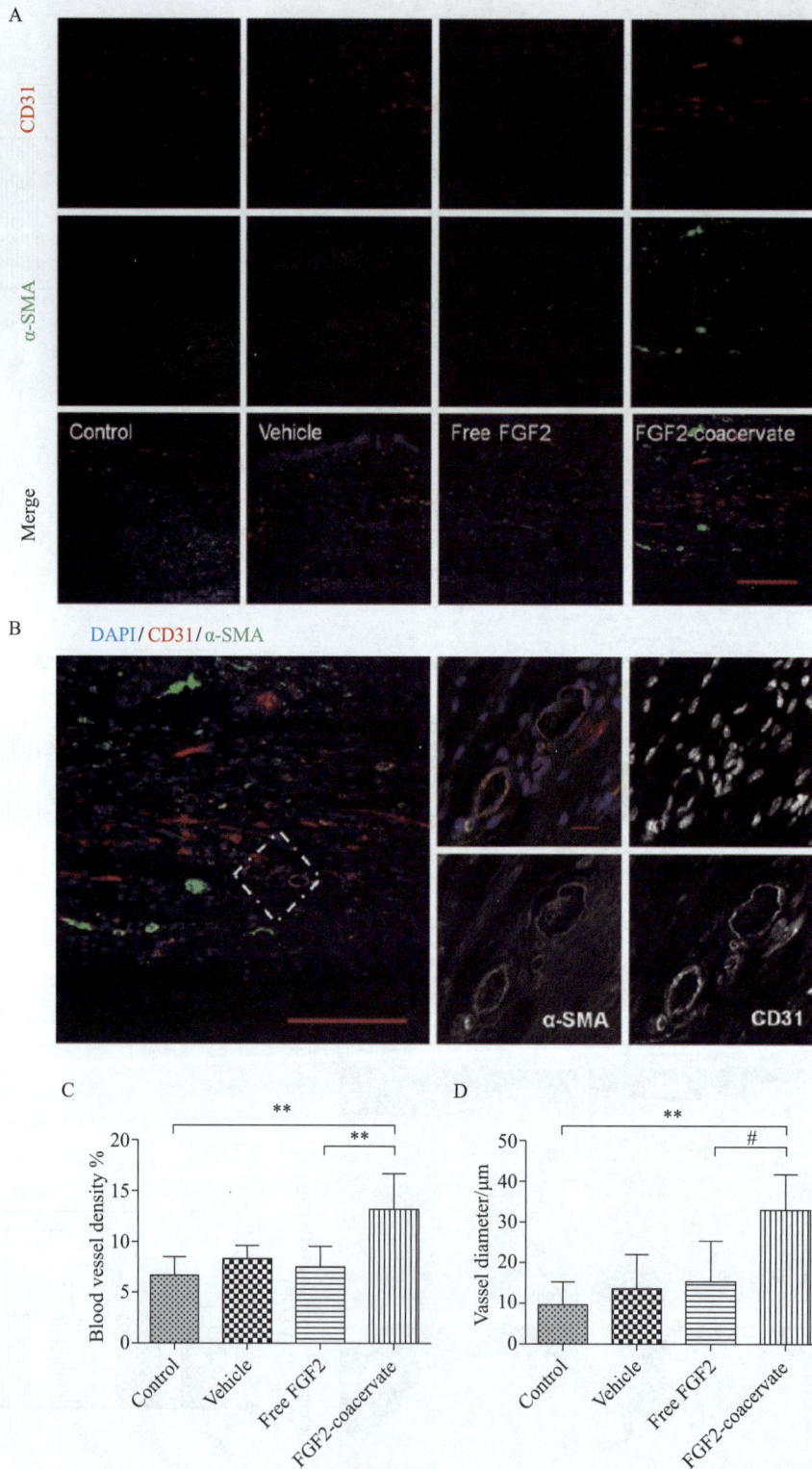

Fig. 10. Immunofluorescence detection of CD31 and α-SMA at the wound area on the day 17. (A) Representative confocal images of granulation tissue near the wound margin show endothelial cell (CD31, red) and mural cell (α-smooth muscle actin, green) with DAPI (blue) nuclear staining. Scale bars = 200 μm. (B) High magnification revealed by the colocalization of cells (yellow) as potential mature vessels. The circular vessel-like structures were observed in the wound area. Scale bars = 50 μm. (C) The histogram represents the blood vessel density of the immunofluorescence results. (D) The histogram represents the vessel diameter of the blood vessels. $^{**}P < 0.01$ *vs.* control, $^{#}P < 0.05$ *vs.* free FGF2.

Supporting information

The supporting information is available on the ACS publications website at DOI:10.1021/acs.biomac.6b00398.

References

[1] Clark RA, Ghosh K, Tonnesen MG. Tissue engineering for cutaneous wounds[J]. The Journal of investigative dermatology, 2007, 127(5): 1018-1029.

[2] Gurtner GC, Werner S, Barrandon Y, *et al.* Wound repair and regeneration[J]. Nature, 2008, 453: 314.

[3] Diegelmann RF, Evans MC. Wound healing: an overview of acute, fibrotic and delayed healing[J]. Front Biosci, 2003, 9(71): 283-289.

[4] Sen CK, Gordillo GM, Roy S, *et al.* Human skin wounds: a major and snowballing threat to public health and the economy[J]. Wound repair and regeneration : official publication of the Wound Healing Society [and] the European Tissue Repair Society, 2009, 17(6): 763-771.

[5] Schultz GS, Davidson JM, Kirsner RS, *et al.* Dynamic reciprocity in the wound microenvironment[J]. Wound repair and regeneration : official publication of the Wound Healing Society [and] the European Tissue Repair Society, 2011, 19(2): 134-148.

[6] Risau W. Angiogenic growth factors[J]. Progress in growth factor research, 1990, 2(1): 71-79.

[7] Knighton DR, Phillips GD, Fiegel VD. Wound healing angiogenesis: indirect stimulation by basic fibroblast growth factor[J]. Journal of Trauma & Acute Care Surgery, 1990, 30(12 Suppl): S134.

[8] Werner S, Grose R. Regulation of wound healing by growth factors and cytokines[J]. Physiological reviews, 2003, 83(3): 835-870.

[9] Shirakata Y. Heparin-binding EGF-like growth factor accelerates keratinocyte migration and skin wound healing[J]. Journal of Cell Science, 2005, 118(11): 2363-2370.

[10] Kasuya A, Tokura Y. Attempts to accelerate wound healing[J]. Journal of dermatological science, 2014, 76(3): 169-172.

[11] Bizenjima T, Seshima F, Ishizuka Y, *et al.* Fibroblast growth factor-2 promotes healing of surgically created periodontal defects in rats with early, streptozotocin-induced diabetes *via* increasing cell proliferation and regulating angiogenesis[J]. Journal of clinical periodontology, 2015, 42(1): 62-71.

[12] Penn JW, Grobbelaar AO, Rolfe KJ. The role of the TGF-β family in wound healing, burns and scarring: a review[J]. International Journal of Burns & Trauma, 2012, 2(1): 18.

[13] Losi P, Briganti E, Errico C, *et al.* Fibrin-based scaffold incorporating VEGF- and bFGF-loaded nanoparticles stimulates wound healing in diabetic mice[J]. Acta biomaterialia, 2013, 9(8): 7814-7821.

[14] Shi HX, Lin C, Lin BB, *et al.* The anti-scar effects of basic fibroblast growth factor on the wound repair *in vitro* and *in vivo*[J]. PloS one, 2013, 8(4): e59966.

[15] Robson MC, Phillips LG, Lawrence WT, *et al.* The safety and effect of topically applied recombinant basic fibroblast growth factor on the healing of chronic pressure sores[J]. Annals of surgery, 1992, 216(4): 401-406; discussion 406-408.

[16] Kurita Y, Tsuboi R, Ueki R, *et al.* Immunohistochemical localization of basic fibroblast growth factor in wound healing sites of mouse skin[J]. Archives of dermatological research, 1992, 284(4): 193-197.

[17] Tayalia P, Mooney DJ. Controlled Growth Factor Delivery for Tissue Engineering[J]. Advanced Materials, 2010, 21(32-33): 3269-3285.

[18] Barrientos S, Brem H, Stojadinovic O, *et al.* Clinical application of growth factors and cytokines in wound healing[J]. Wound repair and regeneration : official publication of the Wound Healing Society [and] the European Tissue Repair Society, 2014, 22(5): 569-578.

[19] Aviles RJ, Annex BH, Lederman RJ. Testing clinical therapeutic angiogenesis using basic fibroblast growth factor (FGF-2)[J]. British journal of pharmacology, 2003, 140(4): 637-646.

[20] She Z, Wang C, Li J, *et al.* Encapsulation of basic fibroblast growth factor by polyelectrolyte multilayer microcapsules and its controlled release for enhancing cell proliferation[J]. Biomacromolecules, 2012, 13(7): 2174-2180.

[21] Zomer Volpato F, Almodóvar J, Erickson K, *et al.* Preservation of FGF-2 bioactivity using heparin-based nanoparticles, and their delivery from electrospun chitosan fibers[J]. Acta biomaterialia, 2012, 8(4): 1551-1559.

[22] Reimer K, Vogt PM, Broegmann B, *et al.* An innovative topical drug formulation for wound healing and infection treatment: *in vitro* and *in vivo* investigations of a povidone-iodine liposome hydrogel[J]. Dermatology (Basel, Switzerland), 2000, 201(3): 235-241.

[23] Xiang Q, Xiao J, Zhang H, *et al.* Preparation and characterisation of bFGF-encapsulated liposomes and evaluation of wound-healing activities in the rat[J]. Burns : journal of the International Society for Burn Injuries, 2011, 37(5): 886-895.

[24] Johnson NR, Wang Y. Controlled delivery of heparin-binding EGF-like growth factor yields fast and comprehensive wound healing[J]. Journal of controlled release : official journal of the Controlled Release Society, 2013, 166(2): 124-129.

[25] Walker A, Turnbull JE, Gallagher JT. Specific heparan sulfate saccharides mediate the activity of basic fibroblast growth factor[J]. The Journal of biological chemistry, 1994, 269(2): 931-935.

[26] Chu H, Johnson NR, Mason NS, *et al.* A [polycation:heparin] complex releases growth factors with enhanced bioactivity[J]. Journal of controlled release : official journal of the Controlled Release Society, 2011, 150(2): 157-163.

[27] Chu H, Gao J, Wang Y. Design, synthesis, and biocompatibility of an arginine-based polyester[J]. Biotechnology progress, 2012, 28(1): 257-264.

[28] Chu H, Chen CW, Huard J, *et al.* The effect of a heparin-based coacervate of fibroblast growth factor-2 on scarring in the infarcted myocardium[J]. Biomaterials, 2013, 34(6): 1747-1756.

[29] Davidson JM, Yu F, Opalenik SR. Splinting Strategies to Overcome Confounding Wound Contraction in Experimental Animal Models[J]. Advances in wound care, 2013, 2(4): 142-148.

[30] Zonari A, Martins TM, Paula AC, *et al.* Polyhydroxybutyrate-co-hydroxyvalerate structures loaded with adipose stem cells promote skin healing with reduced scarring[J]. Acta Biomaterialia, 2015, 17: 170-181.

[31] Vulic K, Shoichet MS. Tunable growth factor delivery from injectable hydrogels for tissue engineering[J]. Journal of the American Chemical Society, 2012, 134(2): 882-885.

[32] Al-Qattan MM, Abd-Elwahed MM, Hawary K, *et al.* Myofibroblast Expression in Skin Wounds Is Enhanced by Collagen III Suppression[J]. Biomed Res Int, 2016, 2015: 958695.

[33] Kapoor M, Liu S, Huh K, *et al.* Connective tissue growth factor promoter activity in normal and wounded skin[J]. Fibrogenesis & tissue repair, 2008, 1(1): 3.

[34] Watarai A, Schirmer L, Thönes S, *et al.* TGFβ functionalized star-PEG-heparin hydrogels modulate human dermal fibroblast growth and differentiation[J]. Acta Biomaterialia, 2015, 25: 65-75.

[35] Sellke FW, Laham RJ, Edelman ER, *et al.* Therapeutic Angiogenesis With Basic Fibroblast Growth Factor: Technique and Early Results[J]. Annals of Thoracic Surgery, 1998, 65(6): 1540-1544.

[36] Kroll J, Waltenberger J. Regulation of the endothelial function and angiogenesis by vascular endothelial growth factor-A (VEGF-A[J]. Z Kardiol, 2000, 89(3): 206-218.

[37] Li J, Wei Y, Liu K, *et al.* Synergistic effects of FGF-2 and PDGF-BB on angiogenesis and muscle regeneration in rabbit hindlimb ischemia model[J]. Microvascular research, 2010, 80(1): 10-17.

[38] Komori M, Tomizawa Y, Takada K, *et al.* A Single Local Application of Recombinant Human Basic Fibroblast Growth Factor Accelerates Initial Angiogenesis During Wound Healing in Rabbit Ear Chamber[J]. Anesthesia & Analgesia, 2005, 100(3): 830-834.

[39] Demirdögen B, Elçin AE, Elçin YM. Neovascularization by bFGF releasing hyaluronic acid-gelatin microspheres: *in vitro* and *in vivo* studies[J]. Growth factors (Chur, Switzerland), 2010, 28(6): 426-436.

[40] Duraisamy Y, Slevin M, Smith N, *et al.* Effect of glycation on basic fibroblast growth factor induced angiogenesis and activation of associated signal transduction pathways in vascular endothelial cells: possible relevance to wound healing in diabetes[J]. Angiogenesis, 2001, 4(4): 277-288.

[41] Tonnesen MG, Feng X, Clark RA. Angiogenesis in wound healing[J]. The journal of investigative dermatology. Symposium proceedings, 2000, 5(1): 40-46.

[42] Takamiya M, Saigusa K, Aoki Y. Immunohistochemical study of basic fibroblast growth factor and vascular endothelial growth factor expression for age determination of cutaneous wounds[J]. The American journal of forensic medicine and pathology, 2002, 23(3): 264-267.

[43] Nogami M, Hoshi T, Kinoshita M, *et al.* Vascular endothelial growth factor expression in rat skin incision wound[J]. Medical molecular morphology, 2007, 40(2): 82-87.

[44] DeLisser HM, Christofidou-Solomidou M, Strieter RM, *et al.* Involvement of endothelial PECAM-1/CD31 in angiogenesis[J]. The American journal of pathology, 1997, 151(3): 671-677.

[45] Jain RK. Molecular regulation of vessel maturation[J]. Nature medicine, 2003, 9(6): 685-693.

A thermosensitive heparin-poloxamer hydrogel bridges aFGF to treat spinal cord injury

Qingqing Wang, Xiaokun Li, Jian Xiao

1. Introduction

Spinal cord injury (SCI) is a crippling and severely disabling disease with almost 12 000 new cases occurring annually. SCI causes a significant loss of sensory and motor functions as well as a wide range of disabilities *via* two primary phases.[1] The initial mechanical injury causes a structural disturbance; this is followed by long-term secondary damage comprising inflammation, apoptosis, oxidative stress, and the formation of glial scars.[2] Currently, injury stabilization by decompression surgery, secondary complication prevention, and rehabilitation *via* drug administration are considered essential for functional recovery after SCI. The molecules involved with neurological recovery after SCI are designed to protect surviving tissue against degeneration,[3] inhibit inflammation,[4] promote regenerative growth of lesioned axons,[5] and reduce glial scars,[6,7] all of which are barriers of neuron axon regeneration after SCI.

Acidic fibroblast growth factor (aFGF) is one of the powerful factors involved in the protection and regeneration of the nervous system[8-11] and has been demonstrated as safe and feasible in a clinical trial.[12] A proteomics study indicated that aFGF can reduce the number of apoptotic neurons and the inflammatory reaction after SCI;[13-15] however, as a macromolecular protein, aFGF has poor penetrability of the blood spinal cord barrier (BSCB). Thus, aFGF delivery *via* either subcutaneous or intravenous administration is ineffective in SCI. *In situ* administration can help aFGF bypass the BSCB, but the effects of aFGF are limited due to its limited shelf life and susceptibility to biochemical variations in the body. Therefore, identifying a more effective route of aFGF administration and maintaining aFGF sustained release are urgently needed. Several recent reviews summarized the development of the cells and drugs delivery strategies into the spinal cord and reviewed the role of hydrogel in SCI treatments trategies.[16-18] Many new materials such as three-dimensional (3D) biomimetic hydrogel,[19,20] nanoparticles,[21,22] and novel scaffolds[23] were used to carry substances (drugs,antibodies, peptides, or other proteins) and/or cells for SCI treatment. Besides, with the deep understanding of the mechanisms of SCI, many selective delivery tools that could selectively treat/target the aim cells or tissue have been developed.[24,25] Hydrogels are nontoxic, biodegradable, 3D porous structures that can act as promising protective agents and vehicles to load and deliver biological macromolecules.[20,26] Several growth factor (GF) hydrogel systems have been reported for the treatment of SCI, including a hyaluronan, methylcelluloseand hydrogel, or nanoparticle composite with PDGF,[27,28] a beta hairpin peptide hydrogel containing NGF,[29] a hyaluronic acid hydrogel with BDNF,[30] a HEMA-MOETACL hydrogel containing bFGF,[31] and a VEGF-loaded alginate hydrogel.[32] The most ideal hydrogels for SCI recovery should be thermosensitive, have a high loading capacity, and offer maximal protection of the GFs. However, none of these hydrogels are optimal. Identifying the most appropriate biocompatible material for loading GFs that could act as a scaffold and maximize their potential in promoting a comprehensive recovery of SCI is still a big challenge. In this work, we designed a novel thermosensitive aFGF-infused heparin-poloxamer hydrogel that could load and transfer aFGF to the injured spinal cord in a localized and sustained manner. We infused modified heparin, a sulfated polysaccharide and a representative antithrombotic drug, into a poloxamer hydrogel to bind aFGF and implement controlled-release behaviors as well as maximize the effectiveness of the molecule while minimizing the biochemical modifications that are common of biologically active proteins such as cytokines and GFs, especially aFGF.[33-35] Heparin-containing hydrogels can immobilize and protect high-affinity heparin-bound aFGF from degradation,[36] release GF in a sustained manner,[36-38] enhance the aFGF binding affinity to receptors on the cell surface to activate more intracellular signaling pathways, and increase both the stability and activity of the GF.[33,39] Furthermore, the HP hydrogel has a controlled sol-to-gel transition temperature and is suitable for orthotopic injection. Our results indicate that the aFGF-HP hydrogel has the potential for not only the localized and sustained transmission of aFGF to the injured spinal cord but also comprehensive tissue regeneration and recovery of SCI. Here, we provide extensive evidence that this method may expedite the applications of aFGF in the clinical treatment of SCI.

2. Materials and methods

2.1 Preparation of P and HP hydrogels

Poloxamer 407 was purchased from Badische Anilin Soda Fabrik Ga (Shanghai, China). The synthesis of HP according to 1-ethyl-3-(3-dimethylaminopropyl)-carbodiimide (EDC)/N-hydroxysuccinimide (NHS) method was previously described.[35] First, poloxamer 407 (1 mM) reacted with diaminoethylene (3 mM) to form a monoamine-terminated poloxamer (MATP). Next, 0.5 mM MATP was reacted with 0.5 mM heparin salt by 0.5 mM EDC and 0.25 mM NHS in 0.5 M 4-morpholine ethane sulfonic acid (MES) buffer for 1 d. The amine groups of poloxamer 407 were coupled with carboxyl ones of heparin specifically and resulted in amide bond formation. After that, the mixture was dialyzed for 72 h and lyophilized. Finally, the heparin-poloxamer (HP) was obtained. Lyophilized powder of P or HP was mixed in aFGF solution with modest stirring, and then the mixture was stored at 4 °C overnight to form the aFGF loaded hydrogel method.[40]

2.2 Characterization of aFGF-HP hydrogels

The gelation temperature measurements of the aFGF-HP hydrogel were measured as previously reported.[35] The micromorphology of the prepared aFGF-HP hydrogels was observed by scanning electron microscopy (SEM). The aFGF-HP hydrogels and drug-free HP hydrogels were freeze-dried and sputter-coated with gold followed by scanning observation. Rheological measurements of the aFGF-P and aFGF-HP were performed using the discovery hybrid rheometer. The transition temperature and amplitude sweep were measured using the stainless steel parallel plate flat plates (25 mm). The shear frequency was set to 10 rad/s; shear strain was set to 1%.

2.3 Release profiles of aFGF from aFGF-HP hydrogels

The release profiles of activated aFGF from the aFGF-HP hydrogels were analyzed by adding 100 μl of aFGF-HP hydrogel (containing 100 ng of aFGF) into 500 μl of 0.9% saline and incubating at 37 °C. At specific time points (12 h and 1, 3, 5, 7, 14, 21, and 28 d), the solution was centrifuged for 10 min at 12 000 g, and the supernatant was collected and replaced with the same volume of fresh saline. The aFGF concentration in the supernatant was measured by using an aFGF enzyme-linked immunosorbent assay kit (ELISA, Westang System, Shanghai, China).

2.4 Spinal cord injury model and drug treatment

Adult female Sprague-Dawley rats (220–250 g, $n = 108$) were obtained from the Animal Center of the Chinese Academy of Science (Shanghai, China). The care and use of all animals conformed to guidelines set forth by the Chinese National Institutes of Health. All the rats were housed under controlled environmental conditions. To induce an SCI, all the animals were anesthetized by 8% (w/v) chloral hydrate (3.5 ml/kg, i.p.). The ninth ribs and T9 vertebrae were located using a locating pin and confirmed by an animal digital X-ray machine (Kubtec Model XPERT.8; KUB Technologies Inc.) Afterward, a laminectomy was performed at the T9 vertebrae after the vertebral column was exposed. The spinal cord was fully exposed, and a moderate crushing injury was performed using a vascular clip for 1 min (30 g forces, Oscar, China).[41] After SCI, 10 μl of HP hydrogel, an aFGF solution, or aFGF-HP hydrogel was orthotopically injected (OI) at a dose of 2 μg/μl using a microsyringe. The aFGF solution, which was dissolved in saline (500 μl, 0.04 μg/μl) and intravenously (IV) injected through the tail vein, was set as a control (aFGF IV). Postoperative monitoring included manual bladder emptying three times a day. Subsequently, the rats were sacrificed at 1, 3, 7, 14, 28, or 56 d after treatment.

2.5 Measurement of blood-spinal cord barrier disruption

The integrity of the BSCB was investigated with Evan's Blue dye extravasation assay according to our previous report.[42] Evan's Blue dye solution (2%, 4 ml/kg) was injected through the tail vein at 1 d after inducement of SCI. Two hours later, rats were anaesthetized and sacrificed, and the spinal cords were sectioned with a cryostat 30 μm coronal slices. The fluorescence of Evan's Blue was observed with a confocal fluorescence microscope.

2.6 Transmission electron microscopy

Spinal cord tissues were fixed in 2.5% (w/v) glutaraldehyde solution overnight, postfixed in 2% (v/v) osmium tetroxide, and blocked with 2% (v/v) uranyl acetate. Tissues were embedded in Araldite after dehydration in a series of acetone washes. Semithin section and toluidine blue staining were performed for observation of location. Finally, ultrathin sections of at least six blocks per sample were cut and observed using a TEM.

2.7 Tissue preparation

Animals were anesthetized with 8% (w/v) chloralic hydras (3.5 ml/kg, i.p.) at specific time points after SCI. For Nissl staining, immuno-histochemistry, etc., 0.5 cm section of the spinal cord was dissected out, postfixed by 4% paraformaldehyde for 6 h and then embedded in paraffin. Longitudinal or transverse sections (5 μm thick) were mounted on slides for following staining. For western blot test, a spinal cord segment (0.5 cm length) at the contusion epicenter was dissected and stored at −80 ℃ immediately.

2.8 Western blot

The supernatant of tissue or cells was collected for protein assay. The extracts were first quantified with BCA reagents. Proteins (80 μg) were separated on 10% gels and transferred onto poly(vinylidene difluoride) membrane (Bio-Rad, Hercules, CA, USA). The membrane was blocked with 5% (w/v) milk (Bio-Rad) in tris buffered saline with 0.05% Tween-20 (TBST) for 120 min and incubated with the primary antibody solutions overnight at 4 ℃ followed by treatment with horseradish peroxidase-conjugated secondary antibodies for 60 min. Signals were visualized by Chemi DocXRS$^+$ Imaging System (Bio-Rad). All experiments were repeated three times.

2.9 Histology, immunofluorescence, and immuno-histochemistry

Longitudinal or transverse sections mounted on slides were prepared as described above. Transverse sections for histopathological examination were treated by hematoxylin and eosin staining, Nissl staining, and Luxol fast blue (LFB) staining following the manufacturer's instructions. Brightfield images were acquired using light microscopy. For immunofluorescence, longitudinal sections were treated with primary antibodies targeting the following proteins: NF-200 (1:2 000, Abcam), GFAP (1:2 000, Abcam), microtubule-associated protein 2 (MAP-2, 1:300, Santa Cruz) and CD68 (1:400, Abcam). The transverse sections were treated with primary antibodies targeting NeuN (1:400, Abcam), Claudin5 (1:200, Santa Cruz), and cleaved caspase-3 (1:300, Cell Signaling Technologies). The sections were washed four times with phosphate buffered saline with 0.05% Tween-20 (PBST) and incubated with AlexaFluor 568, AlexaFluor 488, or AlexaFluor 647 donkey antirabbit/mouse secondary antibodies for 1 h at 37 ℃. Afterward, the sections were washed with phosphate-buffered saline (PBS), incubated with 4′,6-diamidino-2-phenylindole for 7 min, rinsed with PBS, and finally sealed with a coverslip. For immuno-histochemistry, the longitudinal sections were treated with primary antibodies targeting the following proteins: myelin basic protein 2 (MBP-2, 1:400, Santa Cruz), Nestin (1:200, Abcam), and GAP-43 (1:200, Cell Signaling Technologies) and followed by incubation with horseradish peroxidase-conjugated secondary antibodies overnight at 4 ℃. Next, the sections were developed with 3,3′-diaminobenzidine and counterstained with hematoxylin. All the images were captured using a confocal fluorescence microscope (Nikon, Japan).

2.10 Locomotion recovery evaluation

Locomotion recovery analyses, including the Basso−Beattie−Bresnahan (BBB) locomotion scale, inclined plane test, and footprint test[43] were performed at 0, 3, 7,14, 21, and 28 d. In brief, the BBB scores range from 0 to 21 points. The inclined plane test[44] was also performed to assess functional improvement at each time point, and the footprint analysis was performed by dipping the animal's hindpaws with red dye as previously described.[45] Outcome measures were obtained by five independent examiners who were blinded to the experimental conditions.

2.11 Statistical analysis

All data were presented as the mean ± standard error of the mean (SEM). Differences between groups in BBB scores and inclined plane test were analyzed with use of generalized linear mixed models. Dynamic interaction between aFGF and HP hydrogel were measured by a 2 × 2 factorial trial. Statistical analysis of the other data was performed using one-way analysis of variance (ANOVA). The P values less than 0.05 were considered statistically significant.

3. Results

3.1 Characterization of the aFGF-HP hydrogel

The relationship between the HP concentration and the gelation temperature is shown in Fig. 1B. Considering the body temperature of animals and humans (37 ℃), the aFGF-HP hydrogel with an HP concentration of 17% was observed to have a suitable gelation temperature. To test the effects of the HP and P hydrogels on aFGF release, the *in vitro* release profile of aFGF from aFGF-HP was recorded. Less than 10% of the aFGF was detected in the supernatant after synthesis of the aFGF-HP and aFGF-P hydrogels, indicating that the loading efficiency of these two hydrogels was greater than 90%. An initial burst release (~ 18%) of aFGF from aFGF-P was observed on day 1, and another ~7% was released over the following 4 d. However, a negligible amount of aFGF was released from the aFGF-P hydrogel after day 5, with ~ 25% of loaded aFGF released by day 28 (Fig. 1C). In contrast, a sustained release behavior of aFGF was observed in the aFGF-HP hydrogel. Approximately 55% of the loaded aFGF was released from the aFGF-HP hydrogel by day 28, which was 2 times greater than that in the aFGF-P hydrogel (Fig. 1C). As shown in Fig. 1D,E, storage modulus (G′) and loss modulus (G″), respectively, represent elastic and viscous behavior of these two gels. Varying temperatures were performed to reveal the gelation process of these two systems (Fig. 1D). Amplitude sweep was conducted to analyze the physical nature of the hydrogels (Fig. 1E). The two systems showed a similar sol-to-gel transition between 21 and 26 ℃. The sol-to-gel transition was moderate, and the transition temperature was similar to room temperature, making the gels suitable for manipulation *in vitro* and applications *in vivo*. The amplitude sweep displayed the similar intersection at moderate strain amplitude of ~ 6.5%. The results indicated that these two hydrogels were both relatively

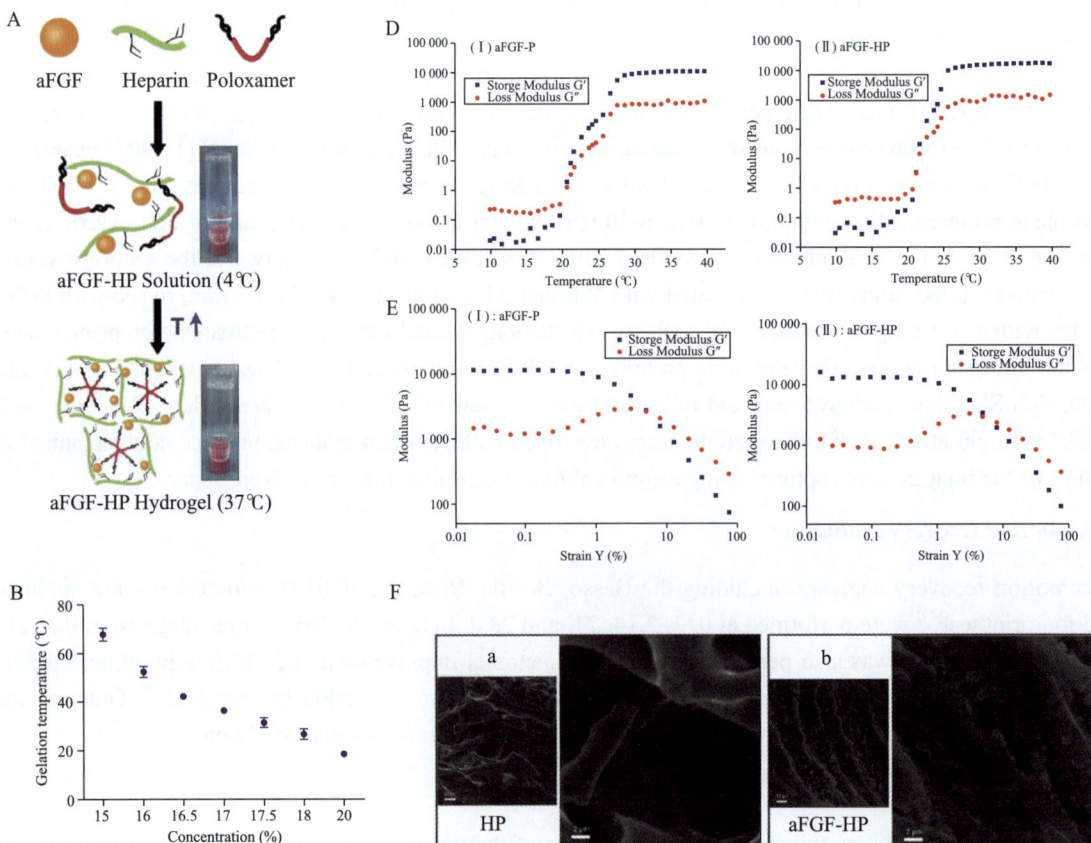

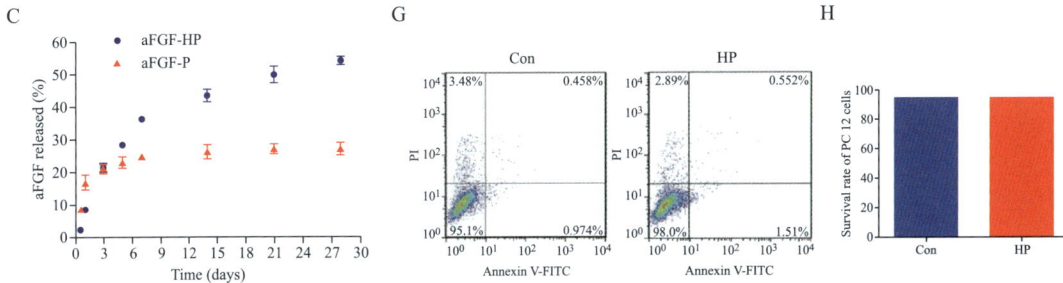

Fig. 1. Characterization of aFGF-HP hydrogel. (A) Schematic of the preparation of aFGF-HP. (B) The gelation temperature of aFGF-HP with different concentration of HP. (C) The release profile of active aFGF fromaFGF-HP and aFGF-P hydrogel. (D) Storage (G′) and loss (G″) moduli of aFGF-P and aFGF-HP hydrogels as a function of temperature from 10 to 40 ℃. (E) Amplitude sweep of aFGF-P and aFGF-HP hydrogels displaying storage modulus (G′) and loss modulus (G″). (F) SEM images of the lyophilized HP hydrogel and aFGF-HP hydrogel. (G) The survival rate of PC12 cells with or without treatment of HP using PI/annexin V-FITC staining. (H) Quantification results of the survival rate of PC12 cells from (E). All experiments were performed in triplicate, and data are presented as mean ± SEM.

soft and suitable for the biological application on the spinal cord. The morphology of the HP and aFGF-HP hydrogels was also observed under SEM. Compared to the smooth surface of the HP hydrogel, the aFGF-HP hydrogel had a porous structure resembling a cribriform plate (Fig. 1F), where the aFGF proteins can be adsorbed. Furthermore, the HP hydrogel itself showed no toxicity in PC12 cells (Fig. 1G,H). On the basis of the characteristics observed, the aFGF-HP hydrogel sustains thermosensitivity feature as well as a 3D porous structure, both of which are favorable for the localized and sustained delivery of aFGF. However, heparin-containing hydrogels can immobilize and protect aFGF from degradation, which allows the release of aFGF in a sustained manner.

3.2 aFGF-HP attenuated BSCB disruption by preventing the loss of tight junction and adherens junction proteins after SCI

BSCB disruption is one of the most serious types of damage from SCI and is maximally disrupted at 24 h post-SCI.[46] To observe the effects of aFGF-HP on BSCB integrity, we examined the permeability of the BSCB at day 1 after SCI injury by using the Evans Blue assay ($n = 5$). As shown in Fig. 2B−D, compared with the sham group, the SCI rats indicated a significant increase in the amount of EB extravasation after SCI. aFGF administration reduced the levels of extravasation to varying degrees, and the levels of EB were lowest in the aFGF-HP group, which were similar to those in the sham group. In addition, the fluorescence intensity of EB was ordered as the aFGF-HP/OI group > aFGF/OI group > aFGF/IV group> HP/OI group (Fig. 3E−H, $P < 0.01$). It is well-accepted that tight junctions (TJs) and adherens junctions (AJs) are involved in maintaining the integrity of the BSCB.[47] Next we examined the effect of aFGF-

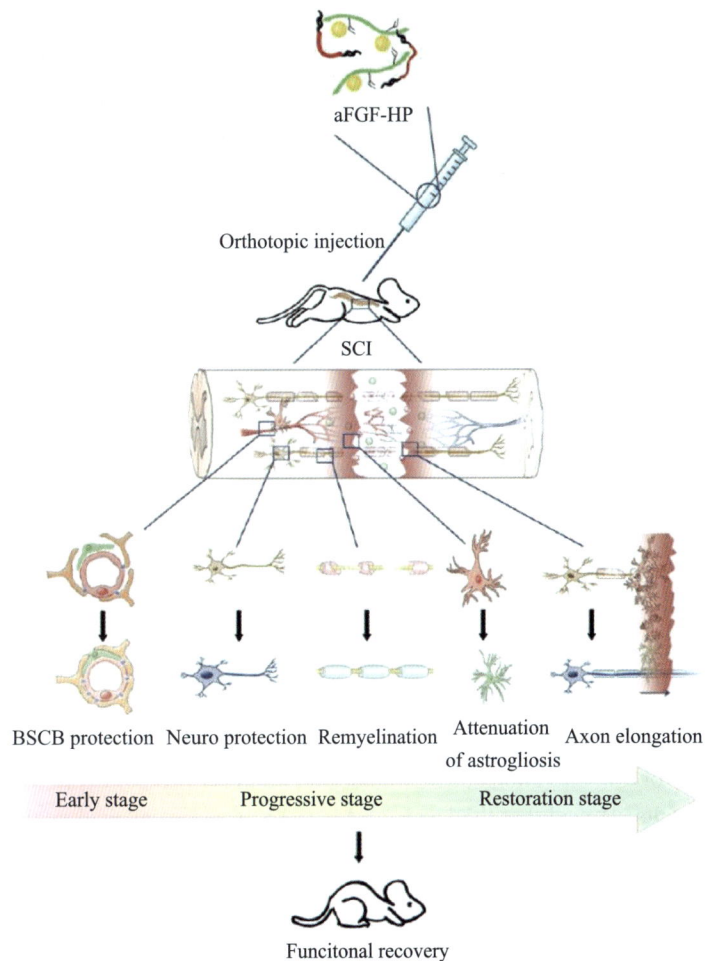

Fig. 2. Schematic of aFGF-HP thermosensitive hydrogels enhance the recovery of SCI. The protection of aFGF-HP containing BSCB protection, neuroprotection, remyelination, attenuation of astrogliosis, axon elongation in three different stages after SCI, which are the main obstacles to recovery of SCI.

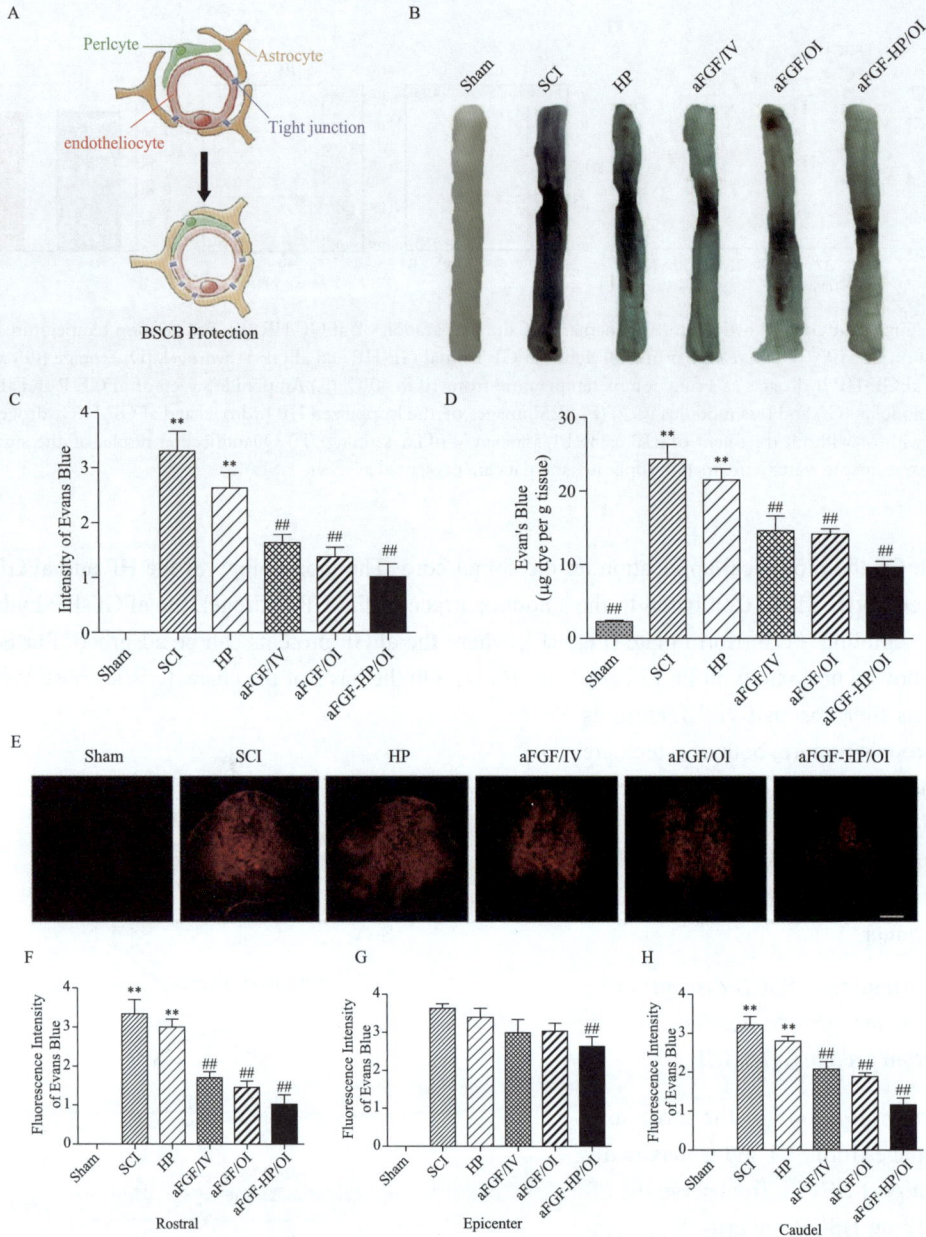

Fig. 3. aFGF-HP attenuates BSCB disruption at 24 h post-SCI. (A) Schematic of the structure of BSCB and the BSCB protection of aFGF-HP. (B) Representative images of whole spinal cords with Evan's Blue dye staining at 24 h post-SCI. (C) Quantification intensity results of Evans Blue from A by software ImageJ. (D) Quantification data of EB content of spinal cord (μg/g). (E) Representative confocal images showing the fluorescence of Evans Blue Dye extravasation from the transverse area of the spinal cord of each group. Scale bar = 1 000 μm. (F−H) Quantification of the fluorescence intensity of Evan's Blue in each group at rostral 5 mm, caudal 5 mm, and lesion site. All data represent mean values ± SEM, $n = 4$. $^{#}P < 0.05$, $^{##}P < 0.01$ *vs.* the SCI group, $^{*}P < 0.05$, $^{**}P < 0.01$ *vs.* the aFGF-HP group.

HP on the alterations of SCI-induced TJ and AJ protein expression by western blotting and immunofluorescence. Our results showed that the levels of AJs (P120-catenin) as well as the TJs (Occludin, Claudin5) were decreased after SCI and that decreases were significantly ameliorated in the aFGF-treated groups, especially in the aFGF-HP/OI group (Fig. 4A−D). To further confirm the effects of aFGF-HP on protecting the BSCB, we applied H_2O_2 to HBMVECs and measured the paracellular permeability of FITC-dextran to evaluate the permeability of the BSCB. As shown in Fig. S2A, compared with the H_2O_2 group, the penetrability to FITC-dextran was decreased most frequently in the aFGF-HP group. Furthermore, the expression levels of proteins associated with AJs (β-catenin) and TJs (Claudin5) were enhanced with aFGF-HP treatment to a greater degree than the levels observed in the other groups (Fig. 2B−D). The results showed that aFGF deters BSCB disruption by inhibiting the degradation of AJ and TJ proteins during the initial stages after SCI.

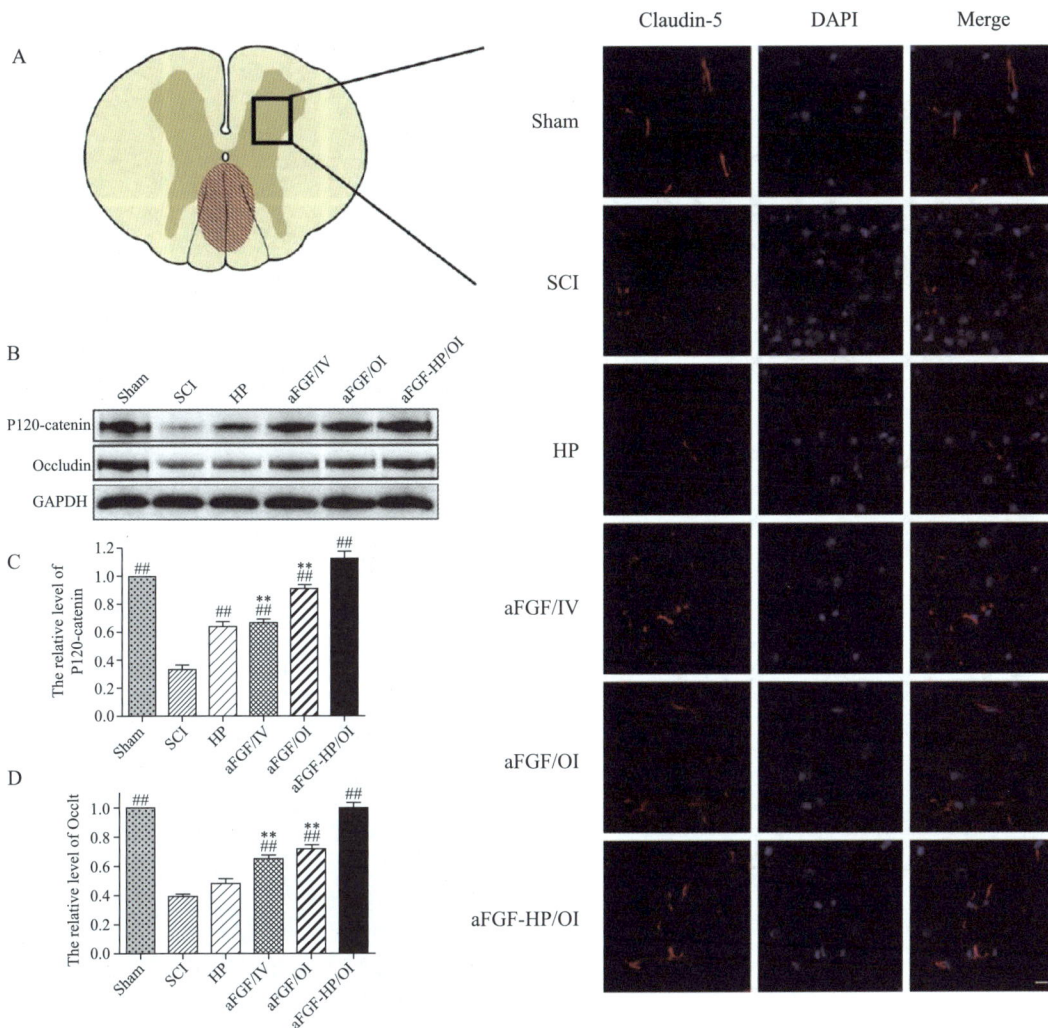

Fig. 4. aFGF-HP attenuates BSCB disruption by preventing loss of TJ and AJ proteins at 24 h after SCI. (A) Immunofluorescence staining of TJ protein Claudin5 (red) in each group. Scale bar = 10 μm. (B) Representative western blots result of AJ protein P120, TJ protein TJ protein. (C, D) Quantification of western blot data from (B). All data represent mean values ± SEM, $n = 5$. $^{#}P < 0.05$, $^{##}P < 0.01$ $vs.$ the SCI group, $^{*}P < 0.05$, $^{**}P < 0.01$ $vs.$ the aFGF-HP group.

In addition, *in situ* administration of aFGF shows a more pronounced protective effect of the BSCB than intravenous administration, and HP enhances this effect of aFGF.

3.3 aFGF-HP reduces the apoptosis of neurons in vivo and in vitro

Cell apoptosis rapidly occurs after the initial trauma, after which a broad and prolonged apoptotic event arises around the epicenter of the contusion.[48,49] To evaluate the role of the aFGF-HP hydrogel in modulating cellular apoptosis after SCI, immuno-histochemistry staining for NeuN (red) and cleaved caspase-3 (green) as well as terminal deoxynucleotidyl transferase (TdT) dUTP Nick-End Labeling (TUNEL) staining were performed on neurons at 7 d post injury (dpi). As shown in Fig. 5A,B and Fig. 6A, the percentage of the cleaved caspase-3-positive neurons and the number of TUNEL-positive cells in the SCI group were noticeably increased. The aFGF treatments reduced the number of apoptotic cells to varying degrees, but the aFGF-HP hydrogel resulted in a more remarkable reduction of neuronal apoptosis. The expression of cleaved caspase-3 was further tested by western blotting in each group at either 7 dpi or 6 h after H_2O_2 treatment. As shown in Fig. 6B,C, and Fig. S3C–E, aFGF-HP substantially inhibited the apoptosis of neurons either caused by SCI in the rats or induced by H_2O_2 in PC-12 cells. The microstructures of these neurons were also examined by transmission electron microscopy (TEM; Fig. 6D). The neurons in the sham group had normal mitochondria and an endoplasmic reticulum (ER) with many ribosomes. However, the organelles in neurons from the SCI group were almost completely disintegrated. The organelles were protected by the aFGF treatments, with few organelles disintegrated

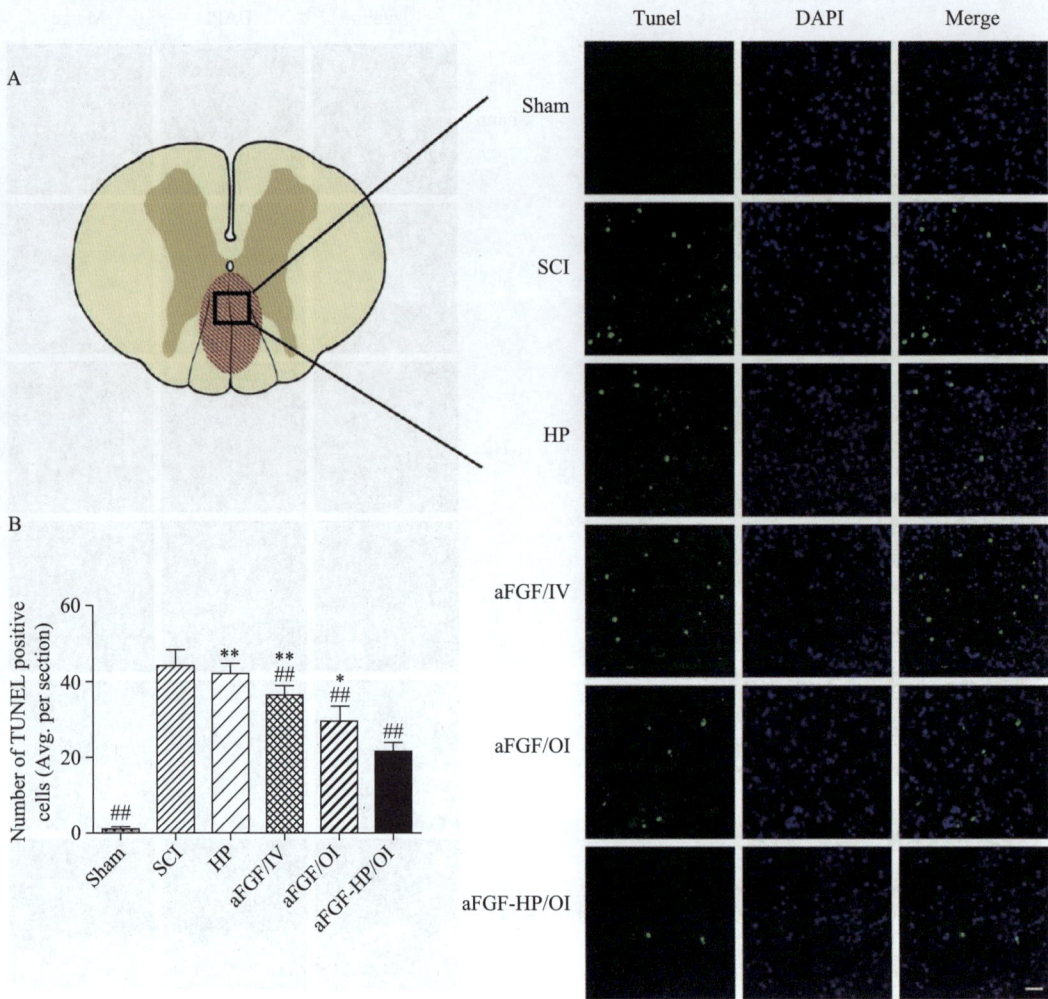

Fig. 5. aFGF-HP reduces cell apoptosis at lesion site at 7 d after injury. (A) Immunofluorescence staining for TUNEL (green) of sections from the injured spinal cord in each group. Scale bar = 50 μm. (B) Quantitative estimation of apoptotic and TUNEL cells from five independent sections between 5 mm from the injury epicenter. All data represent mean values ± SEM, $n = 5$. $^{\#}P < 0.05$, $^{\#\#}P < 0.01$ *vs.* the SCI group, $^{*}P < 0.05$, $^{**}P < 0.01$ *vs.* the aFGF-HP group.

in the aFGF-HP/OI group, suggesting that HP protects aFGF from modifications. Taken together, these data revealed the hierarchy of the effects on reducing neuronal apoptosis to the benefit of the functional recovery of SCIas follows: aFGF-HP/ OI group > aFGF/OI group > aFGF/IV group> HP/OI group.

3.4 aFGF-HP promotes the rehabilitation of the neurons in vivo and in vitro

To further test the effects of aFGF-HP on promoting neuronal rehabilitation, the expression levels of GAP-43 and Nestin, which are two classic indicators of neural regeneration, were tested in each group by western blotting and immuno-histochemistry at 7 dpi. As shown in Fig. 7A–C, minimal GAP-43 and Nestin were expressed in the sham group. In contrast, the expression levels of GAP-43 and Nestin in the presence of aFGF treatment were significantly increased. Among all the groups, the aFGF-HP/ OI group showed the highest GAP-43 and Nestin levels. These results in the aFGF-HP/OI group were confirmed by immuno-histochemistry, providing further evidence of the effect of aFGF-HP on neuronal rehabilitation (Fig. 7D–F). Finally, the histological morphology in each group was evaluated using-HE and Nissl stain at 5 mm rostral and 5 mm caudal of the spinal cord. As shown in Fig. 8A–C, in contrast to the sham group, severe damage to the central gray matter and dorsal white matter was obvious in the SCI rats. The aFGF-treated groups presented decreased damage to varying degrees the quantitative results indicated that the aFGF-HP/OI group showed the highest percentage of preserved tissue than the other aFGF treatment groups. The number of ventral motor neurons (VMNs) was counted. As shown in Fig. 8A,D,E, a great loss of VMNs after SCI; however, aFGF (especially the aFGF-

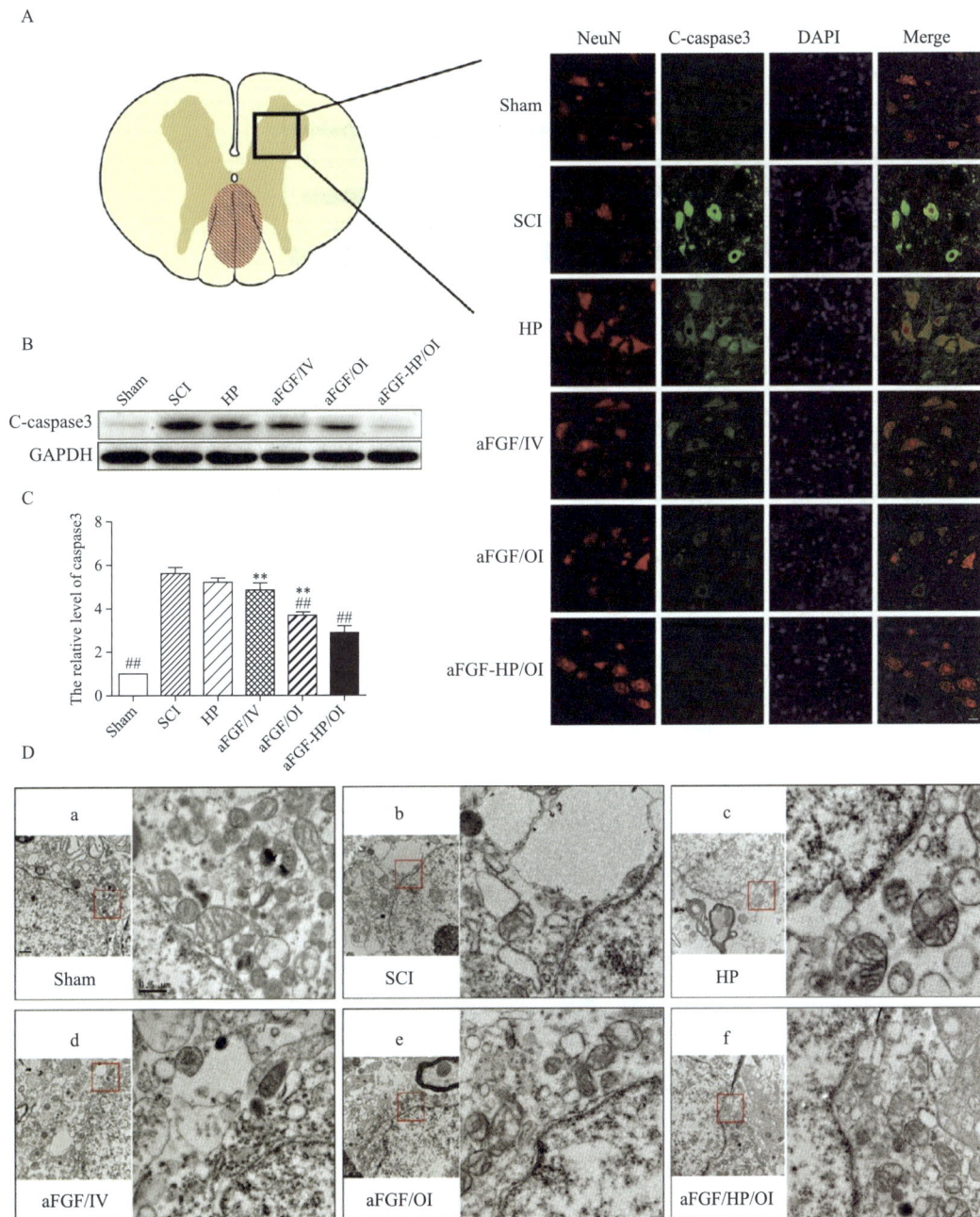

Fig. 6. aFGF-HP reduces neuron apoptosis at 7 d after SCI. (A) Immunofluorescence images show that C-caspase3 (green) colocalize in neuron (NeuN, red) in each group. Scale bar = 20 μm. (B) Protein expressions of C-caspase3 in the spinal cord segment at the contusion epicenter. GAPDH was used as the control and band density normalization. (C) The optical density analysis of C-caspase3 proteins. (D, a–f) TEM images show the microstructure of the neurons in each group. Values were expressed as the mean ± SEM, $n = 5$ per group. $^{#}P < 0.05$, $^{##}P < 0.01$ vs. the SCI group, $^{*}P < 0.05$, $^{**}P < 0.01$ vs. the aFGF-HP group.

HP hydrogel) significantly mitigated the loss of VMNs. The results demonstrated that the aFGF-HP hydrogel can reduce neuron loss and ameliorate the pathological morphology of the injured tissues. Collectively, the aFGF-HP hydrogel combined with an *in situ* injection revealed the best protective effects to neurons by reducing neuron apoptosis and promoting neuron rehabilitation.

3.5 aFGF-HP promotes remyelination and axonal rehabilitation in vivo and in vitro

Remyelination and axonal regeneration is a critical aspect of sensory and motor function recovery after SCI.[50-53] To determine the effect of the aFGF-HP hydrogel on remyelination, the degree of myelin sheath destruction was assessed

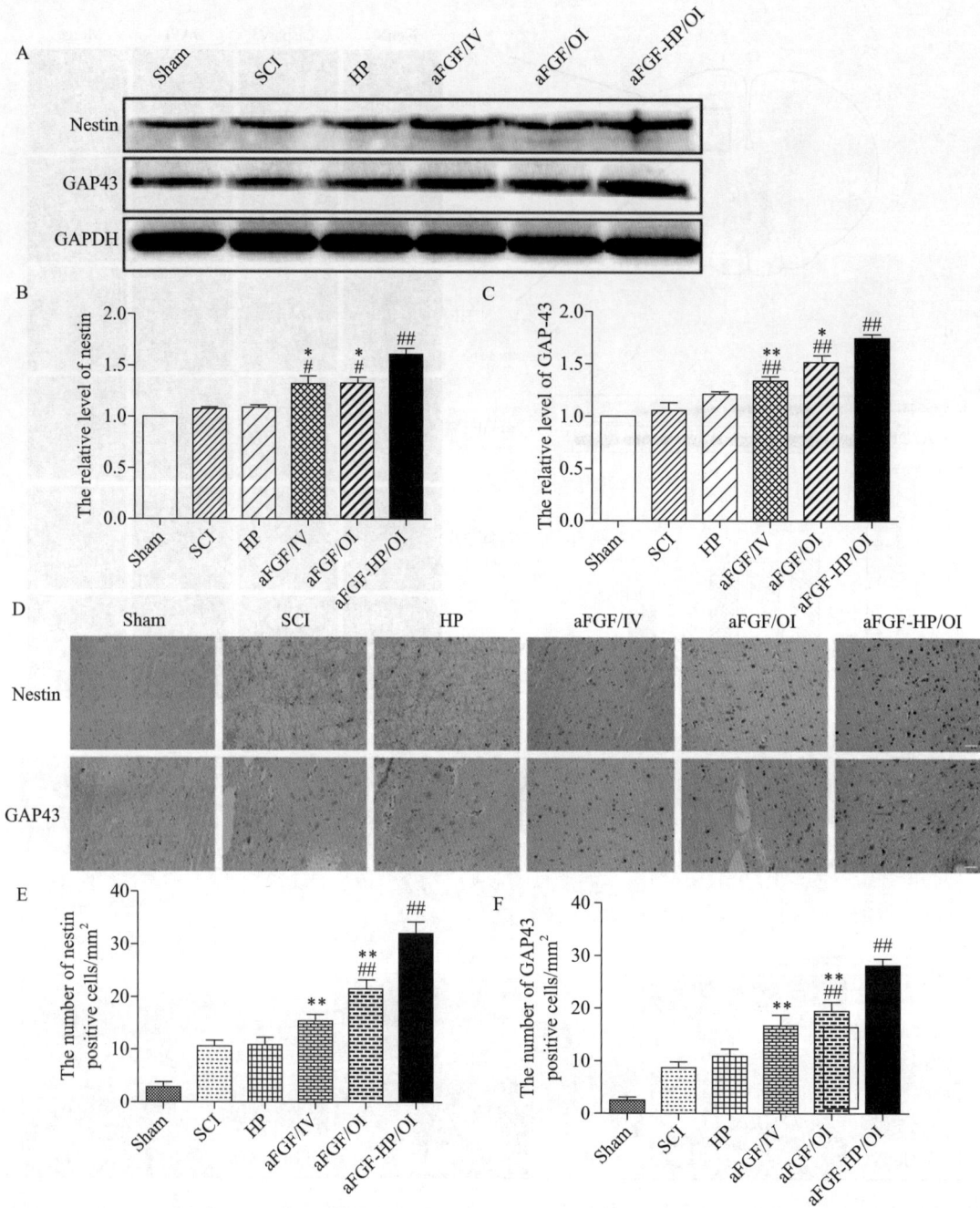

Fig. 7. aFGF-HP enhances neuron restoration at 7 d after SCI. (A) Protein expressions of GAP-43 and Nestin in each group. (B, C) Quantification of western blot data from (B). (D−F) Immuno-histochemisty staining and quantification data of GAP-43 and Nestin in each group. Scale bar = 50 μm. Values were expressed as the mean ± SEM, $n = 5$ per group. $^{\#}P < 0.05$, $^{\#\#}P < 0.01$ vs. the SCI group, $^{*}P < 0.05$, $^{**}P < 0.01$ vs. the aFGF-HP group.

using LFB staining at 28 dpi. As shown in Fig. 9A,B, the hierarchy of the amount of LFB-positive myelin was as follows: aFGF-HP/OI group > aFGF/ OI group > aFGF/IV group > HP/OI group. The micro-structure of the myelin was also examined by TEM (Fig. 9A). In the sham group, the structure of the myelin sheath was clear, and the layers were closely packed with a large number of microtubules in the axon. However, the myelin sheath in the SCI group presented vacuolar changes, acantholysis and a loss of microtubules. The degree of myelin sheath destruction was reduced after the aFGF treatmbts, with the aFGF-HP/OI group showing an obvious and more pronounced effect on myelin sheath restoration than the other treatment groups. Furthermore, we examined the expression of myelin basic proteins (MBPs),

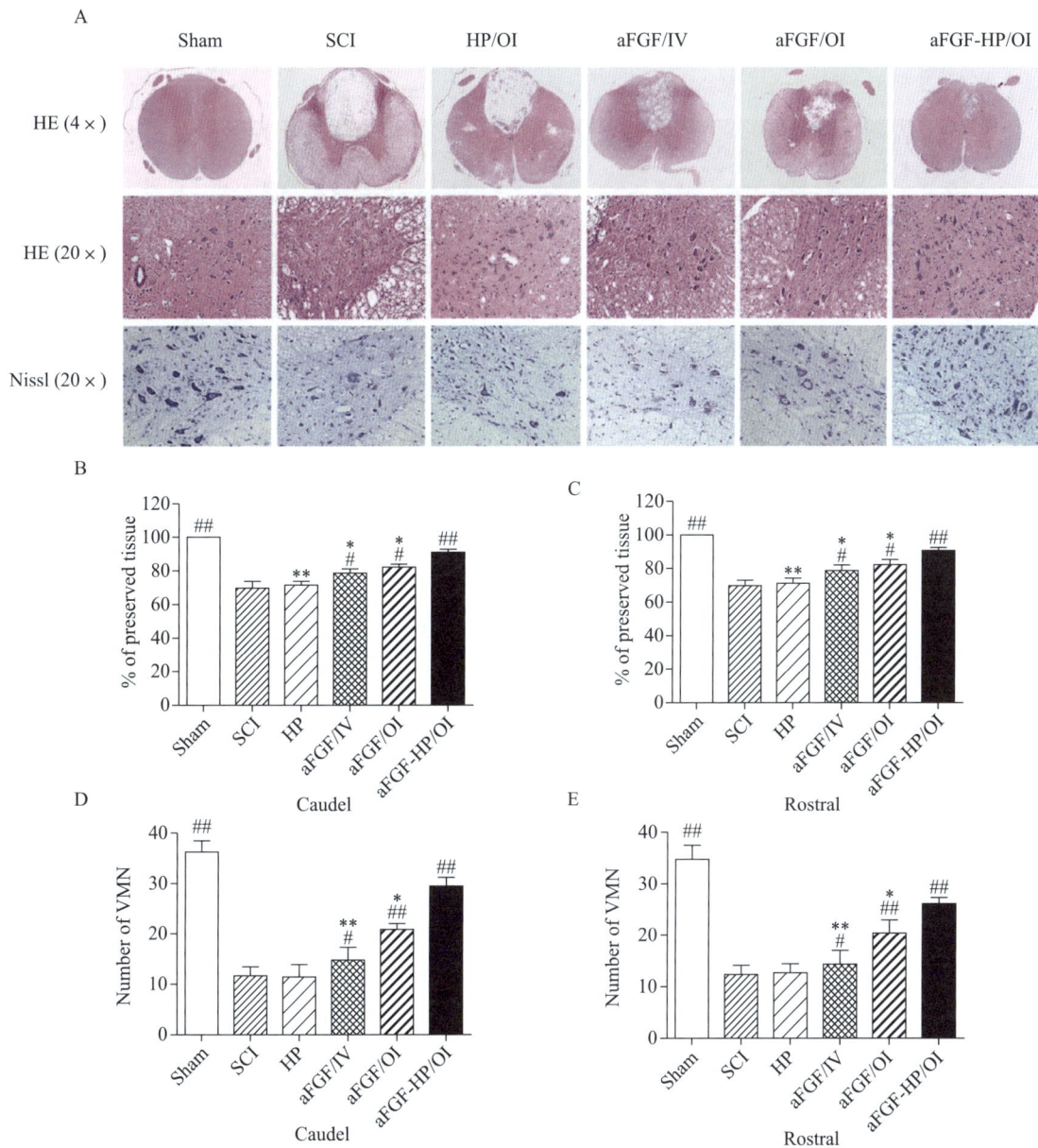

Fig. 8. aFGF-HP decreases the damage of tissue structure and the loss of neurons at 28 d after SCI. (A) Representative images from HE, Nissl staining at 28 dpi. (B, C) Quantification of the percent of preserved tissue at rostral 5 mm, caudal 5 mm of the spinal cord. (D, E) Counting analysis of VMN at rostral 5 mm, caudal 5 mm of the spinal cord. Values were expressed as the mean ± SEM, $n = 5$ per group. $^{\#}P < 0.05$, $^{\#\#}P < 0.01$ *vs.* the SCI group, $^{*}P < 0.05$, $^{**}P < 0.01$ *vs.* the aFGF-HP group.

which are structural proteins and constituents of the myelin sheath, in each group *in vivo* and *in vitro* by western blotting and immuno-histochemistry (Fig. 9C−F and Fig. S4C,E). The results revealed that MBP protein expression was significantly decreased after SCI but that aFGF treatment increased the expression with the following hierarchy: aFGF-HP/OI group > aFGF/OI group > HP/OI group. Additionally, to determine the effects of aFGF-HP on axonal rehabilitation, we examined the expression of MAP-2, which is a structural protein and a constituent of axon microtubules, in each group by immunofluorescence and western blotting (Fig. 10A,B). The results revealed that the number of MAP-2-positive axons in the SCI group was significantly decreased and disorganized at 28 dpi; however, compared to the SCI group, the

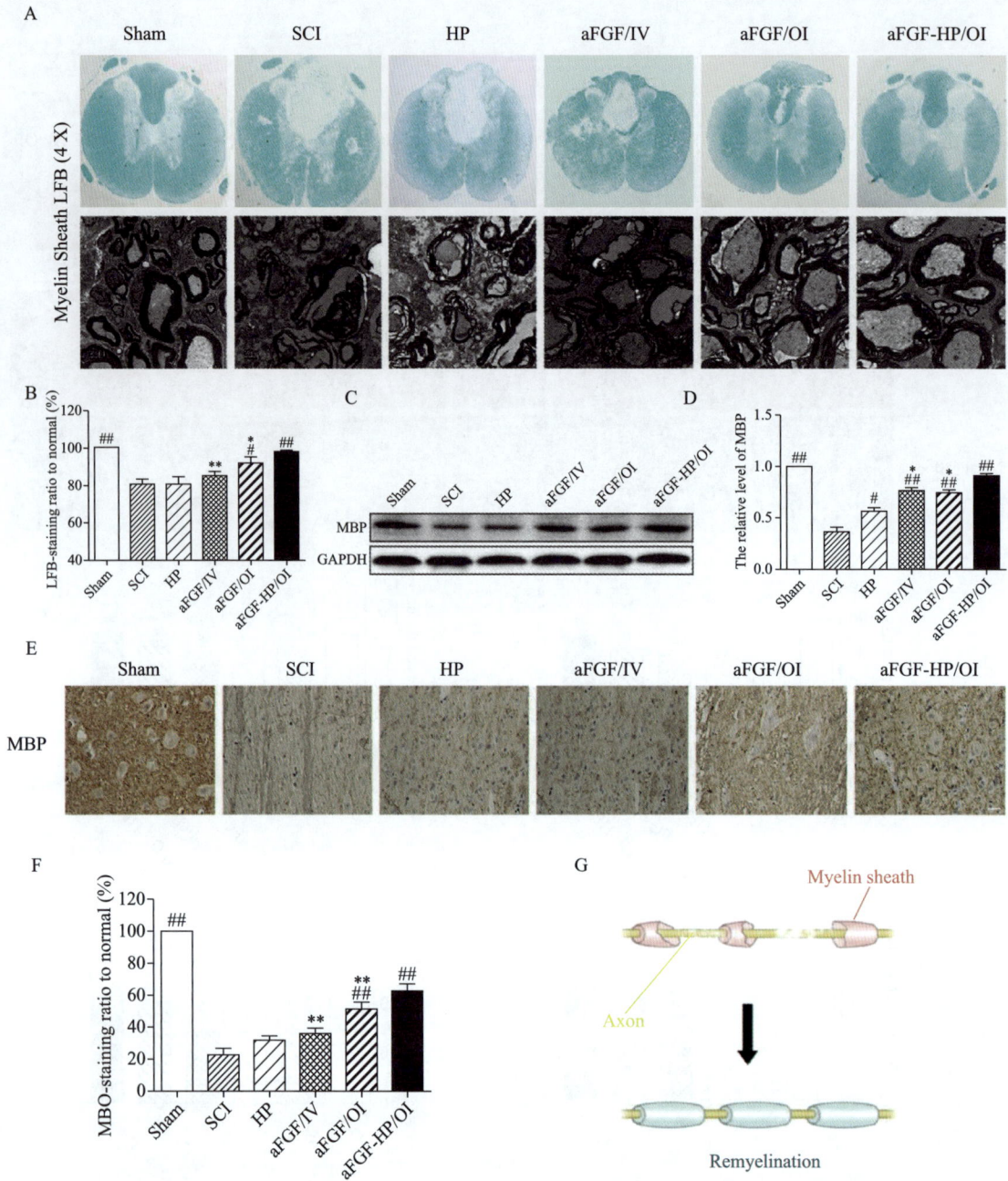

Fig. 9. aFGF-HP promotes remyelination at 28 d after SCI. (A) Representative images of white matter with LFB staining and TEM images of the myelin sheath at 28 dpi. (B) Quantification of LFB staining ratio of normal. (C, D) Protein expressions and quantification data of MBP in each group. (E, F) Immuno-histochemisty staining and quantification data of MBP in each group. Scale bar = 50 μm. (G) Schematic of aFGF-HP on promoting remyelination. Values were expressed as the mean ± SEM, n = 5 per group. [#]$P < 0.05$, [##]$P < 0.01$ $vs.$ the SCI group, [*]$P < 0.05$, [**]$P < 0.01$ $vs.$ the aFGF-HP group.

aFGF-HP/OI group presented tighter and more continuous MAP-2-positive axons, which was similar to the observed morphology in the sham group. The results were further confirmed by western blotting to detect MAP-2 both $in\ vivo$ and $in\ vitro$ (Fig. 10C,D and Fig. S4C,D). In addition, Fig. S4A,B show the neurite length of the PC12 cells. Compared to the control group, the neurite length was reduced in the H_2O_2 group but was increased in the aFGF-HP group. The hierarchy of the neurite length was as follows: aFGF-HP/OI group > aFGF/OI group > aFGF/IV group> HP/OI group. Taken together, aFGF exerted an effect on promoting axonal growth and remyelination, and the aFGF-HP hydrogel can maximize this effect.

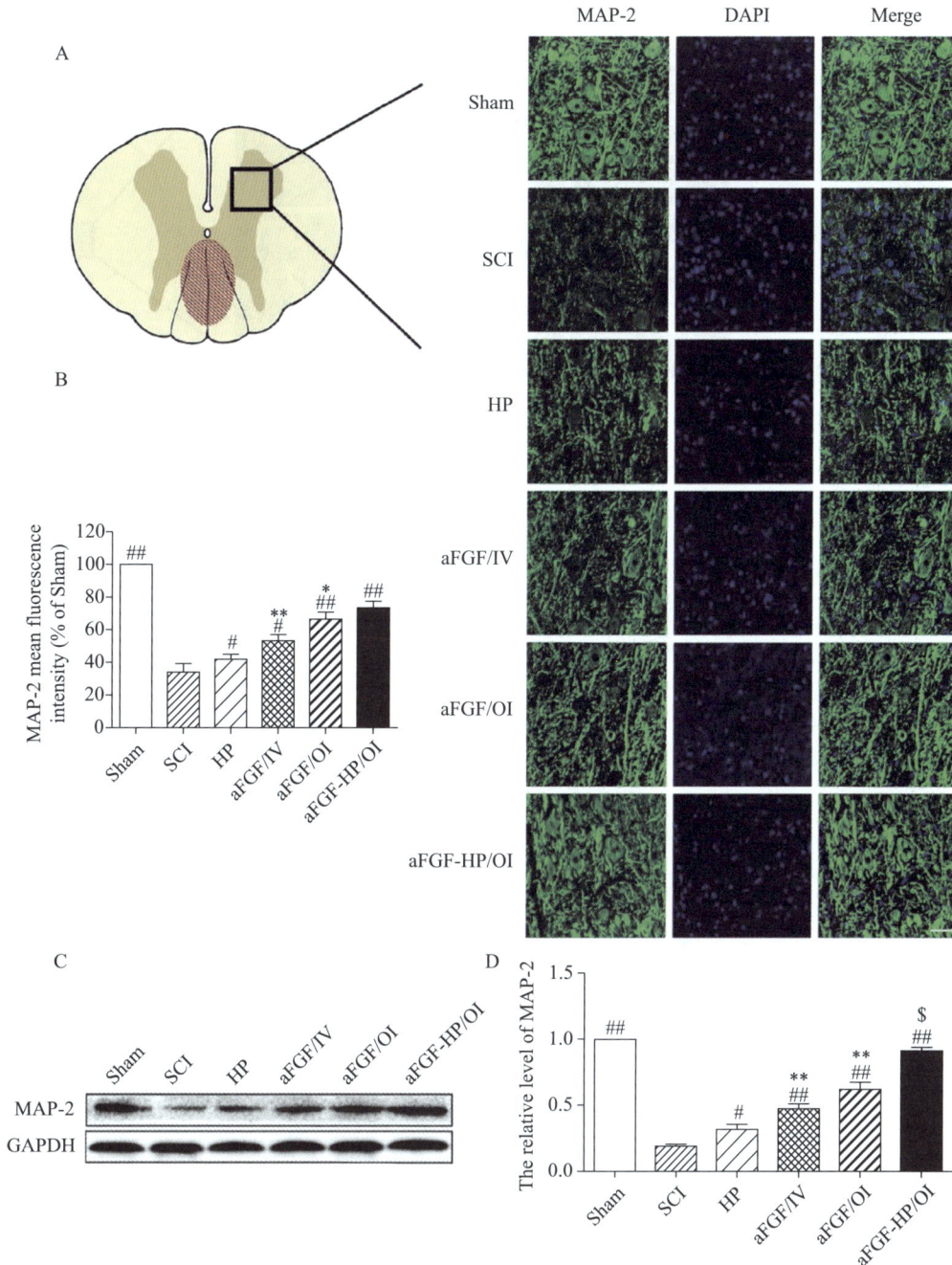

Fig. 10. aFGF-HP enhances axonal reparation at 28 d after SCI. (A) Fluorescence images of axon shows the expressions of MAP-2 in each group. Scale bar = 50 μm. (B) Quantification of fluorescence intensity from (B). (C, D) Protein expressions and quantification data of MBP in each group. Values were expressed as the mean ± SEM, $n = 5$ per group. $^{#}P < 0.05$, $^{##}P < 0.01$ *vs.* the SCI group, $^{*}P < 0.05$, $^{**}P < 0.01$ *vs.* the aFGF-HP group.

3.6 aFGF-HP attenuates the reactive astrogliosis after SCI and prevents scattering of inflammatory cells

Although the relationship between glial scar formation (mainly formed by activated astrocytes) and axonal regeneration is still debated,[54,55] it is widely accepted that glial scars provide a vital role in the recovery after SCI.[56,57] To this end, the effects of the aFGF-HP hydrogel on glial scars were tested. We first measured the expression of GFAP (a marker of astrocyte activation) at 1, 3, 7, 14, 28, and 56 dpi by using immunofluorescence. As shown in Fig. 11B,C, the astrogliosis presented hypertrophy and hyperplasia at 7 dpi and appeared as broad bundles interlacing and blending with the neighboring neurons at 14 dpi. A glial scar was formed at 28 dpi and did not significantly change after this. On

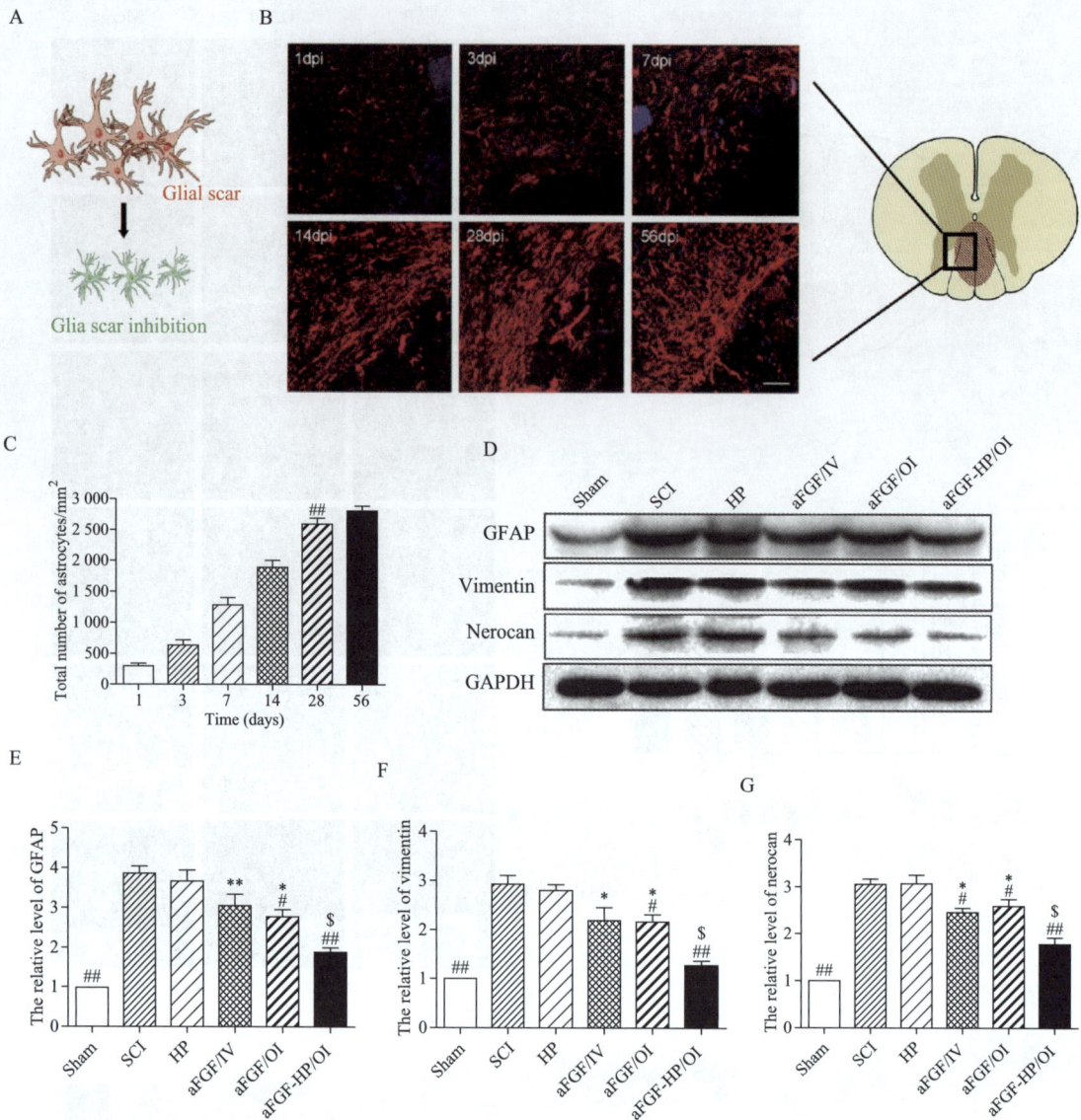

Fig. 11. aFGF-HP attenuates the reactive astrogliosis at 28 d after SCI. (A) Schematic of aFGF-HP on attenuating the reactive astrogliosis. (B) Im-munofluorescence staining of GFAP on the 1, 3, 7, 14, 28, 56 dpi. Scale bar = 50 μm. (C) Quantitative analyses the number of reactive astrogliosis around the lesion site. (D) Western blots results show the expressions of GFAP, Neurocan, and vimentin in each group. (E−G) Quantification of western blot data from (D). Values are expressed as the mean ± SEM, $n = 5$ per group. $^{\#}P < 0.05$, $^{\#\#}P < 0.01$ $vs.$ the SCI group, $^{*}P < 0.05$, $^{**}P < 0.01$ $vs.$ the aFGF-HP group.

the basis of these results, 28 dpi was selected for evaluating the degree of astrogliosis. We examined the expression of GFAP and vimentin (a marker of reactive astrocytes) *in vivo* and *in vitro* by western blotting (Fig. 11D,E and Fig. S5A−C). A marked increase in the levels of these two proteins was observed in the SCI group than in the sham group; however, the aFGF-HP hydrogel treatment reduced the protein levels of GFAP and vimentin significantly. The chondroitin sulfate proteoglycans (CSPGs) secreted from astrocytes is the primary inhibitor of axonal regeneration. Neurocan, a glial scar-related CSPG, was markedly increased after injury but significantly inhibited after aFGF-HP hydrogel treatment both *in vivo* and *in vitro* (Fig. 11D,G and Fig. S5A,D). These results were further confirmed by immunofluorescence staining. As shown in Fig. 12A−C, the crush injury around the lesion site led to highly reactive astrogliosis and the formation of a glial scar. Immunofluorescence revealed that aFGF-HP significantly reduced GFAP expression, downregulated the number of reactive astrocytes, and reversed their morphological alterations while concomitantly reducing the thick-ness of scar. Furthermore, it has been reported that glial scars can limit inflammation and inhibit the proliferation of inflammatory cells. Therefore, double staining for GFAP (red) and CD68 (green) was performed to observe the glial scar and inflammatory cells. As shown in Fig. 12A, inflammatory cells were present and scattered after SCI. The aFGF-

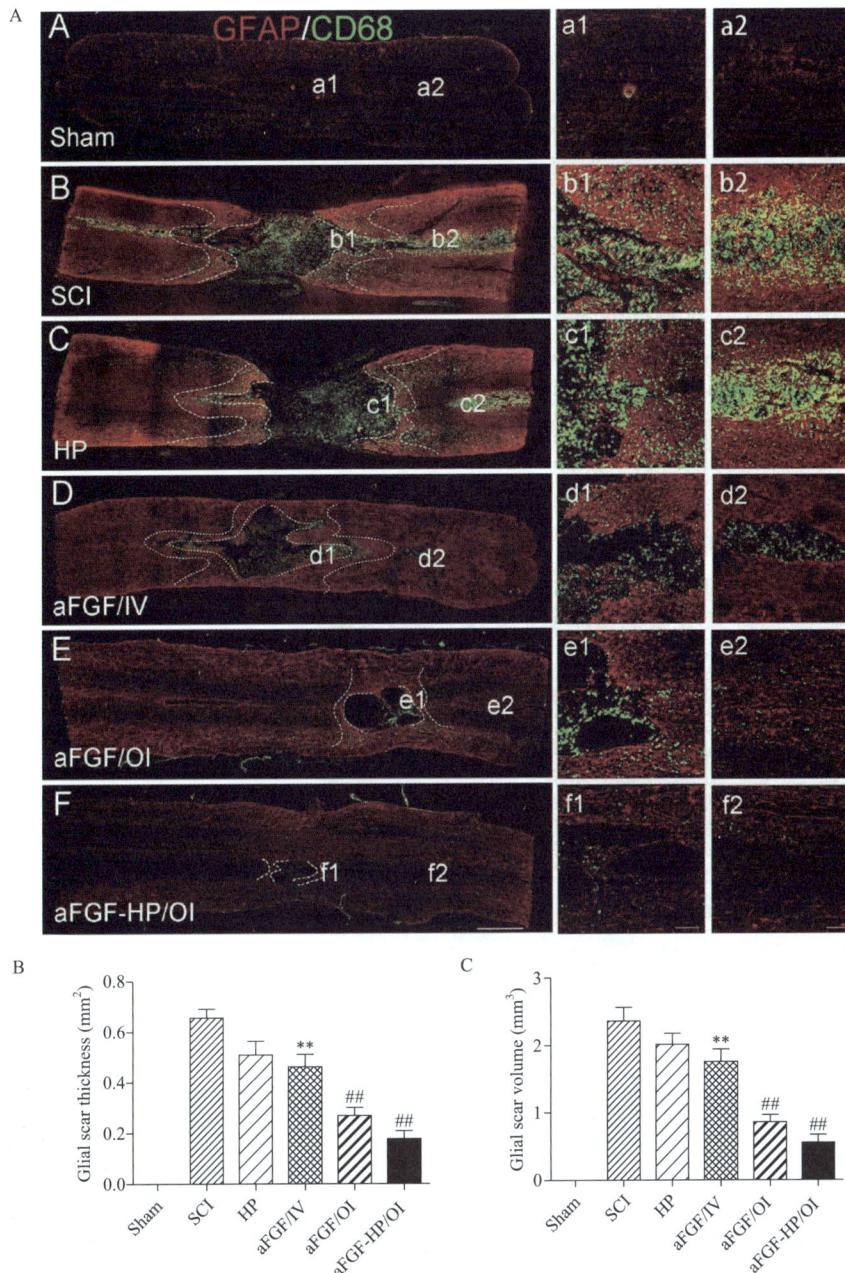

Fig. 12. aFGF-HP attenuates the reactive astrogliosis and inhibits the spread of inflammatory cells at 28 d after SCI. (A, A−F) Immunofluorescence images of the whole spinal cord shows the relationship of astrogliosis (red), which contain glial scar (dotted lines) and leukocytes (CD68, green) in each group; (A, a1−f1) enlarged image at the edge of lesion cites in each group; (A, a2−f2) enlarged image at 5 mm caudal from the lesion cite in each group. Scale bar = 1000 μm. (B) Quantitative analyses of glial scar thickness. (C) Quantitative analyses of glial scar volume. Values are expressed as the mean ± SEM, $n = 5$ per group. $^{\#}P < 0.05$, $^{\#\#}P < 0.01$ vs. the SCI group, $^{*}P < 0.05$, $^{**}P < 0.01$ vs. the aFGF-HP group.

HP hydrogel treatment markedly reduced the number of CD68+ cells and prevented inflammatory cell scattering. These results showed that aFGF-HP can weaken the glial scar and prevent inflammatory cell scattering. In addition, the effect of aFGF-HP on attenuating reactive astrogliosis and preventing inflammatory cell scattering was better than that of the other treatment groups ($P < 0.05$).

3.7 aFGF-HP promotes axonal generation across the glial scar

Whether the axons above the injured site can cross the scar in the injured area has become the focus of SCI repair in recent years.[54,58] Double staining for GFAP (red) and NF-200 (green) was performed to observe whether neurofilaments can across the glial scar surrounding the lesion site (Fig. 12A,B). In the SCI group, the neurofilaments were completely lost in the injury epicenter. The HP-and aFGF/IV-treated animals showed only a mild increase in the number of NF-200-positive axons that passed through the scar. By contrast, the aFGF-HP treatment group presented a pronounced number of NF-200-labeled fibers around the lesion site that had grown beyond the glial scar to a greater degree than the aFGF/OI group. Biotinylated dextran amine is an effective anterograde tracing neural tracer that is an important tool for detection of axonal growth.[59] To provide further evidence that the aFGF-HP hydrogel can promote axonal growth across the scar, frozen sections of the T12-L1 plane (under the injured site) were tested using BDA staining. As shown in Fig. 13C,D, the number of BDA-positive axons was abundant in the normal sham rats but sharply decreased in the SCI group. The aFGF-HP hydrogel treatment increased the number of BDA-positive fibers ~ 8-to 10-fold over the number in the SCI group, which was an additional 2-to 3-fold over the levels observed in aFGF/ OI group. The hierarchy of therapeutic activity in the regeneration process of SCI was as follows: aFGF-HP/OI group > aFGF/OI group > aFGF/ IV group> HP/OI group. These data indicated that the aFGF-HP hydrogel can promote axonal growth across the scar, which is of great benefit for the functional recovery of SCI.

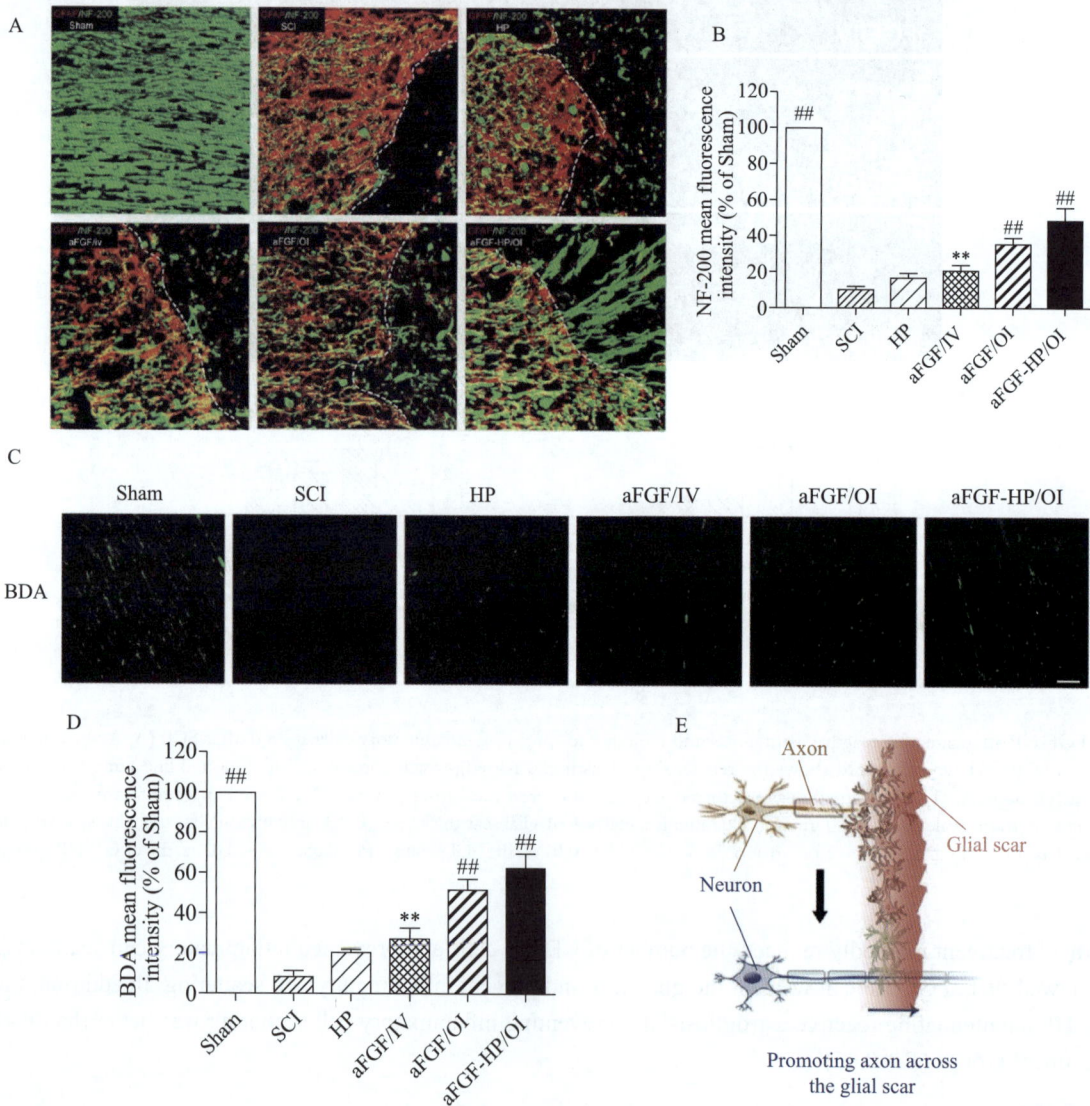

Fig. 13. aFGF-HP promotes axons across the scar at 28 d after SCI. (A) Representative images containing astrocytic fronts (dashed lines) and neurofilament (NF-200) immunofluorescence on spinal cord sections. Scale bar = 50 μm. (B) Quantitative analysis of NF-200 staining intensity. (C) The expression of BDA protein in the immunofluorescence staining at caudal 5 mm of the spinal cord on the 28th d after SCI. (D) Quantitative analysis of BDA results. (E) Schematic of aFGF-HP on promoting axons across the scar. Values were expressed as the mean ± SEM, $n = 5$ per group. #$P < 0.05$, ##$P < 0.01$ vs. the SCI group, *$P < 0.05$, **$P < 0.01$ vs. the aFGF-HP group.

3.8 aFGF-HP promotes the motor function after SCI

aFGF-HP exerted a positive effect on BSCB protection, neuroprotection, remyelination, and axonal rehabilitation as well as attenuated reactive astrogliosis and promoted axonal growth across the scar. Whether these effects can be translated into motor function recovery requires further examination. We use three behavioral tests, namely, the inclined plane test, the BBB locomotion scale test, and footprint test, to measure functional recovery. The hind legs of all the rats lost function immediately after SCI and showed restoration in a time-dependent manner. The results showed significant differences in the recovery of motor function among the experimental groups. By estimating the BBB score and the angle of incline, the aFGF-HP/OI group showed the most significant effect followed by the aFGF/OI group (Fig. 14A,B). The footprint test can intuitively show the restoration of hind leg movement at 28 dpi. The rats treated with the aFGF-HP hydrogel exhibited coordinated crawling with the tail raised and almost achieved the functional levels of the control group, whereas rats in the SCI group were still dragging their hind legs (Fig. 14C). All these data indicate that the aFGF-HP/OI group showed maximum improvements regarding functional recovery to a higher degree than the aFGF/OI group, aFGF/IV group, HP/OI group, and SCI group. Furthermore, the dynamic interaction between aFGF and the HP hydrogel as measured by a 2 × 2 factorial trial can enhance the motor function recovery ($P < 0.01$). By comparison, the effect of the aFGF/OI group was shown to be better than that of the aFGF/IV group, indicating that an *in situ* injection is the preferred administration method for these drugs ($P < 0.01$). Taken together, the aFGF-HP hydrogel in association with an *in situ* injection could effectively improve motor function recovery after SCI.

3.9 aFGF-HP inhibits the ER stress signaling pathway

Our previous reports indicated that the ER stress signal contributes to the induction of apoptosis in neuronal injury diseases.[60,61] To determine the relationship between aFGF-HP and the regulation of ER stress *in vivo*, we detected proteins involved in the ER stress-induced apoptosis signaling pathway by western blotting and immunofluorescence staining. As shown in Fig. 15A, immunofluorescence staining revealed that the number of cells positive for CHOP, the most significant ER stress-induced apoptosis protein, was increased in spinal cord lesions in the SCI group. However, the number of positive cells was reduced in the aFGF-treated groups, particularly in the aFGF-HP/OI group. In addi-

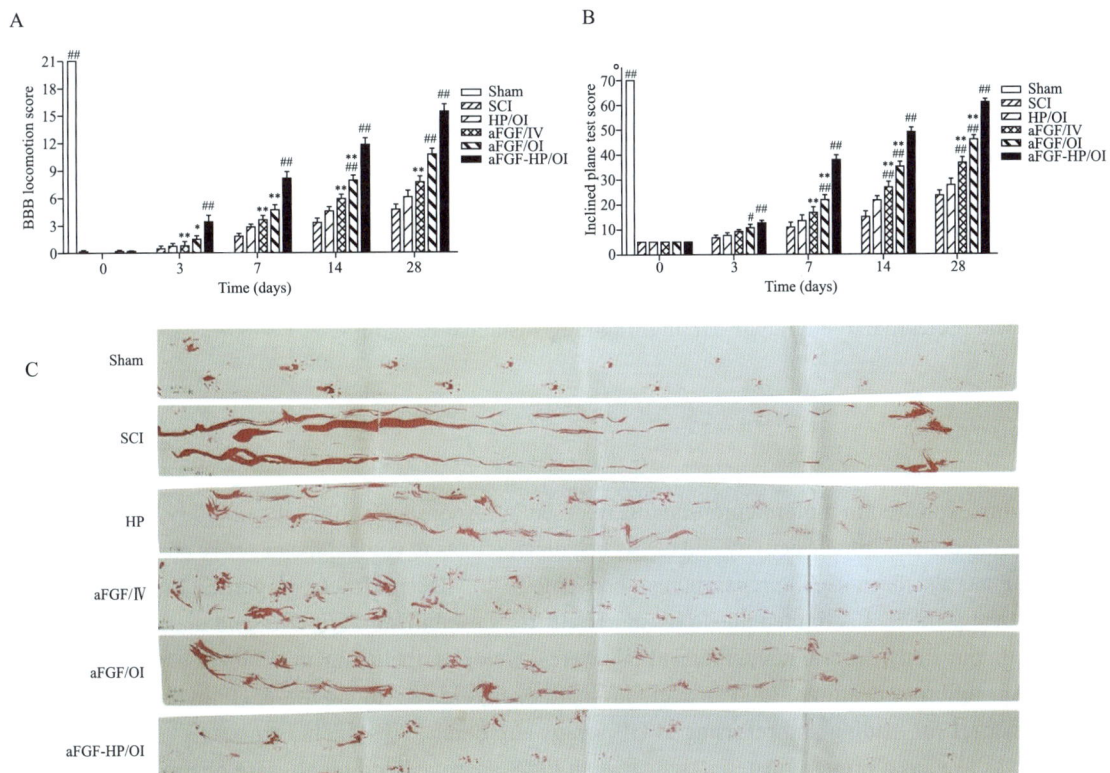

Fig. 14. aFGF-HP improves the motor function recovery of SCI rat. (A) The BBB locomotion scores and (B) the inclined plane test scores of the different groups. (C) Footprint analyses of the different groups. Values were expressed as the mean ± SEM, $n = 12$ per group. $^{#}P < 0.05$, $^{##}P < 0.01$ *vs.* the SCI group, $^{*}P < 0.05$, $^{**}P < 0.01$ *vs.* the aFGF-HP group.

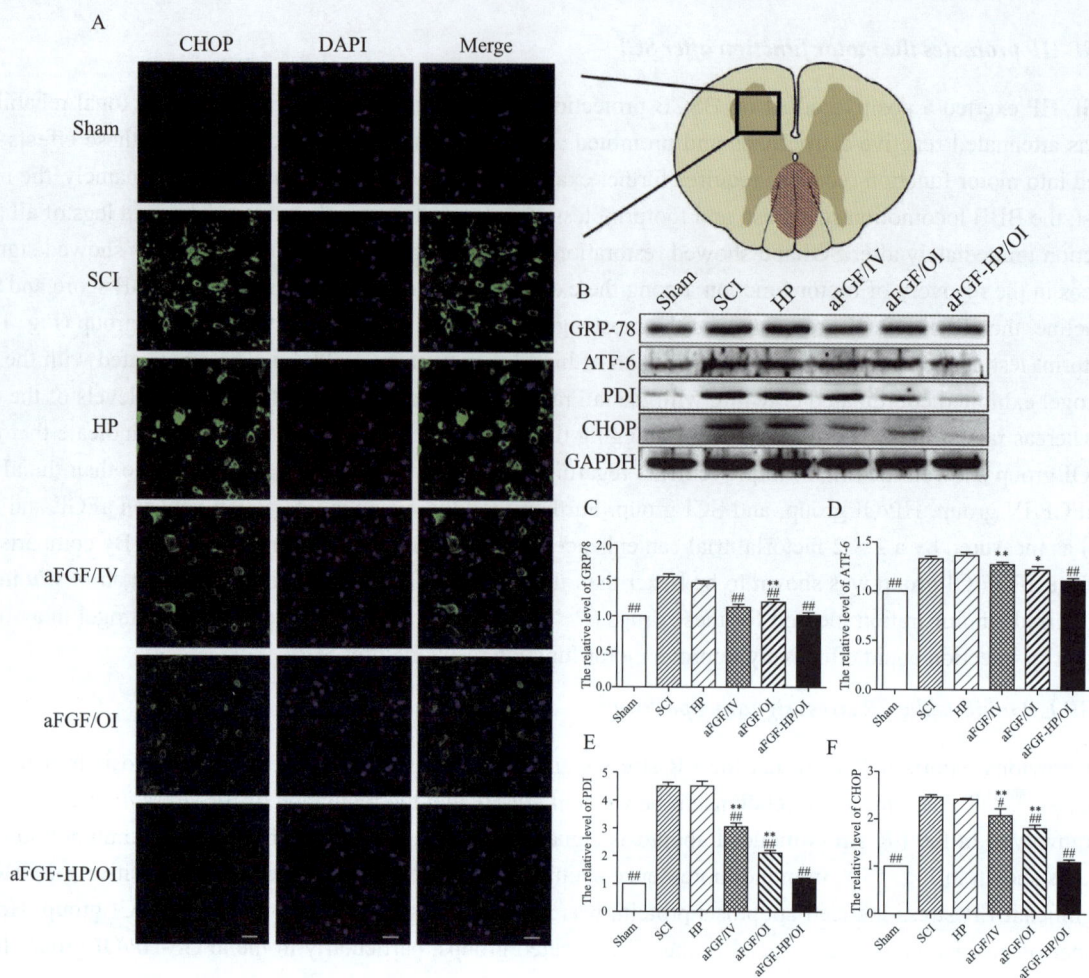

Fig. 15. aFGF-HP inhibits the activation of ER stress *in vivo* at 7 d after SCI. (A) Fluorescence images of spinal cord shows the expressions of CHOP in each group. Scale bar = 50 μm. (B) Protein expressions of GRP78, ATF-6, PDI, and CHOP of segments from the injured spinal cord in different group at 7 d after SCI. (C–F) Quantification of western blot data from (B). Values were expressed as the mean ± SEM, $n = 5$ per group. $^{#}P < 0.05$, $^{##}P < 0.01$ *vs.* the SCI group, $^{*}P < 0.05$, $^{**}P < 0.01$ *vs.* the aFGF-HP group.

tion, the levels of ER stress-related proteins (GRP78, ATF-6, PDI, and CHOP) were significantly increased at 7 dpi but decreased after aFGF treatment; furthermore, the protein levels in the aFGF-HP-treated rats were much lower than those in the aFGF group, which was in accordance with the immunofluorescence staining results (Fig. 15B–F). All these data revealed the critical protective role of aFGF-HP in mitigating sustained ER stress.

4. Discussion

aFGF is highly expressed in motor neurons and is released in response to sublethal cell injury.[62,63] It is well-accepted that aFGF has direct neurotrophic activity and exerts beneficial effects to combat the negative consequences of SCI.[9,64] Exogenous aFGF has also been used to repair human nonacute SCI.[12] Despite these properties, the practical therapeutic use of aFGF to treat acute SCI is limited due to its short half-life, destabilization *in vivo*, and undesirable effects at high systemic levels. In our study, several novel biomaterials were developed, including an HP thermosensitive hydrogel,[35,65] a H_2S-releasing nanofibrous coating,[66] and an acellular matrix scaffold.[67] Among these, HP hydrogel was found to exert the best properties for loading and releasing aFGF *versus* any other FGFs, including bFGF.[65] In our HP-hydrogel, the poloxamer was used as a primary material, which is an FDA-approved and highly safe pharmaceutical adjuvant for venous injection with heparin to load aFGF. On the one hand, unlike other positively charged FGFs, HP and aFGF are negatively charged, which allows for relatively easy release of aFGF from HP hydrogels.[65] On the other hand, compared with poloxamer alone, HP can load a much higher amount of aFGF and release it in a slow and sustained manner, which can be beneficial for SCI repair. This phenomenon could be largely attributed to heparin, which can conjugate with the hydrogel though its −COOH and −OH groups and bind to the GF with its −SH group.[33] In addition, heparin can protect aFGF from acid or thermal inactivation, and protease degradation as well as stabilize the conformation, thereby effectively protecting aFGF activity.[36,38,68] With these advantages, HP is a promising candidate for delivering aFGF for SCI therapy.

In addition, the lack of a comprehensive method to evaluate the effects of therapeutics on human SCI hinders the development of new therapies. Previous studies found that the BSCB disruption,[69] neuron loss,[3] demyelination,[70] axonal impairment,[55] and astrocytic gliosis[57] are common indicators that reflect the neurological damage of SCI. In these years, a lot of biological materials were developed for SCI treatment. Some of them were especial for providing the best environment for adhesion and proliferation of cells.[71,72] Some of them were designed to achieve the drug target and controlled release delivery.[29,31] Each material had its own characteristics. To the best of our knowledge, we provided the first multifaceted evidence that a novel aFGF-loaded HP hydrogel administered *via in situ* injection (which can bypass the BSCB more efficiently than intravenous injection) could effectively promote the neuroprotective effect and recovery after SCI.

BSCB integrity plays a crucial role in sustaining the function of the spinal cord. Sarah A *et al.* showed that the BSCB was disrupted within 1 h after injury and remained open for 5 d, with maximum permeability observed at 24 h post injury.[73] In the current study, we first discovered that aFGF treatment decreased the extravasation of EB dye at 1 dpi as well as reduced the penetrability of an H_2O_2-treated cell monolayer to FITC-dextran. Another interesting finding was that the reduction of TJ and AJ proteins such as β-catenin and claudin-5 was inhibited, which is closely related to the penetrability of the BSCB during SCI. Those results suggested that aFGF could prevent BSCB disruption. Regarding the effects of the different administration routes, our results showed that the aFGF/OI group had a better effect on BSCB protection than the aFGF/IV group, which suggested that *in situ* administration of aFGF can bypass the BSCB and more effectively concentrate the drug at the lesion site than intravenous administration. In addition, the aFGF-HP/OI group had a more pronounced effect than the aFGF/OI group, which exhibited less release of aFGF. This result can be explained by the protective effect of HP on aFGF, which creates a synergistic effect. In conclusion, we discovered that aFGF-HP exerted a better protective effect in preserving the BSCB during the early stage of SCI at 1 dpi.

Previous studies have reported that aFGF exerts direct and potent neurotrophic activity and promotes axonal growth.[10,11] In this study, our results showed that aFGF can reduce the level of neural apoptosis and increase the expression of GAP43 and Nestin, all of which are associated with neural restoration. In addition, we showed that aFGF reduced white matter injury in the spinal cord by inhibiting acantholysis of the myelin sheath and the reduced MBP expression. Lastname *et al.* found that microtubule stabilization can promote axon growth;[74] our results expanded on this notion by showing that aFGF facilitated the axon regeneration *in vivo* and *in vitro* and increased the expression of MAP-2, indicating that the positive effect of aFGF on axonal growth was associated with microtubule stabilization. In addition, the aFGF-HP/OI group exhibited a better effect than either the aFGF/OI or aFGF/IV groups, suggesting that the slow and sustained release of aFGF from the aFGF-HP hydrogel can significantly promote the neuroprotective effect. In conclusion, the potential of aFGF on preventing neuron cell death as well as promoting neuronal axon regeneration after SCI can be achieved upon *in situ* administration of the aFGF-HP hydrogel.

It is widely regarded that excessive scar tissue formation is a major factor for inhibiting axonal regeneration;[75] furthermore, it has been verified that preventing the proliferation of scar-forming astrocytes or removing the inhibitory CSPGs secreted from reactive astrocytes could effectively improve functional deficiency after SCI.[57,76] However, Mark A. Anderson *et al.* recently found that preventing astrocyte scar formation failed to produce spontaneous regrowth of the axons through the lesions.[56] In contrast, our results showed that both the physical and chemical barriers, including astroglial proliferation, glial scar formation, and Neurocan secretion from reactive astrocytes, were markedly reduced after aFGF treatment both *in vivo* and *in vitro*. Moreover, more NF-200-positive fibers were detected at the lesion site after SCI. Current studies have revealed that reactive astrogliosis limits the inflammatory response, and reducing astrocyte scar formation induced the widespread infiltration of inflammatory cells.[77] However, our data indicated that aFGF treatment did not induce infiltration of CD68+ (a marker of macrophages) cells but rather reduced the number of CD68+ cells. In summary, our results suggest that administration of aFGF ameliorated the barriers induced by reactive astrocytes and confined the inflammatory region, which can also support axonal regrowth beyond the glial scars. In addition, sustained local delivery of aFGF-HP *via in situ* injection locally and continuously released aFGF, which exerted better effects than the other tested administration routes of aFGF, suggesting that aFGF treatment *via* a slow-release carrier might be a more valid method for providing nerve regeneration during the later stages of SCI.

Previous studies have shown that aFGF plays vital neuro-protective and neuroregenerative roles through the PI3K/Akt and MAPK/ERK pathways;[13,78,79] however, the detailed mechanism is still unclear. Our previous reports have suggested that the ER stress-signaling pathway may play a direct role in inducing apoptosis in neuronal injury diseases.[80,81] Our study is the first to demonstrate that ER stress-associated proteins, including GRP78, ATF-6, caspase 12, PDI, and CHOP, were obviously increased after SCI and were decreased after treatment with the aFGF-HP hydrogel *in vivo*. Our results showed that the aFGF-HP hydrogel treatment exerted neuroprotective and neuroregenerative effects and improved functional recovery after SCI in part by inhibiting ER stress-induced apoptosis.

5. Conclusions

A novel aFGF heparin-poloxamer thermosensitive hydrogel was shown to be the optimal formulation for loading and releasing aFGF *versus* other FGFs based on data in clinical trials. The aFGF-HP hydrogel, when administered *via in situ* injection, effectively enhanced the recovery of SCI. aFGF-HP exerted neuroprotective effects and created advantageous conditions for BSCB protection, neuroprotection, axonal regeneration, reactive astrogliosis suppression, and functional restoration by inhibiting ER stress. In addition, the positive effects of aFGF-HP were better achieved by *in situ* administration to bypass the BSCB. The aFGF-HP hydrogel could facilitate and prolong aFGF delivery to the damaged spinal cord and maximize the effects of aFGF while minimizing the adverse effects (such as carcinogenicity or tumorigenicity). aFGF-HP, as a slow-release carrier, represents a more effective approach for neuro-protection and could be a clinically feasible therapeutic approach for patients suffering from SCI.

Supporting Information

The supporting information is available on the ACS Publications website at DOI: 10.1021/acsami.6b13155.

References

[1] Saunders LL, Clarke A, Tate DG, *et al.* Lifetime prevalence of chronic health conditions among persons with spinal cord injury[J]. Archives of physical medicine and rehabilitation, 2015, 96(4): 673-679.

[2] Penas C, Guzmán MS, Verdú E, *et al.* Spinal cord injury induces endoplasmic reticulum stress with different cell-type dependent response[J]. Journal of neurochemistry, 2007, 102(4): 1242-1255.

[3] Zhang HY, Wang ZG, Wu FZ, *et al.* Regulation of autophagy and ubiquitinated protein accumulation by bFGF promotes functional recovery and neural protection in a rat model of spinal cord injury[J]. Molecular neurobiology, 2013, 48(3): 452-464.

[4] Allison DJ, Thomas A, Beaudry K, *et al.* Targeting inflammation as a treatment modality for neuropathic pain in spinal cord injury: a randomized clinical trial[J]. Journal of neuroinflammation, 2016, 13(1): 152.

[5] Kawabata S, Takano M, Numasawa-Kuroiwa Y, *et al.* Grafted Human iPS Cell-Derived Oligodendrocyte Precursor Cells Contribute to Robust Remyelination of Demyelinated Axons after Spinal Cord Injury[J]. Stem cell reports, 2016, 6(1): 1-8.

[6] Xue F, Wu EJ, Zhang PX, *et al.* Biodegradable chitin conduit tubulation combined with bone marrow mesenchymal stem cell transplantation for treatment of spinal cord injury by reducing glial scar and cavity formation[J]. Neural regeneration research, 2015, 10(1): 104-111.

[7] Chung J, Kim MH, Yoon YJ, *et al.* Effects of granulocyte colony-stimulating factor and granulocyte-macrophage colony-stimulating factor on glial scar formation after spinal cord injury in rats[J]. Journal of neurosurgery. Spine, 2014, 21(6): 966-973.

[8] Lee YS, Hsiao I, Lin VW. Peripheral nerve grafts and aFGF restore partial hindlimb function in adult paraplegic rats[J]. Journal of neurotrauma, 2002, 19(10): 1203-1216.

[9] Lee LM, Huang MC, Chuang TY, *et al.* Acidic FGF enhances functional regeneration of adult dorsal roots[J]. Life sciences, 2004, 74(15): 1937-1943.

[10] Tsai MJ, Tsai SK, Huang MC, *et al.* Acidic FGF promotes neurite outgrowth of cortical neurons and improves neuroprotective effect in a cerebral ischemic rat model[J]. Neuroscience, 2015, 305: 238-247.

[11] Lee YS, Baratta J, Yu J, *et al.* AFGF promotes axonal growth in rat spinal cord organotypic slice co-cultures[J]. Journal of neurotrauma, 2002, 19(3): 357-367.

[12] Wu JC, Huang WC, Chen YC, *et al.* Acidic fibroblast growth factor for repair of human spinal cord injury: a clinical trial[J]. Journal of neurosurgery. Spine, 2011, 15(3): 216-227.

[13] Vargas MR, Pehar M, Cassina P, *et al.* Fibroblast growth factor-1 induces heme oxygenase-1 *via* nuclear factor erythroid 2-related factor 2 (Nrf2) in spinal cord astrocytes: consequences for motor neuron survival[J]. The Journal of biological chemistry, 2005,

280(27): 25571-25579.

[14] Burgess WH, Friesel R, Winkles JA. Structure-function studies of FGF-1: dissociation and partial reconstitution of certain of its biological activities[J]. Molecular reproduction and development, 1994, 39(1): 56-60; discussion 60-51.

[15] Ma C, Xu J, Cheng H, et al. A neural repair treatment with gait training improves motor function recovery after spinal cord injury. In: International Conference of the IEEE Engineering in Medicine & Biology Society IEEE Engineering in Medicine & Biology Society Conference, Vol. 2010, 2010: 5553-5556.

[16] Tsintou M, Dalamagkas K, Seifalian AM. Advances in regenerative therapies for spinal cord injury: a biomaterials approach[J]. Neural regeneration research, 2015, 10(5): 726-742.

[17] Silva NA, Sousa N, Reis RL., et al. From basics to clinical: A comprehensive review on spinal cord injury[J]. Progress in Neurobiology, 2014, 114(1): 25-57.

[18] Perale G, Rossi F, Santoro M, et al. Multiple drug delivery hydrogel system for spinal cord injury repair strategies[J]. Journal of controlled release : official journal of the Controlled Release Society, 2012, 159(2): 271-280.

[19] Caron I, Rossi F, Papa S, et al. A new three dimensional biomimetic hydrogel to deliver factors secreted by human mesenchymal stem cells in spinal cord injury[J]. Biomaterials, 2016, 75: 135-147.

[20] Oliveira AL, Sousa EC, Silva NA, et al. Peripheral mineralization of a 3D biodegradable tubular construct as a way to enhance guidance stabilization in spinal cord injury regeneration[J]. Journal of materials science. Materials in medicine, 2012, 23(11): 2821-2830.

[21] Papa S, Caron I, Erba E, et al. Early modulation of pro-inflammatory microglia by minocycline loaded nanoparticles confers long lasting protection after spinal cord injury[J]. Biomaterials, 2016, 75: 13-24.

[22] Caron I, Papa S, Rossi F, et al. Nanovector-mediated drug delivery for spinal cord injury treatment[J]. Wiley Interdiscip Rev Nanomed Nanobiotechnol, 2014, 6(5): 506-515.

[23] Cerqueira SR, Oliveira JM, Silva NA, et al. Microglia Response and In Vivo Therapeutic Potential of Methylprednisolone-Loaded Dendrimer Nanoparticles in Spinal Cord Injury[J]. Small, 2016, 12(8): 972.

[24] Chen Z, Wu D, Li L, et al. Apelin/APJ System: A Novel Therapeutic Target for Myocardial Ischemia/Reperfusion Injury[J]. DNA Cell Biol, 2016, 35(12): 766-775.

[25] Mann AP, Scodeller P, Hussain S, et al. A peptide for targeted, systemic delivery of imaging and therapeutic compounds into acute brain injuries[J]. Nat Commun, 2016, 7: 11980.

[26] Perale G, Rossi F, Sundstrom E, et al. Hydrogels in spinal cord injury repair strategies[J]. ACS Chem Neurosci, 2011, 2(7): 336-345.

[27] Fuhrmann T, R Y Tam, Ballarin B, et al. Injectable hydrogel promotes early survival of induced pluripotent stem cell-derived oligodendrocytes and attenuates longterm teratoma formation in a spinal cord injury model[J]. Biomaterials, 2016, 83: 23-36.

[28] Donaghue IE, Shoichet MS. Controlled release of bioactive PDGF-AA from a hydrogel/nanoparticle composite[J]. Acta Biomater, 2015, 25: 35-42.

[29] Lindsey S, Piatt JH, Worthington P, et al. Beta Hairpin Peptide Hydrogels as an Injectable Solid Vehicle for Neurotrophic Growth Factor Delivery[J]. Biomacromolecules, 2015, 16(9): 2672-2683.

[30] Fuhrmann T, Obermeyer J, Tator CH, et al. Click-crosslinked injectable hyaluronic acid hydrogel is safe and biocompatible in the intrathecal space for ultimate use in regenerative strategies of the injured spinal cord[J]. Methods, 2015, 84: 60-69.

[31] Chen B, He J, Yang H, et al. Repair of spinal cord injury by implantation of bFGF-incorporated hema-moetacl hydrogel in rats[J]. Sci Rep, 2015, 5: 9017.

[32] des Rieux A, De Berdt P, Ansorena E, et al. Vascular endothelial growth factor-loaded injectable hydrogel enhances plasticity in the injured spinal cord[J]. J Biomed Mater Res A, 2014, 102(7): 2345-2355.

[33] Rubin JS, Day RM, Breckenridge D, et al. Dissociation of heparan sulfate and receptor binding domains of hepatocyte growth factor reveals that heparan sulfate-c-met interaction facilitates signaling[J]. J Biol Chem, 2001, 276(35): 32977-32983.

[34] Nie T, Baldwin A, Yamaguchi N, et al. Production of heparin-functionalized hydrogels for the development of responsive and controlled growth factor delivery systems[J]. J Control Release, 2007, 122(3): 287-296.

[35] Tian JL, Zhao YZ, Jin Z, et al. Synthesis and characterization of Poloxamer 188-grafted heparin copolymer[J]. Drug Dev Ind Pharm, 2010, 36(7): 832-838.

[36] Yoon JJ, Chung HJ, Lee HJ, et al. Heparin-immobilized biodegradable scaffolds for local and sustained release of angiogenic growth factor[J]. J Biomed Mater Res A, 2006, 79(4): 934-942.

[37] Ishihara M, Obara K, Ishizuka T, et al. Controlled release of fibroblast growth factors and heparin from photocrosslinked chitosan hydrogels and subsequent effect on in vivo vascularization[J]. J Biomed Mater Res A, 2003, 64(3): 551-559.

[38] Sakiyama-Elbert SE, Hubbell JA. Development of fibrin derivatives for controlled release of heparin-binding growth factors[J]. J Control Release, 2000, 65(3): 389-402.

[39] Taguchi T, Kishida A, Sakamoto N, et al. Preparation of a novel functional hydrogel consisting of sulfated glucoside-bearing polymer: activation of basic fibroblast growth factor[J]. J Biomed Mater Res, 1998, 41(3): 386-391.

[40] Yong CS, Choi JS, Quan QZ, et al. Effect of sodium chloride on the gelation temperature, gel strength and bioadhesive force of poloxamer gels containing diclofenac sodium[J]. Int J Pharm, 2001, 226(1-2): 195-205.

[41] Zhou KL, Zhou YF, Wu K, et al. Stimulation of autophagy promotes functional recovery in diabetic rats with spinal cord injury[J]. Sci Rep, 2015, 5: 17130.

[42] Zheng B, Ye L, Zhou Y, et al. Epidermal growth factor attenuates blood-spinal cord barrier disruption via PI3K/Akt/Rac1 pathway after acute spinal cord injury[J]. J Cell Mol Med, 2016, 20(6): 1062-1075.

[43] Basso DM, Beattie MS, Bresnahan JC. A sensitive and reliable locomotor rating scale for open field testing in rats[J]. J Neurotrauma, 1995, 12(1): 1-21.

[44] Rivlin AS, Tator CH. Objective clinical assessment of motor function after experimental spinal cord injury in the rat[J]. J Neurosurg, 1977, 47(4): 577-581.

[45] de Medinaceli L, Freed WJ, Wyatt RJ. An index of the functional condition of rat sciatic nerve based on measurements made from walking tracks[J]. Exp Neurol, 1982, 77(3): 634-643.

[46] Figley SA, Khosravi R, Legasto JM, et al. Characterization of vascular disruption and blood-spinal cord barrier permeability following traumatic spinal cord injury[J]. J Neurotrauma, 2014, 31(6): 541-552.

[47] Bernacki J, Dobrowolska A, Nierwińska K, et al. Physiology and pharmacological role of the blood-brain barrier[J]. Pharmacological reports : PR, 2008, 60(5): 600-622.

[48] Bethea JR, Dietrich WD. Targeting the host inflammatory response in traumatic spinal cord injury[J]. Curr Opin Neurol, 2002, 15(3): 355-360.

[49] Sakurai M, Nagata T, Abe K, et al. Survival and death-promoting events after transient spinal cord ischemia in rabbits: induction of Akt and caspase3 in motor neurons[J]. J Thorac Cardiovasc Surg, 2003, 125(2): 370-377.

[50] Warden P, Bamber NI, Li H, et al. Delayed glial cell death following wallerian degeneration in white matter tracts after spinal cord dorsal column cordotomy in adult rats[J]. Exp Neurol, 2001, 168(2): 213-224.

[51] Xie XM, Shi LL, Shen L, et al. Co-transplantation of MRF-overexpressing oligodendrocyte precursor cells and Schwann cells promotes recovery in rat after spinal cord injury[J]. Neurobiol Dis,

2016, 94: 196-204.

[52] Gao R, Li X, Xi S, *et al.* Exogenous Neuritin Promotes Nerve Regeneration After Acute Spinal Cord Injury in Rats[J]. Hum Gene Ther, 2016, 27(7): 544-554.

[53] Santos D, Giudetti G, Micera S, *et al.* Focal release of neurotrophic factors by biodegradable microspheres enhance motor and sensory axonal regeneration *in vitro* and *in vivo*[J]. Brain Res, 2016, 1636: 93-106.

[54] Huang Z, Gao Y, Sun Y, *et al.* NB-3 signaling mediates the crosstalk between post-traumatic spinal axons and scar-forming cells[J]. Embo j, 2016, 35(16): 1745-1765.

[55] Shao WY, Liu X, Gu XL, *et al.* Promotion of axon regeneration and inhibition of astrocyte activation by alpha A-crystallin on crushed optic nerve[J]. Int J Ophthalmol, 2016, 9(7): 955-966.

[56] Anderson MA, Burda JE, Ren Y, *et al.* Astrocyte scar formation aids central nervous system axon regeneration[J]. Nature, 2016, 532(7598): 195-200.

[57] Zhao YY, Yuan Y, Chen Y, *et al.* Histamine promotes locomotion recovery after spinal cord hemisection *via* inhibiting astrocytic scar formation[J]. CNS Neurosci Ther, 2015, 21(5): 454-462.

[58] Mukhamedshina YO, Garanina EE, Masgutova GA, *et al.* Assessment of Glial Scar, Tissue Sparing, Behavioral Recovery and Axonal Regeneration following Acute Transplantation of Genetically Modified Human Umbilical Cord Blood Cells in a Rat Model of Spinal Cord Contusion[J]. PLoS One, 2016, 11(3): e0151745.

[59] Chen P, Goldberg DE, Kolb B, *et al.* Inosine induces axonal rewiring and improves behavioral outcome after stroke[J]. Proc Natl Acad Sci U S A, 2002, 99(13): 9031-9036.

[60] Zhang H, Wu F, Kong X, *et al.* Nerve growth factor improves functional recovery by inhibiting endoplasmic reticulum stress-induced neuronal apoptosis in rats with spinal cord injury[J]. J Transl Med, 2014, 12: 130.

[61] Zhou Y, Ye L, Zheng B, *et al.* Phenylbutyrate prevents disruption of blood-spinal cord barrier by inhibiting endoplasmic reticulum stress after spinal cord injury[J]. Am J Transl Res, 2016, 8(4): 1864-1875.

[62] Shin JT, Opalenik SR, Wehby JN, *et al.* Serum-starvation induces the extracellular appearance of FGF-1[J]. Biochim Biophys Acta, 1996, 1312(1): 27-38.

[63] Mouta Carreira C, Landriscina M, Bellum S, *et al.* The comparative release of FGF1 by hypoxia and temperature stress[J]. Growth Factors, 2001, 18(4): 277-285.

[64] Cuevas P, Carceller F, Gimenez-Gallego G. Acidic fibroblast growth factor prevents death of spinal cord motoneurons in newborn rats after nerve section[J]. Neurol Res, 1995, 17(5): 396-399.

[65] Wu J, Zhu J, He C, *et al.* Comparative Study of Heparin-Poloxamer Hydrogel Modified bFGF and aFGF for *in Vivo* Wound Healing Efficiency[J]. ACS Appl Mater Interfaces, 2016, 8(29): 18710-18721.

[66] Wu J, Li Y, He C, *et al.* Novel H2S Releasing Nanofibrous Coating for *In Vivo* Dermal Wound Regeneration[J]. ACS Appl Mater Interfaces, 2016, 8(41): 27474-27481.

[67] Xu HL, Mao KL, Lu CT, *et al.* An injectable acellular matrix scaffold with absorbable permeable nanoparticles improves the thera-

peutic effects of docetaxel on glioblastoma[J]. Biomaterials, 2016, 107: 44-60.

[68] Tanihara M, Suzuki Y, Yamamoto E, *et al.* Sustained release of basic fibroblast growth factor and angiogenesis in a novel covalently crosslinked gel of heparin and alginate[J]. J Biomed Mater Res, 2001, 56(2): 216-221.

[69] Bartanusz V, Jezova D, Alajajian B, *et al.* The blood-spinal cord barrier: morphology and clinical implications[J]. Ann Neurol, 2011, 70(2): 194-206.

[70] Kurita N, Kawaguchi M, Kakimoto M, *et al.* Reevaluation of gray and white matter injury after spinal cord ischemia in rabbits[J]. Anesthesiology, 2006, 105(2): 305-312.

[71] Ji WC, Zhang XW, Qiu YS. Selected suitable seed cell, scaffold and growth factor could maximize the repair effect using tissue engineering method in spinal cord injury[J]. World J Exp Med, 2016, 6(3): 58-62.

[72] Kabu S, Gao Y, Kwon BK, *et al.* Drug delivery, cell-based therapies, and tissue engineering approaches for spinal cord injury[J]. J Control Release, 2015, 219: 141-154.

[73] Lee JY, Kim HS, Choi HY, *et al.* Fluoxetine inhibits matrix metalloprotease activation and prevents disruption of blood-spinal cord barrier after spinal cord injury[J]. Brain, 2012, 135(Pt 8): 2375-2389.

[74] Ruschel J, Hellal F, Flynn KC, *et al.* Axonal regeneration. Systemic administration of epothilone B promotes axon regeneration after spinal cord injury[J]. Science, 2015, 348(6232): 347-352.

[75] Rodriguez-Grande B, Swana M, Nguyen L, *et al.* The acute-phase protein PTX3 is an essential mediator of glial scar formation and resolution of brain edema after ischemic injury[J]. J Cereb Blood Flow Metab, 2014, 34(3): 480-488.

[76] Hayashi N, Miyata S, Kariya Y, *et al.* Attenuation of glial scar formation in the injured rat brain by heparin oligosaccharides[J]. Neurosci Res, 2004, 49(1): 19-27.

[77] Wanner IB, Anderson MA, Song B, *et al.* Glial scar borders are formed by newly proliferated, elongated astrocytes that interact to corral inflammatory and fibrotic cells *via* STAT3-dependent mechanisms after spinal cord injury[J]. J Neurosci, 2013, 33(31): 12870-12886.

[78] Alam J, Wicks C, Stewart D, *et al.* Mechanism of heme oxygenase-1 gene activation by cadmium in MCF-7 mammary epithelial cells. Role of p38 kinase and Nrf2 transcription factor[J]. J Biol Chem, 2000, 275(36): 27694-27702.

[79] Ryter SW, Xi S, Hartsfield CL, *et al.* Mitogen activated protein kinase (MAPK) pathway regulates heme oxygenase-1 gene expression by hypoxia in vascular cells[J]. Antioxid Redox Signal, 2002, 4(4): 587-592.

[80] Zhang HY, Zhang X, Wang ZG, *et al.* Exogenous basic fibroblast growth factor inhibits ER stress-induced apoptosis and improves recovery from spinal cord injury[J]. CNS Neurosci Ther, 2013, 19(1): 20-29.

[81] Wang Z, Zhang H, Xu X, *et al.* bFGF inhibits ER stress induced by ischemic oxidative injury *via* activation of the PI3K/Akt and ERK1/2 pathways[J]. Toxicol Lett, 2012, 212(2): 137-146.

Dual delivery of NGF and bFGF coacervater ameliorates diabetic peripheral neuropathy *via* inhibiting schwann cells apoptosis

Rui Li, Xiaokun Li, Jian Xiao

1. Introduction

Diabetic peripheral neuropathy (DPN) as one kind of the most common and chronic complications of diabetes mellitus occur in approximately 50% of all diabetic patients [1, 2]. It results in pain, paraesthesia, and decreased sensation, and can negatively influence quality of life [3]. Currently, there are no specific therapies to successfully prevent DPN except glycemic control [4]. Nevertheless, maintaining stable blood glucose is often difficult to achieve in many patients. Therefore, it needs to further explore the better treatment for DPN.

Recent evidence has indicated that endoplasmic reticulum stress (ERS) exerts an essential role in the onset and progression of DPN [5]. ERS is being increasingly considered as one of the main molecular mechanisms underlying DPN [6]. The endoplasmic reticulum (ER) is a sophisticated membrane system which exerts a vital role in the process of newly proteins synthesis and folding, and the storage of calcium. Pathological cellular stressors that disrupt ER homeostasis such as nutrient deficiency, oxidative stress, perturbation of calcium homeostasis, and increase of unsaturated fatty acids or cholesterol, can all induce ERS [7, 8]. As counter measures for ERS, cells carry out unfolding protein response (UPR) that includes: reducing the excessive folding of proteins, up-regulating the synthesis of related-chaperones and enzymes. These measures promote the ability of proteins to fold properly, and reinforce the self-repair ability of the ER [9, 10]. Effective new treatment methods for DPN must thus target the ERS-UPR pathway.

Basic fibroblast growth factor (bFGF), a neurotrophic factor, can play the part of a crucial regulator for neuroprotection, neurogenesis and angiogenesis from various insults [11]. Nerve growth factor (NGF), the first discovered neurotrophin, has been extensively shown to promote survival and maintain neuronal function [12]. Both factors subserve the maintenance and development of neurons and facilitate neural repair in the peripheral nervous system (PNS). It has been reported that diabetes significantly reduced the production and secretion of bFGF and NGF in sciatic nerve tissue, and exogenously administered either of these two neurotrophic factors (NTFs) improved morphological and functional recovery [13-15]. However, a therapeutic strategy for DPN, based on a single growth factor (GF), may not be sufficient to provide robust neuroprotective effects because neural network comprises different neurons that requires different NTFs [16].

In a previous study, we developed an injectable coacervate, made of a polycation, poly (ethylene arginyl aspartate diglyceride) (PEAD) and GF-binding heparin, which easily bound a various of growth factors (GFs) and controlled its release in a steady way [17-19]. Here, we investigated whether use of bFGF and NGF in combination could prevent the progression or promote the recovery of diabetic neuropathy in streptozotocin (STZ)-induced diabetic rats. Since both of these two GFs are proteins, they are unstable and degrade rapidly *in vivo* [20, 21], thus it would be ideal to control co-delivery of these two GFs for promoting nerve repair.

In our current study, we had developed an injectable GFs coacervate with bFGF and NGF, and tried to reveal whether GFs coacervate exerts a better protective role on DPN. Additionally, we also explored the molecular mechanism underlying the protective role of GFs coacervate on DPN, aiming to provide the theoretical basis for treatment of DPN.

2. Materials and methods

2.1 Reagents and antibodies

Recombinant human bFGF was purchased from Grost (Grost Biotechnology, Zhejiang, China). NGF, heparin and streptozotocin (STZ) were purchased from Sigma (Sigma–Aldrich, St. Louis, MO, USA). PEAD was a gift from University of Pittsburgh. Hematoxylin and eosin were purchased from Beycotime Biotechnology. NGF and bFGF enzyme linked immunosorbent assay (ELISA) kits were purchased from Elabscience Biotechnology. Dulbecco's modified Eagle's medium (DMEM) and fetal bovine serum (FBS) were purchased from Invitrogen (Carlsbad, CA, USA). Antibodies against GRP-78, ATF-6, ATF-4 and Caspase-12 were purchased from Abcam Biotechnology (Cambridge, MA, USA). Anti-CHOP and anti-XBP-1 were purchased from Santa Cruz Biotechnology (Santa Cruz, CA, USA). Anti-GAPDH was purchased from Bioworld Biotechnology.

2.2 Growth Factor release assay

Poly (ethylene argininylaspartate diglyceride) (PEAD) was synthesized as previously described [22]. PEAD, heparin, NGF and bFGF were seriatim dissolved in 0.9% normal saline to obtain 10 mg/ml solutions and sterilized using 0.22 μm Millipore filter. The release assay *in vitro* ($n = 3$) was performed using 1 μl of NGF and 1 μl of bFGF combined together, then mixed with 10 μl of heparin followed lastly by the addition of 50 μl of PEAD solution. On Day 1, 4, 7, 14, 21, 28 and 35, the coacervate was gently mixed and centrifuged at 12 000 g for 10 min. Then, the supernatant was collected and stored, and 50 μl of fresh saline was added to the pellet. According to the ELISA kit manufacturer's instructions, the collected supernatant was measured by ELISA to detect the amount of released growth factor.

2.3 Induction of DPN and drug treatment

Eight-week old male Wistar rats (200–220 g) were purchased from the Animal Center of the Chinese Academy of Sciences in Shanghai, China. The protocol for animal care and use was conformed to the Guide for the Care and Use of Laboratory Animals from the National Institutes of Health and was approved by the Animal Care and Use Committee of Wenzhou Medical University. Animals were maintained in an aseptic animal room at least 1 week before the experiment with a temperature of 20–24 ℃ on a 12-h light/dark cycle and free access to food and water. Diabetes was induced by intraperitoneally injecting STZ with a dose of 65 mg/kg in phosphate-buffered saline (PBS). Control group received an equal volume of PBS. After 48 h, rats were detected the blood glucose, and the concentrations ≥16.7 mmol/L were considered as diabetes [23, 24]. After 8 weeks, diabetic rats were randomly divided into three groups: STZ-induced diabetes, free GFs (NGF + bFGF) and GFs coacervate ([PEAD:heparin: NGF + bFGF]). Each groups contained eight rats. For the GFs coacervate group, 0.1 ml saline solution (60 μg NGF, 60 μg bFGF, 1.2 mg heparin and 6 mg PEAD) was injected into the right thigh and soleus muscles through a 1.0 ml syringe only once. However, for the free GFs group, the dosages of NGF and bFGF were decided according to Mika's report [14], in which animals were administered intramuscular 20 μg NGF and 20 μg bFGF once daily for 3 consecutive days. STZ-induced diabetes group was administrated with the same volume of saline and control animals did not receive any treatment. After 30 days, the rats were anesthetized with 4% choral hydrate (10 ml/kg IP) and then perfused with 0.9% NaCl. The sciatic nerves from both sides were dissected out and harvested, and the pathology index was assessed.

2.4 Hot plate test

Hot plate test was to evaluate the sensory functional recovery of animals by measuring hind paw's licking and shaking. The test was conducted by two independent examiners who were blinded to remedy and to record sensory recovery on weekly bases after drug administration. Briefly, a hot plate at 55 ℃ ± 1 ℃ was prepared for the test, and the animals were positioned to stand with the operated hind paw on the hot plate. Thermal withdrawal reflex (TWRL) was measured by recording the time between placing in the hot plate and shaking or licking the paws. The cut-off time was set at 20 s to minimize skin injury. All tests were repeated for 4 times with a 5 min interval. If no hind paw withdraw was observed after 20 s, the TWRL was considered as 20 s.

2.5 Walking track analysis

Walking track analysis was carried out each week after treatment to assess motor functional recovery, and the sciatic function index (SFI) value was calculated using the method proposed by Bain et al [25]. The formula for calculation is as follows:

$$\text{SFI} = -38.3 \times (\text{EPL}-\text{NPL})/\text{NPL} + 109.5 \times (\text{ETS}-\text{NTS})/\text{NTS} + 13.3 \times (\text{EIT}-\text{NIT})/\text{NIT} - 8.8$$

E represented DPN group, N represented normal group. PL is the distance between the third toe and heel, TS is the distance between the first and fifth toes. IT is the distance between the second and fourth toes. Generally, a SFI value around 0 indicated normal nerve function, and a value around 100 indicated total dysfunction. SFI was a negative value and a higher SFI meant the better function of the sciatic nerve. All experiments were repeated by at least two separate investigators and the person who performed the surgeries never participated in the behavioral experiments.

2.6 Cell culture and treatment

RSC 96 cells (a rat Schwann cell line) were obtained from ScienCell Research Laboratories. They were cultured in Dulbecco's modified Eagle Medium (DMEM) containing 5.5 mM D-glucose supplemented with 100 U/ml penicillin, 100 mg/ml streptomycin and 10% fetal bovine serum, and incubated in a humidified atmosphere containing 5% CO_2 at 37℃. After two passages, RSC96 cells were plated at a density of 5000 per well in a 96-well plate for the MTT assay. For protein extraction and apoptosis assay, cells were seeded at a density of $(1-5) \times 10^5$/ml in 6-plate well and permitted to attach and grow for 24 h. The RSC96 cells in each experiment were divided into four groups: (1) the control group; (2) the high glucose (HG) group (30 mM high glucose DMEM); (3) the HG (30 mM) + Free GFs (Each GF was added at a final 50 ng/ml) group; and (4) the HG (30 mM) + GFs coacervate (the same concentration of GFs) group. All treatments lasted for 24 h.

2.7 Western blot analysis

For protein analysis of *in vivo* samples, the frozen sciatic nerves were homogenized in lysis buffer containing 137 mM NaCl, 20 mM Tris-HCl (pH 7.5), 1% NP40 and a protease inhibitor cocktail (10 μl/ml; GE Healthcare Biosciences, Pittsburgh, PA, USA). The complex was then centrifuged at 12 000 rpm, and the supernatant was obtained for protein assay. For *in vitro* samples, SCs were lysed in RIPA buffer (25 mM Tris-HCl, 150 mM NaCl, 1% Nonidet P-40, 1% sodium deoxycholate, and 0.1% sodium dodecyl sulfate) with protease and phosphatase inhibitors. Protein concentrations were quantified using a BCA Protein Assay Kit (Thermo, Rockford, IL, USA). The equivalent of 80 μg of total protein was loaded onto SDS-PAGE and transferred to PVDF membrane (Bio-Rad), and the membrane was blocked with 5% non fat-milk in TBS with 0.05% Tween 20 (TBST) for 1.5 h. Primary antibodies were incubated overnight at 4℃ with the following optimized dilutions: GRP78 (1:1 000), ATF-6 (1:1 000), XBP-1 (1:300), ATF-4 (1:1 000), Caspase-12 (1:1 000), CHOP (1:300) and GAPDH (1:10 000). The membranes were washed with TBST 3 times and incubated with horseradish peroxidase-conjugated secondary antibodies (1:10 000) for 1 h at room temperature. Signals were visualized using the ChemiDocTM XRS +Imaging System (Bio-Rad). The intensity of immunoreactivity was quantified using Java's freely available NIH Image J software. Experiments were repeated three times. GAPDH was used as an internal control.

2.8 Immunohistochemistry and histology

The collected sciatic nerve tissue was post-fixed in cold 4% paraformaldehyde overnight, and embedded in paraffin. Transverse sections of 5-μm thickness were cut, and the lesion epicenter stained with hematoxylin and eosin (HE). To determine the CHOP and Caspase-12 activities, the slides were incubated with 0.3% H_2O_2 in methanol for 30 min, followed by incubating with 10% normal donkey serum for 1 h at room temperature in PBS containing 0.1% Triton X-100. Next, the sections were incubated at 4℃ overnight with a primary antibody against Caspase-12 (1:1 000) and CHOP (1:100). After primary antibody incubation, sections were washed three times for 10 min with PBS and then incubated with Alexa Fluor 488 (1:1 000) or TR-conjugated secondary antibodies for 1 h at room temperature. Sections were rinsed three times with PBS and incubated with 4,6-diamidino-2-phenylindole (DAPI) for 5 min and finally washed with PBS and sealed with a coverslip. The images were captured using a Nikon ECLPSE 80i microscope.

2.9 Apoptosis assay

DNA fragmentation in longitudinal paraffin-cut sections (5 μm) of sciatic nerves at the lesion site was detected using the TUNEL apoptosis assay kit (Beyotime Institute of Biotechnology) according to the manufacturer's protocol. Sections were counter-stained with DAPI (blue color), Images were taken at × 400 and the number of TUNEL-positive cells in each section was counted through Image-Pro Plus software. Apoptosis in cultured RSC 96 cells was assessed by FACScan flow cytometer (Becton Dickinson, Franklin Lakes, NJ, USA) as the manual description flow-cytometry using a PI/Annexin V-FITC kit (Invitrogen, Carlsbad, CA, USA). Early and late apoptosis were evaluated by the ratio of fluorescence 2 (for propidium iodide) intensity *versus* fluorescence 1 (for annexin) intensity plots. The percentage of cells stained by annexin V alone was recorded as early apoptosis, whereas the percentage of cells stained by both annexin V and propidium iodide was recorded as late apoptosis.

2.10 Statistical analysis

The data were expressed as the mean ± SD. Statistical differences were evaluated using One-way analysis of variance (ANOVA) followed by Tukey's test with GraphPad Prism 5 software (GraphPad Software Inc., La Jolla, CA, USA). For all comparisons, values of $P < 0.05$ were considered statistically significant.

3. Results

3.1 Release of GFs bound to coacervate

To investigate the amount of GFs that was sequestered into the coacervate, we immersed the GFs-coacervate in saline buffer and measured the release rates of bFGF and NGF by ELISA on Day 1, 4, 7, 14, 21, 28 and 35. As showed in Fig. 1, the release rate of NGF is faster than bFGF. At the 1st day, the coacervate released about 1,520 ng NGF, which was more than the bFGF whose release quantity was about 480 ng. Afterwards, both of GFs release curve showed nearly linear and sustained trend. Until the day 35, about 66.4% of bFGF still retained on the coacervate, but NGF is only about 33.1%. Considering the dissociation constant (Kd) of bFGF (2 nM) and NGF (600 nM), it is easily to understand that the binding property of bFGF to heparin-PEAD is more stronger than NGF, leading to different release rate. Because the release rate of incorporated GFs *in vivo* is also influenced by enzymes such as heparinase or erepsin, one would expect a faster rate of release *in vivo*. Next, we would systematically evaluate the role of GFs coacervate for DPN restoration in diabetic rats.

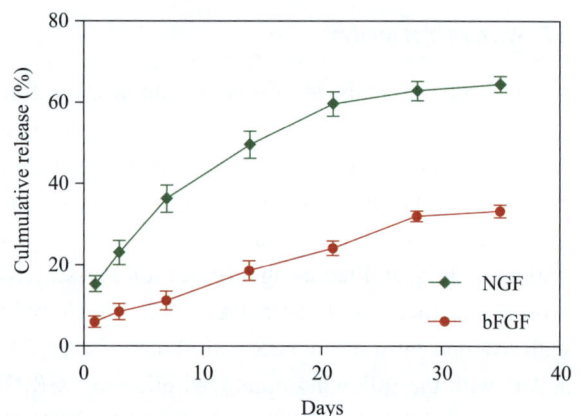

Fig. 1. The coacervate *in vitro* controls the release of bFGF and NGF for 35 days in a steady fashion. Equal amount of bFGF and NGF were combined, then mixed with heparin followed by PEAD to form coacervate. After centrifuged, supernatant was collected. The amount of released bFGF and NGF was measured by ELISA at day 1, 4, 7, 14, 21, 28, and 35, Data were presented as means ± SD (*n*= 3 per group).

3.2 GFs coacervate prevents progression of motor and sensory neural dysfunction with no influence on body weight and blood glucose

We then used the walking track analysis and hot plate test to compare the efficacy of two different treatment approaches: free GFs *versus* GFs coacervate, as potential intervention therapies for DPN. We divided the STZ-induced rats into three groups (STZ-diabetes, free GFs, GFs coacervate) and there was no significant difference among the three groups prior to drug treatments. These rats were then treated and tested, as described, for up to 5 weeks.

Our results showed that the free GFs treatment at Day 7 significantly increased the hindlimb locomotor function and withdrawal latency, even better than the GFs coacervate treated group (Fig. 2B, C). 14 days after treatment, the SFI value and the withdrawal threshold of the free GFs group was similar to that in GFs coacervate group. However, from

A

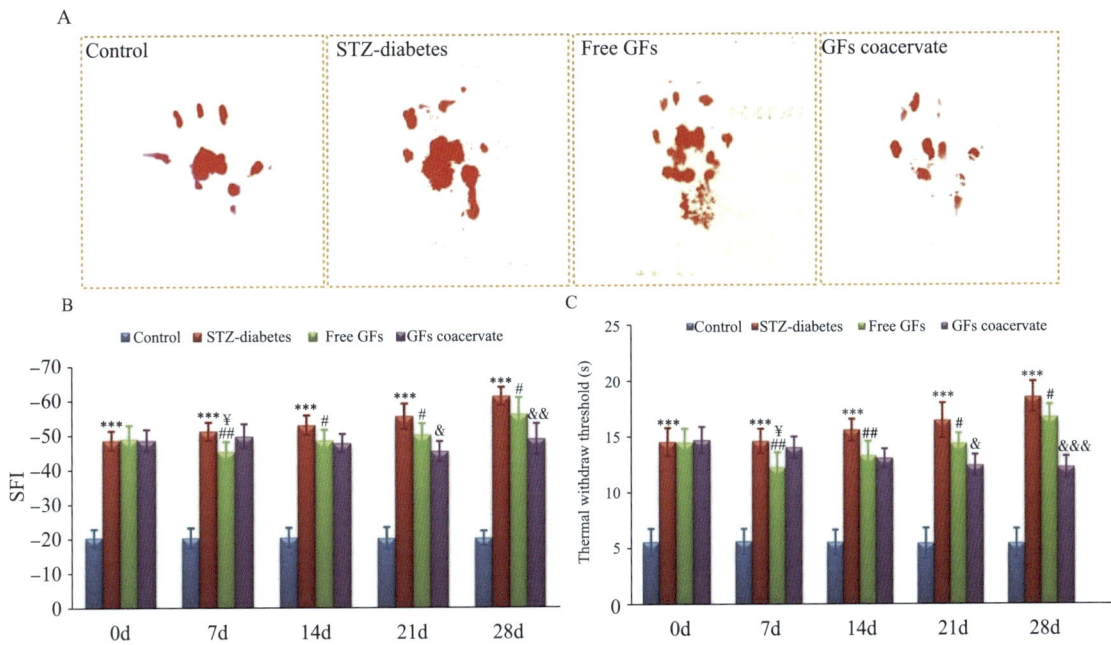

Fig. 2. The recovery of motor and sensory function was evaluated by walking track analysis and hot plate test. (A) Photographs of the rats' footprints in each group at 30 days after treatment. (B), (C) Statistical analysis of sciatic function index (SFI) value and thermal withdraw threshold. ***$P < 0.001$ vs. control group, #$P < 0.05$, ##$P < 0.01$ vs. STZ-diabetes group, &$P < 0.05$, &&$P < 0.01$, &&&$P < 0.001$ vs. the free GFs group, ¥$P < 0.05$ vs. the GFs coacervate group. Data are the mean values ± SD, $n = 8$.

day 21 on, these two parameters exhibited significant differences among the three diabetic groups; the free GFs group showed a distinct recovery in motor and sensory function compared to the STZ-diabetes group, but inferior to that in GFs coacervate group ($n = 8$, $P < 0.05$). This different became even more noticeable at day 28.

All animals were measured for their blood glucose level and for their body weight at 8 weeks before drug treatment, and at sacrificed time following drug treatment. All STZ-received rats showed significantly higher blood glucose levels than those of control groups but weren't different in themselves. Interestingly, the blood glucose level of DPN rats remained unchanged after they injected with Free GFs or GFs coacervate (Table 1). The changes in body weight in all groups showed a trend similar to the plasma glucose change. These results suggest that GFs coacervate can effectively promote functional improvement of motor and sensory recovery without affecting plasma glucose levels and body weight in DPN rats.

Table 1. Body weights and blood glucose concentrations in nondiabetic and STZ diabetic rats treating with free GFs or GFs coacervate

Group	Body weight (g)		Blood glucose (mmol/L)	
	0 day	30 days	0 day	30 days
Control	422±15	437±13	6.5±0.5	6.5±0.6
STZ-diabetes	230±11**	219±13**	20.9±2.1***	22.6±2.3***
Free GFs	231±14	227±11	21.0±2.3	20.8±2.8
GFs coacervate	227±18	229±15	20.2±2.0	20.3±2.2

Data are expressed as mean ± SD, $n = 8$ per group. **$P < 0.01$, ***$P < 0.001$ vs. the control group.

3.3　GFs coacervate ameliorates neurological morphology in DPN rats

At 30 days after treatment, demyelination and fiber irregularity of sciatic nerve were evaluated by H&E staining. Axonal atrophy with irregularity of neuropile and unclear boundary in myelin sheaths were seen in sciatic nerves of STZ-diabetes group. In contrast, this change appeared to be mild in free GFs-treated group, mainly with nerve fibers of

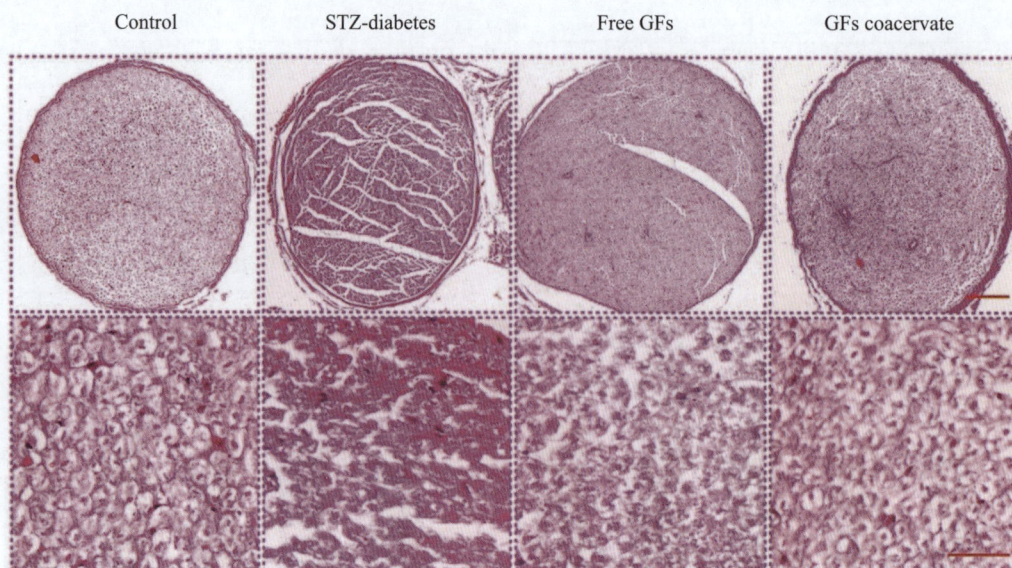

Fig. 3. HE staining results of cross-sectional tissue slices of control, STZ-diabetes, free GFs, and GFs coacervate group respectively. The above magnification was 10× and the below magnification was 40×.

ordered arrangement and myelin sheaths of extensive regeneration. Yet, the GFs coacervate group had the best regularity of arranged nerve fibers, and the boundary of myelin sheaths evidently clear (Fig. 3). These results indicated that GFs coacervate was able to counteract against the morphology changes associated with diabetic neuropathy of the sciatic nerve.

3.4 GFs coacervate decreases cells apoptosis in the sciatic nerve with diabetic neuropathy

As a measure of DNA fragmentation, TUNEL staining with sections of sciatic nerves were obtained in each group at day 30 after treatment. As shown in Fig. 4A, the number of TUNEL-positive cells in diabetic sciatic nerve without drug administration was significantly increased, when compared with those in the control animals ($P < 0.001$). On the contrary, the number of increased apoptotic cell in diabetic sciatic nerve considerably reduced when treated with free GFs or GFs coacervate. Interestingly, the reverse effect of the GFs coacervate group was better than the free GFs group, nearly reached the same as control tissue ($P < 0.05$, Fig. 4B). These results demonstrated that GFs coacervate exhibited significantly protective effects on sciatic nerve of DPN rats with fewer apoptotic cells.

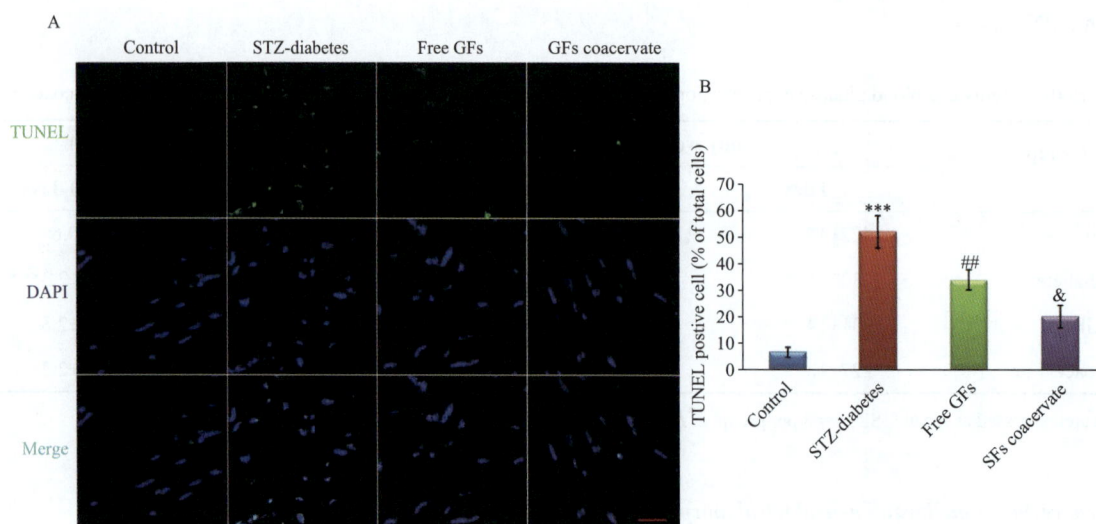

Fig. 4. GFs coacervate decreases the level of apoptosis in sciatic nerve lesions. (A) Representative micrographs showing immunofluorescence with TUNEL (green). Nuclei are labeled with DAPI (blue), Scale bars=50 μm. (B) The percentage of TUNEL-positive cells in the sciatic nerve microsection of four groups. ***$P <0.001$ vs. the control group, ##$P < 0.01$ vs. the STZ-diabetes group, &$P < 0.05$ vs. the free GFs group. Results are mean ± SD of three independent experiments.

3.5 GFs coacervate inhibits excessive ERS in the DPN rats

ERS activation is related to DPN [5, 26]. To test whether or not ERS is involved in neuroprotective role of GFs on DPN, we firstly investigated the expression level of ERS in neural tissues of STZ diabetic rats after treating with free GFs or GFs coacervate. In samples from rats with a 12-week post diabetes induction, Western blot results revealed a clear upregulation of GRP-78, ATF-6, XBP-1, ATF-4, CHOP and Caspase-12, all well-recognized markers for ERS, suggesting that ERS is involved in DPN development and progression.

With free GFs treatment, the rise in these stress markers expression was decreased. In addition, the levels of these stress markers in GFs coacervate group were significantly lower than those in free GFs group, this trend also corresponded with the statistical analysis (Fig. 5A, B). To further confirm the role of GFs coacervate on ERS, CHOP and Caspase-12 expression in sciatic nerve sections of DPN rats were detected by immunofluorecent staining analysis. In the line of Western blot changes, the CHOP and Caspase-12 positive red or green signals in the free GFs group were significantly less than the control group, but more than GFs coacervate (Fig. 5C), which suggests that GFs coacervate has a better capacity of inhibiting excessive ERS in sciatic nerves of DPN rats than free GFs groups. Taken together, these results strongly suggest that GFs coacervate is more efficacious in attenuating ERS response after DPN.

3.6 GFs coacervate reduces the HG-induced apoptosis of RSC96 cells in vitro

To further ensure the remarkable protective function of GFs coacervate, we tested its impact on hyperglycaemia-induced apoptosis in a cellular model, RSC96 cells. The cells were cultured in 30 mM HG with or without GFs coacervate treatment. Based on our results of MTT assays, HG-induced apoptosis was markedly decreased after treating with GFs coacervate (Fig. 6 A), and it was better than only free GFs treatment. We then used fluorescence activated cell sorting analysis to distinguish and measure viable, early apoptotic, late apoptotic or necrotic cells to further demonstrate the antiapoptotic effect of GFs coacervate on RSC96 cells. Our results showed that both GFs coacervate and free GFs clearly inhibited the apoptotic cells as compared to HG group (Fig. 6 B, C), and GFs coacervate was more effective than the free GFs. Collectively, these data indicate that GFs coacervate is very effective in inhibiting HG-induced apoptosis.

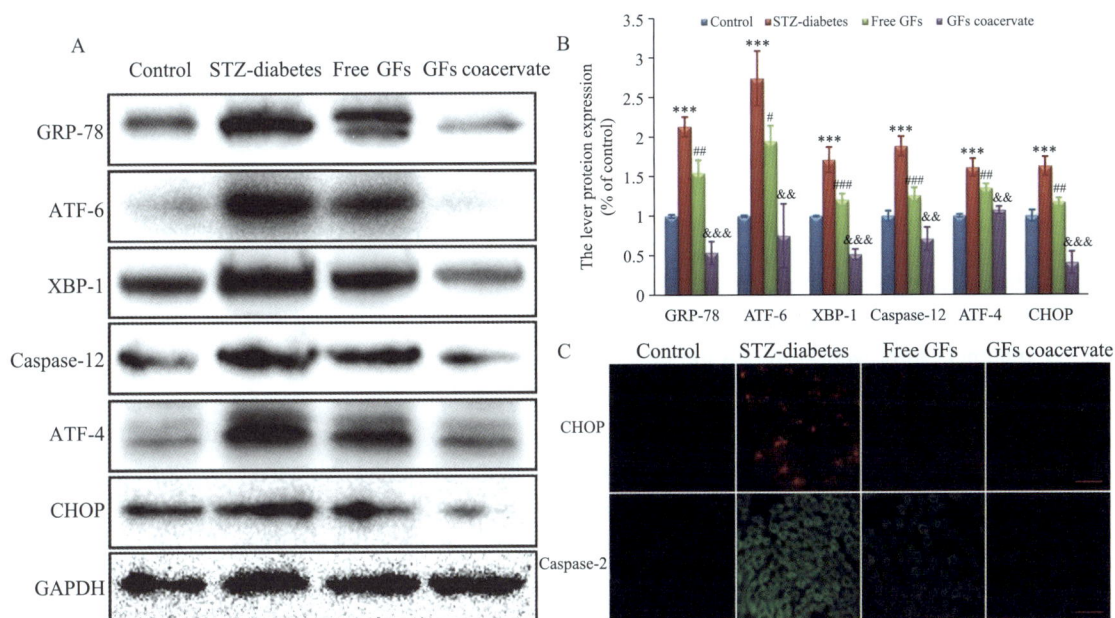

Fig. 5. GFs coacervate administration inhibits excessive ERS in the DPN rats. (A) Sciatic nerve tissues samples were analyzed with Western Blotting for the expression of GRP-78, ATF-6, XBP-1, ATF-4, CHOP and Csapase-12. GAPDH was used for band density normalization. (B) The optical density analysis of GRP-78, ATF-6, XBP-1, ATF-4, CHOP and Csapase-12. ***$P < 0.001$ vs. the control group, #$P < 0.05$, ##$P < 0.01$, ###$P < 0.001$ vs. the STZ-diabetes group, &&$P < 0.01$, &&&$P < 0.001$ vs. the free GFs group. Mean values ± SD, $n=8$. (C) Immunofluorescent staining of CHOP and caspase-12 in each group. Scale bars=50 μm.

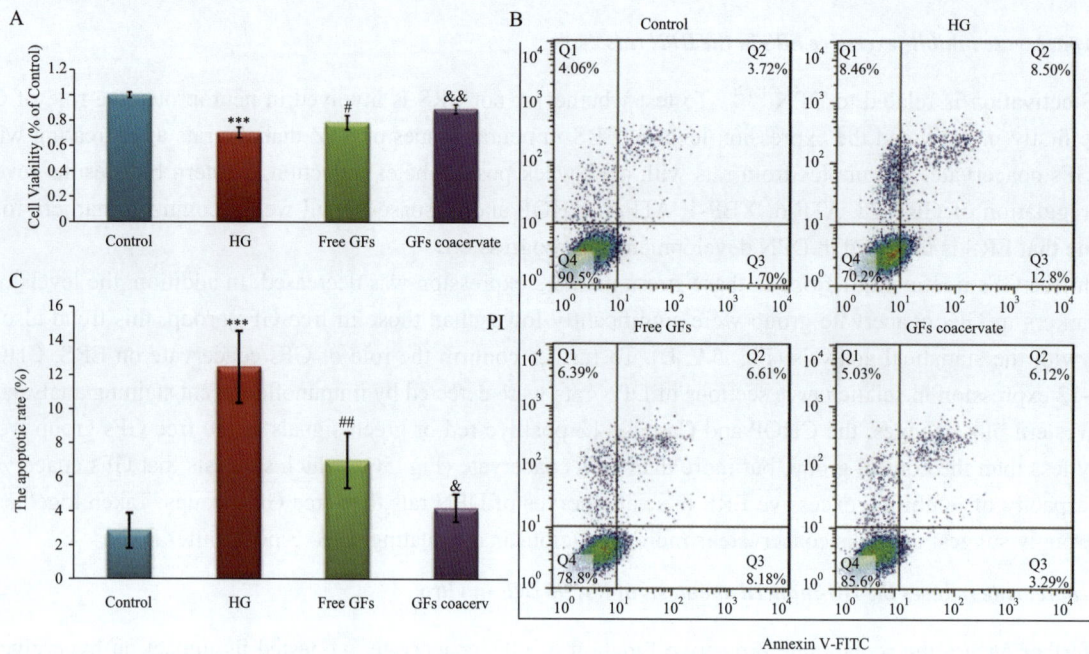

Fig. 6. GFs coacervate suppresses HG-induced apoptosis in SCs. (A) SCs were treated with free GFs or GFs coacervate for 24 h under HG conditions and then cell viability was assessed by MTT assay. (B) Flow cytometry result of PI/Annexin V-FITC staining for cell apoptosis analysis. (C) Quantitative analysis of the early apoptotic rates from three separate experiments. $^{***}P < 0.001$ *vs.* the control group, $^{#}P < 0.05$, $^{##}P < 0.01$ *vs.* the HG group, $^{&}P < 0.05$, $^{&&}P < 0.01$ *vs.* the free GFs group.

3.7 GFs coacervate protects HG-cultured RSC96 cells by inhibiting excessive ERS in vitro

To determine whether suppression of chronic ERS is involved in GFs coacervate mediated antiapoptotic effect, we detected the levels of the ERS response proteins including GRP-78, ATF-6, XBP-1, Caspase-12, ATF-4 and CHOP in RSC96 cells by Western blot methods. Consistent with the data *in vivo*, HG treatment induced significant increases in the levels of GRP-78, ATF-6, XBP-1, Caspase-12, ATF-4 and CHOP expression. Although treatment with free GFs reversed the up-regulation of these protein levels, GFs coacervate treatment was more effective in these measures (Fig. 7A, B). Taken together, these results suggested that GFs coacervate treatment reduced ERS, resulting in the suppression of SCs apoptotic under HG condition.

4. Discussion

DPN is a chronic complication that seriously affects the quality of life of diabetes person and occurs in 60%-70% of patients [27] with symptoms including spontaneous pain, hyperalgesia, and diminished sensation [28]. Currently, the only effective treatment to prevent or retard the development of DPN and alleviate symptoms is glucose control and pain management [4]. However, its role in recovery of the structure and function for nervous system in established DPN is controversial. Unfortunately, present drug therapy for DPN are mainly including aldose reductase inhibitor (ARI), B vitamins, essential fatty acids γ-linolenic acid and the antioxidant a-lipoic acid. Moreover, many of them just provide symptomatic treatment; even some of them show adverse side effects [29]. For example, Tolrestate is a kind of ARI compound that can action on DPN, but showed disappointed clinical efficacy [30]. Thus, seeking for new therapeutic strategies on DPN becomes necessary.

NTFs, including bFGF and NGF, provide trophic and tropic support that are vital for PNS development and function. NGF regulates intraneural homeostasis during development by providing neurotrophic and regulating intracellular pathways to promote neuronal sprouting [31]. bFGF is a mitogenic cationic polypeptide that can facilitate neurite extension and stimulate SCs proliferation, as well as inducing angiogenesis [32]. Both exogenous NGF and bFGF have been shown to have protective effects in rodents with DPN [14, 33]. Furthermore, a deficiency of those two GFs may cause neu-

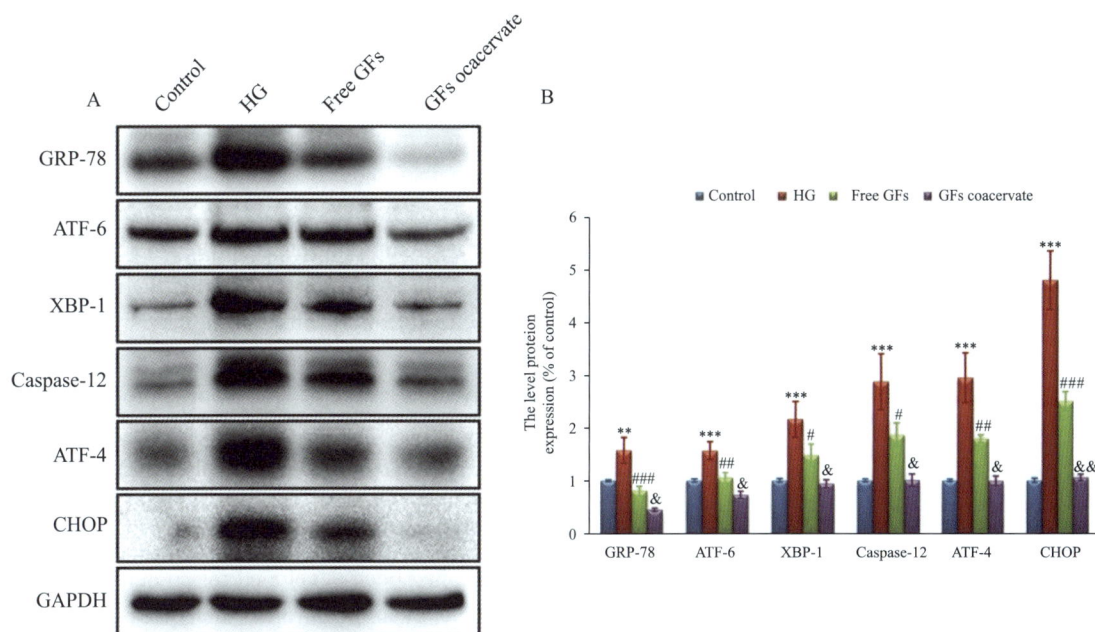

Fig. 7. GFs coacervate attenuates HG-induced ERS in SCs. (A) Representative western blot results of ERS markers: GRP-78, ATF-6, XBP-1, ATF-4, CHOP and Csapase-12 in each group. (B) Quantification of western blot data from A. $^{**}P < 0.05$, $^{***}P < 0.001$ $vs.$ the control group, $^{#}P < 0.05$, $^{##}P < 0.01$, $^{###}P < 0.001$ the HG group, $^{&}P < 0.05$, $^{&&}P < 0.01$ $vs.$ the free GFs group. All data are represent as mean values ± SD, n = 3.

ron susceptible to injury and death [34, 35]. A number of studies are mainly focus on administrating only one kind of those two cytokines to investigate the therapeutic effectiveness. Since they have the synergistic effect on DPN, why not combine them together? This combinatorial therapy on NGF and bFGF in our work is distinguished from all the moment research. However, as the kind of protein component, free GFs have a short circulating half-life and degrade easily in body fluids [20, 21]. So it is difficult for GFs to be retained at lesion sites. Seeking for a controlled delivery system that can preserve their processibility and biocompatibility would be particularly attractive for biomedical applications. Thus, we used a coacervate protein delivery platform that consists of native heparin and a novel polycation, poly (ethylene argininylaspartate diglyceride) (PEAD), to deliver GFs. As demonstrated on Fig. 1, this [PEAD:heparin] coacervate not only combined bFGF and NGF in a massive loading capability but also persistently and steadily controlled their release for at least 35 days. Our study revealed that only single administration of the GFs coacervate was sufficient for the persistent reparation of diabetic neuropathy. Moreover, GFs delivered by the coacervate promotes better nerve recovery than dual therapy with free GFs.

In DPN model of diabetic rats, we firstly assessed functional recovery of sensory and motor systems after treating with GFs using walking track analysis and hot plate test. Free bFGF and NGF treatment induced a transient improvement in these behavioural tests, however, sustained improvement over four weeks was observed with the combined bFGF and NGF coacervate treatment relative to the untreated diabetic group. Additionally, GFs coacervate was also found to improve sciatic nerve morphology including ameliorating unclear boundary in myelin sheaths, and reducing the loss of nerve fibers, as well as significantly reducing SCs apoptosis (Fig. 3 and 4). Interestingly, the body weight and blood glucose level in DPN rats remained unchanged after treating with free GFs or GFs coacervate, indicating that the neuroprotective effect of GFs or GFs coacervate on DPN doesn't depend on the regulation of glucose level and body weight.

The pathophysiological mechanisms of DPN are multifactorial, which includes enhanced polyol pathway activities, increased advanced glycation end products, altered hexosamine pathways, and producted massive free radical. ERS, as a momentous mechanism for metabolic diseases, have been reported extensively [36, 37], especially for DPN. Lupachyk et al found that proteins implicated in ERS were overexpressed in spinal cord and sciatic nerve of STZ-induced diabetic rodents. And administration of ERS inhibitors could suppress the levels of GRP78, GRP94, ERO1α and CHOP expression, accompanied by the recovery of neurological function [6]. They also observed that sciatic nerve dysfunction and glucose intolerance were alleviated in high-fat diet mice and Zucker (fa/fa) rats when treated with trimethylamine oxide, a selective inhibitor of eukaryotic initiation factor-2alpha (eiF2α) [26]. In the present study, the change levels of ERS response proteins including GRP-78, ATF-6, XBP-1, ATF-4, CHOP and Csapase-12 were tested to confirm whether ERS is involved in the beneficial role of GFs coacervate on DPN [5]. As shown in Fig. 5, GFs coacervate treatment significantly reduced upregulation of ERS proteins in the STZ-diabetic rats more than those in treated with free GFs. This result was also confirmed by immunofluorescence analysis. Taken together, these data suggest that GFs coacervate may be related to the inhibition of ERS, consequently suppressing SCs apoptosis.

As spongiocyte in the PNS, SCs exert a pivotal role in supporting axon outgrowth and regeneration, and forming myelin sheath to help repair damaged nerves [38]. Under HG condition, the SCs' injury was earlier than ongoing myelinic denaturation and axonal atrophy [39-41]. Because of the similar characteristics on primary SCs, the cultured rat Schwann cell line-RSC 96 cells in 30 mM high-glucose (HG) medium were able to mimic metabolic changes of diabetic patients with DPN. As shown in Fig. 6, 7, SCs in HG induced a significantly high level of ERS response proteins and caused a higher apoptotic rate compared to the control group. This apoptotic activity was suppressed by both free GFs or GFs coacervate treatment, however, the inhibitory effect of GFs coacervate was significantly greater than that of free GFs. Indeed, the current research has verified that GFs coacervate plays a vital role in anti-apoptosis by inhibiting excessive ERS activation of SCs under the hyperglycemic condition.

In conclusion, as shown in Fig. 8, this heparin-based coacervate had been developed for co-delivery of bFGF and NGF, which shown its property to combine GFs with high load efficiency and controlled their release at least 35 days. GFs coacervate recovered the function and structure of sciatic nerve by improved motor and sensory with more ordered nerve fibers and regenerated myelin sheath as well as suppressed apoptosis of SCs in DPN rats. Moreover, the inhibition of ERS-induced apoptosis is the molecular mechanism of the GFs coacervate protective effect on DPN, highlighting protective role of GFs coacervate in ERS and apoptosis of Schwann cell may be a useful therapeutic strategy for DPN. Further experimental and clinical studies will focus on evaluating its efficacy and long-term safety, which may promote the application of GFs coacervate as a treatment modality for diabetic neuropathy.

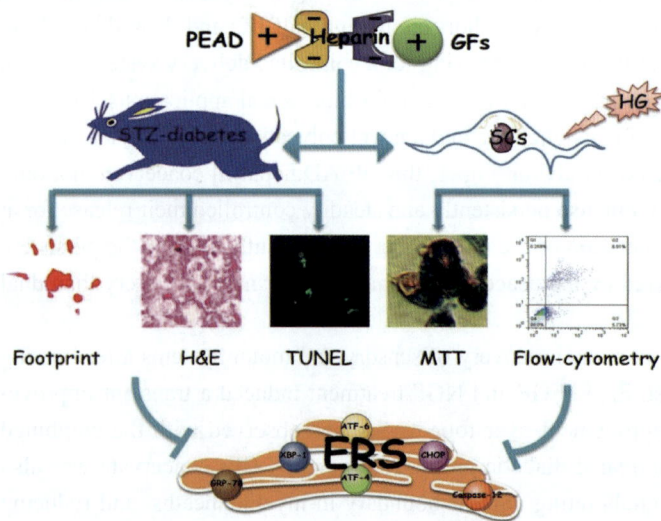

Fig. 8. Illustrating the therapeutic effect of NGF+bFGF : heparin : PEAD coacervate on DPN-rats and HG-SCs and its mechanism. For the STZ-induced diabetic rats, GFs coacervate mediated nerve regeneration and functional recovery by improved motor and sensory with more ordered nerve fibers and regenerated myelin sheath as well as suppressed apoptosis of SCs. Furthermore, the molecular mechanism of the GFs coacervate protective effect is involved in inhibiting excessive ERS-induced SCs apoptosis.

References

[1] Sinnreich M, Taylor BV, Dyck PJ. Diabetic neuropathies. Classification, clinical features, and pathophysiological basis[J]. Neurologist, 2005, 11(2): 63-79.

[2] Singh R, Kishore L, Kaur N. Diabetic peripheral neuropathy: current perspective and future directions[J]. Pharmacol Res, 2014, 80: 21-35.

[3] Tesfaye S, Boulton AJ, Dyck PJ, et al. Diabetic neuropathies: update on definitions, diagnostic criteria, estimation of severity, and treatments[J]. Diabetes Care, 2010, 33(10): 2285-2293.

[4] Callaghan B, Cheng H, Hartsfield C, et al. Diabetic neuropathy: clinical manifestations and current treatments[J]. The Lancet. Neurology, 2012, 11(6): 521-534.

[5] O'Brien PD, Hinder LM, Sakowski SA, et al. ER stress in diabetic peripheral neuropathy: A new therapeutic target[J]. Antioxid Redox Signal, 2014, 21(4): 621-633.

[6] Lupachyk S, Watcho P, Stavniichuk R, et al. Endoplasmic reticulum

stress plays a key role in the pathogenesis of diabetic peripheral neuropathy[J]. Diabetes, 2013, 62(3): 944-952.

[7] Hotamisligil GS. Endoplasmic reticulum stress and the inflammatory basis of metabolic disease[J]. Cell, 2010, 140(6): 900-917.

[8] Eizirik DL, Cardozo AK, Cnop M. The role for endoplasmic reticulum stress in diabetes mellitus[J]. Endocr Rev, 2008, 29(1): 42-61.

[9] Hotamisligil GS. Endoplasmic reticulum stress and atherosclerosis [J]. Nat Med, 2010, 16(4): 396-399.

[10] Zhang HY, Wang ZG, Lu XH, et al. Endoplasmic reticulum stress: relevance and therapeutics in central nervous system diseases[J]. Mol Neurobiol, 2015, 51(3): 1343-1352.

[11] Andrades JA, Wu LT, Hall FL, et al. Engineering, expression, and renaturation of a collagen-targeted human bFGF fusion protein[J]. Growth Factors, 2001, 18(4): 261-275.

[12] Lane JT. The role of retinoids in the induction of nerve growth factor: a potential treatment for diabetic neuropathy[J]. Transl Res, 2014, 164(3): 193-195.

[13] Hellweg R, Raivich G, Hartung HD, et al. Axonal transport of endogenous nerve growth factor (NGF) and NGF receptor in experimental diabetic neuropathy[J]. Exp Neurol, 1994, 130(1): 24-30.

[14] Nakae M, Kamiya H, Naruse K, et al. Effects of basic fibroblast growth factor on experimental diabetic neuropathy in rats[J]. Diabetes, 2006, 55(5): 1470-1477.

[15] Tomlinson DR, Fernyhough P, Diemel LT. Role of neurotrophins in diabetic neuropathy and treatment with nerve growth factors[J]. Diabetes, 1997, 46 Suppl 2: S43-49.

[16] Chen SQ, Cai Q, Shen YY, et al. Combined use of NGF/BDNF/bFGF promotes proliferation and differentiation of neural stem cells in vitro[J]. Int J Dev Neurosci, 2014, 38: 74-78.

[17] Wu J, Ye J, Zhu J, et al. Heparin-Based Coacervate of FGF2 Improves Dermal Regeneration by Asserting a Synergistic Role with Cell Proliferation and Endogenous Facilitated VEGF for Cutaneous Wound Healing[J]. Biomacromolecules, 2016, 17(6): 2168-2177.

[18] Chen WC, Lee BG, Park DW, et al. Controlled dual delivery of fibroblast growth factor-2 and Interleukin-10 by heparin-based coacervate synergistically enhances ischemic heart repair[J]. Biomaterials, 2015, 72: 138-151.

[19] Awada HK, Johnson NR, Wang Y. Dual delivery of vascular endothelial growth factor and hepatocyte growth factor coacervate displays strong angiogenic effects[J]. Macromol Biosci, 2014, 14(5): 679-686.

[20] Poduslo JF, Curran GL. Permeability at the blood-brain and blood-nerve barriers of the neurotrophic factors: NGF, CNTF, NT-3, BDNF[J]. Brain Res Mol Brain Res, 1996, 36(2): 280-286.

[21] Yuge T, Furukawa A, Nakamura K, et al. Metabolism of the intravenously administered recombinant human basic fibroblast growth factor, trafermin, in liver and kidney: degradation implicated in its selective localization to the fenestrated type microvasculatures[J]. Biol Pharm Bull, 1997, 20(7): 786-793.

[22] Chu H, Johnson NR, Mason NS, et al. A [polycation:heparin] complex releases growth factors with enhanced bioactivity[J]. J Control Release, 2011, 150(2): 157-163.

[23] Coppey LJ, Gellett JS, Davidson EP, et al. Effect of antioxidant treatment of streptozotocin-induced diabetic rats on endoneurial blood flow, motor nerve conduction velocity, and vascular reactiv-

ity of epineurial arterioles of the sciatic nerve[J]. Diabetes, 2001, 50(8): 1927-1937.

[24] Schmeichel AM, Schmelzer JD, Low PA. Oxidative injury and apoptosis of dorsal root ganglion neurons in chronic experimental diabetic neuropathy[J]. Diabetes, 2003, 52(1): 165-171.

[25] Bain JR, Mackinnon SE, Hunter DA. Functional evaluation of complete sciatic, peroneal, and posterior tibial nerve lesions in the rat[J]. Plast Reconstr Surg, 1989, 83(1): 129-138.

[26] Lupachyk S, Watcho P, Obrosov AA, et al. Endoplasmic reticulum stress contributes to prediabetic peripheral neuropathy[J]. Exp Neurol, 2013, 247: 342-348.

[27] Deli G, Bosnyak E, Pusch G, et al. Diabetic neuropathies: diagnosis and management[J]. Neuroendocrinology, 2013, 98(4): 267-280.

[28] Vinik AI, Park TS, Stansberry KB, et al. Diabetic neuropathies[J]. Diabetologia, 2000, 43(8): 957-973.

[29] Bosi E, Conti M, Vermigli C, et al. Effectiveness of frequency-modulated electromagnetic neural stimulation in the treatment of painful diabetic neuropathy[J]. Diabetologia, 2005, 48(5): 817-823.

[30] Pfeifer MA, Schumer MP, Gelber DA. Aldose reductase inhibitors: the end of an era or the need for different trial designs?[J]. Diabetes, 1997, 46 Suppl 2: S82-89.

[31] Skaper SD. The neurotrophin family of neurotrophic factors: an overview[J]. Methods Mol Biol, 2012, 846: 1-12.

[32] Fujimoto E, Mizoguchi A, Hanada K, et al. Basic fibroblast growth factor promotes extension of regenerating axons of peripheral nerve. In vivo experiments using a Schwann cell basal lamina tube model[J]. J Neurocytol, 1997, 26(8): 511-528.

[33] Aloe L, Rocco ML, Bianchi P, et al. Nerve growth factor: from the early discoveries to the potential clinical use[J]. J Transl Med, 2012, 10: 239.

[34] Hellweg R, Hartung HD. Endogenous levels of nerve growth factor (NGF) are altered in experimental diabetes mellitus: a possible role for NGF in the pathogenesis of diabetic neuropathy[J]. J Neurosci Res, 1990, 26(2): 258-267.

[35] Dobrowsky RT, Rouen S, Yu C. Altered neurotrophism in diabetic neuropathy: spelunking the caves of peripheral nerve[J]. J Pharmacol Exp Ther, 2005, 313(2): 485-491.

[36] Ozcan U, Cao Q, Yilmaz E, et al. Endoplasmic reticulum stress links obesity, insulin action, and type 2 diabetes[J]. Science, 2004, 306(5695): 457-461.

[37] Xu C, Bailly-Maitre B, Reed JC. Endoplasmic reticulum stress: cell life and death decisions[J]. J Clin Invest, 2005, 115(10): 2656-2664.

[38] Bhatheja K, Field J. Schwann cells: origins and role in axonal maintenance and regeneration[J]. Int J Biochem Cell Biol, 2006, 38(12): 1995-1999.

[39] Eckersley L. Role of the Schwann cell in diabetic neuropathy[J]. Int Rev Neurobiol, 2002, 50: 293-321.

[40] Gumy LF, Bampton ET, Tolkovsky AM. Hyperglycaemia inhibits Schwann cell proliferation and migration and restricts regeneration of axons and Schwann cells from adult murine DRG[J]. Mol Cell Neurosci, 2008, 37(2): 298-311.

[41] Bestetti G, Rossi GL, Zemp C. Changes in peripheral nerves of rats four months after induction of streptozotocin diabetes. A qualitative and quantitative study[J]. Acta Neuropathol, 1981, 54(2): 129-134.

Chapter 7
Bioreactor and Engineering

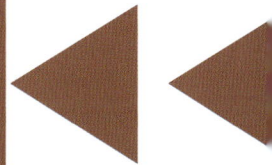

Increased production of human fibroblast growth factor 17 in *Escherichia coli* and proliferative activity in NIH3T3 cells

Meiyu Wu, Xiaokun Li, Haijun Wang

1. Introduction

The human fibroblast growth factors (FGFs) protein family consists of 22 members, which share a high affinity for heparin, as well as high-sequence homology within a central core domain of 120 amino acids [1]. FGFs are essential in biological functions, such as angiogenesis, mitogenesis, cell differentiation and wound repair. FGF17 is a member of the heparin binding growth factor family [2], which is structurally the most homologous to FGF8 and FGF18. FGF8, FGF17 and FGF18 are highly conserved between human and mice, sharing 93% identity [2,3]. Mouse FGF17 has three isoforms, while human FGF17 has just two: FGF17a and FGF17b, the latter of which has been selected as the canonical sequence [4]. FGF17 is preferentially expressed in the embryonic brain and is highly associated with the nervous system [5].

Numerous studies have indicated that FGF17 may serve as a therapeutic agent to potentially treat certain types of disease. There is an increasing demand in the market to produce the FGF17 protein, and the large-scale production of bioactive human FGF17 is a challenging rate-limiting step. Given these factors, the development of a process that may enable significant preparation of sufficient, highly bioactive recombinant human (rh)FGF17 is considered to be a high priority for further investigations of the underlying mechanisms and clinical pathology. With the development of bio-technology, various expression systems are currently being used for expressing recombinant proteins for industrial pro-duction, as well as in research for structural and biochemical studies [6]. *Escherichia coli*, with a short growth cycle, low cost, high stability and high transformation efficiency, is suitable for large-scale manufacture [7]. In addition, *E. coli* are the most frequently used expression system for high-scale production of recombinant proteins [8-10].

As human(h)FGF17 is an important growth factor and, to the best of our knowledge, its non-tag expression in *E. coli* has not been reported, an rhFGF17 expression vector pET3a-rhFGF17, with a high expression level of rhFGF17 protein with soluble protein and inclusion bodies, was constructed in the present study. Furthermore, the high purity of rhFGF17 protein was obtained *via* heparin affinity and SP Sepharose Fast Flow chromatography. In addition, the bio-logical activity of rhFGF17, which may significantly increase the proliferative activity of NIH3T3 cells was examined. This novel expression strategy markedly enhanced the yield of rhFGF17 with high biological activity, which may meet the demand for fundamental research and therapeutic applications.

2. Materials and methods

2.1 Reagents and bacterial strain

The PCR purification, gel extraction and plasmid miniprep kits, and DNA Marker were purchased from Takara Biotechnology Co., Ltd. (Dalian, China). Goat anti-FGF17 polyclonal antibody (cat. no. sc-16826) and mouse anti-goat IgG-HRP (cat. no. sc-2354) were purchased from Santa Cruz Biotechnology, Inc. (Dallas, TX, USA). Heparin Sepha-rose column, SP Sepharose Fast Flow and AKTA purifier were purchased from GE Healthcare Life Sciences (Shanghai, China). The *E. coli* DH5α and BL21(DE3)pLysS component cells were purchased from Beijing Solarbio Science & Technology Co., Ltd. (Beijing, China).

2.2　Construction of rhFGF17 expression vector

The coding sequence of rhFGF17 (GenBank reference, NM_001304478.1) was obtained from the pUC57-FGF17 vector, previously constructed by our lab (unpublished data), using a Veriti™ Thermal Cycler (cat. no. 4375786; Thermo Fisher Scientific, Inc., Waltham, MA, USA) with Phusion® High-Fidelity PCR Master Mix (cat. no. M0531S; New England BioLabs, Inc., Ipswich, MA, USA). Amplification conditions were as follows: Initial denaturation at 98℃ for 30 sec, followed by 30 cycles at 98℃ for 10 sec, at 65℃ for 20 sec and at 72℃ for 20 sec, with a final extension step at 72℃ for 10 min. The DNA fragment rhFGF17 was subsequently cloned into pET3a vector, using the *Nde*I and *Bam*HI restriction enzymes, to create the recombinant expression vector, pET3a-hFGF17, according to the manufacturer's protocol. *Nde*I (cat. no. R0111S) and *Bam*HI (cat. no. R0136S) were purchased from New England BioLabs, Inc.

2.3　Production of rh FGF17

The recombinant vector pET3a-hFGF17 was transformed into BL21(DE3)PLysS component cells. Briefly, 50 ng pET3a-hFGF17 vector were added to 100 μl thawed BL21(DE3)PLysS component cells. Cells were incubated for 30 min on ice, heat shocked at 42℃ for 90 sec, and then plated on a pre-warmed LB agar plate for further culture. The transformed colonies were cultured in 5 ml LB medium (tryptone 10 g/L, yeast extract 5 g/L, NaCl 5 g/L, in ddH$_2$O) containing 100 μg/ml ampicillin and 35 μg/ml chloramphenicol at 37℃. When the optical density $(OD)_{600}$ reached 0.6–0.8, isopropyl β-D-1-thiogalactopyranoside (IPTG) was added to a final concentration of 1 mM. The cultures were incubated at 37℃ for 4 h under agitation (speed, 200 rpm). The colony with the greatest expression level was selected as the seed strain in subsequent experiments.

2.4　Optimizing the expression conditions for rhFGF17

The IPTG concentration for rhFGF17 expression yield was evaluated at 37℃ and 16℃. Detection of soluble rhF-GF17 was performed as follows: The seed strain was cultured overnight with agitation at 200 rpm in 20 ml LB medium containing 10 μg/ml ampicillin and 35 μg/ml chloramphenicol at 37℃. Subsequently, the culture (6 ml) was transferred into two bottles, each containing 600 ml fresh LB medium with 100 μg/ml ampicillin and 35 μg/ml chloramphenicol for further growth. When OD_{600} reached 0.6–0.8, the IPTG was added to final concentrations of nd 1 mM, and cultured for 4 h at 37℃ (speed, 200 rpm) and 24 h at 16℃ (speed, 180 rpm). Cells were collected by centrifugation at 15 000 g for 20 min at 4℃. The cell pellets were resuspended in improved lysis buffer [20 mM Tris-HCl, 200 mM Nacl, 1% Triton X-100, 0.2% deoxysodium cholate, 1 mM EDTA, 5% glycerol, 0.2 M sucrose and 1 mM phenyl-methylsulfonyl fluoride (PMSF; pH 7.5)]. Cells were lysed by sonication for 10 min in an ice bath. Following centrifugation at 15 000 g for 20 min at 4℃, the sediment and the supernatant were separated by 12% SDS-PAGE and the protein expression levels of rhFGF21 were determined, using western blot analysis.

2.5　Purification of soluble rhFGF17

The bacteria cells were harvested and lysed in lysis buffer (pH 7.5) containing 50 mM Tris-HCl, 2 mM EDTA, 300 mM NaCl, 1% Triton X-100, 0.2% deoxysodium cholate, 5%–10% glycerol, 0.01 M sucrose and 1 mM PMSF. Supernatants were collected for subsequent purification. The following steps were all performed at 4℃: First, the heparin-sepharose column was equilibrated with five bed volumes of binding buffer (20 mM Tris-HCl buffer, 25 mM NaCl and 1 mM EDTA; pH 7.5) at a rate of 1 ml/min. Subsequently, the supernatant was applied to the column. Following binding, the column was washed with binding buffer with gradients of 0.4, 0.6, 0.8 and 1.0 M NaCl. Further purification was performed using an SP Sepharose Fast Flow, where the methodology was the same as the heparin-sepharose purification. Finally, fractions were collected from the column according to the ultraviolet absorption peaks and conductivity curve. Then the elution fractions were determined using 12% SDS-PAGE.

2.6　Isolation and refolding of rhFGF17 inclusion bodies

Following fermentation, bacteria were harvested by centrifugation at 10 000 g at 4℃ for 15 min, and wet bacteria (1 g) was resuspended in 20 ml lysis buffer. The inclusion bodies were collected following centrifugation at 10 000 g at 4℃ for 15 min and resuspended in wash buffer (20 mM Tris-HCl, 200 mM NaCl, 1% Triton X-100 and 1 mM EDTA; pH10) by centrifugation at 10 000 g at 4℃ for 15 min after ultrasonication in an ice bath. Subsequently, inclusion bodies (1 g) were resuspended in 20 ml denaturing buffer (8 M urea, 20 mM Tris, 150 mM Nacl, 3 mM EDTA, 5 mM DTT and 0.5 M arginine; pH 7.5). The protein was then refolded by a combination of dialysis and slow dilution. First, the denaturing buffer was dialyzed in dialysis buffer (20 mM Tris, 50 mM NaCl, 15% glycerol, 0.5 M arginine and 4 M urea; pH 7.5) until the urea concentration reached 4 M; subsequently, the buffer in the dialysis bag were collected by centrifugation at 10 000 g at 4℃ for 15 min and then slowly diluted into appropriate volumes of renaturing buffer (20 mM Tris-HCl, 50 mM NaCl, 30% glycerol and 0.5 M arginine; pH 7.5). Following centrifugation at 15 000 g at 4℃ for 20 min, the supernatant was retained and prepared for inclusion in the heparin-sepharose column. Refolding of the protein was performed at 4℃.

2.7 Purification of rhFGF17 inclusion bodies

According to the heparin affinity of rhFGF17, a heparin-sepharose column was selected for the purification. Purification procedures were the same as soluble rhFGF17. Refolding rhFGF17 protein was loaded onto the column that was equilibrated with wash buffer (the same as the soluble fraction) at a speed of 1 ml/min. The flow-through was collected. The protein was subsequently eluted using 0.4–1.0 M NaCl gradient in wash buffer at a speed of 1 ml/min. The elution fractions were collected and determined by Coomassie blue staining of 12% SDS-PAGE.

2.8 Western blot analysis

Protein concentration was determined using the Lowry protein assay. Purified rhFGF17 proteins (50 ng) were separated by 12% SDS-PAGE and transferred onto polyvinylidene difluoride membranes. The membranes were blocked with 5% non-fat milk for 20 min at room temperature, and then incubated with primary antibodies at 4℃ overnight, followed by incubation with the secondary antibody at room temperature for 30 min. Protein bands were visualized by enhanced chemiluminescence using the ChemiDoc™ MP Imaging System (Bio-Rad Laboratories, Inc., Hercules, CA, USA). Goat anti-FGF17 polyclonal anti-body served as the primary antibody (dilution, 1:1 000) and mouse anti-goat IgG-HRP was used as the secondary anti-body (dilution, 1:8 000). The molecular sizes of the obtained protein were verified by comparison with the migration of pre-stained protein markers (cat. no. 26616; Thermo Fisher Scientific, Inc.).

2.9 Mitogenic activity of rhFGF17 assay

NIH3T3 cells (2×10^3 cells/well) were cultured in Dulbecco's modified Eagle's medium (DMEM) containing 10% fetal bovine serum (Thermo Fisher Scientific, Inc.) in a 96-well plate at 37℃ for 24 h. The medium was then replaced with DMEM supplemented with 1% FBS and cells were starved overnight. The cells were treated with different concentrations of rhFGF17 or commercial rhFGF17 (R&D Systems China Co., Ltd., Shanghai, China) for 48 h and the number of viable cells was determined by adding 25 µl MTT (5 mg/ml) per well for 4 h. Finally, the medium was discarded and 150 µl dimethyl sulfoxide was added to each well to dissolve the crystals by agitation at room temperature for 10 min; the absorbance was immediately measured at a wavelength of 600 nm using the GENESYS™ 10 S UV-Vis Spectrophotometer (Thermo Fisher Scientific, Inc.).

3. Results

3.1 Construction of the rhFGF17 expression vector

To produce the rhFGF17 protein, an expression vector containing the optimized hFGF17 gene was constructed. The hFGF17 fragment was obtained (Fig. 1A), then digested with *NdeI* and *Bam*HI and cloned into the pET3a vector to create the pET3a-rhFGF17 recombinant plasmids, which were then confirmed by restriction enzymatic analysis (Fig. 1B, C) and automated DNA sequencing.

3.2 Expression of rhFGF17 in BL21(DE3)pLysS

The recombinant plasmid was transformed into BL21(DE3)pLysS. The SDS-PAGE demonstrated that rhFGF17 was induced by 1 mM IPTG and the apparent molecular band was ~23 kDa, corresponding to the predicted molecular weight (22.6 kDa; Fig. 2A). The greatest expression level of rhFGF17 was ~30% of total protein.

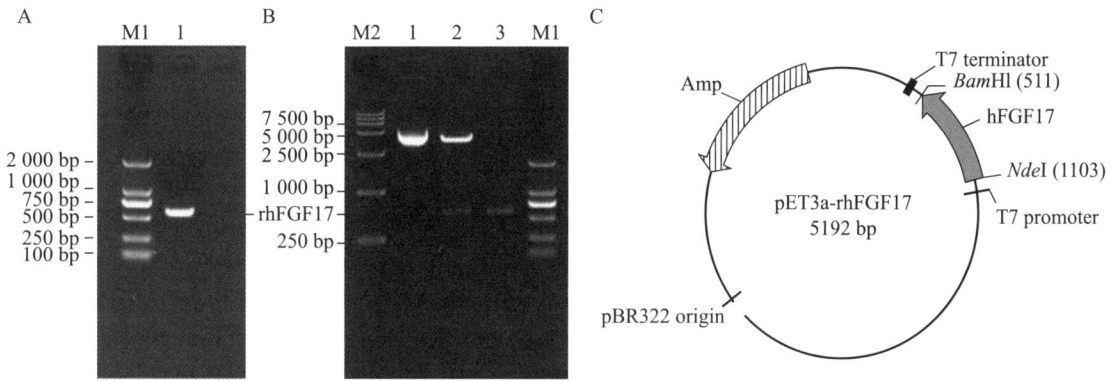

Fig. 1. Construction of the pET3a-rhFGF17 expression vector. (A) rhFGF17 fragment obtained from pUC57-FGF17 by polymerase chain reaction amplification. Lane 1, FGF17 (597 bp); lane M1, DNA marker 1. (B) Identification of recombinant plasmid by enzyme digestion (*Nde*I and *Bam*HI); Lane 1, pET3a-rhFGF17; lane 2, restriction products of recombinant plasmid pET3a-rhFGF17; lane 3, rhFGF17 fragment control; lane M1, DNA marker 1; lane M2 DNA marker 2. (C) Structure of the pET3a-rhFGF17 vector. rhFGF17, recombinant human fibroblast growth factor 17.

3.3　Optimizing the expression of soluble rhFGF17

To establish the optimal culture conditions, the following concentrations of IPTG were evaluated: 0.2, 0.4, 0.8 and 1.0 mM at 37℃ or 16℃, under agitation at 180 rpm. When rhFGF17 was induced by 0.4 mM IPTG at 37℃ or 0.8 mM IPTG at 16℃, the rhFGF17 yield reached the highest level with ratios of ~30% and ~20% of the total protein, respectively according to the SDS-PAGE results (Fig. 2B). Following fermentation in a 2-liter flask under the above-mentioned optimized conditions, the yield of bacteria was ~9 g/l at 37℃ and 6 g/l at 16℃. Soluble detection was performed by lysis. SDS-PAGE analysis of the lysate supernatant and sediment indicated that the recombinant protein was marginally soluble at 16℃, but inclusion bodies appeared to be formed at 37℃ (Fig. 2C).

3.4　Purification of soluble rhFGF17

The soluble product was purified with improved lysis buffer and more soluble proteins were obtained with almost no sediment (Fig. 3A). Heparin-affinity column chromatography combined with SP-Sepharose column chromatography was used for purification of the soluble fraction of proteins. rhFGF17 was eluted with 1.0 M NaCl in elution buffer from the two columns (Fig. 3B, C), and the yield was 1 mg/g (1 mg rhFGF17 from 1 g bacteria cells).

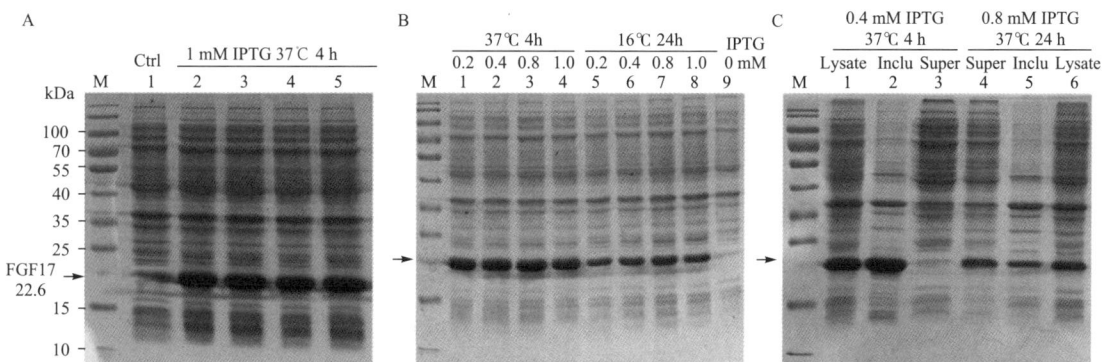

Fig. 2. Optimizing the expression conditions of rhFGF17. (A) SDS-PAGE analysis of rhFGF17 expression in BL21(DE3)PLysS induced by 1 mM IPTG for 4 h at 37℃. Lane 1, served as a control and was not induced with IPTG; lanes 2-5, induced with IPTG; (B) Optimizing the expression conditions of rhFGF17. Lanes 1-4 and 5-8: 0.2, 0.4, 0.8, 1.0 mM IPTG induced at 37℃ for 4 h and 16℃ for 24 h, respectively. (C) Distribution of rhFGF17. Lanes 1-3, 37℃ culture (lane 1, induced BL21(DE3)PLysS/pET3a-rhFGF17; lane 2, inclusion bodies of bacteria following ultrasonication; and lane 3, supernatant). Lanes 4-6, 16℃ culture (lane 4, supernatant of bacteria following ultrasonication; lane 5, inclusion bodies; and lane 6, induced BL21(DE3)PLysS/pET3a-rhFGF17. rhFGF17, recombinant human fibroblast growth factor 17; IPTG, isopropyl β-D-1-thiogalactopyranoside; Ctrl, control.

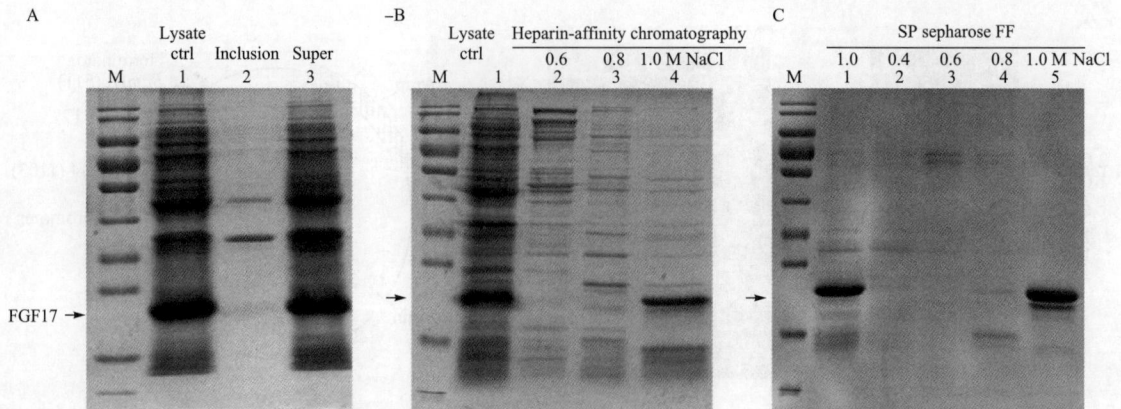

Fig. 3. SDS-PAGE analysis of the purification of soluble rhFGF17 using improved lysis buffer. (A) Lane 1, lysate control; lane 2, inclusion bodies of bacteria following ultrasonication; lane 3, supernatant. (B) Purification of soluble rhFGF17 with heparin-affinity chromatography (lanes 2-4). Lane 1, supernatant of bacteria after ultrasonication; lane 2-4 eluted with 0.6, 0.8, 1.0 M NaCl from heparin-affinity chromatography, (C) Lanes 1-5, SP Sepharose Fast Flow of rhFGF17 eluted with different NaCl concentrations. Lane1 and 5, 1.0 M NaCl; lanes 2-4, 0.4, 0.6 and 0.8 M NaCl. The arrow indicates the rhFGF17 band site. rhFGF17, recombinant human fibroblast growth factor 17; Ctrl, control; FF, fast flow.

3.5 Purification and identification of rhFGF17 inclusion bodies

rhFGF17 inclusion bodies were predominantly produced from the culture condition of 37℃ for 4 h. rhFGF17 was denatured by urea and refolded in the dialysis buffer by dialysis and then renaturing buffer by dilution at pH 7.5 (Fig. 4A). As indicated in Fig. 4A denaturing buffer dissolved the majority of the rhFGF17. The concentration of total protein in the denaturing buffer was ~41 mg/ml and in the renaturing buffer prior to applying it to the heparin-sepharose column, total protein was decreased to ~2 mg/ml. As demonstrated in Fig. 4B the fractions containing rhFGF17 were finally eluted by heparin affinity chromatography using 20 mM Tris-HCl containing 1.0 M NaCl. The purified rhFGF17 protein yield reached 8 mg/g (8 mg rhFGF17 from 1 g bacteria cells).

The purified soluble rhFGF17 and rhFGF17 inclusion bodies were homogenous and their purity was >95%. Western blot analysis demonstrated that the purified rhFGF17 had good immunoreactivity with the anti-human FGF17 antibody (Fig. 4C).

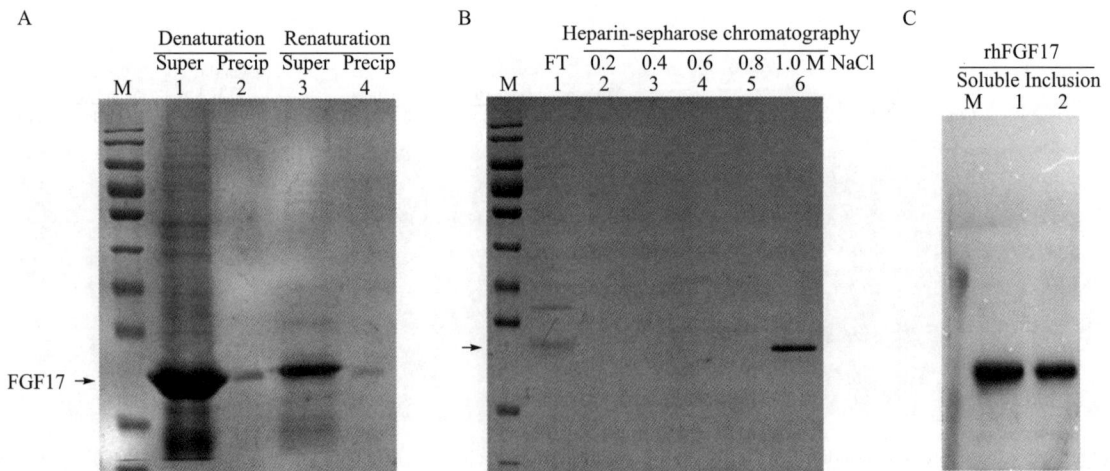

Fig. 4. SDS-PAGE analysis of the purification of rhFGF17 inclusion bodies. (A) Lanes 1 and 3, Supernatant rhFGF17 and precipitation rhFGF17 in denaturation and renaturation buffer; lanes 2 and 4, Precipitation rhFGF17 in denaturation and renaturation buffer. (B) Heparin-sepharose chromatography. Lane 1, FT; lanes 2-6, eluted rhFGF17 with 20 mM Tris-HCl containing 0.2, 0.4, 0.6, 0.8 and 1.0 M NaCl, respectively. (C) Western blot analysis of rhFGF17. Lane 1, purified soluble rhFGF17; lane 2, purified rhFGF17 inclusion bodies. rhFGF17, recombinant human fibroblast growth factor 17; FT, flow through.

3.6 Mitogenic activity of rhFGF17

To assess the biological activity of purified rhFGF17, the proliferative effect of rhFGF17 was determined using a standard MTT assay on NIH3T3 cells and compared with commercial rhFGF17 (the positive control). As shown in Fig. 5, the two purified soluble forms and inclusion bodies of rhFGF17 demonstrate similar mitogenic activity in NIH3T3 cells, which is consistent with the findings of a previous study [11]. Additionally, compared with the commercial rhFGF17, the rhFGF17 protein formed during the present study exhibited improved biological activity. Furthermore, rhFGF17 was found to have a dose-dependent effect on the viability of NIH3T3 cells, whereas the negative control did not. Finally, the results demonstrated that the soluble and inclusion body forms of rhFGF17 had a marked biological effect on NIH3T3 cells.

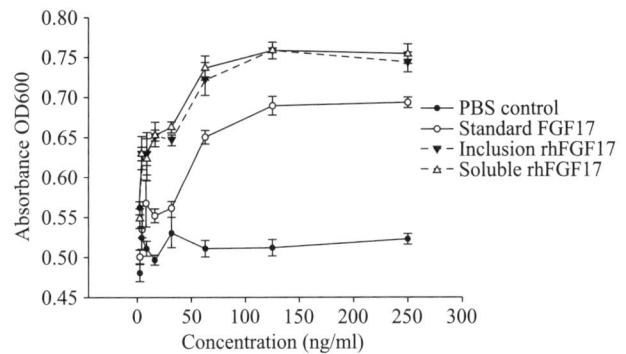

Fig. 5. Mitogenic activity of rhFGF17 on NIH3T3 cells. Data are expressed as the mean ± standard deviation. rhFGF17, recombinant human fibroblast growth factor 17; OD, optical density; PBS, phosphate-buffered saline.

4. Discussion

As a novel member of the FGF family, numerous pharmacological studies have demonstrated that FGF17 is a key factor in neuropsychiatric diseases due to its important roles in the patterning of the cerebellum and cortex [12]. As a potential carcinogen, FGF17 is predominantly associated with prostate cancer [13] and hematopoietic tumors [14]. Therefore, it is necessary to investigate FGF17 and develop strategies for abundant production of FGF17 with high bioactivity. As reported previously, the recombinant form of FGF17 protein was produced using insect cells; however, compared with prokaryotic expression systems, eukaryotic systems are considered unsuitable for large-scale purification [15]. To date, there are few reports regarding the expression of hFGF17, particularly in E. coli expression systems. The low level of soluble production and difficulty purifying inclusion bodies, particularly denaturing and refolding, has restricted further research and application. There are certain methods used to overcome these limitations, including fusion systems to enhance target protein expression, such as Halo-tag fusion [16]. However, the method for obtaining target protein requires that the fused tag must be removed, which involves an expensive cleavage restriction enzyme and may impact the bioactivity of the target protein.

Low temperatures increase the expression levels of soluble proteins and reduce the aggregation of recombinant proteins, thus reducing the formation of inclusion bodies [17]. In addition, low agitation speeds will reduce the speed of bacteria proliferation, but increase the amount of soluble proteins. Therefore, in the current study, the culture conditions at 37℃ and 200 rpm, and 16℃ and 180 rpm would yield high levels of inclusion bodies and soluble proteins, respectively. To further improve the production levels of the target protein, the expression conditions were optimized according to the IPTG concentration, thus the expression level of inclusion bodies and soluble protein reached >30% and >20% of total protein, respectively with 0.4 mM IPTG for 4 h at 37℃ and 1 mM IPTG for 24 h at 16℃. Meanwhile, the lysis buffer was improved by the addition of more Tris, glycerol and sucrose; thus, a soluble protein was obtained with almost no sediment (Fig. 3A). Taken together, the conditions were improved and high production levels of target protein were achieved for purification.

Based on an isoelectric point of 10.43 and the heparin binding ability for rhFGF17, the non-fusion rhFGF17 protein was efficiently separated by heparin-sepharose chromatography and SP Sepharose Fast Flow [18,19]. The purified rhFGF17 proteins were biologically active in vitro and exerted a dose-dependent effect on the proliferation of NIH3T3 cells; inclusion-bodies were demonstrated to have a biological activity similar to the soluble proteins. Thus, the soluble proteins and inclusion bodies obtained using the culture conditions at 37℃ and 200 rpm, and 16℃ and 180 rpm, respectively, are efficiently produced and are characterized by high levels of bioactivity. Furthermore, FGF17 has previously been reported to be involved in Kallmann syndrome [20] and causes tamoxifen resistance in vitro [21]. Therefore, whether there is a direct association between FGF17 and breast cancer requires further investigation.

In conclusion, soluble and inclusion bodies of rhFGF17 were successfully expressed in *E. coli*. The current study indicates that the non-tagged expression of either soluble proteins or inclusion bodies of rhFGF17 is simple, viable and highly effective, making it convenient for high-efficiency expression and purification of proteins, whilst preserving the high biological activity levels.

References

[1] Ornitz DM, Itoh N. The Fibroblast Growth Factor signaling pathway[J]. Wiley Interdisc Rev Dev Biol, 2015, 4(3): 215-266.

[2] Hoshikawa M, Ohbayashi N, Yonamine A, et al. Structure and expression of a novel fibroblast growth factor, FGF-17, preferentially expressed in the embryonic brain[J]. Biochem Biophys Res Commun, 1998, 244(1): 187-191.

[3] Ohbayashi N, Hoshikawa M, Kimura S, et al. Structure and expression of the mRNA encoding a novel fibroblast growth factor, FGF-18[J]. J Biol Chem, 1998, 273(29): 18161-18164.

[4] Xu J, Lawshe A, MacArthur CA, et al. Genomic structure, mapping, activity and expression of fibroblast growth factor 17[J]. Mech Dev, 1999, 83(1-2): 165-178.

[5] O'Leary DD, Chou SJ, Sahara S. Area patterning of the mammalian cortex[J]. Neuron, 2007, 56(2): 252-269.

[6] Dong X, Tang B, Li J, et al. Expression and purification of intact and functional soybean (Glycine max) seed ferritin complex in Escherichia coli[J]. J Microbiol Biotechnol, 2008, 18(2): 299-307.

[7] Jana S, Deb JK. Strategies for efficient production of heterologous proteins in Escherichia coli[J]. Appl Microbiol Biotechnol, 2005, 67(3): 289-298.

[8] Derynck R, Roberts AB, Winkler ME, et al. Human transforming growth factor-alpha: precursor structure and expression in E. coli[J]. Cell, 1984, 38(1): 287-297.

[9] Verdon J, Girardin N, Marchand A, et al. Purification and antibacterial activity of recombinant warnericin RK expressed in Escherichia coli[J]. Appl Microbiol Biotechnol, 2013, 97(12): 5401-5412.

[10] Ajikumar PK, Xiao WH, Tyo KE, et al. Isoprenoid pathway optimization for Taxol precursor overproduction in Escherichia coli[J]. Science, 2010, 330(6000): 70-74.

[11] Song L, Huang Z, Chen Y, et al. High-efficiency production of bioactive recombinant human fibroblast growth factor 18 in Escherichia coli and its effects on hair follicle growth[J]. Appl Microbiol Biotechnol, 2014, 98(2): 695-704.

[12] Tabares-Seisdedos R, Rubenstein JL. Chromosome 8p as a potential hub for developmental neuropsychiatric disorders: implications for schizophrenia, autism and cancer[J]. Mol Psychiatry, 2009, 14(6): 563-589.

[13] Heer R, Douglas D, Mathers ME, et al. Fibroblast growth factor 17 is over-expressed in human prostate cancer[J]. J Pathol, 2004, 204(5): 578-586.

[14] Nezu M, Tomonaga T, Sakai C, et al. Expression of the fetal-oncogenic fibroblast growth factor-8/17/18 subfamily in human hematopoietic tumors[J]. Biochem Biophys Res Commun, 2005, 335(3): 843-849.

[15] Hoshikawa M, Ohbayashi N, Yonamine A, et al. Structure and expression of a novel fibroblast growth factor, FGF-17, preferentially expressed in the embryonic brain[J]. Biochem Biophys Res Commun, 1998, 244(1): 187-191.

[16] Hoshikawa M, Ohbayashi N, Yonamine A, et al. Structure and Expression of a Novel Fibroblast Growth Factor, FGF-17, Preferentially Expressed in the Embryonic Brain[J]. Biochemical & Biophysical Research Communications, 1998, 244(1): 187-191.

[17] Sun C, Li Y, Taylor SE, et al. HaloTag is an effective expression and solubilisation fusion partner for a range of fibroblast growth factors[J]. PeerJ, 2015, 3: e1060.

[18] de Groot NS, Ventura S. Effect of temperature on protein quality in bacterial inclusion bodies[J]. FEBS Lett, 2006, 580(27): 6471-6476.

[19] Berman B, Ostrovsky O, Shlissel M, et al. Similarities and differences between the effects of heparin and glypican-1 on the bioactivity of acidic fibroblast growth factor and the keratinocyte growth factor[J]. J Biol Chem, 1999, 274(51): 36132-36138.

[20] Lee YF, Schmidt M, Graalfs H, et al. Modeling of dual gradient elution in ion exchange and mixed-mode chromatography[J]. J Chromatogr A, 2015, 1417: 64-72.

[21] Miraoui H, Dwyer AA, Sykiotis GP, et al. Mutations in FGF17, IL17RD, DUSP6, SPRY4, and FLRT3 are identified in individuals with congenital hypogonadotropic hypogonadism[J]. Am J Hum Genet, 2013, 92(5): 725-743.

[22] Meijer D, Sieuwerts AM, Look MP, et al. Fibroblast growth factor receptor 4 predicts failure on tamoxifen therapy in patients with recurrent breast cancer[J]. Endocr Relat Cancer, 2008, 15(1): 101-111.

Application of oleosin-flanked keratinocyte growth factor-2 expressed from *Arabidopsis thaliana* promotes hair follicle growth in mice

Min Liu, Xiaokun Li

1. Introduction

The hair follicle is the most dynamic mini-organ that undergoes life-long cycles of rapid growth (anagen), regression (catagen) and resting periods (telogen). Hair follicles are composed of epidermal (epithelial) and dermal (mesenchymal) compartments, and their interaction plays an important role in the morphogenesis and growth of the follicle. In particular, mesenchyme-derived dermal papilla (DP) cells, located at the base of the hair follicles and surrounded by the hair matrix (HM), release a series of signals that directly influences the whole follicular epithelium and regulates hair growth. Therefore, the dermal papilla cells (DPCs) are considered to be inducers in the process of hair growth. DPCs lose some intrinsic properties, especially their hair-inductive capacity, during *in vitro* culture and this is accompanied by significant changes in gene expression profile, such as the lysozyme gene which is down-regulated in cultured DPCs.

Keratinocyte growth factor-2 (KGF-2) is found in dermal papilla fibroblasts and its receptor, fibroblast growth factor receptor 2 (FGFR2), in the neighboring outer root sheath of keratinocytes. Administration of recombinant human KGF-2% (rhKGF-2) at 10 ng/ml significantly stimulated human hair-follicle cell proliferation in organ culture (26%–35%), and rhKGF-2 expressed in *Escherichia coli* has biological activity in promoting human hair growth (Jang, 2005). ker-atinocyte growth factor 2 (KGF2) has a wide range of target cells and, through combination with specific receptors and epithelial cells, to promote cell proliferation, differentiation and migration of epithelial cells (Streatfield, 2007).

The demand for recombinant therapeutic molecules for clinical applications is increasing. Plant seeds are associated with protein synthesis and storage, and thus have high protein contents, low protease activities, and low water contents (Muntz, 1998; Ma *et al.*, 2003). Various strategies have been developed to maximize the yield of recombinant proteins in seeds (Kim *et al.*, 2013; Shigemitsu *et al.*, 2013). Oleosin fusion polypeptides retain their native targeting to oil bodies *in vivo* and fractionate with oil bodies following aqueous extraction and separation (Nykiforuk *et al.*, 2006; van Rooijen and Moloney, 1995). The fused product is correctly targeted into the oil body and retains its functional capacity and therefore the native conformational folding of the protein (Banilas *et al.*, 2011). For seed oil bodies, in particular, the level of recombinant protein accumulation is the most crucial factor for increased productivity (Huang, 1996; Scott *et al.*, 2010). The key element for accumulation and stability is the oleosin molecule itself (Li *et al.*, 2002).

The protein-rich cereal crops, grain legumes and oil seeds are attractive seed-based platforms for the production of recombinant proteins. On the other hand, due to its easy transformation and short regeneration time, *Arabidopsis thaliana* has also been used as a model to express pharmaceutical proteins before administering to crops for large-scale field application (Downing *et al.*, 2006).

Banilas *et al.* (2011) has shown that dimeric oleosin fusions followed by or flanking a green fluorescent protein (GFP) have a higher level of accumulation compared with single-oleosin-based constructs, and that stable associations of oleosin-oligomeric fusions with oil bodies retain the native conformation of the GFP. In order to avoid the high cost of expressed in *E. coli* and purification of KGF2, we have examined an efficient expression system in plants. We have investigated the properties of two different constructs, employing a dimeric oleosin-flanked KGF2 peptide with the two oleosins on either the same or different sides. We also analyzed whether these constructs can improve accumulation or affect the biological activity of KGF2 on hair follicle growth compared with the effects of a single-oleosin-based construct.

2. Materials and methods

2.1 Expression vector construction and plant transformation

The sequence of human KGF2 (GenBankaccession number KP866148) was optimized according to the amino acid sequence of human Fgf10 (GenBank accession number NP004456). The T-DNA region of the pCAMBIA1301-OK2 plasmid contained a phaseolin promoter (phaP) with a double enhancer, oleosin-gene, *KGF2* gene, phaseolin terminator (phaT), a cauliflower mosaic virus 35S promoter sequence, *bar* gene and a nopaline synthase terminator (Engineering Research Center of Bioreactor and Pharmaceutical Development, Ministry of Education, Jilin Agricultural University, China) (Fig. 1A).

We generated synthetic DNA sequences, designated as Oleosin–Oleosin::KGF2 and Oleosin::KGF2-Oleosin, by modifying the pCAMBIA1301-OK2 vector (Fig. 1A). To create the O–O:: KGF2 expression cassette, *Oleosin* gene (GenBank accession number NM113682) was inserted at the *Nco*I site between phaP and the *Oleosin* gene of O::KGF2, with the newly inserted *Oleosin* in-frame to the pre-existing one. The O::KGF2-O cassette contained an *Oleosin* gene following O::KGF2, which was inserted in-frame at the *Hind*III site next to the pre-existing KGF2. Consequently, the resulting O–O::KGF2 and O::KGF2-O constructs both contained two sequential inframe copies of *Oleosin*.

Orientations and copy numbers of the inserted oleosin genes were checked by dual-enzyme digestion of plasmid DNA with *Nco*I and *Hind*III restriction enzymes, with further confirmation carried out by DNA sequencing. The complete expression cassettes between the right and left borders of the T-DNA are annotated in Fig. 1A.

The pCAMBIA1301 O–O:: KGF2 and O::KGF2-O plasmids were introduced independently into *Agrobacterium tumefaciens* strain LBA4404 by the freeze–thaw transformation method (Logemann *et al.*, 2006; Sambrook and Gething, 1989). *Arabidopsis thaliana* (L.) Heyhn.ecotype Columbia 0 was then transformed by the floral dip technique (Clough and Bent, 1998; Zhang *et al.*, 2006) *via Agrobacterium tumefaciens*-mediated transformation. The T1 seeds were sown onto ½ strength Murashige and Skoog medium (PhytoTechnology Laboratories, Shawnee, KS, USA) containing 1% (*w/v*) agar and 10 mg Basta herbicide/ml, then the positive transgenic plants transplanted into soil to generate T_2 seeds, and analyzed.

2.2 PCR amplification of genomic DNA

Genomic DNA was isolated from fresh leaf tissue of transgenic and non-transgenic plants using a DNA extraction kit (BioTeke, Beijing, China). To confirm the insertion of recombinant genes, PCR amplification of *KGF2* gene was performed using the primer pairs as shown in Supplementary Table 1. PCR conditions consisted of 30 cycles of 94℃ for 30 s and 55℃ for 30 s, with a final step of 72℃ for 10 min. Expected sizes of O–O::*KGF2* and O::*KGF2*-O DNA products were both1, 272 bp (Fig. 1B).

2.3 Purification of oil bodies

T_3 transgenic *A. thaliana* seeds (25 mg) were ground in 1.5 ml centrifuge tubes with a pestle in 50 μl precooled sodium phosphate buffer (PBS, pH 7.5) (Tzen *et al.*, 1997), centrifuged at 12 000×*g* and 4℃ for 20 min to obtain the floating oil bodies fraction. Oil bodies were washed twice with 50 μl PBS and centrifuged as before. Precipitated material and buffer under the oil bodies was removed and the oil body fraction (80 μl) was collected. It was stored at 4℃ until needed.

2.4 SDS-PAGE and immunoblot analysis

Seeds (1 mg) of O::KGF2, O–O::KGF2, and O:: KGF2-O transgenic (T_3) and wild-type *Arabidopsis thaliana* plants were ground with a pestle in 1.5 ml centrifuge tubes containing 100 μl precooled Tris/HCl (50 mM, pH 8.0). Loading buffer (5 ×) was then added into the slurry and mixed. After boiling for 10 min, the mixtures were centrifuged for 10 min. Supernatants were analyzed *via* SDS-PAGE under reducing conditions using two 12% (*w/v*) polyacrylamide gels that were subsequently stained overnight with Coomassie Blue.

Following SDS-PAGE, the gels were electroblotted onto 0.45 μm PVDF membranes and immunoblotting was

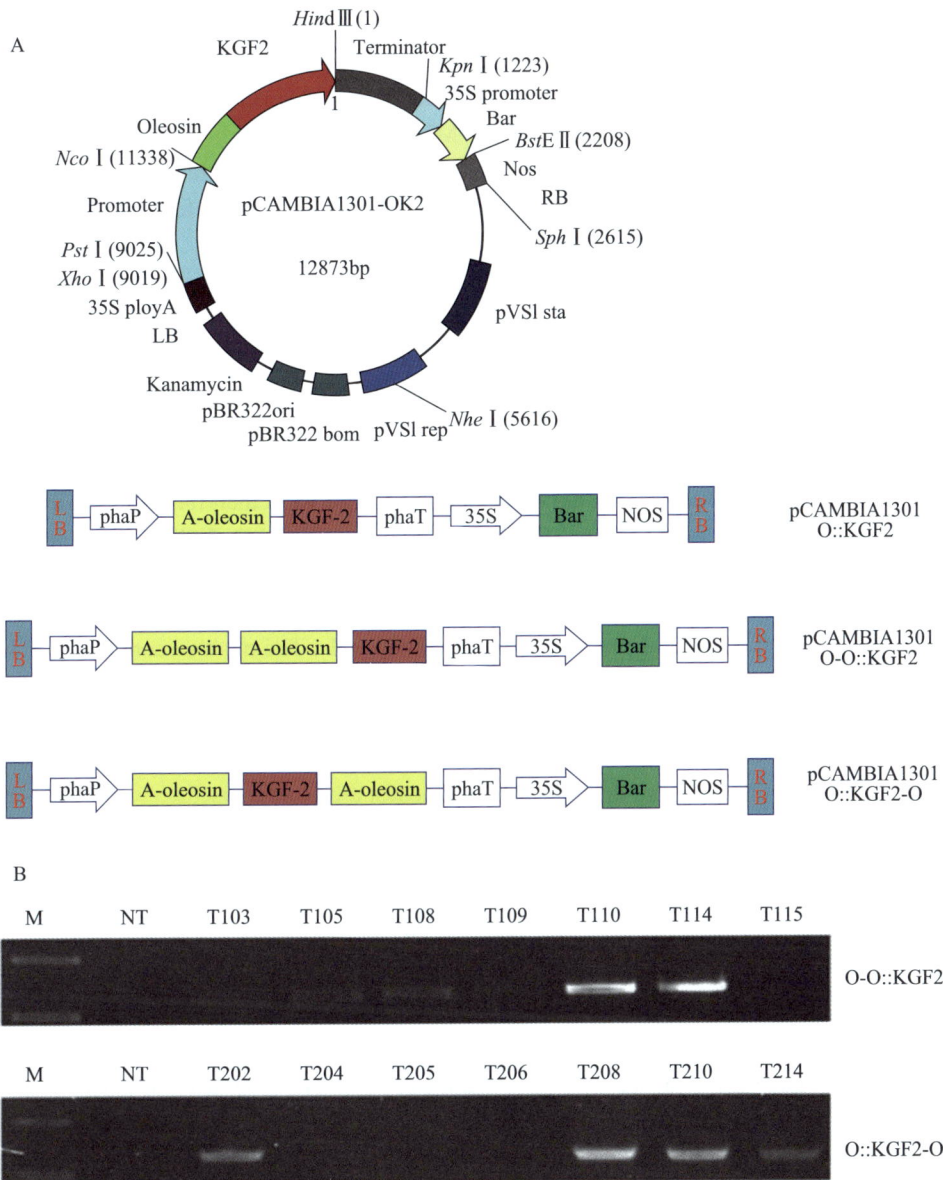

Fig. 1. Construction of vector for plant transformation. (A) Schematic diagram of oleosin-KGF2 fusion constructs used. The pCAMBIA1301 plant expression vector encodes an *Arabidopsis* oleosin fused to KGF2. O::KGF2 (single-oleosin-fused KGF2), O–O::KGF2, and O::KGF2-O are designations for the cassettes within the pCAMBIA1301 vectors. *LB* left border, *PhaP* phaseolin promoter, *A-oleosin* 18-kDa *Arabidopsis* oleosin, *PhaT* phaseolin terminator, *35S* cauliflower mosaic virus 35S promoter, *Bar* bar herbicide-resistance gene, *RB* right border. (B) Results of PCR analysis of genomic DNA from transgenic plants. Genomic DNA was extracted from O–O::KGF2-(1 272 bp) and O::KGF2-O-(1 272 bp) trans-genic plants. *M* DL-15 000 DNA marker, *NT* genomic DNA from non-transgenic *Arabidopsis* plants (negative control).

performed using a monoclonal anti-KGF2 antibody (1:2 000; R&D Systems, Shanghai, China). The membranes were washed and then incubated with anti-mouse IgG-HRP (1:8 000; Santa Cruz Biotech-nology, USA). Proteins were de-tected using a Beyo ECL Plus kit (Beyotime, China) on a Bio-Rad ECL system. The results were analyzed and quanti-fied with Quantity One software.

2.5 *In vitro assay of O::KGF2, O–O::KGF2, and O::KGF2-O biological activity*

The epithelial cells, FGFR2 III b-BaF3, were used to determine the activity of the three recombinant oleosin-fused KGF2 polypeptides (O::KGF2, O–O::KGF2, and O::KGF2-O) that were expressed in plant seed oil bodies. Prolifera-tion of FGFR2 III b-BaF3 cells was determined by the MTT method (see Ornitz *et al.*, 1996). First, the FGFR2 III b-BaF3 cells were grown in RPMI 1640 medium supplemented with 10% (*v/v*) fetal bovine serum, 10% (*v/v*) conditioned medium from WEHI-3 cells, L-glutamine, and antibiotics (100 IU/ml each of penicillin and streptomycin) until the culture reached the mid-logarithmic growth phase. The cultures were then transferred to a 96-well plate (10^5 cells per well) and treated for 48 h with KGF2 from *E. coli* (Abcam, Hong Kong) or recombinant oleosin-fused KGF2 proteins at 0.1–200 ng/ml. The cells in each well were incubated with 25 µl MTT (5 mg/ml) for 4 h. The medium was removed, 150 µl DMSO was added to each well to dissolve the crystals with shaking at room temperature for 10 min and the absorbance of the solution was immediately measured at 570 nm in a micro-plate reader using a reference wavelength of 630 nm.

2.6 In vivo analysis of O::KGF2, O–O::KGF2, and O::KGF2-O activity

To characterize the effects of recombinant oleosin-fused KGF2 (O::KGF2, O–O::KGF2, and O::KGF2-O) protein on hair growth *in vivo*, we essentially followed the protocol developed by Kawano *et al.* (2005). All procedures involved 8-week-old C57BL/6 male mice (20 ± 2 g), whose care was approved by the Institutional Animal Care and Use Committee of Wenzhou Medical University, China. The procedures were performed in accordance with institutional guidelines for animal experiments. After 2 days of conditioning, 30 mice were anesthetized, their dorsal hair gently cut short with a trimmer, and photographed using a digital camera. The mice were then randomly divided, five individuals per group, into six groups: three treatment groups (O::KGF2, O–O::KGF2, and O::KGF2-O), a negative control group (normal saline), a positive control group (KGF2 from *E. coli* and a blank control group (wild-type *Arabidopsis* seed protein). Crude proteins extracted from transgenic and wild-type plant seeds were smeared onto the skin of individuals in the three treatment groups and the blank control group, respectively. The positive control group was treated with KGF2 solution (500 µg/ml), and the negative control group was treated with an equivalent volume of normal saline. All six groups were dosed at a rate of 2 ml/kg body weight, which was administered once daily for 12 days. The mice were maintained on a standard laboratory diet and acidified water ad libitum. On day 13, they were anesthetized, photographed, and killed, and the full thickness of the dorsal skin in the test area was excised.

2.7 HE staining

The harvested samples were fixed and embedded in paraffin, and the embedded skin samples were cut into 4 µm thick sections using standard procedures (Paus *et al.*, 1999). Finally, the sections were stained with hematoxylin and eosin and observed under a microscope.

2.8 Statistical analysis

Data are expressed as the mean ± standard error of the mean (SEM) of at least three independent experiments *in vitro*. All statistical analyses were performed with Graphpad Prism software. For comparison of more than two groups, one-way ANOVA followed by a Bonferroni-Dunn test was used. Statistical significance was considered to be a *P* value < 0.05.

3. Results

3.1 Construction of the vector and transgenic plant for expression of O–O::KGF2 and O::KGF2-O

Synthetic DNA sequences designated as O–O:: KGF2 and O::KGF2-O was generated by modifying the pCAMBIA1301-OK2 vector (Fig. 1A). Both O–O:: KGF2 and O::KGF2-O constructs contained two sequential in-frame copies of *Oleosin*.

Orientations and copy numbers of the inserted oleosin genes were checked and confirmed by DNA sequencing. The complete expression cassettes between the right and left borders of the T-DNA are annotated in Fig. 1A.

Arabidopsis thaliana was transformed with the pCAMBIA1301 plant binary expression vectors. Concatamers of two oleosin molecules constituted the polypeptide. Nine independent transgenic lines (T_0) were obtained by screening on Basta herbicide. After self-pollination and subsequent screening on Basta-supplemented medium, eight independent homozygous lines (T_2) were obtained for further analyses of the expected constructs. To confirm the presence of transgenes in the regenerated plants, we carried out PCR analysis of genomic DNA from eight randomly selected transgenic lines derived from each type of vector (Fig. 1B). The transgenic plant lines with O–O::KGF2 and O::KGF2-O exhibited the expected 1272-bp amplification bands. An analysis of oleosin-fused KGF2 expression in the different constructs was conducted using mature T_3 seeds. Oil-body-associated seed proteins were analyzed to determine expression levels and targeting of the different fusion proteins.

3.2 Expression of KGF2 in the oil bodies isolated from transgenic plants with single-oleosin-fused KGF2 (O::KGF2), and double-oleosin-fused KGF2 (O–O::KGF2 and O::KGF2-O)

To determine the specificity of oleosin-fused polypeptide targeting, oil bodies isolated from wild-type, single-oleosin-fused KGF2 (O::KGF2), and double-oleosin-fused KGF2 (O–O::KGF2 and O::KGF2-O) transgenic plants were subjected to SDS-PAGE (Fig. 2A). Transgenic lines harboring the O–O::KGF2 and O::KGF2-O constructs displayed protein bands of approx. 53 and 54 kDa, respectively. According to SDS-PAGE and western blot analysis, the two constructs exhibited a higher average recombinant polypeptide accumulation than that of O::KGF2 control, with O::KGF2-O appearing to have the highest expression (Fig. 3B). The expression of O–O::KGF2 and O::KGF2-O constructs is 1.6-fold and 2.3-fold compared with O::KGF2, respectively (Fig. 2B). After appropriate normalization of band intensities and accounting for molecular masses of the different oleosin-fused KGF2 s, the relative mean values of recombinant protein accumulation in O–O::KGF2 and O::KGF2-O transformed lines were respectively 1.9-fold and 4.1-fold higher than that of s O::KGF2 (Fig. 2C). A ratio of 3:1 in T1 generation transgenic plants expressed the KGF2, suggesting that transgenic integration took place at a single locus, or several closely linked loci.

3.3 O–O::KGF2 and O::KGF2 promote cell proliferation in FGFR2b-BaF3 cells

To evaluate the effectiveness of recombinant oleosin-fused KGF2 bioactivity, the proliferative effect of O–O::KGF2, O::KGF2-O, and single-oleosin-fused KGF2 were determined on FGFR2IIIb-BaF3 epithelial cells using a standard MTT assay and compared with that of KFG2 from *E. coli* (positive control) and wild-type *Arabidopsis* (negative control). As shown in Fig. 3, *E. coli* KGF2, O–O::KGF2, and O::KGF2 induced a comparable miltonic response in FG-FR2IIIb-BaF3 cells, with the activity of O::KGF2-O being slightly lower. Furthermore, O–O::KGF2 and O::KGF2 had a dose-dependent effect on stimulated FGFR2b-BaF3 cells whereas O::KGF2-O, similar to the negative control, had no distinct effect (Fig. 3). We therefore conclude that both O–O::KGF2 and O::KGF2 promotes cell proliferation in FGFR2b-BaF3 cells.

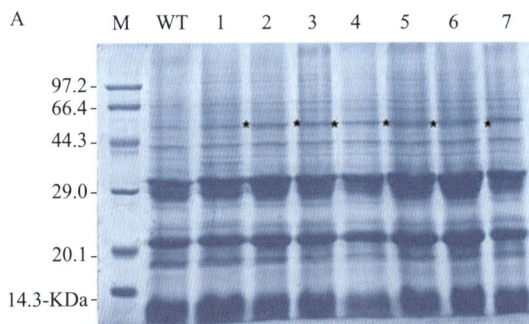

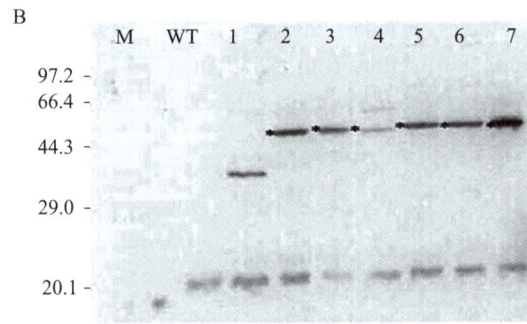

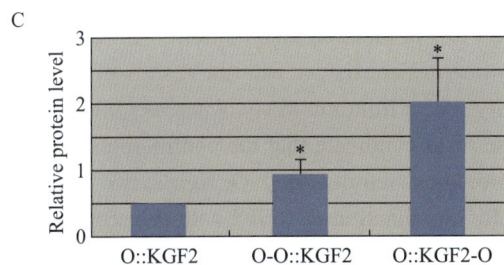

Fig. 2. Fused oleosin-KGF2 protein levels in different transgenes. (A) Representative SDS-PAGE gel of oil-body-associated proteins showing the variation in accumulation levels of recombinant polypeptides from different plant lines compared with the wild type and KGF2 from *E. coli*. Molecular weights (kDa) of recombinant peptides are indicated. *WT* wild type, *Lane 1* single-oleosin-fused KGF2 (O::KGF2; described in Fig. 1), *Lanes 2–4* O–O::KGF2 (53 kDa) transformed plants T3#5, T3#13, and T3#20, *Lanes 5–7* O::KGF2-O (54 kDa) transformed plants T3#4, T3#11, and T3#25. *Asterisks* indicate expected recombinant proteins of appropriate size that were confirmed by immunoblot analysis (B, C) Ratios of accumulation levels of O–O:: KGF2 and O::KGF2-O relative to single-oleosin-fused KGF2 (O::KGF2) after normalization of different molecular weights. Values are mean ± SEM of at least five biological replicates. The statistical significance is indicated with *asterisks* (*). *$P < 0.05$ *vs.* O::KGF2.

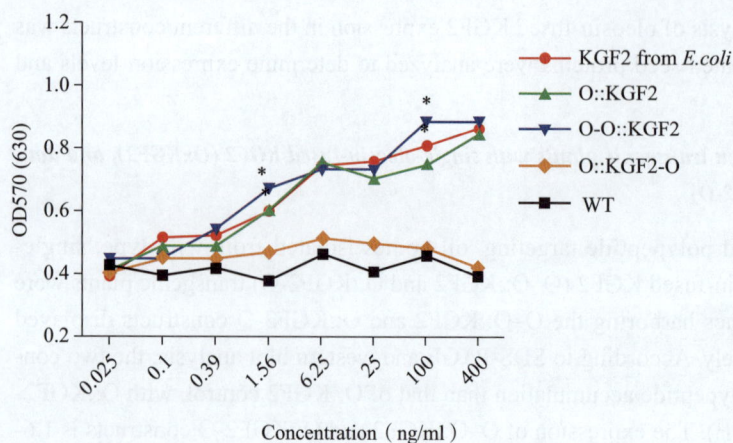

Fig.3. Effects of different concentrations of O::KGF2, O–O::KGF2, and O::KGF2-O on cell proliferation in FGFR2IIIb-BaF3 cells. KGF2 from *E. coli* was used as a positive control (KGF-2 from *E. coli*), wild-type (WT), and the groups treated with O::KGF2, O–O::KGF2, and O::KGF2-O, respectivly. Proliferation was quantified by measuring absorbance at 570 nm. Values are mean ± SEM of at least five biological replicates. The statistical significance is indicated with *asterisks* (*). *P < 0.05 *vs.* KFG2 (from *E. coli*) or O::KGF2.

3.4 Recombinant KGF2 oil-body protein stimulates hair follicle growth in mice

To further evaluate the biological activity of O–O::KGF2, O::KGF2-O, and single-oleosin-fused KGF2, subcutaneous administration to male C57BL/6 mice was used to analyze the effect of these proteins on hair growth. Twelve days after treatment with crude oil-body protein from O–O::KGF2, O::KGF2-O, and O::KGF2 transgenic plant seeds, different levels of hair growth were observed on the exterior surfaces of mouse dorsal skin over the entire test area; this growth was vigorous compared with that of the blank control group (Fig. 4A). Examination of the reverse side of the skin revealed different degrees of extensive anagen hair follicle growth in mice with pigmentation or hair growth (in Fig. 4A, black spots indicate anagen hair follicles). The effects of oil-body protein from O–O::KGF2, O::KGF2-O, or O::KGF2 transgenic plant seeds were more obvious than those from wild-type plants. Both O–O::KGF2 and O::KGF2 had a more obvious stimulating effect than did that of O::KGF2-O, with O–O::KGF2 having a slightly stronger effect than KGF2 from *E. coli* (Fig. 4). Furthermore, the skin of five of the six mice treated with recombinant oleosin-fused KGF2 protein showed apparent changes, whereas none of the skin samples from the six normal-saline control mice exhibited hair growth or strong pigmentation, and only a slight effect was observed in mice treated with oil-body protein from wild-type *A. thaliana* plant seeds. Examination of the reverse side of control skin samples revealed few or no anagen hair follicles, as indicated by their white color in Fig. 4A. These results were further confirmed by histological examination of skin sections (Fig. 4B). When O–O::KGF2, O::KGF2-O, and O::KGF2 were administered topically to the skin of mice in the same telogen state, anagen hair growth among *E. coli* KFG2-treated, saline-treated, and wild-type mice was comparable (Fig. 4C).

4. Discussion

Transgenic plants as bioreactors are an attractive option for high-yield economic production of recombinant proteins. We found that the O::KGF2-O construct had the highest expression but very little biological activity, whereas the O–O::KGF2 expression cassette showed more obvious activity but slightly less production than that of O–O::KGF2. At the protein expression level, our data from SDS-PAGE and western blotting are consistent with the results of Banilas *et al.* (2011). Interestingly, however, O–O::KGF2 exhibited ideal activity in the miltonic assay, whereas O::KGF2-O showed none; similar results were seen in the animal experiment. These results indicate that the configuration of the oleosin bonding site relative to KGF2 exerts a tremendous influence on biological activity. In O–O::KGF2, two oleosins are on the same side of the target gene, which we suspect is convenient for combination of KGF2 with its receptors; in O::KGF2-O, in contrast, the oil inclusion body structure prevents exposure to KGF2, with KGF2 consequently unable to combine with the receptors. The performance of O–O::KGF2, both with respect to protein expression and activity, was superior to that of the single-oleosin-fused gene. The phenotype of these transgenic lines was not observed under standard growth conditions. We have demonstrated an efficient strategy to express high levels of oleosinfused KGF2. In addition, consistent with our goal of finding a topically applied, skin-penetrating drug delivery system, plant seed oil can

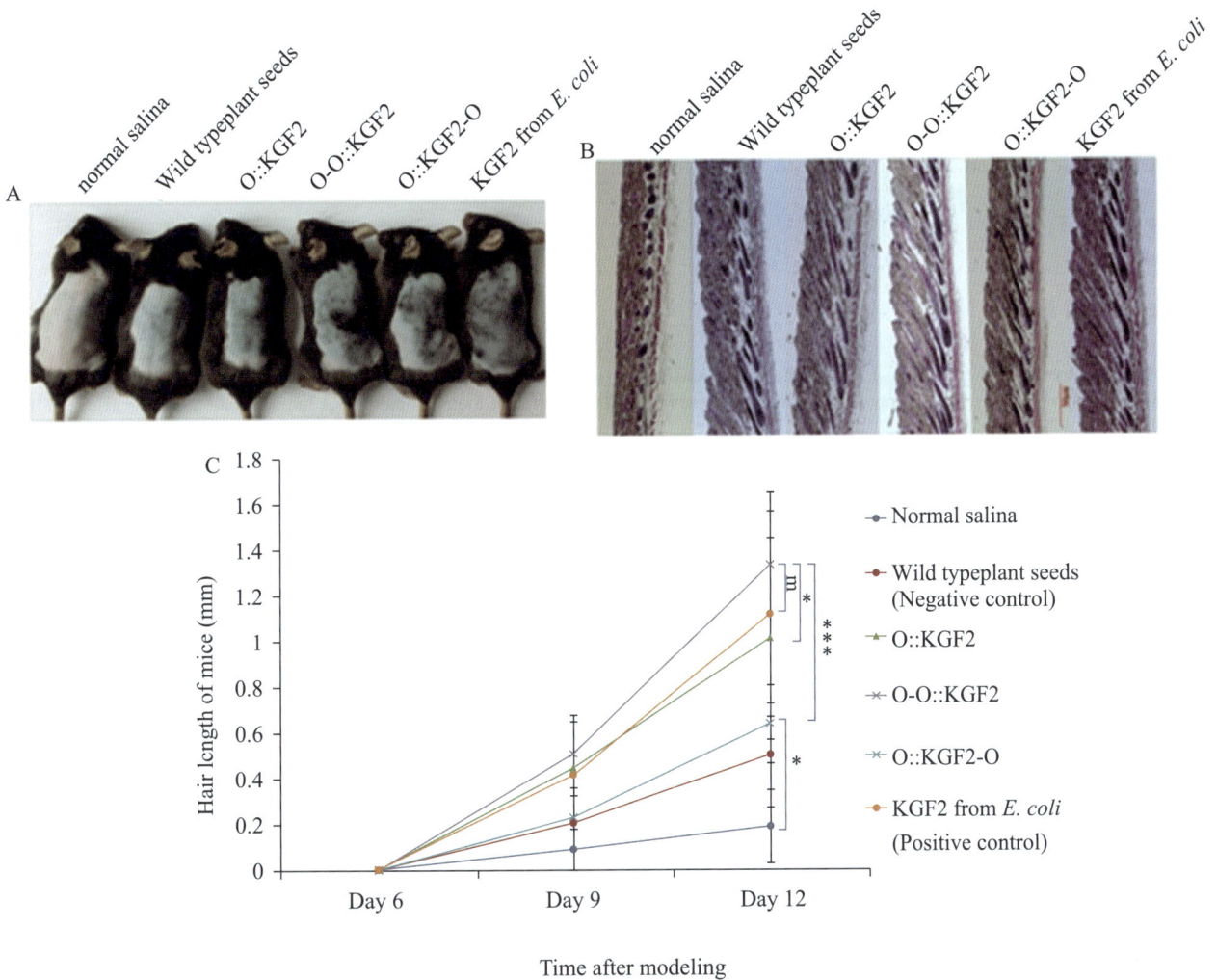

Fig. 4. Induction of hair growth by oil-body protein from single-oleosin-fused KGF2 (O::KGF2), O–O::KGF2, and O::KGF2-O in mice with telogen-stage hair follicles. Thirty 55-day-old male C57BL/6 mice were anesthetized and their dorsal hair gently cut short. Crude proteins extracted from transgenic or wild-type plant seeds were applied to the skin of individuals, with the negative control group treated with normal saline. On day 12, mice were anesthetized and killed, and the full thickness of the dorsal skin in the test area was excised. (A) Representative mice from each treatment are shown ($n = 6$). (B) Histology of hair follicles in mice from each treatment group (Scale bars = 50 μm). Mouse skin was embedded in paraffin, sectioned, stained with hematoxylin and eosin, and photographed. (C) The length of randomly plucked hairs was measured at different time intervals (6, 9 and 12 days) after topical application. Values are the mean ± SD of five mice. $^{ns}P > 0.05$, $^{*}P < 0.05$, $^{***}P < 0.01$ (one-way ANOVA, Tukey's test).

increase the permeability of drugs and thus lead to better drug effectiveness and safety. Plant oil body structures consist of an oleosin embedded within the phospholipid monolayer separating the triacylglycerol storage site of embryo-located subcellular particles (Hsieh and Huang, 2004; Murphy, 1990; Siloto *et al.*, 2006). Consequently, oleosin-rich oil bodies remain stable and small, providing a high surface-to-volume ratio and facilitating their recovery in large amounts from dried, stored oilseeds. Oil bodies can be easily separated from most other seed cell components by flotation centrifugation, and also contains a relatively small number of different proteins (Abell *et al.*, 1997; van Rooijen and Moloney, 1995).

We have characterized over-expression of KGF-2 in an oil body as a promising agent for development of agents for human hair loss treatments. However, KGF-2 is not an only factor capable of promoting hair growth. Many growth factors are also responsible for promoting hair follicle growth such as HGF, IGF, and EGF. Development of use of these growth factors would be another approach for hair growth improvement. Taken together, the present study analyzed the consequences of rhKGF-2 treatment on the human hair follicles. We showed the stimulatory effect of rhKGF-2 on hair growth. Our findings suggest that rhKGF-2 expressed in plant oil seeds has biological activity for promoting mice hair growth.

Supplementary material

Electronic supplementary material to this article can be found in the online version (doi:10.1007/s10529-016-2119-y).

References

Abell BM, Holbrook LA, Abenes M, *et al.* Role of the proline knot motif in oleosin endoplasmic reticulum topology and oil body targeting[J]. Plant Cell, 1997, 9(8): 1481-1493.

Banilas G, Daras G, Rigas S, *et al.* Oleosin di-or tri-meric fusions with GFP undergo correct targeting and provide advantages for recombinant protein production[J]. Plant Physiol Biochem, 2011, 49(2): 216-222.

Clough SJ, Bent AF. Floral dip: a simplified method for Agrobacterium-mediated transformation of Arabidopsis thaliana[J]. Plant J, 1998, 16(6): 735-743.

Downing WL, Galpin JD, Clemens S, *et al.* Synthesis of enzymatically active human alpha-L-iduronidase in Arabidopsis cgl (complex glycan-deficient) seeds[J]. Plant Biotechnol J, 2006, 4(2): 169-181.

Hsieh K, Huang AH. Endoplasmic reticulum, oleosins, and oils in seeds and tapetum cells[J]. Plant Physiol, 2004, 136(3): 3427-3434.

Huang AH. Oleosins and oil bodies in seeds and other organs[J]. Plant Physiol, 1996, 110(4): 1055-1061.

Jang JH. Stimulation of human hair growth by the recombinant human keratinocyte growth factor-2 (KGF-2)[J]. Biotechnol Lett, 2005, 27(11): 749-752.

Kim HU, Jung SJ, Lee KR, *et al.* Ectopic overexpression of castor bean LEAFY COTYLEDON2 (LEC2) in Arabidopsis triggers the expression of genes that encode regulators of seed maturation and oil body proteins in vegetative tissues[J]. FEBS Open Bio, 2013, 4: 25-32.

Li M, Murphy DJ, Lee KH, *et al.* Purification and structural characterization of the central hydrophobic domain of oleosin[J]. J Biol Chem, 2002, 277(40): 37888-37895.

Logemann E, Birkenbihl RP, Ulker B, *et al.* An improved method for preparing Agrobacterium cells that simplifies the Arabidopsis transformation protocol[J]. Plant Methods, 2006, 2: 16.

Ma JK, Drake PM, Christou P. The production of recombinant pharmaceutical proteins in plants[J]. Nat Rev Genet, 2003, 4(10): 794-805.

Muntz K. Deposition of storage proteins[J]. Plant Mol Biol, 1998, 38(1-2): 77-99.

Murphy DJ. Storage lipid bodies in plants and other organisms[J]. Prog Lipid Res, 1990, 29(4): 299-324.

Nykiforuk CL, Boothe JG, Murray EW, *et al.* Transgenic expression and recovery of biologically active recombinant human insulin from Arabidopsis thaliana seeds[J]. Plant Biotechnol J, 2006, 4(1): 77-85.

Ornitz DM, Xu J, Colvin JS, *et al.* Receptor specificity of the fibroblast growth factor family[J]. J Biol Chem, 1996, 271(25): 15292-15297.

Paus R, Muller-Rover S, Van Der Veen C, *et al.* A comprehensive guide for the recognition and classification of distinct stages of hair follicle morphogenesis[J]. J Invest Dermatol, 1999, 113(4): 523-532.

Sambrook J, Gething MJ. Protein structure. Chaperones, paperones[J]. Nature, 1989, 342(6247): 224-225.

Scott RW, Winichayakul S, Roldan M, *et al.* Elevation of oil body integrity and emulsion stability by polyoleosins, multiple oleosin units joined in tandem head-to-tail fusions[J]. Plant Biotechnol J, 2010, 8(8): 912-927.

Shigemitsu T, Masumura T, Morita S, *et al.* Accumulation of rice prolamin-GFP fusion proteins induces ER-derived protein bodies in transgenic rice calli[J]. Plant Cell Rep, 2013, 32(3): 389-399.

Siloto RM, Findlay K, Lopez-Villalobos A, *et al.* The accumulation of oleosins determines the size of seed oilbodies in Arabidopsis[J]. Plant Cell, 2006, 18(8): 1961-1974.

Streatfield SJ. Approaches to achieve high-level heterologous protein production in plants[J]. Plant Biotechnol J, 2007, 5(1): 2-15.

Tzen JT, Peng CC, Cheng DJ, *et al.* A new method for seed oil body purification and examination of oil body integrity following germination[J]. J Biochem, 1997, 121(4): 762-768.

van Rooijen GJ, Moloney MM. Plant seed oil-bodies as carriers for foreign proteins[J]. Biotechnology (N Y), 1995, 13(1): 72-77.

Zhang X, Henriques R, Lin SS, *et al.* Agrobacterium-mediated transformation of Arabidopsis thaliana using the floral dip method[J]. Nat Protoc, 2006, 1(2): 641-646.

Expression of functional recombinant human fibroblast growth factor 8b and its protective effects on MPP+-lesioned PC12 cells

Nazi Chen, Jisheng Ma, Xiaokun Li

1. Introduction

Fibroblast growth factor 8 (FGF8) is a member of the FGF family and shares 30% – 40% amino acid sequence identity with other family members (Tanaka *et al.*, 1992). FGF8 was initially cloned from the Shionogi mouse mammary carcinoma cell line (SC-3) (Lorenzi *et al.*, 1995) and was identified as an androgen-induced growth factor. The human FGF8 gene is localized to chromosome 10q24 (Payson *et al.*, 1996) and consists of three exons (Crossley and Martin, 1995). An interesting aspect of FGF8 in human is that its messenger RNA (mRNA) can be alternatively spliced to generate four potential protein isoforms designated as FGF8a, b, e, and f (Gemel *et al.*, 1996). FGF8b appears to be the predominantly expressed species in prostate cancer and breast cancer (Gnanapragasam *et al.*, 2003; Tanaka *et al.*, 1998). FGF8b has been shown to be the most transforming isoform in experiments with NIH3T3 cells (Ghosh *et al.*, 1996). FGF8 plays a critical role in multiple physiological functions, including cellular proliferation and differentiation, embryonic development (Crossley and Martin, 1995; Heikinheimo *et al.*, 1994; Sun *et al.*, 1999), tissue repair, tumor growth (Kwabi-Addo *et al.*, 2004; Uchii *et al.*, 2008; Zhong *et al.*, 2006), metastatic progression, and angiogenesis (Mattila *et al.*, 2001). Moreover, FGF8 is able to nourish neural stem cells and induce DA neurons (Tanaka *et al.*, 2001; Ye *et al.*, 1998), which indicates that FGF8 can be directly used for the treatment of degenerative diseases.

Parkinson's disease (PD) is the second most common neurodegenerative disease and is caused by the progressive and selective loss of mesencephalic dopaminergic neurons of the nigrostriatal pathway (Aarsland *et al.*, 2012; Schapira and Olanow, 2004). With regard to its clinical manifestations, distinguishing characteristics include motor (resting tremor, rigidity, brady- and hypokinesia, and postural instability) and non-motor (cognitive, psychiatric, autonomic, olfactory, and sleeping disturbances) symptoms (Aarsland *et al.*, 2012; Rodriguez-Oroz *et al.*, 2009). While the etiology of the degeneration of SNpc cells remains unknown, mechanisms that lead to neuronal cell death have been elucidated, including oxidative stress, apoptosis, inflammation, mitochondrial dysfunction, and misfolded protein accumulation (Pluquet *et al.*, 2015; Shrivastava *et al.*, 2013). Accumulation of misfolded proteins is a distinguishing aspect of Parkinson's disease (Baba *et al.*, 1998), which causes endoplasmic reticulum (ER) stress and activates unfolded protein responses (UPR), which eventually initiates cell apoptosis (Hetz *et al.*, 2013; Volmer *et al.*, 2013). Most of the available treatment options are aimed at restoration of the physiological dopaminergic activity. FGF8 exhibits a multitude of activities on nervous tissue, which include promoting neuronal survival and neurite outgrowth, and improving development and function of dopaminergic neurons (Tanaka *et al.*, 2001; Ye *et al.*, 1998). Thus, we considered that FGF8b may have a cytoprotective effect against Parkinson's disease and hypothesized that FGF8b might affect ER stress genes, including cysteinyl aspartate specific proteinase 12 (Caspase12) and glucose-regulated protein 78 (GRP78), and thereby suppress dopaminergic neuronal cell death. Although FGF8b protein expression and purification have been reported previously (Huang *et al.*, 2013; Potula *et al.*, 2008), the protein yield was low or barely detectable in some cases.

With the development of biotechnology, a variety of alternative expression systems are now being used for expressing recombinant proteins for industrial production as well as in research for structural and biochemical studies (Dong *et al.*, 2008). Compared with other systems, the insect cell-baculovirus expression system (IC-BEVS) has several advantages including similar posttranslational modifications as those in mammalian cells and high levels of efficient expression. There is also inherent safety during manufacture and for the final product because insect cells are free of human pathogens and can be cultivated easily in serum- and protein-free media (Carinhas *et al.*, 2009; Drugmand *et al.*, 2012). In addition, the IC-BEVS can produce single and large multimeric proteins with molecular weights of several hundred kilodaltons, as the baculoviral genome can accommodate large fragments of heterologous DNA (Trowitzsch *et al.,* 2010). Thus, we used a IC-BEVS to produce a sufficient amount of FGF8b protein to meet the demands for biological activity evaluation and potential use in preclinical studies.

As clinical applications of FGF8b are worthy of investigation, but its yield is limited, we constructed an optimum recombinant human FGF8b Baculovirus vector (bacmid-rhFGF8b) and used *Spodoptera frugiperda* 9 (Sf9) cells to successfully express high levels of rhFGF8b. Furthermore, we undertook purification of rhFGF8b protein using heparin-affinity chromatography and obtained high purity for the homogenous rhFGF8b protein. Importantly, the produced rhFGF8b was found to have a significant mitogenic effect on NIH3T3 cells and prevented necrosis and apoptosis of 1-METHYL-4-phenyl pyridine (MPP$^+$)-treated PC12 cells. We also demonstrated that rhFGF8b suppressed dopaminergic neuronal cell death against ER stress induced by MPP$^+$ in PC12 cells. The results suggest that FGF8b may be a promising candidate therapeutic drug for neurodegenerative diseases related to ER stress.

2. Materials and methods

2.1 Materials

The Bac-to-Bac® Baculovirus Expression System (cat. no. 10359-016), which consists of MAX Efficiency® DH-10Bac™ Competent *Escherichia coli*, the pFastBac™ Vector, and Cellfectin® II Transfection Reagent, was purchased from Invitrogen (Carlsbad, USA). Sf9 cells, GIBCO™ SF-900II SFM cell culture products, and Dulbecco's modified Eagle medium (DMEM) were also purchased from Invitrogen. TaKaRa Ex *Taq*, r*Taq* polymerase, restriction enzymes *Bam*HI and *Hin*dIII, DL2 000 DNA Marker and DL15 000 DNA Marker, gel extraction kit, and plasmid miniprep kit were purchased from TaKaRa Company (Dalian, China). PageRuler Prestained Protein Ladder was purchased from Thermo Scientific (Lithuania). The bicinchoninic acid (BCA) kit, ECL chemiluminescence kit, and phenylmethanesulfonyl fluoride (PMSF) were purchased from Beyotime Institute of Biotechnology. Heparin Sepharose column and AKTA purifier were purchased from GE Healthcare (Piscataway, NJ, USA). All primers were synthesized by Invitrogen (Shanghai, China). Rabbit anti-human FGF8b and mouse anti-β-actin antibodies, donkey anti-rabbit, and donkey anti-mouse IgG-HRP were purchased from Santa Cruz Biotechnology (Heidelberg, Germany). Rabbit anti-Caspase12, rabbit anti-Caspase3, and rabbit anti-GRP78 antibodies were purchased from Abcam, Inc. (Abcam, Cambridge, MA, USA). Methylthiazol tetrazolium (MTT) and MPP$^+$ were purchased from Sigma (USA). PC12 cells were purchased from the Institutes of Biomedical Sciences (IBS), Fudan University (Shanghai, China). The *E. coli* DH5α and NIH3T3 cells were obtained from the Wenzhou Medical University Zhejiang Provincial Key Laboratory of Biotechnology Pharmaceutical Engineering.

2.2 Construction of bacmid-FGF8b recombinant plasmid

The coding sequence of human FGF8b (GenBank accession number NM006119) was optimized according to *S. frugiperda MNPV* codon usage (http://www.kazusa.or.jp/codon). The DNA fragment (GenBank accession number KT359345) was then cloned into the *Bam*HI and *Hin*dIII restriction enzyme sites of the pUC57-FGF8b plasmid (BGI, Beijing, China). The primary FGF8b translation product contains a 39-amino acid signal sequence in the hydrophobic *N*-terminal region, which is not present in the mature FGF8b molecule. PUC57-FGF8b and pFastBac transfer vector were digested with *Bam*HI and *Hin*dIII, respectively, and then ligated to create pFastBac-FGF8b constructs. The constructs were transformed into *E. coli* DH5α. Correct insertion of the genes was confirmed by restriction enzymatic analysis and automated DNA sequencing. The accurate transfer vector was transfected into competent *E. coli*. DH10Bac containing a helper plasmid to assist transposition of the recombinant Tn7 sequence into the bacmid DNA. Recombinant bacmid-FGF8b was selected and identified by PCR with the appropriate primers to recognize human FGF8b as follows: forward, 5′-CCCAAGCTTAGCGGGGCTCAGGAG-3′; reverse, 5′-CGCGGATCCATGCAGGTCACCGTG-3′. PCR was conducted with 50 μl of reaction mixture containing 0.5 μl TaKaRa Ex Taq (5 U/μl), 5 μl 10× Ex *Taq* buffer (Mg^{2+} Plus), 4 μl dNTPs (each 2.5 mM), and 2 μl each of the forward and reverse primers (each 20 μM). The thermocycling parameters used for PCR were as follows: 2 min at 98℃ for denaturation, 30 cycles of 30 s at 98℃, 30 s at 55℃, and 45 s at 72℃. Recombinant bacmid-FGF8b were extracted following the manufacturer's instructions of the Bac-to-Bac

Baculovirus Expression System and stored for up to 2 weeks at 4℃.

2.3 Sf9 cell culture and recombinant baculovirus production

Sf9 cells (GIBCO, USA) were maintained in 125-ml shaker flasks containing 40 ml SF900II serum-free medium (GIBCO). The cells were incubated at 27.3℃ in a nonhumidified orbital shaker at 115 rpm. When cell density reached $2×10^6$ viable cells/ml, Sf9 cells were subcultured by seeding $(3–5)×10^5$ viable cells/ml in new flasks containing a growth medium. For rhFGF8b protein production, we used suspension cultures in 500-ml shaker flasks containing 125 ml growth medium at a density of $2×10^6$ viable cells/ml.

Transfection of Sf9 cells was performed in a six-well plate. Sf9 cells in the mid-logarithmic time ($1.5×10^6$–$2.5×10^6$ viable cells/ml) were transferred to a six-well plate ($8×10^5$/well) and allowed to attach for 30 min at room temperature. Transfection was performed with Cellfectin® II Reagent according to the manufacturer's protocol. The cells were incubated at 27.3℃ for 84 h, and then cellular debris was removed by centrifugation at $500×g$ for 5 min. The supernatant was designated as the P1 viral stock and stored in 2% fetal bovine serum at 4℃ while being protected from light. Baculoviral stock amplification was performed by further transfected insect cell, and the titer was determined by a viral plaque assay.

2.4 Production optimization and purification of rhFGF8b

To determine the optimal condition for FGF8b expression, multiplicity of infection (MOI), cell density, and harvest time were investigated in 125-ml shaker flasks containing 40 ml culture medium at 27.3℃ and 115 rpm. The harvest time was evaluated at an MOI of 2 and cells were collected at 24, 36, 48, 60, 72, 84, 96, 108, and 120 h postinfection. Cell pellets were resuspended and incubated in RIPA lysate buffer (Beyotime, China) with 1% PMSF (Beyotime, China) for 10 min on ice. The supernatant was collected and protein samples were analyzed by Coomassie blue staining of 12% (v/v) sodium dodecyl sulfate polyacrylamide gel electrophoresis (SDS-PAGE). Proteins were transferred to PVDF membranes, and immunoblotting was performed using a peroxidase conjugated rabbit polyclonal anti-human FGF8b antibody (1:1000; Santa Cruz Biotechnology, USA). The membranes were washed and then incubated with horse radish peroxidase (HRP) conjugated donkey anti-rabbit IgG (1:8000; Santa Cruz Biotechnology, USA). Proteins were detected by the Beyo ECL Plus Kit (Beyotime, China) in the Bio-Rad ECL system. The results were analyzed and quantified by Quantity One software.

Sf9 cells were centrifuged at $500×g$ for 5 min to collect the cells. Cell pellets were resuspended in 50 mM phosphate buffer (pH 7.2) and lysed by sonication at 200 W for 5 s with an interval time of 5 s for 30 cycles. The resulting cell lysate was cleared of debris by ultracentrifugation, and then passed through a 0.22-μm filter. The purification was performed with a Heparin Sepharose affinity chromatography. The samples flow through the Heparin Sepharose resin (GE, USA) with binding buffer (50 mmol/L phosphate, pH 7.2) at 1 ml/min using the AKTA purifier system. rhFGF8b protein was collected from the column with stepwise gradients of 0.6, 1.2, and 2.0 M NaCl. The elution fractions were collected and assessed by Coomassie blue staining of 12% (v/v) SDS-PAGE. Fractions containing FGF8b were concentrated with a Millipore filter, and the concentration was evaluated with a BCA kit, and then the purified rhFGF8b fractions were stored at −80℃ to retain biological activity.

2.5 Mitogenic activity of rhFGF8b assay

We used the NIH 3T3 cell line (American Type Culture Col-lection, Rockville, MD) to determine the activity of the rhFGF8b that was expressed in BEVS. First, the cells were maintained in DMEM supplemented with 10% fetal bovine serum (FBS), 100 U/ml penicillin, and 100 mg/ml streptomycin until the culture reached the mid-logarithmic time, then detached and reseeded in a 96-well plate ($8×10^3$/well), and incubated at 37℃ for 24 h. The cells were serum-starved overnight prior to stimulation with either rhFGF8b or human bFGF protein for 48 h, and the cells were then incubated with 25 μl/well (5 mg/ml) MTT for 4 h. Finally, the medium was removed and 150 μl/well of DMSO was added to dissolve the crystals by shaking at room temperature for 10 min; the absorbance was immediately measured at 490 nm using a microplate reader.

2.6 PC12 cell culture and cell model of Parkinson's disease

The rat pheochromocytoma PC12 was maintained in DMEM supplemented with 10% FBS, 100 U/ml penicillin, and 100 mg/ml streptomycin at 37℃ in a 5% CO_2 humidified incubator. The culture medium was changed every 2 days. Cells in the mid-logarithmic time were transferred to a 96-well plate (5×10^3/well) and incubated at 37℃ for 24 h. The cells were serum-starved overnight prior to treatment with final concentrations of 200–2 000 μmol/L MPP^+ for 48 h. After the treatment, the cells cultured in 96-well plates were used for MTT assay to measure cell viability.

2.7 Cytoprotection of rhFGF8b in vitro

The neuroprotection of rhFGF8b on PC12 cells was evaluated using the MPP^+-induced model of PD. PC12 cells were divided into four experimental groups: control, injury group, rhFGF8b, and bFGF treatment groups. Cells were transferred to either 96-well plates (2×10^3 per well) or six-well plates (2.0×10^5 per well) and incubated at 37℃ for 24 h. The cells were serum-starved overnight prior to treatment with MPP^+ (500 μmol/L) for 48 h, followed by a 2-h stimulation with either rhFGF8b or bFGF. Cells treated with MPP^+ only for 48 h were used as injury group, and the same volumes of medium only were added to the control group. After the treatment, the cells cultured in 96-well plates were used for MTT assay to measure cell viability, and those in six-well plates were assessed by an Annexin-V/PI double staining kit (Becton-Dickinson) using flow cytometry.

2.8 rhFGF8b protection against ER stress in vitro

Total RNA obtained from PC12 cells in six-well plates from the injury group and rhFGF8b treatment group was extracted using TRIzol reagent (Invitrogen, Carlsbad, CA) according to manufacturer's instructions. cDNA sequences were generated by reverse transcriptase-polymerase chain reaction (RT-PCR) using the SuperScript pre-amplification system according to the manufacturer's protocol (Promega, Madison, MI). Quantitative PCR was performed with CFX96 Touch™ Real-Time PCR Detection System (Bio-Rad) with SYBR® Premix Ex Taq™ GC (Perfect Real Time) (Takara, Dalian, PR China) in volume of 15 μl. The primers used for PCR amplification were as follows: Caspase12 (sense: 5′-AATGGAGGTAAATGTTGGAGTG-3′, antisense: 5′-CTCTTCTGCCCTTTCTGTCTTC-3′); GRP78 (sense: 5′-CTGAAGACAAAGGGACAGGA-3′, antisense: 5′-CTCAATTTTCTCCCAACGAA-3′); Caspase3 (sense: 5′-TGC-GGCGTTACACGACCTT-3′, antisense: 5′-CAAAGCCAGTGGCACTCATTCTC-3′); Bcl-xl (sense: 5′-AGGCTG GCGATGAGTTT G-3′, antisense: 5′-CGGCTCTCGGCTGCTGCATT-3′); bax (sense: 5′-TGGTTGCCCTTTTC-TACTTTG-3′, antisense: 5′-GAAGTAGGAAAGGAGGCCATC-3′); and β-actin (sense: 5′-ATTTGCACCACACTTTC-TACA-3′, antisense: 5′-TCACGCACGATTTCCCTCTCAG-3′). β-actin was used as internal standard for quantifying mRNA. Typical PCR parameters were 50℃ for 2 min and 95℃ for 2 min, followed by 40 cycles of 95℃ for 15 s, 55℃ for 15 s, 72℃ for 20 s, followed by a final extension step at 72℃ for 10 min. Reactions were run in triplicate and data were normalized to a calibrator sample using the $2^{-\Delta\Delta ct}$ method with correction for amplification efficiency (Pfaffl 2001).

PC12 cells from the injury group and rhFGF8b treatment group were homogenized in lysis buffer as described above, and the cell lysate samples were centrifuged (12 000 g, 4℃) for 30 min. Total protein concentration was determined by BCA kit. Western blot analysis was performed as described in detail previously. Membranes were incubated with antibodies against GRP78 (1:1 000; Abcam, Cambridge, MA, USA), Caspase12 (1:1 000; Abcam, Cambridge, MA, USA), Caspase3 (1:1 000; Abcam, Cambridge, MA, USA), and actin (1:1 000; Abcam, Cambridge, MA, USA). Proteins were detected with HRP conjugated secondary antibodies (Santa Cruz Biotechnology, USA), and immunoreactive protein bands were visualized using the Bio-Rad ECL system and quantified by optical densitometry.

2.9 Statistical analysis

All data are presented as the means±standard error of mean (SEM). One-way ANOVA followed by a *post hoc* Turkey's test was used for determining the statistical differences between groups. For all analyses, a P value less than 0.05 was considered statistically significant. All experiments were performed in triplicates and repeated at least three times.

3. Results

3.1 Recombinant bacmid-FGF8b construction and baculovirus generation

To produce recombinant hFGF8b protein, recombinant plasmids bearing the optimized hFGF8b gene were con-

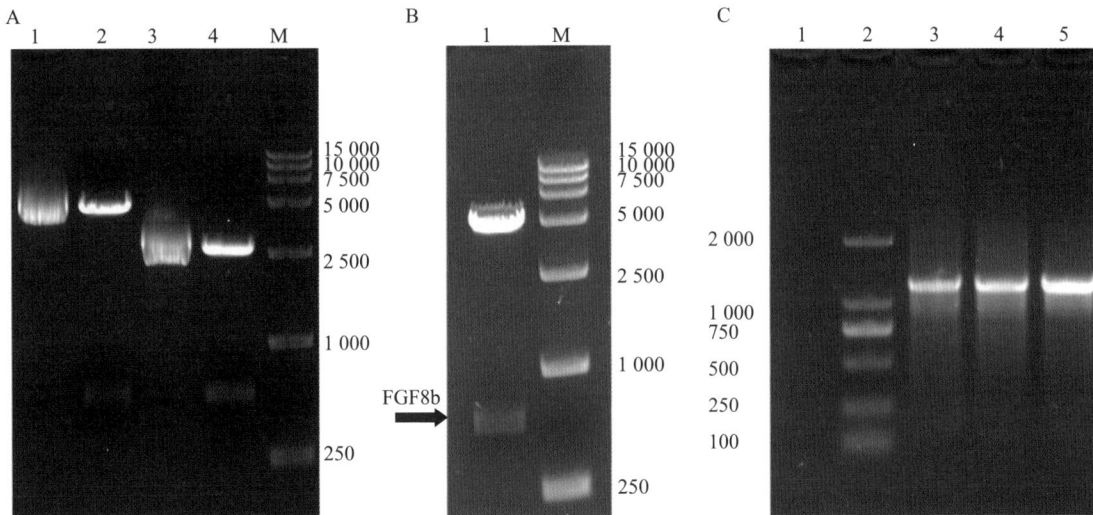

Fig. 1. Agarose gel electrophoresis was undertaken to analyze enzyme-digested products. The strategy for construction of pFastbac-FGF8b is described in "materials and methods." The molecular weight of the enzyme digestion (*Bam*HI and *Hin*dIII) fragments are shown in (A) *lanes 1* and *3* PUC57-rhFGF8b and pFastbac-KGF1, *lanes 2* and *4* restriction products of PUC57-rhFGF8b and pFastbac-KGF1, respectively. Identification of recombinant plasmid by enzyme digestion (*Bam*HI and *Hin*dIII) is shown in (B) *lane 1* restriction products of pFastbac-FGF8b. The bacmid-FGF8b PCR amplification analysis. is shown in (C) *lane 1* negative control, *lane 2* DNA Marker DL 2000, *lanes 3, 4* and *5* bacmid transposed with pFastBac-FGF8b.

structed. DNA sequence encoding of the optimized human FGF8b was excisable with *Bam*HI and *Hin*dIII (Fig. 1A) from the pUC57-FGF8b vector, and it was around 600 bp. The aim gene was cloned in the transfer vector pFastBac and further confirmed by restriction enzymatic analysis (Fig. 1B) and DNA sequencing. The results of the sequences of rhFGF8b (595 bp) conformed to the desired sequence. The correct transfer vectors were transformed into DH10 Bac *E. coli*, and white-blue plaque selection was conducted. White colonies were PCR amplified by gene special primers (Fig. 1C), and the right recombinant bacmid-FGF8b was transfected into Sf9 cells by liposomes to collect the baculovirus stock. The construction strategy and detailed procedure are described in "materials and methods".

3.2　Expression and optimization of rhFGF8b production in Sf9 cells

To determine the optimal condition for FGF8b expression, the expression was monitored by Western blot. Fig. 2 shows the Western blot results of the rhFGF8b proteins at various time points postinfection in cell lysates. rhFGF8b protein bands were clearly recognized by the antibody, and the sizes of rhFGF8b protein bands were consistent and as expected at around 23 kDa. FGF8b was detectable in cell lysates at around 36 h and reached a maximum at 60 h. Additionally, MOI of 8 pfu/ml was suitable for harvest. However, rhFGF8b proteins at various time points postinfection in medium supernatants were instable (data not shown), possibly because cell lysis occurring at the end of the cultivation could compromise the quantity and quality of the rhFGF8b produced (by release of proteases or other factors).

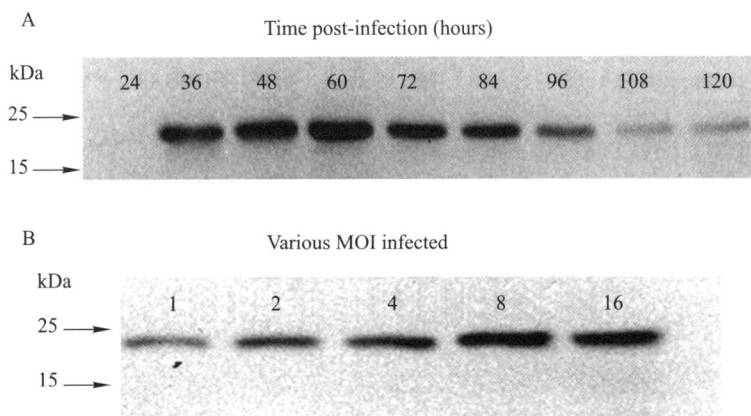

Fig. 2. Western blot analyses of recombinant FGF8b expression in different infection time and MOI. Detailed steps are provided in "material and methods". The molecular size of rhFGF8b is approximately 23 kDa (A, B) as expected. A polyclonal antihFGF8b antibody was used for the Western blot analysis.

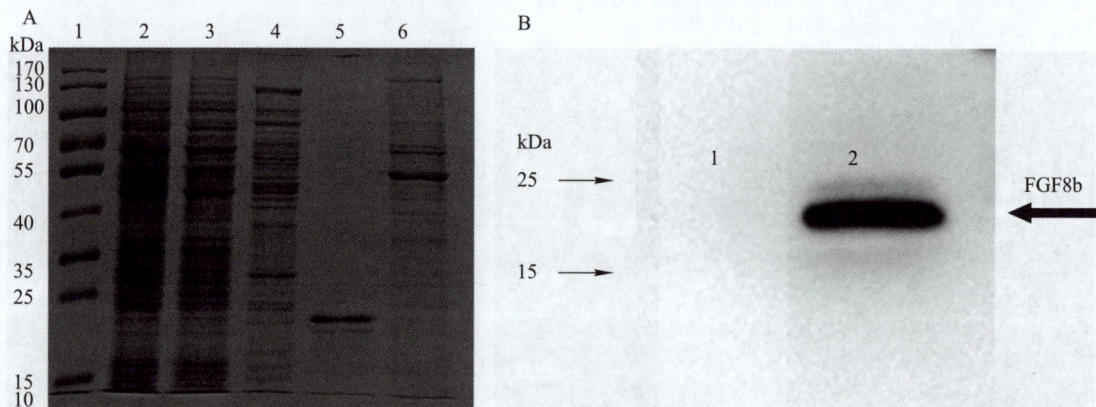

Fig. 3. SDS-PAGE analysis of purification of rhFGF8b and its characterization by Western blotting. (A) SDS-PAGE analysis of the fraction collected from heparin-affinity chromatography. *Lane 1* cell lysates, *lane 2* flow though, *lane 3* 0.6 M NaCl-eluted fraction, *lane 4,* 1.2 M NaCl-eluted fraction, *lane 5* 2.0 M NaCl-eluted fraction, *lane M* protein Ladder. (B) Western blot analysis of individual fractions. *Lane 1* 0.6 M NaCl-eluted fraction, *lane 2* 1.2 M NaCl-eluted fraction. A polyclonal anti-hFGF8b antibody was used for the Western blot analysis.

3.3 Purification and identification of rhFGF8b

Next, the soluble fraction of proteins from the cell lysates were purified as described in "materials and methods". As shown in Fig. 3, the fractions containing rhFGF8b were finally eluted by heparin-affinity chromatography in a single major peak using 50 mM PB containing 1.2 M NaCl (Fig. 3A). The recovered rhFGF8b was homogenous, with a purity of over 90%, as analyzed by SDS-PAGE (Fig. 3A). Western blotting analysis (Fig. 3B) with a specific anti-human FGF8b antibody showed a good immunoreactivity with the target protein.

3.4 Mitogenic activity of recombinant hFGF8b

The biological activity of purified recombinant hFGF8b was tested on stimulating proliferation of NIH3T3 cells using a standard MTT assay and compared with human bFGF (positive control, Sino Biological Inc, Beijing) because it has been well confirmed that bFGF can strongly influence active DNA synthesis in NIH3T3 cells and exhibit relatively good neuroprotective effects (de Oliveira *et al.,* 2010; Litteljohn and Hayley, 2012). As shown in Fig. 4, similar to bFGF, the purified rhFGF8b was able to stimulate the proliferation of NIH3T3 cells in a dose-dependent manner, ranging from 0.5–64 nM, which is consistent with the findings of previous studies (Ghosh *et al.,* 1996; Ohuchi *et al.,* 1994). Thus, we speculate that rhFGF8b produced with this method had a remarkable mitogenic effect on NIH3T3 cells.

3.5 Neuroprotective activity of rhFGF8b in PC12 cells

PC12 cells treated with different concentrations of MPP$^+$ for 48 h exhibited attenuated cell viability in a dose-dependent manner (Fig. 5A). As shown in Fig. 5A, B, treatment with 500 μmol/L MPP$^+$ significantly decreased the sur-

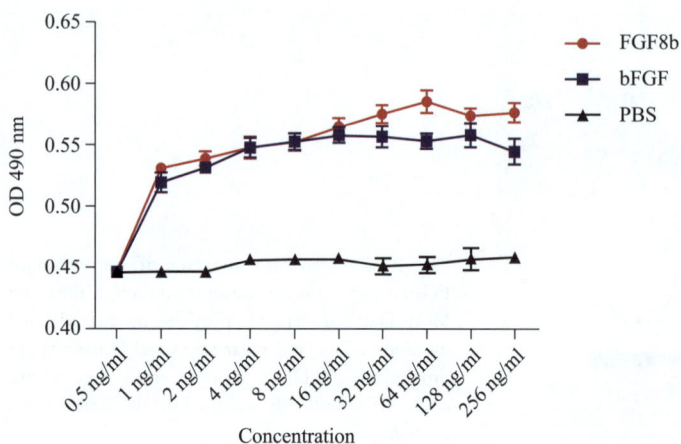

Fig. 4. Mitogenic activity analysis of different concentrations of rhFGF8b and bFGF on NIH3T3 cells *in vitro.* Cells were treated as described in "materials and methods". Cell proliferation was determined by the MTT method. PBS was used as a negative control.

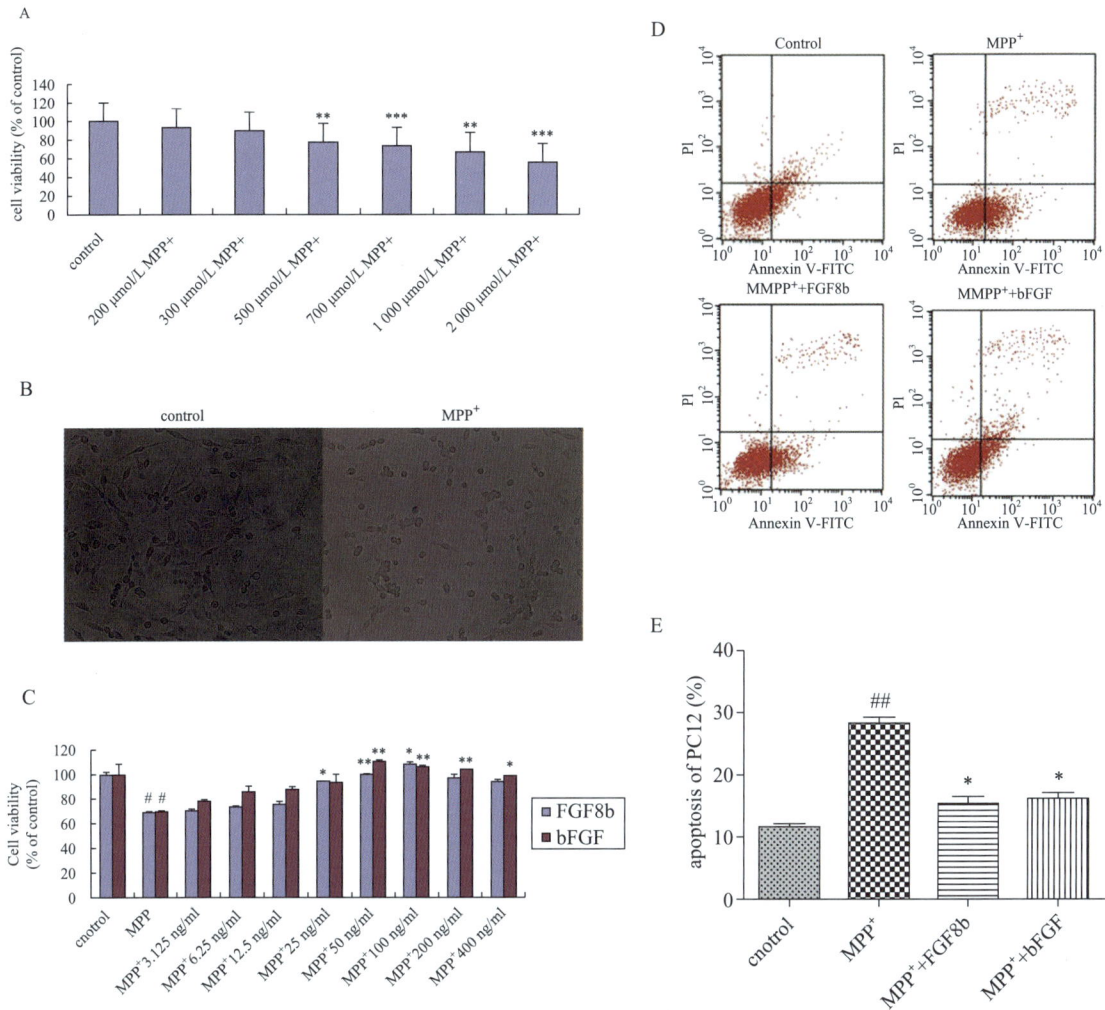

Fig. 5. Neuroprotective activity of rhFGF8b in PC12 cells. (A) Cell model of Parkinson's disease. MPP$^+$-induced PC12 cell injury observed by the MTT method. (B) Microscope observed MPP$^+$-induced PC12 cell injury. Scale bars 100 μm. (C) Proliferation promotion effect of FGF8b on the cell model of PD. Cells were treated as described in "materials and methods". Cell viability was determined by the MTT method. (D) Protection effect of rhFGF8b on PC12 cells was further analyzed by Annexin-V/PI double staining. (E) Quantitative evaluation of cell apoptosis. All data are presented as mean±SEM. $^*P<0.05$, $^{**}P<0.01$, $^{***}P<0.001$ compared with the control group; $^#P<0.05$, $^{##}P<0.01$ compared with the injury group.

vival of PC12 cells and inhibited neurite outgrowth compared with that by PBS treatment. Next, the protective effects of rhFGF8b and bFGF were examined by pretreatment for 2 h prior to MPP$^+$ administration. The results showed that similar to bFGF, the purified rhFGF8b significantly protected the cells against neuronal injury, and stimulation of cell proliferation reached maximum for FGF8b at approximately 100 ng/ml (Fig. 5C). To identify whether anti-apoptotic activity contributed to the neuroprotective action of rhFGF8b, we examined the effect of rhFGF8b and bFGF on MPP$^+$-induced apoptosis in PC12 cells. Annexin-V/PI double staining indicated that the protective effects of rhFGF8b (100 ng/ml) prevented necrosis and inhibited apoptosis as well as bFGF (50 ng/ ml) (Fig. 5D, E).

3.6 rhFGF8b protection against ER stress in vitro

To preliminarily explore the molecular mechanisms of FGF8b, the effect of FGF8b on mRNA levels of apoptosis and ERS-related genes was investigated by qRT-PCR during MPP$^+$-induced PC12 cell injury. Bcl-xl, Caspase3, and bax are important markers for apoptosis. The fate of cells is thought to be determined by the balance between proapoptotic and anti-apoptotic genes. FGF8b (100 ng/ml) significantly increased anti-apoptotic gene Bcl-xl mRNA levels after a pre-treatment for 2 h prior to MPP$^+$ (500 μmol/L) administration (Fig. 6A). FGF8b also suppressed increased levels of proapoptotic genes Caspase3 and bax that were induced by MPP$^+$ (Fig. 6A).

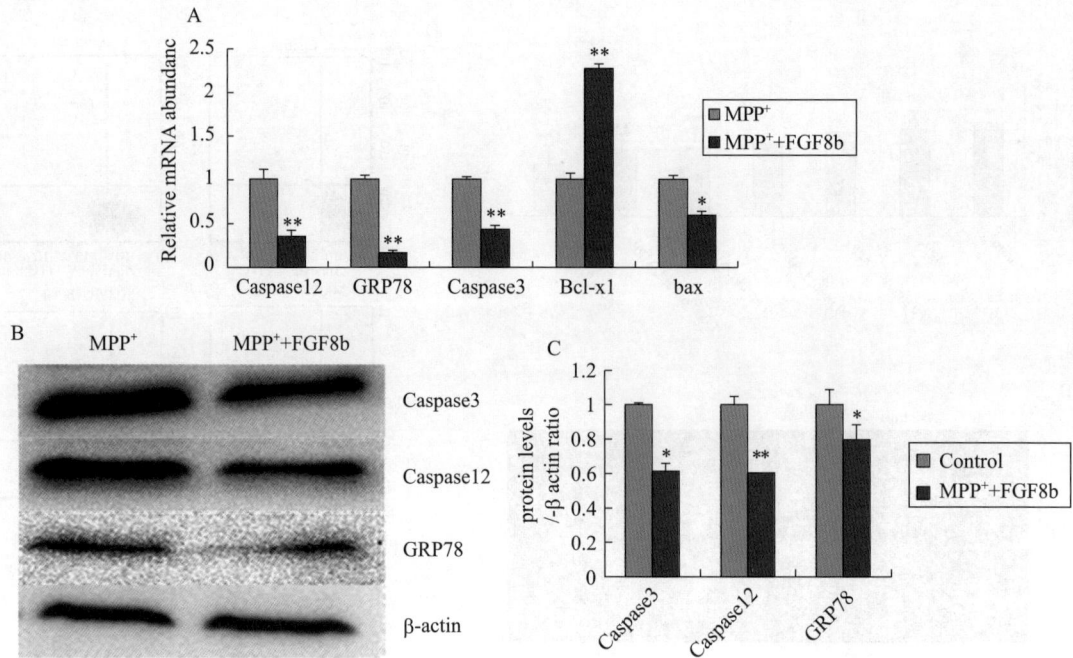

Fig. 6. The molecular mechanisms of the neuroprotective activity of FGF8b in PC12 cells. (A) Effect of FGF8b on mRNA expression levels of Caspase12, GRP78, Caspase3, Bcl-xl, and bax. Cells were treated as described in "materials and methods". Abundance of mRNA was measured by real-time PCR. (B) Western blot analysis of Caspase3, Caspase12, GRP78, and actin (loading control) proteins. Cells were treated as described in "materials and methods". (C) Quantitative evaluation of Caspase3, Caspase12, and GRP78 expression. β-actin was used as an internal standard. All data are presented as mean±SEM. $^*P<0.05$, $^{**}P<0.01$ compared with the injury group.

Glucose-regulated protein (GRP78) plays an important role in ER stress response by activating molecules like IRE1, PERK, and ATF6, which result in unfolded protein response (UPR). Overexpression of GRP78 occurs during MPP$^+$ injury, and upregulated expression of GRP78 can restore proteins to their correct conformation and provide protection for cell survival (Liu et al., 1997). However, if the ER stress is prolonged, then UPR activates apoptotic signaling (Pluquet et al., 2015). As shown in Fig. 6, mRNA levels of Caspase12 and GRP78 (ER stress-associated apoptosis factor and ER stress-inducible molecular chaperone, respectively) were reduced by FGF8b (Fig. 6A). The result indicated that FGF8b might protect PC12 cells against ER stress induced by MPP$^+$.

To confirm that FGF8b could inhibit apoptosis and protect against ER stress, the expression levels of the proapoptotic protein Caspase3 and ER stress markers, Caspase12 and GRP78, were analyzed by immunoblotting. In agreement with the real-time PCR data, FGF8b (100 ng/ml) caused significant decreases in protein levels of Caspase3, Caspase12, and GRP78 (Fig. 6B, C). These results indicated that FGF8b could protect PC12 cells against ER stress induced by MPP$^+$.

4. Discussion

A wealth of pharmacological studies have previously demonstrated that FGF8 is a promising therapeutic candidate for neurodegenerative diseases because of its multitude of activities on nervous tissue and its role in improving development and function of dopaminergic neurons (Roussa and Krieglstein, 2004). In addition, FGF8 is considered to have an important biological role during embryonic development, especially in brain development, gastrulation, and limb morphogenesis (Heikinheimo et al., 1994; Ohuchi et al., 1994). In particular, with regard to mesencephalic development, FGF8 is expressed in cardiac mesoderm underlying the mesencephalic/metencephalic region (Crossley and Martin 1995; Heikinheimo et al., 1994; Mahmood et al., 1995). As such, it is necessary to develop methods that allow for abundant production of FGF8 with high bioactivity for future specific treatment of FGF8-related diseases. As the predominantly expressed species, although recombinant FGF8b has been expressed previously, the low level of expression and difficulty in producing highly bioactive protein has restricted further research and application. A widely used method to evade these limitations is the fusion strategy expression of target protein, such as His6-tagged, GST-tagged, and Halotagged. However, these methods have shortcomings in terms of efficient soluble expression and bioactivity (Sun *et al.,* 2015). Specifically, to achieve release of a target protein, the removal of the fused tag must be performed. However, the cleavage reaction is expensive and may impact the bioactivity of the target protein. Here, we report a rapid and efficient strategy to express and purify high levels of recombinant hFGF8b.

In our experiments, we successfully expressed rhFGF8b in Sf9 cells. The IC-BEVS not only is very simple and rapid but also enables efficient purification of proteins from cell lysate supernatant. More importantly, by optimizing the gene sequence and expression conditions, we obtained mature rhFGF8b with the removed signal peptide. Like other fibroblast growth factors, FGF8b had a strong affinity to heparin. In addition, Heparin Sepharose chromatography has been routinely used for the separation and purification of some therapeutic proteins (Berman *et al.,* 1999; Huang *et al.,* 2012; Kenig *et al.,* 2008). Therefore, we used Heparin Sepharose to efficiently separate rhFGF8b from undesirable impurities of the cell lysate supernatant. The molecular size of purified rhFGF8b was a little higher than that expressed in an *E. coli* expression system (Huang *et al.,* 2013), which may be caused by distinct modifications in insect cells. The purified recombinant human FGF8b protein was biologically active *in vitro*. Like bFGF, FGF8b could significantly stimulate the proliferation of NIH3T3 cells in a dose-dependent manner, which is consistent with the finding of previous studies (Ghosh *et al.,* 1996). Interestingly, rhFGF8b expressed in Sf9 cells displayed better biological activity than that of prokaryotic expression (Huang *et al.,* 2013). Thus, FGF8b expression in IC-BEVS not only is efficient but also results in high biological activity.

As described previously, FGF8 is able to nourish the neural stem cells and induce DA neurons (Tanaka *et al.,* 2001; Ye *et al.,* 1998). Thus, we considered that FGF8b may have neuroprotective effects for neurodegenerative diseases. The PC12 cell line, the classic cell model for neuroprotective assays relevant to PD, was chosen to assess the neuroprotective activity and molecular mechanism of FGF8b. MPP^+ is a classic neurotoxin that is commonly used for induction of Parkinsonism and testing of therapeutic candidates. Hence, we used a MPP^+-induced cell model of PD to investigate the neuroprotective effects of FGF8b. MPP^+ treatment of PC12 cells caused extensive necrosis and apoptosis, and induced a significant decline in the concentrations of striatal monoamine neurotransmitters and their metabolites (DA, HVA and DOPAC). In addition, MPP^+ exposure increased the expression of ER stress markers, Caspase12 and GRP78, indicating that MPP^+ induced ER stress activation (Omura *et al.,* 2012). However, similar to bFGF, pretreatment with FGF8b for 2 h efficiently protected cells from MPP^+-induced cell death by preventing apoptosis (Fig. 5).

ER stress is one of the causative factors in the development of PD (Lindholm *et al.,* 2006; Yoshida, 2007). It has been demonstrated that MPP^+, which is used experimentally to create models of sporadic PD, induces ER stress (Omura *et al.,* 2012). Thus, we hypothesized that the molecular site of FGF8b action would be related to ER stress. First, we confirmed that treatment with MPP^+ and FGF8b decreased mRNA levels of ER stress markers, Caspase12 and GRP78, and proapoptotic genes, Caspase3 and bax (Fig. 6A). We also observed that the anti-apoptotic gene, Bcl-xl mRNA levels were significantly upregulated after FGF8b exposure (Fig. 6A). Consistent with this mRNA result, decreased protein levels of Caspase12 and GRP78, and Caspase3 were observed 48 h after FGF8b exposure (Fig. 6B, C). These results indicate that FGF8b exerts a protective function by alleviating ER stress.

In summary, mature recombinant human FGF8b was successfully expressed in Sf9 cells by baculoviral vectors from a codon-optimized FGF8b gene. Purification was undertaken using heparin-affinity chromatography, and the identity of the purified protein was confirmed by Western blot analysis. The rhFGF8b could significantly stimulate proliferation of NIH3T3 cells. *In vitro*, FGF8b efficiently maintains cell survival and decreases the amount of cell apoptosis and necrosis in a MPP^+-induced cell model of PD. FGF8b exerts neuroprotective effects by alleviating ER stress during PD. This study demonstrates that rhFGF8b expression in IC-BEVS is a viable and convenient method to achieve highly efficient expression and purification of FGF8b with high bioactivity preserved, and FGF8b may have therapeutic potential for the treatment of PD and neurodegenerative disorders related to ER stress.

References

Aarsland D, Pahlhagen S, Ballard CG, *et al.* Depression in Parkinson disease--epidemiology, mechanisms and management[J]. Nat Rev Neurol, 2011, 8(1): 35-47.

Baba M, Nakajo S, Tu PH, *et al.* Aggregation of alpha-synuclein in

Lewy bodies of sporadic Parkinson's disease and dementia with Lewy bodies[J]. Am J Pathol, 1998, 152(4): 879-884.

Berman B, Ostrovsky O, Shlissel M, *et al.* Similarities and differences between the effects of heparin and glypican-1 on the bioactivity of acidic fibroblast growth factor and the keratinocyte growth factor[J]. J Biol Chem, 1999, 274(51): 36132-36138.

Carinhas N, Bernal V, Yokomizo AY, et al. Baculovirus production for gene therapy: the role of cell density, multiplicity of infection and medium exchange[J]. Appl Microbiol Biotechnol, 2009, 81(6): 1041-1049.

Crossley PH, Martin GR. The mouse Fgf8 gene encodes a family of polypeptides and is expressed in regions that direct outgrowth and patterning in the developing embryo[J]. Development, 1995, 121(2): 439-451.

de Oliveira GP, Duobles T, Castelucci P, et al. Differential regulation of FGF-2 in neurons and reactive astrocytes of axotomized rat hypo-glossal nucleus. A possible therapeutic target for neuroprotection in peripheral nerve pathology[J]. Acta Histochem, 2010, 112(6): 604-617.

Dong X, Tang B, Li J, et al. Expression and purification of intact and functional soybean (Glycine max) seed ferritin complex in Esch-erichia coli[J]. J Microbiol Biotechnol, 2008, 18(2): 299-307.

Drugmand JC, Schneider YJ, Agathos SN. Insect cells as factories for biomanufacturing[J]. Biotechnol Adv, 2012, 30(5): 1140-1157.

Gemel J, Gorry M, Ehrlich GD, et al. Structure and sequence of human FGF8[J]. Genomics, 1996, 35(1): 253-257.

Ghosh AK, Shankar DB, Shackleford GM, et al. Molecular cloning and characterization of human FGF8 alternative messenger RNA forms[J]. Cell Growth Differ, 1996, 7(10): 1425-1434.

Gnanapragasam VJ, Robinson MC, Marsh C, et al. FGF8 isoform b expression in human prostate cancer[J]. Br J Cancer, 2003, 88(9): 1432-1438.

Heikinheimo M, Lawshe A, Shackleford GM, et al. Fgf-8 expression in the post-gastrulation mouse suggests roles in the development of the face, limbs and central nervous system[J]. Mech Dev, 1994, 48(2): 129-138.

Hetz C, Chevet E, Harding HP. Targeting the unfolded protein response in disease[J]. Nat Rev Drug Discov, 2013, 12(9): 703-719.

Huang Z, Ye C, Liu Z, et al. Solid-phase N-terminus PEGylation of re-combinant human fibroblast growth factor 2 on heparin-sepharose column[J]. Bioconjug Chem, 2012, 23(4): 740-750.

Huang P, Wang Z, Tian H, et al. The Constructing and Purification of Recombinant Human Fibroblast Growth Factor 8b Expressed Vector[J]. China Biotechnology, 2013, 33(1): 14-19.

Kenig M, Gaberc-Porekar V, Fonda I, et al. Identification of the heparin-binding domain of TNF-alpha and its use for efficient TNF-alpha purification by heparin-Sepharose affinity chromatography[J]. J Chromatogr B Analyt Technol Biomed Life Sci, 2008, 867(1): 119-125.

Kwabi-Addo B, Ozen M, Ittmann M. The role of fibroblast growth fac-tors and their receptors in prostate cancer[J]. Endocr Relat Cancer, 2004, 11(4): 709-724.

Lindholm D, Wootz H, Korhonen L. ER stress and neurodegenerative diseases[J]. Cell Death Differ, 2006, 13(3): 385-392.

Litteljohn D, Hayley S. Cytokines as potential biomarkers for Parkin-son's disease: a multiplex approach[J]. Methods Mol Biol, 2012, 934: 121-144.

Liu H, Bowes RC, 3rd, van de Water B, et al. Endoplasmic reticulum chaperones GRP78 and calreticulin prevent oxidative stress, Ca^{2+} disturbances, and cell death in renal epithelial cells[J]. J Biol Chem, 1997, 272(35): 21751-21759.

Lorenzi MV, Long JE, Miki T, et al. Expression cloning, developmen-tal expression and chromosomal localization of fibroblast growth factor-8[J]. Oncogene, 1995, 10(10): 2051-2055.

Mahmood R, Bresnick J, Hornbruch A, et al. A role for FGF-8 in the initiation and maintenance of vertebrate limb bud outgrowth[J]. Curr Biol, 1995, 5(7): 797-806.

Mattila MM, Ruohola JK, Valve EM, et al. FGF-8b increases angiogenic capacity and tumor growth of androgen-regulated S115 breast can-cer cells[J]. Oncogene, 2001, 20(22): 2791-2804.

Ohuchi H, Yoshioka H, Tanaka A, et al. Involvement of androgen-

induced growth factor (FGF-8) gene in mouse embryogenesis and morphogenesis[J]. Biochem Biophys Res Commun, 1994, 204(2): 882-888.

Omura T, Asari M, Yamamoto J, et al. HRD1 levels increased by zonisamide prevented cell death and caspase-3 activation caused by endoplasmic reticulum stress in SH-SY5Y cells[J]. J Mol Neurosci, 2012, 46(3): 527-535.

Payson RA, Wu J, Liu Y, et al. The human FGF-8 gene localizes on chromosome 10q24 and is subjected to induction by androgen in breast cancer cells[J]. Oncogene, 1996, 13(1): 47-53.

Pfaffl MW. A new mathematical model for relative quantification in real-time RT-PCR[J]. Nucleic Acids Res, 2001, 29(9): e45.

Pluquet O, Pourtier A, Abbadie C. The unfolded protein response and cellular senescence. A review in the theme: cellular mechanisms of endoplasmic reticulum stress signaling in health and disease[J]. Am J Physiol Cell Physiol, 2015, 308(6): C415-C425.

Potula HH, Kathuria SR, Ghosh AK, et al. Transient expression, puri-fication and characterization of bioactive human fibroblast growth factor 8b in tobacco plants[J]. Transgenic Res, 2008, 17(1): 19-32.

Rodriguez-Oroz MC, Jahanshahi M, Krack P, et al. Initial clinical mani-festations of Parkinson's disease: features and pathophysiological mechanisms[J]. Lancet Neurol, 2009, 8(12): 1128-1139.

Roussa E, Krieglstein K. Induction and specification of midbrain dopa-minergic cells: focus on SHH, FGF8, and TGF-beta[J]. Cell Tissue Res, 2004, 318(1): 23-33.

Schapira AH, Olanow CW. Neuroprotection in Parkinson disease: mys-teries, myths, and misconceptions[J]. Jama, 2004, 291(3): 358-364.

Shrivastava P, Vaibhav K, Tabassum R, et al. Anti-apoptotic and anti-inflammatory effect of Piperine on 6-OHDA induced Parkinson's rat model[J]. J Nutr Biochem, 2013, 24(4): 680-687.

Sun X, Meyers EN, Lewandoski M, et al. Targeted disruption of Fgf8 causes failure of cell migration in the gastrulating mouse embryo[J]. Genes Dev, 1999, 13(14): 1834-1846.

Sun C, Li Y, Taylor SE, et al. HaloTag is an effective expression and sol-ubilisation fusion partner for a range of fibroblast growth factors[J]. PeerJ, 2015, 3: e1060.

Tanaka A, Miyamoto K, Minamino N, et al. Cloning and characterization of an androgen-induced growth factor essential for the androgen-dependent growth of mouse mammary carcinoma cells[J]. Proc Natl Acad Sci U S A, 1992, 89(19): 8928-8932.

Tanaka A, Furuya A, Yamasaki M, et al. High frequency of fibroblast growth factor (FGF) 8 expression in clinical prostate cancers and breast tissues, immunohistochemically demonstrated by a newly established neutralizing monoclonal antibody against FGF 8[J]. Cancer Res, 1998, 58(10): 2053-2056.

Tanaka A, Kamiakito T, Hakamata Y, et al. Extensive neuronal localiza-tion and neurotrophic function of fibroblast growth factor 8 in the nervous system[J]. Brain Res, 2001, 912(2): 105-115.

Trowitzsch S, Bieniossek C, Nie Y, et al. New baculovirus expression tools for recombinant protein complex production[J]. J Struct Biol, 2010, 172(1): 45-54.

Uchii M, Tamura T, Suda T, et al. Role of fibroblast growth factor 8 (FGF8) in animal models of osteoarthritis[J]. Arthritis Res Ther, 2008, 10(4): R90.

Volmer R, van der Ploeg K, Ron D. Membrane lipid saturation acti-vates endoplasmic reticulum unfolded protein response transducers through their transmembrane domains[J]. Proc Natl Acad Sci U S A, 2013, 110(12): 4628-4633.

Ye W, Shimamura K, Rubenstein JL, et al. FGF and Shh signals con-trol dopaminergic and serotonergic cell fate in the anterior neural plate[J]. Cell, 1998, 93(5): 755-766.

Yoshida H. ER stress and diseases[J]. FEBS J, 2007, 274(3): 630-658.

Zhong C, Saribekyan G, Liao CP, et al. Cooperation between FGF8b overexpression and PTEN deficiency in prostate tumorigenesis[J]. Cancer Res, 2006, 66(4): 2188-2194.

High production in *E. coli* of biologically active recombinant human fibroblast growth factor 20 and its neuroprotective effects

Haishan Tian, Xiaokun Li

1. Introduction

Fibroblast growth factor (FGF) 20 is a paracrine member of the FGF family (Kirikoshi *et al.*, 2000) and is predominantly expressed in the brain, with much lower expression in other tissues (Jeffers *et al.*, 2002; Jeffers *et al.*, 2001; Maclachlan *et al.*, 2005; Ohmachi *et al.*, 2000). Previous work has shown that FGF20 is an endogenous neurotrophic factor expressed in dopaminergic neurons within the substantia nigra pars compacta (Ohmachi *et al.*, 2000), where it can enhance their survival (Ohmachi *et al.*, 2003). In later work (Takagi *et al.*, 2005), FGF20 was shown to promote the differentiation of monkey embryonic stem cells into dopaminergic neurons, which when injected into the brain of monkeys with experimental Parkinson's disease, it alleviated some of the symptoms of the disease. Genetic analyses have suggested a link between a polymorphism in *fgf20* and Parkinson's disease. For example, analysis of 644 families (van der Walt *et al.*, 2004) showed a highly significant association of Parkinson's disease single nucleotide polymorphisms located in intronic and the 3′ regulatory region of *fgf20*. Although not all subsequent studies agree (de Mena *et al.*, 2010), the current balance of evidence is that at least some of these polymorphisms underlie the disease process (Ma *et al.*, 2015; Zhu *et al.*, 2014). At a mechanistic level, it has been found that the rs12720208 single nucleotide polymorphism results in a switch of miRNA binding, which appears to be a potential driver of the disease (Wang *et al.*, 2008). Further work has shown that FGF20 promotes differentiation of human embryonic stem cells into dopaminergic neurons and that in the rat, it has similar protective effects to those found in monkey (Shimada *et al.*, 2009; Sleeman *et al.*, 2012). These data demonstrate that the levels of FGF20 must be appropriately controlled to maintain brain homeostasis and that FGF20 has the potential to be used in treating some neurodegenerative diseases due to its capacity to induce dopaminergic neuron differentiation from embryonic stem cells and its neuroprotective activity.

Some neurodegenerative diseases have been shown to result in endoplasmic reticulum stress (ER stress), causing neuronal apoptosis (Swietnicki, 2006). ER stress is one of the causative factors in the development of Alzheimer's disease (Ansari and Khodagholi, 2013). It has been demonstrated that the amyloidogenic Aβ25–35 peptide, which is used experimentally to create models of Alzheimer's disease, induces ER stress (Liu *et al.*, 2009). Thus, it is of interest to determine if the neuroprotective effects of FGF20 extend to reducing or preventing ER stress caused by Aβ25–35, since this would increase the therapeutic possibilities of FGF20. Establishing the therapeutic potential of FGF20 will require large amounts of active protein for biological, preclinical, and eventual clinical studies.

As the first step in the evaluation of FGF20's therapeutic possibilities, we have developed a means to produce large amounts of biologically active recombinant human FGF20 (rhFGF20). We constructed an optimized recombinant human FGF20 expression vector (pET3a-rhFGF20) and used *E. coli* BL21(DE3)pLysS to successfully express high levels of rhFGF20, which was insoluble. The rhFGF20 was efficiently refolded and purified in a single step by an on-column heparin affinity approach. The rhFGF20 was found to have a mitogenic activity in both NIH 3T3 cells and PC-12 cells and protected the latter from Aβ25–35-induced apoptosis, an established *in vitro* model of this aspect of Alzheimer's disease. RT-PCR and Western blot analyses indicated that the rhFGF20-mediated protection mechanism operated *via* an ER stress anti-apoptotic mechanism. Thus, the rhFGF20 has high activity and substantial promise for fundamental research that may lead to the development of therapeutic applications.

2. Materials and methods

2.1 Reagents and bacterial strain

The gel extraction kit, bicinchoninic acid (BCA) kit, plasmid miniprep kit, RNAiso Plus, realtime PCR reagent kit, and restriction enzymes *Nde* I and *Bam*H I were all purchased from TaKaRa Company (Dalian, China). The lactate dehydrogenase (LDH) kit was purchased from Nanjing Jiancheng Company (Nanjing, China). SYBR was purchased from Roche Company (Roche, Germany). Isopropyl-β-D-thiogalactoside (IPTG) and methylthiazol tetrazolium (MTT) were purchased from Bio-Tech (Gold Bio-Technology, MO). Dulbecco's modified Eagle's medium (DMEM) and fetal bovine serum (FBS) were purchased from Invitrogen (Carlsbad, CA). Aβ25–35 was purchased from Sigma-Aldrich (Sigma, USA). PC-12 cells and NIH 3T3cells were purchased from the library of the Shanghai Institute of Cell Biology Institute library (Shanghai, China). The HiTrap heparin Sepharose was purchased from GE Healthcare (Piscataway, USA). Rabbit anti-human FGF20 polyclonal antibody, rabbit antirat caspase 12 polyclonal antibody, rabbit antirat GRP78 polyclonal antibody, and goat antirat β-actin polyclonal antibody were all purchased from Abcam Inc. (Abcam, USA). The expression vectors pET3a, *E. coli* DH5α, and BL21(DE3)pLysS were obtained from our own laboratory (Wenzhou Medical University, China).

2.2 Construction of rhFGF20 expression vector

The coding sequence of *hFGF20* (corresponding to the amino acid sequence of human FGF20, GenBank accession number NM-019851.2) was enzymatically digested with *Nde* I and *Bam*H I (TaKaRa) and then ligated into the previously digested pET3a expression vector to produce the pET3a-rhFGF20 construct. The construct was then transformed into *E. coli* DH5α. The correct insertion of the cDNA into the plasmid was validated by restriction enzyme analysis.

2.3 rhFGF20 induction and expression

The expression vector pET3a-rhFGF20 was transformed into *E. coli* BL21(DE3)pLysS. Colonies were picked and grown in 5 ml of LB medium both containing 100 μg/ml of ampicillin and 34 μg/ml of chloramphenicol at 37 ℃ until the A_{600} reached 0.6–0.8. IPTG (Bio-Tech) was then added to a final concentration of 1 mM, and the culture was incubated at 37 ℃ for 4 h. The protein from samples of each culture was analyzed by 12% (*v/v*) SDS-PAGE, and rhFGF20 levels were determined by densitometric scanning. Finally, the colony with the highest expression level was used as the seed strain for subsequent high-density fermentation.

2.4 Large-scale fermentation of rhFGF20

The seed strain pET3a-rhFGF20-BL21(DE3)pLysS was cultivated in 100 ml LB medium with ampicillin (100 μg/ml) and chloramphenicol (34 μg/ml) with rotation at 200 rpm and 37 ℃. When A_{600} reached 0.8–1.2, the culture was transferred into 1 000 ml of the modified medium containing tryptone (10 g/L), yeast extract (10 g/L), KH_2PO_4 (2.5 g/L), K_2HPO_4 (1 g/L), NaCl (4 g/L), and glycerol (6 g/L), pH 7.5, and incubated with shaking at 180 rpm and 37 ℃. When A_{600} reached 3–5, the culture was transferred to a 30-L fermenter containing fermentation medium composed of tryptone (16 g/L), yeast extract (16 g/L), KH_2PO_4 (2.5 g/L), K_2HPO_4 (1 g/L), NaCl (4 g/L), and sugarcane molasses (5 ml/L). After being cultured for 2 h, the trophic medium including $MgSO_4$ (1 g/L), glucose solution (50%), and cultivation solution (10 g/L tryptone, 10 g/L yeast extract, 2.5 g/L KH_2PO_4, 1.0 g/L K_2HPO_4, and 4 g/L NaCl) was added by turns. The culture was kept under this condition until A_{600} reached 18–22, at which point it was fed IPTG to a final concentration of 1 mM to begin induction. After induction for 4 h, cells were harvested *via* centrifugation at 9 000 rpm for 10 min at 4 ℃, and the cell pellet was frozen at −80 ℃. As shown in Table 1, we summarized the fermentation parameters of three batches.

2.5 Isolation of inclusion bodies

Soluble detection of rhFGF20 was performed as follows. The resulting frozen cell pellet was thawed and resuspended in ice-cold 20 mM Tris-Cl buffer (pH 7.5), which contained 5 mM EDTA–2Na, 1% (*v/v*) Triton-X-100, and 150 mM NaCl at a ratio of 1 g cell pellet to 10 ml Tris-Cl buffer. The cell suspension was sonicated in an ice bath, and

Table 1.　The fermentation parameters of three batches

	Before induction					After induction			
Time (h)	1	2	3	4	4.5	1	2	3	4
Temperature (℃)	37.00 ± 0.01	37.02 ± 0.02	36.99 ± 0.02	37.01 ± 0.01	37.00 ± 0.02	35.00 ± 0.02	35.00 ± 0.01	34.97 ± 0.03	34.99 ± 0.01
pH	6.92 ± 0.05	6.95 ± 0.03	6.97 ± 0.04	6.96 ± 0.03	6.98 ± 0.02	7.15 ± 0.03	7.21 ± 0.02	7.18 ± 0.04	7.20 ± 0.03
Oxygen level (%)	80.5 ± 2.13	65.1 ± 1.97	36.5 ± 2.30	28.2 ± 1.21	25.5 ± 1.72	25.3 ± 2.90	28.5 ± 1.88	40.8 ± 1.22	53.4 ± 1.92
A_{600}	1.02 ± 0.10	249 ± 0.16	5.15 ± 0.63	13.14 ± 0.51	21.32 ± 0.69	34.14 ± 1.45	40.13 ± 1.39	43.15 ± 1.06	45.12 ± 1.25
rotation	200	300	650	650	650	650	650	550	450

Data are presented as the mean ± SDs of three batches.

insoluble material was collected by centrifugation at 20 000 rpm for 30 min at 4℃.

2.6　Washing of the inclusion body protein

The resulting pellet comprised the inclusion body protein, which was washed using wash buffer I (20 mM Tris-Cl, 2 mM EDTA-2Na, 0.2% (w/v) sodium deoxycholate, 1% (v/v) Triton X-100, pH 7.5) and resuspended and centrifuged at 20,000 rpm for 30 min at 4℃. The pellet was then washed twice with wash buffer II (20 mM Tris-Cl, 2 mM EDTA-2Na, 1% (v/v) Triton X-100, pH 7.5), and the final pellet was washed in wash buffer III (20 mM Tris-Cl, 2 mM EDTA-2Na, 2 M urea, pH 7.5).

2.7　Solubilization and refolding of the inclusion body protein

The inclusion body proteins were dissolved in buffer A (20 mM Tris-Cl, 2 mM EDTA-2Na, 8 M urea, 5 mM dithiothreitol, pH 7.5) at 4℃ for 15 h before being centrifuged at 20 000 rpm for 30 min. A HiTrap heparin Sepharose column (20 ml) was preequilibrated with ten volumes of buffer B (20 mM Tris-Cl, 2 mM EDTA-2Na, 8 M urea, 5 mM dithiothreitol, pH 7.5), and 600 ml (containing 546 mg total protein) denatured protein supernatant was applied to it, followed by extensive washes with ten volumes of buffer B. Further three-step washes with ten volumes of buffer B mixed with buffer C (20 mM Tris-Cl, 2 mM EDTA-2Na, 1 M urea, 5 mM dithiothreitol, pH 7.5) (B:C = 7:3, 4:6 and only buffer C, respectively) were performed overnight to ensure the maximal refolding of the protein and to remove impurities. All the above procedures were performed under gravity at 4℃.

2.8　rhFGF20 purification

Bound refolding protein was eluted with ten volumes of buffer D (20 mM Tris-Cl, 2 mM EDTA-2Na, 0.6 M NaCl, pH 7.5), buffer E (20 mM Tris-Cl, 2 mM EDTA-2Na, 0.9 M NaCl, pH 7.5), buffer F (20 mM Tris-Cl, 2 mM EDTA-2Na, 1.2 M NaCl, pH 7.5), and buffer G (20 mM Tris-Cl, 2 mM EDTA-2Na, 2 M NaCl, pH 7.5). The elution fractions were collected and analyzed by 12% (v/v) SDS-PAGE. Fractions containing rhFGF20 were concentrated by ultrafiltration on a Millipore filter (3 000 kDa), and then protein was measured using a BCA kit (TaKaRa). All purification procedures were carried out at 4℃, and purified rhFGF20 protein was stored at −80℃.

2.9　Western blot analysis

Western blot analysis was used to identify rhFGF20, caspase12, GRP78, and β-actin. Briefly, protein samples were subjected to 12% (v/v) SDS-PAGE and then transferred onto a polyvinylidene fluoride membrane for antibody probing. The membrane was blocked in TBST (8 g/L NaCl, 0.2 g/L KCl, 3 g/L Tris-Cl, 0.1% (v/v) Tween 20, pH = 7.4) containing 5% (w/v) nonfat dry milk with shaking for 2 h and was incubated with mouse anti-hFGF20, rabbit anti-rat caspase12, rabbit anti-rat GRP78, or goat anti-rat β-actin monoclonal antibody (1:800) overnight at 4℃ (Abcam). After washes with TBST, membranes were incubated with a peroxidase-conjugated rabbit anti-mouse or goat anti-rabbit secondary antibody for 90 min (all 1:8 000). After three washes with TBST, polypeptide bands were visualized using an enhanced-chemiluminescence kit (Abcam), according to the manufacturer's instructions.

2.10 MTT growth assay

NIH 3T3 and PC-12 ccells (Shanghai Institute of Cell Biology Institute library) were used to determine the activity of rhFGF20 compared to two classic standard FGFs, FGF1 and FGF2, that were expressed in *E. coli* BL21(DE3)pLysS. Cells RT-PCR analysis of cell were grown in 96-well tissue culture plates with DMEM (Invitrogen) supplemented with 10% (*v/v*) FBS (Invitrogen,). The cells were serum-starved for 24 h by culture in DMEM alone, treated with various concentrations of rhFGF20, FGF1, and FGF2 for 48 h. The number of cells was then determined with MTT. Briefly, 20 μl of MTT (Bio-Tech) (5 mg/ml) was added to each well followed by 4-h incubation. The medium was then removed and replaced with 150 μl DMSO. Finally, the absorbance was measured at A_{570} nm for signal detection and at A_{690} nm for a background reading.

2.11 Toxicity of Aβ25–35 on PC-12 cells

Aβ25–35 (Sigma) was diluted with distilled water to a final concentration of 1000 μM and stored at −20 °C. At the time of experimentation, Aβ25–35 was diluted in PBS to the required concentration and incubated for 7 days at 37 °C. PC-12 cells were grown in a 96-well tissue culture plate with DMEM supplemented with 10% (*v/v*) FBS. The cells were serum-starved for 24 h and then treated for 48 h with various concentrations of Aβ25–35, as indicated in the figure legends.

2.12 Different concentrations of rhFGF20, FGF1, and FGF2 in a model of Aβ25–35 induced apoptosis on PC-12 cells

PC-12 cells were subjected to an initial incubation of 2 h with 20 μM Aβ25–35, and then rhFGF20, FGF1, and FGF2 were added for 48 h. The number of viable cells was determined by measuring MTT incorporation, as described for proliferation assays.

2.13 Detection of LDH in culture medium

Using a commercially available lactate dehydrogenase (LDH) kit (Nanjing Jiancheng), we measured the activity of LDH in the culture medium according to the manufacturer's instructions. LDH rate was calculated as follows: Cell LDH $(U/L) = (A_{sample} - A_{contrast}) / (A_{standard} - A_{blank}) \times 2 \times 1\,000$.

2.14 RT-PCR analysis of cell apoptosis-related genes

To measure the mRNA levels of caspase12, GRP78, caspase3, Bcl-xl, Bcl-2, and Bax, we used a commercially available RT-PCR kit (TaKaRa) according to the manufacturer's instructions. We normalized all resulting values to the housekeeping gene, β-actin. RNA was isolated from the control group (Aβ25–35-treated) and the rhFGF20 group using the kit's TRIzol reagent method and according to the manufacturer's instructions. cDNA was synthesized using PCR, and the resulting cDNAwas used for RT-PCR. The primers used were as follows:

caspase12	sense primer: 5′-AATGGAGGTAAATGTTGGAGTG-3′
	antisense primer: 5′-CTCTTCTGCCCTTTCTGTCTTC-3′
GRP78	sense primer: 5′-CTGAAGACAAAGGGACAGGA-3′
	antisense primer: 5′-CTCAATTTTCTCCCAACGAA-3′
caspase 3	sense primer: 5′-TGCGGCGTTACACGACCTT-3′
	antisense primer: 5′-CAAAGCCAGTGGCACTCATTCTC-3′
Bcl-xl	sense primer: 5′-AGGCTGGCGATGAGTTTG-3′
	antisense primer: 5′-CGGCTCTCGGCTGCTGCATT-3′
Bcl-2	sense primer: 5′-GGCATCTTCTCCTTCCAG-3′
	antisense primer: 5′-ATCCCAGCCTCCGTTAT-3′
Bax	sense primer: 5′-TGGTTGCCCTTTTCTACTTTG-3′
	antisense primer: 5′-GAAGTAGGAAAGGAGGCCATC-3′
β-actin	sense primer: 5′-ATTTGCACCACACTTTCTACA-3′
	antisense primer: 5′-TCACGCACGATTTCCCTCTCAG-3'

PCR consisted of an initial denaturation cycle of 37℃ for 15 min, which was ramped up to 95℃ for 5 s. A 15-μl PCR reaction was run, which contained 7.5 μl SYBR Green Supermix, 1 μl each of the forward and reverse primers, and 1.5 μl each of the cDNA template and 4 μl RNase/ DNase free water. All reactions were performed in triplicate, and the experiment was repeated three times. The real-time PCR detection system was run with the following cycle parameters: 1 cycle at 3 min and 95℃, 40 cycles at 10 s and 95℃, 10 s at 58℃, 1 min at 68℃, and finally, a melt curve to assess uniform product formation. A standard curve using a tenfold serial dilution of a non-template control was used to determine amplification efficiency and relative expression levels.

3. Results

3.1 Plasmid construction and expression of rhFGF20

The insertion of a cDNA encoding *fgf20* into pET3a was demonstrated by enzymatic digestion with *Nde* I and *Bam*H I, which produced two bands: one at 5 000 bp, corresponding to pET3a and the other at 630 bp, corresponding to the *fgf20* cDNA (Supplementary Fig. S1). DNA sequencing confirmed the correct insertion of the cDNA encoding *fgf20*. The expression plasmid was then transformed into *E. coli* BL21(DE3)/ pLysS. Protein expression was induced by 1 mM IPTG and 12% (*v/v*) SDS-PAGE, and Western blot demonstrated the presence of an immunoreactive polypeptide corresponding to rhFGF20 of the appropriate molecular weight, 23.5 kDa. In the absence of IPTG induction, the protein was virtually undetectable (Fig. 1A, B).

After IPTG induction, cells were sonicated in lysis buffer and then centrifuged. Fig. 2A shows that almost all rhFGF20 was present in the pellet, indicating that rhFGF20 was expressed in inclusion bodies. Attempts to produce soluble FGF20 by varying the temperature and the concentration of IPTG were not successful, which is consistent with previous work (Sun *et al.*, 2015). Therefore, the solubilization and refolding of FGF20 in inclusion bodies was undertaken.

3.2 Solubilization and purification of rhFGF20 from inclusion bodies

The inclusion body protein was successively washed with wash buffers, resuspended, and was centrifuged at 20 000 rpm for 30 min at 4℃, yielding a pellet after each centrifugation. The protein profile of each supernatant and precipitate was analyzed by 12% (*v/v*) SDS-PAGE (Fig. 2B). The inclusion body protein was solubilized at 4℃ by stirring in buffer A for 15 h. After centrifugation, the supernatant was found to contain FGF20. The renaturation took advantage of the fact that FGF paracrines bind to heparin and that their primary heparin binding site consists of amino acids that are proximate in the folded protein but distant in sequence (Xu *et al.*, 2013). Renaturation on a column of heparin Sepharose was performed by stepwise changes of buffers to ensure correct folding of the protein. After complete refolding, the heparin affinity column contained the refolded protein (Fig. 3A). Next, the FGF20 bound to the heparin column was subjected by heparin affinity chromatography, a common means to purify FGFs (Song *et al.*, 2014). As shown in Fig.

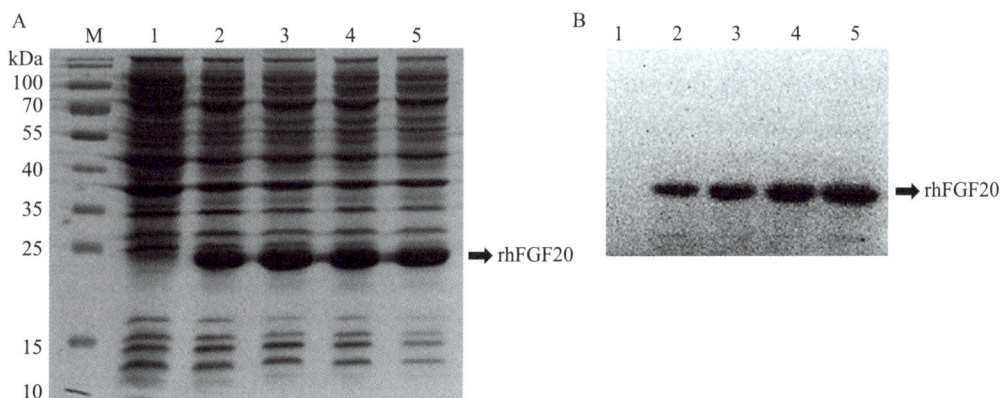

Fig. 1. Cloning of cDNA encoding FGF20 and its expression. (A) Expression of rhFGF20 induced in BL21(DE3)pLysS and analyzed by 12% (*v/v*) SDS-PAGE. Lane 1: uninduced; lanes 2, 3, 4, 5: induction of different clones; lane M: molecular weight marker. (B) Expression of rhFGF20 analyzed by Western blot. Lane 1: uninduced; lanes 2, 3, 4, and 5: induced of different clones; lane M: molecular weight marker.

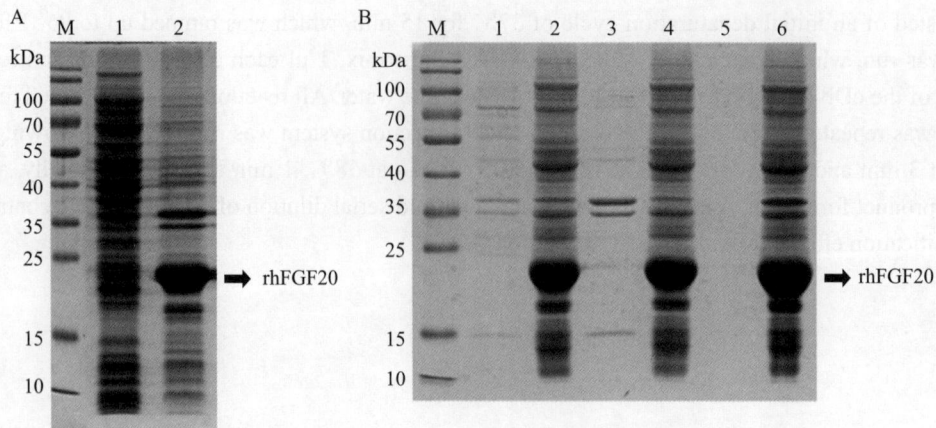

Fig. 2. Identification and washing of the inclusion body protein. (A) Detection of rhFGF20 in the soluble and insoluble fractions of BL21(DE3) pLysS following cell lysis and centrifugation, analyzed by 12% (*v/v*) SDS-PAGE. Lane 1: supernatant; lane 2: pellet; lane M: molecular weight marker. (B) Washing of the inclusion body protein. Lane 1: washed supernatant using wash buffer I; lane 2: washed pellet using wash buffer I; lane 3: washed supernatant using wash buffer II; lane 4: washed pellet using wash buffer II; lane 5: washed supernatant using wash buffer II; lane 6: washed pellet using wash buffer II; lane M: molecular weight marker.

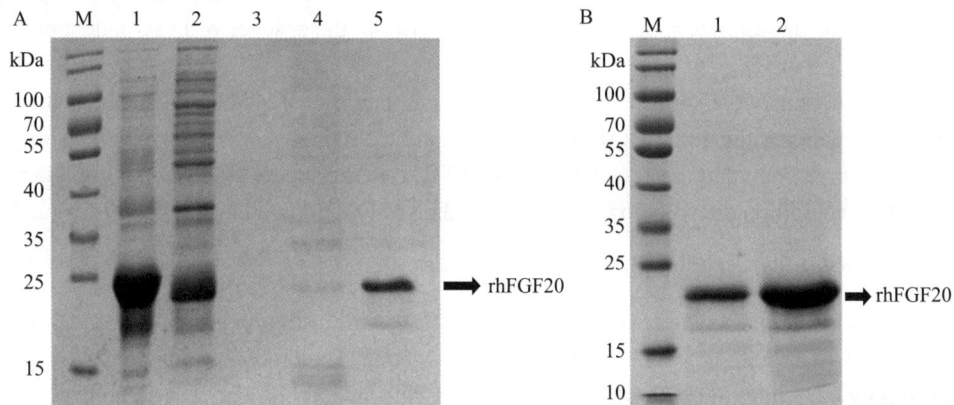

Fig. 3. Heparin Sepharose column refolding and purification of rhFGF20 analyzed by 12% (*v/v*) SDS-PAGE. (A) *Lane 1*: supernatant following centrifugation of solubilized inclusion bodies; lane 2: flow through fraction from heparin Sepharose; lane 3: washed with ten volumes of 0.6 M NaCl (buffer D); lane 4: washed with ten volumes of 0.9 M NaCl (buffer E); lane 5: elution with ten volumes of 1.2 M NaCl (buffer F); lane M: molecular weight marker. (B) Fractions containing rhFGF20 were concentrated with Millipore filter. Lane 1: before ultrafiltration; lane 2: after ultrafiltration; lane M: molecular weight marker

3A, the fractions containing rhFGF20 were finally eluted by heparin affinity chromatography using 20 mM Tris-Cl, 2 mM EDTA-2Na, 1.2 M NaCl, which is similar to that obtained by others with smaller amounts of soluble FGF20 (Sun *et al.* 2015). Fractions containing rhFGF20 were then concentrated using a Millipore filter (Fig. 3B). Quantification of the results from the solubilization of the inclusion body protein and purification of rhFGF20 shows that after processing the inclusion body protein, the target protein was purified by heparin affinity chromatography with a resulting rhFGF20 purity higher than 96%, and the yield was 218 mg/100 g wet cells (Table 2).

Table 2. Summary of the purification of rhFGF20

	Purification inclusion body protein weight (g)	Volume (ml)	Protein concentration (mg/ml)	Total protein (mg)	Purity (%)	Yield (mg/100 g wet bacteria)
Protein solubilization	54	600	0.91	546	58%	317
Heparin affinity		247	0.92	227	96%	218

Data present was the average of three batches. Total protein was determined by BCA method. The amount of target proteins was estimated by densitometry analysis of the protein band in SDS-PAGE gels. Total protein = protein concentration (mg/ml) × volume (ml). Yield = total protein (mg) × purity (%).

3.3 Mitogenic activity of rhFGF20, FGF1 and FGF2 on NIH 3T3 and PC-12 cells

To evaluate the activity of rhFGF20, we used an MTT assay to analyze the proliferative effects of rhFGF20 on NIH 3T3 and PC-12 cells. The activities of FGF1 and FGF2 which have well established growth promoting activities in these cells (Boilly *et al.*, 2000) were used as positive controls. As shown in Fig. 4 and similar to both FGF1 and FGF2, purified rhFGF20 was able to induce a mitogenic response on NIH 3T3 cells, although this was of lower magnitude than seen with FGF1 and FGF2. Furthermore, rhFGF20 was found to have a dose-dependent effect on the proliferation of NIH 3T3 cells, with a half maximal stimulatory effect seen at around 2 ng/ml, comparable to FGF1 and FGF2 (Fig. 4). Thus, the rhFGF20 solubilized from inclusion bodies and then refolded produced a substantial mitogenic effect on NIH 3T3 cells.

To ensure that the activity of rhFGF20 was not restricted to just one cell type, we then evaluated its growth stimulatory effect on PC-12 cells, which have properties analogous to neurons for which they are a convenient, albeit simplified, model. Again, the activities of FGF1 and FGF2 were used as a benchmark. The purified rhFGF20 induced a mitogenic response on PC-12 cells comparable to that of FGF2 (Fig. 5). In contrast, FGF1 stimulated the proliferation of PC-12 cells to a lesser extent. The dose dependence of the stimulation of cell growth by rhFGF20 and FGF2 was similar, and they had a half-maximal effect at around 4 ng/ml. The lower activity of FGF1 may reflect its lower thermal stability at 37 °C (Xu *et al.*, 2013) compared to that of FGF2 and rhFGF20 (Fan *et al.*, 2007).

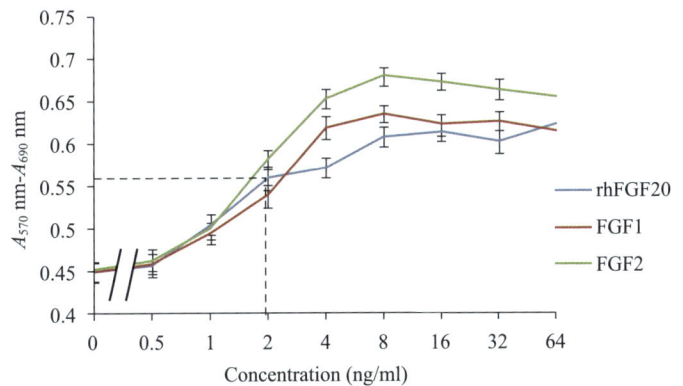

Fig. 4. Mitogenic activity of rhFGF20, FGF1, and FGF2 on NIH 3T3 cells. Cells were plated into 96-well plates and after 24 h, were serum-starved for 24 h, and then the rhFGF20, FGF1, and FGF2 were added for 48 h, after which MTT incorporation was measured, as described in the "materials and methods" section. PBS (the vehicle) was used as a negative control. Results are the SD± of triplicate wells from five experiments.

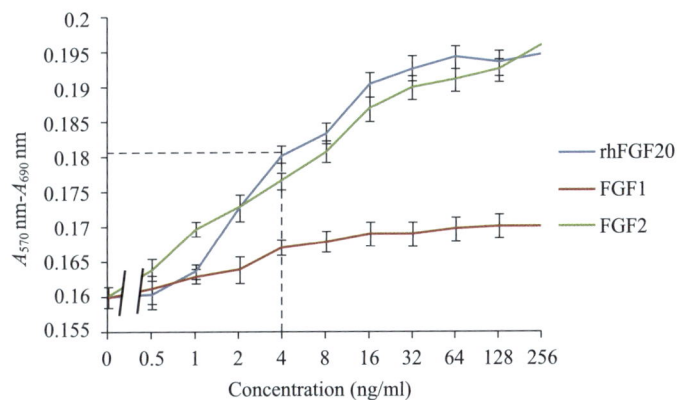

Fig. 5. Mitogenic activity of rhFGF20, FGF1 and FGF2 on PC-12 cells. Cells were plated into 96-well plates and after 24 h, were serum-starved for 24 h, and then the rhFGF20, FGF1, and FGF2 were added for 48 h, after which MTT incorporation was measured, as described in the "materials and methods" section. PBS (the vehicle) was used as a negative control. Results are the SD± of triplicate wells from five experiments. PBS was used as a negative control.

3.4 Protective effect of rhFGF20 on PC-12 cells treated with Aβ25–35

PC-12 cells, though originating from the adrenal gland, have neuronal characteristics and are used as a model for Aβ25–35 toxicity. PC-12 cells were treated with different concentrations of Aβ25–35 for 48 h. Since the MTT assay measures the mitochondrial membrane electrochemical gradient, it provides a measure of both cell proliferation (more cells, more mitochondria) and of cell viability, so it was used here as an indicator of the latter. As shown in Fig. 6A, as the concentration of Aβ25–35 increased, cellular viability measured by MTT incorporation decreased. When compared to the control (no Aβ25–35), cells exposed to Aβ25–35 at 20 μM had a cell survival rate of 61%. We then used microscopy to analyze cell morphological changes, where we saw that normal PC-12 cells had nerve cell-like morphology and strong refraction (Fig. 6B). When PC-12 cells were treated with 20 μM Aβ25–35, there was evidence for a reduction in cellular protrusions, resulting in swelling, as well as rounder cells, shrinkage, a decrease in refraction, and partially adherent cells (Fig. 6B, C). Above this concentration, we saw significant cytotoxicity. Given this restriction, we chose to use Aβ25–35 at a concentration of 20 μM.

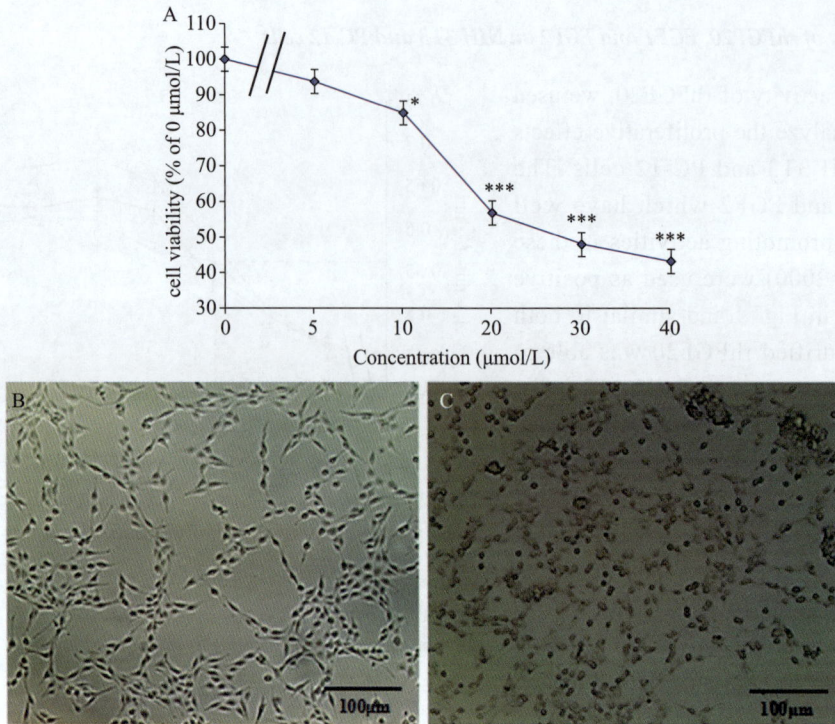

Fig. 6. (A) The viability of PC-12 cells treated with Aβ25–35. PC-12 cells were plated into 96-well plates for 24 h and then serum starved for 48 h. Aβ25–35 was then added for a further 48 h, after which the incorporation of MTT into cells was measured. Results are the SD± of triplicate wells from five experiments and a *T* test performed. *P < 0.05, **P < 0.01, ***P < 0.001 for cells with Aβ25–35 compared to untreated cells. (B, C) Morphological changes of PC-12 after treatment with Aβ25–35. Scale bars = 100 μm. (B) The normal PC-12 cells, (C) PC-12 cells treated with Aβ25–35.

Fig. 7 shows the protective effect of rhFGF20 on PC-12 cells treated with Aβ25–35 cells, and rhFGF20 had a protective effect at a concentration range between 16 and 256 ng/ml). FGF2 also had a protective effect, whereas FGF1 did not.

An LDH assay was then used to quantify directly the level of cell damage, since this relates directly to LDH release from the cytosol to the culture medium. Compared to untreated cells, cells treated with Aβ25–35 had a significant increase in LDH release, indicating that cellular damage or death was occurring (Fig. 8). When rhFGF20 at a concentration of 64 ng/ml was applied with Aβ25–35, LDH release was significantly lower than the cells treated with Aβ25–35 alone. FGF2, but not FGF1, elicited a similar response to rhFGF20.

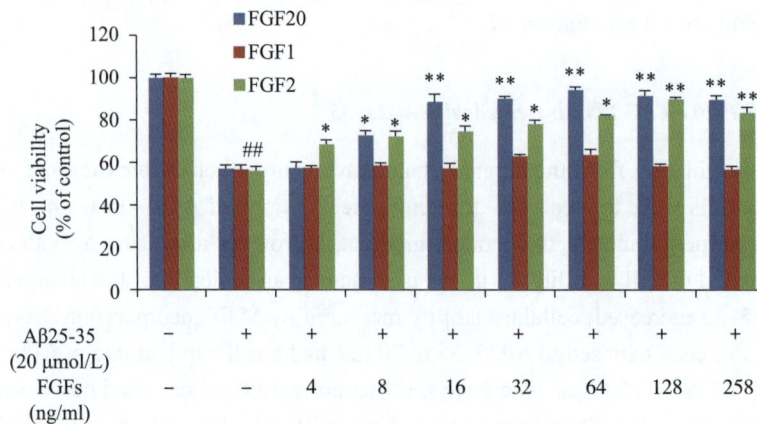

Fig. 7. Effect of rhFGF20, FGF1, and FGF2 on PC-12 cells treated with Aβ25–35. PC-12 cells were plated into 96-well plates for 24 h and then serum starved for 48 h. Aβ25–35 was then added, in some instances with 64 ng/ml rhFGF20, FGF1, or FGF2 for a further 48 h, after which the incorporation of MTT into cells was measured. Results are the SD± of triplicate wells from five experiments and a *t* test performed. *P < 0.05, **P < 0.01 with the Aβ25–35 group; ##P < 0.01 with the control.

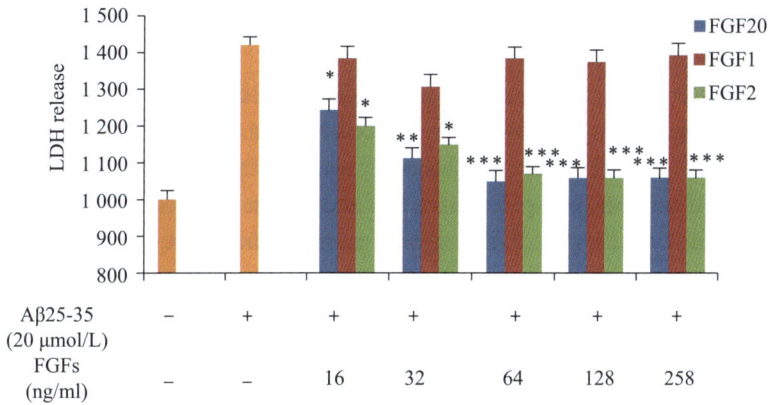

Fig. 8. LDH release by PC-12 cells treated with Aβ25–35 and rhFGF20. PC-12 cells were measured for the activity of LDH in the culture medium according to the manufacturer's instructions. $^{***}P < 0.001$ with the Aβ25–35 group.

3.5 RT-PCR and Western blot analysis of cell apoptosis-related genes

Since Aβ25–35 cytotoxicity on PC-12 cells has been shown to be mediated by ER stress and apoptosis (Xian *et al.*, 2012), key mRNAs that mark these events were measured by RT-PCR. Thus, changes in the levels of mRNAs encoding the apoptosis-related protein caspase12, caspase3, GRP78, Bcl-xl, Bcl-2, and Bax were quantified using RT-PCR in cells treated with Aβ25–35 and with both rhFGF20 and Aβ25–35 (64 ng/ml) (Fig. 9A). It is well known that caspase12, caspase3, GRP78, and Bax are pro-apoptotic genes, while Bcl-xl and Bcl-2 are anti-apoptotic genes (Banhegyi *et al.*, 2007; Hotamisligil, 2010). The results show that the expression levels of pro-apoptotic caspase12, caspase3, GRP78, and Bax were all decreased, while expression of anti-apoptotic Bcl-xl and Bcl-2 was significantly increased in the cells

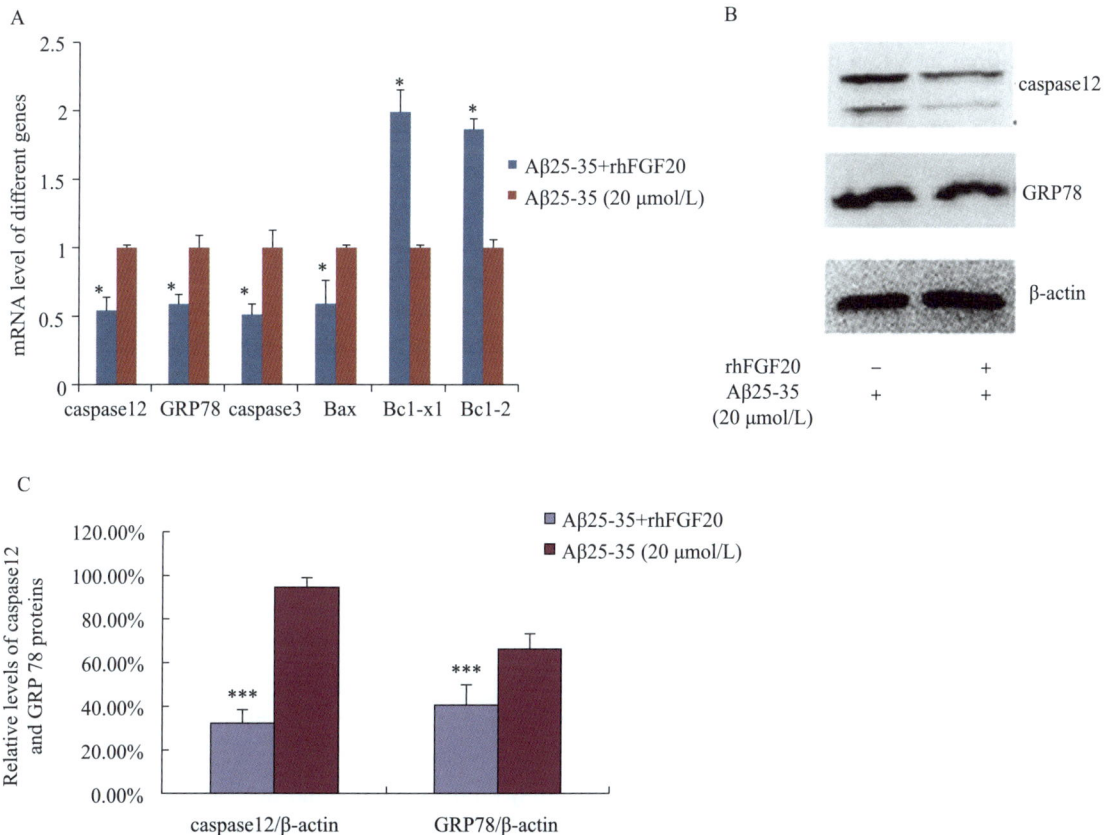

Fig. 9. Expression of mRNAs and proteins associated with ER stress following treatment of PC12 cells with Aβ25–35 and rhFGF20. (A) Total RNA was extracted from different groups and subjected to real-time PCR quantification as described under the "materials and methods" section. $^{*}P < 0.05$. (B) Western blot analysis for caspase12 and GRP78 in the endoplasmic reticulum (ER) membrane fraction of the different group. The upper trace of each panels have shown representative blots of the respective protein in the Aβ25–35 group (*left hand*) and rhFGF20 group (*right hand*). (C) The lower panels show the bar graphs summarizing the Western blot data. $^{**}P < 0.01$, $^{***}P < 0.001$.

treated with 64 ng/ml rhFGF20 and Aβ25–35 (Fig. 9A). These results indicate that treatment with rhFGF20 in this cellular model of Aβ25–35-induced cytotoxicity leads to cellular resistance to apoptosis.

Western blots were performed to determine if at least some of the changes in mRNA were also occurring at the protein level. Caspase12 is an ER stress-associated apoptosis factor, and GRP 78 is an ER stress-inducible molecular chaperone. Exposure to Aβ25–35 increased the expression of ER stress markers, caspase12 and GRP 78 (Fig. 9B), indicating directly that Aβ25–35 induced ER stress activation. When rhFGF20 (64 ng/ml) was added with Aβ25–35, there was a significant decrease in the levels of caspase 12 and GRP 78 (Fig. 9B, C). These results demonstrate that treatment with rhFGF20 leads to the reduction of two key pro-apoptotic proteins, caspase 12 and GRP 78 (as a marker for ER stress), that are induced by Aβ25–35.

4. Discussion

FGF20 is expressed preferentially in the brain where it has been found to enhance the survival of dopaminergic neurons and to upregulate dopamine biosynthesis (Grothe and Timmer, 2007; Ohmachi *et al.*, 2000). Moreover, genetic studies have suggested a link between single nucleotide polymorphisms in *fgf20* and Parkinson's disease (Foo *et al.*, 2014; Maclachlan *et al.*, 2005; Zhu *et al.*, 2014).Thus, FGF20 may be a candidate for the treatment of some diseases such as Parkinson's. This will require substantial biological and preclinical studies followed by clinical trials. The first step in the evaluation and development of a protein drug is its large-scale production, which is the aim of the present work.

Despite optimizing codon usage to that of *E. coli*, rhFGF20 was mainly expressed as an inclusion body protein. One reason for the production of insoluble protein is that the FGF20 expression yield was too high. Such levels would exceed the normal metabolism of *E. coli*, as protein synthesis would occur so quickly that there was not sufficient time for folding (Baneyx and Mujacic, 2004; Swietnicki, 2006). An advantage of this is that the expression levels are high, and purification from inclusion bodies is generally simpler since there are fewer endogenous *E. coli* proteins present (Garcia-Fruitos *et al.*, 2012). Therefore, we increased the production scale by using a nutrient fed-batch mode to maintain oxygen levels in the fermentation broth, to extend the engineered bacteria's logarithmic phase, and to increase product volume and expression. This yielded a high density of expression rhFGF20 (Table 2).

Despite high protein yields of insoluble protein, there remains a substantial challenge of solubilization and refolding of the protein. In the case of FGF20, this is compounded by the fact that the active protein is a dimer (Fan *et al.*, 2007). In early experiments, a conventional solubilization–dilution approach was used. However, this was lengthy and diluted the FGF20 substantially, which made subsequent purification more difficult (Supplementary Figs. S2 and S3; Table S1). Therefore, an alternative approach was tested, which takes advantage of the fact that FGF20 is both very basic and binds with high affinity to heparin. The interaction of native FGFs with the polysaccharide is driven by ionic bonding but demonstrates substantial specificity, both in terms of the structures recognized by the FGF in the polysaccharide and in terms of the binding sites of the latter in the protein (Xu *et al.*, 2013). It is also established that peptides corresponding to the core of the primary heparin-binding site of at least FGF2 bind heparin specifically (Kinsella *et al.*, 1998). Therefore, the solubilized and denatured FGF20 was loaded onto a heparin affinity column in the absence of electrolytes. The FGF20, which has a basic PI (PI = 7.9) would bind to the heparin by at least ion exchange. Given the likely higher affinity of the amino acids in the core of the primary heparin-binding site, which are contiguous in sequence, it is likely that these would engage with heparin preferentially. During the refolding process, binding to heparin will encourage the formation of a full heparin-binding site, which from sequence alignment with FGF9 (Xu *et al.*, 2013) also contains amino acids that are distant in sequence but physically adjacent in the folded protein. This may also align the protein so that dimerisation can occur. The washing of the inclusion bodies produced FGF20 that was 60% pure. The affinity on column refolding was then followed by affinity chromatography on the same column, which produced FGF20 at a final protein purity of more than 96% and a yield of 218 mg/100 g wet cells. Given the large number of extracellular heparin-binding proteins with important regulatory roles in health and disease (Ori *et al.*, 2011), the heparin affinity refolding and chromatography procedure developed here may have widespread application.

The successful refolding of the FGF20 is indicated by its requiring 1.2 M NaCl to be eluted from the heparin affinity column, since the primary heparin binding site of FGFs con-sists of a group of amino acids that are adjacent in sequence around beta strands 11–12, as well as amino acids that are distant in sequence (Xu *et al.,* 2013). However, this is not sufficient evidence, particularly as FGF20 exists as a dimer, which is required for its activity (Fan *et al.,* 2007). Therefore, the biological activity of the FGF20 was measured. As for other paracrine FGFs, this requires an interaction with the cognate receptor tyrosine kinase (FGFR) and the heparan sulfate (HS) co-receptor; the formation of the ternary complex with the FGF ligand requires the different binding surfaces of the latter to be correctly oriented with respect to each other (Schlessinger *et al.,* 2000), which can only occur in a folded protein requires.

Initial experiments were performed in NIH 3T3 cells to detect the stimulation of proliferation by rhFGF20 using the MTT incorporation assay. The positive controls consisted of FGF1 and FGF2, which both have strong growth stimulatory effects on these cells. The results show that purified rhFGF20 had a dose-dependent stimulatory effect on the proliferation of NIH 3T3 cells (Fig. 4). However, the magnitude of the stimulation of proliferation was not as substantial as that of FGF1 or FGF2 (Fig. 4). One explanation is that NIH 3T3 cells only have FGFR1 and FGFR2 (Li *et al.,* 1994), to which FGF1 and FGF2 can bind with high affinity, whereas FGF20 preferentially binds FGFR3 (Zhang and Kaufman, 2008).

The stimulation of fibroblast proliferation by rhFGF20 indicates that the protein is active, but its function in cells closer to the neuronal phenotype would require interaction with HS co-receptor structures and FGFRs closer to those found in brain. Consequently, we investigated the neurotrophic ability of rhFGF20 in PC-12 cells. In these cells, the activity of rhFGF20 relative to FGF1 and FGF2 was more substantial than in NIH 3T3 fibroblasts. In terms of establishing the activity profile of the rhFGF20, it was of interest to determine if it had any neuroprotective effects. To do this, PC-12 cells were challenged with the Aβ25–35 peptide, a key molecular component of Alzheimer's disease. FGF1 and FGF2 were again used as comparators, since they have been previously reported to have protective effects in this context (Chen *et al.,* 2007; Kiyota *et al.,* 2011). The results show that rhFGF20 provides very effective protection against Aβ25–35-mediated apoptosis in PC-12 cells (Fig. 7), which occurs, at least in part, by mitigating the ER stress caused by Aβ25–35 This was evidenced by the decrease in mRNAs encoding caspase12, GRP78, caspase3, and Bax, increases in those encoding Bcl-xl and Bcl-2 (Fig. 9A), and decreased protein levels of caspase12 and GRP78 (Fig. 9B, C), indicating a protective role for rhFGF20 mediated by decreasing ER stress on this cellular model of Aβ25–35 toxicity.

In summary, the experiments collectively establish a procedure for rhFGF20 high density culture fermentation as well as the solubilization of inclusion body protein and its subsequent refolding and purification on a single heparin affinity column, which may be a useful strategy for other heparin-binding proteins. The work also establishes that the rhFGF20 has full biological activity and a novel effect of the protein in protecting cells against apoptotic effects of Aβ25–35, which indicates that FGF20 may have applications in Alzheimer's disease, as well as in Parkinson's disease.

Supplementary material

Electronic supplementary material to this article can be found in the online version (doi:10.1007/s00253-015-7168-y).

References

Ansari N, Khodagholi F. Molecular mechanism aspect of ER stress in Alzheimer's disease: current approaches and future strategies[J]. Curr Drug Targets, 2013, 14(1): 114-122.

Baneyx F, Mujacic M. Recombinant protein folding and misfolding in Escherichia coli[J]. Nat Biotechnol, 2004, 22(11): 1399-1408.

Banhegyi G, Baumeister P, Benedetti A, *et al.* Endoplasmic reticulum stress[J]. Ann N Y Acad Sci, 2007, 1113: 58-71.

Boilly B, Vercoutter-Edouart AS, Hondermarck H, *et al.* FGF signals for cell proliferation and migration through different pathways[J]. Cytokine Growth Factor Rev, 2000, 11(4): 295-302.

Chen H, Tung YC, Li B, *et al.* Trophic factors counteract elevated FGF-2-induced inhibition of adult neurogenesis[J]. Neurobiol Aging, 2007, 28(8): 1148-1162.

de Mena L, Cardo LF, Coto E, *et al.* FGF20 rs12720208 SNP and mi-croRNA-433 variation: no association with Parkinson's disease in Spanish patients[J]. Neurosci Lett, 2010, 479(1): 22-25.

Fan H, Vitharana SN, Chen T, *et al.* Effects of pH and polyanions on the thermal stability of fibroblast growth factor 20[J]. Mol Pharm, 2007, 4(2): 232-240.

Foo JN, Tan LC, Liany H, *et al.* Analysis of non-synonymous-coding variants of Parkinson's disease-related pathogenic and susceptibility genes in East Asian populations[J]. Hum Mol Genet, 2014, 23(14): 3891-3897.

Garcia-Fruitos E, Vazquez E, Diez-Gil C, *et al.* Bacterial inclusion bodies: making gold from waste[J]. Trends Biotechnol, 2012, 30(2): 65-70.

Grothe C, Timmer M. The physiological and pharmacological role of basic fibroblast growth factor in the dopaminergic nigrostriatal system[J]. Brain Res Rev, 2007, 54(1): 80-91.

Hotamisligil GS. Endoplasmic reticulum stress and the inflammatory basis of metabolic disease[J]. Cell, 2010, 140(6): 900-917.

Jeffers M, McDonald WF, Chillakuru RA, et al. A novel human fibroblast growth factor treats experimental intestinal inflammation[J]. Gastroenterology, 2002, 123(4): 1151-1162.

Jeffers M, Shimkets R, Prayaga S, et al. Identification of a novel human fibroblast growth factor and characterization of its role in oncogenesis[J]. Cancer Res, 2001, 61(7): 3131-3138.

Kinsella TJ, Kunugi KA, Vielhuber KA, et al. Preclinical evaluation of 5-iodo-2-pyrimidinone-2'-deoxyribose as a prodrug for 5-iodo-2'-deoxyuridine-mediated radiosensitization in mouse and human tissues[J]. Clin Cancer Res, 1998, 4(1): 99-109.

Kirikoshi H, Sagara N, Saitoh T, et al. Molecular cloning and characterization of human FGF-20 on chromosome 8p21.3-p22[J]. Biochem Biophys Res Commun, 2000, 274(2): 337-343.

Kiyota T, Ingraham KL, Jacobsen MT, et al. FGF2 gene transfer restores hippocampal functions in mouse models of Alzheimer's disease and has therapeutic implications for neurocognitive disorders[J]. Proc Natl Acad Sci U S A, 2011, 108(49): E1339-1348.

Li Y, Basilico C, Mansukhani A. Cell transformation by fibroblast growth factors can be suppressed by truncated fibroblast growth factor receptors[J]. Mol Cell Biol, 1994, 14(11): 7660-7669.

Liu R, Gao M, Qiang GF, et al. The anti-amnesic effects of luteolin against amyloid beta(25-35) peptide-induced toxicity in mice involve the protection of neurovascular unit[J]. Neuroscience, 2009, 162(4): 1232-1243.

Ma ZG, Xu J, Liu TW. Quantitative assessment of the association between fibroblast growth factor 20 rs1721100 C/G polymorphism and the risk of sporadic Parkinson's diseases: a meta-analysis[J]. Neurol Sci, 2015, 36(1): 47-51.

Maclachlan T, Narayanan B, Gerlach VL, et al. Human fibroblast growth factor 20 (FGF-20; CG53135-05): a novel cytoprotectant with radioprotective potential[J]. Int J Radiat Biol, 2005, 81(8): 567-579.

Ohmachi S, Mikami T, Konishi M, et al. Preferential neurotrophic activity of fibroblast growth factor-20 for dopaminergic neurons through fibroblast growth factor receptor-1c[J]. J Neurosci Res, 2003, 72(4): 436-443.

Ohmachi S, Watanabe Y, Mikami T, et al. FGF-20, a novel neurotrophic factor, preferentially expressed in the substantia nigra pars compacta of rat brain[J]. Biochem Biophys Res Commun, 2000, 277(2): 355-360.

Ori A, Wilkinson MC, Fernig DG. A systems biology approach for the investigation of the heparin/heparan sulfate interactome[J]. J Biol Chem, 2011, 286(22): 19892-19904.

Schlessinger J, Plotnikov AN, Ibrahimi OA, et al. Crystal structure of a ternary FGF-FGFR-heparin complex reveals a dual role for heparin in FGFR binding and dimerization[J]. Mol Cell, 2000, 6(3): 743-750.

Shimada H, Yoshimura N, Tsuji A, et al. Differentiation of dopaminergic neurons from human embryonic stem cells: modulation of differentiation by FGF-20[J]. J Biosci Bioeng, 2009, 107(4): 447-454.

Sleeman IJ, Boshoff EL, Duty S. Fibroblast growth factor-20 protects against dopamine neuron loss in vitro and provides functional protection in the 6-hydroxydopamine-lesioned rat model of Parkinson's disease[J]. Neuropharmacology, 2012, 63(7): 1268-1277.

Song L, Huang Z, Chen Y, et al. High-efficiency production of bioactive recombinant human fibroblast growth factor 18 in Escherichia coli and its effects on hair follicle growth[J]. Appl Microbiol Biotechnol, 2014, 98(2): 695-704.

Sun C, Li Y, Taylor SE, et al. HaloTag is an effective expression and solubilisation fusion partner for a range of fibroblast growth factors[J]. PeerJ, 2015, 3: e1060.

Swietnicki W. Folding aggregated proteins into functionally active forms[J]. Curr Opin Biotechnol, 2006, 17(4): 367-372.

Takagi Y, Takahashi J, Saiki H, et al. Dopaminergic neurons generated from monkey embryonic stem cells function in a Parkinson primate model[J]. J Clin Invest, 2005, 115(1): 102-109.

van der Walt JM, Noureddine MA, Kittappa R, et al. Fibroblast growth factor 20 polymorphisms and haplotypes strongly influence risk of Parkinson disease[J]. Am J Hum Genet, 2004, 74(6): 1121-1127.

Wang G, van der Walt JM, Mayhew G, et al. Variation in the miRNA-433 binding site of FGF20 confers risk for Parkinson disease by overexpression of alpha-synuclein[J]. Am J Hum Genet, 2008, 82(2): 283-289.

Xian YF, Ip SP, Lin ZX, et al. Protective effects of pinostrobin on beta-amyloid-induced neurotoxicity in PC12 cells[J]. Cell Mol Neurobiol, 2012, 32(8): 1223-1230.

Xu X, Wang N, Xu H, et al. Fibroblast growth factor 20 polymorphism in sporadic Parkinson's disease in Northern Han Chinese[J]. J Clin Neurosci, 2013, 20(11): 1588-1590.

Zhang K, Kaufman RJ. From endoplasmic-reticulum stress to the inflammatory response[J]. Nature, 2008, 454(7203): 455-462.

Zhu R, Zhu Y, Liu X, et al. Fibroblast growth factor 20 (FGF20) gene polymorphism and risk of Parkinson's disease: a meta-analysis[J]. Neurol Sci, 2014, 35(12): 1889-1894.

Expression of bioactive recombinant human fibroblast growth factor 10 in *Carthamus tinctorius* L. seeds

Jian Huang , Xiaokun Li

1. Introduction

FGF10, also referred to as keratinocyte growth factor 2 (KGF2), is a member of the FGF superfamily. The superfamily contains 22 members in human [1] and belongs to the FGF7 subfamily, which includes FGF3/7/10/22. FGF10 was initially identified in rat (*Rattus norvegicus*), in 1996, as encoding a typical secreted protein of 215 amino acids containing an N-terminal signal sequence [2]. In 1997, human FGF10 was isolated from the lung; it encodes a protein of 208 amino acids weighing approximately 19 kDa, and is located on 5p13-p12; it shares 95.6% sequence identity to rat FGF10 [3]. FGF10 is an epithelialemesenchymal signaling molecule [4], and mediates biological responses by activating FGF receptor 2b (FGFR 2b) with heparin sulfate in a paracrine manner [5].

FGF10, exhibiting diverse biological functions, regulates early development and organogenesis in the lung, limb, white adipose tissue, heart, liver, brain, kidney, cecum, ocular glands, thymus, inner ear, tongue, trachea, eye, stomach, prostate, salivary gland, mammary gland, and whiskers [6]. FGF10 disorders are related to many diseases, including aplasia of lacrimal and salivary glands (ALSG), lacrimo-auriculo-dento-digital syndrome (LADD), limb deficiencies (LDs), cleft lip and palate (CLP), chronic obstructive pulmonary disease (COPD), autism spectrum disorder (ASD) [6], rotator cuff disease (RCD) [7], hypospadias [8], slit-eye [9], and extreme myopia [10]. FGF10 produced from tumor cells, plays important roles in tumor growth, by both paracrine and autocrine manners [11], including pancreatic cancer, breast cancer, lung cancers [6], ameloblastoma [12], skin papillomas [13], and bladder cancer [14].

The applications of FGF10 are varied, which stimulate hair growth *in vitro* [15], play important roles in tissue repair [16], burn wounds [1], corneal epithelial wounds, and acute lung injury [16]; furthermore FGF10 induces differentiation of embryonic stem cells into a gut-like structure, cardiomyocytes, and hepatocytes [6]. Thus, exploration of a cheap, safe, and efficient method to produce this protein is essential. The oilbody-oleosin technology could express recombinant proteins in seed oil bodies, which target recombinant proteins to the surface of oil bodies through covalent fusions with oleosin [17]. Oil bodies are discrete storage organelles found in oil seeds, comprising a hydrophobic triacylglycerol core surrounded by a half-unit phospholipid membrane and an outer shell of specialized proteins known as oleosins [18].

After consideration of many of the following factors, the oil bodies of safflower (*Carthamus tinctorius* L.) were chosen for production of rhFGF10. Safflower is self-pollinating with low out-crossing habits, and is well adapted to the semi-arid conditions of the tropics and subtropics [19], which facilitate to manufacture on a large scale with high yield, and safflower seeds facilitate to transport in room temperature. Moreover, safflower seeds contain low amounts of water and protein kinase, facilitating maintenance of heterogonous protein stability. Safflower seeds contain a large amount of oil bodies (OBs). These OBs can easily be separated from cell components in seeds by centrifugation, and furthermore, they contain relatively few different proteins [20]. This helps to reduce purification steps and costs associated with using oil bodies to produce heterogonous proteins. Here, we expressed rhFGF10 in safflower using oilbody-oleosin technology and analyzed bioactivity by stimulating BaF3 cells proliferation.

2. Materials and methods

2.1 Construction of rhFGF10 expression vectors

The pOTBar expression vector [21] used in this study was supplied by the Jilin Agricultural University, China. The

T-DNA region of the pOTBar plasmid contains a phaseolin promoter, phaseolin terminator, 35S promoter, *bar* gene, and *Nos* gene. The *rhFGF10* coding sequence was sourced from GenBank (GenBank: AF508782.1) and modified by codon optimization according to the codon use table of plant. The gene was then synthesized by Genewiz (Jiang Su, China). *Oleosin* and *rhFGF10* were amplified from the plasmids pUC19-oleosin (Supplied by the Jilin Agricultural University, China) and pUC19-rhFGF10, respectively, using the following appropriate primers: forward, 5′-CCATGGCGGATA-CAGCTAGAGGAACCCATCA-3′; reverse, 5′-CATGTCCTGACCAAGGG-CAGTAGTGTGCTGGC-3′; and forward, 5′-GCCAGCACACTACTGCCCTTGGTCAGGACATG-3′; reverse, 5′-CCCAAGCTTCTATTATGAGTGTACCAC-CATTGGAAGAAAG-3′. Fusion PCR was used to amplify the *oleosin-rhFGF10* fusion gene, which was cloned into the pOTBar expression vector to construct the recombinant plasmid pOTBar-oleosin-rhFGF10. The expression vector pOTBar-oleosin-rhFGF10 was further assessed by PCR and restriction enzymatic analysis. The freezee-thaw method was used to transfer plasmid pOTBar-oleosin-rhFGF10 into *Agrobacterium tumefaciens* EHA105, and its success assessed by PCR.

2.2 Agrobacterium-mediated transformation of safflower and efficient recovery of transgenic plants via grafting

Seeds of safflower JI HONG YI HAO (supplied by the Jilin Agricultural University, China) were used for this study. Seeds were sterilized with 0.1% $HgCl_2$ for 10–15 min with shaking, subsequently rinsed with sterile distilled water three times, each time for 5 min. Sterilized seeds were germinated aseptically on seed germination medium (Table 1S1) and incubated in the dark at 25 ℃ for 3 days (Fig. 1A). Approximately 20 days before grafting, mature seeds were sown into a pot (soil:vermiculite is 3:1) for producing rootstocks.

One day prior to transformation, 50 μl of *Agrobacterium* harboring plasmid pOTBar-oleosin-rhFGF10 was added to 50 ml of liquid YEP media containing 50 mg/ml kanamycin and 25 mg/ml rifampicin (Sigma, Hong Kong, China), and grown overnight at 28 ℃ with agitation at 180 rpm until the OD_{600} reached 0.6–0.8. Freshly isolated cotyledons from germinated safflower seeds were infected with 50 ml *Agrobacterium* culture, with 100 μM AS (Acetosyringone) added, for 15 min (Fig. 1B); a gentle agitation was performed during the infection. Explants infected with *Agrobacterium* were laid on sterile filter paper to remove excess *Agrobacterium* and transferred to co-cultivation media (Table 1S2; Fig. 1C). All plates were sealed with parafilm to avoid contamination, and incubated in the dark at 25 ℃ for 3 days.

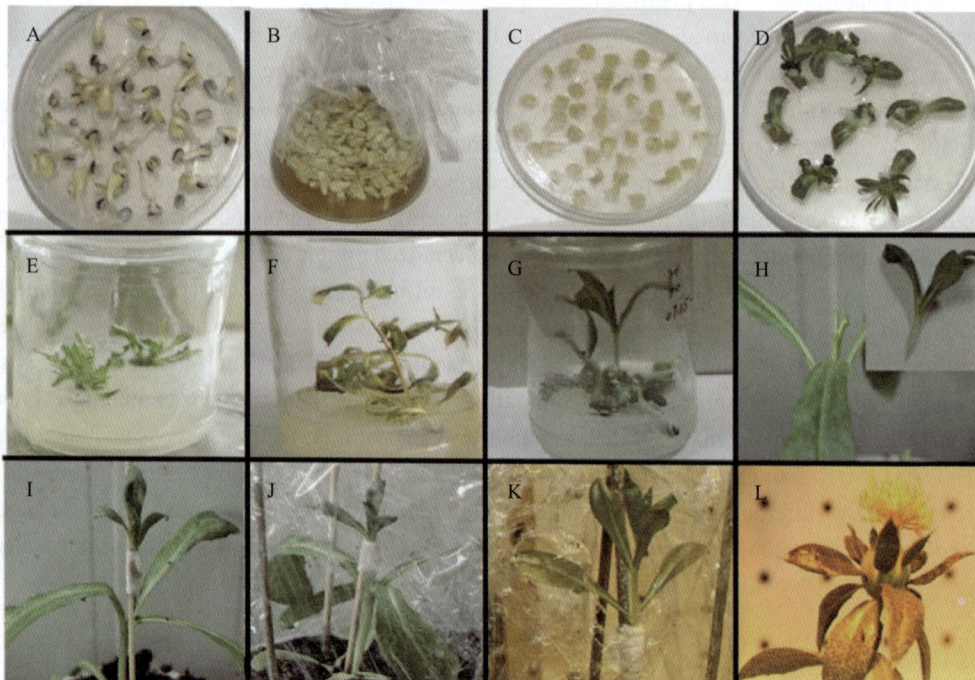

Fig. 1. Agrobacterium-mediated transformation of safflower *via* tissue culture and grafting of transgenic seedlings on to rootstocks of safflower. (A) Seeds germination. (B) Infection with Agrobacterium. (C) Co-cultivation. (D) Shots initiation. (E) Seedlings elongation. (F and G) Seedlings elongation with glufosinate ((F) showing withered and yellow, (G) exhibiting strong). (H) V-shaped transgenic scion and rootstock. (I) Parafilm holding the scion and rootstock. (J) The pot with grafted plantlets covering with preservative film. (K) The successful grafted plant. (L) The mature T_0 transgenic plant.

Table 1.　Composition of media for tissue culture of safflower

Component (mg/l)	Media			
	S1	S2	S3	S4
	Seed germination	Co-cultivation	Shoot initiation	Seedling elongation
Murashige and Skoog basal medium with vitamins	4 330	4 330	4 330	4 330
Thiamine. HCl	0.4	0.4	0.4	0.4
Pyridoxine. HCl	0.5	0.4	0.4	0.4
Nicotinic acid	0.2	0.4	0.4	0.4
Glycine	2	2	2	2
Inositol	100	100	100	100
Sucrose	20 000	30 000	30 000	10 000
1-Naphthaleneacetic acid	0	1.5	1.5	0
6-Benzylaminopurine	0	0.5	0.5	0
AS	0	19.62	0	0
KNO_3	0	0	0	3 800
Agar	8 000	8 000	8 000	8 000
Ceftriaxone sodium	0	0	100	200
Carbenicillin	0	0	200	100

(1)　The media pH should be regulated between 5.8 and 6.0 before adding the agar.

(2)　All the agents were obtained from Phyto Technology Laboratories, USA.

Three days after *Agrobacterium* infection, explants were transferred to shoot initiation media (Table 1S3) and grown at 25 ℃ under a 16/8-h (day/night) regime. After 15 days, once regeneration shoots had become strong and touched the cover of the plate (Fig. 1D), explants were excised and regeneration shoots cultured on seedlings elongation media (Table 1S4) at 25 ℃ under 16/8-h (day/night) conditions (Fig. 1E). Seven days after seedlings had emerged, they were moved to a selection media containing 0.1% (*w/v*) glufosinate (Boehringer Mannheim Corporation, Mannheim, Germany). Regenerated seedlings exhibiting strong growth were considered to be putatively transgenics (Fig. 1H), while the withered and yellow seedlings were designated as escapes and discarded (Fig. 1F). After 7 days, seedlings (approximately 3 cm with 2–3 true leaves) were collected and used for grafting (Fig. 1G).

Rootstocks with strong growth (6–8 true leaves) were deemed suitable for grafting. Rootstock seedlings were sliced horizontally using an operating knife blade, retaining two true leaves and approximately 5 cm stem. Next, a vertical cut 3 mm deep was made in the stem. Suitable regenerated seedlings could be used as scions, and were cut to create matching V-shape (Fig. 1H), and inserted in the prepared rootstock. Parafilm (Penchiney, USA) was used to hold scion and root stock tightly at the grafting point (Fig. 1I). Pots with grafted plantlets were covered with preservative film to maintain a humid environment, and grown at 21 ℃ under an 8.5-klux 16/8-h (day/night) regime (Fig. 1J). After about 1 week, when 2–3 new leaves had grown from the scion, grafted plantlets had reached a stage at which they could survive; to allow surviving grafted plantlets to adapt to the external environment, a hole was torn in the preservative film (Fig. 1K). After a further 7 days, the covering preservative film was removed from successful grafts, and unsuccessful grafts discarded.

2.3　PCR detection of rhFGF10 in successful graft safflowers

Total DNA was extracted from 100 mg of successful graft and wild-type (WT) young safflower leaf tissue using a Plant Genomic DNA Extraction kit (BioTeke, Beijing, China). PCR amplification was performed using successful graft safflower leaf total DNA as template. WT safflower leaf total DNA served as the negative control; ddH$_2$O served as the blank control; and plasmid pOTBar-oleosin-rhFGF10 as the positive control. The thermal profile of the PCR program was: initial denaturation at 94℃ for 15 min; 35 cycles of 92℃ for 30 s, 52℃ for 30 s, 72℃ for 1 min; and a final extension at 72℃ for 10 min. Amplified products were size fractionated on a 1.0% *w/v* agarose gel.

2.4 Oil bodies purification and protein analysis of oleosin-rhFGF10

Transgenic and WT safflower seeds (with pericarp removed) were fully crushed in 200 μl phosphate buffered saline (PBS) in a 1.5 ml centrifuge tube with a pestle and centrifuged at 12 000 *g* and 4℃ for 5 min. The floating oil bodies fraction was collected in a new 1.5 ml centrifuge tube and the residue were crushed again to collect oil bodies. Oil bodies were washed twice with 50 μl PBS and stored at 4℃ for further use. Oil bodies concentration was measured using a BCA protein assay kit (BioTeke).

The oil bodies that expressed oleosin-rhFGF10 and WT oil bodies were diluted to 3 μg/μl by PBS and separated by 15% SDSePAGE (10 μl sample per lane). Following electrophoresis, proteins were transferred to PVDF membranes (PerkinElmer, Boston, MA, USA) using a Transfer Cell (Bio-Rad Laboratories, Hercules, CA, USA), and the PVDF membranes were incubated with primary antibodies against FGF10 (1:200 dilution, rabbit, Bioss, Beijing, China). Membranes were washed with TBST buffer and incubated with alkaline phosphatase-conjugated goat anti-rabbit IgG/AP antibody (Bioss) according to the manufacturer's protocol. Antibody immunodetection was performed using Western Blue Stabilized Substrate for Alkaline Phosphatase (Promega).

2.5 Cellular proliferation assay

BaF3 cells (Supplied by Wenzhou medical university, Zhejiang, China) were expanded in corning flasks (25 cm², Corning, USA) at 37℃, 5% CO₂; growth medium was composed of RPMI 1640 (Hyclone, Thermo Fisher Scientific, USA), 10% fetal calf serum (FBS, Lanzhou Baling Biotechnology, China), penicillin/streptomycin solution (100 U/ml and 50 μg/ml, respectively; Hyclone), and 10% interleukin-3-conditioned medium (IL-3, PEPROTECH, Rocky Hill, USA). Experiments were conducted in 96-well plates (Costar, Thermo Fisher Scientific, USA), in which was added 90 μl basal medium (RPMI 1640, 10% FBS, penicillin/streptomycin), 30 μl standard rhFGF10 (positive control, expressed in *Escherichia coli*, supplied by the Wenzhou medical university, Zhejiang, China), and the oil bodies that expressed oleosin-rhFGF10, respectively, with a final concentration of 50 ng/ml, and then diluted four times well by well. WT safflower oil bodies served as the negative control. Before the experiments, cells were centrifuged at 1 000 g for 10 min, and resuspended in the basal medium at a final concentration of 6×10⁵ cells/ml in a final volume of 50 μl/well. Cells were incubated for 72 h at 37℃ and 20 ml 0.4% (*w/v*) MTT (Methylthiazol tetrazolium, Gold Biotechnology, St. Louis, MO, USA) solution added to each well, and then incubated for a further 4 h at 37℃. Finally, 10% SDS was added to each well and incubated for 10 h at 37℃. The plates were analyzed at 570/630 nm to obtain absorbance values using a Microplate Reader model 450 (Bio-Rad Company).

3. Results

3.1 Construction of rhFGF10 expression vectors

Expression vectors bearing the *oleosin-rhFGF10* gene were constructed to produce oleosin-rhFGF10 fusion proteins (Fig. 2). The *oleosin* and *rhFGF10* genes were obtained by PCR respectively, and the *oleosin-rhFGF10* gene obtained by fusion PCR. The recombinant plasmid pOTBar-oleosin-rhFGF10 was further assessed by PCR and restriction enzymatic analysis, and the fragment size and quality checked using 1.0% *w/v* agarose gel electrophoresis.

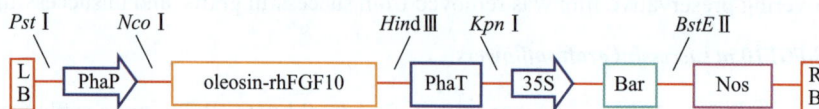

Fig. 2. Schematic map of recombinant plasmid pOTBar-oleosin-rhFGF10. The T-DNA region of pCAMBI A-1301 was replaced by *Pst*I and *Bst*EII between T-Border (LB) and Nos. The 35S-bar gene was inserted into T-DNA region by *Knp*I and *Bst*EII. The *oleosin-rhFGF10* gene was inserted in T-DNA region by *Nco*I and *Hin*dIII. The recombinant plasmid was named pOTBar-oleosin-rhFGF10. PhaP: phaseolin promoter, PhaT: phaseolin terminator, 35S: CaMV35S promoter, Bar: *bar* gene, Nos: Nopaline synthase terminator.

3.2 Agrobacterium-mediated transformation of safflower and efficient recovery of transgenic plants via grafting

Safflower cotyledon explants were chosen as the target tissue for genetic modification. The pOTBar-oleosin-rhFGF10 plasmid was transformed into safflower using *A. tumefaciens* transformation methodology *via* tissue culture, and mature safflower plants were obtained by grafting (Fig. 1). The plants through critical steps of the transformation protocol and the number of successful transgenic plants are presented in Table 2. A data set generated from 20 different infections that produced 11 mature transgenic safflower plants. Transformation efficiency was 0.3%.

Table 2. The plants through critical steps of the transformation protocol and the number of successful transgenic plants

Cotyledons co-cultivated with Agrobacterium	Seedlings ready for graft obtained	Successful grafts	Successful transgenic plants	Transformation efficiency*
3 640	237	96	11	0.3%

* The transformation efficiency was calculated as the (successful transgenic plants/infected cotyledons) × 100%.

3.3 PCR detection of rhFGF10 in successful graft safflowers

To confirm *oleosin-rhFGF10* had invaded in safflower, PCR amplification was carried out using genomic DNA from T_0 plants (successful grafts) as template. Gel electrophoresis revealed 11 lines of successful transgenic plants (Fig. 3). PCR was performed on T_1 and T_2 plants to measure Mendel segregation, and plants not containing the T-DNA insert were discarded.

3.4 Protein analysis of oleosin-rhFGF10

To confirm oleosin-rhFGF10 was expressed in safflower seeds, oil bodies extracted from transgenic T_3 and WT safflower seeds were analyzed by SDSePAGE (Fig. 4A) and Western blotting (Fig. 4B). This revealed the oleosin-rhFGF10 fusion protein band was approximately 46.7 kDa, the WT seeds protein had no band present at this position. And a schematic which represented the procedure of expression and targeting of oleosin-rhFGF10 on oil bodies using oilbody-oleosin technology was displayed in Fig. 5.

3.5 Cellular proliferation assay

To evaluate the bioactivity of the oil bodies that expressed oleosin-rhFGF10, oil bodies extracted from transgenic safflower T_3 seeds were analyzed using a standard MTT assay on BaF3 cells, and compared with standard rhFGF10 and oil bodies extracted from WT safflower seeds. Similar to the positive control, oil bodies that expressed oleosin-rhFGF10 could stimulate BaF3 cell proliferation (Fig. 6). Furthermore, oil bodies that expressed oleosin-rhFGF10 had a dose-dependent effect on the viability of BaF3 cells; the negative control also had some affirmative effects, but not as

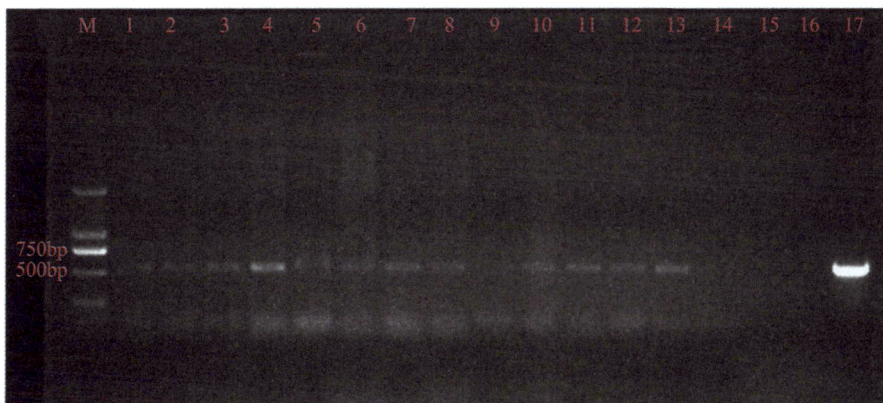

Fig. 3. Agarose gel for PCR amplification of genomic DNA from T_0 plants. Lane 1–14: PCR products generated from successful graft plants. Lane 15: negative control (wild type safflower). Lane 16: bank control (ddH₂O). Lane 17: positive control (plasmid pOTBar-oleosin-rhFGF10).

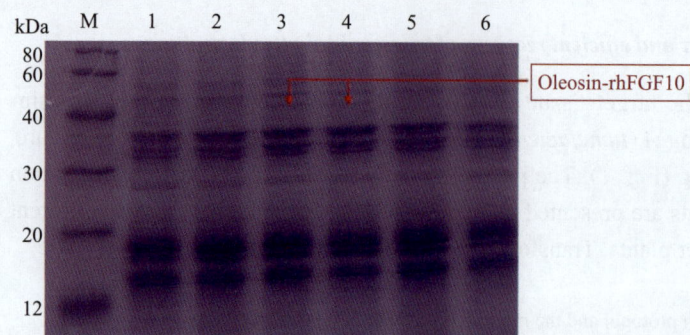

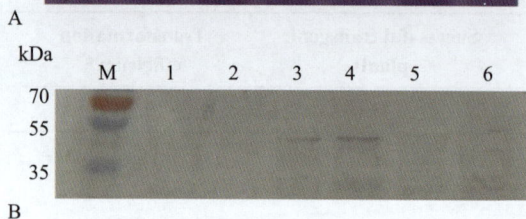

Fig. 4. Protein analysis of oleosin-rhFGF10 by SDS–PAGE and Western blotting. (A) Coomassie-stained SDS–PAGE of the oil bodies that expressed oleosin-rhFGF10 from transgenic safflower. (B) Detection on oleosin-rhFGF10 protein from the transgenic safflower by Western blotting. M: protein marker. Lane 1–5: the transgenic safflower (T3) oil bodies. Lane 6: the wild-type (WT) safflower oil bodies.

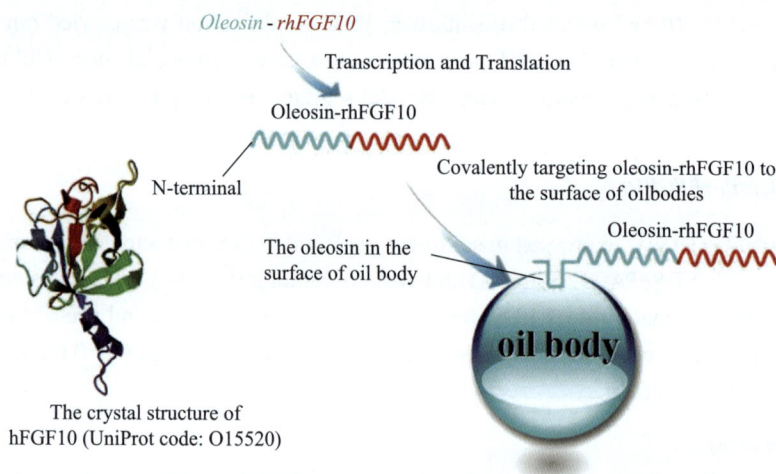

Fig. 5. Schematic representation of expression and targeting of oleosin-rhFGF10 on oil bodies using oilbody-oleosin technology.

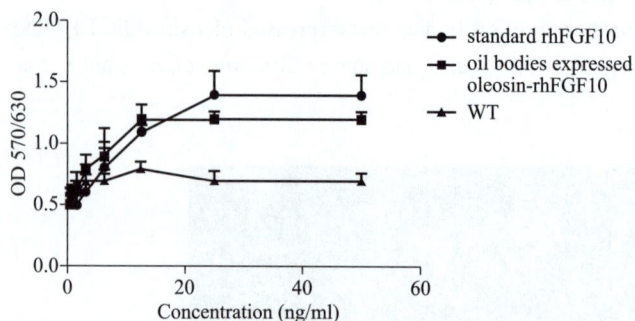

Fig. 6. Activity analysis of the oil bodies that expressed oleosin-rhFGF10 in the transgenic safflower seeds on BaF3 cells *in vitro*. Increasing concentrations of oil bodies that expressed oleosin-rhFGF10 or standard rhFGF10 (positive control) were added. Oil bodies from wild-type safflower were used as a negative control. Proliferation was quantified by measuring the absorbance at 570/630 nm ($n = 6$).

significant as the standard rhFGF10 and oil bodies that expressed oleosin-rhFGF10. Thus, this single experiment found that oil bodies expressed oleosin-FGF10 fusion had a dose-dependent effect on cellular proliferation.

4. Discussion

Recombinant human FGF10 has been expressed in crop including *Arabidopsis thaliana* [22] and *Brassica napus* L. [23]. *A. thaliana* expression platforms offer the potential for safe production for oleosin-rhFGF10. However, the *A. thaliana* seeds were small and easy to break off in the natural condition. The *Brassica napus* L. seeds are main food and feed crops which can lead to genetic pollution. So, the *C. tinctorius* L. were chosen for production of oleosin-rhFGF10 because safflower is self-pollinating, well adapted to the semi-arid conditions, containing low amounts of water and protein kinasege. Oleosins are unique proteins with natural surfactant properties derived from alternating amphipathic and lipo-philic domains. The central domain of oleosins is highly lipophilic, tightly anchoring the protein within the neutral lipid core of the oilbody. The amphipathic N- and C-termini interact with the phospholipids membrane forming a network that surrounds the oilbody in an amphipathic shell. The resulting structure is a highly stable [17]. According to the properties of oleosin, various economically and scientifically important proteins have been obtained at a lower cost of production by using oilbody-oleosin technology. This technology fuses heterogonous proteins to the N- or C-terminus of oleosin at the oil body surface. Human precursor insulin, human EGF, ApoA1 [20], human aFGF [21], and hyaluronidase PH-20 [24] have all been expressed using this technology and demonstrated to show biological activity.

In this study, oleosin-rhFGF10 was successfully expressed in safflower seeds using oilbody-oleosin technology. Step 1: expression of oleosin-rhFGF10 with the rhFGF10 fused to the C-terminus of oleosin and expressed under the control of a seed-specific promoter. Step 2: oleosin-rhFGF10 is targeted to oil body membrane through covalent fusions with oleosin. The plant expression vector, pOTBar-oleosin-rhFGF10, was constructed and transformed into safflower using *A. tumefaciens* transformation methodology, *via* tissue culture. Safflower roots *in vitro* are so weak that fail to survive the transfer from tissue culture media to soil [19]. Therefore, grafting method was used to obtain regenerated transgenic plants. Eleven successful transgenic plants were obtained. PCR was performed on T_0, T_1, and T_2 plants to confirm successful transgenic plants and discard plants losing the T-DNA insert through Mendel separation. Oleosin-rhFGF10 fusion proteins were then analyzed by SDSePAGE and Western blotting, demonstrating that oleosin-rhFGF10 was successfully expressed in safflower seeds, and the expression levels was 0.14% of total seed proteins; 135.45 g rhFGF10 protein could be produced in 1 hectare of GM safflower (the production of safflower were 4500 kg per hectare and the levels of total seed proteins were 2.15% of safflower seeds). The results of BaF3 cells analysis demonstrated that oil bodies expressed oleosin-rhFGF10 from the transgenic safflower seeds had a proliferation effect on BaF3 cells. This study demonstrated that using oilbody-oleosin technology to express rhFGF10 is simple, viable, economic, which might be useful for the mass production of FGF10.

References

[1] Plichta JK, Radek KA. Sugar-coating wound repair: a review of FGF-10 and dermatan sulfate in wound healing and their potential application in burn wounds[J]. J Burn Care Res, 2012, 33(3): 299-310.

[2] Yamasaki M, Miyake A, Tagashira S, *et al.* Structure and expression of the rat mRNA encoding a novel member of the fibroblast growth factor family[J]. J Biol Chem, 1996, 271(27): 15918-15921.

[3] Emoto H, Tagashira S, Mattei MG, *et al.* Structure and expression of human fibroblast growth factor-10[J]. J Biol Chem, 1997, 272(37): 23191-23194.

[4] Zhang X, Ibrahimi OA, Olsen SK, *et al.* Receptor specificity of the fibroblast growth factor family. The complete mammalian FGF family[J]. J Biol Chem, 2006, 281(23): 15694-15700.

[5] Ohta H, Konishi M, Itoh N. FGF10 and FGF21 as regulators in adipocyte development and metabolism[J]. Endocr Metab Immune Disord Drug Targets, 2011, 11(4): 302-309.

[6] Itoh N, Ohta H. Fgf10: a paracrine-signaling molecule in development, disease, and regenerative medicine[J]. Curr Mol Med, 2014,

14(4): 504-509.

[7] Motta Gda R, Amaral MV, Rezende E, *et al.* Evidence of genetic variations associated with rotator cuff disease[J]. J Shoulder Elbow Surg, 2014, 23(2): 227-235.

[8] Carmichael SL, Ma C, Choudhry S, *et al.* Hypospadias and genes related to genital tubercle and early urethral development[J]. J Urol, 2013, 190(5): 1884-1892.

[9] Puk O, Esposito I, Soker T, *et al.* A new Fgf10 mutation in the mouse leads to atrophy of the harderian gland and slit-eye phenotype in heterozygotes: a novel model for dry-eye disease?[J]. Invest Ophthalmol Vis Sci, 2009, 50(9): 4311-4318.

[10] Yoshida M, Meguro A, Okada E, *et al.* Association study of fibroblast growth factor 10 (FGF10) polymorphisms with susceptibility to extreme myopia in a Japanese population[J]. Mol Vis, 2013, 19: 2321-2329.

[11] Sugimoto K, Yoshida S, Mashio Y, *et al.* Role of FGF10 on tumorigenesis by MS-K[J]. Genes Cells, 2014, 19(2): 112-125.

[12] Nakao Y, Mitsuyasu T, Kawano S, *et al.* Fibroblast growth factors

7 and 10 are involved in ameloblastoma proliferation *via* the mitogen-activated protein kinase pathway[J]. Int J Oncol, 2013, 43(5): 1377-1384.

[13] Hertzler-Schaefer K, Mathew G, Somani AK, *et al*. Pten loss induces autocrine FGF signaling to promote skin tumorigenesis[J]. Cell Rep, 2014, 6(5): 818-826.

[14] Chung SS, Koh CJ. Bladder cancer cell in co-culture induces human stem cell differentiation to urothelial cells through paracrine FGF10 signaling[J]. *In Vitro* Cell Dev Biol Anim, 2013, 49(10): 746-751.

[15] Jang JH. Stimulation of human hair growth by the recombinant human keratinocyte growth factor-2 (KGF-2)[J]. Biotechnol Lett, 2005, 27(11): 749-752.

[16] Steiling H, Werner S. Fibroblast growth factors: key players in epithelial morphogenesis, repair and cytoprotection[J]. Curr Opin Biotechnol, 2003, 14(5): 533-537.

[17] Markley N, Nykiforuk C, Boothe J, *et al*. Producing proteins using transgenic oilbody-oleosin technology[J]. Biopharm international, 2006, 19(6).

[18] Nykiforuk CL, Boothe JG, Murray EW, *et al*. Transgenic expression and recovery of biologically active recombinant human insulin

from Arabidopsis thaliana seeds[J]. Plant Biotechnol J, 2006, 4(1): 77-85.

[19] Belide S, Hac L, Singh SP, *et al*. Agrobacterium-mediated transformation of safflower and the efficient recovery of transgenic plants *via* grafting[J]. Plant Methods, 2011, 7: 12.

[20] Bhatla SC, Kaushik V, Yadav MK. Use of oil bodies and oleosins in recombinant protein production and other biotechnological applications[J]. Biotechnol Adv, 2010, 28(3): 293-300.

[21] Yang J, Guan L, Guo Y, *et al*. Expression of biologically recombinant human acidic fibroblast growth factor in Arabidopsis thaliana seeds *via* oleosin fusion technology[J]. Gene, 2015, 566(1): 89-94.

[22] Wang L, Wang D, Yang J, *et al*. Expression of oleosin-KGF2 in Arabidopsis thaliana *via* oleosin fusion technology. In: Colloquium of 2013 National Congress of Plant Biology, 2013.

[23] Pan G, Zhang S, Liu X, *et al*. Cloning of keratinocyte growth factor 2 gene (KGF2) and its transformation to Brassica napus L[J]. Sheng Wu Gong Cheng Xue Bao, 2010, 26(6): 767-771.

[24] Li H, Yang J, Chen Y, *et al*. Expression of a functional recombinant oleosin-human hyaluronidase hPH-20 fusion in Arabidopsis thaliana[J]. Protein Expr Purif, 2014, 103: 23-27.

Expression of bioactive recombinant human fibroblast growth factor 9 in oil bodies of *Arabidopsis thaliana*

Shanyong Yi , Xiaokun Li , Chao Jiang

1. Introduction

Fibroblast growth factor 9 (FGF9) is present in various human body tissues where it effectively promotes mitosis and cell growth. FGF9 is involved in bone development, angiogenesis, embryonic development, damage repair, cell apoptosis, nerve regeneration, hair growth, and other physiological and pathological processes. The *hFGF9* gene is tightly on clustered chromosome 13q11–q12, whereas ox *FGF9* is tightly clustered on chromosome 12 and mouse *FGF9* is tightly clustered on chromosome 14 [1]. The coding sequence of *hFGF9* is well conserved, exhibiting 94.9% and 88.7% identity to the ox and mouse variants, respectively. There is a potential polyadenylation site in the 3'-untranslated region of *hFGF9* mRNA, and a high G/C area in the 5'-untranslated region [2].

FGF9 adopts a pyramid-like structure, with the N- and C-terminal regions lying outside the trefoil core region being ordered and forming 2 α-helices and 12 β-strands in the crystallographic dimer [3,4]. FGF9, FGF16, and FGF20 form a subfamily based on similarities in sequence and phylogeny [5]. Proteins within this subfamily do not possess the amino-terminal export sequence typical of FGFs, and are secreted through the traditional endoplasmic reticulum (ER)–golgi secretory pathway [6,7].

Diverse functions of the FGF ligands have been identified by binding and activating the FGFR family of tyrosine kinase receptors in a dependent manner [8]. There are four *FGFR* genes (*FGFR1–4*) that encode receptors comprising three extracellular immunoglobulin domains (D1–3), a single-pass transmembrane domain, and a cytoplasmic tyrosine kinase domain [9]. Given the biological role of FGF9 in important processes including ovarian cancer progression, bone development, nerve regeneration, and gonadal differentiation, studies have focused on identifying mechanisms underlying these effects. Enhanced understanding of the role of FGF9 may aid the diagnosis of ovarian cancer, treatment of carti-lage disorders, and study of gonadal differentiation.

Plants have been studied extensively for their utility as an inexpensive and scalable alternative to common expression systems for the production of exogenous proteins. Plant-based expression systems offer multiple advantages over microbial or mammalian host systems, including cost effectiveness, storage and transportation convenience, genetic stability, and high yield potential [10]. Furthermore, plants possess all of the cellular machinery required for post-translational modifications of proteins, and they are intrinsically safe.

Oil bodies are maintained as small individual units with diameters of 0.5–2.0 μm, and are surrounded by a phospholipid monolayer containing multiple proteins, most of which are oleosins [11]. Low-molecular-weight oleosins are hydrophobic plant membrane proteins that cover the entire surface of oil bodies [12]. Oil body size is determined by oleosin accumulation [13]. Oleosins adopt a unique structural configuration that comprises poorly conserved amphipathic N- and C-terminal domains, and a highly conserved central hydrophobic domain [14,15]. Moreover, oleosins appear to act as a natural emulsifying and stabilizing agents at oil–water interfaces [16]. Therefore, oleosins possess potential biotechnological applications as emulsion stabilizers in various cosmetic and cosmeceutical products [17,18].

Oleosins have been employed as carrier molecules in the expression and purification of recombinant pharmaceutical peptides and industrial enzymes [19,20]. The process of oleosin fusion involves fusion of heterologous proteins to the N- or C-terminus of oleosin and subsequent expression of the recombinant protein under the control of an *oleosin* gene promoter or other seed-specific promoter [21,22]. This fusion technology extends the protein half-life, and allows easy transportation and storage [23]. Moreover, oleosin fusion has been widely used to express foreign proteins. The Sem-BioSys biotechnology company constructed a plant expression vector pSBS4405 and transformed it into *Arabidopsis thaliana* for production of human insulin [24]. Additionally, SemBioSys has successfully used the safflower oil body to express human insulin and achieved commercial production standards. Human epidermal growth factor fused to oleosin has also been expressed in *A. thaliana* and an accumulation level of 0.12% was achieved [25]. Our laboratory has produced functional recombinant oleosin–human hyaluronidase and biologically active, recombinant human acidic fibroblast growth factor in *A. thaliana* seeds [26,27].

Many exogenous proteins have been expressed in transgenic plants since the first successful production of a mouse monoclonal antibody in plants [28]. We report the construction of the expression vector pOTB–rhFGF9 and subsequent expression of rhFGF9 in the *A. thaliana* oil bodies. Expression of the oleosin–rhFGF9 fusion protein was confirmed by SDS-PAGE and Western blotting. Moreover, the oil bodies expressed oleosin–rhFGF9 from transgenic *A. thaliana* seeds could stimulate NIH/3T3 cell proliferation.

2. Materials and methods

2.1 Materials

Plasmids and strains: the plasmid pOTB possesses a basic skeleton, a phaseolin promoter/terminator, the *A. thaliana* oleosin gene, a 35S promoter, the *bar* gene, and a Nos terminator. *Escherichia coli* DH5α and *Agrobacterium tumefaciens* EHA105 cells were obtained from the Ministry of Education Engineering Research Center of Bioreactor and Pharmaceutical Development, Jilin Agricultural University. The coding sequence of rhFGF9 was sourced from GenBank (Gene ID: 2254) and modified by codon optimization according to the codon use table of *A. thaliana*. The gene was then synthesized by Genewiz (Jiang Su, China).

Test material: mature *A. thaliana* seeds.

Enzymes and reagents: Ex *Taq*, polymerase chain reaction (PCR) purification kit, gel extraction kit, and a plasmid miniprep kit were all purchased from Takara (Dalian, China). Restriction enzymes *Nco*I and *Hin*dIII, *pfu*DNA polymerase, and T4 DNA ligase were also purchased from Takara. All DNA primers were synthesized and sequenced by Sangon Bioengineering Co. Ltd. (Shanghai, China). Kanamycin and rifampicin were purchased from Sigma (Hong Kong, China). Glufosinate was purchased from the Boehringer Mannheim Corporation (Mannheim, Germany). Dulbecco's modified Eagle medium (DMEM) was purchased from Invitrogen (Carlsbad, CA, USA). Methylthiazol tetrazolium (MTT) was obtained from Gold Biotechnology (St. Louis, MO, USA).

2.2 Methods

2.2.1 Construction of the pOTB–rhFGF9 vector

The pOTB plasmid was digested with *Nco*I and *Hin*dIII. The *rhFGF9* gene was extracted from pUC-rhFGF9 (Genewiz Biotech) and by digestion with *Nco*I and *Hin*dIII. This *rhFGF9* fragment was inserted into the cleaved pOTB plasmid by incubation with T4 DNA ligase at 4℃ for 10 h. The new recombinant plasmid pOTB–rhFGF9 was transformed into DH5α competent cells and amplified. pOTB–rhFGF9 was then transformed into EHA105 competent cells using the freeze–thaw method [29]. The positive colonies were identified by RT-PCR using rhFGF9-specific primers (forward: 5'-C TACTTCGGAGTTCAGGATGC-3'; reverse: 5'-CACCT TATCAGGGTCCACAG-3').

2.2.2 A. thaliana transformation

A. thaliana ecotype Columbia specimens were selected for floral dip when a pot of healthy plants contained approximately 20–30 inflorescences and some maturing siliques. Siliques are routinely clipped off in our lab [30]. Floral-dip liquid medium contained 100 g/L sucrose, 1% B5 (200×) basal medium, 2 mg/L 6-BA, 1 M sodium hydroxide, and 200 μl surfactant Silwet L-77, and was prepared as previously described [31]. Plants were inverted and their aerial parts dipped in EHA105-containing floral-dipping medium for 5 min, followed by wrapping in plastic film to maintain a high humidity for 16–24 h. Plastic covers were then removed and plants grown in a growth chamber until drying and harvesting of seeds (T_1) with a sample bag.

2.2.3 Selection of transgenic A. thaliana

T_1 seeds were grown in sterilized soil until they had grown six leaves. Then, primary transformants were selected using 0.5% glufosinate, spraying once every other day for a total of three times, but their cotyledons became chlorotic and bleached within 3–5 days. Resistant seedlings grew healthy green leaves. The selected lines were confirmed to contain the rhFGF9 sequence by PCR, using genomic DNA as a template and rhFGF9 gene-specific primers. Additionally, many homozygous T_3 seeds werc obtained by further reproduction. These T_3 seed lines were used for protein expression analysis and activity assays.

2.2.4 Oil bodies purification

Wild-type and T_3 transgenic *A. thaliana* seeds (20 mg) were fully ground in 1.5 ml centrifuge tubes with apestle in 50 μl precooled sodium phosphate buffer (PBS, pH 7.5) [32]. Then, the mixtures were spun at 12 000 *g* and 4℃ for 20 min to obtain the floating oil bodies fraction. Oil bodies were washed twice with 50 μl PBS and spun as before. Precipitated material and buffer under the oil bodies was then removed, the oil bodies fraction was collected, the volume was 80 μl and stored at 4℃ until further use.

2.2.5 Protein analysis of oleosin–rhFGF9

Thereafter, 20 μl loading buffer (250 mM Tris–HCl (pH 6.8), 10% (*w/v*) sodium dodecyl sulfate (SDS), 0.5% (*w/v*) bromophenol blue, 50% (*v/v*) glycerol, 5% (*v/v*) β-mercaptoethanol) and 80 μl PBS was added to the oil bodies, mixed and boiled for 10 min, and then the mixtures were analyzed *via* 10% SDS-PAGE (10 μl sample per lane). Gels were stained with coomassie blue overnight and destained using coomassie blue destainer. Proteins on additional gels were transferred to polyvinylidene difluoride membranes (Whatman, Maidstone, UK) using a SEMIDRY Transfer Cell (Bio-Rad Laboratories, Hercules, CA, USA). Electroblotting was performed at 300 mA for 90 min. Then, the membranes were blocked with 100 ml Tris-buffered saline (8.8 g/L NaCl, and 20 mM Tris–HCl, pH 8.0) containing 5% skim milk and 0.05% Tween-20 overnight at 4℃. Membranes were immuno-blotted with a rabbit anti-hFGF9 polyclonal antibody (Bioss, Beijing, China) and incubated with alkaline phosphatase-conjugated goat anti-rabbit IgG/AP antibody (Bioss) according to the manufacturer's protocol. Antibody immunodetection was performed using Western Blue Stabilized Substrate for Alkaline Phosphatase (Promega).

2.2.6 Activity assay for the oil bodies that expressed oleosin–rhFGF9

The oil bodies that expressed oleosin–rhFGF9 were purified from *A. thaliana* seeds and were prepared as "oil bodies purification method". The oil bodies that expressed oleosin–rhFGF9 could stimulate cell proliferation by the MTT assay in NIH/3T3 cells (American Type Culture Collection, Rockville, MD, USA). Cells were cultured in DMEM containing 10% fetal bovine serum (FBS), 100 U/ml ampicillin and 100 U/ml streptomycin until the midlogarithmic phase. Next, cells were seeded into a 96-well plate (5×10^3 cells/well), and cultured in 100 μl DMEM low-sugar medium with 0.4% FBS at 37℃ for 24 h. Cells were then incubated with different concentrations of the oil bodies that expressed oleo-sin–rhFGF9 and bFGF protein (positive control, Abcam, Hong Kong) for 48 h, followed by addition of 20 μl MTT (5 mg/ml) to each well and incubation for 4 h at 37℃. The culture medium was discarded and 100 μl DMSO was added to each well. After incubation for 10 min at room temperature, absorbance at 570/630 nm was assessed using a Microplate Reader model 450 (Bio-Rad Company).

3. Results

3.1 Construction of rhFGF9 expression vectors

The phaseolin promoter of pOTB regulates tissue-specific expression of the transgene during seed development. We constructed an *rhFGF9* gene expression cassette for insertion on pOTB (Fig. 1). This enabled specific expression of rhFGF9 in *A. thaliana* seeds and enabled it to be anchored at oil body surfaces.

3.2 RT-PCR detection of rhFGF9 in transgenic A. thaliana

The presence of *rhFGF9* in T_3 independent glufosinate-resistant lines was confirmed by RT-PCR using total RNA as the template. Six of 12 glufosinate-resistant lines yielded bands of the expected 574 bp (Fig. 2) by the random primer of *rhFGF9* sequence. These six independent T_3 lines (T_3–2, T_3–4, T_3–5, T_3–8, T_3–10, and T_3–12) were used for subsequent analyses.

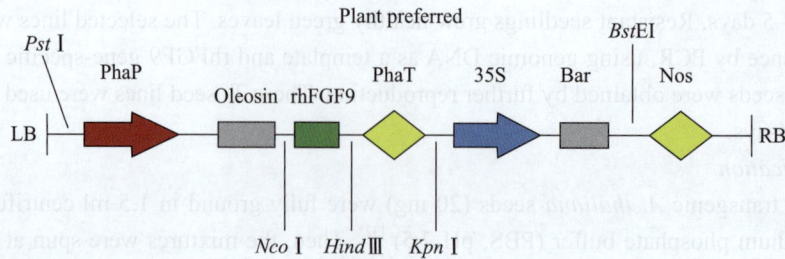

Plant preferred

Fig. 1. Schematic map of recombinant plasmid pOTB–rhFGF9. The T-DNA region of pCAMBI A-1301 was replaced by *Pst*I and *Bst*ÆII between T-Border (LB) and Nos. The 35S-bar gene was insert into T-DNA region by *Pst*I and *Bst*EI. The *oleosin* gene was fused with the phaseolin promoter, then fusion gene was insert into T-DNA region by *Pst*I and *Nco*I. The *rhFGF9* gene was linked to the 3′ -end of *oleosin* gene in T-DNA region by *Nco*I and *Hind*III, generating an 41.5 kDa fusion protein. The recombinant plasmid was named pOTB–rhFGF9. The T-DNA of the pOTB–rhFGF9 vector included a phaseolin promoter/terminator, an *Arabidopsis thaliana oleosin* gene, *rhFGF9* gene, the 35S promoter, the *bar* gene and Nos terminator. PhaP: phaseolin promoter, Oleosin: *Arabidopsis thaliana* oleosin gene, rhFGF9: recombinant human fibroblast growth factor 9, PhaT: phaseolin terminator, 35S: CaMV35S promoter, Bar: the glufosinate resistance gene, Nos: Nopaline synthase terminator.

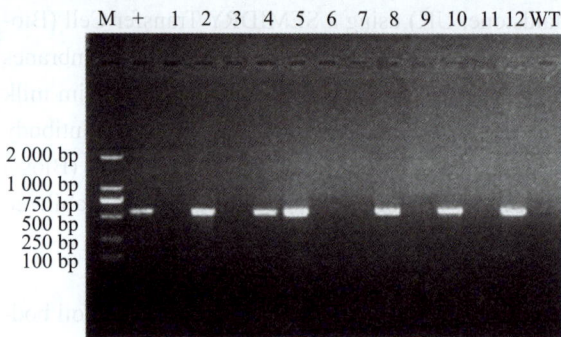

Fig. 2. Agarose gel for screening positive transgenic lines by RT-PCR amplification. Lane +: positive control (pOTB–rhFGF9 plasmid); lane 1– lane 12: the transgenic *Arabidopsis thaliana* T_3–1, T_3–2, T_3–3, T_3–4, T_3–5, T_3–6, T_3–7, T_3–8, T_3–9, T_3–10, T_3–11, T_3–12; lane WT: the wild-type *Arabidopsis thaliana*.

3.3 Expression of oleosin–rhFGF9 fusion protein in transgenic A. thaliana seeds

Expression of the oleosin–rhFGF9 fusion protein was evaluated by extraction of the oil bodies from seeds of the six independent transgenic T_3 lines harboring rhFGF9 DNA, followed by SDS-PAGE and Western blotting. Only an approximate quantification of the fusion protein levels was possible because the accumulation of oleosin–rhFGF9 fusion protein in the oil bodies of transgenic seeds was not accurately quantified and ELISA is not suitable for determining fusion protein concentrations in oil bodies. The oleosin–rhFGF9 fusion protein was predicted to have a molecular weight of 41.5 kDa, and Western blotting analysis of oil bodies from transgenic *A. thaliana* revealed an rhFGF9-positive signal of this size. Consistently, no band was present at this position in wild-type seed samples (Figs. 3 and 4). Amongst the six transgenic lines, levels of oleosin–rhFGF9 in *A. thaliana* seeds ranged from 3.00 to 32.9 µg/mg. The line T_3–4 was determined with the highest expression level, which was approximately 32.9 mg rhFGF9 protein per gram of seeds.

3.4 Activity analysis of the oil bodies that expressed oleosin–rhFGF9

Line T_3–4 was chosen to evaluate the bioactivity of the oil bodies that expressed oleosin–rhFGF9. The cell-proliferative effect of the oil bodies that expressed oleosin–rhFGF9 was determined using a standard MTT assay in NIH/3T3 cells. Cellular response to the oil

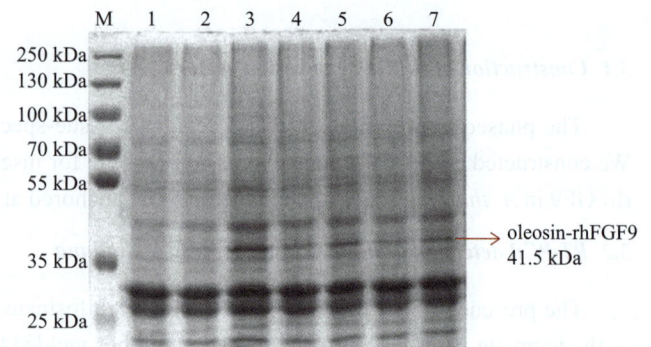

Fig. 3. Identification by SDS–PAGE of oleosin–rhFGF9 expressed in oil bodies from transgenic *Arabidopsis thaliana*. M: protein marker; lane 1: the wild-type (WT) *Arabidopsis thaliana* oil bodies; lane 2–lane 7: the oleosin–rhFGF9 expressed in oil bodies from T_3 transgenic *Arabidopsis thaliana* T_3–2, T_3–4, T_3–5, T_3–8, T_3–10 and T_3–12.

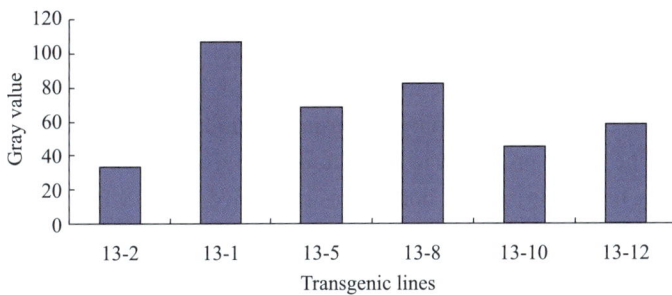

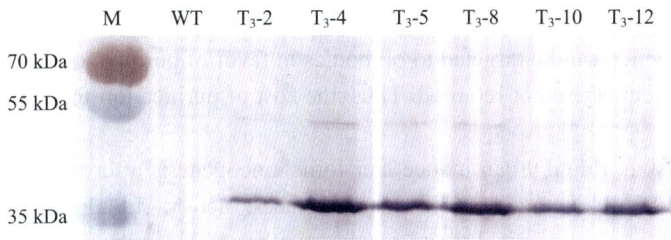

Fig. 4. Detection on oleosin–rhFGF9 protein of the transgenic *Arabidopsis thaliana* by Western blotting and the gray value analysis. M: protein marker; lane 1: the wild-type (WT) *Arabidopsis thaliana* oil bodies; lane 2–lane 7: the oleosin–rhFGF9 expressed in oil bodies from T_3 transgenic *Arabidopsis thaliana* T_3–2, T_3–4, T_3–5, T_3–8, T_3–10 and T_3–12.

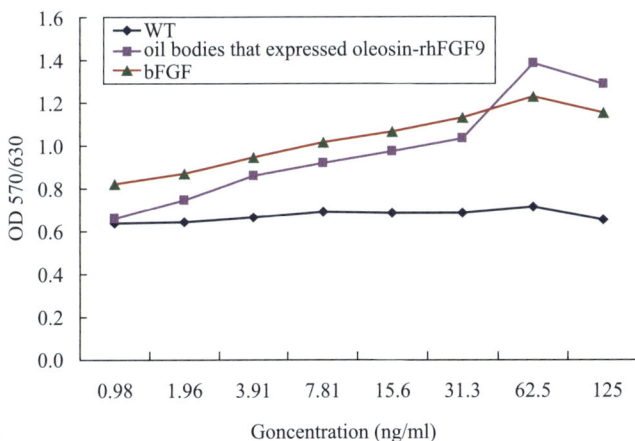

Fig. 5. Proliferation activity analysis of different concentrations of oil bodies that expressed oleosin–rhFGF9 in the transgenic *Arabidopsis thaliana* seeds on NIH/3 T3 cells *in vitro*. Increasing concentrations of oil bodies that expressed oleosin–rhFGF9 (solid circle) or bFGF (solid triangles) were added. Oil bodies from wild-type *Arabidopsis thaliana* were used as a negative control (solid diamond). Proliferation was quantified by measuring the absorbance at 570/630 nm.

bodies that expressed oleosin–rhFGF9 was compared with that of standard bFGF protein. Standard bFGF was used because bFGF can strongly stimulate proliferation in NIH/3T3 cells [33]. A gradient of bFGF concentrations (0.98–125 ng/ml) was used (Fig. 5). The proliferative response of NIH/3T3 cells to the oil bodies that expressed oleosin–rhFGF9 was comparable to the response to standard bFGF. Furthermore, the oil bodies that expressed oleosin– rhFGF9 was found to have a dose-dependent effect on the viability of NIH/3T3 cells. This finding suggests that the oil bodies expressed oleosin–rhFGF9 from the transgenic line T_3–4 had a remarkable proliferation effect on NIH/3 T3 cells.

4. Discussion and conclusion

The use of transgenic plants as bioreactors is an attractive option for high-yield economic production of recombinant proteins. We successfully constructed the plant binary expression vector pOTB–rhFGF9. Codons were optimized for expression in *A. thaliana*. Transgenic *A. thaliana* accumulated oleosin–rhFGF9 within seeds, and homozygotes (T_3) were also obtained. Our study further supports the use of oleosin-fusion technology as an attractive method for protein expression, with advantages in product quality, cost effectiveness, and safety [34,35]. Oleosin-fusion technology has distinct advantages, including the ability for long storage of exogenous proteins in the oil bodies, easy transportation, and a lack of reaction with endogenous proteins and pathogens such as that which occurs with proteins produced in animal cell systems [36]. Additionally, purification process which purified rhFGF9 in *E. coli* was more complex than oil body system. The rhFGF9 fused to the C-terminus of oleosin which can be targeted to oil bodies in favor of purification. The purification process was simpleness and refolding of proteins were not required. Thus, the cost of purification from oil body expression system should be less than other systems.

Many polypeptide growth factors are expressed in skin. rhFGF9 can induce hair follicle neogenesis after wounding [37]. As oleosins can act as a natural emulsifying and stabilizing agent at oil/water interfaces, oleosin–rhFGF9 has a potential application in promoting hair growth. The ability to economically and reliably synthesize bioactive oleosin–rhFGF9 is required to evaluate the practicality of such treatment, and to increase scale of production should it be warranted.

The oleosin–rhFGF9 fusion protein was expressed in *A. thaliana* for the first time and demonstrated that the oil bodies expressed oleosin–rhFGF9 exhibited the expected activity. Oil bodies that expressed oleosin–rhFGF9 were purified from *A. thaliana* seeds and the oil bodies were purification by gradient centrifugation method. However, the target protein was gave play to the function by oil bodies. The oil bodies have a biological structure similar to liposomes. So the oil bodies have increased stability of target protein. The target protein was fused to oleosin C-terminal, set in the oil body surface with no need for purification. The identity of the purified oil bodies was confirmed by SDS-PAGE and Western blotting. The oil bodies that expressed oleosin–rhFGF9 could significantly promote proliferation of NIH/3T3 cells. The rhFGF9 protein was set in the surface of oil bodies and all rhFGF9 protein can give full play to their function. The position control (bFGF) was 125 ng/ml and the oil bodies that expressed oleosin–rhFGF9 was also 125 ng/ml according to the Western blot semi-quantitative method. The extraction quantity of the wild type oil bodies was similar to oil bodies that expressed oleosin–rhFGF9 (the oil bodies were extracted from 20 mg seeds). Our data demonstrate the potential for mass production of rhFGF9 and provide a basis for development of external applications for oleosin–rhFGF9 protein. This study demonstrated that the oil body expression system can be used effectively for the production of rhFGF9.

Supplementary data

Supplementary data associated with this article can be found, in the online version, at http://dx.doi.org/10.1016/j.pep.2015.08.006.

References

[1] Mattei MG, Penault-Llorca F, Coulier F, *et al.* The human FGF9 gene maps to chromosomal region 13q11-q12[J]. Genomics, 1995, 29(3): 811-812.

[2] Colvin JS, Feldman B, Nadeau JH, *et al.* Genomic organization and embryonic expression of the mouse fibroblast growth factor 9 gene[J]. Dev Dyn, 1999, 216(1): 72-88.

[3] Eriksson AE, Cousens LS, Weaver LH, *et al.* Three-dimensional structure of human basic fibroblast growth factor[J]. Proc Natl Acad Sci U S A, 1991, 88(8): 3441-3445.

[4] Plotnikov AN, Eliseenkova AV, Ibrahimi OA, *et al.* Crystal structure of fibroblast growth factor 9 reveals regions implicated in dimerization and autoinhibition[J]. J Biol Chem, 2001, 276(6): 4322-4329.

[5] Miyamoto M, Naruo K, Seko C, *et al.* Molecular cloning of a novel cytokine cDNA encoding the ninth member of the fibroblast growth factor family, which has a unique secretion property[J]. Mol Cell Biol, 1993, 13(7): 4251-4259.

[6] Revest JM, DeMoerlooze L, Dickson C. Fibroblast growth factor 9 secretion is mediated by a non-cleaved amino-terminal signal sequence[J]. J Biol Chem, 2000, 275(11): 8083-8090.

[7] Nickel W. Unconventional secretory routes: direct protein export across the plasma membrane of mammalian cells[J]. Traffic, 2005, 6(8): 607-614.

[8] Beenken A, Mohammadi M. The FGF family: biology, pathophysiology and therapy[J]. Nat Rev Drug Discov, 2009, 8(3): 235-253.

[9] Mohammadi M, Olsen SK, Ibrahimi OA. Structural basis for fibroblast growth factor receptor activation[J]. Cytokine Growth Factor Rev, 2005, 16(2): 107-137.

[10] Bhatla SC, Kaushik V, Yadav MK. Use of oil bodies and oleosins in recombinant protein production and other biotechnological applications[J]. Biotechnol Adv, 2010, 28(3): 293-300.

[11] Jolivet P, Roux E, D'Andrea S, *et al.* Protein composition of oil bodies in Arabidopsis thaliana ecotype WS[J]. Plant Physiol Biochem, 2004, 42(6): 501-509.

[12] Xu M, Liu D, Li G. Cloning of Soybean 24 kDa oleosin gene and its transient expression as a carrier for forgeign protein[J]. Agricultural sciences in China, 2004, 3(5): 321-329.

[13] Siloto RM, Findlay K, Lopez-Villalobos A, *et al.* The accumulation of oleosins determines the size of seed oilbodies in Arabidopsis[J]. Plant Cell, 2006, 18(8): 1961-1974.

[14] Li W, Li LG, Sun XF, *et al.* An oleosin-fusion protein driven by the CaMV35S promoter is accumulated in Arabidopsis (Brassicaceae) seeds and correctly targeted to oil bodies[J]. Genet Mol Res, 2012, 11(3): 2138-2146.

[15] Huang CY, Chung CI, Lin YC, *et al.* Oil bodies and oleosins in

Physcomitrella possess characteristics representative of early trends in evolution[J]. Plant Physiol, 2009, 150(3): 1192-1203.

[16] Liu Q, Sun Y, Su W, et al. Species-specific size expansion and molecular evolution of the oleosins in angiosperms[J]. Gene, 2012, 509(2): 247-257.

[17] Moloney MM, Joseph B, Deckers HM. Oil body based personal care products. United States patent US 6582710[p]. 2001.

[18] Moloney MM, Joseph B, Deckers HM. Products for topical applications comprising oil bodies, United States patent US 6582710[P]. 2003.

[19] Parmenter DL, Boothe JG, van Rooijen GJ, et al. Production of biologically active hirudin in plant seeds using oleosin partitioning[J]. Plant Mol Biol, 1995, 29(6): 1167-1180.

[20] van Rooijen GJ, Moloney MM. Plant seed oil-bodies as carriers for foreign proteins[J]. Biotechnology (N Y), 1995, 13(1): 72-77.

[21] Stoger E, Ma JK, Fischer R, et al. Sowing the seeds of success: pharmaceutical proteins from plants[J]. Curr Opin Biotechnol, 2005, 16(2): 167-173.

[22] Boothe J, Nykiforuk C, Shen Y, et al. Seed-based expression systems for plant molecular farming[J]. Plant Biotechnol J, 2010, 8(5): 588-606.

[23] Bhatla SC, Kaushik V, Yadav MK. Use of oil bodies and oleosins in recombinant protein production and other biotechnological applications[J]. Biotechnol Adv, 2010, 28(3): 293-300.

[24] Giddings G, Allison G, Brooks D, et al. Transgenic plants as factories for biopharmaceuticals[J]. Nat Biotechnol, 2000, 18(11): 1151-1155.

[25] Moloney MM, van Rooijen G. Expression of epidermal growth factor in plant seeds, United States Patent US 7091401[P]. 2006.

[26] Li H, Yang J, Chen Y, et al. Expression of a functional recombinant oleosin-human hyaluronidase hPH-20 fusion in Arabidopsis thaliana[J]. Protein Expr Purif, 2014, 103: 23-27.

[27] Yang J, Guan L, Guo Y, et al. Expression of biologically recombinant human acidic fibroblast growth factor in Arabidopsis thaliana seeds via oleosin fusion technology[J]. Gene, 2015, 566(1): 89-94.

[28] Twyman RM, Stoger E, Schillberg S, et al. Molecular farming in plants: host systems and expression technology[J]. Trends Biotechnol, 2003, 21(12): 570-578.

[29] Hofgen R, Willmitzer L. Storage of competent cells for Agrobacterium transformation[J]. Nucleic Acids Res, 1988, 16(20): 9877.

[30] Zhang X, Henriques R, Lin SS, et al. Agrobacterium-mediated transformation of Arabidopsis thaliana using the floral dip method[J]. Nat Protoc, 2006, 1(2): 641-646.

[31] Weigel D, Glazebook J. Arabidopsis: A Laboratory Manual, 2002: 165-165.

[32] Tzen JT, Peng CC, Cheng DJ, et al. A new method for seed oil body purification and examination of oil body integrity following germination[J]. J Biochem, 1997, 121(4): 762-768.

[33] Gospodarowicz D. Localisation of a fibroblast growth factor and its effect alone and with hydrocortisone on 3T3 cell growth[J]. Nature, 1974, 249(453): 123-127.

[34] Streatfield SJ. Approaches to achieve high-level heterologous protein production in plants[J]. Plant Biotechnol J, 2007, 5(1): 2-15.

[35] Fischer R, Stoger E, Schillberg S, et al. Plant-based production of biopharmaceuticals[J]. Curr Opin Plant Biol, 2004, 7(2): 152-158.

[36] Larrick JW, Thomas DW. Producing proteins in transgenic plants and animals[J]. Curr Opin Biotechnol, 2001, 12(4): 411-418.

[37] Gay D, Kwon O, Zhang Z, et al. FgF9 from dermal gammadelta T cells induces hair follicle neogenesis after wounding[J]. Nat Med, 2013, 19(7): 916-923.

Expression of biologically recombinant human acidic fibroblast growth factor in *Arabidopsis thaliana* seeds *via* oleosin fusion technology

Jing Yang, Xiaokun Li

1. Introduction

Human acid fibroblast growth factor (aFGF), also called FGF-1, the physiological form of which contains 154 amino acids (Zazo *et al.*, 1992) is a heparin binding protein. It was involved in a variety of biological processes, including angiogenesis, cell proliferation, and differentiation (Kenneth and Guillermo, 1986; Jose Feito *et al.*, 2011). The aFGF protein is an important member of the growth factor families. The aFGF were originally identified as peptides with mitogenic activity for fibroblasts. The aFGF has regenerative capabilities when administered after focal cerebral ischemia in different species (Mitani *et al.*, 1992; Sasaki *et al.*, 1992), so it may have broad prospects for the treatment of acute focal cerebral ischemia (Jose Feito *et al.*, 2011). The aFGF also has fortissimo tissue-injury repair properties that might be relevant for medical applications.

Disputes about the safety of using aFGF in the human body have badly slowed down its therapeutic development. Except for the topical application of aFGF to treat burn wounds in China, no other pharmacological application of FGF has been approved (Wu *et al.*, 2005). Lozano *et al.* (2000) showed that a shortened form of aFGF including amino acids 20–154 of the full-length sequence was high-level expressed and purified in *Escherichia coli* and the expression level was up to 150 mg/L. The biological activity showed that a shortened form of aFGF including amino acids 20–154 has no significant differences. Three groups of test results showed that the degradation problem of N-terminus was solved and dimer formation is decreased obviously. So we chose a shortened form of aFGF including amino acids 20–154. We modified the N-terminus of the aFGF gene by eliminating residues 1–19, which weakened its mitogenic properties and preserved its non-mitogenic properties.

The need for cheap production of a mass of proteins has led to a new industry for producing recombinant proteins in transgenic plants. The potential of molecular pharming, using transgenic plants as bioreactors can produce therapeutic proteins. Plants as vehicle provide an attractive expression system for many proteins (Richter *et al.*, 2000; Petolino *et al.*, 2000; Tacket *et al.*, 1998). The expression of therapeutic proteins in plant has a safe and low-cost advantage, and process post-translational modifications. However, the expression level and stability of recombinant proteins in plants especially in plant seeds are influenced by several factors for example the cis-regulatory elements, mRNA stability and final site of protein accumulation in plant cells or tissues (Doran, 2006). Oil bodies (OBs) are lipid-storage organelles in plant seeds that provide energy for seedlings during germination (Huang, 1996). OBs are composed of a TAG core surrounded by a phospholipid (PL) monolayer that contains oleosins, caleosins and steroleosins including several that stabilize the organelle. OBs can be easily separated from the cell components in seeds by flotation centrifugation and contain relatively few different proteins (van Rooijen and Moloney, 1995). When used to recover oil body-associated recombinant proteins, this process greatly enriches for the target protein and can reduce purification steps.

Because of the oil body's peculiar structure, a novel technology named oil body fusion technology has been developed in which heterologous proteins are fused to the N- or C-terminus of oleosin in oil body surface and expressed under the control of an oleosin gene promoter or seed-specific promoter (Stoger *et al.*, 2005; Boothe *et al.*, 2010). It is one of the most popular methods because it can extend protein half-life, and allows easy transportation and storage (Bhatla *et al.*, 2010). There have been many reports of oleosin-fusion technology being used with heterologous proteins. Recombinant human precursor insulin fused with oleosin has been expressed in *Arabidopsis* and shown biological activity (Nykiforuk, 2006). Human epidermal growth factor (hEGF) fused with oleosin has also been expressed in *Arabidopsis* and an accumulation level of 0.12% was achieved (Moloney *et al.*, 2006; Bhatla *et al.*, 2010). The fusion protein Oleosin-ApoA1 has been expressed in *Arabidopsis* and *Carthamus tinctorius* L. and reached commercial production standards (Moloney *et al.*, 2004; Bhatla *et al.*, 2010). Many heterologous proteins have been expressed in transgenic plants since the successful production of a mouse monoclonal antibody in plants (Twyman *et al.*, 2003; Jung *et al.*, 2010). Here, we expressed aFGF in the oil body of *Arabidopsis* through the construction of the plant expression vector pKO-aFGF. The expression of the oleosin-aFGF fusion protein was checked by SDS-PAGE and the antigenicity was detected by Western blot. The aFGF protein expressed in transgenic *A. thaliana* seeds stimulated NIH/3T3 cell proliferation activity.

2. Materials and methods

2.1 Materials

Plasmids and strains: The plasmid pKO for transformation was constructed using the pCAMBIA1301 plasmid as a basic skeleton, and contained the phaseolin promoter/terminator (Patent PCT/US01/ 47495), the *A. thaliana oleosin* gene (*AtOLE*, GenBank accession no. X62353.1) 35S promoter (GenBank accession no. AF21 8816.1), *bar* gene (GenBank accession AF218816.1) and terminator of nos (GenBank accession AF234307), *aFGF* gene (GenBank accession no. BC03 2697.1). *E. coli* DH5α and *Agrobacterium tumefaciens* EHA105 were obtained from the laboratory of the Engineering Research Center of Bioreactor and Pharmaceutical Development, Ministry of Education, Jilin Agricul-tural University, China.

Test material: mature seeds of A. thaliana.

Enzymes and reagents: The restriction enzymes *Nco*I and *Hin*dIII, *pfu*DNA polymerase and T4 DNA ligase were purchased from Takara (Dalian, China). All primers were synthesized and sequenced by Sangon Bioengineering Co., Ltd. (Shanghai, China). Kanamycin (Kan), streptomycin (Str) and rifampicin (Rif) were purchased from Sigma (Hong Kong, China). Glufosinate was purchased from the Boehringer Mannheim Corporation (Mannheim, Germany). Rabbit anti-aFGF polyclonal antibody was purchased from Abcam, Inc. (Cambridge, MA, USA). Isopropyl-β-D-thiogalactoside (IPTG) and methylthiazol tetrazolium (MTT) were obtained from Gold Biotechnology (St. Louis, MO, USA). Dulbecco's modified Eagle medium (DMEM) was purchased from Invitrogen (Carlsbad, CA, USA).

2.2 Construction of the pKO-aFGF vector

The recombinant plasmid skeleton was derived from pCAMBIA1301 plasmid vector. The T-DNA region of pCAMBIA1301 was replaced by *pst*I and *Bst*EII between T-Border (LB) and Nos. The *35S-bar* gene was amplified by PCR from pEGAD plasmid using the forward primer with *Pst*I, *Nco*I, *Hin*dIII, *Kpn*I (CCCTGCA GCCATGGTCTAGAGG-*TACC*ATCCGTCAACAT GGTGG) and the reverse primer with *Bst*EII (GGG*TTACC*TCAGATCTCG GTGACGGGC). The 35S-bar gene was inserted into pCAMBIA1301-revised by *Pst*I and *Bst*EI and resulted in pCAMBIA1301-35S-bar. The phaseolin promoter was amplified by PCR from *Phaseolus vulgaris* genome (the forward primer: CG*CTGCAG*-GAATTCATTGTACTCCCAG, the reverse primer: CCTCTAGCTGTATCCGCCATAGTAGAGTAGTATTGAATAT GAG). The RNA from *Arabidopsis thaliana* seeds was extracted and reversed transcription into cDNA. The *A. thaliana* oleosin gene was amplified by PCR from *A. thaliana* cDNA (the forward primer: CTCATATTCAAT ACTACTCTAC-TATGGCGGATACAGCTAGA GGAAC, the reverse primer: CATG*CCATGG*TAGTAGTGTGCTGGCCACCACG). The *A. thaliana* oleosin gene was fused with the phaseolin promoter by fusion PCR method (the forward primer: CG*CTGCAG*GAATTCATTGTACTCCCAG,the reverse primer: CATG*CCATGG*TAGTAGTGTGCTGGCCACCACG). The fusion gene was inserted into pCAMBIA1301-35S-bar vector by *Pst*I and *Nco*I, named pCAMBIA 1301-F-B. The phaseolin terminator was amplified by PCR from *Phaseolus vulgaris* genome. It was inserted into pCAMBIA1301-F-B vector by *Hin*dIII and *Kpn*I, named pKO vector (Fig. 1).

The *aFGF* gene was transformed with plant-preferred codons. Then, the pUC57-aFGF vector with unique *Nco*I and *Hin*dIII sites was synthesized by Sangon Biotech. The pKO plasmid was extracted from *E. coli* and double restriction enzyme digested with *Nco*I and *Hin*dIII. The aFGF gene was inserted into the pKO plasmid. The new recombinant plas-

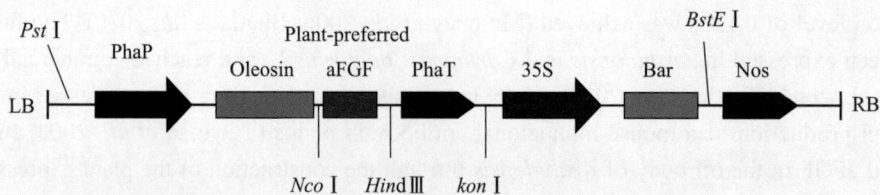

Fig. 1. Schematic map of recombinant plasmid pKO-aFGF. The T-DNA region of pCAMBI A-1301 was replaced by *Pst*I and *Bst*EII between T-Border (LB) and Nos. The 35S-bar gene was inserted into the T-DNA region by *Pst*I and *Bst*EI. The oleosin gene was fused with the phaseolin promoter, then fusion gene was inserted into T-DNA region by *Pst*I and *Nco*I. The aFGF gene was linked to the 3'-end of oleosin gene in T-DNA region by *Nco*I and *Hind*III. The recombinant plasmid was named pKO-aFGF. The T-DNA of the pKO-aFGF vector included a phaseolin promoter/terminator, an *A. thaliana* oleosin gene, *aFGF* gene, the 35S promoter, the *bar* gene and nos gene terminator. PhaP: phaseolin promoter, Oleasin: *A. thaliana* oleosin gene, aFGF: acidic fibroblast growth factor, PhaT: phaseolin terminator, 35S: CaMV35S promoter, Nos: Nopaline synthase terminator gene.

mid named pKO-aFGF was transformed into *E. coli* DH5α competent cells. The pKO-aFGF recombinant plasmid was extracted from *E. coli* DH5α and tested by PCR and digestion. Then, it was transformed into *Agrobacterium* EHA105 competent cells using the freeze–thaw method (Höfgen and Willmitzer, 1988). Positive colonies were identified by PCR with aFGF-specific primers: F1 (5 -ATGGCTAACTACAAGAAG-3; forward) and R1 (5 -TTAATCAGAAGAA ACTG-GCAA T-3; reverse). ExTaq DNA polymerase (Takara Bio, Dalian, China) was used in the PCR reaction system. A total of 30 cycles were performed with a denaturation step at 94 ℃ for 30 s, an annealing step at 60 ℃ for 45 s and an elongation step at 72 ℃ for 90 s.

2.3 Transformation into A. thaliana

A. thaliana Columbia ecotype (4–5 weeks old, containing numerous unopened floral buds) was chosen as the transformation host. Preparation of liquid medium containing *A. tumefaciens*, 5% sucrose, 0.1% B5, 0.001% 6-BA, 0.009% 1 M sodium hydroxide and 400 μl/L of the surfactant Silwet L-77 was performed according to the *Arabidopsis* test manual (Weigel and Glazebook, 2004). Unopened *A. thaliana* floral buds were infiltrated for 7 min, and the plants were laid flat under a plastic dome and cultured in the dark for 24–48 h after inoculation. Then, the infected *A. thaliana* plants were transferred to normal lighting conditions and grown until seeds were collected (T$_1$).

2.4 Selection of transgenic A. thaliana

The T$_1$ transgenic seeds were stratificated at 4 ℃ for 2 days, Primary transformant (T$_1$) seeds were screened on 1/2 Murashige and Skoog (MS) basal plates supplemented with 11 mg/mL Basta. The independent Basta-resistant lines were transferred to soil after screening on culture medium and were further screened in the soil [vermiculite: soil (V:V) 7:3] with 1% Basta. *A. thaliana* plants were further grown until collected T$_2$ seeds. The T$_2$ seeds were screened by Basta and then collected T$_3$ seeds. The seeds from independent homozygous T$_3$ lines were used for protein expression analysis and activity assay.

2.5 Oil purification

Oil bodies were purified using the method described by Tzen *et al.* (1997). Twenty milligrams of seeds were ground in 200 μl sodium phosphate buffer (pH 7.5). The suspension was spun at 10 000×g and 4 ℃ for 30 min. The floating oil body fraction was collected, resuspended in 200 μl sodium phosphate buffer (pH 7.5), and spun as before. After centrifugation and removal of the upper buffer, the oil body fraction was collected and stored at 4 ℃ until further use.

2.6 Analysis of aFGF protein linked to oil body

Twenty milligrams of seeds were ground in 200 μl sodium phosphate buffer (pH 7.5). The loading quantity of sample was 10 μl crude oil body and it was separated by 12% acrylamide in SDS-PAGE. The proteins were transferred onto Immobilon-P polyvinylidene difluoride (PVDF) membranes (PerkinElmer, Boston, MA, USA) using a SEMI-DRY Transfer Cell (Bio-Rad Laboratories, Hercules, CA, USA), and immunoblotted with a rabbit anti-aFGF polyclonal antibody (Abcam) according to the manufacturer's protocol. Immunoreactive bands were checked with western blotting luminal reagents.

2.7 Activity assay of aFGF

To verify that the aFGF produced and purified from *A. thaliana* had a stimulatory effect on the proliferation of NIH/3T3 cells, an MTT assay was performed. NIH/3T3 cells were seeded in flat-bottomed, 96-well plates at an initial density of 5×10^4 cells per ml (100 μl per well) and cultured in DMEM low-sugar medium for 24 h at 37 ℃. After 3 days of incubation with aFGF, 20 μl MTT solution was added to each well. The cells were then incubated for a further 4 h at 37 ℃, the culture medium included the MTT solution in the wells was removed, and 150 μl DMSO was added to each well and mixed thoroughly to dissolve the crystals. The plates were read at 570/630 nm in a Microplate Reader model 450 to obtain absorbance values.

3. Results and discussion

3.1 Construction of a plant oil body expression vector

The T-DNA region of the pKO plasmid contained a phaseolin promoter, oleosin gene, phaseolin terminator, 35S promoter, *bar* gene and *nos* gene. The phaseolin promoter controls tissue-specific transgene expression during seed development. For the pKO-aFGF plasmid, we constructed an *aFGF* gene expression cassette (Fig. 1) containing the *aFGF* gene under the control of the phaseolin seed-specific promoter (phaP)/terminator (phaT). This construct enabled specific expression in *A. thaliana* seeds. The oleosin gene was as signal peptide to carry aFGF anchoring in oil body surface.

3.2 RT-PCR detection of recombinant aFGF transcripts in transgenic Arabidopsis

The pKO-aFGF plasmid was transformed into *A. thaliana* by a floral dip method. Primary transformant seeds were screened on 1/2 MS basal plates supplemented with 11 mg/ml Basta. The independent Basta-resistant lines were transferred into soil to continue to screen and were further confirmed using the *aFGF* cDNA as a template. The aFGF transcripts were detected by RT-PCR. Of the eleven analyzed transgenic plants, six exhibited clear bands. A specific 423 bp PCR product was generated. The six lines showed the target bands among twelve independent Basta-resistant lines and the positions of the target bands were expected at 423 bp (Fig. 2). Therefore, the aFGF proteins were expressed at the transcriptional level.

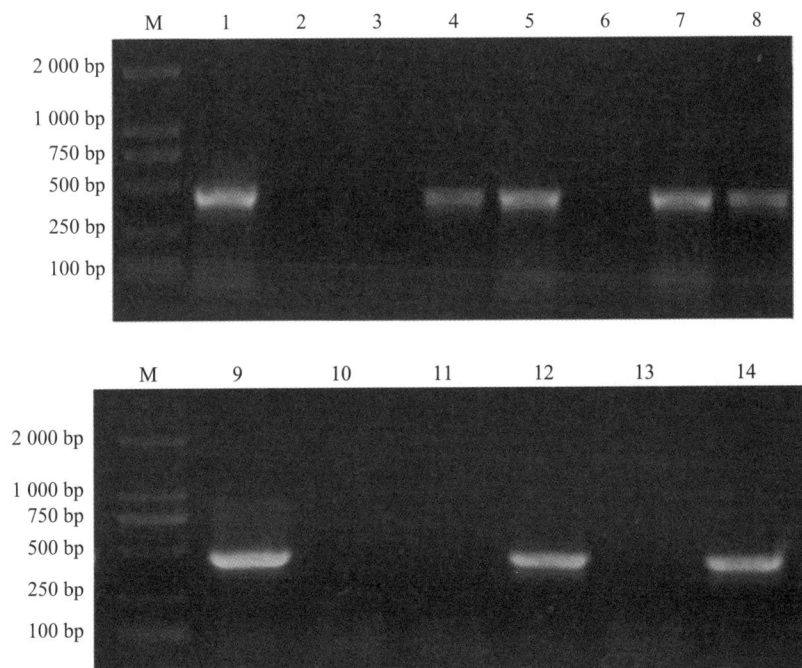

Fig. 2. Agarose gel for screening positive transgenic lines by RT-PCR amplification. Lane 1 and lane 9: positive control (aFGF plasmid); lane 2–lane 8: the transgenic *A. thaliana* T_3-1,T_3-2,T_3-3, T_3-4, T_3-5, T_3-6 and T_3-7; lane 10–lane 12: the transgenic *A. thaliana* T_3-8,T_3-9 and T_3-10; lane 13: the wild-type *A. thaliana*; lane 14: T_3-11.

3.3 Expression of recombinant aFGF protein in transgenic A. thaliana

To evaluate the accumulation of the oleosin-aFGF fusion protein in pKO-aFGF transformants, the crude oil body was extracted and oil body-associated proteins of transgenic (T_3-3, T_3-4, T_3-6, T_3-7, T_3-10, T_3-11) and wild-type A. thaliana plants were analyzed by SDS-PAGE and western blotting. The aFGF gene was predicted to encode 135 amino acids. Determination of the crude oil body extracts from the pKO-aFGF-transformed plants showed an immunoreactive protein with a molecular weight of 33.5 kD, which is identical size to oleosin-aFGF fusion protein, suggesting that the oleosin precursor was properly assembled in the transgenic A. thaliana oil body. The six pKO-aFGF-transformed lines also exhibited positive signals in seeds.

However, the accumulation of oleosin-aFGF fusion protein in the oil body of transgenic lines was not accurately quantified, because ELISA method was not suited for testing fusion protein in the oil body. So the fusion protein was roughly quantified by western blot method. There was no band at this position in the wild-type seeds (Figs. 3 and 4). Then there were more oil body-associates observed in transgenic lines 7, 10, and 11 and WT than the others. Furthermore, these differences may have come from the purification efficiency during oil body preparation.

3.4 NIH/3T3 activity analysis of plant oil bodies containing the aFGF protein

The NIH/3T3 cell line is generally used for evaluation of the biological activity of aFGF. To evaluate the biological activity of different transgenic lines (T_3-3, T_3-4, T_3-6, T_3-7, T_3-10, T_3-11), NIH/3T_3 cells were used to test the stimulation

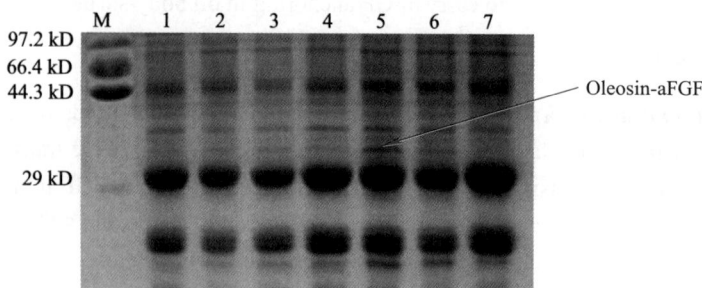

Fig. 3. Identification of SDS-PAGE of crude oil bodies in transgenic *Arabidopsis thaliana*. M: protein marker; lane 1–lane 6: the crude oil body from T_3 transgenic A. *thaliana* T_3-3, T_3-4, T_3-6, T_3-7, T_3-10 and T_3-11; lane 7: the crude oil body from wild-type (WT) A. *thaliana*.

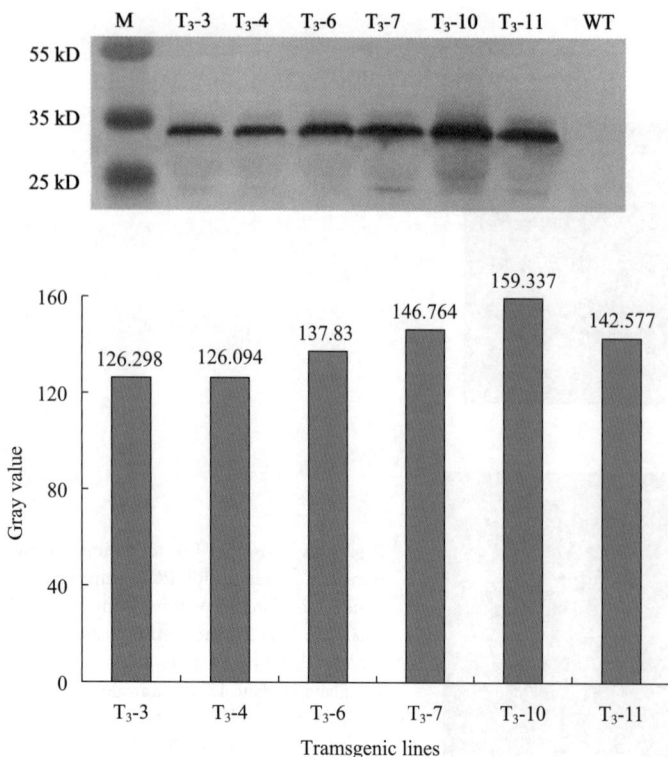

Fig. 4. Detection on aFGF protein of the transgenic *Arabidopsis thaliana* by Western blot and the gray value analysis of lane 1–lane 6: the crude oil body from T_3 transgenic A. *thaliana* T_3-3, T_3-4, T_3-6, T_3-7, T_3-10, and T_3-11; lane 7: the crude oil body from wild-type (WT) A. *thaliana*.

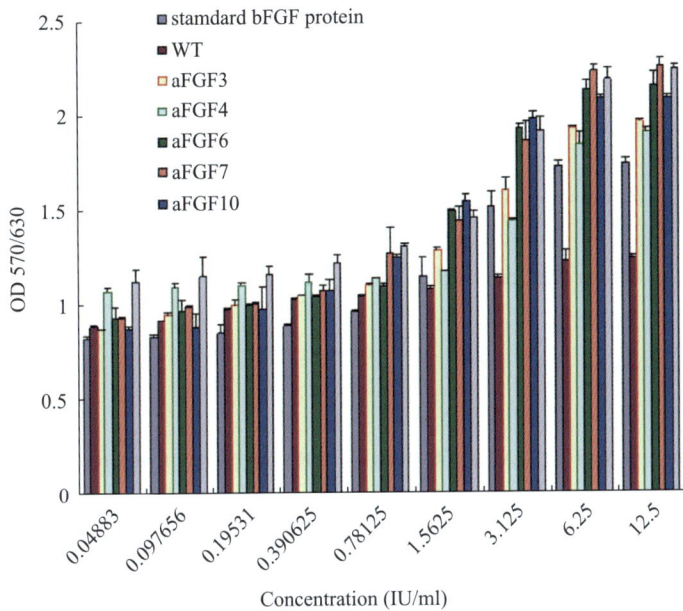

Fig. 5. The activities assay of aFGF protein in the transgenic *Arabidopsis thaliana* seeds. Dose–response curves for proliferation activity. Increase of NIH/3T3 fibroblast cells were expressed as the percentage increases in absorbance (570/630 nm). The test sample included the standard bFGF protein (■), oil body from wild-type *A. thaliana* (■), aFGF3 (□), aFGF4 (□), aFGF6 (■), aFGF7 (■), aFGF10 (■), aFGF11 (–).

of cell proliferation. As shown in Fig. 5, the standard bFGF concentration was set as a gradient from 0.04883 to 12.5 IU/ml. The results suggested that aFGF proteins from the T_3 different transgenic lines had a dose-dependent cell proliferative effect on the NIH/3 T3 cells. The oil bodies with aFGF from different lines had stimulation of cell proliferation activity that was higher than the bFGF standard protein.

Oil body-based pharmaceutical formulations include therapeutic, diagnostic and delivery agents. Oil body-based emulsions can be used as adjuvants in pharmaceutical protein base for dermatological products, components for orally administered medicines, etc. In these products oil bodies may also carry an active ingredient to be delivered to host, if needed. Personal care products wherein oil body-based emulsions may be used include various cosmetic and cosmeceutical products such as creams, lotions and makeup products, hair care products, and bath products such as soaps, washes and cleansers (Deckers *et al.*, 2001, 2003). In products like toothpaste, oil bodies may also serve as carriers of components such as flavoring agent, fluoride, silicas, chelating agents, and sweetener. The recombinant proteins expressed in the oil body can be stored for longer periods than those obtained from other sources. GUS enzyme has been reported to remain active for more than one year when expressed as oleosin fusion in seeds (van Rooijen and Moloney, 1995). Moreover, recombinant seeds can be easily transported. Furthermore, proper refolding of proteins takes place spontaneously when expressed on oil bodies (Nykiforuk *et al.*, 2005). Recombinant proteins can be expressed in the oilseeds themselves, or otherwise the protein can be expressed in any system of choice. It can then be targeted to oil bodies for purification and refolding. So the oil body expression system was the better option than the other different expression systems. The aFGF fused to the C-terminus of oleosin and expressed under the control of a seed-specific promoter. Thus, expensive steps needed for purification and refolding of proteins are not required. The expression of aFGF with plant organelle signaling sequences need to purify aFGF protein, thus the purification cost of products should be increased. The oil body linked to aFGF was applied in many fields. Many researches were done in SemBioSys Genetics Inc. The oil body was suitable for expressing FGF protein.

4. Conclusions

Here, an *aFGF* gene was expressed by *A. thaliana* and accumulated in the transgenic seeds. We successfully constructed the plant binary expression vector pKO-aFGF and T_3 transgenic homozygotes were obtained. The oil body-associated proteins were analyzed by SDS-PAGE and western blotting, and the results showed that the T_3-3 and T_3-4 transgenic plants expressed the recombinant protein at relatively low levels, while the T_3-10 line expressed it at relatively high levels. The results of NIH/3T3 cell analysis demonstrated that the activity of aFGF from the transgenic *A. thaliana* seeds was higher than that of bFGF standard protein. This is the first trial of aFGF production in an oil body expression system, and the recombinant protein exhibited typical activity. This result might be useful for the mass production of aFGF. We have confirmed that the oil body expression system can be used effectively for the production of aFGF.

Supplementary data

Supplementary data to this article can be found online at http://dx. doi.org/10.1016/j.gene.2015.04.036.

References

Bhatla SC, Kaushik V, Yadav MK. Use of oil bodies and oleosins in recombinant protein production and other biotechnological applications[J]. Biotechnol Adv, 2010, 28(3): 293-300.

Boothe J, Nykiforuk C, Shen Y, et al. Seed-based expression systems for plant molecular farming[J]. Plant Biotechnol J, 2010, 8(5): 588-606.

Deckers HM, Van Rooijen G, Boothe J, et al. Oil body based personal care products. United States patent US 6183762.

Deckers HM, Van Rooijen G, Boothe J, et al. Products for topical applications comprising oil bodies. United States patent US 6582710.

Doran PM. Foreign protein degradation and instability in plants and plant tissue cultures[J]. Trends Biotechnol, 2006, 24(9): 426-432.

Hofgen R, Willmitzer L. Storage of competent cells for Agrobacterium transformation[J]. Nucleic Acids Res, 1988, 16(20): 9877.

Huang AH. Oleosins and oil bodies in seeds and other organs[J]. Plant Physiol, 1996, 110(4): 1055-1061.

Feito MJ, Jimenez M, Fernandez-Cabrera C, et al. Strategy for fluorescent labeling of human acidic fibroblast growth factor without impairment of mitogenic activity: a bona fide tracer[J]. Anal Biochem, 2011, 411(1): 1-9.

Jung Y, Jung MY, Park JH, et al. Production of human hyaluronidase in a plant-derived protein expression system: plant-based transient production of active human hyaluronidase[J]. Protein Expr Purif, 2010, 74(2): 181-188.

Thomas KA, Gimenez-Gallego G. Fibroblast growth factors: broad spectrum mitogens with potent angiogenic activity[J]. Trends in Biochemical Sciences, 1986, 11(2): 81-84.

Lozano RM, Pineda-Lucena A, Gonzalez C, et al. 1H NMR structural characterization of a nonmitogenic, vasodilatory, ischemia-protector and neuromodulatory acidic fibroblast growth factor[J]. Biochemistry, 2000, 39(17): 4982-4993.

Mitani A, Oomura Y, Yanase H, et al. Acidic fibroblast growth factor delays in vitro ischemia-induced intracellular calcium elevation in gerbil hippocampal slices: a sign of neuroprotection[J]. Neurochem Int, 1992, 21(3): 337-341.

Moloney MM, van Rooijen G. Preparation of heterologous proteins on oil bodies.United States patent US 6753167, 2004-06-22.

Moloney MM, van Rooijen G. 2006. Expression of epidermalgrowth factor in plant seeds, United States patent US 7091401.

Nykiforuk CL, Boothe JG, Murray EW, et al. Transgenic expression and recovery of biologically active recombinant human insulin from Arabidopsis thaliana seeds[J]. Plant Biotechnol J, 2006, 4(1): 77-85.

Petolino JF, Young S, Hopkins N, et al. Expression of murine adenosine deaminase (ADA) in transgenic maize[J]. Transgenic Res, 2000, 9(1): 1-9.

Richter LJ, Thanavala Y, Arntzen CJ, et al. Production of hepatitis B surface antigen in transgenic plants for oral immunization[J]. Nat Biotechnol, 2000, 18(11): 1167-1171.

Sasaki K, Oomura Y, Suzuki K, et al. Acidic fibroblast growth factor prevents death of hippocampal CA1 pyramidal cells following ischemia[J]. Neurochem Int, 1992, 21(3): 397-402.

Stoger E, Ma JK, Fischer R, et al. Sowing the seeds of success: pharmaceutical proteins from plants[J]. Curr Opin Biotechnol, 2005, 16(2): 167-173.

Tacket CO, Mason HS, Losonsky G, et al. Immunogenicity in humans of a recombinant bacterial antigen delivered in a transgenic potato[J]. Nat Med, 1998, 4(5): 607-609.

Twyman RM, Stoger E, Schillberg S, et al. Molecular farming in plants: host systems and expression technology[J]. Trends Biotechnol, 2003, 21(12): 570-578.

Tzen JT, Peng CC, Cheng DJ, et al. A new method for seed oil body purification and examination of oil body integrity following germination[J]. J Biochem, 1997, 121(4): 762-768.

van Rooijen GJ, Moloney MM. Plant seed oil-bodies as carriers for foreign proteins[J]. Biotechnology (NY), 1995, 13(1): 72-77.

Weigel, D, Glazebook, J. Arabidopsis: a laboratory manual, 2004: 7-17.

Wu X, Su Z, Li X, et al. High-level expression and purification of a nonmitogenic form of human acidic fibroblast growth factor in Escherichia coli[J]. Protein Expr Purif, 2005, 42(1): 7-11.

Zazo M, Lozano RM, Ortega S, et al. High-level synthesis in Escherichia coli of shortened and full-length human acidic fibroblast growth factor and purification in a form stable in aqueous solutions[J]. Gene, 1992, 113(2): 231-238.

Highly efficient expression of functional recombinant human keratinocyte growth factor 1 and its protective effects on hepatocytes

Ping Xue, Xiaokun Li

1. Introduction

Keratinocyte growth factor 1 (KGF1), also known as fibroblast growth factor (FGF)7, is a member of the FGF family and was initially purified from the conditioned medium of M426 human embryonic lung fibroblasts (Rubin *et al.*, 1989). KGF1 has a wide range of biological activities, but unlike other FGF members, KGF1 is specific for epithelial cells in various tissues, such as alveolar epithelial cells (Deimling *et al.*, 2007), liver parenchymal cells (Steiling *et al.*, 2004), gastrointestinal cells (Housley *et al.*, 1994), urinary tract epithelial cells (Yi *et al.*, 1995), and a variety of squamous epithelial cells (Fuchs, 1993). In addition to its mitogenic function, KGF1 has been identified as a potent survival factor for various types of epithelial cells *in vitro* and *in vivo* (reviewed by Werner, 1998; Finch and Rubin, 2004) by protecting these cells from various insults (Finch and Rubin, 2004). The effects of KGF1 on tissue repair and cytoprotection, and its mechanisms of action in keratinocytes been reviewed elsewhere (auf dem Keller *et al.*, 2004). Encouragingly, the first drug derived from KGF1 (palifermin) has been approved by the FDA for the treatment of oral mucositis. There are also potential applications of KGF1 in chronic liver injury (Steiling *et al.*, 2004), liver regeneration (Tsai and Wang, 2011), diabetic wound healing (Peng *et al.*, 2011), acute lung injury (Ulrich *et al.*, 2005), and fetal lung hypoplasia (Teramoto *et al.*, 2003), indicating that KGF1 is a valuable growth factor to develop further.

Acute liver injury is one of the most challenging gastrointestinal emergencies encountered (Shakil *et al.*, 2000), and it is difficult to treat and has a high mortality rate in clinical practice (Bernal *et al.*, 2010). Extensive necrosis and apoptosis of hepatocytes is a major pathological feature in acute liver injury (Zou *et al.*, 2013). Therefore, increasing the anti-apoptotic properties of hepatocytes is a new approach for treating acute liver injury (Zou *et al.*, 2013). KGF1 is not only a strong candidate for the niche signal of liver progenitor cells that support liver regeneration (Takase *et al.*, 2013) but also protects murine hepatocytes from tumor necrosis factor-induced apoptosis *in vivo* and *in vitro* (Senaldi *et al.*, 1998). Thus, we considered that KGF1 may have a cytoprotective effect against liver cell damage. In addition, KGF1 protects pulmonary epithelial cells from oxidative stress *via* the Akt pathway (Ray, 2005). Although KGF1 protein expression and purification have been reported previously (Ron *et al.*, 1993; Spahr *et al.*, 1997; Hsu *et al.*, 1998; Luo *et al.*, 2004), the protein yield is low or barely detectable in some cases. Furthermore, KGF1 is unstable during purification and storage processes. An aggregation pathway of KGF1 and its stabilization was studied by physical changes (Chen *et al.*, 1994a, b). KGF1 stability enhanced by mutagenesis (Osslund *et al.*, 1998; Hsu *et al.*, 2006) has been studied in an *Escherichia coli* system. In Chinese hamster ovary (CHO) cells, KGF1 has been expressed as two isoforms, KGF-a containing a post-translation modification by *N,O*-glycanase and KGF-b with a 23-amino acid N-terminal deletion without post-translation modification (Hsu *et al.*, 1998). Luo *et al.*, (2004) showed a simple improvement of recombinant KGF1 production in the BL21 (DE3) pLysS strain expressing a GST-FGF7 fusion protein by addition of $MgCl_2$ and achieved the highest yield of a KGF1 fusion protein reported thus far. However, fusion proteins need to be recovered, resulting in increased costs of the final product. Obtaining a high yield of native KGF1 using an *E. coli* expression system still remains a challenge. In this study, we used a baculovirus expression system to produce a sufficient amount of KGF1 protein to meet the demands for biological activity evaluation and potential use in preclinical studies.

For biomanufacturing, insect cells were first used to express human β-interferon (Smith *et al.*, 1983). Thus far, there have been thousands of exogenous genes expressed using the baculovirus expression system, including those encoding recombinant pharmaceutical proteins and vaccines (Drugmand *et al.*, 2012). Although the KGF receptor has been expressed in *Spodoptera frugiperda* 9 (Sf9) cells (Liu *et al.,* 1998), there are no reports of KGF1 expression in insect cells. Compared with other systems, the insect cell-baculovirus expression system (IC-BEVS) has several advantages including similar post-translational modifications as those in mammalian cells and high levels of expression. Two of the highest reported yields using the IC-BEVS in industrial application are 300 mg/L human collagenase using *Trichoplusia nicells* cells and 80 mg/L human porapolipoprotein AI using SF cells (George *et al.,* 1997; Pyle *et al.,* 1995). There is also inherent safety during manufacture and for the final product because insect cells are free of human pathogens and can grow in serum-free media (Galbraith, 2002). In addition, the IC-BEVS can produce single and large multimeric proteins with molecular weights of several hundred kilodaltons (Trowitzsch *et al.,* 2010).

As clinical applications of KGF1 are worthy of investigation, but the yield is limited, it is necessary to establish an efficient expression system to produce sufficient quantities of recombinant KGF1 to meet the need for preclinical and commercial applications. We previously reported recombinant human (rh)KGF1$_{163}$ and rhKGF$_{140}$ expression in Sf9 cells (Zhu *et al.,* 2013; Xue *et al.,* 2012) and rhKGF1$_{163}$ effects on follicle regeneration (Zhu *et al.,* 2013). In this study, we compared the expression and bioactivity of the KGF1 precursor, rhKGF1$_{163}$ and rhKGF$_{140}$. We also investigated the cytoprotective effects of these forms of KGF1 on HL7702 liver cells and mice with CCl$_4$-induced liver injury.

2. Materials and methods

2.1 Materials

The *E. coli* TOP10 strain and HaCaT cells were obtained from the Wenzhou Medical University Zhejiang Provincial Key Laboratory of Biotechnology Pharmaceutical Engineering. The Bac-to-Bac® Baculovirus Expression System (cat. no. 10359-016), which consists of MAX Efficiency® DH10Bac™ Competent *E. coli*, the pFastBac™ Vector, and Cellfectin® II Transfection Reagent, was purchased from Invitrogen (Carlsbad, USA). Sf-9 cells, GIBCO™ SF-900II SFM cell culture products, and RPMI 1640 medium were also purchased from Invitrogen. The pMD-18 T vector, ExTaq polymerase, rTaq polymerase, T4 DNA ligase, restriction endonucleases, and DL2000 DNA Marker were purchased from TAKARA Biotechnology (Dalian). HyClone DMEM and fetal bovine serum were purchased from Thermo Scientific (Beijing, China). PageRuler Prestained Protein Ladder was purchased from Thermo Scientific (Lithuania). ProtecBlock™ was purchased from Fermentas Biotechnology (Lithuania). The Bradford protein concentration assay kit and ECL chemiluminescence kit were purchased from Beyotime Institute of Biotechnology. Human KGF1 MAb (clone 29568) and mouse IgG1 were purchased from R&D Systems (USA). Donkey anti-mouse IgG-HRP was purchased from Santa Cruz Biotechnology (Heidelberg, Germany). Polyvinylidene fluoride (PVDF) membranes (0.22 μm) were purchased from Millipore. Dimethyl sulfoxide (DMSO) and 3-[4,5-dimethyl-thiazol-2-yl]-2,5 diphenyl tetrazolium bromide (MTT) were purchased from Sigma (USA).

2.2 Gene optimization and recombinant bacmid DNA generation

A schematic of the recombinant bacmid DNA of kgf1 is shown in Fig. 1. The coding sequence of human KGF1 (GenBank accession no. KF840563), which is a 585 bp open reading frame encoding a 194-amino acid polypeptide with a calculated molecular size of 22 512 Da (Gene ID, 2252) (Finch *et al.,* 1989), was optimized according to *Spodoptera frugiperda MNPV* codon usage (http://www.kazusa.or.jp/ codon). The DNA fragment was then cloned into the *Not*I and *Pst*I restriction enzyme sites of the pUC57-KGF$_1$ plasmid (Inovogen, Beijing, China). The primary KGF1 translation product contains a 31-amino acid signal sequence in the hydrophobic N-terminal region, which is not present in the mature KGF1 molecule. Moreover, as the native sequence of KGF1 is unstable, Hsu *et al.,* (2006) investigated several KGF1 analogs and found that the analog with deletion of 23 N-terminal amino acids has the highest stability and retention of activity. Therefore, we investigated the expression of three forms of human KGF1 in Sf9 cells, namely the KGF1 precursor, KGF1, and D23-KGF1 encoding 194, 163, and 140 aa, respectively (referred to as KGF1$_{194}$, KGF1$_{163}$, and KGF1$_{140}$). Genes encoding the KGF1 precursor, KGF1, and D23-KGF1 were amplified from pUC57-KGF$_1$ by PCR using the following primers: forward, KGF1$_{194}$ 5'-GC^GGCCGC <u>ATG</u> CAC AAA TGG-3', KGF1$_{163}$ 5'-GC^GGCCGC <u>ATG</u> TGC AAC GAC ATG-3', and KGF1$_{140}$ 5' GC^GGCCGC <u>ATG</u> TCT TAC GAC TAC-3' (start codon is underlined); reverse, 5'-CTGCA^G <u>TTA</u> GGT GAT AGC CAT-3' (stop codon is underlined). Forward and reverse primers contained

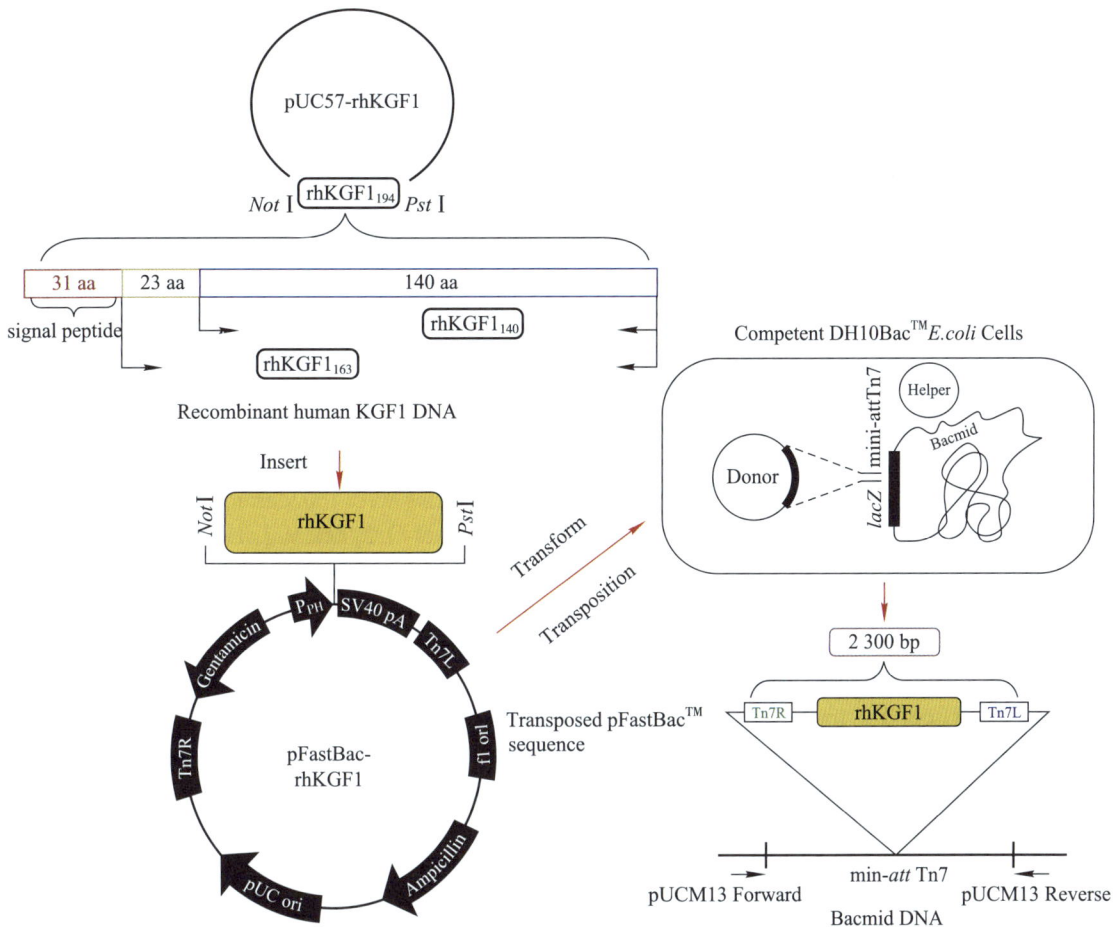

Fig. 1. Schematic of the recombinant bacmid DNA of kgf1. Based on the human KGF1 mRNA coding sequence and insect-preferred codons, a full-sequence *kgf1* gene (*rhKGF1~194~*) was designed and synthesized. rhKGF1$_{163}$ and rhKGF1$_{140}$ were synthesized by PCR amplification. *rh-KGF1* genes were inserted into the pFastBac vector and then transfected into the DH10Bac bacterial strain containing a helper plasmid to assist transposition of the recombinant Tn7 sequence into the bacmid DNA. The detailed steps are provided in "Materials and methods".

*Not*I and *Pst*I sites, respectively. PCR was conducted in a 50 μl reaction mixture containing 0.25 μl Ex *Taq* polymerase (5 U/μl), 5 μl 10×Ex *Taq* buffer (plus Mg^{2+}), 4 μl dNTP (2.5 mM each), 37.75 μl ddH$_2$O, 1 μl template plasmid, and 1 μl of each primer (20 μM). The PCR parameters were 30 cycles of 30 s at 94℃, 30 s at 50℃, and 1 min at 72℃. The PCR products were ligated into the T vector to create T-rhkgf163 and T-rhkgf140 constructs. DH5α *E. coli* were then transformed with the constructs. Correct insertion of the genes was confirmed by DNA sequencing. rhkgf1$_{194}$, rhkgf1$_{163}$, and rhkgf1$_{140}$were digested with *Not*I and *Pst*I from pUC57-KGF1, T-kgf163, and T-kgf140, respectively, and then ligated into the pFastBac transfer vector to create pFastBac-kgf1 (194, 163, and 140) constructs. The three transfer vectors were transfected into competent *E. coli*. DH10Bac containing the parent bacmid bMON14272 and helper plasmid pMON7124. As shown in Fig. 1, recombinant bacmid-kgf1 (194, 163, and 140) were selected and kgf1 (194, 163, and 140) were amplified by PCR. Recombinant Bacmid-kgf1 (194, 163, and 140) were extracted following the manufacturer's instructions of the Bac-to-Bac Baculovirus Expression System and stored for up to 2 weeks at 4℃.

2.3 Cell culture and recombinant baculovirus production

Sf9 cells (GIBCO, USA) were cultured in 125 ml shaker flasks containing 27 ml pre-warmed SF900II serum-free medium (GIBCO). The cells were incubated at (28±0.5)℃ in a nonhumidified orbital shaker at 125 rpm. At >2×10^6 viable cells/ml, Sf9 cells were subcultured by seeding (3–5)×10^5 viable cells/ml in new flasks containing pre-warmed growth medium. For rhKGF1 protein production, we used suspension cultures in 500 ml shaker flasks containing 125 ml growth medium at a density of 2×10^6 viable cells/ml.

Transfection of Sf9 cells was performed in a 6-well plate. Sf9 cells in the log phase of growth [(1.5–2.5)×10^6 cells/ml] with >95% viability were seeded at 8×10^5 cells per well in 2 ml medium and allowed to attach for 15 min at room temperature. Transfection was performed with Cellfectin® II Reagent according to the manufacturer's instructions. The cells were incubated at 27°C for 72 h, and then cellular debris was removed by centrifugation at $500 \times g$ for 5 min. The supernatant was designated as the P1 viral stock and stored in 1% fetal bovine serum at 4°C while being protected from light. Baculoviral stock amplification was performed by following standard procedures, and the titer was determined by a viral plaque assay.

2.4 Production optimization and purification of rhKGF1

To determine the optimal condition for KGF1 expression, multiplicity of infection (MOI), cell density, and harvest time were investigated in 125 ml shaker flasks containing 30 ml culture medium at 27°C with shaking at 115 rpm. The harvest time was evaluated at an MOI of 2 and cells were collected at 12, 24, 36, 48, 60, 72, 84, and 96 h postinfection. Cell pellets were re-suspended and incubated in RIPA lysate buffer (Beyotime, China) with 1% ProtecBlock™ (Fermentas, Lithuania) for 10 min. The supernatant was collected and protein samples were separated by 15% sodium dodecyl sulfate polyacrylamide gel electrophoresis (SDS-PAGE). Proteins were transferred to PVDF membranes, and immunoblotting was performed using a monoclonal anti-FGF7 anti-body (1:2 000; R & D Systems). The membranes were washed and then incubated with anti-mouse IgG-HRP (1:5 000; Santa Cruz Biotechnology, USA). Proteins were detected by the Beyo ECL Plus Kit (Beyotime, China) in the Bio-Rad ECL system. The results were analyzed and quantified by Quantity One software.

Purification of KGF1 has been described previously (Rubin *et al.*, 1989; Ron *et al.*, 1993; Hsu *et al.*, 1998). Sf9 cells were centrifuged at $500 \times g$ for 10 min to collect the cells and culture supernatants. Cell pellets were re-suspended in 50 mM phosphate buffer (pH 7.5) and lysed by sonication at 200 W for 5 s with an interval time of 10 s for 20 cycles. The lysate was centrifuged to remove debris and then passed through a 0.45 μm filter. The culture supernatant was also centrifuged and filtered. Heparin-sepharose affinity chromatography and cation exchange chromatography were used for purification. The samples were loaded onto a column containing 25 ml heparin-sepharose resin (GE, USA) that had been equilibrated in 50 mmol/L phosphate buffer (pH 7.2) at 1 ml/min using the Acta purifier system. The column was washed with a linear-step gradient of increasing NaCl concentrations, and selected fractions were further separated by SP-FF cation exchange chromatography (GE, USA) using a NaCl elution gradient from 0.3 to 1.2 M. Fractions containing rhKGF1 were applied to 10 kDa Millipore ultrafiltration for protein concentration. Finally, protein concentrations were evaluated with a Bradford protein concentration assay kit, and then the protein samples were freeze dried and stored at −80°C.

2.5 In vitro assay of rhKGF1 biological activity

An *in vitro* mitogenic bioassay was used to determine the biological activity of rhKGF1 in BaF3 cells by the MTT method which were described previously (Ornitz *et al.*, 1996). FGFR2IIIb-BaF3 cells were maintained in RPMI 1 640 medium supplemented whit 10% fetal bovine serum, 10% conditioned media from WEHI-3 cells, L-glutamine, and anti-biotics (100 IU/ml each of penicillin and streptomycin). Cells were seeded in 96-well plates (1×10^5/well) and treated with final concentrations of 0.1–200 ng/ml rhKGF1 for 48 h. The cells were then incubated with 25 μl/well (5 mg/ml) MTT for 4 h. The medium was removed and 150 μl/well DMSO was added to dissolve the crystals by shaking at room temperature for 10 min. Absorbance values were measured at 570 nm with a reference wavelength of 630 nm.

2.6 Cytoprotection of rhKGF1 in vitro

The protective effect of rhKGF1 on liver cells was evaluated using the human normal hepatocyte line HL7702. HL7702 cells were evaluated as four experimental groups: control, injury group, rhKGF1$_{163}$ and rhKGF1$_{140}$ treatment groups. For treatment groups, 5×10^5 cells were seeded in 6-mm dishes with rhKGF1$_{163}$ or rhKGF1$_{140}$ (100 ng/ml). After 2 h of incubation, 6.25 mmol/L CCl$_4$ was added to the cultures follow by a further 6 h of incubation. The injury group was treated with CCl$_4$ only for 6 h, and the same volumes of medium only were added to the control group. Cell viability was then assessed by an Annexin-V/PI double staining kit (Becton-Dickinson) using flow cytometry.

2.7 rhKGF1 protection against acute liver injury in vivo

Thirty-five 7-week-old male ICR mice were randomly divided into seven groups with five mice for each treatment. CCl$_4$ was administered at 0, 0.031 2, 0.062 5, 0.125, 0.25, 0.5, and 1 % in 0.1 ml sesame oil/10 g body weight by intraperitoneal injection. Blood samples were drawn from the mouse eye socket at 24 h after CCl$_4$ injection and 12 h of starvation. The mice were sacrificed and their livers were removed and rinsed in 0.9 % NaCl. The left hepatic lobe was removed, fixed in 4% paraformaldehyde, and then stained with hematoxylin–eosin (H & E). Alanine aminotransferase (ALT) and aspartate aminotransferase (AST) levels in the serum were measured by MINDRAY BS300 Biochemical Analyzer at 340 nm. Superoxide dismutase (SOD) and malondialdehyde (MDA) in liver homogenates were measured by enzyme-linked immunosorbent assays according to the manufacturer's instructions. Kits for ALT, AST, SOD, and MDA measurement were purchased from Nanjing Jiancheng Bioengineering Institute.

Twenty ICR mice were randomly divided into four groups with five mice in each group: control, injury group, rhKGF1$_{163}$ and rhKGF1$_{D23}$ treatment groups. Treatment groups were pretreated with rhKGF1$_{163}$or rhKGF1$_{D23}$ at 2 μg/g body weight by subcutaneous injection. After 24 h, the injury group and treatment groups were intraperitoneally injected with 1% CCl$_4$. The control group was untreated. Samples were collected and analyzed as described above.

2.8 Statistics

All values are expressed as the means ± standard error. Comparisons between groups were performed by the Tukey test with a 95% confidence interval using Graphpad Prism software. Significance was accepted at $P<0.05$. Samples were analyzed in triplicate. All experiments were repeated at least three times.

3. Results

3.1 Recombinant bacmid-KGF1 construction and baculovirus generation

We previously failed to obtain high-level expression of KGF1 in *E. coli* or plants. This promoted us to try the insect cell-baculovirus expression system as an alternative, as the insect cell-baculovirus expression system has been used successfully for the expression of a wide variety of eukaryotic proteins (Contrerasómez *et al.*, 2013; Drugmand *et al.*, 2012; van Oers, 2011). KGF1$_{194}$ was the entire coding region, including the native signal peptide. We choose to express the precursor of KGF1 because there is evidence that the signal peptide could assistant foreign protein secretion in insect cells, and there are so many advantages to secret a protein into media for high level accumulation and easy purification. The mature form of KGF1 is unstable, deletion of 23 amino acid in N-terminal could make rhKGF1$_{140}$ more stable than the mature or other analogies. Therefore we designed these three forms to test in sf9 cells. The rhKGF1$_{194}$ gene was excisable with *Not* I and *Pst*I (Fig. 2A, picture 2) from the pUC57-KGF1 vector, and rhKGF1$_{163}$ and rhKGF1$_{140}$ were amplified from the pUC57-KGF1 too (Fig. 2B, C, picture 1), and they were around 600, 500, and 450 bp, respectively. The

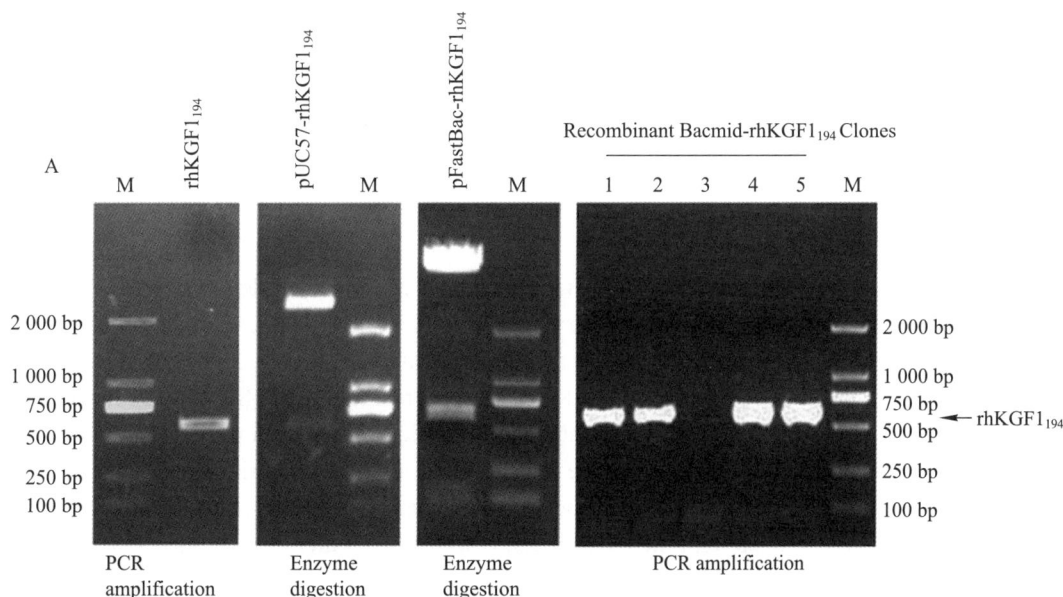

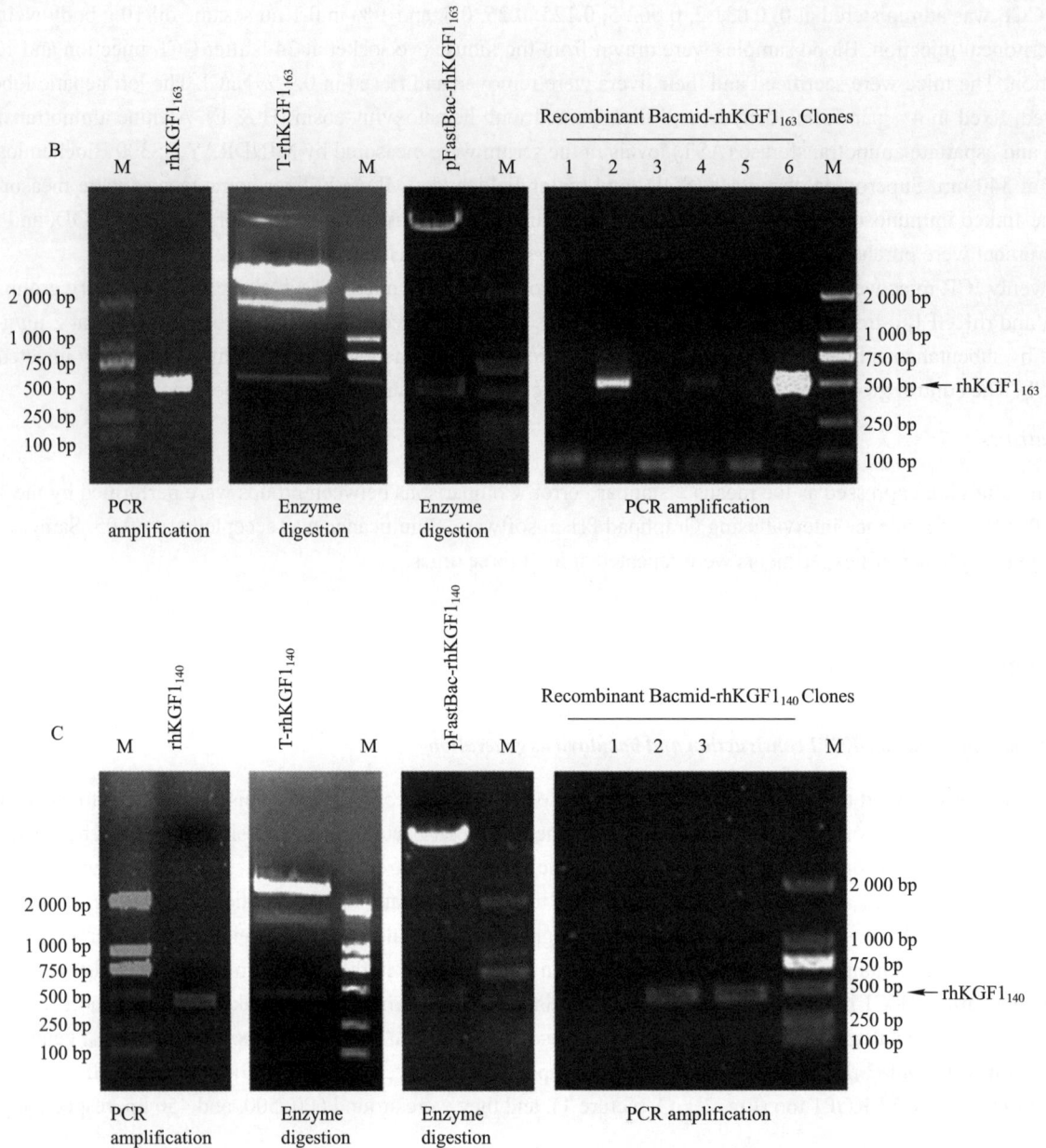

Fig. 2. Agarose gel electrophoresis was undertaken to analyze the PCR and enzyme-digested products during recombinant bacmid DNA construction. Recombinant bacmid-rhKGF1$_{194}$, bacmid-rhKGF1$_{163}$, and bacmid-rhKGF1$_{140}$ were constructed and identified in (A–C), respec-tively. The first picture of (A) is rhKGF1$_{194}$ gene PCR analysis, the second is the gene digested by NotI and PstI from pUC57-KGF1 plasmid, the third is transfer vector of pFastbac-KGF1$_{194}$ gene identification by NotI and PstI digesting, and the last one is Bacmid-kgf1$_{194}$ PCR amplification analysis. The similar order for (B, C) and the detailed steps are provided in "Materials and methods".

aim genes were needed to insert the transfer vector pFastBac and further confirmed by designing and DNA sequencing (Fig. 2A–C, third picture). The correct transfer vectors were transformed into DH10 Bac E. coli, and blue/white selective was conducted. White colonies were PCR amplified by gene special primers (Fig. 2A–C, last picture), the right recombinant bacmid-KGF1$_{194}$, bacmid-KGF1 and bacmid-KGF1$_{140}$ were transfected into Sf9 cells by liposomes respectively. Once the transfected cells appeared the signs of late stage infection (about 72 h post-transfection), collect the medium containing virus from each well (~ 2 ml). Remove cells and large debris by centrifugation, transfer the clarified supernatant to fresh 15 ml snap-cap tubes. The P1 viral stock were obtained, but for large-scale expression foreign protein we need further transfected insect cell until the P4 viral stock, which had a titer of more than 1×10^8 as determined by a viral plaque assay.

3.2 *Expression of rhKGF1 in Sf9 cells*

Fig. 3 shows the Western blot results of the three KGF1 proteins at various time points postinfection in cell lysates and medium supernatants. rhKGF1 protein bands were clearly recognized by the antibody. The sizes of rhKGF1$_{194}$ and rhKGF1$_{163}$ protein bands were very similar and as expected at around 20 kDa, indicating that the signal peptide was removed by the signal peptidase in Sf9 cells. rhKGF1$_{140}$ showed the expected band at 17 kDa. The molecular sizes were lower than that of the wide-type KGF1 at 28 kDa, which has been isolated from human fibroblasts (Rubin *et al.*, 1989) and CHO cells (Hsu *et al.*, 1998). KGF1$_{194}$ was detectable in the medium at around 36 h, and rhKGF1$_{163}$ and rhKGF1$_{140}$ were detectable in the medium beginning at 60 h.

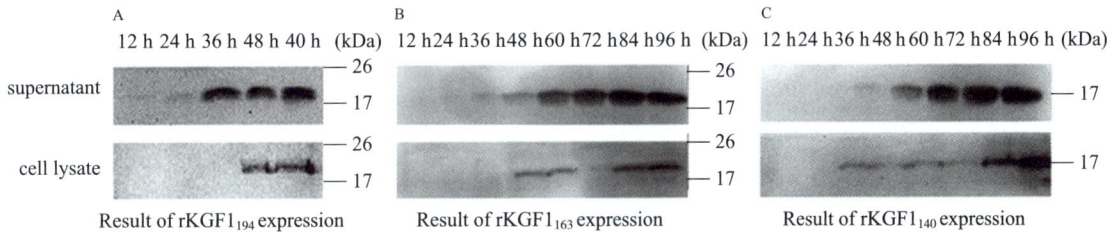

Fig. 3. Western blot analyses of recombinant KGF1$_{194}$, KGF1$_{163}$, and KGF1$_{140}$ expressions in (A–C), respectively (culture supernatant and intracellular). rhKGF1$_{194}$ containing the signal peptide was expressed from postinfection of 36 h and earlier than rhKGF1$_{163}$ and rhKGF1$_{140}$ which were from 60 h. The molecular sizes of rhKGF1$_{194}$ and rhKGF1$_{163}$ proteins were approximately 20 kDa (A, B), which was higher than that of the rhKGF1$_{140}$ (C). Large-scale cultures were harvested at 60, 96, and 96 h for rhKGF1$_{194}$, rhKGF1$_{163}$, and rhKGF1$_{140}$, respectively. A monoclonal anti-hKGF1 antibody was used for the Western blot analysis.

3.3 *Purification of rhKGF1*

As shown the Fig. 4, heparin-affinity chromatography combined with SP-sepharose chromatography were used for purification from cell lysates or medium supernatants from 1 000 ml cultures. The collected elution fractions were analyzed by SDS-PAGE (Fig. 4A, C, E) and Western blotting (Fig. 4B, D, F) to detect the three forms of the protein. Western blot analysis indicated that the target protein was eluted with 0.6 M NaCl from the heparin column and 0.45 M NaCl from the SP-sepharose column (Fig. 4). However, western blotting showed rhKGF1$_{194}$ and rhKGF1$_{163}$ as a single protein and rhKGF1$_{140}$ migrated as two bands near 17 kDa. The two migrated bands of rhKGF1$_{140}$ were analyzed by MALDI-TOF mass spectrometry, and the results indicated that they were both KGF1 with different modifications.

3.4 *Mitogenic activity assay*

KGF1 is a human mitogen that is specific for epithelial cells (Finch *et al.*, 1989), it plays an important role in the regulation of embryonic development, cell proliferation and cell differentiation. However, unlike other FGF members, KGF1 is specific for epithelial cells because receptor (FGFR2IIIb) binding specificity is an essential mechanism for regulating its activity (Ornitz *et al.*, 1996; Zhang *et al.*, 2006). Fig. 5 illustrates the response curves of mitogenic activity in cultured FGFR2IIIb-BaF3 cells induced by rhKGF1. rhKGF1$_{194}$, rhKGF1$_{163}$, and D23-KGF1 stimulated BaF3 cell proliferation in a dose-dependent manner. Stimulation of cell proliferation reached the half maximal rate for D23-KGF1 at approximately 1–2 ng/ml. By contrast, rhKGF1$_{194}$ and rhKGF1$_{163}$ displayed lower mitogenic activities, possibly because of their instability. We incubated equal amounts of rhKGF1$_{194}$, rhKGF1$_{163}$, and D23-KGF1 at 4℃ in PBS for 60 h. Western blot analysis showed that rhKGF1 migrated to 17 kDa, whereas D23-KGF1 was relatively more stable (data not shown). Thus, rhKGF1$_{194}$, rhKGF1$_{163}$, and D23-KGF1 had a remarkable mitogenic effect on BaF3 cells, and D23-KGF1 had more biological activity and stability than rhKGF1$_{194}$ and rhKGF1$_{163}$.

3.5 *rhKGF1 protection of hepatocytes against damage by CCl$_4$ in vitro*

As shown in Fig. 6, treatment with 6.25 mmol/L CCl$_4$ significantly decreased the survival of HL7702 cells compared with that by DMSO treatment. Next, the protective effects of rhKGF1$_{163}$ and rhKGF1$_{140}$ were evaluated by pretreatment for 2 h prior to CCl$_4$ administration. The results showed that either rhKGF1$_{163}$ or rhKGF1$_{140}$ protected the cells

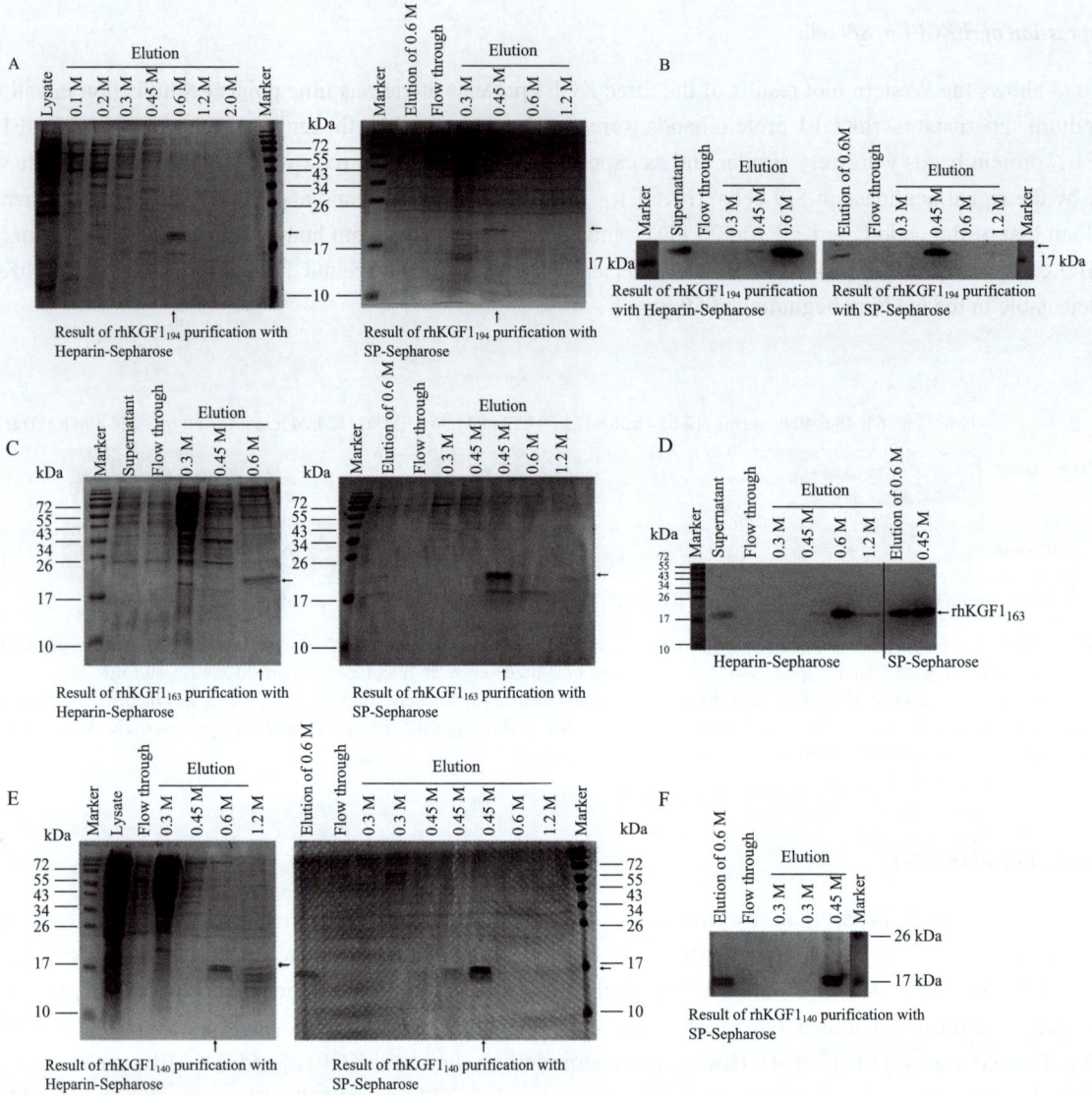

Fig. 4. Purification of recombinant KGF1 proteins. (A) Analysis of rhKGF1₁₉₄ purified from cell lysates by SDS-PAGE and Coomassie blue staining. (B) Western blot analysis of individual fractions. (C) SDS-PAGE analysis of rhKGF1₁₆₃ purified from supernatants of Sf9 cells that were infected with the recombinant bacmid-rhKGF1₁₆₃ baculovirus. (D) Western blot of (C). (E) SDS-PAGE analysis of rhKGF1₁₄₀ purified from cell lysates. (F) Western blotting of SP-sepharose fractions. We used 15 % polyacrylamide gels for all analyses. A monoclonal anti-hKGF1 antibody was used for Western blot analysis.

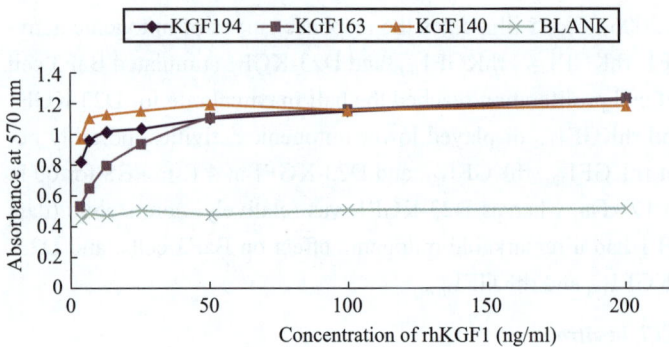

Fig. 5. Mitogenic activity of rhKGF1₁₆₃ and rhKGF1₁₄₀ in BaF3 cells. Cells were treated as described in "materials and methods." Cell proliferation was determined by the MTT method. A blank containing the same volume of medium was used for the negative control.

against damage by CCl$_4$ (Fig. 6C). Annexin-V/PI double staining indicated that the protective effects of rhKGF1$_{163}$ and rhKGF1$_{140}$ prevented necrosis and inhibited apoptosis (Fig. 6D). Fig. 6B shows that rhKGF1$_{163}$ or rhKGF1$_{140}$ did not stimulate HL7702 cell proliferation during CCl$_4$-induced damage, suggesting that rhKGF1 maintained HL7702 cell survival.

3.6 rhKGF1 prevents CCl$_4$-induced acute liver injury in vivo

In acute liver injury induced by 1 % CCl$_4$ administration to ICR mouse, a large number of liver cells underwent necrosis, ALT decreased gradually, and the bilirubin level was higher, indicating the "bilirubin transaminase separation" phenomenon which is a sign of hepatic necrosis. To elucidate rhKGF1 protection in this liver injury model, mice were pretreated with rhKGF1 prior to CCl$_4$ administration. rhKGF1$_{163}$ and rhKGF1$_{140}$ elevated the serum levels of ALT and AST, and alleviated liver injury to some extent. Compared with the CCl$_4$ group, rhKGF1$_{163}$ and rhKGF1$_{140}$ significantly elevated ALT and AST levels (Fig. 7B, C; $^*P<0.05$; $^{**}P<0.01$; and $^{***}P<0.001$). In addition, rhKGF1$_{163}$ and rhKGF1$_{140}$ increased the activity of SOD significantly (Fig. 7E; $^*P<0.05$ and $^{**}P<0.01$ $vs.$ the CCl$_4$ group) and decreased the amount of MDA to protect cells from oxidative damage but without a significant difference (Fig. 7F).

In tissue sections, necrosis and apoptosis were observed by H&E staining. Apoptotic cells show chromatin condensation and nuclear fragmentation. Necrotic tissue was red dye-free structure of homogeneous material, and nuclei disap-

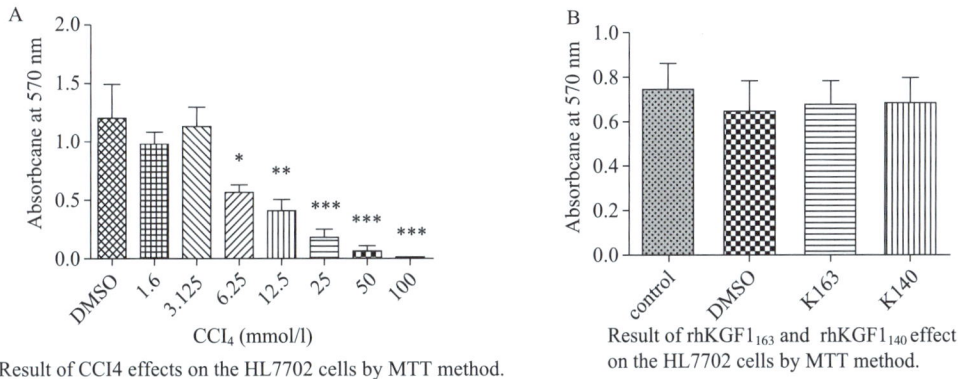

Result of CCl4 effects on the HL7702 cells by MTT method.

Result of rhKGF1$_{163}$ and rhKGF1$_{140}$ effect on the HL7702 cells by MTT method.

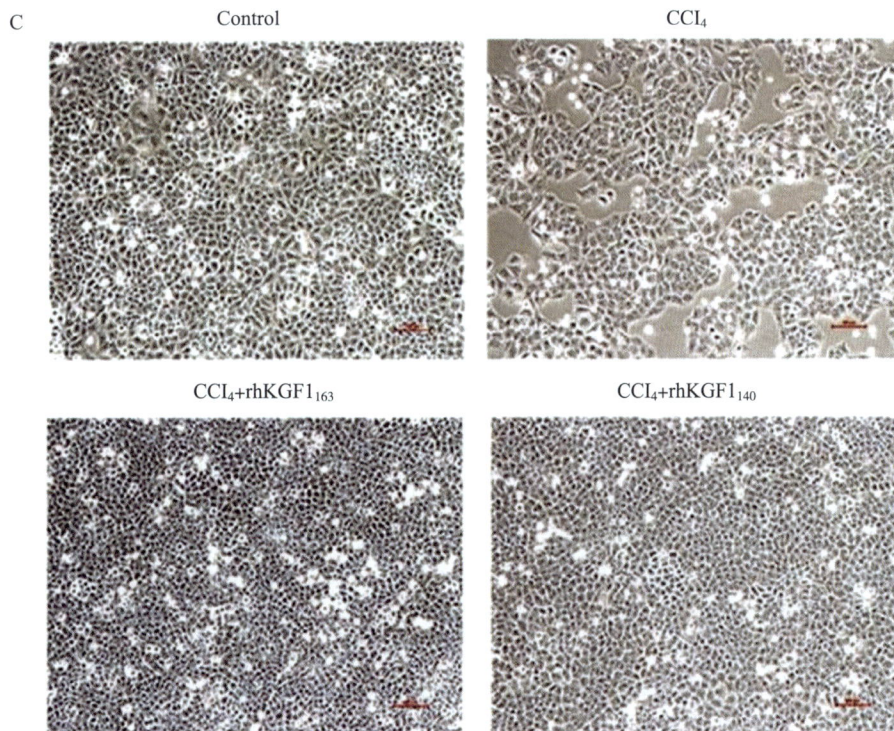

Microscope observed rhKGF1$_{163}$ and rhKGF1$_{140}$ effect on the CCl$_4$ induced HL7702 cells injury.

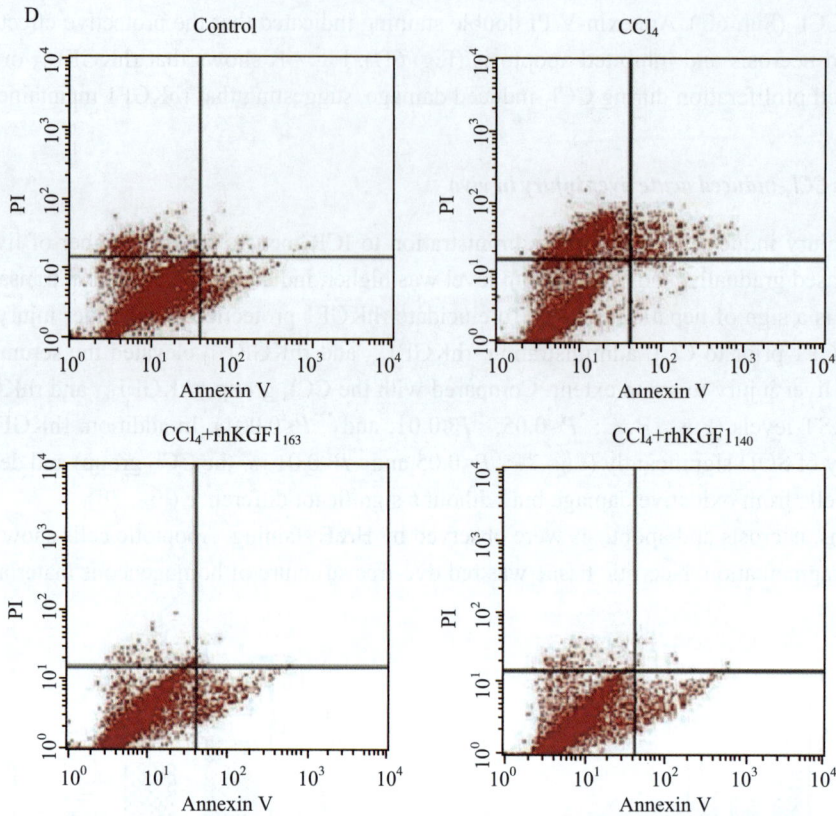

Analysis the effect of rhKGF1$_{163}$ and rhKGF1$_{140}$ on CCl$_4$ induced HL7702 cells injury by FCM.

Fig. 6. CCl$_4$-induced HL7702 cell injury observed by the MTT method (A). Treatment with 6.25 mmol/L CCl$_4$ resulted in a significant decrease of cell survival compared with that in the DMSO group. (B) rhKGF1$_{163}$ or rhKGF1$_{140}$ (100 ng/ml) did not promote HL7702 cell proliferation. However, pretreatment with rhKGF1$_{163}$ or rhKGF1$_{140}$ (100 ng/ml) for 2 h before 1 % CCl$_4$ administration prevented cell injury (C). The effect of rhKGF1 on HL7702 cells was further analyzed by Annexin-V/PI double staining. (D) rhKGF1$_{163}$ and rhKGF1$_{140}$ protected HL7702 cells from CCl$_4$-induced necrosis and apoptosis.

peared. Both rhKGF1$_{163}$ and rhKGF1$_{140}$ decreased the number of necrotic and apoptotic liver cells, but rhKGF1$_{140}$ was obviously more efficient (Fig. 7G).

4. Discussion

In this present study, we successfully expressed rhKGF1 in Sf9 cells. Although recombinant KGF1 has been expressed previously, the yield is very low. Ron *et al.* (1993) expressed recombinant KGF1 in BL21 (DE3) pLysS *E. coli* and characterized some of the KGF biological functions. However, KGF1 is highly toxic to these cells and inhibits their growth by comprising 1% ~ 2% of the total cellular protein. Chen *et al.* (1994a) reported the mechanism of rhKGF1 aggregation and stabilization, which was expressed in *E. coli*, but did not mention the expression level. Bare *et al.* (1994) reported the effect of cysteine substitutions on the activity and stability of bacterially derived KGF. Ptitsyn *et al.* (1998) reported synthesis of the gene encoding human KGF and construction of vectors for cytoplasmic production of rhKGF in *E. coli*. The level of recombinant protein expression was 1%–1.5% of total cellular protein. To study the biochemical and structural characteristics of KGF1 in detail, Hsu *et al.* (1998) expressed and isolated two human KGF isoforms produced in CHO cells. The yield of the KGF1 isoforms was 3.1 mg/L. These yields do not meet the need for applications in research and clinical trials, which require large quantities of purified high quality KGF1 with high biological activity. Luo *et al.* (2004) reported a simple improvement to the cost effectiveness of recombinant KGF1 production in the BL21 (DE3) pLysS strain expressing a GST-FGF7 fusion protein by addition of MgCl$_2$. The yield of GST-KGF1 was 17±1.4 mg/L, which was about 50% of the amount of GST-FGF1 produced by the same method (Luo *et al.*, 2004). The

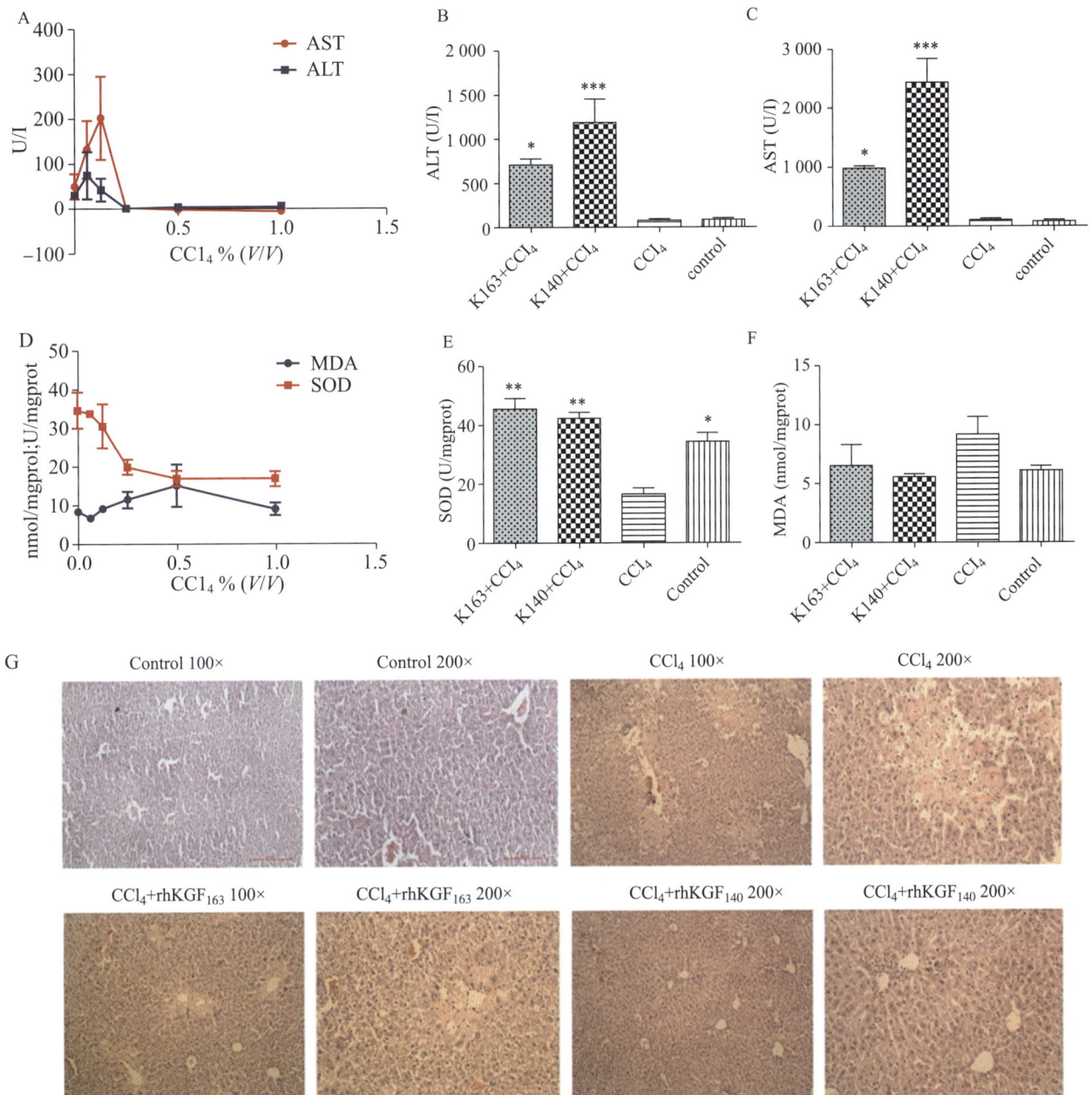

Fig. 7. Protection against CCl_4-induced acute liver injury in mice by rhKGF1. Thirty-five 7-week-old male ICR mice were intraperitoneally injected with various concentrations of CCl_4. Serum levels of ALT and AST and SOD and MDA levels in liver tissues are shown in (A) and (D), respectively. Twenty ICR mice were divided into four groups as described in "materials and methods." In acute liver injury induced by 1% CCl_4, ALT, AST, SOD, and MOD levels in $rhKGF1_{163}$ and $rhKGF1_{140}$ pre-treatment groups *vs.* the CCl_4 group are shown in (B), (C), (E), and (F), respectively. Liver tissues from the different treatments were stained with H & E (G).

yield of GST-KGF1 and subsequent recovery of mature ^{54}ser-KGF1 (4.8±0.5 mg/L) was more than five times higher than that produced without $MgCl_2$ addition. Despite this increase of fusion protein yield, to isolate the KGF1 portion, fusion products need to be subjected to trypsin treatment. To increase the yield of nonfused KGF1, we used an IC-BEVS. The yields of purified $rhKGF1_{194}$, $rhKGF1_{163}$, and D23-KGF1 were between the yields of KGF1 derived from the bacterial BL21 (DE3) pLysS strain and CHO cells (data not shown). The IC-BEVS is not only very simple and fast but also enables efficient purification of proteins from the culture medium. More importantly, by optimizing the gene sequence and expression conditions, we obtained mature rhKGF1 and D23-KGF1.

Considering the heparin-binding ability of KGF1, we combined the use of heparin-sepharose affinity chromatography and SP-FF cation exchange chromatography. In the Sf9-baculovirus expression system, the signal peptide of rhK-

GF1 was removed because the molecular size of rhKGF1$_{194}$ was similar to that of mature rhKGF1$_{163}$. However, whether the N-terminal is removed correctly still needs to be verified. The molecular sizes of rhKGF1$_{194}$ nor rhKGF1$_{163}$ were both lower than the 28-kDa human KGF1 isolated from a human embryonic lung fibroblast cell line (Rubin *et al.*, 1989) and KGF-a expressed in CHO cells (Hsu *et al.*, 2006). This result may be caused by distinct modifications between insect and mammal cells. For example, *N*-glycanase digestion to release Asn-linked carbohydrates (Hsu *et al.*, 2006) results in 20 – 22 kDa KGF1 proteins. Further deglycosylation with neuraminidase and *O*-glycanase to remove O-linked carbohydrates results in deglycosylated KGF-a that migrates as a 20-kDa protein band similar to that observed for *E. coli* and insect-derived KGF1. More interestingly, rhKGF1$_{140}$ has two distinct bands of equal intensity at around 17 kDa, similar to KGF-b expressed in CHO cells, which is KGF-a processed by removal of 23 amino acids from its N-terminal to remove post-translational modification sites. Mass spectroscopic analysis of the two bands of rhKGF1$_{140}$ showed a 100% score for KGF1. In addition, the higher band had 58 carbamidomethyls more than the lower band that contained 20 carbamidomethyls, which may have caused the 2 088 Da difference between them. The protein sequence and structural properties of these KGF1 s require further analysis.

KGF1 has five cysteinyl residues at positions 1, 15, 40, 102, and 106, including two disulfide loops between Cys^1-Cys^{15} and Cys^{102}-Cys^{106}, and Cys^{40} as free cysteinyl residues (Bare *et al.*, 1994; Hsu *et al.*, 1998). Mutagenesis and truncation analysis of the amino terminus of KGF1 revealed that the first 23 residues of the native KGF1 polypeptide can be removed without reducing its mitogenic activity (Osslund *et al.*, 1998). In this study, both rhKGF1$_{163}$ and D23-KGF1 isoforms were biological activity in BaF3 cells, despite a notable difference between their protein sequences. This result indicates that the N-terminal disulfide loop is not important for maintaining the biological activity and molecular stability of KGF1 (Hsu *et al.*, 1998). Furthermore, D23-KGF1 displayed more activity than that of rhKGF1$_{163}$ in stimulating cell proliferation. Moreover, the stability of D23-KGF1 was higher than that of rhKGF1$_{163}$. Therefore, D23-KGF1 expression in Sf9 cells by the baculovirus system is not only efficient but also results in high biological activity.

KGF1 has been shown to protect the lung from a variety of oxidative insults (Ray, 2005). Thus, we considered that KGF1 has cytoprotection effects on liver cells against CCl$_4$-induced oxidative injury caused by reactive oxygen species. To determine whether rhKGF1$_{163}$ and D23-KGF1 had protective effects on hepatocytes, we used the human normal liver cell line HL7702. CCl$_4$ treatment of HL7702 cells caused extensive necrosis and apoptosis. However, pretreatment with rhKGF1$_{163}$ or D23-KGF1 for 2 h efficiently protected cells from CCl$_4$-induced cell death *in vitro* (Fig. 6) and *in vivo* (Fig. 7). In future studies, we are interested in determining the relationship of rhKGF1 structure and function, and elucidating the molecular mechanism of liver protection by KGF1.

In summary, mature rhKGF1, its precursor, and an N-terminal deletion analog were successfully expressed in Sf9 cells by baculoviral vectors from a codon-optimized *KGF1* gene. The signal peptide of the *KGF1* precursor is removed in Sf9 cells because the molecular sizes of mature *KGF1* and its precursor are similar at around 20 kDa. D23-*KGF1* shows two distinct bands of equal intensity at 17 kDa, which are similar to KGF-b expressed in CHO cells without glycanase modification and 23-amino acid N-terminal deletion. Purification was performed by heparin-affinity and SP-FF cation exchange chromatography. The purified proteins were identified by Western blot analysis. rhKGF1$_{194}$, rhKGF1$_{163}$, and D23-KGF1 significantly stimulate proliferation of BaF3 cells, and D23-KGF1 is more biologically active and stable than the other recombinant KGF1s. *In vitro*, rhKGF1$_{163}$ and D23-KGF1 maintain cell survival during CCl$_4$-induced damage. *In vivo*, rhKGF1 regulates ALT, AST, SOD, and MDA levels, alleviates liver cell damage, and decreases the amount of liver cell apoptosis and necrosis. This study demonstrates that rhKGF1 expression in Sf9 cells is a viable method to achieve highly efficient expression and purification of KGF1 with high bioactivity.

References

auf dem Keller U, Krampert M, Kumin A, *et al.* Keratinocyte growth factor: effects on keratinocytes and mechanisms of action[J]. Eur J Cell Biol, 2004, 83(11-12): 607-612.

Bare LA, Brown M, Goyal S, *et al.* Effect of cysteine substitutions on the mitogenic activity and stability of recombinant human keratinocyte growth factor[J]. Biochem Biophys Res Commun, 1994, 205(1): 872-879.

Bernal W, Auzinger G, Dhawan A, *et al.* Acute liver failure[J]. Lancet, 2010, 376(9736): 190-201.

Chen BL, Arakawa T, Hsu E, *et al.* Strategies to suppress aggregation of recombinant keratinocyte growth factor during liquid formulation development[J]. J Pharm Sci, 1994, 83(12): 1657-1661.

Chen BL, Arakawa T, Morris CF, *et al.* Aggregation pathway of recombinant human keratinocyte growth factor and its stabilization[J].

Pharm Res, 1994, 11(11): 1581-1587.

Contreras-Gomez A, Sanchez-Miron A, Garcia-Camacho F, *et al.* Protein production using the baculovirus-insect cell expression system[J]. Biotechnol Prog, 2014, 30(1): 1-18.

Deimling J, Thompson K, Tseu I, *et al.* Mesenchymal maintenance of distal epithelial cell phenotype during late fetal lung development[J]. Am J Physiol Lung Cell Mol Physiol, 2007, 292(3): L725-741.

Drugmand JC, Schneider YJ, Agathos SN. Insect cells as factories for biomanufacturing[J]. Biotechnol Adv, 2012, 30(5): 1140-1157.

Finch PW, Rubin JS. Keratinocyte growth factor/fibroblast growth factor 7, a homeostatic factor with therapeutic potential for epithelial protection and repair[J]. Adv Cancer Res, 2004, 91: 69-136.

Finch PW, Rubin JS, Miki T, *et al.* Human KGF is FGF-related with properties of a paracrine effector of epithelial cell growth[J]. Science, 1989, 245(4919): 752-755.

Fuchs E. Epidermal differentiation and keratin gene expression[J]. J Cell Sci Suppl, 1993, 17: 197-208.

Galbraith D. Regulatory aspects of recombinant protein products by baculovirus expression systems[J]. Bioproc J, 2002, 1(2): 47-51.

George HJ, Marchand P, Murphy K, *et al.* Recombinant human 92-kDa type IV collagenase/gelatinase from baculovirus-infected insect cells: expression, purification, and characterization[J]. Protein Expr Purif, 1997, 10(1): 154-161.

Housley RM, Morris CF, Boyle W, *et al.* Keratinocyte growth factor induces proliferation of hepatocytes and epithelial cells throughout the rat gastrointestinal tract[J]. J Clin Invest, 1994, 94(5): 1764-1777.

Hsu YR, Hsu EW, Katta V, *et al.* Human keratinocyte growth factor recombinantly expressed in Chinese hamster ovary cells: isolation of isoforms and characterization of post-translational modifications[J]. Protein Expr Purif, 1998, 12(2): 189-200.

Hsu E, Osslund T, Nybo R, *et al.* Enhanced stability of recombinant keratinocyte growth factor by mutagenesis[J]. Protein Eng Des Sel, 2006, 19(4): 147-153.

Liu JJ, Shay JW, Wilson SE. Characterization of a soluble KGF receptor cDNA from human corneal and breast epithelial cells[J]. Invest Ophthalmol Vis Sci, 1998, 39(13): 2584-2593.

Luo Y, Cho HH, Jones RB, *et al.* Improved production of recombinant fibroblast growth factor 7 (FGF7/KGF) from bacteria in high magnesium chloride[J]. Protein Expr Purif, 2004, 33(2): 326-331.

Ornitz DM, Xu J, Colvin JS, *et al.* Receptor specificity of the fibroblast growth factor family[J]. J Biol Chem, 1996, 271(25): 15292-15297.

Osslund TD, Syed R, Singer E, *et al.* Correlation between the 1.6 A crystal structure and mutational analysis of keratinocyte growth factor[J]. Protein Sci, 1998, 7(8): 1681-1690.

Peng C, Chen B, Kao HK, *et al.* Lack of FGF-7 further delays cutaneous wound healing in diabetic mice[J]. Plast Reconstr Surg, 2011, 128(6): 673e-684e.

Ptitsyn LR, Al'tman IB, Gurov MV, *et al.* Production of recombinant human keratinocyte growth factor in Escherichia coli cells[J]. Bioorg Khim, 1998, 24(7): 523-529.

Pyle LE, Barton P, Fujiwara Y, *et al.* Secretion of biologically active human proapolipoprotein A-I in a baculovirus-insect cell system: protection from degradation by protease inhibitors[J]. J Lipid Res, 1995, 36(11): 2355-2361.

Ray P. Protection of epithelial cells by keratinocyte growth factor signaling[J]. Proc Am Thorac Soc, 2005, 2(3): 221-225.

Ron D, Bottaro DP, Finch PW, *et al.* Expression of biologically active recombinant keratinocyte growth factor. Structure/function analysis of amino-terminal truncation mutants[J]. J Biol Chem, 1993, 268(4): 2984-2988.

Rubin JS, Osada H, Finch PW, *et al.* Purification and characterization of a newly identified growth factor specific for epithelial cells[J]. Proc Natl Acad Sci U S A, 1989, 86(3): 802-806.

Senaldi G, Shaklee CL, Simon B, *et al.* Keratinocyte growth factor protects murine hepatocytes from tumor necrosis factor-induced apoptosis *in vivo* and *in vitro*[J]. Hepatology, 1998, 27(6): 1584-1591.

Shakil AO, Kramer D, Mazariegos GV, *et al.* Acute liver failure: clinical features, outcome analysis, and applicability of prognostic criteria[J]. Liver Transpl, 2000, 6(2): 163-169.

Smith GE, Summers MD, Fraser MJ. Production of human beta interferon in insect cells infected with a baculovirus expression vector[J]. Mol Cell Biol, 1983, 3(12): 2156-2165.

Spahr CS, Narhi LO, Speakman J, *et al.* The effects of *in vitro* methionine oxidation on the bioactivity and structure of human keratinocyte growth factor[J]. Techniques in Protein Chemistry, 1997, 8(97): 299-308.

Steiling H, Muhlbauer M, Bataille F, *et al.* Activated hepatic stellate cells express keratinocyte growth factor in chronic liver disease[J]. Am J Pathol, 2004, 165(4): 1233-1241.

Takase HM, Itoh T, Ino S, *et al.* FGF7 is a functional niche signal required for stimulation of adult liver progenitor cells that support liver regeneration[J]. Genes Dev, 2013, 27(2): 169-181.

Teramoto H, Yoneda A, Puri P. Gene expression of fibroblast growth factors 10 and 7 is downregulated in the lung of nitrofen-induced diaphragmatic hernia in rats[J]. J Pediatr Surg, 2003, 38(7): 1021-1024.

Trowitzsch S, Bieniossek C, Nie Y, *et al.* New baculovirus expression tools for recombinant protein complex production[J]. J Struct Biol, 2010, 172(1): 45-54.

Tsai SM, Wang WP. Expression and function of fibroblast growth factor (FGF) 7 during liver regeneration[J]. Cell Physiol Biochem, 2011, 27(6): 641-652.

Ulrich K, Stern M, Goddard ME, *et al.* Keratinocyte growth factor therapy in murine oleic acid-induced acute lung injury[J]. Am J Physiol Lung Cell Mol Physiol, 2005, 288(6): L1179-1192.

van Oers MM. Opportunities and challenges for the baculovirus expression system[J]. J Invertebr Pathol, 2011, 107 Suppl: S3-15.

Werner S. Keratinocyte growth factor: a unique player in epithelial repair processes[J]. Cytokine Growth Factor Rev, 1998, 9(2): 153-165.

Xue P, Zhu XJ, Liu XJ, *et al.* Expression of recombinant truncated human keratinocyte growth factor 1 in insect cells[J]. Journal of Jilin University, 2012, 38(4): 633-639.

Yi ES, Shabaik AS, Lacey DL, *et al.* Keratinocyte growth factor causes proliferation of urothelium *in vivo*[J]. J Urol, 1995, 154(4): 1566-1570.

Zhang X, Ibrahimi OA, Olsen SK, *et al.* Receptor specificity of the fibroblast growth factor family. The complete mammalian FGF family[J]. J Biol Chem, 2006, 281(23): 15694-15700.

Zhu X, Jiang C, Xue P, *et al.* Expression and Purification of Biological-active Recombinant Human Keratinocyte Growth Factor-1 Base on Baculovirus Expression Vector System[J]. China Biotechnology, 2013, 33(3): 47-53.

Zou SS, Yang W, Yan HX, *et al.* Role of beta-Catenin in regulating the balance between TNF-alpha- and Fas-induced acute liver injury[J]. Cancer Lett, 2013, 335(1): 160-167.

High-efficiency production of bioactive recombinant human fibroblast growth factor 18 in *Escherichia coli* and its effects on hair follicle growth

Lintao Song, Xiaokun Li

1. Introduction

Fibroblast growth factor 18 (FGF18) belongs to the heparin-binding growth factor family, and it was first identified in 1998 (Ohbayashi *et al.*, 1998). Full-length human FGF18 consists of 207 amino acids containing two potential *N*-linked glycosylation domains (Katoh, 2005) and is structurally most homologous to FGF8 and FGF17 among the FGF family (Hu *et al.*, 1998; Ohbayashi *et al.*, 1998). FGF18 is expressed predominantly in the adult lungs and kidneys (Ohbayashi *et al.*, 1998), as well as in several discrete regions during embryonic development (Dichmann *et al.*, 2003; Ohuchi *et al.*, 2000; Sato *et al.*, 2004; Usui *et al.*, 2004). It plays critical roles in multiple physiological functions, including skeletal growth and development (Liu *et al.*, 2002; Long and Ornitz, 2013), hair growth and skin maintenance (Greco *et al.*, 2009; Kawano *et al.*, 2005; Kimura-Ueki *et al.*, 2012; Plikus, 2012), cortical neuron activity (Hasegawa *et al.*, 2004), and morphogenesis and angiogenesis (Ishibe *et al.*, 2005). It has been tested both in experimental models of alopecia (Kimura-Ueki *et al.*, 2012) and clinically in patients for the treatment of osteoarthritis (Beyer and Schett, 2010; Vincent, 2012). Intraperitoneal administration of recombinant FGF18 induces significant weight gain of the liver and intestine in mice (Hu *et al.*, 1998). Like other FGFs (Arakawa *et al.*, 1989; Ghosh *et al.*, 1996; Xu *et al.*, 1999; Zhan *et al.*, 1992), FGF18 stimulated proliferation of NIH3T3 cells in a heparin sulfate-dependent manner (Hu *et al.*, 1998). In addition, FGF18 has been extensively investigated as a factor of bone growth and development (endochondral ossification) *via* the regulation of chondrogenesis and osteogenesis (Behr *et al.*, 2011; Ellsworth *et al.*, 2002; Liu *et al.*, 2002; Moore *et al.*, 2005). FGF18 also contributes to the control of mature chondrocytes and their progenitors and is an important regulator of limb development (Behr *et al.*, 2011). Notably, Kimura-Ueki *et al.* (2012) reported that FGF18 might be clinically applicable as a potent therapeutic agent for alopecia.

It is well accepted that FGF18 has an important role in the physiological regulation of bone development and the hair cycle and has pharmacological significance in the pathogenesis of human disease. There is a remarkable demand in the market for production of this protein. However, therapeutic applications of hFGF18 have been restricted by its low level of expression and difficulty in producing highly bioactive protein. Given these limiting factors, high priority should be given to the development of strategies that could enable significant preparation of sufficient, highly bioactive hFGF18 for further mechanisms and pharmacological research. Hu *et al.* (1999) expressed FLAG-tagged FGF18 in mammalian cells; however, several mammalian cell expression systems are more complicated and costly, making this strategy difficult to use in the development of large-scale fermentation processes. Moreover, the preparation of sufficient amounts of virus for large-scale expression is time consuming. Recently, Jeon *et al.* (2012) expressed His6-tagged FGF18 in *Escherichia coli* TOP 10 cells. However, higher levels of expression were not achieved, and the resulting hexahistidine-tagged FGF18 had higher immunogenicity and lower bioactivity, and it has more difficulty to be an effective therapeutic drug. It has been previously reported that therapeutic peptides/proteins, which express non-fusion genes, exhibit clinical properties superior to those of their corresponding tagged protein molecules (Huang *et al.*, 2008), and addition of fusion tags to the recombinant protein is a key factor that affects the formation of inclusion bodies (Zhu *et al.*, 2013). Therefore, using the structural properties of the target protein, such as disulfide bond formation and heparin-binding ability, could be an intelligent choice for expression and purification. Accumulating reports have shown the successful expression and purification of bioactive human proteins such as FGF1 (Wu *et al.*, 2005), FGFR (Ryu *et al.*, 2006), and KGF2 (Wu *et al.*, 2009) utilizing this strategy.

With the development of biotechnology, a variety of alternative expression systems are now being used for expressing recombinant proteins for industrial production, as well as in research for structural and biochemical studies (Dong *et al.,* 2008). However, the *E. coli* expression system is the most frequently practice used for high-level production of recombinant protein (Ajikumar *et al.,* 2010; Derynck *et al.,* 1984; Quick and Wright, 2002; Verdon *et al.,* 2012). It is low cost and has high transformation efficiency, quick growth, and suitability for large-scale manufacture, which contribute to the selection of *E. coli* as an expression host (Jana and Deb, 2005).

Since hFGF18 is an important growth factor and its non-fusion expression in *E. coli* has not been reported, we constructed an optimum recombinant human FGF18 expression vector (pET3c-rhFGF18), and used *E. coli* strain Origima (DE3) cells to successfully express high levels of rhFGF18. Because it could eliminate both active thioredoxin and reductase expression, it may thus facilitate cytoplasmic disulfide bond formation necessary for the correct folding of the protein (Prinz *et al.,* 1997). Furthermore, we undertook purification of rhFGF18 protein using a CM Sepharose FF and heparin affinity chromatography and obtained high purity of the homogenous rhFGF18 protein. Importantly, the produced rhFGF18 was found to have a significant mitogenic effect on NIH3T3 cells and influenced hair follicle growth *in vivo*. This is the first report regarding the expression and purification of non-tagged active rhFGF18 in *E. coli* and the resultant expressed recombinant protein with relatively high activity for fundamental research and therapeutic applications.

2. Materials and methods

2.1 Reagents and bacterial strain

TaKaRa Ex *Taq*, polymerase chain reaction (PCR) purification kit, gel extraction kit, bicinchoninic acid (BCA) kit, and plasmid miniprep kit were purchased from TaKaRa Company (Dalian, China). Restriction enzymes *Nde*I and *Bam*HI were purchased from NEB (Ipswich, MA, USA). Isopropyl-β-D-thiogalactoside (IPTG) and methylthiazol tetrazolium (MTT) was obtained from Bio-Tech (Gold BioTechnology, St. Louis, MO). Dulbecco's modified Eagle medium (DMEM) was purchased from Invitrogen (Carlsbad, CA). CM Sepharose FF, Heparin-Sepharose column, and AKTA purifier were purchased from GE Healthcare (Piscataway, NJ, USA). All primers were synthesized by Invitrogen (Shanghai, China). Rabbit anti-FGF18 polyclonal antibody was purchased from Abcam, Inc. (Abcam, Cambridge, MA, USA). The expression vectors pET22b and pET3c, *E. coli* DH5α, and Origami (DE3) and BL21 (DE3)PlysS were obtained from the laboratory (Engineering Research Center of Bioreactor and Pharmaceutical Development, Ministry of Education, Jilin Agricultural University, China).

2.2 Construction of rhFGF18 expression vector

The coding sequence of *hFGF18* (the amino acid sequence of human FGF18, GenBank accession number NP003853) was amplified from a T vector containing the sequence of human FGF18 (GenBank accession number KC778400) optimized according to the codon usage table of *E. coli* (http://www.kazusa.or.jp/codon/) by PCR with the appropriate primers to recognize human FGF18, as follows: forward, 5′-GGA ATT CCA TAT GTA CAG CGC ACC TAG CGC ATG-3′; reverse, 5′-CGC GGA TCC TTA GGC CGG GTG TGT CGG-3′. The forward primer and reverse primers contained *Nde*I and *Bam*HI sites, respectively. PCR was conducted with 50 μl of reaction mixture containing 0.25 μl TaKaRa Ex *Taq* (5 U/μl), 5 μl 10× Ex *Taq* buffer (Mg²⁺ Plus), 4 μl dNTPs (each 2.5 mM), and 1 μl each of the forward and reverse primers (each 20 μM). The thermocycling parameters used for PCR were as follows: 0.5 min at 94℃ for denaturation, 0.5 min at 55℃ for annealing, and 1 min at 72℃ for extension. After 30 cycles, the amplified PCR products was digested with *Nde*I and *Bam*HI and then ligated into the previously digested pET22b and pET3c expression vectors to create the pET22b-rhFGF18 and pET3c-rhFGF18 constructs. The constructs were transformed into *E. coli* DH5α. The accurate insertion of the gene into the plasmid was confirmed by automated DNA sequencing. The expression vectors (pET22b-rhFGF18 and pET3c-rhFGF18) were further assessed by restriction enzymatic analysis and transformed into competent cells of *E. coli* strains Origima (DE3) and BL21 (DE3) PlysS.

2.3 Production and soluble screening of rhFGF18

For promoting the best expression of rhFGF18, the recombinant *E. coli* Origima (DE3) or BL21 (DE3)PlysS harboring the accurate sequence of hFGF18 was shaker-cultured at 37 ℃ and 180 rpm in 5 ml Luria-Bertani (LB) medium containing 2 % glucose and 100 μg/ml ampicillin until the cell density reached an OD_{600} of 0.6. The cells were initiated with a final concentration of 1 mM IPTG as inducer and incubated at 37 ℃ for 4 h with shaking at 180 rpm. The expression of each culture was analyzed by Coomassie blue staining of 12 % (*v/v*) sodium dodecyl sulfate polyacrylamide gel electrophoresis (SDS-PAGE), and the expression level of rhFGF18 was determined by densitometry. The highest expression of rhFGF18 transformant was used in subsequent experiments.

Thereafter, we analyzed IPTG concentration, temperature, and time after induction factors for rhFGF18 expression yield and production of soluble rhFGF18 in Origima (DE3)/pET3c-rhFGF18. The bacteria were harvested by centrifugation at 5 000×*g* for 10 min at 4 ℃, and the cell pellet was then resuspended in 20 mM Tris–HCl (pH 6.5) buffer containing 1 mM ethylene diamine tetraacetic acid, 1 mM phenylmethylsulfonyl fluoride, 0.05% Tween80, and 5 mM β-mercaptoethanol. Then, the cells were lysed by sonication for 10 min in an ice bath. The cells lysates were prepared by centrifugation for 10 min at 12 000×*g* at 4 ℃, and the supernatant was transferred to a fresh tube.

2.4 Purification and identification of rhFGF18

According to the isoelectric point of target protein, CM Sepharose FF was chosen for the purification of rhFGF18. First, the CM cation exchange column was equilibrated with ten bed volumes of binding buffer (20 mM PB, pH 6.5, 25 mM NaCl) at a rate of 1 ml/min. Subsequently, the soluble cell extract was applied to the column. After binding, the column was further washing with binding buffer, and then eluted with binding buffer containing different concentrations of NaCl. Then, further purification was performed with a heparin-sepharose column pre-equilibrated with binding buffer until the OD_{280} of the effluent reached base line. Finally, rhFGF18 protein was collected from the column with stepwise gradients of 0.3, 0.8, and 1.5 M NaCl. The elution fractions were collected and determined by Coomassie blue staining of 12% (*v/v*) SDS-PAGE. Fractions containing rhFGF18 were concentrated with a Millipore filter, and the concentration was evaluated with a BCA kit. Importantly, all purification procedures were carried out at 4 ℃ and purified rhFGF18 fractions were stored at −80 ℃ to retain biological activity.

The purity of rhFGF18 was further examined by HPLC analysis, and the sample loaded onto a C18 column. The HPLC was operated on Agilent 1 260 Infinity equipped with C18 column from Agilent. The elution was conducted using a linear gradient of 0–90% acetonitrile at a flow rate of 0.5 ml/min in the presence of 0.1% trifluoroacetic acid. The absorbance was measured continuously at 280 nm.

Western blotting was performed using a peroxidase-conjugated rabbit polyclonal anti-human FGF18 antibody for further identification according to the manufacturer's protocol. The molecular sizes of the obtained protein were verified by comparison with the migration of pre-stained protein markers electrophoresed in parallel lanes.

2.5 Mitogenic activity of rhFGF18 assay

We used the NIH 3T3 cell line (American Type Culture Collection, Rockville, MD) to determine the activity of the rhFGF18 that was expressed in *E. coli* Origima (DE3). First, the cells were grown in DMEM containing 10% fetal bovine serum (FBS), 100 U/ml ampicillin, and 100 U/ml streptomycin until the culture reached the mid-logarithmic time, then transferred to a 96-well plate (5×10^3/well), and incubated at 37 ℃ for 24 h. The medium was then replaced with DMEM supplemented with 0.4% FBS, and the cells were serum starved for 24 h. Next, the cells were treated with different concentrations of rhFGF18 and human FGF1 protein for 48 h, and the number of viable cells was determined by adding 20 μl MTT (5 mg/ml) per well for 4 h. Finally, the medium was discarded and 150 μl of DMSO was added to each well. After incubation for 30 min at room temperature, the absorbance was immediately measured at 600 nm using a microplate reader.

2.6 In vivo analysis of rhFGF18 activity

To characterize the effects of the purified rhFGF18 on hair growth *in vivo*, we essentially followed the protocol developed by Kawano *et al.* (2005). All procedures involving 56-day-old C57BL/6 male mice (18–22 g), and their cares were approved by the Institutional Animals Care and Use Committee at Jilin Agricultural University, China, and performed in accordance with institutional guidelines for animal experiments. After conditioning for 2 days, 16 mice (C57BL/6) were then anesthetized, and their dorsal hair was gently cut short with a trimmer and photographed using a digital camera. Following this, the mice were randomly divided into the treatment group (FGF18, n=8) and negative control group (phosphate-buffered saline (PBS), n=8). Then, eight mice were injected subcutaneously with rh-FGF18 solution (1 mg/ml) into their backs at a dose of 1 mg/kg body weight, while the remaining eight received PBS at a corresponding volume. Thereafter, rhFGF18 and PBS were administered once daily for 14 days. The mice were then maintained for selected numbers of days on a standard laboratory diet and acidified water ad libitum. On day 15, they were anesthetized, photographed, and killed, and the full-thickness of the dorsal skin in the test area was excised. The harvested samples were fixed and embedded in paraffin, and then, the embedded skin samples were cut into 4 μm-thick sections using standard procedures (Paus *et al.,* 1999). Finally, the sections were stained with hematoxylin and eosin (H & E) and observed under a microscope.

3. Results

3.1 Construction of hFGF18 expression vectors

To produce recombinant hFGF18 protein, expression vectors bearing the optimized *hFGF18* gene were constructed. The construction strategy and detailed procedure are described in "Materials and methods." The final product (full-length hFGF18) was obtained by PCR (Fig. 1A), then digested with *Nde*I and *Bam*HI, and cloned into the expression vectors (pET22b and pET3c) to create the recombinant plasmids pET22b-rhFGF18 and pET3c-rhFGF18, which were confirmed by automated DNA sequencing and restriction enzymatic analysis (Fig. 1B). The results of the sequences of hFGF18 (643 bp) were conformed to the desired sequence.

3.2 Expression screening and optimization of soluble rhFGF18 production

To elucidate the optimal production method of rhFGF18, we utilized Origima (DE3) and BL21 (DE3)PlysS bacteria and two kinds of recombinant plasmid for expression screening. Here, we performed several small-scale expression experiments. The results showed that, except for the combination of Origima (DE3)/pET3c-rhFGF18, all other combinations resulted in target protein being greatly lower expressed (Fig. 2).

The combination of Origima (DE3)/pET3c-rhFGF18 was used for optimization of induction conditions for improved production of soluble rhFGF18. The recombinant was shaker-cultured at 37℃ and 180 rpm in LB medium until the culture reached mid-logarithmic growth (OD_{600}=0.6). Next, *E. coli* cells harboring hFGF18 were treated with 1 mM

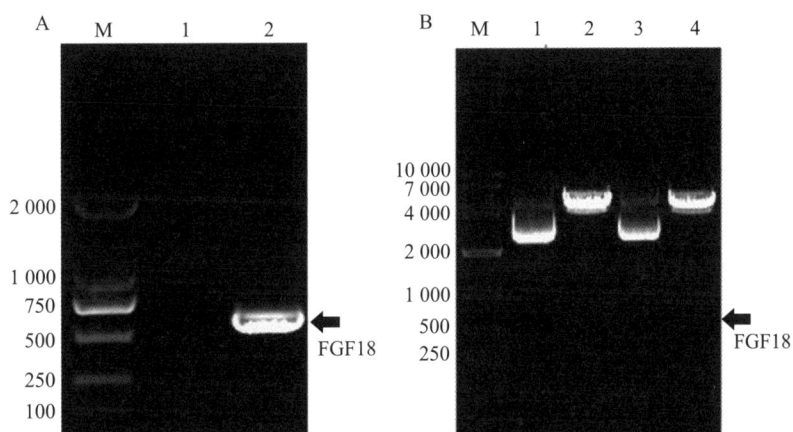

Fig. 1. Synthesis of FGF18 by PCR and identification by restriction enzymatic analysis. The strategy for synthesizing FGF18 is described in "material and methods." The molecular weight of the PCR fragment containing FGF18 is shown in (A) *Lane 1* negative control (without template vector), *lane 2* FGF18 fragment (643 bp). Identification of recombinant plasmid by enzyme digestion (*Nde*I and *Bam*HI) is shown in (B) *Lanes 1 and 3* pET3c-rhFGF18 and pET22b-rhFGF18, respectively; *lanes 2 and 4* restriction products of recombinant plasmid pET3c-rhFGF18 and pET22b-rhFGF18, respectively.

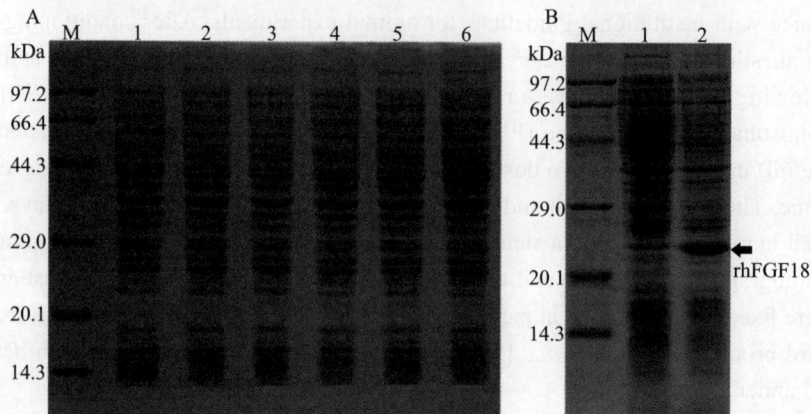

Fig. 2. SDS-PAGE analysis of rhFGF18 expression screening and optimization of induction conditions for production of soluble rhFGF18. Two kinds of recombinant plasmid were transformed into E. coli strain Origima (DE3) and BL21 (DE3)PlysS for expression screening. The results showed that the Origima (DE3)/pET3c-rhFGF18 transformant was effective for expression of target protein. (A) Lane M molecular weight standards; lanes 1, 3, and 5 uninduced BL21 (DE3)PlysS/pET22b-rhFGF18, BL21 (DE3)PlysS/pET3c-rhFGF18, and Origima (DE3)/ pET22b-rhFGF18, respectively; lanes 2, 4, and 6 induced BL21 (DE3)PlysS/pET22b-rhFGF18, BL21 (DE3)PlysS/pET3c-rhFGF18, and Origima (DE3)/ pET22b-rhFGF18, respectively. (B) Lane M molecular weight standards, lanes 1 and 2 uninduced and induced Origima (DE3)/ pET3c-rhFGF18. The bacteria containing Origima (DE3)/pET3c-rhFGF18 were induced by 1 mM IPTG for 10 h at 25℃.

IPTG for 10 h at 25℃ and then collected and lysed. The average bacterial yield of three batches was more than 652 g in a 30-L fermentor. SDS-PAGE analysis of the lysate supernatant showed that the recombinant protein was expressed as a soluble product with a molecular weight of about 23 kDa corresponding to the target protein of rhFGF18 (Fig. 2B). Densitometry scanning revealed that the amount of expressed recombinant hFGF18 was more than 30% of the total cellular protein at 10 h after induction. Simultaneously, we found that the rhFGF18 protein was expressed in inclusion bodies at 37℃ (data not shown).

3.3 Purification and identification of rhFGF18

Next, the soluble product was purified as described in "Materials and methods." As demonstrated in Fig. 3A, the fractions containing rhFGF18 were finally eluted by heparin-affinity chromatography using 20 mM PB containing 0.8 M NaCl. The purified rhFGF18 protein yield was 155 mg/L. And the recovered rhFGF18 was homogenous, and its purity was over 90%, as estimated by HPLC, with a retention time of 14.959 min (Fig. 4). Western blotting analysis with a specific anti-human FGF18 antibody showed a specific reaction with the target protein, and revealed part of the rhFGF18 protein was degraded (Fig. 3B).

3.4 Mitogenic activity of recombinant hFGF18

To evaluate the effectiveness of recombinant hFGF18 bioactivity, the proliferative effect of rhFGF18 was deter-

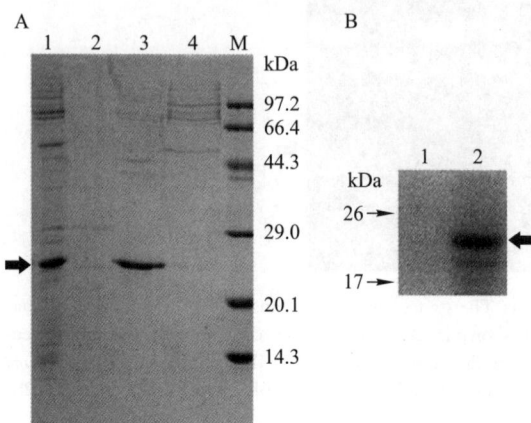

Fig. 3. SDS-PAGE analysis of purification of rhFGF18 and its characterization by Western blotting. (A) SDS-PAGE analysis of the fraction collected from CM Sepharose FF (lane 1) and heparin-affinity chromatography (lanes 2–4), respectively. Lane 1 fraction eluted with 0.5 M NaCl from CM Sepharose FF, lane 2 0.3 M NaCl-eluted from heparin-sepharose chromatography, lane 3 0.8 M NaCl-eluted fraction, lane 4 1.5 M NaCl-eluted fraction, lane M molecular weight standards. (B) Western blotting analysis of the rhFGF18. Lane 1 bacterial lysate of transformants uninduced by IPTG as negative control, lane 2 the bacterial lysate of transformants induced by 1 mM IPTG.

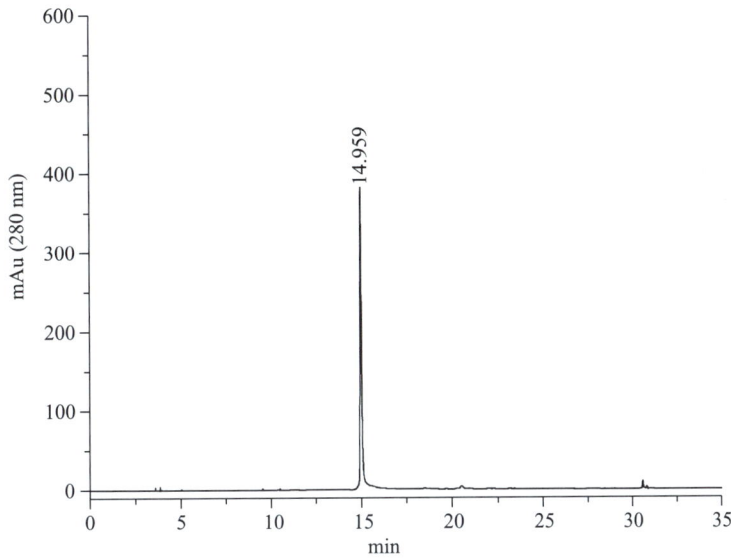

Fig. 4. HPLC analysis of the purified rhFGF18. The purity of rhFGF18 eluted from a heparin-affinity column was further evaluated by HPLC analysis using a C18 column. As seen from the chromatogram, the y-axis indicates the absorbance (280 nm, mAu), while the x-axis elution time (minutes). The main peak was observed at 14.959 min. The purity of purified rhFGF18 was more than 90%.

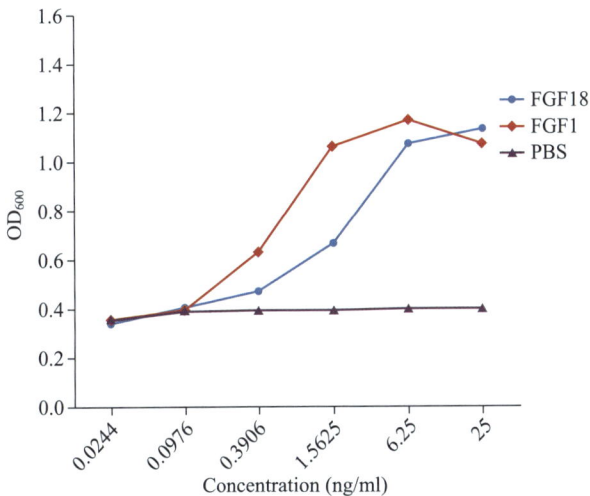

Fig. 5. Mitogenic activity analysis of different concentrations of rhFGF18 and FGF1 on NIH3T3 cells *in vitro*. Cell cultures were prepared as in "materials and methods." Increasing concentrations of FGF18 (*solid circle*) or FGF1 (*solid diamond*) were added. PBS was used as a negative control (*solid triangles*). Proliferation was quantified by measuring the absorbance at 600 nm.

mined using a standard MTT assay on NIH3T3 cells and compared with human FGF1 (positive control, Abcam, Hong-Kong) because it has been well confirmed that FGF1 can strongly active DNA synthesis in NIH3T3 cells (Gospodarowicz, 1974). As shown in Fig. 5, similar to FGF1 the purified rhFGF18 induced a comparable mitogenic response in NIH3T3 cells, which is consistent with the findings of previous studies (Hu *et al.,* 1999). Furthermore, rhFGF18 was found to have a dose-dependent effect on the viability of NIH3T3 cells, and the negative control did not have any affirmative effect (Fig. 5). Thus, we speculate that rhFGF18 produced with this method had a remarkable mitogenic effect on NIH3T3 cells.

3.5 *In vivo bioactivity of rhFGF18*

To evaluate further the biological activity of rhFGF18, the effect of the rhFGF18 on hair growth was analyzed by subcutaneous administration of male C57BL/6 mice. In our experiments, 14 days after treatment with rhFGF18 protein, the exterior surface of the dorsal skin of the mice exhibited vigorous hair growth throughout the entire test area (Fig. 6A). Examination of the reverse side of the skin revealed extensive growth of anagen hair follicles in the mice with pigmentation or hair growth (black spots indicate anagen hair follicles) (Fig. 6A). Furthermore, the skin from one of the eight mice that received FGF18 showed no apparent changes, whereas none of the skin samples from the eight control

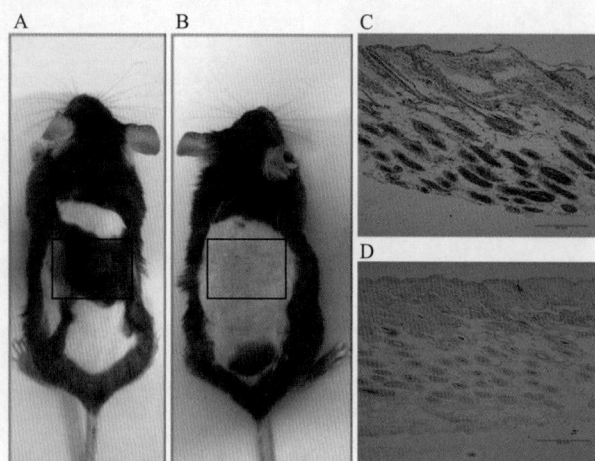

Fig. 6. Induction of hair growth by rhFGF18 protein in mice with telogen stage hair follicles. Sixteen 56-day-old male C57BL/6 mice were anesthetized and their dorsal hair was gently cut short, and rhFGF18 was administered subcutaneously into the dorsal test area (*n*= 16). The squared area is the test area. (A) After 14 days, the mice that received rhFGF18 showed vigorous hair growth. (B) As a control, another group of mice received PBS. Representative mice for each treatment are shown. On day 15, they were anesthetized and killed, and the full-thickness of the dorsal skin in the test area was excised. A representative result is shown. (C) Histology of the hair follicles from mice administered with FGF18. (D) Histology of the hair follicles from mice administered with PBS. The skin from the mice in a and b was embedded in paraffin, sectioned, stained with H&E, and photographed. Scale bars=50 μm.

mice exhibited hair growth or strong pigmentation. Examination of the reverse side of control skin revealed little or no anagen hair follicles, as is indicated by their white color (Fig. 6B). Meanwhile, these results were further confirmed by histological examination of skin sections (Fig. 6C, D). When rhFGF18 was administered subcutaneously to mice in a uniform telogen state, anagen hair growth was compared between the FGF18-and PBS-administered mice. Our findings suggest that the rhFGF18 expressed using this method is important for the regulation of hair growth and the maintenance of skin in adult mice and may be an effective approach to stimulate hair growth.

4. Discussion

A wealth of pharmacological studies has previously shown that FGF18, a member of the FGF family, has a high therapeutic potential for cartilage repair in preclinical and clinical cartilage disorders (Moore *et al.*, 2005). In addition, several *in vivo* studies using different animal models have shown that recombinant human FGF18 could regulate hair growth and skin maintenance and have possibilities for alopecia therapies in humans (Greco *et al.*, 2009; Kimura-Ueki *et al.*, 2012). It is necessary to develop methods for abundant production of FGF18 with high bioactivity for specific treatment of FGF18-related diseases in the future. However, the low level of expression and difficulty in producing highly bioactive homogeneous protein has restricted its therapeutic applications. A widely used method to evade these limitations is the fusion strategy expression of target protein, such as His$_6$-tagged, glutathione-*S*-transferase and thioredoxin, but these methods have shortcomings in terms of efficient soluble expression, bioactivity, and immunogenicity (Terpe, 2003). Specifically, to achieve release of target protein, the cleavage reaction must be performed. Most importantly, the removal of the fused tag is expensive and may impact on the bioactivity of the target protein. This may restrict development of any therapeutic proteins including rhFGF18 because higher biological activity, lower expenditure, and manufacturing reproducibility are essential for regulatory approval. We have reported a rapid and efficient strategy to express and purify high levels of recombinant hFGF18.

In our experiments, we used the most commonly used *E. coli* expression system for high-level expression of heterologous proteins due to its well-established, fast growth rate, resulting high yields of protein expression. However, the structural features of hFGF18 pose quite a challenge for its production by genetic engineering in *E. coli*. The difficulties primarily stem from the activity-dependent conformation and potential toxicity of this peptide. To eliminate the adverse effect of expression levels of rhFGF18, preferential codons of *E. coli* were introduced into the coding sequence of rhFGF18(ESM Fig. S1). Origima (DE3) was chosen as the expression host strain because it could eliminate both active thioredoxin and reductase expression and thus may facilitate cytoplasmic disulfide bond formation necessary for the correct folding of the protein (Prinz *et al.*, 1997). Taken together, for efficient protein expression both were indispensable. To further improve the production level of the target protein, we successively optimized several pivotal factors of expression conditions (IPTG concentration, temperature, and time after induction) (ESM Fig. S2). It has been previously reported that stress conditions and high rates of protein synthesis are the main causes of the formation of inclusion bodies (Gatti-Lafranconi *et al.,* 2011). Under optimal expression conditions, the high soluble expression level of rhFGF18 reached more than 30 % of total protein after treatment with 1 mM IPTG for 10 h at 25 ℃ in Origima (DE3) host strain. Actually, the use of a lower temperature (25 ℃) to increase soluble protein levels and reduce the aggregation of recombinant proteins, thus reducing the inclusion bodies formed, is quite prevalent (de Groot and Ventura 2006). In addition, a long induction period is also necessary.

Because of the fact that the heparin binging ability of hFGF18 could be specifically captured by heparin-sepharose, the non-fusion rhFGF18 protein was efficiently separated from undesirable impurities of *E. coli* lysate supernatant by a heparin-affinity chromatograph. In addition, heparin-sepharose chromatography has been routinely used for the separation and purification of some therapeutic proteins (Berman *et al.,* 1999; Huang *et al.,* 2012; Kenig *et al.,* 2008). Therefore, heparin-sepharose may provide an environment favorable for maintaining hFGF18 bioactivity during purification. Using the heparin-sepharose strategy, we successfully purified the rhFGF18 and produced highly bioactive homogeneous rhFGF18. We utilized its heparin binging ability to generate a non-fusion expression vector to produce rhFGF18 that is able to retain more bioactivity because of avoiding cleavage of the fusion-tagged protein. Unfortunately, the rhFGF18 was very sensitive to the environmental temperature and degraded in the short term (Fig. 3B). Like other FGFs, sensitivity to temperature and proteolytic enzymes significantly impedes its clinical applications. Fortunately, poly(ethylene glycol) (PEG) has been extensively used to improve protein biostabilities and to increase the half-life time of protein *in vivo* (Caliceti and Veronese, 2003; Veronese and Pasut, 2005). Therefore, our research placed emphasis on the PEG modification of rhFGF18 to increase its *in vivo* biostability and therapeutic potency.

Certainly, the purified recombinant human FGF18 protein was biologically active *in vitro*. Like FGF1, FGF18 had a dose-dependent effect on the proliferation of NIH3T3 cells, demonstrating that the rhFGF18 expressed from *E. coli* Origima (DE3) is more favorable for retaining heparin-binding ability leaving an intact functional complex comprising FGF, FGFRs, and heparin. Thus, we speculate that FGF18 has a mitogenic effect on NIH3T3 cells, which is consistent with the finding of previous studies (Hu *et al.,* 1999). Interestingly, rhFGF18 produced by the non-fusion method had better biological activity than FLAG-tagged hFGF18 (Hu *et al.,* 1999). We speculate that the FLAG tag may lead to lower bioactivity. Meanwhile, its specific activity on NIH3T3 cells was of a lesser magnitude than that of FGF1. This result suggests that FGF18 may be less potent than FGF1 in fibroblasts. A possible explanation of this effect could be that fibroblasts may not be the primary physiological target cell type for FGF18. Interestingly, Shimoaka *et al.* (2002) suggested that the mitogenic activity of FGF18 is more specific to bone and cartilage cells than FGF1 and FGF2. Furthermore, FGF18 has been previously reported to activate the proliferation of different cell types, such as human dermal papilla cells, epidermal keratinocytes, vascular endothelial cells, hepatic parenchymal cells, and pancreatic ductal epithelium (Hu *et al.,* 1999; Kawano *et al.,* 2005; Ohbayashi *et al.,* 2002; Smith *et al.,* 2007).

A variety of polypeptide growth factors, including various members of the fibroblast growth factor family, are expressed in skin. As reported previously, FGF18 mRNA is strongly expressed in telogen hair follicles (Kawano *et al.,* 2005). When male C57BL/6 mice were subcutaneously administered with FGF18 during telogen, hair growth occurred in the FGF18 treatment group earlier than the PBS control group. Reportedly, FGF18 was delivered subcutaneously during anagen, and matrix cell proliferation was immediately inhibited, leading to strong suppression of hair follicle growth (Kimura-Ueki *et al.,* 2012). rhFGF18 protein has contrasting pharmacological effects on hair growth in mice, depending on the hair cycle stage of the follicles. Furthermore, the anagen-promoting effects of FGF7 and FGF10 are very different to the activity of FGF18 (Greco *et al.,* 2009). It is likely that FGF7 and FGF10 activate FGFR2b, an epithelial-specific FGF receptor subtype; in contrast, FGF18 activates FGFR3c and FGFR4 (Zhang *et al.,* 2006). While signaling through FGFR2b results in epithelial cell proliferation, signaling through FGFR3c and FGFR4 induces a complex phenotype that is sometimes inhibitory (Iwata *et al.,* 2000; Ornitz and Marie, 2002). This probably explains why the biological effects of FGF18 and FGF7/FGF10 differ significantly. In our studies, we also observed significant hair follicle growth after subcutaneously injecting rhFGF18 for 14 days during the telogen stages of the hair growth cycle, compared to the negative control (PBS). However, Kimura-Ueki *et al.,* (2012) reported that FGF18 might be performed the inhibition of rhFGF18 on anagen progression by hair follicle. The only certainty is that the effects of rhFGF18 on hair follicle growth could be applied in further research and therapeutic applications.

In summary, recombinant human FGF18 was successfully expressed in the *E. coli* strain Origima (DE3) from optimized non-fusion FGF18 gene. Purification was undertaken using CM Sepharose FF and heparin affinity chromatography, the identity of the purified protein was confirmed by Western blotting, and its purity was determined by HPLC analysis. The rhFGF18 could significantly promote proliferation of NIH3T3 cells. *In vivo*, subcutaneous administration with rhFGF18 during telogen of the hair growth cycle could remarkably regulate hair growth in C57BL/6 mice. This study demonstrated that non-tagged expression of optimal rhFGF18 is simple, viable, and highly effective, making it convenient for high level expression and purification of protein with high bioactivity preserved.

Supplementary material

Electronic supplementary material to this article can be found in the online version (doi:10.1007/s00253-013-4929-3).

References

Ajikumar PK, Xiao WH, Tyo KE, *et al.* Isoprenoid pathway optimization for Taxol precursor overproduction in Escherichia coli[J]. Science, 2010, 330(6000): 70-74.

Arakawa T, Hsu YR, Schiffer SG, *et al.* Characterization of a cysteine-free analog of recombinant human basic fibroblast growth factor[J]. Biochem Biophys Res Commun, 1989, 161(1): 335-341.

Behr B, Sorkin M, Manu A, *et al.* Fgf-18 is required for osteogenesis but not angiogenesis during long bone repair[J]. Tissue Eng Part A, 2011, 17(15-16): 2061-2069.

Berman B, Ostrovsky O, Shlissel M, *et al.* Similarities and differences between the effects of heparin and glypican-1 on the bioactivity of acidic fibroblast growth factor and the keratinocyte growth factor[J]. J Biol Chem, 1999, 274(51): 36132-36138.

Beyer C, Schett G. Pharmacotherapy: concepts of pathogenesis and emerging treatments. Novel targets in bone and cartilage[J]. Best Pract Res Clin Rheumatol, 2010, 24(4): 489-496.

Caliceti P, Veronese FM. Pharmacokinetic and biodistribution properties of poly(ethylene glycol)-protein conjugates[J]. Adv Drug Deliv Rev, 2003, 55(10): 1261-1277.

de Groot NS, Ventura S. Effect of temperature on protein quality in bacterial inclusion bodies[J]. FEBS Lett, 2006, 580(27): 6471-6476.

Derynck R, Roberts AB, Winkler ME, *et al.* Human transforming growth factor-alpha: precursor structure and expression in E. coli[J]. Cell, 1984, 38(1): 287-297.

Dichmann DS, Miller CP, Jensen J, *et al.* Expression and misexpression of members of the FGF and TGFbeta families of growth factors in the developing mouse pancreas[J]. Dev Dyn, 2003, 226(4): 663-674.

Dong X, Tang B, Li J, *et al.* Expression and purification of intact and functional soybean (Glycine max) seed ferritin complex in Escherichia coli[J]. J Microbiol Biotechnol, 2008, 18(2): 299-307.

Ellsworth JL, Berry J, Bukowski T, *et al.* Fibroblast growth factor-18 is a trophic factor for mature chondrocytes and their progenitors[J]. Osteoarthritis Cartilage, 2002, 10(4): 308-320.

Gatti-Lafranconi P, Natalello A, Ami D, *et al.* Concepts and tools to exploit the potential of bacterial inclusion bodies in protein science and biotechnology[J]. Febs j, 2011, 278(14): 2408-2418.

Ghosh AK, Shankar DB, Shackleford GM, *et al.* Molecular cloning and characterization of human FGF8 alternative messenger RNA forms[J]. Cell Growth Differ, 1996, 7(10): 1425-1434.

Gospodarowicz D. Localisation of a fibroblast growth factor and its effect alone and with hydrocortisone on 3T3 cell growth[J]. Nature, 1974, 249(453): 123-127.

Greco V, Chen T, Rendl M, *et al.* A two-step mechanism for stem cell activation during hair regeneration[J]. Cell Stem Cell, 2009, 4(2): 155-169.

Hasegawa H, Ashigaki S, Takamatsu M, *et al.* Laminar patterning in the developing neocortex by temporally coordinated fibroblast growth factor signaling[J]. J Neurosci, 2004, 24(40): 8711-8719.

Hu MC, Qiu WR, Wang YP, *et al.* FGF-18, a novel member of the fibroblast growth factor family, stimulates hepatic and intestinal proliferation[J]. Mol Cell Biol, 1998, 18(10): 6063-6074.

Hu MC, Wang YP, Qiu WR. Human fibroblast growth factor-18 stimulates fibroblast cell proliferation and is mapped to chromosome 14p11[J]. Oncogene, 1999, 18(16): 2635-2642.

Huang Y, Rao Y, Feng C, *et al.* High-level expression and purification of Tat-haFGF19-154[J]. Appl Microbiol Biotechnol, 2008, 77(5): 1015-1022.

Huang Z, Ye C, Liu Z, *et al.* Solid-phase N-terminus PEGylation of recombinant human fibroblast growth factor 2 on heparin-sepharose column[J]. Bioconjug Chem, 2012, 23(4): 740-750.

Ishibe T, Nakayama T, Okamoto T, *et al.* Disruption of fibroblast growth factor signal pathway inhibits the growth of synovial sarcomas: potential application of signal inhibitors to molecular target therapy[J]. Clin Cancer Res, 2005, 11(7): 2702-2712.

Iwata T, Chen L, Li C, *et al.* A neonatal lethal mutation in FGFR3 uncouples proliferation and differentiation of growth plate chondrocytes in embryos[J]. Hum Mol Genet, 2000, 9(11): 1603-1613.

Jana S, Deb JK. Strategies for efficient production of heterologous proteins in Escherichia coli[J]. Appl Microbiol Biotechnol, 2005, 67(3): 289-298.

Jeon E, Yun YR, Kang W, *et al.* Investigating the role of FGF18 in the cultivation and osteogenic differentiation of mesenchymal stem cells[J]. PLoS One, 2012, 7(8): e43982.

Katoh M, Katoh M. Comparative genomics on FGF8, FGF17, and FGF18 orthologs[J]. Int J Mol Med, 2005, 16(3): 493-496.

Kawano M, Komi-Kuramochi A, Asada M, *et al.* Comprehensive analysis of FGF and FGFR expression in skin: FGF18 is highly expressed in hair follicles and capable of inducing anagen from telogen stage hair follicles[J]. J Invest Dermatol, 2005, 124(5): 877-885.

Kenig M, Gaberc-Porekar V, Fonda I, *et al.* Identification of the heparin-binding domain of TNF-alpha and its use for efficient TNF-alpha purification by heparin-Sepharose affinity chromatography[J]. J Chromatogr B Analyt Technol Biomed Life Sci, 2008, 867(1): 119-125.

Kimura-Ueki M, Oda Y, Oki J, *et al.* Hair cycle resting phase is regulated by cyclic epithelial FGF18 signaling[J]. J Invest Dermatol, 2012, 132(5): 1338-1345.

Liu Z, Xu J, Colvin JS, *et al.* Coordination of chondrogenesis and osteogenesis by fibroblast growth factor 18[J]. Genes Dev, 2002, 16(7): 859-869.

Long F, Ornitz DM. Development of the endochondral skeleton[J]. Cold Spring Harb Perspect Biol, 2013, 5(1): a008334.

Moore EE, Bendele AM, Thompson DL, *et al.* Fibroblast growth factor-18 stimulates chondrogenesis and cartilage repair in a rat model of injury-induced osteoarthritis[J]. Osteoarthritis Cartilage, 2005, 13(7): 623-631.

Ohbayashi N, Hoshikawa M, Kimura S, *et al.* Structure and expression of the mRNA encoding a novel fibroblast growth factor, FGF-18[J]. J Biol Chem, 1998, 273(29): 18161-18164.

Ohbayashi N, Shibayama M, Kurotaki Y, *et al.* FGF18 is required for normal cell proliferation and differentiation during osteogenesis and chondrogenesis[J]. Genes Dev, 2002, 16(7): 870-879.

Ohuchi H, Kimura S, Watamoto M, *et al.* Involvement of fibroblast growth factor (FGF)18-FGF8 signaling in specification of left-right asymmetry and brain and limb development of the chick embryo[J]. Mech Dev, 2000, 95(1-2): 55-66.

Ornitz DM, Marie PJ. FGF signaling pathways in endochondral and intramembranous bone development and human genetic disease[J]. Genes Dev, 2002, 16(12): 1446-1465.

Paus R, Muller-Rover S, Van Der Veen C, *et al.* A comprehensive guide for the recognition and classification of distinct stages of hair follicle morphogenesis[J]. J Invest Dermatol, 1999, 113(4): 523-532.

Plikus MV. New activators and inhibitors in the hair cycle clock: targeting stem cells' state of competence[J]. J Invest Dermatol, 2012, 132(5): 1321-1324.

Prinz WA, Aslund F, Holmgren A, *et al.* The role of the thioredoxin and glutaredoxin pathways in reducing protein disulfide bonds in the Escherichia coli cytoplasm[J]. J Biol Chem, 1997, 272(25): 15661-15667.

Quick M, Wright EM. Employing Escherichia coli to functionally express, purify, and characterize a human transporter[J]. Proc Natl Acad Sci U S A, 2002, 99(13): 8597-8601.

Ryu EK, Cho KJ, Kim JK, *et al.* Expression and purification of recombinant human fibroblast growth factor receptor in Escherichia coli[J]. Protein Expr Purif, 2006, 49(1): 15-22.

Sato T, Joyner AL, Nakamura H. How does Fgf signaling from the isthmic organizer induce midbrain and cerebellum development?[J]. Dev Growth Differ, 2004, 46(6): 487-494.

Shimoaka T, Ogasawara T, Yonamine A, *et al.* Regulation of osteoblast, chondrocyte, and osteoclast functions by fibroblast growth factor (FGF)-18 in comparison with FGF-2 and FGF-10[J]. J Biol Chem, 2002, 277(9): 7493-7500.

Smith SM, West LA, Hassell JR. The core protein of growth plate perlecan binds FGF-18 and alters its mitogenic effect on chondrocytes[J]. Arch Biochem Biophys, 2007, 468(2): 244-251.

Terpe K. Overview of tag protein fusions: from molecular and biochemical fundamentals to commercial systems[J]. Appl Microbiol Biotechnol, 2003, 60(5): 523-533.

Usui H, Shibayama M, Ohbayashi N, *et al.* Fgf18 is required for embryonic lung alveolar development[J]. Biochem Biophys Res Commun, 2004, 322(3): 887-892.

Verdon J, Girardin N, Marchand A, *et al.* Purification and antibacterial activity of recombinant warnericin RK expressed in Escherichia coli[J]. Appl Microbiol Biotechnol, 2013, 97(12): 5401-5412.

Veronese FM, Pasut G. PEGylation, successful approach to drug delivery[J]. Drug Discov Today, 2005, 10(21): 1451-1458.

Vincent TL. Explaining the fibroblast growth factor paradox in osteoarthritis: lessons from conditional knockout mice[J]. Arthritis Rheum, 2012, 64(12): 3835-3838.

Wu X, Su Z, Li X, *et al.* High-level expression and purification of a non-mitogenic form of human acidic fibroblast growth factor in Escherichia coli[J]. Protein Expr Purif, 2005, 42(1): 7-11.

Wu X, Tian H, Huang Y, *et al.* Large-scale production of biologically active human keratinocyte growth factor-2[J]. Appl Microbiol Biotechnol, 2009, 82(3): 439-444.

Xu J, Lawshe A, MacArthur CA, *et al.* Genomic structure, mapping, activity and expression of fibroblast growth factor 17[J]. Mech Dev, 1999, 83(1-2): 165-178.

Zhan X, Hu X, Friedman S, *et al.* Analysis of endogenous and exogenous nuclear translocation of fibroblast growth factor-1 in NIH 3T3 cells[J]. Biochem Biophys Res Commun, 1992, 188(3): 982-991.

Zhang X, Ibrahimi OA, Olsen SK, *et al.* Receptor specificity of the fibroblast growth factor family. The complete mammalian FGF family[J]. J Biol Chem, 2006, 281(23): 15694-15700.

Zhu S, Gong C, Ren L, *et al.* A simple and effective strategy for solving the problem of inclusion bodies in recombinant protein technology: His-tag deletions enhance soluble expression[J]. Appl Microbiol Biotechnol, 2013, 97(2): 837-845.

Oil body bound oleosin-rhFGF9 fusion protein expressed in safflower (*Carthamus tinctorius* L.) stimulates hair growth and wound healing in mice

Jingbo Cai, Xiaokun Li, Chao Jiang

1. Background

Fibroblast growth factor 9 (FGF9), also known as Glia-activating factor (GAF), was originally isolated from human glioma cells [1, 2]. FGF9, FGF16 and FGF20 are similar in structure and comprise the FGF9 subfamily of the fibroblast growth factor (FGF) superfamily. Full-length human FGF-9 is a 208 amino acid polypeptide lacking a typical signal sequence. Accordingly, the secretion of FGF9 is mediated by an N-linked carbohydrate chain and occurs *via* the constitutive endoplasmic reticulum/Golgi secretory pathway [2, 3]. The human *FGF9* gene is located on chromosome 13q11-q12, whereas mouse *FGF9* is located on chromosome 14; the human and mouse coding sequences exhibit 88.7% identity [4, 5]. There are four tyrosine kinase fibroblast growth factor receptors (FGFR1–4), which undergo alternative splicing to produce isoforms with high affinity, ligand-dependent responses to different FGFs. The specificity of FGF ligand receptor interaction is augmented by heparin, heparin sulfate, or other glycosaminoglycan chains to ensure stable binding and to activate diverse physiological functions. FGF9 can bind and activate FGFR3IIIc, FGFR3IIIb and FGFR2IIIc, but can also activate other receptors with lower affinity, such as FGFR1IIIc and FGFR4; FGF9 has highest affinity to bind and activate FGFR3 but shows no activity toward FGFR1b or -2b [6, 7].

FGF9 is found in a wide variety of tissues and organs and has multiple physiological functions. It is an indispensable growth factor for human development. FGF9 contributes to bone development and repair, angiogenesis, embryonic development, cell apoptosis, nerve regeneration, and hair follicle regeneration [8–10]. In addition, FGF9 participates in the development of heart, brain, kidney, muscle, joint and other tissues [11].

The deletion or overexpression of FGF9 causes many related diseases, such as major depressive disorder [12], multiple synostoses syndrome [13], elbow knee synostosis [14], disorders of sex development, primary synovial chondromatosis, Dupuytren's disease [15], skeletal dysplasia, and colorectal, endometrial and ovarian carcinoma [16]. The widespread biological functions of FGF9 have drawn significant attention to its potential for clinical application, which has been addressed in many studies.

In particular, previous reports have focused on cancers or tumors, the treatment of bone related disorders, wound healing, and the exploration of hair regeneration. In light of ongoing research into applications of FGF9, there is a demand to produce this protein at low expense, and high efficiency and safety.

Plant expression systems and the oil body oleosin technology provide a convenient method for the production of exogenous recombinant fusion proteins in a large-scale, reliable, cheap, safe, effective and short-term manner. Oil bodies are simple storage organelles found in oil seeds, with a diameter of 0.5–2.0 μm, comprising a triacylglycerol matrix enclosed by a monolayer of phospholipids and structural oil body membrane proteins, principally oleosins [17]. Markley et al. [18] used this approach to express recombinant proteins in the oil bodies of transgenic seeds. Recombinant proteins were targeted to the surface of oil bodies through covalent fusion with oleosin.

The oil bodies of safflower (*Carthamus tinctorius* L.) were chosen for the production of rhFGF9. Safflower is a small acreage crop that is largely self-pollinating with low out-crossing habits and genetic stability, and is well adapted to the semiarid conditions of the tropics and subtropics [18, 19]. An annual plant from the family Compositae, safflower can be grown counter-seasonally with cost-effective large-scale production, allowing maximum flexibility for the management of seed transport and storage at normal atmospheric temperature. As an important oil seed crop, safflower contains high oil content in seeds, ranging from 28% to 30%, which is increased 5%–8% in improved varieties [20].2The seeds contain a large number of oil bodies but small amounts of water, which ensures oil body stability. The oil bodies can easily be extracted from seeds by grinding, separating by centrifugation and then purifying by washing, to provide an economical, convenient and fast procedure for obtaining exogenous proteins.

Hair loss (alopecia) is a common phenomenon and can be emotionally troubling to affected people. Minoxidil and finasteride are currently used to treat alopecia. Both slow the progression of hair loss but do not regenerate new hair, and both can cause side effects. Growth factors are potential therapeutic agents that could reduce side effects and create the possibility of hair regrowth, leading to studies of their functions and mechanisms of action. Gay and colleagues [9] studied the molecular mechanisms of hair follicle regeneration in a wound-induced hair neogenesis model, suggesting that FGF9 from γδ T cells modulates hair follicle regeneration and triggers Wnt expression and subsequent Wnt activation in wound fibroblasts through a unique feedback mechanism. Treatment with a growth factor cocktail including FGF9, delivered by microneedling, was effective and safe, and seemed to be more effective than a growth factor cocktail lacking FGF9 [21]. It has been reported that FGFs stimulate hair growth through β-catenin and Sonic hedgehog (Shh) expression [22]. Martz et al. [23] revealed that the FGF9-mediated promotion of hair regeneration is related to the Wnt pathway. In addition, FGF9 is secreted by both mesothelial and epithelial cells, and plays important roles in organ development [24, 25]. In young mice, FGF9 mRNAs were increased on day 2 after wounding compared with day 0, and were significantly upregulated at other times during wound healing [26]. Evaluation of FGF9 expression during the healing of mouse and adult human skin following laser ablation showed that the expression of FGF9 protein and mRNA were up-regulated [27]. Thus, FGF9 has potential therapeutic application for promoting both hair growth and wound healing.

2. Results

2.1 Construction of rhFGF9 expression vector

The rhFGF9 expression vector was constructed and showed as previously report [8]. And clones carrying the desired expression vector were identified by PCR to evaluate insert size and verified by restriction enzyme digestion.

2.2 Safflower transformation and transgenic plant regeneration via grafting

The pOTBar-oleosin-rhFGF9 plasmid was transformed into the safflower genome using the *Agrobacterium tumefaciens*-mediated infection method, and grafted transgenic safflower plants were obtained (Fig. 1). The numbers of plants transformed and grafted at major steps in the procedure are listed in the animation (Table 1). The transformation rate was 0.75%.

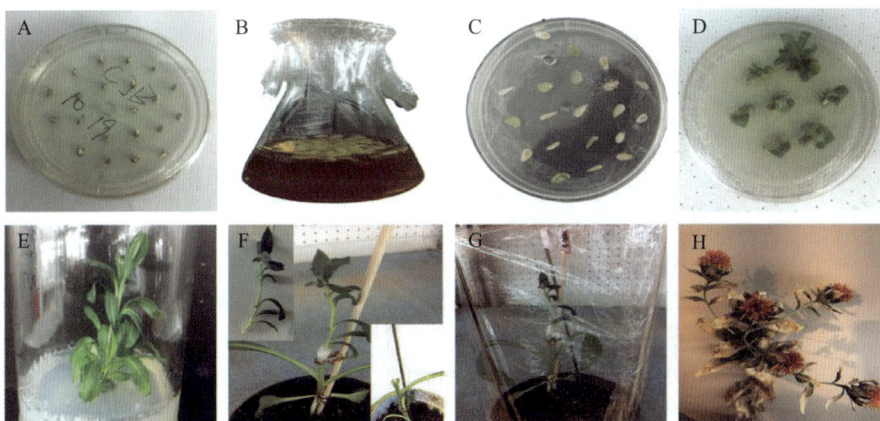

Fig. 1. *Agrobacterium-mediated* transformation of safflower and transgenic plants of safflower *via* tissue culture and grafting. (A) Seeds germination. (B) Infection with Agrobacterium. (C) Co-cultivation. (D) Shots initiation. (E) Seedlings elongation. (F) grafted plantlets with parafilm holding V-shaped transgenic scion and rootstock by grafting. (G) The successful grafted plant in pot through covering with preservative film. (H) The mature T_0 transgenic plant.

Table 1. Plants transformation and grafting of significant steps and quantity statistics

Cotyledon explants	Shoots as scions	Survived grafts	Transgenic plants	Transformation efficiency[a]
1 869	242	86	14	0.75%

[a]The transformation efficiency was calculated as the (transgenic plants/cotyledons) × 100%.

Successfully grafted T_0 safflower plants were identified by PCR analysis of genomic DNA to determine whether oleosin-rhFGF9 had integrated into the genome. Fourteen transgenic safflower plant lines were identified and harvested from 15 independent infections (Fig. 2). T_1 and T_2 plants were produced in agreement with Mendel's law of segregation. Plants without the oleosin-rhFGF9 gene, identified by PCR, were discarded.

2.3 Protein analysis of oleosin-rhFGF9

The oil body-bound oleosin-rhFGF9 fusion protein expressed in transgenic T_3 safflower seeds was evaluated by SDS-PAGE and western blotting (Fig. 3). A band of 41.5 kDa was seen for transgenic T_3 safflowers but not for WT (wild type) safflowers. The molecular weight and position of this band corresponded to an FGF9-positive band identified by western blotting. And according to BCA and ELISA assay, the results show that the level of oil body protein was 2.4% of safflower seeds, and the expression level of oleosin-rhFGF9 was 0.14% of oil body protein.

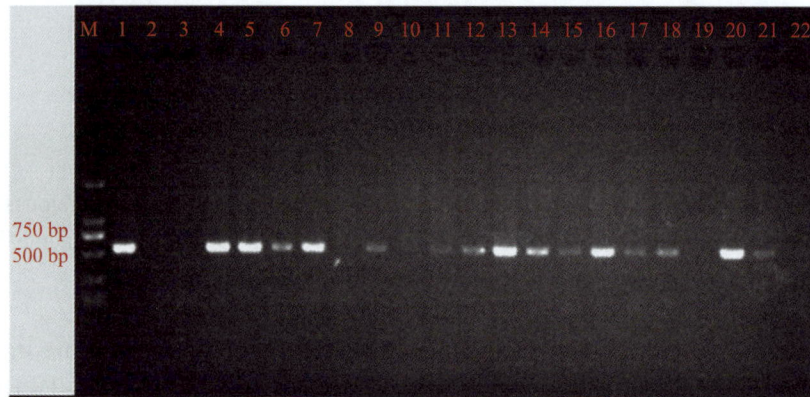

Fig. 2. T_0 safflower plants PCR amplification products of genomic DNA for 1% agarose gel. M: 2000 DNA maker. Lane 1: positive control (plasmid pOTBar-oleosin-rhFGF9). Lane 2: blank control (ddH₂O). Lane 3: negative control (wild-type safflower). Lane 4–22: PCR amplification products of successful grafted safflower plants.

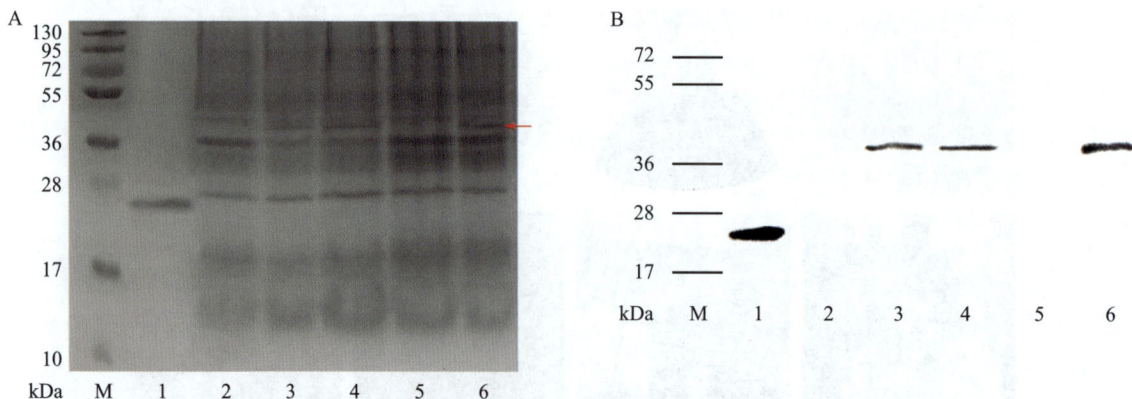

Fig. 3. SDS-PAGE and Western blotting of protein analysis of oleosin-rhFGF9. (A) Identification of oleosin-rhFGF9 from transgenic safflower by SDS-PAGE. M: protein marker. Line 1: purified rhFGF9. Lane 2: oil body protein of the wild-type (WT) safflower. Lane 3–6: oil body protein of the transgenic safflower (T_3-2, T_3-4, T_3-10, T_3-17). (B) Western blotting analysis on oleosin-rhFGF9 from the transgenic safflower. M: protein marker. Line 1: purified rhFGF9. Lane 2: oil body protein of the wild-type (WT) safflower. Lane 3–6: oil body protein of the transgenic safflower (T_3-2, T_3-4, T_3-10, T_3-17).

2.4 Mitogenic activity of oleosin-rhFGF9

The effect of oil body bound oleosin-rhFGF9 from transgenic T_3 safflowers on NIH/3 T3 cell proliferation was examined using a standard MTT method. The proliferative activity induced by oil body bound oleosin-rhFGF9 was comparable with that induced by the positive control (purified rhFG9) (Fig. 4). Furthermore, a dose-dependent effect of oil body bound oleosin-rhFGF9 on cell proliferation was seen. The oil bodies of wild-type (WT) safflower also increased proliferation, but this effect was not statistically significant. Only rhFGF9 and oil body bound oleosin-rhFGF9 significantly increased the proliferation of NIH/3 T3 cells.

2.5 In vivo analysis of oleosin-rhFGF9 activity

C57BL/6 mice were used to investigate the effects of oil body bound oleosin-rhFGF9 on both hair growth and wound healing. At the beginning of the experiments,

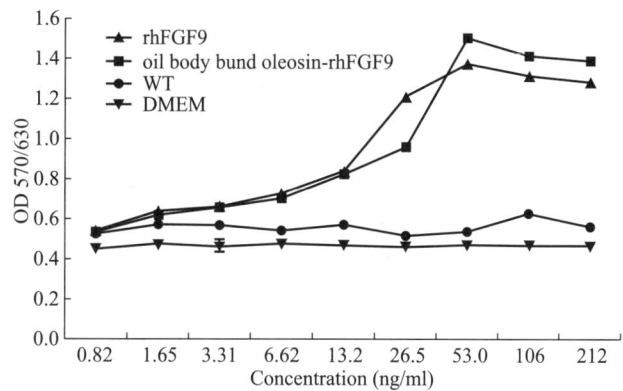

Fig. 4. The effect of oil body bound oleosin-rhFGF9 of transgenic safflower was analyzing the activity of NIH/3 T3 cells. Various concentrations (0.82–212 ng/ml) of wild-type (WT) and oil body bound oleosin-rhFGF9 or rhFGF9 (FGF9 from E.coli) were used in NIH/3 T3 cells. DMEM was used as a blank control. Proliferation was quantified by measuring the absorbance at 570/630 nm.

the hair follicles of depilated dorsal skin were in the resting phase of the hair cycle (telogen), and so the skin was glossy and pink. After 15 days of treatment, oil body bound oleosin-rhFGF9 showed obvious effects in both the hair regeneration (Fig. 5) and wound healing experiments (Fig. 6). In the hair regeneration experiment, dorsal skin had darkened on day 5, indicating that the growth phase of the hair cycle (anagen) had begun. The skin was gray with extremely short hair shafts emerging on day 10. The skin was black with many new hairs visible on day 15. Overall, the positive control group and the two oil body bound oleosin-rhFGF9 treated groups exhibited more visible hair growth over several days compared with the blank control group and the negative control group. Moreover, the high dose of oil body bound oleosin-rhFGF9 (50 μg/μl) had a greater effect on hair growth than rhFGF9 (0.07 μg/μl) or the low dose of oil body bound oleosin-rhFGF9 (10 μg/μl). Hair regrowth was slow in the blank control and negative control groups. The numbers of regenerating of hair follicles seen in H&E stained sections were consistent with the macroscopically-observed hair regrowth results (Fig. 5B, C). The expression of β-catenin in skin was localized to hair follicles (Fig. 6B). Stronger β-catenin staining was seen following treatment with oil body bound oleosin-rhFGF9 (50 μg/μl) compared with the other groups.

In the wound healing experiment, healing had obviously begun on day 5, the wounds were almost completely healed on day 10, and the wounds were fully healed with a small white scar visible on day 15. Overall, the positive control group and the two oil body bound oleosin-rhFGF9 treated groups exhibited faster wound healing compared with the blank control and negative control groups. The high dose of oil body bound oleosin-rhFGF9 (50 μg/μl) had a greater effect on wound healing than rhFGF9 (0.07 μg/μl) or the low dose of oil body bound oleosin-rhFGF9 (10 μg/μl). This difference was significant on day 5, but the difference to rhFGF9 was not significant on day 10 and 15. The blank control and negative control groups showed slow wound healing. The degree of wound healing seen in H&E and Masson's trichrome stained sections was consistent with the results described above (Fig. 6B). The rates of wound healing are shown in Fig. 6C.

3. Discussion

Clinical applications of FGFs have been extensively studied, including FGF9, and there is a need for a suitable supply of recombinant FGF proteins. At present, three major expression systems are used to produce proteins, *Escherichia coli*, insect cells and animal cells, but all have important limitations. Plant expression systems offer distinct advantages, including economy, time savings, convenience, safety, long storage, easy transportation and high yield [28]. The use of safflower as a plant expression system for the production of a oleosin-rhFGF9 fusion protein offers maximum benefit. Moreover, transgenic oil body-oleosin technology is already widely employed in the model plant, *Arabidopisis thaliana*

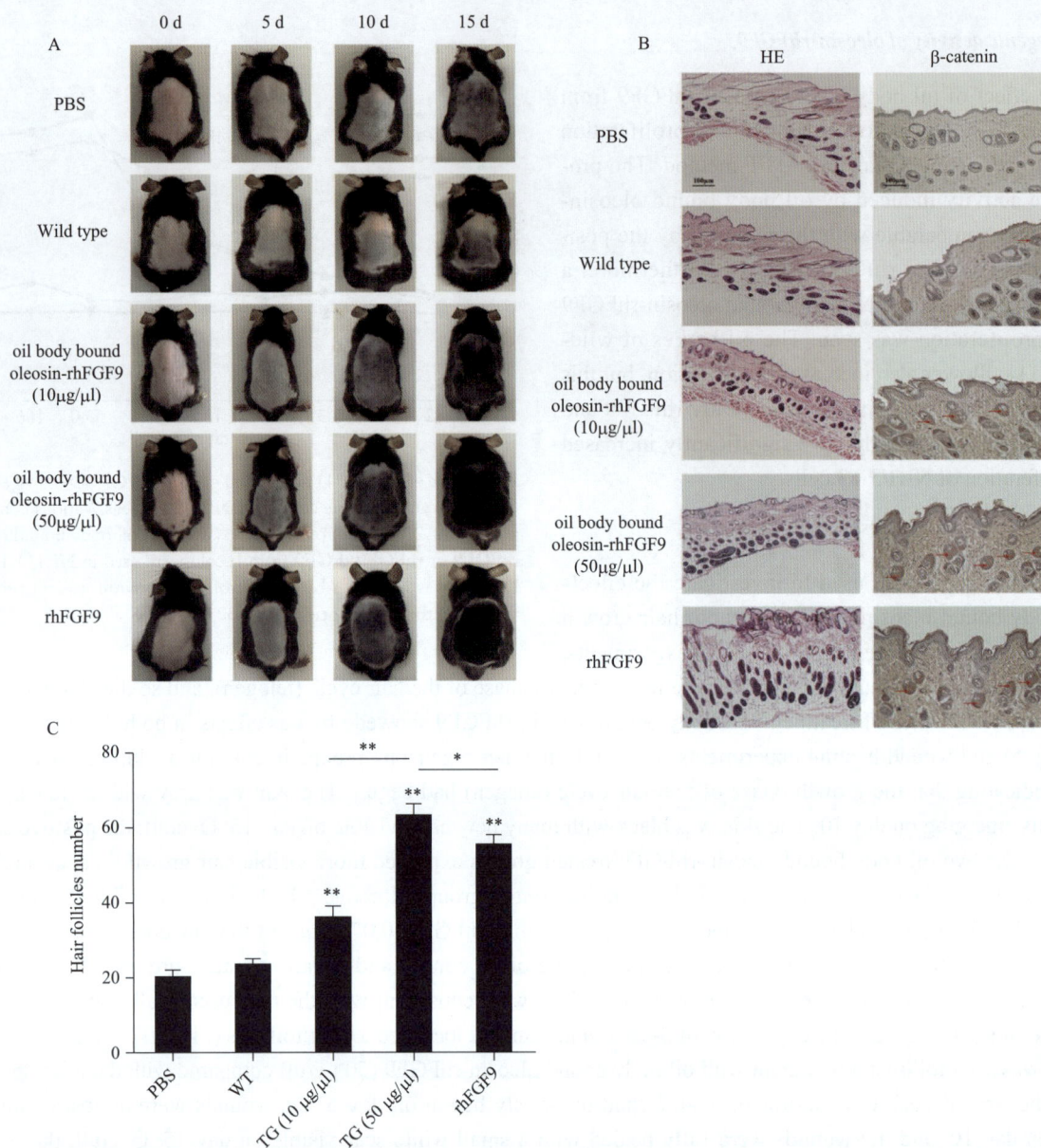

Fig. 5. The effect of the oil body bound oleosin-rhFGF9 of transgenic safflower induces hair growth after depilation when hair follicle was telogen. (A) Oil body bound oleosin-rhFGF9 was daubed on the dorsal skin of C57BL/6 mice (6-week-old). On every 0, 5, 10, 15 day, C57BL/6 mice was taken photographs and observed hair growth status. (B) Sections of dorsal skin were stained by HE and the expression of β-catenin was detected by immunohistochemical staining. Brown represents positive result with red arrow. Scale bars = 100 μm. (C) The number of hair follicles in skin. Data are the mean ± SD, $^*P < 0.05$, $^{**}P < 0.01$ compare to blank control group. TG represents treated group with oil body bound oleosin-rhFGF9.

and in safflower [18]. Without the need for tedious, difficult purification, fusion proteins in oil bodies are easily ac-cessible for topical application to the skin.

In this study, we successfully constructed an oleosin-rhFGF9 expression vector, transformed safflower using the *Agrobacterium tumefaciens*-mediated method, and expressed oleosin-rhFGF9 in the oil bodies of transgenic seeds. According to BCA and ELISA assay, the results show that the level of oil body protein was 2.4% of safflower seeds, and the expression level of oleosin-rhFGF9 was 0.14% of oil body protein; 140.66 g oleosin-rhFGF9 can be produced in 1 ha of transgenic safflowers, and 4 200 kg of safflower per hectare. The oil body bound oleosin-rhFGF9 was biologically active. We found that it had notable, dose-dependent mitogenic activity towards NIH/3 T3 cells. The greatest mitogenic activity was seen at a concentration of 53 ng/ml. Importantly, the oil body bound oleosin-rhFGF9 also had significant effects on hair growth and wound healing, and appeared to induce hair growth through the up-regulation of β-catenin.

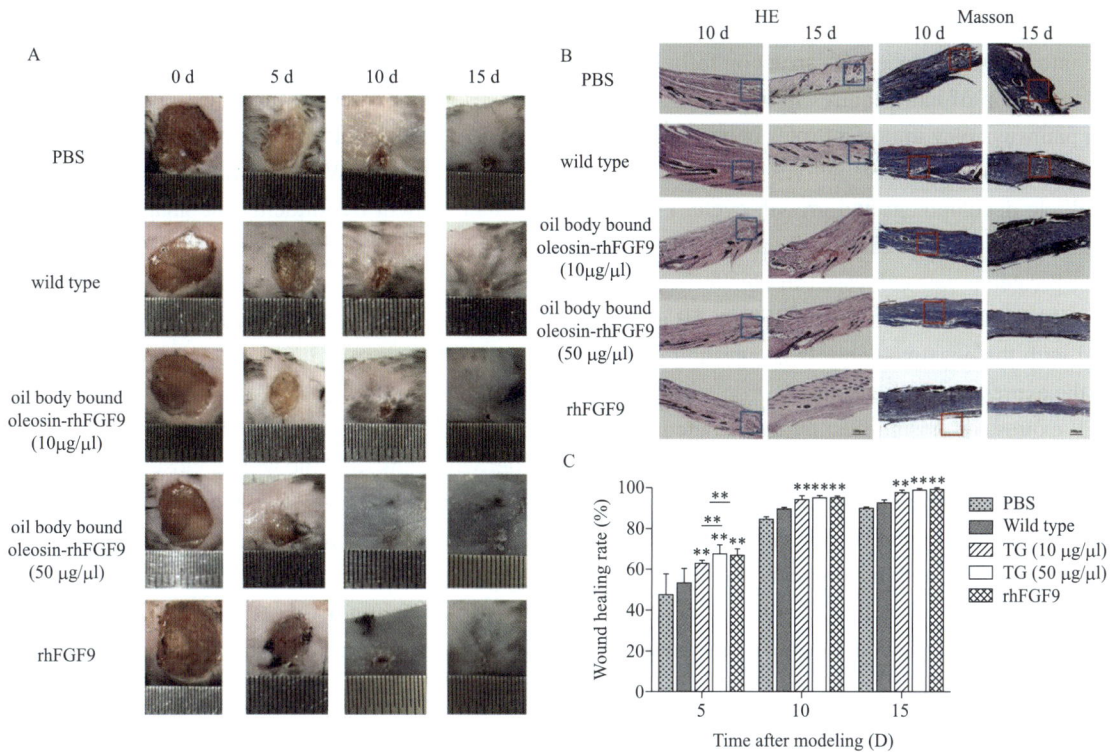

Fig. 6. The effect of the oil body bound oleosin-rhFGF9 of transgenic safflower induces wound healing. (A) Oil body bound oleosin-rhFGF9 was daubed on the wound skin of C57BL/6 mice (6-week-old). On every 0, 5, 10, 15 day, C57BL/6 mice was taken photographs and observed wound healing rate. (B) Sections of dorsal skin were stained by HE and Masson. Scale bars = 100 μm. (C) The rate of wound healing in skin. Data are the mean ± SD, $^*P < 0.05$, $^{**}P < 0.01$ compare to blank control group. TG represents treated group with oil body bound oleosin-rhF-GF9.

As an appendageal organ of skin, hair plays an important role in temperature regulation and physical protection. The hair follicle, a unique, characteristic organ of mammals, represents a stem cell-rich, prototypic neuroectodermal-mesodermal interaction system. The hair follicle is composed of epidermis and dermis, which contain the root sheaths and dermal papilla respectively. The regrowth of hair requires signaling between the epidermal and dermal components [29]. An increasing number of people are affected by serious skin diseases such as alopecia, cracked skin and varying degrees of burns. FGF9 is secreted by both mesothelial and epithelial cells, and only is expressed in the epithelium. It is involved in the early differentiation of epithelial cell layers, in epithelial invagination and ectodermal organogenesis (ectodermal organs include hair, feathers, scales, teeth, beaks, nails, horns and several eccrine glands) [27, 30]. In hair follicles, FGF9 mRNA expression is highest in telogen, at 22 days after depilation, at approximately 300 mRNA copy numbers per cell; FGFR2 and FGFR3 are abundantly expressed in anagen VI (at 18 days), at approximately 10 000 and 28 000 mRNA copy numbers per cell respectively [31]. Compared with other FGFs (FGF1, 2, 5, 7, 10, 13, and 22), FGF9 is expressed in skin at a relatively low mRNA copy number. However, FGF9 from dermal γδ T cells induces hair follicle neogenesis after wounding, and activates Wnt expression in the wound through a unique feedback mechanism to promote skin regeneration [9]. FGF9 may induce hair growth from follicles by binding FGFR2 and FGFR3, activating downstream signaling pathway proteins, and stimulating the follicles to initiate hair regeneration. In addition, FGF9 plays a role in wound healing, and its expression is up-regulated in laser-induced wounds [27]. Thus, FGF9 has a positive effect on both hair growth and wound healing through one or two signaling pathways.

Other FGFs have previously been expressed in plant oil bodies. For example, recombinant KGF2 has been expressed in *Arabidopsis thaliana* oil bodies, and has effects on hair growth in mice [32]. FGFs stimulate hair growth in C57BL/6 mice at a concentration of 500 μg/ ml [33]. When we treated mouse dorsal skin with oil body bound oleosin-rhFGF9 at 50 μg/μl and 10 μg/μl, the high dose had a notable effect on hair growth, slightly greater than that of rhFGF9 (0.07 μg/μl). Oil bodies help to maintain protein stability. The surfactant properties of oleosins and the non-coalescing nature of oil bodies mean they act as emulsifying agents, enhancing their potential for biotechnological applications [28, 34]. The absorption of topically-applied oil body bound oleosin-rhFGF9 may have been accelerated because of this emulsifying property. Abundant oil body bound oleosin-rhFGF9 can be absorbed to concentrate in the epidermis, and then penetrate into the dermis where it can act on follicles to induce hair growth.

The formation of hair requires intercellular signaling to trigger gene expression changes in the follicle. The Wnt signaling pathways play important roles in hair follicle development. Specific Wnts maintain anagen-phase gene expression *in vitro* and hair-inductive activity in a skin reconstitution assay [35]. The Wnt signaling pathways that are active in hair follicle development and growth cycle. FGFs promoted hair growth by inducing the anagen phase in telogen C57BL/6 mice, and FGF treatment induces the expression of β-catenin and Shh in hair follicles [33]. In this study, we found that β-catenin was expressed in hair follicles and was associated with newly growing hairs. Treatment with rh-FGF9 or oil body bound oleosin-rhFGF9 (at 50 μg/μl or 10 μg/μl) resulted in stronger immunohistochemical staining compared with the negative controls, suggesting that oil body bound oleosin-rhFGF9 may promote hair growth by increasing the expression of β-catenin.

FGF9 expression is significantly upregulated at various times during wound healing in young mice, but is low in healthy skin. In particular, FGF9 mRNA is increased on day 2 after wounding, and the wound closure of aged (35-week-old) hairless mice is substantially slower than young adult (8-week-old) mice [26]. When we treated mouse dorsal skin wounds with oil body bound oleosin-rhFGF9 at 50 μg/μl and 10 μg/μl, the results were similar to the hair growth experiment. Macroscopic and histological observations indicated that the high dose of oil body bound oleosin-rhFGF9 had a notable effect on wound healing, slightly greater than that of rhFGF9 (0. 07 μg/μl).

Hence, the oil body-bound oleosin-FGF9 fusion protein appears to accelerate wound healing as well as promoting hair growth.

4. Conclusions

In this study, we constructed an optimized rhFGF9 expression vector (pOTB-oleosin-rhFGF9) and subsequently expressed oleosin-rhFGF9 in safflower oil bodies. Importantly, the oil body-bound oleosin-rhFGF9 produced from transgenic safflower seeds were found to have a significant mitogenic effect on NIH3T3 cells, and also to promote hair growth and wound healing. Furthermore, we undertook immunohistochemistry of β-catenin to investigate whether its expression was upregulated after treatment with oil body bound oleosin-rhFGF9 to regrow new hair. This is the first report regarding the expression of active, oil body-bound oleosin-rhFGF9 for topical application to promote hair growth and wound healing, providing a data basis for the development of therapeutic applications.

5. Methods

5.1 Reagents and bacterial strains

TaKaRa LA *Taq* polymerase, the restriction enzymes, NcoI and HindIII, pfu DNA polymerase, and T4 DNA ligase were all purchased from Takara (Dalian, China). A polymerase chain reaction (PCR) purification kit, gel extraction kit, plasmid miniprep kit, plant genomic DNA extraction kit and bicinchoninic acid (BCA) kit were all purchased from Bio TeKe Corporation (Beijing, China). Kanamycin and rifampicin were purchased from Sigma (Hong Kong, China). Dulbecco's modified Eagle medium (DMEM) was purchased from Hyclone (Logan, UT, USA). Methylthiazol tetrazolium (MTT) was obtained from Gentihold (Beijing, China). All primers and gene coding sequences were synthesized by Genewiz (Jiang Su, China). The expression vector, pOTBar, and the plasmids, pUC19-oleosin, *Escherichia coli* DH5α and *Agrobacterium tumefaciens* EHA105 were obtained from the Ministry of Education Engineering Research Center of Bioreactor and Pharmaceutical Development, Jilin Agricultural University.

5.2 Construction of rhFGF9 expression vector

The pOTBar plasmid was used for the construction of rhFGF9 expression vector and the same method as previous report [8]. The Oleosin and rhFGF9 primers as following: oleosin forward, 5′-CCATGGCGGATACAGC TAGAGGAACC-3′; oleosin reverse, 5′-CTCTCCCA AAGGAGCCATAGTAGTGTGCTGGC-3′; rhFGF9 forward,

5′-GCCAGCACACTACTATGGCTCCTTTGGG AGAG-3′; rhFGF9 reverse, 5′-CCCAAGCTTAAGATT GAGA-AAGGATATCCTTGT-3′.

5.3　Safflower transformation and transgenic plant regeneration via grafting

Agrobacterium tumefaciens-mediated transformation of safflower and grafting of regenerated seedlings has been reported previously [19, 36]. The safflower seeds, JI HONG YI HAO, used in this study had been certified, and were supplied by the Ministry of Education Engineering Research Center of Bioreactor and Pharmaceutical Development, Jilin Agricultural University. Prior to germination, seeds were surface sterilized by soaking in 0.1% $HgCl_2$ solution, and then handling under sterile conditions, by shaking for 10 min, and rinsing five times for 1 min each with sterile distilled water soon afterwards. The surface-sterilized seeds were germinated aseptically on seed germination medium as shown in the animation (see additional file 1, Table R1, S1) [36]and incubated at 25℃, in 24 h darkness, for 3–4 days (Fig. 1A). Wild safflower seeds to use as rootstocks were cultivated in a pot that included soil and vermiculite (three times as much soil as vermiculite by volume) for 20 days before grafting.

The day before transformation, 100 μl of *Agrobacterium* harboring the recombinant plasmid pOTBar-oleosin-rhFGF9 was taken from −80℃ storage and added directly to 100 ml liquid YEP medium containing 50 mg/ml kanamycin and 25 mg/ml rifampicin, and was then grown overnight at 28℃ with agitation at 180 rpm. The *Agrobacterium* bacterial culture for infecting safflower was adjusted to $OD_{600} = 0.6–0.8$. Next, cotyledonary explants were isolated and inoculated by exposing them for 15 min to 100 ml *Agrobacterium* culture (Fig. 1B) with gentle agitation during the infection. The bacterial fluid was then discarded, and infected explants were blotted dry on sterile filter paper and transferred to co-cultivation medium (see additional file 1, Table R1, S2; Fig. 1C) enriched with 100 μM acetosyringone. All plates were placed in a cultivation incubator at 25℃, in darkness, for 3 days.

Three days after co-cultivation, explants were transferred to bud initiation medium (see additional file 1, Table R1, S3) and grown at 25℃ under the cycle of 16 h day alternating with 8 h night. After approximately 15 days, when regeneration shoots become sufficiently strong and could touch the plate cover (Fig. 1D), excised explants of the regeneration shoots were placed on seedling elongation medium (see additional file 1, Table R1, S4) and cultured at 25℃ under a cycle of 16 h day alternating with 8 h night. Before grafting, they were screened on the same medium with 0.1% glufosinate. After several days, regenerated plantlets that emerged and were growing well were tentatively judged to be transgenic candidates, and were grafted and grown until approximately 3–4 cm long (Fig. 1E).

Prepared rootstocks were grown in pots for 14 days until they had 4–6 true leaves. To prepare scions, 3–4 cm long regenerated seedlings with a strong stem were cut with a thin knife blade on both sides of the stem, at 45° angles to form a V-shape, and were then placed in distilled water to retain moisture. Suitable rootstocks were horizontally transected above the two true leaves, and the stem was then vertically slit down the center to a depth matching the V-shaped scions. A prepared scion was inserted into the rootstock and the junction between them was wrapped using parafilm, with the necessary degree of tightness to hold them together (Fig. 1F). Grafted seedlings were grown in pots made airtight by covering with a preservative film to maintain humidity, in an environment of 21℃, 8.5 klux, 16 h day and 8 h night. After 3–4 days' growth, plantlets were hardened by making a hole in the preservative film to enable exposure to the external environment while simultaneously retaining the moisture required for survival, and were then grown for a further 7 days (Fig. 1 G). Once the scion of grafted seedlings had grown several new leaves, the preservative film covering the pots was removed. Unsuccessful grafts were discarded, and successfully grafted T_0 transgenic plants were ultimately harvested (Fig. 1 H).

5.4　PCR validation of transgenic safflowers

Transgenesis of successfully grafted safflower plants was verified by PCR amplification of the *rhFGF9* gene. Total genomic DNA that was extracted from young leaf tissue using a rapid plant genomic DNA extraction kit was used as template with the specific primers (forward: 5'-CTTTGGGAGAGGTGGGAAACTACTT-3'; reverse: 5′-CACCTGGGACTATTCCACGGACTCG-3). The positive, negative and blank controls were the pOTBar-oleosin-rhFGF9 plasmid, WT safflower leaf total DNA and double-distilled H_2O, respectively. The thermal profile of the PCR was: initial denaturation at 94℃ for 7 min; 30 cycles of amplification at 94℃ for 30 s, 55℃ for 45 s, and 72℃ for 90 s; and finally, extension at 72℃ for 7 min. After PCR amplification, the products were evaluated by electrophoresis in 1% agarose gels.

5.5 Oil body extraction, purification and protein analysis

For both WT and transgenic safflower plants, the shells were stripped from two or three seeds, and they were thoroughly ground using a pestle in a 1.5 ml centrifuge tube with 200 μl phosphate buffer saline (PBS, pH 7.5). The tubes were then centrifuged at 12 000×g for 5 min, and the supernatant and floating oil body phase were transferred to a new 1.5 ml centrifuge tube. The above procedure was repeated twice. The oil bodies were then washed three times with 200 μl PBS, centrifuging as above to finally collected the purified oil bodies. A BCA protein assay kit was used to measure oil body protein concentration, and then the oil bodies were stored at 4 ℃ for further use.

Electrophoresis loading buffer and PBS were added to the oil bodies to a protein concentration of 3.5 μg/μl, and then boiled for 10 min to denature the protein. The oil body-bound oleosin-rhFGF9 was analyzed by 12% sodium dodecyl sulfate–polyacrylamide gel electrophoresis (SDS-PAGE) using 10 μl samples per lane. Gels were visualized by Coomassie brilliant blue staining and subjected to further analysis by western blotting. Proteins were transferred to polyvinylidene fluoride membranes, blocked with blocking liquid, incubated with a rabbit anti-hFGF9 polyclonal primary antibody (1 : 500 dilution, Bioss, Beijing, China) and a horseradish peroxidase (HRP)-conjugated secondary antibody (1 : 2000, Abcam, Cambridge, MA, USA), and ultimately showed by enhanced chemiluminescence. A Human FGF9 ELISA Kit (Bioss) was used to measure oleosin-rhFGF9 concentration in the oil body protein, according to the manufacturer's protocol.

5.6 Mitogenic activity of oleosin-rhFGF9

The NIH/3 T3 cell line (American Type Culture Collection, Rockville, MD) was used to detect the mitogenic activity of oil body bound oleosin-rhFGF9. Briefly, cells were grown in a culture flask containing DMEM, 10% fetal bovine serum (FBS), and ampicillin and streptomycin (both 100 U/ml). Cells at the appropriate growth phase were seeded into a 96-well plate (5×10^3 cells per well), cultivated under normal or cell starvation conditions for 24 h, and then treated for 48 h with oil body bound oleosin-rhFGF9 or rhFGF9 (purified rhFGF9 from E. coli) at various concentrations from 0.82–212 ng/ml. The cells were then incubated with 20 μl MTT for 4 h, the culture medium was added to 100 μl dimethyl sulfoxide and mixed to homogeneity by shaking, and optical absorbance values at 570/630 nm were measured using a microplate reader.

5.7 In vivo analysis of oleosin-rhFGF9 activity

All animal experimentation investigation conforms with the Guide for the Care and Use of Laboratory Animals published by the US National Institutes of Health (NIH Publication No. 85–23, revised 1996). The experiment was authorized by Jilin Agricultural University ethical committee. Mice were purchased from Changchun Billion Biotechnology Limited Liability Company (Changchun, China) and allowed to adapt to their new environment with free access to water and food for 1 week. Healthy 6-week-old male C57BL/6 mice (18–22 g) were randomly assigned to either the hair regeneration or the wound healing experiment. For each experiment, six of heathy male C57BL/6 mice were randomly assigned to each of five treatment groups: a blank control group (treated with PBS), a negative control group (50 μg/μl WT safflower oil body protein), a positive control group (0.07 μg/μl of purified rhFGF9 from E. coli, provided by the School of Pharmaceutical Science, Key Laboratory of Biotechnology and Pharmaceutical Engineering, Wenzhou Medical College), a high-dose group (50 μg/μl of oil body bound oleosin-rhFGF9), and a low-dose group (10 μg/μl of oil body bound oleosin-rhFGF9). All mice were anesthetized, their dorsal hair was clipped with a shaver, and then residual hair was completely removed using a depilatory paste. For the wound healing experiment, surgical scissors were used to make two 1-cm-diameter full thickness wound, one on each side of the dorsal skin. Oil bodies were extracted every second day, and the protein concentration in each preparation was measured using the BCA protein assay kit, as above. Treatments were applied by every second day daubing 100 μl onto the dorsal skin, working from the centerline outwards. The dorsal skin was subsequently photographed. On day 15, mice were sacrificed by cervical dislocation, and the dorsal skin was collected for histological analysis. Skin samples were fixed in 4% paraformaldehyde, embedded in paraffin, serially sectioned, stained with hematoxylin and eosin (H & E, Solarbio, Beijing, China) or Masson's trichrome (Solarbio), and observed by microscopy.

5.8　Immunohistochemistry

Skin sections were incubated in 3% peroxidase for 10 min, rinsed twice in PBS for 3 min, heated in citrate buffer to induce epitope retrieval, blocked in bovine albumin 20 for min at room temperature, and then incubated with a rabbit anti-β-catenin antibody (1:200, Bioss) at 4℃ over night. The following day, sections were incubated with a HRP-conjugated secondary antibody (1: 1 000, Abcam, Cambridge, MA, USA) for 30 min, and then stained with a diaminobenzidine chromogen kit (Solarbio) until they showed a palpable brown color.

5.9　Statistical analysis

Results are presented as mean ± standard deviation (SD). Data were analyzed by GraphPad Prism, version 6.01 software (GraphPad Software Inc., La Jolla, CA, USA), and ImageJ software (Rawak Software, Inc., Munich Stuttgart, Germany). One-way ANOVA was used to compare multiple groups at the $P < 0.05$ level of significance.

Supplementary data

Supplementary data to this article can be found in the online version (doi:10.1186/s12896-018-0433-2).

References

[1] Naruo K, Seko C, Kuroshima K, *et al.* Novel secretory heparin-binding factors from human glioma cells (glia-activating factors) involved in glial cell growth. Purification and biological properties[J]. J Biol Chem, 1993, 268(4): 2857-2864.

[2] Miyamoto M, Naruo K, Seko C, *et al.* Molecular cloning of a novel cytokine cDNA encoding the ninth member of the fibroblast growth factor family, which has a unique secretion property[J]. Mol Cell Biol, 1993, 13(7): 4251-4259.

[3] Revest JM, DeMoerlooze L, Dickson C. Fibroblast growth factor 9 secretion is mediated by a non-cleaved amino-terminal signal sequence[J]. J Biol Chem, 2000, 275(11): 8083-8090.

[4] Mattei MG, De Moerlooze L, Lovec H, *et al.* Mouse fgf9 (fibroblast growth factor 9) is localized on chromosome 14[J]. Mamm Genome, 1997, 8(8): 617-618.

[5] Mattei MG, Penault-Llorca F, Coulier F, *et al.* The human FGF9 gene maps to chromosomal region 13q11-q12[J]. Genomics, 1995, 29(3): 811-812.

[6] Zhang X, Ibrahimi OA, Olsen SK, *et al.* Receptor specificity of the fibroblast growth factor family. The complete mammalian FGF family[J]. J Biol Chem, 2006, 281(23): 15694-15700.

[7] Yayon A. FGF9 as a specific ligand for FGFR3[J]. 1996.

[8] Yi S, Yang J, Huang J, *et al.* Expression of bioactive recombinant human fibroblast growth factor 9 in oil bodies of Arabidopsis thaliana[J]. Protein Expr Purif, 2015, 116: 127-132.

[9] Gay D, Kwon O, Zhang Z, *et al.* Fgf9 from dermal gammadelta T cells induces hair follicle neogenesis after wounding[J]. Nat Med, 2013, 19(7): 916-923.

[10] Behr B, Leucht P, Longaker MT, *et al.* Fgf-9 is required for angiogenesis and osteogenesis in long bone repair[J]. Proc Natl Acad Sci U S A, 2010, 107(26): 11853-11858.

[11] Chen XY, Xiao-Lin WU, Ming-Min GU, *et al.* Investigation on function and tissue expression profile of transgenic mice with mutated FGF9 gene[J]. Journal of Diagnostics Concepts & Practice, 2009.

[12] Aurbach EL, Inui EG, Turner CA, *et al.* Fibroblast growth factor 9 is a novel modulator of negative affect[J]. Proc Natl Acad Sci U S A, 2015, 112(38): 11953-11958.

[13] Tang L, Wu X, Zhang H, *et al.* A point mutation in Fgf9 impedes joint interzone formation leading to multiple synostoses syndrome[J]. Hum Mol Genet, 2017, 26(7): 1280-1293.

[14] Murakami H, Okawa A, Yoshida H, *et al.* Elbow knee synostosis (Eks): a new mutation on mouse Chromosome 14[J]. Mamm Genome, 2002, 13(7): 341-344.

[15] Forrester HB, Temple-Smith P, Ham S, *et al.* Genome-wide analysis using exon arrays demonstrates an important role for expression of extra-cellular matrix, fibrotic control and tissue remodelling genes in Dupuytren's disease[J]. PLoS One, 2013, 8(3): e59056.

[16] Krejci P, Prochazkova J, Bryja V, *et al.* Molecular pathology of the fibroblast growth factor family[J]. Hum Mutat, 2009, 30(9): 1245-1255.

[17] Liu WX, Liu HL, Qu le Q. Embryo-specific expression of soybean oleosin altered oil body morphogenesis and increased lipid content in transgenic rice seeds[J]. Theor Appl Genet, 2013, 126(9): 2289-2297.

[18] Markley N, Nykiforuk C, Boothe J, *et al.* Producing proteins using transgenic oilbody-oleosin technology[J]. Biopharm International, 2006, 19(6): 34-42.

[19] Belide S, Hac L, Singh SP, *et al.* Agrobacterium-mediated transformation of safflower and the efficient recovery of transgenic plants *via* grafting[J]. Plant Methods, 2011, 7: 12.

[20] Gupta SK. Brassicas[A]. In: *Technological Innovations in Major World Oil Crops, Volume 1: Breeding* (Gupta SK, ed). New York, NY: Springer New York, 2012: 53-83.

[21] Lee SY, Chun SW, Kim JB, *et al.* P085 therapeutic effects of growth factor cocktail including FGF9 scalp application in patients with androgenetic alopecia[J]. 프로그램북 (구초록집), 2016, 68(2): 377-378.

[22] Lin WH, Xiang LJ, Shi HX, *et al.* Fibroblast growth factors stimulate hair growth through beta-catenin and Shh expression in C57BL/6 mice[J]. Biomed Res Int, 2015, 2015: 730139.

[23] Martz L. FGF9 for baldness[J]. Science-Business eXchange, 2013, 6(24): 590-590.

[24] Yin Y, Wang F, Ornitz DM. Mesothelial- and epithelial-derived FGF9 have distinct functions in the regulation of lung development[J]. Development, 2011, 138(15): 3169-3177.

[25] Korf-Klingebiel M, Kempf T, Schluter KD, *et al.* Conditional trans-

genic expression of fibroblast growth factor 9 in the adult mouse heart reduces heart failure mortality after myocardial infarction[J]. Circulation, 2011, 123(5): 504-514.

[26] Komi-Kuramochi A, Kawano M, Oda Y, et al. Expression of fibroblast growth factors and their receptors during full-thickness skin wound healing in young and aged mice[J]. J Endocrinol, 2005, 186(2): 273-289.

[27] Zheng Z, Kang HY, Lee S, et al. Up-regulation of fibroblast growth factor (FGF) 9 expression and FGF-WNT/beta-catenin signaling in laser-induced wound healing[J]. Wound Repair Regen, 2014, 22(5): 660-665.

[28] Bhatla SC, Kaushik V, Yadav MK. Use of oil bodies and oleosins in recombinant protein production and other biotechnological applications[J]. Biotechnol Adv, 2010, 28(3): 293-300.

[29] Andl T, Reddy ST, Gaddapara T, et al. WNT signals are required for the initiation of hair follicle development[J]. Dev Cell, 2002, 2(5): 643-653.

[30] Tai YY, Chen RS, Lin Y, et al. FGF-9 accelerates epithelial invagination for ectodermal organogenesis in real time bioengineered organ manipulation[J]. Cell Commun Signal, 2012, 10(1): 34.

[31] Kawano M, Komi-Kuramochi A, Asada M, et al. Comprehensive analysis of FGF and FGFR expression in skin: FGF18 is highly expressed in hair follicles and capable of inducing anagen from telogen stage hair follicles[J]. J Invest Dermatol, 2005, 124(5): 877-885.

[32] Liu M, Chu S, Ai J, et al. Application of oleosin-flanked keratinocyte growth factor-2 expressed from Arabidopsis thaliana promotes hair follicle growth in mice[J]. Biotechnol Lett, 2016, 38(9): 1611-1619.

[33] Lin WH, Xiang LJ, Shi HX, et al. Fibroblast growth factors stimulate hair growth through beta-catenin and Shh expression in C57BL/6 mice[J]. Biomed Res Int, 2015, 2015: 730139.

[34] D'Andrea S, Jolivet P, Boulard C, et al. Selective one-step extraction of Arabidopsis thaliana seed oleosins using organic solvents[J]. J Agric Food Chem, 2007, 55(24): 10008-10015.

[35] Kishimoto J, Burgeson RE, Morgan BA. Wnt signaling maintains the hair-inducing activity of the dermal papilla[J]. Genes Dev, 2000, 14(10): 1181-1185.

[36] Huang J, Yang J, Guan L, et al. Expression of bioactive recombinant human fibroblast growth factor 10 in Carthamus tinctorius L. seeds[J]. Protein Expr Purif, 2017, 138: 7-12.

Two-hundred-liter scale fermentation, purification of recombinant human fibroblast growth factor-21, and its anti-diabetic effects on ob/ob mice

Qi Hui, Xiaokun Li, Xiaojie Wang

1. Introduction

Fibroblast growth factor-21 (FGF-21) is a cytokine that is a member of the FGF-19 subfamily. It regulates lipid and glucose metabolism (Fukumoto, 2008; Kharitonenkov *et al.*, 2005). FGF-21 is produced primarily in liver (Nishimura *et al.*, 2000), and is also found in adipocytes (Hondares *et al.*, 2011), skeletal muscle (Hojman *et al.*, 2009; Ribas *et al.*, 2014), pancreas (Wente *et al.*, 2006) and hypothalamus (Bookout *et al.*, 2013). FGF-21 has shown its effects in decreasing plasma glucose and triglyceride levels, improving insulin sensitivity (Kim *et al.*, 2013), lowering low-density lipoprotein cholesterol, increasing high-density lipoprotein cholesterol (Kharitonenkov *et al.*, 2005) and ameliorating hepatic steatosis (Coskun *et al.*, 2008). The human FGF-21 protein comprises 209 amino acids with a high structure similarity to the mouse FGF-21 protein (75% amino acid identity) (Nishimura *et al.*, 2000). The C and N termini of FGF-21 interact with FGF receptors and β-klotho, respectively, both of which are critical for complete FGF-21 functionality (Yie *et al.*, 2009).

Escherichia coli (*E. coli*) expression system saves time and cost in producing exogenous proteins including interferons (Vu *et al.*, 2016), interleukins (Dagar *et al.*, 2017), granulocyte colony-stimulating factor (Vemula *et al.*, 2015), and fibroblast growth factors (Lee *et al.*, 2017; Wang *et al.*, 2017; Ye *et al.*, 2016). Thus, *E. coli* has been widely used for therapeutic protein production on laboratory and industrial scales.

Recently, several studies have demonstrated that FGF-21 is a safe and effective agent to treat obesity and type II diabetes mellitus with its complications (Huang *et al.*, 2017; Wente *et al.*, 2006; Xu *et al.*, 2009), such as fast blood absorption and lentemente elimination in systematic circulation (He *et al.*, 2018). However, studies regarding large-scale expression of bioactive recombinant human FGF-21 (rhFGF-21) are scarce. Wang *et al.* and Zhang *et al.* expressed hFGF-21 in *E. coli* in a soluble form using the molecular chaperone small ubiquitin-related modifier (SUMO) (Wang *et al.*, 2010) and pET3c (Zhang *et al.*, 2012) vectors, respectively. Nevertheless, the high expense of SUMO protease, target protein degradation as well as high time consumption limited both strategies in terms of large-scale production. It is necessary to establish pilot-scale production of FGF-21 because of the need for long-term administration and the wide use of FGF-21 (Cao *et al.*, 2017; Chiavaroli *et al.*, 2017; Pan *et al.*, 2017). Therefore, in this study, to meet the increasing requirements of experimental research as well as clinical applications, high cell density fermentation, expression, renaturation, and purification of rhFGF-21 were conducted on the 30-L and 200-L scale. Subsequently, we determined the characteristics and biological activity of purified rhFGF-21 expressed in 200-L scale fermentation *in vitro* as well as its anti-diabetic effects on ob/ob mice *in vivo*.

2. Materials and methods

2.1 Materials

Tryptone and yeast extract were purchased from Oxoid Co., Ltd. (Hampshire, England). Restriction enzymes, Pyrobest DNA polymerase, gel extraction kit, PCR purification kit, and plasmid mini-prep kit were purchased from Dalian Takara Company (Dalian, China). DEAE sepharose, phenyl sepharose-6, and the Sephadex G-25 column were purchased from GE Company (USA). Isopropyl-1-thio-β-galactopyranoside (IPTG) was purchased from Beijing D ingguo Changsheng Biotechnology Co., Ltd. (Beijing, China). Quick Start™ Bradford 1x Dye Reagent was purchased from Bio-Rad (USA). Monoclonal mouse anti-human FGF-21 antibody was purchased from R&D systems (Minneapolis, MN, USA). Polyclonal monkey anti-human FGF-21 antibody was purchased from Santa Cruz Biotechnology (USA). The human hepatic cells HL-7702 were obtained from the Cell Bank of the Chinese Academy of Sciences (Shanghai, China). Additionally, human FGF-21 standard was identified by Shanghai Institutes for Biological Sciences, Chinese Academy of Sciences.

2.2 Construction of pET3c-rhFGF-21 expression vector

According to the natural gene sequence of *human FGF-21* (GenBank accession number AB021975.1) and the codon preference of *E. coli*, we designed an optimized gene sequence of *FGF-21* (GenBank accession number MH628650) whose mRNA accession number was BAA99415.1. The optimized gene sequence of *FGF-21 was* synthesized by Tsingke Biological Technology Co., Ltd. (Hangzhou, China). The forward and reverse primers for human FGF-21 (forward, 5′-CGC CAT ATG CAC CCC ATC CCT GAC-3′; reverse, 5′-GAG GAT CCT CAG GAA GCG TAG-3′) contained *Nde* I and *Bam*H I sites, respectively. PCR experiment was performed following the protocol: (1) 1 cycle at 94℃ for 3 min; (2) 30 cycles at 94℃ for 30 s, 59℃ for 30 s, 72℃ for 42 s; and (3) 1 cycle at 72℃ for 5 min. Eventually, the amplified fragments that were cut with restriction enzymes *Nde* I and *Bam*H I were purified with a gel extraction kit followed by ligation into pre-digested pET3c vectors.

The accuracy of integrated genes was validated by Tsingke Biological Technology Co., Ltd. (Hangzhou, China) using automated DNA sequencing. The expression vector pET3c-rhFGF-21 was transformed into *E. coli* strain BL21 (DE3, Catalog No. CD601, Transgen Biotechnology Co., Ltd., Beijing, China).

2.3 Induction and expression of rhFGF-21

Based on the culturing conditions including temperature, pH, dissolved oxygen, induced concentration, and induction times of IPTG in the shake flask, we found that the average expression level of rhFGF-21 was maximum after 4 h of induction. The transformed *E. coli* cells were grown by inoculating 0.3 ml culture in 30-ml sterile LB Petri dish containing 100 µg/ml ampicillin, at 37℃ and 150 rpm. Subsequently, the culture (0.3 ml) was transferred into another sterile LB medium (30 ml) containing 100 µg/ml ampicillin, at 37℃ and 200 rpm. The 30 ml culture (pH 7.2) was then dispensed into a 250-ml flask when A_{600} was at 0.8 to 1.2; then, IPTG was added to reach the concentration of 0.5 mM. Lastly, the culture was incubated in a shaker at 37℃ for 4 h at 200 rpm.

2.4 Fermentation of rhFGF-21

The seed strain of rhFGF-21 was transferred into a 250-ml flask containing 100 ml sterile LB medium (1:100, v/v) consisting of 10.0 g/L tryptone, 100 µg/ml ampicillin, 10.0 g/L NaCl, and 5.0 g/L yeast extract at pH 6.8 to 7.0 and rotated at 200 rpm, 37℃. The culture was then transferred into 1000 ml of a modified sterile medium containing 10 g/L yeast extract, 10 g/L tryptone, 4.0 g/L NaCl, 3.0 g/L K_2HPO_4, and 1.0 g/L KH_2PO_4 (pH 6.8 to 7.0 and at A_{600} = 0.8 to 1.2), and the culture was incubated at 37℃ and shaken at 150 rpm. At A_{600} range between 3.0 to 5.0, the culture was transferred to fermentation medium (1:10, v/v; containing 17.0 g/L tryptone, 23.0 g/L yeast extract, 4.0 g/L NaCl, 3.0 g/L K_2HPO_4, 1.0 g/L KH_2PO_4, 4.0 g/L NH_4Cl, 5.0 g/L glucose and pH 6.8 to 7.0) in a 30-L fermenter (BIOTECH-30JS, Shanghai Baoxing Bio-Engineering Equipment Co., Ltd). $MgSO_4$ (0.6 g/L), $CaCl_2$ (1.3×10^{-2} g/L), and vitamin B1 (5×10^{-3} g/L) were also added into the fermentation medium after sterilization. The agitation speed and fermentation tank ventilation were set at 200 rpm and 1.0 (air volume/culture volume/min, v/v/m), respectively. During cultivation, it was essential to keep the dissolved oxygen level above 20% of air while the pH level was stabilized between 6.8 to 7.0 by adding 25% (v/v) ammonia solution. When A_{600} was between 15 and 17, IPTG was added to a final concentration of 0.5 mM/L. The agitation speed and fermentation tank ventilation were to 300 rpm and 2.0 (v/v/m), respectively. Protein expression level and the cell density in the culture were measured at regular intervals. During induction process, the pH was stabilized at 7.0 to 7.2 by adding 5 g/L glucose solution using a glucose-pH-stat strategy. After induction for 1 h, 1 L nitrogen source (containing 17.0 g/L tryptone, 4.0 g/L NaCl, 23.0 g/L yeast extract, 3.0 g/L K_2HPO_4, 4.0 g/L $MgSO_4$ and 1.0 g/L KH_2PO_4) was added. After 3 h, the cells were collected by centrifuging at 16 000 rpm for 30 min at 4℃, and the pellets were stored in the freezer at −80℃. Scale-up of 200-L scale fermentation (BIOTECH-200JS, Shanghai BaoXing

Bio-Engineering Equipment Co., Ltd) was performed using 84 L fermentation medium with the same formula as the 30-L scale fermentation. The addition volume of nitrogen source was adjusted to 7 L. The formula of fermentation medium and nitrogen source in 200-L scale fermentation were consistent with the formula of the 30-L scale fermentation.

2.5 Preparation, denaturation, and renaturation of inclusion bodies of rhFGF-21

We retrieved the stored pellets, thawed at room temperature, and resuspended in ice-cold 25 mM Tris-HCl buffer (pH 8.0). The buffer contained NaCl and EDTA-2Na with concentrations of 150 mM and 10 mM, respectively. The pellet was mixed with Tris-HCl buffer in a ratio of 1 g to 10 ml. Lysozyme and DNase were then added to the cell suspensions at a scale of 100 g pellet to 0.1 g lysozyme and 1×10^{-3} g DNase. The cell suspensions were stirred and stored at room temperature overnight. After centrifugation at a setting of 9 000 rpm for 30 min at 4℃, the insoluble pellet was collected. The pellet was washed at a ratio of 1 g to 15 ml buffer I (25 mM Tris-HCl, 150 mM NaCl, 10 mM EDTA-2Na, 0.2% (w/v) sodium deoxycholate and pH 8.0). After washing, the pellet was centrifuged at 9 000 rpm for 15 min at 4℃ and recollected at the bottom of the tube. Then, the pellet was washed at a ratio of 1 g cell pellet to 20 ml buffer II (25 mM Tris-HCl, 150 mM NaCl, 10 mM EDTA-2Na, 0.2% (w/v) Triton X-100 and pH 8.0). The sample was centrifuged at a speed of 9 000 rpm for 10 min at 4℃, and the inclusion bodies were collected at the bottom of the tube.

The inclusion bodies were dissolved in denaturation buffer containing 25 mM Tris-HCl, 2.0 mM EDTA-2Na and 8.0 M urea (pH 8.9). The inclusion bodies were mixed with the denaturation buffer in a ratio of 1 g to 15 ml and agitated at 4℃ until dissolved completely. The sample was centrifuged at 9 000 rpm for 30 min at 4℃, the supernatant was dialyzed in renaturation buffer (2 mM EDTA-2Na, 25 mM Tris-HCl, pH 8.9) at a ratio of 1 g inclusion bodies to 200-ml renaturation buffer and stirred at 4℃ over night. After a dialysis bag (molecular weight cutoff 7 000 D, Solarbio Co., Ltd., China) floated in the renaturation buffer, the renatured protein supernatants were collected after centrifugation at a speed of 9 000 rpm for 30 min at 4℃.

2.6 Purification of rhFGF-21

All purification procedures were performed at 4℃. To separate the renatured proteins, the researchers applied supernatant to a DEAE sepharose column (20×50 cm, 6 300 ml of bed volume, flow rate 120 ml/min) after the column was pre-balanced with three bed volumes of buffer (containing 25 mM Tris-HCl, 2.0 mM EDTA-2Na and 30 mM NaCl, pH 8.9). Then, proteins were eluted with the elution buffer I (containing 25 mM Tris-HCl, 2.0 mM EDTA-2Na and 0.1 mM NaCl, pH 8.9) at 150 ml/min flow rate. Pooled protein solution was diluted with buffer (containing 25 mM Tris-HCl, 2.0 mM EDTA-2Na and 4.0 M NaCl, pH 8.9) in the ratio of 1:1 (v/v). We applied diluted solution to a phenyl sepharose-6 column (7.5×60 cm, 1 800 ml of bed volume, flow rate 45 ml/min) after the phenyl sepharose-6 column was pre-balanced with three bed volumes of buffer (25 mM Tris-HCl, 2.0 M NaCl, pH 8.9). Subsequently, the column was washed with three bed volumes of buffer (25 mM Tris-HCl, 2.0 mM EDTA-2Na and 0.1 M NaCl, pH 8.9) at 45 ml/min flow rate until the baseline was stable. The bound proteins were eluted with buffer II (containing 25 mM Tris-HCl, 2.0 mM EDTA-2Na and 0.1 M NaCl, pH 8.9) at 45 ml/min flow rate. Eventually, the purified proteins were desalinated on a Sephadex G-25 column (8.0×100 cm, 4300 ml bed volume), and then were washed with 20 mM PBS (pH 7.0) that contained 50 mM NaCl. The concentration of rhFGF-21 was measured using the Bradford protein assay method (Coomassie blue R-250 staining). The authenticity of rhFGF-21 was confirmed by Western blotting (polyclonal monkey anti-human FGF-21 antibody, Santa Cruz Biotechnology, USA) and MALDI-TOF/MS. Further examination of the purified rhFGF-21 from 200-L scale fermentation was done by SDS-PAGE and RPC-HPLC (4.5×150 mm, 5 μm and Agilent C18) analyses. The isoelectric point of rhFGF-21 was analyzed by an iso-electric focusing electrophoresis apparatus that was purchased from Beijing Liuyi Biological Technology Co., Ltd. (Beijing, China). The purified rhFGF-21 was lyophilized and stored at −20℃. The N-terminal sequencing and molecular peptide mapping of rhFGF-21 stock solution (batch number C20161101) were tested by Shanghai Zhongke New Life Biotechnology Co., Ltd.

2.7 CD spectroscopy

To determine the secondary protein structure of rhFGF-21, circular dichroism (CD) spectroscopy (JASCO 715, JASCO) was used with spectral parameters: room temperature, 0.1 cm cell length, 1 nm bandwidth, scanning rate of 50 nm/min, 4 s response time, and a measurement range of 190–250 nm. For the CD measurement, the purified protein concentration was chosen to be 0.2 mg/ml. Additionally, software Jwstda32 was used for noise reduction.

2.8 Bioactivity assay of purified rhFGF-21 activity

HL-7702 cells were seeded at $1.5–1.8×10^5$ cells/well density on 96-well plates in RPMI-1640 medium consisting of 1% (v/v) penicillin/streptomycin and 10% (v/v) fetal bovine serum (Gibco) and incubated at 37℃ with 5% CO_2. After incubating for 24 h, we replaced the medium with RPMI-1640 medium of 100 μl that contained 0.5% (v/v) FBS, 100 μg/ml streptomycin and 100 U/ml penicillin (maintaining medium) and re-incubated for 24 h. The maintaining medium was refreshed by adding 90 μl per well. Subsequently, 30 μl standard solution (80 IU/ml) and rhFGF-21 stock solution from 200-L scale fermentation were added, followed by four-fold gradient dilution. Each well was made in triplicate. After incubating for 2 days, biological activity of rhFGF-21 was determined *via* glucose oxidase activity assay kit (Changchun Huili Biotech Co., Ltd., China). The concentration of rhFGF-21 stock solution was measured by BCA protein assay kit (Beyotime, China). The activity of rhFGF-21 stock solution was calculated according to the following formula: activity (IU/mg) = biological activity (IU/ml)/concentration of rhFGF-21 (mg/ml).

2.9 Animals and treatment

Male mice weighing 32.0 to 42.3 g, ob/ob, and 19.1 to 25.4 g, C57BL/6J, were obtained from the National Resource Center of Model Mice (NRCMM) of Nanjing University, China. All animals were kept at 20–26℃ and 40–70% humidity with a reverse phase 12-h light/12-h dark cycle and were handled in accordance with Institutional Animal Care and Use Committee (IACUC) guidelines of Wenzhou Medical University (Zhejiang, China), complying with National Institutes of Health (NIH) guidelines for the care and use of laboratory animals. Mice were provided with either standard laboratory chow or 10% high-fat diet and water ad libitum (ad-lib). Ob/ob mice received once-daily s.c. injections of 0.9% (w/v) normal saline (NS, model group), rhFGF-21 (12.5, 37.5, and 112.5 μg/ml) or insulin R (1 IU/ml; Eli Lilly and Company, USA) to achieve a dose of 10 ml/kg body weight. C57BL/6J mice also received once-daily s.c. injections of NS (control group).

2.10 Random blood glucose and fasting blood glucose determinations

At the beginning of the experiment, random blood glucose and fasting blood glucose were measured without any administration of drug. Random blood glucose was measured after 1 h of NS, rhFGF-21 or insulin R treatment at days 3, 7, and 12 of experiment using a blood glucose monitoring system (Accu-Chek; Roche Diagnostics). Administration of NS, rhFGF-21 or insulin R was performed after 4-h fasting on days 4, 7, and 12. An hour later, fasting blood glucose was determined as described above. In addition, random blood glucose was measured the next day after the last administration during the 14-day treatment period.

2.11 OGTT

Ob/ob and C57BL/6J mice were fasted for 3.5 h before the oral glucose tolerance test (OGTT) at 9 d. After 0.5 h of subcutaneous administration of vehicle control (NS), rhFGF-21 or insulin R, oral administration of glucose solution (1.5 g of glucose per kilogram of body weight) *via* gavage was performed. Tail vein plasma was collected at various time points, 0, 30, 60, and 120 min, by measuring blood glucose. Blood glucose concentration was calculated based on the trapezoidal rule of the area under the blood glucose concentration-time curve (AUC).

2.12 i.p. ITT

At 9 days, after 3.5 h of fasting and 30 min of subcutaneous injections of NS, rhFGF-21, or insulin R, we injected the ob/ob intraperitoneally with insulin R (0.5 IU per kilogram of body weight) at time 0. The blood glucose was measured at various time points: 0, 30, 60, and 120 min, and blood glucose concentration was expressed as the area under the blood glucose concentration-time curve (AUC) with the trapezoidal rule.

2.13 Statistical method and analysis

The experiment results were expressed in the form of mean ± standard deviation. The statistical methods including Student t test and one-way and two-way ANOVA were conducted using GraphPad Prism 5.0. The P value < 0.05 was considered as a significant difference.

3. Results

3.1 Plasmid construction and expression of rhFGF-21

Human FGF-21 gene was cloned in pET3c vector with the digestion of restriction enzymes *Nde* I and *Bam*H I and automated DNA sequencing was conducted to confirm the accuracy of the *rhFGF-21* sequence. Subsequently, the pET3C-rhFGF-21 plasmid was transformed into *E. coli* BL21 (DE3) cells. SDS-PAGE analysis was performed on pET3c-rhFGF-21 expression levels, which showed that the recombinant human FGF-21 was induced by 0.5 mM IPTG at 37℃. The molecular weight of the protein was roughly 23 kDa, which is consistent with the expected molecular weight. Additionally, western blotting demonstrated that the target rhFGF-21 protein reacted with anti-human FGF-21 monoclonal antibody (Fig. 1A).

3.2 Pilot-scale fermentation of rhFGF-21

To establish the optimal conditions for improved production of rhFGF-21, a 200-L fermenter was used, based on the abovementioned fermentation parameters with modest modifications. Three fermentation batches were prepared. For pilot-scale fermentation, the conditions were determined to achieve optimal production, which are; during the cultivation process, the pH was stabilized at 6.8 to 7.0 by adding 25% (*v/v*) ammonia solution, and cell growth temperature was 37℃; fermentation tank ventilation was set at 4.0 (*v/v/m*), and the dissolved oxygen level was kept above 20% of air. After growing cells for 4 h, IPTG was added to the fermentation medium at a concentration of 0.5 mM when the A_{600} was between 15 and 17. When the induction period began, fermentation tank ventilation was adjusted to 6.0 (*v/v/m*). During the period of induction, the pH was stabilized at 7.0 to 7.2 by adding glucose solution. One hour after the induction, the nitrogen source was added. By maintaining optimal fermentation conditions, 4 h after the induction, the wet cell weight reached 42.1 ± 0.9 g/L and 38.9 ± 0.6 g/L at the 30-L and 200-L scales, respectively (Tables S1 and S2). Meanwhile, most of the target protein was expressed in inclusion body form and the average expression level of rhFGF-21 was up to 27.6 ± 0.9% (Fig. 1B, D) and 30.9 ± 0.7% (Fig. 1C, D), respectively. Various parameters in pilot-scale production of rhFGF-21 are shown in Fig. 1E, F.

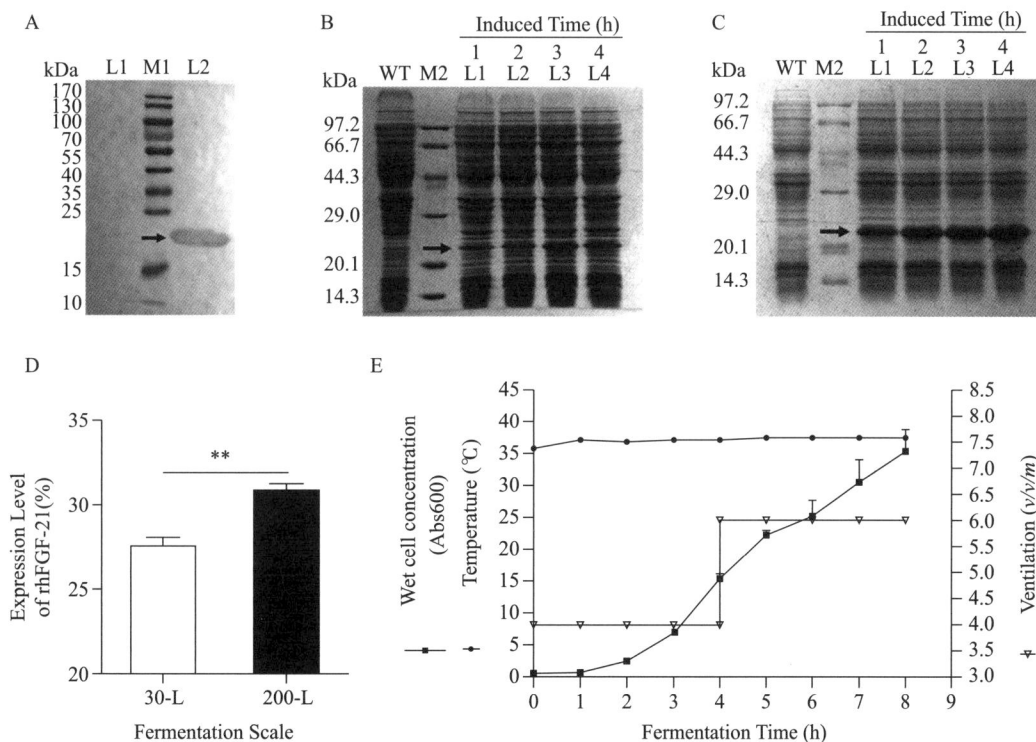

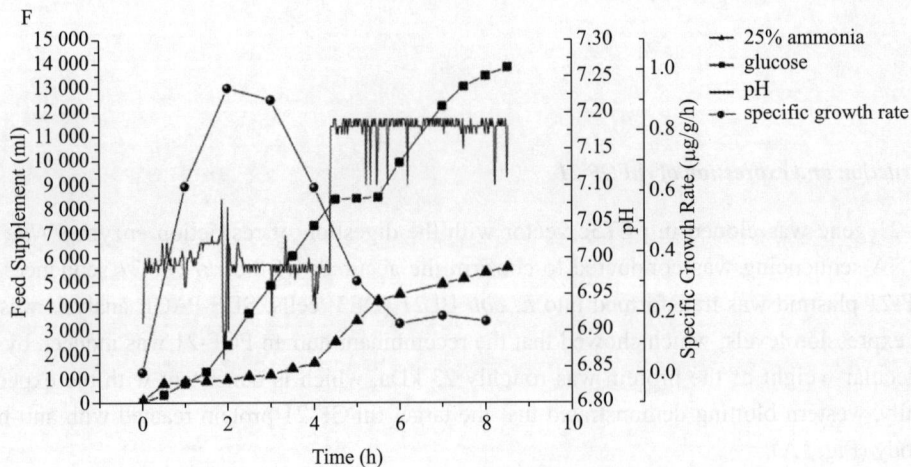

Fig. 1. Expression of recombinant human FGF-21. (A) Western blot analysis rhFGF-21 in shake-flask process. Lane 1, uninduced; lane M1: molecular weight markers 1; lane 3, induced for 4 h. (B), (C) rhFGF-21 expression SDS-PAGE analysis in the 30-L and 200-L fermentor, respectively. WT, uninduced; M2, molecular weight marker 2; lane 1–4, induced for 1 h, 2 h, 3 h, and 4 h, respectively. The above arrow indicates the rhFGF-21. (D) The expression levels of rhFGF-21 at 30-L and 200-L scale fermentor. $^{**}P < 0.01$ for 30-L $vs.$ 200-L ($n = 3$). (E) Variation of parameters in the rhFGF-21 pilot-scale production, which includes wet cell concentration (A_{600}), temperature, fermentor ventilation in 200-L fermentation process. (F) The relation curve of specific growth rate, glucose addition, pH, and ammonia consumption with time, in 200-L fermentation process.

3.3 rhFGF-21 recovery from inclusion bodies

Inclusion bodies were obtained from cell pellets using lysozyme and DNase. The insoluble pellet of centrifuged crude lysates, washed cell suspensions and washed inclusion bodies were evaluated by SDS-PAGE (Fig. 2A). Many other proteins were effectively eliminated after applying 0.2% (w/v) sodium deoxycholate and 0.2% (w/v) Triton X-100 for washing the insoluble pellet (Table S3). Denaturation and renaturation operations were essential steps for converting aggregated target protein to bioactive form. Thus, the inclusion bodies were denatured employing a high concentration of urea (8 M). Thereafter, dialysis was conducted for renaturation of the recombinant human FGF-21.

3.4 Pilot-scale purification and identification of recombinant human FGF-21

To purify the soluble portion of rhFGF-21 (Fig. 2B and Online Resource: Table S3), DEAE sepharose column chromatography was used. The pooled fractions were then purified using phenyl sepharose-6 column chromatography (Fig. 2C). Eventually to desalinate the purified proteins, SDS-PAGE and sephadex G-25 column chromatography was ap-

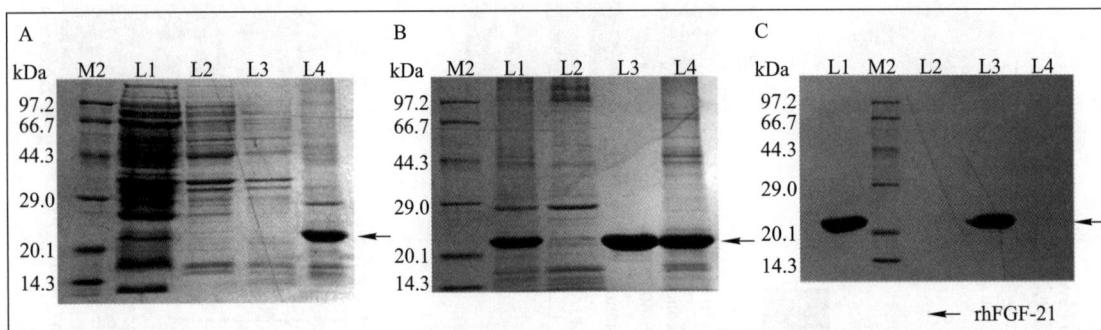

Fig. 2. SDS-PAGE analysis of the inclusion body and purification process of rhFGF-21. (A) The inclusion body washing process was analyzed by SDS-PAGE. Lane M2, molecular weight marker 2; lane 1, the pellet of centrifuged crude lysates; lane 2, washed by washing buffer I; lane 3, washed by washing buffer II; lane 4, eluted inclusion bodies. The arrow indicates the inclusion bodies of rhFGF-21. (B), (C) Proteins purified through DEAE sepharose column chromatography (B) and phenyl sepharose-6 column chromatography (C), respectively. (B) Lane M2, molecular weight marker 2; lane 1, loading samples; lane 2, flow through fraction; lane 3–4, eluted with 0.1 and 2 mol/L NaCl in elution buffer; lane 5: fractions eluted with 2 M NaCl in elution buffer. c Lane M2, molecular weight marker 2; lane 1, loading samples; lane 2: flow through fraction; lane 3, eluted with 0.1 M NaCl in elution buffer; lane 4, washed by distilled water. The arrow indicates the rhFGF-21.

plied (Fig. 3A, B). The purity of rhFGF-21 was higher than 98%, and its retention time was about 20.354 min (Fig. 3B). The arrow indicates the peak of rhFGF-21. The final production of purified rhFGF-21 was 71.1 ± 13.9 mg/L. In addition, the authenticity of rhFGF-21 was confirmed by Western blotting (Fig. 3C) and MALDI-TOF/MS (Fig. 3D). As shown in Fig. 3D, the molecular weight of the rhFGF-21 protein was 19,517.6230 Da, which was consistent with the expected molecular weight. The main isoelectric band of rhFGF-21 was 5.2 to 5.5 (Fig. 3E). CD spectroscopy analysis of purified rhFGF-21 showed that there were 0.0% alpha helix, 10.6% turn, 34.5% beta sheet, and 54.9% random (Fig. 3F).

We performed the N-terminal sequencing and molecular peptide mapping, and the final 15 amino acid sequence of N-terminal was MHPIPDSSPLLQFGG, which was matched with the 15 amino acid sequence of the rhFGF-21 N terminus in the NCBI database. After ultra-performance liquid chroma-tography (UPLC) desalting and separation, the mass spectrometric analysis was performed using a XevoG2-XS QT of mass spectrometer (Waters Co., Ltd., USA). The trypsin and chymotrypsin cleavage coverage of the test samples were 94% and 98%, respectively (Fig. 3G). Considered together the above results, molecular peptide mapping coverage of rhFGF-21 were 100%.

Target protein content, biological activity, and activity of rhFGF-21 stock solution were reached to 10.27 ± 1.46 mg/ml, 702.0 ± 120.13 IU/ml, and 68.67 ± 8.74 IU/mg, respectively.

3.5 Chronic administration of rhFGF-21 lowered blood glucose in ob/ob mice

To assess the effect of rhFGF-21 on glucose level, the researchers recorded random and fasting blood glucose levels in ob/ob and C57BL/6J mice. The results showed that in male ob/ob mice, the blood glucose levels of random group that was treated with rhFGF-21 was much lower than those of the control group (Fig. 4A, $^*P < 0.05$ or $^{**}P < 0.01$). Moreover, we observed that rhFGF-21 had the potential to reduce the fasting blood glucose levels compared to those of the model group (Fig. 4B, $^*P < 0.05$).

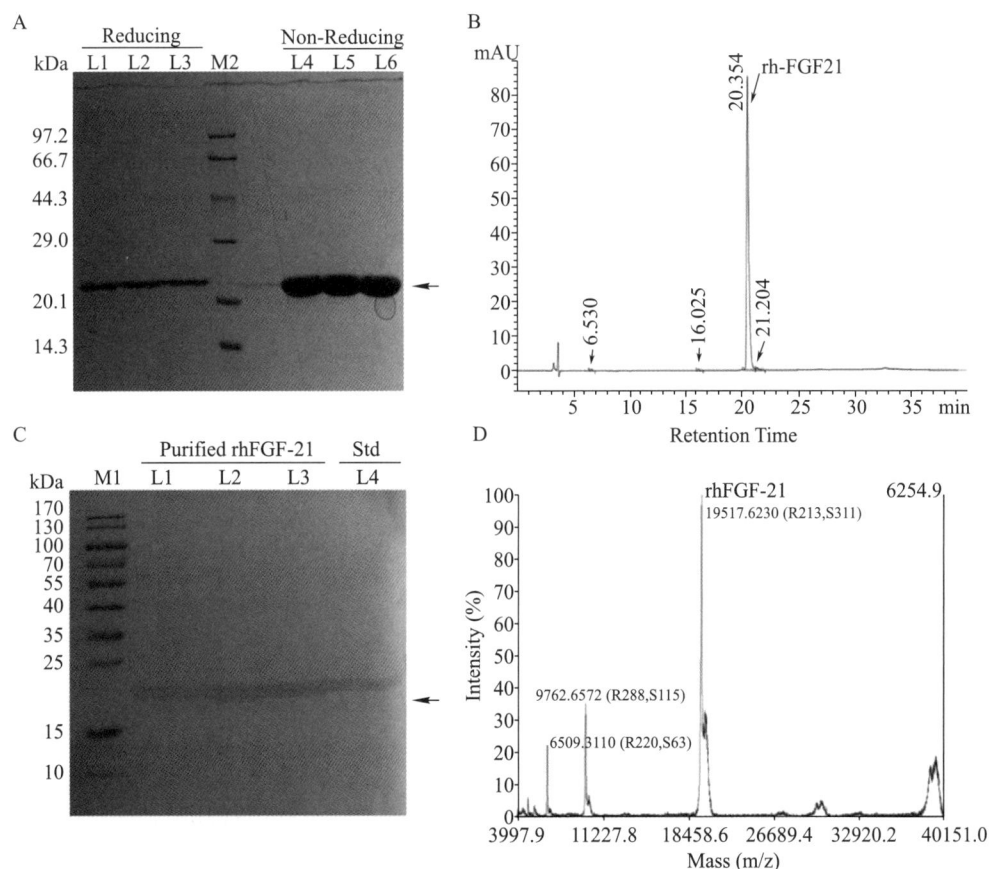

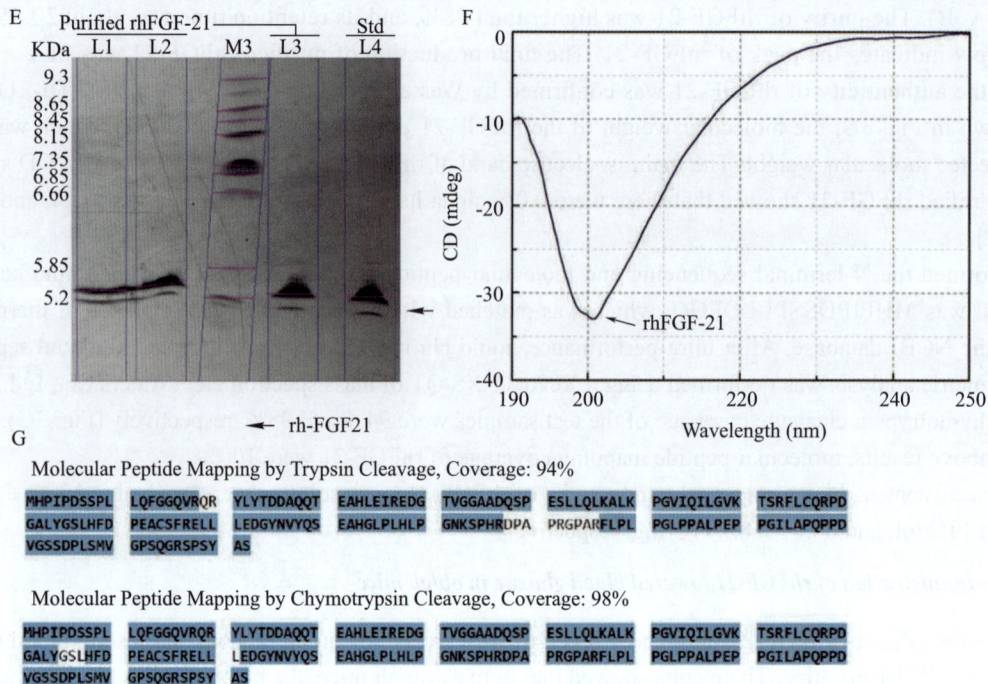

Fig. 3. Identification of purified rhFGF-21. (A) Reducing and non-reducing SDS-PAGE analysis of purified rhFGF-21. Lane 1–3, reduced purified rhFGF-21 from three batches; lane M2, molecular weight marker 2. Lane 4–6, non-reduced purified rhFGF-21 from three batches. (B) HPLC analy- sis of purified rhFGF-21. (C) Western blotting analysis of purified rhFGF-21. Lane M1, molecular weight marker 1; lane 1–3, purified samples from three batches; lane 4: identified human FGF-21 standard. (D) Results of MALDI-TOF/MS. (E) Isoelectric points of purified rh-FGF-21. Lane 1–3, purified rhFGF-21 from three batches. Lane M3, broad pI calibration kit. Lane 4, identified human FGF-21 standard. (F) Far-UV circular dichroism spectrum of rhFGF-21. The protein secondary structure was predicted using structural analysis software. (G) Molecular peptide mapping coverage of rhFGF-21. The matched amino acids were marked in blue background.

3.6 Prolonged subcutaneous injection of rhFGF-21 improves insulin sensitization in ob/ob mice

After 9 days of rhFGF-21 treatment, tolerance tests: OGTT and insulin tolerance test (ITT) were performed on the ob/ob mice (Fig. 4C–F). Glucose tolerance level of male ob/ob mice that were treated with rhFGF-21 increased (Fig. 4C, D, $^*P < 0.05$ or $^{**}P < 0.01$) compared to that of the control group. Furthermore, the test results showed that rh-FGF-21 treated mice were more insulin sensitive (Fig. 4E, F, $^{**}P < 0.01$). The AUCs are shown in Fig. 4D, F.

4. Discussion

Several studies demonstrated that FGF-21 had positive effects on type II diabetes mellitus, regulating lipid and glucose metabolism and increasing insulin sensitivity (Gaich et al., 2013; Goto et al., 2017; Holland et al., 2013; Kharitonenkov et al., 2005). Additionally, evidence demonstrates that FGF-21 ameliorates atherosclerosis (Jin et al., 2016; Kwok and Lam, 2017), cardiovascular diseases (Domouzoglou et al., 2015), protects cerebral ischemia (Yang et al., 2018), and may even increase life expectancy (Xie and Leung, 2017). Recently, the production of FGF-21 has transformed from laboratory-scale to pilot-scale. Thus, the development of high-efficiency and pure bioactive FGF-21 production methods to meet the increasing demands of experimental research and clinical applications have become increasingly important.

Controlling factors for microbial fermentation processes include medium concentration, temperature, pH, dissolved oxygen, etc. Optimizing these factors would create an optimum environment for the growth of rhFGF-21 engineered bacteria and the expression of the desired product so that the target product could be obtained in high amount. Glucose is cheap and easy to measure, so it is a common carbon source for high-density fermentation of recombinant E. coli.

However, high concentrations of glucose in the medium may induce the more side productions of metabolites such

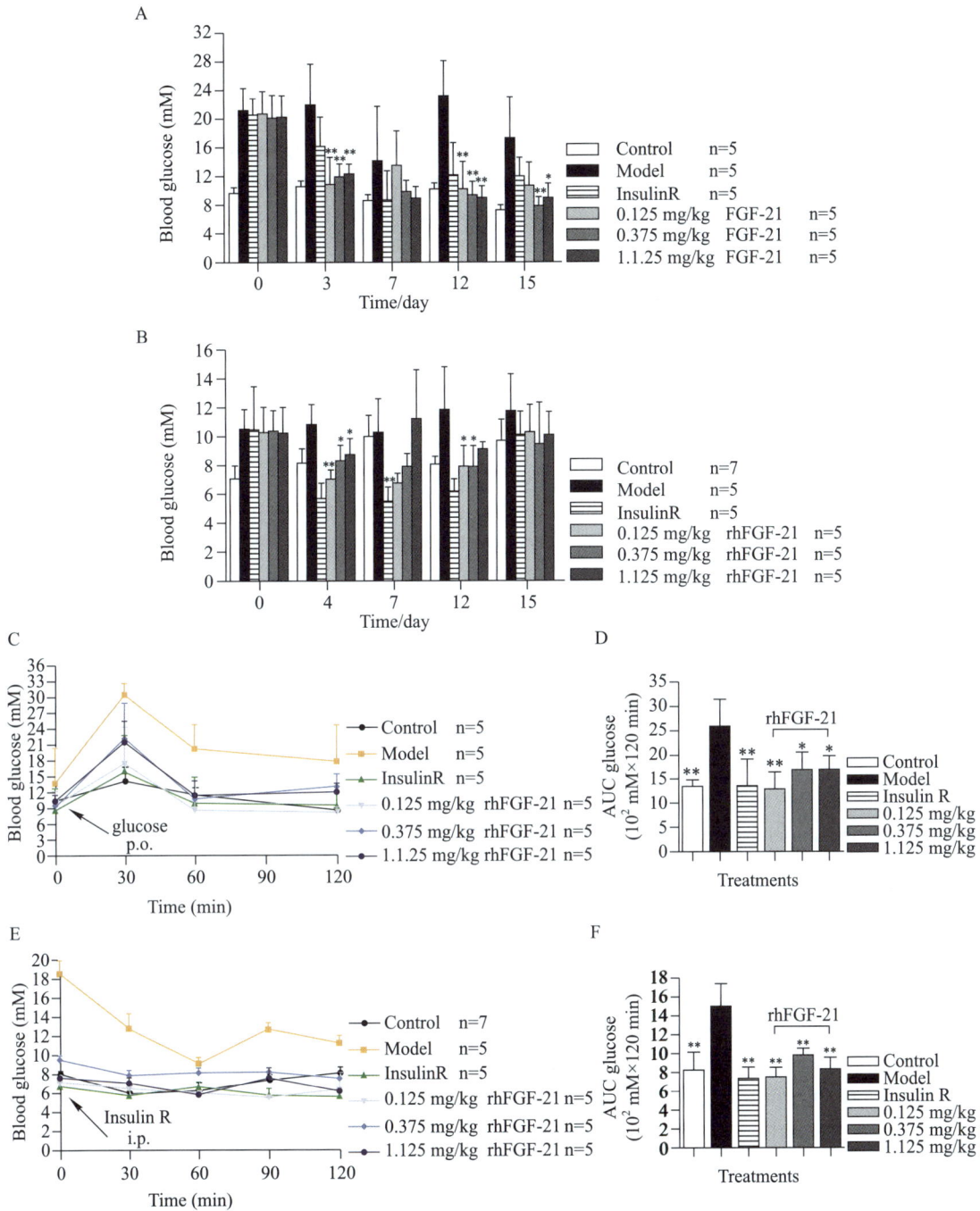

Fig. 4. *In vivo* anti-diabetic effects of purified rhFGF-21. (A) Random blood glucose levels of ob/ob mice. (B) Fasting groups whose blood glucose levels of ob/ob mice. (C) Oral glucose tolerance test (OGTT, 1.5 g glucose/kg body weight). (D) Area under the curve (AUC) in OGTT text. (E) Intraperitoneal insulin tolerance test (i.p. ITT, 0.5 IU/kg body weight). (F) Area under the curve (AUC) in ITT text. $^{*}P < 0.05$, $^{**}P < 0.01$ *vs.* model group.

as acetic acid, which is harmful for high-density fermentation of the cells. The accumulation of acetate can be reduced by controlling addition of glucose and specific growth rate of the *E. coli*. In this study, fermentation feedback parameter pH was taken as the control object, which was associated with glucose flow addition to limit the glucose concentration and specific growth rate in a low level (Fig. 1F), so as to control the production of acetate. As shown in Fig. S1, the specific growth rate and the supplemental glucose curve were divided into two parts. During the growth stage of the bacteria, the specific growth rate of bacteria increased with the increase of glucose addition before 3 h to produce enough bacteria. Thereafter, it was shown in the expression phase of rhFGF-21 (after 4 h of fermentation) that the specific growth rate of bacteria decreased with the decrease of the glucose addition rate, leading to reduction in the accumulation of acetate. In addition, we previously investigated the effects of different glucose concentrations on the culture density and expression of rhFGF-21 engineering bacteria. The results showed that the highest expression of rhFGF-21 and the best cell density were obtained when bacteria were fermented within 5 g/L glucose. During fermentation, the medium pH value is a comprehensive indicator of the metabolic activity of microorganisms under certain environmental conditions. It is an important fermentation parameter and has a great influence on the growth of bacteria and the accumulation of products. Therefore, it is very important to have a perfect control of pH during the fermentation process. In industrial production, the method of pH adjustment is not only acid-base neutralization since acid-base neutralization can neutralize the excess acid and base present in the medium, but it is not able to prevent the constant acid-base changes in the metabolic process. The pH value changes during fermentation is depends on microbial metabolites, then fundamental measure for controlling pH should consider the ratio of physiologically acidic substances to physiologically basic substances in the medium. The best way of pH control should be performed by intermediate feeding. The glucose, as well known which could produce acidic substances during the fermentation process, was added to neutralize the alkaline substances produced by the fermentation. There are actually bunch of equipment which functional like that were available in markets. During the fermentation process, the equipment we used can be automatically adjust the glucose supplement feed rate according to the pH change of the fermentation broth. Our research shows that for the rhFGF-21 engineering strain, the most suitable pH value for the cell growth is 7.0 while for the product expression, it is 7.2. We optimized pH value by combining glucose feed control and acid-base neutralization in the process of rhFGF-21 engineering strain fermentation process. As shown in the Fig. 1F, the supplemental glucose curve is divided into two parts. During the growth stage of the bacteria, there is more physiological alkaline substance produced. The glucose supplementation rate is characterized by uniform acceleration accordingly. Thereafter, at the initial stage of product expression, the bacteria growth became slow in result of physiological alkaline substances reduced. The constant-speed supplemental glucose characteristic curve is observed. In the middle and late stages of product expression, the glucose supplementation rate is characterized by a uniform rate, which is slower than the bacterial growth period. In the process of batch fermentation, nutrients are constantly consumed and a large number of intermediates are produced, which restricts the growth of *E. coli* and the synthesis of rhFGF-21 proteins. In this study, during the fed-batch culture, pH value was used as the control indicator to control the amount of glucose, effectively improving the yield of rhFGF-21. For example, in 200-L fermentation, the medium for fed-batch fermentation or batch fermentation cost about $450. In 200-L scale fed-batch fermentation, the density of bacteria was up to 38.9 ± 0.6 g/L (Table S2), while for batch fermentation, the density of bacteria was only 25.3 ± 0.8 g/L (data not shown).

In this study, the most important challenge was performing efficient renaturation of inclusion bodies *in vitro*. In the preparation of inclusion bodies, we added surfactants for preliminary purification followed by polishing purification *via* chromatography. According to our previous studies, 0.2% (*w/v*) sodium deoxycholate (an ionic surfactant mainly used to solubilize the impurities in precipitates and promote cell lysis) and 0.2% (*w/v*) Triton X-100 (a non-ionic surfactant that is mainly used to solubilize the membrane proteins in the precipitates) were added to the washing buffer I and the washing buffer II, respectively, which were applied to wash the inclusion bodies. The target protein was extracted from dissolved inclusion bodies in mild denaturing conditions (8 M urea). Dilution and dialysis are two classic renaturation methods. We chose the dilution renaturation method because the experimental operation process was simple and low cost. The cost of dialysis method is largely the cost of dialysis bag. During the pilot purification of rhFGF-21, we denatured 658.7 ± 5.4 g (Table S3) of inclusion body each time and obtained 10 L of denatured liquid of rhFGF-21. It takes $340 to purchase dialysis bag with a trapped molecular weight of 3500 Da. Tris-HCl and EDTA-2Na were used as the buffer of renaturation and cost about $40. It could be seen that renaturation of rhFGF-21 inclusion bodies is relatively cost-effective. DEAE is a commonly used weak anion exchange filler whose adsorption affinity is affected by pH. DEAE column chromatography results showed that target protein bound to the anionic filler and most rhFGF-21 was eluted by 0.1 M NaCl (Fig. 2B). The target protein in the regenerating solution was removed because of its low purity, volume and protein content, which was about 10% of the loading sample. Combined with hydrophobic chromatography, endotoxin was efficiently removed, meeting the injection demand (Table S4). The expression of rhFGF-21 in form of inclusion body effectively avoided degradation effects, which occur during expression in soluble form (Wang *et al.*, 2010). In addition, the inclusion body expression strategy required less fermentation time than did soluble form expression (Zhang *et al.*, 2012).

To test the anti-diabetic effect of rhFGF-21 that was purified from the pilot-scale production, rhFGF-21 was administrated to mice subcutaneously for 2 weeks. The blood glucose levels of random and fasting groups that treated with rhFGF-21 were much lower than the control group, avoiding the risk of hypoglycemia. In addition, in ob/ob mice, the prolonged administration of rhFGF-21 increased glucose tolerance level as well as the insulin sensitivity, which suggested that the biological activity of rhFGF-21 was ensured by the expression process of inclusion bodies.

In conclusion, we have established a fermentation process for large-scale production of rhFGF-21. The expression of rhFGF-21 accounts for $30.8 \pm 0.6\%$ of the total bacterial protein, and the bacterial density is up to 38.9 ± 0.6 g/L. About 17.95 ± 0.69 mg purified rhFGF-21 can be obtained for each gram of inclusion body, and about 11.82 ± 0.46 g purified rhFGF-21 can be obtained for a pilot-scale purification. This production process laid the foundation for the clinical application of rhFGF-21 in type 2 diabetes.

Supplementary material

Electronic supplementary material to this article can be found in the online version (doi:10.1007/s00253-018-9470-y).

References

Bookout AL, de Groot MHM, Owen BM, *et al.* FGF21 regulates metabolism and circadian behavior by acting on the nervous system[J]. Nature Medicine, 2013, 19(9): 1147-1152.

Cao F, Liu X, Cao X, *et al.* Fibroblast growth factor 21 plays an inhibitory role in vascular calcification *in vitro* through OPG/RANKL system[J]. Biochemical And Biophysical Research Communications, 2017, 491(3): 578-586.

Chiavaroli A, Recinella L, Ferrante C, *et al.* Effects of central fibroblast growth factor 21 and irisin in anxiety-like behavior[J]. Journal Of Biological Regulators And Homeostatic Agents, 2017, 31(3): 797-802.

Coskun T, Bina HA, Schneider MA, *et al.* Fibroblast Growth Factor 21 Corrects Obesity in Mice[J]. Endocrinology, 2008, 149(12): 6018-6027.

Dagar VK, Adivitiya, Khasa YP. High-level expression and efficient refolding of therapeutically important recombinant human Interleukin-3 (hIL-3) in E-coli[J]. Protein Expression And Purification, 2017, 131: 51-59.

Domouzoglou EM, Naka KK, Vlahos AP, *et al.* Fibroblast growth factors in cardiovascular disease: The emerging role of FGF21[J]. American Journal Of Physiology-Heart And Circulatory Physiology, 2015, 309(6): H1029-H1038.

Fukumoto S. Actions and mode of actions of FGF19 subfamily members[J]. Endocrine Journal, 2008, 55(1): 23-31.

Gaich G, Chien JY, Fu H, *et al.* The Effects of LY2405319, an FGF21 Analog, in Obese Human Subjects with Type 2 Diabetes[J]. Cell Metabolism, 2013, 18(3): 333-340.

Goto T, Hirata M, Aoki Y, *et al.* The hepatokine FGF21 is crucial for peroxisome proliferator-activated receptor-alpha agonist-induced amelioration of metabolic disorders in obese mice[J]. Journal Of Biological Chemistry, 2017, 292(22): 9175-9190.

He Y, Li Y, Wei Z, *et al.* Pharmacokinetics, tissue distribution, and excretion of FGF-21 following subcutaneous administration in rats[J]. Drug Testing And Analysis, 2018, 10(7): 1061-1069.

Hojman P, Pedersen M, Nielsen AR, *et al.* Fibroblast Growth Factor-21 Is Induced in Human Skeletal Muscles by Hyperinsulinemia[J]. Diabetes, 2009, 58(12): 2797-2801.

Holland WL, Adams AC, Brozinick JT, *et al.* An FGF21-Adiponectin-Ceramide Axis Controls Energy Expenditure and Insulin Action in Mice[J]. Cell Metabolism, 2013, 17(5): 790-797.

Hondares E, Iglesias R, Giralt A, *et al.* Thermogenic Activation Induces FGF21 Expression and Release in Brown Adipose Tissue[J]. Journal Of Biological Chemistry, 2011, 286(15): 12983-12990.

Huang Z, Xu A, Cheung BMY. The Potential Role of Fibroblast Growth Factor 21 in Lipid Metabolism and Hypertension[J]. Current Hypertension Reports, 2017, 19(4).

Jin L, Lin Z, Xu A. Fibroblast Growth Factor 21 Protects against Atherosclerosis *via* Fine-Tuning the Multiorgan Crosstalk[J]. Diabetes & Metabolism Journal, 2016, 40(1): 22-31.

Kharitonenkov A, Shiyanova TL, Koester A, *et al.* FGF-21 as a novel metabolic regulator[J]. Journal Of Clinical Investigation, 2005, 115(6): 1627-1635.

Kim HW, Lee JE, Cha JJ, *et al.* Fibroblast Growth Factor 21 Improves Insulin Resistance and Ameliorates Renal Injury in db/db Mice[J]. Endocrinology, 2013, 154(9): 3366-3376.

Kwok KHM, Lam KSL. Fibroblast Growth Factor 21 Mimetics for Treating Atherosclerosis[J]. Endocrinology And Metabolism, 2017, 32(2): 145-151.

Lee JH, Lee JE, Kang KJ, *et al.* Functional efficacy of human recombinant FGF-2s tagged with (His)(6) and (His-Asn)(6) at the N- and C-termini in human gingival fibroblast and periodontal ligament-derived cells[J]. Protein Expression And Purification, 2017, 135: 37-44.

Nishimura T, Nakatake Y, Konishi M, *et al.* Identification of a novel FGF, FGF-21, preferentially expressed in the liver[J]. Biochimica Et Biophysica Acta-Gene Structure And Expression, 2000, 1492(1): 203-206.

Pan ZC, Wang SP, Ou TT, *et al.* A study on the expression of FGF-21 and NF-kappa B pathway in the tissues of atherosclerotic mice[J]. European Review for Medical And Pharmacological Sciences, 2017, 21: 102-107.

Ribas F, Villarroya J, Hondares E, *et al.* FGF21 expression and release in muscle cells: involvement of MyoD and regulation by mitochondria-driven signalling[J]. Biochemical Journal, 2014, 463: 191-199.

Vemula S, Thunuguntla R, Dedaniya A, *et al.* Improved Production and Characterization of Recombinant Human Granulocyte Colony Stimulating Factor from *E-coli* under Optimized Downstream Processes[J]. Protein Expression And Purification, 2015, 108: 62-72.

Vu TT, Jeong B, Krupa M, *et al.* Soluble Prokaryotic Expression and Purification of Human Interferon Alpha-2b Using a Maltose-Binding Protein Tag[J]. Journal Of Molecular Microbiology And Biotechnology, 2016, 26(6): 359-368.

Wang H, Xiao Y, Fu L, *et al.* High-level expression and purification of soluble recombinant FGF21 protein by SUMO fusion in Escherichia coli[J]. Bmc Biotechnology, 2010, 10.

Wang S, Lin H, Zhao T, *et al.* Expression and purification of an FGF9 fusion protein in E-coli, and the effects of the FGF9 subfamily on human hepatocellular carcinoma cell proliferation and migration[J]. Applied Microbiology And Biotechnology, 2017, 101(21): 7823-7835.

Wente W, Efanov AM, Brenner M, *et al.* Fibroblast growth factor-21 improves pancreatic beta-cell function and survival by activation of extracellular signal-regulated kinase 1/2 and Akt signaling pathways[J]. Diabetes, 2006, 55(9): 2470-2478.

Xie T, Leung PS. Fibroblast growth factor 21: a regulator of metabolic disease and health span[J]. American Journal Of Physiology-Endocrinology And Metabolism, 2017, 313(3): E292-E302.

Xu J, Lloyd DJ, Hale C, *et al.* Fibroblast Growth Factor 21 Reverses Hepatic Steatosis, Increases Energy Expenditure, and Improves Insulin Sensitivity in Diet-Induced Obese Mice[J]. Diabetes, 2009, 58(1): 250-259.

Yang X, Hui Q, Yu B, *et al.* Design and Evaluation of Lyophilized Fibroblast Growth Factor 21 and Its Protection against Ischemia Cerebral Injury[J]. Bioconjugate Chemistry, 2018, 29(2): 287-295.

Ye X, Qi J, Yu D, *et al.* Pilot-scale production and characterization of PEGylated human FGF-21 analog[J]. Journal Of Biotechnology, 2016, 228: 8-17.

Yie J, Hecht R, Patel J, *et al.* FGF21 N- and C-termini play different roles in receptor interaction and activation[J]. Febs Letters, 2009, 583(1): 19-24.

Zhang M, Jiang X, Su Z, *et al.* Large-scale expression, purification, and glucose uptake activity of recombinant human FGF21 in Escherichia coli[J]. Applied Microbiology And Biotechnology, 2012, 93(2): 613-621.

Chapter 8
FGFR and Inhibitors

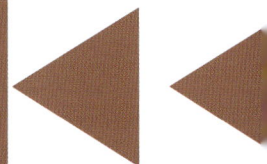

Influenza virus infects epithelial stem/progenitor cells of the distal lung: impact on Fgfr2b-driven epithelial repair

Jennifer Quantius, Xiaokun Li, Saverio Bellusci

1. Introduction

Influenza viruses (IV) may cause primary viral pneumonia in humans with rapid progression to lung failure and fatal outcome, and treatment options for this sometimes devastating disease are limited [1, 2]. Histopathology and clinical features of IV-induced lung injury in humans resemble those of other forms of ARDS (acute respiratory distress syndrome) and are characterized by apoptotic and necrotic airway and alveolar epithelial cell death, loss of pulmonary barrier function and severe hypoxemia [1, 3, 4]. IV primarily infect cell subsets of the upper and lower respiratory tract. In the latter, these are particularly ciliated and goblet cells, club cells and alveolar epithelial cells type II (AECII) [5–7]. Injury of lung epithelial cells is induced by both direct viral cytopathogenicity and unbalanced immune responses [8–11]. The initiation of well-coordinated programs of inflammation termination and of regeneration of the injured distal lung epithelium are a prerequisite for the re-establishment of proper gas exchange. Absence or imbalance of these responses may at best result in chronically organizing infiltrates and aberrant or excess remodeling with tissue fibrosis, associated with long-term pulmonary organ dysfunction in ARDS survivors [12, 13], or in fatal outcome at worst. However, the cellular communication patterns and molecular networks underlying regeneration of the distal lung compartment after severe pathogen-associated injury are incompletely understood to date. In particular, the distinct mechanisms of interaction between injury-causing pathogens with components of regenerative signaling pathways within the lung stem cell niche, determining outcome of the repair response, have not been studied in detail.

Alveolar re-epithelialization after injury was shown to involve different populations of endogenous, organ-resident stem/progenitor cells, which express lineage markers of distal lung epithelium such as club cell-specific protein (CC10/ scgb1a1) or surfactant protein C (SPC/ sftpc), are quiescent under normal conditions and proliferate during repair [14]. More recent reports revealed that intrinsically committed distal airway stem cells (DASC) expressing keratin 5 (krt5) and the transcription factor p63 were found to contribute to *de novo* generation of both bronchiolar and alveolar tissue after formation of cell "pods" in a murine model of IV infection [15, 16]. Vaughan *et al.* defined lineage-negative, integrin(β4)$^+$CD200$^+$ epithelial progenitors as the source of p63/krt5$^+$ amplifying cells regenerating airways and alveoli, highlighting integrin(β4)$^+$CD200$^+$ epithelial cells as important progenitors regenerating the distal lung following IV-induced injury [17].

During regeneration processes, the lung stroma likely plays a key role by maintaining the distinct microenvironment of the stem cell niche, involving extracellular matrix, direct cell-cell contacts and autocrine or paracrine mediators. These signals initiate and co-ordinate self-renewal, fate determination and terminal differentiation of stem/progenitor cells. Different subsets of resident lung stromal/mesenchymal cells have been attributed a role in these processes, including parabronchial smooth muscle cells [18], Sca-1 ^{high} lung mesenchymal cells [19, 20] or a human vimentin$^+$ lung fibroblast population [21]. Signals involved in these cross-talk events include, among others, the paracrine fibroblast growth factors (Fgfs), which regulate cell survival, proliferation, differentiation, and motility. In particular, Fgf7 and Fgf10 and their common tyrosine kinase receptor Fgfr2b (fibroblast growth factor receptor 2b), are indispensable for distal lung development including branching morphogenesis [19, 22–24]. Fgfr2b signaling is also re-activated in stem cell niches of the adult lung after different forms of injury to regenerate the epithelium [23, 25, 26]. The regulation of ligand and receptor expression of the Fgf7/10-Fgfr2b network in the context of lung repair after infectious injury, however, is not well understood.

In the current study, we demonstrate that a highly proliferating EpCam^{high}CD24^{low}integrin (α6β4)^{high} CD200$^+$ distal lung epithelial cell population represents a primary target of pathogenic IV. This population highly enriched cells expressing key characteristics of distal lung epithelial stem/progenitor cells mediating bronchiolar and alveolar repair. Of note, IV tropism to these cells significantly reduced their regeneration capacity by impairment of β-catenin dependent Fgfr2b signaling. These data for the first time demonstrate that the extent of lung stem/ progenitor cell infection by IV is a hallmark of pathogenicity as it critically impacts on lung regeneration capacity after severe IV injury. Moreover, IV-induced regeneration failure could be counteracted by intratracheal application of excess recombinant Fgf10, suggesting recruitment of the non-infected Fgfr2b^{high} stem cell fraction for repair as putative novel treatment strategy to drive organ regeneration in patients with IV-induced ARDS.

2. Results

2.1 *Influenza viruses target epithelial cell subsets of the distal murine lung to different extent after intratracheal infection*

It is well established that IV infect different subsets of the airways and alveoli, particularly ciliated and goblet cells, club cells and AECII [5–7]. However, recent advances in the field resulted in the definition of more specialized subsets of lung epithelial cells, some of which display stem/progenitor cell characteristics and contribute to repair of the injured organ [17, 19, 27]. To address which of these epithelial cell compartments were infected by IV, we fractionated distal lung epithelial cells into different subsets, after dissection of large airways and vessels and depletion of leukocytes and endothelial cells, according to surface expression levels of EpCam and integrin α6 [19], and the lineage markers CD24 (differentiated airway epithelial cells) [19], CC10 (club cells), pro-SPC (AEC II) and T1α (AEC I), by flow cytometry. We identified a high-frequent EpCam^{low}α6^{low} fraction (91.3% ± 1.8%) and a low frequent EpCam^{high}α6^{high} fraction, the latter of which consisted of a CD24^{low} and CD24^{high} population (1.7% ± 0.3% and 6.3% ± 1.8%, respectively, Fig. 1A). The majority of the most abundant EpCam^{low}α6^{low} cells showed a granular cytoplasm typically observed in AEC II, with approximately 95% of the cells expressing the AEC II signature pro-SPC^{high}T1α^{neg} and around 5% expressing an AEC I signature (SPC^{neg}T1α^{+}) (Fig. 1B). EpCam^{high}α6^{high}CD24^{high} cells contained pro-SPC^{neg}CC10^{neg} differentiated small airway epithelial cells (SAEC, 70%), composed of both β-tubulin^{+} ciliated and mucin5AC^{+} goblet cells, and pro-SPC^{neg}CC10^{+} club cells (30%) (Fig. 1C). EpCam^{high}α6^{high}C-D24^{low} cells were cells of homogeneous morphology and stained positive for the stem cell antigen Sca-1^{+} (Fig. 1D).

To analyse which of these epithelial cell subset were targeted by IV, we infected C57BL/6 mice using 500pfu of IV strains of increasing pathogenicity, *i.e.* low-pathogenic H3N2 (x-31), pandemic pH1N1 strain (A/Hamburg/04/09), causing mild to moderate lung injury at this dose in mice, and the highly pathogenic mouse-adapted PR/8 strain [28, 29]. Quantification of the infection rates by staining for IV nucleoprotein (NP) revealed that EpCam^{low}α6^{high} CD24^{high} and EpCam^{low}α6^{low} cells were infected with a frequency of ~ 11% and ~ 6%, respectively, by d4 pi after PR/8 infection, a time point where PR/8 replication in the lung reaches a peak [28]. Subfractionation into differentiated alveolar and airway epithelial cells revealed that rates of PR/8 infection in AEC I and AEC II ranged at ~ 8% and ~ 4%, whereas club cells and ciliated/goblet cells displayed similar PR/8 infection rates of ~ 10%. Of note, EpCam^{high} α6^{high}CD24^{low} cells were infected by IV to high amounts (around 15% of all EpCam^{high} α6^{high}CD24^{low} after PR/8 infection), and the proportion of infected epithelial cell subsets at d4 pi correlated with the level of pathogenicity of the IV strain used (Fig. 1E, F). To further address whether PR/8 revealed increased tropism to EpCam^{high}α6^{high}CD24^{low} cells, AEC, SAEC and EpCam^{high}α6^{high}CD24^{low} cells were flow-sorted, seeded into culture plates at equal numbers and infected *ex vivo* with x-31, PR/8 and pH1N1 at an MOI of 2, respectively. After one replication cycle (6 h), excluding *de novo* infection by progeny virions, the infection rate was determined, reflecting the capacity of each virus strain to infect the respective cell population. Similar to our *in vivo* results, we observed that PR/8 reveals an enhanced tropism to EpCam^{high}α6^{high}CD24^{low} cells (Fig. S1).

2.2 *Highly infectable EpCam^{high}α6^{high}CD24^{low}Sca-1^{pos} cells reveal epithelial stem cell characteristics and generate lung-like organoids in an Fgf10-dependent manner*

Given that the EpCam^{high}α6^{high}CD24^{low}Sca-1^{pos} cells which revealed the highest rates of infection were previously described as epithelial stem/progenitor population giving rise to airway and alveolar epithelium [19], we aimed to further characterize their phenotype and stemness properties. Further analyses using established stem cell

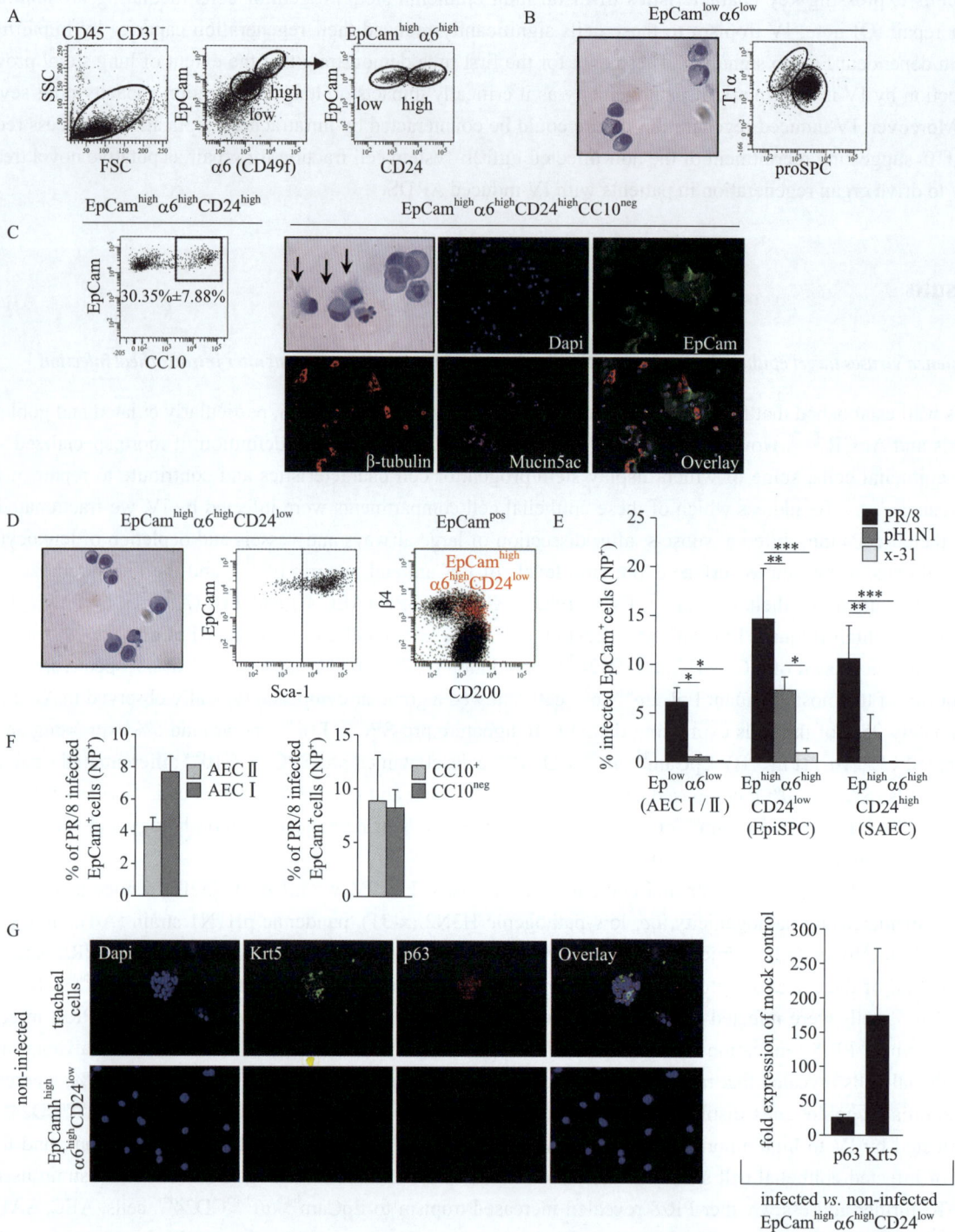

Fig. 1. Characterization of distal lung epithelial cell subpopulations and analysis of their infection rates *in vivo*. (A) Gating strategy of three epithelial cell subsets in CD31 and CD45 depleted lung homogenates of WT mice according to the expression of EpCam, α6 integrin and CD24. (B) Pappenheim stained cytospins of flow-sorted EpCam^{low}α6^{low} epithelial cells and flow cytometric subgating of this fraction with proSPC and T1α. (C) Characterization of the EpCam^{high}α6^{high}CD24^{high} subpopulation by flow cytometry reveals a CC10$^+$ and a CC10^{neg} fraction. Pappenheim stained cytospins of flow-sorted EpCam^{high}α6^{high}CD24^{high}CC10^{neg} epithelial cells (arrows indicate ciliated cells) and immunofluorescence stainings of this cell subset with mucin5ac and β-tubulin after 4 d of culture. (D) Flow-sorted and Pappenheim stained cytospins of the EpCam^{high}α6^{high}CD24^{low} epithelial cell population (left). Further flow cytometric phenotype characterization of the EpCam^{high}α6^{high}CD24^{low} population revealed that it is Sca-1$^+$ (middle) and localizes to the β4 integrin$^+$ and CD200$^+$ fraction of EpCam$^+$ cells (right, EpCam^{high}α6^{high}CD24^{low} population depicted in red). (E, F) WT mice were infected with 500 pfu of the indicated influenza virus strains and the fractions of influenza virus infected (nucleoprotein$^+$, NP$^+$) cells of the different EpCam$^+$ subpopulations were determined by FACS at d4 pi. (G) Cytospins of the flow-sorted EpCam^{high}α6^{high}CD24^{low} population or of tracheal digests (positive control) from uninfected mice were stained for krt5 and p63 (left). Quantification of p63 and krt5 mRNA levels of flow-sorted EpCam^{high}α6^{high}CD24^{low} at d14 pi from PR/8 infected mice (right). Bar graphs represent fold induction compared to mock-infected controls. Bar graphs represent means ± SD of n = 4 independent experiments; $^*P<0.05$; $^{**}P<0.01$; $^{***}P<0.001$.

markers [17] revealed that they were integrin β4+CD200+, a signature which has been confined to a distal lung stem cell phenotype known to engage the krt5/p63 regeneration program [17] (Fig. 1D). In accordance, these cells were negative for krt5 and p63 in healthy lungs, but highly upregulated krt5 and p63 gene expression after IV-induced injury (Fig 1G), suggesting that they contain epithelial stem/progenitor cells (EpiSPC).

To verify these stem/progenitor cell characteristics *ex vivo*, EpCam+ cell fractions were flow-sorted and seeded in organotypic 3D cultures [30]. As opposed to AEC I/II, and SAEC/club cells, EpiSPC developed typical large organoid spheres with cystic or saccular outgrowth in the presence of the growth factors Fgf10 and Hgf (hepatocyte growth factor), a characteristic feature of lung stem/progenitor cells [19] (Fig. S2A). A robust clonogenic potential of EpiSPC was demonstrated by repetitive cycles of serial passaging of digested organospheres by single-cell sorting and detection of *de novo* sphere formation after one week, respectively (Fig. S2B), and by use of clonality assays where tdtomato+ Epi-SPC were mixed with wildtype (WT) EpiSPC at a defined ratio and cultured in matrix, resulting in pure tdtomato+ and tdtomato-neg colonies indicative of clonal expansion (Fig. S2C).

Given that Fgf10-Fgfr2b signaling is indispensable for epithelial stem cell outgrowth *ex vivo* [18, 23, 30], we aimed to further define whether EpiSPC expansion and differentiation were Fgf10-dependent. To understand cellular cross-talk mechanisms involved in activation of the regenerative Fgfr2b axis after IV-induced lung injury we sought to define the predominant cellular source of Fgfr2b ligands, Fgf7 and 10 under homeostatic conditions and in the acute phase of IV-induced lung injury, at the peak of EpiSPC proliferation (d7 pi). Lung digests of mock-or PR/8-infected mice (d7 pi) were therefore fractionated by FACS sorting into four main lineages, including endothelial cells (CD31+CD45-negEpCam-neg, R1), leukocytes (CD31-negCD45+EpCam-neg, R2), epithelial cells (CD31-negCD45-negEpCam+, R3) and CD31-negCD45-negEpCam-negSca-1 high cells (Fig. S3A, left, R4). mRNA expression of Fgfr2b ligands in these four populations revealed that both Fgf7 and Fgf10 expression was significantly increased in the R4 fraction (CD31-negCD45-negEpCam-negSca-1 high) compared to the other three major lineages of the lung (endothelial cells, epithelial cells, leukocytes), independent of IV infection (Fig. S3A, right). Previous data suggested that Sca-1 high expression in EpCam&cells was associated with the fibroblast lineage [20]. To address whether Fgf10-expressing resident mesenchymal cells (rMCs) would support organosphere generation, flow-sorted EpiSPC and rMC were co-cultured for several days in absence of growth factor supplementation. As shown in S3B Fig, presence of rMC was sufficient to drive early organosphere formation at d5 of culture. Furthermore, rMCs mediated saccular outgrowth of EpiSPC spheres at d10 and formation of lung-like structures at d16 of culture, as compared to EpiSPC mono-cultures in supplemented medium, and this response was abrogated early in the cystic phase when Fgf10 was blocked by neutralizing antibodies (Fig. S3D). Of note, co-culture of EpiSPC with either flow-sorted CD45+ (R2) or CD31+ (R1) cells did not result in organosphere formation (Fig. S3C). Finally, lung-like structures derived from EpiSPC-rMA co-cultures significantly upregulated markers of terminal airway and alveolar cell differentiation, such as T1α and β-tubulin (Fig. S3E). Together, these data indicate that EpiSPC both self-renew and differentiate to distal lung epithelial cell subsets in an Fgf10-dependent manner during organotypic culture.

2.3　High renewal capacity of EpiSPC after IV-induced lung injury is mediated by the Fgf10-Fgfr2b axis

Analyses of the proliferative response of various distal lung epithelial cell populations after PR/ 8 infection revealed that the EpiSPC population showed the highest proliferation capacity compared to the AEC and SAEC subsets between d7 to d14 after injury (Fig. 2A and S4). Of note, comparison of EpiSPC and AEC proportions under homeostatic conditions and at d7 pi revealed an increase of the EpiSPC pool from 1.7% ± 0.3% to 5.7% ± 1.8% after IV-infection, whereas the high frequent AEC pool is reduced from 91.3% ± 1.8% to 84.7% ± 4.4%. Quantification of phosphatidylserine externalization by Annexin V expression of non-infected and PR/8 infected WT mice at d7 pi, a time point where apoptotic epithelial injury is most prominent in the lungs [8, 28], revealed that EpiSPC were resistant to IV-induced apoptosis, whereas the other EpCam+ populations showed high levels of apoptosis in response to infection (Fig. 2B). These findings suggest that a damage-resistant cell population with high proliferative capacity is contained in the EpiSPC fraction, which might contribute to renewal of both bronchiolar and alveolar epithelial tissue [19].

Given that Fgf10 is an indispensable growth factor for EpiSPC outgrowth *ex vivo* and that genetic deletion of Fgf10 or of the Fgf10 receptor Fgfr2b results in failure of embryonic lung development [25], we speculated that this pathway might be reactivated to drive EpiSPC proliferation for epithelial regeneration after infectious injury in adult mice. In fact, Fgfr2b surface expression was significantly upregulated on EpiSPC in the course of severe PR/8 infection compared to mock-infected mice, most prominent at d7 post infection (pi) when the proliferative response was highly

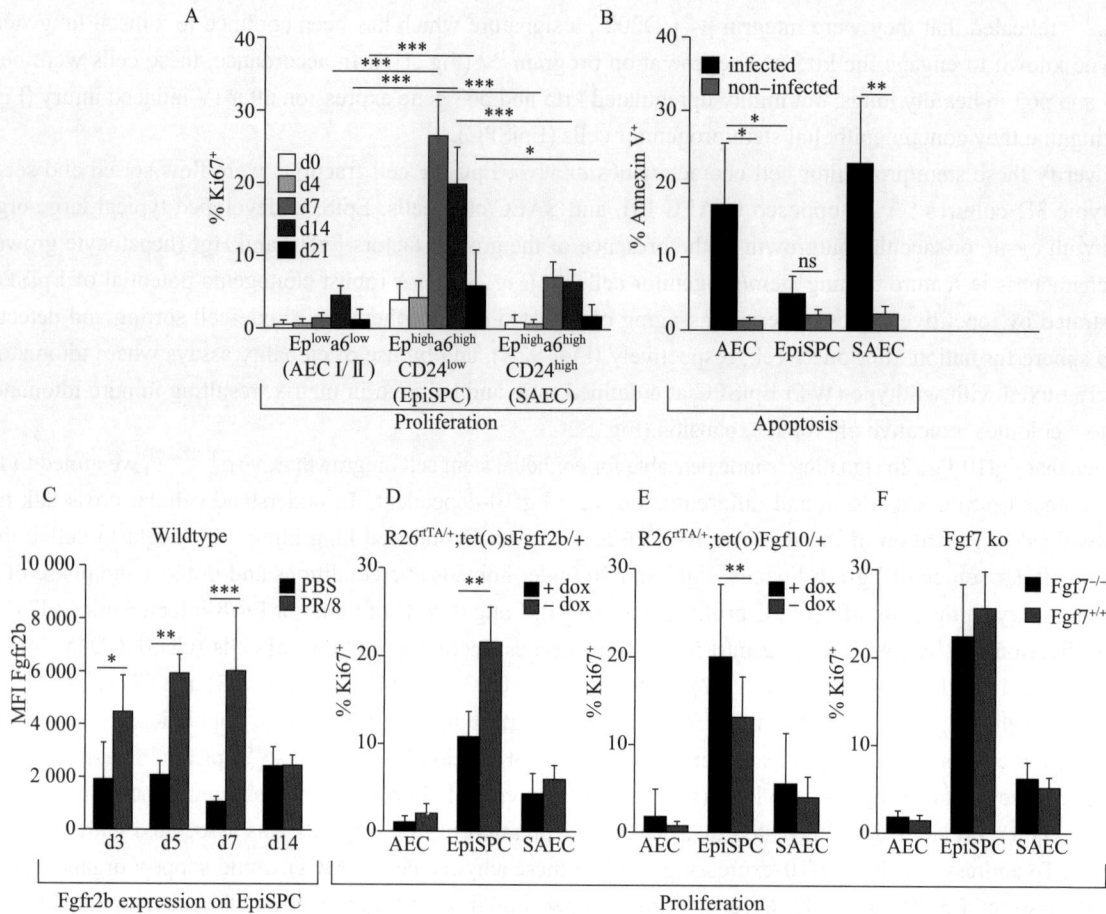

Fig. 2. EpiSPC are resistant to apoptosis and show a high proliferative response after PR/8 infection which is mediated by Fgf10/Fgfr2b signaling. (A) Proliferation rates of the given epithelial cell subsets was analysed in PR/8 infected WT mice by FACS quantification of Ki67$^+$ cells at the indicated time points pi. (B) Apoptosis of each EpCam$^+$ subset was quantified by FACS (Annexin V$^+$ proportions) at d7 post PR/8 infection and of non-infected WT mice. (C) Expression of Fgfr2b on EpiSPC at the given time points post PR/8 or mock infection was quantified by FACS and is given as MFI (median fluorescence intensity) of Fgfr2b ab minus MFI of matched isotype control. The proliferative response of the EpCam$^+$ cell subsets was quantified by FACS at d7 pi in *Rosa26r$^{rTA/+}$;tet(O)sFgfr2b/* + (D) *Rosa26$^{rTA/+}$;tet(O)Fgf10/* + mice (E) and *Fgf7-/-*mice (F) compared to non-dox-induced or WT littermates. Bar graphs represent means ± SD of $n = 4$–6 independent experiments; $^*P<0.05$; $^{**}P<0.01$; +dox, doxycycline food; -dox, normal diet.

increased (Fig. 2C). To decipher the functional role of Fgfr2b and its ligands Fgf10 and Fgf7 in this EpiSPC renewal response, transgenic mice with inducible over-expression of either soluble dominant negative Fgfr2b or overexpression of the ligand Fgf10, were PR/8-infected and proliferation of all EpCam$^+$ subsets was quantified at d7 pi. Attenuation of Fgfr2b signaling by doxycycline induction of a dominant-negative Fgfr2b (scavenging soluble Fgf10) resulted in significant impairment of EpiSPC proliferation capacity compared to non-induced littermates, whereas AEC and SAEC revealed no or little, Fgfr2b-independent proliferation (Fig. 2D). Similarly, the proliferating proportion of EpiSPC was significantly increased in mice with induced overexpression of Fgf10 at d7 pi, compared to non-induced litters (Fig. 2E). Of note, *Fgf7$^{-/-}$*mice exhibited only slightly but not significantly reduced EpiSPC proliferation in comparison to *Fgf7$^{+/+}$* mice (Fig. 2F). To verify that the Fgf10-Fgfr2b axis is indeed a key pathway in the epithelial regenerative response of the distal lung following IV-induced injury, we determined re-establishment of barrier function and outcome in doxycycline (dox)-induced *versus* non-induced *Rosa26$^{rTA/+}$;tet(O)sFgfr2b/+* mice. Blockade of Fgfr2b signaling resulted in significantly increased lung permeability (as determined by alveolar albumin leakage) during the repair phase at d14 pi (Fig. S5A), indicating that this pathway is crucial for re-establishment of gas exchange function. Concomitantly, the surviving sFgfr2b overexpressing mice showed decreased body weight compared to controls during the regeneration phase at d11 to d20 pi, and did not fully regain weight until d21 (Fig. S5B). Together, these findings demonstrate that IV infection induces activation of an Fgfr2b-dependent signaling pathway, which largely mediates the EpiSPC proliferative response and barrier repair after IV-induced injury.

2.4 Highly pathogenic IV inhibit Fgfr2b-dependent renewal in EpiSPC by blockade of β-catenin mediated transcription

Given that the EpiSPC cell fraction harbored stem/progenitor cells crucial for Fgfr2b-driven lung repair and at the same time represented primary targets of high pathogenic PR/8 in the distal lung, we sought to address whether infection of these cells would result in an impaired renewal response. We therefore infected C57BL/6 mice using 500 pfu of IV strains of increasing pathogenicity, *i.e.* x-31, pH1N1, and the highly pathogenic PR/8 [28, 29]. After 21 days, when mice had apparently recovered from IV infection, x-31 and pH1N1 infected mice showed a restored distal lung epithelial architecture, whereas mice infected with the highly pathogenic PR/8 still presented with thickened alveolar walls and incomplete re-epithelialization (Fig. 3A), suggesting that IV of high pathogenicity impaired the regenerative response of the lung. Quantification of Ki67+ fractions in infected (NP+) *versus* non-infected (NPneg) EpiSPC within the same PR/8 infected lungs revealed that the proliferative response was lost in infected EpiSPC (Fig. 3B), associated with loss

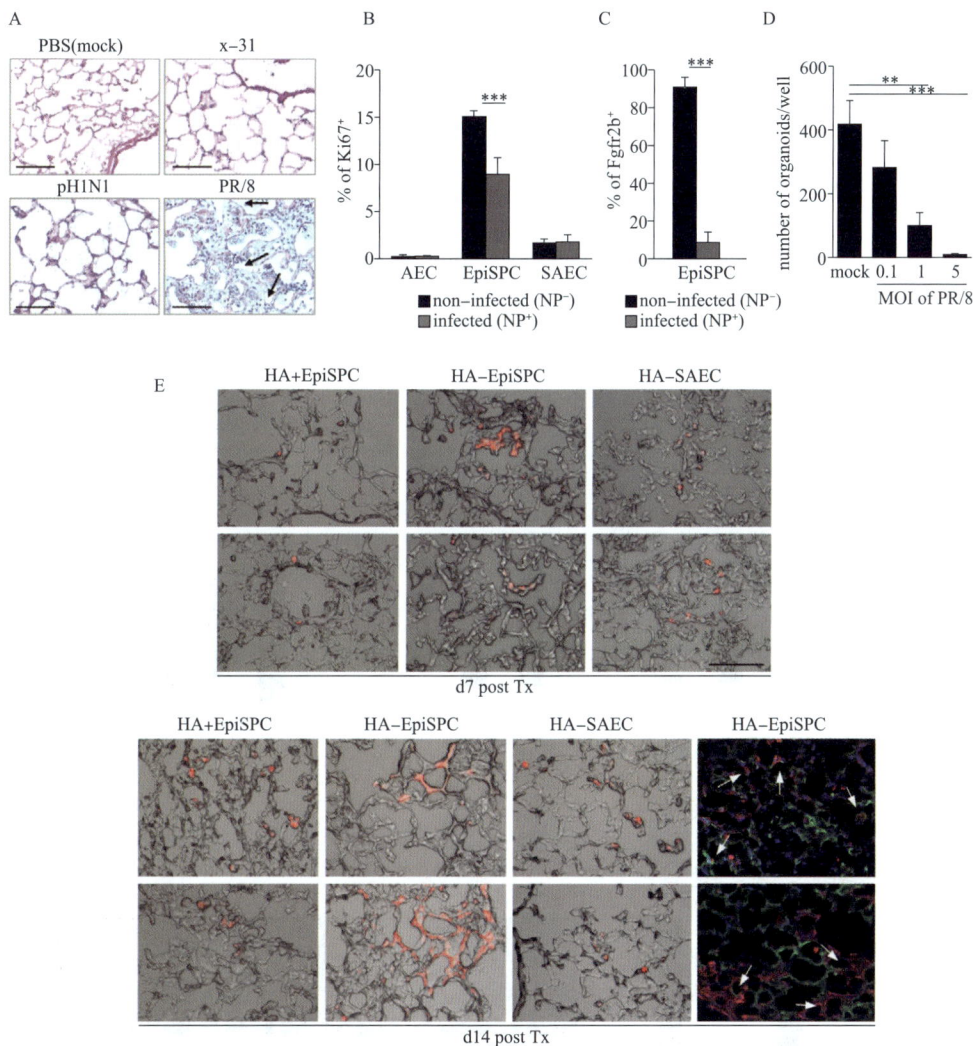

Fig. 3. Influenza virus infected EpiSPC are impaired in their regenerative response due to restricted Fgfr2b expression. (A) WT mice were infected with 500 pfu of the indicated influenza virus strains, or mock-infected, and lung sections were stained with hematoxylin-eosin at d21 pi (arrows indicate areas of non-epithelialized tissue). (B) Infected and non-infected epithelial cell subsets of PR/8 infected WT mice were quantified by flow cytometry for their proliferative response. (C) Quantification of Fgfr2b expression in infected (NP+) and non-infected (NP) EpiSPC by flow cytometry at d4 pi. (D) Flow-sorted EpiSPC were *ex vivo* infected with the indicated MOI of PR/8 and seeded in matrix for 3D cultures. At d6 of culture, the number of formed organoids was quantified. (E) Infected (hemagglutinin+; HA+) or non-infected (hemagglutininneg; HA) EpiSPC or control HA-SAEC were flow-sorted from the lungs of PR/8-infected tdtomato+ mice at d4 pi for intrapulmonary transplantation into 7 d PR/8-infected WT mice. Lung sections were obtained at d7 and d14 after transplantation. Representative micrographs show overlays of brightfield and red staining of tdtomato+ transplanted cells. Overlay of tdtomato+ transplanted cells (red) and the type I AEC cell marker T1α (green) is shown in the right panels (arrows indicate co-expression of T1α and tdtomato); bars = 100 μm. Bar graphs represent means ± SD of n= 3–4 independent experiments; *P<0.05; **P<0.01; ***P<0.001; HA, hemagglutinin; Tx, transplantaion.

of Fgfr2b upregulation in NP⁺ EpiSPC (Fig. 3C). Finally, infection of flow-sorted EpiSPC *ex vivo* with increasing doses of PR/8 followed by organotypic culture resulted in significantly reduced formation of organospheres depending on the multiplicity of infection (MOI) applied (Figs. 3D and S6). This was not due to infection-induced death of EpiSPC (as analysed by live/dead staining). Importantly and in line with these data, intratracheal transplantation of non-infected (viral hemagglutinin-neg; HA^neg) EpiSPC, flow-sorted from the lungs of IV-infected tdtomato⁺ mice, into IV-infected wildtype mice, resulted in integration into and in *de novo* generation of distal lung tissue (including AEC I) between d7-d14 post transplantation, whereas infected (HA⁺) EpiSPC or SAEC showed incorporation into distal lung tissue, but only limited expansion and did not give rise to distal lung tissue (Figs. 3E, S7A and S7B). These data indicate that EpiSPC indeed contain precursors of alveolar tissue *in vivo*, and IV infection of the EpiSPC niche results in defective tissue repair after IV-induced injury (Figs. 3E and S7B). Of note, transplanted flow-sorted EpiSPC of non-infected tdtomato⁺ mice can be visualized at d14 post transplantation in the lung tissue of IV-infected WT mice, but do not expand to generate tissue *de novo* (Fig. S7B, C), suggesting that factors expressed within the stem cell niche during IV-induced injury play a crucial role in early activation of quiescent EpiSPC for tissue repair (*e.g. via* IV-induced upregulation of the p63/krt5 regeneration program, Fig. 1G).

We next addressed the putative mechanism of inhibition of Fgfr2b upregulation in infected EpiSPC. Previous data revealed that Fgfr2b expression is dependent on Wnt/β-catenin signaling in the developing lung [31]. Indeed, conditional knockout of β-catenin by tamoxifen treatment in adult distal lung epithelial cells from Rosa26^ERTCre/ERTCre;Ctnnb1^flox/flox mice grown *ex vivo* (Fig. 4A, left) resulted in impaired upregulation of *fgfr2b* mRNA expression after PR/8 infection (Fig. 4A, right). Recent data suggest that β-catenin is involved in expression of interferon-dependent genes and that IV block β-catenin transcriptional activity *in vitro* as part of an antiviral escape strategy [32]. In fact, activation of the Wnt/β-catenin pathway by LiCl resulted in widely reduced IV replication in *ex vivo* cultured distal lung epithelial cells, whereas inhibition increased replication, as demonstrated by immunofluorescence and quantification of the viral *m segment* expression (Fig. 4B). Concomitantly, expression of the β-catenin target genes *Axin* and *Ccnd1*, and of *Fgfr2b*, was reduced by ~ 50 to 100-fold in infected (HA⁺) compared to non-infected (HA^neg) EpiSPC flow-sorted from PR/8-

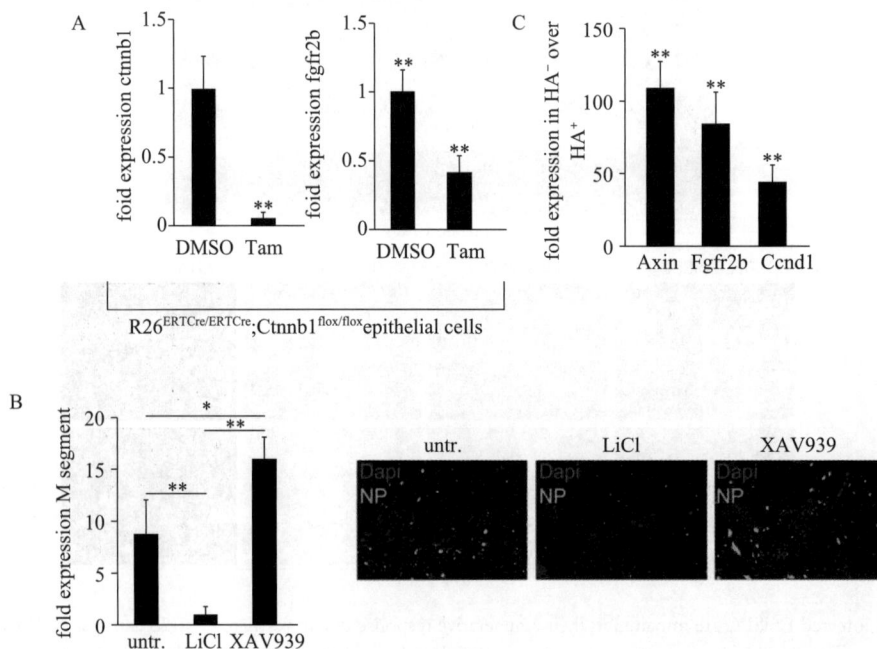

Fig. 4. β-catenin dependent transcription mediates upregulation of *Fgfr2b* expression, which is inhibited in PR/8-infected, but not in non-infected lung epithelial cells. (A) EpCam⁺ lung epithelial cells derived from *Rosa26*^ERTCre/ERTCre;*Ctnnb1*^flox/flox mice were grown to confluency and treated with tamoxifen or DMSO control prior to infection with PR/8 (MOI = 0.1; 24 h). mRNA expression of β-catenin (*Ctnnb1*) (left) or of *Fgfr2b* (right) was quantified and normalized to values of DMSO-treated control. (B) WT distal lung epithelial cells in confluent culture were PR/8-infected (MOI 0.1) and treated with an activator (LiCl) or inhibitor (XAV939) of β-catenin signaling. Expression of the viral M segment was quantified at 16 h pi and normalized to LiCl-treated cultures (left). The right plot shows representative photomicrographs of these cultures stained for IV nucleoprotein (NP) after 6 h of PR/8 infection. (C) WT mice were infected with PR/8 for 7 d and infected (IV hemagglutinin⁺, HA⁺) *vs.* non-infected (HA-) EpCam⁺ cells were flow-sorted. Expression of the β-catenin-dependent transcripts *Axin2*, *Fgfr2b*, and *Ccnd1* was quantified in HA⁻cells and normalized to values from HA⁺ cells. All bar graphs represent means ± SD of n = 3–4 independent experiments; *P<0.05; **P<0.01; Tam, tamoxifen.

challenged mice at d7 pi (Fig. 4C). These data indicate that EpiSPC tropism of IV represents a key factor of pathogenicity. IV interfere with β-catenin-dependent gene transcription in infected EpiSPC, likely to escape β-catenin anti-viral properties, which results in impaired Fgfr2b expression and reduced renewal capacity in infected EpiSPC.

2.5 Exogenous application of excess Fgf10 compensates impaired regeneration of the lung epithelial barrier and improves outcome after severe IV infection

To evaluate whether alveolar deposition of excess Fgf10 would counteract the impaired Fgfr2b-mediated renewal response in IV infected mice by increased recruitment of the non-infected Fgfr2b^{high} EpiSPC, we applied recombinant Fgf10 or PBS to IV-infected C57BL/6 mice at d6 pi. Indeed, Fgf10 treatment resulted in significantly increased proliferation of EpiSPC compared to PBS-treated mice at d7 pi (Fig. 5A). IV-infected mice showed a severely disturbed lung architecture with distinct cellular infiltrates, areas of extensive atelectasis and loss of epithelial cells at d10 pi, which was partially reverted by Fgf10 treatment (Fig. 5B, left). By d21, Fgf10-treated mice revealed an almost normal lung structure with re-epithelialized bronchioli and alveoli (Fig. 5B, right, arrowheads), whereas PBS-treated controls still presented with areas of atelectasis, cellular infiltrates and epithelial injury, indicating failure of epithelial renewal and persisting injury-associated inflammatory responses (Fig. 5B, right, arrows). To verify that Fgf10 indeed impacted re-

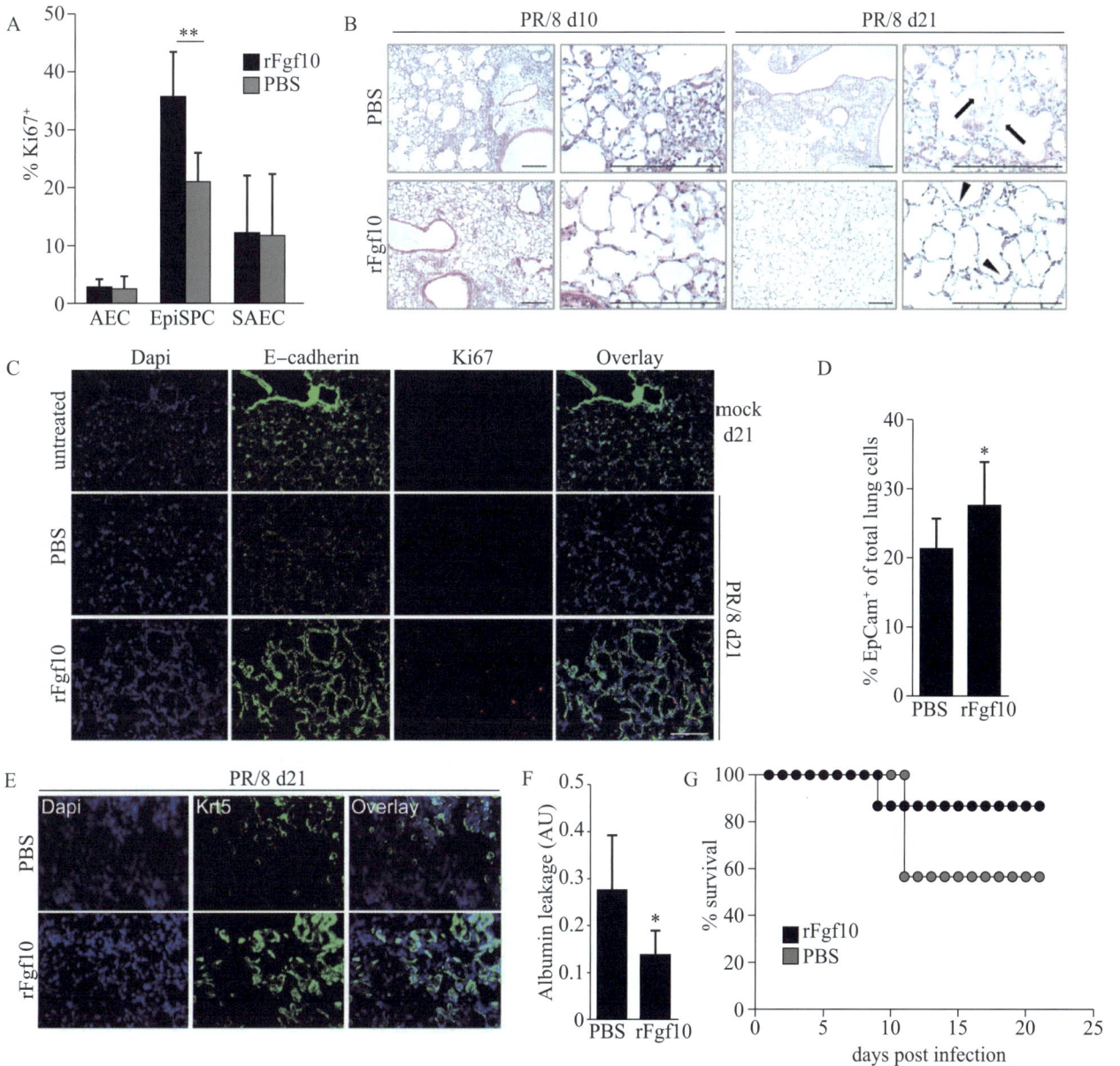

H

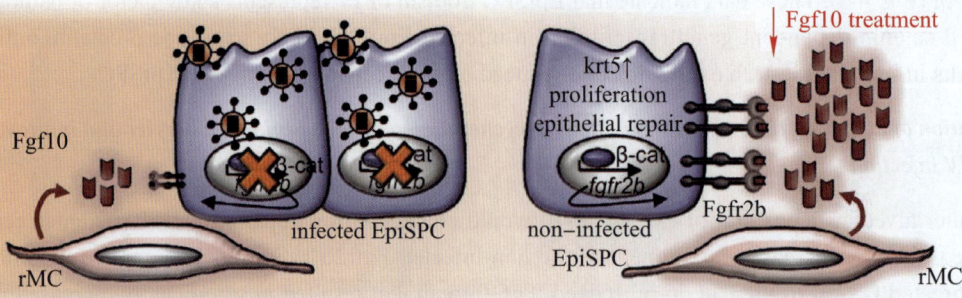

Fig. 5. Therapeutic treatment with recombinant Fgf10 improves influenza virus-induced lung injury and improves re-epithelialization and barrier repair. WT mice were infected with PR/8 and treated with a single dose of either 5 µg recombinant Fgf10 (rFgf10) or diluent (PBS$^{-/-}$) at d6 pi. (A) The proliferative response of EpCam$^+$ epithelial cell subsets was determined by flow cytometry at d7 pi. (B) Lung sections were stained with hematoxylin-eosin at d10 and d21 pi. Arrows depict non-epithelialized alveolar tissue; arrowheads depict areas of ongoing re-epithelialization. (C) Immunofluorescence staining of lung sections for E-cadherin (green), Ki67 (red), and Dapi (blue) at d21 pi. The top row shows lung tissue from mock-infected, untreated mice at d21. (D) Quantification of total lung epithelial cells (EpCam$^+$) in lung homogenates at d14 pi. (E) Lung sections were stained for krt5 (green) and Dapi (blue) at d21 pi. (F) Lung barrier function was analysed by quantification of alveolar leakage of FITC-labeled albumin at d14 pi. Values are given in arbitrary units (AU) and represent ratios of FITC fluorescence in BALF and serum. (G) Survival of $n = 8$ mice per treatment group was analysed until d21 pi. Bar graphs represent means ± SD of $n = 5$–6 independent experiments; $^*P<0.05$; $^{**}P<0.01$. Photomicrographs are representative for $n = 3$–4 independent experiments; bars = 200 µm. (H) Summary: IV with high pathogenicity infect a substantial fraction of EpiSPC, resulting in inhibition of β-catenin-dependent Fgfr2b upregulation and impaired epithelial repair mediated by rMC-expressed Fgf10. Therapeutic application of excess Fgf10 antagonizes IV-induced regeneration failure by engagement of non-infected, Fgfr2bhigh EpiSPC.

establishment of bronchiolar and alveolar epithelial structures, E-cadherin stainings of lung sections were performed and revealed that Fgf10 treatment resulted in complete re-establishment of the epithelium at d21 pi, associated with increased numbers of Ki67$^+$ proliferating cells, whereas PBS-treated mice showed only partial epithelial renewal (Fig. 5C). These findings were confirmed by quantification of the total numbers of EpCam$^+$ cells in these treatment groups (Fig. 5D). Of note, Fgf10-treated murine lungs showed increased expression of krt5, a marker of stem cell-induced repair, at d21 pi (Fig. 5E) [16, 17]. Finally, Fgf10-mediated epithelial repair resulted in improved barrier function at d14 pi, and improved survival until d21 compared to controls (Fig. 5F, G), highlighting the therapeutic potential of Fgf10 to improve EpiSPC-dependent epithelial regeneration.

3. Discussion

Repair of the injured lung epithelium including structural and functional re-establishment of alveolar barrier function after severe IV pneumonia is crucial for recovery and survival. In this study, we demonstrate that a fraction of distal lung epithelial cells phenotyped as EpCam^{high}-α6β4^{high}CD24^{low}Sca-1^{high}CD200$^+$ EpiSPC drive epithelial renewal processes involving Fgf10/ Fgfr2b-mediated signaling. Of note, the impaired alveolar regeneration after infection with highly pathogenic IV observed in mice and reported in humans [3] was associated with increased viral infection rates of EpiSPC in the distal lung compared to AEC and SAEC, and IV-induced inhibition of β-catenin-dependent gene transcription impaired regenerative Fgfr2b-signaling in these progenitor cells. Whereas transplantation of non-infected EpiSPC isolated from murine lungs, resulted in integration into lung tissue and *de novo* generation of distal lung epithelium including AEC I, previously infected EpiSPC did not give rise to lung tissue in the distal lung. These data highlight that tropism of IV to subsets of the lung stem cell niche may be a crucial determinant of IV pathogenicity resulting in severe impairment of Fgfr2b-mediated lung regeneration, and likely persistent failure of barrier function and worsened outcome.

Regeneration of the epithelial compartment of the distal lung was shown to involve different stem/progenitor cell populations, including p63$^+$krt5$^+$ lineage-negative, β4$^+$ epithelial progenitors or distal airway stem cells (DASC$^{p63/krt5}$) [16, 17], α6β4 high alveolar cells, and more line-age-committed CC10$^+$ or SPC$^+$ populations [14, 17, 33, 34]. Our data show that the EpiSPC population phenotyped as EpCam^{high}α6β4^{high}CD24^{low}Sca-1$^+$CD200$^+$ [19, 35] contained cells with stem characteristics as verified by organoid outgrowth in 3D cultures, and clonogenic potential in presence of growth factors including Fgf10. Furthermore, EpiSPC gave rise to cells expressing markers of terminally differentiated airway and alveolar epithelium in matrigel, suggesting that they are precursors of bronchiolar and alveolar epithelium. EpiSPC displayed high proliferation capacity after bronchio-alveolar injury caused by IV infection, as opposed to other distal lung epithelial cell populations. This renewal response was associated with strong induction of the p63/krt5 regeneration program, found to be crucial for distal lung repair [17, 36]. Furthermore, Fgf10-treated mice increased krt5 expression in their lungs, suggesting that the cells we identify as EpiSPC contribute to the p63/krt5 pool, and that expansion or generation of krt5+ cells is dependent on Fgf10. Conflicting data exist on the capacity of lineage-committed cells to be progenitors of differentiated distal lung cells [17, 37, 38]. Zheng *et al.* suggested that most of the newly induced p63+ cells in the IV-damaged distal lung compartment might be derived from CC10+ cells, whereas a recent report defined them as lineage-negative [17, 39], highlighting that the contribution of different stem/progenitor populations to alveolar repair may be injury-specific, dependent on the region and extent of injury, and on microenvironmental factors regulated in the context of defined types of damage. With respect to recent data highlighting the AEC II pool as stem cell niche of the alveolar epithelium, we found that the EpCam^{low}α6^{low} AEC II fraction proliferated only to a limited extent after IV infection *in vivo*. However, our data do not fully exclude contribution of an AEC II progenitor to the alveolar regeneration process, as demonstrated for bleomycin-induced damage [33], particularly as AECII constitute a highly abundant cell population of the lung, and even a small proliferating AECII fraction could still contribute to epithelial repair.

Clearly, EpiSPC proliferation after IV-induced injury largely depended on Fgfr2b and its ligand Fgf10, as demonstrated by use of *Rosa26$^{rtTA/+}$;tet(O)sFgfr2b/+*, and *Rosa26$^{rtTA/+}$;tet(O) Fgf10/+* mice, whereas Fgf7 did not substantially contribute. Given that *fgf7$^{-/-}$* mice are viable and do not display gross lung abnormalities as compared to *Fgf10$^{-/-}$* and *Fgfr2b$^{-/-}$* mice [25], and given that organoid formation from EpiSPC *ex vivo* is strictly dependent on Fgf10 but does not require Fgf7 [30], we conclude that Fgf10 rather than Fgf7 mediates EpiSPC renewal, although both ligands share the same receptor. A recent report highlights different functions of these ligands with respect to Fgfr2b processing and recycling [40], suggesting that the pro-longed proliferative response observed after exogenous Fgf10 application at d21 pi might be associated with Fgf10-induced maintenance of Fgfr2b expression on EpiSPC. With respect to cellular origin of Fgfr2b ligands within the stem/progenitor cell niche, an EpCam^{neg}Sca-1^{high} cell population of non-leukocyte and non-endothelial lineage [24] was found to be the primary source and supported for lung organoid formation in 3D culture. The lung mesenchyme is known to be the cellular origin of Fgf10 during lung organogenesis and postnatally [23, 24], and therefore represents a key orchestrator of the EpiSPC niche. Cellular responses of Fgf10 in the developing lung include epithelial progenitor cell maintenance and prevention of epithelial differentiation [41]. Our data confirm a central role of Fgf10 in survival and proliferation in adult lung EpiSPC *ex vivo* and *in vivo*, and demonstrate that neutralization of Fgf10 in EpiSPC-mesenchymal cell co-cultures results in inhibition of sphere outgrowth at a very early stage.

Canonical β-catenin signaling was found to induce expression of the *Fgfr2b* gene in the developing lung epithelium [31]. A key finding reported here is that IV infect EpiSPC and interfere with β-catenin-dependent gene transcription of Fgfr2b, resulting loss of Fgfr2b upregulation in the infected fraction of EpiSPC, which are thus unable to proliferate to promote repair. It has been recently demonstrated that β-catenin is indispensable for expression of type I interferon in response to IV infection in different cell lines. Many viruses have evolved gene products during co-evolution with their hosts by which they can induce and control various responses of their host cell, in particular early innate immune pathways. Mechanistically, a direct interaction of the viral NS1 protein, a potent antagonist of host innate antiviral responses [42], with the Wnt receptor *frizzled* upstream of canonical β-catenin signaling was discussed [43]. More recent publications suggest an interaction of Influenza or Sendai Virus-induced host cell components of the NF-κB pathway or of IRF3, respectively, with nuclear β-catenin to repress β-catenin-dependent gene transcription [32, 44]. Additionally, another report suggests that expression of the pandemic 1918 IV polymerase subunit PB2 increases virulence by inhibition of the Wnt signaling cascade which impacts on regeneration of the inflamed lung tissue [45]. Our own data clearly support the concept that the canonical β-catenin pathway is anti-viral, as demonstrated in studies using primary distal lung epithelial cells *ex vivo* infected with IV in presence of a β-catenin activator or inhibitor. This suggests that inhibition of β-catenin-dependent gene transcription is a conserved strategy of viral immune escape, which additionally results in blockade of renewal programs in EpiSPC. Our data furthermore provide a comprehensive, FACS-based quantification of infection rates of various lung epithelial cell compartments of the distal murine lung, and particularly indicate that the extent of EpiSPC infection by different IV strains represents an important, previously undefined factor of viral pathogenicity. In addition, the finding that EpiSPC as opposed to differentiated epithelium[10] are not subjected to infection-associated apoptosis but survive (likely due to constitutive expression of maintenance/renewal-associated survival pathways), raises the question whether viral ´imprinting´ will cause changes of transcriptional or epigenetic programs of stem cell plasticity resulting in long-term epithelial dysfunction.

Altogether, we provide evidence that pathogens such as IV severely affect the progenitor cell-mediated, Fgfr2b-dependent repair of the distal lung epithelium, and that intratracheal treatment of pathogen-injured lungs with excess Fgf10, to recruit the non-infected, Fgfr2bhigh EpiSPC fraction, promoted epithelial renewal without inducing aberrant repair [46] at the dose used. Fgf10 might therefore represent a putative treatment option to foster organ repair and re-establish gas exchange function after IV-induced and possibly other forms of ARDS.

4. Materials and methods

4.1 Mice

Wildtype C57BL/6 mice were purchased from Charles River Laboratories. *CMV-Cre* mice [47] were crossed with *rtTA*^{flox} mice [48] to generate mice expressing *rtTA* under the ubiquitous *Rosa26* promoter. This constitutive *Rosa26*$^{rtTA/rtTA}$ mouse line was then crossed with *tet(O) sFgfr2b/+* or *tet(O)Fgf10/+* responder lines to generate *Rosa26*$^{rtTA/+}$;*tet(O)sF-gfr2b/+* and *Rosa26*$^{rtTA/+}$;*tet(O)Fgf10/+* double heterozygous animals on a mixed genetic background, allowing ubiquitous expression of dominant-negative soluble Fgfr2b [49, 50] or of Fgf10 [18, 46] by administration of doxycycline-containing normal rodent diet with 0.0625% doxycycline (Harlan Teklad). Mice were genotyped as described previously [46, 50–52]. *Fgf7*$^{-/-}$ mice were obtained from Jackson Laboratory and backcrossed for several generations on a C57BL/6 background (strain #4161). B6.129(Cg)-*Gt(ROSA)26Sor*$^{tm4(ACTB-tdTomato,-EGFP)Luo}$/J (mTmG) mice in C57BL/6 genetic background, a tamoxifen-responsive driver mouse line, and *Ctnnb1*$^{flox/flox}$ mice were obtained from Jackson Laboratory (strains #7676, #3309 and #4152) and the latter bred to generate homozygous *Rosa26*$^{ERTCre/ERTCre}$;*Ctnnb1*$^{flox/flox}$ mice on a C57BL/6 background allowing induction of a β-catenin knockout by application of tamoxifen. Mice were housed under pathogen-free conditions and experiments were performed according to the regional institutions guidelines.

4.2 Reagents

The following antibodies were used for flow cytometric analyses, cell sorting or immunofluores-cence: CD49f PE or Pacific Blue (clone: GoH3), CD326 (EpCam) APC-Cy7 or FITC (clone G8.8), CD24 PE-Cy7 (clone: M1/69), Ly-6A/E (Sca-1) PerCP/Cy5.5 or Pacific Blue (clone: D7), CD31 Alexa fluor 488 or PE (clone: MEC13.3), CD45 FITC or APC-Cy7 (clone: 30-F11), CD200 PE (clone: OX-90), T1α/podoplanin APC (clone: 8.1.1.) and corresponding isotype controls syrian hamster IgG (clone SHG-1); all Biolegend. Influenza A virus nucleoprotein (NP) FITC (clone: 431, Abcam), Fgfr2b (clone: 133730) and corresponding isotype control IgG2a (clone: 54447, both R&D Systems), p63 (Life Span Biotechnology), CC10 (clones T-18 and S-20) and isotype-matched normal goat IgG (Santa Cruz Biotechnology), CD104 Alexa fluor 647 (clone: 346-11A, AbD SeroTec), Ki67 FITC or PE (clone: B56) and corresponding isotype control IgG1κ FITC or PE (clone: MOPC-21, both BD Bioscience), Annexin V Alexa fluor 647 (Invitrogen), E-cadherin (clone: DECMA-1, Abcam), p63 Alexa fluor 555 (clone: P51A, Bioss), Podoplanin (clone: RTD4E10, Abcam) or corresponding isotype control syrian hamster IgG (clone: SHG-1, Abcam), beta IV tubulin (clone: ONS.1A6) and corresponding isotype control IgG1 (clone: CT6, both Abcam), cytokeratin 5 FITC (Bioss), Uteroglobin (clone: EPR12008, abcam) and isotype-matched monoclonal rabbit IgG (abcam), purified Ki67 (Thermo Scientific), purified pro-surfactant protein C (Millipore), biotinylated mucin 5AC (clone: 45M1, Abcam), anti-influenza NP (clone: 1331, Meridian Life Science). Secondary antibodies used were anti-Streptavidin APC (Becton Dickinson), anti-rabbit Alexa fluor 488/555, anti-goat Alexa fluor 647, anti-mouse Alexa fluor 555/647, anti-rat Alexa fluor 488/647, anti-hamster Alexa fluor 488 (all Molecular Probes). Magnetic separation was performed using bio-tinylated rat anti-mouse CD45, CD16/32 and CD31 mAb (BD Bioscience, Pharmingen). For *ex vivo* neutralization assays anti-fgf10 (clone: C-17) or normal goat IgG (Santa Cruz Biotechnology) were used at a concentration of 5 μg/ml. For flow cytometric analyses, cells were routinely stained with 7-AAD (Biolegend) or fixable live/dead stain reagents (Molecular Probes) for dead cell exclusion.

4.3 In vivo treatment protocols

Mice were anaesthesized and intratracheally inoculated with 500 pfu (plaque forming units) of A/PR/8/34 (H1N1, mouse-adapted), A/x-31 (H3N2), or A/Hamburg/5/09 (pandemic H1N1), grown and quantified in Madin Darby Canine Kidney (MDCK) cells (obtained from American Type Culture Collection) and diluted in a total volume of 70 μl in sterile PBS$^{-/-}$. In the treatment approach, 5 μg recombinant Fgf10 (R&D Systems) dissolved in sterile PBS$^{-/-}$or PBS$^{-/-}$alone were intratracheally applied to IV infected mice. Venous blood and BALF were collected as described previously [53]. Lung permeability was determined by i.v. injection of 100 μl FITC-labeled albumin (Sigma-Aldrich) and quantification of FITC fluorescence ratios in BALF and serum with a fluorescence reader (FLX800, Bio-Tek instruments) as described elsewhere [28]. In selected experiments, 20,000 flow-sorted HA^{+} or HA^{neg} EpiSPC from IV infected mTmG mice were intratracheally applied into IV infected WT mice at d7 pi. Virus titers from BALF were determined by immunohistochemistry-based plaque assay on confluent MDCK cells in 6-well plates in duplicates as previously described [54]. Infected mice were monitored 1–3 times per day and a morbidity score was calculated from weight loss, general appearance, breathing frequency/dyspnea, and body temperature. Mice with a score $\geq$ 20 were moribund, sacrificed and classified as dead in mortality studies.

4.4 Isolation of murine distal lung cells

Lung homogenates of distal lung cell suspensions were obtained by instillation of dispase (BD Biosciences) and 0.5 ml low-melting agarose (Sigma) through the trachea into the HBSS (Gibco) perfused lung, followed by incubation in dispase for 40 min as previously described [55]. After gelling of the agarose and removal of the agarose-filled trachea and proximal bronchial tree, the lung was homogenized (GentleMACS, MACS Miltenyi Biotech) in DMEM/2.5% HEPES with 0.01% DNase (Serva) and filtered through 100 μm and 40 μm nylon filters. Cell suspensions were incubated with biotinylated rat anti-mouse CD45, CD16/32 and CD31 mAb for 30 min at 37℃ followed by incubation with biotin-binding magnetic beads and magnetic separation to deplete leukocytes and endothelial cells prior to flow cytometric analysis and cell sorting or to further culture.

4.5 Flow cytometry and cell sorting

Multicolor flow cytometry or high speed cell sorting was performed with an LSR Fortessa or an Aria III cell sorter using DIVA software (BD Bioscience). For analytical measurements 1–5x 10^{5} cells were freshly stained with fluorochrome-labeled antibodies for 20 min at 4℃ in BD FACS buffer. For intracellular stainings (NP, proSPC), permeabilization of cells was achieved by previous incubation with 0.2% saponin in PBS$^{-/-}$ for 15 min at 4℃, followed by incubation with anti-NP FITC, anti-proSPC, or respective isotype control mAbs for 20 min at 4℃. When non-labeled primary mAb were used, a fluorescent labeled secondary Ab was added and incubated for 20 min at 4℃ in FACS buffer. Doublets and dead cells were routinely excluded from the analyses (the latter by using 7AAD). Annexin V staining was performed on fresh, non-permeabilized cells. Prior to antibody incubation, cells were washed and resuspended in Annexin V buffer (BD Bioscience) and incubated with Annexin V 647 and further mAbs in Annexin V buffer for 20 min at 4℃. The stained cells were washed and resuspended in Annexin V buffer. Cell sorting was performed with an 85 or 100 μm nozzle. Single cell sorting was performed using the automated cell deposition unit (ACDU) with a 24-well plate and 12 mm cell culture inserts (0.4 μm pore size, Millipore). Purity of flow-sorted cells was always > 95%.

4.6 Culture of flow-sorted lung cells in matrix and clonogenic assays

Mono-or co-culture of EpiSPC and rMC was performed as described previously [30]. In brief, flow sorted cells were counted, resuspended and mixed with growth factor reduced matrix (BD Biosciences) diluted with EpiSPC medium (α-MEM, 10% FCS, 1× pen/strep, 1× insulin/transferrin/selenium, 2 mM L-glutamine, 0.0002% heparin) at a 1 : 1 ratio. Cell suspensions were seeded in 12 mm cell culture inserts (0.4 μm pore size, Millipore) in a 24-well plate and incubated for 5 min at 37℃, 5% CO$_2$ to allow gelling. EpiSPC medium was then added to the bottom wells of the plate. In selected experiments, 50 ng/ml recombinant Fgf10 and 30 ng/ml recombinant Hgf (both R&D systems) or anti-Fgf10 or control Ab were added to the medium at day 2 of culture. For matrix digestion a preheated dispase/collagenase I (Boehringer, Gibco) mixture (3 mg/ml) was added and a single cell suspension was obtained for re-seeding or single-cell sorting. Images were taken with a DM IL LED microscope and a corresponding camera MC170 HD (Leica).

4.7 Immunofluorescence and immunohistochemistry

To obtain lung cryosections, lungs were perfused with HBSS and filled with 1.5 ml TissueTek (Sakura) mixed with

PBS$^{-/-}$ at a 1 : 1 ratio as described [56]. Lungs were removed, snap-frozen and 4–10 μm sections were prepared using a Leica cryotome. In selected experiments, lungs were filled with a TissueTek/PBS$^{-/-}$ mixture containing 1% paraformalde-hyde and were incubated in 1% paraformaldehyde after removal. Lung cryosections were stained with Hematoxylin-Eo-sin or fixed with 4% paraformaldehyde for 20 min, blocked with 0.05% Tween 20, 5% BSA, 5% horse serum in PBS$^{-/-}$ for 30 min and stained with fluorochrome-labeled mAb diluted in PBS$^{-/-}$, 0.1% BSA, 0.2% Triton X-100 for 2 h. After washing, secondary mAbs were added for 2 h, followed by mounting with Dapi containing mounting medium (Vecta-shield, Vector Labs). Epithelial or mesenchymal cells cultured in chamber slides (Nunc) were fixed in a 1 : 1 ratio of cold acetone/methanol for 5 min and blocked with 3% BSA in PBS for 30 min prior to staining. Cytospins were addi-tionally stained with Pappenheim stain. Analysis was performed with a Leica DM 2 000 or with the Evos Fl Auto (Invit-rogen) microscope.

4.8 Ex vivo infection of primary cells

Primary murine distal lung cells contained >90% epithelial cells as determined by FACS. Cells were grown in 24-well plates (Greiner) or in chamber slides (Nunc) in DMEM enriched with HEPES, L-Glutamine, FCS, and pen/strep, until confluency and infected with PR/8 at the indicated MOI, as described previously [55]. PR/8 was diluted in PBS$^{-/-}$ containing BSA and pen/strep and added to the cells for 1 h, until the inoculum was removed and changed to infection medium (DMEM supplemented with BSA, pen/strep, L-Glutamine and trypsin) for further incubation. For inhibition of β-catenin, isolated distal lung epithelial cells of *Rosa26$^{ERTCre/ERTCre}$*: *Ctnnb1$^{flox/flox}$* mice were treated with 1 μM tamoxifen (Sigma-Aldrich) for 24 hours prior to PR/8 infection. Wildtype cells were treated with either 50 mM LiCl (Abcam) or 10 μM XAV939 (Abcam) directly after PR/8 infection, followed by RNA extraction or immunofluorescence staining. For infection of FACS-sorted lung cells (AEC, EpiSPC, SAEC), the cells were counted, seeded in wells or infected in tubes for 1 hour with the given virus strain and MOI, and were either seeded in matrix, or further incubated at 37 ℃, 5% CO$_2$ with EpiSPC medium and processed for FACS analysis at the given time point pi.

4.9 Quantitative real-time PCR

RNA from sorted or cultivated cells was isolated using RNeasy Kit (Qiagen) according to manufacturer's manual. cDNA synthesis was performed, as described previously [56] or with RiboSPIA kit (NuGen) according to manual. Actin or ribosomal protein subunit S-18 (RPS-18) expression served as normalization controls for the qRT-PCR, and the reac-tions were performed with SYBR green I (Invitrogen) in the AB Step one plus Detection System (Applied Bioscience). The following intron spanning primers were used: *Actin* (FP, 5′-ACCCTAAGGC-CAACCGTGA-3′; RP, 5′-CAGAG-GCATACAGGGACAGCA-3′), *Rps-18* (FP, 5′-CCGCCATGTCTCTAGTGATCC-3′; RP, 5′-TTGGTGAGGTCGAT-GTCTGC-3′), *p63* (FP, 5′-CAAAGAACGGCGATGGTACG-3′; RP 5′-CCTCTCACTGGTAGGTACAGC-3′), *Krt5* (FP, 5′-CCTTCGAAACACCAAGCACG-3′; RP 5′-AGGTTGGCACACTGCTTCTT-3′), β-*tubb* (FP, 5′-CCACCACCATGC-GGGAAA-3′; RP, 5′-CTGATGACCTCCCAGAACTT G-3′), *Fgf10* (FP, 5′-CCATGAACAAGAAGGGGAAA-3′; RP 5′-CCATTGTGCTGCCAGTTAAA-3′), *Fgf7* (FP, 5′-TCGCACCCAGTGGTACCTG-3′; RP, 5′-ACTGCCACGGTCCT-GA TTTC-3′), *Axin2 (FP,* 5′-AAGCCCCATAGTGCCCAAAG-3′; RP, 5′-GGGTCCTGGGTAAA TGGGTG-3′), *Fgfr2b* (FP, 5′-AAGAGGACCAGGGATTGGCA-3′; RP, 5′-GTACGGTGCTC CTTCTGGTTC-3′), *Ctnnb1* (FP, 5′-ACTTGC-CACACGTGCAATTC-3′; RP, 5′-ATGGTGCG TACAATGGCAGA-3′), *Ccnd1* (FP, 5′-GCGTACCCTGACACCAAT-3′; RP, 5′-GGTCTCCT CCGTCTTGAG-3′), *Pdpn* (FP, 5′ CCCCAATAGAGATAATGCAGGGG-3′; RP, 5′-GCCAAT GGCTAACAAGACGC-3′), *Influenza Virus M segment* (5′-GGACTGCAGCGTAGACGC-3′; 5′-CATCCTGTTG-TATATGAG-3′; 5′-CATTCTGTTGTATATGAG-3′). The relative gene abundance compared to the reference gene *Actin* or *Rps-18*) was calculated as dCt value (Ct$_{reference}$–Ct$_{target}$). Data are presented as dCT, ddCt (dCt$_{reference}$—dCt$_{target}$) or fold change of gene expression (2^{ddCt}).

4.10 Ethics statement

Animal experiments performed at the UGMLC were approved by the regional authorities of the State of Hesse (Regierungspräsidium Giessen; reference numbers 100–2012, 48–2013, 26–2013, 09–2009) and conducted according to the legal regulations of the German federal animal protection law (Tierschutzgesetz).

4.11 Statistics

All data are given as mean ± SD. Statistical significance between 2 groups was estimated using the unpaired Student's *t* test or ANOVA and post-hoc Tukey for comparison of 3 groups and calculated with GraphPadPrism. A *P* value less than 0.05 was considered significant.

Supporting information

Supporting information to this article can be found online at https://doi.org/10.1371/journal.ppat.1005544.

References

[1] Jain S, Kamimoto L, Bramley AM, *et al.* Hospitalized Patients with 2009 H1N1 Influenza in the United States, April-June 2009[J]. New England Journal of Medicine, 2009, 361(20): 1935-1944.

[2] Jefferson T, Jones MA, Doshi P, *et al.* Neuraminidase inhibitors for preventing and treating influenza in healthy adults and children[J]. Cochrane Database of Systematic Reviews, 2014, (4).

[3] Mauad T, Hajjar LA, Callegari GD, *et al.* Lung Pathology in Fatal Novel Human Influenza A (H1N1) Infection[J]. American Journal of Respiratory and Critical Care Medicine, 2010, 181(1): 72-79.

[4] Short KR, Kroeze EJBV, Fouchier RAM, *et al.* Pathogenesis of influenza-induced acute respiratory distress syndrome[J]. Lancet Infectious Diseases, 2014, 14(1): 57-69.

[5] Weinheimer VK, Becher A, Toennies M, *et al.* Influenza A Viruses Target Type II Pneumocytes in the Human Lung[J]. Journal of Infectious Diseases, 2012, 206(11): 1685-1694.

[6] Matrosovich MN, Matrosovich TY, Gray T, *et al.* Human and avian influenza viruses target different cell types in cultures of human airway epithelium[J]. Proceedings of the National Academy of Sciences of the United States of America, 2004, 101(13): 4620-4624.

[7] Heaton NS, Langlois RA, Sachs D, *et al.* Long-term survival of influenza virus infected club cells drives immunopathology[J]. Journal of Experimental Medicine, 2014, 211(9): 1707-1714.

[8] Hoegner K, Wolff T, Pleschka S, *et al.* Macrophage-expressed IFN-beta Contributes to Apoptotic Alveolar Epithelial Cell Injury in Severe Influenza Virus Pneumonia[J]. Plos Pathogens, 2013, 9(2).

[9] Brandes M, Klauschen F, Kuchen S, *et al.* A Systems Analysis Identifies a Feedforward Inflammatory Circuit Leading to Lethal Influenza Infection[J]. Cell, 2013, 154(1): 197-212.

[10] Herold S, Ludwig S, Pleschka S, *et al.* Apoptosis signaling in influenza virus propagation, innate host defense, and lung injury[J]. Journal of Leukocyte Biology, 2012, 92(1): 75-82.

[11] Hillaire MLB, Rimmelzwaan GF, Kreijtz JHCM. Clearance of influenza virus infections by T cells: risk of collateral damage?[J]. Current Opinion in Virology, 2013, 3(4): 430-437.

[12] Herridge MS, Tansey CM, Matte A, *et al.* Functional Disability 5 Years after Acute Respiratory Distress Syndrome[J]. New England Journal of Medicine, 2011, 364(14): 1293-1304.

[13] Dos Santos CC. Advances in mechanisms of repair and remodelling in acute lung injury[J]. Intensive Care Medicine, 2008, 34(4): 619-630.

[14] Leeman KT, Fillmore CM, Kim CF. Lung Stem and Progenitor Cells in Tissue Homeostasis and Disease[A]. In: *Stem Cells in Development and Disease* (Rendl M, ed), Vol. 107, 2014: 207-233.

[15] Kumar PA, Hu Y, Yamamoto Y, *et al.* Distal Airway Stem Cells Yield Alveoli *In Vitro* and during Lung Regeneration following H1N1 Influenza Infection[J]. Cell, 2011, 147(3): 525-538.

[16] Zuo W, Zhang T, Wu DZA, *et al.* p63Krt5 distal airway stem cells are essential for lung regeneration[J]. Nature, 2015, 517(7536): 616-620.

[17] Vaughan AE, Brumwell AN, Xi Y, *et al.* Lineage-negative progenitors mobilize to regenerate lung epithelium after major injury[J]. Nature, 2015, 517(7536): 621-625.

[18] Volckaert T, Dill E, Campbell A, *et al.* Parabronchial smooth muscle constitutes an airway epithelial stem cell niche in the mouse lung after injury[J]. Journal of Clinical Investigation, 2011, 121(11): 4409-4419.

[19] McQualter JL, Yuen K, Williams B, *et al.* Evidence of an epithelial stem/progenitor cell hierarchy in the adult mouse lung[J]. Proceedings of the National Academy of Sciences of the United States of America, 2010, 107(4): 1414-1419.

[20] McQualter JL, Brouard N, Williams B, *et al.* Endogenous Fibroblastic Progenitor Cells in the Adult Mouse Lung Are Highly Enriched in the Sca-1 Positive Cell Fraction[J]. Stem Cells, 2009, 27(3): 623-633.

[21] Ruiz EJ, Oeztuerk-Winder F, Ventura J-J. A paracrine network regulates the cross-talk between human lung stem cells and the stroma[J]. Nature Communications, 2014, 5.

[22] McQualter JL, McCarty RC, Van der Velden J, *et al.* TGF-beta signaling in stromal cells acts upstream of FGF-10 to regulate epithelial stem cell growth in the adult lung[J]. Stem Cell Research, 2013, 11(3): 1222-1233.

[23] Volckaert T, De Langhe S. Lung epithelial stem cells and their niches: Fgf10 takes center stage[J]. Fibrogenesis & Tissue Repair, 2014, 7.

[24] El Agha E, Herold S, Al Alam D, *et al.* Fgf10-positive cells represent a progenitor cell population during lung development and postnatally[J]. Development, 2014, 141(2): 296-306.

[25] Fairbanks TJ, Kanard RC, De Langhe SP, *et al.* A genetic mechanism for Cecal atresia: the role of the Fgf10 signaling pathway[J]. Journal of Surgical Research, 2004, 120(2): 201-209.

[26] Shyamsundar M, McAuley DF, Ingram RJ, *et al.* Keratinocyte Growth Factor Promotes Epithelial Survival and Resolution in a Human Model of Lung Injury[J]. American Journal of Respiratory and Critical Care Medicine, 2014, 189(12): 1520-1529.

[27] Kotton DN, Morrisey EE. Lung regeneration: mechanisms, applications and emerging stem cell populations[J]. Nature Medicine, 2014, 20(8): 822-832.

[28] Herold S, Steinmueller M, von Wulffen W, *et al.* Lung epithelial apoptosis in influenza virus pneumonia: the role of macrophage-expressed TNF-related apoptosis-inducing ligand[J]. Journal of Experimental Medicine, 2008, 205(13): 3065-3077.

[29] Otte A, Gabriel G. 2009 pandemic H1N1 influenza A virus strains display differential pathogenicity in C57BL/6J but not BALB/c mice[J]. Virulence, 2011, 2(6): 563-566.

[30] Bertoncello I, McQualter J. Isolation and clonal assay of adult lung epithelial stem/progenitor cells[J]. Curr Protoc Stem Cell Biol, 2011, Chapter 2: Unit 2G.1.

[31] Shu WG, Guttentag S, Wang ZS, et al. Wnt/beta-catenin signaling acts upstream of N-myc, BMP4, and FGF signaling to regulate proximal-distal patterning in the lung[J]. Developmental Biology, 2005, 283(1): 226-239.

[32] Hillesheim A, Nordhoff C, Boergeling Y, et al. beta-catenin promotes the type I IFN synthesis and the IFN-dependent signaling response but is suppressed by influenza A virus-induced RIG-I/NF-kappa B signaling[J]. Cell Communication and Signaling, 2014, 12.

[33] Barkauskas CE, Cronce MJ, Rackley CR, et al. Type 2 alveolar cells are stem cells in adult lung[J]. Journal of Clinical Investigation, 2013, 123(7): 3025-3036.

[34] Desai TJ, Brownfield DG, Krasnow MA. Alveolar progenitor and stem cells in lung development, renewal and cancer[J]. Nature, 2014, 507(7491): 190-194.

[35] McQualter JL, Bertoncello I. Concise Review: Deconstructing the Lung to Reveal Its Regenerative Potential[J]. Stem Cells, 2012, 30(5): 811-816.

[36] Chapman HA, Li X, Alexander JP, et al. Integrin alpha 6 beta 4 identifies an adult distal lung epithelial population with regenerative potential in mice[J]. Journal of Clinical Investigation, 2011, 121(7): 2855-2862.

[37] Rock JR, Barkauskas CE, Cronce MJ, et al. Multiple stromal populations contribute to pulmonary fibrosis without evidence for epithelial to mesenchymal transition[J]. Proceedings of the National Academy of Sciences of the United States of America, 2011, 108(52): E1475-E1483.

[38] Rawlins EL, Okubo T, Xue Y, et al. The Role of Scgb1a1(+) Clara Cells in the Long-Term Maintenance and Repair of Lung Airway, but Not Alveolar, Epithelium[J]. Cell Stem Cell, 2009, 4(6): 525-534.

[39] Zheng D, Yin L, Chen J. Evidence for Scgb1a1(+) Cells in the Generation of p63(+) Cells in the Damaged Lung Parenchyma[J]. American Journal of Respiratory Cell and Molecular Biology, 2014, 50(3): 595-604.

[40] Francavilla C, Rigbolt KTG, Emdal KB, et al. Functional Proteomics Defines the Molecular Switch Underlying FGF Receptor Trafficking and Cellular Outputs[J]. Molecular Cell, 2013, 51(6): 707-722.

[41] Volckaert T, Campbell A, Dill E, et al. Localized Fgf10 expression is not required for lung branching morphogenesis but prevents differentiation of epithelial progenitors[J]. Development, 2013, 140(18): 3731-3742.

[42] Wolff T, Ludwig S. Influenza Viruses Control the Vertebrate Type I Interferon System: Factors, Mechanisms, and Consequences[J]. Journal of Interferon and Cytokine Research, 2009, 29(9): 549-557.

[43] Shapira SD, Gat-Viks I, Shum BOV, et al. A Physical and Regulatory Map of Host-Influenza Interactions Reveals Pathways in H1N1

Infection[J]. Cell, 2009, 139(7): 1255-1267.

[44] Baril M, Es-Saad S, Chatel-Chaix L, et al. Genome-wide RNAi Screen Reveals a New Role of a WNT/CTNNB1 Signaling Pathway as Negative Regulator of Virus-induced Innate Immune Responses [J]. Plos Pathogens, 2013, 9(6):e1003416.

[45] Forero A, Tisoncik-Go J, Watanabe T, et al. The 1918 Influenza Virus PB2 Protein Enhances Virulence through the Disruption of Inflammatory and Wnt-Mediated Signaling in Mice[J]. J Virol, 2015, 90(5): 2240-2253.

[46] Clark JC, Tichelaar JW, Wert SE, et al. FGF-10 disrupts lung morphogenesis and causes pulmonary adenomas in vivo[J]. American Journal of Physiology-Lung Cellular and Molecular Physiology, 2001, 280(4): L705-L715.

[47] Sauer B. Inducible gene targeting in mice using the Cre/lox system[J]. Methods, 1998, 14(4): 381-392.

[48] Gossen M, Bujard H. Tight control of gene expression in mammalian cells by tetracycline-responsive promoters[J]. Proceedings of the National Academy of Sciences of the United States of America, 1992, 89(12): 5547-5551.

[49] Parsa S, Kuremoto K-i, Seidel K, et al. Signaling by FGFR2b controls the regenerative capacity of adult mouse incisors[J]. Development, 2010, 137(22): 3743-3752.

[50] Hokuto I, Perl AKT, Whitsett JA. Prenatal, but not postnatal, inhibition of fibroblast growth factor receptor signaling causes emphysema[J]. Journal of Biological Chemistry, 2003, 278(1): 415-421.

[51] Schwenk F, Baron U, Rajewsky K. A cre-transgenic mouse strain for the ubiquitous deletion of loxP-flanked gene segments including deletion in germ cells[J]. Nucleic Acids Research, 1995, 23(24): 5080-5081.

[52] Belteki G, Haigh J, Kabacs N, et al. Conditional and inducible transgene expression in mice through the combinatorial use of Cre-mediated recombination and tetracycline induction[J]. Nucleic Acids Research, 2005, 33(5):e51.

[53] Herold S, Tabar TS, Janssen H, et al. Exudate Macrophages Attenuate Lung Injury by the Release of IL-1 Receptor Antagonist in Gram-negative Pneumonia[J]. American Journal of Respiratory and Critical Care Medicine, 2011, 183(10): 1380-1390.

[54] Unkel B, Hoegner K, Clausen BE, et al. Alveolar epithelial cells orchestrate DC function in murine viral pneumonia[J]. Journal of Clinical Investigation, 2012, 122(10): 3652-3664.

[55] Herold S, von Wulffen W, Steinmueller M, et al. Alveolar epithelial cells direct monocyte transepithelial migration upon influenza virus infection: Impact of chemokines and adhesion molecules[J]. Journal of Immunology, 2006, 177(3): 1817-1824.

[56] Cakarova L, Marsh LM, Wilhelm J, et al. Macrophage Tumor Necrosis Factor-alpha Induces Epithelial Expression of Granulocyte-Macrophage Colony-stimulating Factor Impact on Alveolar Epithelial Repair[J]. American Journal of Respiratory and Critical Care Medicine, 2009, 180(6): 521-532.

Peptidomimetic suppresses proliferation and invasion of gastric cancer cells by fibroblast growth factor 2 signaling cascade blockage

Wulan Li, Guang Liang and Xiaokun Li

1. Introduction

The incidence of gastric cancer (GC) has dramatically decreased over the past several decades, but it remains the second most common type of cancer worldwide [1]. Therefore, identifying a potent therapeutic target for GC and relative targeted drugs is important. Previous publications implicated cytokines (CKs) in tumorigenesis, development, metastasis, and recurrence in GC [2]. A better understanding of the CK network can provide an effective therapeutic target for GC. For instance, vascular endothelial growth factor (VEGF) is a potent target for GC therapy [3,4]. VEGF inhibitors, such as bevacizumab, have been applied for clinical use in several other cancers, such as colorectal cancer, non-small-cell lung cancer, breast cancer, and glioblastoma [5]. Thus, CKs have been the focus of studies on GC therapy.

Basic fibroblast growth factor (FGF2) is a member of the FGF family that belongs to CKs. It can intensify fibroblast growth factor receptor substrate2 (FRS2) and then activate extracellular regulated protein kinases (ERK1/2, including ERK1 and ERK2), protein kinases B (PKB or AKT), and phosphatidylinositol 3-kinase (PI3K) by binding with fibroblast growth factor receptors (FGFR), which result in its pluripotency *in vivo* [6]. Aberrant FGF2 signaling can promote tumorigenesis, progression, migration, and tumor angiogenesis [7]. Numerous studies have reported that FGF2 is closely associated with several common malignancies, such as lung cancer [8,9], bladder cancer [10], ovarian cancer [11], and hepatocellular carcinoma [12]. Consequently, FGF2 is considered a potential target for tumor treatment.

In the stomach, FGF2 can significantly promote the proliferation of rat gastric epithelial RGM-1 cells by upregulating FGFR1 or FGFR2 and activating the ERK1/ERK2 signal transduction pathway [13]. Furthermore, other studies highlighted that FGF2 overexpression was detected in GC, and FGF2 mRNA expression could be used as a parameter to evaluate the GC prognosis [14]. Some studies reported that FGF2 is a key factor in the advanced stage of diffuse-type gastric carcinomas and may serve as a therapeutic target for GC [15].

Reported FGF2 inhibitors mainly include oligonucleotide carbohydrate inhibitors (PI-88) [16–18] and negatively charged organic small molecules (suramin) [19]. Most of these compounds exhibit a depressant effect through their charge interaction with FGF2. The poor targeting selection attributed to this characteristic results in numerous adverse events; thus, no FGF2 inhibitors are applied for clinical use [7]. By contrast, peptide antagonists with several features containing high activity, low toxicity, and minimal consumption have been emphasized in the field of tumor research [20].

In an earlier work, we isolated a short peptide (called P7) from a phage display heptapeptide library [21]. Meanwhile, we verified that P7 can suppress FGF2-induced breast cancer cell [22], melanoma cell [23], and K562 cell (chronic myeloid leukemia cell line) proliferation [24]. However, as a natural peptide, P7 is susceptible to degradation (data not shown), resulting in its limited clinical application. Given this defect, we modified P7 and presented a stable peptidomimetic (called P29), which possesses low toxicity and better antitumor effect.

2. Materials and methods

2.1 Cell culture

MGC803 (Shanghai Institute of Biosciences and Cell Resources Center) and KATO III (Xiangya Cell Center of

Central South University) were grown in RMPI-1640 media (Gibco, Eggenstein, Germany) supplemented with 10% fetal bovine serum (FBS) (Gibco) and 1% penicillin streptomycin (Gibco) in a humidified ThermoForma (Thermo Fisher Scientific, Waltham, Massachusetts, USA) containing 5% CO_2 at 37℃. Balbc 3T3 cells (Cell Bank of Chinese Academy of Sciences) were maintained in Dulbecco's modified Eagle's medium (4.5 g/L D-glucose, L-glutamine, 110 mg/L sodium pyruvate) (Gibco) with 10% FBS in a ThermoForma.

2.2 Real-time surface plasmon resonance

The ProteOn-XPR36 system (Bio-Rad, Hercules, California, USA) was used to measure the binding affinity of peptidomimetic P29 [Pro – (D – Leu) – Leu – Gln – Ala – Thr – Leu – Gly – Gly – Gly – Ser – NH_2, purity > 95%, the configuration of D – Leu is 'D', other chiral amino acid residues are all 'L', from China Peptides Company, Shanghai, China] (Supplementary Fig. S1, Supplemental digital content 1, *http:// links.lww.com/ACD/A124*) with purified FGF2 (PeproTech EC) at 25℃. FGF2 (purity > 95%) was immobilized onto a GLH sensor surface following the manufacturer's instructions. The peptidomimetics were diluted in running buffer (0.005% Tween-20, 10 mmol/L PBS, pH 7.4) and injected into the sensor chip at a range of concentrations(25, 50, 100, 200, and 400 μmol/L), and flow speed was set at 30 μl/min. Finally, the ProteOn imaging system and related software tools were used to monitor the response units. Signals were normalized using the appropriate controls.

2.3 Stability assay

P29 (1 mmol/L, 60 μl) was incubated with 140 μl of plasma at 37℃ in various durations. The incubation reaction was ended by adding 5% acetic acid. The solid-phase extraction technology and freeze-drying method were applied to obtain high-purity peptidomimetic powder from the P29–plasma intermixture. The powder was lysed in 100 μl of sterile water. The peptide concentration of this lysate was detected with high performance liquid chromatography (Agilent Technologies Inc., Santa Clara, California, USA). The high performance liquid chromatography conditions were as follows: column, ZORBAX SB-C18 (4.6 × 150 mm); elution, H_2O containing 0.05% trifluoroacetic acid and 100% MeCN containing 0.05% trifluoroacetic acid; flow rate, 1 ml/ min; and detective wavelength, 214 nm. The Cot curve was plotted using GraphPad Prism software, 5.0 (GraphPad, San Diego, California, USA).

2.4 Western blot assay

Starved cells were pretreated with serially diluted peptides (1, 4, and 16 μmol/L) plus FGF2, FGF2 alone, or sterile water. Subsequently, the cellular proteins were extracted, subjected to 10% SDS-PAGE, and then transferred to PVDF membrane (Millipore, Billerica, Massachusetts, USA). The membrane was blocked with 5% nonfat dry milk (Bio-Rad) at room temperature for 90 min with gentle rotation. After the milk had been rinsed with TBST, the membrane was incubated with primary antibody [an anti-phospho-ERK1/2 mouse mAb (E-4) (1 : 300, sc-7383; Santa Cruz Biotechnology Inc., Santa Cruz, California, USA), an anti-ERK1/2 rabbit mAb (H-72) (1 : 300, sc-292838; Santa Cruz Biotechnology Inc.), an anti-phospho-FRS2 rabbit mAb (Y196) (1 : 1 000, #3864; Cell Signaling Technology, Beverly, Massachusetts, USA), an anti-FRS2 rabbit mAb (H-91) (1 : 300, sc-8318; Santa Cruz Biotechnology Inc.), an anti-phospho-AKT rabbit mAb (Ser473) (D9E) (1 : 1 000, #4046; Cell Signaling Technology), an anti-AKT goat mAb (C-20) (1 : 300, sc-1618; Santa Cruz Biotechnology Inc.), an anti-cyclin D1 rabbit mAb (H-295) (1 : 300, sc-753; Santa Cruz Biotechnology Inc.), or an anti-GAPDH mAb (FL-335) (1 : 1 000, sc-25778; Santa Cruz Biotechnology Inc.)] overnight at 4℃, followed by a donkey anti-rabbit (1 : 3 000, sc-2313; Santa Cruz Biotechnology Inc.) or a donkey anti-goat (1 : 3 000, sc-2020; Santa Cruz Biotechnology Inc.) or a goat anti-mouse IgG HRP-linked antibody (1 : 3 000, sc-2005; Santa Cruz Biotechnology Inc.) for 1 h. The unconjugated secondary antibody was eluted by TBST before the blots were visualized using an ECL detection kit (Bio-Rad) according to the manufacturer's instructions. The results were analyzed using Quantity One software (Bio-Rad) to determine the relative ratio.

2.5 Cell cycle analysis

Starved cells were treated with FGF2 plus serial dilution peptides (1, 4, and 16 μmol/L), FGF2 alone, or sterile water (blank) for 48 h. The cells were washed with PBS (HyClone, Logan, Utah, USA) twice, collected, fixed in 75% ice-cold ethanol, and stained with 500 μl of propidium iodide (PI) (Becton Dickinson and Company, BD Biosciences, San Jose, California, USA) for 10 min at 4℃ in the dark. The suspension was filtered using a 200-mesh gauze and then subjected to FACSCalibur (BD Biosciences Clontech, BD Biosciences) flow cytometric analysis. Data were analyzed using the ModFit DNA analysis program.

2.6 Cell viability assay

Cells were seeded in 96-well plates at densities of 3×10^3 cells per well and then allowed to attach overnight. After starved cultivation in RMPI-1640 with non-FBS for 24 h, the cells were treated with 20 ng/ml FGF2 plus serial dilution peptides (0.25, 1, 4, and 16 µmol/L), FGF2 alone, or sterile water (blank group) for 48 h. Cell viability was determined by MTT colorimetric assay as described. In brief, 25 µl of MTT (Solarbio Life Sciences, Beijing, China) was added to each well and incubated with cells for 4 h. After the medium had been removed, 150 µl of dimethylsulfoxide (Sigma, St Louis, Missouri, USA) was added to each well. Absorbance was then measured at 490 nm to detect the number of viable cells.

2.7 Colony formation assay

Cells were seeded in six-well plates at densities of 1500 cells per well. After being allowed to adhere to the wells, cells were starved in RMPI-1640 with 0% FBS for 24 h. The starved cells were then treated with the indicated treatment for 48 h. The medium with the indicated treatment was removed and replaced with fresh medium with 10% FBS. After 1 week, adherent macroscopic colonies were washed with PBS, fixed with 4% paraformaldehyde for 10 min, stained with crystal violet solution (C0121; Beyotime Biotechnology, Nantong, China) for 30 min, and then counted visually.

2.8 Transwell migration assay

Starved cells (5×10^4) were plated in the upper chamber of a 24-well BioCoat Matrigel invasion chamber (BD Biosciences) previously coated with 500 µl of RMPI-1640 containing 10% FBS used as a chemoattractant in the lower chamber. The upper and lower chambers were treated with sterile water, FGF2 alone, or FGF2 plus serial dilution P29 (1, 4, and 16 µmol/L). After incubation for 24 h, cells that passed through the membrane filter were fixed and stained with crystal violet solution for 15 min and then placed on a microslide. The number of invading cells was counted using a fluorescence microscope (Nikon Corporation, Tokyo, Japan) in five random × 20 fields.

2.9 Statistical analysis

GraphPad Prism software, 5.0 was used to analyze the experimental data. Student's *t*-test was performed to compare data between two groups, and one-way analysis of variance followed by Tukey's multiple comparison tests was used to analyze the multiple comparison data. *P* less than 0.05 was considered statistically significant.

3. Results

3.1 P29 strongly combines with FGF2

To compare the binding affinity between P29 and FGF2, we used surface plasmon resonance to monitor the P29–ligand interaction signal. Figure 1 shows that P29 could bind to the immobilized FGF2 at concentrations of 25, 50, 100, 200, and 400 µmol/L. Subsequently, global fitting of the kinetic data was applied to calculate the KD value from various concentrations of P29 using 1 : 1 Langmuir binding. As shown in the data, FGF2 exhibited the highest binding affinity to P29 with a KD value of $1.17E - 08M$, whereas the binding capacities of FGF-21, FGF1, and KFG-2 were lower with KD values of $8.18E - 01M$, $9.62E - 01M$, and $3.94E - 05M$ (Fig. 1, Supplementary Table S1), respectively.

3.2 P29 has a longer half-time in plasma in vitro

A series of techniques were used to investigate the stability of P29 in plasma *in vitro*. Fig. 2A and Supplementary Fig. S2A show that the concentration had better linearity with peak area ($R^2 = 0.9998$) and was proportional to the peak area. A favorable result was also obtained, with the half-time of P29 reaching up to 10 h (Fig. 2B, Supplementary Fig. S2B).

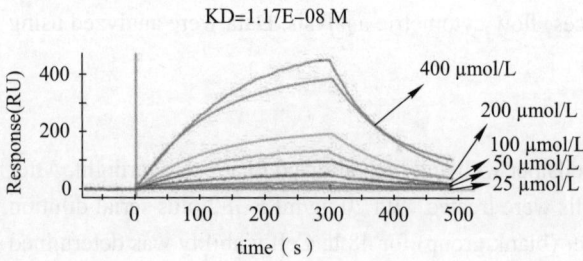

KD=1.17E−08 M

Fig. 1. P29 interacts with FGF2 in a dose-dependent manner. Interaction between FGF2 and P29 was revealed using the surface plasmon resonance technique. FGF2 immobilized on a GLM sensor surface was exposed to P29 at various concentrations as indicated.

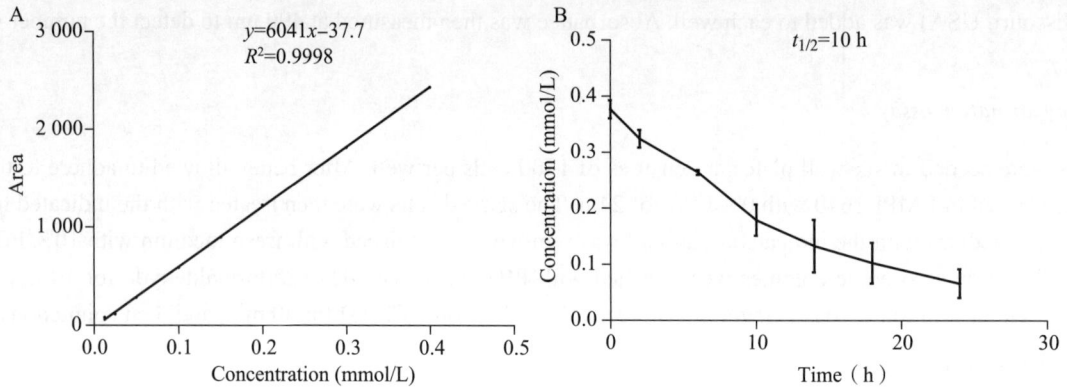

$y=6041x-37.7$
$R^2=0.9998$

$t_{1/2}=10$ h

Fig. 2. Half-time of peptidomimetic P29 in human plasma *in vitro*. (A) P29 was diluted into various concentrations (0.4, 0.3, 0.2, 0.15, 0.1, 0.05, 0.025, and 0.0125 μmol/L) and analyzed by high performance liquid chromatography. *y*-Axis and *x*-axis indicate the peak area of analysis and the mean sample concentration, respectively. (B) P29 incubated with plasma for 0, 2, 6, 10, 14, 18, and 24 h as indicated. *y*-Axis and *x*-axis indicate the concentration of P29 and time, respectively.

3.3 P29 blocks FGF2/FGFR signaling

We investigated whether P29 could affect the phosphorylation of some proteins (FRS2, AKT, and ERK). Western blot assay was performed to detect the level of phosphorylated FRS2 (p-FRS2), phosphorylated AKT (p-AKT), and phosphorylated ERK1/2 (p-ERK1/2). Fig. 3 shows that, in KATO III and MGC803 cells, treatment with FGF2 for 10 min upregulated the phosphorylation of FRS2, AKT, and ERK1/2, whereas pretreatment with P29 for 10 min before stimulation with FGF2 evidently inhibited the activation of these proteins. Moreover, 4 μmol/L P29 completely suppressed the activation of FGF signaling.

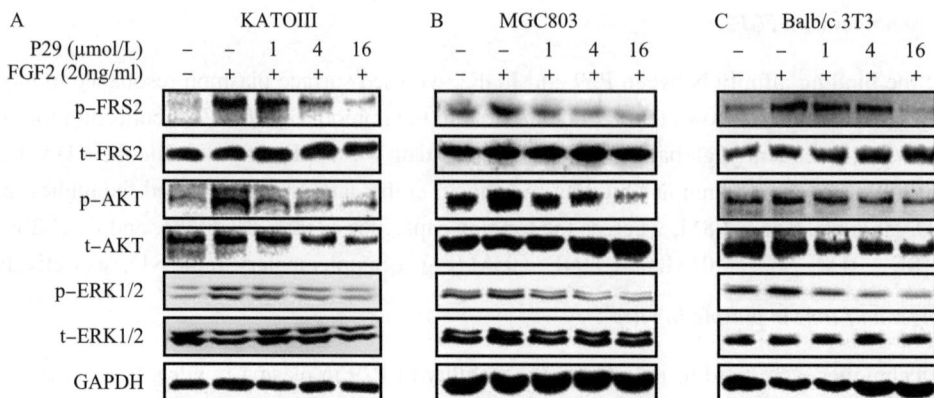

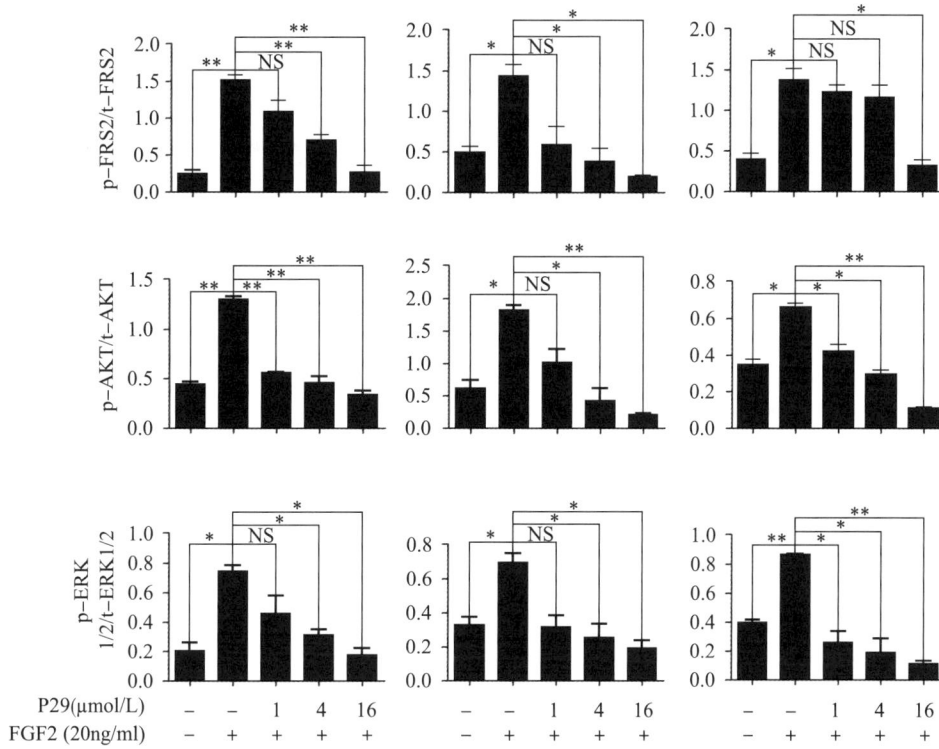

Fig. 3. Effect of peptidomimetic P29 on cellular protein activation triggered by FGF2 signal. Starved KATO III cells (A) and MGC803 (B) cells were treated with serially diluted P29 (1, 4, and 16 μmol/L) for 10 min before stimulation with 20 ng/ml FGF2 for 10 min or treated with 20 ng/ml FGF2 alone for 10 min. Starved Balb/c 3T3 cells (C) were treated with various P29 concentrations for 10 min and then stimulated with 20 ng/ml FGF2 for 15 min or treated with 20 ng/ml FGF2 alone for 15 min. Starved cells treated with sterile water served as control. Phosphory-lated levels of FRS2, ERK, and AKT were detected by western blot assay. Images shown are representative of one of two independent experiments. NS indicates no statistical significance. $^{*}P < 0.05$, $^{**}P < 0.01$, and $^{***}P < 0.001$. FGF2, fibroblast growth factor 2.

3.4 P29 arrests FGF2-induced cells at the G0/G1 phase

Owing to the close connection between cell proliferation and cell cycle, flow cytometry combined with PI stain-ing contributed to the identification of cell cycle distribution of GC. Fig. 4A shows that FGF2 decreased the G0/G1 phase cell ratio from 63.52% ± 0.42% to 55.16% ± 0.32% but increased the S phase cell ratio from 28.48% ± 0.42%

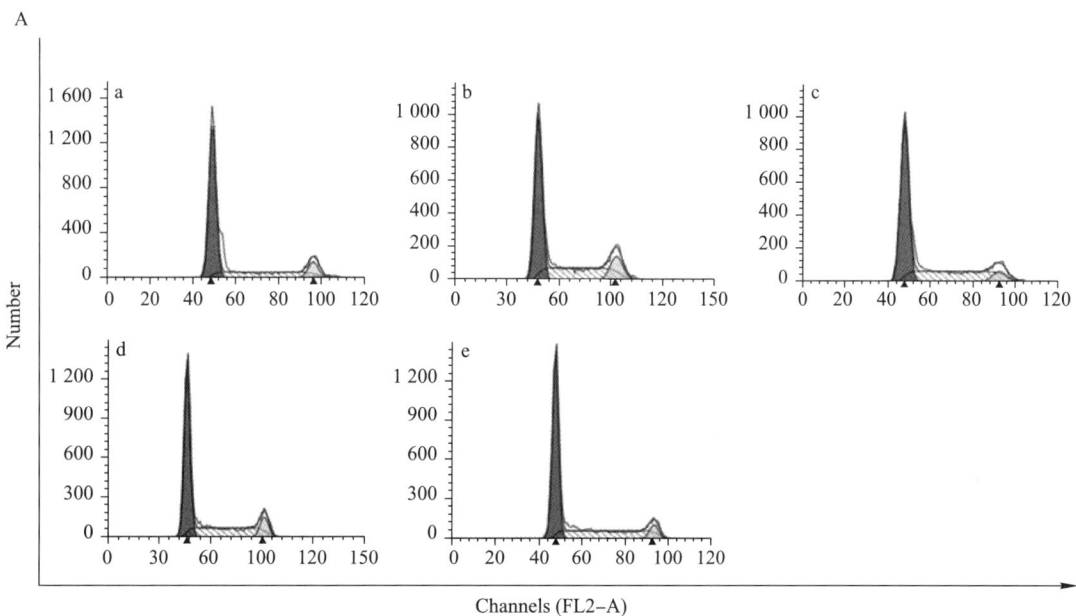

B

Group	G0/G1 (%)	G2/M (%)	S (%)
a	63.52 ± 0.42	8.00 ± 0.32	28.48 ± 0.42
b	55.16 ± 0.32	8.00 ± 0.02	36.84 ± 0.19
c	55.28 ± 0.01	8.00 ± 0.12	36.72 ± 0.10
d	58.07 ± 0.30	8.00 ± 0.28	33.93 ± 0.30
e	59.94 ± 0.06	8.00 ± 0.42	32.06 ± 0.09

C

D

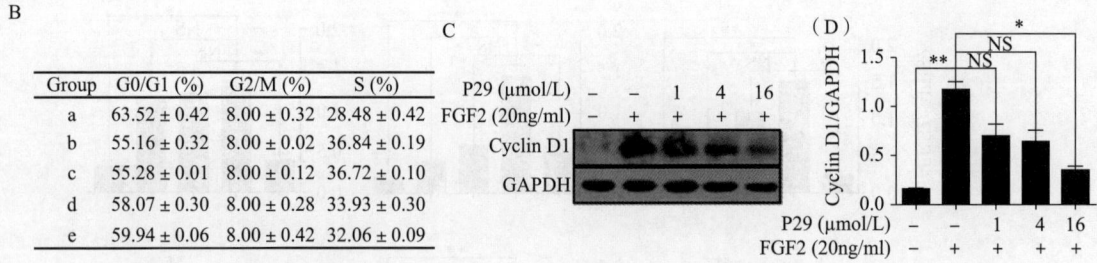

Fig. 4. Effect of peptidomimetic P29 on the cell cycle in FGF2-stimulated KATO III cells. (A) Cells were starved for 24 h and then treated with 20 ng/ml FGF2 (B) or 20 ng/ml FGF2 plus various concentrations of P29 (C–E: 1, 4, and 16 μmol/L, respectively) for 48 h. The control group (A) was not treated with FGF2 or P29. Representative images are from one of the three independent experiments. (B) Cell cycle distribution of the control and treated cells. Data are presented as the mean ± SD of three independent experiments. (C) Cells were starved for 24 h and then treated with 20 ng/ml FGF2 or 20 ng/ml FGF2 plus indicated concentrations of P29 for 24 h. (D) P29 reversed FGF2-induced alteration of cyclin D1. Data are mean and SEM. $^{**}P < 0.01$. FGF2, fibroblast growth factor 2; NS, nonsignificant.

to 36.84% ± 0.19%. P29 could significantly counteract this effect of FGF2 and thereby result in cell cycle arrest at the G0/G1 phase. To further examine the association of cell cycle regulatory proteins, western blot analysis was conducted with the treatment of P29. It was observed that cyclin D1 was significantly suppressed with 16 μmol/ L P29 treatment for 24 h (Fig. 4C). These phenomena suggest that P29 decreased cell proliferation by reversing the regulation effect of FGF2 on the cell cycle.

3.5 P29 suppresses the FGF2-induced proliferation of GC cells

MTT colorimetric assay was performed to determine the effects of P29 on cell proliferation. As shown in Fig. 5A, P29 had a dose-dependent inhibitory effect on cell proliferation (including KATO III and MGC803) induced by FGF2. The 50% inhibition of proliferation on MGC803 and KATO III was 0.7 and 3.2 μmol/L, respectively. Furthermore, the colony formation assay shows that P29 significantly reduced the number of KATO III colonies formed after 7 days of culture compared with FGF2-treated control (Fig. 5B).

3.6 P29 suppresses cell migration

The effect of P29 on cell migration was assessed by the Transwell migration assay. Figure 6 shows that FGF2 evidently strengthened the invasive capability of MGC803cells. P29 could inhibit the invasiveness of MGC803 cells in a dose-dependent manner. Statistical analysis showed that 4 μmol/L P29 caused a distinct inhibition of cell migration.

4. Discussion

GC is a common disease that is difficult to treat [1]. Current approaches for GC patients, including the reform of surgical operation and the optimization of radiation and chemotherapy, remain insufficient to reduce GC mortality. In GC

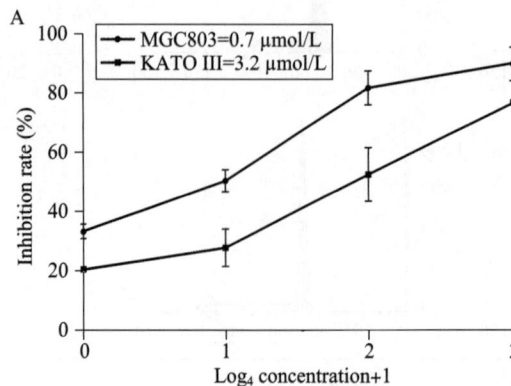

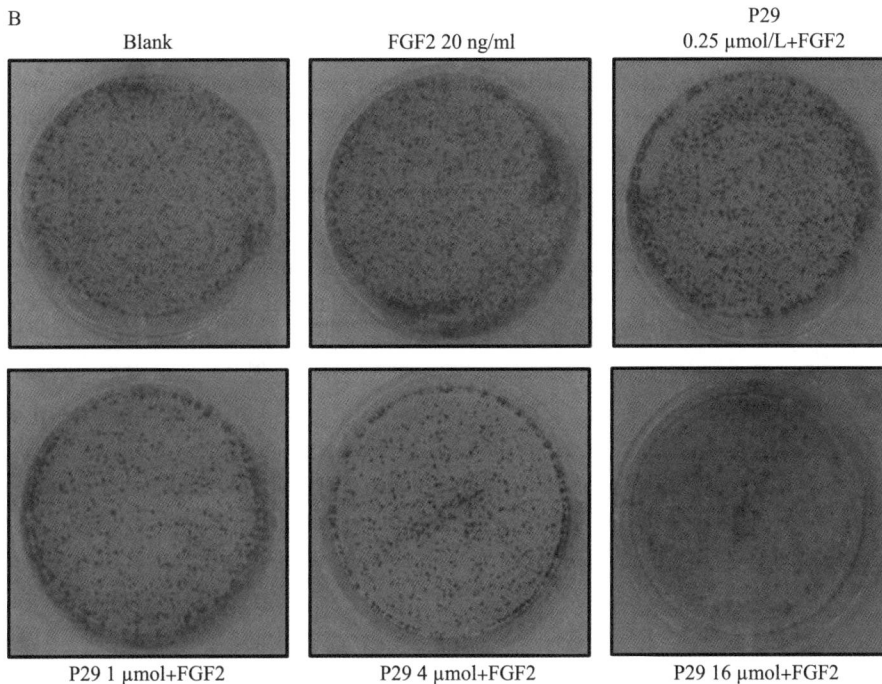

Fig. 5. Effect of peptidomimetic P29 on FGF2-stimulated proliferation of KATO III and MGC803 cells. (A) Two types of cells were treated with 20 ng/ml FGF2 plus P29 at various concentrations (0.25, 1, 4, and 16 μmol/L) after starving for 24 h. Cell proliferation was measured 48 h later by means of MTT assay. Data are presented as the mean ± SD of three independent experiments performed in triplicate. (B) P29 suppressed FGF2-induced colony formation of KATO III cells. FGF2, fibroblast growth factor 2.

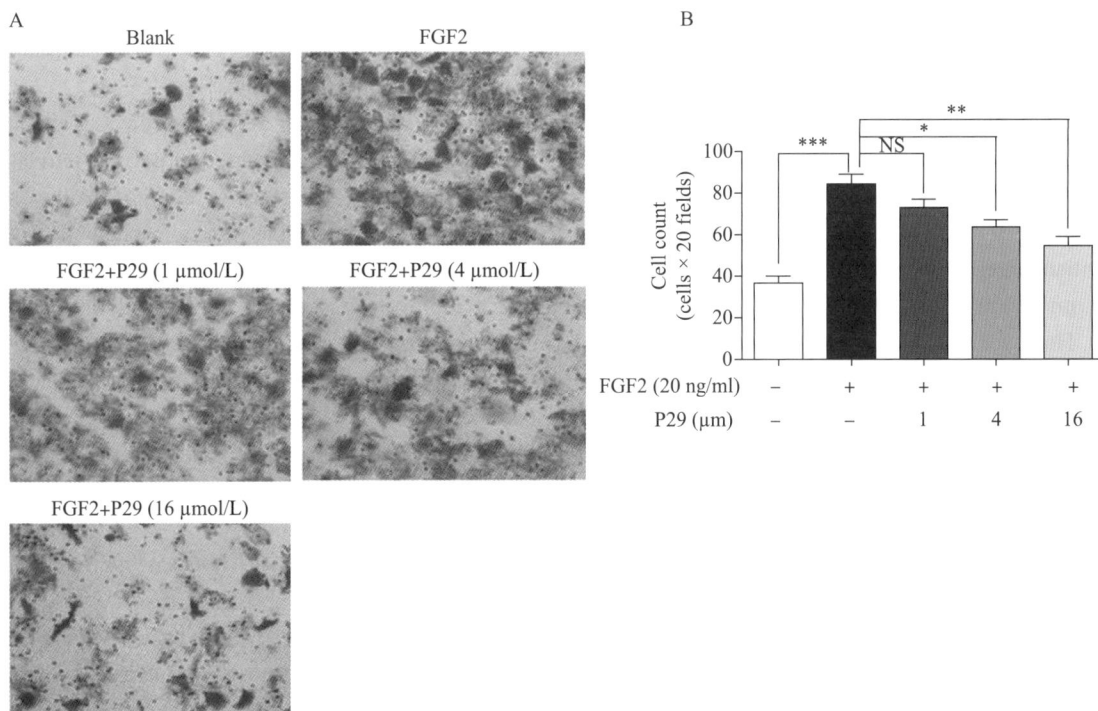

Fig. 6. Effect of peptidomimetic P29 on FGF2-stimulated invasion of MGC803 cells. (A) Starved cells were treated with 20 ng/ml FGF2 plus P29 at the indicated concentrations or with 20 ng/ml FGF2 alone for 24 h. A blank group treated with sterile water served as the control group. Harvested cells were placed on a slide and counted using a fluorescence microscope in 20 × 20 fields. (B) Statistical analysis of the cell amount of each group in 20 × 20 fields. Bars are mean values ± SD from 90 cells from three independent experiments. $^*P < 0.05$, $^{**}P < 0.01$, $^{***}P < 0.001$. FGF2, fibroblast growth factor 2; NS, nonsignificant.

comprehensive treatment, chemotherapy serves a crucial function [25]. However, cytotoxic agents, such as paclitaxel and 5-fluorouracil, which can cause numerous severe adverse effects, have been applied as chemotherapeutics for most GC patients [26]. In addition, target therapy has been used in oncotherapy over the past decades. CKs are closely associated with tumorigenesis, and GC development and can thus be a potent therapeutic target for GC [2,3]. For instance, VEGF expression can indicate a poor prognosis of GC [27], and VEGF can serve as an efficient therapeutic target for GC [4]. Moreover, c-met [28] and HER2 [29] are identified as potent targets for GC treatment. As a type of CK, FGF2 is a potential therapeutic target for GC [15].

FGF2 is a member of the FGF family and is involved in the development, angiogenesis, and metastasis of diverse tumor types [8,10–12]. FGF2 can distinctly enhance the proliferation and angiogenesis of the oophoroma [11]. Overexpression of FGF2 is frequently observed in squamous cell carcinoma, and the abnormal activation of FGF2 signals may provide a novel method for the early diagnosis of squamous cell carcinoma [8]. In non-small-cell lung cancer, FGF2 is perceived as an indicator of metastasis-free survival or overall survival, and high plasma FGF2 level is closely related to poor outcomes [9]. FGF2 level is associated with higher tumor micro-vessel density in liver cancer [12]. For GC, a previous study highlighted that FGF2 mRNA expression was observed in 64% of cancerous tissues but in only 10% of noncancerous tissues. The expression level of FGF2 mRNA can also be a useful parameter for patient prognosis [30]. Another article indicated that FGF2 can accelerate the proliferation and angiogenesis of GC and be involved in GC invasion and metastasis [31].

In this study, we confirmed that FGF2 accelerated the proliferation of GC cells and strengthened the invasive capability of GC cells. We analyzed the functional mechanism of FGF2 in GC and found that FGF2 could activate ERK1/2 or AKT and promote a change in the cell cycle from the G0/G1 phase to the S phase by upregulation of cyclin D1. The ERK1/2 signaling pathway is known to be involved in cell proliferation, whereas the AKT signaling pathway mediates cell survival. It suggests that FGF2 is a potential target for GC treatment. The FGF2 inhibitor suramin exhibited an inhibitory effect on the growth of GC cells and a promoting effect on the differentiation of GC cells [32]. Nevertheless, further research on suramin and GC was not conducted, and few studies reported a drug specifically targeting FGF2 for GC. Hence, a working drug specifically targeting FGF2 for GC therapy is necessary. In this study, P29 decreased MAPK signaling by blocking the phosphorylation of FRS2, decreasing the level of cyclin D1, and arresting the cell cycle at the G0/G1 phase, thereby resulting in the inhibitory effect on GC cell proliferation and colony formation. P29 can downregulate the activation of AKT, consequently weakening the survival capability of GC cells. P29 can also inhibit GC cell invasion. Therefore, P29 is expected to be a promising drug targeting FGF2 for GC therapy.

Given the importance of FGF2 in cancers, studies on FGF2 antagonists have been receiving considerable attention in the field of oncotherapy. Suramin is a well-known FGF2 inhibitor that has been reported in several articles for its good antitumor effect and has been used in clinical trials for multiple cancers [19]. PI-88 is an inhibitor that has a highly reproducible sulfonated oligosaccharide mixture and can compete with heparin sulfate in binding to FGF to execute potent antiangiogenic and antimetastatic effects [17]. A phase I clinical trial on PI-88 in melanoma provided adequate evidence to proceed to a phase II clinical trial [16]. A phase II trial on melanoma suggested that further study is warranted for PI-88 [18]. However, the studies on PI-88 in melanoma are terminated in phase II trials. In addition to the aforementioned types of antagonists, other inhibitors, such as thalidomide [33] and 5′-O-tritylinosine (KIN59, a thymidine phosphorylase inhibitor) [34], are also available. However, no FGF2 antagonists have been applied in the clinic because of their toxicity in experiments, poor target selection, and other limitations. Peptide reagents have been considered a viable therapeutic option in cancer therapy over the past few decades for their low toxicity, high activity, and low dose [20], but no study has reported on the peptide inhibitors of FGF2 in GC. Compared with the above inhibitors, P29 is a peptide antagonist that barely kills normal hepatocytes (Supplementary Fig. S3, Supplemental digital content 5, *http://links.lww.com/ACD/A128*).

Our research has focused on the FGF2/FGFR signaling transduction pathway for several years. We used the phage display technique and isolated a heptapeptide called P7 [21]. P7 can inhibit FGF2-induced cell proliferation by arresting the cell cycle at the G0/G1 phase and blocking MAPK signaling in the MDA-MB-231 breast cancer cell line [22], as well as in the melanoma cell line B16-F10 [23] and in K562 cells [24]. However, as a natural peptide, P7 is extremely unstable. Previous literature has suggested that modifying peptides enhances their stability [35]. Accordingly, we modified the second amino acid residue of P7 from L-type to D-type to achieve the optimization of the lead peptide, and we obtained the peptidomimetic P29. Compared with P7, P29 exhibited a longer half-time of ~ 10 h and was more stable.

5. Conclusion

FGF2, as a significant CK in GC, could accelerate GC cell proliferation and migration. However, P29, as a peptidomimetic derived from P7, could block the effect of FGF2 and induce an enhanced antitumor effect in GC *in vitro*. As a modified peptidomimetic, P29 is not only stable but is also nontoxic to normal cells. This study provides sufficient evidence that FGF2 could be regarded as a therapeutic target for GC and that P29 may be a novel approach for GC treatment.

Supplemental digital content

Supplemental digital content to this article can be found on the journal's website (doi: 10.1097/CAD.0000000000000312).

References

[1] Alberts SR, Cervantes A, van de Velde CJH. Gastric cancer: epidemiology, pathology and treatment[J]. Annals of Oncology, 2003, 14: 31-36.

[2] Tahara E. Abnormal Growth Factor/Cytokine Network in Gastric Cancer[J]. Cancer Microenvironment, 2008, 1(1): 85-91.

[3] Amram ML, Benamran DA, Roth AD. Targeted therapies in digestive oncology[J]. Revue medicale suisse, 2011, 7(296): 1131-1132, 1134-1136.

[4] Fushida S, Oyama K, Kinoshita J, et al. VEGF is a target molecule for peritoneal metastasis and malignant ascites in gastric cancer: prognostic significance of VEGF in ascites and efficacy of anti-VEGF monoclonal antibody[J]. Oncotargets and Therapy, 2013, 6: 1445-1451.

[5] Liu MY, Wang WF, Hou YT, et al. Fibroblast growth factor (FGF)-21 regulates glucose uptake through GLUT1 translocation[J]. African Journal of Microbiology Research, 2012, 6(10): 2504-2511.

[6] Beenken A, Mohammadi M. The FGF family: biology, pathophysiology and therapy[J]. Nature Reviews Drug Discovery, 2009, 8(3): 235-253.

[7] Manetti F, Corelli F, Botta M. Fibroblast growth factors and their inhibitors[J]. Current Pharmaceutical Design, 2000, 6(18): 1897-1924.

[8] Behrens C, Lin HY, Lee JJ, et al. Immunohistochemical Expression of Basic Fibroblast Growth Factor and Fibroblast Growth Factor Receptors 1 and 2 in the Pathogenesis of Lung Cancer[J]. Clinical Cancer Research, 2008, 14(19): 6014-6022.

[9] Rades D, Setter C, Dahl O, et al. Fibroblast growth factor 2 – a predictor of outcome for patients irradiated for stage II-III non-small-cell lung cance[J]. International Journal of Radiation Oncology Biology Physics, 2012, 82(1): 442-447.

[10] Marzioni D, Lorenzi T, Mazzucchelli R, et al. Expression of basic fibroblast growth factor, its receptors and syndecans in bladder cancer[J]. International Journal of Immunopathology and Pharmacology, 2009, 22(3): 627-638.

[11] Lin W, Peng Z-l, Zheng A, et al. The effect of basic fibroblast growth factor in ovarian cancer growth and angiogenesis[J]. Chinese J Med Genet, 2003, 20(6): 532-535.

[12] El-Assal ON, Yamanoi A, Ono T, et al. The clinicopathological significance of heparanase and basic fibroblast growth factor expressions in hepatocellular carcinoma[J]. Clinical Cancer Research, 2001, 7(5): 1299-1305.

[13] Luo J-C, Lin H-Y, Lu C-L, et al. Dexamethasone inhibits basic fibroblast growth factor-stimulated gastric epithelial cell proliferation[J]. Biochemical Pharmacology, 2008, 76(7): 841-849.

[14] Ueki T, Koji T, Tamiya S, et al. Expression of basic fibroblast growth factor and fibroblast growth factor receptor in advanced gastric carcinoma[J]. Journal of Pathology, 1995, 177(4): 353-361.

[15] Noda M, Hattori T, Kimura T, et al. Expression of fibroblast growth factor 2 mRNA in early and advanced gastric cancer[J]. Acta Oncologica, 1997, 36(7): 695-700.

[16] Basche M, Gustafson DL, Holden SN, et al. A phase I biological and pharmacologic study of the heparanase inhibitor PI-88 in patients with advanced solid tumors[J]. Clinical Cancer Research, 2006, 12(18): 5471-5480.

[17] Chow LQM, Gustafson DL, O'Bryant CL, et al. A phase I pharmacological and biological study of PI-88 and docetaxel in patients with advanced malignancies[J]. Cancer Chemotherapy and Pharmacology, 2008, 63(1): 65-74.

[18] Lewis KD, Robinson WA, Millward MJ, et al. A phase II study of the heparanase inhibitor PI-88 in patients with advanced melanoma[J]. Investigational New Drugs, 2008, 26(1): 89-94.

[19] Ord JJ, Streeter E, Jones A, et al. Phase I trial of intravesical Suramin in recurrent superficial transitional cell bladder carcinoma[J]. British Journal of Cancer, 2005, 92(12): 2140-2147.

[20] Ho HK, Yeo AHL, Kang TS, et al. Current strategies for inhibiting FGFR activities in clinical applications: opportunities, challenges and toxicological considerations[J]. Drug Discovery Today, 2014, 19(1): 51-62.

[21] Wu X, Yan Q, Huang Y, et al. Isolation of a novel basic FGF-binding peptide with potent antiangiogenetic activity[J]. Journal of Cellular & Molecular Medicine, 2010, 14(1-2): 351-356.

[22] Li Q, Gao S, Yu Y, et al. A novel bFGF antagonist peptide inhibits breast cancer cell growth[J]. Molecular Medicine Reports, 2012, 6(1): 210-214.

[23] Yu Y, Gao S, Li Q, et al. The FGF2-binding peptide P7 inhibits melanoma growth *in vitro* and *in vivo*[J]. Journal of Cancer Research and Clinical Oncology, 2012, 138(8): 1321-1328.

[24] Wang C, Yu Y, Li Q, et al. P7 peptides suppress the proliferation of K562 cells induced by basic fibroblast growth factor[J]. Tumor Biology, 2012, 33(4): 1085-1093.

[25] Cervantes A, Roda D, Tarazona N, et al. Current questions for the treatment of advanced gastric cancer[J]. Cancer Treatment Reviews, 2013, 39(1): 60-67.

[26] Fujitani K. Overview of Adjuvant and Neoadjuvant Therapy for

Resectable Gastric Cancer in the East[J]. Digestive Surgery, 2013, 30(2): 119-129.

[27] Yin L, Wang X, Luo C, *et al*. The Value of Expression of M2-PK and VEGF in Patients with Advanced Gastric Cancer[J]. Cell Biochemistry and Biophysics, 2013, 67(3): 1033-1039.

[28] Teng L, Lu J. cMET as a potential therapeutic target in gastric cancer[J]. International Journal of Molecular Medicine, 2013, 32(6): 1247-1254.

[29] Bouche O, Penault-Llorca F. HER2 and gastric cancer: a novel therapeutic target for trastuzumab[J]. Bulletin Du Cancer, 2010, 97(12): 1429-1440.

[30] Zhang W, Chu Y-Q, Ye Z-Y, *et al*. Expression of Hepatocyte Growth Factor and Basic Fibroblast Growth Factor as Prognostic Indicators in Gastric Cancer[J]. Anatomical Record-Advances in Integrative Anatomy and Evolutionary Biology, 2009, 292(8): 1114-1121.

[31] Ru G-Q, Zhao Z-S, Tang Q-L, *et al*. mRNA expression of basic fibroblast growth factor and hepatocyte growth factor in gastric car-

cinoma and significance thereof[J]. Zhonghua yi xue za zhi, 2008, 88(29): 2030-2035.

[32] Choe G, Kim WH, Park J-G, *et al*. Effect of suramin on differentiation of human stomach cancer cell lines[J]. Journal of Korean Medical Science, 1997, 12(5): 433-442.

[33] Mei S-C, Wu R-T. The G-rich promoter and G-rich coding sequence of basic fibroblast growth factor are the targets of thalidomide in glioma[J]. Molecular Cancer Therapeutics, 2008, 7(8): 2405-2414.

[34] Liekens S, Bronckaers A, Belleri M, *et al*. The Thymidine Phosphorylase Inhibitor 5 '-O-Tritylinosine (KIN59) Is an Antiangiogenic Multitarget Fibroblast Growth Factor-2 Antagonist[J]. Molecular Cancer Therapeutics, 2012, 11(4): 817-829.

[35] Gentilucci L, de Marco R, Cerisoli L. Chemical Modifications Designed to Improve Peptide Stability: Incorporation of Non-Natural Amino Acids, Pseudo-Peptide Bonds, and Cyclization[J]. Current Pharmaceutical Design, 2010, 16(28): 3185-3203.

Attenuating endogenous Fgfr2b ligands during bleomycin-induced lung fibrosis does not compromise murine lung repair

BreAnne MacKenzie, Xiaokun Li,Saverio Bellusci

The interstitial lung disease idiopathic pulmonary fibrosis (IPF) occurs between the sixth and seventh decades of life at a rate of 2–4/10 000 [21]. The 5-year survival rates approximate just 10%–15% [21]. The pathomechanism of IPF is not yet fully understood; however, it is thought to occur as a result of chronic epithelial injury or stress, resulting in the accumulation of myofibroblasts that express high levels of extracellular matrix [19]. Genetic manipulation of lung development pathways in the context of bleomycin-lung injury, including Notch, transforming growth factorβ (Tgfβ), bone morphogenetic protein (Bmp), Sonic hedgehog (Shh), fibroblast growth factors (Fgfs), epidermal growth factor (Egf), and winglesstype MMTV integration site family (Wnt), combined with results based on studies using IPF patient materials, have led to the development of potential therapeutic treatments for IPF [31, 38].

Fgf7 and Fgf10 signal in a paracrine fashion *via* epithelially expressed Fgfr2b receptor [43]. The signal results in a phosphorylation cascade, mediated by fibroblast growth factor receptor substrate (Frs2), which activates PI3K-and MAPKsignaling pathways and/or activation of phospholipase Cγ (Plcγ). Depending on the cell type and context, Fgfr2b signaling culminates in survival, growth, and differentiation of epithelial cells. Fgf10/Fgfr2b signaling is critical for murine lung development whereas Fgf7 is dispensable [3, 16, 27]. Fgfs have been reported to act upstream of Wnt signaling [23]. Interestingly, bleomycin-injured mice with epithelial-specific deletion of β-catenin signaling, a downstream target of both Fgf[23] and Wnt signaling [26], suffered increased fibrosis [37]. Although Wnt signaling was previously thought to play an exclusively profibrotic role by mediating epithelial-to-mesenchymal transition (EMT), this report revealed the importance of β catenin-mediated protection of epithelial cells against bleomycin injury.

In the bleomycin mouse model, past studies have focused primarily on the beneficial effect of prophylactic treatment with palifermin, a pharmacological agent composed of a truncated form of keratinocyte growth factor (KGF), also known as FGF7 [7, 36]. Although palifermin demonstrated a protective, prophylactic effect, genetic *Fgf10* expression postbleomycin injury [11] resulted in increased survival as well as prevention and accelerated resolution of lung fibrosis in mice. Although current therapies target tyrosine kinases for the treatment of IPF [2], whether endogenous FGF signaling plays a protective, pathogenic, or ambivalent role in IPF is still unknown. Given the beneficial effects of exogenous Fgfr2b ligands on lung repair, the authors hypothesized that endogenous Fgfr2b ligands play a critical role in repair following bleomycin injury. However, endogenous Fgfr2b ligands as well as Fgfr2b receptor expression, were decreased following bleomycin injury in wild-type mice. Thus, unsurprisingly, attenuating endogenous Fgfr2b ligands during bleomycin-induced lung injury did not lead to significantly increased fibrosis or decreased survival. In summary, although endogenous Fgfr2b ligand signaling failed to play a critical role in limiting fibrosis, these results do not negate the potential benefit of exogenously stimulating developmental pathways to protect against lung fibrosis.

1. Methods

1.1 Animal care

All experiments were performed in accordance with the National Institutes of Health Guidelines for the Use of Laboratory Animals. Animal experiments were approved by the Institutional Animal Care and Use Committee at Children's Hospital Los Angeles protocol 193-12 and the Federal Authorities for Animal Research of the Regierungspraesidium Giessen, Hessen, Germany, protocols 72/ 2012 and 73/2012.

1.2 Generation of mice

CMV-Cre mice [33] were crossed with *rtTA^flox^* mice [4] to generate mice expressing *rtTA* under the ubiquitous *Rosa26* promoter. This constitutive *Rosa26^rtTA/+^* mouse line was then crossed with the *tet(O)solFgfr2b/+* responder line to generate *Rosa26^rtTA/+^;tet(O)sFgfr2b/+* double-heterozygous animals, allowing ubiquitous expression of dominant-negative soluble Fgfr2b (28). All mice were generated on a CD1 mixed background. Attenuation of Fgfr2b ligand activity was achieved by administration of doxycyclinecontaining food; normal rodent diet with 0.0625% doxy-cycline (Har-lan Teklad). *Tet(O)Cre* [*B6.Cg-Tg(tetO-cre)1Jaw/J*] [30] and *Tomatof^lox/flox^* reporter mice [*B6;129S6-Gt(ROSA)26Sortm9(CAG-tdTomato) Hze/J*] [24] were purchased from Jackson Laboratory. Mice were genotyped as described previously [4, 12, 34].

1.3 Bleomycin administration

Female mice 10–14 wk old were anesthetized with a mixture of 0.6 µl/g ketamine 10% (100 mg/ml) and 0.3 µl/g Domitor 10% (0.5 mg/ml) dissolved in 0.7% saline. A microsprayer (PennCentury) was used to administer an intratracheal dose of either 0.7% saline or bleomycin (1.0–3.0 U/kg) (Hexal or SigmaAldrich). Weight, activity, respiration, and temperature was monitored daily and mice were euthanized if they showed a significant decline in health parameters.

1.4 Lung compliance measurement

Mice were deeply anesthetized with a mixture of 1.2 µl/g ketamine 10% (100 mg/ml, Bela Pharm), 0.6 µl/g Domitor 10% (0.5 mg/ml; Orion), 1 : 4 parts heparin, and dissolved in saline. Lung function was measured by using the SCIREQ flexiVent forced-oscillation plethysmograph to give an overall readout of lung function. Mice were intubated transtracheally and ventilated at a rate of 150 breaths/min with a positive end-expiratory pressure (PEEP) between 1 and 3 cmH$_2$O. PEEP was calculated automatically by flexiVent 7 software and was dependent on the weight of the animal. After stable ventilation was achieved (spontaneous breathing ceased as the heart continued to beat), a 3 s, weightdependent, fixed-volume waveform was initiated every 15–20 s, eight times. During this perturbation, "snapshots" of respiratory compliance were taken and the average of eight measurements represented the value of one biological sample.

1.5 Left lobe perfusion and isolation

The left lobe was perfused from 22–24 cm above the mouse for 1 min with PBS followed by 2 min with 4% para-formaldehyde (PFA). The trachea was tied off with a string, and the lung was removed and placed in 4% PFA for at least 24 h at room temperature or up to 1 wk at 4℃. Lungs were then embedded with a Leica embedding machine (EG 1150C). Paraffin blocks were kept cold and 3-to 4-µm sections were cut.

1.6 Hematoxylin and eosin

Three-to 4-µm sections were deparaffinized, dipped in water, and stained in Mayer's hematoxylin solution for 1–3 min and washed under running tap water for up to 10 min. Slides were monitored under the microscope for staining progression. Slides were then incubated for 2 min in eosin dye and brought back through increasing gradients of ethanol and xylene, then coverslipped with Pertex mounting medium.

1.7 Masson's trichrome stain

Three-to 4-µm sections were deparaffinized and stained with Gomori's Green Trichrome Stain Kit (Dako AR166) according to manufacturer's protocol.

1.8 Lung morphometry

For alveolar morphometry, lungs were flushed with PBS at a vascular pressure of 20 cmH$_2$O. Then PBS was infused *via* the trachea at a pressure of 20 cmH$_2$O and fixed with 4% paraformaldehyde in PBS (pH 7.0) *via* the trachea at a pressure of 20 cmH$_2$O. Investigations were performed with 5-µm sections of paraffin-embedded left lobe of the lungs. The mean linear intercept, mean air space, and mean septal wall thickness were measured after staining with hematoxylin and eosin (H/E). Total scans from the left lobe were analyzed by using a Leica DM6000B microscope with an automated stage according to the procedure previously described [25, 42] which was implemented into the Qwin V3 software (Leica, Wetzlar, Germany). Horizontal lines (distance 40 μm) were placed across each lung section. The number of times the lines cross alveolar walls was calculated by multiplying the length of the horizontal lines and the number of lines per section then dividing by the number of intercepts. Bronchi and vessels above 50 μm in diameter were excluded prior to the computerized measurement. The air space was determined as the nonparenchyma, nonstained area. The septal wall thickness was measured as the length of the line perpendicularly crossing a septum. From the respective measurements, mean values were calculated.

1.9 Fibrosis quantification on histological sections

Ashcroft scoring was performed blinded by using a modified Ashcroft scoring protocol (as described in Ref. 14) on H/E-stained sections of murine left lobes. Traditionally, multiple ×20 images are scored; however, we imaged stained left lobes with light microscopy at the lowest objective (×1.25), which allowed for visualization of the entire section. ImageJ software was used to measure the area of the lung that was covered in confluent fibrotic mass (data are presented as % confluent fibrosis per total area of the section). Sections were measured blindly, a total of three times, and scores were averaged.

1.10 Hydroxyproline assay

QuickZyme total collagen assay was performed according to manufacturer's instructions. Briefly, either cranial and accessory or caudal and medial lobes were extracted, rinsed briefly in PBS, and dried overnight in a ventilated hood. Lungs were weighed and 6 M HCl was added for a final concentration of 50 mg tissue/ml. Lungs and collagen standards were then incubated for 20 h overnight at 95 ℃ and cooled to room temperature. Next, tubes were centrifuged at 13 000 g for 10 min. Hydrolyzed supernatant was diluted 10-fold with 4 M HCl and used for the assay. A microplate reader (Tecan Infinite 200 PRO) was used for color detection. A standard curve was calculated from the collagen standards and the total hydroxyproline content was assessed.

1.11 RNA extraction

After lung function measurements were taken, the right bronchus was clamped and either cranial and accessory or caudal and medial lobes were removed, placed in TRIzol, homogenized in GentleMACs, and frozen in liquid nitrogen for RNA extraction. Next, transcardiac perfusion of the left lobe was performed with a 20-G needle and 15 ml PBS.

1.12 Western blot

Loading buffer was added to protein samples from cell extracts (5% SDS in bromophenol blue and β mercaptoethanol) denatured for 5 min at 95 ℃ and cooled on ice. At least 10 μg of sample was loaded on a 10% polyacrylamide gel and run at 25 mA per gel for ~2 h. Samples were then electrically transferred to a polyvinylidene fluoride membrane (Amersham) by semidry electroblotting (70 mA per gel; gel size 7 × 9 cm) for 90 min. The membrane was blocked with 5% milk in Tris-buffered saline (TBS) blocking buffer at room temperature on shaker for 1 h followed by incubation with primary antibody: COL1a1 (Meridian no. T47770R), FGF1 (Abcam no. ab9588 1 : 2 000), FGF7 (Santa Cruz no. sc27126 1 : 200), FGF10 (Abcam no. ab71794, 1 : 200), Col1a1 (Meridian no. T40777R, 1 : 1 000, 8% gel), SPRY2 (Santa Cruz no. sc10082, 1 : 200), SPRY4 (Santa Cruz no. sc30051, 1 : 200), FGFR1 (Santa Cruz no. sc-121, 1 : 200), FGFR2 (Santa Cruz no. sc-122, 1 : 200), p-ERK1/2 (Cell Signaling no. 4370S; 1 : 1 000), total ERK1/2 (Cell Signaling no. 9102S; 1 : 1 000), p-Akt total (Cell Signaling no. 4060S, 1 : 1 000), total-Akt (Cell Signaling no. 4691S, 1 : 3 000), βactin (Abcam no. ab8227; 1 : 30 000), and GAPDH (Cell Signaling no. cs2118, 1 : 1 000) overnight at 4 ℃. After washing with 1× TBS and Tween 20 (TBS-T) four times for 15 min each, the membrane was incubated with swine antirabbit horseradish peroxidase (Dako no. P0217) secondary antibody (dilution 1 : 2 000) at room temperature for 1 h followed by four times washing with 1× TBS-T buffer for 15 min each. The protein bands were detected by ECL (Enhanced Chemiluminescence, Amersham) treatment, followed by exposure of the membrane.

1.13 Quantitative PCR

RNA was reverse transcribed (Qiagen QuantiTect Reverse Transcription Kit, no. 205313). cDNA was diluted to a concentration between 20 ng/μl. Primers were designed by use of Roche Applied Sciences online Assay Design Tool. All primers were designed to span introns and were blasted by using NCBI software for specificity. SYBRGreen Master

Mix (Applied Biosciences 4309155) was used for RT-PCR with a Roche LightCycler 480 machine. Samples were run in triplicate with *Hprt* as reference genes for mouse samples.

1.14 FACS

Accessory and caudal lobes were isolated in ice-cold Hanks' balanced salt solution (HBSS). Next, lobes were chopped finely using sterile razor blades and transferred to a 10-ml solution of 0.5% collagenase in HBSS. Then solution was heated to 37°C on a hot plate and stirred on high for 60 min. Next the dissociated homogenate was passed through 18-G, 20-G, 24-G needles, respectively, then filtered through 70-μm and 40-μm filters. One volume HBSS was added to dilute collagenase and homogenates were centrifuged at 1 500 rpm for 5 min to remove the enzyme solution. Cells were then resuspended in 500 μl 0.5% FCS in PBS and stained with anti-red fluorescent protein (RFP) pAb rabbit, Life Technologies, R10367 (1 : 200) for 20 min at 4°C, followed by washing and flow cytometric analysis with LSR Fortessa equipped with FACSDiva software (BD Bioscience).

1.15 Statistical analyses

One-way ANOVA was performed on densitometry plots of Western blots followed by a Dunnett's test of significance. A Student's *t*-test was performed on the log-transformed value of the qPCR fold changes as well as compliance, hydroxyproline, and confluent areas of fibrosis measurements. For FACS analyses, *t*-tests were performed on the probit values. A binomial significance test was used to determine the statistical significance of soluble Fgfr2b detection. Conformity of the data with the assumptions of the tests was checked with residual analysis.

2. Results

2.1 Modest recruitment of the Fgf-signaling pathway during spontaneous repair initiated by bleomycin-induced lung injury in mice

To investigate whether the endogenous Fgf-signaling pathway is recruited during bleomycin-induced lung injury, CD1 mice were given 1 U/kg bleomycin or saline intratracheally. This bleomycin dose generates robust fibrosis and gives a survival rate of 100% at 28 dpi in CD1 mice (Fig. 1A). Mice were euthanized at given time points according to weight loss to ensure maximal survival to 28 dpi (Fig. 1B). Injury was confirmed in each mouse by lung compliance measurements (Fig. 1C), calculation of confluent fibrotic areas of H/E-stained left lobes (Fig. 1D), hydroxyproline deposition (Fig. 1E), Masson's trichrome staining (Fig. 1, F–J), and Col1a1 Western blotting of whole lung homogenate (Fig. 1K, L). In this model, bleomycin-induced lung injury peaked between 14 and 21 days postinjury (dpi). An additional model using historical controls (5 U/kg, C57BL/6 females) was also used to comparatively evaluate Fgf-signaling targets and mRNA expression, and similar results were obtained (data not shown).

Next, Western blots were performed on Fgfr2b ligands, receptors, and downstream signaling targets on lung homogenate lysates isolated from animals 7, 14, 21, and 28 days after bleomycin injury or 2 wk after saline administration. Col1a1 expression was used as an indicator of fibrotic injury and most strongly expressed at 14 dpi and slightly reduced thereafter (Fig. 1K, L). Fgf ligands were decreased for the most part following injury with the exception of Fgf10, which was slightly elevated compared with Fgf1 and Fgf7 at 14 dpi (Fig. 1K, L). Fgfr1 and Fgfr2 expression increased significantly following injury. Importantly, qPCR analyses indicated that Fgfr11b, Fgfr2c, and Fgfr1c isoforms were increased although Fgfr2b remained decreased (Fig. 1M). Spry2, a negative regulator of MAPK signaling in the epithelium was decreased following injury, though expression was increased at 28 dpi (Fig. 1K, L). Spry4, a negative regulator of MAPK signaling in the cells of mesenchymal origin (lung fibroblasts) was slightly elevated at 21 and 28 dpi (Fig. 1K, L). Etv-4, a downstream target of Fgf10 signaling, also known as Pea-3, was strongly induced following injury (Fig. 1K, L). Lastly, general MAPK-signaling targets, which are also targets of Fgf signaling were evaluated. At 7 dpi, p-Akt was slightly increased and again strongly activated at 28 dpi (Fig. 1K, L). The marker p-Erk1 peaked at 14 dpi and decreased at 28 dpi (Fig. 1K, L), whereas p-Erk2 was not significantly regulated (Fig. 1K, L). Compared with mice injured with a higher dose of bleomycin (5 U/kg, data not shown), p-Akt signaling was similarly regulated. It was strongly induced 3–4 wk following injury (Fig. 1K, L). In addition, p-Erk1 and p-Erk2 were moderately regulated in both models.

In summary, during spontaneous repair after bleomycin injury in wild-type mice, Fgf10 expression was moderately increased along with receptor Fgfr1b and downstream targets Spry2, Etv4, and p-Akt at 28 dpi. The endogenous epithelial-expressed Fgfr2b receptor was drastically reduced following bleomycin injury (Fig. 1M) and began to recover expression at 21 dpi, whereas c-isoform expression remained significantly elevated. The significance and contribution of the Fgf10/ Fgfr1b-signaling axis to lung repair is still elusive and will require further investigation.

2.2　Validation of the Rosa26$^{rtTA/+}$;tet(O)sFgfr2b/+ transgenic line

To test whether the attenuation of all Fgfr2b ligands would result in increased fibrosis, the Rosa26$^{rtTA/+}$;tet(O)sFgfr2b/+; in this study referred to as the double-transgenic (DTG) mouse line was used [28] (Fig. 2A). The Rosa26 promoter drives ubiquitous expression of reverse tetracycline transactivator, which in the presence of doxycycline (dox) binds a tetracycline response sequence. Binding results in the activation of a cytomegalovirus (CMV) promoter, which drives

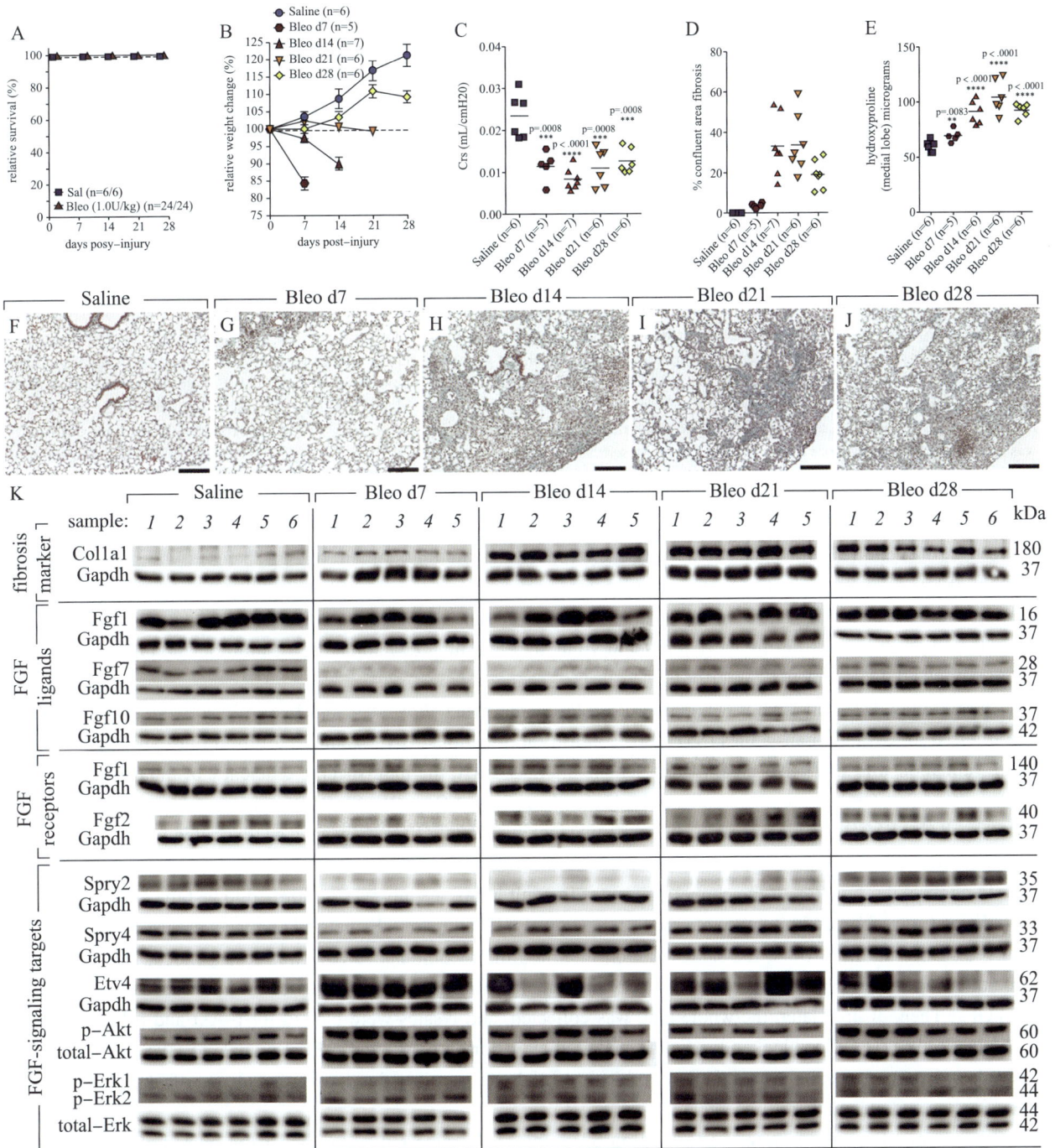

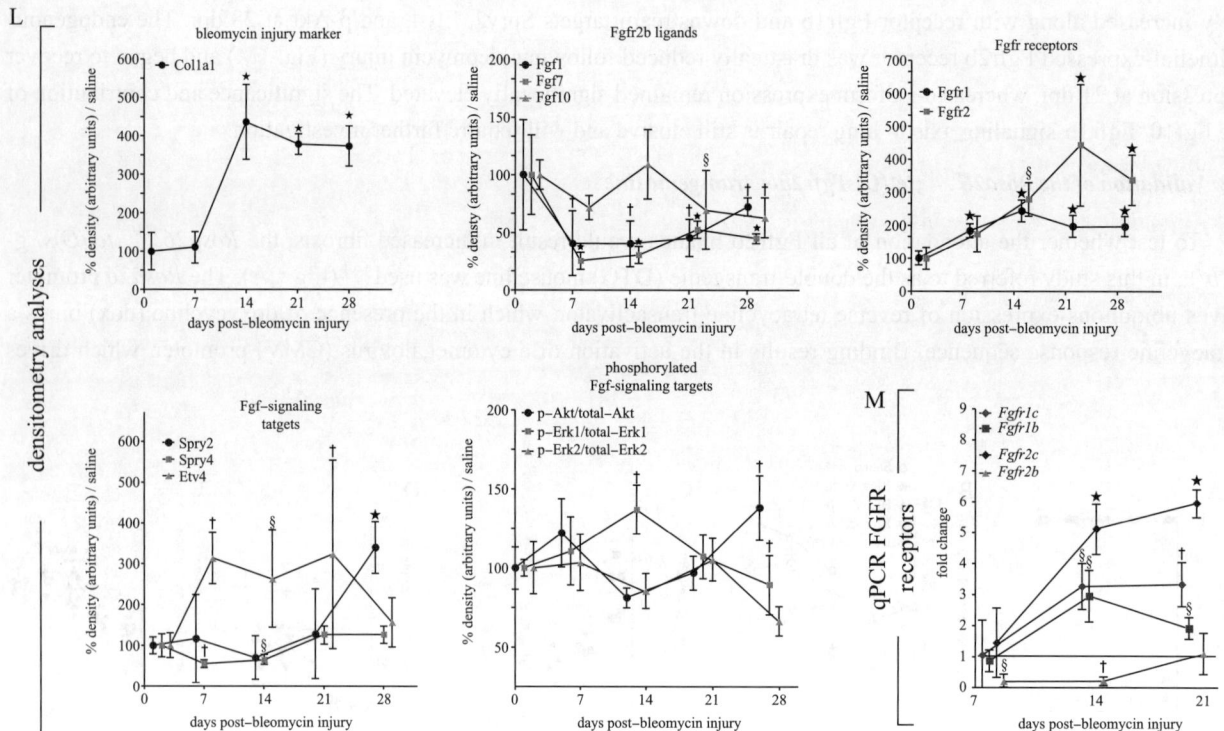

Fig. 1. Fibrosis injury (1 U/kg) peaked between 14 and 21 days postinjury (dpi) in CD1 female, wild-type mice, moderate recruitment of Fgfr2b signaling following injury (Fgfs). (A): survival curve. (B): relative weight change. (C): compliance. (D): quantification of confluent fibrotic areas in hematoxylin and eosin (H/E) stains of left lobes. E: hydroxyproline content of medial lobes. (F)–(J): Masson's trichrome stain of representative time points following injury. (K): Western blots for Fgf-signaling pathway members of saline or bleomycin-treated mice. (L): quantification of blot densities normalized to saline controls (gene of interest divided by control gene) and represented as percent of saline expression. (M): since the Western blot antibodies used do not distinguish between receptor isoforms, qPCR was performed on epithelial (b-isoforms) and mesenchymal cisoforms of Fgfr1 and Fgfr2 receptor. Already at 7 dpi, *Fgfr2b* was significantly reduced and remained so until 21 dpi. At 14 dpi, c-isoforms of both receptors were increased, as well as Fgfr1b. The c-isoforms remained elevated at 21 dpi, while *Fgfr1b* returned to saline levels. One-way ANOVA was performed against control values and error bars represent 95% confidence intervals; $^{§}P < 0.05$; $^{†}P < 0.005$; $^{★}P < 0.0001$. Scale bars: 100 μm.

expression of a chimeric transgene containing the extracellular binding domain of Fgfr2b fused with the heavy chain domain of IgG (Fig. 2A). The line was previously used in the context of naphthalene and hyperoxia lung injury to demonstrate the critical role of Fgfr2b ligands in the lung repair process [12, 13, 39]. In addition, this line was also used to define the role of Fgfr2b ligands during early lung embryonic and late lung development [12], limb development [6], postnatal mammary gland development [29], incisor homeostasis [28], and gut homeostasis [1].

In this study, DTG littermates lacking the *Rosa26^{rtTA/+}* construct [*Rosa26^{+/+};tet(O)sFgfr2b/+*] were used as controls, and referred to as single transgenics (STG). To confirm the functionality of soluble Fgfr2b in our experimental conditions, validation was also performed in adult female animals. First, the lung-specific efficiency of the driver was tested in *Rosa26^{rtTA/+};tet(O)Cre/+;Tomat^{ofl/+}* mice fed +doxfood for 7 days (Fig. 2E, F). RFP expression was detected in ~25% of total cells by FACS and in none of the cells in mice lacking the *tet(O)Cre* transgene as illustrated by fluorescence stereomicroscopy (Fig. 2, B–E″).

To confirm the function of the chimeric receptor in adult lungs, a study was performed to test the ability of induced DTG lungs (+dox food ad libitum) to attenuate exogenous FGF7 signaling. Female STG mice were used as controls and received PBS with 0.1% BSA, the same solution in which the recombinant FGF7 was resuspended. DTG mice were fed either normal food or +dox food for 1 wk. Next, females from each group received an intratracheal dose of 10 μg of rFGF7. Then, 30 min later, the whole lung was collected, and lysates were blotted for p-Akt and p-Erk1/2 signals. Although +dox DTG mice blocked the FGF7-mediated elevation in p-Akt and p-Erk1-signals to levels of PBS-treated controls, p-Erk2 remained elevated. Failure to block p-Erk2 was possibly due to overabundance of FGF7 and resultant signaling *via* endogenous Fgfr2 receptors (Fig. 2, F–H′).

Morphometric analyses were performed on STG and DTG mice fed +dox food from postnatal days (PN) 1 to

PN105(Fig. 2, I–L). The chimeric transcript was detected only in DTG mice (Fig. 2I) and lung compliance remained un-af-fected (Fig. 2J). In concurrence with previous studies [12], morphometric analyses revealed no significant differences in mean linear intercept, air space, or septal wall thickness in DTG mice (Fig. 2K–M). Although no lung defects were present, DTG mice fed +dox food from PN28 to PN88 showed characteristic inhibition of maxillary incisor regeneration (Fig. 2P, P′) [28].

2.3   *Attenuation of Fgfr2b ligands during fibrosis formation postbleomycin injury did not result in increased fibrosis.*

To determine whether endogenous Fgfr2b ligands expedite fibrosis resolution, a relatively low dose of bleomycin (1 U/kg it), which generated between 80 and 100% survival and mild fibrosis at 28 dpi, was used. First, Fgfr2b ligands were attenuated from 6 to 14 dpi (Fig. 3) and next during fibrotic resolution (14 –28 dpi) (Fig. 4). Fgfr2b ligands attenuation had no impact on relative survival (Fig. 3A) though a trend toward delayed weight recovery in DTG mice was observed (Fig. 3B). Specific soluble *Fgfr2b* expression in DTG was confirmed (Fig. 3C). A slight increase in lung compliance was measured at 28 dpi in DTG *vs.* STG (Fig. 3D). Upon histological examination both STG and DTG lungs showed areas of fibrosis (Fig. 3, E and F). However, quantification of the confluent areas of fibrosis in the left lobe did not reveal any difference between DTG and STG (Fig. 3G). In agreement with these results, no differences were observed for total hydroxyproline (Fig. 3H). Together, these results indicate that attenuation of Fgfr2b ligands following bleomycin injury (6–28 dpi) had no impact on fibrosis resolution by 28 dpi.

Although downstream targets were just moderately engaged in wild-type mice injured with either 1.0 U/kg or 5.0 U/kg bleomycin doses, a slightly higher bleomycin dose (2 U/kg it) was administered to our genetically modified mice to test whether endogenous Fgfr2b ligands would play an important role in lung repair following more severe injury. To focus on the contribution of Fgfr2b ligands to the resolution phase, ligands were attenuated from 14 through 28 dpi. No difference in survival rate (Fig. 4A) was observed. The relative weight change between DTG and STG were similar (Fig. 4B). The expression of soluble *Fgfr2b* was detected only in DTG as previously reported (Fig. 4C). No difference in lung function was observed (Fig. 4D). No difference for hydroxyproline deposition between DTG and STG (Fig. 4H) was

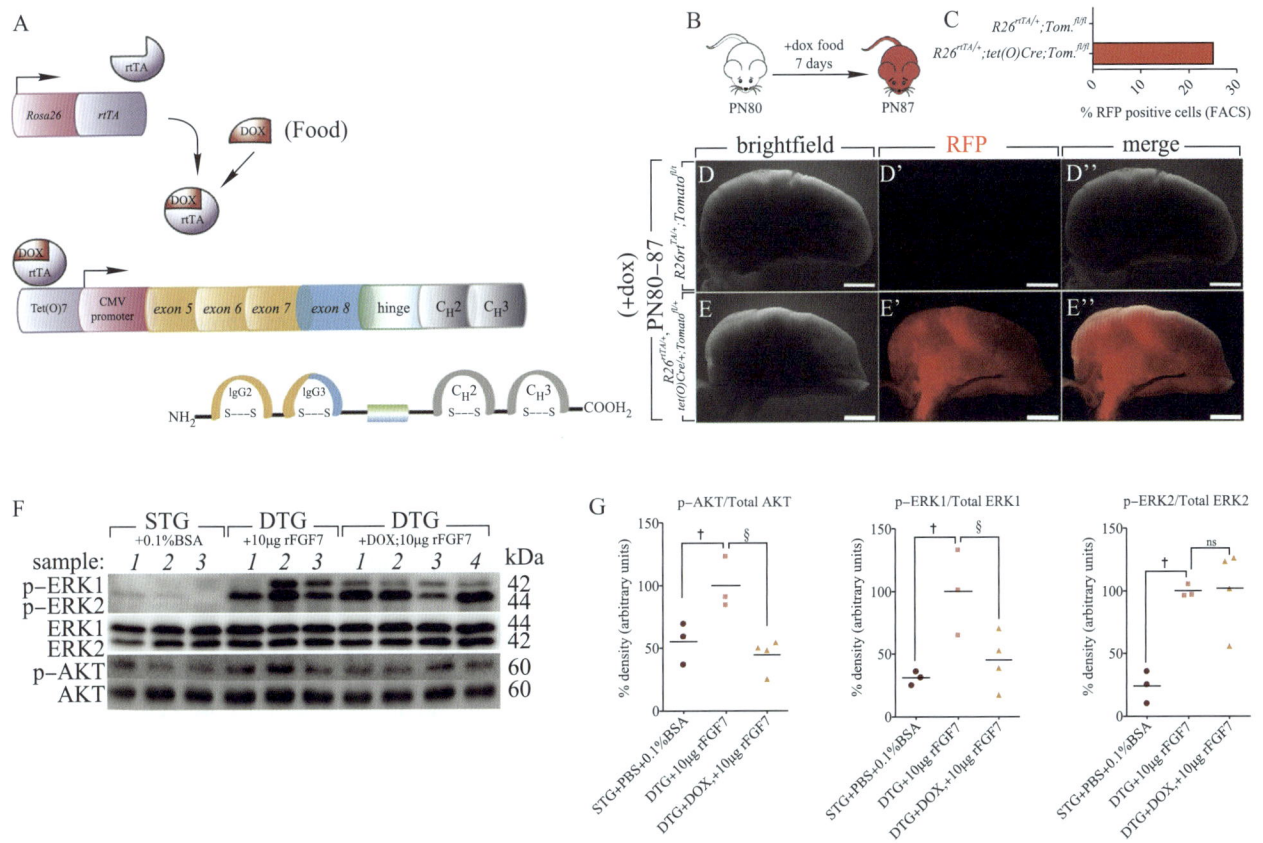

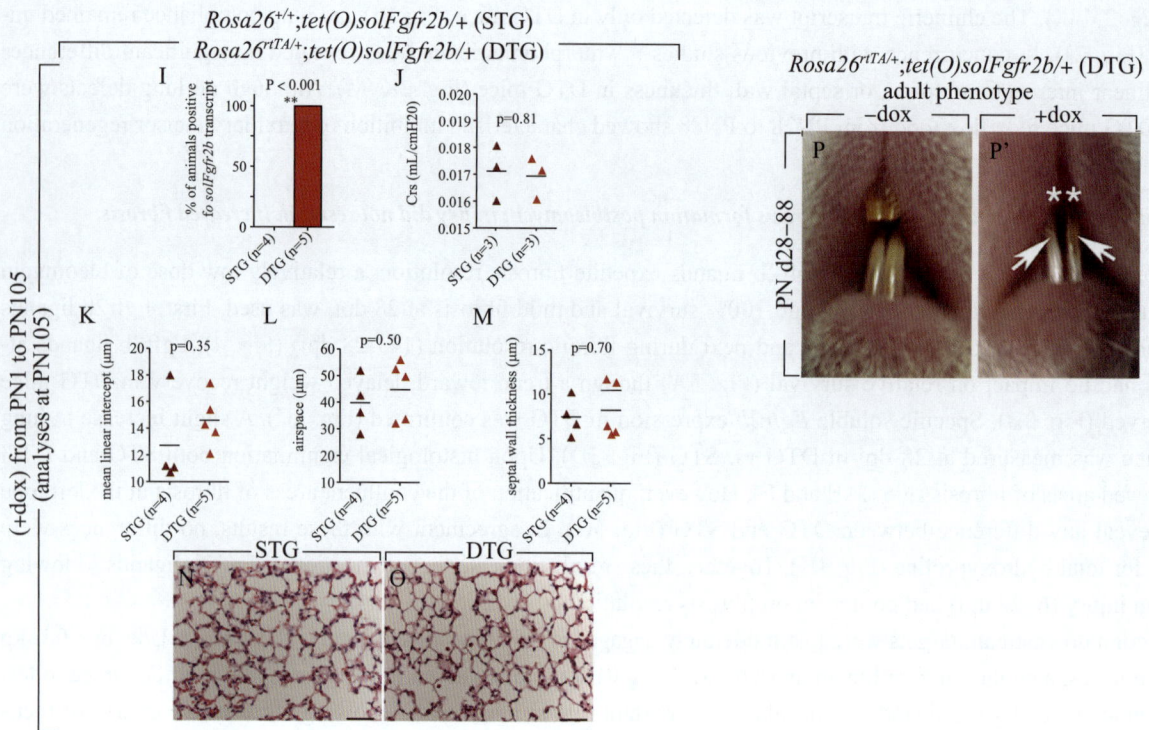

Fig. 2. Validation of *Rosa26^{rtTA/+};tet(O)sFgfr2b/+* [double-transgenic (DTG)] mice. The *Rosa26* promoter drives ubiquitous expression of reverse tetracycline transactivator (rtTA), which in the presence of doxycycline (dox) binds a tetracycline response sequence. Binding results in the activation of a CMV promoter, which drives expression of a chimeric transgene containing the extracellular binding domain of Fgfr2b fused with the heavy chain domain of IgG (A). Lung-specific efficiency of *Rosa26* promoter was tested in *Rosa26^{rtTA/+};tet(O)Cre/+;Tomato^{fl/+}* mice fed +dox-food for 7 days (B and C). Red fluorescent protein (RFP) expression was detected in ~25% of total cells by FACS and in none of the cells in mice lacking the *tet(O)Cre* transgene as illustrated by fluorescence stereomicroscopy (D–E″). Single-transgenic (STG) mice ($n = 3$) received 50 μl of PBS with 0.1% BSA; DTG mice were fed normal food ($n = 3$) or +dox food ($n = 4$) for 1 wk and were given an intratracheal dose of 10 μg of FGF7. At 30 min later, the lysates were collected and blotted for p-Akt and p-Erk1/2 signals (F). +dox DTG mice blocked FGF7-mediated p-Akt (G) and p-Erk1 signals (H), p-ERK2 (H′) remained elevated (F–H′). †Significant; §very significant. The chimeric transcript was detected only in DTG mice (I) and lung compliance was not changed in DTG mice fed +dox food from postnatal day (PN) 1 to PN105 (J). **Very significant. K–O: morphometric analyses were performed on these mice, and in concurrence with previous studies no significant differences in mean linear intercept, air space, or septal wall thickness were observed in DTG mice. Adult DTG mice fed +dox food from PN28-88 failed to regenerate maxillary incisors (P–P').

observed. In summary, attenuation of Fgfr2b ligands post-bleomycin injury following the peak of fibrosis (14 –28 dpi) does not have any impact on the extent of fibrosis at 28 dpi.

2.4 Attenuation of Fgfr2b ligands immediately following bleomycin injury did not result in increased fibrosis

Attenuating Fgfr2b ligands at later stages following injury (6–28 and 1–28 dpi) had no effect on the level of bleomycin-induced lung injury incurred. Because Fgfr2b ligands are known to have a protective effect on lung epithelium, next it was tested whether attenuation of endogenous Fgfr2b ligands signaling immediately afterward and throughout injury impacts the extent of fibrosis incurred at 28 dpi. Fgfr2b ligands were attenuated throughout injury (0–28 dpi). With the exception of one STG animal, all animals survived until euthanized at 28 dpi (Fig. 5A). No significant differences in relative weight change were observed, although as in Fig. 5B, a trend toward delayed weight recovery in DTG mice was observed (Fig. 5B). Specific soluble *Fgfr2b* expression in DTG was confirmed (Fig. 5C). No significant change in lung compliance was measured at 28 dpi in DTG *vs.* STG (Fig. 5D). Upon histological examination both STG and DTG had areas of fibrosis (Fig. 5, E and F). However, quantification of the confluent fibrosis areas did not reveal any difference between DTG and STG lungs (Fig. 5G). In agreement with these results, no differences were observed for total hydroxyproline (Fig. 5H). Attenuation of Fgfr2b ligands in DTG mice for the duration of the injury did not lessen fibrosis incurred at 28 dpi.

In an attempt to further engage endogenous repair mechanisms, 3.0 U/kg it of bleomycin was used in the final ex-

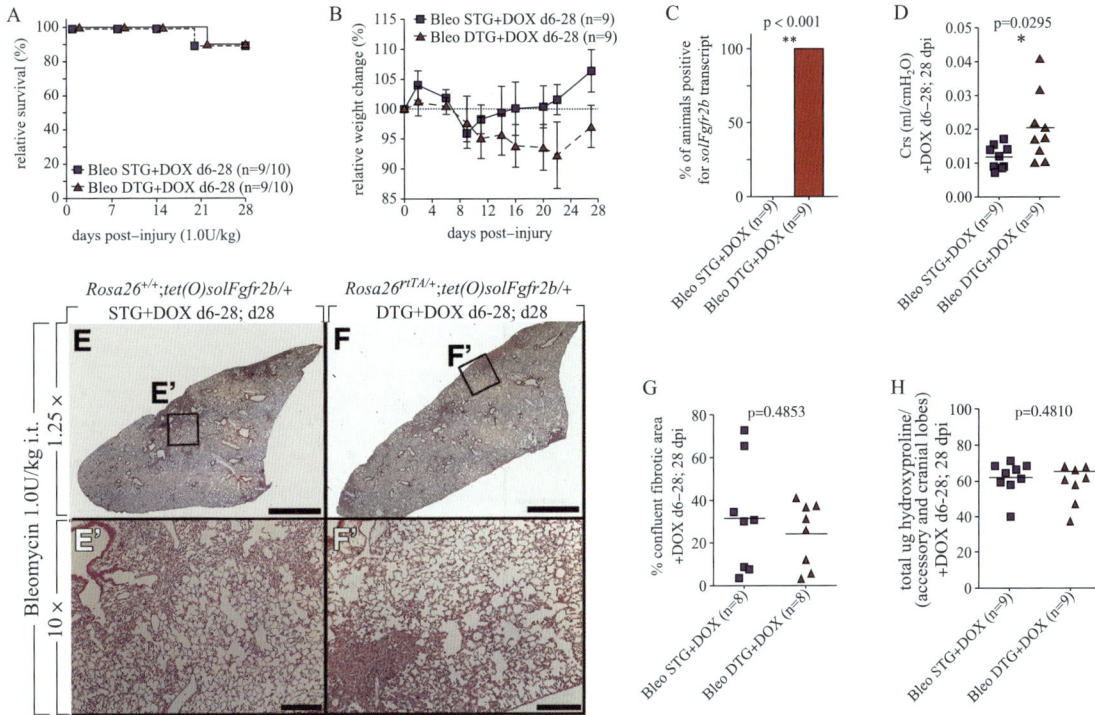

Fig. 3. Lack of endogenous *Fgfr2b* ligands signaling during injury (6–28 dpi) did not lead to increased bleomycin-induced lung injury (28 dpi). (A): survival curve. (B): relative weight change. (C): all DTG mice tested positive for *solFgfr2b* transcript at 28 dpi. **Very significant. (D): compliance. *Significant. E–F': low and high magnification of H/E staining of STG control mice (E and E') and DTGs fed doxycycline food from 6 to 28 dpi (F and F'). (G): quantification of confluent fibrotic areas in H/E stains of left lobes. *H*: hydroxyproline content of accessory and medial lobes. Scale bars *E* and *F*: 2 mm; (E') and (F'): 200 μm.

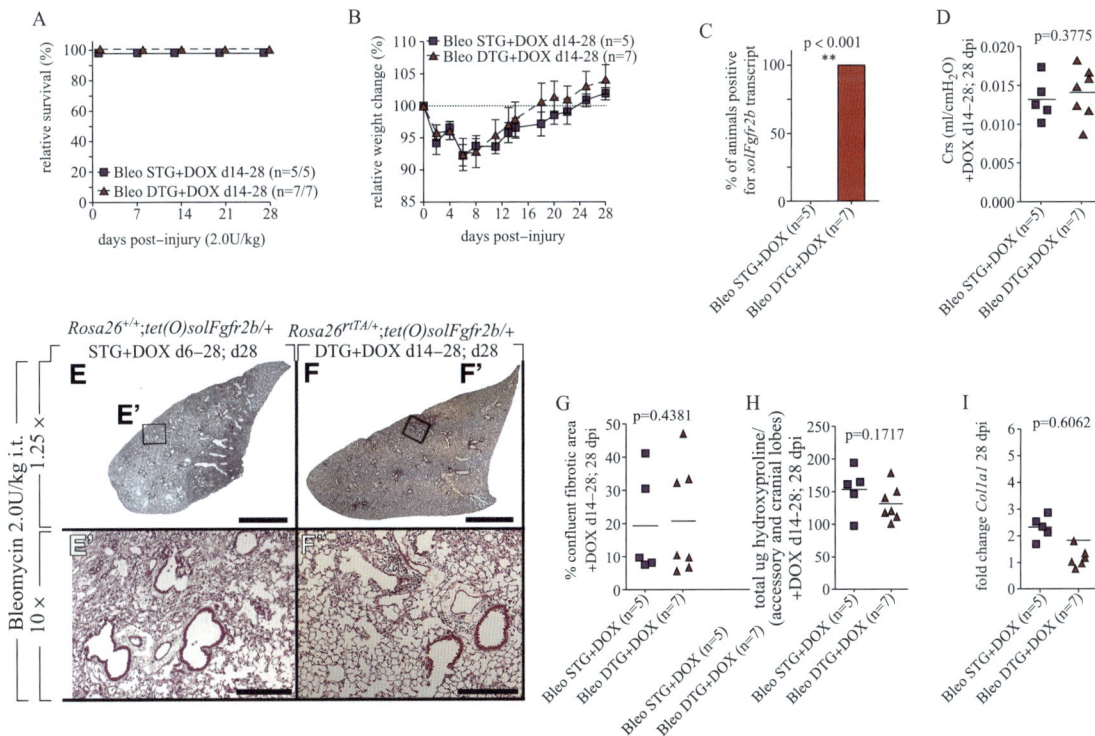

Fig. 4. Lack of endogenous *Fgfr2b* ligands signaling during injury (14 –28 dpi) did not lead to increased bleomycin-induced lung injury (28 dpi). (A) survival curve. (B) relative weight change. (C) all DTG mice tested positive for *solFgfr2b* transcript at 28 dpi. (D) compliance. (*E–F'*) low and high magnification of H/E staining of STG control mice (E and E') and DTGs fed doxycycline food from 14 to 28 dpi (F and F'). (G) quantification of confluent fibrotic areas in H/E stains of left lobes. (H) hydroxyproline content of accessory and medial lobes. (I) *Col1a1* expression. Scale bars (E) and (F): 2 mm; (E') and (F'): 200 μm.

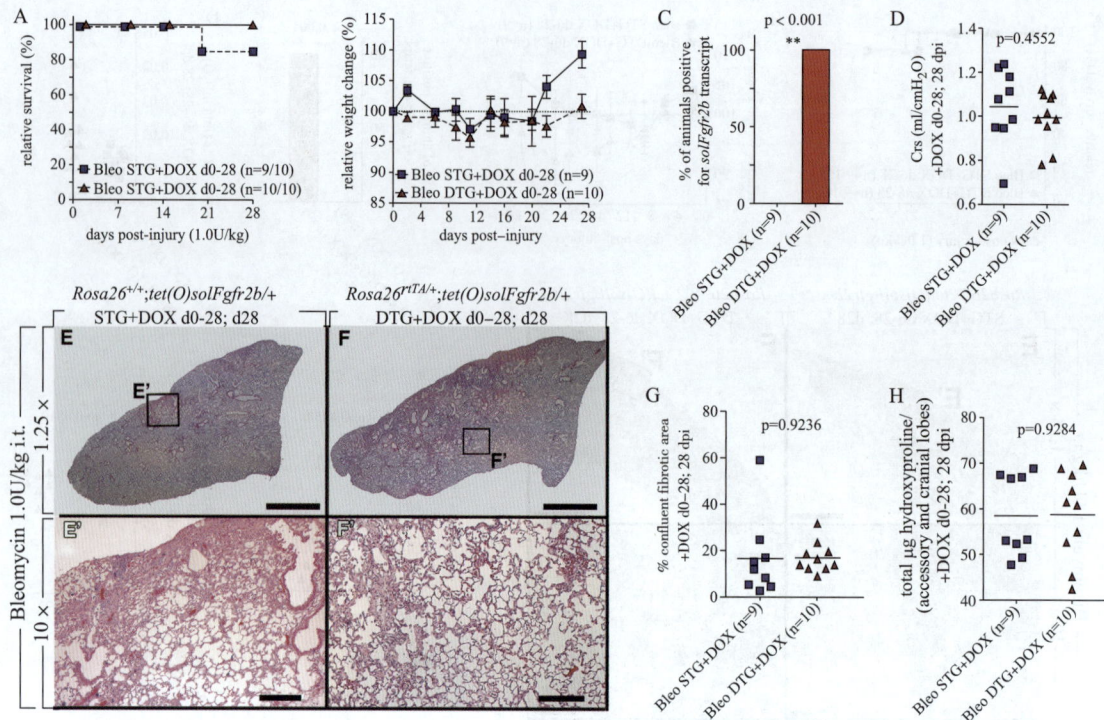

Fig. 5. Lack of endogenous *Fgfr2b* ligands signaling during injury (0 –28 dpi) did not lead to increased bleomycin-induced lung injury (28 dpi). (A): survival curve. (B): relative weight change. (C): all DTG mice tested positive for *solFgfr2b* transcript at 28 dpi. **, Very significant. (D): compliance. (E–F'): low and high magnification of H/E staining of STG control mice (E and E') and DTGs fed doxycycline food from 0 to 28 dpi (F and F'). (G): quantification of confluent fibrotic areas in H/E stains of left lobes. (H): hydroxyproline content of accessory and medial lobes. Scale bars (E) and (F): 2 mm; (E') and (F'): 200 μm.

periment (Fig. 6). The soluble receptor was induced from the day of bleomycin injury until the day of euthanasia; between 6 and 11 dpi (Fig. 6). Although the initial aim of this study was to analyze the extent of fibrosis at 28 dpi, 3.0 U/kg it of bleomycin was too severe for CD1 mice. Therefore mice were euthanized and analyzed at earlier time points. Five mice from both the STG and the DTG groups were removed at 6 dpi for analyses based on weight-loss criteria (< 20% of initial weight, data not shown). The other mice (STG; $n = 3$ and DTG; $n = 4$) were analyzed at 1 dpi. Induction of the soluble receptor was detected in DTG mice (Fig. 6A). A trend toward increased weight loss for DTG mice that survived to 1 dpi was observed (Fig. 6B). Although some variability in measurements occurred due to differences in the day of euthanasia (6 –11 dpi), no differences between STGs and DTGs were detected at any time point in regards to compliance (Fig. 6C), hydroxyproline (Fig. 6D), and the confluent fibrotic areas (Fig. 6G). In wild-type mice, bleomycin injury compared with noninjured mice triggered decreased *Sftpc* expression at 7 dpi and *Scgb1a1* at 14 dpi (data not shown). Therefore, expression of AECII cell-specific transcript *Sftpc*, *Scgb1a1* for club cells, and the general epithelial marker *EpCam* was measured in animals euthanized at 6 dpi. However, no differences in marker expression were observed between DTG and STG lungs (Fig. 6H–J).

3. Discussion

3.1 *Fgfr2b ligand signaling is important for lung development and repair*

Fgfs play pleiotropic roles both during organogenesis and homeostasis [15]. Fgfr2b ligands are part of a family of 22 identified members. Fgf10 is required for lung formation and loss of *Fgf10* leads to lung agenesis, whereas loss of *Fgf1* and *Fgf7* during development does not result in a lung phenotype in mice. The cellular and molecular bases for differences between Fgf7 and Fgf10 signaling are still unclear. Recently, mass spectrometry-based proteomics revealed that

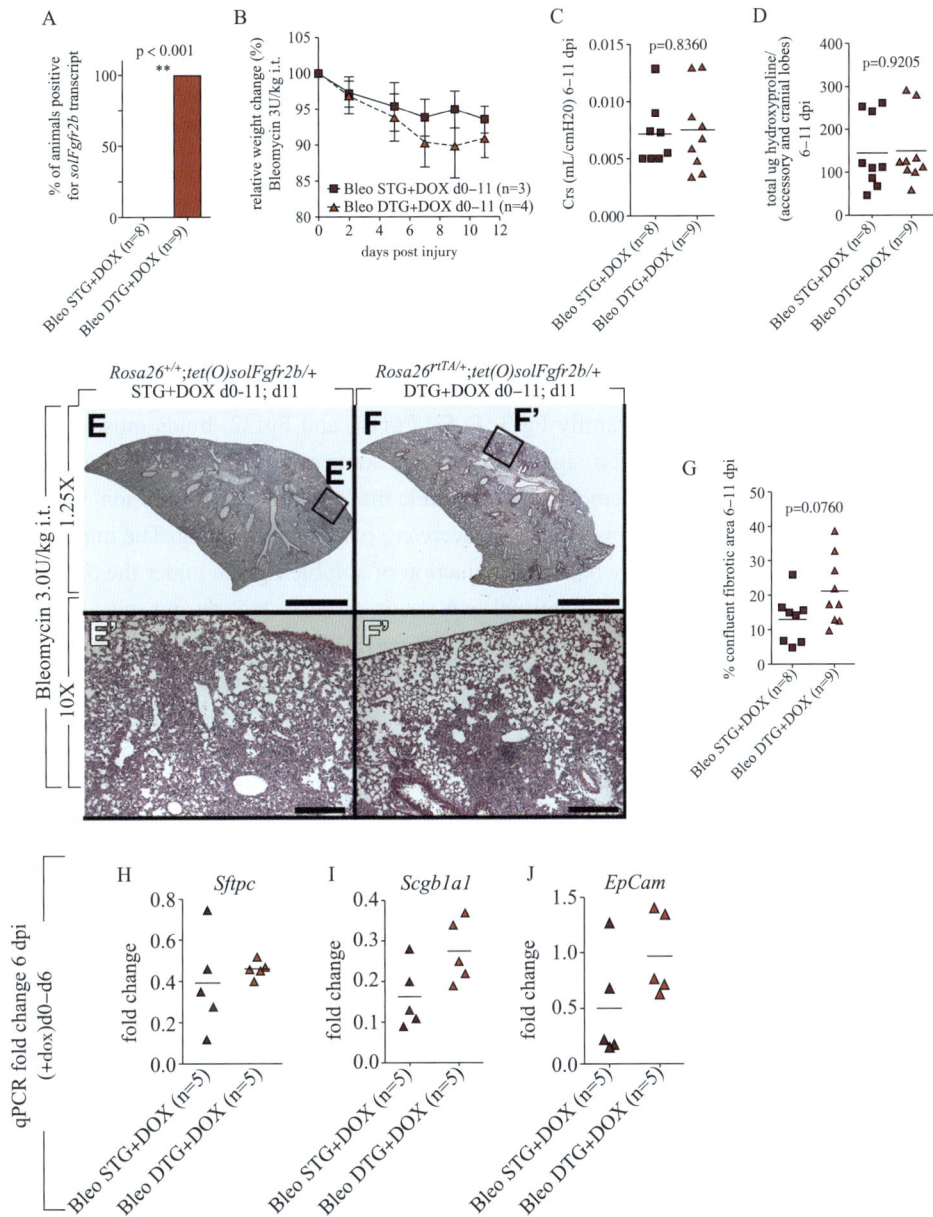

Fig. 6. Lack of endogenous *Fgfr2b* ligands signaling during injury (6 –11 dpi) did not lead to increased bleomycin-induced lung injury (6 –11 dpi). (A): all DTG mice tested positive for *solFgfr2b* transcript at 28 dpi. **Very significant. (B): relative weight change in mice that survived until 11 dpi (3/8 STG) and (4/9 DTG). (C): compliance. (D): hydroxyproline content of accessory and medial lobes. (E–F'): low and high magnification of H/E staining of STG control mice at 11 dpi (E and E') and DTGs fed doxycycline food from 0 to 11 dpi (F and F'). (G): quantification of confluent fibrotic areas in H/E stains of left lobes. (H–J): no decreases in epithelial marker expression were detected in injured 6 dpi DTG mice *vs.* STG; qPCR for *Sftpc, Scgb1a1, EpCam*; corresponding saline controls normalized to 1 (data not shown). Scale bars (E') and (F'): 2 mm; (E') and (F'): 200 μm.

Fgf7 and Fgf10 elicit distinct biochemical response downstream of the Fgfr2b receptor. In particular, Fgf7 leads to rapid but transient phosphorylation of Akt and Shc whereas Fgf10 leads to the progressive and sustained phosphorylation of these mediators. In addition, Fgf10 triggers phosphorylation of tyrosine 734 and the associated recruitment of SH3bp4, a relatively novel adaptor protein. It has been proposed that Fgf10 leads to increased recycling of Fgfr2b at the cell surface whereas Fgf7 results in transient signaling [8]. Unlike Fgf7 and Fgf10, which act mostly through Fgfr2b, Fgf1 acts *via* all Fgf receptor isoforms. Fgf10 appears to be critical not only for the survival and proliferation of the distal epithelial lung progenitors [35] but also for the repair of the bronchiolar epithelium following naphthalene exposure [39]. Lung epithelial cell-specific overexpression of *Fgf10* in mice during the first, second, or third week postbleomycin injury was both protective and therapeutic as characterized by increased survival and attenuated lung fibrosis [11]. Administration of

Fgf7 or palifermin, a pharmacological agent composed of a truncated form of Fgf7, also reduced fibrosis and increased survival in both rats and mice [7, 10, 22, 32]. In humans, haploinsufficiency for *FGF10* is associated with chronic obstructive pulmonary disease (COPD) [18]. Likewise, in humans, SNPs in *FGF7* correlate with increased risk for developing COPD [5].

In contrast to previous studies that used exogenous Fgfr2b ligands to attenuate bleomycin-induced lung injury, this study first assessed the activation of endogenous Fgfr2b ligands in injured wild-type mice and then attenuated Fgfr2b ligands following bleomycin injury to assess their contribution to lung repair. Given the significant reduction in Fgfr2b receptor expression following bleomycin injury, it was not surprising that attenuation of endogenous Fgfr2b ligands had no effect on fibrosis outcome.

3.2 DTG mice efficiently attenuate endogenous Fgfr2b ligands

The $Rosa26^{rtTA/+};tet(O)sFgfr2b/+$ (DTG) mouse line was used to ubiquitously trap all Fgfr2b ligands during injury. Fgf1, in addition to ligands of the Fgf7 subfamily Fgf3, Fgf7, Fgf10, and Fgf22, binds most strongly to Fgfr2b [43]. Although Fgf10 contains a nuclear localization signal and may in some contexts act in an intracrine fashion [20], the $Rosa26^{rtTA/+};tet(O)sFgfr2b/+$ model has been demonstrated to mimic the loss of *Fgf10* expression during development [35], demonstrating that Fgf10's activity in the lung is mainly *via* secreted, paracrine signaling. The impact of trapping Fgfr2b ligands during lung injury has been previously reported. Induction of soluble Fgfr2b under the *SpC-rtTA/+* promoter in adult mice subjected to hyperoxia injury led to abnormal expression of surfactant during injury, which contributed to increased lethality [13]. A similar result was obtained in $Rosa26^{rtTA/+};tet(O)sFgfr2b/+$ neonates exposed to hyperoxia (Chao and Bellusci, unpublished results). Furthermore, in the context of naphthalene injury [39] as well as H1N1 influenza virus infection (Quantius *et al.*, unpublished results), lung injury was increased in DTG animals. Mice used in this study were thoroughly validated and demonstrated both the embryonic and adult phenotypes characteristic of this line.

3.3 Attenuation of endogenous Fgfr2b ligands during bleomycin injury did not result in increased fibrosis

Doxycycline-fed bleomycin-injured $Rosa26^{rtTA/+};tet(O)sFgfr2b/+$ (DTG) mice did not incur increased fibrosis compared with injured STG mice. There are several explanations for the lack of increased injury in DTG mice following bleomycin injury. First, the weak recruitment of Fgf ligands in this injury model indicated an insignificant contribution of endogenous Fgfr2b ligands to the repair process. Second, although solFgfr2b traps both Fgf7 and Fgf10 ligands, which have been shown to convey protective signals to the injured epithelium, it also traps Fgf1, which binds to all Fgfrs. Although its effects are not well characterized, Fgf1 signaling is potentially ambivalent in the context of bleomycin lung injury. As Fgf1 signals to cells of both epithelial and mesenchymal origins, blocking an Fgf1-mediated survival signal to fibroblasts following bleomycin injury, especially following 14 dpi, when fibroblasts are most abundant, may be beneficial. Moreover, in a study using a soluble, dominant-negative Fgfr2c-isoform construct, it was demonstrated that blocking mesenchymal Fgfr2c mediated signaling following bleomycin injury attenuated fibrosis [17]. Third, although FACS analyses of $Rosa26^{rtTA/+};Tomato^{fl/+}$ mice revealed that doxycycline induced *rtTA* expression in 25% of the lung cells, for maximal ligand attenuation during bleomycin injury a lung-specific driver may be required. Lastly, compensation by other endogenous repair pathways such as Wnt [37] may adequately compensate for the attenuation of Fgf signaling. In the future, lung cell type-specific models targeting specific ligands and receptors are needed to more accurately dissect the role of Fgf signaling in lung repair.

3.4 Tyrosine kinase inhibitors demonstrate therapeutic effects in bleomycin-treated mice, further suggesting endogenous Fgfr2b ligand signaling is dispensable for repair

Tyrosine kinase receptors mediate a variety of growth factor signaling pathways. High levels of MAPK and ERK phosphorylation are associated with IPF. Three major tyrosine kinase pathways relevant for lung disease have been described: the VEGFR, PDGFR, and FGFR pathways. The tyrosine kinase inhibitor BIBF1120 blocks these pathways and has demonstrated a protective and therapeutic in the bleomycin model [40]. In addition, phase III clinical trials demonstrated that BIBF1120 treatment both decreased the rate of decline in forced vital capacity and reduced the number of acute exacerbations in IPF patients [41]. In mouse models, just as enhanced activation of the epithelial receptor tyrosine kinase Fgfr2b-isoform *via* exogenous Fgfr2b ligands leads to epithelial protection and lessens fibrosis, attenuation of Fgfr2c-isoform signaling also attenuates fibrosis. These results suggest that enhanced Fgfr2b-isoform signaling expedites lung protection and repair, whereas Fgfr2c-isoform ligand signaling (*via* Fgf1, Fgf2, Fgf9) may fuel the fibrosis fire by relaying survival signals to fibroblasts. In conclusion, although global tyrosine kinase inhibitors such as BIBF1120 likely inhibit FGFR2b signaling, the contribution of VEGF, PDGF, and FGFR2(c) to fibrosis formation may be far greater. Whether exogenously stimulating Fgfr2b signaling following treatment with tyrosine kinase inhibitors further attenuates bleomycin-induced fibrosis injury remains to be investigated.

References

[1] Al Alam D, Danopoulos S, Schall K, *et al.* Fibroblast growth factor 10 alters the balance between goblet and Paneth cells in the adult mouse small intestine[J]. American Journal of Physiology-Gastrointestinal and Liver Physiology, 2015, 308(8): G678-G690.

[2] Antoniu SA. Nintedanib (BIBF 1120) for IPF: a tomorrow therapy?[J]. Multidisciplinary Respiratory Medicine, 2012, 7.

[3] Bellusci S, Grindley J, Emoto H, *et al.* Fibroblast Growth Factor 10(FGF10) and branching morphogenesis in the embryonic mouse lung[J]. Development, 1997, 124(23): 4867-4878.

[4] Belteki G, Haigh J, Kabacs N, *et al.* Conditional and inducible transgene expression in mice through the combinatorial use of Cre-mediated recombination and tetracycline induction[J]. Nucleic Acids Research, 2005, 33(5) e51.

[5] Brehm JM, Hagiwara K, Tesfaigzi Y, *et al.* Identification of FGF7 as a novel susceptibility locus for chronic obstructive pulmonary disease[J]. Thorax, 2011, 66(12): 1085-1090.

[6] Danopoulos S, Parsa S, Al Alam D, *et al.* Transient Inhibition of FGFR2b-Ligands Signaling Leads to Irreversible Loss of Cellular beta-Catenin Organization and Signaling in AER during Mouse Limb Development[J]. Plos One, 2013, 8(10).

[7] Deterding RR, Havill AM, Yano T, *et al.* Prevention of bleomycin-induced lung injury in rats by keratinocyte growth factor[J]. Proceedings of the Association of American Physicians, 1997, 109(3): 254-268.

[8] Francavilla C, Rigbolt KTG, Emdal KB, *et al.* Functional Proteomics Defines the Molecular Switch Underlying FGF Receptor Trafficking and Cellular Outputs[J]. Molecular Cell, 2013, 51(6): 707-722.

[9] Gossen M, Bujard H. Tight control of gene expression in mammalian cells by tetracycline-responsive promoters[J]. Proceedings of the National Academy of Sciences of the United States of America, 1992, 89(12): 5547-5551.

[10] J G, ES Y, AM H, *et al.* Intravenous keratinocyte growth factor protects against experimental pulmonary injury[J]. The American journal of physiology, 1998, 275(null): L800-805.

[11] Gupte VV, Ramasamy SK, Reddy R, *et al.* Overexpression of Fibroblast Growth Factor-10 during Both Inflammatory and Fibrotic Phases Attenuates Bleomycin-induced Pulmonary Fibrosis in Mice[J]. American Journal of Respiratory and Critical Care Medicine, 2009, 180(5): 424-436.

[12] Hokuto I, Perl AKT, Whitsett JA. Prenatal, but not postnatal, inhibition of fibroblast growth factor receptor signaling causes emphysema[J]. Journal of Biological Chemistry, 2003, 278(1): 415-421.

[13] Hokuto I, Perl AKT, Whitsett JA. FGF signaling is required for pulmonary homeostasis following hyperoxia[J]. American Journal of Physiology-Lung Cellular and Molecular Physiology, 2004, 286(3): L580-L587.

[14] Huebner R-H, Gitter W, El Mokhtari NE, *et al.* Standardized quantification of pulmonary fibrosis in histological samples[J]. Biotechniques, 2008, 44(4): 507-511, 514-517.

[15] Itoh N, Ornitz DM. Fibroblast growth factors: from molecular evolution to roles in development, metabolism and disease[J]. Journal of Biochemistry, 2011, 149(2): 121-130.

[16] Izvolsky KI, Shoykhet D, Yang Y, *et al.* Heparan sulfate-FGF10 interactions during lung morphogenesis[J]. Developmental Biology, 2003, 258(1): 185-200.

[17] Wang J, Yu Z, Zhou Z, *et al.* Inhibition of alpha-SMA by the Ectodomain of FGFR2c Attenuates Lung Fibrosis[J]. Molecular Medicine, 2012, 18(6): 992-1002.

[18] Klar J, Blomstrand P, Brunmark C, *et al.* Fibroblast growth factor 10 haploinsufficiency causes chronic obstructive pulmonary disease[J]. Journal of Medical Genetics, 2011, 48(10): 705-709.

[19] Korfei M, Ruppert C, Mahavadi P, *et al.* Epithelial endoplasmic reticulum stress and apoptosis in sporadic idiopathic pulmonary fibrosis[J]. American Journal of Respiratory and Critical Care Medicine, 2008, 178(8): 838-846.

[20] Kosman J, Carmean N, Leaf EM, *et al.* Translocation of fibroblast growth factor-10 and its receptor into nuclei of human urothelial cells[J]. Journal of Cellular Biochemistry, 2007, 102(3): 769-785.

[21] Lewis D, Scullion J. Palliative and end-of-life care for patients with idiopathic pulmonary fibrosis: challenges and dilemmas[J]. International Journal of Palliative Nursing, 2012, 18(7): 331-337.

[22] Liu C-J, Ha X-Q, Jiang J-J, *et al.* Keratinocyte Growth Factor (KGF) Gene Therapy Mediated by an Attenuated Form of Salmonella typhimurium Ameliorates Radiation Induced Pulmonary Injury in Rats[J]. Journal of Radiation Research, 2011, 52(2): 176-184.

[23] Lu JN, Izvolsky KI, Qian J, *et al.* Identification of FGF10 targets in the embryonic lung epithelium during bud morphogenesis[J]. Journal of Biological Chemistry, 2005, 280(6): 4834-4841.

[24] Madisen L, Zwingman TA, Sunkin SM, *et al.* A robust and high-throughput Cre reporting and characterization system for the whole mouse brain[J]. Nature Neuroscience, 2010, 13(1): 133-140.

[25] McGrath-Morrow SA, Cho C, Soutiere S, *et al.* The effect of neonatal hyperoxia on the lung of p21(Waf1/Cip1/Sdi1)-deficient mice[J]. American Journal of Respiratory Cell and Molecular Biology, 2004, 30(5): 635-640.

[26] Nelson WJ, Nusse R. Convergence of Wnt, beta-catenin, and cadherin pathways[J]. Science, 2004, 303(5663): 1483-1487.

[27] Ohuchi H, Hori Y, Yamasaki M, *et al.* FGF10 acts as a major ligand for FGF receptor 2 IIIb in mouse multi-organ development[J]. Biochemical and Biophysical Research Communications, 2000, 277(3): 643-649.

[28] Parsa S, Kuremoto K-i, Seidel K, *et al.* Signaling by FGFR2b controls the regenerative capacity of adult mouse incisors[J]. Development, 2010, 137(22): 3743-3752.

[29] Parsa S, Ramasamy SK, De Langhe S, *et al.* Terminal end bud maintenance in mammary gland is dependent upon FGFR2b signaling[J]. Developmental Biology, 2008, 317(1): 121-131.

[30] Perl AKT, Tichelaar JW, Whitsett JA. Conditional gene expression in the respiratory epithelium of the mouse[J]. Transgenic Research, 2002, 11(1): 21-29.

[31] Rafii R, Juarez MM, Albertson TE, *et al.* A review of current and novel therapies for idiopathic pulmonary fibrosis[J]. Journal of Thoracic Disease, 2013, 5(1): 48-73.

[32] Sakamoto S, Yazawa T, Baba Y, *et al.* Keratinocyte Growth Factor Gene Transduction Ameliorates Pulmonary Fibrosis Induced by Bleomycin in Mice[J]. American Journal of Respiratory Cell and Molecular Biology, 2011, 45(3): 489-497.

[33] Sauer B. Inducible gene targeting in mice using the Cre/lox

system[J]. Methods, 1998, 14(4): 381-392.

[34] Schwenk F, Baron U, Rajewsky K. A cre-transgenic mouse strain for the ubiquitous deletion of loxP-flanked gene segments including deletion in germ cells[J]. Nucleic Acids Research, 1995, 23(24): 5080-5081.

[35] Sekine K, Ohuchi H, Fujiwara M, et al. Fgf10 is essential for limb and lung formation[J]. Nature Genetics, 1999, 21(1): 138-141.

[36] Sugahara K, Iyama KI, Kuroda MJ, et al. Double intratracheal instillation of keratinocyte growth factor prevents bleomycin-induced lung fibrosis in rats[J]. Journal of Pathology, 1998, 186(1): 90-98.

[37] Tanjore H, Degryse AL, Crossno PF, et al. beta-Catenin in the Alveolar Epithelium Protects from Lung Fibrosis after Intratracheal Bleomycin[J]. American Journal of Respiratory and Critical Care Medicine, 2013, 187(6): 630-639.

[38] Verkaar F, Zaman GJR. New avenues to target Wnt/beta-catenin signaling[J]. Drug Discovery Today, 2011, 16(1-2): 35-41.

[39] Volckaert T, Dill E, Campbell A, et al. Parabronchial smooth muscle constitutes an airway epithelial stem cell niche in the mouse lung after injury[J]. Journal of Clinical Investigation, 2011, 121(11): 4409-4419.

[40] Wollin L, Maillet I, Quesniaux V, et al. Antifibrotic and Anti-inflammatory Activity of the Tyrosine Kinase Inhibitor Nintedanib in Experimental Models of Lung Fibrosis[J]. Journal of Pharmacology and Experimental Therapeutics, 2014, 349(2): 209-220.

[41] Woodcock HV, Molyneaux PL, Maher TM. Reducing lung function decline in patients with idiopathic pulmonary fibrosis: potential of nintedanib[J]. Drug Design Development and Therapy, 2013, 7: 503-510.

[42] Woyda K, Koebrich S, Reiss I, et al. Inhibition of phosphodiesterase 4 enhances lung alveolarisation in neonatal mice exposed to hyperoxia[J]. European Respiratory Journal, 2009, 33(4): 861-870.

[43] Zhang X, Ibrahimi OA, Olsen SK, et al. Receptor specificity of the fibroblast growth factor family - The complete mammalian FGF family[J]. Journal of Biological Chemistry, 2006, 281(23): 15694-15700.

The therapeutic potential of a novel non-ATP-competitive fibroblast growth factor receptor 1 inhibitor on gastric cancer

Chaochao Xu, Guang Liang and Xiaokun Li

1. Introduction

The incidence of gastric cancer (GC) has decreased markedly worldwide. However, 989 600 new cases of stomach cancer (8% of the total new cancer cases) and 738 000 deaths (10% of the total deaths) have occurred in the past 7 years [1]. Surgical techniques and postoperative adjuvant chemotherapies have improved, but the total survival rate of GC remains unsatisfactory. Therefore, understanding the molecular mechanisms of GC and developing new targeted therapies to improve the survival rate of GC patients are important.

Investigation of targeted inhibitors of receptor tyrosine kinases (RTKs) is currently one of the prevalent topics of cancer treatment research; many inhibitor drugs, including EGFR and VEGFR inhibitors, are used clinically [2,3]. For GC, some studies report that there are gene amplification, mutations, and rearrangements of RTKs; RTK inhibition might be a new therapeutic strategy for GC. For example, foretinib (GSK1363089), imatinib, regorafenib, and other RTK inhibitors have shown great therapeutic potential against GC [4-6]. FGFR, which is an RTK, can activate downstream signaling pathways, including FRS2α, PI3K/AKT, and ERK1/2 pathways, after ligand [fibroblast growth factor 2 (FGF2)] binding [7]. Overexpression of fibroblast growth factor receptors (FGFRs) extensively involves the regulation of physiological and pathological functions, including cell proliferation, apoptosis, metastasis, and angiogenesis [8]. In GC, FGFRs are overactivated by several mechanisms, including gene amplification, chromosomal translocation, and mutation [9]. Compared with other FGFRs, FGFR1 expression is amplified in GC cell lines and tissues [10]. The development of targeted inhibitors of FGFR1 may be a promising therapeutic strategy for GC.

Nordihydroguaiaretic acid (NDGA) is a novel non-ATP-competitive FGFR inhibitor [11]. In our previous study, we designed and obtained a novel non-ATP-competitive FGFR1 inhibitor L6123. L67123 showed better inhibitory activity on the level of FGFR1 kinases than NDGA, which was used as a positive control (Fig. 1). L6123 was identified as a selective FGFR1 inhibitor with therapeutic potential in nonsmall cell lung cancer *in vivo* and *in vitro* (data not shown). Therefore, we hypothesized that L6123 has therapeutic potential in FGFR1-overexpressing GC cells. The results obtained were in agreement with our hypothesis that L6123 showed excellent anti-GC activity by inhibiting the FGFR signaling pathway.

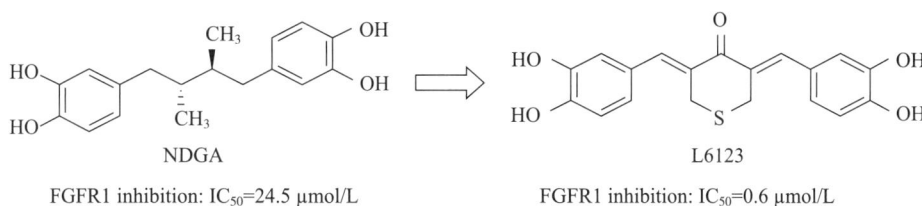

FGFR1 inhibition: IC_{50}=24.5 μmol/L   FGFR1 inhibition: IC_{50}=0.6 μmol/L

Fig. 1. Structures of L6123 and NDGA. The IC_{50} of FGFR1 inhibition: 0.6 μmol/L for L6123; 24.5 μmol/L for NDGA. FGFR1, fibroblast growth factor receptor 1; NDGA, nordihydroguaiaretic acid.

2. Methods

2.1 Cell lines, compounds, and reagents

Human GC cells MGC-803, SGC-7901, and BGC-823 were purchased from the Shanghai Institute of Biosciences and Cell Resources Center (Chinese Academy of Sciences, Shanghai, China), Wuhan Boster Biological Engineering Co. Ltd (Wuhan, People's Republic of China), and the Xiangya Cell Center of Central South University (Changsha, China), respectively. SGC-7901, BGC-823, and MGC-803 cells were maintained in RPMI 1640 medium with 10% fetal bovine serum (FBS) and 1% penicillin. The wild-type mouse embryonic fibroblast (MEF^{-WT}) and MEF$^{-FGFR1-FGFR2-FRS2\alpha-KO}$ (FGFR1, FGFR2, and FRS2α gene knockout) cell lines were kindly provided by Fen Wang (Professor), Texas A&M University, and were cultured in Dulbecco's modified Eagle's medium with 1% penicillin and 10% FBS (Gibco, Eggenstein, Germany). All cells were incubated at 37℃ in an atmosphere of 5% CO_2. L6123 was synthesized and purified in our laboratory, and the purity was 98.0%. NDGA was purchased from Sigma (St Louis, Missouri, USA). Recombinant human FGF2 was purchased from the Institute of Biological and Natural Product, Wenzhou Medical University, Wenzhou, China.

2.2 Cell proliferation assay

An MTT assay was performed to evaluate the antiproliferative activity of the compound L6123 against the GC cell lines SGC-7901, BGC-823, and MGC-803, and the MEF^{-WT} and MEF$^{-FGFR1-FGFR2-FRS2\alpha-KO}$ cells. All cells (4000 cells/well) were seeded in a 96-well plate. After 24 h, the culture medium was removed and all cells were treated with increasing concentrations (20/27, 20/9, 20/3, 20, and 60 μmol/L) of compound L6123 for 72 h. NDGA was used as a positive control. After treatment, the viability of the cells was tested using an MTT assay.

2.3 Antibodies and western blotting assay

All antibodies, including the goat anti-rabbit immunoglobulin G (IgG)-horseradish peroxidase (HRP) and mouse anti-goat IgG-HRP antibodies, were purchased from Santa Cruz Biotechnology (Santa Cruz, California, USA). Anti-pFRS2α and anticleaved-caspase-3 were purchased from Cell Signaling Technology (Beverly, Massachusetts, USA). The western blot was operated by standard means. After washing with PBS, 60 μl/well cell lysates were added to a six-well plate at 4℃ for 3 min. Then, cell lysates were collected and centrifuged to remove the insoluble components. The supernatant was run on 10% SDS-PAGE and then transferred to a PVDF membrane. After blocking with 5% nonfat dry milk in TBST, the membrane was incubated with the primary antibodies (anti-pFGFR1, anti-FGFR1, anti-pFRS2α, anti-FRS2α, anti-pERK1/2, anti-ERK1/2, anticleaved-caspase-3, anti-pro-caspase-3, anti-Bcl-2, anticleaved-PARP, and anti-GAPDH) overnight and subsequently incubated with goat anti-rabbit IgG or mouse anti-goat IgG HRP-linked antibody. The blots were detected using an ECL detection kit (Bio-Rad, Hercules, California, USA) according to the manufacturer's procedure. The results were analyzed using Quantity One software (Bio-Rad) to determine the relative band density ratio.

2.4 Cell apoptosis assay

The percentage of apoptotic cells was detected by flow cytometry using the annexin V and propidium iodide (PI) staining. SGC-7901 cells were exposed to different compound concentrations (5, 10, and 20 μmol/L) for 48 h and were subsequently harvested. NDGA was used as a positive control. Finally, cells were incubated with 1 × binding buffer, annexin V (5 μl), and PI (1 μl) in a dark room for 15 min. Cells were analyzed by FACScalibur Flow Cytometry (BD Biosciences, San Jose, California, USA).

2.5 Hoechst assay

SGC-7901 cells (4×10^5 cells/well) were exposed to different L6123 concentrations (5, 10, and 20 μmol/L) for 48 h before staining with Hoechst 33 342 dye (Beyotime Biotech, Nantong, China). NDGA (20 μmol/L) was used as a positive control. The stained cells were observed under a fluorescence microscope (Nikon, Tokyo, Japan). Images were viewed under a × 200 objective.

2.6 Transwell invasion assay

SGC-7901 cell migration was performed in Corning Transwell insert chambers (8.0 μm pore size) according to the manufacturer's instructions. SGC-7901 cells (1×10^5) were paved in 200 μl of serum-free RPMI 1640 medium in the upper well (precoated with diluted Matrigel) before incubation with various concentrations (5, 10, and 20 μmol/L) of L6123 for 24 h. RPMI 1640 medium (500 μl) with 10% FBS was added to the lower chambers. After 24 h at 37℃, cells were removed from the upper surface of the membrane by a cotton swab. The membranes were cut from the chamber and fixed with 4% paraformaldehyde for 15–20 min. The membranes were stained with crystal violet for 25–30 min. Finally, cells that adhered to the lower surface of the membranes were counted and imaged by phase microscopy. Images were observed under a × 200 objective.

2.7 Statistical analysis

All data were assayed in triplicate ($n = 3$) and were represented as mean ± SEM. Statistical analyses were calculated using Student's t-test and one-way analysis of variance using GraphPad Prism 5.0 (GraphPad, San Diego, California, USA). A P value of less than 0.05 was considered statistically significant.

3. Results

3.1 L6123 suppressed the growth of GC cell lines

On the level of FGFR1 kinases, L6123 showed better inhibitory activity than NDGA (FGFR1 inhibition IC_{50} of 0.6 μmol/L for L6123 and 24.5 μmol/l for NDGA). FGFR1 was highly expressed in the GC cell lines SGC-7901, BGC-823, and MGC-803. The proliferation and colony formation of GC cells were inhibited by silencing FGFR1 [10]. The antitumor effect of L6123 and NDGA on GC cells was tested using an MTT assay. All GC cell lines were treated with various concentrations of L6123 and NDGA for 72 h. L6123 had lower IC_{50} than NDGA in SGC-7901, BGC-823, and MGC-803 (Fig. 2A). Therefore, L6123 showed better antitumor effect than NDGA. To de-

A

Compound	IC$_{50}$ (μmol/L)		
	BGC-823	MGC-803	SGC-7901
L6123	36.8 ± 2.1	12.1 ± 2.4	12.3 ± 0.5
NDGA	74.7 ± 2.0	72.2 ± 2.0	52.9 ± 0.9

B

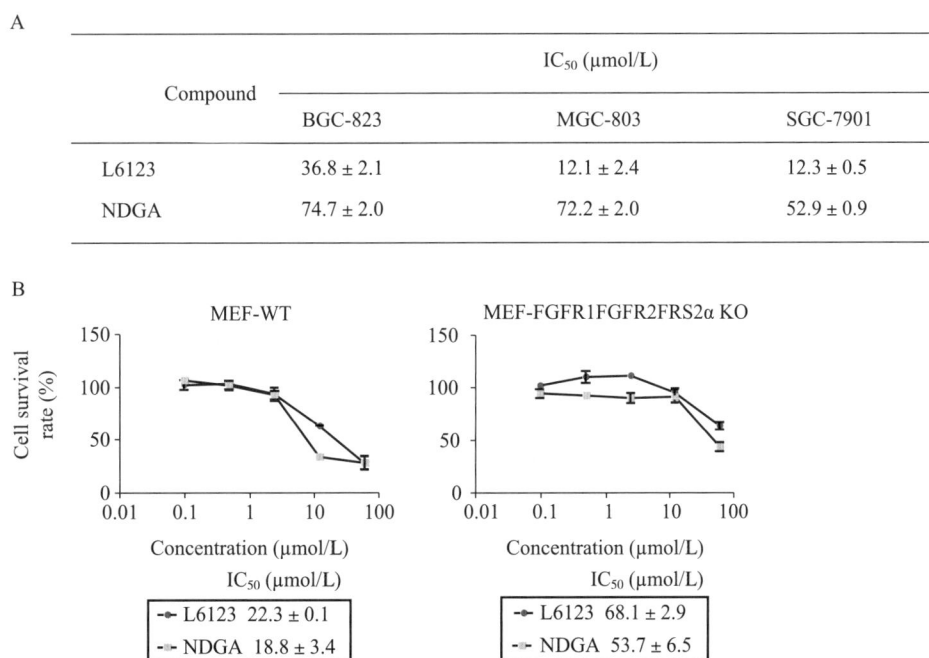

Fig. 2. Compounds L6123 and NDGA inhibited cell proliferation. (A) The IC_{50} of L6123 and NDGA inhibiting GC cells (SGC-7901, BGC-823, and MGC-803) proliferation. (B) L6123 and NDGA all showed better inhibitory effect on MEF[WT] cells than that of MEF[FGFR1-FGFR2-FRS2α-KO] cells. NDGA, nordihydroguaiaretic acid.

tect the target selectivity of L6123, the antiproliferative activity of L6123 on MEF^{-WT} and MEF$^{-FGFR1-FGFR2-FRS2\alpha-KO}$ cells was studied using an MTT assay. MEF^{-WT} and MEF$^{-FGFR1-FGFR2-FRS2\alpha-KO}$ cells were treated with various concentrations of L6123 or NDGA for 72 h. L6123 showed better inhibitory activity against MEF^{-WT} than MEF$^{-FGFR1-FGFR2-FRS2\alpha-KO}$ cells (Fig. 2B). FGFR1 knockout inhibited the antiproliferative activity of L6123. Moreover, L6123 showed higher IC$_{50}$ than NDGA in MEF$^{-FGFR1-FGFR2-FRS2\alpha-KO}$ cells (IC$_{50}$: 68.1 ± 2.9 µmol/L for L6123 and 53.7 ± 6.5 µmol/L for NDGA).

3.2 L6123 downregulated the phosphorylation of FGFR1 and downstream signaling pathways

In GC cell lines, L6123 had better antitumor activity than NDGA, but the mechanism remains unclear. The expression of FGFR1 protein in SGC-790 was the highest [10] among the GC cell lines (SGC-7901, BGC-823, and MGC-803), which was consistent with our findings (data not shown). Meanwhile, L6123 and NDGA showed the best inhibitory activity against SGC-790. Hence, SGC-7901 was used to investigate (by western blot analysis) whether L6123 could downregulate FGFR1 and its downstream signaling pathways. L6123 induced an evident and dose-dependent decrease in FGF2-induced phosphorylation of FGFR1, FRS2α, and ERK1/2 (Fig. 3). Therefore, L6123 showed significant antitumor activity by downregulating the FGFR1/ FRS2α/ERK1/2 pathway in GC cells. NDGA could exert an antitumor effect by inhibiting RTK activity [11–13], which is in agreement with our finding that NDGA (20 µmol/L) could arrest the FGFR1/FRS2α/ERK1/2 pathway (Fig. 3).

3.3 Compound L6123 enhanced apoptosis in the GC cells

The effects of L6123 on cell apoptosis were analyzed by flow cytometry, Hoechst staining, and western blot. We investigated whether the mitochondria-mediated apoptotic pathway was involved in L6123 induced apoptosis. The apop-

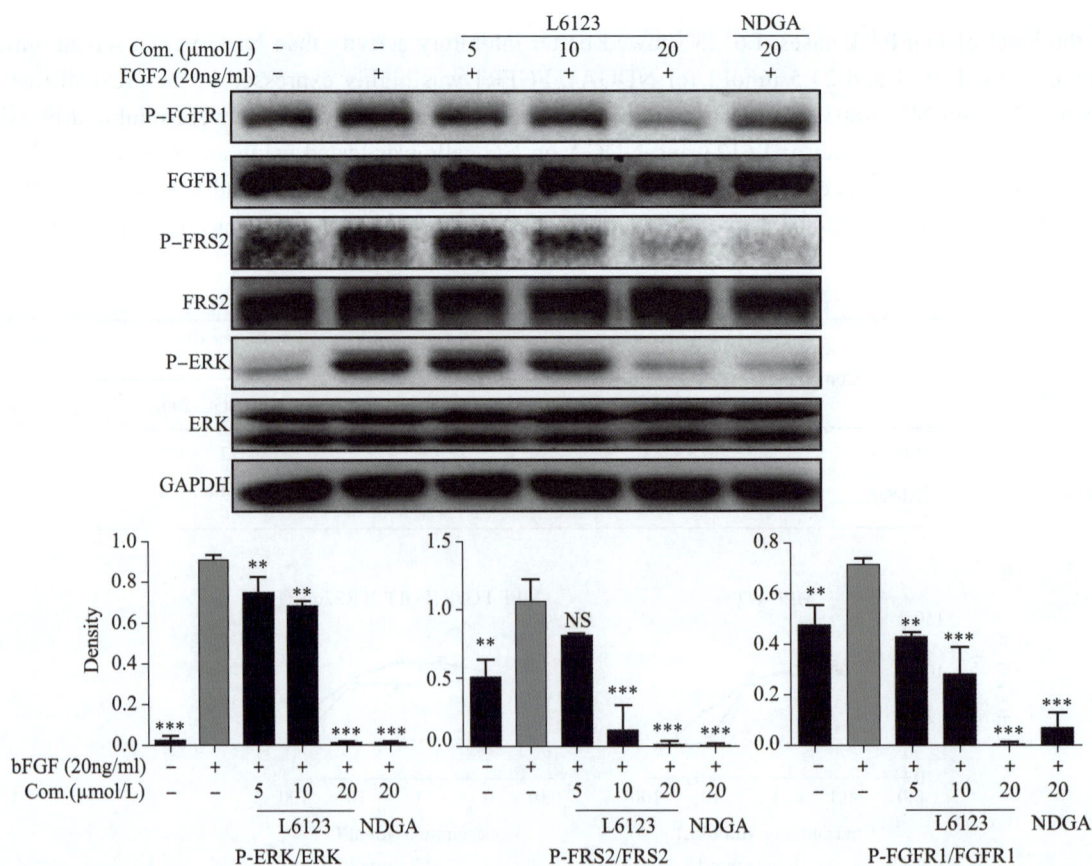

Fig. 3. Compound L6123 suppressed FGF2-induced phosphorylation of FGFR1, FES2α, and ERK1/2 in a dose-dependent manner. SGC-7901 cell was treated with compound L6123 (5, 10 and 20 µmol/L) for 1 h, starved for 24 h, and then stimulated with FGF2 (20 ng/ml) for 10 min; cell lysates was collected and the phosphorylation levels of FGFR1, FRS2α, and ERK1/2 were tested using a western blotting assay. NDGA (20 µmol/L) was used as a positive control. The column figure was the normalized optical density as a percentage of the relevant total protein. Data are presented as the mean ± SD of three independent experiments conducted in triplicate.**$P < 0.01$; ***$P < 0.001$. Com., compound; FGF, fibroblast growth factor; FGFR, fibroblast growth factor receptor 2; NDGA, nordihydroguaiaretic acid; NS, not significant.

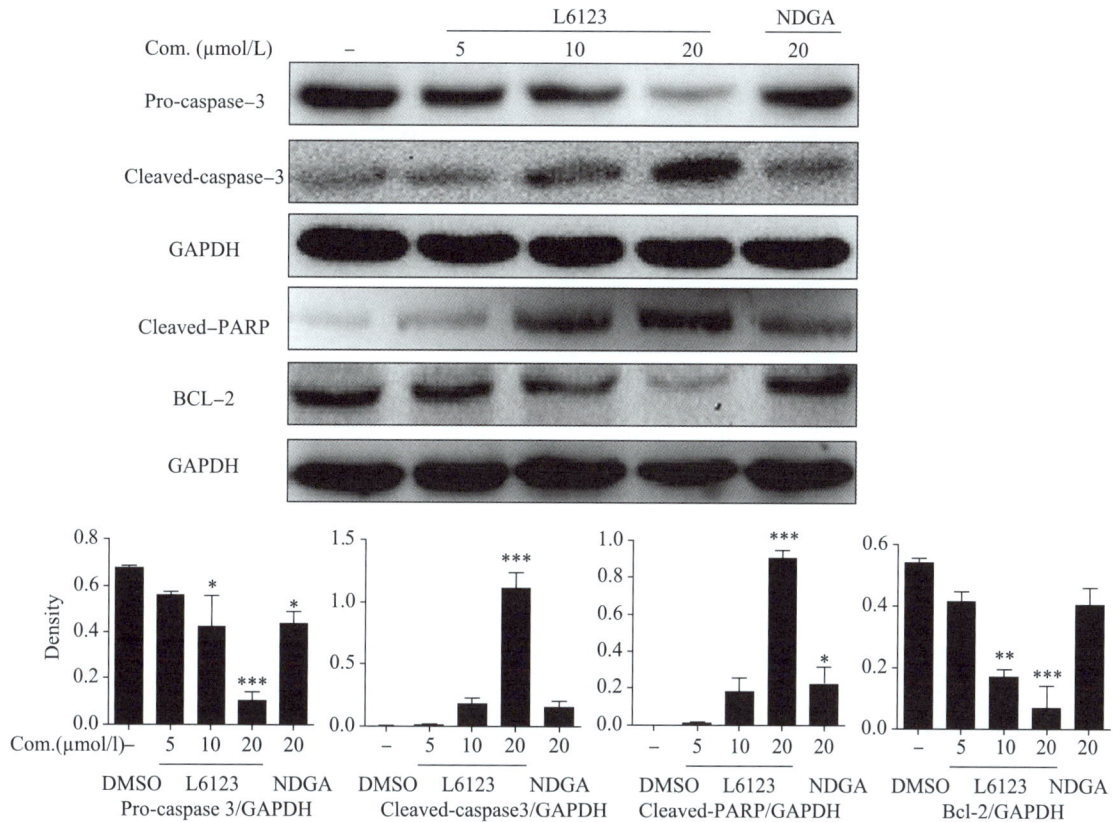

Fig. 4. Compound L6123 activated caspase-3 and PARP and suppressed Bcl-2 in a dose-dependent manner in SCG-7901 cells. SCG-7901 cells were exposed to L6123 or NDGA at indicated concentrations for 48 h. The levels of Bcl-2, cleaved-caspase-3, pro-caspase-3, and cleaved-PARP were detected by western blot analysis. GAPDH was used as a criterion. Data are presented as the mean ± SD of three independent experiments conducted in triplicate. $^{*}P < 0.05$; $^{**}P < 0.01$; $^{***}P < 0.001$. Com., compound; DMSO, dimethyl sulfoxide; GAPDH, glyceraldehyde 3-phosphate dehydrogenase; NDGA, nordihydroguaiaretic acid.

tosis-related molecules, namely, Bcl-2, cleaved-caspase-3, pro-caspase-3, and cleaved-PARP, were used to evaluate the apoptotic ability of SGC-7901 cells treated with varying concentrations of L6123. The expression of cleaved-caspase-3, pro-caspase-3, and Bcl-2 decreased, and cleaved-PARP expression increased in SGC-7901 cells after pretreatment with varying concentrations of L6123. However, the effect of NDGA on cell apoptosis was not obvious (Fig. 4). The result of flow cytometry using the annexin V-PI dual-labeling technique showed that L6123 increased the number of apoptotic SGC-7901 cells to 0.7, 2.9, and 14.1% at concentrations of 5, 10, and 20 μmol/L, respectively. However, the total apoptotic cell percentage was only 1.8% after pretreatment with NDGA (20 μmol/L) (Fig. 5A). The same result was found in Hoechst staining. SGC-7901 cell number increased after pretreatment with different concentrations of L6123 for 48 h, and nuclear schizolysis and condensations occurred in a dose-dependent manner (Fig. 5B). Thus, L6123 could induce GC cell apoptosis.

3.4 Compound L6123 inhibited cell invasion

We detected the invasion ability of SGC-7901 cells treated with varying concentrations of L6123. The cell invasion capacity was measured using a Transwell invasion assay with diluted Matrigel chamber precoating. SGC-7901 cells (1×10^5) were paved in 200 μl of serum-free RPMI 1640 medium in the upper well, and were treated or not treated with various concentrations of L6123. Cells that passed through the Matrigel and Transwell membrane were stained. The results of the Transwell cell invasion are presented in Fig. 6. The addition of L6123 (at 5, 10, and 20 μmol/L) in the upper well downregulated the invading cell numbers in a dose-dependent manner. In addition, NDGA (20 μmol/L) failed to reduce the number of invading cells.

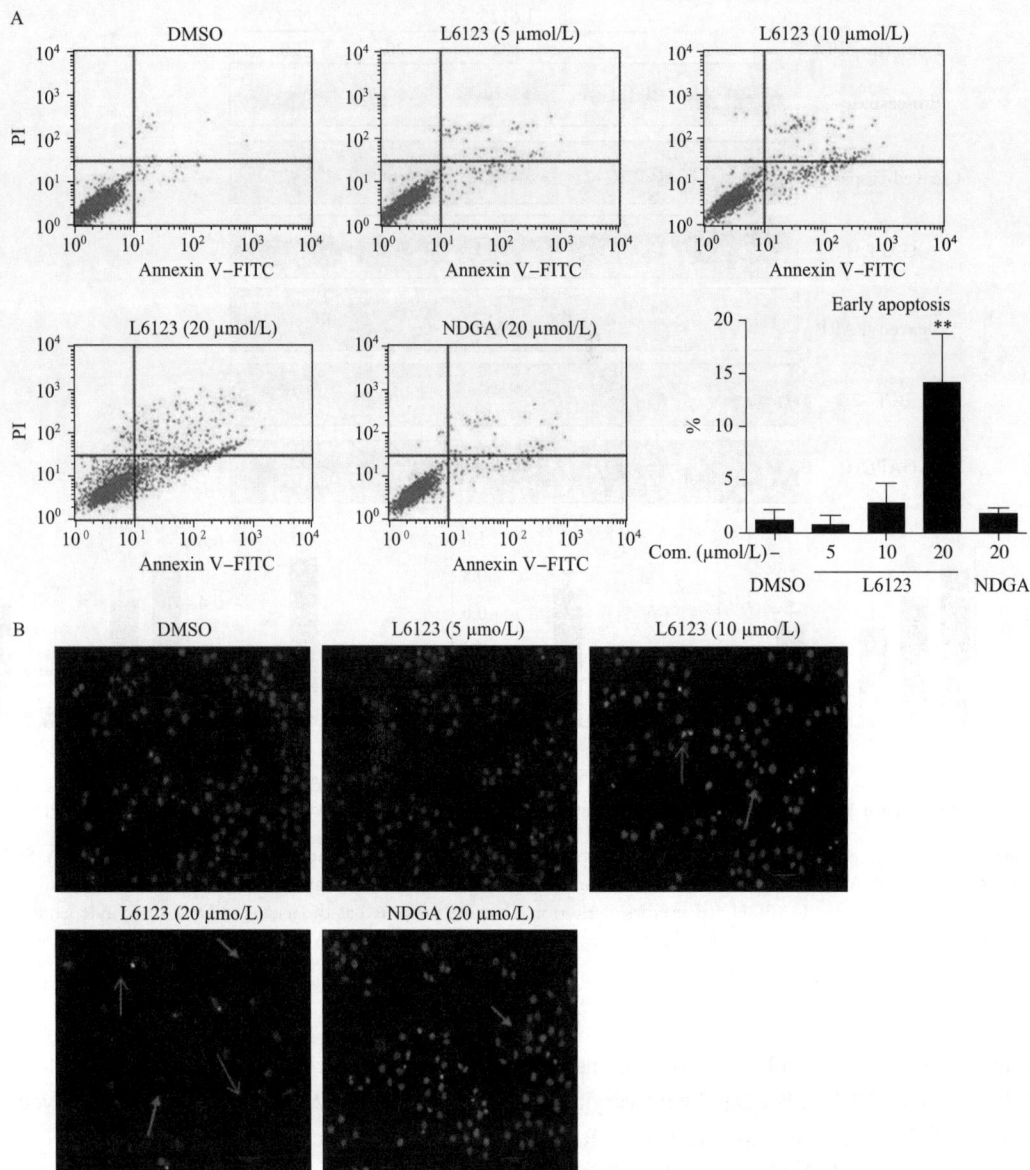

Fig. 5. Compound L6123 induced SCG-7901 cells apoptosis. (A) SGC-7901 cells were incubated with indicated concentrations for 48 h and then stained with annexin V and PI. The number of apoptotic cells was detected by flow cytometry. The figures were representative of three separate experiments. (B) Hoechst staining and morphological changes was observed in SCG-7901 cells cultured with L6123 (5, 10, and 20 μmol/L) or NDGA (20 μmol/L) for 48 h. Figures (×200) were representative of more than three separate experiments.**$P < 0.01$. Com., compound; DMSO, dimethyl sulfoxide; FITC, fluorescein isothiocyanate; NDGA, nordihydroguaiaretic acid; PI, propidium iodide.

4. Discussion

In recent years, genetic amplifications of FGFR family members have been discovered in GC. Many researchers found FGFR2 amplification in about 4%–10% of GCs; FGFR2 amplification was associated with depth of invasion, lymph node metastasis, distant metastasis, and TMN staging, but was not associated with age, sex, and degree of differentiation of GC patients [14–16]. Targeted FGFR2 inhibitors, such as GP369, Ki23057, and FGFR2 monoclonal antibodies, could effectively inhibit GC growth and enhance the chemosensitivity of drugresistant GC cells [17–20]. By detecting FGFR1 in GC tissue specimens, Oki *et al.* [21] found that FGFR1 expression was amplified, and the overexpression was related closely to EphA4 expression; both FGFR1 and EphA4 expressions play an important role in GC. Wen *et al.* [10] also found that FGFR1 was amplified not only in gastric tissue samples but also in a variety of GC cell lines; when the FGFR1 was silenced by miR-133b, the growth of GC cell lines was inhibited. FGFR1 might be a promising target in the

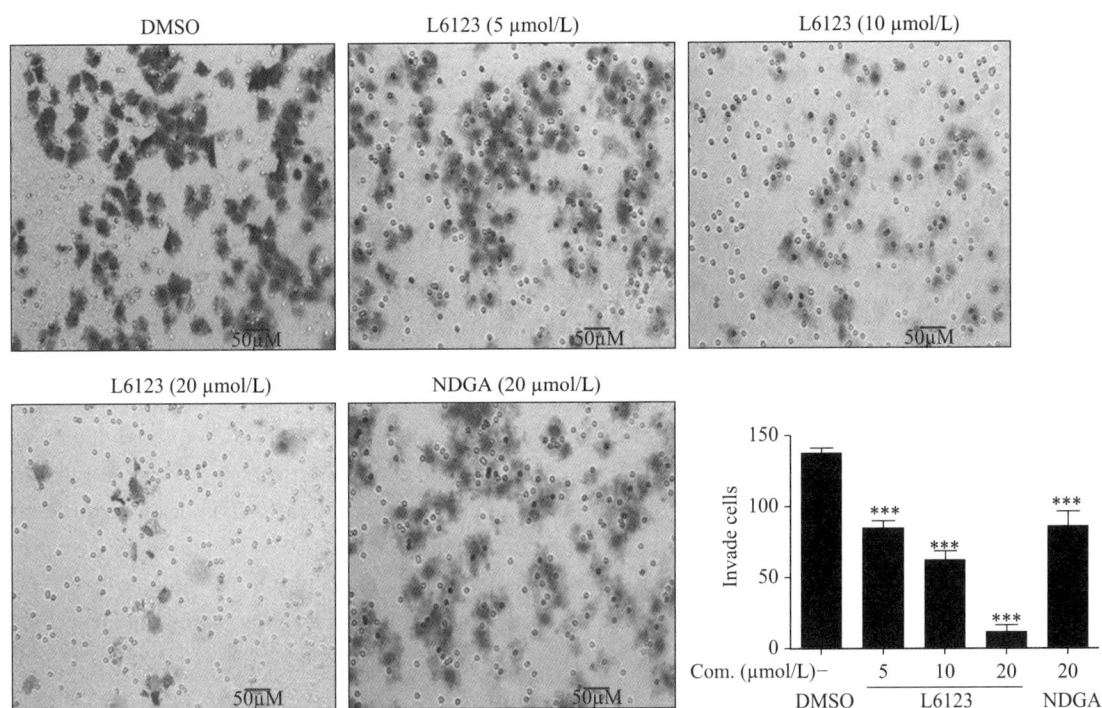

Fig. 6. Compound L6123 suppressed the invasion ability of SGC-7901 cells in a dose-dependent manner. After incubation with compound L6123 (5, 10, and 20 μmol/L) for 24 h, the invasion ability was test using a Transwell invasion assay. NDGA (20 μmol/L) was used as a positive control. Figures (×200) were representative of three separate experiments. Com., compound; DMSO, dimethyl sulfoxide; NDGA, nordihydroguaiaretic acid.

therapy of GCs. Targeting FGFR1 inhibitors with minimal side effects and low cell toxicity is important in GC therapy.

Because of multiple targets and the limited selectivity of the ATP-competitive inhibitor, we attempted to discover a novel kinase inhibitor. Non-ATP-competitive inhibitors may show targeted selectivity; the research and development of non-ATP-competitive inhibitors has become the focus of research [22,23]. However, except for ARQ 069 [24], information on other non-ATP-competitive FGFR1 inhibitors is limited. NDGA is a non-ATP-competitive FGFR3 kinase inhibitor that inhibits FGFR3 autophosphorylation and downstream signaling in multiple myeloma *in vitro* and *in vivo* [11]. We found that NDGA showed better selective inhibitory effect against FGFR1 than against FGFR3. Hence, using NDGA as a positive control, we successfully designed a series of novel non-ATP-competitive FGFR1 kinase inhibitors, which showed better inhibition activity against FGFR1 than NDGA [25]. Among the active FGFR1 inhibitors, the compound L6123 showed significant inhibitory activity against FGFR1 (IC_{50}: 0.6 μmol/L). Thus, the antitumor activity of L6123 on GC was explored. L6123 showed a good antiproliferative effect on GC cell lines, including SGC-7901, BGC-823, and MGC-803, in which FGFR1 was overexpressed. The activity of L6123 against three GC cell lines was better than that of NDGA, and this finding was in agreement with the activities of L6123 and NDGA against FGFR1 kinase. Thus, compound L6123 showed better activity than NDGA not only at the level of FGFR1 kinases but also at the cellular level.

Target selectivity is very important for a kinase inhibitor. The antiproliferative activities of L6123 against MEF-FGFR1-FGFR2-FRS2α-KO (FGFR1 knockout) and MEF-WT were detected using an MTT assay, and the results were compared. L6123 showed higher inhibitory effect against MEF-WT than against MEF-FGFR1-FGFR2-FRS2α-KO. FGFR1 knockout downregulated the antiproliferative activity of L6123 and L6123 showed an antitumor effect by targeting FGFR1, at least partly. Similar to ATP-competitive FGFR1 inhibitors AZD4547 [26] and BGJ398 [27] and non-ATP-competitive FGFR1 inhibitor ARQ 069 [24], L6123 showed a satisfactory inhibitory effect on FGFR2 and FGFR3 (data not shown). Thus, the target selectivity of L6123 needs improvement. We are designing novel analogs with L6123 as the leading compound.

ERKs are members of the MAPK superfamily that play a major role in cell proliferation. In many cancers, ERK1/2 functions as a downstream signaling molecule of FGFRs [22]. FRS2α, which is a substrate of FGFR1, can induce the activation of ERK1/2 and FRS2α and is vital for the FGF/FGFR pathway [28]. FGFR1/FRS2α/ERK1/2 signaling has not been investigated previously in GC cell lines. We confirmed that FGF2 can activate the FGFR1/FRS2α/ERK1/2 pathway. L6123 showed inhibitory effects on the growth of GC cells by inhibiting this signal pathway. Recently, Zhao *et al.* [29] confirmed that FGF signaling regulates cell survival and migration by the regulation of NFκB and CXCL4-SDF1 pathways. Further studies are required to determine whether L6123 suppresses cell survival and migration by the NFκB and CXCL4-SDF1 pathways.

Bcl-2, caspase-3, and PARP are apoptosis-related molecules that participate in the mitochondria-mediated apoptotic pathway. siRNA silencing of FGFR expression in the human GC cell line MGC-803 induced the activity of the apoptosis pathway by the upregulation of Bax and caspase-3 [30]. Moreover, FGFR inhibitor PD173074 caused apoptotic death by decreasing the expression of Bcl-2, survivin, and Mcl-1 and by increasing the expression of Bax [31]. L6123 enhanced apoptosis of the GC cells in response to FGFR1 downregulation, as confirmed by the change in apoptosis-related molecules Bcl-2, cleaved-caspase-3, pro-caspase-3, and cleaved-PARP. The epithelial–mesenchymal transition (EMT) is a core process in tumor progression and its deregulation is associated with the cancer cell's ability to invade stromal tissues and migrate to other regions [32]. The FGFR1 inhibitor PD173074 induces EMT transition through the transcription factor AP-1 in head and neck squamous cell carcinoma [33]. L6123 could prohibit gastric cell invasion. Further studies are required to determine whether L6123 could induce EMT and to elucidate the mechanism underlying this activity.

FGFR1-targeted therapy is a promising strategy for the treatment and diagnosis of GC. In this study, we proved that L6123 inhibits the phosphorylation of FGFR1 and its downstream signaling molecules at the cellular level. L6123 significantly repressed proliferation, inhibited invasion, and induced apoptosis in FGFR1-overexpressing GC cells.

References

[1] Jemal A, Bray F, Center MM, *et al.* Global Cancer Statistics[J]. Ca-a Cancer Journal for Clinicians, 2011, 61(2): 69-90.

[2] Zamecnikova A. Novel approaches to the development of tyrosine kinase inhibitors and their role in the fight against cancer[J]. Expert Opinion on Drug Discovery, 2014, 9(1): 77-92.

[3] Judson I, Scurr M, Gardner K, *et al.* Phase II Study of Cediranib in Patients with Advanced Gastrointestinal Stromal Tumors or Soft-Tissue Sarcoma[J]. Clinical Cancer Research, 2014, 20(13): 3603-3612.

[4] Kataoka Y, Mukohara T, Tomioka H, *et al.* Foretinib (GSK1363089), a multi-kinase inhibitor of MET and VEGFRs, inhibits growth of gastric cancer cell lines by blocking inter-receptor tyrosine kinase networks[J]. Investigational New Drugs, 2012, 30(4): 1352-1360.

[5] Wang C, Zheng B, Chen Y, *et al.* Imatinib as preoperative therapy in Chinese patients with recurrent or metastatic GISTs[J]. Chinese Journal of Cancer Research, 2013, 25(1): 63-70.

[6] Overton LC, Heinrich MC. Regorafenib for treatment of advanced gastrointestinal stromal tumors[J]. Expert Opinion on Pharmacotherapy, 2014, 15(4): 549-558.

[7] Katoh M, Katoh M. FGF signaling network in the gastrointestinal tract (Review)[J]. International Journal of Oncology, 2006, 29(1): 163-168.

[8] Beenken A, Mohammadi M. The FGF family: biology, pathophysiology and therapy[J]. Nature Reviews Drug Discovery, 2009, 8(3): 235-253.

[9] Wesche J, Haglund K, Haugsten EM. Fibroblast growth factors and their receptors in cancer[J]. Biochemical Journal, 2011, 437: 199-213.

[10] Wen D, Li S, Ji F, *et al.* miR-133b acts as a tumor suppressor and negatively regulates FGFR1 in gastric cancer[J]. Tumor Biology, 2013, 34(2): 793-803.

[11] Meyer AN, McAndrew CW, Donoghue DJ. Nordihydroguaiaretic acid inhibits an activated fibroblast growth factor receptor 3 mutant and blocks downstream signaling in multiple myeloma cells[J]. Cancer Research, 2008, 68(18): 7362-7370.

[12] Zavodovskaya M, Campbel MJ, Maddux BA, *et al.* Nordihydroguaiaretic acid (NDGA), an inhibitor of the HER2 and IGF-1 receptor tyrosine kinases, blocks the growth of HEF12-overexpress-

ing human breast cancer cells[J]. Journal of Cellular Biochemistry, 2008, 103(2): 624-635.

[13] Youngren JF, Gable K, Penaranda C, *et al.* Nordihydroguaiaretic acid (NDGA) inhibits the IGF-1 and c-erbB2/HER2/neu receptors and suppresses growth in breast cancer cells[J]. Breast Cancer Research and Treatment, 2005, 94(1): 37-46.

[14] Matsumoto K, Arao T, Hamaguchi T, *et al.* FGFR2 gene amplification and clinicopathological features in gastric cancer[J]. British Journal of Cancer, 2012, 106(4): 727-732.

[15] Jung E-J, Jung E-J, Min SY, *et al.* Fibroblast growth factor receptor 2 gene amplification status and its clinicopathologic significance in gastric carcinoma[J]. Human Pathology, 2012, 43(10): 1559-1566.

[16] Deng N, Goh LK, Wang H, *et al.* A comprehensive survey of genomic alterations in gastric cancer reveals systematic patterns of molecular exclusivity and co-occurrence among distinct therapeutic targets[J]. Gut, 2012, 61(5): 673-684.

[17] Bai A, Meetze K, Vo NY, *et al.* GP369, an FGFR2-IIIb-Specific Antibody, Exhibits Potent Antitumor Activity against Human Cancers Driven by Activated FGFR2 Signaling[J]. Cancer Research, 2010, 70(19): 7630-7639.

[18] Qiu H, Yashiro M, Zhang X, *et al.* A FGFR2 inhibitor, Ki23057, enhances the chemosensitivity of drug-resistant gastric cancer cells[J]. Cancer Letters, 2011, 307(1): 47-52.

[19] Zhao W-M, Wang L, Park H, *et al.* Monoclonal Antibodies to Fibroblast Growth Factor Receptor 2 Effectively Inhibit Growth of Gastric Tumor Xenografts[J]. Clinical Cancer Research, 2010, 16(23): 5750-5758.

[20] Yashiro M, Shinto O, Nakamura K, *et al.* Synergistic antitumor effects of FGFR2 inhibitor with 5-fluorouracil on scirrhous gastric carcinoma[J]. International Journal of Cancer, 2010, 126(4): 1004-1016.

[21] Oki M, Yamamoto H, Taniguchi H, *et al.* Overexpression of the receptor tyrosine kinase EphA4 in human gastric cancers[J]. World Journal of Gastroenterology, 2008, 14(37): 5650-5656.

[22] Liang G, Liu Z, Wu J, *et al.* Anticancer molecules targeting fibroblast growth factor receptors[J]. Trends in Pharmacological Sciences, 2012, 33(10): 531-541.

[23] Fang Z, Gruetter C, Rauh D. Strategies for the Selective Regulation

of Kinases with Allosteric Modulators: Exploiting Exclusive Structural Features[J]. Acs Chemical Biology, 2013, 8(1): 58-70.

[24] Eathiraj S, Palma R, Hirschi M, *et al.* A Novel Mode of Protein Kinase Inhibition Exploiting Hydrophobic Motifs of Autoinhibited Kinases discovery of ATP-independent inhibitors of fibroblast growth factor receptor[J]. Journal of Biological Chemistry, 2011, 286(23): 20677-20687.

[25] Wu J, Ji J, Weng B, *et al.* Discovery of novel non-ATP competitive FGFR1 inhibitors and evaluation of their anti-tumor activity in non-small cell lung cancer *in vitro* and *in vivo*[J]. Oncotarget, 2014, 5(12): 4543-4553.

[26] Gavine PR, Mooney L, Kilgour E, *et al.* AZD4547: An Orally Bioavailable, Potent, and Selective Inhibitor of the Fibroblast Growth Factor Receptor Tyrosine Kinase Family[J]. Cancer Research, 2012, 72(8): 2045-2056.

[27] Guagnano V, Furet P, Spanka C, *et al.* Discovery of 3-(2,6-Dichloro-3,5-dimethoxy-phenyl)-1-{6- 4-(4-ethyl-piperazin-1-yl)-p henylamino -pyrimidin-4-yl}-1-methyl-urea (NVP-BGJ398), A Potent and Selective Inhibitor of the Fibroblast Growth Factor Receptor Family of Receptor Tyrosine Kinase[J]. Journal of Medicinal Chemistry, 2011, 54(20): 7066-7083.

[28] Sato T, Gotoh N. The FRS2 family of docking/scaffolding adaptor proteins as therapeutic targets of cancer treatment[J]. Expert Opinion on Therapeutic Targets, 2009, 13(6): 689-700.

[29] Zhao M, Ross JT, Itkin T, *et al.* FGF signaling facilitates postinjury recovery of mouse hematopoietic system[J]. Blood, 2012, 120(9): 1831-1842.

[30] Zhou D, Jiang X, Ding W, *et al.* RETRACTED: siRNA-participated chemotherapy: an efficient and specific therapeutic against gastric cancer (Retracted article. See vol. 141, pg. 2069, 2015)[J]. Journal of Cancer Research and Clinical Oncology, 2013, 139(12): 2057-2070.

[31] Ye T, Wei X, Yin T, *et al.* Inhibition of FGFR signaling by PD173074 improves antitumor immunity and impairs breast cancer metastasis[J]. Breast Cancer Research and Treatment, 2014, 143(3): 435-446.

[32] Angela Nieto M. Epithelial Plasticity: A Common Theme in Embryonic and Cancer Cells[J]. Science, 2013, 342(6159): 1234850

[33] Nguyen PT, Tsunematsu T, Yanagisawa S, *et al.* The FGFR1 inhibitor PD173074 induces mesenchymal-epithelial transition through the transcription factor AP-1[J]. British Journal of Cancer, 2013, 109(8): 2248-2258.

Discovery and anti-cancer evaluation of two novel non-ATP-competitive FGFR1 inhibitors in non-small-cell lung cancer

Jianzhang Wu, Xiaokun Li, Guang Liang

1. Background

Lung cancer is the most common cause of death from cancer worldwide, and non-small-cell lung cancer (NSCLC) accounts for 85% of the total incidence [1]. Recently, molecular targeted chemotherapy with RTK inhibitors has been used in clinics for the treatment of NSCLC because of the importance of a series of receptor tyrosine kinases (RTKs) in the development of NSCLC [1,2]. Small-molecule inhibitors of epidermal growth factor receptor (EGFR), such as gefitinib and erlotinib, have been approved by the U.S. Food and Drug Administration (FDA) for the treatment of NSCLC [3,4]. Unfortunately, NSCLC treatment remains challenging because of some problems, including adverse effects and drug resistance associated with the ATP-competitive kinase inhibition mode of the majority of RTK inhibitors [5-7]. The ATP-binding pocket is highly conserved among members of the kinase family, and it is difficult to find selective agents [7,8]. Moreover, the ATP-competitive inhibitors must compete with high intracellular ATP levels leading to a discrepancy between IC_{50}s measured by biochemical *versus* cellular assays. The non-ATP-competitive inhibitors, called type II or type III inhibitors, offer the possibility of overcoming these problems [7,9]. Thus, the development of RTK inhibitors that do not compete with ATP is an urgent need for the treatment of NSCLC.

Fibroblast growth factor receptors (FGFRs) belong to the family of RTK superfamily, and FGFRs, especially FGFR1, was reported to be highly related to the development and progress of NSCLC [1,10-17]. Amplification and activating mutations of FGFR1 have been observed in NSCLC [13,14,17], while silencing the expression of FGFR1 by siRNA or pharmacological inhibition of FGFR1 by small molecules suppresses the development of NSCLC [11,12,16,17]. These observations make FGFRs increasingly a attractive target for the therapeutic intervention in cancer. Two FGFR inhibitors, namely AZD4547 and BGJ398, have entered phase II clinical trials, while more small-molecule inhibitors, such as SU5402, PD173074, TKI-258, and SU6668, have failed in clinical trials due to various complications associated with the side effects caused by the ATP-competitive inhibition mode [8]. To date, only five non-ATP-competitive FGFR inhibitors have been identified, including nordihydroguaiaretic acid (NDGA) [18], NF449 [19], ARQ069 [20], and recently reported A114 and A117 [21]. Despite advances in the field, identifying highly-selective, small-molecule inhibitors that target an inactive conformation or a new domain of FGFR continues to be a significant challenge.

In this report, we characterize two nordihydroguaiaretic acid (NDGA) analogs, i.e., Ad23 and Af23, as two kinase inhibitors that effectively target FGFR1 (Fig. 1A). Furthermore, we provide data that indicates these kinase inhibitors have a distinct ATP-independent mode of action. Furthermore, these two compounds have shown excellent anti-cancer activity against NSCLC H460 cells both *in vitro* and *in vivo*. These data further confirm that bisaryl-1,4-dien-3-one structures could be used as non-ATP-competitive FGFR1 inhibitors for the treatment of NSCLC.

2. Methods

2.1 Cell lines, compounds, and reagents

NSCLC cell line, H460, was purchased from ATCC (*Manassas, VA*). FGFR1-overexpressing HEK 293 cell lines were kindly gifted by the Institute of Materia Medical, Xi'an Jiaotong University. Various compounds were designed and synthesized in our laboratory, including Af23 (3,5-bis(3,4-dihydroxybenzylidene)-tetrahydropyran-4-one) and Ad23

(3,5-bis(3,4-dihydroxybenzylidene)-tetra-hydrothiopyran-4-one) (Fig. 1A). Their purity was detected by HPLC (>98.0%) before they were used in biological experiments. The compounds were dissolved in DMSO solution for *in vitro* assay. Their water-soluble formulations for *in vivo* studies were prepared using the pharmaceutical method described previously [22]. All the antibodies were purchased from Santa Cruz Biotechnology (*Santa Cruz, CA*). Hoechst staining kit was purchased from Beyotime Biotech (*Nantong, China*). Recombinant FGFR1 proteins were obtained from Carna Biosciences, Inc. (*Kobe, Japan*).

2.2　Cell-free FGFR1 kinase assays

Using the method described previously in Ref. [21], the FGFR1 kinase inhibition assay of NDGA and its analogs were performed by Caliper Mobility Shift Assay with ATP concentration at its Km value (262 μM). Staurosporine was used as a positive control. For the determination of IC_{50}, the compounds were tested in duplicate at 10 concentrations, ranging from 5 nM to 100 μM. Then, conversion data were collected on Caliper EZ reader (*Hopkinton, MA*). The IC_{50} values were obtained by GraphPad Prism 5 (*GraphPad, San Diego, CA*).

2.3　ATP competitive inhibition assay

This experiment was performed to test the relationship between the compounds and ATP in which the concentration of the substrate was constant, while the concentrations of ATP were set at 4192, 2096, 1048, 524, 262, 131, 66, and 33 μM. The global competitive inhibition fit for the compounds was performed based on percent conversion = $(Vmax*X)/\{km*[(1 + I/Ki)^n] + X\}$, where X is the ATP concentration, and n is the Hill coefficient. Specific details of this method were presented in a previous report [21].

2.4　MTT assay

The anti-proliferative activities of compounds were detected by MTT assay. H460 cells were seeded in a 96-well plate with RPMI-1640 medium that contained 0.1% FBS for 24 h. Then, the cells were treated with the compounds at the indicated concentrations (0.74, 2.22, 6.67, 20, and 60 μM) for 72 h. The proliferation of the H460 cells was detected through MTT assay, and the IC_{50} values were calculated by GraphPad software.

2.5　Western blot analysis

Cells or homogenated tumor tissues were lysated. Protein concentrations in all the samples were determined by using the Bradford protein assay kit (*Bio-Rad, Hercules, CA*). The lysates were separated by SDS-PAGE electro-phoresis, and electro-transferred to a 0.22-μm polyvinyldene difluoride membrane. After blocking with TBS that contained 5% non-fat milk for 1.5 h at room temperature, the membranes were incubated with different primary antibodies overnight at 4℃. Following the TBST wash, immuno-reactive bands were detected by incubating with respective secondary antibody conjugated with horseradish peroxidase for 1 h. Immuno-reactive bands were visualized by using an ECL kit (*Bio-Rad, Hercules, CA*).

2.6　Hoechest staining

After the H460 cells were incubated with the compounds for 72 h, cells were stained with Hoechst 33342 dye according to the protocol provided with the kit (*Beyotime Biotech, Nantong, China*). The cells were imaged under fluorescent microscope (*Nikon, Tokyo, Japan*), and the pictures were taken at 200× objective.

2.7　Analysis of cell apoptosis

H460 cells were placed in 60-mm plates for 12 h and then treated with NDGA, Ad23, or Af23 at the indicated concentrations for 24 h. Then, the cells were harvested and stained with annexin V and propidium iodide (PI) in the presence of 100 mg/mL of RNAse and 0.1% Triton X-100 for 30 min at 37℃. Flow-cytometric analysis was performed using FACS calibur (*BD Sciences, CA*).

2.8　In vivo anti-tumor study

All animal experiments complied with the Wenzhou Medical College Policy on the Care and Use of Laboratory Animals (Wenzhou Medical College Animal Policy and Welfare Committee, Document ID: 201100103). Five to six-week-old athymic nu/nu female BALB/cA mice (18–22 g) were purchased from the Animal Center of the China Pharmaceutical University (Nanjing, China). The animals were housed at a constant room temperature with a 12:12-hr (light: dark) cycle and fed a standard rodent diet and water. H460 cells were harvested and mixed with Matrigel at proportions of 1:1. Then, the cells were injected subcutaneously into the right flank (2×10^6 cells in 200 μl of PBS) of 7-week-old, BALB/cA nude mice. Two days after the H460 cells were injected, the mice were injected intraperitoneally (i.p.) with a water-soluble preparation of either compound Ad23 or compound Af23 in PBS at a dosage of 5 mg/kg/day for 28 days, whereas the control mice were injected with the liposome vehicle in PBS (n = 10 in each group). The volume of the tumors were determined by measuring their length (l) and width (w) and calculated using the formula; $V = 0.52 \times l \times w^2$. The weight of the tumors were recorded on the day the mice were killed.

2.9 Immunohistochemistry analysis

On day 30 after tumor induction, the mice were killed in a CO_2 chamber, and the tumor tissues were dissected and weighed. Some of the tissues were lysed for protein isolation and then processed for the determination of signaling pathway proteins using Western blot method. A part of harvested tumor tissues were fixed in 10% formalin at room temperature overnight, processed, and embedded in paraffin. The paraffin-embedded tissues were sectioned (5-μm thick) followed by staining with primary antibodies. The signal was detected by biotinylated secondary antibody and developed with 3,3-diaminobenzidine (DAB).

2.10 Statistical analysis

All *in vitro* experiments were repeated at least three times. Data were presented as means ± SD or mean ± SEM. The statistical significance of differences between groups was obtained by the *student's t test* or ANOVA multiple comparisons in GraphPad Prism 5 (License Number: GPW5-415777-RAG-2191, *GraphPad Software Inc., San Diego, CA*). P values less than 0.05 ($P < 0.05$) were considered to be significant.

3. Results

3.1 Af23 and Ad23 inhibits FGFR1 kinase *via* a non-ATP dependent manner

The leading compound NDGA is a natural product isolated from creosote bush. It exhibits multiple pharmacological effects, such as anti-oxidation, anti-inflammation, and anti-tumor [18,23]. Recently, Meyer *et al.* found that NDGA could inhibit the autophosphorylation of FGFR3 kinase both *in vitro* and *in vivo* [18]. In our previous cell-free assay, we found that the IC_{50} values of NDGA against FGFR1 and FGFR3 were 24.5 and 72.4 μM, respectively, indicating that NDGA exhibits better inhibitory activity against FGFR1 than FGFR3 (Fig. 1A). Therefore, using NDGA as a leading compound, we designed and synthesized a series of structural analogs (Fig. 1A). Next, we tested the inhibitory activity of synthetic NDGA analogs against FGFR1 kinase by mobility shift assay.

The inhibitory potency of 72 bisaryl-1,4-dien-3-one compounds against FGFR1 kinase was evaluated by *in vitro* kinase assays. Out of the 72 compounds, Ad23 and Af23 were found to exhibit much stronger inhibition against FGFR1 kinase activity than NDGA and other analogs (IC_{50}: Ad23,0.6 μM; Af23,1.4 μM) (Fig. 1A). Thus these two were chosen for further studies. Subsequently, the kinase inhibition modes of both Ad23 and Af23 were studied. As shown in Figure 1B, the velocity of FGFR1 substrate phosphorylation without inhibitors increases as the ATP concentration increased, and it was reached to the peak at an ATP concentration of 2000 μM. At concentrations greater than the IC_{50} value (1.4 μM for Ad23; 1.88 μM for Af23; 100 μM for NDGA), the kinase activity was decreased by more than 90%, and further increases in the concentration of ATP, even up to 4190 μM, had no effect on the inhibitory potency of the compounds (Fig. 1B). These results showed that the inhibition of FGFR1 kinase activity by Ad23, Af23, and NDGA was not dependent on the concentration of ATP. Thus, we obtained two novel non-ATP-competitive FGFR1 inhibitors, i.e., Ad23 and Af23, from the leading NDGA.

3.2 Ad23 and Af23 inhibits the cellular FGFR1 phosphorylation

The inhibitory effects of these two compounds on FGFR1 activation were determined in FGFR1-overexpressing

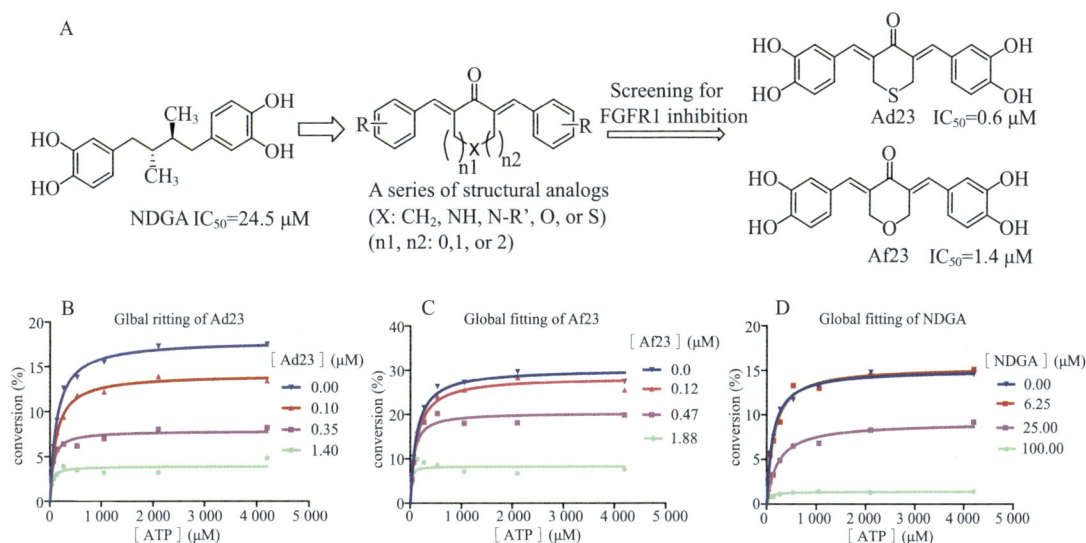

Fig. 1. NDGA analogs Af23 and Ad23 inhibited FGFR1 activities in a non-ATP competitive manner. (A) The profile of design and FGFR1 kinase inhibition assay of NDGA analogs. FGFR1 kinase inhibition rates of the compounds were evaluated by caliper mobility shift assay, and IC_{50} values were calculated using conversion rates. The data were shown as a mean of 3–5 independent tests. (B) Af23 and Ad23 inhibit FGFR1 through a mechanism that is independent of the concentration of ATP. Selective ATP-competitive kinase assay of compounds Ad23 (B), Af23 (C), and NDGA (D) with FGFR1 was carried out through caliper mobility shift assay. The conversion data were fitted with Graphpad for global fitting, using "mixed model inhibition".

293 cells and human NSCLC H460 cells. As shown in Figures 2A and B, pre-treatment with Ad23 or Af23 dose-dependently reduced the bFGF-induced phosphorylation of FGFR1 in both the cell lines. Also, both Ad23 and Af23 inhibited the phosphorylation of FRS2, a proliferative substrate of FGFR1, in a dose-dependent manner in H460 cells (Fig. 2C). Consistent with the cell-free results, Ad23 and Af23 had greater activity than NDGA, and Ad23 showed stronger inhibition than Af23 against cellular FGFR1 phosphorylation.

3.3 Ad23 and Af23 inhibited the proliferation and induced the apoptosis of H460 cell line

Next, the growth inhibition of H460 cells by NDGA, Ad23, and Af23 was studied by MTT assay. Our data showed that Af23, Ad23, and NDGA exhibited marked inhibitory effects against H460 cells (Fig. 3A). The inhibitory potencies (IC_{50} values) of Af23 and Ad23 were much greater when compared to NDGA. Further, Western blot analysis showed that the cleavage of caspase-3 and caspase-9 increased after treatment with Ad23 or Af23, indicating that these compounds could induce apoptosis in H460 cells after a 12-h treatment (Fig. 3B). Further, Hoechst staining was performed 12 h after treatment with the compounds (Fig. 3C). A concentration-dependent increase in the number of cells with nuclear condensation and fragmentation was observed in both the groups. Next, we assessed the effects of Ad23 and Af23 on the induction of apoptosis in H460 cells by flow cytometric analysis. Fig. 3D shows that both Ad23 and Af23 dose-dependently increased the H460 apoptosis after 24-h treatment. At a concentrations of 20 μM, both Ad23-treated group (Annexin V^+/PI^+, 44.8% ± 7.07%) and Af23-treated group (48.2% ± 11.12%) induced a greater rate of cell apoptosis than NDGA (27.2% ± 5.27%). We have also tested the growth inhibition of Ad23 and Af23 against human liver cells HL7702 and human fetal lung cell line MRC-5 which expresses low level of FGFR1. The results showed that all the IC_{50} values of Ad23, Af23, and NDGA against HL7702 or MRC-5 cells were greater than 30 μM (Fig. 3A).

3.4 Ad23 and Af23 significantly suppressed the H460 tumor growth in xenograft mouse model

In order to further assess the anti-tumor activities of the NDGA analogs, we tested the efficacies of Af23 and Ad23 in the H460 xenograft mouse model. Treatment with Af23 or Ad23 for 28 days resulted in significant reduction in tumor volume (Fig. 4A). The weight of the tumors were also reduced markedly in the Af23-treated and Ad23-treated groups, with the inhibition rate of 67.4% and 75.8%, respectively (Fig. 4B). To evaluate whether the inhibition of tumor growth by Ad23 or Af23 was associated with the inhibition of FGFR1 activity *in vivo*, we analyzed the expression of p-FGFR1 in the tumor tissues. As shown in Fig. 4C, Ad23 and Af23 exhibited a significant increased inhibitory effect on FGFR1

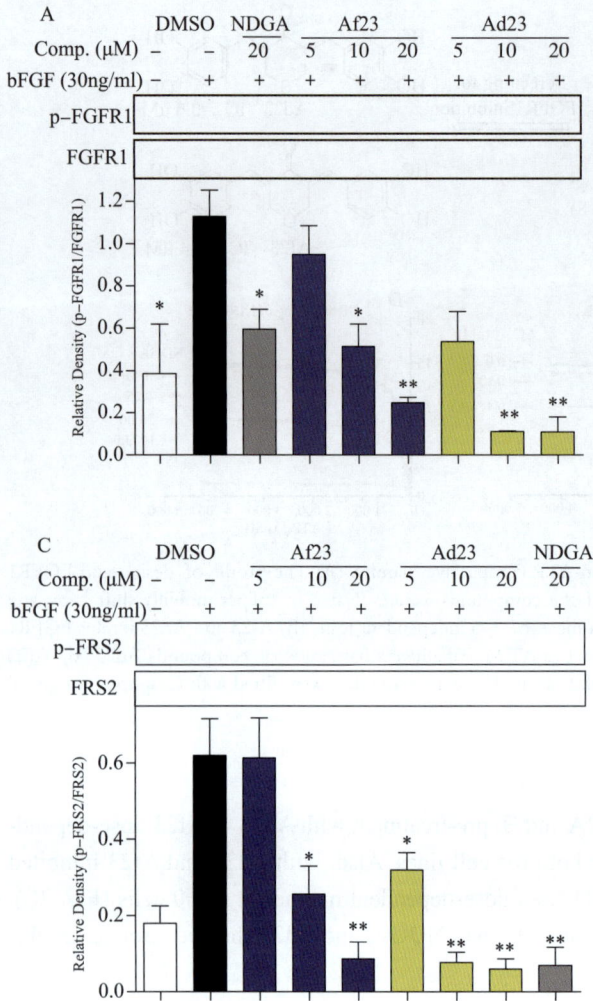

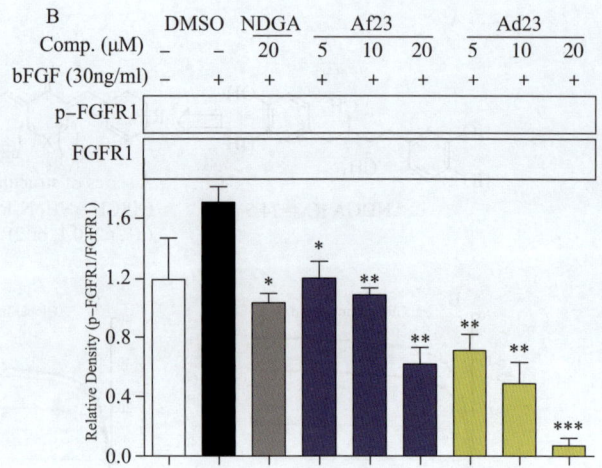

Fig. 2. Compounds Ad23 and Af23 inhibited intracellular FGFR1/ FRS2 phosphorylation. FGFR1 over-expression 293 cells (A) or H460 cells (B and C) were pretreated with compounds at indicated concentrations or vehicle (0.1% DMSO), respectively. Then, cells were stimulated with bFGF (30 ng/ml) for 10 min, and the phosphorylation levels of FGFR1 (A and B) and FRS2 (C) in cell lysates was measured by western blot analysis. The figures were representative of 3 separate experiments. The column figures show the normalized optical density as a percentage of total protein control. Bars represent the mean ± SEM of 3 independent experiments. Statistical significance relative to bFGF alone group was expressed, *P <0.05, **P < 0.01, ***P < 0.001.

phosphorylation in H460 tumor xenografts than the vehicle control tumors. Also, no obvious toxicity was observed in the Af23-treated group or the Ad23-treated group, evidenced by no obvious loss of weight among the two groups during the period of treatment (Fig. 4D).

Prior studies have revealed that phosphorylation of FGFR1 can lead to the activation of downstream signaling cascades including ERK and AKT, which plays an important role in the proliferation and survival of cancer cells. Thus, the phosphorylation of ERK and AKT in tumor samples was tested by immunohistochemical assays (Fig. 4E). Similarly, these compounds inhibited the FGFR1-downstream ERK and AKT phosphorylation. Finally, the immunochemical data also showed that the expression of Bcl-2, Cyclin D1 and COX-2 was reduced to a far greater extent in the Ad23-treated group and the Af23-treated group than compared to the vehicle-treated group (Fig. 4E), indicating that these two FGFR1 inhibitors also induced tumor-cell apoptosis in H460 xenografts.

4. Discussion

FGFR1 is highly related to the development of lung cancer [10,12-15,17,24]. Ren et al. identified four NSCLC cell lines and two, newly-established primary lung-cancer cultures that showed high FGFR1 expression levels [24]. They also found that treatment with ponatinib, an FGFR1 inhibitor, could inhibit cell growth in NSCLC cell lines [24]. Terai et al. revealed that the activation of the FGF2-FGFR1 autocrine pathway may be a novel mechanism of acquired resistance to the EGFR inhibitor, gefitinib, in NSCLC [12]. There has been increasing evidence indicating that FGFR1 inhibitors could be a promising candidate for the treatment of NSCLC in clinics. Although a variety of ATP-competitive FGFR1

A

Comp.	H460	HL7702	MRC–5
Af23	9.9 ± 1.2	87.8 ± 18.2	33.6 ± 5.1
Ad23	6.7 ± 0.9	> 100	54.7 ± 6.9
NDGA	15.8 ± 1.2	> 100	32.2 ± 7.4

B

C

D

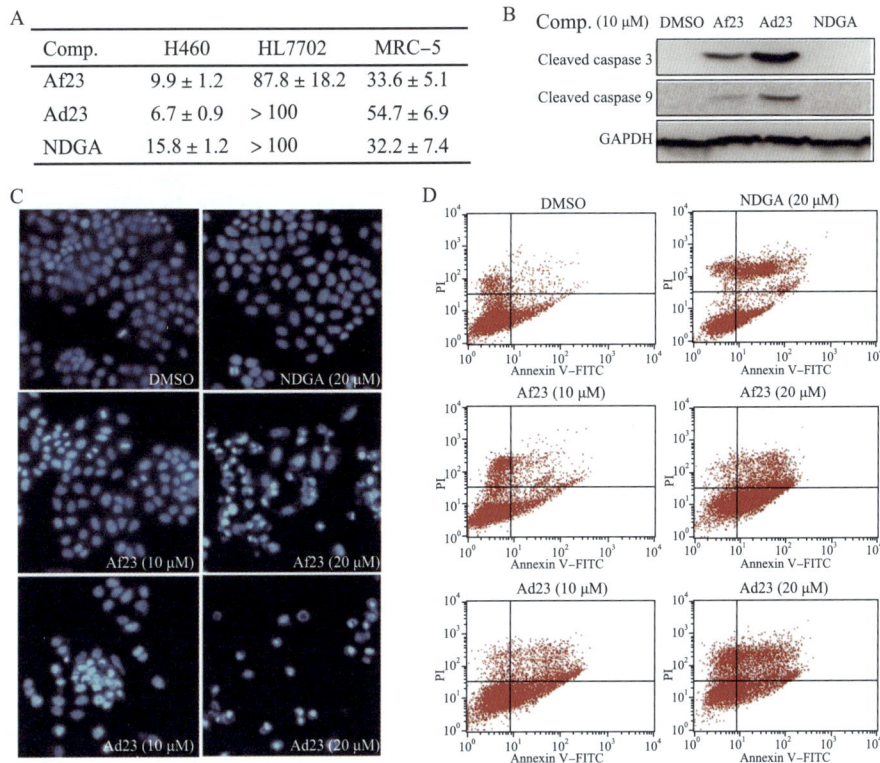

Fig. 3. Af23 and Ad23 inhibited proliferation and induced apoptosis in H460 cells. (A) H460 cells were treated with Af23, Ad23 or NDGA at different concentration (0.74, 2.22, 6.67, 20, and 60 μM) for 72 h. The viability of H460 cells were detected by MTT assay, and the IC_{50} values of compounds were fitted with GraphPad. (B) Effects of Af23 and Ad23 on caspase activation in H460 cells. H460 cells were harvested and lysated after incubated with Af23 (10 μM), Ad23 (10 μM), or NDGA (10 μM) for 12 h. The levels of cleaved caspase-3 and cleaved caspase-9 were determined by western blot analysis. (C) Morphological changes and hoechst staining were observed in H460 cells cultured with and without Af23, Ad23, or NDGA at indicated concentrations for 12 h (200×). The figures were representative of more than three separate experiments. (D) Af23 and Ad23 induced cell apoptosis in H460 cells. H460 cells were treated with Af23, Ad23, or NDGA at indicated concentrations for 24 h, and then stained with Annexin V and PI, followed by detection using flow cytometry. The representative pictures are shown.

inhibitors with therapeutic prospects for lung cancer have been identified, most of them failed in pre-clinical or clinical studies because of their low efficacy or high toxicity. At present only two selective FGFR1 inhibitors, i.e., AZD4547 and BGJ398, are being studied in clinical trials (phase II) [8]. The ATP-competitive FGFR1 inhibitors functions by targeting the ATP-binding pocket of FGFR1, which may lead to a decrease in their efficiency when high physiological or intracellular concentrations of ATP exist [8]. In addition, since the ATP-binding site is highly conserved in RTKs, most inhibitors exhibit limited selectivity within RTKs, which induces side effects during treatment, such as nausea, weakness, and elevated blood pressure [25]. For instance, PD173074 and SU5402 failed to enter phase II clinical trials due to their high toxicities [25]. Therefore, the exploration of non-ATP-competitive FGFR1 inhibitors has attracted extensive attention in recent years.

NDGA was reported previously to inhibit FGFR3 kinase [18]. In this study, we found that NDGA exhibited better inhibitory activity against FGFR1 than FGFR3. Using NDGA as a leading compound, we designed and synthesized several NDGA analogs with the basic skeleton of bisaryl-1,4-dien-3-one (Fig. 1A). After screening for kinase inhibition, we obtained two FGFR1 inhibitors (Ad23 and Af23) that had inhibitory activities better than compared to NDGA. Interestingly, NDGA and its analogs retained their potency for the inhibition of kinase activity when the concentration of ATP increased, suggesting that the inhibitory effects of these compounds were independent of the concentration of ATP (Fig. 1B). So far, ARQ069 is the only published molecule that inhibits FGFR1/2 in a manner that does not compete with ATP. ARQ069 exhibits FGFR1/2 kinase inhibition with IC_{50} values of 0.84 and 1.23 μM, respectively [20]. Although the IC_{50} values of Ad23, Af23, and ARQ069 are at micromolar concentration levels, the observation that the inhibition of FGFR1 autophosphorylation (Fig. 2) and the inhibition of the direct FGFR1 downstream substrate (Fig. 1A) occur at different dose levels was consistently detectable. A literature search on kinase inhibitors yielded several reports

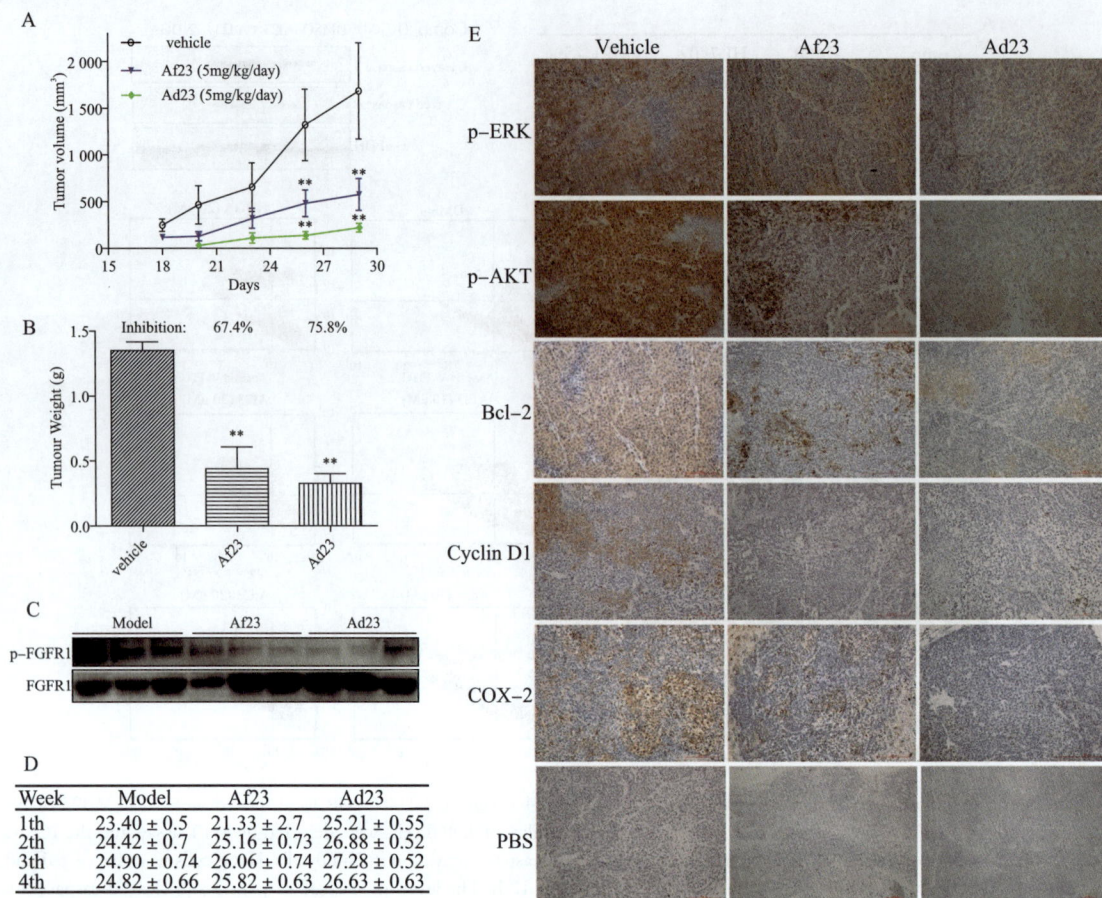

Fig. 4. Anti-tumor effects of compounds Af23 and Ad23 in H460 xenograft models. Xenografts were established in nude mice. Two days after the mice were treated with liposome vehicle (once daily, i.p.), Af23 (once daily, i.p., 5 mg/kg/day) or Ad23 (once daily, i.p., 5 mg/kg/day) for 28 days ($n = 10$ in each group). (A) Tumor volume (mm³) and (B) Tumor weight (g) were recorded ($n = 10$). Points, mean of 10 mice; bars, SD. **$P < 0.01$. (C) pFGFR1 expressions in tumor tissues were detected by Western Blot with FGFR1 as internal control (3 mice in each group were used); (D) Body weight of each group was recorded ($n = 10$ in each group); (E) The levels of p-ERK, p-AKT, Bcl-2, CyclinD1, and COX-2 in tumor tissues were detected by immunohistochemical staining (6 mice in each group were used). Representative pictures are shown.

describing that non-ATP-competitive kinase inhibitors may not display identical IC$_{50}$ values with that of classic ATP-competitive inhibitors for the inhibition of both kinase autophosphorylation and downstream signaling pathways [20,24]. Our novel NDGA analogs (Ad23 and Af23) also showed micromole-grade FGFR1 inhibitory effects in a manner that was independent of ATP.

Figure 2 further revealed the anti-FGFR1 ability of Ad23 and Af23 in the cellular levels using FGFR1-overexpressed 293 cells and NSCLC H460 cells. These two compounds also dose-dependently inhibited FRS2 phosphorylation in H460 cells. These data led us to investigate the anti-cancer efficacy of Ad23 and Af23 further. We evaluated the anti-proliferative effects of Ad23 and Af23 in vitro. As shown in Figure 3, Ad23 and Af23, as well as NDGA, inhibited cell growth and induced cell apoptosis in NSCLC H460 cells; they also had low toxicities against normal MRC-5 cells and normal human liver cells (HL-7702 cells). Further, we showed the potent anti-tumor ability of these two inhibitors in the H460 xenograft mouse model. Previously, studies on ARQ069, a non-ATP-competitive inhibitor, did not report the in vivo anti-tumor activity. In the present study, the data revealed that the compounds Ad23 and Af23 suppressed the phosphorylation of FGFR1 in H460 tumor tissues, thereby inhibited the downstream phosphorylation of ERK and AKT, and reduced the expression of BCL-2, COX-2, and Cyclin D1 (Fig. 4). At the same time, we observed that Ad23 and Af23 exhibited high safety in vivo (Fig. 4D). As already known, the ATP-competitive inhibitory mode leads to the biggest problems (toxicity and side effects) of current FGFR1 inhibitors. Our findings for Ad23 and Af23 indicated that the non-ATP-competitive FGFR1 inhibition might be a new cancer therapeutic alternative with much lower toxicity in vivo. However, continued research is needed to examine the underlying FGFR1-binding mechanism and preclinical evaluation of these two compounds. In spite of the predicted "DFG-OUT" docking model, it is unclear how Ad23/Af23 exactly binds to the FGFR1 kinase domain or other domains, which needs to be demonstrated by X-ray diffraction-based structural biology study. Also, it is important to test the RTK-inhibitory selectivity of these two compounds at both molecular and cellular levels in the future.

5. Conclusion

Given the critical importance of FGFR1 in the pathogenesis and development of NSCLC, this study identified two novel, non-ATP-competitive inhibitors of FGFR1 kinase, *i.e.*, Ad23 and Af23, both of which exhibited good anti-tumor activity *in vitro* and *in vivo*. These two compounds were shown to have the potential to be developed as novel agents for the treatment of NSCLC. The results of the present study indicate that Ad23 and Af23deserve further studies both in the pre-clinical evaluation and in the field of medicinal chemistry for developing structurally different and more effective bisaryl-1,4-dien-3-one-containing FGFR1 inhibitors.

References

[1] Kono SA, Marshall ME, Ware KE, *et al.* The fibroblast growth factor receptor signaling pathway as a mediator of intrinsic resistance to EGFR-specific tyrosine kinase inhibitors in non-small cell lung cancer[J]. Drug Resistance Updates, 2009, 12(4-5): 95-102.

[2] Saijo N. Tyrosine-kinase inhibitors-new standard for NSCLC therapy[J]. Nature Reviews Clinical Oncology, 2010, 7(11): 618-619.

[3] Sordella R, Bell DW, Haber DA, *et al.* Gefitinib-sensitizing EGFR mutations in lung cancer activate anti-apoptotic pathways[J]. Science, 2004, 305(5687): 1163-1167.

[4] Horn L, Sandler A. Epidermal Growth Factor Receptor Inhibitors and Antiangiogenic Agents for the Treatment of Non-Small Cell Lung Cancer[J]. Clinical Cancer Research, 2009, 15(16): 5040-5048.

[5] Zhou W, Ercan D, Chen L, *et al.* Novel mutant-selective EGFR kinase inhibitors against EGFR T790M[J]. Nature, 2009, 462(7276): 1070-1074.

[6] Hammerman PS, Jaenne PA, Johnson BE. Resistance to Epidermal Growth Factor Receptor Tyrosine Kinase Inhibitors in Non-Small Cell Lung Cancer[J]. Clinical Cancer Research, 2009, 15(24): 7502-7509.

[7] Zhang J, Yang PL, Gray NS. Targeting cancer with small molecule kinase inhibitors[J]. Nature Reviews Cancer, 2009, 9(1): 28-39.

[8] Liang G, Liu Z, Wu J, *et al.* Anticancer molecules targeting fibroblast growth factor receptors[J]. Trends in Pharmacological Sciences, 2012, 33(10): 531-541.

[9] Fang Z, Gruetter C, Rauh D. Strategies for the Selective Regulation of Kinases with Allosteric Modulators: Exploiting Exclusive Structural Features[J]. Acs Chemical Biology, 2013, 8(1): 58-70.

[10] Kohler LH, Mireskandari M, Knoesel T, *et al.* FGFR1 expression and gene copy numbers in human lung cancer[J]. Virchows Archiv, 2012, 461(1): 49-57.

[11] Dutt A, Ramos AH, Hammerman PS, *et al.* Inhibitor-Sensitive FGFR1 Amplification in Human Non-Small Cell Lung Cancer[J]. Plos One, 2011, 6(6): e20351.

[12] Terai H, Soejima K, Yasuda H, *et al.* Activation of the FGF2-FGFR1 Autocrine Pathway: A Novel Mechanism of Acquired Resistance to Gefitinib in NSCLC[J]. Molecular Cancer Research, 2013, 11(7): 759-767.

[13] Tran TN, Selinger CI, Kohonen-Corish MRJ, *et al.* Fibroblast growth factor receptor 1 (FGFR1) copy number is an independent prognostic factor in non-small cell lung cancer[J]. Lung Cancer, 2013, 81(3): 462-467.

[14] Preusser M, Berghoff AS, Berger W, *et al.* High rate of FGFR1 amplifications in brain metastases of squamous and non-squamous lung cancer[J]. Lung Cancer, 2014, 83(1): 83-89.

[15] Heist RS, Mino-Kenudson M, Sequist LV, *et al.* FGFR1 Amplification in Squamous Cell Carcinoma of The Lung[J]. Journal of Thoracic Oncology, 2012, 7(12): 1775-1780.

[16] Yang J, Zhao H, Xin Y, *et al.* MicroRNA-198 Inhibits Proliferation and Induces Apoptosis of Lung Cancer Cells *Via* Targeting FGFR1[J]. Journal of Cellular Biochemistry, 2014, 115(5): 987-995.

[17] Zhang J, Zhang L, Su X, *et al.* Translating the Therapeutic Potential of AZD4547 in FGFR1-Amplified Non-Small Cell Lung Cancer through the Use of Patient-Derived Tumor Xenograft Models[J]. Clinical Cancer Research, 2012, 18(24): 6658-6667.

[18] Meyer AN, McAndrew CW, Donoghue DJ. Nordihydroguaiaretic acid inhibits an activated fibroblast growth factor receptor 3 mutant and blocks downstream signaling in multiple myeloma cells[J]. Cancer Research, 2008, 68(18): 7362-7370.

[19] Krejci P, Murakami S, Prochazkova J, *et al.* NF449 Is a Novel Inhibitor of Fibroblast Growth Factor Receptor 3 (FGFR3) Signaling Active in Chondrocytes and Multiple Myeloma Cells[J]. Journal of Biological Chemistry, 2010, 285(27): 20644-20653.

[20] Eathiraj S, Palma R, Hirschi M, *et al.* A Novel Mode of Protein Kinase Inhibition Exploiting Hydrophobic Motifs of Autoinhibited Kinases: discovery of atp-independent inhibitors of fibroblast growth factor receptor[J]. Journal of Biological Chemistry, 2011, 286(23): 20677-20687.

[21] Wang Y, Cai Y, Ji J, *et al.* Discovery and identification of new non-ATP competitive FGFR1 inhibitors with therapeutic potential on non-small-cell lung cancer[J]. Cancer Letters, 2014, 344(1): 82-89.

[22] Wu J, Li J, Cai Y, *et al.* Evaluation and Discovery of Novel Synthetic Chalcone Derivatives as Anti-Inflammatory Agents[J]. Journal of Medicinal Chemistry, 2011, 54(23): 8110-8123.

[23] Lue J-M, Nurko J, Weakley SM, *et al.* Molecular mechanisms and clinical applications of nordihydroguaiaretic acid (NDGA) and its derivatives: An update[J]. Medical Science Monitor, 2010, 16(5): RA93-RA100.

[24] Ren M, Hong M, Liu G, *et al.* Novel FGFR inhibitor ponatinib suppresses the growth of non-small cell lung cancer cells overexpressing FGFR1[J]. Oncology Reports, 2013, 29(6): 2181-2190.

[25] Liang G, Chen G, Wei X, *et al.* Small molecule inhibition of fibroblast growth factor receptors in cancer[J]. Cytokine & Growth Factor Reviews, 2013, 24(5): 467-475.

DFG-out mode of inhibition by an irreversible type-1 inhibitor capable of overcoming gate-keeper mutations in FGF receptors

Zhifeng Huang, Xiaokun Li, Moosa Mohammadi

The FGF family of ligands consists of 18 structurally related polypeptides that signal in paracrine or endocrine fashion through four FGFRs (FGFR1-FGFR4) and their alternatively spliced isoforms to regulate a myriad of biological processes in human development, metabolism, and tissue homeostasis.[1,2] FGFs bind and dimerize the extracellular domains of FGFRs in concert with heparan sulfate glycosaminoglycans or single-pass klotho coreceptor proteins positioning the cytoplasmic kinase domains in proper proximity/orientation for transphosphorylation on A-loop tyrosines.[3,4] This event elevates the intrinsic kinase activity of FGFRs leading to subsequent autophosphorylation on tyrosines in the flanking juxtamembrane (JM) and C-tail regions that mediate recruitment and phosphorylation of a distinct set of intracellular effector proteins by the activated FGFR evoking activation of intracellular signaling pathways.[4-6]

Uncontrolled activation of FGF signaling due to gain-of-function mutations in FGFRs, FGFR gene fusions involving various dimerizing partners, or overexpression/misexpression of FGFs and FGFRs contributes to a number of developmental disorders and cancer.[7-10] Gain-of-function mutations in FGFRs were initially discovered in human congenital craniosynostosis and dwarfism syndromes. Later studies showed that the very same mutations occur somatically in diverse cancers, including multiple myeloma,[12] bladder cancer,[13] endometrial cancer,[14] glioblastoma,[15] lung cancer,[16] adenoid cystic carcinoma,[17] and benign skin cancer.[18] FGFR gene fusions, originally found in the 8p11 myeloproliferative syndrome (an aggressive atypical stem cell myeloproliferative disorder),[7,19] have since been extended to glioblastoma, bladder, and lung cancers.[20,21] Overexpression of FGFs and FGFRs has been documented in breast, prostate, and bladder cancers.[22] Single nucleotide polymorphism in FGFR2 has been linked with susceptibility to breast cancer,[23] and SNP in FGFR4 has been associated with resistance to chemotherapy.[24] In light of these data, FGFRs are now considered major targets for cancer drug discovery.

Indeed, several small molecule ATP-competitive inhibitors are being pursued in the clinic for FGFR-associated cancers including endometrial and prostate cancer. These include dovitinib,[25] ponatinib,[26,27] brivanib,[28] multitargeted RTK inhibitors with coverage of FGFRs, and AZD4547,[29] which has a more restricted FGFR target specificity profile. In addition, there are historical FGFR inhibitors such as PD173074,[30] SU5402,[31] and FIIN-1[32] which have been extensively used as pharmacological probes. All of these inhibitors are reversible ATP-competitive inhibitors with the exception of FIIN-1, which covalently targets an unusual cysteine located in the glycine-rich loop of FGFR1−4. These inhibitors exhibit differential activity profiles with most acting primarily on the autoinhibited FGFRKs, while others also show activity against FGFR kinases carrying gain-of-function mutations. However, these inhibitors are ineffective against gate-keeper mutations,[33,34] a mechanism that has been well documented to confer resistance in the clinic to many drugs targeting oncogenic kinases such as Bcr-Abl (T315I), EGFR (T790M), PDGFR (T674I), and c-Kit (T670I).

There is a major impetus to elucidate the structure−function relationships of FGFR kinases including the mechanisms of action of gain-of-function mutations and inhibitors as such data can provide crucial information to guide the development of inhibitors with improved selectivity and potency toward FGFR isoforms. To date, crystal structures of FGFR1−3 kinases in an autoinhibited state or in an activated state induced either by A-loop phosphorylation or by gain-of-function mutations have been determined.[35-37] In addition, for FGFR1 and FGFR2 kinases, crystal structures exist of inhibitor bound forms.[38-40] These structural data have guided the discovery of inhibitors with narrowed specificity toward FGFR kinases. Notably, the FGFR1K−PD173074 structure[40] was used as template to develop FIIN-1[32] and FIIN-2, pyridopyrimidine-based irreversible inhibitors that exhibit greater specificity toward FGFRs. These inhibitors carry a reactive acrylamide group that is capable of forming a covalent bond with the thiol group of a cysteine uniquely present in the glycine-rich loop of FGFRs. Importantly, FIIN-2 shows activity against the FGFR kinase harboring gate-keeper mutation.

Rhabdomyosarcoma is the most common soft tissue sarcoma in children. [8] FGFR4 activation due to overexpression or gain-of-function mutations in the FGFR4 kinase domain has been correlated with advanced-stage cancer and poor survival. [8,41] FGFR4 inhibition has been shown to stop growth of rhabomyosarcoma cell lines and cause tumor shrinkage in xenograft studies[41,42] supporting the notion that these mutations play causal roles in tumorigenesis. To facilitate the ongoing drug discovery for rhabdomyosarcoma, we solved the first crystal structures of FGFR4K alone and in complex with ponatinib and FIIN-2. These structures provide the first examples for a DFG-out mode of inhibition of FGFRK by an ATP-competitive inhibitor. Remarkably, FIIN-2 also binds in the DFG-out mode despite not conforming to the pharmacophore required for this binding mode. [44]In addition, the FIIN-2 gate-keeper mutant complex demonstrates how the internal rotational flexibility allows this compound to adapt to the bulkier side chains at the gate-keeper location, thus retaining its inhibitory activity. These findings have general implications for the structure-guided design of inhibitors that can overcome the gate-keeper mutation in FGFR and likely other kinases.

1. Results

1.1 Crystal structure of autoinhibited FGFR4 kinase

As expected, the FGFR4 kinase domain (FGFR4K) adopts the canonical bilobate fold of protein kinases with the smaller N-terminal lobe exhibiting the characteristic twisted five-stranded β sheet and the αC helix and the larger C-terminal lobe consisting of mainly α helices (Fig. 1A). Both the A-loop and the loop connecting αD and αE helices, referred to as the kinase insert, are fully ordered. The ordering of the A-loop is due to the intramolecular contacts between the loop and the rigid body of the C-lobe. By contrast, the observed conformation of the kinase insert is solely attributable to favorable crystal lattice contacts. The kinase insert region of FGFR4K bulges out of the main body of the kinase domain and, unlike FGFR1−3 kinases, lacks tyrosine autophosphorylation sites (Fig. S1A).

The unphosphorylated FGFR4K is in an autoinhibited catalytically incompetent state, as evidenced by its comparison with the published crystal structures of unphosphorylated auoinhibited FGFR1−2 kinases, and activated FGFR1−3 kinases either by A-loop tyrosine phosphorylation or by pathogenic gain-of-function mutations (Fig. S2). As in FGFR1−3 kinases, FGFR4K auto-inhibition is principally governed by a network of inhibitory hydrogen bonds at the kinase hinge region termed the molecular brake (Fig. 1C). This network, which is mediated by a triad of residues consisting of Asn-535, Glu-551, and Lys-627 in FGFR4K, restrains the N-lobe movement toward the C-lobe that accompanies kinase activation. Reminiscent of the unphosphorylated FGFR1K structure, an additional constraint is provided by the DFGLAR motif at the beginning of the A-loop, whose conformation physically interferes with N-lobe rotation. [36] In fact, as in the unphosphorylated FGFR1K and FGFR2K structures, FGFR4K also contains the catalytically important salt bridge between Lys-503 and Glu-520 (αC), which is known to help orient Lys to coordinate α and β phosphates of ATP (Fig. 1B). Last, as in FGFRK1,[36] the FGFR-invariant Arg-650 at the C-terminal end of the A-loop makes bidentate hydrogen bonds with Asp-612 (the general base) from the catalytic loop, thereby directly blocking the access of substrate into the active site (Fig. 1D).

1.2 The FGFR4K gate-keeper mutations confer resistance to ponatinib but are sensitive to FIIN-2

As alluded to previously, ponatinib (previously AP24534; Fig. S3A) is a multitargeted RTK inhibitor with coverage of FGFR kinases that is currently being evaluated in clinical trials for several cancers including endometrial cancer and rhabdomyosarcoma. [27,45] Importantly, we have recently shown that, in contrast to other FGFR inhibitors including dovitinib and PD173074, ponatinib is capable of effectively targeting not only the autoinhibited FGFR2 kinases but also FGFR2K that has undergone activation by gain-of-function mutations with the exception of gate-keeper mutation[33] Using the FGFR1K−PD173074 complex structure as a template, we have recently developed an irreversible covalently acting inhibitor, termed FIIN-2 (Fig. S3B), that is capable of targeting FGFRKs harboring gate-keeper mutations.

To date, four oncogenic FGFR4 mutations have been identified in rhabdomyosarcoma tumors including N535K, N535D, V550L, and V550E. [8] According to our structure, the N535K or N535D mutations confer gain-of-function by disengaging the autoinhibitory molecular brake at the kinase hinge region. By contrast, the mechanism by which the V550L and V550E mutations confer gain-of-function is not fully understood. These mutations affect the gate-keeper

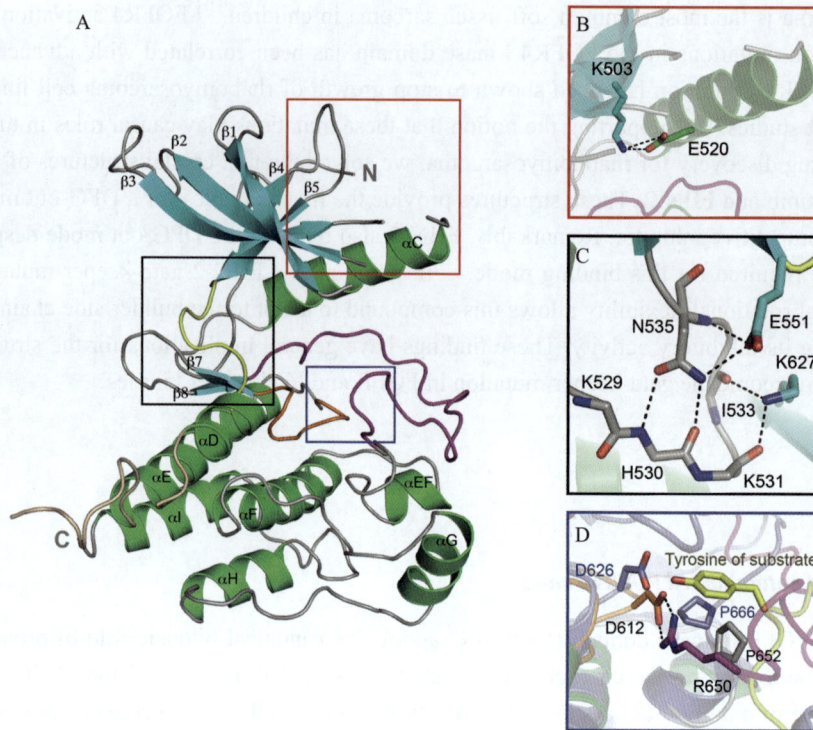

Fig. 1. The crystal structure of wild-type FGFR4 kinase. (A) Ribbon diagram of the wild-type FGFR4K structure. β strands and α helices are colored cyan and green, respectively. The A-loop, catalytic loop, kinase insert, and kinase hinge are colored magenta, orange, wheat, and yellow, respectively. (B) Close-up view of the N-lobe showing formation of the catalytically critical salt bridge between K503 and E520. (C) Close-up view of the molecular brake at the kinase hinge region. (D) Close-up view of the active site of FGFR4K[WT] and activated FGFR2K (in slate) complexed with peptide (in yellow sticks) following superimposition of these two structures. Note that bidentate hydrogen bonds between R650 and D612 (the general base) block the access of substrate tyrosine into the active site of FGFR4K. The side chain of R650 in the FGFR4K structure occupies roughly the same space as the substrate tyrosine in the FGFR2K−peptide complex structure. In all figures, side chains of selected residues are shown as sticks, and atom colorings are as follows: oxygens in red, nitrogens in blue, and coloring of carbons follow the coloring scheme of the specific region of the kinase from which they derive. The hydrogen bonds are shown as black dashed lines.

residue of FGFR4 kinase that is known to control the access of ATP-competitive inhibitors to the rear hydrophobic pocket in the ATP binding cleft. We first assessed the kinase activities of oncogenic FGFR4K variants harboring the V550E, V550L, N535D, or N535K rhabomyosarcoma mutations using an *in vitro* peptide phosphorylation assay. Consistent with the published cell-based data, [8] all four mutants exhibited elevated kinase activity compared to wild-type kinase as evident by the rapid completion of substrate monophosphorylation and appearance of diphosphorylated substrate peaks in the mass spectra of the oncogenic variants (Fig. 2).

Next, the abilities of ponatinib and FIIN-2 to inhibit wild-type FGFR4K and its four oncogenic variants were examined. The data showed that ponatinib inhibited not only the wild-type FGFR4K (Fig. 3A, left panel) but also FGFR4Ks that have undergone activation either by A-loop phosphorylation (Fig. S4) or by gain-of-function mutations (N535K or N535D; Supporting Information Fig. S5). The V555L and V550E gate-keeper mutants were resistant to inhibition by ponatinib, however (Figs. 3A and S5). By contrast, FIIN-2 effectively inhibited the substrate phosphorylation ability of all mutants including the V550L gate-keeper mutant (Fig. 3B). To understand the molecular basis for the differential sensitivity of the FGFR4K gate-keeper mutations to ponatinib and FIIN-2, we decided to determine the crystal structures of wild-type FGFR4K bound to ponatinib, the FGFR4K[V550L] gate-keeper mutant alone, and in complex with FIIN-2.

1.2 Ponatinib inhibits FGFR4K by inducing a dFG-in → DFG-out rearrangement

The FGFR4K−ponatinib complex crystallized under identical conditions to the free FGFR4K, yielding crystals that were isomorphous to the free FGFR4K crystals. As anticipated, ponatinib binds into the ATP binding pocket between the N and C lobes (Fig. 4A). Drug binding does not induce any significant change in the interlobe angle. The C-alpha atoms of FGFR4K−ponatinib and apo-FGFR4K structures superimpose very well (RMSD of 0.2 Å) with the exception

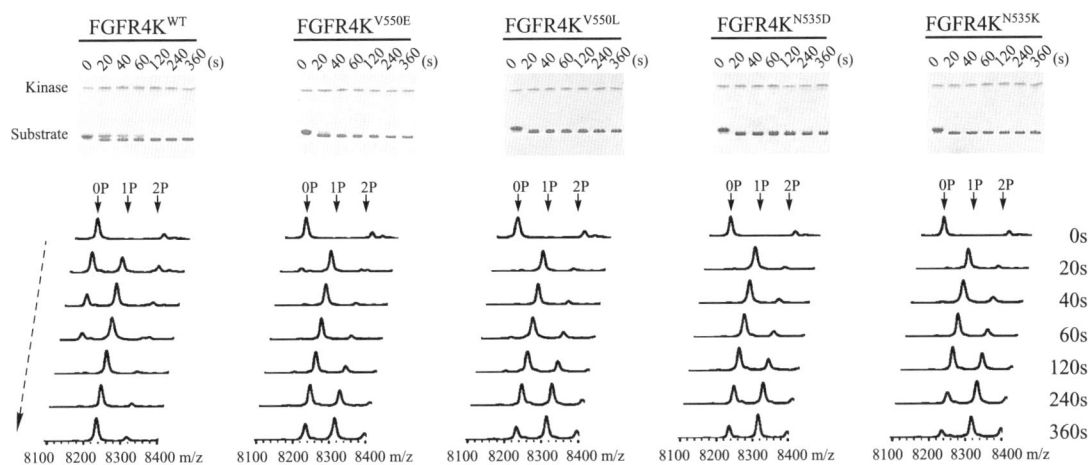

Fig. 2. FGFR4K mutants harboring rhabdomyosarcoma mutations exhibiting elevated kinase activity. The substrate phosphorylation activities of FGFR4K^{WT}, FGF4K^{N535K}, FGFR4K^{N535D}, FGFR4K^{V550L}, and FGFR4K^{V550E} were compared using native-PAGE (upper panel) coupled with time-resolved MALDI-TOF MS (lower panel). 0P, 1P, and 2P indicate the positions of the unphosphorylated, monophosphorylated, and dephosphorylated substrate peptide.

of the DFG motif at the beginning of the A-loop, which undergoes a dramatic DFG-in → DFG-out rearrangement in response to ponatinib binding (Figs. 4A and S6A).

Ponatinib consists of an imidazo$^{[1,2-b]}$pyridazine heterocyclic scaffold that is linked *via* an acetylene group to a methylphenyl ring that in turn is joined *via* an amide bond to a trifluoromethylphenyl aromatic ring (Fig. 4A). A methylpiperazine ring has been appended *via* methyl linkage to the trifluoromethylphenyl aromatic ring to aid in penetration of the drug into cells. Ponatinib binds into the ATP binding cleft in an extended conformation. The methylphenyl and trifluoromethylphenyl rings are almost coplanar and have a 90° interplanar angle with the (imidazo[1,2-*b*]pyridazine) bicyclic aromatic ring. Ponatinib engages a vast area that stretches from the kinase hinge region at the back of the kinase all the way to the catalytic pocket at the front end of the kinase.

The aromatic rings of the drug engage three sites within the ATP binding cleft (Fig. 4A). At site 1, the imidazo[1,2-*b*]pyridazine scaffold occupies approximately the same space as the adenine ring of ATP and makes a single hydrogen bond with the backbone amide nitrogen atom of Ala-553 in the kinase hinge region (Fig. 4A, middle panel). Reminiscent of ATP binding, the imidazo[1,2-*b*]pyridazine aromatic ring is sandwiched between hydrophobic residues from N- and C-lobes of the kinase. The rigid acetylene linkage directs the remaining portion of the drug deep toward the rear corner of the ATP binding pocket where the methylphenyl and 3-trifluoromethylphenyl aromatic rings of the inhibitor engage sites 2 and 3, respectively (Fig. 4A, middle panel). Importantly, these aromatic rings induce two significant conformational changes in the ATP binding cleft including (I) displacement of the catalytic Lys-503 side chain in site 2 and (II) an outward flipping of the DFG motif in site 3 (Fig. 4A, right panel). These structural rearrangements are necessary to alleviate steric conflicts with the compound ultimately optimizing binding interactions of the inhibitor.

At site 2, the methylphenyl group pushes the side chain of catalytic Lys-503, which along with Val-550, the gatekeeper residue, and Met-524 from the αC helix form a hydrophobic pocket that binds the methylphenyl aromatic ring. The displacement of Lys-503 indirectly helps the catalytic Glu-520 from the αC helix to make a direct hydrogen bond with the amide linkage between aromatic rings of the drug (Fig. 4A, middle panel). At site 3, the 3-trifluoromethylphenyl moiety expels the DFG phenylalanine out of the cleft and occupies the hydrophobic pit that becomes vacant upon outward movement of the phenylalanine (Fig. 4A, right panel). The displaced phenylalanine side chain is now in position to engage in favorable hydrophobic contacts with the scaffold and the acetylene linker (Fig. 4A, middle panel). As another important consequence of phenylalanine displacement, Asp-630 from DFG is also forced into a catalytically incompetent orientation where the backbone atoms of Asp-630 gain the ability to make hydrogen bonds with the amide linkage between the aromatic rings of the inhibitor. Interestingly, even the piperazine moiety of the drug contributes to drug binding affinity. The piperazine ring falls in the vicinity of the catalytic loop where it engages in hydrogen bonds with the loop (Fig. 4A, middle panel). The overall binding mode of ponatinib in the FGFR4K−ponatinib structure resembles that observed in the Abl−Ponatinib complex structure where the DFG-out mode of inhibition was initially observed.[46]

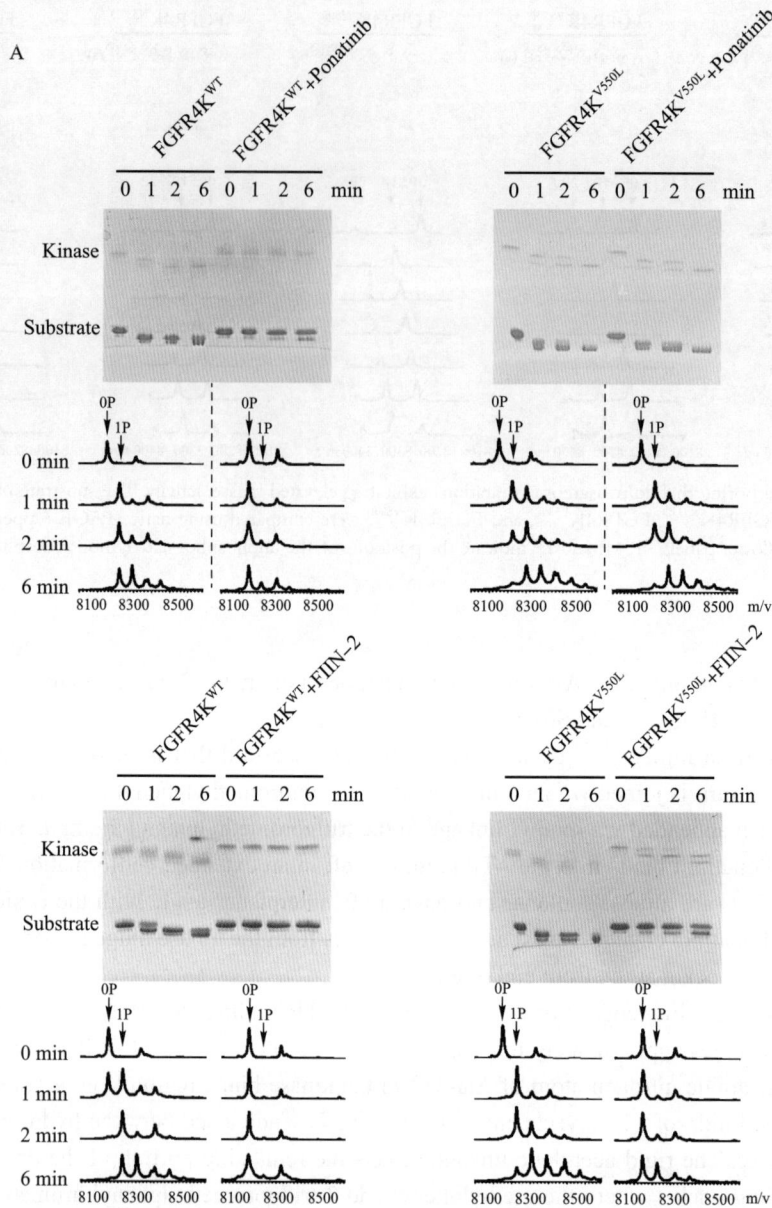

C

Table 1. Antiproliferattive activity of FGFR lnhibitors on Ba/F3 Cells

Ba/F3 Cell lines	IC50 (nM)	
	Ponatinib	FIIN-2
Parental	> 3 300	> 3 300
FGFR4K^{WT}	452	32
FGFR4K^{V550L}	> 3 300	482

Fig. 3. The V550L gate-keeper mutation conferring resistance to ponatinib but not to FIIN-2. The abilities of ponatinib (A) and FIIN-2 (B) to inhibit substrate phosphorylation activities of FGFR4K^{WT} and the FGFR4K^{V550L} (gate-keeper mutant) were compared using native-PAGE (upper panel) and time-resolved MALDI-TOF MS (lower panel). 0P, 1P, and 2P indicate the positions of the unphosphorylated, monophosphorylated, and dephosphorylated substrate peptide. (C) Antiproliferative activity of ponatinib and FIIN-2 on transformed Ba/F3 cells.

A

B

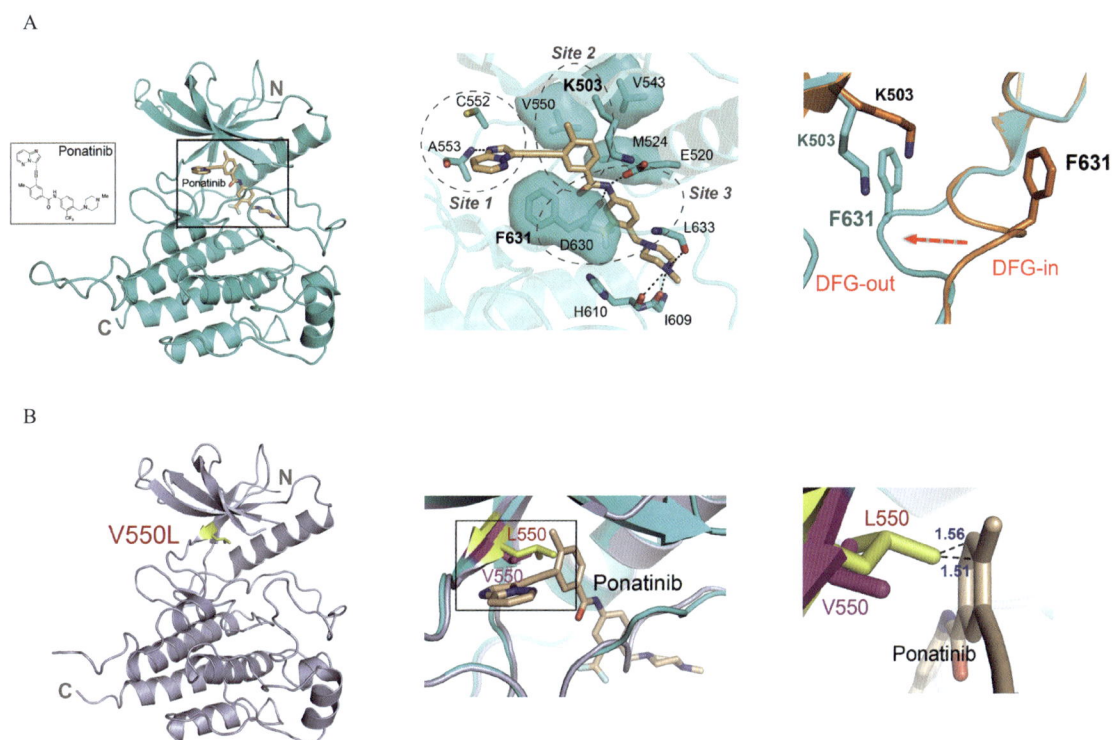

Fig. 4. Structural basis for FGFR4K^{WT} inhibition by ponatinib and resistance caused by the V550L gate-keeper mutation. (A) Ribbon diagram of the FGFR4K^{WT}−ponatinib cocrystal structure. The middle panel shows the close-up view of the main interactions between FGFR4K^{WT} and ponatinib. The hydrogen bonds are indicated as black dashed lines, and the hydrophobic interactions are shown as surface. The right panel shows a close-up view of the DFG motif in the FGFR4K^{WT} (in orange) and FGFR4K^{WT}−ponatinib (in cyan) following superimposition of the two structures. Note that ponatinib forces the DFG out of the ATP binding pocket. The phenylalaninein DFG region and K503 are rendered as orange and cyan sticks and labeled in black and cyan, respectively. (B) Ribbon diagrams of the FGFR4K^{V550L} structure. Superimposition of the FGFR4K^{WT}− ponatinib complex structure onto FGFR4K^{V550L} reveals steric clashes between the added methyl group in Leu-550 and the imidazo [1,2-b]pyridazine scaffold of ponatinib which underlie the resistance of the FGFR4K^{V550L} to ponatinib. The V550 in FGFR4K^{WT} and L550 in FGFR4K^{V550L} are shown in pink and yellow sticks, and labeled in pink and red, respectively. In all the structures, the ponatinib is rendered as sticks and labeled in black.

Unlike Abl−Ponatinib, however, the glycine-rich loop of FGFR4 does not partake in ponatinib recognition.

1.3 Gate-keeper mutations confer resistance to ponatinib inhibition by introducing a steric clash with the inhibitor

As shown in Supporting Information Fig. S5, ponatinib is capable of silencing all the FGFR4 pathogenic mutations with the exception of the V550L and V550E gate-keeper mutations. To understand the molecular basis for how these mutations render the kinase refractory to inhibition, we also solved the crystal structure of FGFR4K harboring the V550L gate-keeper mutation (Fig. 4B). Superimposition of the FGFR4K−ponatinib complex structure onto FG-FR4K^{V550L} reveals steric clashes between the added methyl group in Leu-550 and the imidazo[1,2-b]pyridazine scaffold of ponatinib which underlie the resistance of the FGFR4K^{V550L} to ponatinib (Fig. 4B).

1.4 Crystal structure of FGFR4K^{V550L} complexed with FIIN-2

As shown in Fig. 3, unlike ponatinib, FIIN-2 is capable of inhibiting the gate-keeper V550L mutant. To understand how FIIN-2 is capable of overcoming gate-keeper mutations, the crystal structure of the FGFR4K^{V550L} mutant in complex with FIIN-2 was solved. FIIN-2 is a PD173074-based compound in which the cyclic urea N of the pyridopyrimidine scaffold has been derivatized with an acrylamidobenzyl substituent possessing a reactive acrylamide in the para position (Figs. 5A and S3B). The benzyl moiety serves as a spacer to position the acrylamide, the electrophilic center of the compound in the vicinity of the thiol group of a unique cysteine in the glycine-rich loop of FGFRs (Fig. S1C) allowing for formation a covalent bond via a Michael addition reaction. To this end, we first used mass spectrometry to demonstrate that FIIN-2 irreversibly reacts with Cys-477 (in the glycine-rich loop) in both FGFR4K^{WT} and FG-FR4K^{V550L}. To do so, FGFR4K^{WT} and FGFR4K^{V550L} were incubated with FIIN-2 and digested with trypsin, and adduct formation between the tryptic peptide containing Cys-477 and FIIN-2 was analyzed by tandem mass spectrometry. As shown in Fig. 5B, in the presence of FIIN-2, the mass of the tryptic peptide containing the Cys-477 increased by 634.3 Da, corresponding to the mass of the drug, confirming that FIIN-2 can irreversibly inhibit both FGFR4K^{WT} and FG-FR4K^{V550L}.

The FGFR4K^{V550L}−FIIN-2 complex structure shows that like ponatinib, FIIN-2 binding does not affect the kinase interlobe angle (Figs. 5C and S7A). The C-alpha atoms of FGFR4K^{V550L}−FIIN-2 and apo-FGFR4K^{V550L} match closely with the exceptions of the glycine-rich loop and the DFG motif, both of which undergo major conformational rearrangements in response to drug binding (Fig. 5C,D,E and S7B). Remarkably, the DFG motif undergoes an outward transition reminiscent of that seen in the FGFR4K−ponatinib structure (Fig. 5E). This is rather surprising because FIIN-2, like its parent molecule PD173074, lacks a functional group necessary to actively force the DFG out of the ATP binding cleft. As detailed below, this unusual property of FIIN-2, a type-I inhibitor, to bind FGFR4K like a type-II inhibitor is a direct consequence of the covalent bonding between FIIN-2 to FGFR4K.

The pyridopyrimidine scaffold of FIIN-2 occupies roughly the same space as the bicyclic ring of ponatinib (site 1)

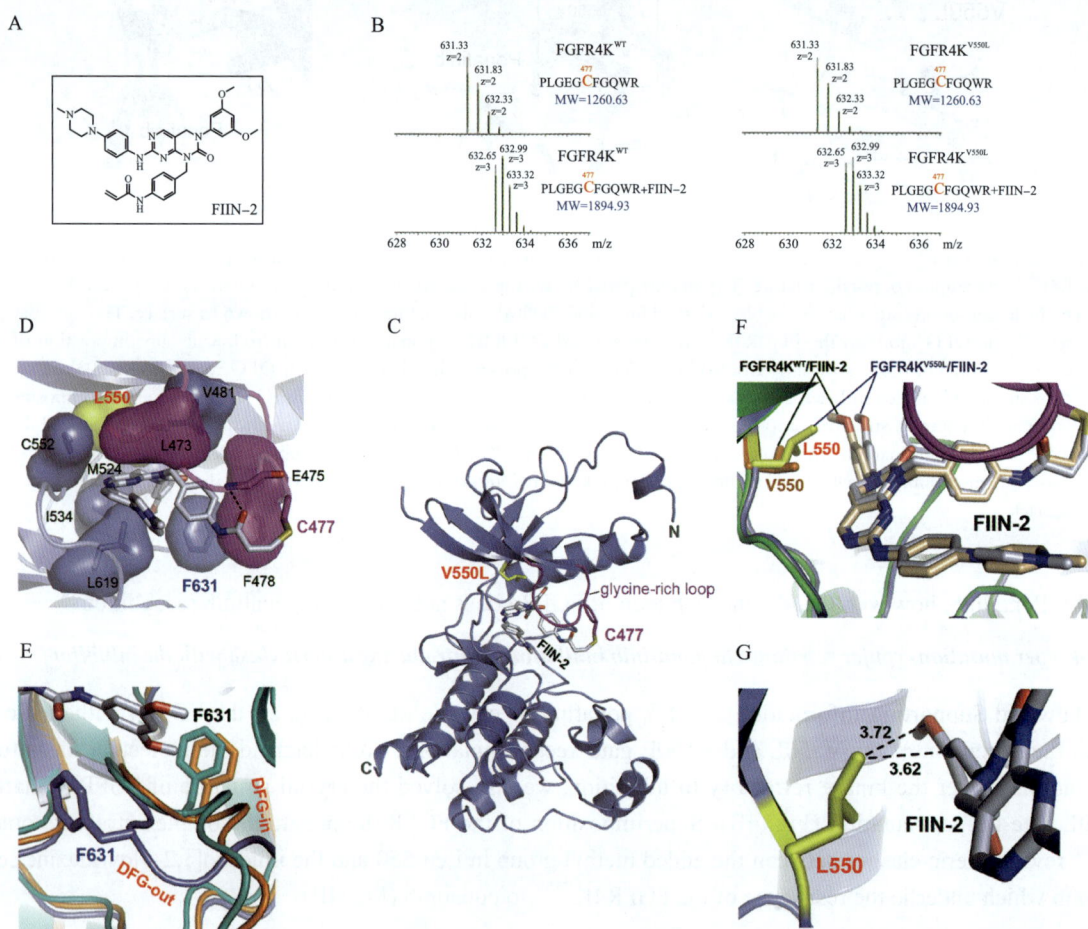

Fig. 5. Structural basis for the inhibition of FGFR4K^{V550L} gate-keeper mutant by FIIN-2. (A) The chemical structure of FIIN-2. (B) The LC-MS/MS spectra of the kinase peptide (Pro42-Arg53) from FGFR4K^{WT} and FGFR4K^{V550L} with and without FIIN-2. The reacting Cys477 from the glycine-rich loop of the kinase is highlighted in red color. (C) Ribbon diagram of the FGFR4K^{V550L}−FIIN-2 cocrystal structure. (D) The close-up view of the main interactions between FGFR4K^{V550L} and FIIN-2. The hydrogen bonds are indicated as black dashed lines, and the hydrophobic interactions are shown as surface. (E) Close-up view of the DFG motif conformation in the FGFR4K^{WT} (in orange), FGFR4K^{V550L} (in teal), and FGFR4K^{V550L}−FIIN-2 (in blue) structures following superimposition of the three structures. Note that FIIN-2 also binds to the ATP-binding site of FGFR4K in DFG-out mode. The phenylalanines in the DFG region of FGFR4K^{WT}, FGFR4K^{V550L}, and the FGFR4K^{V550L}−FIIN-2 complex are rendered as orange, teal, and blue sticks and labeled in black and blue, respectively. (F) Superimposition of the FGFR4K^{WT}−FIIN-2 complex structure onto the FGFR4K^{V550L}−FIIN-2 structure. Note that rotational freedom around the single bond linking the scaffold and dimethoxyphenyl of FIIN-2 allows for small structural adjustments to bypass any potential steric clash with the bulkier side chain of L550. The V550 in FG-FR4K^{WT} and L550 in FGFR4K^{V550L} are shown in orange and yellow sticks, and labeled in orange and red, respectively. (G) The distances between L550 of the FGFR4K^{V550L} gate-keeper mutant and FIIN-2 are shown as dashed lines and labeled in a black color. In all of the structures, the FIIN-2 is rendered as sticks and labeled in black.

and is sandwiched by hydrophobic residues from the N and C lobes of kinase (Fig. 5C,D). Likewise, the dimethoxyphenyl ring, the key determinant of selectivity of PD173074 and likewise FIIN-2 for FGFRs, penetrates deep into the back pocket of the cleft engaging the same site as the methylphenyl ring of ponatinib (site 2). The acrylamidobenzyl group protrudes out of the ATP-binding pocket and places its a,b-unsaturated acrylamide, the electrophilic center of the drug, in the vicinity of nucleophilic thiol group of Cys-477, resulting in a covalent bond formation *via* a Michael addition reaction (Fig. 5). This covalent bonding pulls the glycine-rich loop toward the compound enabling additional contacts between the compound and the glycine-rich loop to form. Specifically, the phenylalanine from the glycine-rich loop makes hydrophobic contacts with the acrylamidobenzyl ring of drug and backbone amid nitrogens of the glycine-rich loop form a hydrogen bond with the carbonyl group of acrylamide of the drug (Fig. 5D). In addition to causing the observed conformational change of the glycine-rich loop, the covalent bond between FIIN-2 and the glycine-rich loop cysteine is ultimately responsible for the DFG-flip seen in the structure. Specifically, the altered conformation of the glycine-rich loop creates favorable p–p stacking contacts between the Phe-478 from the glycine-rich loop and the Phe-631 from the DFG motif (Fig. 5D), which stabilizes the DFG-out conformation enabling the Phe-631 to also contribute to inhibitor binding.

Comparison of the FGFR4K^{V550L}–FIIN-2 and FGFR4K^{WT}–ponatinib structures explains the molecular basis for the differential sensitivity of these two inhibitors toward the V550L gate-keeper mutation. While the added methyl group in Leu-550 introduces steric clash with the imidazo[1,2-*b*]pyridazine scaffold of ponatinib (Fig. 4B, right panel), Leu-550 is still able to make favorable hydrophobic contacts with the dimethoxyphenyl ring of FIIN-2 (Fig. 5D). It is noteworthy that the rigidity of the acetylene linkage is disadvantageous as it precludes any structural adjustment of the methylphenyl moiety of ponatinib (Fig. S3A) to alleviate this steric clash. In contrast, rotational freedom around the single bond linking the scaffold and dimethoxyphenyl of FIIN-2 (Fig. S3B) would allow for small structural adjustments to bypass any potential steric clash with the bulkier side chain of L550. Indeed, an overlay of the crystal structure of the FGFR4K^{WT}–FIIN-2 complex onto the FGFR4K^{V550L}–FIIN-2 structure shows that the dimethoxyphenyl ring in the FGFR4K^{V550L}–FIIN-2 complex undergoes slight rotation around the single bound linker to accommodate for the bulkier leucine side chain in the gate-keeper mutant (Fig. 5F,G).

2. Discussion

In this report, we elucidated the molecular bases for FGFR4 kinase autoinhibition, inhibition by ponatinib and FIIN-2, and drug resistance caused by gate-keeper mutations. The FGFR4K–ponatinib and FGFR4K–FIIN-2, reported here, are the first examples of FGFR–inhibitor complexes featuring a DFG-out mode of inhibition. In fact, only a tiny fraction of published tyrosine kinase-inhibitor structures depict a DFG-out mode of inhibition. Among RTKs, KIT, TIE2, MET, and VEGFR2 are the only examples that have been shown so far to bind inhibitors in a DFG-out fashion. [47-49]

Previously, crystal structures of FGFR1 and FGFR2 kinases in complex with inhibitors bearing oxyindole and pyridopyrimidine and quinazolin as scaffolds have been solved. [38,39,50] In none of these structures, however, does the inhibitor penetrate deep enough to access site 3, and accordingly the DFG motif remains in its original "in" conformation. In fact, the oxyindoles do not even make use of site 2, although they can induce conformational changes in the glycine-rich loop to create hydrophobic contacts between conserved phenylalanine from the glycine-rich loop and the drug contributing to drug affinity. The FGFR4K–ponatinib (Fig. 4) and FGFR4K–FIIN-2 (Fig. 5) complex structures elegantly demonstrate that these two inhibitors attain their superior inhibitory potency against FGFR kinases by binding the kinase *via* a DFG-out mechanism. In addition, the FGFR4K–FIIN-2 structure, the first structure of an FGFR kinase with a covalently acting inhibitor (Fig. 5), shows how this compound takes advantage of a unique cysteine in the glycine-rich loop of FGFRs to achieve FGFR target specificity.

Interestingly, in contrast to FGFRs, where the DFG-out conformation has never been visualized in the previously published apo crystal structures, there are structures of unliganded KIT and Abl that display a DFG-out conformation in the absence of an inhibitor. [51,52] These data imply that in FGFRs, the DFG motif rarely transitions into the out conformation, whereas the DFG-out conformation can occur with significant frequencies in these other RTKs. Since the relative distribution of the DFG-in/DFG-out states will dictate the energetics of drug binding, future efforts should be directed toward exploring the dynamics of this transition in solution. Taken together, comparison of FGFR4K–ponatinib and FGFR4K-FIIN-2 complex structures with previous FGFRK-inhibitor complexes showcases a substantial degree of conformational heterogeneity both in the DFG motif and glycine-rich loop that should be harnessed when tailoring more efficacious FGFRK inhibitors. The structural data provide roadmaps for the design of novel inhibitors for FG-FRKs which incorporate the salient inhibitory features of ponatinib and FIIN-2. In the FGFR4K−FIIN-2 structure, the hydrophobic pocket (site 3) that becomes vacant upon outward flipping of the DFG phenylalanine remains unutilized. Hence, the inhibitory potency of FIIN-2 may be significantly improved by derivatizing it with an aromatic ring such that it gains the ability to engage this hydrophobic pocket as it occurs in the FGFR4K−ponatinib structure. Likewise, the structural data pinpoint two unique cysteines, one in the catalytic loop of all four FGFRKs[35] and the other in the hinge region of FGFR4K (Fig. 1B) that can be exploited for the design of more selective covalent inhibitors for FGFR4K and other FGFRs.

3. Methods

Please refer to the Supporting Information for full details.

3.1 Protein expression and purification

The human FGFR4 kinase domains FGFR3K$^{445-753}$, including its mutated forms, and the C-terminal tail peptide of FGFR2 kinase (FGFR2K$^{761-821}$) were all expressed using pET bacterial expression vectors with an N-terminal 6XHis-tag to aid in protein purification.

3.2 Crystallization and structure determination

All the crystals were grown by hanging drop vapor diffusion method either at 4 ℃ (FGFR4K^{WT}, FGFR4K^{V550L}, and FGFR4K^{WT}−ponatinib) or 18 ℃ (FGFR4K$^{V550L/Cys477}$−FIIN-2). FGFR4K^{WT} crystallized in a buffer composed of 0.1 M MES (pH 5.5), 20% (w/v) PEG 4 000, 0.2 M Li$_2$SO$_4$, and 0.01 M taurine. Crystals of the FGFR4K^{V550L} were obtained using a crystallization buffer composed of 0.1 M Tris (pH 7.5), 20% (w/v) PEG 1 500, and 0.2 M (NH$_4$)$_2$SO$_4$. The FG-FR4K^{WT}−ponatinib complex was crystallized using a crystallization buffer composed of 0.1 M MES (pH 5.5), 25% (w/v) PEG 4 000, 0.15 M (NH$_4$)$_2$SO$_4$, and 4% (v/v) formamide. The FGFR4K$^{V550L/C477}$−FIIN-2 complex was crystallized using a crystallization buffer composed of 0.1 M HEPES (pH 7.5), 1.0 – 1.2 M (NH$_4$)$_2$SO$_4$, and 10 mM yttrium(III) chloride hexahydrate. All diffraction data were processed using the HKL2000 suite, [53] and the crystal structures were solved using maximum likelihood molecular replacement program Phaser in the PHENIX software suite. [54] The crystal structure of wild-type FGFR2 kinase (PDB ID: 2PSQ) [35] was used as the search model. Model building was carried out using Coot, [55] and refinements were done using phenix.ref ine in the PHENIX suite. [54] Data collection and structure refinement statistics are listed in Table 1.

Table 1.   X-ray data collection and refinement statistics

construct	FGFR4K^{apo}	FGFR4K-Ponatinib	FGFR4K^{V550L}	FGFR4K^{V550L}-FIIN-2
data collection				
resolution (Å)	50.0−1.50 (1.53−1.50)	50−1.90 (1.93−1.90)	50−1.68 (1.71−1.68)	50−2.2 (2.24−2.20)
space group	$P2_1$	$P2_1$	$P2_1$	$R3$
unit cell parameters (Å, deg)	$a = 42.384$	$a = 42.722$	$a = 42.671$	$a = 139.599$
	$b = 61.336$	$b = 61.593$	$b = 61.472$	$b = 139.599$
	$c = 61.084$	$c = 60.311$	$c = 61.819$	$c = 49.660$
	$\alpha = 90.00$	$\alpha = 90.00$	$\alpha = 90.00$	$\alpha = 90.00$
	$\beta = 99.01$	$\beta = 97.94$	$\beta = 99.43$	$\beta = 90.00$
	$\gamma = 90.00$	$\gamma = 90.00$	$\gamma = 90.00$	$\gamma = 120.00$
content of the asymmetric unit	1	1	1	1

Continued Table

construct	FGFR4K^{apo}	FGFR4K-Ponatinib	FGFR4K^{V550L}	FGFR4K^{V550L}-FIIN-2
measured reflections (#)	348260	182746	243115	88774
unique reflections (#)	49375	24319	34654	18138
data redundancy	7.1 (6.0)	7.5 (7.7)	7.0 (5.4)	4.9 (2.4)
data completeness (%)	100 (100)	99.2 (98.1)	96.6 (94.2)	99.1 (90.1)
R_{sym} (%)	5.8 (19.5)	7.5 (30.3)	5.2 (16.7)	10.2 (34.4)
I/sig refinement	53.6 (8.6)	41.8 (7.4)	50.2 (10.0)	13.5 (1.7)
R factor/R free	22.2/24.8	17.8/21.2	23.5/26.9	19.3/23.4
number of protein atoms	2204	2317	2242	2139
number of nonprotein/solvent atoms	10	44	5	47
number of solvent atoms	0	49	0	0
RMSD bond length (Å)	0.005	0.015	0.006	0.008
RMSD bond angle (deg)	1.04	1.61	1.00	1.23
PDB ID	4QQT	4QRC	4QQJ	4QQ5

[a]Numbers in parentheses refer to the highest resolution shell.

[b]$R_{sym} = \Sigma|I - <I>|\Sigma I$, where I is the observed intensity of a reflection, and $<I>$ is the average intensity of all the symmetry related reflections.

3.3 Peptide substrate phosphorylation assay by native gel and MALDI-TOF mass spectrometry

Peptide substrate phosphorylation activities of wild-type and pathogenic mutated FGFR4 kinases (FGFR4K^{WT}, FGFR4K^{N535K}, FGFR4K$^{N535\ D}$, FGFR4K^{V550L}, FGFR4K^{V550E}) and the inhibitory efficiency of ponatinib or FIIN-2 were analyzed by native gel electrophoresis and positive ion MALDI-TOF MS (Bruker Autoflex MALDI-TOF, Bruker Daltonics) in linear mode.

3.4 Inhibition of kinase autophosphorylation by ponatinib

The autophosphorylation of the wild-type FGFR4 kinase and its pathogenic variants (FGFR4K^{WT}, FGFR4K^{N535K}, FGFR4K^{N535D}, FGFR4K^{V550L}, FGFR4K^{V550E}) inhibited by ponatinib were analyzed by native gel electrophoresis and LTQ Orbitrap (Thermo Electron) LC-MS/MS.

3.5 BaF3 Cell Viability Assay

TEL-FGFR4-transformed BaF3 cells were seeded in a 96 well plate and treated with the indicated concentration of the compounds. After 72 h, cell viability was assessed by MTS assay. The IC$_{50}$ values were calculated using GraphPad Prism version 5.0 (GraphPad Software Inc.). To generate the FGFR4^{V550L} expressing BaF3 cell line, the V550L mutation was introduced into the Tel-FGFR4^{WT} chimera, which had been subcloned into the retroviral expression vector, using site-directed mutagenesis (Agilent) and was tranduced into BaF3 cell line using retroviral infection.

3.6 Analysis of covalent bond formation between FIIN-2 and FGFR4K by LC-MS/MS

To test if FIIN-2 can form a covalent bond with Cys477 in the glycine-rich loops, FGFR4K$^{WT/C477}$ and FGFR4K$^{V550L/C477}$ were incubated with FIIN-2 overnight at 4 ℃, digested with trypsin, and analyzed by LC-MS/MS. The spectral region corresponding to the kinase tryptic peptide (Pro42−Arg53), which contains the reactive Cys477, was extracted from the raw data and was used to show the mass shift of the peptide in the presence of FIIN-2.

The coordinates and structure factors have been deposited in the RCSB Protein Data Bank under PDB IDs 4QQT, 4QRC, 4QQJ, and 4QQ5 and will be immediately released upon publication.

Supporting information

Supporting information to this article can be found on the journal's website (doi: 10.1021/cb 5006745).

References

[1] Beenken A, Mohammadi M. The FGF family: biology, pathophysiology and therapy[J]. Nature Reviews Drug Discovery, 2009, 8(3): 235-253.

[2] Itoh N, Ornitz DM. Fibroblast growth factors: from molecular evolution to roles in development, metabolism and disease[J]. Journal of Biochemistry, 2011, 149(2): 121-130.

[3] Goetz R, Mohammadi M. Exploring mechanisms of FGF signalling through the lens of structural biology[J]. Nature Reviews Molecular Cell Biology, 2013, 14(3): 166-180.

[4] Lemmon MA, Schlessinger J. Cell Signaling by Receptor Tyrosine Kinases[J]. Cell, 2010, 141(7): 1117-1134.

[5] Pawson T. Specificity in signal transduction: From phosphotyrosine-SH2 domain interactions to complex cellular systems[J]. Cell, 2004, 116(2): 191-203.

[6] Schlessinger J, Lemmon MA. SH2 and PTB domains in tyrosine kinase signaling[J]. Science's STKE : signal transduction knowledge environment, 2003, 2003(191): RE12-RE12.

[7] Roumiantsev S, Krause DS, Neumann CA, et al. Distinct stem cell myeloproliferative/T lymphoma syndromes induced by ZNF198-FGFR1 and BCR-FGFR1 fusion genes from 8p11 translocations[J]. Cancer Cell, 2004, 5(3): 287-298.

[8] Taylor JG, Cheuk AT, Tsang PS, et al. Identification of FGFR4-activating mutations in human rhabdomyosarcomas that promote metastasis in xenotransplanted models[J]. Journal of Clinical Investigation, 2009, 119(11): 3395-3407.

[9] Chen H, Huang Z, Dutta K, et al. Cracking the Molecular Origin of Intrinsic Tyrosine Kinase Activity through Analysis of Pathogenic Gain-of-Function Mutations[J]. Cell Reports, 2013, 4(2): 376-384.

[10] Webster MK, Donoghue DJ. FGFR activation in skeletal disorders: Too much of a good thing[J]. Trends in Genetics, 1997, 13(5): 178-182.

[11] Wilkie AOM. Bad bones, absent smell, selfish testes: The pleiotropic consequences of human FGF receptor mutations[J]. Cytokine & Growth Factor Reviews, 2005, 16(2): 187-203.

[12] Chesi M, Nardini E, Brents LA, et al. Frequent translocation t(4;14)(p16.3;q32.3) in multiple myeloma is associated with increased expression and activating mutations of fibroblast growth factor receptor 3[J]. Nature Genetics, 1997, 16(3): 260-264.

[13] Cappellen D, de Oliveira C, Ricol D, et al. Frequent activating mutations of FGFR3 in human bladder and cervix carcinomas[J]. Nature Genetics, 1999, 23(1): 18-20.

[14] Pollock PM, Gartside MG, Dejeza LC, et al. Frequent activating FGFR2 mutations in endometrial carcinomas parallel germline mutations associated with craniosynostosis and skeletal dysplasia syndromes[J]. Oncogene, 2007, 26(50): 7158-7162.

[15] Rand V, Huang JQ, Stockwell T, et al. Sequence survey of receptor tyrosine kinases reveals mutations in glioblastomas[J]. Proceedings of the National Academy of Sciences of the United States of America, 2005, 102(40): 14344-14349.

[16] Grose R, Dickson C. Fibroblast growth factor signaling in tumorigenesis[J]. Cytokine & Growth Factor Reviews, 2005, 16(2): 179-186.

[17] Frierson HF, Jr., Moskaluk CA. Mutation signature of adenoid cystic carcinoma: evidence for transcriptional and epigenetic reprogramming[J]. Journal of Clinical Investigation, 2013, 123(7): 2783-2785.

[18] Logie A, Dunois-Larde C, Rosty C, et al. Activating mutations of the tyrosine kinase receptor FGFR3 are associated with benign skin tumors in mice and humans[J]. Human Molecular Genetics, 2005, 14(9): 1153-1160.

[19] Reiter A, Sohal J, Kulkarni S, et al. Consistent fusion of ZNF198 to the fibroblast growth factor receptor-1 in the t(8;13)(p11;q12) myeloproliferative syndrome[J]. Blood, 1998, 92(5): 1735-1742.

[20] Wu Y-M, Su F, Kalyana-Sundaram S, et al. Identification of Targetable FGFR Gene Fusions in Diverse Cancers[J]. Cancer Discovery, 2013, 3(6): 636-647.

[21] Singh D, Chan JM, Zoppoli P, et al. Transforming Fusions of FGFR and TACC Genes in Human Glioblastoma[J]. Science, 2012, 337(6099): 1231-1235.

[22] Chaffer CL, Dopheide B, Savagner P, et al. Aberrant fibroblast growth factor receptor signaling in bladder and other cancers[J]. Differentiation, 2007, 75(9): 831-842.

[23] Fletcher MNC, Castro MAA, Wang X, et al. Master regulators of FGFR2 signalling and breast cancer risk[J]. Nature Communications, 2013, 4:2464.

[24] Sugiyama N, Varjosalo M, Meller P, et al. Fibroblast Growth Factor Receptor 4 Regulates Tumor Invasion by Coupling Fibroblast Growth Factor Signaling to Extracellular Matrix Degradation[J]. Cancer Research, 2010, 70(20): 7851-7861.

[25] Andre F, Bachelot T, Campone M, et al. Targeting FGFR with Dovitinib (TKI258): Preclinical and Clinical Data in Breast Cancer[J]. Clinical Cancer Research, 2013, 19(13): 3693-3702.

[26] Quintas-Cardama A. Ponatinib in Philadelphia Chromosome-Positive Leukemias[J]. New England Journal of Medicine, 2014, 370(6): 577-577.

[27] Gozgit JM, Wong MJ, Moran L, et al. Ponatinib (AP24534), a Multitargeted Pan-FGFR Inhibitor with Activity in Multiple FGFR-Amplified or Mutated Cancer Models[J]. Molecular Cancer Therapeutics, 2012, 11(3): 690-699.

[28] Llovet JM, Decaens T, Raoul J-L, et al. Brivanib in Patients With Advanced Hepatocellular Carcinoma Who Were Intolerant to Sorafenib or for Whom Sorafenib Failed: Results From the Randomized Phase III BRISK-PS Study[J]. Journal of Clinical Oncology, 2013, 31(28): 3509-3516.

[29] Gavine PR, Mooney L, Kilgour E, et al. AZD4547: An Orally Bioavailable, Potent, and Selective Inhibitor of the Fibroblast Growth Factor Receptor Tyrosine Kinase Family[J]. Cancer Research, 2012, 72(8): 2045-2056.

[30] Nguyen PT, Tsunematsu T, Yanagisawa S, et al. The FGFR1 inhibitor PD173074 induces mesenchymal-epithelial transition through the transcription factor AP-1[J]. British Journal of Cancer, 2013, 109(8): 2248-2258.

[31] Grand EK, Chase AJ, Heath C, et al. Targeting FGFR3 in multiple myeloma: inhibition of t(4;14)-positive cells by SU5402 and PD173074[J]. Leukemia, 2004, 18(5): 962-966.

[32] Zhou W, Hur W, McDermott U, et al. A Structure-Guided Approach to Creating Covalent FGFR Inhibitors[J]. Chemistry & Biology, 2010, 17(3): 285-295.

[33] Byron SA, Chen H, Wortmann A, *et al.* The N550K/H Mutations in FGFR2 Confer Differential Resistance to PD173074, Dovitinib, and Ponatinib ATP-Competitive Inhibitors[J]. Neoplasia, 2013, 15(8): 975-988.

[34] Blencke S, Zech B, Engkvist O, *et al.* Characterization of a conserved structural determinant controlling protein kinase sensitivity to selective inhibitors[J]. Chemistry & Biology, 2004, 11(5): 691-701.

[35] Chen H, Ma J, Li W, *et al.* A molecular brake in the kinase hinge region regulates the activity of receptor tyrosine kinases[J]. Molecular Cell, 2007, 27(5): 717-730.

[36] Bae JH, Boggon TJ, Tome F, *et al.* Asymmetric receptor contact is required for tyrosine autophosphorylation of fibroblast growth factor receptor in living cells[J]. Proceedings of the National Academy of Sciences of the United States of America, 2010, 107(7): 2866-2871.

[37] Huang Z, Chen H, Blais S, *et al.* Structural Mimicry of A-Loop Tyrosine Phosphorylation by a Pathogenic FGF Receptor 3 Mutation[J]. Structure, 2013, 21(10): 1889-1896.

[38] Mohammadi M, McMahon G, Sun L, *et al.* Structures of the tyrosine kinase domain of fibroblast growth factor receptor in complex with inhibitors[J]. Science, 1997, 276(5314): 955-960.

[39] Eathiraj S, Palma R, Hirschi M, *et al.* A novel mode of protein kinase inhibition exploiting hydrophobic motifs of autoinhibited kinases: discovery of ATP-independent inhibitors of fibroblast growth factor receptor [J]. Journal of Biological Chemistry, 2011, 286(23): 20677-20687.

[40] Mohammadi M, Froum S, Hamby JM, *et al.* Crystal structure of an angiogenesis inhibitor bound to the FGF receptor tyrosine kinase domain[J]. Embo Journal, 1998, 17(20): 5896-5904.

[41] Ezzat S, Zheng L, Zhu XF, *et al.* RETRACTED: Targeted expression of a human pituitary tumor-derived isoform of FGF receptor-4 recapitulates pituitary tumorigenesis (Retracted article. See vol. 125, pg. 3303, 2015)[J]. Journal of Clinical Investigation, 2002, 109(1): 69-78.

[42] Ye Y-W, Hu S, Shi Y-Q, *et al.* Combination of the FGFR4 inhibitor PD173074 and 5-fluorouracil reduces proliferation and promotes apoptosis in gastric cancer[J]. Oncology Reports, 2013, 30(6): 2777-2784.

[43] Ho HK, Nemeth G, Ng YR, *et al.* Developing FGFR4 Inhibitors As Potential Anti-Cancer Agents *Via* In Silico Design, Supported by *In Vitro* and Cell-Based Testing[J]. Current Medicinal Chemistry, 2013, 20(10): 1203-1217.

[44] Liu Y, Gray NS. Rational design of inhibitors that bind to inactive kinase conformations[J]. Nature Chemical Biology, 2006, 2(7): 358-364.

[45] Li SQ, Cheuk AT, Shern JF, *et al.* Targeting Wild-Type and Mutationally Activated FGFR4 in Rhabdomyosarcoma with the Inhibitor Ponatinib (AP24534)[J]. Plos One, 2013, 8(10): e76551.

[46] Zhou T, Commodore L, Huang W-S, *et al.* Structural Mechanism of the Pan-BCR-ABL Inhibitor Ponatinib (AP24534): Lessons for Overcoming Kinase Inhibitor Resistance[J]. Chemical Biology & Drug Design, 2011, 77(1): 1-11.

[47] Leproult E, Barluenga S, Moras D, *et al.* Cysteine Mapping in Conformationally Distinct Kinase Nucleotide Binding Sites: Application to the Design of Selective Covalent Inhibitors[J]. Journal of Medicinal Chemistry, 2011, 54(5): 1347-1355.

[48] Kharitonenkov A, Shanafelt AB. FGF21: A novel prospect for the treatment of metabolic diseases[J]. Current Opinion in Investigational Drugs, 2009, 10(4): 359-364.

[49] Simard JR, Getlik M, Gruetter C, *et al.* Fluorophore Labeling of the Glycine-Rich Loop as a Method of Identifying Inhibitors That Bind to Active and Inactive Kinase Conformations[J]. Journal of the American Chemical Society, 2010, 132(12): 4152-4160.

[50] Liang G, Liu Z, Wu J, *et al.* Anticancer molecules targeting fibroblast growth factor receptors[J]. Trends in Pharmacological Sciences, 2012, 33(10): 531-541.

[51] Mol CD, Dougan DR, Schneider TR, *et al.* Structural basis for the autoinhibition and STI-571 inhibition of c-Kit tyrosine kinase[J]. Journal of Biological Chemistry, 2004, 279(30): 31655-31663.

[52] Levinson NM, Kuchment O, Shen K, *et al.* A Src-like inactive conformation in the Abl tyrosine kinase domain[J]. Plos Biology, 2006, 4(5): 753-767.

[53] Otwinowski Z, Minor W. Processing of X-ray diffraction data collected in oscillation mode[J]. Macromolecular Crystallography, Pt A, 1997, 276: 307-326.

[54] Adams PD, Grosse-Kunstleve RW, Hung LW, *et al.* PHENIX: building new software for automated crystallographic structure determination[J]. Acta Crystallographica Section D-Biological Crystallography, 2002, 58: 1948-1954.

[55] Emsley P, Cowtan K. Coot: model-building tools for molecular graphics[J]. Acta Crystallographica Section D-Biological Crystallography, 2004, 60: 2126-2132.

A novel FGF2 antagonist peptide P8 with potent antiproliferation activity

Lei Fan, Guang Liang, Xiaokun Li

1. Introduction

The family of fibroblast growth factors (FGFs) plays an important role in several biological processes such as cellar proliferation, survival, migration, invasion, and differentiation [1]. Their activities are mediated by FGF receptor-dependent pathways following the phosphorylation of relevant receptors [2]. Tyrosine-phosphorylated fibroblast growth factor receptor substrate2α (FRS2α) serves as a site for recruitment of multiple Grb2/SOS complexes, leading to activation of the Ras/ mitogen-activated protein kinase (MAPK) signaling pathway crucial for cell proliferation [3, 4]. Recently, accumulated evidences demonstrate that abnormal FGF signaling accelerates tumor development by promoting cancer cell proliferation and survival [5]. One of the members in FGF family fibroblast growth factor 1 (FGF1) is related to angiogenesis and the growth of new blood vessels. Furthermore, overexpression of FGF1 is detected in tumors and correlates with malignancy [6]; fortunately, a novel single-chain variable fragment antibody against FGF1 inhibits the growth of breast carcinoma cells [5]. In addition, keratinocyte growth factor 2 (KGF2) selectively induces epithelial cell proliferation, differentiation, and migration, and it is reported that KGF2 is related to bladder cancer and prostate adenocarcinoma [7, 8].

Simultaneously, it has been reported that fibroblast growth factor 2 (FGF2) is commonly upregulated in a variety of malignant tumors and contributes to tumorigenesis and progression [9]. Therefore, FGF2 is viewed as one of the potential targets for cancer therapy [10, 11]. The FGF2 antagonists are mainly small-molecule inhibitors such as PI-88 [12], Suramin [13, 14], and PNU145156E [15], which are proved to break the FGF2 signal transduction *via* simulating the structure of heparin to form a hydrogen bond with the basic amino acids of FGF2 [16]. However, these heparin-simulated compounds also bind to the positively charged residues on the surface of a variety of proteins and interfere with the physiological functions of the proteins *in vivo*, resulting in potentially harmful side effects [17, 18].

In the previous study, we isolated a high-affinity FGF2-binding peptide P7 with strong inhibitory effects against FGF2-induced cell proliferation and angiogenesis by phage display technology [6, 19–21]. Like other short peptides, sensitivity to proteolytic enzymes significantly impedes its clinical applications. In order to identify the nonfunctional amino acid residues of P7 peptide, alanine scanning was carried out. In the process of alanine-scanning mutagenesis, a peptide with Leu-7 substituted by alanine (P8, PLLQATAGGGS-NH$_2$) was found to have potentials of binding to FGF2 and antiproliferation activity of Balb/c3T3 cells. Herein, we attempt to investigate the antitumor effects of the isolated novel peptide on the tumor cells and provide experimental foundation for further developing a FGF2-targeted strategy contributing to antitumor therapy.

2. Materials and methods

2.1 Materials

A novel peptide (P8, PLLQATAGGGS-NH$_2$) was synthesized by SBS Company (Beijing, China) with purity higher than 95%. Recombinant human FGF2, KGF2, and FGF1 were purchased from PeproTech Inc. (Rocky Hill, NJ, USA). The medium of dulbecco's modified eagle's medium (DMEM) and RPMI-1640 were purchased from Invitrogen (CA, USA). Fetal bovine serum (FBS) and 0.25% trypsin (containing EDTA) were obtained from HyClone (Logan , U

T, USA). Methylthiazoletetrazolium (MTT) and dimethylsulfoxide (DMSO) were from Sigma-Aldrich (St. Louis, MO, USA). Nuclear and Cytoplasmic Protein Extraction Kit was the product of Boster (Wuhan, China). Protease phosphatase inhibitor mixture was obtained from Applygen (Beijin, China). Forty percent acrylamide, Coomassie Brilliant Blue, TEMED, Tris, glycine, sodium dodecyl sulfate (SDS), pre-stained protein marker, and nonfat dry milk were from Bio-Rad (Germany). p-FRS2α (Tyr 196) was purchased from Cell Signaling Technology (Beverly, MA, USA). p-ERK1/2, ERK2, FRS2, and GAPDH were obtained from Santa Cruz Biotechnology, Inc. (CA, USA).

2.2　Cell lines

SGC7901 (The Type Culture Collection of Wuhan University) and NCI-H460 (American Type Culture Collection, USA) were cultured in RMPI-1640 with 10% FBS. Balb/c 3T3 and B16-F10 (The Type Culture Collection of the Chinese Academy of Sciences, Shanghai, China) were grown in DMEM (high glucose) supplemented with 10% FBS, while NIH3T3 (The Type Culture Collection of the Chinese Academy of Sciences, Shanghai, China) was in DMEM (low glucose) supplemented with 10% FBS.

2.3　Cell viability assay

Cells were seeded in 96-well plates with 5×10^3 cells per well. After starved cultivation for 24 h with the medium containing 0.1% FBS, cells were treated with FGF2 alone, or FGF2 plus peptides for certain time. The number of viable cells was then detected by MTT method. Briefly, 20 μl of MTT (5 g/L) was added into each well and incubated for 4 h in the incubator at 37℃ with 5% CO_2. After removal of the medium, 150 μl of DMSO was added into each well and the plate was shaken at room temperature for 10 min. The absorbance was immediately measured at 490 nm to determine the number of viable cells.

2.4　Western blot analysis

Starved cells were pretreated with serially diluted peptides for 5 min before stimulation with FGF2. Cells were collected and lysed in 1× SDS-polyacrylamide gelelectrophoresis(SDS-PAGE) loading buffer. The lysate was boiled and centrifuged at 12 000×g for 10 min at 4℃ to remove the insoluble components. The supernatant was run on 10% SDS-PAGE gel followed by being transferred to a PVDF membrane. After being blocked with 5% nonfat dry milk in TBST for 1.5 h, the membrane was incubated with the primary antibody (an anti-phospho-FRS2α rabbit mAb or an anti-phospho-ERK1/2 rabbit mAb) overnight followed by incubation with goat anti-rabbit IgG, HRP-linked antibody for 1 h. The blots were detected with an ECL detection kit according to the manufacturer's procedure. Nonphosphorylated FRS2α or ERK1/2 was used as the reference control. The results were analyzed by Quantity One software to determine the relative ratio.

2.5　Cell cycle analysis

Cells were seeded in 60-mm plates with 3×10^4 cells per plate. After being starved for 24 h, these were treated with 20 ng/ml FGF2 alone or 20 ng/ml FGF2 plus serially diluted peptides for 48 h. Cells were collected and fixed with 70% ice-cold ethanol for 12 h at −20℃, then stained with 50 μg/ml propidium iodide (PI) for 30 min, and then subjected to FACS Calibur flow cytometer analysis with excitation at 488 nm and emission at 560–640 nm (FL2 mode). Data were analyzed with the FlowJo analysis program.

2.6　Colony formation assay

Freshly resuspended tumor cells B16-F10 (1×10^3/well) were plated in a six-well plate and cultured overnight, starved for 24 h, and treated with 20 ng/ml FGF2 alone or 20 ng/ml FGF2 plus serially diluted peptides for 1 week. Surviving colonies were counted after staining with crystal violet solution and photographed. Each experiment was done in triplicate and performed for three times.

2.7　Cell morphology analysis

Cells were seeded in 96-well plates with 4 000 cells per well overnight and treated with peptide at the final concentrations of 0.25, 1, 4, and 16 μmol/L. Cells cultured with complete medium were used as the control. The cell morphology was observed under an inverted microscope.

2.8 Statistical analysis

All experiments were repeated at least three independent times. Statistical differences between the groups were determined with one-way ANOVA (SPSS 13.0). A value of $P < 0.05$ was considered statistically significant.

3. Results

3.1 P8 peptide inhibits FGF2-stimulated proliferation and activation of FRS2α in Balb/c3T3 cells

MTT colorimetric method was applied to detect the effects of P8 peptide on FGF2-stimulated proliferation of Balb/c 3T3 cells with abundant FGF2 receptors. As shown in Fig. 1A, P8 peptide has a significant dose-dependent inhibitory effect on the proliferation of Balb/c 3T3 cells induced by FGF2 during the range of the detected concentrations. The complete inhibitory effect on FGF2-induced proliferation by P8 peptide was observed at about 4 μM.

To further investigate the initial mechanism for the effect of P8 peptide on FGF2-induced proliferation in Balb/c 3T3 cells, Western blotting was applied to detect the effect of P8 peptide on the activation of FGF2 triggering signal transduction. Our setting was to further evaluate the effect of P8 peptide on FGF2-induced FRS2α phosphorylation in Balb/c 3T3 cells. The results demonstrated that FGF2 indeed triggered intense phosphorylation of FRS2α, but pretreatment of cells with P8 peptide (4 μM) for 5 min before stimulation with FGF2 resulted in significant blockage of FRS2α activation, just as P7 peptide did (Fig. 1B).

3.2 The influence of P8 peptide on FGF2-stimulated proliferation of tumor cells

MTT assay was also used to detect the effect of P8 peptide on FGF2-induced proliferation of tumor cells including B16-F10, NCI-H460, and SGC7901. The results showed that P8 peptide could inhibit the proliferation of tumor cells induced by FGF2 in a dosedependent (Fig. 2A–C) and time-dependent (Fig. 2D) manners. Administration of P8 peptide at the concentration of 4 μM suppressed more than 90% of FGF2-induced proliferation in all detected tumor cells.

3.3 P8 peptide blocks FGF2-induced phosphorylation of FRS2α and MAP kinase in tumor cells

FGF2 binding induces phosphorylation of FGFRs, which subsequently activates FRS2α and the downstream MEK/ERK signaling pathway involved in cell proliferation. The effect of P8 peptide on FGF2-stimulated activation of FRS2α

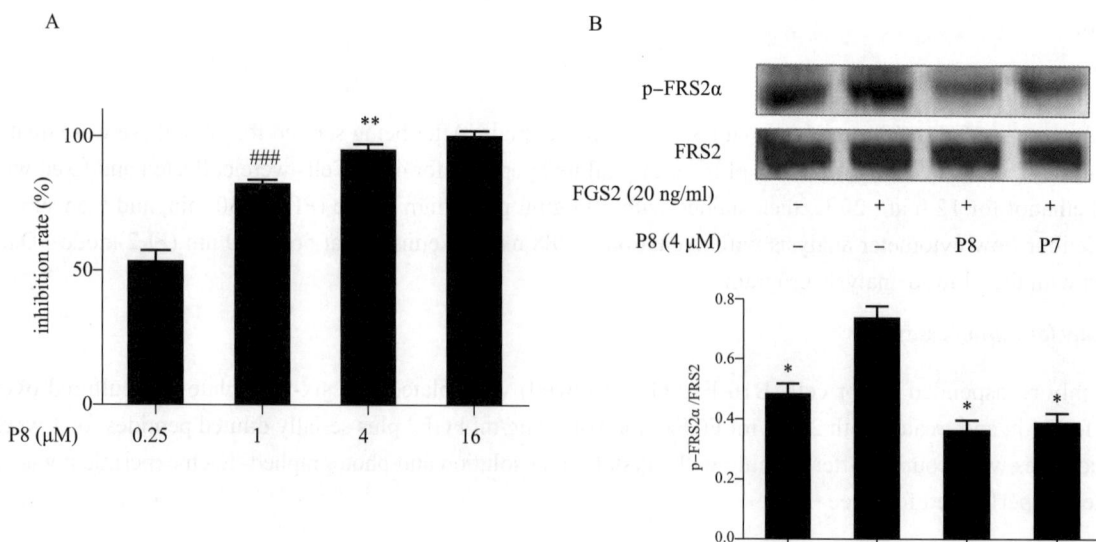

Fig. 1. P8 suppresses proliferation and activation of FRS2α of Balb/c3T3 cells. (A) Starved cells were treated with 20 ng/ml FGF2 alone and 20 ng/ml FGF2 plus P8 at the indicated concentrations, and cell proliferation was measured 48 h later with MTT assay. Data are presented as the mean±SD of three independent experiments performed in triplicate. (B) Cells were pretreated with P8 (4 μM) and P7 (4 μM) for 5 min before stimulation with 20 ng/ml FGF2 for 20 min. The phosphorylated and total levels of FRS2α were determined by Western blot analysis. *Bar groups* represent means±SD. $^{###}P < 0.001$ vs. the 0.25 μmol/L group; $^{**}P < 0.01$ vs. the 1 μmol/L group; $^{*}P < 0.05$ vs. the FGF2 group.

A

B

C

D

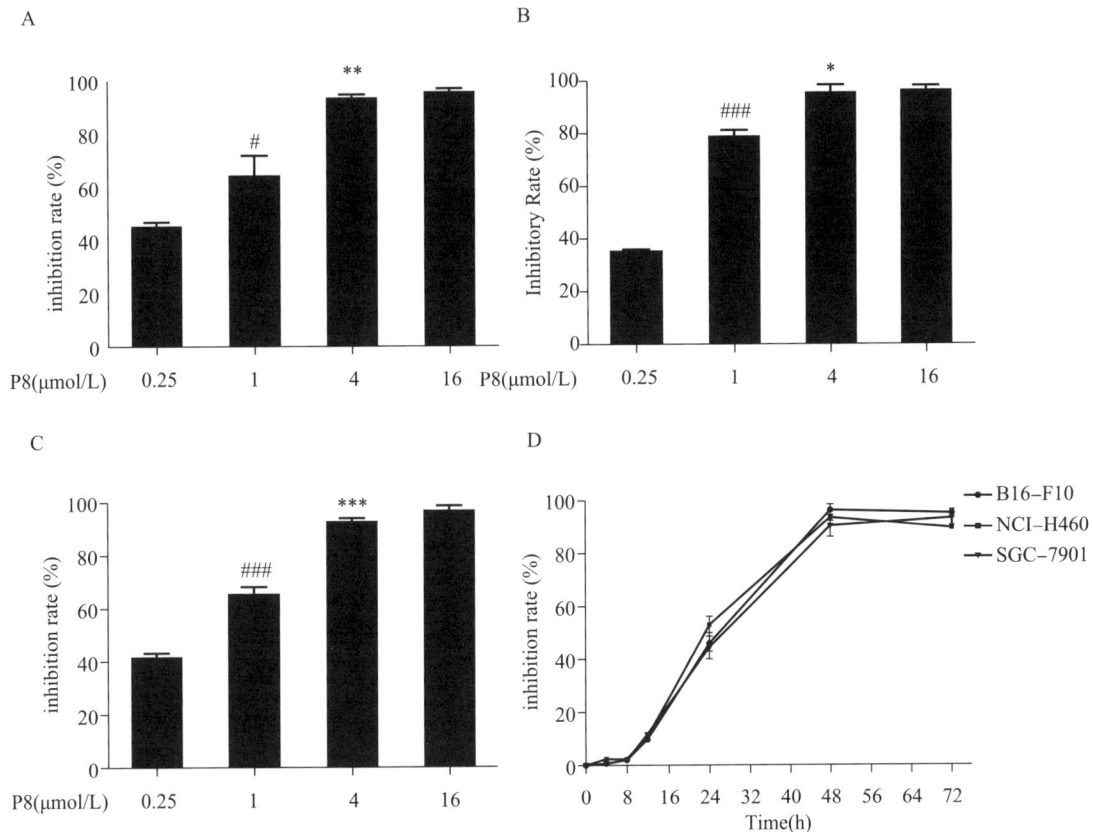

Fig. 2. P8 peptide suppresses FGF2-stimulated proliferation in tumor cells including B16-F10, NCI-H460, and SGC7901 in dose-dependent (A–C) and time-dependent (D) manners. A–C Starved cells were treated with 20 ng/ml FGF2 alone and 20 ng/ml FGF2 plus P8 at the indicated concentrations (0.25, 1, 4, and 16 μM), and cell proliferation was measured 48 h later by MTT assay. D Starved cells were treated with FGF2 alone, or FGF2 plus P8 peptide (4 μM) for 4, 8, 12, 24, 48, and 72 h. The number of viable cells was then detected by MTT method. Data are presented as the mean±SD of three independent experiments performed in triplicate. [#]$P<0.001$ and [###]$P<0.05$ *vs.* the 0.25 μmol/L group; [*]$P<0.05$, [**]$P<0.01$, and [***]$P<0.001$ *vs.* the 1 μmol/L group.

and ERK1/2 in B16-F10, NCI-H460, and SGC7901 cells was analyzed by Western blot. As shown in Fig. 3, FGF2 stimulation significantly enhanced the phosphorylation of FRS2α and ERK1/2, whereas pretreatment with P8 peptide (0.25–16 μM) for 5 min resulted in dose-dependent blockage of FRS2α and ERK1/2 activation. P8 peptide at the concentration of 4 μM suppressed the activation of the detected signal molecules in three types of tumor cells.

3.4 P8 peptide arrests FGF2-induced cells at the G0/G1 phase in B16-F10 cells by flow cytometry analysis

Cell cycle analysis by flow cytometry was performed to further understand the effect of P8 peptide on FGF2-induced cell cycle progression of B16-F10 cells. The results shown in Fig. 4 indicated that FGF2-treated cells presented an increased G0/G1-phase population compared with the control and P8 peptide decreased the G0/G1-phase population, suggesting that P8 peptide inhibited FGF2-stimulated cell proliferation by changing the cell cycle distribution.

3.5 P8 peptide inhibits FGF2-stimulated proliferation in B16-F10 cells by colony formation assay

The colony formation assay was used to identify the effect of the antiproliferation on B16-F10 cells. The results showed an increased number of colonies treated with FGF2 compared with the control, but P8 peptide obviously decreased the number of colonies of B16-F10 at 4 μM (Fig. 5).

3.6 P8 Peptide inhibits KGF2-, FGF1-, and FGF2-stimulated FRS2α activation of SGC7901 cells

FRS2α is the common substrate of all kinds of FGFRs, and its phosphorylation represents the activation of FGF-triggered signaling pathway. In this setting, Western blot was applied to detect the effect of P8 peptide. The results demonstrated that these three FGFs triggered intense phosphorylation of FRS2α in the SGC7901 cells (Fig. 6). However,

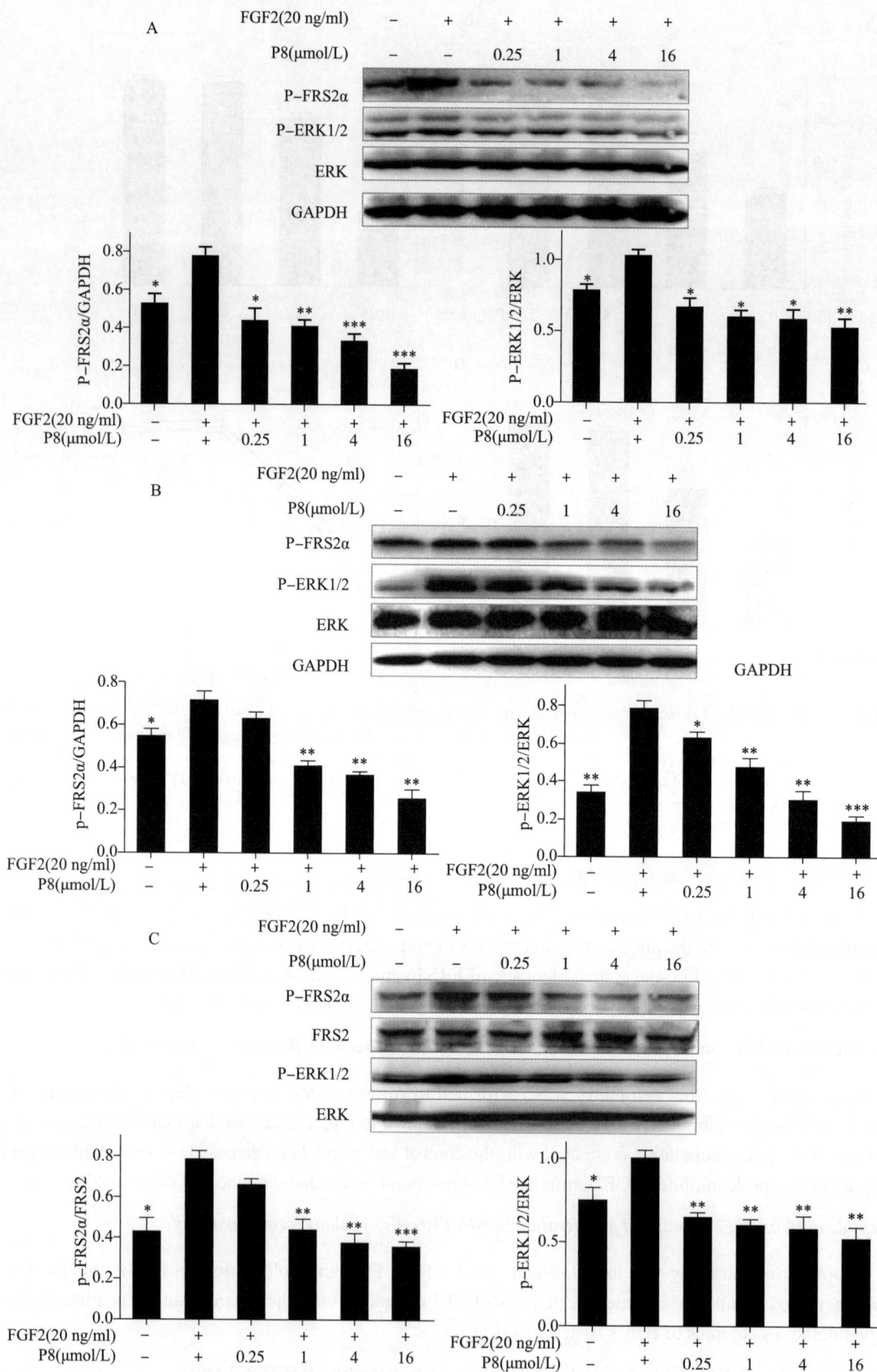

Fig. 3. The effect of P8 on FGF2-stimulated activation of FRS2α and ERK1/2 in B16-F10 (A), NCI-H460 (B), and SGC7901 (C) cells. Cells were pretreated with serially diluted P8 peptide (0.25, 1, 4, and 16 μM) for 5 min before stimulation with 20 ng/ml FGF2 for 10 min (B16-F10), 20 min (NCI-H460), and 10 min (SGC7901), and subjected to Western blot analysis of the phosphorylated and total levels of FRS2α, ERK1/2 and GAPDH. Results are expressed as means±SD. $^{*}P < 0.05$, $^{**}P < 0.01$, and $^{***}P < 0.001$ $vs.$ FGF2 group.

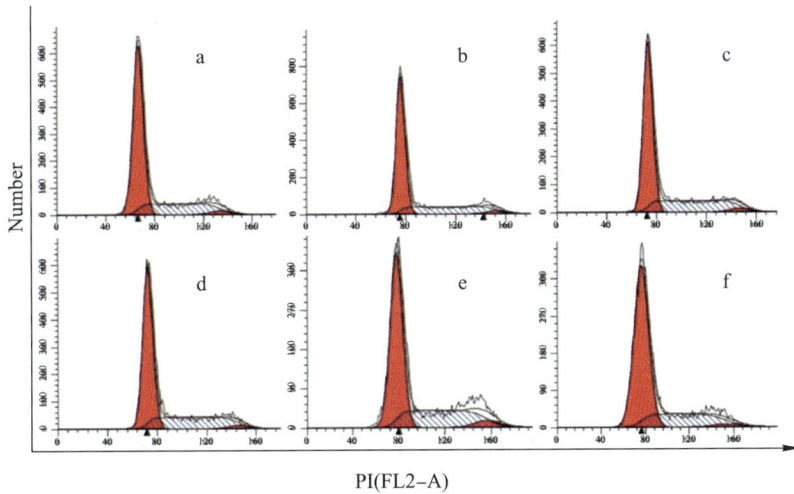

Flow cytomerty analysis of the effect of synthesized P8
peptides on cell cycle

Group	G0/G1(%)	G2/M(%)	S(%)
a	69.92 ± 0.95	2.92 ± 0.53	27.17 ± 0.42
b	52.03 ± 1.22	1.87 ± 2.37	45.85 ± 1.52
c	64.06 ± 1.20	3.11 ± 0.16	32.84 ± 1.03
d	65.88 ± 0.65	3.31 ± 0.98	30.96 ± 1.17
e	67.64 ± 0.34	3.67 ± 0.52	28.70 ± 0.18
f	69.33 ± 2.06	3.47 ± 1.27	27.10 ± 1.64

Fig. 4. P8 peptide alters the cell cycle distribution of FGF2-stimulated B16-F10 cells: (a) control group; (b) 20 ng/mL FGF2-treated group; and (c–f) groups treated with 20 ng/ml FGF2 plus various concentrations of P8 peptide (0.25, 1, 4, and 16 μM, respectively). Data shown are the representative pictures of three independent experiments.

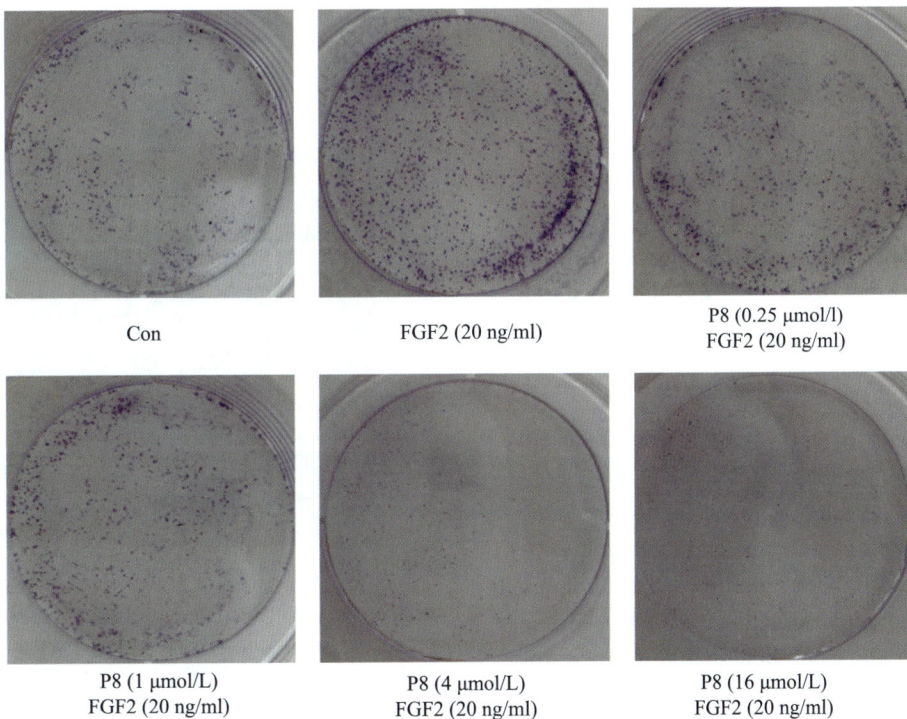

Con

FGF2 (20 ng/ml)

P8 (0.25 μmol/l)
FGF2 (20 ng/ml)

P8 (1 μmol/L)
FGF2 (20 ng/ml)

P8 (4 μmol/L)
FGF2 (20 ng/ml)

P8 (16 μmol/L)
FGF2 (20 ng/ml)

B

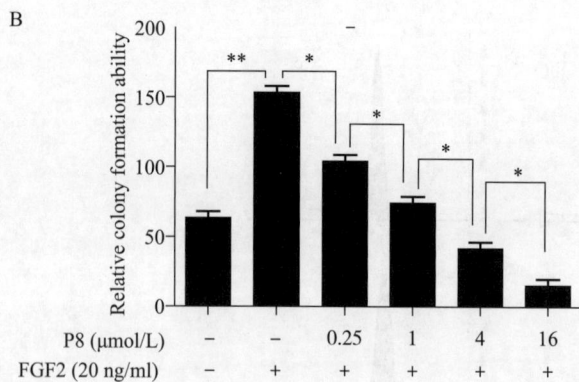

Fig. 5. P8 peptide inhibits FGF2-stimulated proliferation in B16-F10 cells by colony formation assay. Starved cells were treated with 20 ng/ml FGF2 alone and 20 ng/ml FGF2 plus P8 at the indicated concentrations (0.25, 1, 4, and 16 μM) for 1 week. Data are presented as the mean±SD of three independent experiments performed in triplicate. $^{**}P<0.01$ and $^{*}P<0.05$.

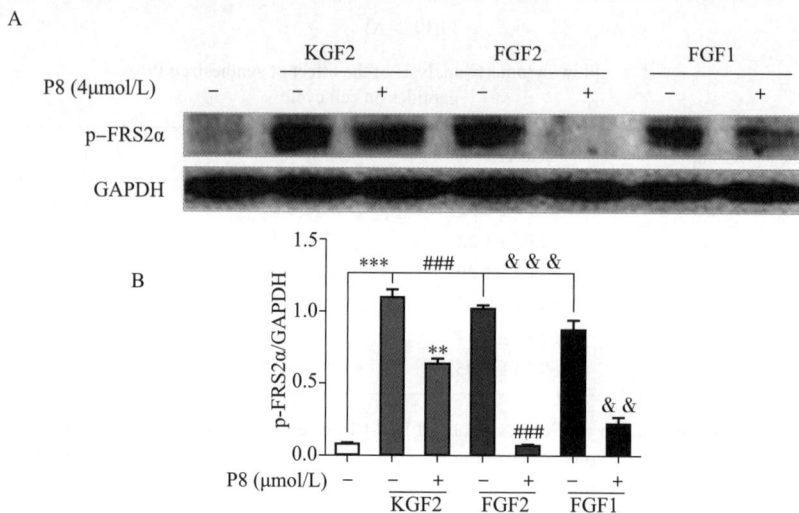

A

B

Fig. 6. Western blot assay was used to detect the target of P8 peptide. P8 peptide was pretreated for 5 min on starved cells SGC7901, and KGF-2 (100 ng/ml), FGF1 (100 ng/ml) with heparin (50 μg/ml), and FGF2 (20 ng/ml) were applied as different stimuli. *Bar groups* represent means±SD. $^{***}P<0.001$ *vs.* control group, $^{**}P<0.01$ *vs.* KGF2 group; $^{###}P<0.001$ *vs.* control group, $^{###}P<0.01$ *vs.* FGF1 group; $^{&&&}P<0.001$ *vs.* control group, $^{&&}P<0.01$ *vs.* FGF2 group.

in the pretreatment of SGC7901 cells with P8 peptide (4 μM) before stimulation with KGF2, FGF1, and FGF2, the activation of FRS2α was all suppressed in varying degrees and the inhibition on FGF2 was found to be preeminent. So, we supposed that P8 might be used as a multi-target antagonist.

3.7 The effect of P8 peptide on cell morphology

The morphology of cells treated with different concentrations of P8 peptide was observed under the inverted microscope. Compared with the control group, no significant effect of P8 peptide on cell morphology was observed at the detected concentrations. Cells remain in normal shape and good refraction even when treated with 16 μM P8 peptide, suggesting that P8 peptide was noncytotoxic on Balb/c 3T3, B16-F10, NCI-H460, and SGC7901 cells (Fig. 7).

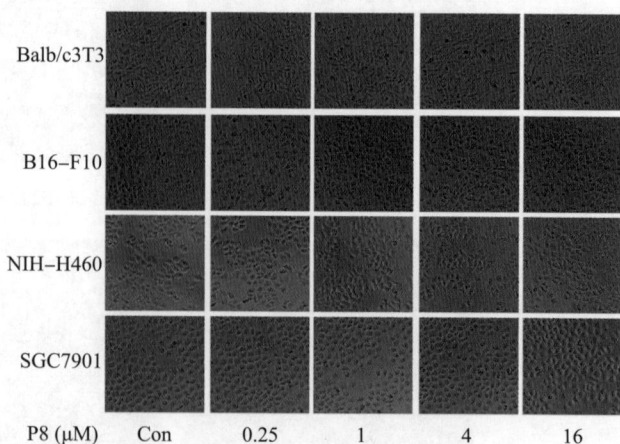

Fig. 7. The effect of P8 on cell morphology. Cells were seeded in 96-well plates and treated with P8 peptide at the final concentrations of 0.25, 1, 4, and 16 μM. Cells cultured with complete medium were used as the control.

4. Discussion

A wealth of pharmacological studies has previously shown that FGF2 is widely upregulated in malignant tumors and contributes to tumorigenesis and progression [1]. And there is increasing evidence showed that FGF2 is viewed as one of the potential targets for cancer therapy [10, 11]. Previously, we had showed that the specific FGF2-binding peptide P7 with strong inhibitory effects on cell proliferation and angiogenesis with FGF2-stimulation may have potential in cancer therapy [6, 19–21]. In this study, we developed a biopanning strategy using phage display technology and alanine scanning for identifying a novel FGF2-binding peptide, named P8.

Furthermore, fibroblast growth factor receptors have been shown to act as a driving oncogene in certain cancers to maintain the malignant properties of tumor cell *via* a cell autonomous manner [22]. In our study, the novel P8 peptide significantly inhibited the proliferation of Balb/c 3T3 cells, which highly express FGF2 receptors, induced by FGF2 in a dose-dependent manner. In addition, three tumor cells B16-F10, NIH-H460, and SGC7901 related to the overexpression of FGF2 have been used to study with FGF antagonists [21, 23, 24].

It has been reported that FGF2 promotes cancer cell proliferation through the activation of the Ras/Raf/MEK/ERK pathway [25–28]. In order to determine which MAPK pathway involved in mediating the inhibitory effect of P8 on FGF2-induced proliferation, phosphorylation of ERK1/2 was detected by Western blot. As shown in Fig. 3, P8 suppressed FGF2-induced ERK1/2 phosphorylation in a dose-dependent manner. The effects on FGF2-stimulating proliferation of cancer cell lines demonstrated that P8 peptide inhibited FGF2-induced proliferation and downregulated the activation of FRS2α/ERK cascade in B16-F10, NIH-H460, and SGC7901 cells through MAPK signaling pathway. And cell proliferation is regulated during the G0/G1 phase in the cell cycle [29]. FGF2 promotes the expression of cell cycle regulatory proteins involved in cell cycle entry and progression through the G1 and S phases [18, 30]. The results of cell cycle showed that P8 peptide significantly arrested the cycle at the G0/G1 phase in FGF2-induced B16-F10 cells. The results of MTT assay showed that P8 peptide suppressed the cell proliferation in dose-dependent and time-dependent manners. The results of colony formation assay showed that P8 peptide inhibited the cell proliferation in a dose-dependent manner. Therefore, the novel peptide (P8) may exert inhibitory effects on FGF2-stimulated proliferation in tumor cells by suppressing the ability of FGF2-stimulated cell cycle through the cell phase from G0/G1 to S phase. Besides, the cytotoxicity of P8 peptide was evaluated by observation of the effect of P8 peptide on cell morphology. Cells treated with P8 peptide displayed a similar shape and refraction to the cells treated without P8 peptide, ruling out the possibility that P8 peptide inhibited cell proliferation *via* the cytotoxicity, which is superior to other small-molecule inhibitors [17, 18]. These implied that P8 peptide had the potential of antitumor activity *via* binding to FGF2 with no toxicity.

Among the other FGF-induced tumors, it has been reported that FGF1 is overexpressed in carcinoma and *via* interactions with fibroblast growth factor receptors to promote the grade of the diseases [31]. KGF2 is a growth factor that selectively induces epithelial cell proliferation, differentiation, and migration [12]. Both of FGFs serve as the targets in cancer therapy [2]. Interestingly, our results showed that P8 peptide not only availably inhibited the phosphorylation of FRS2α stimulated by FGF2 but also FGF1 and KGF2, which is different from P7 peptide. It suggested that P8 peptide not only targets FGF2, but also FGF1 and KGF2. It seems reasonable to speculate that P8 peptides may develop as a multi-target antagonist peptide contributing to the tumor treatment, which is currently being addressed in our laboratory.

In summary, our results demonstrate that the novel FGF2-binding P8 peptide provides an effective FGF2 antagonist and may have potential application for the treatment of proliferative disorders, including a variety of tumor with upregulation of FGF1, FGF2, and KGF2. Further studies will be aimed at characterizing its potential therapeutic role in tumor and the multi-target antagonist.

References

[1] Powers CJ, McLeskey SW, Wellstein A. Fibroblast growth factors, their receptors and signaling[J]. Endocrine-Related Cancer, 2000, 7(3): 165-197.

[2] Goldfarb M. Fibroblast growth factor homologous factors: Evolu-

tion, structure, and function[J]. Cytokine & Growth Factor Reviews, 2005, 16(2): 215-220.

[3] Turner N, Grose R. Fibroblast growth factor signalling: from development to cancer[J]. Nature Reviews Cancer, 2010, 10(2): 116-129.

[4] Zhang J, Yang PL, Gray NS. Targeting cancer with small molecule kinase inhibitors[J]. Nature Reviews Cancer, 2009, 9(1): 28-39.

[5] Shi H-L, Yang T, Deffar K, et al. A Novel Single-chain Variable Fragment Antibody Against FGF-1 Inhibits the Growth of Breast Carcinoma Cells by Blocking the Intracrine Pathway of FGF-1[J]. Iubmb Life, 2011, 63(2): 129-137.

[6] Wang C, Yu Y, Li Q, et al. P7 peptides suppress the proliferation of K562 cells induced by basic fibroblast growth factor[J]. Tumor Biology, 2012, 33(4): 1085-1093.

[7] Memarzadeh S, Xin L, Mulholland DJ, et al. Enhanced paracrine FGF10 expression promotes formation of multifocal prostate adenocarcinoma and an increase in epithelial androgen receptor[J]. Cancer Cell, 2007, 12(6): 572-585.

[8] Chung SS, Koh CJ. Bladder cancer cell in co-culture induces human stem cell differentiation to urothelial cells through paracrine FGF10 signaling[J]. In Vitro Cellular &Developmental Biology-Animal, 2013, 49(10): 746-751.

[9] Facchiano A, Russo K, Facchiano AM, et al. Identification of a novel domain of fibroblast growth factor 2 controlling its angiogenic properties[J]. Journal of Biological Chemistry, 2003, 278(10): 8751-8760.

[10] Rusnati M, Presta M. Fibroblast growth Factors/Fibroblast growth factor receptors as targets for the development of anti-angiogenesis strategies[J]. Current Pharmaceutical Design, 2007, 13(20): 2025-2044.

[11] Acevedo VD, Ittmann M, Spencer DM. Paths of FGFR-driven tumorigenesis[J]. Cell Cycle, 2009, 8(4): 580-588.

[12] Cochran S, Li CP, Fairweather JK, et al. Probing the interactions of phosphosulfomannans with angiogenic growth factors by surface plasmon resonance[J]. Journal of Medicinal Chemistry, 2003, 46(21): 4601-4608.

[13] Takano S, Gately S, Neville ME, et al. Suramin, an anticancer and angiosuppressive agent, inhibits endothelial cell binding of basic fibroblast growth factor, migration,proliferation, and induction of urokinase-type plasminogen activator[J]. Cancer Research, 1994, 54(10): 2654-2660.

[14] Danesi R, Delbianchi S, Soldani P, et al. Suramin inhibits bFGF-induced endothelial cell proliferation and angiogenesis in the chick chorioallantoic membrane[J]. British Journal of Cancer, 1993, 68(5): 932-938.

[15] Sola F, Capolongo L, Moneta D, et al. The antitumor efficacy of cytotoxic drugs is potentiated by treatment with PNU 145156E, a growth-factor-complexing molecule[J]. Cancer Chemotherapy and Pharmacology, 1999, 43(3): 241-246.

[16] Wu J, Liang G, Wu X, et al. Progress of Inhibitors Targeting Fibroblast Growth Factor[J]. Chemistry, 2010.

[17] Manetti F, Corelli F, Botta M. Fibroblast growth factors and their inhibitors[J]. Current Pharmaceutical Design, 2000, 6(18): 1897-1924.

[18] Fan HK, Zhou H, Li W. The interaction of fibroblast growth factor/fibroblast growth factor receptor and FGF inhibitors[J]. Progress in Biochemistry & Biophysics, 2001, 28(3): 338-341.

[19] Wu X, Yan Q, Huang Y, et al. Isolation of a novel basic FGF-binding peptide with potent antiangiogenetic activity[J]. Journal of Cellular and Molecular Medicine, 2010, 14(1-2): 351-356.

[20] Wang C, Lin S, Nie Y, et al. Mechanism of antitumor effect of a novel bFGF binding peptide on human colon cancer cells[J]. Cancer Science, 2010, 101(5): 1212-1218.

[21] Yu Y, Gao S, Li Q, et al. The FGF2-binding peptide P7 inhibits melanoma growth in vitro and in vivo[J]. Journal of Cancer Research and Clinical Oncology, 2012, 138(8): 1321-1328.

[22] Knights V, Cook SJ. De-regulated FGF receptors as therapeutic targets in cancer[J]. Pharmacology & Therapeutics, 2010, 125(1): 105-117.

[23] Wang R, Luo W, He D, et al. Inhibition of Proliferation of Non-small Cell Lung Cancer Cells by a bFGF Antagonist Peptide[J]. International Journal of Peptide Research and Therapeutics, 2014, 20(1): 109-115.

[24] Wu X, Huang H, Wang C, et al. Identification of a novel peptide that blocks basic fibroblast growth factor-mediated cell proliferation[J]. Oncotarget, 2013, 4(10): 1819-1828.

[25] Smalley KSM. A pivotal role for ERK in the oncogenic behaviour of malignant melanoma?[J]. International Journal of Cancer, 2003, 104(5): 527-532.

[26] Nesbit M, Nesbit HKE, Bennett J, et al. Basic fibroblast growth factor induces a transformed phenotype in normal human melanocytes[J]. Oncogene, 1999, 18(47): 6469-6476.

[27] Lazar-Molnar E, Hegyesi H, Toth S, et al. Autocrine and paracrine regulation by cytokines and growth factors in melanoma[J]. Cytokine, 2000, 12(6): 547-554.

[28] Lefevre G, Babchia N, Calipel A, et al. Activation of the FGF2/FGFR1 Autocrine Loop for Cell Proliferation and Survival in Uveal Melanoma Cells[J]. Investigative Ophthalmology & Visual Science, 2009, 50(3): 1047-1057.

[29] Neary JT, Kang Y, Shi Y-F. Cell cycle regulation of astrocytes by extracellular nucleotides and fibroblast growth factor-2[J]. Purinergic Signalling, 2005, 1(4): 329-336.

[30] Pages G, Lenormand P, Lallemain G, et al. Mitogen-activated protein kinases p42mapk and p44mapk are required for fibroblast proliferation[J]. Proceedings of the National Academy of Sciences of the United States of America, 1993, 90(18): 8319-8323.

[31] Dai X, Cai C, Xiao F, et al. Identification of a novel aFGF-binding peptide with anti-tumor effect on breast cancer from phage display library[J]. Biochemical and Biophysical Research Communications, 2014, 445(4): 795-801.

Discovery and identification of new non-ATP competitive FGFR1 inhibitors with therapeutic potential on non-small-cell lung cancer

Yi Wang, Xiaokun Li, Guang Liang

1. Introduction

Fibroblast growth factor receptors (FGFRs) belong to a sub-family of the receptor tyrosine kinase superfamily (RTKs). After ligand binding, FGFRs activate a series of downstream signaling pathways, such as the mitogen-activated protein kinase (MAPK) and the phosphoinositide-3-kinase (PI3K)/Akt pathways [1,2]. When functuion mutations or over-expression are gained, activation of the FGFR signaling system can lead to excessive cell proliferation, angiogenesis, and other pathophysiological changes, culminating in the development of cancer or other diseases [3]. Studies in the last few years have uncovered increasing evidence that FGFRs are driving oncogenes in certain cancers and act in a cell autonomous fashion to maintain the malignant properties of tumour cells [4]. Given the important role of FGFRs in the development and progression of tumors, FGFRs gradually have become an important target of cancer treatment [2,5]. At present, several small-molecule, FGFR inhibitors are being tested in clinical trials as anti-tumor drug candidates [6,7]. Many other small-molecule inhibitors are being assessed in pre-clinical studies [3,4,8].

Generally, small molecules of FGFR inhibitors are achieved by targeting the ATP-binding domain and the competition with ATP to lock the kinase into an inactive state [8]. Most of the current, small-molecule, FGFR inhibitors are structural analogs or derivatives of ATP. However, approximately 518 RTKs are encoded by the human genome, and they all share a similar ATP-binding structure characterized by two lobes connected by a hinge region [9]. Therefore, most inhibitors bind to the relatively-conserved, ATP-binding domain in RTKs and lack kinase selectivity, which gives rise to a variety of side effects and toxic effects in clinical and pre-clinical studies [8]. Kinase inhibitors that target the non-ATP-binding domain are attractive because that form is more likely to represent a distinct conformation that may, in turn, lead to the identification of more selective inhibitors. It also is particularly important to look for inhibitors that specifically inhibit FGFRs [3]. However, despite advances in the field, identifying highly-selective, small-molecule inhibitors that target an inactive conformation or a new domain of FGFR continues to be a significant challenge [3,7].

In this study, we identified two, novel, non-ATP-competitive, irreversible FGFR inhibitors, i.e., (2-oxocyclopentane-1,3-diylidene)bis(methanylylidene))bis(2-methoxy-4,1-phenylene) dipropionate (A114) and (2-oxocyclopentane-1,3-diylid-ene)bis(methanylylidene))bis(2-methoxy-4,1-phenylene) diisobutyrate (A117), *via* kinase inhibitory assay of a chemical bank that contained 156 bisaryl-1,4-dien-3-one compounds, and these two compounds significantly inhibited the growth of tumors by specifically targeting FGFR1. Our data suggest that these novel FGFR1 inhibitors may be a potential therapy for treatment of non-small-cell, lung-cancer cells (NSCLC) and provide a new structural lead for selective FGFR1 inhibitors.

2. Materials and methods

2.1 Cell lines, compounds, and reagents

Human lung carcinoma cell line H460 was purchased from ATCC (Manassas, VA). Human lung (bronchial) epithelial cell line BEAS-2B was purchased from the Cell Library Committee of the Chinese Academy of Sciences (*Shanghai, China*). FGFR1-overexpressing 293 cells were given to us by the Institute of Materia Medica, Xi'an Jiaotong University. A bank of 156 compounds was established by our laboratory [10–12]. Before being used in the biological experiments, the compounds were purified by re-crystallization or silica gel chromatography to attain purities greater than 97%. The general chemical structure of these compounds is shown in Fig. 1A. In our *in vitro* studies, these compounds were used in DMSO solution. In the *in vivo* studies, a water-soluble preparation of compound A114 or A117 was prepared using the previously-described pharmaceutical method [13]. Anti-p-FGFR1, anti-FGFR1, anti-p-AKT, anti-AKT, anti-p-ERK, anti-ERK, anti-GAPDH, anti-Actin, anti-Bcl-2, anti-Cyclin D1, anti-COX-2, goat anti-rabbit IgG-HRP, and mouse anti-goat IgG-HRP antibodies were purchased from Santa Cruz Biotechnology (*Santa Cruz, CA*); anti-cleavaged caspase-3 antibody was purchased from Cell Signaling Technology, Inc. (*Danvers, MA*), and a Hoechst staining kit was purchased from Beyotime Biotech (*Nantong, China*). PI/RNase staining buffer was purchased from *BD* Bioscience (*Franklin Lakes, NJ*), and recombinant FGFR1, FGFR2, FGFR3, EGFR, c-MET, and PDGFR-β proteins were obtained from Carna Biosciences, Inc. (*Kobe, Japan*). Staurosporine, DMSO, and ATP were purchased from Sigma (*St. Louis, MO*). Peptide FAM-P22 was purchased from GL Biochem (*Shanghai, China*).

2.2 Kinase inhibition assays

The activities of the tyrosine kinase were detected by Caliper Mobility Shift Assay on EZ Reader (*Caliper Life Sciences, MA*) according to the instructions provided. The ATP concentration was set at the K_m value of FGFR1, 262 μM. For the determination of IC_{50}, the compounds were tested in duplicate at 10 concentrations, ranging from 5 nM to 100 μM. Specific details of each assay are available in the Supporting information. In the electrophoretic mobility shift assays, product accumulation was expressed as percentage conversion, product peak height/(product peak height + substrate peak height). In the experiments for testing the relationship between the compounds and ATP, the concentration of the substrate was constant, while the concentration of ATP was set at 4192, 2096, 1048, 524, 262, 131, 66, and 33 μM. The global competitive inhibition fit for the compounds was performed based on% conversion = $(V_{max} \times X)/\{K_m \times [(1 + I/K_i)^n] + X\}$, where X is the ATP concentration and n is the Hill coefficient. For analysis of receptor tyrosine kinase phosphorylation and downstream signal transduction pathways in human cancer cells, starved cells were treated with compounds for 4 h and stimulated with bFGF (20 ng/ml) for 10 min; then, the cells were collected and processed for Western blot analysis. Details of this assay are available in the Supporting information.

2.3 Inhibition dynamics test

The association rate constant (K_{on}) value of compound A117 on FGFR1 with an ATP concentration of km was detected *in vitro* by Caliper Mobility Shift Assay. The compounds were tested in duplicate for 10 different concentrations. Specific details of each assay are available in the Supporting information. Details of this assay are available in the Supporting information.

2.4 Reversibility assay

The rapid dilution experiment, as described previously [14], was used to demonstrate the binding mode of A117 to FGFR1. FGFR1 kinase was pre-incubated with and without A117 ($10 \times IC_{50}$, 20 μM) at room temperature for 30 min. Then, the enzyme mix and the substrate mix were transferred to the 384-well assay plate, and the Caliper EZ Reader was used to assay the kinase activity of this mixture. Specific details of each assay are available in the Supporting information. Details are available in the Supporting information.

2.5 Molecular docking simulation

The docking simulation of the indicated compound with protein was conducted with Tripos' molecular modeling package, *i.e.,* Sybyl-2.0 (*Tripos, St. Louis, MO*). The crystal structure of FGFR1 was obtained from the Protein Data Bank (*PDB ID*: 3RHX). The ligand-binding groove on the proteins was kept rigid, whereas all torsible bonds of the ligands were set free to allow flexible docking to produce more than 100 structures. The final, docked conformations were obtained when ligand poses with the lowest binding energy, and then the conformations were used to analyze the interaction mode between the ligand and its target.

2.6 Cell proliferation assay

Compounds were assayed for their anti-proliferative activities against H460 and BEAS-2B cells using the MTT assay. In brief, the BEAS-2B and H460 cells were cultured with A114 and A117 (10 μM), respectively, for 0, 12, 24, 36, 48, and 72 h, while DMSO was used as the vehicle control. After treatment, the proliferation of the cells was determined by MTT assay.

2.7 Cell cycle analysis

H460 cells were treated with A114 or A117 in various doses (0, 1, 5 and 20 μM) for 12 and 24 h, and then they were trypsinized, washed in PBS, and fixed in 75% ethanol/PBS. The DNA was labeled with propidium iodide. Cells were detected by flow cytometry analysis, and cell-cycle profiles were determined using ModFit LT software (*Becton Dickinson, San Diego, CA*).

2.8 Hoechst staining

H460 cells treated with A114 and A117 (0, 5, and 10 μM) for 72 h were stained with Hoechst 33342 dye (*Beyotime Biotech, Nantong, China*). The cells were imaged with the dye using a fluorescent microscope (*Nikon, Tokyo, Japan*) with 20× amplification.

2.9 In vivo anti-tumor study

All animal experiments complied with the Wenzhou Medical College's Policy on the Care and Use of Laboratory Animals. Five-week-old to six-week-old athymic nu/ nu female BALB/cA mice (18–22 g) were purchased from the Animal Center of the China Pharmaceutical University (Nanjing, China). The animals were housed at a constant room temperature with a 12 : 12-h (light:dark) cycle and fed a standard rodent diet and water. H460 cells were harvested and mixed with Matri Gel at proportions of 1 : 1. Then, the cells were injected subcutaneously into the right flank (2×10^6 cells in 200 μl of PBS) of 7-week-old female BALB/cA nude mice. Two days after the H460 cells were injected, the mice were injected intraperitoneally (i.p.) with a water-soluble preparation of either compound A114 or A117 in PBS at dosage of 10 mg/kg/day for 28 days, whereas the control mice were injected with the liposome vehicle in PBS ($n = 10$ in each group). The volumes of the tumors were determined by measuring their length (*l*) and width (*w*) and calculating their volume as $V = 0.52 \times l \times w^2$. The weights of the tumors were recorded on the day the mice were killed.

2.10 Tissue immunoblot and immunohistochemistry

On day 30 after tumor induction, the mice were killed in a CO_2 chamber, and the tumor tissues were dissected. Some of the tissues were lysed for protein isolation and then processed for the determination of signaling pathway phosphorylation using the western blot method. Other harvested tumor tissues were fixed in 10% formalin at room temperature overnight, processed, and embedded in paraffin. The paraffin-embedded tissues were sectioned (5-μm thick). Tissue sections were stained primarily with antibodies. The signal was detected by biotinylated secondary antibody and developed with 3,3-diaminobenzidine (DAB). Quantitative assays of the immunochemistry data were obtained with Image-Pro Plus 6.0 (*Media Cybernetics, Inc., Bethesda, MD*).

2.11 Statistical analysis

All *in vitro* experiments were performed in triplicate ($n = 3$). The data were expressed as means ± SEM. All statistical analyses were performed using GraphPad Prism 5.0 (*GraphPad, San Diego, CA*). The Student's *t*-test and two-way ANOVA were used to analyze the differences between the sets of data. A *P* value of <0.05 was considered significant.

3. Results

3.1 A114 and A117 selectively inhibit FGFR1 kinase

The inhibitory potency of 156 bisaryl-1,4-dien-3-one compounds against FGFR1 kinase was evaluated by *in vitro* kinase assays. Out of the 156 compounds (Fig. 1A), A114 and A117 were found to have high affinities for FGFR1 (IC$_{50}$: 3.0 ± 1.0 μM for A114; 2.6 ± 0.4 μM for A117). To test the specificity of A114 and A117, we further evaluated their inhibition against other RTKs, including PDGFR-β, FGFR3, FGFR2, EGFR, and c-MET. As shown in Fig. 1B, A114

A

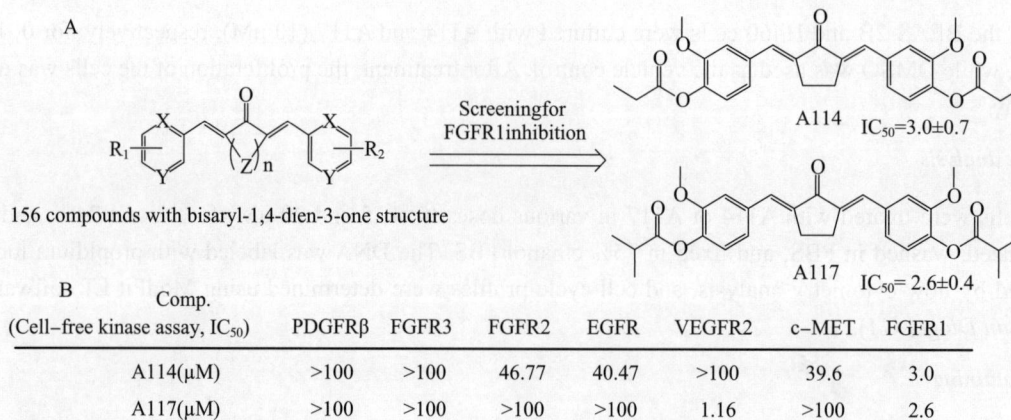

Screening for
FGFR1 inhibition

156 compounds with bisaryl-1,4-dien-3-one structure

A114 IC$_{50}$=3.0±0.7

A117 IC$_{50}$= 2.6±0.4

B

Comp. (Cell–free kinase assay, IC$_{50}$)	PDGFRβ	FGFR3	FGFR2	EGFR	VEGFR2	c–MET	FGFR1
A114(µM)	>100	>100	46.77	40.47	>100	39.6	3.0
A117(µM)	>100	>100	>100	>100	1.16	>100	2.6

Fig. 1. FGFR1 kinase inhibition assay of 156 synthetic bisaryl-1,4-dien-3-one-containing compounds. (A) Structural skeleton of 156 tested compounds and structures of A114 and A117; (B) A114 and A117 selectively inhibit FGFR1. Compounds were performed with Caliper Mobility Shift Assay for RTK inhibition. Conversion data were copied from the Caliper program. Inhibition rate,% = (max-conversion)/(max–min)*100. "Max" stands for DMSO control; "min" stands for low control. The data were fitted with GraphPad to obtain the IC$_{50}$ values. The data shown represent the means of 3–5 independent tests.

exhibited a modest inhibition of FGFR2 (IC$_{50}$: 46.77 µM), EGFR (IC$_{50}$: 40.47 µM), and c-MET (IC$_{50}$: 39.6 µM), while A117 only inhibited FGFR1. These data suggested that A114 and A117 exhibit potent and selective inhibition against FGFR1.

3.2 A114 and A117 inhibit FGFR1 through a mechanism that is ATP independent

To test the inhibitory kinetics and mode of the compounds, we evaluated the effect of the concentration of ATP on the apparent potency of the inhibition of the activation of FGFR1 by A114 and A117. In the absence of inhibitors, the velocity of the phosphorylation of the FGFR1 substrate increased as the concentration of ATP increased, and it became constant when the concentration of ATP reached 1 048 µM (Fig. 2A–C). At compound concentrations of about three times the IC$_{50}$ values (16.4 µM for A114; 6.9 µM for A117), more than 90% of the kinase activity was abolished, and further increases in ATP concentration, even up to 4.19 mM, had no effect on the inhibitory potency of the compounds (Fig. 2A, B). PD173074, a previously-characterized, ATP-competitive, FGFR1 inhibitor, was used as a comparison. As shown in Fig. 2C, the velocity was affected markedly in the PD173074-treated group by increases in the concentration of ATP. When the potency of the inhibition of kinase activity (IC50) of each compound was plotted as a function of the concentration of ATP, the inhibition was shown to be independent of the concentration of ATP (Fig. 2D, E). In contrast, it was observed that the IC$_{50}$ values of PD173074 were affected significantly by the concentration of ATP (Fig. 2F). These results showed that the inhibition of FGFR1 kinase activity by A114 and A117 was not dependent on the concentration of ATP even at physiological concentrations of ATP.

3.3 A114 and A117 are predicted to recognize the inactive conformation of FGFR1

The observation that A114 and A117 inhibited FGFR1 potently, selectively, and without competition from ATP, prompted us to conduct further investigation of the modes by which these two compounds bind to their target. Using a molecular docking method and a previously-described molecular model of FGFR1 with ARQ069, which is an inhibitor that does not compete with ATP (FGFR1-ARQ069 complex structure, PDB Code: 3RHX [15]), we docked A114 and A117 with the inactive conformation of FGFR1 kinase. The bisphenylenyl cyclopentanone core of A114/A117 is sandwiched in a hydrophobic cleft. As shown in Fig. 2G, one propionyl group of A114 makes two hydrogen-bond interactions with the hinge region, while the other propionyl group forms one hydrogen bond with Ala640. In Fig. 2H, the carbonyl oxygen in the propionyl group of A117 forms a hydrogen bond with R646. Importantly, the comparison of the modeling of FGFR1-A114/ A117 with previously-solved FGFR1-ARQ069 showed a similar mode for A114/A117 and ARQ069 binding to the inactive and auto-inhibitory conformation of FGFR1. Fig. 2G and H shows that the phenylalanine (Phe489) of the glycine-rich loop made a downward movement and established van der Waals interactions with the phenyl ring and/or cyclopentanone ring of A114/A117. The interaction between A114/A117 and the phenyl ring of the

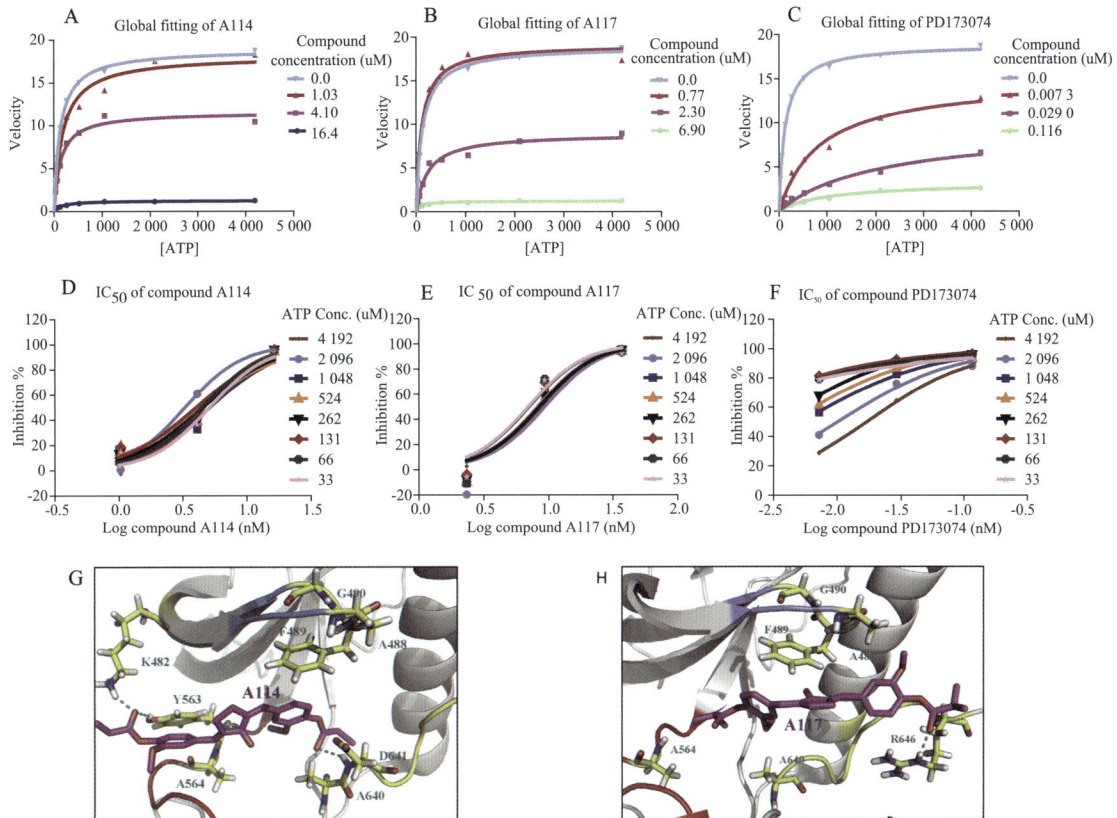

Fig. 2. A114 and A117 inhibit FGFR1 through a mechanism that is independent of the concentration of ATP. Selective ATP-competitive kinase assay of compounds A114 (A), A117 (B), and PD173074 (C) with FGFR1 through Caliper Mobility Shift Assay. The conversion data were fitted with Graphpad for global fitting, using "mixed model inhibition". (D–F) The data were fitted with GraphPad to obtain the IC_{50} values. Molecular docking simulation of A114 (G) or A117 (H) with FGFR1 protein was conducted with Tripos' molecular modeling package, Sybyl-x.v1.1.083.

glycine-rich loop serves as an anchor to stabilize the conformation of the glycine-rich loop and contributes to the preference of A114/A117 for the inactive form of FGFR1.

3.4 A117 shows a slow-binding and irreversible inhibition on FGFR1

To clarify the binding profile, the K_{on} value of representative A117 on FGFR1 kinase with the ATP concentration at the km value was detected *in vitro* by Caliper Mobility Shift Assay. As shown in Fig. 3A, the conversion of the substrate was increased significantly when the reaction time was prolonged in the fast phase K_{obs} of A117, whereas the increase tended to be steady in the slow phase K_{obs}. This suggested that A117 is slow to bind to FGFR1. The binding measurements provided a K_{on} of 0.0000111 mol/s and confirmed the slow interaction of A117 with FGFR1 (Fig. 3B). To further verify the intrinsic property of A117, we determined the reversibility of its binding with FGFR1 using a dilution method [15]. In this approach, an amount of kinase that was 75 times the normal amount was used in a pre-incubation reaction for 30 min (A117 with pre-incubation group) or 0 min (A117 without the pre-incubation group) with a concentration of A117 that was 10 times greater than the IC_{50} value. After incubation, the reaction buffer plus ATP and substrate were added to the enzyme/inhibitor mixture, and receptor kinase activity was measured continuously. In general, a reversible inhibitor dissociates quickly, allowing immediate recovery of enzymatic activity, whereas a slowly-reversible inhibitor allows a gradual increase in activity. In contrast, an irreversible inhibitor prevents recovery of enzymatic activity. As shown in Fig. 3C, about half of the FGFR1 activity was inhibited after incubation with A117, demonstrating that A117 is an irreversible inhibitor of FGFR1. In addition, the group of A117 without pre-incubation did not show significant inhibition of FGFR1 activity, also suggesting a slow binding of A117 to FGFR1.

3.5 A114 and A117 inhibit the phosphorylation of FGFR1 and downstream signaling molecules

Activation of FGFR1 and its downstream signaling molecules has been verified to correlate with tumor growth and

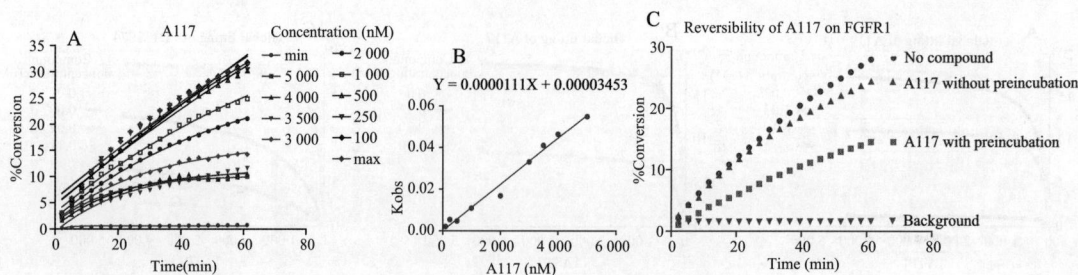

Fig. 3. A117 shows a slow-binding and irreversible inhibition on FGFR1. (A) The substrate conversion of A117 on kinase FGFR1 with ATP concentration at km was measured by Caliper Mobility Shift Assay *in vitro* with the prolongation of reaction time. (B) After the conversion data were copied from the Caliper program, the conversion and concentrations of the compound were fitted in GraphPad to get association rate constant (K_{on}) and initial rate constant (K_{obs}). (C) A rapid dilution experiment was used to demonstrate the reversible binding of A117 to FGFR1. FGFR1 kinase (75×) was incubated with and without A117 (10 × IC_{50}, 20 μM) at room temperature for 30 min. Then, the enzyme mix and the substrate mix were transferred to the 384-well assay plate, and Caliper EZ Reader was used to assay the enzyme activity of this mixture.

angiogenesis in a number of different cancers [8]. The effects of compounds A114 and A117 on the activation of FGFR1 and its downstream signaling pathways were determined in human lung cancer H460 cells (Fig. 4A) and FGFR1-over-experssing 293 cells (Fig. 4B) by the western blot analysis. The results showed that the bFGF in-duced phosphorylation of FGFR1 was reduced significantly in a concentration-dependent manner after pretreatment of compounds A114 and A117 for 2 h in both cell lines. Phosphorylation of FGFR1 triggered downstream proliferative signaling, including AKT and ERK [8]. Then, we tested the effects of these compounds on the activation of ERK1/2 and AKT in H460 cells. As shown in Fig. 4A, A114 and A117 caused a marked, concentration-dependent decrease in bFGF-induced phosphorylation of both ERK1/2 and AKT in cancer cells, and the band almost disappeared when the concentrations of the compounds reached 10 μM.

3.6 A114 and A117 inhibit lung cancer cell proliferation and induce cell cycle arrest and apoptosis

Next, we determined the effects of A114 and A117 on the proliferation of H460 cells. Human lung (bronchial) epithelial cell line, BEAS-2B, which showed relatively low FGFR1 expression (Fig. 4C), was used to determine whether the compounds had effects on normal lung cells, Our data found that A114 and A117 at concentrations of 7.57 μM and 6.45 μM, respectively, exhibited their IC_{50} against H460, while they had much higher IC_{50} values toward BEAS-2B cells (Fig. 4D). In time-based experiments, they suppressed the proliferation of the cancer cell line significantly at 10 μM within a 72 h period (Fig. 4E).

To determine whether the growth inhibition of H460 cells by the compounds was accompanied with arresting the cell cycle or apoptosis, the H460 cells were treated with A114 or A117 at the indicated concentrations for 12–72 h. Then, the cells were fixed or harvested, and the cell cycle populations were determined by flow cytometry, and cell apoptosis was analyzed by Hoechst staining and the western blot method. The results showed that A114 induced G0/G1 arrest in a concentration-dependent manner at 12 h, and a similar result was found in the A117-treated group at 24 h (Fig. 4F), which suggested that the inhibition of cell proliferation by A114 and A117 was associated with the induction of the arrest of the G0/G1 phase. In addition, the analysis demonstrated that cleavage of caspase-3 became more intense with increased concentrations of A114 and A117, indicating that these two compounds could induce H460 cell apoptosis after a 48-h treatment (Fig. 4G). Further, Hoechst staining were performed 72 h after the treatment with the compounds, and it indicated that there was a concentration-dependent increase in the number of cells with nuclear condensation and fragmentation (strong blue fluorescence) (Fig. 4H–L). These results showed that the inhibition of H460 cell growth that was induced by FGFR1 inhibitors A114 and A117 was associated with the arrest of the cell cycle arrest and cell apoptosis.

3.7 A114 and A117 potently inhibit H460 tumor growth in xenograft models

To assess their potential clinical utility, we evaluated the *in vivo* efficacies of A114 and A117 in H460 cell tumor xenograft models using BALB/cA nude mice. As shown in Fig. 5A, treatment with A114 or A117 for 28 days resulted in significant reduction in the volume of the tumors. The weights of the tumors weight also were reduced significantly in the groups treated with A114 and A117 with inhibitions of 54.0% and 55.3%, respectively (Fig. 5B). In addition, the

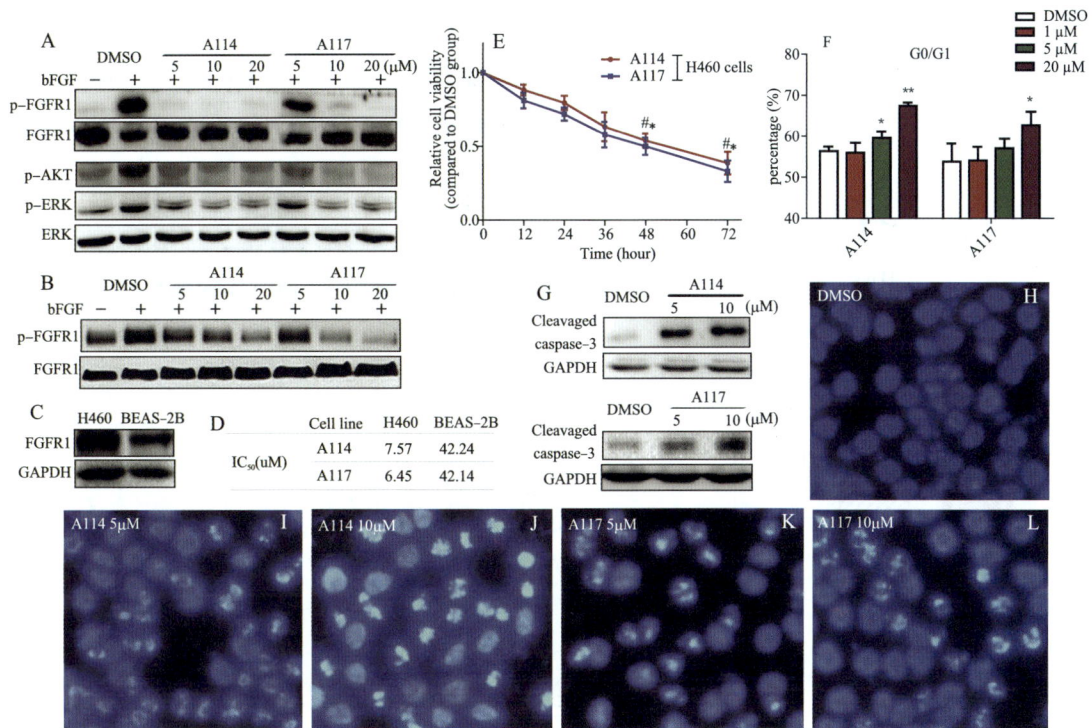

Fig. 4. Compounds A114 and A117 inhibited cell cycle and apoptosis in H460 cells by inhibiting the phosphorylation of FGFR1, AKT, and ERK: (A, B) compounds A114 and A117 inhibited bFGF-stimulated phosphorylations of FGFR1, AKT, and ERK by a concentration-dependent manner. H460 cells (A) or FGFR1 over-expressing 293 cells (B) were pretreated with compound A114 (5, 10, and 20 μM), A117 (5, 10, and 20 μM) or DMSO, respectively. Then, the cells were stimulated with bFGF (20 ng/ml) for 5 min, and the phosphorylation of FGFR1, AKT, and ERK was measured (C–E). Compounds A114 and A117 inhibited the proliferation of lung cancer cells. The H460 and BEAS-2B cells (5×10^3 cells/well; 96-well plates) were plated in RPMI-1640 medium with 10% FBS with A114 or A117 (10 μM) for 0, 12, 24, 36, 48, and 72 h. DMSO was used as the vehicle control. The expression of FGFR1 in H460 and BEAS-2B cells was confirmed by the western blot method (C). The proliferation of the H460 and BEAS-2B cells was detected through an MTT assay (D, E). (F) Compounds A114 and A117 induced cell cycle arrest at the G0/G1 phase in H460 cells. H460 cells were treated with A114 and A117 (0, 1, 5, and 20 μM) for 12 and 24 h. The distribution of the cycle of the cells was detected by flow cytometry. The figures were representative of three separate experiments. (G) Effect of A114 and A117 on the activation of caspase-3 in H460 cells. H460 cells were incubated with A114 and A117 (0, 5, and 10 μM, respectively) for 48 h. The caspase activation after administration was assayed by the western blot method. (H–L) Morphological changes and Hoechst staining were observed in H460 cells cultured with and without A114 or A117 (0, 5, and 10 μM) for 72 h (200×). The figures were representative of more than three separate experiments.

body weights of the mice decreased by less than 10% during the treatment (no significant difference, data not shown). To assess whether the inhibition of tumor growth by A114 and A117 was due to the inhibition of FGFR1 *in vivo*, we analyzed the tumor samples for the effects of the molecules on the levels of p-FGFR1, p-ERK, and p-AKT. A114 and A117 exhibited a marked inhibition of FGFR1 phosphorylation in H460 tumor xenografts compared to that in the ve-hicle-treated tumors (Fig. 5C). Similarly, these two molecules inhibited ERK and AKT phosphorylation (Fig. 5C). The inhibition of FGFR1 and downstream signaling phosphorylation by these two compounds was correlated with its attenu-ation of tumor growth (Fig. 5A, B).

Given the importance of cell cycle arrest and apoptosis in the *in vitro* inhibition of A114-and A117-induced growth (Fig. 4E–K), we detected the expression of three related markers, *i.e.*, Bcl-2 (for anti-apoptosis), Cyclin D1 (for cell cycle), and Cox-2 in tumor tissues using immunohistochemical analysis. As shown in Fig. 5D and E, the expression of these three proteins was decreased significantly in the A114-and A117-treated groups compared to the vehicle-treated group ($^*P < 0.01$ or $^{**}P < 0.05$), which was consistent with the *in vitro* findings in that it indicated that these two FGFR1 inhibitors may attenuate the growth of H460 xenografts *via* blocking the downstream induction cell cycle and apoptosis.

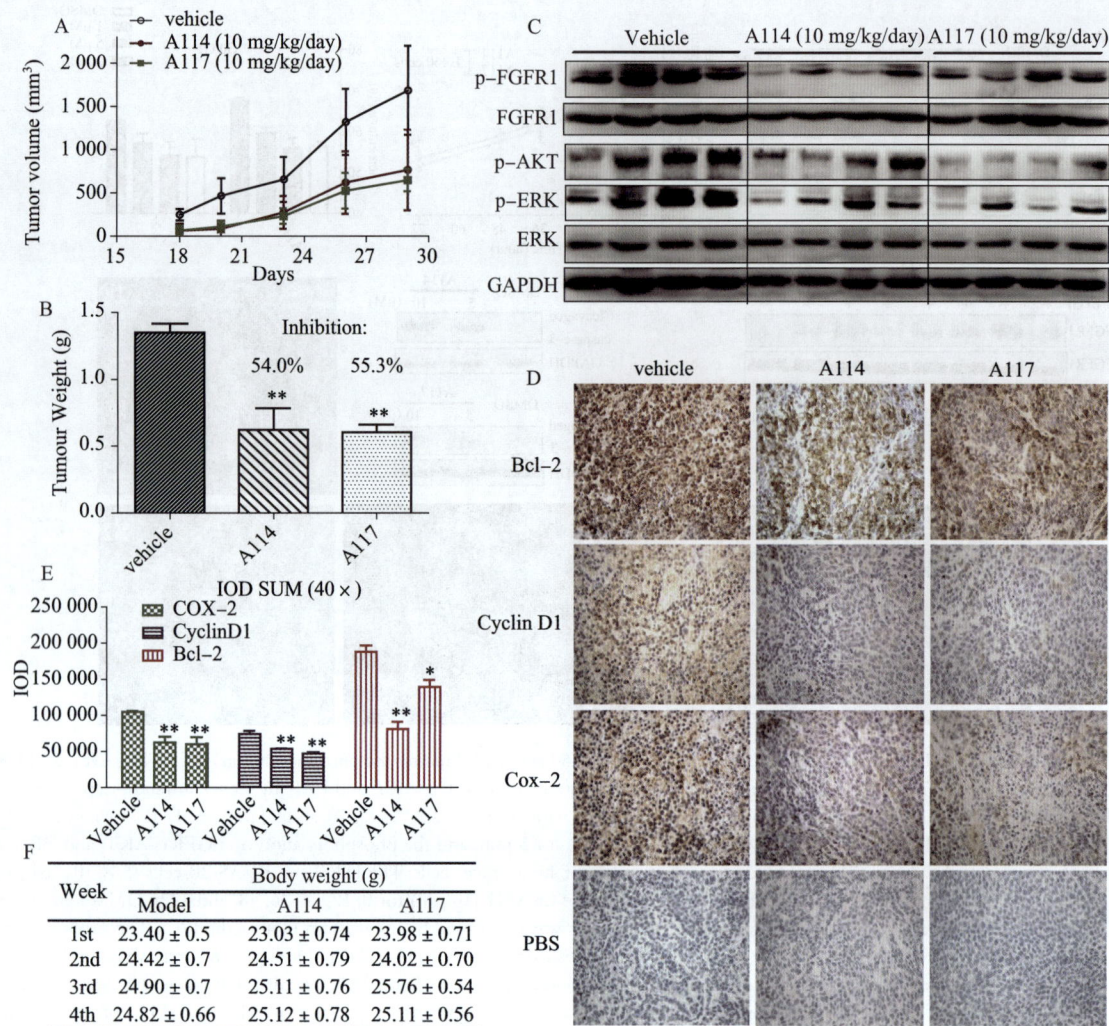

Fig. 5. Anti-tumor effects of compounds A114 and A117 on xenograft tumor growth: Xenografts were established in nude mice. Two days after the mice were injected with H460 cells, they were given a daily injection of compound A114 or A117 (10 mg/kg) or vehicle (saline) for 28 days. (A) Tumor volume (mm^3) and (B) Tumor weight (g) were recorded. Points, mean of 4–5 mice; bars, SD. $^{**}P < 0.01$. (C) pFGFR1, p-AKT, p-ERK expressions in tumor tissues, FGFR1, ERK and GADPH were detected as internal control; (D) Bcl-2, cyclin D1, Cox-2 in tumor tissues, representative pictures are shown; (E) Quantity assays of the immunochemistry data were obtained. Points, mean of 4–5 mice; bars, SD. $^{*}P < 0.05$, $^{**}P < 0.01$ and (F) body weight of each group was recorded.

4. Discussion

Studies of the development of FGFR-targeted, anti-cancer drugs still emphasize inhibitors that are competitive with ATP [3]. Although several such inhibitors, including NP603 [16], AZD4547 [17], BGJ398 [18], PD173074 [5], and acenaphtho[1,2-b]pyrrole derivatives [19] show partial selectivity for FGFRs, two major problems remain to be resolved. First, such inhibitors may lose their efficiency in clinical studies due to the high physiological or intracellular concentrations of ATP [3]. Second, adverse reactions and toxicity of low-selective, ATP-competitive inhibitors remain a challenge [3,20]. PD173074 and SU5402 failed to enter phase II clinical trials due to their high toxicity [3]. Other FGFR inhibitors that have entered clinical trials may generate nausea, weakness, elevated blood pressure, and other adverse reactions due to their concurrent inhibition of other RTKs. Thus, their clinical efficacy is limited [3,8]. Recently, in an attempt to increase the efficiency, specificity, and selectivity of FGFR inhibitors, researchers have investigated non-ATP-competitive inhibitors. By optimizing the binding between chemicals and the non-conserved, inactive, conformation regions, Eathiraj *et al.* found a small molecule, ARQ069, with FGFR1/2 kinase inhibition and an IC_{50} of 0.84 and 1.23 μM, respectively [15]. So far, ARQ069 is the only reported molecule that inhibits FGFR1/2 in a non-ATP-competitive manner, and its efficacy is not affected by high intracellular concentrations of ATP. In fact, crystal X-ray structural analysis showed that ARQ-069 also acts on the ATP-binding pocket, but it combines with an inactive ATP binding site ("DFG-OUT" conformation), thereby inducing a conformation shift that is quite different from that of the active, ATP-binding site ("DFG-IN" conformation) [15]. This conformational change causes the kinase to expose an additional hydrophobic pocket, known as the allosteric site, which has considerable sequence variation across different receptor kinases and contributes to the kinase selectivity of ARQ-069 [15]. In addition, Pavel *et al.* reported another class of new Suramin analogues, and the representative compound, NF449, also exhibited non-ATP-competitive inhibition of FGFR3 [21]. Nevertheless, its specific binding site remains unclear.

In this study, we identified two potent FGFR1 inhibitors with new structural skeletons *via* cell-free kinase-inhibitory screening (Fig. 1). The observation that A114 and A117 inhibited FGFR1 potently, selectively, and without competing with ATP (Figs. 1, 2) prompted us to further investigate the mode by which A114 and A117 bind to their targets. We performed the docking of A114 & A117 with the FGFR1 kinase domain. The results showed that A114/A117 may possess an FGFR1-binding mechanism that is similar to that of ARQ069. The hydrophobic residue, Phe489, whose phenyl ring makes a downward movement under the interactions with A114/A117 and then leads to the stabilization of the inactive conformation of FGFR1, is critical for the non-ATP-competitive interaction of A114/A117 (Fig. 2G, H). This structural difference could contribute to the selectivity of A114/ A117 for the inactive forms of FGFR1. A similar downward glycine-rich loop conformation has, however, been observed in several other kinase-inhibitor complexes, and it has been suggested that this conformation has a role in stabilizing the inactive state of kinases [22–25]. Although a number of small-molecule, FGFR inhibitors have been reported, this is the second time that the non-ATP-competitive inhibitors have been described through the "DFG-OUT" conformation, and A114 and A117, especially, represent a new kind of lead structure that is totally different from ARQ069.

Another important property of these inhibitors is the irreversibility of the FGFR1 inhibition (Fig. 3C). Small-molecule kinase inhibitors can bind to kinases in a reversible or an irreversible fashion. Reversible kinase inhibitors typically bind to the ATP site with the kinase in an active conformation or an inactive conformation. Irreversible inhibitors usually possess electrophilic functional groups, such as α,β-unsaturated carbonyls, that react with the nucleophilic sulfhydryl functional group of an active-site cysteine. By forming covalent bonding between a Michael acceptor and Cys486, Gray *et al.* designed and developed a class of small-molecule, irreversible inhibitors of FGFR1, which are represented by FIIN1 [26]. Interestingly, although A117 contains two α,β-unsaturated carbonyl groups, the molecular docking does not undergo the Michael reaction with a certain cysteine in the FGFR1 kinase domain. The mechanism for irreversible inhibition of A114/A117 is still unclear. In addition, the inhibition of FGFR2 by ARQ069 follows a slow dissociation mechanism [15], which could contribute to the observed non-competitive kinetics. Despite the fact that the computer-assistant analysis contributed to the prediction of the binding mode between A117 and FGFR1 kinase, the exact mechanism should be demonstrated by X-ray crystallographic studies in the future.

Non-small cell lung cancer H460 cells in people are characterized by amplification of the *FGFR1* gene [27]. Since A114 and A117 have been well demonstrated to inhibit FGFR1 kinase activity, we examined the inhibitory effects of A114 and A117 on the growth of H460 cells (Fig. 4). The compounds showed considerable inhibitory activity against phosphorylation of FGFR1 in bFGF-stimulated H460 cells and FGFR1-overexpressing 293 cells (Fig. 4A, B). In addition, these two compounds inhibited the concentration-dependent phosphorylation of the two major signaling pathways downstream of FGFR1, including ERK and/or AKT (Fig. 4A, B). And A114 and A117 showed less influence on the proliferation of BEAS-2B cells without FGFR1 amplification (Fig. 4D). In the *in vivo* study, p-ERK and p-AKT expression also were decreased in A114-treated and A117-treated tumors, compared with the control tumors (Fig. 5C). These findings suggest that A114 and A117 may exert a significant effect against H460 cells by affecting the FGFR1-ERK/ AKT pathways. ERK and AKT are the main pathways responsible for the inhibition of apoptosis and the proliferation of cells. Treatment of H460 cells with A114 and A117 increased apoptosis in a concentration-dependent manner (Fig. 4G–L). Inhibition of the MAPK or PI3K pathways by A114 and A117 may be responsible for the apoptosis observed at 24–72 h after treatment because these pathways collaborate in regulating the cycle of the cells and controlling their survival. The use of A114 and A117 to modulate these critical, regulatory molecules also results in arresting the cycle of the cells in a relatively early state (Fig. 4F). The inhibition of the FGFR1 signaling pathway in cancer cells provide the possibility of extending therapeutic options for bisaryl-1,4-dien-3-ones in cancer treatment. Indeed, in addition to the cellular effects, we have shown that A114 and A117 are highly effective in inhibiting tumor growth in a H460 xenograft mouse model, accompanied with a decrease in FGFR1 phosphorylation and an increase in the downstream markers for arresting the cycle of the and apoptosis in treated tumor tissues (Fig. 5). At the same time, we obtained evidence that A114 and A117 were very safe to use (data not shown).

Given the critical importance of FGFR1 in maintaining the neoplastic properties of a variety of cancers and the need for improved, more-effective medical treatments of cancer [1,2], the results of the present study indicate that A114 and A117 deserve further study in the interest of developing structurally-different, more-effective bisaryl-1,4-dien-3-one-containing kinase inhibitors, especially in the context of human tumors that over express FGFR1 and/ or harbor secondary mutations in their FGFR1. To the best of our knowledge, this is the first time that bisaryl-1,4-dien-3-ones have been reported to be non-ATP-competitive, FGFR1 inhibitors. The "DFG-OUT," inactive, conformation-binding mode of the bisaryl-1,4-dien-3-one scaffold and its irreversible binding contribute to a high FGFR1-inhibitory selectivity of these compounds. Further X-ray crystallographic studies are underway and will demonstrate the detailed binding mechanism of A117 with FGFR1 kinase, which may provide an exact binding mechanism and structural lead for the design of drugs that feature non-ATP-competitive, irreversible FGFR1 inhibitors.

Supplementary material

Supplementary data associated with this article can be found, in the online version, at http://dx.doi.org/10.1016/j.canlet.2013.10.016.

References

[1] Turner N, Grose R. Fibroblast growth factor signalling: from development to cancer[J]. Nature Reviews Cancer, 2010, 10(2): 116-129.

[2] Wesche J, Haglund K, Haugsten EM. Fibroblast growth factors and their receptors in cancer[J]. Biochemical Journal, 2011, 437: 199-213.

[3] Kumar SBVS, Narasu L, Gundla R, et al. Fibroblast Growth Factor Receptor Inhibitors[J]. Current Pharmaceutical Design, 2013, 19(4): 687-701.

[4] Hadden MK, Lemieux S. Targeting the Fibroblast Growth Factor Receptors for the Treatment of Cancer[J]. Anti-Cancer Agents in Medicinal Chemistry 2013, 13(5): 748-761.

[5] Norman RA, Schott A-K, Andrews DM, et al. Protein-Ligand Crystal Structures Can Guide the Design of Selective Inhibitors of the FGFR Tyrosine Kinase[J]. Journal of Medicinal Chemistry, 2012, 55(11): 5003-5012.

[6] Gavine PR, Mooney L, Kilgour E, et al. AZD4547: An Orally Bioavailable, Potent, and Selective Inhibitor of the Fibroblast Growth Factor Receptor Tyrosine Kinase Family[J]. Cancer Research, 2012, 72(8): 2045-2056.

[7] Guagnano V, Furet P, Spanka C, et al. Discovery of 3-(2,6-Dichloro-3,5-dimethoxy-phenyl)-1-{6- 4-(4-ethyl-piperazin-1-yl)-p henyl-amino -pyrimidin-4-yl}-1-methyl-urea (NVP-BGJ398), A Potent and Selective Inhibitor of the Fibroblast Growth Factor Receptor Family of Receptor Tyrosine Kinase[J]. Journal of Medicinal Chemistry, 2011, 54(20): 7066-7083.

[8] Liang G, Liu Z, Wu J, et al. Anticancer molecules targeting fibroblast growth factor receptors[J]. Trends in Pharmacological Sciences, 2012, 33(10): 531-541.

[9] Fabbro D, Cowan-Jacob SW, Moebitz H, et al. Targeting Cancer with Small-Molecular-Weight Kinase Inhibitors[A]. In: Kinase Inhibitors: Methods and Protocols (Kuster B, ed), Vol. 795, 2012: 1-34.

[10] Zhao C, Cai Y, He X, et al. Synthesis and anti-inflammatory evaluation of novel mono-carbonyl analogues of curcumin in LPS-stimulated RAW 264.7 macrophages[J]. European Journal of Medicinal Chemistry, 2010, 45(12): 5773-5780.

[11] Liang G, Zhou H, Wang Y, et al. Inhibition of LPS-induced production of inflammatory factors in the macrophages by mono-carbonyl analogues of curcumin[J]. Journal of Cellular and Molecular Medicine, 2009, 13(9B): 3370-3379.

[12] Liang G, Li X, Chen L, et al. Synthesis and anti-inflammatory activities of mono-carbonyl analogues of curcumin[J]. Bioorganic & Medicinal Chemistry Letters, 2008, 18(4): 1525-1529.

[13] Wang Y, Xiao J, Zhou H, et al. A Novel Monocarbonyl Analogue of Curcumin, (1E,4E)-1,5-Bis(2,3-dimethoxyphenyl)penta-1,4-dien-3-one, Induced Cancer Cell H460 Apoptosis via Activation of Endoplasmic Reticulum Stress Signaling Pathway[J]. Journal of Medicinal Chemistry, 2011, 54(11): 3768-3778.

[14] Wood ER, Truesdale AT, McDonald OB, et al. A unique structure for epidermal growth factor receptor bound to GW572016 (Lapatinib): Relationships among protein conformation, inhibitor off-rate, and receptor activity in tumor cells[J]. Cancer Research, 2004, 64(18): 6652-6659.

[15] Eathiraj S, Palma R, Hirschi M, et al. A novel mode of protein kinase inhibitionexploiting hydrophobic motifs of autoinhibited kinases: discovery of ATP-independent inhibitors of fibroblast growth factor receptor [J]. Journal of Biological Chemistry, 2011, 286(23): 20677-20687.

[16] Kammasuda N, Boonyarat C, Tsunoda S, et al. Novel inhibitor for fibroblast growth factor receptor tyrosine kinase[J]. Bioorganic & Medicinal Chemistry Letters, 2007, 17(17): 4812-4818.

[17] Zhang J, Zhang L, Su X, et al. Translating the Therapeutic Potential of AZD4547 in FGFR1-Amplified Non-Small Cell Lung Cancer through the Use of Patient-Derived Tumor Xenograft Models[J]. Clinical Cancer Research, 2012, 18(24): 6658-6667.

[18] Guagnano V, Kauffmann A, Woehrle S, et al. FGFR Genetic Alterations Predict for Sensitivity to NVP-BGJ398, a Selective Pan-FGFR Inhibitor[J]. Cancer Discovery, 2012, 2(12): 1118-1133.

[19] Chen Z, Wang X, Zhu W, et al. Acenaphtho 1,2-b pyrrole-Based Selective Fibroblast Growth Factor Receptors 1 (FGFR1) Inhibitors: Design, Synthesis, and Biological Activity[J]. Journal of Me-

dicinal Chemistry, 2011, 54(11): 3732-3745.

[20] Carmi C, Mor M, Petronini PG, *et al.* Clinical perspectives for irreversible tyrosine kinase inhibitors in cancer[J]. Biochemical Pharmacology, 2012, 84(11): 1388-1399.

[21] Krejci P, Murakami S, Prochazkova J, *et al.* NF449 Is a Novel Inhibitor of Fibroblast Growth Factor Receptor 3 (FGFR3) Signaling Active in Chondrocytes and Multiple Myeloma Cells[J]. Journal of Biological Chemistry, 2010, 285(27): 20644-20653.

[22] Nolen B, Taylor S, Ghosh G. Regulation of protein kinases: Controlling activity through activation segment conformation[J]. Molecular Cell, 2004, 15(5): 661-675.

[23] Johnson LN. Protein kinase inhibitors: contributions from structure to clinical compounds[J]. Quarterly Reviews of Biophysics, 2009, 42(1): 1-40.

[24] Gajiwala KS, Wu JC, Christensen J, *et al.* KIT kinase mutants show unique mechanisms of drug resistance to imatinib and sunitinib in gastrointestinal stromal tumor patients[J]. Proceedings of the National Academy of Sciences of the United States of America, 2009, 106(5): 1542-1547.

[25] Taylor SS, Yang J, Wu J, *et al.* PKA: a portrait of protein kinase dynamics[J]. Biochimica Et Biophysica Acta-Proteins and Proteomics, 2004, 1697(1-2): 259-269.

[26] Zhou W, Hur W, McDermott U, *et al.* A Structure-Guided Approach to Creating Covalent FGFR Inhibitors[J]. Chemistry & Biology, 2010, 17(3): 285-295.

[27] Drilon A, Rekhtman N, Ladanyi M, *et al.* Squamous-cell carcinomas of the lung: emerging biology, controversies, and the promise of targeted therapy[J]. Lancet Oncology, 2012, 13(10): E418-E426.

FGFR4 and TGF-β1 expression in hepatocellular carcinoma: correlation with clinicopathological features and prognosis

Zhixin Chen, Xiaokun Li, Lin Cai

1. Introduction

Hepatocellular carcinoma (HCC), which is the sixth most common cancer in terms of its incidence rate and the third most common cause of cancer-related deaths globally, is responsible for about 600 000 deaths annually [1]. The five-year survival rate of this cancer is merely 7%. Curative therapies of surgical treatment, including hepatic resection and liver transplantation, improve the chances of survival of patients with HCC [2-4]. However, a limited number of patients can be treated with surgery because of the damage to liver function. The prognosis for most patients remains poor after surgery for multicentric recurrence and extrahepatic metastasis [5-6]. This disappointing outcome clearly indicates that the current knowledge regarding diagnosis, prevention, and treatment of liver cancer is insufficient, which strongly suggests a pressing need for further innovative research to control this devastating disease.

Transforming growth factor-β1 (TGF-β1) has been described as a prototypical multifunctional cytokine, participating in the regulation of vital cellular processes such as cell proliferation, differentiation and angiogenesis as well as a number of basic physiological functions including tissue development, immunosuppression and extracellular matrix formation. Recently, another essential function of TGF-β1 that has come to light is its role as a tumor suppressor in various types of cells. Research has demonstrated that TGF-β1 plays a dual role in mouse skin carcinogenesis as well as in other human and murine cancer models [7-11]. However, TGF-β1 has also been shown to facilitate the epithelial-to-mesenchymal transition of hepatocytes that in turn participates in the progression of liver fibrosis [12]. The effect of TGF-β1 in different tumors and tumor cell strains is complex due to the specific environment of the cell and the underlying mechanisms are unclear.

Members of the FGF receptor (FGFR) family of receptor tyrosine kinases are of tremendous significance in a variety of human cancers. FGFR4 is over-expressed in malignant melanoma [13], breast cancer [14], renal cell carcinoma [15] and hepatocellular carcinoma (HCC) [16]. Although its role in oncogenesis remains to be fully elucidated, several findings provide evidence for a modulatory role of FGFR4 in HCC development and progression. FGFR4 is the predominant FGFR isoform present in human hepatocytes [17]. High FGFR4 transcript levels have also been previously reported in liver tissue [18]. Together, these findings suggest that FGFR4 may be a novel therapeutic target in the diagnosis and treatment of this disease.

Both TGF-β1 and FGFR4 could promote the invasiveness and metastasis of tumor only under the specific cell surroundings. Whether or not these two molecules exist some relationship, there have no report about it. In the present study, we first hypothesized the role of combined expression of two kinds of oncoproteins, TGF-β1 and FGFR4, in the genesis and development of liver cancer. This study was designed to determine the expression levels of TGF-β1 and FGFR4 in HCCs and adjacent normal tissues by immunohistochemistry in order to assess their relationship. We further investigated the relationship be-tween TGF-β1 and FGFR4 expression and the presence of clinicopathological pathological features. At the same time we sought to predict the prognosis of HCC from the results.

2. Materials and methods

2.1 Patients and specimens

Cancerous tissues and surrounding noncancerous hepatic parenchyma were obtained from 126 primary HCC patients who underwent curative resection surgery at the Second Affiliated Hospital of Wenzhou Medical College Yuying Children's Hospital, from January 2002 to December 2007. Approval for all studies was obtained from the Second Affiliated Hospital of Wenzhou Medical College, Yuying Children's Hospital Ethics Committee. Informed consent was obtained from all patients prior to sample collection. For inclusion, patients required suitable formalin-fixed, paraffin-embedded tissue specimens and complete clinicopathologic and follow-up data. Samples were obtained from 92 men and 34 women aged 29–80 years. Tumors were staged according to the tumor, lymph node, and metastasis (TNM) classi-fication system of the 2002 International Union against Cancer. The histologic grade of tumor differentiation was assigned using the Edmondson grading system. Tumor size was based on the largest dimension of the tumor specimen. Vascular invasion was determined by microscopic examination of the re-sected specimen. In the corresponding noncancerous parenchyma, cirrhosis was found in 50 patients (40%). Detailed clinicopathologic features of the HCC cases are shown in Table 1.

Table 1.　Correlations between of TGF-β1 and FGFR4 expression and clinicopathologic features

Clinicopathological parameters	n	Expression of TGF-β1				Expression of FGFR4			
		positive (n=106)	negative (n=20)	χ^2	P	positive (n=94)	negative (n=32)	χ^2	P
Age (55.83±12.97)									
< 56 years	58	46	12	1.867	0.172	40	18	1.803	0.179
≥ 56 years	68	60	8			54	14		
Gender									
Male	92	81	11	3.916	0.048	72	20	2.407	0.121
Female	34	25	9			22	12		
Tumor size									
< 5 cm	75	61	14	1.083	0.298	52	23	2.716	0.099
≥ 5 cm	51	45	6			42	9		
AFP									
< 20 ng / ml	93	80	13	0.954	0.329	70	23	0.083	0.773
≥ 20 ng /ml	33	26	7			24	9		
Tumor Differentiation									
Well	41	32	9	2.196	0.334	30	11	2.674	0.263
Moderately	61	52	9			43	18		
Poorly	24	22	2			21	3		
lymph node metastasis									
Present	24	23	1	1.661	0.197	19	5	0.326	0.568
Absent	102	93	19			75	27		
Vascular invasion									
Present	35	33	2	3.745	0.053	28	7	0.745	0.388
Absent	91	73	18			66	25		
TNM stage									
I-II	78	59	19	10.954	0.001	53	25	4.747	0.029
III-IV	48	47	1			41	7		

2.2 Immunohistochemical staining

An immunohistochemical analysis was performed on paraffin-embedded sections using the Elivision plus system (Maixin Bio, Fuzhou, China) following the manufacturer's instructions. The sections were boiled in retrieval solution to expose the antigens. Rabbit anti-human TGF-β1 polyclonal antibody (Maixin Bio, Fuzhou, China), rabbit anti-human FGFR4 polyclonal antibody and mouse anti-human FGF19 monoclonal antibody (Santa Cruz Biotechnology, Santa Cruz, CA, USA) were applied as primary antibodies to the sections at a dilution of 1:50. The section slides were incubated with primary antibodies overnight at 4℃ and then washed to remove excess antibody with phosphate-buffered saline (PBS). The Elivision plus system was used to detect bound antibodies. Reaction products were visualized by incubation with 3, 3'-diaminobenzidine. Sections were dehydrated, counterstained with hematoxylin, and mounted. Negative controls were treated identically except that the primary antibody was replaced by PBS.

2.3 Immunohistochemical scoring

Immunohistochemical results for TGF-β1 and FGFR4 were evaluated by two investigators separately in all the specimens in a blinded manner. The positive signals of TGF-β1 and FGFR4 expression stained yellow or brown, mainly in the cytoplasm. Buffy staining of the cell membrane, cytoplasm or nuclei was positive for each of them. We randomly selected ten high-power fields (magnification, ×400; 100 cells/high-power field) and counted 1 000 cells in each core [20]. The percentage of positive tumor cells was determined by each observer, and the average of the two scores was calculated. In this study, the percentage of positive cells expressing TGF-β1 and FGFR4 were categorized as follows: < 10% (-) and ≥ 10% (+) for TGF-β1 [21], < 30% (-) and ≥ 30% (+) for FGFR4 [22].

2.4 Statistical analysis

The Pearson Chi-square test or Fisher's exact test was used to compare categorical variables; and correlation between TGF-β1 and FGFR4 was evaluated using the Spearman rank correlation coefficient test. Using the method described by Kaplan-Meier, overall survival curves were obtained from the date of operation to the last visit or death. A Cox proportional hazards regression model was used for multivariate analysis of survival. All statistical analyses were performed with SPSS 15.0 software (SPSS Inc, Chicago, IL, USA). P values of less than 0.05 were considered statistically significant.

3. Results

3.1 Clinicopathological data

Among the 126 patients studied, 92 (73%) were men and 34 (27%) were women, with a mean age of 55.8 years (range, 29 to 80 years). 41 (32.5%) of the studied tumors were classified as well differentiated HCC, 61 (48.4%) as moderately differentiated, and 24 (19.1%) as poorly differentiated. There were 24 cases (19%) of lymph node metastasis and 35 cases (27.8%) of vascular invasion. 78 cases (61.9%) had TNM stage I-II, and 48 cases (38.1%) had TNM stage III – IV. Based on the MRI examination, 75 cases were categorized as small tumor (tumor size < 5 cm) and 51 were large tumor (tumor size ≥ 5 cm). The follow-up period was defined as the interval from the date of operation to that of the last visit or the patient's death. Deaths from other causes were treated as censored cases.

3.2 Immunohistochemical analysis

TGF-β1 and FGFR4 were localized mainly in the cytoplasm of tumor cells or hepatocytes. Most of the stroma cells were negative for anti-TGF-β1 and anti-FGFR4 staining, although sporadic positive staining on these cells was also observed (Fig. 1C, F). TGF-β1 was also partly expressed in fibroblastic cells. Of the 126 samples, 106 (84.1%) samples showed high intratumoral and 81 (64.3%) samples high peritumoral TGF-β1 expression (Table 2). There was intratumoral FGFR4 expression in 94 (74.6%) samples and peritumoral expression in 72 (57.1%) samples (Table 3). Both Fig. 1 and Fig. 2 show the results of TGF-β1 and FGFR4 staining, respectively, of intratumoral and peritumoral tissue. The expression of TGF-β1 and FGFR4 in the carcinoma tissues was significantly higher than that in peritumoral liver tissues ($P < 0.05$).

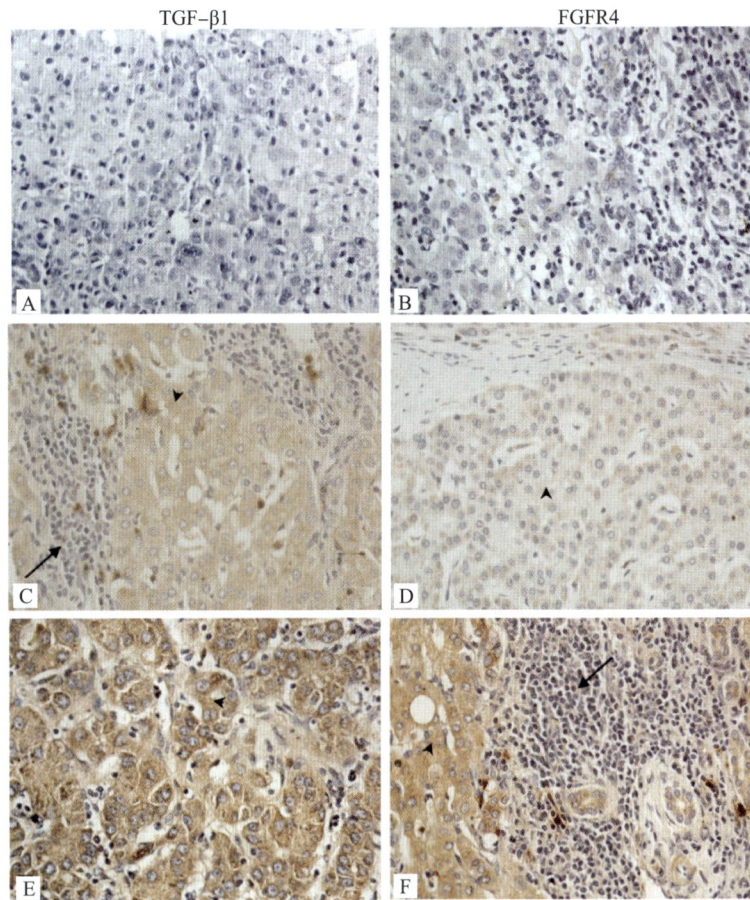

Fig. 1. Immunohistochemical staining of TGF-β1 and FGFR4 in liver cancer tissues. No staining was detected for (A) TGF-β1 and (B) FGFR4 in the blank control group. (C) Weak cytoplasmic staining of TGF-β1 in tumor cells and some stromal cells. (D) Weak FGFR4 staining in tumor cells. (E) High TGF-β1 staining in tumor cells. (F) High FGFR4 staining in tumor cells and weak staining in stromal cells. (Arrowhead indicated the tumor cells and arrow indicated the stromal cells). (All photos are shown at × 400 magnification).

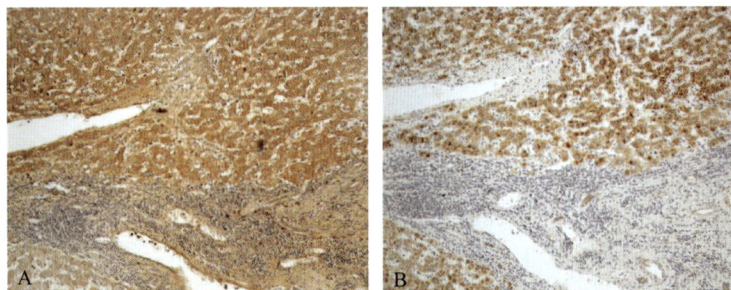

Fig. 2. Comparison of the immunostaining patterns between (A) TGF-β1 and (B) FGFR4 in liver cancer tissues (× 100).

Table 2.　Expression of TGF-β1 in cancer tissues and paracancer tissues

Group	n	Positive	Negative	Positive rate(%)	χ^2	P
Paracancer Tissues	126	81	45	64.29	12.958	0.000
Cancer Tissues	126	106	20	84.13		

Table 3. Expression of FGFR4 in cancer tissues and paracancer tissues

Group	n	Expression of FGFR4			χ^2	P
		Positive	Negative	Positive rate (%)		
Paracancer Tissues	126	72	54	57.14	8.544	0.003
Cancer Tissues	126	94	32	74.60		

3.3 Correlations between TGF-β1 and FGFR4 expression and clinicopathologic features

Univariate analysis suggested that staining with TGF-β1 bore no relation to age and sex ($P > 0.05$); while the expression of FGFR4 also showed no significantly higher levels in older patients than in younger patients ($P > 0.05$). We also found that TGF-β1 and FGFR4 had no significant correlation with other prognostic factors, such as tumor size, serum AFP level, tumor differentiation, lymph node metastasis and vascular invasion ($P > 0.05$). In contrast, an association was apparent between TGF-β1 and FGFR4 staining and disease stage (Table 1). Tumors of patients with high TGF-β1 and FGFR4 expression levels were more likely to be at a higher TNM stage ($P = 0.001$ and 0.029, respectively).

3.4 Correlations between TGF-β1 and FGFR4 expression and prognosis

The five year survival rate for TGF-β1 negative expression was 45.6%, median survival time was 50.4 months. The five year survival rate for TGF-β1 positive expression was 8.5%, median survival time was 32.3 months. Patients with positive TGF-β1 expression had shorter OS compared to those with negative TGF-β1 expression according to the Kaplan-Meier analyses ($P < 0.05$) (Fig. 3A).

The five year survival rate for FGFR4 negative expression was 70.1%, median survival time was 51.2 months. The five year survival rate for FGFR4 positive expression was 8.3%, median survival time was 29.4 months. Survival analyses using the Kaplan-Meier method showed that patients with positive FGFR4 expression had shorter overall survival (OS) compared to those with negative FGFR4 expression ($P < 0.05$) (Fig. 3B).

3.5 Multivariate analysis of clinicopathological paramaters and prognosis

The factors with possible prognostic effects in hepatocarcinoma were analyzed by Cox regression analysis. The study revealed that vascular invasion ($P = 0.003$), expression of TGF-β1 ($P = 0.002$) and FGFR4 ($P = 0.001$) were independent prognostic factors of patients with hepatocarcinoma (Table 4). However, age, sex, tumor size, serum AFP level, tumor differentiation, lymph node metastasis, and TNM stage had no prognostic value.

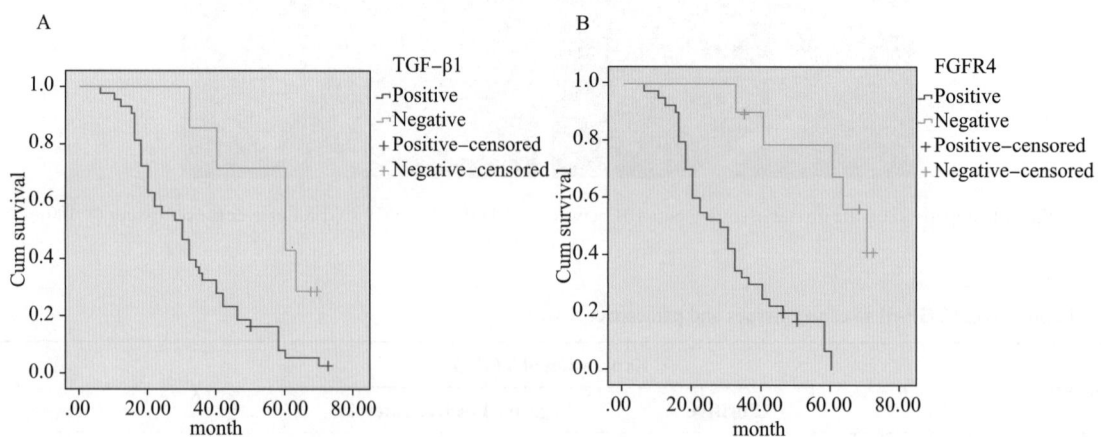

Fig. 3. Kaplan-Meier curves with univariate analyses (log-rank) for patients with (A) negative TGF-β1 expression *versus* positive TGF-β1 expression and (B) negative FGFR4 expression *versus* positive FGFR4 expression in hepatocarcinoma patients.

Table 4. Multivariate analysis of hepatocarcinoma patients prognosis

	B	SE	Wald	df	Sig	Exp (B)
Vasular invasion	2.014	0.320	8.217	1	0.003	8.115
TGF-β1	3.313	0.786	11.841	1	0.002	10.226
FGFR4	2.616	0.687	10.624	1	0.001	9.337

3.6 Association among expression of TGF-β1 and FGFR4

Ninety one hepatocarcinoma cases had positive expression of both TGF-β1 and FGFR4, and seventeen hepatocarcinoma cases had negative expression of both TGF-β1 and FGFR4. Correlation analysis of these potential biomarkers revealed that intratumoral FGFR4 correlated with high intratumoral TGF-β1 expression ($r = 0.595$, $P < 0.05$) (Table 5). We also detected the outcomes of TGF-β1-positive/ FGFR4-positive, TGF-β1-positive/FGFR4-negative, TGF-β1-negative/FGFR4-positive, and TGF-β1-negative/FGFR4-negative hepatocarcinoma patients, and we found that there was a significant difference in overall comparisons ($X^2 = 34.7$, $P = 0.000$, Fig. 4). The mean survival time were 30.2±1.76 months for TGF-β1-positive/FGFR4-positive group, 43.3±5.44 months for TGF-β1-positive/FGFR4-negative, 39.5±3.32 months for TGF-β1-negative/FGFR4-positive, 50.2±3.91 months for TGF-β1-negative/ FGFR4-negative, respectively.

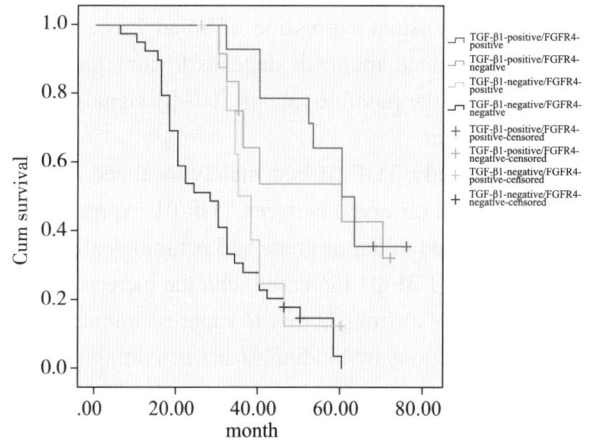

Fig. 4. Kaplan-Meier curves with univariate analyses (log-rank) for patients with TGF-β1-positive/FGFR4-positive, TGF-β1-positive/ FGFR4-negative, TGF-β1-negative/FGFR4-positive, and TGF-β1-negative/FGFR4-negative hepatocarcinoma patients.

Table 5. The relationship between TGF-β1 and FGFR4 expression in HCCs

	n	FGFR4 expression		r**	P*
		Positive (n=94)	Negative (n=32)		
TGF-β1 expression					
Positive	106	91	15	0.595	0.000
Negative	20	3	17		

* χ^2 test; ** Spearman rank correlation coefficient.

4. Discussion

HCC has the worst prognosis among all major cancers. This could be due to the fact that no effective methods of early diagnosis are currently available as well as the lack of effective therapies, resulting in high mortality of patients diagnosed with HCC. Recent molecular investigations have suggested that molecular targeting can be a powerful therapeutic device for treating human malignancies, including liver cancer. Molecular targeting medicines appear to hold great potential in treating liver cancer [19]. We show here that the expression of TGF-β1 and FGFR4 is elevated in liver cancer, as compared to normal tissues. These findings provide evidence for the modulatory roles of TGF-β1 and FGFR4 in HCC progression and suggest that TGF-β1 and FGFR4 may be important and novel therapeutic targets in treating HCC.

Transforming growth factor β (TGFβ) is a multifunctional cytokine that regulates the proliferation and differentiation of various types of cells. Three subtypes of TGF-β receptor, including TβR-1, TβR-2 and TβR-3, have been identified. TGF-β binds to TβRs (serine/threonine kinase receptors), which mediate the intracellular activation of signal transduction pathways through Smad proteins. Studies demonstrated that the TGF-β and its receptor are associated with tumors, and TGF-β1, as a prototypic member of the TGF-β superfamily of signaling molecules, is involved in the regulation of cell growth and differentiation, angiogenesis, immunosuppression, extracellular matrix formation, fibrogenesis, and tumorigene-sis [23-24]. The effect of TGF-β1 in tumors is complex, TGF-β1 is considered as a tumor suppressor gene in the initial stage of tumorigenesis, and growth inhibition by the TGF-β1 has been extensively studied in diverse cell types. TGF-β1 can selectively induce tumor cell-cycle arrest and apoptosis in hepatic cells [25-27]. However, TGF-β1 can enhance growth in the progression of late stage tumors and the possible mechanisms for these growth-enhancing effects includes induced immunosuppression, enhanced angiogenesis, and increased peritumoral stroma formation. Li *et al* reported that TGF-β1 affects both proliferation and apoptosis of GC cells through the regulation of p15 and p21, and induces the transient expression of Smad 7 as a negative feedback modulation of TGF-β1 signaling [28]. The ability of TGF-β1 to induce apoptosis depends to some extent upon the cellular concentration of various TGF-β1 receptors [29]. Nevertheless, the possible role of TGF-β1 signaling in the simultaneous modulation of HCC proliferation and apoptosis remains unclear.

In our study, TGF-β1 was mainly localized in the cytoplasm of HCC cells, staining yellow or brown. A significant difference was observed between TGF-β1 expressions levels in HCC and matched peritumoral tissues. TGF-β1 expression was related to tumor grade and pathological stage, but not to age, sex and tumor size. These results showed that the expression of TGF-β1 increased with the increase of tumor grade. Hence, TGF-β1 is not only a growth suppression factor but also has a strong ability to suppress immunity. Fibroblast growth factors (FGFs) orchestrate a variety of signaling molecule functions by binding to and activating their transmembrane tyrosine kinase receptors (FGFRs). FGFRs have a conserved structure comprising three extracellular immunoglobulin (Ig) domains, a single-pass transmembrane domain and a cytoplasmic tyrosine kinase domain [30]. The FGF/FGFR signaling system plays important roles in cell proliferation, migration, differentiation, morphogenesis, and angiogenesis. FGFR4 is one of the members of the FGFR family that is associated with tumor. Several lines of evidence support this hypothesis that FGFR4 may play an important role in hepatocellular carcinoma. FGFR4 is the predominant FGFR isoform present in human hepatocytes [17]. FGF19 as a high affinity, heparin-dependent ligand for FGFR4 shows exclusive binding to FGFR4. FGF19-induced hepatocyte proliferation has been reported to be uniquely mediated by FGFR4 [31]. It is suggested that FGF19/FGFR4 system plays a critical role in HCC progression [32]. Our findings also showed that the expression of FGFR4 correlate with the prognosis of hepatocarcinoma. We estimated that the detailed mechanism by which FGF19/FGFR4 contributes to the poor prognosis of patients with HCC maybe correlate with TGF-β1 signaling. Previous research reported that liver tissue has the highest FGFR4 and KLB transcript levels, and both of these proteins are essential for ligand-stimulated activity by this signaling system [18]. But the role of FGFR4 in oncogenesis is controversial. Some researchers have reported that FGFR4 contributes significantly to HCC progression by modulating α-fetoprotein (AFP) secretion, proliferation, and anti-apoptosis [16]. However in this study, the expression of FGFR4 in HCCs was not significantly correlated to serum AFP levels. Other lines of evidence suggest that the resident hepatocyte FGFR4 is a candidate for limiting hepatoma progres-sion rather than promoting it. The overexpression of FGFR4 is related to an increase in apoptosis and better prognosis [33]. It is possible that contextual factors including the identity and concentration of ligand, as well as the levels of FGFRs and co-receptor expression, might modulate the role of FGFR4 in tumorigenesis.

In particular, our study provides correlations between FGFR4 and TGF-β1 in hepatocarcinoma tissues. Positive expression of FGFR4 or TGF-β1 could affect the survival of HCC patients. Univariate and multivariate analyses revealed both TGF-β1 and FGFR4 to be the independent prognostic factors in HCCs. It is reported that NSCLC cell lines which induced by TGF-β could exhibit FGFR1 expression [34]. Here we estimated the crosstalk between FGFR4 and TGF-β1 in hepatocarcinoma. The molecular rationale under the connection need to be further explored.

On the whole, we have demonstrated that intratumoral TGF-β1 and FGFR4 expression may be correlated with postoperative survival and relapse in patients with HCC. Our findings suggest that these two proteins may be potential targets for adjuvant therapy. Because the present study was retrospective, the results need to be further validated in future prospective studies.

References

[1] Parkin DM, Bray F, Ferlay J, *et al.* Global cancer statistics, 2002[J]. Ca-a Cancer Journal for Clinicians, 2005, 55(2): 74-108.

[2] Lau W-Y, Lai ECH. Hepatocellular carcinoma: current management and recent advances[J]. Hepatobiliary & Pancreatic Diseases International, 2008, 7(3): 237-257.

[3] Bruix J, Sherman M. Management of hepatoceullular carcinoma[J]. Hepatology, 2005, 42(5): 1208-1236.

[4] El-Serag HB, Rudolph L. Hepatocellular carcinoma: Epidemiology and molecular carcinogenesis[J]. Gastroenterology, 2007, 132(7): 2557-2576.

[5] Chen YJ, Yeh SH, Chen JT, *et al.* Chromosomal changes and clonality relationship between primary and recurrent hepatocellular carcinoma[J]. Gastroenterology, 2000, 119(2): 431-440.

[6] Imamura H, Matsuyama Y, Tanaka E, *et al.* Risk factors contributing to early and date phase intrahepatic recurrence of hepatocellular carcinoma after hepatectomy[J]. Journal of Hepatology, 2003, 38(2): 200-207.

[7] Caulin C, Scholl FG, Frontelo P, *et al.* Chronic exposure of cultured transformed mouse epidermal cells to transforming growth factor-beta 1 induces an epithelialmesenchymal transdifferentiation and a spindle tumoral phenotype[J]. Cell Growth & Differentiation, 1995, 6(8): 1027-1035.

[8] Cui W, Fowlis DJ, Bryson S, *et al.* TGF beta 1 inhibits the formation of benign skin tumors, but enhances progression to invasive spindle carcinomas in transgenic mice[J]. Cell, 1996, 86(4): 531-542.

[9] Portella G, Cumming SA, Liddell J, *et al.* Transforming growth factor beta is essential for spindle cell conversion of mouse skin carcinoma *in vivo*: Implications for tumor invasion[J]. Cell Growth & Differentiation, 1998, 9(5): 393-404.

[10] Frontelo P, Gonzalez-Garrigues M, Vilaro S, *et al.* Transforming growth factor beta(1) induces squamous carcinoma cell variants with increased metastatic abilities and a disorganized cytoskeleton[J]. Experimental Cell Research, 1998, 244(2): 420-432.

[11] Romero D, Iglesias M, Vary CPH, *et al.* Functional blockade of Smad4 leads to a decrease in beta-catenin levels and signaling activity in human pancreatic carcinoma cells[J]. Carcinogenesis, 2008, 29(5): 1070-1076.

[12] Zeisberg M, Yang C, Martino M, *et al.* Fibroblasts derive from hepatocytes in liver fibrosis *via* epithelial to mesenchymal transition[J]. Journal of Biological Chemistry, 2007, 282(32): 23337-23347.

[13] Streit S, Mestel DS, Schmidt M, *et al.* FGFR4 Arg388 allele correlates with tumour thickness and FGFR4 protein expression with survival of melanoma patients[J]. British Journal of Cancer, 2006, 94(12): 1879-1886.

[14] Roidl A, Berger H-J, Kumar S, *et al.* Resistance to Chemotherapy Is Associated with Fibroblast Growth Factor Receptor 4 Up-Regulation[J]. Clinical Cancer Research, 2009, 15(6): 2058-2066.

[15] Takahashi A, Sasaki H, Kim SJ, *et al.* Identification of receptor genes in renal cell carcinoma associated with angiogenesis by differential hybridization technique[J]. Biochemical and Biophysical Research Communications, 1999, 257(3): 855-859.

[16] Ho HK, Pok S, Streit S, *et al.* Fibroblast growth factor receptor 4 regulates proliferation, anti-apoptosis and alpha-fetoprotein secretion during hepatocellular carcinoma progression and represents a potential target for therapeutic intervention[J]. Journal of Hepatology, 2009, 50(1): 118-127.

[17] Kan M, Wu XC, Wang F, *et al.* Specificity for fibroblast growth factors determined by heparan sulfate in a binary complex with the receptor kinase[J]. Journal of Biological Chemistry, 1999, 274(22): 15947-15952.

[18] Lin BC, Wang M, Blackmore C, *et al.* Liver-specific activities of FGF19 require Klotho beta[J]. Journal of Biological Chemistry, 2007, 282(37): 27277-27284.

[19] Furukawa T. Molecular targeting therapy for pancreatic cancer: current knowledge and perspectives from bench to bedside[J]. Journal of Gastroenterology, 2008, 43(12): 905-911.

[20] vanDiest PJ, vanDam P, HenzenLogmans SC, *et al.* A scoring system for immunohistochemical staining: consensus report of the task force for basic research of the EORTC-GCCG[J]. Journal of Clinical Pathology, 1997, 50(10): 801-804.

[21] Saito H, Tsujitani S, Oka S, *et al.* The expression of transforming growth factor-beta 1 is significantly correlated with the expression of vascular endothelial growth factor and poor prognosis of patients with advanced gastric carcinoma[J]. Cancer, 1999, 86(8): 1455-1462.

[22] Motoda N, Matsuda Y, Onda M, *et al.* Overexpression of fibroblast growth factor receptor 4 in high-grade pancreatic intraepithelial neoplasia and pancreatic ductal adenocarcinoma[J]. International Journal of Oncology, 2011, 38(1): 133-143.

[23] Ueno T, Hashimoto O, Kimura R, *et al.* Relation of type II transforming growth factor-beta receptor to hepatic fibrosis and hepatocellular carcinoma[J]. International Journal of Oncology, 2001, 18(1): 49-55.

[24] Zhang L, Yuan S-Z. Expression of c-erbB-2 oncogene protein, epidermal growth factor receptor, and TGF-beta1 in human pancreatic ductal adenocarcinoma[J]. Hepatobiliary & pancreatic diseases international : HBPD INT, 2002, 1(4): 620-623.

[25] Masuhara M, Yasunaga M, Tanigawa K, *et al.* Expression of hepatocyte growth factor, transforming growth factor alpha, and transforming growth factor beta(1) messenger RNA in various human liver diseases and correlation with hepatocyte proliferation[J]. Hepatology, 1996, 24(2): 323-329.

[26] Fan GS, Ma XM, Kren BT, *et al.* The retinoblastoma gene product inhibits TGF-beta 1 induced apoptosis in primary rat hepatocytes and human HuH-7 hepatoma cells[J]. Oncogene, 1996, 12(9): 1909-1919.

[27] Zong L, Qu Y, Xu M, *et al.* 18 alpha-Glycyrrhetinic Acid Down-Regulates Expression of Type I and III Collagen *via* TGF-B1/Smad Signaling Pathway in Human and Rat Hepatic Stellate Cells[J]. International Journal of Medical Sciences, 2012, 9(5): 370-379.

[28] Li X, Zhang Y-Y, Wang Q, *et al.* Association between endogenous gene expression and growth regulation induced by TGF-beta 1 in human gastric cancer cells[J]. World Journal of Gastroenterology, 2005, 11(1): 61-68.

[29] Lu Y, Wu L-Q, Li C-S, *et al.* Expression of transforming growth factors in hepatocellular carcinoma and its relations with clinicopathological parameters and prognosis[J]. Hepatobiliary & Pancreatic Diseases International, 2008, 7(2): 174-178.

[30] Eswarakumar VP, Lax I, Schlessinger J. Cellular signaling by fibroblast growth factor receptors[J]. Cytokine & Growth Factor Reviews, 2005, 16(2): 139-149.

[31] Xie MH, Holcomb I, Deuel B, *et al.* FGF-19, a novel fibroblast growth factor with unique specificity for FGFR4[J]. Cytokine, 1999, 11(10): 729-735.

[32] Miura S, Mitsuhashi N, Shimizu H, *et al.* Fibroblast growth factor 19 expression correlates with tumor progression and poorer prognosis of hepatocellular carcinoma[J]. Bmc Cancer, 2012, 12.

[33] Huang X, Yang C, Jin C, *et al.* Resident Hepatocyte Fibroblast Growth Factor Receptor 4 Limits Hepatocarcinogenesis[J]. Molecular Carcinogenesis, 2009, 48(6): 553-562.

[34] Thomson S, Petti F, Sujka-Kwok I, *et al.* Kinase switching in mesenchymal-like non-small cell lung cancer lines contributes to EGFR inhibitor resistance through pathway redundancy[J]. Clin Exp Metastasis, 2008, 25(8): 843-854.

Transient inhibition of FGFR2b-ligands signaling leads to irreversible loss of cellular β-catenin organization and signaling in AER during mouse limb development

Soula Danopoulos, Xiaokun Li, Saverio Bellusci

1. Introduction

Congenital anomalies of the limb occur between 1 in 500 to 1 in 1 000 live human births [1]. They are often the result of a complex interaction of multiple minor genetic abnormalities with environmental risk factors. Intrauterine disruption of limb development by exposure of the fetus to teratogens, usually between the third and eighth week of gestation, can also *per se* lead to anomalies of the limb. The precise molecular and cellular bases of these anomalies are still largely unknown and require a better understanding of normal limb development.

The growth and patterning of vertebrate limbs is regulated by epithelial-mesenchymal cell interactions, involving a diverse array of signaling pathways. In mouse, limb development along the body flank is initiated with the formation of forelimb buds at embryonic day 9.5 (E9.5) followed 12 hours later by hindlimb buds. The early limb bud is composed of mesenchymal cells derived from the lateral plate mesoderm, covered by ectoderm cells, a subset of which converge at the dorso-ventral border of limb buds to form a pluristratified structure termed the Apical Ectodermal Ridge (AER) [2]. As simple as the anatomy of the limb bud appears, it is composed of many signaling zones that control the temporal and spatial specification of the mesenchymal progenitors in the limb. These signaling zones determine the three different axes of the mature limb: proximal-distal (PD), anterior-posterior (AP) and dorso-ventral (DV). Along the PD axis, the skeletal elements of mature limbs can be divided into three domains: the proximal stylopod (humerus/femur), the zeugopod (radius/tibia and ulna/fibula) and the distal autopod (carpal/tarsal, metacarpal/metatarsal, phalanges).

The AER is the earliest signaling domain to be induced during limb bud formation. It is formed by the action of FGF10, produced by lateral plate mesoderm, on Fibroblast Growth Factor Receptor 2b (FGFR2b), expressed by ectoderm cells [3-4]. FGF10 also induces the expression of *Fgf8* in the AER, which in turn acts on the underlying mesenchymal cells located in the putative "undifferentiated zone" (UZ) thus allowing the amplification of the different skeletal progenitors of the limb [5] (for review see [6]).

Using a non targeted transgenic approach to express constitutively and ubiquitously a soluble form of FGFR2b acting as a dominant negative receptor, it was reported that mutant embryos at E18.5 display a large variety of defects including complete limb agenesis or agenesis of the hindlimb associated with truncated forelimb with missing autopod [7]. Further investigations of the role of FGFR2b signaling in limb development have confirmed the previous results and produced some interesting but conflicting results. Using a *Msx2-Cre* driver line to abrogate FGFR2b function in the AER after forelimb AER formation but before hindlimb AER formation, Lu *et al.* [8] reported decreased *Fgf8* expression and loss of AER, resulting in the complete loss of the autopod skeletal elements in the forelimb as well as hindlimb agenesis. However, no changes in cell proliferation or cell death were observed in the distal mesenchyme of the forelimb bud. Yu and Ornitz [9] used the same transgenic approach to discover reduced mesenchymal cell proliferation at E10.5–E11 but not E10.0, with no impact on cell death. Analysis of *Hoxa13* expression, a marker of autopod progenitors, showed that *Msx2-Cre*-mediated targeting of *Fgfr2*, reduces the pool of autopod progenitors [8]. Since developmental events occur at a rapid pace in the developing limbs, one drawback of using a Cre line to delete *Fgfr2* expression is that it will not abrogate the activity of the endogenous FGFR2b protein present prior to the complete inactivation of the conditional *Fgfr2* allele. Therefore, upon Cre activation, the precise analysis of the resulting phenotype and the associated primary defects are limited by the presence of a residual FGFR2 activity which persistence will depend on its stability. In addition, as the deletion of *Fgfr2* in the AER is irreversible, it is difficult to investigate whether restoring FGFR2 signaling in the

AER is sufficient to re-induce AER formation.

Here, we report the use of a novel approach to robustly target signaling induced by FGFR2b-ligands interaction within a relatively narrow window of time at desired developmental time points, in order to investigate its role/s at later stages on limb outgrowth and patterning, as well as on AER morphology and cell behavior. In this model, soluble dominant-negative FGFR2b molecules are generated by administration of doxycycline to mice harboring a dox/transactivator tet(O)-responsive transgene. We find that transient FGFR2b-ligands signaling inhibition leads to permanent disorganization of β-catenin, a cellular component critical for both cell adhesion and signaling. In harmony with this result, restoration of FGFR2b-ligands signaling after a 24-hour inhibition period is not sufficient to trigger *de novo* AER formation. We also demonstrate that interruption of FGFR2b-ligands signaling affects distinct elements of the limb skeleton in a time and dose-dependent manner.

2. Results

2.1 FGFR2b-ligands signaling controls progressive limb growth along the proximal-distal axis

We have previously reported that we could use a double transgenic (DTG) [$R26^{rtTA+/-}$;*TetOsFgfr2b*/+] (also called [$R26^{rtTA/+}$;*Tg*/+]) *in vivo* system to inducibly and reversibly attenuate FGFR2b-ligands signaling in the post-natal mouse [10]. The *Rosa26*$^{rtTA/+}$ line allows the ubiquitous expression of the transactivator rtTA. The *tetOsFgfr2b*/+ line contains a construct allowing the expression of a secreted fusion protein composed of the extracellular part of FGFR2b fused with the heavy chain domain of immunoglobulin. Upon exposure to doxycycline, the transactivator rtTA is activated and will induce the expression of this fusion protein, which will be transported outside the cell. We therefore expect this fusion protein to act in a non-cell autonomous fashion as a decoy receptor for FGFR2b-ligands.

We first aimed to validate the use of our double transgenic mice in the context of limb development. Pregnant females carrying both DTG heterozygous and control embryos were placed on Doxycycline containing (Dox) food between E8.5 and E13.5, corresponding to the pre-induction, induction and post-induction stages of mouse limb buds. DTG embryos (n = 5 out of 5, the phenotypes described thereafter are always 100% penetrant) exposed to Dox food from E8.5 (pre-induction) to E13.5 failed to generate limbs (Fig. 1A, B). Skeletal preparation of these embryos sacrificed at E18.5 indicates a complete failure of limb development phenocopying *Fgfr2b* null embryos [5] (data not shown). By contrast, exposure at E10.5 (early limb bud), 24 hours after forelimb induction and only 12 hours after hindlimb induction, resulted in shorter forelimbs and very rudimentary hindlimbs in DTG embryos (n = 15, Fig. 1C, D). Dox treatment from E11.5 (late limb bud) to E13.5 led to the absence of autopod in both forelimb and hindlimb in the DTG embryos (n = 11, Fig. 1E– G). Dox treatment from E13.0 to E16.5 led to defective separation of the digits (Fig. 1H–K). To better visualize the impact on cartilage condensations, DTG embryos carrying an additional *Topgal* allele [11] were used (Fig. 1H–K). Dox treatment from E13.5 to E16.5 led to shortening of all five digits in both forelimbs and hindlimbs (ratio digit length in DTG *versus* control HL: 78.5% ± 7.3%, FL: 84.3% ± 6.4%) with digits 1 and 5 being more severely affected (n = 20). Skeleton staining was carried out to better visualize this phenotype and examine the affected cartilage condensations, only to discover shorter phalanx 1 and 2 as well as the specific absence of the third phalanx in the hindlimb (Fig. 1P–S) (ratio phalanx length in DTG *versus* control limbs P1: HL: 88.5% ± 3.1%, FL: 86.8% ± 9.1%, P2: HL: 72% ± 8.5%, FL: 77% ± 16.7%, P3: HL: 0%, FL: 47% ± 0.7%). In conclusion, the brachydactyly phenotype is associated with defective proximal-distal growth of the digits with completely missing phalange 3 in the HL. This phenotype is reminiscent of the digit defects (ranging from aplasia to hypoplasia), which most often involved the thumbs in patients with hypomorphic *FGF10* mutations [12]. Interestingly, the forelimbs are slightly less affected than the hindlimbs, indicating that the asynchrony in mouse fore- and hindlimb development continues well into E13.5. No obvious limb defects were observed in DTG heterozygous embryos exposed to Dox food from E14 onwards (n = 17, data not shown). However, we cannot exclude a role for FGFR2b-ligands signaling in limb development beyond E14, which, if any, is likely to involve ossification rather than specification and patterning of the skeleton. The postnatal functionality of limbs in Dox-treated DTG embryos is difficult to analyze because they all die at birth from abnormal lung development (Al Alam and Bellusci, unpublished observation).

Taken together, these data validate the use of DTG mice to attenuate specifically FGFR2b-ligands signaling in the

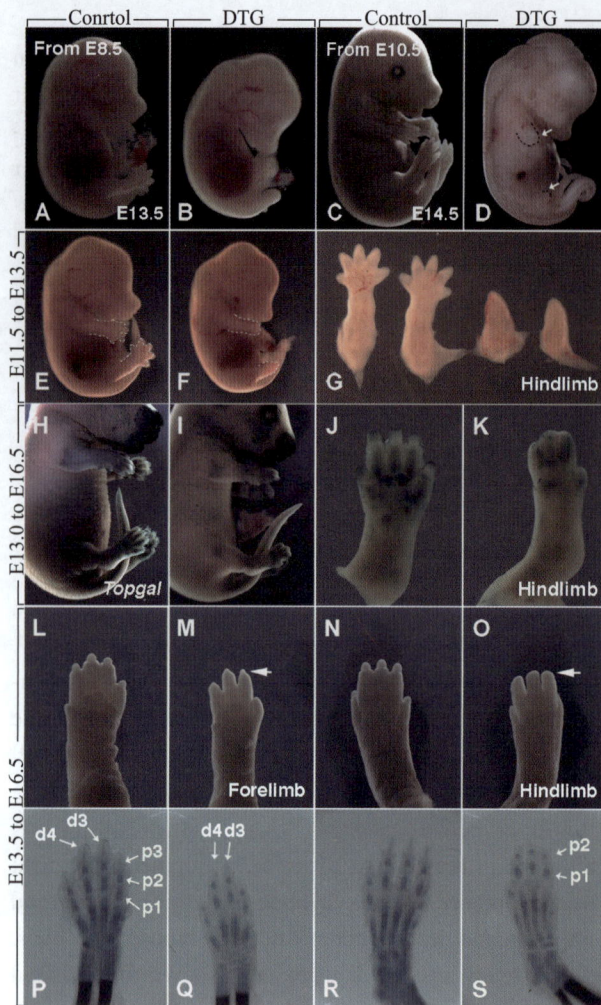

Fig. 1. Signaling induced by FGFR2b-ligands interaction controls progressive limb growth along the proximal-distal axis. Pregnant females carrying [R26^rtTA/+;Tg/+] double transgenic (DTG) embryos and single transgenic [R26^rtTA/+ or Tg/+] control embryos were treated continuously with Doxycycline food starting at different developmental stages; (A,B) Treatment at E8.5, before limb induction: loss of both hindlimbs and forelimbs in E13.5 DTG embryos. (C,D) Treatment at E10.5, after limb bud induction: Formation of rudimentary forelimbs and almost complete absence of hindlimbs in E14.5 DTG embryos. (E–F) Treatment at E11.5: Absence of autopod in both hindlimbs and forelimbs of E13.5 DTG embryos. (G) Dissected hindlimbs in DTG and controls shown in (E,F). (H–I) Treatment at E13.0: control (H) and DTG (I) embryos at E16. Note that the *Topgal* allele was introduced in DTG and control embryos to visualize the extent of mesenchymal condensation in the limb. (J,K) Dissected left hindlimbs from embryos shown in H and I displaying failure of separation of the digits in DTG hindlimb. (L–O) Treatment at E13.5: truncation of the digits in both forelimbs and hindlimbs. (P–S) Alcian blue/alizarin red staining indicates the reduction in the size of the P3 phalange in the forelimb and complete loss of the P3 phalange in the hindlimb of DTG embryos treated from E13.5 to E16.5. d, digits; p, phalanges.

developing limbs and show that the role of FGFR2b-ligands is not confined to the induction and autopod initiation phases, as previously described (E8.5 to E13.5) [5,8,9]. Rather, FGFR2b signaling continues to play a role in digit outgrowth.

2.2 Impact of transient FGFR2b-ligands attenuation before and after limb bud induction on the formation of the skeletal elements along the Proximal/Distal axis

To examine the impact of transient FGFR2b-ligands signaling attenuation on the formation of the limb skeleton, pregnant females carrying DTG and control embryos were given a single Dox-IP dose at E8.5, E9.5, E10.5 and E11.5 and their embryos were collected and analyzed at E18.5. We also used different allelic combination of R26^rtTA and Tg to determine the impact of the gene dosage on the severity of the limb phenotype. Double heterozygous transgenic embryos ([R26^rtTA/+;Tg/+]) exposed to Dox-IP at E8.5 (1–1.5 days before forelimb and hindlimb induction, respectively) displayed shorter forelimbs but quasinormal hindlimbs (n = 7, Fig. 2A and B, left embryo). This result supports our claim that inducible inhibition of FGFR2b-ligands signaling is indeed reversible, as the sustained blockade of FGFR2b-ligands signaling between E8.5 and E13.5 led to limb agenesis (Fig. 1A,B). However, double homozygous transgenic embryos [R26^rtTA/rtTA;Tg/Tg] did not produce forelimbs and had severely truncated hindlimbs (n = 10, Fig. 2A and B, right embryo). Double heterozygotes (Fig. 2C) showed normal scapula but reduced stylopod (humerus) and zeugopod (radius and ulna) (n = 7). Interestingly, the right limbs were more severely affected, with a near absence of right humerus and shortened femur, and the complete absence of right ulna and fibula. Furthermore, the autopodal digits had formed in both fore and hindimbs, but these were fewer on the right side. By comparison, the double homozygous DTGs had much shorter femur and no elements beyond a rudimentary tibia. Unexpectedly, double homozygous DTG embryos exposed to Dox-IP at E9.5, at the time of forelimb induction but 12 hours before hindlimb formation, displayed a complete absence of both forelimbs and hindlimbs (n = 13, Fig. 2E,F) suggesting that FGFR2b-ligands attenuation at E9.5 leads to irreversible loss of the AER.

We next examined the consequences of inhibiting FGFR2b-ligands signaling at E10.5, 24 and 12 hours after forelimb and hindlimb induction, respectively. Mutant forelimbs displayed a progressive loss of distal skeletal elements as a function of the genotype (Fig. 2G). [$R26^{rtTA/+}$; $Tg/+$] embryos (n = 11) displayed only a truncation of the digits, whilst in [$R26^{rtTA/+}$; Tg/Tg] embryos (n = 9) the autopod was completely absent, as previously shown in Fig. 1. In [$R26^{rtTA/rtTA}$; Tg/Tg] embryos (n = 14), the entire autopod and the bulk of zeugopod failed to develop. The corresponding phenotypes were more severe in the hindlimbs (Fig. 2H). For example, [$R26^{rtTA/rtTA}$; Tg/Tg] embryos failed to generate any hindlimbs (n = 14, data not shown) and the [$R26^{rtTA/+}$; Tg/Tg] embryos displayed an aborted zeugopod but a normal stylopod (n = 9). These data are consistent with an irreversible loss of the AER from a single Dox-IP injection at E10.5. The level of inhibition of FGFR2b-ligands signaling at this time point and its subsequent impact on the amplification of the mesenchymal progenitors that will later form skeletal elements in the zygopod and autopod correlates with the genotype. Our results also indicate that at E10.5, the mesenchymal progenitors that will later contribute to the stylopod (humerus and femur in fore and hindlimb, respectively) do not require FGFR2b-ligands signaling for their specification and amplification.

Finally, the inhibition of FGFR2b-ligands signaling at E11.5, 48 and 36 hours after forelimb and hindlimb induction, respectively led only to digit defects in the forelimb of both [$R26^{rtTA/+}$; Tg/Tg] (n = 13) and [$R26^{rtTA/rtTA}$; Tg/Tg] (n = 16) embryos (Fig. 2I and Fig. S1). The [$R26^{rtTA/rtTA}$; Tg/Tg] hindlimbs (n = 13) exhibited an almost complete absence of autopod while in the [$R26^{rtTA/+}$; Tg/Tg] hindlimb (n = 16) it was normal (Fig. 2J). Interestingly the truncation of the autopod appears to form with a distal to proximal gradient suggesting that the AER did not recover from transient FGFR2b-ligands inhibition at E11.5.

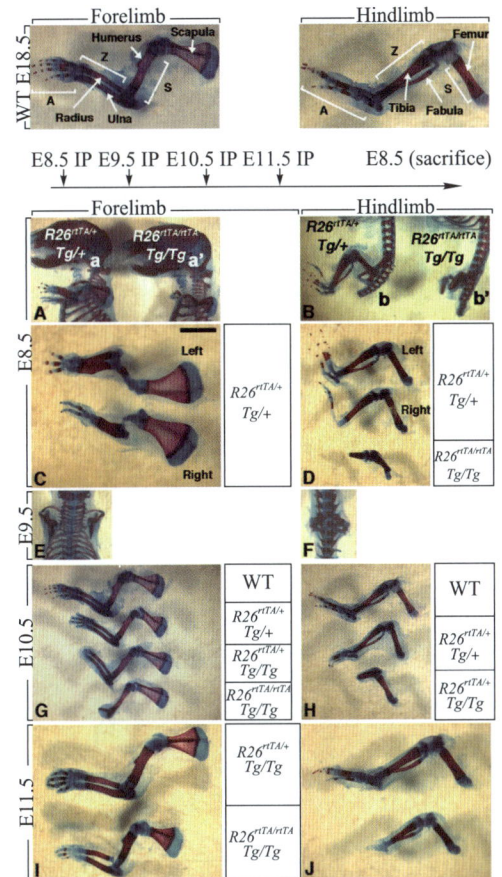

Fig. 2. Transient attenuation of FGFR2b-ligands signaling, before and after limb bud induction, affects different skeletal elements along the A/P axis. Alcian blue/alizarin red staining of embryos was used to visualize the bone *versus* cartilage respectively. Images of E18.5 embryos which were exposed to Dox at E8.5 (A–D), E9.5 (E–F), E10.5 (G,H) and E11.5 (I–J). Hindlimbs demonstrate more drastic defects than forelimbs. Also, homozygous *vs.* heterozygous embryos and right *vs.* left limbs are differently affected.

These results indicate that at all of the post-limb bud induction time-points studied-E9.5, E10.5 and E11.5-the AER does not recover from transient attenuation of FGFR2b-ligands signaling. Hence, we next aimed to define the role of FGFR2b-ligands signaling on AER morphology and cell behavior.

2.3 Dynamics of soluble Fgfr2b expression and activity in vivo after single Dox-IP administration at E11

The initial experiments shown in Fig. 1 relied on sufficient uptake of Dox-containing food over a period of days by pregnant females carrying DTG heterozygous embryos. However, the fate of mesenchymal progenitors is determined within narrow time windows between E9.5 to E11.5. Therefore, to be able to pinpoint the role/s of FGFR2b-ligands signaling in different developmental processes, we refined our experimental approach by delivering a single dose of Doxycycline (1.5 mg/kg/body weight) intraperitoneally (Dox-IP) at different time points (Fig. 2). In order to determine the time frame during which we can characterize the primary consequences of FGFR2b attenuation, we aimed to define the level of soluble *Fgfr2b* expression at different time points after a single Dox-IP administration in pregnant females carrying E11 [$R26^{rtTA/rtTA}$; Tg/Tg] homozygous embryos (Fig. 3A). We isolated the right forelimbs of DTG embryos at 0.5, 1, 2, 4, 6, 12 and 24 hours after Dox-IP and measured soluble *Fgfr2b* expression in each limb independently (n = 3) by qRT-PCR using specific primers which do not recognize the *endogenous Fgfr2b* transcripts (Fig. 3B). Our results indicate that *sFgfr2b* expression is detected as early as 30 minutes after Dox IP and reaches a maximum of expression at 6 hours followed by a steep decline at 24 hours. Interestingly, the levels of *sFgfr2b* expression at 24 hours in double ho-

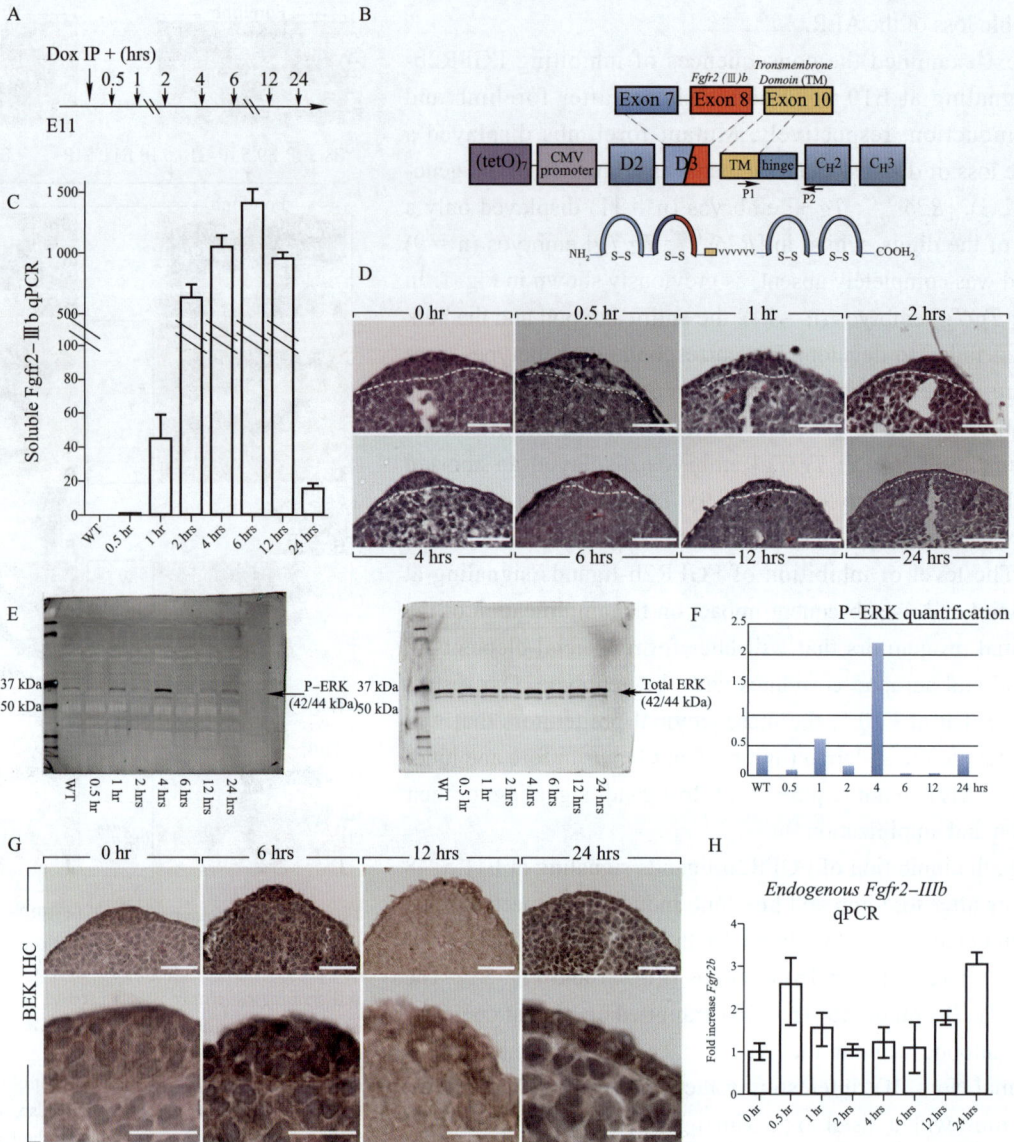

Fig. 3. Dynamics of soluble *Fgfr2b* expression and impact on AER maintenance after a single Dox-IP injection. (A) Embryos were collected at 0.5, 1,2,4,6,12 and 24 h after Dox IP at E11. (B) Schematic of the *soluble Fgfr2b* structure indicating the position of the specific primers P1 and P2 used to detect *sFgfr2b* expression. (C) Quantification of *soluble Fgfr2b* by qRT-PCR indicating a peak of expression at 6 h and a steep decrease at 24 hrs. (D) Analysis of the AER at these different time points showing a progressive diseappearance of the AER. (E) Western blot from whole E11 embryos exposed to Dox at different time points. Significant decrease in P-ERK levels is observed after 4 hrs. (F) Quantification of the P-ERK/Total ERK ratio at the different time points. (G) BEK (FGFR2) expression by IHC indicating that FGFR2 is still expressed in the rudimentary AER at 24 h post Dox-IP. (H) qRT-PCR for endogenous *Fgfr2b* expression supporting the IHC results. Scale bar D: 50 μm; G-upper panels: 50 μm; G-lower panels: 25 μm.

mozygous embryos are still 10 times higher compared to the ones observed at 30 minutes (Fig. 3C). Histological analysis of the corresponding left forelimbs (n = 3) showed progressive AER disappearance (Fig. 3D) with no visible AER at 24 hours post Dox-IP while an ectodermal thickening is still observed in the corresponding time-matched controls (data not shown). Inhibition of FGFR2b-ligands activity was investigated by western blot using p-ERK antibodies on whole embryo extracts (n = 1 per well) collected at different time points after Dox-IP at E11. The western blot was repeated 2 more times using independent embryos. We consistently found (n = 3) that during the first 4 hours after Dox-IP, p-ERK is increased suggesting the involvement of compensatory mechanisms upon FGFR2b signaling attenuation. However, between 4 and 24 hours, p-ERK expression is almost completely extinct only to be found re-induced at 24 hours (Fig. 3E, F). Interestingly, endogenous FGFR2 expression in the epithelium investigated using BEK Antibodies (recognizing an epitope localized in the C-terminal cytoplasmic domain of FGFR2 which is common to the epithelial and mesenchymal isoforms of FGFR2) is maintained in the AER/ectoderm of the forelimb over time after Dox-IP administration (Fig. 3G, n = 5). This result was confirmed by qRT-PCR using specific primers for endogenous *Fgfr2b* (Fig. 3H, n = 4).

2.4 Loss of Fgf8 expression in DTG AER after Dox-IP injection

To test AER functionality, we checked the expression of *Fgf8* by WMISH at t = 0 (control), 1 hour and 2 hours post Dox-IP delivery to E11 *R26^{rtTA/rtTA}*; *Tg/Tg* homozygous embryos. *Fgf8* expression is strongly expressed in the AER of control limbs (Fig. 4A,B). Moreover, the AER can be easily visualized as an elevated ridge at the interface between the dorsal and ventral limb by Scanning Electron Microscopy (SEM) (Fig. 4B′–B″). Only one hour post Dox-IP injection, DTG AERs showed abnormal *Fgf8* expression (Fig. 4C, n = 8) with defects ranging from absence of *Fgf8* expression along the limb (n = 3 out of 8 DTG embryos) to gaps in *Fgf8* expression in the AER (n = 5 out of 8 DTG embryos). However, close up examination of the forelimbs indicated that in our experimental conditions, the AER, expressing *Fgf8*, was detaching (inset in Fig. 4D). Interestingly, SEM indicated that the AER is still present in the limb 1 hour after Dox-IP (Fig. 4D–D″) suggesting that the lack of *Fgf8* expression at 1 hour post Dox-IP is due to the physical de-

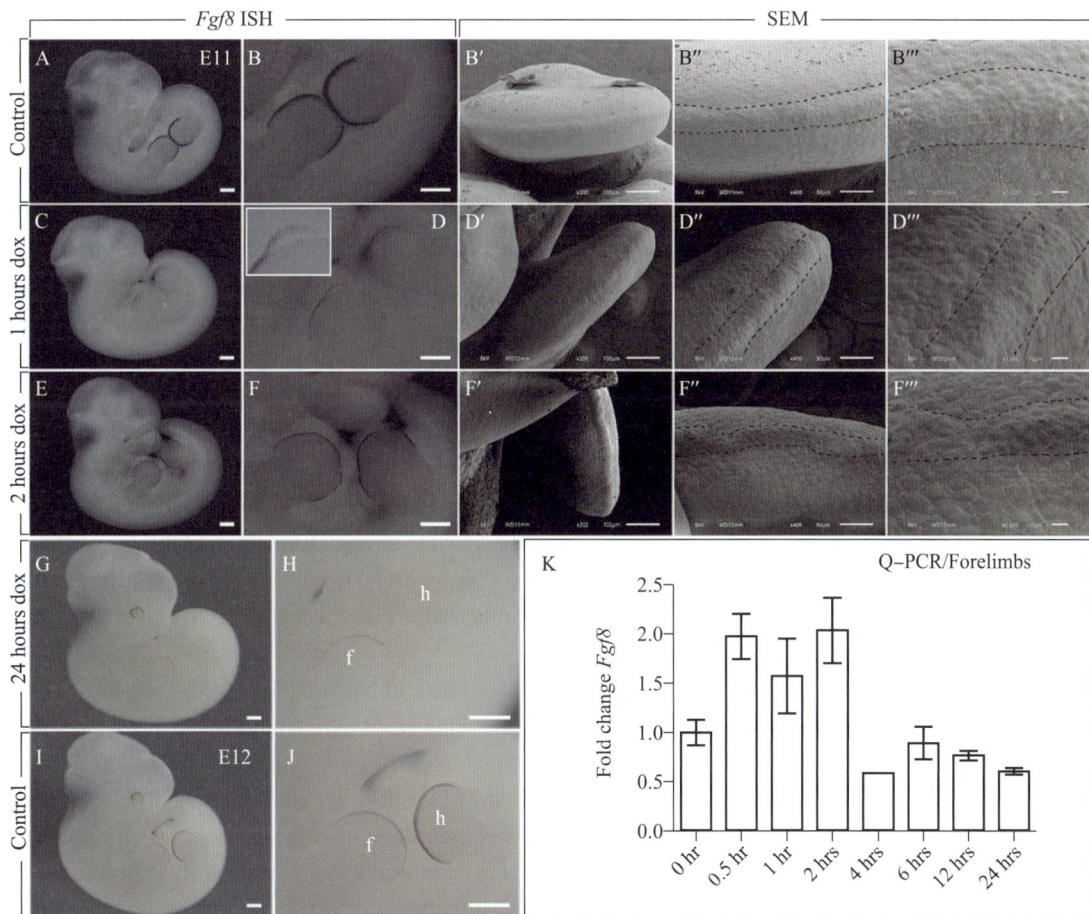

Fig. 4. Expression of *Fgf8* in the AER following Dox-IP. (A–F) WMISH for *Fgf8* in control (A,B), *Rosa26^{rtTA/rtTA}*; *Tg/Tg* embryo after 1 hour Dox-IP injection (C,D) and 2 hours after Dox-IP injection (E,F). B,D,F are high magnification of A,C,E. (C,D) *Fgf8-AER* expression is decreased at 1 hour after Dox-IP injection. (inset in D) Close up examination of the limb shows that the AER is detaching. (E,F) *Fgf8-AER* is significantly expressed 2 hours after Dox-IP injection. However, note that the expression at 2 hours is still lower than the one observed in the control and still exhibits gaps in *Fgf8* expression indicating defective AER at this time point. (B′–B‴,D′–D‴,F′–F‴) SEM images of control (B′–B‴), 1 hour Dox-IP (D′–D‴) and 2 hours Dox-IP (F′–F‴) embryos showing that the AER is still present at 1 and 2 h after Dox-IP. (G,H) *Fgf8* expression at 24 h post Dox-IP showing complete absence of *Fgf8* expression in the hindlimb and a residual expression in the forelimb. (K) Quantification of *Fgf8* expression by qRT-PCR in the forelimbs at different times post Dox-IP. Note that *Fgf8* expression is still present at 1 hr post Dox-IP supporting the hypothesis that the lack of *Fgf8* expression at 1 Dox-IP by WMISH is due to the physical loss of the AER. Scale bar A,C,E,G,I: 500 μm; B,D,F,H,J: 300 μm; B′,D′,F′: 100 mm; B″,D″,F″: 50 μm; B‴,D‴,F‴: 10 μm.

tachment of the AER as the likely consequence of decreased cell adhesion rather than decreased *Fgf8* RNA level. We propose that such decrease in cell adhesion is particularly apparent following enzymatic treatment during the WMISH procedure. Supporting a transient change in the cell adhesion status at 1 hour post Dox-IP, *Fgf8*-AER expression was almost normal at 2 hours after Dox-IP, bar a few localized domains (Fig. 4E–F). Like for the 1 hour post Dox-IP time point, SEM analysis at 2 hours post Dox-IP indicated the presence of a structurally defined AER (Fig. 4F′–F″). Interestingly, after 24 hours post Dox-IP, *Fgf8* expression is almost completely absent in the hindlimb but still present in the forelimb (Fig. 4G,H) compared to the corresponding E12 control limbs (Fig. 4I,J). We also measured directly *Fgf8* expression in dissected FL by qPCR over time (Fig. 4K).

Our results indicated increased *Fgf8* expression within the first 2 hours following Dox-IP delivery, confirming that the absence or decreased expression of *Fgf8* after 1 hour Dox-IP observed by WMISH is due to the detachment of the AER and not to the loss of *Fgf8* expression *per se*. From 4 hours onwards, *Fgf8* expression is reduced confirming the progressive loss of a functional AER.

2.5 Cellular and Molecular defects in the AER appear shortly after attenuation of FGFR2b-ligands signaling

To further study the cellular and molecular defects in the AER of double homozygous DTG [*R26*$^{rtTA/rtTA}$; *Tg/Tg*] embryos, we injected pregnant females with a single dose of Dox-IP at E11 and examined the cellular structure of the AER 1 and 2 hours later by Transmission Electron Microscopy (TEM). Analysis of semi-thin sections showed that wild type AER (n = 4) is normally composed of three to four layers of polystratified epithelial cells with smooth and round nuclei (Fig. 5A), and covered by periderm, a thin monolayer of elongated squamous like cells (Fig. 5B,C). The border between the AER and the adjacent squamous epithelium was also clearly visible (black arrows in Fig. 5A). However, one hour after Dox-IP (n = 5), this border is no longer visible, the epithelial cells in the AER are no longer compactly arranged at the rim and some of the nuclei became irregular in shape (Fig. 5D–F). Two hours after Dox-IP (n = 4), the appearance of the superficial peridermal cells is abnormal while the cells in the AER appear again more compacted (Fig. 5H–I).

The cellular changes in the AER could result from the dispersion of the AER cells into the adjacent squamous epithelium following changes in their cell adhesion status or amplified cell death. To investigate whether these are due to a reduction in the cohesive properties of the AER cells, we first examined the levels of β1-integrin, the transcription factor P63 and E-cadherin, which are known to regulate cell adhesion [13–16]. Levels of β1-integrin showed a marked decrease within 1 and 2 hours post Dox-IP injection in DTG-AER (n = 4 for each time point) (Fig. 5M,P) compared to the control-AER (n = 5) (Fig. 5J). This decrease also occurred in the underlying mesenchyme. A transient reduction in P63 was observed 1-hour post Dox-IP injection (n = 3) (Fig. 5K,N) but this was partially restored within the following hour (n = 4) (Fig. 5Q *vs.* K). E-cadherin expression was decreased at 1 and 2 hours post Dox-IP (n = 5 for each time point) (Fig. 5O, R) compared to the E11 control AER (n = 4) (Fig. 5L) confirming the cell adhesion defects upon FGFR2b-ligands signaling attenuation. We also measured the expression of β1-integrin and P63 by qRT-PCR in FL at different times after Dox-IP (Fig. 5S,T) (n = 3 for each time point). Our results indicate a compensatory increase at the RNA level of the expression of these two genes during the first 0.5–1 hour of Dox treatment.

Examination of cell death levels by TUNEL staining showed a transient but significant reduction in AER cell death, 1 hour post Dox-IP injection (n = 5), compared to the control (n = 5) (Fig. 5U,V). Apoptosis levels were subsequently increased in the AER 2-hours after Dox-IP injection (n = 5)(Fig. 5W).

Based on these observations, we propose that upon inhibition of FGFR2b-ligands signaling at E11, the multistratified and tightly-compacted epithelial cells in the AER lose their cell-cell and/or cell-matrix adhesion to resemble their neighboring squamous epithelial cells. Also, apoptosis, which is a feature of a functional AER, is decreased as an immediate response to attenuation of FGFR2b-ligands signaling. Altogether, our results indicate that the AER does not recover at the structural, cellular and molecular level from a single dose of Dox-IP.

2.6 Transient loss of AER function affects mesenchymal cell proliferation but not cell death

We next investigated the impact of FGFR2b-ligands attenuation on cell proliferation and apoptosis in the AER and the adjacent mesenchyme by carrying out double immunolabeling for E-cadherin in combination with either Phospho-histone H3 or cleaved Caspase 3, on DTG homozygous embryos (n = 5) exposed to a single Dox-IP injection at E10.5 and examined 24 hours later. E11.5 limbs were used as controls (n = 5). We found a significant decrease in cell proliferation in both the AER and the adjacent mesenchyme (Fig. 6A,B *vs.* C,D,I). As suggested from Fig 2G,H, the AER did

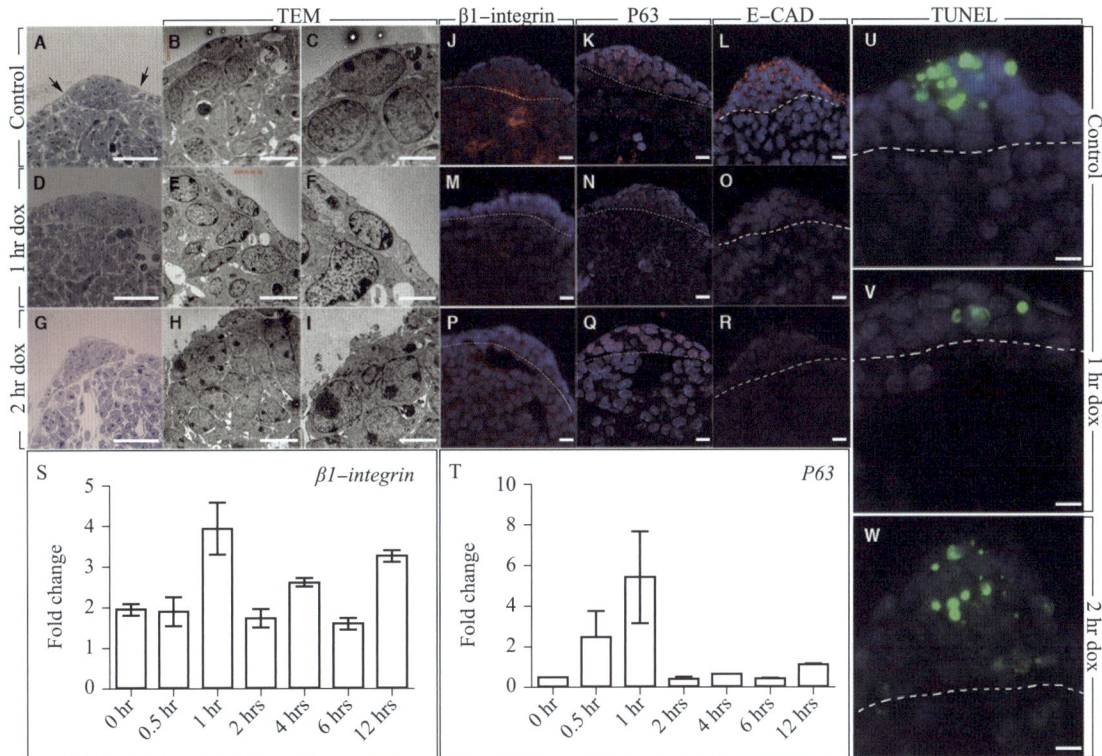

Fig. 5. Cell adhesion and cell death are reduced in the AER after attenuation of FGFR2b-ligands signaling. Histology (A, D, G) and TEM (B, C, E, F, H, I) images of the AER at E11, E11+ 1 hr and E11+ 2 h post Dox-IP. (D) Note that at 1 hr the AER is spreading and no longer a compact pseudostratified epithelium like in the control (A). SEM analysis does not indicate major changes except for irregularly shaped nuclei. (G–I) after 2 h Dox-IP, the AER seemingly reformed as a compact structure (G) but SEM analysis indicated that the most superficial layer, the periderm is missing. (J–R) Cell-cell adhesion was tested by IF for b1-integrin (J,M,P), P63 (K,N,Q) and E-Cadherin (L,O,R) expression. β1-integrin expression is reduced in DTG-AER 1 and 2 hours after Dox-IP (M, P) in comparison to the control AER at E11 (J). P63 expression is reduced in DTG-AER 1 hours after Dox-IP (N) compared to the control AER at E11 (K). No significant difference is observed at 2 hours after Dox-IP (Q) compared to the control AER. E-cadherin expression is reduced in DTG-AER 1 and 2 hours after Dox-IP (O,R) in comparison to the control AER at E11 (L). (U–W) TUNEL staining for control AER at E10.5 (U), DTG-AER 1 hour after Dox-IP (V) and 2 hours after Dox-IP (W) demonstrate reduction in cell death at 1 hour after Dox-IP in the DTG-AER. (S and T) Quantification by q-PCR of *β1-integrin* and *P63* expression. Scale bar A,D,G: 25 μm; B,E,H: 5 μm; C,F,I: 2 μm; J–R: 20 μm; U–W: 20 μm.

not recover from FGFR2b-ligands attenuation at E10.5. In order to quantify the defects in the AER, we considered the single layer of epithelium, stained positive for E-cadherin at the very tip of the limb, as the rudimentary AER in the mutants and examined proliferation and cell death in this structure. In the controls, 14.1% of the cells in the AER stained positive for PHH3 while only 0.9% were positive in the AER of the DTG ($P = 0.0103$; Fig. 6I; n = 5). Similarly, in the adjacent mesenchyme, 11.2% of cells were proliferating in the controls *versus* 4.2% in the DTG ($P = 0.041$; Fig. 6I, n = 5). As expected and due to the quasiabsence of AER, a significant decrease in cell death was observed in the DTG AER (Fig. 6G, H) as compared to control AER (Fig. 6E, F; 0.08%); 4.26% *vs.* 0.08%, respectively ($P = 0.0084$; Fig. 6J, n = 5). No significant change in cell death was observed in the DTG mesenchyme (Fig. 6G, H) as compared to the controls (Fig. 6E, F): 1.4% in the DTG *vs.* 0.8% in the control ($P = 0.24$; Fig. 6J, n = 5).

2.7 *The vascular system in the limb is conserved following FGFR2b-ligands signaling attenuation*

Abnormal limb development has recently been connected with impaired vascular formation [17]. We therefore examined the integrity of the vascular system in the E11 limbs at 6 hours post Dox-IP by anti-PECAM immunofluorescence labeling, and validated our results by qRT-PCR, quantifying the expression of *Pecam* and *Vegfa*. Our results indicated no significant differences in PECAM expression between control (Fig. S2A,B) and experimental limbs (Fig. S2C,D). In both cases, endothelial cells were found to be abundant in the limb mesenchyme. Interestingly, PECAM expression is not enriched at the level of the AER suggesting that, unlike other organs such as the lung, the endothelial cells do not interact directly with the AER for its maintenance *via* the secretion of angiocrine factors. The quantification of *Pecam*

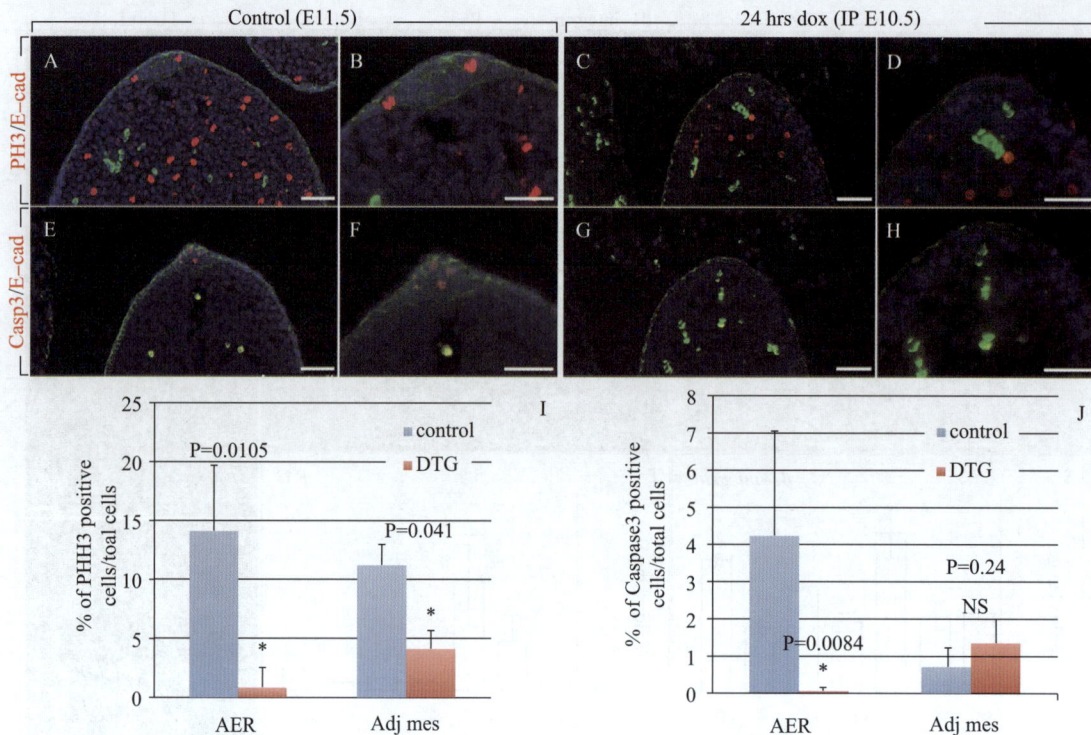

Fig. 6. FGFR2b-ligands signaling controls cell proliferation in the mesenchyme of the limb bud. (A–D) Phosphohistone H3 and E-cadherin double IF staining in control E11.5 (A,B) and DTG [$R26^{rtTA/rtTA}$; Tg/Tg] (C,D) limb bud exposed to Dox-IP at E10.5 and analyzed at E11.5 demonstrate significant reduction in cell proliferation of both the AER and the adjacent mesenchyme. (E–H) Caspase 3 IF staining for cell death in control limb bud at E11.5 (E,F) and DTG (G,H) limb buds exposed to Dox-IP at E10.5 and analyzed at E11.5 display significant decrease in apoptosis of the rudimentary AER, there is no change in the apoptosis of the adjacent mesenchyme. (Adj mesenchyme = Adjacent mesenchyme). (I) Quantification of PHH3 positive cells. (J) Quantification of caspase 3 positive cells. Bars represent the mean 6 s.e.m. of at least 5 independent samples of each. Mann-whitney non-parametric test was performed. *$P \leqslant 0.05$. Scale bar A–H: 50 µm.

expression by qRT-PCR (Fig. S2E) indicated a slight increase in *Pecam* expression in the mutant limbs over the time period considered (0.5–24 hours) while *Vegfa* expression did not change significantly (Fig. S2F). Overall, we did not observe major impairment of the vascular system upon inhibition of FGFR2b-ligands signaling.

2.8 Impact of FGFR2b-ligands attenuation on mesenchymal progenitor differentiation

The transcription factors *Meis1*, *Hoxa11* and *Hoxa13* have been previously reported as specific markers for the stylopod, zeugopod and autopod [8]. We measured the level and pattern of expression of these genes by qRT-PCR at different times after Dox-IP treatment (0, 0.5, 1, 2, 4, 6, 12, 24 hrs; 3 independent limbs were used for each time point) and by WMISH 2 hours after Dox-IP (n = 3; Fig. 7), respectively in double homozygous embryos. We found that the expression of the stylopod marker *Meis1* is drastically increased by qRT-PCR upon FGFR2b-ligands attenuation (Fig. 7A). This increase was confirmed by WMISH (Fig. 7G–I *vs.* D–F). The expression of the zeugopod marker *Hoxa11* showed a decrease by WMISH (Fig. 7M–O *vs.* J–L) but this was not found significant by qRT-PCR (Fig. 7B). The autopod marker *Hoxa13* was decreased between 1 and 6 h post Dox-IP (Fig. 7C). This last result was also confirmed by WMISH (Fig. 7S–U *vs.* P–R). Overall these results support that FGFR2b-ligands signaling acts indirectly to control the formation of the mesenchymal progenitors in the autopod domain. However, as the overall pattern of gene expression by WMISH at E11 plus 2 hours is not drastically perturbed, this result indicates that the observed distal limb truncations upon inhibition of FGFR2b-ligands interaction is due to cell death or/and reduced proliferation but not to proximalization (change in cell fate) of the mesenchymal progenitors.

2.9 Loss of canonical WNT signaling in the AER after attenuation of FGFR2b-ligands signaling

Females carrying triple heterozygous transgenic embryos (DTG [$R26^{rtTA/+}$; $Tg/+$], as well as *Topgal*, a reporter for

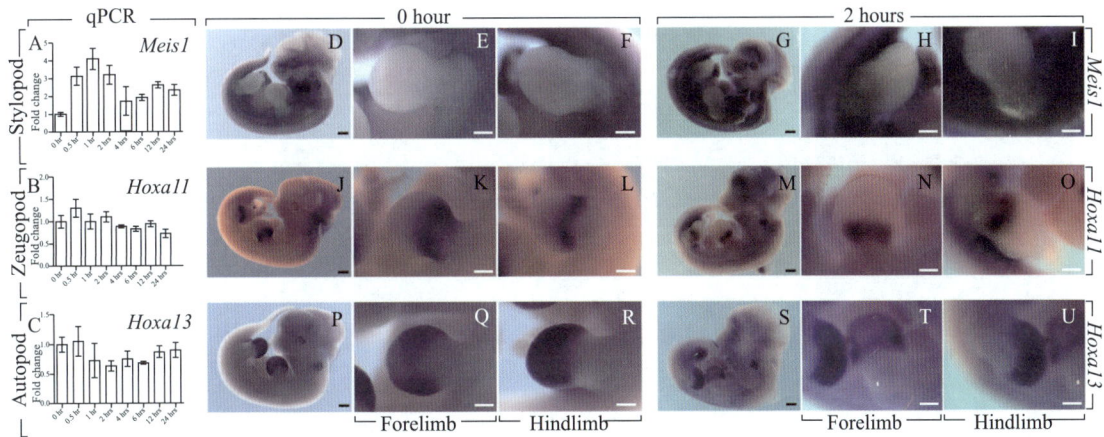

Fig. 7. Fate of the mesenchymal progenitors upon FGFR2b-ligands inactivation. (A–C) Quantification by qRT-PCR of *Meis1*, *Hoxa11* and *Hoxa13* expression in the developing forelimb at different time-points after Dox injection at E11. (D–U) WMISH at 0 hr (D–F; J–L; P–R) and 2 hours Dox-IP (G–I; M–O; S–U) for *Meis1* (D–I), *Hoxa11* (J–O) and *Hoxa13* (P–U). Note the increase in the expression of proximal/stylopod progenitor marker *Meis1* at the expense of the distal/autopod marker *Hoxa13*. Scale bars: D,J,P,G,M,S: 500 μm; E,F,K,L,Q,R,H,I,N,O,T,U: 300 μm.

WNT signaling [11] that is strongly expressed in the AER [18], were injected with Dox-IP at E11 and embryos were harvested one hour later and stained with X-gal substrate. As evidenced in Fig. 8A–B, control embryos (n = 5) showed a robust and specific expression of LacZ (Topgal) in the AER of their fore-and hindlimb buds. A few Topgal-positive cells were found in the adjacent dorsal and ventral ectoderm. By contrast, in DTG herozygous embryos (n = 7) the level of Topgal expression was drastically reduced in the AER (Fig. 8C,D), more so in the hindlimb compared to the forelimb buds (Fig. 7D). Similar results were observed 2 hours (n = 5, Fig. 8E,F) as well as 12 and 24 hours after Dox-IP (Fig. S3). These results indicate that FGFR2b-ligands attenuation has a rapid impact on WNT signaling in the AER. To seek further evidence that WNT signaling is reduced in AER of Dox-IP treated ([$R26^{rtTA/rtTA}$; Tg/Tg]) homozygous embryos, and assess its impact, we measured the level of Serine 552 phosphorylation on β-catenin protein (Fig. 8G,H). A significant decrease in the number of S552-β-catenin positive cells was noted both in the AER and the mesenchyme upon FGFR2b-ligands attenuation (3.9% *vs.* 1.3% in the AER and 5.4% *vs.* 3.3% in the mesenchyme, $P = 0.025$ and 0.028, respectively, n = 4 for each genotype). To determine the potential cause of this decrease in canonical WNT signaling, we examined *Dkk1* expression by WMISH, a known WNT signaling inhibitor, only to find a significant up-regulation in the AER of homozygous [$R26^{rtTA/rtTA}$; Tg/Tg] (n = 7) embryos when compared to controls (n = 6) (Fig. 8J,K). We also investigated the expression of *Dkk1*, *Wnt3*, *Wnt3a*, *Axin2* and *Fgf10* expression by qRT-PCR. *Dkk1* expression is increased at 0.5–2 hours confirming the WMISH result but then decreases progressively to very low levels in the following 4–24 hours Dox-IP period (Fig. 8L) making it unlikely that the sustained inhibition of WNT signaling following FGFR2b-ligands attenuation is due to this known WNT signaling inhibitor. We also found that *Wnt3*, a ligand expressed in the epithelium and critical for AER maintenance, is decreased between 2 and 12 hours only to reach normal levels at 24 hours (Fig. 8M). The expression of *Wnt3a*, expressed in the mesenchyme in mice progressively increases over time (Fig. 8N). Interestingly, levels of *Axin2* expression, used as a read out for global WNT signaling in the epithelium and mesenchyme fluctuated overtime (Fig. 8O), a likely reflection of the compensatory mechanisms at work following FGFR2b inactivation. Finally, the expression of *Fgf10* is quite stable for the time frame considered (Fig. 8P). To further determine which WNT signaling component were being altered, we performed a limited WNT signaling pathway qRT-PCR array in forelimbs of one E11 DTG embryos following 6 hours Dox-IP compared to 0 hr. We identified potential genes of interest that are up-regulated such as *Frzb*, *Pitx2, and Wnt8a* or down-regulated such as *Wnt2b*, *Wnt3a*, *Wnt3*, *Wnt7a*, *Wnt7b*, *Wnt16*, *Fzd4*, *Fzd8*, *Fzd9*, *Wif1*, and *Wisp1*. The expression of these genes was then carefully assessed by qRT-PCRs using individual forelimbs of four independent embryos in the control (0 hr) and experimental (6 h Dox-IP) group. The changes in all the above genes were statistically validated as shown in Table S2. Interestingly, *Wnt3*, *Wnt7a* and *Wnt7b* are all ligands expressed in the ectoderm [19] and could therefore account for the decreased WNT-AER signaling. In addition, other *Wnt* ligands are such as *Wnt2b*, *Wnt16* as well as the *Wnt* receptors *Fzd4*, *8*, *9* and the *Wnt* negative regulators *Wif1* and *Wisp1* are expressed mostly in the proximal mesenchyme during early limb development (see Table S2 and [19]

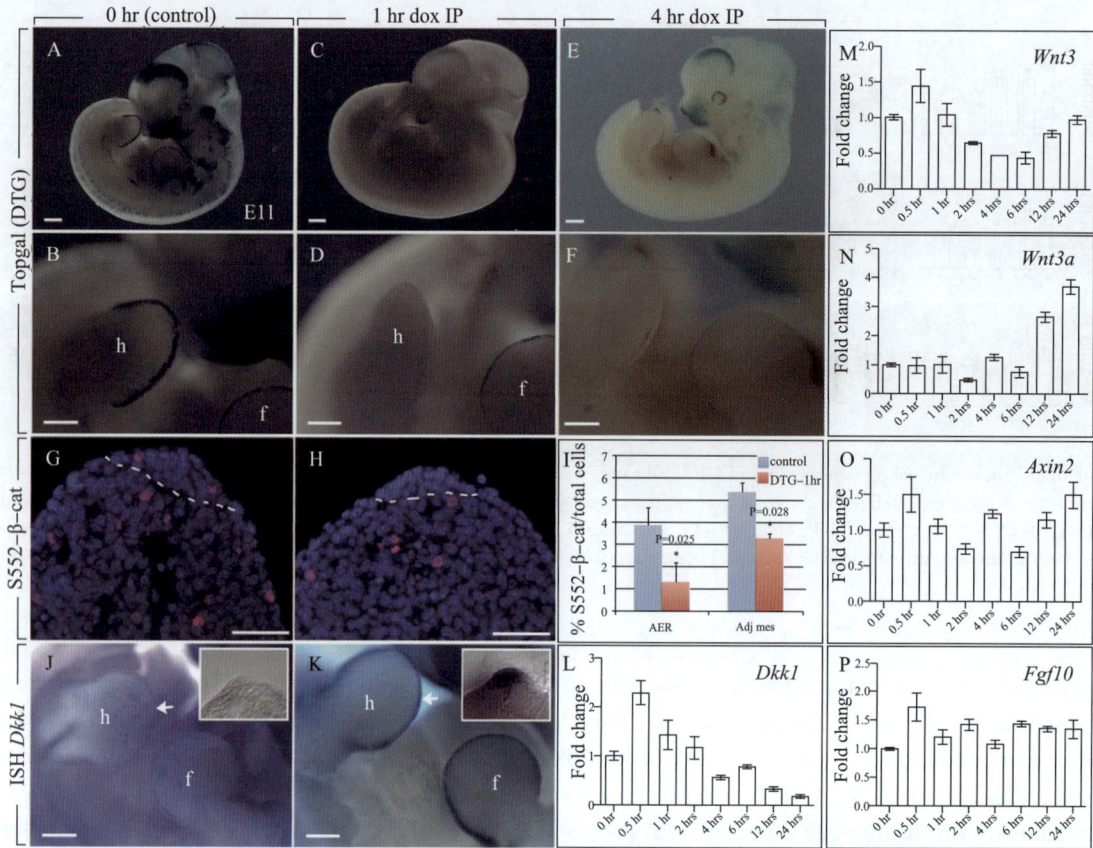

Fig. 8. Loss of canonical WNT signaling in the AER after attenuation of FGFR2b-ligands signaling. (A,B) *Topgal*, a WNT signaling reporter shows strong expression in the AER of both fore-and hind-limbs of the control embryos at E11. (C,F) *Topgal* expression is mostly lost in the AER of DTG embryos 1 hour (C,D) and 4 h (E,F) after Dox-IP injection at E11. (G–H) IF for the activated form of β-catenin in control (G) and DTG one hour after Dox-IP at E11 (H). Note the strong reduction in β-catenin positive cells in the AER and in the adjacent mesenchyme confirming the *Topgal* results. (I) Quantification of G and H. Bars represent the mean ± s.e.m. of at least 5 independent samples of each. Mann-Whitney non-parametric test was performed; *$P \leq 0.05$. (J,K) WMISH for *Dkk1* indicating robust up-regulation of the WNT inhibitor 1 hour after Dox-IP (K) compared to the control limbs (J). Insets in J and K are corresponding vibratome cross sections through the limb focusing on the AER. (B,D,F are high magnification of A,C,E respectively). (L–P) Quantification by qRT-PCR of *Dkk1* (L), *Wnt3* (M), *Wnt3a* (N), *Axin2* (O) and *Fgf10* (P) at different time points after single Dox-IP injection at E11. h, hindimb; f, forelimb. Scale bar A,C: 170 μm; B,D,H,I: 50 μm; E,F: 50 μm.

suggesting that transient inhibition of FGFR2b-ligands signaling has a profound impact on WNT signaling arising from both the epithelium and the mesenchymal compartment.

2.10 FGF10 directly activates β-catenin signaling

To confirm that FGF10 directly activates WNT/β-catenin, cells transfected with the β-catenin reporter TOPFLASH, were treated with FGF10, WNT3A or LiCl for 1 and 6 h (Fig. S4, n = 3 for each time point and condition). As expected, stimulation of cells with known WNT/β-catenin agonists (WNT3A and LiCl) led to an increase in activity. FGF10 treatment resulted in a 1.6 fold increase in β-catenin activity after 1 hr. Interestingly, this increased activity appeared transient since we did not observe an increase in β-catenin activity after 6 h of treatment. Stimulation of cells with both FGF10 and WNT3A together did not lead to a further increase in β-catenin whilst cells transfected with the control plasmid TOPFLASH were unresponsive to all growth factors (Data not shown).

2.11 Attenuation of FGFR2b-ligands signaling leads to cellular disorganization of β-catenin

The loss of WNT signaling in the AER led us to further examine the cellular localization of β-catenin. It has been reported previously that inactivation of β-catenin in the AER leads to the loss of this structure [20]. Examination of total β-catenin by western blot (n = 3 using independent embryos for each time point) in the whole embryo between 0 and

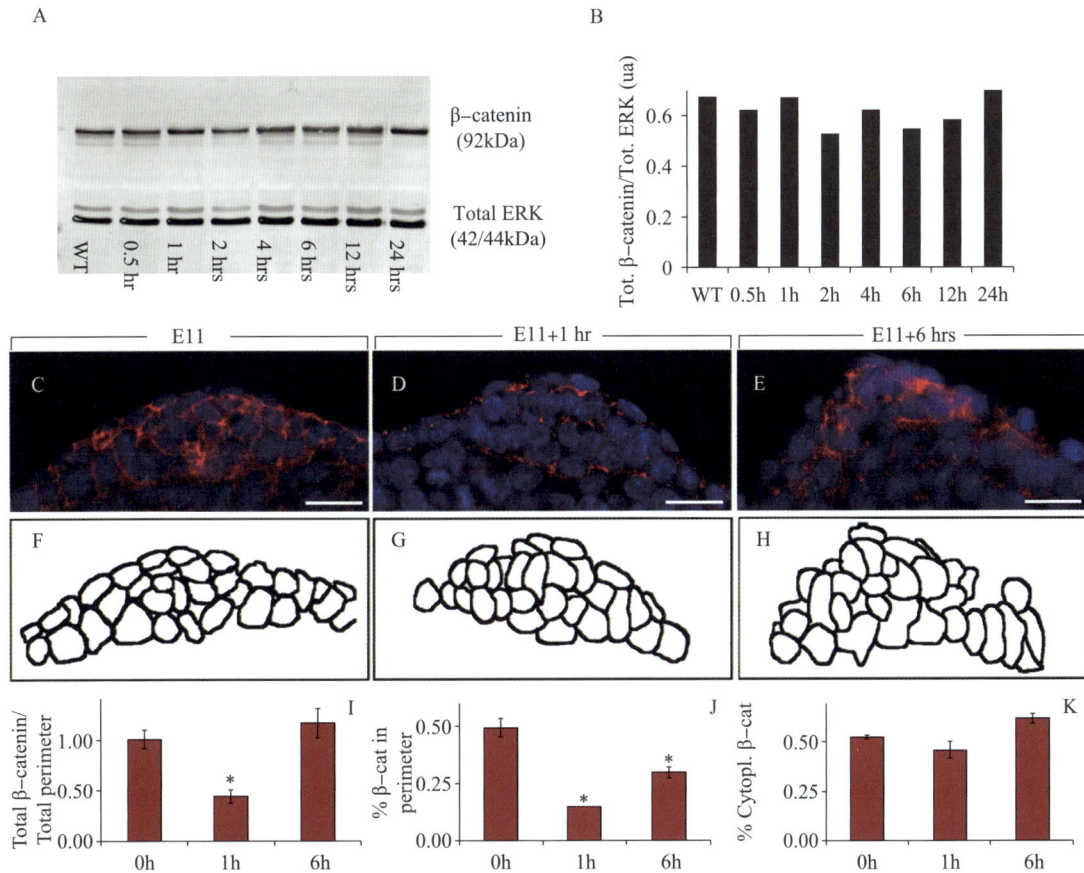

Fig. 9. Attenuation of FGFR2b-ligands signaling leads to cellular disorganization of β-catenin. (A) Western blot of total β-catenin using protein extract from whole embryo isolated at different time-points after a single Dox-IP injection at E11. (B) Quantification of the western blot shown in A. (C–E) IF for β-catenin in the AER of E11 forelimbs at 0 hr, (C), 1 h (D) and 6 h (E) after Dox-IP injection. (F–H) Schematic representation of the individual cells corresponding to the images shown in (C–E). (I–K) Quantification of total β-catenin in the AER (I), total β-catenin at the plasma membrane (J) and total β-catenin in the cytoplasmic compartment (K). Scale bars: A,C,E: 500 μm; B,D,F,F,J: 300 μm; C–E: 20 μm. doi:10.1371/journal.pone.0076248.g009

24 h (n = 1 for each time point) after Dox-IP showed that total β-catenin is not drastically affected over this time period (Fig. 9A,B) even though a trend towards a decrease in global β-catenin expression was observed after 2 h Dox-IP. Careful examination of β-catenin expression by IF at the level of the AER at 0, 1 and 6 h after Dox-IP (n = 3 for each time point) revealed significant changes in cellular localization of β-catenin (Fig. 9C–E). Quantification of the IF signal in the AER between 1 h Dox-IP and 0 h (n = 3 for each time point) indicated decrease in total β-catenin expression (measured as the ratio of total β-catenin per AER divided by total perimeter) (0.44±0.06 *vs.* 1.01±0.09, P = 0.005, Fig. 9I). This global decrease was associated with specific decrease in β-catenin expression at the membrane (measured as the ratio of β-catenin in the perimeter over total perimeter) (14%±0% *vs.* 49%±4%, P = 0.005 Fig. 9J) but unchanged total β-catenin in the cytoplasm (measured as the ratio of cytoplasmic β-catenin over total β-catenin) (0.46±0.04 *vs.* 0.53±0.01, P = 0.20; Fig. 9K). Altogether, these data are in harmony with impaired β-catenin signaling following massive β-catenin destabilization. Quantification of these parameters at 6 h (n = 3) indicated a restoration of the total level of β-catenin compared to 0 h (Fig. 9I). However, the presence of β-catenin in the plasma membrane pool is still reduced (30%±2% *vs.* 49%±4%, P = 0.005 Fig. 9J) while the percentile of cytoplasmic pool is unchanged (Fig. 9K) suggesting that the adhesive properties of the AER cells are still perturbed at 6 h Dox-IP.

3. Discussion

3.1 FGFs play important roles in vertebrate limb development

Fgf10 is the main *Fgfr2b ligand* expressed in the limb between E10.5 and E12.5 (Fig. S5) suggesting that our transgenic system allows addressing specifically the early role of FGF10 signaling to the Apical Ectodermal Ridge *via* FGFR2b. Indeed, FGFR2b acts as the main receptor for FGF10 during limb development as evidenced by the absence of limbs in both *Fgf10* and *Fgfr2b* null embryos [5,21,22]. Previous studies using [*Msx2-cre*; *Fgfr2*fl/fl] mouse to conditionally delete *Fgfr2* in the AER reported the loss of autopod in the forelimbs, and agenesis of hindlimbs [8–9]. However, these studies failed to delineate the role of FGFR2b signaling at different stages during the pre and post-limb bud induction, since the authors did not use an inducible Cre system. Here we show that these are rendered possible by the use of an inducible and reversible mouse model in which signaling induced by FGFR2b-ligands interaction is inhibited after exposure to Doxycycline. In this *in vivo* model, a transactivator rtTA is expressed constitutively from the ubiquitous *Rosa26 (R26)* locus, leading to the ubiquitous expression of soluble dominant-negative FGFR2b molecules. These act by sequestering all FGFR2b-activating ligands, including FGF10, away from cell surface-expressed FGFR2b. Indeed, soluble FGFR2b molecules are as effective as genetic ablation of *Fgfr2b* and *Fgf10* [3–5,10].

3.2 Attenuation of FGFR2b-ligands interaction using the DTG system is fully reversible

During previous studies of postnatal mammary gland and adult tooth, we found that our DTG system to attenuate FGFR2b-ligands signaling is not leaky and fully reversible [10,23]. The present results also support reversibility in soluble *Fgfr2b* expression and activity during embryonic development. First, Dox-IP administration to $R26^{rtTA/rtTA}$;Tg/Tg embryos at E11 leads to a peak in *soluble Fgfr2b* expression 6 hours later with a return to almost base line level at 24 hours. When the injection occurs at E8.5, this translates into inhibition of the AER in the forelimb (which is formed at E9.5, 24 h after the Dox-IP injection) and partially disrupted AER in the hindlimb (which is formed at E10, 36 h after the Dox-IP injection). We therefore conclude that the activity of the soluble FGFR2b protein in this particular allelic combination, which allows for the highest level of soluble FGFR2b expression, lasts around 36 hours. Second, Dox-IP administration to [$R26^{rtTA/rtTA}$; Tg/Tg] embryos at E7.5 leads to completely normal limb formation at E18.5 (data not shown), which is consistent with the 36 hours inhibition period ending at E9.0, 12 h and 24 h before the induction of the AER in the forelimb and hindlimb, respectively. Third, Dox-IP administration to [$R26^{rtTA/+}$; Tg/+] embryos at E8.5, an allelic combination which allows for the lowest level of soluble FGFR2b, leads to relatively mild forelimb defects (missing stylopod) and a nearly normal hindlimb (Fig. 10B) suggesting that the activity of soluble FGFR2b is minimal at 24 hours post Dox injection (at the time of forelimb AER induction) and absent at 36 hours post Dox-IP (at the time of hindlimb induction). We can therefore conclude that the expression of soluble *Fgfr2b* in our transgenic system is not leaky and is inducible and reversible. In addition, the different allelic combinations allow for a temporal inhibition of FGFR2b signaling up to 24 hours for the lower doses of *sFgfr2b* or up to 36 hours for the higher doses of *sFgfr2b* following a single Dox-IP injection. Interestingly, the comparison of the different phenotypes in heterozygous *versus* homozygous between transient (Fig. 2) and sustained (Fig. 1) FGFR2b-ligands attenuation suggests that as the dose of soluble FGFR2b increases, more proximal truncations are generated (Fig. 10B). This is the likely consequence of defective mesenchymal expansion occurring at the time of soluble FGFR2b induction. It seems therefore that soluble FGFR2b dosage is translated into a temporal factor that corresponds to the amplitude and duration of FGFR2b inhibition (Fig. 10C).

3.3 Inducible FGFR2b-ligands signaling attenuation allows the characterization of the early changes impacting the AER at the cellular and molecular levels

The rapid disappearance of the AER in response to FGFR2b-ligands signaling attenuation *via* the DTG system allows for fine dissection of the mechanisms by which interaction of FGFR2b with its ligands impacts the AER and its knock-on effects on adjacent mesenchymal cell population. The timing of FGFR2b-ligands inactivation in the DTG system is fundamentally different from the one aiming to conditionally delete *Fgfr2* expression using the *Cre/Lox* technol-

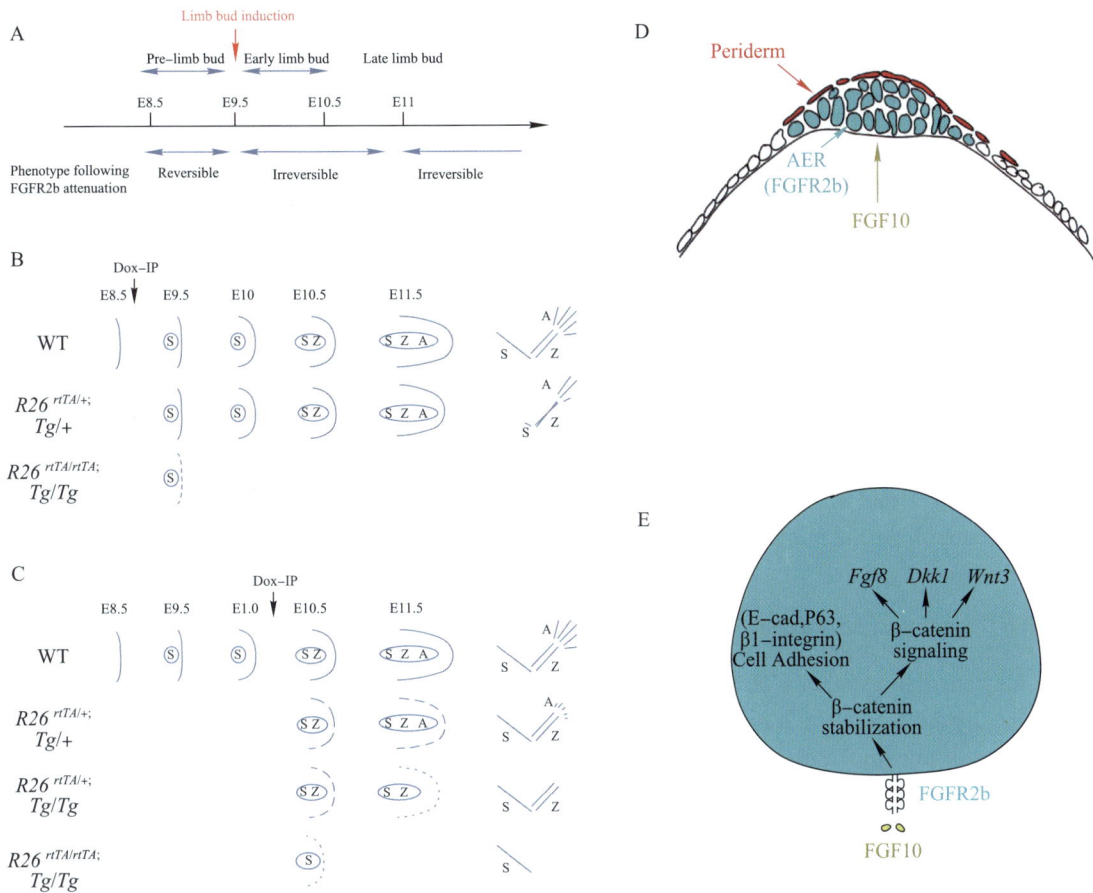

Fig. 10. Signaling induced by FGFR2b-ligands interactionplays a critical function to control the amplification of the mesenchymal progenitors throughout limb development. (A) FGFR2b-ligands signaling plays a major function in the amplification of the mesenchymal cells that will give rise to the stylopod prior to limb bud induction. Transient inhibition of FGFR2b-ligands signaling at E8.5 is compatible with limb induction while inhibition at E9.5, 10.5 and E11.5 leads to the irreversible loss of the AER. (B) Consequences of Dox-IP at E8.5. In double heterozygous embryos, the mesenchymal progenitors that are specified to give rise to the stylopod are not amplified but the AER is induced at E9.5 allowing the formation and amplification of the mesenchymal progenitors for the *zeugopod* and autopod. Note that in our model the efficiency of the AER may not be the same as in WT as progenitors for Z and A are not amplified at the same rate leading to corresponding skeletal defects. In double homozygous embryos, the stylopod progenitors are not amplified and the AER is not functional (dotted line) leading to limb agenesis. (C) Consequences of Dox-IP at E10/E10.5. In double heterozygous embryos, the AER is lightly affected at E10.5 (dotted lined with big distances between gaps) the progenitors for the autopod are partially amplified leading to shorter digits. In [$R26^{rTA/+}$; *Tg/Tg*] embryos, the AER is mildly affected at E10.5 (dotted line with smaller distance between gaps) the progenitors for the autopod are not amplified at all leading to absence of autopod. In double homozygous embryos, the AER is no longer functional at E10.5 (dotted line) and leads to absence of amplification of the mesenchymal progenitors for the zeugopod and autopod). (C) Schematic representation of the AER showing the superficial layer of periderm cells covering the compact AER cells expressing FGFR2b. FGFR2b ligand, FGF10 is expressed in the underlying mesenchyme. (D) FGFR2b signaling in the AER cells allows β-catenin stabilization. Such stabilization downstream of FGFR2b signaling, allows β-catenin function in cell adhesion and in signaling, *Fgf8*, *Dkk1* and *Wnt3* are known downstream targets.

ogy [8] [9]. In the latter, the function of existing FGFR2 molecules is unperturbed at the onset of genetic ablation. Thus, for example, it takes at least 24 hours, from the onset of Cre expression in the AER using the *Msx2-Cre* driver line, to see the complete disappearance of the AER (from stage 29 through 45 roughly corresponding to E10.5 through E11.5 [8]). The presented phenotypes therefore depend not only on the timing of Cre expression but also on the stability and turnover of the pre-existing FGFR2b molecules.

Previous reports have described the mechanism of AER formation; In particular Altabef *et al* [24–25] have shown that AER is formed by the convergence of ectodermal cells at the presumptive dorso-ventral boundary of developing limb buds. This convergence suggests that the AER-fated ectodermal cells acquire adhesive characteristics that distinguish them from their neighbors to eventually form a compact multistratified epithelium. The formation of protein complexes containing cytoskeletal proteins, receptor tyrosine kinase and extracellular ligands is often organized around Integrins and Cadherins [26]. Our study is the first to analyze the process of AER maintenance downstream of FGFR2b-ligands signaling. We found that β1-integrin, E-cadherin and P63 expression were reduced upon blockade of FGFR2b-ligands and this was accompanied by a relatively rapid and dramatic remodeling of the multilayered AER epithelium (Fig. 10E). It remains to be determined whether the AER cells lose their identity and become fully incorporated into the overlying ectoderm, or retain some of their original characteristics. Interestingly, embryos that are deficient in both α3 and α6-integrins exhibit a flattened ridge containing cells that lack the usual columnar morphology. In addition, epithelial cell proliferation was reduced in the AER and alterations of the basal lamina underlying the ectoderm were observed [27]. Overall, these results suggest that integrins are required for the organization and/or compaction of the ectodermal cells in the AER. Our results indicate that FGFR2b-ligands signaling to the AER potentially works upstream of integrins to control the formation and maintenance of such a distinctly differentiated structure. Rapid changes in cell morphology are usually caused by remodeling of cell cytoskeleton (e.g. microtubule reassembly) and so FGFR2b-ligands signaling could also lay directly upstream of these mechanisms.

In terms of appearance and structure, AER cells appear to recover 2 hours after a single Dox-IP dose at E11.0. However, data in Fig. 2, 3 and S2 indicate that this apparently "recovered" AER is not functional. The cellular and molecular processes controlling the initial recovery of the AER (2–4 h time point) during development are unknown and will require further investigation.

3.4 FGF and WNT signaling control de novo AER induction

Our data indicate that restoration of FGFR2b-ligands signaling alone is not sufficient to induce de novo AER signaling. Using the Topgal reporter as a read out for WNT signaling at different times after Dox-IP, we show that WNT-AER signaling is still impaired at the 24 hour time point, where soluble FGFR2b activity is negligible or absent. We propose that this is likely the underlying cause of lack of de novo AER induction. Interestingly, using the Msx2-Cre driver line, Lu et al. [8] reported that the impact of Fgfr2 deletion on the maintenance of the AER could be rescued by the concomitant expression of a stable form of β-catenin. Even though this rescue experiment does not allow us to conclude that WNT signaling activation after a transient inhibitory period (24 hour) is sufficient to induce de novo AER formation, it is likely that the stabilization of β-catenin at significant levels is the limiting factor for de novo AER formation (Fig. 10E). Furthermore it indicates that FGFR2b-ligands signaling to the AER, even though it is per se capable of directly activating β-catenin signaling, is not enough to provide sufficient activation of this pathway to re-engage the cellular and molecular mechanisms in the ectodermal cells to reform the specialized AER structure. In support of this conclusion, it has recently been shown that AER can be 're-induced' by insertion of WNT2b and FGF10-expressing cells into wounded chick limbs [28]. Interestingly, the AER can be re-induced only in wounded limbs but not in intact limbs. The molecular basis for this difference is unclear. Thus, FGF signaling in combination with WNT signaling are likely to be instructive in this process of de novo AER formation. However, our data also indicates a strict requirement for FGFR2b-ligands signaling in the maintenance of the AER throughout the bud stage of limb development (Fig. 2–3).

3.5 A series of WNT ligands are involved in WNT-AER signaling

Conclusions regarding the respective importance of FGF vs. β-catenin signaling in the AER can be drawn based on the limb phenotype of [Msx2-Cre; Fgfr2$^{flox/flox}$] vs. [Msx2-Cre; β-cat$^{flox/flox}$] mutant embryos, with the latter being more severe than the former. While both mutants exhibit hindlimb agenesis, the forelimbs are differently affected. [Msx2-Cre; Fgfr2f$^{lox/flox}$] exhibit autopod agenesis while [Msx2-Cre; β-cat$^{flox/flox}$] mutant forelimbs fail to form the zygopod (ulna radius) and the autopod. Our results indicate that FGF10/FGFR2b signaling can directly activate β-catenin signaling in HEK293T cell line. We believe that even if this is the case during limb development, other growth factors, such as WNT ligands, are also contributing to WNT-AER signaling. Wnt3 in mouse has been identified as a critical gene for AER maintenance during limb development [20]. The limb phenotype of [Msx2-Cre; Wnt3$^{flox/flox}$] animals ranged from completely normal to completely absent hindlimb, with most of the hindlimbs exhibiting mild to severe autopod defects or more extensive truncations that extended into more proximal segments of the limb. Interestingly, these mutant embryos exhibited seemingly normal forelimb, suggesting that other WNT ligands are at work to compensate for the lack of Wnt3 in the forelimb or that FGF10/FGFR2b signaling in the forelimb is enough to compensate the loss of Wnt3 expression. Suggesting slightly different activities for FGFR2b signaling in the hindlimb vs. forelimb during development, we found that Fgf8 expression is still maintained in the forelimb 24 h Dox-IP (Fig. 4H) while it is completely absent in the hindlimb at this stage. This conclusion appears to also apply for *Wnt3*. However, our *Wnt* qRT-PCR array showed that many proximal mesenchymal *Wnt* target genes are affected when FGFR2b-ligands signaling is hindered. The changes in these different genes disrupts β-catenin signaling, thus preventing the maintenance of the AER.

3.6 FGFR2b-ligands signaling is not sufficient to induce de novo AER formation after transient FGFR2b-ligands inactivation

Figure 8P indicated that the endogenous *Fgf10* expression level is not changed upon FGFR2b-ligands inactivation and Figure 3H shows that the expression of endogenous *Fgfr2b* is increased at 24 hours following Dox-IP administration. In addition, the analysis of the E18.5 limb phenotype following a single IP injection in pregnant females carrying E8.5 [$R26^{rtTA/+}$; *Tg/+*] embryos suggest that the expression/activity of soluble *Fgfr2b* is very low at the 24 hours time point (which corresponds to the induction of the AER in the forelimb at E9.5) and negligible at the 36 hours time point (which corresponds to the induction of the AER in the hindlimb at E10). Altogether these results are pointing out to a scenario where both FGF10 and FGFR2b are expressed normally 24 hours after Dox-IP with a residual presence of soluble FGFR2b at 24 h and complete absence of the inhibitor at 36 hrs. We conclude that the activation of the endogenous FGFR2b/FGF10 pathway is restored 24 h after Dox IP but that this is not sufficient for *de novo* AER formation. Interestingly, our results indicated that the WNT pathway is still inhibited after 24 h (Fig. S3) suggesting that one or several critical elements of the WNT pathway is/are missing at this stage, in spite of the restoration of the endogenous FGF10/FGFR2b pathway. In addition to the *Wnt* ligands described in the previous section, our results point out to irreversible cellular localization defects in β-catenin *per se* in the AER cells correlating with the continuous lack of β-catenin signaling observed in our studies. This is likely the main reason underlying the lack of *de novo* AER formation. The fate of these β-catenin-impaired AER cells is still unclear. It is possible that these cells are now incorporated as part of the squamous epithelium. At this point, restoration of endogenous FGF10/FGFR2b signaling during embryonic limb development is not sufficient to change the fate of these squamous epithelial cells back to the AER fate.

In conclusion, our findings show that FGFR2b-ligands signaling has critical stage-specific roles in maintaining the AER during limb development

4. Materials and methods

4.1 Ethics statement

Animal experiments were performed under the research protocols (31-08 and 31-11) approved by the Animal Research Committee at Children's Hospital Los Angeles and in strict accordance with the recommendations in the Guide for the Care and Use of Laboratory Animals of the National Institutes of Health. The approval identification for Children's Hospital Los Angeles is AAALAC A3276-01.

4.2 Animals

To generate the inducible mouse model, which expresses soluble FGFR2b, *CMV-Cre* mice were first crossed with $rtTA^{flox}$ mice [29]. The resulting $Rosa26^{rtTA/+}$ ($R26^{rtTA/+}$) mice were crossed with *tet(O)sFgfr2b* (*Tg*) mice [30] for several generations on a mixed background. Different allelic combinations for the $R26^{rtTA}$ and the *tet(O)Fgfr2b (Tg)* transgene ([$R26^{rtTA/+}$; *Tg/+*], [$R26^{rtTA/+}$; *Tg/Tg*] and [$R26^{rtTA/rtTA}$; *Tg/Tg*]) were generated to allow the expression of different levels of soluble FGFR2b following doxycycline (Dox) treatment. These mice are called DTG for simplification but the exact genotype is specified. The control embryos are the wild type and single transgenic littermates of the DTG embryos. The *Topgal* mouse model was previously described by DasGupta and Fuchs [11]. Animals were crossed and time pregnant females were either put on Dox food (Rodent diet with 0.0625% Dox, Harlan Teklad TD01306, Hayward, CA, USA) for several days or injected intraperitoneally (IP) with a single dose of Dox (1.5 mg/kg of mouse in PBS) at a specific developmental stage. Pregnant females were euthanized to collect embryos at different stages. All samples were fixed in 4% Paraformaldehyde (PFA) and dehydrated in successive batches of increasing ethanol concentration for further studies.

4.3 β-galactosidase staining

β-galactosidase/LacZ staining was performed as previously described [32,31]. Briefly, control-*Topgal* and DTG-*Top-*

gal embryos were fixed one hour in 4% PFA. Following the fixation, the embryos were washed in PBS and incubated overnight at 37 ℃ with the LacZ buffer solution containing 40 mg/ml of X-gal (rpi research products, Mount Prospect, IL, USA).

4.4 Bone and cartilage staining

Staining of the skeletons was carried out using minor modifications of a previously described protocol [32]. Embryos were collected at various stages, skinned and eviscerated. The samples were fixed in 95% ethanol for three days, changing ethanol every day and subsequently, stained for cartilage in 0.3% alcian blue 8GS in freshly prepared staining solution at room temperature for two days. Embryos were then washed in distilled water for two hours and stained in 0.2% alizarin red S in 0.5% KOH for several hours at room temperature. Samples were then washed for several days in 0.5% KOH to remove excess color and transferred to 0.5% KOH/20% glycerol and photographed under a Stemi2000 Zeiss microscope. For long-term storage, samples were transferred to 80% glycerol 0.5% KOH.

4.5 Immunofluorescence

Limb buds were embedded in paraffin sectioned and stained for various analyses. Apoptotic cells were detected by incorporation of terminal deoxynucleotidyltransferase mediated UTP nick-end labeling (TUNEL) using the "*In Situ* Cell Death Detection, Fluorescein kit (Roche Applied Science, Indianapolis, IN, USA) as recommended by the manufacturer or by immunofluorescent staining with cleaved caspase 3 antibody (1:100, cell signaling, Danvers, MA, USA). The total number of cells was scored in five photomicrographs (40× magnification) of four independent control and mutant limbs. A total number of 100 cells were counted per sample. For immunofluorescence staining, paraffin sections were stained with primary antibodies against mouse P63 (1:200, D9, Santa Cruz Biotechnologies, Santa Cruz, CA, USA) and β1 integrin (1:100, Millipore, Billerica, MA, USA), E-cadherin (1:100, BD Biosciences, Franklin Lakes, NJ, USA), Phosphohistone H3 (1:200, Cell signaling, Danvers, MA, USA) and β-catenin (1:200, BD Biosciences, San Jose, CA, USA). FITC-and Cy3-conjugated secondary antibodies (1:200, Jackson Immunor-esearch Laboratories, Inc., West Grove, PA, USA) were used; the slides were then mounted with Vectashield containing DAPI. Fluorescent images were acquired using a Leica monochrome camera attached to a Leica DM4000B microscope.

4.6 Quantification of fluorescence signal for β-catenin

The AER and cell boundaries were delineated manually with single-pixel lines using the pencil tool in Photoshop (Adobe Systems Inc., San Jose, CA). Then, internal and peripheral β-catenin signal were quantified using Fiji ImageJ [33] by first expanding the lines with 2 iterations of a morphological dilate operation and then measuring integrated intensity of the red channel that coincides with the expanded lines. Total integrated red intensity within the outer boundaries of the AER was also measured. To quantify the percent distance of cell boundaries covered by β-catenin, all boundary pixels and the pixels containing β-catenin staining above a threshold of 44 were summed separately.

4.7 Scanning electron microscopy

Mouse embryos were extracted quickly from the uteri, washed 6 times in filtered PBS and fixed in a solution of sodium cacodylate 0.1 M pH 7.6/glutaraldehyde 2% at room temperature for 1 hour and then overnight at 4 ℃. They were washed three times in 0.2 M sodium cacodylate for 1 hour at room temperature and transferred in a solution of sodium cacodylate 0.1 M pH7.6/OsO_4 0.1% for 1 hour at room temperature. After a 5-minute wash in distilled water, the embryos were dehydrated in graded ethanols (70% to 100%) and then in amyl acetate (30% to 100%). They were critical point dried in liquid carbon dioxide, mounted on aluminum stubs and coated with gold.

4.8 Transmission electron microscopy

The embryos were fixed with 2% glutaraldehyde in 0.1 M phosphate buffer, post-fixed with 1% OSO_4 in 0.1M phosphate buffer, dehydrated with ethanol, and embedded in Epon with careful orientation. Semi-thin sections were cut and stained with staining solution (azure II, methylene blue, sodium borate, and basic fuscin), and reviewed with a light microscope for selecting the areas of interest for ultrastructural examination. Ultra-thin sections were cut onto the grids and stained with uranyl acetate and a mixture of lead nitrate, lead acetate, and lead citrate. Ultrastructural images were examined with a transmission electron microscope (Morgagni 268), and selected areas were digitally recorded.

4.9　Whole mount in situ hybridization

Embryos were fixed in 4% PFA, washed and dehydrated. *In situ* hybridization was performed with digoxigenin labeled UTP RNA *Fgf8* (a gift from Dr. F. Mariani), *Wnt3* (a gift from Dr. A. McMahon), *Dkk1* (a gift from Dr. C. Niehrs), *Meis 1, Hoxa11, Hoxa13* (gift from Dr. X. Sun) AS probes according to a modified protocol from Bellusci *et al.* [34]. Sense probes were used to verify specific hybridization of the AS probes.

4.10　Real time PCR

RNA was extracted from either hindlimbs or forelimbs of transgenic animals injected with Doxycycline using the iNtRON Biotechnology, Inc. easy-spin™ Total RNA Extraction Kit. RNA (500 ng/ml) was reverse-transcribed into cDNA using Transcriptor First Strand cDNA Synthesis Kit (Roche Applied Science) according to the manufacturer's instructions. cDNA (1 mg) was used for dual color Hydrolysis Probe-Universal probe library based real time PCR, using the LightCycler 480 from Roche Applied Science. *Gapdh* assay commercially available from Roche Applied Science was used as reference gene. See the supplemental data section for the details on the primers and Roche Applied Science Universal probes used for each of the assayed genes (Table S1).

4.11　Statistical analysis

Statistical analyses were performed using Statview software version 4.57.0.0. All data are expressed as means ± SEM. For each of the experiments, at least n = 4 of each condition was used. Comparisons of the changes between controls and DTG were performed using the nonparametric Mann-Whitney test. A $P < 0.05$ was considered significant.

Supporting information

Supporting information to this article can be found online at https://doi.org/10.1371/journal.pone.0076248.

References

[1] Furniss D, Kan SH, Taylor IB, *et al.* Genetic screening of 202 individuals with congenital limb malformations and requiring reconstructive surgery[J]. Journal of Medical Genetics, 2009, 46(11): 730-735.

[2] Saunders JW. The proximo-distal sequence of origin of the parts of the chick wing and the role of the ectoderm[J]. Journal of Experimental Zoology, 1948, 108(3): 363-403.

[3] Sekine K, Ohuchi H, Fujiwara M, *et al.* Fgf10 is essential for limb and lung formation[J]. Nature Genetics, 1999, 21(1): 138-141.

[4] De Moerlooze L, Spencer-Dene B, Revest JM, *et al.* An important role for the IIIb isoform of fibroblast growth factor receptor 2 (FGFR2) in mesenchymal-epithelial signalling during mouse organogenesis[J]. Development, 2000, 127(3): 483-492.

[5] Mariani FV, Ahn CP, Martin GR. Genetic evidence that FGFs have an instructive role in limb proximal-distal patterning[J]. Nature, 2008, 453(7193): 401-405.

[6] Fernandez-Teran M, Ros MA. The Apical Ectodermal Ridge: morphological aspects and signaling pathways[J]. International Journal of Developmental Biology, 2008, 52(7): 857-871.

[7] Celli G, LaRochelle WJ, Mackem S, *et al.* Soluble dominant-negative receptor uncovers essential roles for fibroblast growth factors in multi-organ induction and patterning[J]. Embo Journal, 1998, 17(6): 1642-1655.

[8] Lu P, Yu Y, Perdue Y, *et al.* The apical ectodermal ridge is a timer for generating distal limb progenitors[J]. Development, 2008, 135(8): 1395-1405.

[9] Yu K, Ornitz DM. FGF signaling regulates mesenchymal differentiation and skeletal patterning along the limb bud proximodistal axis[J]. Development, 2008, 135(3): 483-491.

[10] Parsa S, Ramasamy SK, De Langhe S, *et al.* Terminal end bud maintenance in mammary gland is dependent upon FGFR2b signaling[J]. Developmental Biology, 2008, 317(1): 121-131.

[11] DasGupta R, Fuchs E. Multiple roles for activated LEF/TCF transcription complexes during hair follicle development and differentiation[J]. Development, 1999, 126(20): 4557-4568.

[12] Rohmann E, Brunner HG, Kayserili H, *et al.* Mutations in different components of FGF signaling in LADD syndrome[J]. Nature Genetics, 2006, 38(4): 414-417.

[13] Kishimoto TK, Oconnor K, Lee A, *et al.* Cloning of the beta subunit of the leukocyte adhesion proteins: homology to an extracellular matrix receptor defines a novel supergene family[J]. Cell, 1987, 48(4): 681-690.

[14] Carroll DK, Carroll JS, Leong CO, *et al.* p63 regulates an adhesion programme and cell survival in epithelial cells[J]. Nat Cell Biol, 2006, 8(6): 551-561.

[15] Laurikkala J, Mikkola ML, James M, *et al.* p63 regulates multiple signalling pathways required for ectodermal organogenesis and differentiation[J]. Development, 2006, 133(8): 1553-1563.

[16] Rebustini IT, Patel VN, Stewart JS, *et al.* Laminin alpha 5 is necessary for submandibular gland epithelial morphogenesis and influences FGFR expression through beta 1 integrin signaling[J]. Developmental Biology, 2007, 308(1): 15-29.

[17] Therapontos C, Erskine L, Gardner ER, *et al.* Thalidomide induces limb defects by preventing angiogenic outgrowth during early limb formation[J]. Proceedings of the National Academy of Sciences of the United States of America, 2009, 106(21): 8573-8578.

[18] Nam J-S, Park E, Turcotte TJ, *et al.* Mouse R-spondin2 is required for apical ectodermal ridge maintenance in the hindlimb[J]. Developmental Biology, 2007, 311(1): 124-135.

[19] Witte F, Dokas J, Neuendorf F, *et al.* Comprehensive expression analysis of all Wnt genes and their major secreted antagonists during mouse limb development and cartilage differentiation[J]. Gene Expression Patterns, 2009, 9(4): 215-223.

[20] Barrow JR, Thomas KR, Boussadia-Zahui O, *et al.* Ectodermal Wnt3/beta-catenin signaling is required for the establishment and maintenance of the apical ectodermal ridge[J]. Genes & Development, 2003, 17(3): 394-409.

[21] Mailleux AA, Spencer-Dene B, Dillon C, *et al.* Role of FGF10/FG-FR2b signaling during mammary gland development in the mouse embryo[J]. Development, 2002, 129(1): 53-60.

[22] Ohuchi H, Hori Y, Yamasaki M, *et al.* FGF10 acts as a major ligand for FGF receptor 2 IIIb in mouse multi-organ development[J]. Biochemical and Biophysical Research Communications, 2000, 277(3): 643-649.

[23] Parsa S, Kuremoto K, Seidel K, *et al.* Signaling by FGFR2b controls the regenerative capacity of adult mouse incisors[J]. Development, 2010, 137(22): 3743-3752.

[24] Altabef M, Clarke JDW, Tickle C. Dorso-ventral ectodermal compartments and origin of apical ectodermal ridge in developing chick limb[J]. Development, 1997, 124(22): 4547-4556.

[25] Altabef M, Logan C, Tickle C, *et al.* Engrailed-1 misexpression in chick embryos prevents apical ridge formation but preserves segregation of dorsal and ventral ectodermal compartments[J]. Developmental Biology, 2000, 222(2): 307-316.

[26] Juliano RL. Signal transduction by cell adhesion receptors and the cytoskeleton: Functions of integrins, cadherins, selectins, and immunoglobulin-superfamily members[J]. Annual Review of Pharmacology and Toxicology, 2002, 42: 283-323.

[27] De Arcangelis A, Mark M, Kreidberg J, *et al.* Synergistic activities of alpha 3 and alpha 6 integrins are required during apical ectodermal ridge formation and organogenesis in the mouse[J]. Development, 1999, 126(17): 3957-3968.

[28] Satoh A, Makanae A, Wada N. The apical ectodermal ridge (AER) can be re-induced by wounding, wnt-2b, and fgf-10 in the chicken limb bud[J]. Developmental Biology, 2010, 342(2): 157-168.

[29] Belteki G, Haigh J, Kabacs N, *et al.* Conditional and inducible transgene expression in mice through the combinatorial use of Cre-mediated recombination and tetracycline induction[J]. Nucleic Acids Research, 2005, 33(5): e51.

[30] Hokuto I, Perl AKT, Whitsett JA. Prenatal, but not postnatal, inhibition of fibroblast growth factor receptor signaling causes emphysema[J]. Journal of Biological Chemistry, 2003, 278(1): 415-421.

[31] Al Alam D, Green M, Irani RT, *et al.* Contrasting Expression of Canonical Wnt Signaling Reporters TOPGAL, BATGAL and Axin2(LacZ) during Murine Lung Development and Repair[J]. Plos One, 2011, 6(8): e23139.

[32] Hajihosseini MK, Lalioti MD, Arthaud S, *et al.* Skeletal development is regulated by fibroblast growth factor receptor 1 signalling dynamics[J]. Development, 2004, 131(2): 325-335.

[33] Schindelin J, Arganda-Carreras I, Frise E, *et al.* Fiji: an open-source platform for biological-image analysis[J]. Nature Methods, 2012, 9(7): 676-682.

[34] Bellusci S, Henderson R, Winnier G, *et al.* Evidence from normal expression and targeted misexpression that bone morphogenetic protein-4 (Bmp-4) plays a role in mouse embryonic lung morphogenesis[J]. Development, 1996, 122(6): 1693-1702.

Type 1 fibroblast growth factor receptor in cranial neural crest cell-derived mesenchyme is required for Palatogenesis

Cong Wang, Fen Wang, Xiaokun Li

Cleft palate is the most common congenital craniofacial defect in human, which is often associated with cleft lip. It affects about 0.1% newborns in America according to the Center for Diseases Control and Prevention. The palate is formed by fusion of the primary and secondary palates. It consists of two structural parts, the anterior bony hard palate and the posterior muscular soft palate. The primary palate is derived from the posterior protrusion of the medial nasal process, and the secondary palate develops from bilateral outgrowth of the maxillary process [1, 2]. Palate development is a multistep process that involves bilateral palatal shelf growth beside the tongue, elevation of the palatal shelves that grow toward the midline, fusion of palatal shelves at the midline to form the medial edge epithelium (MEE),[5] degeneration of the MEE, and disappearance of the midline epithelial seam [1, 3]. The maxillary shelves are mainly composed of the cranial neural crest (CNC)-derived ecto-mesenchymal cells surrounded by a thin layer of pharyngeal ectoderm-derived epithelial cells [4–7]. The CNC cells are a subset of neural crest cells (NCCs) that are pluripotent and are derived from the lateral ridges of the neural plate during early stages of embryogenesis. During craniofacial development, CNC cells migrate ventrolaterally and populate in the branchial arches, which then contribute extensively to the formation of head and neck mesenchymal structures, including the palate. Defects either in facial mesenchyme patterning and growth or in epithelium fusion result in cleft palate. Several reciprocal epithelial-mesenchymal signaling axes, including the fibroblast growth factor (FGF), bone morphogenetic protein (BMP), Sonic hedgehog (SHH), and Wnt signaling pathways, have been show to play important roles in the migration and proliferation of CNC cells [1, 8–10].

The FGF family consists of 18 tyrosine kinase receptor-mediated members that regulate a broad spectrum of cellular activities [11]. FGF elicits its regulatory signals *via* binding and activating the FGF receptor (FGFR) tyrosine kinases encoded by four highly homologous genes. In the palate, FGF and FGFR isoforms are expressed in a spatiotemporally specific manner and constitute a directional regulatory axis between the stromal and epithelial compartments, regulating palate development [12]. In palate shelves, *Fgf10* expression is restricted to the mesenchyme and *Fgfr2b* expression to the overlying epithelium. Germ line ablation of *Fgf10* or epithelium-specific deletion of *Fgfr2b* leads to cleft palate with impaired palatal shelf outgrowth [13, 14]. Cell proliferation in both epithelium and mesenchyme compartments is reduced in the absence of either *Fgf10* or *Fgfr2b*, suggesting that ablation of the FGF10-FGFR2 signaling axis causes loss of signals from the epithelium back to the underlying mesenchyme, which regulate mesenchymal proliferation. In addition, the FGF signaling intensity during palatogenesis is delicately balanced. Expression of a constitutively active FGFR2 mutant in the epithelium increases palatal shelf mesenchyme proliferation and delays elevation of the shelves, resulting in cleft palate and other craniofacial disorders [15, 16]. Disruption of Sprouty 2 (*Spry2*), a negative feedback regulator of FGF signaling pathways, results in abnormal palate formation [17]. In contrast, ablation of *Fgfr1* in the epithelium with K14 promoter driven *Cre* does not cause major craniofacial defects [18]. The major cell population in the palate shelf mesenchyme is derived from CNC cells, which expresses *Fgfr1* [19]. Although it has been reported that embryos with *Fgfr1* ablation in NCCs have cleft palate [20], no detailed characterization has been done on how ablation of *Fgfr1* in NCCs leads to cleft palate. As FGFR1 is important for patterning in the pharyngeal region [20], its mutations and haploinsufficiency in humans are associated with cleft palate [21–23].

To investigate how mesenchymal FGFR1 regulates craniofacial development, *Fgfr1* alleles were tissue-specifically ablated in NCCs by crossing mice bearing floxed *Fgfr1* (*Fgfr1*flox) and *Wnt1-Cre* (*Wnt1*Cre) transgenic alleles. Ablation of *Fgfr1* in NCCs led to cleft palate, cleft lip, and other severe craniofacial defects. Detailed characterization revealed that ablation of *Fgfr1* in NCCs did not abrogate CNC cell contribution to the palate shelf mesenchyme. However, it upset cell signaling in the medial nasal process and maxillary process areas, and it delayed cell proliferation in both the mesenchyme and epithelium of palatal shelves. The mutant palate shelves failed to elevate during palatogenesis. In addition, although it did not fully prevent the fusion process, it compromised the deterioration of the MEE. Together with the report that loss of the mesenchymal-epithelial FGF10-FGFR2IIIb signaling axis affects cell proliferation in both epithelium and mesenchyme [13], the results indicate that the reciprocal FGF signaling axis between the palate mesenchyme and epithelium is important for the growth and elevation of palate shelves. This is the first report on the mechanism by which mesenchymal FGFR1 signaling regulates palatogenesis.

1. Materials and methods

1.1 Animals and isolation of tissues

All animals were housed at the Program of Animal Resources, Institute of Biosciences and Technology, Texas A&M Health Science Center, and were handled in accordance with the principles and procedures in the Guide for the Care and Use of Laboratory Animals. All experimental procedures were approved by the Institutional Animal Care and Use Committee. Mice carrying the $Wnt1^{Cre}$ transgenic alleles [24], $ROSA26^{lacZ}$ [25] reporter allele, and $Fgfr1^{flox}$ allele [26] were maintained and genotyped as described previously.

1.2 Dissection and in vitro culture of palate shelves

Palatal shelves were dissected from E13.5 embryos. Two palatal shelves were placed on 8-μm-pore size transwell culture plates (BD Biosciences) with their MEE placed in close apposition without apparent distortion of their tissue shape. The paired palate shelves were cultured for 2 days at 37℃ in DMEM supplemented with 1% penicillin/streptomycin [27]. Similar ex vivo cultures were carried with heads without the tongue and mandible from E13.5 embryos [28].

1.3 Histological and immunohistochemical analyses

Prenatal mouse heads were fixed in 4% paraformaldehyde solution for 2 h at 4℃. The fixed tissues were serially dehydrated with ethanol, embedded in paraffin, and sectioned at 5-μm thickness according to standard procedures. Immunohistochemical analyses were performed on paraffin sections mounted on Superfrost/Plus slides (Fisher). Antigens were retrieved by boiling in citrate buffer (10 mM) for 20 min at 100℃ or as suggested by the manufacturers. All sections were incubated with primary antibodies diluted in PBS at 4℃ overnight. The mouse anti-p63 (1:200) and mouse anti-pan-cytokeratin (1:200) antibodies were purchased from Santa Cruz Biotechnology, and rabbit anti-E-cadherin (1:200), rabbit anti-pSmad1/5/8 (1:200), and rabbit anti-vimentin (1:200) antibodies were purchased from Cell Signaling Technology. Specifically bound antibodies were detected with FITC-conjugated secondary antibodies (Invitrogen) and visualized with a Zeiss LSM 510 confocal microscope. To-Pro3 was used for nuclear counterstaining.

For LacZ staining, the tissues were first lightly fixed with 0.2% glutaraldehyde for 30 min and then incubated overnight with 1 mg/ml X-Gal at room temperature. The tissues were post-fixed with 4% paraformaldehyde at room temperature for 1 h after a 10-min PBS wash. The tissues were then dehydrated, paraffinembedded, and sectioned according to regular procedures.

1.4 Gene expression analysis

Total RNA was extracted with the RiboPure RNA isolation reagent (Ambion, TX). Reverse transcription was carried out with SuperScript III (Invitrogen) and random primers. Real time PCR was performed on Mx3000 (Stratagene), using the SYBR Green JumpStart Taq ReadyMix (Sigma) with pairs of primers specific for each transcript and following the manufacturer's protocol. The ratio between expression levels in the two samples was calculated by relative quantification, using β-actin as a reference transcript for normalization. The primer sequences are listed in Table 1.

For in situ hybridization, paraffin-embedded tissue sections were rehydrated followed by digestion with 20 μg/ml protease K for 7 min at room temperature. After prehybridization at 65℃ for 2 h, the hybridization was carried out by overnight incubation at 65℃ with 0.5 μg/ml digoxigenin-labeled RNA probes for the indicated genes. Nonspecifically bound probes were removed by washing four times with 0.1× digoxigenin washing buffer at 60℃ for 30 min. Specifically bound probes were later detected using alkaline phosphatase-conjugated anti-digoxigenin antibody (Roche Applied Science).

Table 1.　Primer sequences for real time RT-PCR

Gene	Forward primer	Reverse primer
Shh	5'-ACATCCACTGTTCTGTGAAAGCA-3'	5'-TCTCGATCACGTAGAAGACCTTCTTG-3'
Ptch	5'-TCAACCCAGCCGACCCAGATT-3'	5'-CCCTGAAGTGTTCATACATTTGCT-3'
Wnt1	5'-CATTTGCACTCTTGGCGCAT-3'	5'-AAGATCGTCAACCGAGGCTG-3'
Notch1	5'-CCCACTGTGAACTGCCCTAT-3'	5'-CACCCATTGACACACACACA-3'
Gli1	5'-GAAGGAATCCGTGTGCCATT-3'	5'-GGATCTGTGTAGCGCTTGGT-3'
Gli2	5'-GGCACCAACCCTTCAGACTA-3'	5'-CTGAGCTGCTCCTGGAGTTG-3'
Gli3	5'-GTCAGCCCTGCGGAATACTA-3'	5'-GGAACCACTTGCTGAAGAGC-3'
BMP2	5'-AAGGAGGAGGCGAAGA-3'	5'-CTGAGTGCCTGCGGTACAGAT-3'
BMP4	5'-AGGAGGAGGAGGAAGAGCAG-3'	5'-TGTGATGAGGTGTCCAGGAA-3'
BMP7	5'-ACCTGGGCTTACAGCTCTCTG-3'	5'-CGGAAGCTGACGTACAGCTCATG-3'
TGFþ	5'-CTAATGGTGGACCGCAACAA-3'	5'-GTACAACTCCAGTGACGTCA-3'
CK14	5'-CTTCCCAATTCTCCTCATCC-3'	5'-GGGCTCTTCCAGCAGTATCT-3'
Jagged1	5'-GCACCCGCGACGAGTGTGAT-3'	5'-TCCCAGGCCTCCACCAGCAA-3'
Wnt3a	5'-CGATCTGGTGGTCCTTGGCTGT-3'	5'-AGCGGAGGCGATGGCATGGA-3'
Msx1	5'-CTCTCGGCCATTTCTCAGTC-3'	5'-TACTGCTTCTGGCGGAACTT-3'
Ptx1	5'-CTCAACGCTTGCCAGTACAA-3'	5'-GGGTCTGGAAAAAGCAAACA-3'
Etv5	5'-GGGAGAGACAAAAACCACCA-3'	5'-ATGGGTGTGCAGTTTCTTCC-3'

The antisense riboprobe of FGFR1 was generated by *in vitro* transcription using T3 RNA polymerase with the Xba I-linearized pKS+ΔFGFR1 vector (generous gift from Dr. Juha Partanen) [26]. The antisense riboprobe of TGFβ3 was generated by *in vitro* transcription using T3 RNA polymerase with the EcoRI-linearized pSK-TGFβ3 vector (kindly provided by Dr. Rulang Jiang) [29].

2.　Results

2.1　Ablation of Fgfr1 in NCCs causes cleft palate

Mutations in *Fgfr1* have been found to be associated with craniofacial malformation, including cleft palate in human. *Fgfr1* is expressed in CNC-derived mesenchymal cells during palatogenesis [19]. To investigate how FGFR1 signaling in CNC cells affected craniofacial development, the *Fgfr1* alleles were tissue-specifically ablated in NCCs by crossing the mice bearing *Fgfr1^flox* and *Wnt1Cre* alleles. Although they appeared to be morphologically normal at E10.5, *Fgfr1* conditional knock-out (*Fgfr1^cKO*) mutant embryos had a slightly reduced frontonasal prominence and maxillary processes (Fig. 1A). LacZ staining of the *Fgfr1^cKO* and wild type embryos bearing the *ROSA26^lacZ* reporter demonstrated that, compared with the *Fgfr1* wild type control at this stage, the CNC cell participation in the frontonasal prominence was significantly reduced in mutant embryos (Fig. 1B), which was in line with the report that FGFR1 is required for CNC cell patterning [20]. In contrast, LacZ staining of coronal sections of E10.5 embryos showed no difference in *ROSA-26^lacZ* reporter activation between wild type and mutant embryos (Fig. 1B, insets), indicating neural tube formation was not affected in mutant embryos.

The structures constituted by fused midline nasal prominence were missing in mutant embryos at the E14.5 and neonatal stage (Fig. 1C). Completely cleft primary and secondary palates as well as cleft lip were readily seen. Partially formed palate rugae were observed in mutant mice at the neonatal stage. The palatal shelves were widely separated in mutant mice, allowing direct view of the underlying presphenoid bone. In addition, the mutant embryos also exhibited

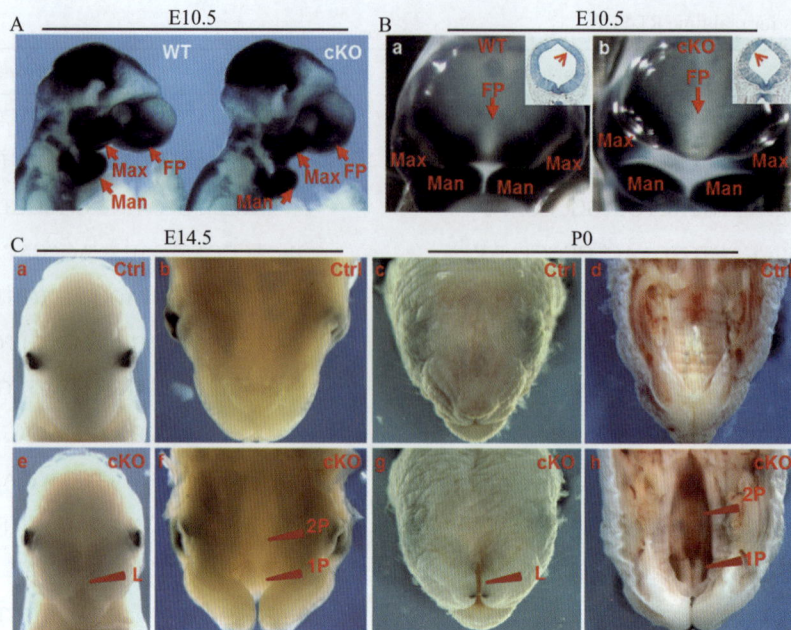

Fig. 1. Ablation of *Fgfr1* in NCCs cells leads to cleft palate. (A) and (B) whole mount lacZ staining showed distribution of *Wnt1^Cre* expressing NCCs in the head of embryonic (E) day 10.5 embryos bearing the *ROSA26^lacZ* reporter and *Wnt1^Cre* alleles. (B) insets in coronal sections of E10.5 embryos bearing the ROSA26 reporter, *Wnt1^Cre*, and the indicated *Fgfr1* alleles were LacZ-stained and eosin-counterstained. (C) mouse heads were collected at E14.5 or postnatal (P) day 0 for frontal facial morphology analyses. *1P*, primary palate; *2P*, secondary palate; *L*, lip; *Man*, mandibular process; *Max*, maxillary process; *MT*, mesencephalic tegmentum; *FP*, frontonasal prominence; *Ctrl*, control; *cKO*, Fgfr1 conditional knock-out; *WT*, Fgfr1 wild type.

other severe orofacial dysformation, including tooth bud defect and micrognathia. Embryos bearing one conditional null *Fgfr1* allele, one or two *Fgfr1flox* alleles without the *Cre* allele, or one *Cre* allele were indistinguishable from wild type embryos, and hereafter were defined as controls.

2.2 Ablation of Fgfr1 in NCCs does not disrupt participation of CNC cells in palate shelves

To characterize the palate defects in *Fgfr1^cKO* embryos, coronal sections of E13.5, E14.5, and E15.5 embryos were H&E-stained for histological analyses. At the stage of E14.5, the anterior portion of the secondary palate in *Fgfr1^flox* embryos was undergoing fusing process, and the MEE was formed, whereas the posterior portion had finished the elevation but was still undergoing expansion processes. The mutant palate shelves, however, were still growing downward at both anterior and posterior positions (Fig. 2A, B). The palate shelves failed to elevate and finish the fusion processes even at E15.5 stages. Although mesoderm-derived mesenchymal cells also contribute to palate shelves as a minor cell population, the majority of palate shelf mesenchymal cells were derived from the CNC [30, 31]. Lineage tracing with the *ROSA26^lacZ* reporter allele revealed that similar to the *Fgfr1^flox* palate shelves, the majority of mesenchymal cells in mutant palate shelves were derived from *Wnt1^Cre*-expressing CNC cells (Fig. 3A, B). However, there were a fraction of cells adjacent to the epithelial cells that were not X-Gal-labeled. The origin of these cells remains to be determined. *In situ* hybridization revealed that *Fgfr1* expression in the palate shelf mesenchyme was diminished (Fig. 3C). In addition, all cells in the mutant palate shelf mesenchyme were vimentin-positive (Fig. 3D), indicating mesenchymal cells.

The size of mutant palate shelves appeared to be smaller than the control at E13.5 (Fig. 2). To determine whether cell proliferation was a causal factor for small palate shelves, BrdU incorporation assays were employed to assess the proliferating cell numbers in palate shelves at the stages of E12.5 to E14.5 (Fig. 4). The results showed that cell proliferation in the epithelium of anterior palate shelves and the mesenchyme at the posterior shelves were reduced at E12.5–13.5, although no differences were found in the anterior mesenchyme and the posterior epithelium in palate shelves (Fig. 4 A, B). However, both the epithelium and mesenchyme of anterior and the mesenchyme of posterior *Fgfr1^cKO* palate shelves had a higher proliferation than control at E14.5, although the posterior epithelium of *Fgfr1^cKO* palate shelves had a similar proliferation activity as the control (Fig. 4C). Thus, it appeared that the cell proliferation in *Fgfr1^cKO* palate shelves was delayed, rather than simply reduced. The data suggest that lack of FGFR1 signals in CNC-derived mesen-

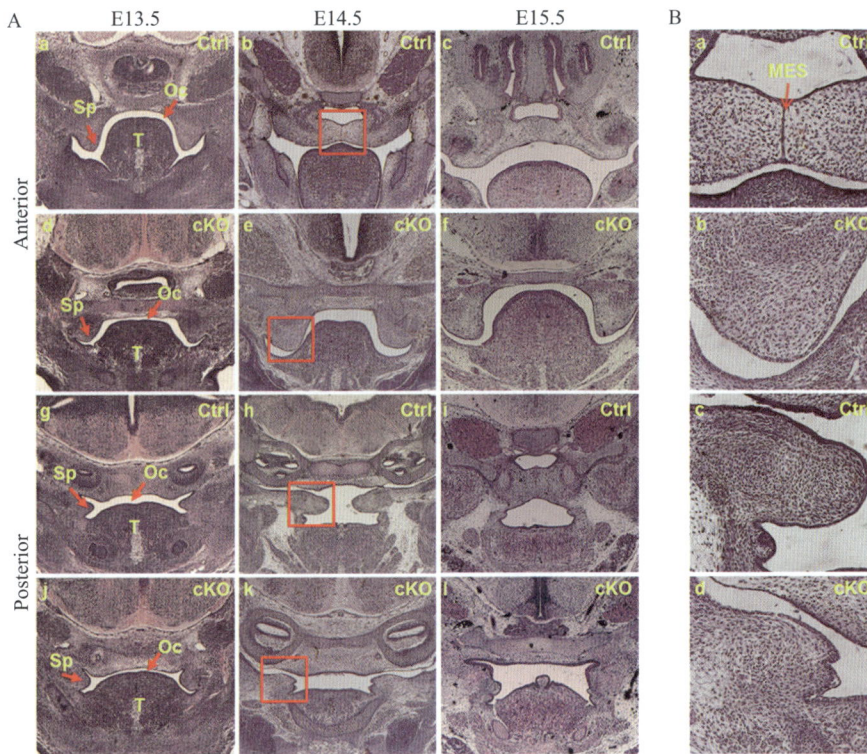

Fig. 2. Failure of palate shelf elevation in *Fgfr1*cKO embryos during palatogenesis. (A) coronal sections of anterior and posterior portions of control or *Fgfr1*cKO embryos collected from the indicated stages were H&E-stained for tissue histological analyses. Unlike control embryos, *Fgfr1*cKO palate shelves failed to elevate and fuse. (B) enlarged pictures of the boxed areas in (A) *Ctrl*, control; *MES*, medline epithelial seam; *Oc*, oral cavity; *Sp*, secondary palate shelf; *T*, tongue.

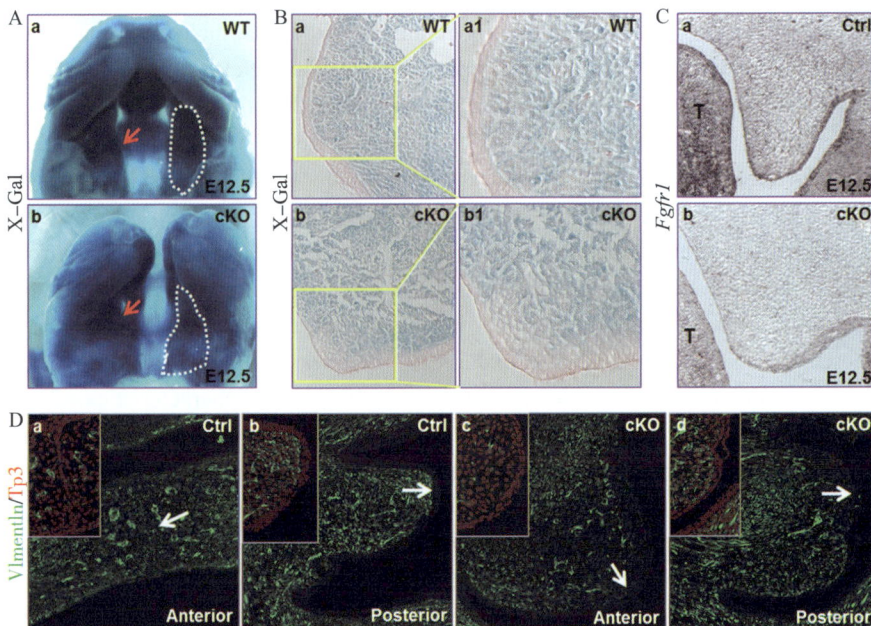

Fig. 3. Ablation of *Fgfr1* in NCC did not affect participation of CNC cells in the palate shelf mesenchyme. (A) whole mount *lacZ* staining showing CNC cells in the palate shelves in E12.5 embryos. (B) same tissue in (A) was paraffin-embedded and sectioned for demonstrating X-Gal-stained cells in the mesen-chyme. (C) *in situ* hybridization showing *Fgfr1* expression in palate shelf mesenchymal cells was diminished in E12.5 *Fgfr1*cKO embryos. (D) coronal sections of E14.5 embryos were immunostained with anti-vimentin antibody. To-Pro3 was used for nuclear counterstaining. Insets were two-channel images of the areas indicated by arrows, showing both the FITC and To-Pro3 signal to demonstrate that the epithelial cells were vimentin-negative.

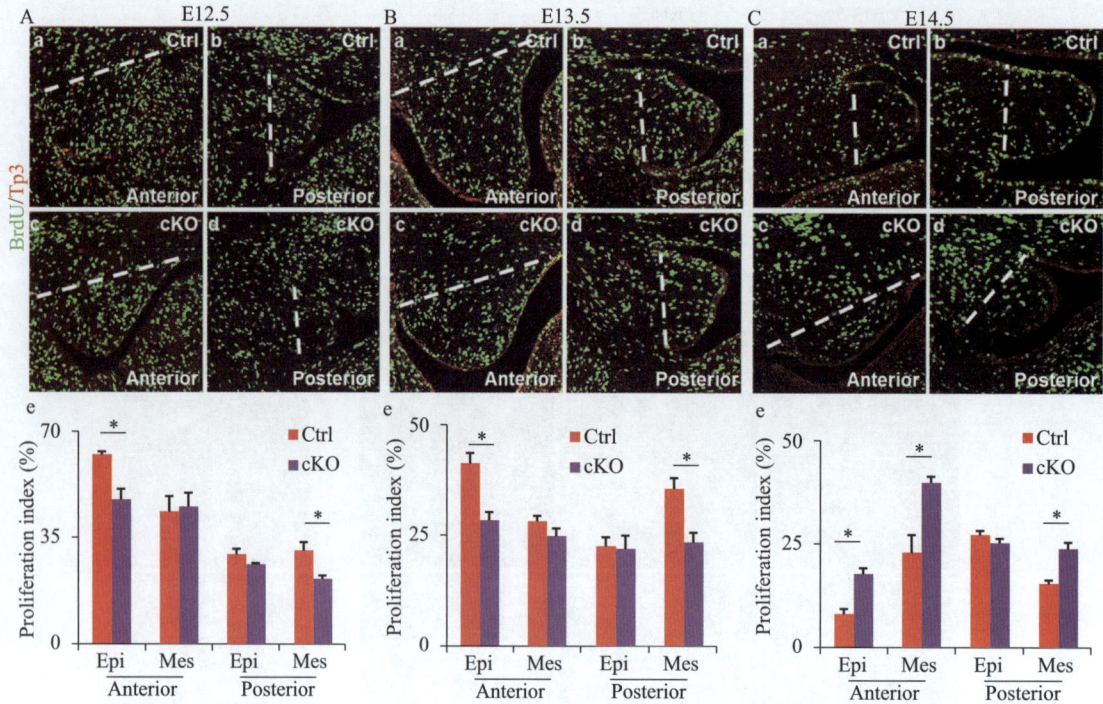

Fig. 4. Delayed cellular proliferation in *Fgfr1^cKO* palate shelves. BrdU incorporation assays demonstrate that *Fgfr1^cKO* palate shelves had compromised proliferation at the E12.5–13.5 (A and B) stages and enhanced proliferation at E14.5 (C) stage. Bottom panels, numbers of labeled cells were scored from three independent samples and expressed as mean ± S.D. *$P < 0.05$; dashed lines indicate the areas where the proliferative cells were counted; *Epi*, epithelium; *Mes*, mesenchyme.

chymal cells in palate shelves results in reduced epithelium proliferation at a non-cell autonomous manner.

2.3 Lacking FGFR1 signals in CNC-derived mesenchymal cells affects degeneration of MEE in palate shelves

During the fusion process of palate shelves, cells in the MEE undergo degeneration and the midline epithelial seam disappears at the end. *Fgfr1^cKO* embryos exhibited multiple craniofacial defects, including micrognathia and heightened tongue, which had been shown to provide a steric hindrance for palate shelf elevation without the fusion process [32–39]. To determine whether lacking mesenchymal FGFR1 affected the fusion directly by compromising epithelial degeneration or indirectly by providing a steric hindrance, E13.5 embryonic heads without the tongue and mandibles were dissected for *ex vivo* cultures for 48 h. Although the palate shelves of both control and *Fgfr1^cKO* embryos did not complete the fusion process, the gap between the two shelves was significantly reduced (Fig. 5A). However, when the two palate shelves were dissected and placed in a proximal apposition, the fusion took place in both control and mutant palate shelves in 2 days (Fig. 5B). H&E staining of the *ex vivo* cultured E13.5 palate shelves showed that both control and *Fgfr1^cKO* palate shelves fused after being cultured for 2 days. However, the gap between the two mutant shelves was not fully filled by mesenchymal cells as the control. In addition, there was still a fraction of midline epithelial seam remained (Fig. 5C). Immunostaining further revealed that expression of epithelial characteristic cytokeratins in the mutant MEE was not eliminated as completely as in controls (Fig. 5D). The results indicate that although it did not abolish the process, ablation of *Fgfr1* in CNC-derived mesenchymal cells compromised the deterioration of MEE cells during the fusion.

p63 is expressed in palate epithelial cells and is often used as an indicator for palate epithelial cell integrity. Immunostaining showed that the MEEs in control palate shelves had a fuzzy E-cadherin staining, which was a sign of deteriorating epithelial cells. The MEE cells in mutant anterior palate shelves also were not intact even though they did not undergo elevation and fusion processes. However, the severity of degeneration was apparently compromised (Fig. 6A). Similarly, E-cadherin staining also showed that, compared with the control, *Fgfr1^cKO* palate shelves had less defused E-cadherin staining in MEE cells at this stage (Fig. 6B). In addition, TUNEL analyses showed that although MEE cells in mutant palate shelves still had apoptotic cells, the numbers were significantly lower than those in control palate shelves (Fig. 6C). Consistently, expression of *Tgfβ3* in MEE cells was reduced in *Fgfr1^cKO* embryos (Fig. 6D), which

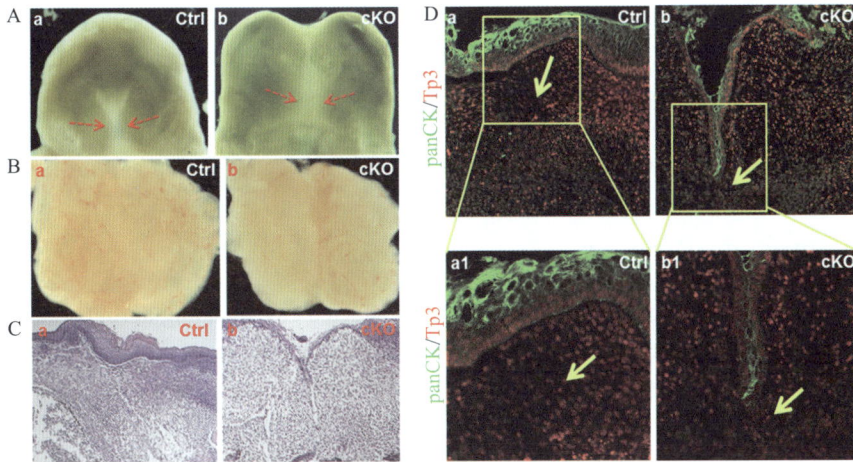

Fig. 5. Ablation of *Fgfr1* in NCCs impairs palate shelf fusion. (A and B) heads without the tongue and mandible or palate shelves dissected from E13.5 embryos were cultured at 37℃ for 48 h showing fusion of the two palate shelves. (C and D) palate tissues in (B) were sectioned and H&E-stained or immunostained with anti-pan-cytokeratin antibodies showing the loss of MEE in fused palate shelves.

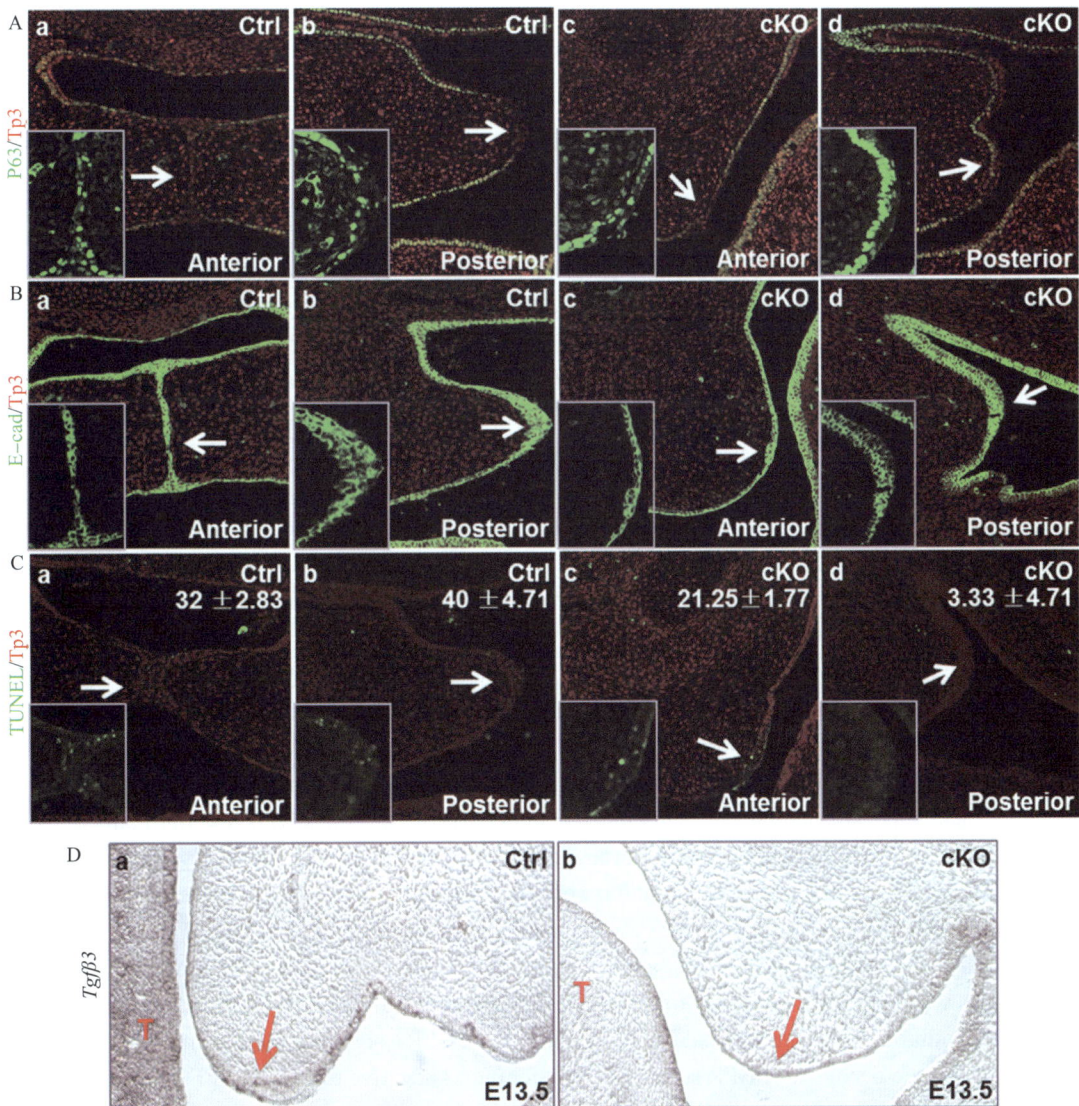

Fig. 6. Compromised deterioration of the MEE cells in *Fgfr1^cKO* palate shelves. (A–C) tissue sections from E14.5 embryos were subjected to immunostaining with anti-p63, E-cadherin (*E-Cad*) antibody, or TUNEL analyses as indicated showing compromised deterioration of epithelial cells in control and *Fgfr1^cKO* palate shelves. Numbers in (C) are average apoptotic epithelial cell numbers in three replicated samples. (D) *in situ* hybridization showing *Tgfβ3* expression in MEE cells in E13.5 embryos.

plays a critical role in promoting fusion of the palatal shelves [40]. Together, the results showed that these characteristic changes in MEE were apparently less obvious in E14.5 *Fgfr1cKO* embryos than those in the control. Therefore, although not essential, FGFR1 signaling in CNC-derived mesenchymal cells is involved in regulating degeneration of the MEE during palate shelf fusion through non-cell autonomous mechanisms. However, the molecular mechanism by which FGFR1 signaling in CNC-derived mesenchymal cells affects MEE cell degeneration and proliferation remains to be characterized.

2.4 Ablation of Fgfr1 in NCCs affects cell signaling in frontofacial tissues

To further characterize how ablation of *Fgfr1* in CNC cells affected cell signaling during craniofacial development, real time RT-PCR analyses were carried out to assess expression of key regulatory molecules in craniofacial development at E10.5 embryos and E14.5 frontofacial tissues. The results clearly demonstrated that expression of *Notch1* and *Bmp4* was increased, and the expression of *Wnt1* was reduced in the E10.5 *Fgfr1cKO* embryos (Fig. 7A). To better assess the FGFR1-regulated gene expression in frontofacial development, the frontofacial part of E14.5 embryos was dissected for real time RT-PCR analyses. The results confirmed that both Wnt and BMP signalings were changed by NCC-specific deletion of *Fgfr1* in E14.5 frontofacial tissues (Fig. 7B). In addition, expression of *Msx1* and *Ptx1* was also reduced in mutant frontofacial tissues. Furthermore, immunostaining showed that phosphorylated Smad1/5/8-positive cells were significantly increased in *Fgfr1cKO* palate shelves, especially in the anterior part at E14.5 stage (Fig. 7C). This further demonstrated increased BMP sig-naling in *Fgfr1cKO* palate shelves.

3. Discussion

The FGF signaling axis is critical for palate development through directional and reciprocal communications between the mesenchyme and epithelium of palate shelves. To date, the majority of studies has been focused on the FGF7/10-FGFR2 signaling axis that directionally mediates the mesenchyme to epithelium communication. How FGF signaling, especially that mediated by FGFR1, in the CNC cells regulates palate formation is not understood. Here, we report that tissue-specific ablation of *Fgfr1* in NCCs with *Wnt1Cre* caused primary and secondary cleft palate, cleft lip, and other craniofacial detects. Detailed analyses revealed that ablation of *Fgfr1* in NCCs did not abrogate patterning of CNC-derived mesenchymal cells in the palate shelves. However, it delayed cell proliferation in both the mesenchyme and epithelium, and impeded development of medial nasal processes and the lift of palate shelves during palatogenesis. In addition, although it did not fully prevent the fusion process of *ex vivo* cultured palate shelves once they were placed in a close contact position, the deterioration of the MEE in mutant palatal shelves was compromised. The detailed mechanism regarding how ablation of *Fgfr1* in the mesenchyme affects cell proliferation in *Fgfr1*-intact epithelial cells remains to be determined, although quantitative RT-PCR analyses showed altered expression of *Bmp*, *Wnt*, and other signaling molecules in the frontofacial tissue of E14.5 *Fgfr1* mutant embryos. In addition, ablation of *Fgfr1* in NCCs affected BMP and Wnt signaling in E10.5 embryos. This further demonstrates the cross-talk between FGF and other signaling pathways during embryonic development.

Palate development is a multifactorial event and is regulated by multiple signaling pathways. The cross-talk of these intertwining pathways is important in regulating palatogenesis [1], and the FGF signaling pathway is no exception. Balance in FGF signaling appears to be important for palate formation. Constitutively activating mutations in FGFR1 and FGFR2 as well as loss of function mutation of FGFR1 lead to cleft palate. Suppression of FGFR signaling *via* FGFR kinase inhibitor causes palate defects [41]. Many sporadic mutations of FGFR1 and FGFR2, as well as FGF3, FGF7, FGF8, FGF10, and FGF18, cause palate malformations in human. These include Kallmann, Pfeiffer, Apert, and Crouzon syndromes where cleft palate is part of a broad craniofacial phenotype [22, 42, 43]. In addition, FGFR1 is widely expressed in the myofibroblasts of injured palate, suggesting that FGFR1 signaling is also important for palate repair during injury [44]. Sprys are decoys for FGFR substrates functioning as negative regulators of FGFR signaling, which are expressed in the FGF signaling domains during mouse craniofacial development [45]. On the one hand, deletion of *Spry2* intensifies FGF signaling intensity, which leads to increased cellular proliferation in the palate shelves and cleft palate [46], without affecting palate shelf fusion in the *in vitro* organ culture system [17]. On the other hand, insufficient FGFR1 sig-naling due to loss-of-function mutations or haploid insufficiency of *Fgfr1* also leads to defects in palatogenesis. Howev-

A

B

C

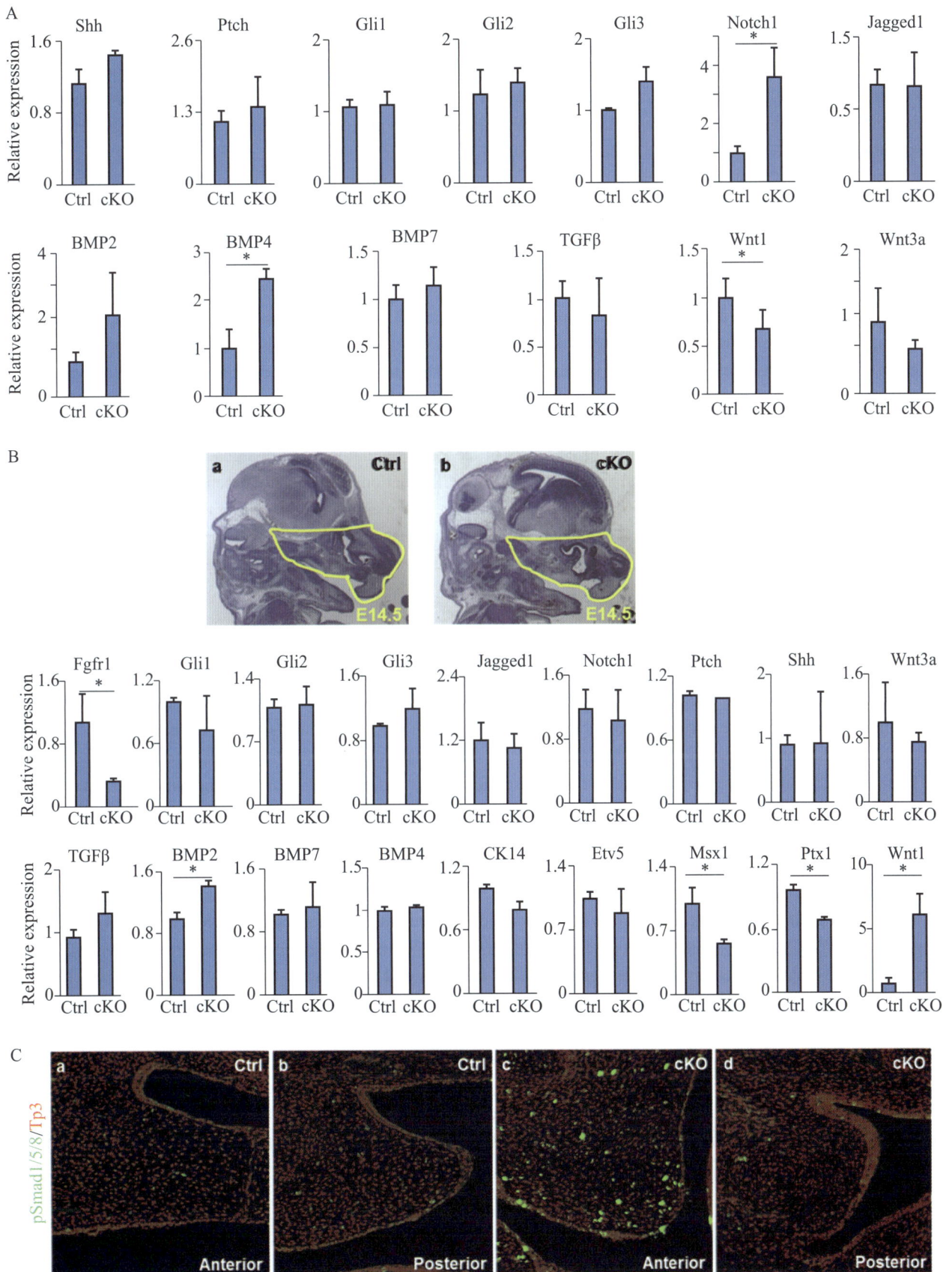

Fig. 7. Ablation of *Fgfr1* in NCCs affects cell signaling in the embryos. (A and B) total RNAs were extracted from E10.5 embryos (A) or E14.5 frontal facial areas defined in panels *a* and *b* (B) for real time RT-PCR analyses of the indicated gene expression. Data are means ± S.D. of three independent analyses. (C) immunostaining of coronal sections of E14.5 embryos with anti-phosphorylated Smad1/5/8 showing increased BMP signaling in *Fgfr1^cKO* palate shelves.

er, how FGFR1 regulates palatogenesis has not been completely clear. Interestingly, our data here showed that although ablation of *Fgfr1* in NCCs did not prevent patterning of CNC cells in palate shelves, it affected cell proliferation and abrogated palate shelf elevation. It did not fully disrupt palate shelf fusion once they were adjacent. Together with the literature, these results suggest that a precise balance of FGFR1 signaling is required for CNC-derived mesenchymal cell proliferation and change in palate shelf conformation. Both excess and deficiency of FGFR1 signaling led to defects in palatogenesis.

As a key step in palatogenesis, the palate shelves changed their conformation and elevated prior to the fusion stage. Ablation of *Fgfr1* in NCCs led to failure in changing palate shelf conformation during palatogenesis (Fig. 2). To date, the mechanism underlying conformational change of palate shelves is not well understood. Several mechanisms have been proposed, which include alteration in cellular proliferation, apoptosis, cell adhesion, or glycosaminoglycan (GAG) content in the extracellular matrix [3]. Our data showed that mesenchymal proliferation was decreased at first and then increased in *Fgfr1* mutant palate shelves, indicating that proliferation was delayed but not disrupted. Therefore, failure of changing palate shelf conformation in *Fgfr1* mutants is not likely due to compromised cell proliferation in the palate shelves. Emerging data show that the composition of GAG in the extracellular matrix varies in different cell types and that the GAG also participates in cell signaling [11]. FGF2 has been shown to modulate GAG expression and stimulate hyaluronan synthase genes *in vitro* [47]. Embryos bearing the *Fgfr2*C342Y mutant show delayed palate elevation and reduced levels of mesenchymal GAGs. Reduced levels of feedback regulators of FGF signaling suggest that this gain-of-function mutation in FGFR2 ultimately resembles loss of FGF function in the palate mesenchyme [15]. Future work to characterize GAG compositions in *Fgfr1*^{cKO} palate shelves is needed to assess the possibility that loss of *Fgfr1* in CNC-derived mesenchymal cells changes GAG compositions and impairs palate shelf elevation required for palate shelf fusion.

In vitro experiments with control and *Fgfr1* mutant palate shelves showed that although mutant palate shelves also fused and formed the MEE when they were placed in a proximal position, the degeneration of MEE cells was compromised (Fig. 5). This indicates that although not essential, FGFR1 signals in CNC-derived mesenchymal cells play an important role in controlling MEE degeneration during palate fusion. The results are different from previous findings that palatal fusion is not affected by the Crouzon gain-of-function FGFR mutation or *Spry2* deficiency[15, 17, 45]. Interestingly, it has been shown that FGF18 from the mesenchyme induces Runx1 that is expressed in the epithelium, which regulates epithelial-mesenchymal transition and morphological changes in the MEE cells during palate fusion [48].

The expression patterns and roles of Msx1, *Bmp2*, and *Bmp4* in palate formation have been extensively studied [49, 50]. Msx1 is expressed in palatal mesenchyme and is required for expression of *Bmp4* in the mesenchyme but not the epithelium. The expression of *Bmp2* can also be indirectly regulated by *Msx1* [49]. *Msx1*-BMP signaling is required for the proliferation of palatal mesenchyme as well as apoptosis of palatal epithelium, [8, 49]. Gain-of-function of BMP signaling due to loss of *Noggin* leads to deregulated cell proliferation, cell death, and changes in gene expression in palate shelves [50]. Wnt signaling also plays critical roles in palate formation [51]. Enhanced cell apoptosis in the palatal epithelium and deregulation of cell proliferation in palatal shelves are associated with increased Bmp signaling intensity[50]. In line with these reports, our RT-PCR analyses showed that ablation of *Fgfr1* in CNC cells led to aberrant expression of *Msx1*, *Bmp2*, *Bmp4*, and *Wnt* signaling components in *Fgfr1*^{cKO} E10.5 embryos and frontofacial tissues of E14.5 embryos (Fig. 7). However, whether changes in expression of the *Msx1-Bmp* axis during E10.5–E14.5 are causal factors of deregulated cell proliferation and apoptosis in *Fgfr1*^{cKO} palatal shelves remains unanswered. Further *ex vivo* or *in vivo* studies are needed to reveal the molecular mechanism by which mesenchymal FGFR1 signals regulate expression of these signaling molecules during palate formation.

In summary, ablation of *Fgfr1* in the NCCs delayed cell proliferation in both mesenchymal and epithelial compartments of palate shelves and abrogated palate shelf elevation; it did not fully disrupt the palate shelf fusion but compromised deterioration of the MEE during the process. This is the first report demonstrating the mechanism by which the FGFR1 signaling in CNC cells regulates palatogenesis.

References

[1] Jiang R, Bush JO, Lidral AC. Development of the upper lip: Morphogenetic and molecular mechanisms[J]. Developmental Dynam-

ics, 2006, 235(5): 1152-1166.

[2] Alappat S, Zhang ZY, Chen YP. Msx homeobox gene family and

craniofacial development[J]. Cell Research, 2003, 13(6): 429-442.

[3] Snyder-Warwick AK, Perlyn CA. Coordinated Events: FGF Signaling and Other Related Pathways in Palatogenesis[J]. Journal of Craniofacial Surgery, 2012, 23(2): 397-400.

[4] Khrapunov SM, Zima VL, Tyulenev VI, et al. Change in conformation of histones F2a and F2b in solutions of different ionic strength[J]. Ukrainskii Biokhimicheskii Zhurnal, 1975, 47(3): 284-289.

[5] Ferguson MWJ. Palate development[J]. Development, 1988, 103: 41-60.

[6] Shuler CF. Programmed cell death and cell transformation in craniofacial development[J]. Critical Reviews in Oral Biology and Medicine, 1995, 6(3): 202-217.

[7] Wilkie AOM, Morriss-Kay GM. Genetics of craniofacial development and malformation[J]. Nature Reviews Genetics, 2001, 2(6): 458-468.

[8] Liu W, Sun XX, Braut A, et al. Distinct functions for Bmp signaling in lip and palate fusion in mice[J]. Development, 2005, 132(6): 1453-1461.

[9] Cobourne MT, Xavier GM, Depew M, et al. Sonic hedgehog signalling inhibits palatogenesis and arrests tooth development in a mouse model of the nevoid basal cell carcinoma syndrome[J]. Developmental Biology, 2009, 331(1): 38-49.

[10] Jin Y-R, Han XH, Taketo MM, et al. Wnt9b-dependent FGF signaling is crucial for outgrowth of the nasal and maxillary processes during upper jaw and lip development[J]. Development, 2012, 139(10): 1821-1830.

[11] McKeehan WL, Wang, F., and Luo, Y. Handbook of Cell Signaling, 2nd Ed.,[J]. Academic/Elsevier Press, New York, 2009, pp. 253–259.

[12] Nie XG, Luukko K, Kettunen P. FGF signalling in craniofacial development and developmental disorders[J]. Oral Diseases, 2006, 12(2): 102-111.

[13] Rice R, Spencer-Dene B, Connor EC, et al. Disruption of Fgf10/Fgfr2b-coordinated epithelial-mesenchymal interactions causes cleft palate[J]. Journal of Clinical Investigation, 2004, 113(12): 1692-1700.

[14] Hosokawa R, Deng X, Takamori K, et al. Epithelial-Specific Requirement of FGFR2 Signaling During Tooth and Palate Development[J]. Journal of Experimental Zoology Part B-Molecular and Developmental Evolution, 2009, 312B(4): 343-350.

[15] Snyder-Warwick AK, Perlyn CA, Pan J, et al. Analysis of a gain-of-function FGFR2 Crouzon mutation provides evidence of loss of function activity in the etiology of cleft palate[J]. Proceedings of the National Academy of Sciences of the United States of America, 2010, 107(6): 2515-2520.

[16] Martinez-Abadias N, Holmes G, Pankratz T, et al. From shape to cells: mouse models reveal mechanisms altering palate development in Apert syndrome[J]. Disease Models & Mechanisms, 2013, 6(3): 768-779.

[17] Matsumura K, Taketomi T, Yoshizaki K, et al. Sprouty2 controls proliferation of palate mesenchymal cells via fibroblast growth factor signaling[J]. Biochemical and Biophysical Research Communications, 2011, 404(4): 1076-1082.

[18] Takamori K, Hosokawa R, Xu X, et al. Epithelial fibroblast growth factor receptor 1 regulates enamel formation[J]. Journal of Dental Research, 2008, 87(3): 238-243.

[19] Lee S, Crisera CA, Erfani S, et al. Immunolocalization of fibroblast growth factor receptors 1 and 2 in mouse palate development[J]. Plastic and Reconstructive Surgery, 2001, 107(7): 1776-1784.

[20] Trokovic N, Trokovic R, Mai P, et al. Fgfr1 regulates patterning of the pharyngeal region[J]. Genes & Development, 2003, 17(1): 141-153.

[21] Kim HG, Herrick SR, Lemyre E, et al. Hypogonadotropic hypogonadism and cleft lip and palate caused by a balanced translocation producing haploinsufficiency for FGFR1[J]. Journal of Medical Genetics, 2005, 42(8): 666-672.

[22] Pitteloud N, Acierno JS, Meysing A, et al. Mutations in fibroblast growth factor receptor 1 cause both Kallmann syndrome and normosmic idiopathic hypogonadotropic hypogonadism[J]. Proceedings of the National Academy of Sciences of the United States of America, 2006, 103(16): 6281-6286.

[23] Sato N, Katsumata N, Kagami M, et al. Clinical assessment and mutation analysis of Kallmann syndrome 1 (KAL1) and fibroblast growth factor receptor 1 (FGFR1, or KAL2) in five families and 18 sporadic patients[J]. Journal of Clinical Endocrinology & Metabolism, 2004, 89(3): 1079-1088.

[24] Danielian PS, Muccino D, Rowitch DH, et al. Modification of gene activity in mouse embryos in utero by a tamoxifen-inducible form of Cre recombinase[J]. Current Biology, 1998, 8(24): 1323-1326.

[25] Soriano P. Generalized lacZ expression with the ROSA26 Cre reporter strain[J]. Nature Genetics, 1999, 21(1): 70-71.

[26] Trokovic R, Trokovic N, Hernesniemi S, et al. FGFR1 is independently required in both developing mid- and hindbrain for sustained response to isthmic signals[J]. Embo Journal, 2003, 22(8): 1811-1823.

[27] Chai Y, Bringas P, Shuler C, et al. A mouse mandibular culture model permits the study of neural crest cell migration and tooth development[J]. International Journal of Developmental Biology, 1998, 42(1): 87-94.

[28] Shiota K, Kosazuma T, Klug S, et al. Developmentof the fetal mouse palate in suspension organ culture[J]. Acta Anatomica, 1990, 137(1): 59-64.

[29] Casey LM, Lan Y, Cho E-S, et al. Jag2-Notch1 signaling regulates oral epithelial differentiation and palate development[J]. Developmental Dynamics, 2006, 235(7): 1830-1844.

[30] Trainor PA, Tan SS, Tam PPL. Cranialparaxialmesoderm: regionalisation of cell fate and impact on craniofacial development in mouse embryos[J]. Development, 1994, 120(9): 2397-2408.

[31] Ito Y, Yeo JY, Chytil A, et al. Conditional inactivation of Tgfbr2 in cranial neural crest causes cleft palate and calvaria defects[J]. Development, 2003, 130(21): 5269-5280.

[32] Song Z, Liu C, Iwata J, et al. Mice with Tak1 Deficiency in Neural Crest Lineage Exhibit Cleft Palate Associated with Abnormal Tongue Development[J]. Journal of Biological Chemistry, 2013, 288(15): 10440-10450.

[33] Bjork BC, Turbe-Doan A, Prysak M, et al. Prdm16 is required for normal palatogenesis in mice[J]. Human Molecular Genetics, 2010, 19(5): 774-789.

[34] Huang X, Goudy SL, Ketova T, et al. Gli3-Deficient Mice Exhibit Cleft Palate Associated With Abnormal Tongue Development[J]. Developmental Dynamics, 2008, 237(10): 3079-3087.

[35] Barrow JR, Capecchi MR. Compensatory defects associated with mutations in Hoxa1 restore normal palatogenesis to Hoxa2 mutants[J]. Development, 1999, 126(22): 5011-5026.

[36] Murray SA, Oram KF, Gridley T. Multiple functions of Snail family genes during palate development in mice[J]. Development, 2007, 134(9): 1789-1797.

[37] Miettinen PJ, Chin JR, Shum L, et al. Epidermal growth factor receptor function is necessary for normal craniofacial development and palate closure[J]. Nature Genetics, 1999, 22(1): 69-73.

[38] Gendronmaguire M, Mallo M, Zhang M, et al. Hoxa-2 mutant mice exhibit homeotic transformation of skeletal elements derived from cranial neural crest[J]. Cell, 1993, 75(7): 1317-1331.

[39] Ricks JE, Ryder VM, Bridgewater LC, et al. Altered mandibular development precedes the time of palate closure in mice homozygous for disproportionate micromelia: An oral clefting model supporting the Pierre-Robin sequence[J]. Teratology, 2002, 65(3): 116-120.

[40] Kaartinen V, Cui XM, Heisterkamp N, et al. Transforming growth factor-beta 3 regulates transdifferentiation of medial edge epithelium during palatal fusion and associated degradation of the basement membrane[J]. Developmental Dynamics, 1997, 209(3): 255-260.

[41] Lee JM, Kim JY, Cho KW, et al. Wnt11/Fgfr1b cross-talk modulates the fate of cells in palate development[J]. Developmental Biology, 2008, 314(2): 341-350.

[42] Alappat SR, Zhang ZY, Suzuki K, et al. The cellular and molecular etiology of the cleft secondary palate in Fgf10 mutant mice[J]. Developmental Biology, 2005, 277(1): 102-113.

[43] Riley BM, Mansilla MA, Ma J, et al. Impaired FGF signaling contributes to cleft lip and palate[J]. Proceedings of the National Academy of Sciences of the United States of America, 2007, 104(11): 4512-4517.

[44] Kanda T, Funato N, Baba Y, et al. Evidence for fibroblast growth factor receptors in myofibroblasts during palatal mucoperiosteal repair[J]. Archives of Oral Biology, 2003, 48(3): 213-221.

[45] Minowada G, Jarvis LA, Chi CL, et al. Vertebrate Sprouty genes are induced by FGF signaling and can cause chondrodysplasia when overexpressed[J]. Development, 1999, 126(20): 4465-4475.

[46] Welsh IC, Hagge-Greenberg A, O'Brien TP. A dosage-dependent role for Spry2 in growth and patterning during palate development[J]. Mechanisms of Development, 2007, 124(9-10): 746-761.

[47] Shimabukuro Y, Ichikawa T, Terashima Y, et al. Basic fibroblast growth factor regulates expression of heparan sulfate in human periodontal ligament cells[J]. Matrix Biology, 2008, 27(3): 232-241.

[48] Charoenchaikorn K, Yokomizo T, Rice DP, et al. Runx1 is involved in the fusion of the primary and the secondary palatal shelves[J]. Developmental Biology, 2009, 326(2): 392-402.

[49] Zhang ZY, Song YQ, Zhao X, et al. Rescue of cleft palate in Msx1-deficient mice by transgenic Bmp4 reveals a network of BMP and Shh signaling in the regulation of mammalian palatogenesis[J]. Development, 2002, 129(17): 4135-4146.

[50] He F, Xiong W, Wang Y, et al. Modulation of BMP signaling by Noggin is required for the maintenance of palatal epithelial integrity during palatogenesis[J]. Developmental Biology, 2010, 347(1): 109-121.

[51] He F, Xiong W, Wang Y, et al. Epithelial Wnt/beta-catenin signaling regulates palatal shelf fusion through regulation of Tgf beta 3 expression[J]. Developmental Biology, 2011, 350(2): 511-519.

Chapter 9
Others

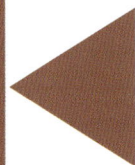

Non-mitogenic form of acidic fibroblast growth factor protects against graft-*versus*-host disease without accelerating leukemia

Yi Wang , Xiaokun Li

1. Introduction

Allogeneic bone marrow transplantation (allo-BMT) is one of the most practical treatments for leukemia patients [1,2]. The therapeutic advantage of this procedure is the ability to mediate graft-*versus*-tumor (GVT) effect. However, its broader clinical application is primarily limited by graft-*versus*-host disease (GVHD). Thus, separation of GVT from GVHD is essential for exploring the full potential of allo-BMT in the treatment of hematologic malignancies.

Acidic fibroblast growth factor (aFGF, also known as FGF-1), a member of the FGF family, is a potent regulator of cell proliferation, differentiation and function. aFGF protects against intestinal injury induced by ischemia and reperfusion *via* regulating P53 and P21 WAF-1 expression [3]. Topical administration of aFGF can also accelerate dermal wound healing in diabetic mice [4]. Although these studies suggest the potential of aFGF to prevent GVHD, the overexpression of FGF receptors in various cancers raises a concern about the safety of using aFGF or other growth factors in cancer patients [5]. We have previously constructed a mutant aFGF by eliminating the N terminal residues 1–27 that are responsible for the mitogenic activity of aFGF, and confirmed that the non-mitogenic form of aFGF (naFGF) has a dramatically decreased mitogenic activity [6], but enhanced anti-apoptotic activity and the ability to protect against ischemia/reperfusion-induced gut epithelium injury [7]. In the present study, we evaluated the effect of naFGF on GVHD and GVT against an aFGF-responsive tumor in comparison with wild-type aFGF in mice after allo-HCT.

2. Materials and methods

2.1 Mice

C57BL/6 (B6, H-2^b) and B6D2F1 (H-2$^{b/d}$) mice were purchased from the Frederick Cancer Research Facility (Frederick, MD), and housed in a specific pathogen-free microisolator environment. Protocols involving animals were approved by the Massachusetts General Hospital Subcom-mittee on Research Animal Care.

2.2 BMT

In the irradiated allo-BMT model, B6D2F1 mice were lethally irradiated (9.5 Gy, ^{137}Cs source) and reconstituted with 8×10^6 BM cells and 2.5×10^7 splenocytes from B6D2F1 or B6 mice within 4–8 h after the irradiation. In the irradiated leukemic allo-BMT model, lethally irradiated B6D2F1 recipients were transplanted with 8×10^6 BM cells and 2.0×10^7 splenocytes from B6D2F1 or B6 mice along with 1×10^4 P815 cells (DBA/2-derived mastocytoma) at the time of BMT. In the nonirradiated syngeneic tumor model, B6D2F1 mice were injected with cyclophosphamide (200 mg/kg) intraperitoneally and reconstituted with 5×10^6 BM cells from B6D2F1 mice and 5×10^3 P815 cells within 24 h. Carcasses were saved in 10% formalin after death for autopsy.

2.3 Growth factor treatment

Recombinant human aFGF or naFGF were prepared as previously described [6]. For radiation allogeneic BMT model, aFGF or naFGF were injected i.p. daily (5 mg/kg) from day − 3 to day 7 with respect to BMT. For the non-radiation syngeneic model, aFGF or naFGF were injected i.p. daily (5 mg/kg) from the day of BMT until death. Control mice were injected with a similar volume of PBS.

2.4 Flow cytometric analysis

Mononuclear cells were prepared from recipient liver, lung, spleen and lymph nodes 4 weeks after BMT. Cells were stained by fluorescence-conjugated anti-mouse CD4, CD8, CD44, and CD62L and assessed using a FACSCalibur flow cytometer (Becton Dickinson, San Jose, CA), in which anti-recipient (H-2D^d) mAb 34-2-12 (BD Pharmingen, San Diego, CA) was used to distinguish between donor and recipient cells.

2.5 Cell proliferation assay

P815 cells were cultured in medium containing aFGF, naFGF or the same volume of PBS for 48 h. Cultures were pulsed with [^{3}H]-thymidine (1 μCi/well) and incorporation was measured 12 h later.

2.6 Statistical analysis

Survival data are presented as Kaplan-Meier survival curves and differences between groups were analyzed by the log-rank test using GraphPad Prism (Dan Diego, CA). Differences between two groups were analyzed by Students' t-test or two-way ANOVA. P values < 0.05 were considered significant.

3. Results

The effect of aFGF and naFGF on GVHD was assessed in a parent-to-F1 (B6 → B6D2F1) allo-BMT model. Compared to PBS-injected controls, mice treated with aFGF or naFGF showed moderate, but significantly prolonged survival (Fig. 1A; $P < 0.05$). No significant difference in GVHD mortality was seen between aFGF-and naFGF-treated recipients. Although the mechanisms remain to be determined, these results indicate that the protective effect of aFGF is mediated predominantly *via* mechanisms independent of its mitogenic activity, presumably through its anti-apoptotic activities, which are preserved in naFGF [7].

We next assessed the effect of aFGF and naFGF on GVT effects against P815 tumor cells (H-2^d) in allo-BMT recipients. Compared to syngeneic controls that all died within 18 days, markedly improved survival was seen in PBS-injected leukemic recipients of allo-BMT (Fig. 1B; $P < 0.000\,1$ *vs.* syngeneic controls). A similar level of protection was detected in naFGF-treated allo-BMT recipients ($P < 0.000\,1$ *vs.* syngeneic controls). Although leukemic recipients treated with naFGF exhibited a similar survival rate as the PBS-injected controls, mice in the former group showed significantly improved body weight recovery (Fig. 1C), which likely reflects naFGF-mediated protection against GVHD. Surprisingly, treatment with aFGF significantly accelerated tumor death in allo-BMT recipients (Fig. 1B; $P < 0.001$ *vs.* allo-BMT recipients treated with naFGF or PBS). Autopsy confirmed the presence of tumors in all aFGF-treated mice (Fig. 1D). These results demonstrate that aFGF treatment can accelerate leukemic death in allo-BMT recipients by its mitogenic activity.

To determine whether aFGF may also affect GVHD and GVT effects by affecting donor T cells, we compared donor T cell activation and expansion in the liver, lung, spleen and lymph nodes between aFGF-treated and PBS-injected allo-BMT recipients. Compared to syngeneic BMT controls, a significant increase in activated (*i.e.*, CD44$^+$ CD62L$^-$) donor T cells, including both CD4$^+$ and CD8$^+$ T cells, was detected in all allo-BMT recipients (Fig. 1E–H). The comparable levels of donor T cell activation between aFGF-treated and control allo-BMT recipients indicate that the observed protection against GVHD and acceleration of tumor death by aFGF is unlikely to be mediated by directly modulating alloreactive T cells.

Furthermore, *in vitro* proliferation of P815 cells was significantly enhanced by aFGF, but not naFGF (Fig. 2A). Similarly, treatment with aFGF, but not naFGF, accelerated death of B6D2F1 mice that received syngeneic BM and P815 cells. As shown in Fig. 2B and C, aFGF-treated leukemic recipients all died within 14 days after tumor induction. Compared to the aFGF-treated group, mice treated with naFGF or PBS showed significantly prolonged survival ($P < 0.0001$ *vs.* the aFGF-treated group). No significant difference in tumor mortality was seen between naFGF-and PBS-treated recipients. Consistent with previously published data [8], P815 cells were found to highly express the genes promoting tumor growth, including FGFR1 (data not shown). Taken together, these data indicate that aFGF may promote

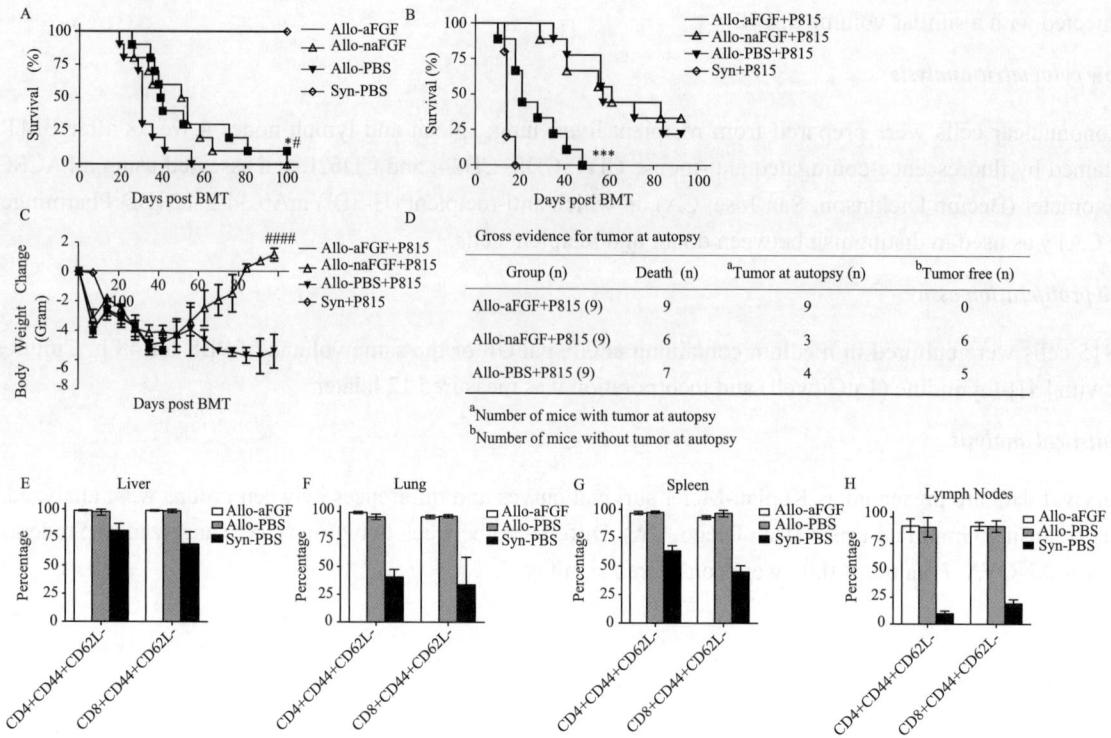

Fig. 1. Effect of aFGF and naFGF on GVHD and GVT. (A) Lethally-irradiated B6D2F1 mice received 8×10^6 BM and 2.5×10^7 spleen cells from syngeneic B6D2F1 or allogeneic B6 mice. Survival rates of 3 representative experiments are shown ($n = 10$/group). Allo-aFGF $vs.$ Allo-PBS, [*]$P < 0.05$; Allo-naFGF $vs.$ Allo-PBS, [#]$P < 0.05$. (B–D) Lethal TBI-treated B6D2F1 mice received 1×10^4 host-type P815 plus 8×10^6 BM and 2×10^7 spleen cells from syngeneic B6D2F1 or allogeneic B6 mice. Representative results of 3 experiments are shown ($n = 9$/group). Shown are survival (B, Allo-aFGF $vs.$ Allo-PBS; [***]$P < 0.001$), body weight changes (C; mean ± SEM; Allo-naFGF $vs.$ Allo-PBS, [####]$P < 0.000\ 1$), and incidence for tumor at autopsy when the mice were dead (D). (E–H): Lethally-irradiated B6D2F1 mice received 8×10^6 BM and 2.5×10^7 spleen cells from syngeneic B6D2F1 or allogeneic B6 mice. At week 4 post-BMT, mice were sacrificed and the percentages of donor $H\text{-}2^{d-}CD4^+CD44^+CD62L^-$ and $H\text{-}2^{d-}CD8^+CD44^+CD62L^-$ effector cells in the liver (E), lung (F), spleen (G), and lymph nodes (H) were determined by FACS. Data are presented as mean ± SD ($n = 3$/group).

tumor growth both *in vitro* and *in vivo*.

4. Discussion

A number of growth factors have been shown to mediate protection against acute and/or chronic GVHD. Vascular endothelial growth factor (VEGF) is a dimeric glycoprotein that increases the vascular permeability and induces the proliferation and migration of endothelial cells to form new blood vessels. Previous studies have shown that vascular endothelial damage is involved in acute GVHD, suggesting that VEGF may ameliorate GVHD. It was reported that patients with low production of VEGF have a higher incidence of acute GVHD and nonrelapse mortality[9]. Kim *et al.* reported that the high circulating levels of VEGF and magnified donor T-cell expansion caused by the blockade of the interaction between VEGF and VEGFR early after allo-HCT are associated with the aggravation of acute GVHD mortality [10]. It was recently reported that blockade of VEGF aggravates the severity of acute GVHD after experimental allogeneic hematopoietic stem cell transplantation[11]. However, VEGF, which is essential for angiogenesis and vascular permeability, also plays a critical role in tumor vascularization and metastasis [12]. Although these studies indicate that VEGF is protective against GVHD, administration of exogenous VEGF may not be an option for controlling GVHD in leukemic recipients. In addition, previous studies have shown that keratinocyte growth factor (KGF, also known as FGF-7)[13] and hepatocyte growth factor (HGF) [14,15] can ameliorate GVHD while preserving the anti-tumor activity of allo-BMT, despite that both factors have the potential to promote cancer development. The KGF receptor is highly expressed in cancer cells, and KGF induces the expression of VEGF that promotes cancer angiogenesis and metastasis [16–18]. HGF/mesenchymal–epithelial transition factor (MET) tyrosine kinase pathway has also been implicated in tumor growth, in-

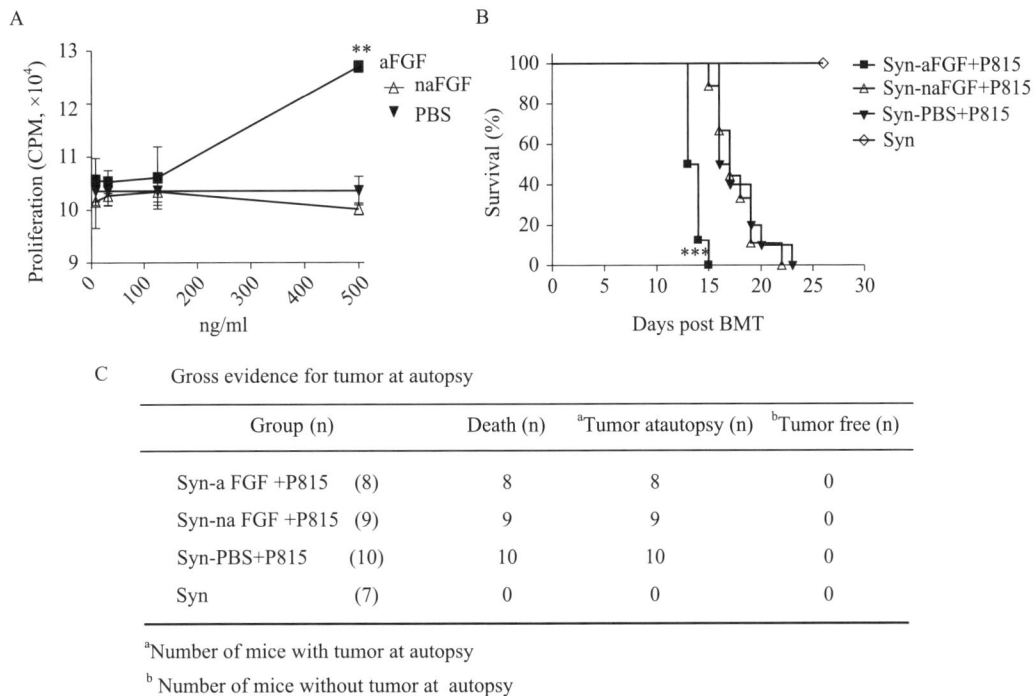

A

B

C Gross evidence for tumor at autopsy

Group (n)		Death (n)	[a]Tumor atautopsy (n)	[b]Tumor free (n)
Syn-a FGF +P815	(8)	8	8	0
Syn-na FGF +P815	(9)	9	9	0
Syn-PBS+P815	(10)	10	10	0
Syn	(7)	0	0	0

[a]Number of mice with tumor at autopsy

[b] Number of mice without tumor at autopsy

Fig. 2. aFGF but not naFGF promotes P815 tumor cell growth both *in vitro* and *in vivo*. (A) P815 cells were incubated in medium containing aFGF or naFGF (at the concentration of 7.81, 31.25, 125 or 500 ng/ml), or the same volume of PBS, and cell proliferation was measured by 3[H] thymidine incorporation. Representative results of 3 experiments are shown and presented as mean ± SEM (CPM) of triplicate cultures. aFGF *vs.* PBS, [**]$P < 0.01$. (B) B6D2F1 mice were injected with cyclophosphamide (200 mg/kg) intraperitoneally and reconstituted within 24 h with 5×10^6 BM cells from B6D2F1 mice and 5×10^3 P815 cells. aFGF or naFGF was injected i.p. daily (5 mg/kg) from the day of BMT until death. Control mice were injected with a similar volume of PBS. Survival rates of 3 representative experiments are shown ($n = 10$). Syn-aFGF + P815 *vs.* Syn-PBS + P815, [***]$P < 0.001$. (C) Incidence for tumor at autopsy when the mice were dead.

vasion and metastasis[19]. It might be possible that the observed anti-tumor effect in these studies was due to the non- or poor responsiveness to KGF or HGF of the tumor cells used.

aFGF, which belongs to the FGF-1 subfamily, is a potent regulator of cell proliferation, differentiation and function. The therapeutic potential of aFGF includes the treatment for cardiovascular disorders [20,21], nerve injuries [22], and wound healing [23]. However, aFGF, whose receptors are highly expressed in cancer cells, has the potential to induce unwanted cancer cell proliferation [24–26]. We have previously constructed a truncated aFGF, which is called the non-mitogenic form of aFGF (naFGF), lacking the mitogen properties by eliminating the first 27 residues from the N terminus [6]. naFGF showed a somewhat attenuated ability to activate intracellular signals downstream of FGF receptors but showed a severe decrease in mitogenic activity [27,28]. Our data proved that administration of recombinant aFGF can attenuate GVHD, but can also accelerate tumor death in allo-BMT recipients. Furthermore, inhibition of GVHD by aFGF, at the dose of 5 mg/kg, is possibly mediated by its effect on the recipient tissues rather than on donor T cells, suggesting that aFGF may synergistically improve the outcome of allo-BMT when used in combination with other GVHD-prophylactic therapies targeting at the donor T cells.

It has been reported that cytokines/cytokine receptors and chemokines/chemokine receptors, such as insulinlike growth factor-1 (IGF-1), FGFR1, interleukin-8 receptor (IL-8R), vascular endothelial growth factor-A (VEGF-A) and VEGF-B, were expressed on P815 tumor cells [8]. All of these genes promote tumor growth both *in vitro* and *in vivo*. aFGF is the ligand for FGFR1, and aFGF has been proved to play potent biological effects in malignant tumor development, including promoting tumor migration and invasion [29]. Also, aFGF can play a role in tumor angiogenesis [24,30]. Therefore, expression of FGFR1 can be a benefit for growth and maintenance of P815 cells. Our data show that the tumor-promoting, but not GVHD-protecting, effect of aFGF is largely dependent on its mitogenic activity, suggesting that the mitogen properties of aFGF could be dissociated from its GVHD protective effects.

In summary, our study showed the first evidence that the use of naFGF may provide a safer approach to inhibiting GVHD in patients with malignancies. In addition, our data also suggest that while not all types of tumors can respond to aFGF or any other growth factors, we need to be cautious when using growth factors in patients with malignant diseases.

References

[1] Sykes M, Spitzer TR. Non-myeloblative induction of mixed hematopoietic chimerism: application to transplantation tolerance and hematologic malignancies in experimental and clinical studies[J]. Cancer treatment and research, 2002, 110: 79-99.

[2] Blazar BR, Murphy WJ. Bone marrow transplantation and approaches to avoid graft-*versus*-host disease (GVHD)[J]. Philosophical Transactions of the Royal Society B-Biological Sciences, 2005, 360(1461): 1747-1767.

[3] Chen W, Fu X-B, Ge S-L, *et al.* Exogenous acid fibroblast growth factor inhibits ischemia-reperfusion-induced damage in intestinal epithelium *via* regulating P53 and P21WAF-1 expression[J]. World Journal of Gastroenterology, 2005, 11(44): 6981-6987.

[4] Mellin TN, Cashen DE, Ronan JJ, *et al.* Acidic Fibroblast Growth Factor Accelerates Dermal Wound Healing in Diabetic Mice[J]. Journal of Investigative Dermatology, 1995, 104(5): 850-855.

[5] Liang G, Liu Z, Wu J, *et al.* Anticancer molecules targeting fibroblast growth factor receptors[J]. Trends in Pharmacological Sciences, 2012, 33(10): 531-541.

[6] Wu XP, Su ZJ, Li XK, *et al.* High-level expression and purification of a nonmitogenic form of human acidic fibroblast growth factor in Escherichia coli[J]. Protein Expression and Purification, 2005, 42(1): 7-11.

[7] Fu XB, Li XK, Wang T, *et al.* Enhanced anti-apoptosis and gut epithelium protection function of acidic fibroblast growth factor after cancelling of its mitogenic activity[J]. World Journal of Gastroenterology, 2004, 10(24): 3590-3596.

[8] Hao S, Bi XG, Su LP, *et al.* Molecular and immunophenotypical characterization of progressive and regressive leukemia cell lines[J]. Cancer Biotherapy and Radiopharmaceuticals, 2005, 20(3): 290-299.

[9] Min CK, Kim SY, Lee MJ, *et al.* Vascular endothelial growth factor (VEGF) is associated with reduced severity of acute graft-*versus*-host disease and nonrelapse mortality after allogeneic stem cell transplantation [J]. Bone Marrow Transplantation, 2006, 38(2): 149-156.

[10] Kim DH, Lee NY, Lee MH, *et al.* Vascular Endothelial Growth Factor Gene Polymorphisms May Predict the Risk of Acute Graft-*versus*-Host Disease following Allogeneic Transplantation: Preventive Effect of Vascular Endothelial Growth Factor Gene on Acute Graft-*versus*-Host Disease[J]. Biology of Blood and Marrow Transplantation, 2008, 14(12): 1408-1416.

[11] Kim AR, Lim JY, Jeong DC, *et al.* Blockade of Vascular Endothelial Growth Factor (VEGF) Aggravates the Severity of Acute Graft-*versus*-host Disease (GVHD) after Experimental Allogeneic Hematopoietic Stem Cell Transplantation (allo-HSCT)[J]. Immune network, 2011, 11(6): 368-375.

[12] Welti J, Loges S, Dimmeler S, *et al.* Recent molecular discoveries in angiogenesis and antiangiogenic therapies in cancer[J]. Journal of Clinical Investigation, 2013, 123(8): 3190-3200.

[13] Krijanovski OI, Hill GR, Cooke KR, *et al.* Keratinocyte growth factor separates graft-*versus*-leukemia effects from graft-*versus*-host disease[J]. Blood, 1999, 94(2): 825-831.

[14] Yoshida Y, Hirano T, Son G, *et al.* Allogeneic bone marrow transplantation for hepatocellular carcinoma: hepatocyte growth factor suppresses graft-*vs.*-host disease[J]. American Journal of Physiology-Gastrointestinal and Liver Physiology, 2007, 293(6): G1114-G1123.

[15] Iwasaki T, Shibasaki S. Hepatocyte Growth Factor Regulates Immune Reactions Caused by Transplantation and Autoimmune Diseases[J]. Yakugaku Zasshi-Journal of the Pharmaceutical Society of Japan, 2013, 133(11): 1159-1167.

[16] Narita K, Fujii T, Ishiwata T, *et al.* Keratinocyte growth factor induces vascular endothelial growth factor-A expression in colorectal cancer cells[J]. International Journal of Oncology, 2009, 34(2): 355-360.

[17] Chang SH, Kanasaki K, Gocheva V, *et al.* VEGF-A Induces Angiogenesis by Perturbing the Cathepsin-Cysteine Protease Inhibitor Balance in Venules, Causing Basement Membrane Degradation and Mother Vessel Formation[J]. Cancer Research, 2009, 69(10): 4537-4544.

[18] Cho K, Matsuda Y, Ueda J, *et al.* Keratinocyte growth factor induces matrix metalloproteinase-9 expression and correlates with venous invasion in pancreatic cancer[J]. International Journal of Oncology, 2012, 40(4): 1040-1048.

[19] Naran S, Zhang X, Hughes SJ. Inhibition of HGF/MET as therapy for malignancy[J]. Expert Opinion on Therapeutic Targets, 2009, 13(5): 569-581.

[20] Belch J, Hiatt WR, Baumgartner I, *et al.* Effect of fibroblast growth factor NV1FGF on amputation and death: a randomised placebo-controlled trial of gene therapy in critical limb ischaemia[J]. Lancet, 2011, 377(9781): 1929-1937.

[21] Zhao T, Zhao W, Chen Y, *et al.* Acidic and basic fibroblast growth factors involved in cardiac angiogenesis following infarction[J]. International Journal of Cardiology, 2011, 152(3): 307-313.

[22] Cheng X, Wang Z, Yang J, *et al.* Acidic fibroblast growth factor delivered intranasally induces neurogenesis and angiogenesis in rats after ischemic stroke[J]. Neurological Research, 2011, 33(7): 675-680.

[23] Xie L, Zhang M, Dong B, *et al.* Improved refractory wound healing with administration of acidic fibroblast growth factor in diabetic rats[J]. Diabetes Research and Clinical Practice, 2011, 93(3): 396-403.

[24] Sugiura K, Ozawa S, Kitagawa Y, *et al.* Co-expression of aFGF and FGFR-1 is predictive of a poor prognosis in patients with esophageal squamous cell carcinoma[J]. Oncology Reports, 2007, 17(3): 557-564.

[25] Cronauer MV, Schulz WA, Seifert HH, *et al.* Fibroblast growth factors and their receptors in urological cancers: Basic research and clinical implications[J]. European Urology, 2003, 43(3): 309-319.

[26] Dai X, Cai C, Xiao F, *et al.* Identification of a novel aFGF-binding peptide with anti-tumor effect on breast cancer from phage display library[J]. Biochemical and Biophysical Research Communications, 2014, 445(4): 795-801.

[27] Lozano RM, Pineda-Lucena A, Gonzalez C, *et al.* H-1 NMR structural characterization of a nonmitogenic, vasodilatory, ischemia-protector and neuromodulatory acidic fibroblast growth factor[J]. Biochemistry, 2000, 39(17): 4982-4993.

[28] Suh JM, Jonker JW, Ahmadian M, *et al.* Endocrinization of FGF1 produces a neomorphic and potent insulin sensitizer[J]. Nature, 2014, 513(7518): 436-439.

[29] Billottet C, Janji B, Thiery JP, *et al.* Rapid tumor development and potent vascularization are independent events in carcinoma producing FGF-1 or FGF-2[J]. Oncogene, 2002, 21(53): 8128-8139.

[30] Aonuma M, Iwahana M, Nakayama Y, *et al.* Tumorigenicity depends on angiogenic potential of tumor cells: dominant role of vascular endothelial growth factor and/or fibroblast growth factors produced by tumor cells[J]. Angiogenesis, 1998, 2(1): 57-66.

Topical application of a new monoclonal antibody against fibroblast growth factor 10 (FGF 10) mitigates propranolol-induced psoriasis-like lesions in guinea pigs

Na Yao, Xiaokun Li

1. Introduction

Psoriasis is a chronic inflammatory skin disease and approximately, affects 2% of the population in the world[1]. It is characterized by excessive growth and aberrant differentiation of keratinocytes in the skin lesions[2]. Currently, numerous therapeutic reagents are available including topical treatments (emollients, tar, dithranol, steroids, and vitamin D analogues), phototherapy (broadband or narrowband ultraviolet radiation B, laser), and systemic agents (anti-metabolites, oral retinoid acids, and immunosuppressants)[3]. However, the therapeutic efficacy of these treatments is limited. Many patients with psoriasis commonly do not respond to or develop tolerance to these therapies. Novel biologic agents such as anti-tumor necrosis factor (TNF) α, TNFα blocker, and anti-IL-12/IL-23, which inhibit autoimmunity and target specific molecular signals in the pathogenesis of psoriasis, are effective in the treatment of severe psoriasis[3]. However, the safety of these therapeutic reagents is of concern.

It is well known that fibroblast growth factor 10 (FGF10) and keratinocyte growth factor (KGF) are crucial growth factors for the proliferation and differentiation of keratinocytes[4]. Among these factors, FGF10 serves as an important mediator of keratinocyte proliferation, differentiation, and migration[5,6]. FGF10 is predominantly secreted by fibroblasts, and it can bind to the IIIb isoform of FGF receptor II. A previous study has shown that the levels of FGF10 expression are elevated in the upper dermis of psoriatic skin and are correlated positively with the numbers of T cell infiltrates and the degrees of keratinocyte proliferation[7]. Moreover, mice with a deficiency in the FGF10 gene have abnormalities in epidermal morphogenesis, a decreased number of proliferating cells in the basal layer, the hypoplastic granular layer, and no distinctive keratohyaline granule and tonofibril[8]. Accordingly, FGF10 is an important factor of keratinocyte proliferation. Therefore, we hypothesized that blockage of FGF10 function by anti-FGF10 could inhibit keratinocyte proliferation and mitigate psoriasis-related inflammation.

In this present study, we generated a novel monoclonal antibody (mAb) against FGF10 (anti-FGF10) and examined the effect of anti-FGF10 in the suppression of keratinocyte proliferation *in vitro* and pathogenic changes in a guinea pig model of topical propranolol-induced psoriasis-like lesions. Our results may provide valuable insights into the role of FGF10 in the pathology of psoriasis and offer a novel approach for disease therapy.

2. Materials and methods

2.1 Ethics statement

Every effort was made to minimize the numbers and suffering of the animals used in the experiments. Animal study was performed in the Laboratory Animal Center, School of Basic Medical Sciences, Jilin University. The animal experiments were approved by the Animal Ethical Committee of the Jilin University.

2.2 Cell culture

Sp2/0 mouse myeloma and human keratinocyte HaCaT cell lines were from the Institute of Biological Products in Changchun, China. Sp2/0 cells were maintained in RPMI-1640 medium (GIBCO, Shanghai, China) containing 10%

fetal bovine serum (FBS, Zhejiang Tianhang Biological Technology, Hangzhou, China) and HaCaT cells were cultured in Dulbecco's Modified Eagle's Medium (DMEM, GIBCO, Carlsbad, CA, USA) containing 20% FBS at 37℃ in a 5% CO_2-humidified incubator.

2.3 Preparation and identification of anti-FGF10

Female BALB/c mice at 6 to 8 weeks of age were obtained from the Institute of Biological Products, Changchun, China. Animals were immunized with 20 μg FGF10 (the Engineering Research Center of Bioreactor and Pharmaceutical Development of Ministry of Education, Jilin Agricultural University, Changchun) in 50% complete Freund's adjuvant (CFA, GIBCO), and two weeks later, the mice were boosted with 20 μg FGF10 in 50% incomplete Freund's adjuvant (IFA, GIBCO) every ten days for two times. Two weeks after the last boosting, the mice were injected intravenously with 10 μg FGF10 and their blood samples were collected for the measurement of anti-FGF10 antibody titers at three days post the last intravenous chanlege. Subsequently, the mice were sacrificed and their splenic mononuclear cells were prepared. The prepared splenic mononuclear cells were fused with Sp2/0 cells at a ratio of 5:1 with polyethylene glycol (PEG) 4000. After the fusion, the cells were cultured in hypoxanthine-aminopterin-thymidine (HAT) medium and the supernatants of cultured hybridomas were harvested for the measurement of anti-FGF10 by enzyme-linked immuno-sorbent assay (ELISA). The positive hybridomas were selected and subjected to further cloning by limited dilution for three times. The generated hybridoma of 2G6 was injected into BALB/c nude mice to generate ascites. The anti-FGF10 antibody of 2G6 in the ascites was purified by affinity chromatography using Protein A beads (Invitrogen, Grand Island, NY, USA). The subclass of mAb of 2G6 was determined by ELISA using an Immunoglobin isotyping ELISA kit, according to the manufacturers' instruction (Sigma, St. Louis, MO, USA), and the purification of 2G6 was identified by sodium dodecyl sulfate-polyacry-lamide gel electrophoresis (SDS-PAGE).

2.4 MTT assay

The impact of anti-FGF10 2G6 on human keratinocyte proliferation was tested by 3-(4,5-dimethylthiazol-2-yl)-2,5-diphenyltetrazolium bromide (MTT) assay. Briefly, HaCaT cells (5×10^4 cells/well) were cultured overnight in a 96-well plate and treated in quintuplicate with FBS-free DMEM medium supplemented with different concentrations of FGF10 alone (10, 50, 100, 200, 400, or 800 ng/ml) or 200 ng/ml of FGF10 and varying concentrations (100, 200, 400, 800, or 1 600 ng/ml) of anti-FGF10 2G6 for 72 hrs. The control cells were cultured in medium alone. The cells were exposed to 20 μl of MTT (5 mg/ml) during the last 4-h incubation. The generated formazan was dissolved in 100 μl of dimethyl sulfoxide (DMSO) and measured for the absorbance at 490 nm (A490) using a microplate spectrophotometer. The average optical density (OD) was calculated.

2.5 Establishment of animal model of psoriasis-like lesions

Male guinea pigs at XX weeks of age were obtained from the Institute of Biological Products in Changchun, China, and housed in a specific pathogen free (SPF) facility with free access to food and water. An animal model of *psoriasis-like lesions* was established, as described previously[9]. At the beginning, six animals were treated topically with 5% propranolol emulsion (10 mg/ml, Shanxi Yunpeng Pharmaceutical, China) on the back of each ear four times per day for three or 21 consecutive days to induce psoriasis-like lesions. The pathological changes in the skin tissues were examined by histology. Subsequently, 45 animals were treated topically with 5% propranolol emulsion (10 mg/ml, Shanxi Yunpeng Pharmaceutical, China) on the back of each ear four times per day for 21 consecutive days to induce psoriasis-like lesions. Another nine animals were treated with phosphate buffered saline (PBS) and used as the healthy controls.

2.6 Treatment

One week after induction, these animals were randomized into six groups (nine animals per group) by a simple random sample using the SPSS software. Animals were treated topically with 100 μl of vehicle PBS as the model group, with 100 mg hydrocortisone butyrate (Tianjin Pharmaceuticals Group, China) as the hydrocortisone group, or with 0.188 mg/ml (high dose group), 0.094 mg/ml (medium dose group), or 0.063 mg/ml (low dose group) of anti-FGF10 2G6 on the back of the ears twice per day for 14 consecutive days. The healthy controls were treated with PBS. The animals were sacrificed one day after the last treatment, and their auricular areas were carefully removed for histological examination.

2.7 Histology

The ear tissues were fixed with buffered formalin, and the paraffin-embedded tissue sections (4 μM) were routinely stained with hematoxylin and eosin (H&E). The sections were examined under a light microscope and scored, according to Baker's score criteria[10] in a blinded fashion. The pathological changes in the corneous layer, epidermis, and dermis of the skin were analyzed and scored separately, as described in Table 1. All the values of individual animals were summarized to obtain a total histopathological score for each animal (maximum score = 10). A lesion with a histopathological score of 4 was defined as a typical psoriasis-like lesion.

2.8 Statistical analysis

Data are presented as the mean ± standard deviation (SD). The difference among the groups was determined using one-way analysis of variance (ANOVA), and the difference between two groups was analyzed by Fisher's least significant difference (LSD) test using the SPSS13.0 software (SPSS Inc., Chicago, IL, USA). A P value of < 0.05 was considered statistically significant.

3. Results

3.1 Anti-FGF10 antagonizes FGF10-stimulated human keratinocyte proliferation in vitro

FGF10 is a crucial growth factor of keratinocyte proliferation. We first tested the role of FGF10 in spontaneous keratinocyte proliferation. Human keratinocyte HaCaT cells were treated with different concentrations of recombinant FGF10 for 72 hrs, and the FGF10-stimulated HaCaT cell proliferation was determined by MTT. As shown in Fig. 1A, treatment with 10–200 ng/mL of FGF10 stimulated HaCaT cell proliferation in a dosedependent manner. Furthermore, we stimulated HaCaT cells with 200 ng/ml of FGF10 in the presence or absence of different concentrations of anti-FGF10 2G6. We found that treatment with different doses of anti-FGF10 2G6 inhibited FGF10-stimulated HaCaT cell proliferation also in a dose-dependent manner (Fig. 1B). Treatment with 100 or 200 ng/ml anti-FGF10 treatment significantly inhibited FGF10-stimulated HaCaT cell proliferation (p <0.05 *vs.* the cells treated with FGF10 alone), and treatment with a higher dose (400, 800, or 1600 ng/ml) of anti-FGF10 resulted in more significant inhibition of HaCaT cell proliferation (p <0.1 *vs.* the cells treated with FGF10 alone). Therefore, the 2G6 mAb has potent anti-FGF10 activity *in vitro*.

Table 1.   Histopathological score criteria

	Pathological change	Score
Corneous layer	Parakeratosis	1.0
	Hyperkeratosis	0.5
	Munro abscess	2.0
Epidermis	Lengthening of rete ridges	0.5–1.5
	Acanthosis	1.0
	Lack of granular layer	1.0
Dermis	Lymphocytic infiltrate	0.5–2.0
	Thinning above papillae	0.5
	Papillary papillae congestion	0.5

3.2 Anti-FGF10 mitigates inflammation and pathogenic changes in chemical-induced psoriasis-like lesions in Guinea Pig

Keratinocyte over-proliferation is associated with the pathogenesis of psoriasis. Next, we tested the hypothesis that treatment with anti-FGF10 2G6 after chemical induction of psoriasis-like lesions could mitigates inflammation and

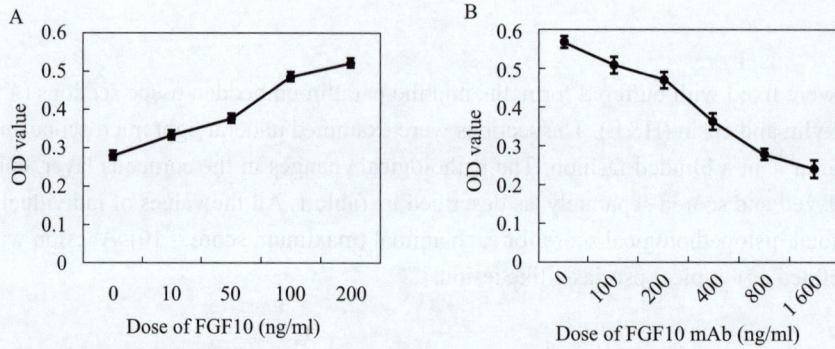

Fig. 1. Anti-FGF10 inhibits HaCaT cell proliferation *in vitro*. HaCaT cells were treated in triplicate with the indicated doses of FGF10 or with 200 ng/ml of FGF10 in the presence or absence of different doses of anti-FGF10 for 72 h. The cell proliferation was measured by MTT assays. The average optical density (OD) value was expressed as the mean ± SEM of each group of cells from five separate experiments. (A) FGF10 stimulated HaCaT cell proliferation *in vitro*. (B) Anti-FGF10 inhibited the FGF10-stimulated HaCaT cell proliferation *in vitro*. $^{*}P < 0.05$, $^{**}P < 0.01$ *vs*. the control cells without FGF10 or without anti-FGF10 treatment.

pathogenic changes in chemical-induced psoriasis-like lesions in guinea pig. Guinea pigs were topically exposed to 5% propranolol emulsion on the back of their ears, and control animals were exposed to control vehicle. We observed that the auricular areas of experimental animals displayed slight desquamation three days after induction, and eschar one week after induction. These areas presented with a typical psoriasis-like lesion and with edema, telangiec-tasia, dry skin/desquamation, and increased skin thickness (Fig. 2A). Histological examination showed increased thickness of epidermis and many inflammatory infiltrates in the lesions at three weeks post induction.

The experimental animals were randomly treated topically with PBS, hydrocortisone butyrate, or different doses of anti-FGF10 daily beginning at one week post induction and continually for two weeks. We found that in comparison with that in the PBS-treated animals, treatment with hydrocortisone butyrate or anti-FGF10 greatly reduced the psoriasiform-related edema, telangiectasia, and dry skin/desquamation in the tested areas at three weeks post induction (Fig. 2B). However, there was no parakeratosis or munro abscess in the lesions of different groups of animals.

Histological analysis indicated that the skin tissues form the healthy controls showed a regular length of rete ridges, granular cell layer (1-3 layers), and acanthosis (3-6 layers) with a few monocytes in the dermis, the tissue samples from the PBS-treated model group of animals displayed hyperkeratosis, reduced numbers of granular cell layers ($\leqslant$ 1 layer),

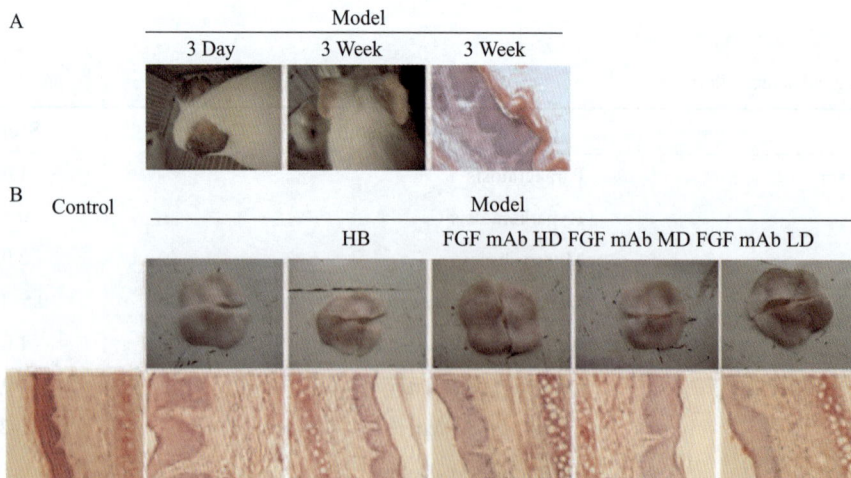

Fig. 2. Pathologic examination of psoriasis-like lesions. Guinea pigs were topically treated with 5% of propranolol emulsion on the back of their ears to induce psoriasis-like lesions and randomly treated topically with PBS, hydrocortisone butyrate, or different doses of anti-FGF10. The pathologic changes and the degrees of inflammation in the auricular areas of individual animals were examined histologically. (A), The morphology of auricular psoriasis-like lesions was examined at 3 days or 3 weeks post propranolol treatment, and tissue sections were examined at 3 weeks post induction (magnification: ×100). (B), The gross and histological examination of psoriasis-like lesions at two weeks post treatment (magnification: ×200). The upper panels (a-e): the gross tissues; The low panels (f-k): histological examination (Magnifi-cation: ×200). HB, hydrocortisone butyrate group; HD, high dose (0.188 mg/ml); MD, medium dose (0.094 mg/ml); LD, low dose (0.063 mg/ml). n = 4-5 for each group at each time point. The monocyte infiltrates are indicated by arrowheads and the thickness of epidermis is indicated by arrows.

increased thickness of acanthosis (13-24 layers) and irregular lengths of rete ridges, accompanied by many inflammatory infiltrates in the dermis, increased thickness of epidermis, and telangiectasia in the lesions (Fig. 2B, Table 2). Quantitative analyses revealed that treatment with hydrocortisone butyrate or anti-FGF10 at any of the doses significantly reduced the thickness of epidermis, the number of inflammatory infiltrates (monocytes) in the dermis, and Baker's scores, as compared with that in the model group ($P < 0.05$, Table 2). It was notable that the numbers of inflammatory infiltrates in the dermis in the anti-FGF10-treated mice were similar to that of the healthy controls ($P > 0.05$), suggesting that anti-FGF10 may suppress the proliferation and migration of inflammatory cells and the release of inflammatory cytokines. These observations indicate that anti-FGF10 mitigates inflammation and pathogenic changes in chemical-induced psoriasis-like lesions in guinea pig.

Table 2.　The pathological changes of the corneous layer, epidermis and dermis in the lesions from different groups of animals

Groups	Baker's Score	The number of monocytes	Thickness of epidermis (mm)
Control	2.25 ± 0.26	76.00 ± 9.82	65.21 ± 11.62
Model	6.31 ± 0.73[**]	114.57 ± 8.77[*]	128.95 ± 10.73[**]
Model + HB	4.53 ± 0.67[**,##]	89.85 ± 12.12[*,##]	97.60 ± 19.56[**,#]
Model + FGF mAb HD	4.83 ± 0.75[**,##]	73.82 ± 8.82[##]	115.26 ± 17.35[**,#]
Model + FGF mAb MD	4.94 ± 0.68[**,##]	90.37 ± 14.84[*,##]	118.52 ± 16.21[**,#]
Model + FGF mAb LD	5.17 ± 0.75[**,##]	97.56 ± 13.62[*,##]	109.40 ± 12.84[**,#]

HB: hydrocortisone butyrate group; HD: high dose (0.188 mg/ml); MD: medium dose (0.094 mg/ml); LD: low dose (0.063 mg/ml). [*]$P < 0.05$, [**]$P < 0.01$ vs. the healthy control; [#]$P < 0.05$, [##]$P < 0.01$ vs. the model group. $n = 9$ for each group.

4. Discussion

It is well known that excessive growth and aberrant differentiation of keratinocytes contribute to the pathological process of psoriasis[2]. Previous studies have shown that FGF10 is an important regulator of keratinocyte proliferation, differentiation, and migration [5,6], and its over-production is associated with the development of psoriasis[11]. To further study the function of FGF10 in keratinocyte proliferation and psoriasis formation, we generated a new mAb against FGF10 with a titer of 1:12 800. The successful production of anti-FGF10 provides a unique reagent for studying the function of FGF10 blockage in keratinocyte proliferation in vitro and the development of psoriasis-like lesions in vivo.

Human keratinocyte line, HaCaT, has been widely used as a model of a highly proliferative epidermis[12], and we cultured HaCaT cells to evaluate the potential effect of anti-FGF10. We found that treatment with different doses of FGF10 stimulated HaCaT cell proliferation in a dose-dependent manner, consistent with previous findings[5,6]. Given that FGF10 is produced by keratinocytes[13], FGF10 may stimulate keratinocyte proliferation in an autocrine fashion. More importantly, we found that treatment with varying doses of anti-FGF10 inhibited the FGF10-stimulated human keratinocyte proliferation also in a dose-dependent manner. These data demonstrated that anti-FGF10 effectively neutralized the activity of FGF10 and inhibited keratinocyte proliferation in vitro.

It is well known that FGF10 expression is up-regulated in the upper dermis of psoriatic skin and that the levels of FGF10 in the lesions are correlated with keratinocyte proliferation and the severity of inflammatory infiltrates in the lesions[7]. On the other hand, FGF10$^{-/-}$ mice display abnormal epidermal morphogenesis[8]. Apparently, FGF10 may promote the growth of keratinocytes in psoriasis and aberrant keratinocyte proliferation contributes to the development of psoriasis-like lesions. We tested the potential therapeutic effect of anti-FGF10 on the propranolol-induced psoriasis-like lesions and we found that treatment with anti-FGF10, like hydrocortisone butyrate, greatly inhibited the severity of psoriasis-like lesions by reducing the Baker's scores, the thickness of epidermis, and the numbers of monocyte infiltrates in the dermis of the animals. To the best of our knowledge, this was the first study to demonstrate that treatment with anti-FGF10 effectively mitigated inflammation and propranolol-induced psoriasis-like lesions in animals. The significant reduction in the numbers of inflammatory infiltrates in the lesions may stem from inhibition of FGF-10-promomted chemokine production and inflammatory cell migration in this model. Indeed, significantly higher levels of serum tumor necrosis factor α (TNF-α), interferon-γ (IFN-γ), interleukin (IL)-6, IL-8, IL-12, and IL-18 are detected in active psoriatic patients, related to that in controls [14].Treatment with anti-TNF-α mAb markedly decreases the clinical activity of psoriasis lesions[15].It is well known that many inflammatory factors contribute to the development and progression of psoriasis and these factors may synergistically promote the development of psoriasis[16]. Indeed, both IL-17a and TNF-α can synergistically induce the production of CXCL8 and β-defensin 2 (BD2) during the development of psoriasis lesions [16]. Treatment with anti-FGF10 alone inhibited inflammation and partially reduced inflammation-related epidermal thickness in this model. It is possible that anti-FGF10 may neutralized FGF10 and inhibit its effect on promoting keratinocyte proliferation, leading to less amount of cytokine and chemokine production. Therefore, anti-FGF10 may be used as an adjuvant therapeutic reagent, in combination with other drugs, such as glucocorticoids and retinoic acids. We are interested in further investigating the combination therapies for the intervention of psoriasis-like lesions, how neutralization of FGF10 by anti-FGF10 affects cytokine and chemokine production in keratinocytes and the potential mechanisms by which anti-FGF10 inhibits inflammatory cell infiltration in the psoriasis-like lesions.

5. Conclusions

We have successfully generated mouse mAb against FGF10 and found that treatment with anti-FGF10 inhibited FHF10-stimulated keratinocyte proliferation in a dose-dependent manner *in vitro*. Furthermore, we found that topical treatment with anti-FGF10 effectively mitigated inflammation and propranolol-induced psoriasis-like lesions in animals. Our findings may provide a proof of principle that the blockage of local FGF10 can inhibit keratinocyte proliferation and mitigate propranolol-induced psoriasis-like lesion. These observations may offer new basis to design new immunotherapies for the intervention of psoriasis in the clinic.

References

[1] Menter A, Gottlieb A, Feldman SR, et al. Guidelines of care for the management of psoriasis and psoriatic arthritis - Section 1. Overview of psoriasis and guidelines of care for the treatment of psoriasis with biologics[J]. Journal of the American Academy of Dermatology, 2008, 58(5): 826-850.

[2] Lowes MA, Bowcock AM, Krueger JG. Pathogenesis and therapy of psoriasis[J]. Nature, 2007, 445(7130): 866-873.

[3] Higgins E, Markham T. Current treatment options in the management of psoriasis[J]. Prescriber, 2010, 21(11): 31-44.

[4] Gibbs S, Pinto ANS, Murli S, et al. Epidermal growth factor and keratinocyte growth factor differentially regulate epidermal migration, growth, and differentiation[J]. Wound Repair and Regeneration, 2000, 8(3): 192-203.

[5] Marchese C, Felici A, Visco V, et al. Fibroblast growth factor 10 induces proliferation and differentiation of human primary cultured keratinocytes[J]. Journal of Investigative Dermatology, 2001, 116(4): 623-628.

[6] Radek KA, Taylor KR, Gallo RL. FGF-10 and specific structural elements of dermatan sulfate size and sulfation promote maximal keratinocyte migration and cellular proliferation[J]. Wound Repair and Regeneration, 2009, 17(1): 118-126.

[7] Kovacs D, Falchi M, Cardinali G, et al. Immunohistochemical analysis of keratinocyte growth factor and fibroblast growth factor 10 expression in psoriasis[J]. Experimental Dermatology, 2005, 14(2): 130-137.

[8] Suzuki K, Yamanishi K, Mori O, et al. Defective terminal differentiation and hypoplasia of the epidermis in mice lacking the Fgf10 gene[J]. Febs Letters, 2000, 481(1): 53-56.

[9] Tuzun BN, Tuzun Y, Gurel N, et al. Psoriasis-like lesions in guinea pigs receiving propranolol[J]. International Journal of Dermatology, 1993, 32(2): 133-134.

[10] Baker BS, Brent L, Valdimarsson H, et al. Is epidermal cell proliferation in psoriatic skin grafts on nude mice driven by T-cell derived cytokines?[J]. British Journal of Dermatology, 1992, 126(2): 105-110.

[11] Albanesi C, De Pita O, Girolomoni G. Resident skin cells in psoriasis: a special took at the pathogenetic functions of keratinocytes[J]. Clinics in Dermatology, 2007, 25(6): 581-588.

[12] Boukamp P, Petrussevska RT, Breitkreutz D, et al. Normal keratinization in a spontaneously immortalized aneuploid human keratinocyte cell line[J]. Journal of Cell Biology, 1988, 106(3): 761-771.

[13] Beer HD, Florence C, Dammeier J, et al. Mouse fibroblast growth factor 10: cDNA cloning, protein characterization, and regulation of mRNA expression[J]. Oncogene, 1997, 15(18): 2211-2218.

[14] Arican O, Aral M, Sasmaz S, et al. Serum levels of TNF-alpha, IFN-gamma, IL-6, IL-8, IL-12, IL-17 and IL-18 in patients with active psoriasis and correlation with disease severity[J]. Mediators of Inflammation, 2005, (5): 273-279.

[15] Oh CJ, Das KM, Gottlieb AB. Treatment with anti-tumor necrosis factor alpha (TNF-alpha) monoclonal antibody dramatically decreases the clinical activity of psoriasis lesions[J]. Journal of the American Academy of Dermatology, 2000, 42(5): 829-830.

[16] Guilloteau K, Paris I, Pedretti N, et al. Skin Inflammation Induced by the Synergistic Action of IL-17A, IL-22, Oncostatin M, IL-1α, and TNF-α Recapitulates Some Features of Psoriasis[J]. Journal of Immunology, 2010, 184(9): 5263-5270.

[17] Garcia-Valladares I, Espinoza LR. Psoriasis pathophysiology[J]. Immunotherapy, 2010, 2(4): 444-445.

A short peptide derived from the gN helix domain of FGF8b suppresses the growth of human prostate cancer cells

Tao Li , Xiaokun Li , Xiaoping Wu

1. Introduction

Prostate cancer is the second most common cause of cancer mortality in men in western countries. Interactions between hormones and growth factors and their receptors play significant roles in the development and progression of prostate cancer. These interactions are involved in the majority of the effects of steroid hormones connected with the growth regulation of hormone-responsive tumors. When hormone-responsive tumors progress to become hormone-independent, their growth is predominantly regulated by growth factors [1,2].

Fibroblast growth factor 8 (FGF8) belongs to the family of FGFs that are known to be involved in fetal central nervous system development, angiogenesis and wound healing [3,4]. Previous studies have demonstrated that FGF8 mRNA is over-expressed in 60–70% of newly diagnosed prostate cancers [5]. The FGF8 gene undergoes alternative splicing, generating four potential isoforms in humans (a, b, e and f) [6], among which FGF8b leads to the greatest transformation and is the major isoform expressed in prostate cancer [7–10]. FGF8b targeted to the prostate epithelium causes prostatic intraepithelial neoplasia (PIN) lesions in transgenic mice [11]. In vitro and in vivo studies have shown that FGF8b accelerates growth, invasion, tumorigenesis, angiogenesis and bone metastasis in prostate cancer [12,13–15]. Therefore, FGF8b has been considered as a potential target for prostate cancer therapy.

Alternative splicing at the N-terminus of FGF8 gives rise to four FGF8 isoforms (a, b, e and f) in humans. FGF8a is the smallest FGF8 isoform and has the common core region of all FGF8 isoforms consisting of 12 anti-parallel β-strands. The remaining isoforms have various lengths and contain additional N-terminal amino acid sequences. The alternatively spliced region of the FGF8b isoform contains 11 N-terminal residues. The FGF8b-FGFR2c structure shows that only the last three residues in the alternatively spliced region of FGF8b, F32, T33, and Q34 are ordered. These three residues combine with the following six residues to form a g helix (gN; residues 32–40), accounting for the higher receptor-binding affinity and FGF8b–FGFR binding specificity toward the "c" isoforms of FGFR1-3 and FGFR4 by inserting F32 and V36 into the vicinity of a hydrophobic groove on receptor D3, implying that the gN helix is a crucial functional domain mediating the specific binding of FGF8b to its receptors.

Schally and coworkers have demonstrated that growth hormone-releasing hormone (GH-RH) serves as an autocrine growth factor in many cancers, and found that synthetic antagonistic analogues of GH-RH inhibit the growth of diverse tumors and show great promise for cancer treatment. Moreover, based on the presence of specific receptors for hypothalamic peptides on human cancers, they developed targeted cytotoxic analogues of luteinizing hormone-releasing hormone (LH-RH) and somatostatin linked to doxorubicin or 2-pyrrolinodoxorubicin. These analogues also inhibit the growth of a variety of tumors, including prostate cancer [16]. Based on sequence alignment and structural analysis, the Facchiano group has also successfully identified a short peptide encompassing residues 48–58 of human FGF2, which is located at the predicted interface of the FGF2 dimer and is potentially involved in FGF2 dimerization, and demonstrated that this peptide strongly inhibits FGF2 activity [17].

According to the above FGF8b-FGFR structural analysis, we speculated that a short peptide containing the amino acid sequence of the gN helix may inhibit the biological activity of FGF8b by disturbing the interaction between FGF8b and its receptors, and thus that it may exert an antitumor effect on prostate cancer. Therefore, in this study we synthesized a gN helix derived short peptide (PNFTQHVREQSLV, referred to as 8b-13) containing a helical secondary structure as predicted by PSIPRED (http://bioinf.cs.ucl.ac.uk/psipred/), and evaluated its therapeutic potential as a potent FGF8b antagonist in prostate cancer.

2. Materials and methods

2.1 Materials

Recombinant human FGF8b was purchased from PeproTechInc (Rocky Hill, NJ, USA). Recombinant human EGF was obtained from the Biopharmaceutical R&D Center of Jinan University (Guangzhou, China). RMPI-1640 and fetal bovine serum (FBS) were purchased from Invitrogen (Carlsbad, CA, USA). The cell proliferation assay reagent MTT was obtained from Roche (Mannheim, Germany). Propidium iodide (PI) was obtained from Sigma (USA). The polyvinylidenedifluoride (PVDF) membrane was obtained from Millipore (Billerica, MA, USA). The enhanced chemiluminescence (ECL) detection kit was purchased from Pierce (Rockford, IL, USA). Anti-phospho-Erk1/2 (catalog no. 4370), anti-Erk1/2 (catalog no. 4695), anti-phospho-P38 (catalog no. 4511), anti-P38 (catalog no. 8690), anti-phospho-Akt (catalog no. 4060), anti-Akt (catalog no. 4691), anti-cyclinD1 (catalog no. 2978), anti-PCNA (catalog no. 2586), anti-GAPDH (catalog no. 2118) antibodies and horseradish peroxidase conjugated goat anti-rabbit secondary antibody were obtained from Cell Signaling Technology (Danvers, MA, USA). Anti-FGF8b antibody (catalog no. MAB323) was purchased from Millipore (Billerica, MA, USA). IPG strips (pH 3–10 nonlinear), SDS, acrylamide, methylenebisacrylamide, TEMED, CHAPS, Bio-Lyte 3–10 ampholyte 40% solution, Tris, glycine, and iodoacetamide were obtained from Bio-Rad (Hercules, CA, USA). Glycerol and ammonium persulfate were purchased from Sigma (St. Louis, MO, USA). DTT and urea were obtained from Promega (Madison, WI, USA). PMSF (catalog no. 36978) was purchased from ThermoFisher. TRIZOL, First-strand cDNA synthesis kit and SYBR green Q-PCR kit were purchased from Bio-Rad (Hercules, CA, USA).

2.2 Cell culture

Human prostate cancer cells (PC-3 and DU-145) were obtained from the Institute of Tissue Transplantation and Immunology of Jinan University and cultured in RMPI-1640 (Invitrogen) containing 10% FBS and maintained in a humidified atmosphere containing 5% CO_2 at 37 °C.

2.3 The synthesis of the 8b-13 and H13 peptides

The 8b-13 peptide (PNFTQHVREQSLV) and its scrambled version H13 (QRVSQFENHPVTL) were synthesized at SBS Genetech (Beijing, China). The purity of the synthetic peptides was assessed by reverse phase high-performance liquid chromatography and was found to be greater than 98%.

2.4 Cell viability assay

PC-3 and DU-145 cells were seeded in 96-well plates at a density of 1×10^3 and 5×10^3 cells per well, respectively, and allowed to attach overnight. After starved cultivation in RMPI-1640 with 0.4% FBS for 24 h, cells were treated with serial dilutions of the 8b-13 or H13 peptides, 40 ng/ml FGF8b alone, or 40 ng/ml FGF8b together with serial dilutions of the 8b-13 or H13 peptides. A neutralizing anti-FGF8b antibody was applied to inhibit endogenous FGF8b to determine whether the endogenous FGF8b expressed by the cells is the reason that 8b-13 inhibits basal cell proliferation. Starved cells were pretreated with the anti-FGF8b antibody (5 µg/ml) for 10 min before the addition of 8b-13 (125 nM). Epidermal growth factor (EGF) was used as an additional proliferation inducing agent to determine whether 8b-13 only inhibits FGF8b-mediated proliferation. Starved cells were treated with 40 ng/ml EGF alone or 40 ng/ml EGF plus serial dilutions of the 8b-13 peptide for 48 h. The number of viable cells was lastly determined by the methylthiazoletetrazolium (MTT) method as previously described [18]. The absorbance was immediately measured at 570 nm to determine the number of viable cells.

2.5 Analysis of endogenous expression of FGF8b in prostate cancer cells

PC-3 and DU-145 cells were plated in 12-well plates at densities of 5×10^4 and 2×10^5 cells per well, respectively, in RMPI-1640 media with 10% FBS and were allowed to attach overnight. The cells were seeded at approximately 80% confluence and lysed with $1 \times$ SDS loading buffer (0.125 M Tris, pH 6.8, 2% sodium dodecyl sulfate, 10% glycerol, 10% β-mercaptoethanol and 0.01% bromophenol blue) containing 1 mM PFSF. The lysate was syringed, boiled for 5 min and subjected to 10% SDS-PAGE followed by transferal to PVDF membranes. The membranes were blocked with 5% non-fat dry milk at room temperature for 1 h and incubated with rabbit monoclonal FGF8b antibody at room temperature for 1 h followed by a horseradish peroxidase conjugated goat anti-rabbit secondary antibody before visualization with ECL reagents. The results were analyzed by Quantity One software to determine the relative ratio and presented in graphs as expression relative to that of GAPDH.

2.6 Cell cycle analysis

PC-3 cells were seeded in 12-well plates at 3×10^4 cells per well, starved for 24 h, and treated with 40 ng/ml FGF8b alone, 40 ng/ml FGF8b plus serial dilutions of the 8b-13 or H13 peptides, or 8b-13 peptides alone for 48 h. The cells were washed twice with PBS, trypsinized and pelleted by centrifugation before suspension in PBS containing 10% FBS. Ice-cold 70% ethanol was added drop wise to the cell suspensions. Samples were kept at 4℃ for 30 min. After three washes with PBS, cells were stained by adding 50 μg/ml propidium iodide (PI). The percentages of cells at various phases of the cell cycle were analyzed using the ModFit DNA analysis program.

2.7 Western blotting analysis of cyclinD1 expression and MAP kinase and AKT activation

PC-3 cells were plated in 12-well plates in RMPI-1640 media as described above. For western blot analysis of cyclinD1 expression, starved cells were pretreated with serial dilutions of peptides for 30 min before stimulation with 40 ng/ml FGF8b for 6 h. For western blot analysis of MAP kinase and AKT activation, starved cells were pretreated with serial dilutions of peptides for 5 min before stimulation with 40 ng/ml FGF8b for 15 min. After washing with cold PBS, cells were lysed in $1 \times$ SDS-PAGE loading buffer. The lysate was syringed, boiled for 5 min, and run on SDS-PAGE gels followed by transferal to PVDF membranes. The membrane was incubated with TBST (25 mM Tris, pH 7.4, 150 mM NaCl and 0.1% Tween-20) containing 5% non-fat dry milk at room temperature for 1 h. After 3 washes with TBST, the membrane was probed with the primary antibodies (an anti-cyclinD1 rabbit mAb, an anti-phospho-Erk1/2 rabbit mAb, an anti-phospho-P38 rabbit mAb, and an anti-phospho-Akt rabbit mAb) at 4℃ overnight followed by incubation with HRP-linked goat anti-rabbit IgG for 1 h at room temperature. The blots were detected with an ECL detection kit according to the manufacturer's procedure. Non-phosphorylated Erk1/2, P38, or Akt were used as the reference controls. The results were analyzed by Quantity One software to determine the relative ratio and presented in graphs as expression relative to GAPDH.

2.8 Sample preparation for two-dimensional gel electrophoresis

PC-3 cells were seeded at approximately 30% confluence and cultured overnight. After starvation for 24 h, cells were treated with 40 ng/ml FGF8b alone or 40 ng/ml FGF8b plus 125 nM 8b-13 for 48 h. Approximately 2×10^7 cells were harvested and lysed in 150 μl lysis buffer that contained 7 M urea, 2 M thiourea, 4% CHAPS, 65 mM DTT, 0.2% pH 3–10 ampholyte, 25 mg/l RNase A, 20 U/ml DNase I, and protease inhibitor cocktail. Samples were incubated at room temperature for 10 min, kept on ice for 2 h, and centrifuged at 12,000 g for 30 min at 4℃. The supernatant was collected and the protein concentrations were determined using the Bradford method [19].

2.9 Two-dimensional gel electrophoresis and image analysis

An equal amount (1 mg) of protein sample was mixed with rehydration buffer (7 M urea, 2 M thiourea, 4% CHAPS, 65 mM DTT, 0.2% pH 3–10 ampholyte and 0.001% bromophenol blue), and loaded on a 17 cm, pH 3–10 nonlinear immobilized pH gradient (IPG) gel strip (Bio-Rad). The IPG strips were then passively rehydrated and subjected to isoelectric focusing followed by equilibration and separation on 12% SDS-PAGE gels as previously described [20].

2.10 Mass spectrometric analysis and database search

The gels were stained with Coomassie G-250 (Bio-Rad) and scanned using a GE-Imagescanner. PDQuest 8.0 software (Bio-Rad) was used to analyze the images. The protein spots were cut, destained in 25 mM NH$_4$HCO$_3$/50% ACN, and then incubated with trypsin at 37℃ overnight. The peptides were extracted, dried in a vacuum concentrator for 3 h, and subjected to tandem time-of-flight mass spectrometry (ABI 4800 TOF-TOF) analysis. Database searches were performed using Mascot software (Matrix science, London, UK), to search NCBI (ncbi.nlm. nih.gov) databases.

2.11 Real-Time quantitative PCR analysis of PAFAH1B2, ESD, CRABP2 and PCNA expression regulated by 8b-13

PC-3 cells were seeded in 6-well plates with 1.5×10^5 cells per well, starved for 24 h and treated with 40 ng/ml FGF8b alone or 40 ng/ml FGF8b plus 125 nM 8b-13 for 48 h. Total RNA was isolated using TRIZOL. Two micrograms of total RNA were reverse-transcribed using the First-Strand cDNA Synthesis Kit according to the manufacturer's instructions. The resulting cDNA was used as a template for quantitative PCR amplification with the SYBR green qPCR Kit. The quantitative PCR was performed using the CFX96 Touch Deep Well real-time PCR Detection System. The sequences of the PCR primers were as follows: PAFAH1B2: 5'-CGGACCCTCTACTTCAGTGT-3'(F) and 5'-CGAACAGTACATCAGGCTCT-3'(R); ESD: 5'-CCTGCACTGTATTGGCTCT-3'(F) and 5'-GCCAAAGTCCCAGCTCTC-3'(R); CRABP2: 5'-CCCAACTTCTCTGGCAAC-3'(F) and 5'-TCCACTGCTGGCTTGGAC-3'(R); PCNA: 5'-TCTGAGGGCTTCGACACCTA-3'(F) and 5'-TACTAGCGCCAAGGTATCCG-3'(R); GADPH: 5'-CCCACT CCTCCACCTTTGAC-3'(F) and 5'-TCTTCCTCTTGTGCTCTTGC-3'(R). The mRNA level of the detected protein was expressed as the relative ratio to the GADPH mRNA level.

2.12 Western blot analysis of PCNA expression regulated by 8b-13

PC-3 cells were seeded in 6-well plates at 1.5×10^5 cells per well. After starvation for 24 h, cells were treated with 40 ng/ml FGF8b alone or 40 ng/ml FGF8b plus 125 nM 8b-13 for 48 h. Samples were separated on a 10% SDS-PAGE gel and transferred to a PVDF membrane. The membrane was blocked with 5% non-fat dry milk and incubated with anti-PCNA antibody (1:4 000 dilution) overnight at 4℃, followed by incubation with HRP-labeled secondary antibody (1:6 000 dilution) for 1 h. Signals were detected by an ECL kit. The results were analyzed by Quantity One software to determine the relative ratio and presented in graphs as expression relative to that of GAPDH.

2.13 Statistical analysis

The statistical analyses were performed using GraphPad Prism software 5.01. The student's t-test was used to compare data between two groups, and a one-way ANOVA followed by Tukey's multiple comparison test was used for multiple comparison data. A P value of <0.05 was considered to be statistically significant.

3. Results

3.1 8b-13 inhibits FGF8b-induced cell proliferation

To investigate the role of 8b-13 in prostate cancer cells, we first evaluated whether the synthetic peptides inhibit the FGF8b-stimulated proliferation of prostate cancer cell lines, including PC-3 and DU-145, using an MTT assay. The results showed that 8b-13 peptides markedly inhibited the induction of proliferation by FGF8b in both cell lines, whereas the scrambled peptide H13 had no suppressive effect on cell growth (Fig. 1A and B). The 8b-13 peptide mediated stronger proliferation inhibition in PC-3 cells than in DU-145 cells, with 50% inhibition (IC50) at approximately 5 nM in PC-3 cells and 25 nM in DU-145 cells (Fig. 1C). The administration of 8b-13 alone also inhibited the growth of two cell lines, both of which express endogenous FGF8b as indicated in Fig. 1D.

To address the issue that the endogenous FGF8b expressed by cells might be the reason that 8b-13 inhibits basal cell proliferation, we used a neutralizing anti-FGF8b antibody to inhibit endogenous FGF8b and then analyzed the effects of 8b-13 on cell proliferation. The results presented in Fig. 1E show that the 8b-13 peptide or anti-FGF8b antibody alone could suppress the cell growth induced by endogenous FGF8b, while the addition of the 8b-13 peptide in the presence of the anti-FGF8b antibody did not further inhibit cell proliferation (8b-13 plus anti-FGF8b antibody group *versus* anti-FGF8b antibody group, $P > 0.05$). This result confirms that 8b-13 inhibits basal cell proliferation by interacting with the endogenous FGF8b expressed by cells. Moreover, we also used an additional proliferation stimulating agent, EGF, to analyze whether 8b-13 inhibits only FGF8b-mediated proliferation. The results indicated that 8b-13 had no inhibitory effect on cell proliferation induced by EGF (Fig. 1F), which when combined with the results of the above MTT assay revealed that 8b-13 exclusively suppressed cell growth mediated by FGF8b.

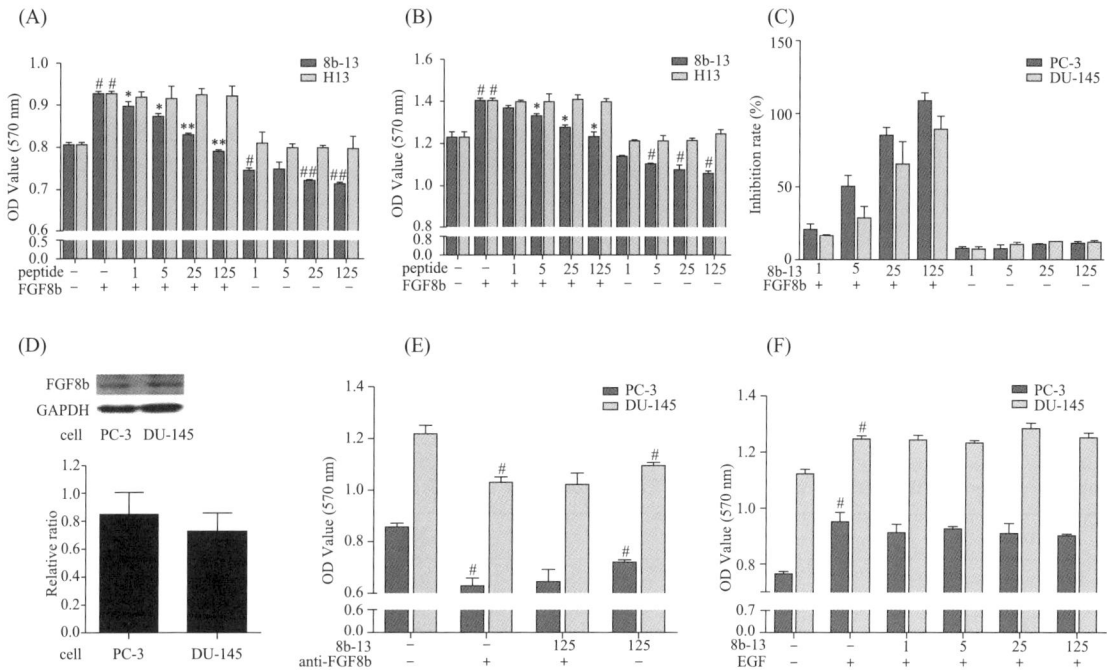

Fig. 1. Effects of the synthetic 8b-13 peptide on FGF8b-stimulated proliferation of PC-3 (A) and DU-145 (B) cells. Starved cells were treated with 40 ng/ml FGF8b plus 8b-13 or the scrambled peptide H13 at the indicated concentrations, and cell proliferation was measured 48 h later using the MTT assay. (C) Comparison of the inhibitory effects of the synthetic 8b-13 peptide on proliferation between PC-3 and DU-145 cells. (D) Analysis of the endogenous FGF8b expression in PC-3 and DU-145 cells by western blotting. (E) Effects of the synthetic 8b-13 peptide on the proliferation of PC-3 and DU-145 cells in the presence of a neutralizing anti-FGF8b antibody. Starved cells were pretreated with the anti-FGF8b antibody (5 μg/ml) for 10 min before 8b-13 (125 nM) was added, and cell proliferation was measured 48 h later using an MTT assay. (F) The effects of the synthetic 8b-13 peptide on the EGF-stimulated proliferation of PC-3 and DU-145 cells. Starved cells were treated with 40 ng/ml EGF alone or 40 ng/ml EGF plus serial dilutions of the 8b-13 peptide for 48 h, followed by the detection of the cell proliferation by an MTT assay. Data are presented as the mean (±SD) of three independent experiments performed in triplicate. $^{\#}P < 0.05$ vs. control group; $^{\#\#}P < 0.01$ vs. control group; $^{*}P < 0.05$ vs. FGF8b group; $^{**}P < 0.01$ vs. FGF8b group.

3.2 The 8b-13 peptide arrests the cell cycle at the G0/G1 phase in PC-3 cells

As cell proliferation depends on cell cycle progress, we further used flow cytometry to determine the effects of the synthetic peptides on the cell cycle progress of PC-3 cells stimulated with FGF8b. As shown in Fig. 2, an increase in the S-phase population and a decrease in the G0/G1-phase population were observed in FGF8b-induced cells compared

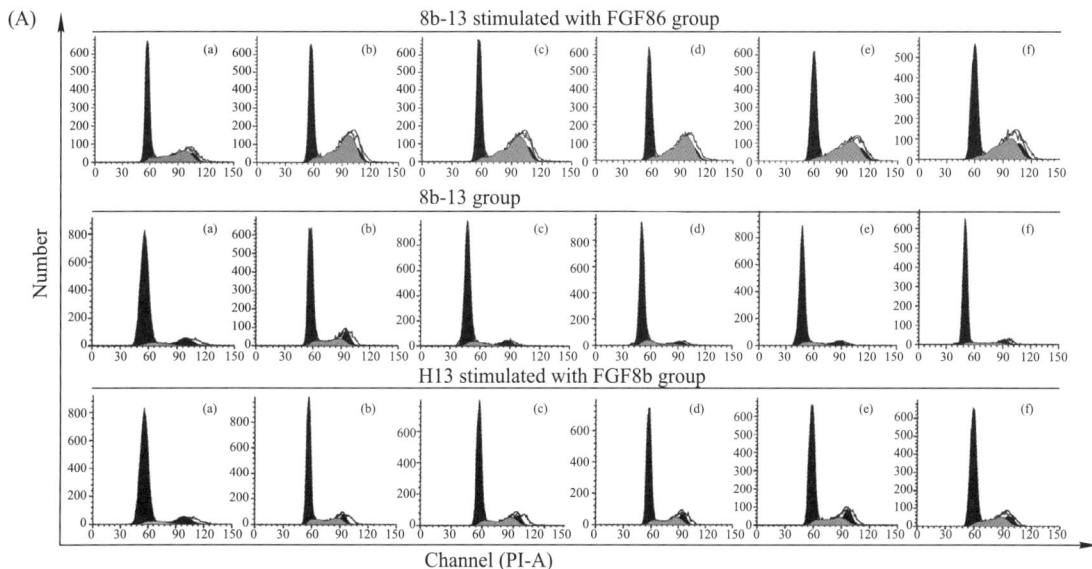

B

Flow cytometry analysis of the effect of synthesized 8b-13 peptides in PC-3 cells stimulated with FGF8b on the cell cycle

Group	G0/G1(%)	G2/M(%)	S(%)
a	62.1±1.92	8.1±0.19	29.8±2.09
b	47.5±3.05	8.9±1.29	43.6±1.85[##]
c	49.5±2.85	8.7±1.79	41.8±1.06
d	51.2±3.44	7.9±1.49	40.9±2.18[*]
e	52.7±2.29	9.0±2.07	38.3±0.23[*]
f	54.8±2.93	11.8±0.89	33.4±2.02[**]

Folw cytometry analysis of the effect of synthesized 8b-13 peptides alone in PC-3 cells on the cell cycle

Group	G0/G1(%)	G2/M(%)	S(%)
a	81.05±0.94	7.81±0.44	11.14±0.5
b	69.46±2.11	10.63±2.31	19.91±0.19[##]
c	83.17±0.38	7.61±0.28	9.22±0.66
d	84.94±0.28	7.17±0.64	7.89±0.38[#]
e	85.66±0.34	6.72±0.21	7.63±0.54[#]
f	86.54±1.21	6.41±0.79	7.05±0.42[#]

Flow cytometry analysis of the effect of synthesized H13 peptides in PC-3 cells stimulated with FGF8b on the cell cycle

Group	G0/G1(%)	G2/M(%)	S(%)
a	81.05±0.94	7.81±0.44	11.14±0.5
b	69.46±2.11	10.63±2.31	19.91±0.19[##]
c	69.79±0.46	8.99±0.19	21.22±0.27
d	70.15±0.09	10.51±0.25	19.34±0.34
e	71.47±1.41	9.63±1.09	18.90±0.32
f	69.23±0.68	8.79±1.11	21.98±1.79

Fig. 2. Inhibition of cell cycle progress in PC-3 cells. (A) PC-3 cells were starved for 24 h and then treated with 40 ng/ml FGF8b (b), 40 ng/ml FGF8b plus various concentrations of 8b-13 or H13, or various concentrations of 8b-13 alone (c-f: 1, 5, 25, and 125 nM). (a) Control cells without FGF8b, 8b-13 or H13. The cells were harvested after a 48 h incubation, stained with propidium iodide, and analyzed using flow cytometry. The images shown here are representative of one of three independent experiments. (B) Cell cycle distribution of the control and treated cells. Data are expressed as the mean ± SD ($n = 3$). [##]$P < 0.01$ vs. control group; [*]$P < 0.05$ vs. FGF8b group; [**]$P < 0.01$ vs. FGF8b group.

with the control. The administration of 8b-13 peptides enhanced the G0/G1 phase percentage and reduced the S-phase percentage of cells stimulated with FGF8b, whereas the scrambled H13 peptides had no effect on FGF8b-induced cell cycle distribution, suggesting that 8b-13 peptides counteracted the regulatory effects of FGF8b on the progress of the cell cycle in a sequence specific manner.

3.3 The 8b-13 peptide suppresses the expression of cyclinD1

CyclinD1, one member of the highly conserved cyclin family involved in cell cycle progress, has been reported to greatly contribute to the G1/S cell cycle transition. Our results showed that 8b-13 peptides suppressed cell cycle progress from the G0/G1 to the S phase in FGF8b-induced cells. We therefore further evaluated whether the synthetic peptides influenced the expression of cyclinD1. As shown in Fig. 3, cyclinD1 was increased by FGF8b stimulation and

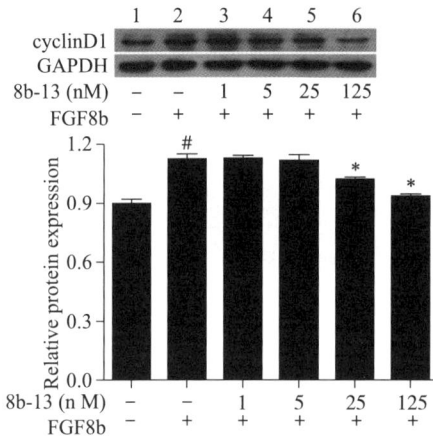

Fig. 3. The synthetic 8b-13 peptide down-regulates the expression of cyclinD1 in PC-3 cells. Starved cells were pretreated with 8b-13 at the indicated concentrations for 30 min before stimulation with 40 ng/ml FGF8b for 6 h. The cell lysates were immunoblotted with cyclinD1 antibody. Data are presented as the mean ($\pm$SD) of three independent experiments. $^{\#}P < 0.05$ *vs.* control group; $^{*}P < 0.05$ *vs.* FGF8b group.

down-regulated by 8b-13 treatment, implying that 8b-13 peptides arrest cells at the G0/G1 phase in part by down-regulating the expression of G1/S-specific cyclinD1.

3.4 The 8b-13 peptide blocks the activation of Akt and MAP kinases

The effects of 8b-13 peptides on FGF8b-induced Akt and MAP kinase activation were assessed by Western blotting. As shown in Fig. 4, FGF8b treatment for 15 min led to intense phosphorylation of Erk1/2, P38, and Akt in PC-3 cells (Fig. 4A, lane 2), whereas pretreatment with the 8b-13 peptide (1–125 nM) for 5 min resulted in significant blockage of Erk1/2, P38 and Akt activation in a dose-dependent manner (Fig. 4A, lanes 3–6). However, compared with the cells stimulated with FGF8b, no significant change was observed in the level of activation of the detected signaling molecules in the cells pretreated with the scrambled peptide H13 (Fig. 4B, lanes 3–6).

3.5 Identification of 8b-13-targeting FGF8b proteins by a proteomic approach

The distinct proteins participating in the effects of 8b-13-targeting FGF8b stimulation on PC-3 cells were further explored by combining two-dimensional electrophoresis and mass spectrometry. We first compared the protein profiles presented in Fig. 5 between control and FGF8b-stimulated cells to determine specific proteins regulated by FGF8b, and then compared the intensities of the selected protein spots between FGF8b-stimulated and 8b-13-treated groups to determine the differentially expressed proteins influenced by 8b-13 targeting FGF8b stimulation. Eight protein spots were identified (Fig. 6), excised from the gels, subjected to trypsin digestion, and analyzed by MALDI-TOF/TOF. Comparison of the data collected from MALDI-TOF/TOF to the NCBI databases using the MASCOT online search tool enabled confident identification of eight proteins as shown in Table 1, among which four proteins (PAFAH1B2, UQCRB, HNRNPC and ESD) were up-regulated and four (CRABP2, CWC15, SNRPF and PCNA) were down-regulated by treatment with the 8b-13 peptide.

3.6 Validation of the expression levels of PAFAH1B2, ESD, CRABP2 and PCNA regulated by 8b-13

To confirm the trends of the expression levels of the proteins identified by the proteomic approach, RT-qPCR was first performed to validate the mRNA levels of the identified proteins, including PAFAH1B2, ESD, CRABP2 and PCNA, which are closely related to cell proliferation. As shown in Fig. 7A, FGF8b stimulation markedly decreased the expression of PAFAH1B2 and ESD and increased the expression of CRABP2 and PCNA, while the addition of 8b-13 peptides up-regulated the expression of PAFAH1B2 and ESD and down-regulated the expression of CRABP2 and PCNA at the transcriptional level. Western blotting was further carried out to confirm the trends of PCNA expression at the translational level. The results also coincided with results from both the proteomic and RT-qPCR analysis (Fig. 7B).

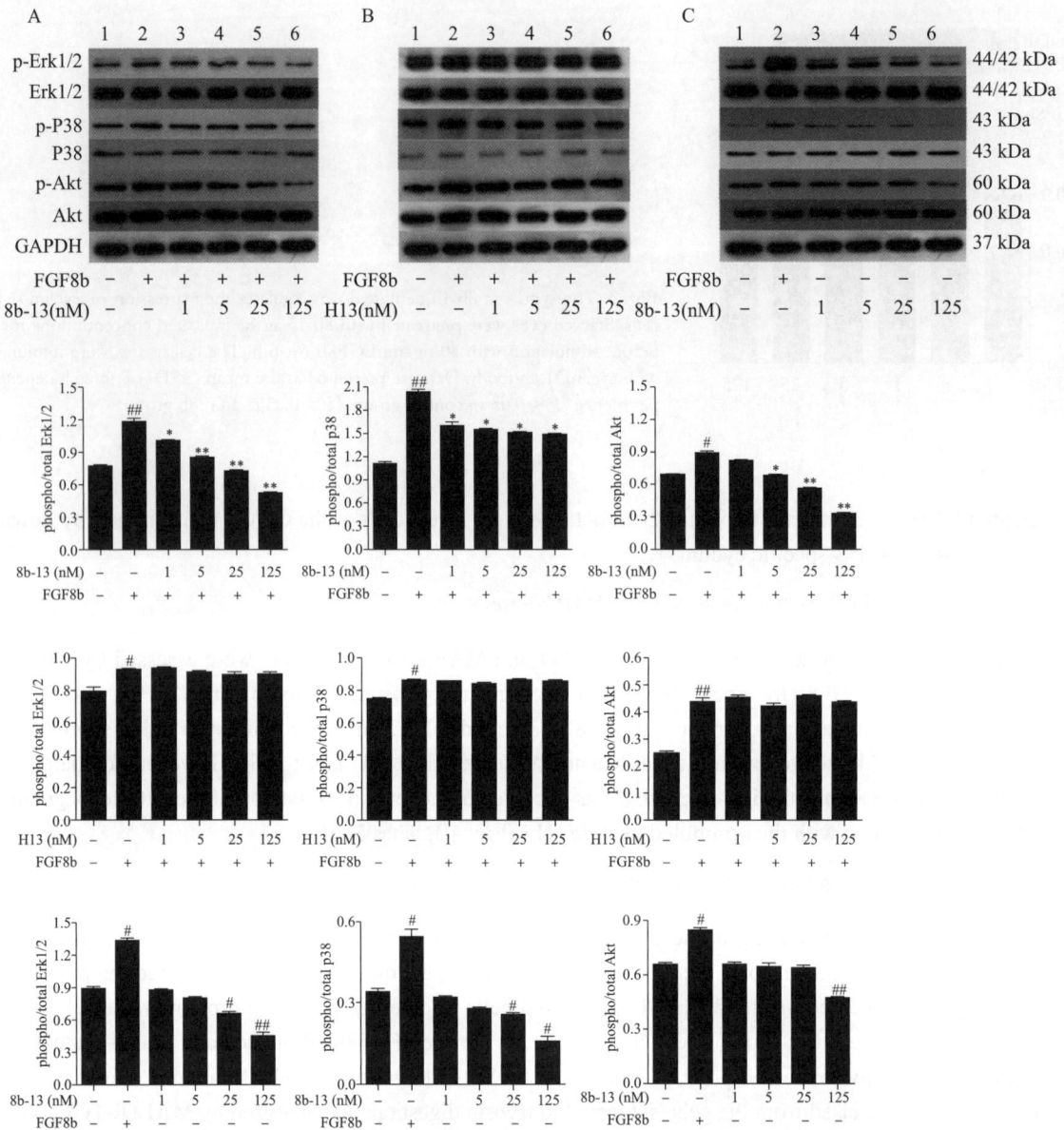

Fig. 4. The synthetic 8b-13 peptide blocks the activation of Akt and MAP kinases. Starved cells were pretreated with serially diluted 8b-13 (A) or the scrambled peptide H13 (B) for 5 min before stimulation with 40 ng/ml FGF8b for 15 min. (C) The cells were treated with 8b-13 peptide alone. The phosphorylated and total levels of Erk1/2, P38 and Akt were determined by western blot analysis. Data are presented as the mean ± SD of three independent experiments. $^{#}P < 0.05$ vs. control group; $^{##}P < 0.01$ vs. control group; $^{*}P < 0.05$ vs. FGF8b group; $^{**}P < 0.01$ vs. FGF8b group.

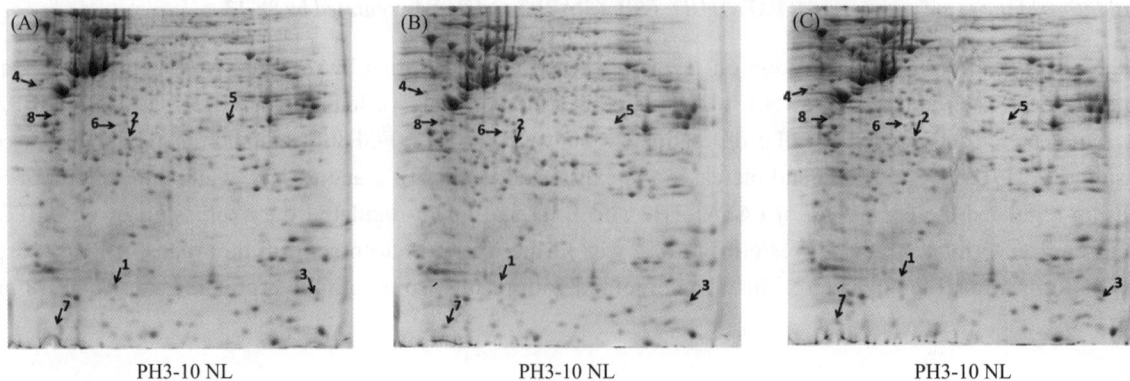

Fig. 5. Comparison of the protein expression patterns between control (A), 40 ng/ml FGF8b-stimulated cells (B), and 40 ng/ml FGF8b plus 125 nM 8b-13 treated cells (C). The proteins were separated by two-dimensional electrophoresis and stained with Coomassie brilliant blue G250. Identified protein spots are indicated by numbers.

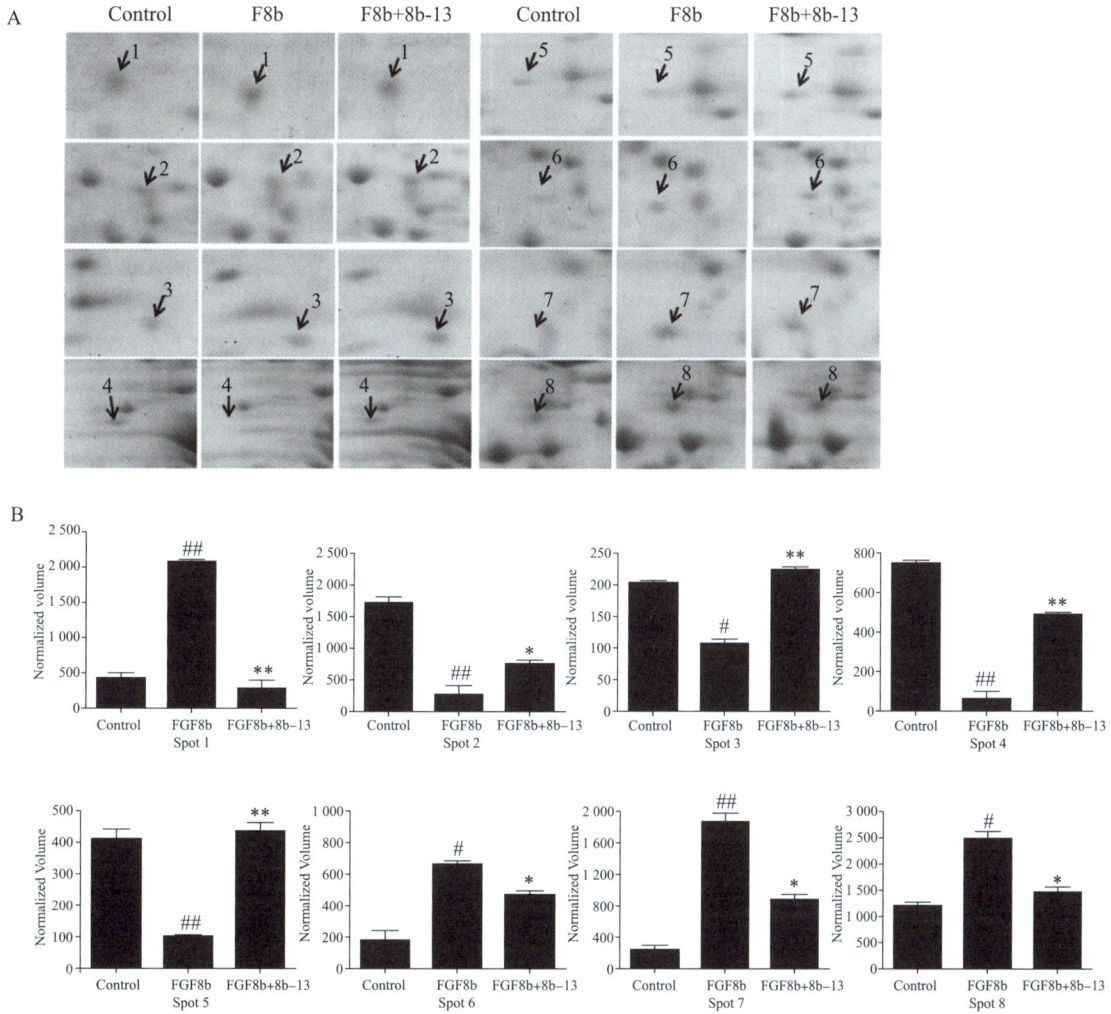

Fig. 6. (A) Enlarged maps of the protein spots differentially expressed between FGF8b-stimulation and 8b-13 treatment. (B) Graphical representation of spot intensities assigned by PDQuest 8.0 software subsequent to normalization. The graphs show the intensities of the protein spots differentially expressed between FGF8b stimulation and 8b-13 treatment. $^{#}P < 0.05$ *vs.* control group; $^{##}P < 0.01$ *vs.* control group; $^{*}P < 0.05$ *vs.* FGF8b group; $^{**}P < 0.01$ *vs.* FGF8b group.

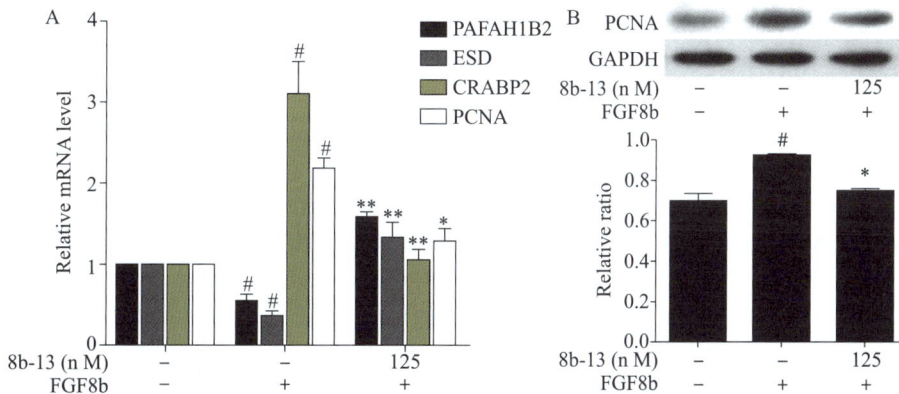

Fig. 7. Validation of the expression levels of the identified proteins. (A) Total RNA was isolated from PC-3 cells treated with 40 ng/ml FGF8b alone or 40 ng/ml FGF8b plus 125 nM 8b-13 for 48 h, and reverse-transcribed for quantitative PCR amplification of PAFAH1B2, ESD, CRABP2 and PCNA. (B) PCNA protein levels were determined in whole cell lysates by western blotting and scanning densitometry. Data are presented as the expression level relative to that of GAPDH. The experiment was repeated once, with similar results. $^{#}P < 0.05$ *vs.* control group; $^{*}P < 0.05$ *vs.* FGF8b group; $^{**}P < 0.01$ *vs.* FGF8b group.

Table 1. MALDI-TOF/TOF results on differentially expressed proteins.

	Protein name	Abbr.	Accession no.	Mw (Da)/PI	Score	CI (%)	Characteristics	Fold
A								
1	Cellular retinoic acid-binding protein 2	CRABP2	IP100216088	15854.1/5.42	387	100	Control of cell proliferation, differentiation, and survival	—6.6
6	Protein CWC15 homolog	CWC15	IP100009009	26665.3/5.55	168	100	Interact with CDC5L	—1.4
7	Small nuclear ribonucleo-protein F	SNRPF	IPI00220528	9775.8/4.7	189	100	Interact with DDX20	—2.1
8	Proliferating cell nuclear antigen	PCNA	IPI0002I700	29092.4/4.57	244	100	An auxiliary and processivity factor for DNA polymerase δ; interact with cyclinD link DNA replication and DNA repair	—1.7
B								
1	Platelet-activating factor acetylhydrolase IB subunit beta	PAFAH1B2	IPI00026546	25724.2/5.57	264	100	Activates cells involved in inflammation; key component of tumor progression	2.9
3	Ubiquinol-cutochrome c reductase binding protein	UQCRB	IPI00798386	11551.9/7.93	353	100	Essential component of the mitochondrial electron transfer system	2.1
4	Heterogeneous nuclear ribonucleoproteins C1/C2	HNRNPC	IPI00216592	32374.9/4.94	219	100	Belongs to the subfamily of ubiquitously expressed hnRNPS processing of pro-mRNA	8.3
5	Esterase D	ESD	IPI00641040	28,607/6.29	245	100	Serving as a genetic marker of retinoblastomas; play a role in detoxification	4.4

"Score" means the similarity between the actual peptide data of the protein obtained from Mass spectrometric analysis and the theoretical peptide data in NCBI databases.

4. Discussion

FGF8b has been shown to function as a potent autocrine growth factor in the stimulation of proliferation of prostate cancer cells.

Furthermore, its paracrine effects including the induction of angiogenesis and osteoblastic differentiation may contribute to tumor progression [21]. FGF family members are known to interact with FGFR as a physiological mechanism to modulate their activities. FGF8b binds to and stimulates mitogenesis in cells containing FGF8b receptors (the "c" isoforms of FGFR1-3 and FGFR4), among which FGFR3c has a much higher affinity for FGF8b than the other three receptors (FGFR3c > FGFR4 > FGFR2c > FGFR1c) [22]. One functional domain of FGF8b, the gN helix, contains the alternatively spliced region accounting for the high affinity and specificity of the ligand to its receptors. A synthetic peptide simulating the structure of the gN helix may bind to FGF8b receptors and interrupt the interaction between FGF8b and it receptors, resulting in an inhibition of FGF8b bioactivity. To evaluate whether the synthetic peptide 8b-13 could function as a potent FGF8b antagonist in prostate cancer cells and could exhibit therapeutic potential in prostate cancer, we first investigated the effects of 8b-13 on the proliferation of PC-3 and DU-145 prostate cancer cell lines. The results of the MTT assay showed that 8b-13 significantly inhibited the growth of the cells stimulated by exogenous and endogenous FGF8b in a dose-dependent manner, which is in agreement with the specific effect of 8b-13 on FGF8b. Moreover, the proliferation inhibition mediated by the 8b-13 peptide was stronger in PC-3 cells than in DU-145 cells. We speculated that the higher inhibitory efficiency of 8b-13 on the proliferation of PC-3 cells is due to differences in FGFR receptor distribution, with the higher affinity FGFR3c and FGFR4 receptors predominant on PC-3 cells while the lower affinity receptor FGFR2c is predominant on DU-145. The prevalence of higher affinity receptors on PC-3 cells may result in stronger 8b-13 mediated inhibitory of proliferation in PC-3 cells than in DU-145 cells [23,24]. As PC-3 cells are more sensitive to 8b-13 treatment, further investigations were carried out with PC-3 cells.

The regulation of cell cycle progression in cancer cells is considered to be a potentially effective mechanism of controlling tumor growth [25,26]. Cell cycle analysis showed that 8b-13 restricted the G1 to S phase progression caused by FGF8b. It is well established that various growth factors, including FGF8b stimuli, can induce cyclinD1 expression *via* the receptor tyrosine kinase-activated Ras/MEK/ERK pathway and Ras/PI3K pathway [27,28]. This results in cell cycle progression through the G1 restriction point to the S phase *via* the formation of active cyclinD1-CDK4/6 complex, which phosphorylates retinoblastoma protein (pRb) and causes its subsequent dissociation from E2F, which are required events for the G1 to S phase progression [29,30]. Our results indicated that the 8b-13 peptide reduced the levels of Erk1/2, P38 and Akt phosphorylation, and down-regulated the expression of cyclinD1 induced by FGF8b. Thus, the mechanisms by which the 8b-13 peptide suppresses the FGF8b-induced growth of prostate cancer cells may be in part by blocking the activation of Akt and MAP kinases, leading to down-regulation of the expression of the G1/S-specific protein cyclinD1, which may provide a molecular target for prostate cancer therapy. Moreover, because the PI3K/Akt pathway is also involved in the regulation of cell survival and apoptosis by FGF8b [28], the potential effects of 8b-13 peptides on cell survival and apoptosis cannot be ruled out.

The proteomic approach was applied to further investigate the mechanisms of the inhibitory effect by which 8b-13 targets FGF8b stimulation on PC-3 cells. Eight differentially expressed proteins influenced by 8b-13 were identified, which are related to the regulation of proliferation, cell cycle, metabolism, and signaling, and may play a role in the mechanisms of the inhibitory effect of 8b-13. For example, one of the down-regulated proteins, proliferating cell nuclear antigen (PCNA), is an auxiliary factor that influences the processivity of DNA polymerase δ. The DNA polymerase δ-PCNA complex is involved in DNA replication and repair. When exposed to antisense oligodeoxynucleotides to PCNA, both DNA synthesis and mitosis in cells were completely suppressed, implying that PCNA is important in cellular DNA synthesis and in cell cycle progression [31]. Analysis of the PCNA structure revealed that the N-terminal region comprising the inner α-helices forms part of the binding site for cyclinD1. Although the nature of the PCNA-cyclinD1 complex remains unclear, the existence of the DNA polymerase δ-PCNA and PCNA-cyclinD1 complexes may link DNA replication and DNA repair with cell cycle control. As our study demonstrated that the 8b-13 peptide reduced the expression of both cyclinD1 and PCNA, it is reasonable to speculate that suppression of DNA synthesis and the G1 to S phase transition caused by down-regulation of PCNA and cyclinD1 in 8b-13 treated cells may contribute to the inhibitory effect of the 8b-13 peptide on cell proliferation.

Another protein is down-regulated by 8b-13, the 15 kDa cellular retinoic acid (RA) binding protein 2 (CRABP2). CRABP2 has been shown to belong to the family of intracellular lipid-binding proteins that bind small hydrophobic molecules, such as retinoids and fatty acids, and it also acts as a co-activator of nuclear retinoid receptors [32,33], increasing the stability of the DNA-bound RXR-RAR complex, and further contributing to the enhancement of RA-mediated transcription of target genes involved in cell proliferation. Moreover, the G1/S-specific cyclinD3, which has been identified as a binding partner of CRABP2, increases the stability of the CRABP2-RAR-RA complex, and thus positively modulates RA-mediated transcription [34]. Therefore, the decreased expression of CRABP2 may influence the regulatory effects of cyclinD3 on RA-mediated transcription and further inhibit cell growth in 8b-13 treated PC-3 cells.

The list of up-regulated proteins in 8b-13 treated PC-3 cells (Table 1) included ESD, HNRNP and UQCRB as well as PAFAH1B2. Platelet activating factor (PAF) is a potent pro-inflammatory phospholipid that activates cells involved in inflammation [35]. The actions of PAF are abolished by hydrolysis of the acetyl residue, a reaction catalyzed by PAF acetylhydrolase (PAFAH) [36]. PAFAH1B is composed of two catalytic alpha subunits, alpha-1 (pafah1b3) and alpha-2 (pafah1b2), and an abeta regulatory subunit (pafah1b1). Both the alpha-2 homodimer and the alpha-1/alpha-2 heterodimer have higher rates of PAF hydrolysis than the alpha-1 homodimer [37,38]. Recent data have expanded on the concept that inflammation is a key component of tumor progression.

Prolonged use of non-steroidal anti-inflammatory drugs (NSAIDs) has been associated with a reduced risk for developing many types of cancers [39]. The up-regulation of PAFAH1B2 by 8b-13 may accelerate the rate of PAF hydrolysis, resulting in blockage of the PAF signal, which is activated by the Ras/MEK/ERK cascade and is involved in inflammation, and thus further suppression of tumor progression.

In conclusion, the present study demonstrated that the synthetic 8b-13 peptide derived from the gN helix domain responsible for receptor-binding affinity and the specificity towards FGF8b predicted by structural analysis suppressed cell proliferation of human prostate cancer cells by arresting the cell cycle at the G0/G1 phase, blocking the activation

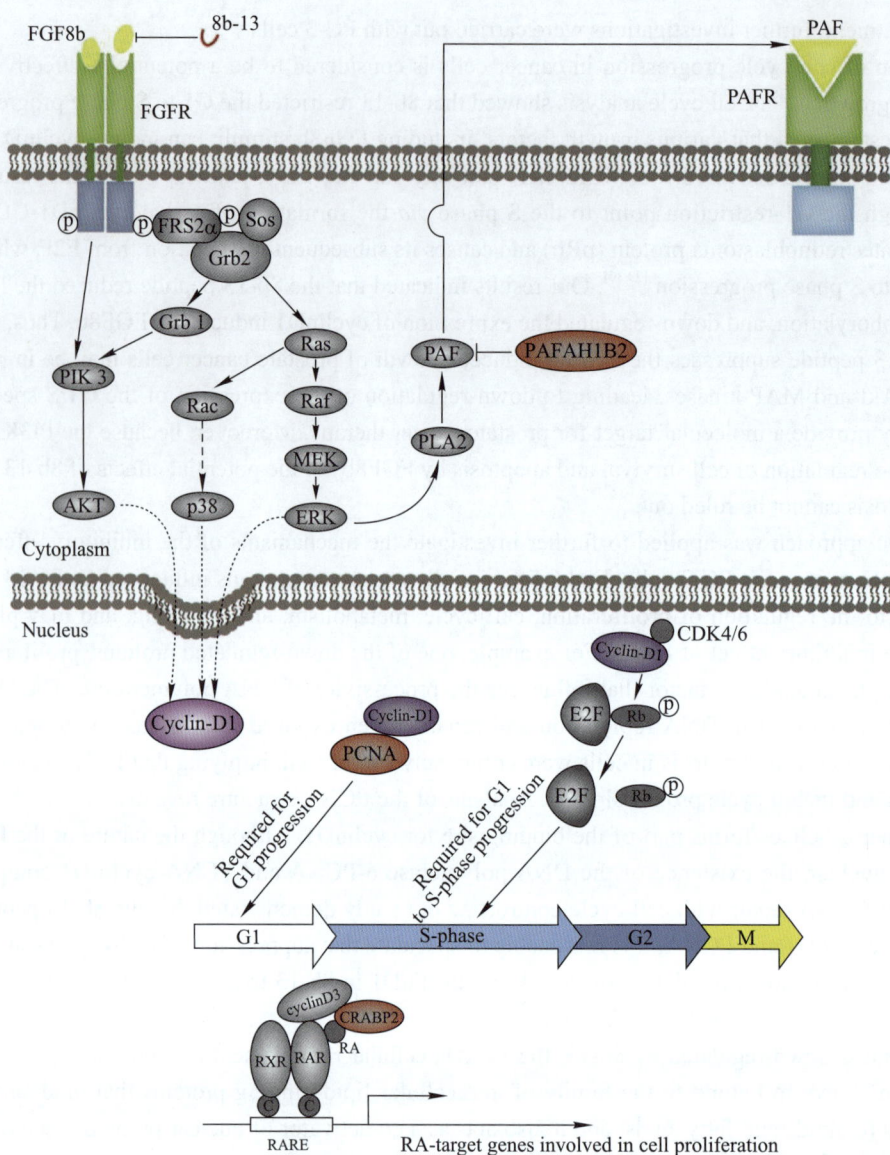

Fig. 8. A model showing the potential mechanisms by which the 8b-13 peptide suppresses the growth of human prostate cancer cells. The synthetic 8b-13 peptides inhibit the cell proliferation of prostate cancer cells by blocking FGF8b-mediated activation of the Erk1/2, P38, and Akt cascades, leading to down-regulation of the expression of G1/S-specific cyclinD1 and cell cycle arrest at the G0/G1 phase. CyclinD1 binds to CDK4/6 to form cyclinD1-CDK4/6 complexes for the phosphorylation of retinoblastoma protein (pRb) and its subsequent dissociation from E2F, which are required for the G1 to S phase progression. Moreover, the synthetic 8b-13 peptide reduces the expression of PCNA and CRABP2, and may subsequently decrease the formation of the PCNA-cyclinD1 complex and the stability of the cyclinD3-CRABP2-RAR-RA complex, resulting in suppression of DNA synthesis, of the G1 to S phase transition, and of the RA-mediated transcription of target genes involved in cell proliferation. The synthetic 8b-13 peptide increases the expression of PAFAH1B2 and may accelerate the rate of PAF hydrolysis, resulting in blockage of the PAF signal, which is activated by the Ras/MEK/ERK cascade and is involved in inflammation and further suppression of tumor progression.

of the Erk1/2, P38, and Akt cascades, and altering the expression of certain proteins involved in the regulation of proliferation and cell cycle progression. These findings suggest that 8b-13 may exert an antitumor effect in prostate cancer and other cancers characterized by abnormally high FGF8b levels. Fig. 8 proposes a model of the potential mechanisms by which 8b-13 suppresses the growth of human prostate cancer cells. Our data also confirm the essential role of the gN helix domain in mediating the activity of FGF8b.

References

[1] Lippman ME, Dickson RB. Mechanisms of growth control in normal and malignant breast epithelium[J]. Recent Prog Horm Res, 1989, 45(1): 383-435.

[2] Ware JL. Growth factors and their receptors as determinants in the proliferation and metastasis of human prostate cancer[J]. Cancer and Metastasis Reviews, 1993, 12(3-4): 287-301.

[3] Crossley PH, Minowada G, MacArthur CA, et al. Roles for FGF8 in the induction, initiation, and maintenance of chick limb development[J]. Cell, 1996, 84(1): 127-136.

[4] Lee SMK, Danielian PS, Fritzsch B, et al. Evidence that FGF8 signalling from the midbrain-hindbrain junction regulates growth and polarity in the developing midbrain[J]. Development, 1997, 124(5): 959-969.

[5] Leung HY, Dickson C, Robson CN, et al. Over-expression of fibroblast growth factor-8 in human prostate cancer[J]. Oncogene, 1996, 12(8): 1833-1835.

[6] Gemel J, Gorry M, Ehrlich GD, et al. Structure and sequence of human FGF8[J]. Genomics, 1996, 35(1): 253-257.

[7] Tanaka A, Furuya A, Yamasaki M, et al. High frequency of fibroblast growth factor (FGF) 8 expression in clinical prostate cancers and breast tissues, immunohistochemically demonstrated by a newly established neutralizing monoclonal antibody against FGF 8[J]. Cancer Research, 1998, 58(10): 2053-2056.

[8] Dorkin TJ, Robinson MC, Marsh C, et al. FGF8 over-expression in prostate cancer is associated with decreased patient survival and persists in androgen independent disease[J]. Oncogene, 1999, 18(17): 2755-2761.

[9] Valve EM, Nevalainen MT, Nurmi MJ, et al. Increased expression of FGF-8 isoforms and FGF receptors in human premalignant prostatic intraepithelial neoplasia lesions and prostate cancer[J]. Laboratory Investigation, 2001, 81(6): 815-826.

[10] Gnanapragasam V, Robinson MC, Marsh C, et al. FGF8 isoform b expression in human prostate cancer[J]. British Journal of Cancer, 2003, 88(9): 1432-1438.

[11] Song ZG, Wu XT, Powell WC, et al. Fibroblast growth factor 8 isoform b overexpression in prostate epithelium: A new mouse model for prostatic intraepithelial neoplasia[J]. Cancer Research, 2002, 62(17): 5096-5105.

[12] Valta MP, Tuomela J, Vuorikoski H, et al. FGF-8b Induces Growth and Rich Vascularization in an Orthotopic PC-3 Model of Prostate Cancer[J]. Journal of Cellular Biochemistry, 2009, 107(4): 769-784.

[13] Song ZG, Powell WC, Kasahara N, et al. The effect of fibroblast growth factor 8, isoform b, on the biology of prostate carcinoma cells and their interaction with stromal cells[J]. Cancer Research, 2000, 60(23): 6730-6736.

[14] Rudra-Ganguly N, Zheng JP, Hoang AT, et al. Downregulation of human FGF8 activity by antisense constructs in murine fibroblastic and human prostatic carcinoma cell systems[J]. Oncogene, 1998, 16(11): 1487-1492.

[15] Valta MP, Tuomela J, Bjartell A, et al. FGF-8 is involved in bone metastasis of prostate cancer[J]. International Journal of Cancer, 2008, 123(1): 22-31.

[16] Schally AV. New approaches to the therapy of various tumors based on peptide analogues[J]. Hormone and Metabolic Research, 2008, 40(5): 315-322.

[17] Aguzzi MS, Faraone D, D'Arcangelo D, et al. The FGF-2-Derived Peptide FREG Inhibits Melanoma Growth In Vitro and In Vivo[J]. Molecular Therapy, 2011, 19(2): 266-273.

[18] Wu X, Yan Q, Huang Y, et al. Isolation of a novel basic FGF-binding peptide with potent antiangiogenetic activity[J]. Journal of Cellular and Molecular Medicine, 2010, 14(1-2): 351-356.

[19] Bradford MM. A rapid and sensitive method for the quantitation of microgram quantities of protein utilizing the principle of protein-dye binding[J]. Analytical Biochemistry, 1976, 72(1-2): 248-254.

[20] Wang C, Lin S, Nie Y, et al. Mechanism of antitumor effect of a novel bFGF binding peptide on human colon cancer cells[J]. Cancer Science, 2010, 101(5): 1212-1218.

[21] Mattila MA, Harkonen PL. Role of fibroblast growth factor 8 in growth and progression of hormonal cancer[J]. Cytokine & Growth Factor Reviews, 2007, 18(3-4): 257-266.

[22] Blunt AG, Lawshe A, Cunningham ML, et al. Overlapping expression and redundant activation of mesenchymal fibroblast growth factor (FGF) receptors by alternatively spliced FGF-8 ligands[J]. Journal of Biological Chemistry, 1997, 272(6): 3733-3738.

[23] Kwabi-Addo B, Ozen M, Ittmann M. The role of fibroblast growth factors and their receptors in prostate cancer[J]. Endocrine-Related Cancer, 2004, 11(4): 709-724.

[24] Valta MP, Tuomela J, Vuorikoski H, et al. FGF-8b induces growth and rich vascularization in an orthotopic PC-3 model of prostate cancer[J]. J Cell Biochem, 2009, 107(4): 769-784.

[25] Pavletich NP. Mechanisms of cyclin-dependent kinase regulation: Structures of Cdks, their cyclin activators, and Cip and INK4 inhibitors[J]. Journal of Molecular Biology, 1999, 287(5): 821-828.

[26] Agarwal R. Cell signaling and regulators of cell cycle as molecular targets for prostate cancer prevention by dietary agents[J]. Biochemical Pharmacology, 2000, 60(8): 1051-1059.

[27] Takuwa N, Takuwa Y. Regulation of cell cycle molecules by the Ras effector system[J]. Molecular and Cellular Endocrinology, 2001, 177(1-2): 25-33.

[28] Nilsson EM, Brokken LJS, Harkonen PL. Fibroblast growth factor 8 increases breast cancer cell growth by promoting cell cycle progression and by protecting against cell death[J]. Experimental Cell Research, 2010, 316(5): 800-812.

[29] Bartek J, Bartkova J, Lukas J. The retinoblastoma protein pathway in cell cycle control and cancer[J]. Experimental Cell Research, 1997, 237(1): 1-6.

[30] Harbour JW, Luo RX, Santi AD, et al. Cdk phosphorylation triggers sequential intramolecular interactions that progressively block Rb functions as cells move through G1[J]. Cell, 1999, 98(6): 859-869.

[31] Jaskulski D, Deriel JK, Mercer WE, et al. Inhibition of cellular proliferation by antisense oligodeoxynucleotides to PCNA cyclin[J]. Science, 1988, 240(4858): 1544-1546.

[32] Napoli JL. Interactions of retinoid binding proteins and enzymes in retinoid metabolism[J]. Biochimica Et Biophysica Acta-Molecular and Cell Biology of Lipids, 1999, 1440(2-3): 139-162.

[33] Delva L, Bastie JN, Rochette-Egly C, et al. Physical and functional interactions between cellular retinoic acid binding protein II and the retinoic acid-dependent nuclear complex[J]. Molecular and Cellular Biology, 1999, 19(10): 7158-7167.

[34] Despouy G, Bastie JN, Deshaies S, et al. Cyclin D3 is a cofactor of retinoic acid receptors, modulating their activity in the presence of cellular retinoic acid-binding protein II[J]. Journal of Biological Chemistry, 2003, 278(8): 6355-6362.

[35] Venable ME, Zimmerman GA, McIntyre TM, et al. Platelet activating factor: a phospholipid autacoid with diverse actions[J]. Journal of Lipid Research, 1993, 34(5): 691-702.

[36] Tjoelker LW, Wilder C, Eberhardt C, et al. Anti-inflammatory properties of a platelet-activating factor acetylhydrolase[J]. Nature,

1995, 374(6522): 549-553.

[37] Ho YS, Swenson L, Derewenda U, *et al.* Brain acetylhydrolase that inactivates platelet-activating factor is a G-protein-like trimer[J]. Nature, 1997, 385(6611): 89-93.

[38] Manya H, Aoki J, Kato H, *et al.* Biochemical characterization of various catalytic complexes of the brain platelet-activating factor

acetylhydrolase[J]. Journal of Biological Chemistry, 1999, 274(45): 31827-31832.

[39] Langman MJS, Cheng KK, Gilman EA, *et al.* Effect of anti-inflammatory drugs on overall risk of common cancer: case-control study in general practice research database[J]. British Medical Journal, 2000, 320(7250): 1642-1646.

Screening a phage display library for a novel FGF8b-binding peptide with anti-tumor effect on prostate cancer

Wenhui Wang, Xiaokun Li, Xiaoping Wu

1. Introduction

Prostate cancer is considered to arise from genetic changes disrupting homeostasis between the cells of prostate epithelial and stromal compartments. Recent data imply that fibroblast growth factors (FGFs) are involved in many of the reciprocal interactions of tumor cells and stromal cells that contribute to prostate tumorigenesis and cancer progression [1–3]. FGFs induce their biological responses by binding to and activating FGFRs (FGFR1–4), a subfamily of cell surface receptor tyrosine kinases (RTKs). The extracellular ligand binding portion of FGFRs is composed of three immunoglobulin-like (Ig-like) domains (D1, D2 and D3) [4–7]. The crystal structure of the ectodomain of the FGFR complex with FGF [8,9] demonstrated that the ligand-binding domain of FGFR involves Ig-like domains II and III, as well as the linker between Ig-like domains II and III.

FGF8 belongs to the fibroblast growth factor family of at least 23 members. Alternative splicing of the human FGF8 gene allows transcription of four different isoforms designated FGF8a, FGF8b, FGF8e, and FGF8f [10]. FGF8b has also been found to have a strongly angiogenic and transforming potential in comparison to FGF8a and FGF8e [11,12]. FGF8b is expressed and secreted by the epithelium, and it signals directionally to mesenchyme by binding FGFR3c, FGFR4, FGFR2c, or FGFR1c, among them FGFR3c is the receptor of FGF8b with much higher affinity than the other three receptors [7,13]. It has been reported that FGF8b is expressed at an increased level in a high proportion of prostate cancers, and correlates with advanced stage and high grade of tumors [14,15] as well as with decreased patient survival [16]. Antagonists targeting FGF8b or its receptors have been considered a potential strategy for prostate cancer therapy by inhibiting cell proliferation and angiogenesis involved in tumor progression. In order to identify peptides that can prevent FGF8b from binding to its receptors, herein, we attempt to isolate a high-affinity FGF8b-binding peptide from a phage display library, and further investigate the functions of the isolated peptide to evaluate its possible therapeutic potential in prostate cancer.

2. Materials and methods

2.1 Materials

Ph.D.-7™ Phage Display Peptide Library Kit (Complexity ~2.8×10^9 transformants) including *Escherichia coli* ER2738 host strain and -96 gIII sequencing primer (5′-^{HO}CCC TCA TAG TTA GCG TAA CG-3′) was purchased from New England Biolabs (Beverly, MA). Recombinant human FGF8b was obtained from PeproTech (Rocky Hill, NJ, USA). HRP-anti-M13 mAb was obtained from Amersham Pharmacia Biotech (Uppsala, Sweden). Dynabeads® M-280 Streptavidin, Dynamag-2 magnet, Dulbecco's modified Eagle's medium (DMEM), RPMI 1640, and fetal bovine serum (FBS) were from Invitrogen (Carlsbad, CA, USA). Propidium iodide (PI) was the product of Sigma (USA). Anti-phospho-Erk1/2, anti-Erk1/2, anti-phospho-Akt, anti-Akt, anti-Cyclin D1, anti-PCNA, anti-GAPDH antibodies, goat anti-rabbit and goat anti-mouse IgG conjugated with horseradish peroxidase (HRP) antibodies were from Cell Signaling Technology (Danvers, MA, USA). Polyvinylidenedifluoride (PVDF) membrane was from Millipore (Billerica, MA, USA). The enhanced chemiluminescence (ECL) detection kit was the product of Pierce (Rockford, IL, USA).

2.2 Phage biopanning

Peptides were selected from a commercially available 7-mer random library that is displayed on phage M13 *via* N-terminal fusion to the minor coat protein, pIII, with a diversity of 2.8×10^9. Individual sterile polystyrene petri dish ($35 \times 10 \text{ mm}^2$) was coated with 10 mg/ml recombinant human FGF8b overnight at 4 ℃ in 0.1 M NaHCO$_3$ (pH 8.6), blocked with bovine serum albumin (BSA) at 5 mg/ml in 0.1 M NaHCO$_3$ for 2 h at room temperature, and washed 6 times (1 min each) with 0.05% Tween-20 in PBS (0.05% PBST). Diluted 10 μl of original library (2×10^{11} plaque-forming units, PFUs) with PBST was added to the dish and incubated for 2 h at room temperature with continuous shaking. To remove unbound phages, the coated dish was washed 10 times (1 min each) with 0.05% PBST, and the phage population remaining attached was eluted with shaking in 1 ml of 0.1 M Glycine-HCl (pH 2.2) for 10 min at room temperature, and neutralized with 100 μl of 1 M Tris-HCl (pH 9.1). The eluate was amplified in *E. coli* ER2738 culture, purified by precipitation with polyethylene glycol PEG/NaCl, titrated as described in the standard protocol (NEB), and used in the next round of screening. Two additional rounds of selection were performed under more stringent conditions. Briefly, plates were coated with less amount of FGF8b and shorter incubation time (5 μg for 1.5 h and 2.5 μg for 1 h in the 2nd and 3rd round, respectively), and washed with higher concentration of PBST (0.1% and 0.3% for 2nd and 3rd round, respectively) for longer time (10×2 min and 10×3 min for 2nd and 3rd round, respectively). After three consecutive rounds of selection, the phage clones were subjected to ELISA analysis.

2.3 Enzyme-linked immunosorbent assay (ELISA) for selecting positive phages

Maxi-sorp 96-well microtiter plates (Nunc) were coated at 4 ℃ overnight with FGF8b and aFGF (as controls), respectively. After the plates were blocked with blocking buffer (PBSM, PBS with 2% dry milk) and washed with 0.05% PBST for 3 times, phage clones (10^{10} pfu/well) and control phage vcsM13 were added and incubated at room temperature for 1 h. With the exception of its wild-type coat protein pIII displaying no N-terminal fusion foreign peptides, phage vcsM13 is identical to those in the phage display heptapeptide library. After washing for 3 times with 0.05% PBST, 200 μl of horseradish peroxidase (HRP)-anti-M13 (1:5 000) was added and the plates were incubated for another hour at room temperature. The plates were washed again with 0.05% PBST and the substrate (50 μl/well of 3,3′,5,5′-tetramethyl-benzidine; TMB) was added. The reaction was terminated 20 min later by adding 50 μl/well of 2 M H$_2$SO$_4$. The absorbance was measured at 450 nm.

2.4 DNA sequencing and peptide synthesis

ssDNA was prepared according to the standard protocol (NEB). DNA sequencing was carried out by Beijing Genomic Institute (Shenzhen, China). The BioEdit Sequence Alignment Editor software and the ProtParam programs (Ibis Biosciences, Carlsbad, CA, USA) were applied to analyze DNA sequence of the positive phage clones.

The Ph.D.-7 Phage Display Peptide Library is a combinatorial library of random peptide 7-mers fused to a minor coat protein (pIII) of M13 Phage. The displayed heptapeptides are expressed at the N-terminus of pIII, and followed by a short spacer (Gly–Gly–Gly–Ser) and then the wild-type pIII sequence, having no free negatively charged carboxylate. When the designed peptides were synthesized at SBS Genetech (Beijing, China), a spacer sequence Gly–Gly–Gly–Ser was added to the C-terminus and the C-terminal carboxylate was amidated to block the negative charge. The P12 peptide was synthesized on solid phase using a rapid and practical Fmoc strategy, and purified by reverse-phase HPLC. High purity grade (> 98%) was obtained after purification. The synthetic peptide was further characterized for its identity by mass spectrometry analysis.

2.5 Cell viability assay

PC-3 and HUVEC cells were seeded in a volume of 200 μl at a density of 1×10^3 cells per well in 96-well plates and allowed to attach overnight, respectively. After starved cultivation in RPMI 1640 and DMEM with 0.4% FBS for 24 h, respectively, cells were treated with serially diluted peptides, FGF8b alone, or FGF8b plus serially diluted peptides for 48 h. The viability of cells was determined by the methylthiazole tetrazolium (MTT) colorimetric assay. Briefly, 20 μl of MTT was added to each well and incubated with cells for 4 h. The absorbance was immediately measured at 490 nm to determine the number of viable cells.

2.6 *Flow cytometric analysis of the cell cycle*

Flow cytometry analysis was carried out to analyze the effect of P12 on the cell cycle progress of FGF8b-stimulated cells. PC-3 and HUVEC cells were seeded in 6-well plates with 8×10^4 cells and 1.2×10^5 cells per well respectively, starved for 24 h, and treated with FGF8b alone or FGF8b plus serially diluted peptides for 48 h. Cells were harvested and fixed in 70% ice-cold ethanol for 6 h at 4 ℃. After being washed with PBS for 3 times, cells were stained for DNA content by using of 300 μl PBS containing 50 μg/ml propidium iodide (PI) and 50 μg/ml preboiled RNase A. The suspension was incubated in dark at room temperature for 30 min and then subjected to FACS Calibur flow cytometer analysis with excitation at 488 nm and emission at 560–640 nm (FL2 mode). Data were analyzed with the ModFit DNA analysis program.

2.7 *Mitogen-activated protein kinase (MAPK) and Akt activation assay*

Starved PC-3 and HUVEC cells were treated with serially diluted peptides for 5 min prior to stimulation with FGF8b for 10 min. After being washed with cold PBS, cells were lysed in $1 \times$ SDS-PAGE loading buffer. The lysate was clarified by centrifugation at 12 000 rpm for 10 min at 4℃ to remove the insoluble components. The samples were separated by 10% SDS-PAGE and transferred to a PVDF membrane (350 mA, 70 min). The membrane was blocked with TBST containing 5% non-fat dry milk (RT, 1 h), and incubated with the primary antibody (an anti-phospho-Erk1/2 rabbit mAb, or an anti-phospho-Akt rabbit mAb) at 4 ℃ overnight, followed by goat anti-rabbit IgG, HRP-linked antibody at RT for 1 h. The blots were detected with an ECL detection kit according to the manu-facturer's procedure. Non-phosphorylated Erk1/2, or Akt was used as the reference control. The results were analyzed by Quantity One 4.6 software to determine the relative ratio.

2.8 *Western blot analysis of expressions of Cyclin D1 and PCNA*

For detecting the expressions of Cyclin D1 in PC-3 and HUVEC, cells were seeded in 6-well plates with 8×10^4 cells and 1.2×10^5 cells per well, starved for 24 h, and treated with serially diluted peptides for 30 min prior to stimulation with FGF8b for 6 h and 12 h, respectively. For assessing the expressions of PCNA in PC-3, cells were seeded in 6-well plates with 8×10^4 cells per well, starved for 24 h, and treated with 40 ng/ml FGF8b alone, or 40 ng/ml FGF8b plus 4 μM P12 peptides for 48 h. Cells were collected and lysed to prepare the samples for electrophoresis on a 10% SDS-PAGE gel followed by transferring to a PVDF membrane. The membrane was incubated with an anti-Cyclin D1 rabbit mAb an anti-PCNA mouse mAb, or an anti-GAPDH rabbit mAb at 4℃ overnight, followed by goat anti-rabbit or goat anti-mouse IgG, HRP-linked antibody at RT for 1 h. The blots were detected with an ECL detection kit according to the manufacturer's procedure. The results were analyzed by Quantity One 4.6 software to determine the relative ratio.

2.9 *Statistical analysis*

Data were presented as mean ± standard deviations (SD) from at least three independent experiments. All statistical analyses were performed by using GraphPad Prism software, version 5.01. Student's *t*-test was used to compare data in two groups, and one-way ANOVA followed by Tukey's multiple comparison test was used for multiple comparison data. A *P* value of <0.05 was considered statistically significant.

3. Results

3.1 *Selection of specific FGF8b-binding phage clones*

Ph.D.-7™ Phage Display Peptide Library was subjected to three rounds of affinity selection with gradually increased stringency of selection. The plates were blocked with different agents (BSA, Non-fat milk, and Gelatin for the 1st, 2nd and 3rd round, respectively), coated with a reduced amount of FGF8b and shorter incubation time (10 μg for 2 h, 5 μg for 1.5 h and 2.5 μg for 1 h in the 1st, 2nd and 3rd round, respectively), and washed with a higher concentration of Tween (0.05%, 0.1% and 0.3% for the 1st, 2nd and 3rd round, respectively). The output phage (*P*) refers to the titer of the phages eluted from FGF8b-coated petri dish, while the output phage of negative control (*N*) means the titer of the phages eluted from the Petri dishes uncoated with FGF8b. The enrichment efficiency of the phages specifically bound to FGF8b was determined by *P/N* value. As shown in Table 1, after three cycles of panning, *P/N* value was increased to 100, suggesting that the phage-displayed peptides specifically bound to FGF8b were successfully enriched.

Table 1. Selective enrichment for FGF8b binding phages

Round	FGF8b (lg)	Input phage (pfu)	Output phage (pfu) P	Output phage (pfu) of negative control N	Recovery (%)	P/N
1	10	2×10^{11}	9×10^5	4×10^5	4.5×10^{-4}	2.25
2	5	4×10^{10}	4×10^5	8×10^4	1×10^{-3}	5
3	2.5	10×10^{10}	1×10^5	1×10^3	1×10^{-4}	100

*pfu, Plaque forming unit.

High-affinity FGF8b-binding clones were further identified from the recovered phage clones by ELISA. Phage vcsM13 was used as the control in the ELISA assay. Phage clones were considered to possess high affinity for FGF8b if their O.D. values were two times greater than that of phage vcsM13. In order to determine binding specificities, we also detected the ability of phage clones binding to aFGF, one member of FGF family with high affinity binding to all isoforms of FGF receptors. As shown in Fig. 1, after three rounds of selection, 12 clones were detected by ELISA, among which seven clones with higher affinity and specificity for FGF8b (clones 4, 6, 7, 8, 10, 11, 12) were selected for sequencing.

3.2 Sequence analysis and property prediction of selected phage clones

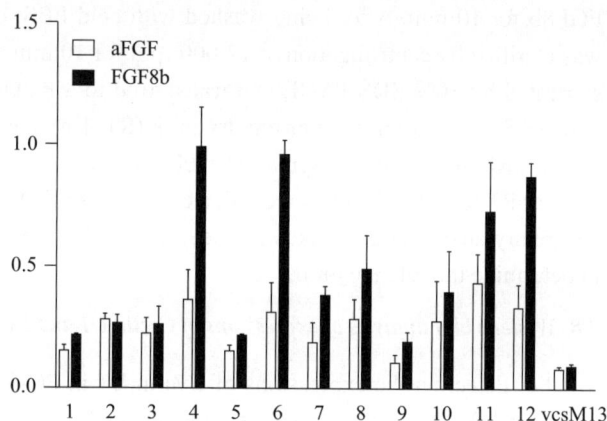

Fig. 1. Specific binding of the positive phage clones to FGF8b. The binding affinity of the 12 positive phage clones and the control vcsM13 to FGF8b and aFGF was determined by ELISA assay. Data presented are the mean O.D. values (±S.D.) of triplicate samples.

The amino acid sequences of the peptides displayed on the selected phages were deduced from the DNA sequences and analyzed using the BioEdit and ProtParam programs (Table 2). FGF8b binds to and stimulates mitogenesis in cells expressing FGFR3c, FGFR4, FGFR2c, or FGFR1c. The affinity of FGF8b binding to FGFR3c is much higher than binding to the other three isoforms [17]. The crystal structure of the ectodomain of the FGFR complex with FGF8b demonstrated that the ligand-binding domains of FGFR involve the highly conserved Ig-like domain 2 and 3, and the linker region between D2 and D3. Therefore, the amino acid sequences of the selected peptides were compared with the motif (151–355 aa) located at D2–D3 of FGF8b high-affinity receptor FGFR3c using BioEdit Sequence Alignment Editor.

Table 2. Properties of peptides displayed by specific FGF8b-binding phages

Heptapeptides	Clone	Sequences	Similarities	Theoretical pI
P4	4	FETLPSR	0.0291262	6
P6	6	NPLLSIQ	0.0291262	5.52
P7	7	LQGAHLR	0.0291262	9.76
P8	8	IPPLYFS	0.0341463	5.52
P10	10	QWPLMTT	0.0291262	5.52
P11	11	WRPPMLV	0.0341463	9.75
P12	12	HSQAAVP	0.0341463	6.74

*pI, Isoelectric point.

Phage clone No. 12 (P12), as well as P8 and P11, showed the highest sequence similarity to D2–D3 of FGFR3c (0.0341463, PAM250 Matrix). P12 (HSQAAVP) contains 3 identical amino acids (AVP) to the authentic FGFR3 D2 sequence aa 163–169 (LLAVPAA), among which L163A165P167 conserved in FGFR2 and FGFR1 directly participates in ligand binding.

In the physiological condition, P12 carries negative charges. Since the motif LLAVPAA (pI 5.52) in D2 of FG-FR3c also carry negative charges, it is likely that P12 may bind to FGF8b by mimicking the electrostatic interaction of the FGF8b binding the corresponding motif of FGFR3c. Taken together, these data suggest that the candidate peptide P12 sharing 3 identical amino acids (AVP) to the ligand binding motif in D2 of FGF8b high affinity receptor may bind FGF8b *via* electrostatic interactions and therefore may have a greater potential to interrupt FGF8b binding to its receptor than other identified heptapeptides do.

3.3 Heptapeptide-library-derived peptide P12 inhibits FGF8b-stimulated cell proliferation

The effects of the synthetic peptide P12 on the proliferation of PC-3 and HUVEC cells were assessed by MTT assay. Starved cells were treated with FGF8b alone, FGF8b plus various concentrations of P12, or P12 peptides alone for 48 h. As shown in Fig. 2, P12 peptides had a dose-dependent inhibitory effect on the proliferation of both PC-3 and HUVEC cells stimulated with FGF8b. Administration of P12 alone suppressed the growth of PC-3 cells expressing endogenous FGF8b, but had little inhibitory effect on HU-VEC cells expressing little endogenous FGF8b, implying that the inhibitory effect of P12 on cell proliferation specifically targets FGF8b.

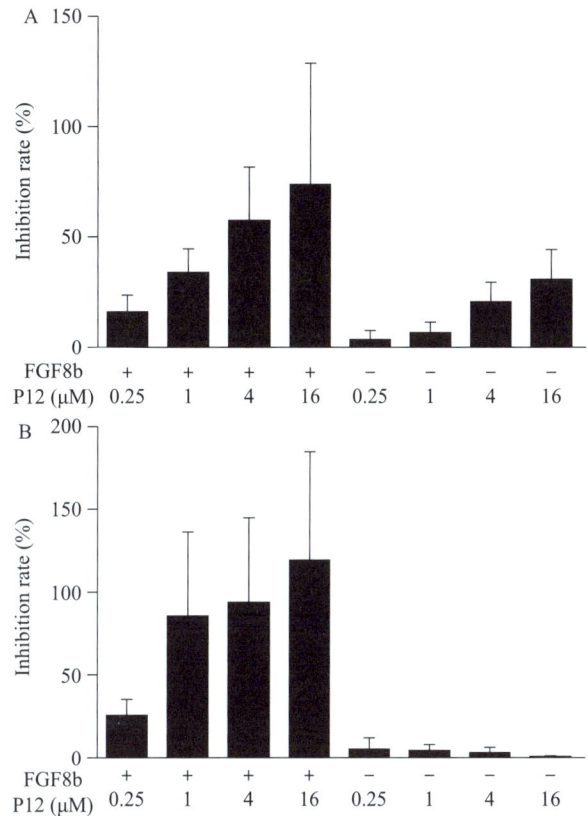

Fig. 2. Effects of synthetic P12 peptides on FGF8b-stimulated cell proliferation. (A) PC-3 cells were treated with 40 ng/ml FGF8b alone, 40 ng/ml FGF8b plus P12 at the indicated concentrations, or P12 alone. (B) HUVEC cells were treated with 20 ng/ml FGF8b alone, 20 ng/ml FGF8b plus P12 at the indicated concentrations, or P12 alone. Cell proliferation was measured 48 h later using MTT assay. Data are presented as the mean±SD of three independent experiments performed in triplicate.

3.4 P12 arrests FGF8b-induced cells at the G0/G1 phase via Cyclin D1

Propidium iodide staining combined with flow cytometry analysis was performed to investigate the effect of the synthetic peptides on cell cycle progression of PC-3 and HUVEC cells induced by FGF8b. The results shown in Fig. 3 indicated that FGF8b-treated cells presented an increased S-phase population and a decreased G0/G1-phase population compared with the control, whereas addition of P12 peptides increased the percentage of FGF8b-induced cell in G0/ G1 phase and decreased the S-phase percentage.

It has been reported that Cyclin D1 is a G1/S-specific regulating protein controlling cell cycle progress. As P12 suppressed the cell cycle transition from G1 to S phase and arrest cell cycle at G0/G1 phase, western blot was further carried out to evaluate the effect of P12 on the expression of Cyclin D1. As shown in Fig. 4, FGF8b significantly increased the expression levels of Cyclin D1 in both PC-3 and HUVEC cells. Pretreatment with P12 peptides (0.25-16 µM) for 30 min before stimulation with FGF8b lead tosignificant decrease in the expression of Cyclin D1, suggesting that P12 peptides arrest cells at G0/G1 phase partly *via* decreasing the expression of G1/S-specific Cyclin D1.

3.5 P12 blocks FGF8b-induced phosphorylation of Akt and MAP kinases

The effects of P12 on FGF8b-triggered signal transduction were determined by detecting its capacity to inhibit FGF8b-induced.

Akt and MAP kinases activation. As shown in Fig. 5, exogenous FGF8b significantly stimulated the phosphorylation of Erk1/2 and Akt in both PC-3 and HUVEC cells. Pretreatment with P12 peptides (0.25–16 µM) for 5 min before

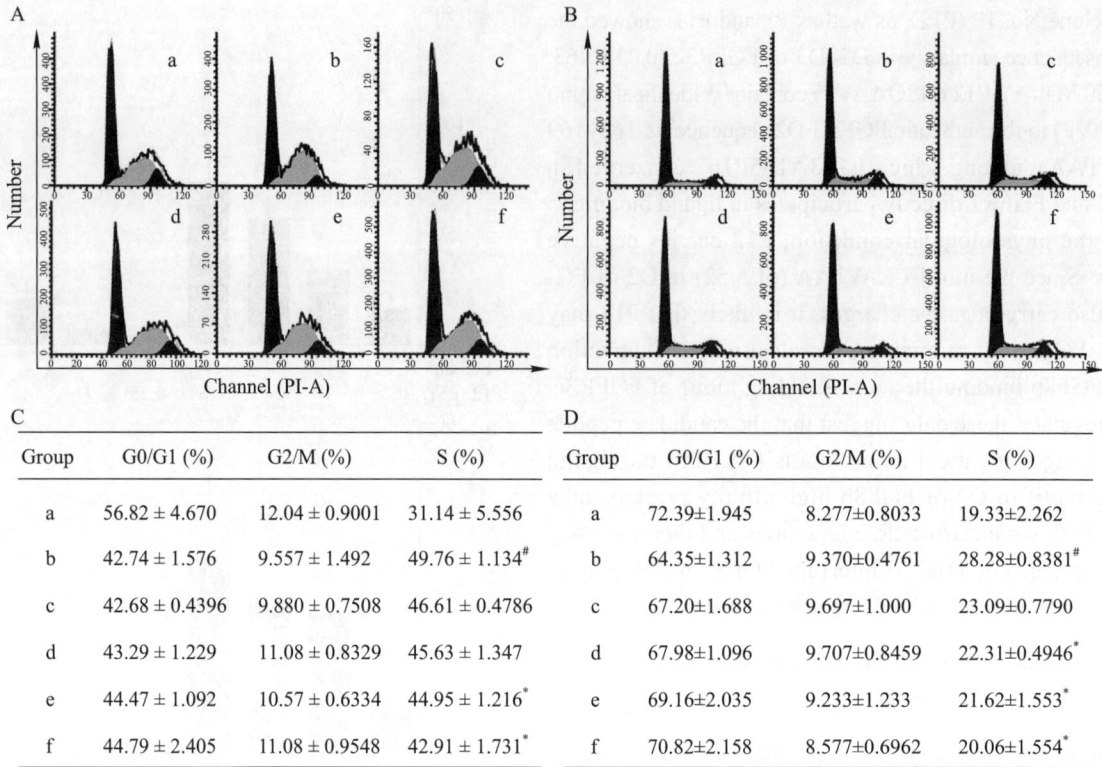

Group	G0/G1 (%)	G2/M (%)	S (%)
a	56.82 ± 4.670	12.04 ± 0.9001	31.14 ± 5.556
b	42.74 ± 1.576	9.557 ± 1.492	49.76 ± 1.134[#]
c	42.68 ± 0.4396	9.880 ± 0.7508	46.61 ± 0.4786
d	43.29 ± 1.229	11.08 ± 0.8329	45.63 ± 1.347
e	44.47 ± 1.092	10.57 ± 0.6334	44.95 ± 1.216[*]
f	44.79 ± 2.405	11.08 ± 0.9548	42.91 ± 1.731[*]

Group	G0/G1 (%)	G2/M (%)	S (%)
a	72.39±1.945	8.277±0.8033	19.33±2.262
b	64.35±1.312	9.370±0.4761	28.28±0.8381[#]
c	67.20±1.688	9.697±1.000	23.09±0.7790
d	67.98±1.096	9.707±0.8459	22.31±0.4946[*]
e	69.16±2.035	9.233±1.233	21.62±1.553[*]
f	70.82±2.158	8.577±0.6962	20.06±1.554[*]

Fig. 3. Flow cytometric analysis of cell cycle using propidium iodide. (A) PC-3 cells were starved for 24 h and then treated with 40 ng/ml FGF8b (b), or 40 ng/ml FGF8b plus various concentrations of P12 (c–f: 0.25, 1, 4, and 16 μM) for 48 h. (a) Control cells without treatment of FGF8b, or P12. (B) HUVEC cells were starved for 24 h and then treated with 20 ng/ml FGF8b (b), or 20 ng/ml FGF8b plus various concentrations of P12 (c–f: 0.25, 1, 4, and 16 μM) for 48 h. (a) Control cells without treatment of FGF8b or P12. (C and D) Cell cycle distribution of the control and treated PC-3 and HUVEC cells. [#]$P < 0.05$ $vs.$ control group; [*]$P < 0.05$ $vs.$ FGF8b group.

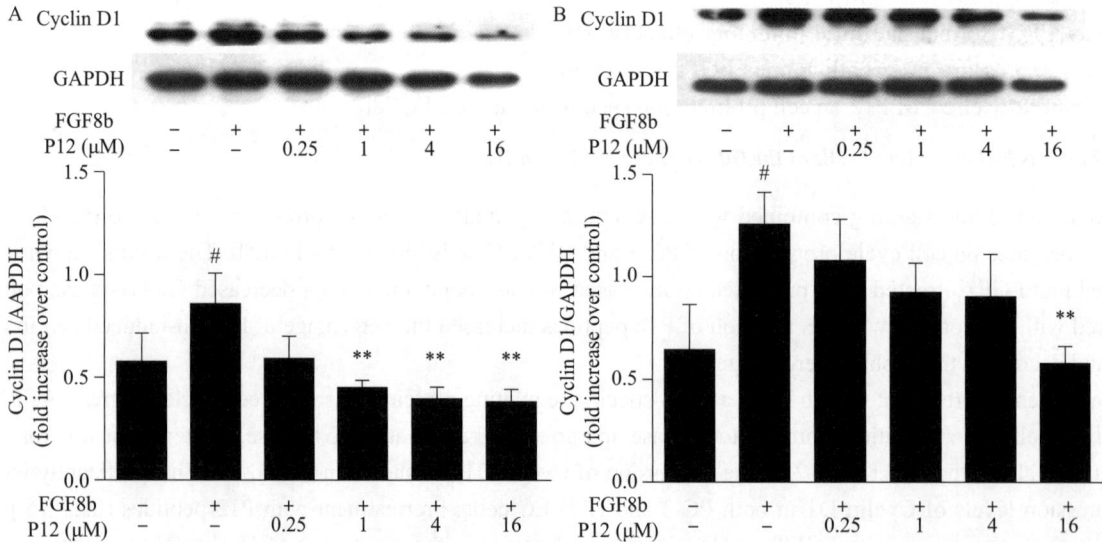

Fig. 4. Synthetic P12 peptides counteracted the regulatory effect of FGF8b on Cyclin D1. (A) PC-3 cells were starved for 24 h and then treated with 40 ng/ml FGF8b or 40 ng/ml FGF8b plus various concentrations of P12 for 6 h. (B) HUVEC cells were starved for 24 h and then treated with 20 ng/ml FGF8b or 20 ng/ml FGF8b plus various concentrations of P12 for 12 h. Sample loadings were controlled by GAPDH protein quantification. [#]$P < 0.05$ $vs.$ control group; [**]$P < 0.01$ $vs.$ FGF8b group.

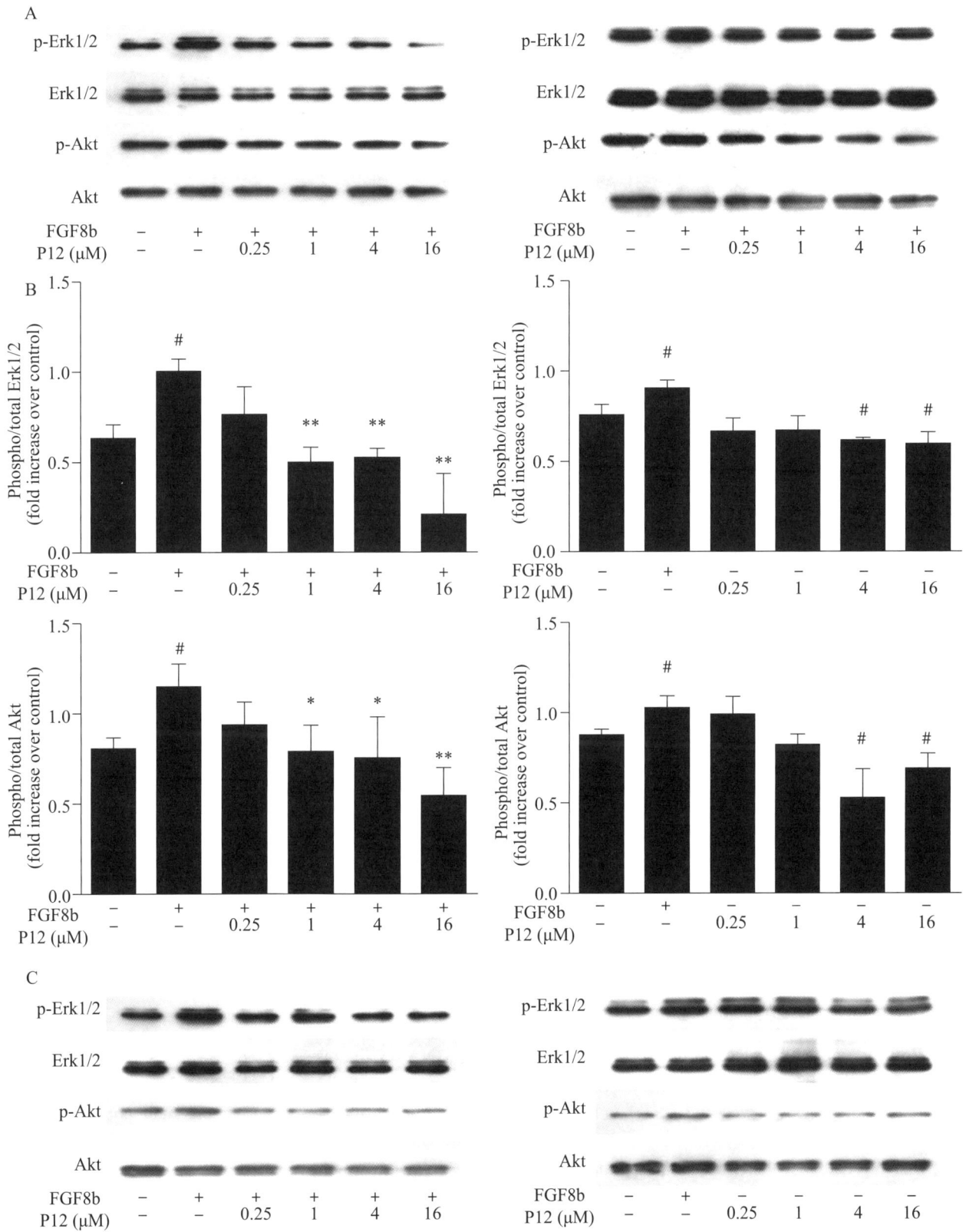

A

B

C

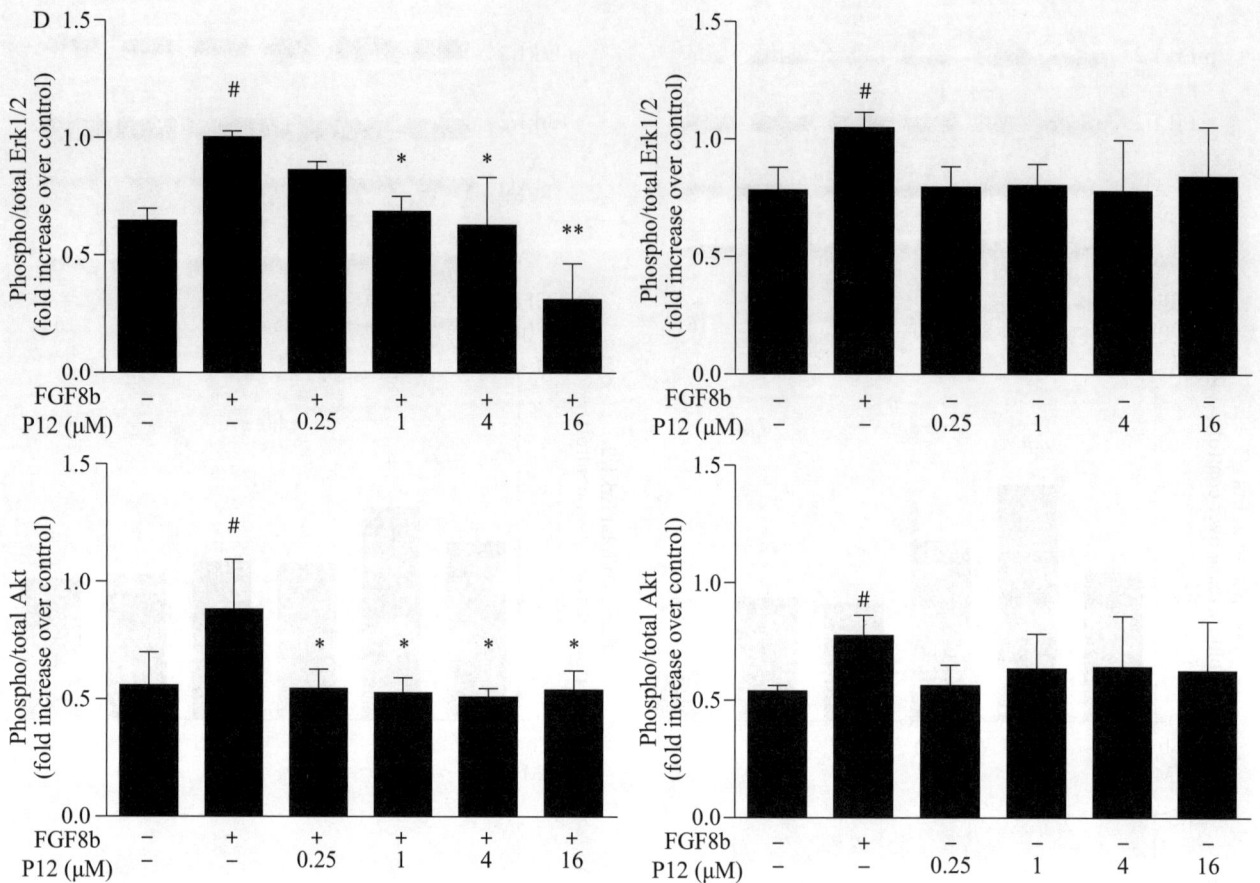

Fig. 5. Synthetic P12 peptides inhibit FGF8b-induced Erk1/2 and Akt activation. (A) PC-3 cells were pretreated with P12 at the indicated concentrations for 5 min before stimulation with 40 ng/ml FGF8b for 10 min (left panel), or treated with P12 alone at the indicated concentrations (right panel). (C) HUVEC cells were pretreated with P12 at the indicated concentrations for 5 min before stimulation with 20 ng/ml FGF8b for 10 min (left panel), or treated with P12 alone at the indicated concentrations (right panel). The phosphorylated and total levels of Erk1/2 and Akt were determined by western blot analysis. (B and D) Density ratios of phosphorylated proteins to total proteins were presented as the mean±SD of three independent experiments. $^{\#}P < 0.05$ vs. control group; $^{*}P < 0.05$, $^{**}P < 0.01$ vs. FGF8b group.

stimulation with FGF8b resulted in significant blockage of the activation of both signal molecules in a dose-dependent manner. Administration of P12 alone also suppressed the phosphorylation of Erk1/2 and Akt induced by endogenous FGF8b in PC-3 cells. However, P12 alone had little effect on the activation of signal molecules in HUVEC cells with little endogenous FGF8b expression.

3.6 P12 counteracts the regulatory effect of FGF8b on PCNA expression

Proliferating cell nuclear antigen (PCNA) is known as a DNA polymerase accessory protein involved in DNA replication, DNA repair, and cell cycle control, and considered to be a marker of cell proliferation in various cancers. Previous studies have showed that FGF8b enhanced the expression level of PCNA in PC-3 cells (data not shown). We speculated that P12 peptides inhibited FGF8b-stimulated proliferation of PC-3 cells possibly via regulation of PCNA expression. Therefore, the effect of P12 on the expression of PCNA was further evaluated by Western blot analysis. As shown in Fig. 6, P12 treatment down-regulated PCNA expression induced by FGF8b, giving a hint that PCNA plays an important role in P12 peptides counteracting the FGF8b-stimulated proliferation in PC-3 cells.

4. Discussion

Preclinical approaches using phage display technology are mainly addressed to find and characterize small molecules such as antibodies and peptides with targeting and in some cases neutralizing activity against various members

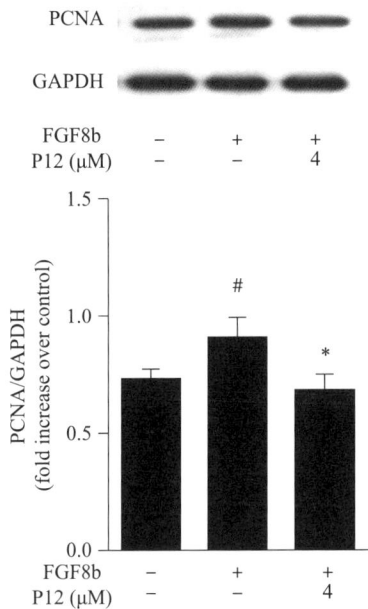

Fig. 6. Synthetic P12 peptides counteracted the regulatory effect of FGF8b on proliferation-associated protein PCNA expression. PC-3 cells were starved for 24 h and then treated with 40 ng/ml FGF8b alone, or 40 ng/ml FGF8b plus 4 μM P12 for 48 h. The expression of PCNA was detected by western blot analysis. Sample loading was controlled by GAPDH protein quantification. [#]$P < 0.05$ *vs.* control group; [*]$P < 0.05$ *vs.* FGF8b group.

of the growth factors and receptor families. The "anti-growth factor approach" addressed to block the ligand-receptor interaction represents a very promising strategy in cancer therapy. FGF8b is the major isoform of FGF8 expressed in prostate cancer, and is the most transforming among the FGF8 isoforms. Accumulating studies have shown that FGF8b is up-regulated in prostate cancer, and accelerates tumor growth and angiogenesis. Therefore, FGF8b has been considered as a potential target for prostate cancer therapy.

In the present study, we screened a phage-displayed heptapeptide library to identify FGF8b antagonists, and obtained seven FGF8b-binding phage clones with significant affinity and specificity. Alignment of the selected peptide sequences with the primary sequences of FGF8b high-affinity receptor, FGFR3c, revealed high sequence homology between P12 and FGFR3c D2–D3. Three amino acids (AVP) of P12 were identical to its corresponding motif in D2 of FGFR3c, FGFR2, and FGFR1. Moreover, P12 and the corresponding motif both carry negative charges. The dominant expressed FGF receptors include FGFR3c in PC-3 cells and FGFR3c, FGFR1c in HUVEC cells [18–20]. Since the affinity of FGF8b for FGFR3c appears to be higher, the preferential receptor for FGF8b in PC-3 and HUVEC cells is probably FGFR3c. Given that D2 is involved in ligand binding of FGFRs, the electrostatic complementarity is important in peptide interactions, and FGFR3c serves as the potential receptor for FGF8b in PC-3 and HUVEC cells, it is reasonable to speculate that P12 may have the capability to bind FGF8b and block the biological activity of FGF8b in PC-3 and HUVEC cells by interrupting its interactions with FGFR3c. Consistent with this possibility, synthetic P12 peptides mediate strong inhibition of cell proliferation, and activations of Erk1/2 and Akt cascades both in PC-3 cells stimulated by either exogenous or endogenous FGF8b, and in HUVEC cells stimulated by exogenous FGF8b, but exert little effect on HUVEC cells with little endogenous FGF8b expression.

It is known that Cyclins and Cdks are two kinds of crucial regulatory molecules determining cell cycle progression [21]. The distinct Cyclin binds to the corresponding activated catalytic partner Cdk resulting in forming the functional Cyclin-Cdk complexes requiring for phosphorylating specific protein substrates to propel cells through the distinct stages of the cell cycle. For instance, Cyclin D1 binding to CDK4/6 forms the active complexes of Cyclin D1-CDK4/6 for phosphorylating of retinoblastoma protein (pRb) and subsequent releasing of E2F transcription factors, resulting in activations of specific gene expressions required for G1 to S phase progression [22]. Moreover, it was reported that FGF8b induced Cyclin D1 expression *via* the receptor tyrosine kinases-activated Ras/MEK/Erk pathway and Ras/PI3K pathway [23]. Cell cycle analysis showed that P12 restricted G1 to S phase progression caused by FGF8b. Further investigation demonstrated that P12 peptides down-regulated the expression of Cyclin D1, and attenuated activations of Erk1/2 and Akt induced by FGF8b. It is reasonable to speculate that the mechanisms of P12 peptides restricting FGF8b-induced G1 to S phase progression may be partly *via* blockage of the Akt and MAP kinase activations, and subsequent down-regulation of the expression of G1/S-specific protein, Cyclin D1.

PCNA is a member of the DNA sliding clamp family of proteins that assist in DNA replication and repair [24]. Multiple proteins involved in DNA replication and repair facilitate fast processing of DNA by binding to PCNA rather than directly associating with DNA [25]. Besides, PCNA also forms complexes with Cyclin-CDK complexes, and acts as a connector between CDK and its substrates, stimulating their phosphorylation, and thus control the cell cycle progression [26,27]. Our results revealed that P12 peptides down-regulated PCNA expression induced by FGF8b, suggesting PCNA may involve in the mechanisms by which P12 counteracts the FGF8b-stimulated proliferation and cell cycle progression.

In summary, we successfully isolated an FGF8b-binding peptide P12 by screening a phage display heptapeptide library with FGF8b, which provides an effective FGF8b/FGFR antagonist, and may have potential application for the treatment of a variety of cancers including prostate cancer characterized by abnormal high expression level of FGF8b.

References

[1] Kwabi-Addo B, Ozen M, Ittmann M. The role of fibroblast growth factors and their receptors in prostate cancer[J]. Endocrine-Related Cancer, 2004, 11(4): 709-724.

[2] Mattila MA, Harkonen PL. Role of fibroblast growth factor 8 in growth and progression of hormonal cancer[J]. Cytokine & Growth Factor Reviews, 2007, 18(3-4): 257-266.

[3] Zhang Y, Zhang J, Lin Y, et al. Role of epithelial cell fibroblast growth factor receptor substrate 2 alpha in prostate development, regeneration and tumorigenesis[J]. Development, 2008, 135(4): 775-784.

[4] Plotnikov AN, Hubbard SR, Schlessinger J, et al. Crystal structures of two FGF-FGFR complexes reveal the determinants of ligand-receptor specificity[J]. Cell, 2000, 101(4): 413-424.

[5] Wang F, Kan M, Xu JM, et al. Ligand-specific structural domains in the fibroblast growth factor receptor[J]. Journal of Biological Chemistry, 1995, 270(17): 10222-10230.

[6] Yeh BK, Igarashi M, Eliseenkova AV, et al. Structural basis by which alternative splicing confers specificity in fibroblast growth factor receptors[J]. Proceedings of the National Academy of Sciences of the United States of America, 2003, 100(5): 2266-2271.

[7] Zhang X, Ibrahimi OA, Olsen SK, et al. Receptor specificity of the fibroblast growth factor family - The complete mammalian FGF family[J]. Journal of Biological Chemistry, 2006, 281(23): 15694-15700.

[8] Pellegrini L, Burke DF, von Delft F, et al. Crystal structure of fibroblast growth factor receptor ectodomain bound to ligand and heparin[J]. Nature, 2000, 407(6807): 1029-1034.

[9] Plotnikov AN, Schlessinger J, Hubbard SR, et al. Structural basis for FGF receptor dimerization and activation[J]. Cell, 1999, 98(5): 641-650.

[10] Ghosh AK, Shankar DB, Shackleford GM, et al. Molecular cloning and characterization of human FGF8 alternative messenger RNA forms[J]. Cell Growth & Differentiation, 1996, 7(10): 1425-1434.

[11] Mattila MMT, Ruohola JK, Valve EM, et al. FGF-8b increases angiogenic capacity and tumor growth of androgen-regulated S115 breast cancer cells[J]. Oncogene, 2001, 20(22): 2791-2804.

[12] Ruohola JK, Viitanen TP, Valve EM, et al. Enhanced invasion and tumor growth of fibroblast growth factor 8b-overexpressing MCF-7 human breast cancer cells[J]. Cancer Research, 2001, 61(10): 4229-4237.

[13] Macarthur CA, Lawshe A, Xu JS, et al. FGF-8 isoforms activate receptor splice forms that are expressed in mesenchymal regions of mouse development[J]. Development, 1995, 121(11): 3603-3613.

[14] Gnanapragasam V, Robinson MC, Marsh C, et al. FGF8 isoform b expression in human prostate cancer[J]. British Journal of Cancer, 2003, 88(9): 1432-1438.

[15] Murphy T, Darby S, Mathers ME, et al. Evidence for distinct alterations in the FGF axis in prostate cancer progression to an aggressive clinical phenotype[J]. Journal of Pathology, 2010, 220(4): 452-460.

[16] Dorkin TJ, Robinson MC, Marsh C, et al. FGF8 over-expression in prostate cancer is associated with decreased patient survival and persists in androgen independent disease[J]. Oncogene, 1999, 18(17): 2755-2761.

[17] Blunt AG, Lawshe A, Cunningham ML, et al. Overlapping expression and redundant activation of mesenchymal fibroblast growth factor (FGF) receptors by alternatively spliced FGF-8 ligands[J]. Journal of Biological Chemistry, 1997, 272(6): 3733-3738.

[18] Antoine M, Wirz W, Tag CG, et al. Expression pattern of fibroblast growth factors (FGFs), their receptors and antagonists in primary endothelial cells and vascular smooth muscle cells[J]. Growth Factors, 2005, 23(2): 87-95.

[19] Kudo K, Arao T, Tanaka K, et al. Antitumor Activity of BIBF 1120, a Triple Angiokinase Inhibitor, and Use of VEGFR2(+)pTyr(+) Peripheral Blood Leukocytes as a Pharmacodynamic Biomarker In Vivo[J]. Clinical Cancer Research, 2011, 17(6): 1373-1381.

[20] Valta MP, Tuomela J, Vuorikoski H, et al. FGF-8b Induces Growth and Rich Vascularization in an Orthotopic PC-3 Model of Prostate Cancer[J]. Journal of Cellular Biochemistry, 2009, 107(4): 769-784.

[21] Israels ED, Israels LG. The cell cycle[J]. The oncologist, 2000, 5(6): 510-513.

[22] Lukas J, Bartkova J, Bartek J. Convergence of mitogenic signalling cascades from diverse classes of receptors at the cyclin D-cyclin-dependent kinase-pRb-controlled G(1) checkpoint[J]. Molecular and Cellular Biology, 1996, 16(12): 6917-6925.

[23] Nilsson EM, Brokken LJS, Harkonen PL. Fibroblast growth factor 8 increases breast cancer cell growth by promoting cell cycle progression and by protecting against cell death[J]. Experimental Cell Research, 2010, 316(5): 800-812.

[24] Kelman Z, Odonnell M. Structural and functional similarities of prokaryotic and eukaryotic DNA polymerase sliding clamps[J]. Nucleic Acids Research, 1995, 23(18): 3613-3620.

[25] Maga G, Hubscher U. Proliferating cell nuclear antigen (PCNA): a dancer with many partners[J]. Journal of Cell Science, 2003, 116(15): 3051-3060.

[26] Koundrioukoff S, Jonsson ZO, Hasan S, et al. A direct interaction between proliferating cell nuclear antigen (PCNA) and Cdk2 targets PCNA-interacting proteins for phosphorylation[J]. Journal of Biological Chemistry, 2000, 275(30): 22882-22887.

[27] Xiong Y, Zhang H, Beach D. D type cyclins associate with multiple protein kinases and the DNA replication and repair factor PCNA[J]. Cell, 1992, 71(3): 505-514.

FGF21 improves cognition by restored synaptic plasticity, dendritic spine density, brain mitochondrial function and cell apoptosis in obese-insulin resistant male rats

Piangkwan Sa-nguanmoo, Xiaokun Li, Siriporn C. Chattipakorn

1. Introduction

Long term consumption of a high fat diet (HFD) has been shown to result in obesity, which then causes insulin resistance (Fung *et al.*, 2001; Riccardi *et al.*, 2004). We previously found that male rats fed with a 12-week HFD not only developed peripheral insulin resistance, but also brain insulin resistance indicated by the impairment of brain insulin signaling and insulin-induced long-term depression (LTD) (Pipatpiboon *et al.*, 2012; Pratchayasakul *et al.*, 2011). In addition, we found that those rats had increased brain oxidative stress, brain mitochondrial dysfunction, decreased synaptic plasticity as well as dendritic spine density in the CA1 region of the hippocampus (Pintana *et al.*, 2012, 2013; Pratchayasakul *et al.*, 2015), which is the region of the brain that involves the learning and memory process. The dysfunction of hippo-campal neurons has been shown to cause a loss of learning and memory (Winocur *et al.*, 2005). Furthermore, other previous studies also demonstrated that long-term HFD consumption significantly increased brain damage, leading to impaired long-term potentiation (LTP), decreased dendritic spine at apical CA1 hippocampus region and resulting in impaired learning and memory (Beilharz *et al.*, 2015; Stranahan *et al.*, 2008).

Several clinical studies demonstrated that overweight or higher body mass index (BMI) is correlated with poor cognition and learning and memory deficits including impaired executive function performance in middle aged adults (Cournot *et al.*, 2006; Elias *et al.*, 2003; Sabia *et al.*, 2009). In addition, longitudinal studies have shown that higher body composition and central obesity are related with cognitive decline, particularly in global cognitive function, executive function, and memory over time (Gunstad *et al.*, 2010). Raji and colleagues also demonstrated that a higher BMI can cause brain atrophy in various regions including the frontal lobe, anterior cingulate gyrus, hippocampus and thalamus, when compared with people with normal BMI (Raji *et al.*, 2010). Furthermore, the impaired memory and executive functioning has been reported in patients with type 1 and type 2 diabetes (Munshi *et al.*, 2006; Northam *et al.*, 2001; Reaven *et al.*, 1990). In addition, Den and colleagues demonstrated that subjects with type 2 diabetes also had hippocampal and amygdala atrophy when compared with control subjects (den Heijer *et al.*, 2003). All of these findings from clinical studies suggest that the implication of hippocampus occur following obese-insulin resistant condition.

Fibroblast growth factor 21 (FGF21) is an endocrine hormone and is mainly expressed in the liver, adipose tissues and pancreas (Kharitonenkov and Shanafelt, 2009; Nishimura *et al.*, 2000). Previous studies found that FGF21 exerts beneficial effects on metabolic regulation such as the controlling of glucose levels and lipid homeostasis (Kharitonenkov *et al.*, 2007; Kim *et al.*, 2013; Lin *et al.*, 2013; Xu *et al.*, 2009a, 2009b). FGF21 activity is mediated by the fibroblast growth factor receptor (FGFR) and β-klotho (KLB), which is an essential co-receptor for FGF21 activity; therefore the cells lacking β-klotho are unable to respond to FGF21 (Adams *et al.*, 2012; Ogawa *et al.*, 2007). When FGF21 binds with those receptors, it causes the activation of downstream targets, including the phosphorylation of fibroblast growth factor receptor substrate 2 (FRS2) and extracellular-signal-regulated kinases (ERK1/2). Previous studies found that administration of FGF21 into ob/ob mice, db/db mice, diet-induced obese (DIO) mice and diabetic monkeys led to improved metabolic parameters such as weight loss promotion, improved insulin sensitivity and lipid profile, reduced blood glucose without hypoglycemia and decreased insulin levels (Kharitonenkov *et al.*, 2007; Kim *et al.*, 2013; Lin *et al.*, 2013; Xu *et al.*, 2009a, 2009b). It has been shown that FGF21 levels were also increased under several pathological conditions including obesity, metabolic syndrome and diabetes (Bobbert *et al.*, 2013; Mashili *et al.*, 2011; Novotny *et al.*, 2014; Zhang *et al.*, 2008). A recent study investigated the effect of LY2405319, an FGF21 analog, in obese humans with type 2 diabetic subjects, and found that FGF21 could improve dyslipidemia, reduce body weight gain, reduce fasting plasma insulin levels and increase adiponectin levels (Gaich *et al.*, 2013).

FGF21 is expressed in the brain and can be produced by glia cells and neurons (Johanna Mäkelä *et al.*, 2014). In addition, FGF21 can cross the blood brain barrier following exogenous application and it has been detected in human cerebrospinal fluid (Hsuchou *et al.*, 2007; Tan *et al.*, 2011). FGF21 exerted neuroprotective effects, which were mediated by an increase in the levels of peroxisome proliferator activated receptor γ coactivator 1α (PGC1-α) and its activity (Johanna Mäkelä *et al.*, 2014). Those events subsequently increased the levels of mitochondrial antioxidant enzymes and improved mitochondrial biogenesis and cell viability (Johanna Mäkelä *et al.*, 2014). Moreover, FGF21 has been shown to preserve cognitive function in D-galactose-induced aging mice (Yu *et al.*, 2015). Despite these beneficial effects of FGF21 on improving metabolic function in obese and diabetic animal models, little is known about its effect on brain function under an obese-insulin resistant condition.

However, the effects of FGF21 on cognitive function, which associated with brain oxidative stress, brain mitochondrial function, brain apoptosis, hippocampal synaptic plasticity and dendritic spine density in obese-insulin resistant male rats have not been investigated. Therefore, in this study, we hypothesized that the prevention of cognitive decline by FGF21 in the obese-insulin resistant male rats is associated with its ability to improve peripheral insulin sensitivity, reduce systemic inflammation, restore brain mitochondrial function, decrease brain oxidative stress, decrease brain cell apoptosis and restore hippocampal synaptic plasticity.

2. Materials and methods

2.1 Animal models and experimental protocols

All experimental protocols were approved by the Faculty of Medicine, Chiang Mai University Institutional Animal Care and Use Committee, in compliance with NIH guidelines. Eighteen male Wistar rats weighing 200–220 g were purchased from the National Animal Center, Salaya Campus, Mahidol University, Thailand. All animals were housed individually in a temperature-controlled environment under a light-dark cycle of 12:12 h. After the rats were acclimatized for one week, they were divided into two groups, one to receive a normal diet (ND; 19.77% E fat), which was a standard laboratory pellet diet (Mouse Feed Food No. 082, C.P. Company, Bangkok, Thailand) ($n = 6$), or a high fat diet (HFD; 59.28% E fat) group ($n = 12$). The HFD contained 59.3% total energy from fat with the major composition of fat being saturated fatty acid from lard as described in our previous study (Pratchayasakul *et al.*, 2011). These diets were given for 12 weeks. At week 13, the HFD-fed rats were subdivided into two subgroups to receive either 0.9% normal saline solution (0.9% NSS; 0.1 mg/kg/day; i.p) as a vehicle (HFV) ($n = 6$) or recombinant human FGF21 (FGF21, 0.1 mg/kg/day; i.p) (HFF) ($n = 6$) for four weeks. We used 0.1 mg/kg/day of FGF 21 in the present study because this dose has been shown to improve peripheral insulin sensitivity in previous studies (Coskun *et al.*, 2008; Zhang *et al.*, 2013). Recombinant human FGF21 (rhFGF21) was obtained from Prof. Dr. Xiaokun Li, Zhejiang Provincial Key Laboratory of Biopharmaceuticals, Wenzhou Medical College, Wenzhou, Zhejiang 325,035, P.R. China. Recombinant human FGF21 (rhFGF21) was produced using *Escherichia coli* and purified to be endotoxin free (Wang *et al.*, 2010). All animals were given ad libitum access to food and water. At the end of protocol, the locomotor activity of each rat was tested by an open field test (OFT). After that, the spatial learning and memory was determined by the Morris water maze (MWM) test. An oral glucose tolerance test (OGTT) was also carried out before the animals were sacrificed by decapitation. Blood samples were collected for determining metabolic parameters. The brain was rapidly removed for electrophysiological and biochemical analysis. For the sample size, we used $n = 6$/group for investigation of metabolic parameters, open field test, Morris water maze test, brain mitochondrial function, LTP and western blot analysis. We also used the separated animals ($n = 6$/group) for investigation of the dendritic spine density. The experimental protocol is shown in Fig. 1.

2.2 Chemical analysis for metabolic parameters

Fasting plasma glucose, cholesterol and triglyceride levels were determined by a colorimetric assay (ERBA diagnostic, Mannheim, Germany). Fasting plasma high-density lipoprotein (HDL) levels were determined by a commercial

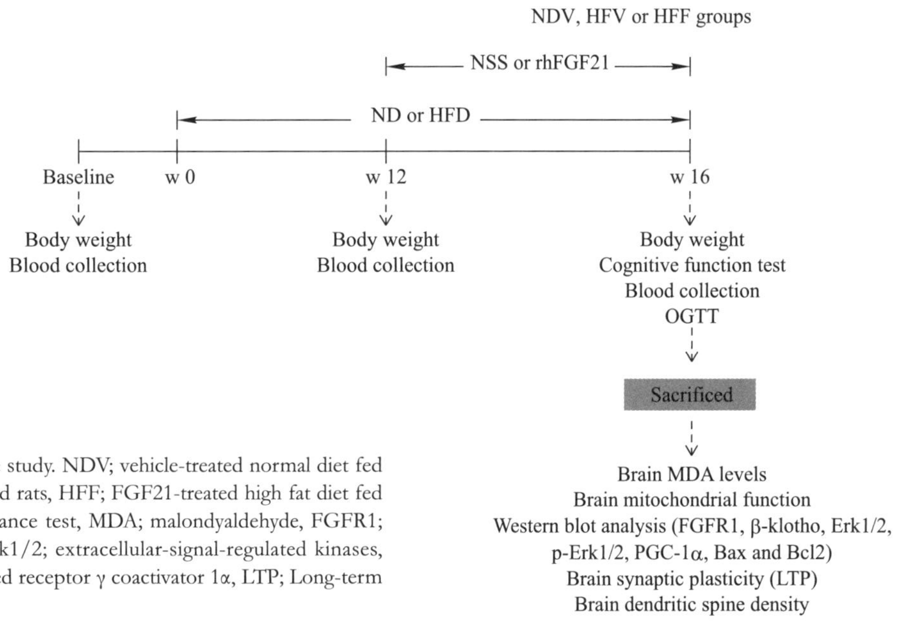

Fig. 1. The experimental protocol of the study. NDV; vehicle-treated normal diet fed rats, HFV; vehicle-treated high fat diet fed rats, HFF; FGF21-treated high fat diet fed rats, w; week, OGTT; oral glucose tolerance test, MDA; malondyaldehyde, FGFR1; fibroblast growth factor receptor 1, Erk1/2; extracellular-signal-regulated kinases, PCG-1α; peroxisome proliferator activated receptor γ coactivator 1α, LTP; Long-term potentiation.

colorimetric assay kit (Biovision, CA, USA). The plasma low-density lipoproteins (LDL) levels were estimated from Friedewald's equation (Friedewald *et al.*, 1972). Previous studies demonstrated that both HDL and LDL levels affected spatial learning and memory in several models such as rats fed with saturated fat, high fat, high cholesterol diet and obese-insulin resistant rats (Granholm *et al.*, 2008; Pratchayasakul *et al.*, 2015; Thirumangalakudi *et al.*, 2008) by increased brain oxidative stress, activated brain microglia and proinflammatory cytokine as well as increased amyloid precursor protein (APP) processing enzyme. Therefore, the present study investigated the effect of a FGF21 on HDL and LDL in obese insulin resistant condition. Fasting plasma insulin levels were evaluated using a sandwich enzyme-linked immunosorbent assay (ELISA) kit (Millipore, MI, USA). The severity of peripheral insulin resistance was assessed by the homeostasis model assessment (HOMA) as described previously (Matthews *et al.*, 1985). An oral glucose tolerance test (OGTT) was performed as described previously (Pratchayasakul *et al.*, 2015). Areas under the curves (AUCs) were calculated to evaluate glucose tolerance.

2.3 Serum TNF-α, adiponectin and plasma FGF21 levels

Serum tumor necrosis factor alpha (TNF-α) levels were determined by a rat TNF-α enzyme-linked immunosorbent assay (ELISA) kit (GE Healthcare, UK). Serum adiponectin levels were determined by a rat adiponectin enzyme-linked immunosorbent assay (ELISA) (Invitrogen, life technologies, Carlsbad, CA, USA). Plasma FGF21 levels were determined by a Mouse/Rat FGF21 enzyme-linked immunosorbent assay (ELISA) kit (R&D systems Inc., Minneapolis, MN, USA).

2.4 Serum and brain malondyaldehylde (MDA) levels

Serum and brain MDA levels are markers of lipid peroxidation levels (Gulbahar *et al.*, 2009). The levels of MDA were determined by high-performance liquid chromatography (HPLC) as described previously (Pintana *et al.*, 2013).

2.5 Cognitive tests

In this study, the open-field test (OFT) was used to evaluate the locomotor activity of the rats. This method was modified from a previous study (Arakawa, 2005). The apparatus consisted of a square-based box opened from above (75 × 75 cm base, 40 cm height). The base was divided into 25 equal squares, each of them sized 15 × 15 cm. Lighting in the testing room was bright (1155 lx). Briefly, the rat was placed into a box, which consisted of white lines, and was observed for 2 min. The numbers of lines that the animals crossed was interpreted as activity (Pintana *et al.*, 2013). To evaluate cognitive function, the protocol of the Morris Water Maze test was used as described previously (Pintana *et al.*,

2012). The MWM set up was a round water pool (diameter 170 cm and height 60 cm) which was assigned with four cardinal points (N = north, S = south, E = east and W = west) and separated into four quadrants (NE = north east, NW = north west, SW = south west and SE = south east). Rats were given four different starting points per day. The round platform (diameter 10 cm) was located in the middle of one of the four quadrants (target quadrant). This protocol evaluated spatial learning and memory ability by two assessments: an acquisition test (hidden platform) and a probe test (removal of the platform from the water pool). Different shaped makers were pasted in the middle of each four quadrants higher than the edge of the pool by about 10 cm. For the acquisition test, rats were tested for five executive days at the same time on each day. The animals rested in the testing room 30 min before the experiment. After 30 min, the animals were placed in the water at one of the randomized starting points, and their time taken to reach the platform was recorded. The rats were left on the platform for 15 s after finding it. After that, the rats were removed from the water and allowed to rest for 15 s before being placed at the other three starting points. In the probe test, at day six, the hidden platform was removed and time spent in the target quadrant was recorded. Data analysis of the MWM test was performed using Smart 3.0 software (Panlab, Harvard Apparatus, Barcelona, Spain).

2.6 Extracellular recordings of hippocampal slices for electrical-induced long-term potentiation (LTP)

At the end of the experiment, animals were anesthetized and decapitated. The hippocampal slices were prepared as previously described (Chattipakorn and McMahon, 2002). Briefly, field excitatory postsynaptic potentials (fEPSPs) were evoked by stimulating the Schaffer collateral-commissural pathway with a bipolar tungsten electrode, whereas fEPSPs recordings were taken from the stratum radiatum of the hippocampal CA1 region with micropipettes (3 MΩ) filled with 2 M NaCl. The LTP protocol is described in a previous study (Sripetchwandee et al., 2014a). Data were filtered at 3 kHz, digitized at 10 kHz, and stored in a computer using pClamp9.2 software (Axon Instruments, CA, USA). The initial slope of the fEPSPs were measured and plotted against time.

2.7 Golgi impregnation and analysis

Previous studies reported that dendritic spine density was related to synaptic plasticity, LTP (Pratchayasakul et al., 2015), therefore we investigated the dendritic spine density in this experimental protocol. After sacrifice by decapitation, brains were removed and rinsed with double distilled water. After that, brain tissue was processed for Golgi staining using a commercially available kit (FD Neurotechnologies kit, PK 401, Ellicott City, USA) as described previously (Pratchayasakul et al., 2015; Sripetchwandee et al., 2016). Briefly, the area of the hippocampus and two segments of pyramidal cell in the CA1 region were randomly examined. Both segments were located on the tertiary apical dendrites. The dendritic spines were viewed through an inverted microscope (IX-81, Olympus, Tokyo, Japan). For the dendritic spine density analysis, two segments from pyramidal cells in the CA1 hippocampus area were randomly measured with 100–200 μm apart from soma and 20 μm in dendritic length. Three neuronal cells per brain slices were chosen for quantitative analysis (3 slices/animals, $n = 6$ animals/group). Therefore, nine neurons from each animal were analyzed. The number of spines was counted using a hand counter, and the dendritic lengths were measured using Xcellence imaging software (Olympus, Tokyo, Japan).

2.8 Immunoblotting

To investigate the expression of fibroblast growth factor receptor 1 (FGFR1), β-klotho, ERK1/2, ERK1/2 phosphorylation (p-Erk1/2), PGC-1α, and brain cells apoptosis markers; Bax and Bcl2, homogenated brain tissues from each subgroup were boiled at 95 °C for 5 min. Then, the proteins were separated by electrophoresis and transferred onto nitrocellulose membranes as previously described (Pipatpiboon et al., 2013). Immunoblotting was conducted with FGFR1, β-klotho, PGC-1α (1:200, Santa Cruz Biotechnology, Inc., Texas, USA), Erk1/2, p-Erk1/2, BAX (1: 1000, Santa Cruz Biotechnology, Inc., Texas, USA) and BCL-2 (1:1 000, Cell Signaling Technology, Danvers, Massachusetts, USA) overnight. The primary antibody was detected by horse anti-mouse IgG conjugate HRP-linked antibody (1:2 000 dilution, Cell Signaling Technology, Danvers, Massachusetts, USA) for β-Actin. Moreover, β-klotho was detected by rabbit anti goat IgG conjugate HRP-linked antibody (1:2000 Santa Cruz Biotechnology, Inc., Texas, USA). FGFR1, Erk1/2, p-Erk1/2, PGC1-α, Bax and BCL-2 was detected by goat anti-rabbit IgG conjugate HRP-linked antibody (1:2000, Cell Signaling Technology, Danvers, Massachusetts, USA). The protein bands were visualized on Amersham hyperfilm ECL using the Amersham ECL western blotting detection reagents system (GE Healthcare, Buckinghamshire, UK). The membranes were developed using the ChemiDoc touch imaging system (Bio-Rad Laboratories, Hercules, California, USA) on chemiluminescence mode and the densitometric analysis was determined by using an image J program. The results are shown as average signal intensity (arbitrary units).

2.9 Brain mitochondrial function

Isolated mitochondria were prepared by using the same method as described in our previous studies (Pintana *et al.*, 2012; Pipatpiboon *et al.*, 2013). To determine brain mitochondrial function, we evaluated brain mitochondrial reactive oxygen species (ROS) production, brain mitochondrial membrane potential ($\Delta\Psi$m) and brain mitochondrial swelling. The mitochondrial function was determined by following the method in our previous studies (Pintana *et al.*, 2012; Pipatpiboon *et al.*, 2013).

2.10 Brain mitochondrial ROS assay

Brain mitochondrial reactive oxygen species (ROS) were determined using dichloro-hydrofluoresceindiacetate (DCFHDA) fluorescent dye. Brain mitochondria (0.4 mg/ml) were incubated with 2-μM DCFHDA at 25°C for 20 min. The fluorescence was determined using a fluorescent microplate reader at the excitation wavelength of 485 nm and emission wavelength of 530 nm (Pipatpiboon *et al.*, 2012). Increased fluorescent intensity indicates increased ROS production.

2.11 Brain mitochondrial membrane potential ($\Delta\Psi$m) assay

Mitochondrial membrane potential changes ($\Delta\Psi$m) were determined using the fluorescent dye 5,5′,6,6′-tetrachloro-1,1′,3,3′-tetraethyl benzimidazolcarbocyanine iodide (JC-1). JC-1 monomer form, green fluorescence, was excited at a wavelength of 485 nm and detected at the emission wavelength of 590 nm. JC-1 aggregate form, red fluorescence, was excited at a wavelength of 485 nm and detected at the emission wavelength of 530 nm. Brain mitochondria (0.4 mg/ml) were incubated with JC-1 dye at 37°C for 15 min. Mitochondrial membrane potential changes were determined by measuring the fluorescent intensity using a fluorescent microplate reader. The change in mitochondrial membrane potential was calculated as the ratio of red to green fluorescent intensity (Pipatpiboon *et al.*, 2012). Decreased red/green fluorescent intensity ratio indicates mitochondrial depolarization.

2.12 Brain mitochondria swelling assay

Brain mitochondrial swelling was determined by measuring the change in the absorbance of the brain mitochondrial suspension. Brain mitochondria (0.4 mg/ml) were incubated in 2-ml respiration buffer. The suspension was read at 540 nm using a microplate reader. Decreased absorbance indicates mitochondria swelling (Pipatpiboon *et al.*, 2012).

2.13 Statistical analysis

Data was expressed as mean ± SEM. Statistical analysis was assessed by using SPSS program (version17; SPSS, Chicago, III., USA). The significance of the differences in all parameters was calculated using one-way ANOVA followed by Tukey's post-hoc test. For the MWM acquisition test, a two-way ANOVA followed by Tukey's post-hoc test was used. For all comparisons, $P < 0.05$ was considered as statistically significant.

3. Results

3.1 Twelve weeks of high-fat diet (HFD) consumption caused obesity and peripheral insulin resistance

After 12 weeks of HFD consumption, 12-week HFD-fed rats had significantly increased body mass, plasma total cholesterol level, plasma LDL level, plasma insulin level, HOMA index and increased plasma glucose area under the curve (AUCg) with no change in plasma glucose level, when compared with 12-week ND-fed rats (for body mass: $F_{(1,10)} = 28.592$, $P < 0.001$, $\eta^2 = 0.74$; for plasma total cholesterol level: $F_{(1,10)} = 40.902$, $P < 0.001$, $\eta^2 = 0.804$; for plasma LDL level: $F_{(1,10)} = 8.621$, $P = 0.015$, $\eta^2 = 0.463$; for plasma insulin level: $F_{(1,10)} = 5.953$, $P = 0.035$, $\eta^2 = 0.373$; for HOMA index: $F_{(1,8)} = 25.261$, $P = 0.001$, $\eta^2 = 0.759$; for plasma AUCg: $F_{(1,8)} = 9.405$, $P = 0.015$, $\eta^2 = 0.540$; Table

1). These findings indicated that 12 weeks of HFD consumption caused obesity and peripheral insulin resistance.

Table 1. Metabolic parameters in rats fed with normal or high fat diet for 12 weeks

Parameters	ND	HFD
Body mass (kg)	468.33 ± 8.33	580.00 ± 19.15[*]
Food intake (g/day)	24.36 ± 4.45	26.56 ± 8.44
Plasma glucose (mg%)	128.48 ± 4.01	130.10 ± 6.65
Plasma total cholesterol (mg/dl)	67.16 ± 2.55	88.00 ± 2.17[*]
Plasma triglyceride (mg/dl)	55.63 ± 6.20	59.44 ± 7.09
Plasma HDL (mg/dl)	29.79 ± 2.02	30.40 ± 3.90
Plasma LDL (mg/dl)	47.95 ± 3.98	62.83 ± 3.14[*]
Plasma insulin (ng/ml)	2.87 ± 0.61	4.99 ± 0.62[*]
HOMA index	17.24 ± 1.90	36.31 ± 3.73[*]
Plasma Glucose AUC (AUCg) (mg/dl × min × 10^4)	4.63 ± 0.71	6.18 ± 0.40[*]

ND; normal diet fed rats, HFD; high fat diet fed rats.

[*] $P < 0.05$ *vs.* ND.

3.2 FGF21 treatment attenuated peripheral insulin resistance, oxidative stress and pro-inflammatory cytokine caused by obesity

After 28 days of vehicle treatment, these HFD-fed rats (HFV) had significantly increased body mass, visceral fat, plasma total cholesterol levels, plasma LDL levels, plasma insulin levels, HOMA index and plasma glucose AUCg without hyperglycemia when compared with vehicle treated ND-fed rats (NDV) (for body mass: $F_{(2,15)} = 61.725$, $P < 0.001$, $\eta^2 = 0.892$; for visceral fat: $F_{(2,15)} = 93.733$, $P < 0.001$, $\eta^2 = 0.926$; for plasma total cholesterol level: $F_{(2,15)} = 16.639$, $P < 0.01$ $\eta^2 = 0.689$; for plasma LDL level: $F_{(2,15)} = 7.857$, $P = 0.005$, $\eta^2 = 0.512$; for plasma insulin level: $F_{(2,15)} = 4.653$, $P = 0.027$, $\eta^2 = 0.383$; for HOMA index: $F_{(2,15)} = 3.224$, $P = 0.05$, $\eta^2 = 0.301$; for plasma AUCg: $F_{(2,22)} = 3.684$, $P = 0.042$, $\eta^2 = 0.251$; Table 2). Moreover, these HFV rats also had significantly increased serum MDA levels when compared with NDV rats ($F_{(2,15)} = 5.379$, $P = 0.017$, $\eta^2 = 0.418$; Table 2). Additionally, HFV rats significantly increased TNF-α level with decreased serum adiponectin level when compared with NDV rats ($F_{(2,15)} = 5.374$, $P = 0.017$, $\eta^2 = 0.417$; Table 2). These findings indicated that the long-term HFD consumption caused peripheral insulin resistance and the occurrence of peripheral insulin resistance was accompanied by an increase in the oxidative stress and pro-inflammatory cytokine in HFV.

Table 2. Effects of FGF21 administration on peripheral insulin sensitivity parameters and MDA levels in HFD-fed rats

Parameters	NDV	HFV	HFF
Body mass (kg)	520.83 ± 10.83	678.33 ± 11.38[*]	556.67 ± 9.19[*,†]
Visceral fat (g)	23.87 ± 1.94	63.94 ± 1.42[*]	50.51 ± 2.74[*,†]
Food intake (g/day)	23.87 ± 1.94	25.78 ± 3.56	23.97 ± 2.95
Plasma glucose (mg%)	127.62 ± 4.05	130.49 ± 6.54	130.03 ± 3.67
Plasma total cholesterol (mg/dl)	77.34 ± 2.25	114.51 ± 7.55[*]	81.51 ± 3.57[†]
Plasma triglyceride (mg/dl)	59.15 ± 4.60	54.62 ± 2.40	56.65 ± 2.58
Plasma HDL (mg/dl)	32.82 ± 1.94	24.52 ± 1.99[*]	31.10 ± 1.71[†]
Plasma LDL (mg/dl)	51.38 ± 2.99	74.39 ± 5.85[*]	55.59 ± 3.75[†]
Plasma insulin (ng/ml)	2.69 ± 0.86	4.96 ± 1.00[*]	2.82 ± 1.98[†]
HOMA index	16.13 ± 1.22	32.82 ± 8.73[*]	17.29 ± 1.76[†]
Plasma glucose AUC (AUCg) (mg/dl × min × 10^4)	5.29 ± 0.29	7.23 ± 0.65[*]	5.50 ± 0.36[†]

Parameters	NDV	HFV	HFF
Plasma adiponectin (ng/ml)	23.00 ± 3.38	$14.67 \pm 2.94^*$	$24.50 \pm 1.69^\dagger$
Plasma TNF-α (pg/ml)	1.11 ± 0.16	$3.05 \pm 0.67^*$	$1.58 \pm 3.07^\dagger$
Serum MDA (μmol/ml)	1.14 ± 0.17	$2.99 \pm 0.76^*$	$1.13 \pm 0.18^\dagger$
Brain MDA (μmol/mg protein)	0.67 ± 1.25	$1.68 \pm 0.22^*$	$0.96 \pm 0.22^\dagger$
Plasma FGF21 levels (pg/ml)	47.94 ± 8.43	$265.69 \pm 30.74^*$	$573.70 \pm 131.10^{*,\dagger}$

NDV; vehicle-treated normal diet fed rats, HFV; vehicle-treated high fat diet fed rats, HFF; FGF21-treated high fat diet fed rats.

$^*P < 0.05$ *vs.* NDV.

$^\dagger P < 0.05$ *vs.* HFV.

After treatment with FGF21 for 28 days, FGF21 treated HFD-fed rats (HFF) showed significantly decreased body mass, visceral fat, plasma total cholesterol levels, plasma LDL levels, decreased plasma insulin levels, HOMA index, plasma glucose AUCg with increased plasma HDL levels when compared with the vehicle treated HFD-fed rats (HFV). Moreover, the HFF rats had significantly decreased serum MDA levels, decreased serum TNF-α and increased adiponectin levels when compared with HFV rats ($P < 0.05$, Table 2). Malondialdehyde (MDA) is the end product of lipid peroxidation levels and is widely used as a biomarker of oxidative stress (Yagi, 1998). Previous studies demonstrated that the increased brain lipid peroxidation caused cell degeneration and cell death. This lead to impaired cognitive function in several models such as patients with amnestic mild cognitive impairment (MCI) (Markesbery *et al.*, 2005) and obese-insulin resistant rats (Pintana *et al.*, 2013). Therefore, the present study investigated the effect of a FGF21 on MDA in rats under an obese-insulin resistant condition. These findings suggested that FGF21 increased peripheral insulin sensitivity, decreased oxidative stress levels as well as reduced systemic inflammation.

3.3 Obesity caused impaired cognitive function, and FGF21 prevented cognitive decline in obese-insulin resistant rats

The open field test was used to determine the locomotor activity of each rat before the MWM test. The number of lines that the rats crossed during the test was not significantly different between groups, indicating that the locomotor activity of all rats after treatment with either the vehicle or FGF21 was similar.

In the MWM test, the time to reach the platform during the acquisition test (day 3 to day 5) in HFV rats was significantly increased, when compared with that of NDV rats ($F(4,22) = 57.719$, $\eta^2 = 0.340$; Fig. 2A). Moreover, the mean time spent in the target quadrant during the probe test (day 6) in HFV rats was significantly decreased, when compared with that of NDV rats ($F(2,21) = 5.404$, $P = 0.013$, $\eta^2 = 0.340$; Fig. 2B). These results suggested that obese-insulin resistant rats exhibited cognitive decline. After treatment with FGF21 for 28 days, HFF rats had a decreased time to reach the platform during the acquisition test (day 3 to day 5) ($F(4,22) = 57.719$, $\eta^2 = 0.340$; Fig. 2A) and an increased mean time spent in the target quadrant during the probe test (day 6) when compared with HFV rats ($F(2,21) = 5.404$, $P = 0.013$, $\eta^2 = 0.340$; Fig. 2B). Moreover, we also found the swim speeds were not significantly different between groups (26.33 ± 3.86, 26.73 ± 3.82 and 30.85 ± 2.63 cm/s, in NDV, HFV and HFF, respectively). Meanwhile, the distance to reach the hidden platform in HFV rats was significantly increased when compared with that of the NDV rats ($F(2,13) = 10.42$, $P = 0.002$, $\eta^2 = 0.616$). Moreover, HFF rats had decreased the distance to reach the hidden platform when compared with that of HFV rats ($F(2,13) = 10.42$, $P = 0.002$, $\eta^2 = 0.616$) (349.40 ± 87.00, 1102.00 ± 226.60 and 347.50 ± 85.51 cm, in NDV, HFV and HFF, respectively). These findings confirmed that the impairment of cognitive function in HFD rats was due to spatial memory deficit, not because of movement related deficits following obesity, and FGF21 attenuated the cognitive impairment.

3.4 Obesity caused the impairment of hippocampal synaptic plasticity, and FGF21 restored this impairment in obese-insulin resistant rats

The degree of electrical-induced LTP of HFV rats significantly decreased when compared with that of NDV rats ($F(2,23) = 3.033$, $P = 0.05$, $\eta^2 = 0.209$; Fig. 2B). In addition, the number of dendritic spines in the CA1 hippocampus of HFV rats was significantly less than that of NDV rats ($F(2,13) = 15.901$, $P < 0.001$, $\eta^2 = 0.710$; Fig. 2D). These findings

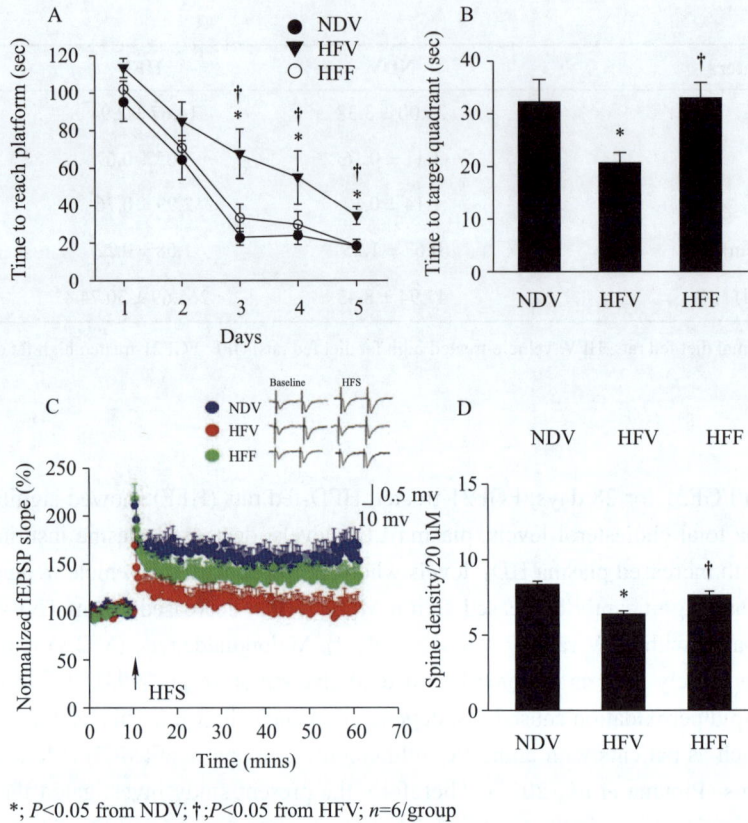

*; $P<0.05$ from NDV; †;$P<0.05$ from HFV; $n=6$/group

Fig. 2. Effects of FGF21 administration on Morris water maze test and hippocampal synaptic plasticity in obese-insulin resistant rats (A) Time to reach the platform in acquisition test and (B) time spent in target quadrant in probe test. (C) The degree of electrical-mediated LTP observed from hippocampal slices and (D) number of dendritic spines on tertiary dendrites in apical dendrite. NDV; vehicle-treated normal diet fed rats, HFV; vehicle-treated high fat diet fed rats, HFF; FGF21-treated high fat diet fed rats. $^*P < 0.05$ *vs.* NDV, $^†P < 0.05$ *vs.* HFV.

suggested that obese-insulin resistant rats had impaired hippocampal synaptic plasticity.

After FGF21 treatment for 28 days, HFF rats had an increase in the degree of electrical-induced LTP when compared with HFV rats ($F(2,23) = 3.033$, $P = 0.05$, $\eta^2 = 0.209$; Fig. 2B).

In addition, the dendritic spine density in CA1 hippocampus of HFF rats significantly increased when compared with that of HFV rats ($F(2,13) = 15.901$, $P < 0.001$, $\eta^2 = 0.710$; Fig. 2D). These findings sug-gested that FGF21 treatment restored hippocampal synaptic plasticity in obese-insulin resistant rats.

3.5 Obesity caused increased plasma FGF21 levels and impaired brain FGF21 signaling

The present study investigated the circulating FGF21 level, the expression of brain FGF21 receptors, including FGFR1 and β-klotho, and brain FGF21 signaling such as Erk1/2, phosphorylated-Erk1/2 (p-Erk1/2) and PGC-1α protein expression. We found that the HFV rats had higher circulating FGF21 levels when compared with NDV rats ($F(2,16) = 12.029$, $P = 0.001$, $\eta^2 = 0.601$; Table 2). The expression of β-klotho and FGFR1 in brain of HFV rats was not significantly different to that of NDV rats (Fig. 3A, B). Interestingly, the level of phosphorylated-FGFR1 (p-FGFR1) expression significantly reduced in HFV rats when compared with NDV rats ($F(2,7) = 18.658$, $P = 0.002$, $\eta^2 = 0.842$; Fig. 3C). Although the expression of total Erk1/2 (t-Erk1/2) expression did not differ between all groups (Fig. 3D) and p-Erk1/2 of HFV rats significantly decreased when compared with those of NDV rats ($F(2,19) = 4.127$, $P = 0.032$, $\eta^2 = 0.303$; Fig. 3E). Moreover, PGC1-α protein expression of HFV was significantly less than that of NDV rats ($F(2,11) = 7.354$, $P = 0.009$, $\eta^2 = 0.512$; Fig. 3F). These findings suggested that the impairment of brain FGF21 signaling occurred in obese-insulin resistant rats.

After FGF21 treatment for 28 days, the highest circulating levels of FGF21 levels were observed in HFF rats when compared with NDV and HFV rats ($F(2,16) = 12.029$, $P = 0.001$, $\eta^2 = 0.601$; Table 2). We did not find a statistically significant difference in β-klotho and FGFR1 expression among all groups (Fig. 3A, B). Moreover, HFF rats had an

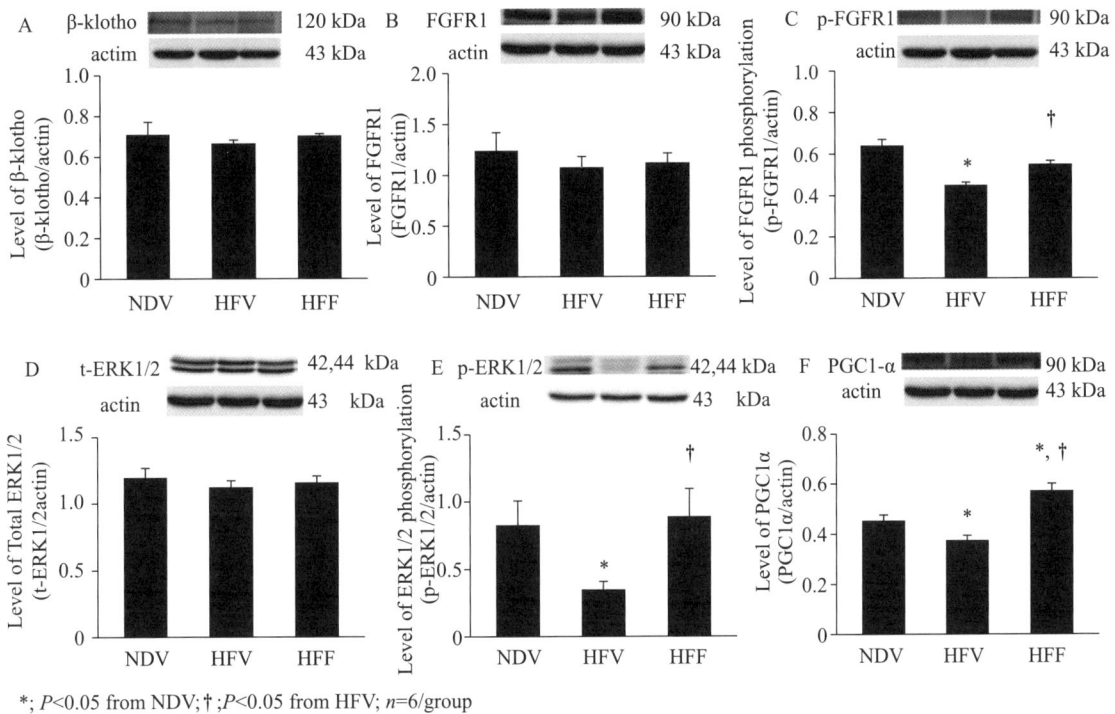

Fig. 3. Effects of FGF21 administration on FGF21 receptor, co-receptor and FGF21 signaling in the brain of obese-insulin resistant rats (A) β-klotho (B) FGFR1 (C) p-FGFR1 (D) t-Erk12 (E) p-Erk1/2 and (D) PGC-1α. NDV; vehicle-treated normal diet fed rats, HFV; vehicle-treated high fat diet fed rats, HFF; FGF21-treated high fat diet fed rats. $^{*}P < 0.05$ $vs.$ NDV, $^{†}P < 0.05$ $vs.$ HFV.

*; $P<0.05$ from NDV; † ;$P<0.05$ from HFV; n=6/group

increase in the expression of p-FGFR1, and p-Erk1/2 protein expression when compared with those of HFV rats (for p-FGFR1: $F(2,7) = 18.658$, $P = 0.002$, $η^2 = 0.842$; for p-Erk1/2: $F(2,19) = 4.127$, $P = 0.032$, $η^2 = 0.303$; Fig. 3C, E). FGF21-treated HFD-fed rats also showed a significant increase in brain PGC-1α expression when compared with NDV and HFV rats ($F(2,11) = 7.354$, $P = 0.009$, $η^2 = 0.512$; Fig. 3F). These findings suggested that FGF21 treatment enhanced FGF21 mediated signaling indicated by the increased p-FGFR1, p-ERK1/2 and PGC1-α levels in obese-insulin resistant rats.

3.6 Obesity caused impaired brain mitochondrial function and increased brain oxidative stress which were attenuated by FGF21 treatment

HFV rats had an increase in brain mitochondrial ROS production, brain mitochondrial membrane potential change (*i.e.* depolarization) as well as brain mitochondrial swelling when compared with NDV rats (for brain mitochondrial ROS production: $F(2,17) = 3.611$, $P = 0.049$, $η^2 = 0.298$; for brain mitochondrial membrane potential change: $F(2,20) = 3.308$, $P = 0.05$, $η^2 = 0.249$; for brain mitochondrial swelling: $F(2,17) = 5.419$, $p = 0.015$, $η^2 = 0.389$; Fig. 4A, B, C).

We also found that the brain MDA level of HFV rats significantly increased when compared with that of NDV rats ($F(2,15) = 7.159$, $P = 0.007$, $η^2 = 0.488$; Table 2). These findings suggested that obese-insulin resistant rats had brain mitochondrial dysfunction with an increase in brain lipid peroxidation levels.

After FGF21 treatment for 28 days, brain mitochondrial ROS production, brain mitochondrial membrane potential change and brain mitochondrial swelling significantly decreased in HFF rats when compared with HFV rats (for brain mitochondrial ROS production: $F(2,17) = 3.611$, $P = 0.049$, $η^2 = 0.298$; for brain mitochondrial membrane potential change: $F(2,20) = 3.308$, $P = 0.05$, $η^2 = 0.249$; for brain mitochondrial swelling: $F(2,17) = 5.419$, $P = 0.015$, $η^2 = 0.389$; Fig. 4A, B, C). Moreover, brain MDA level of HFF rats was lower than that of HFV rats ($F(2,15) = 7.159$, $P = 0.007$, $η^2 = 0.488$; Table 2). In addition, the morphological changes of brain mitochondria were demonstrated by transmission electron microscopy (TEM), and were shown in Fig. 4C. Brain mitochondrial swelling was observed in HFV rats indicated by remarkably unfolded cristae. Brain mitochondrial morphology showed obvious folded cristae in NDV and HFF rats. These findings suggested that FGF21 treatment restored brain mitochondrial function and decreased brain oxidative stress levels in obese-insulin resistant rats.

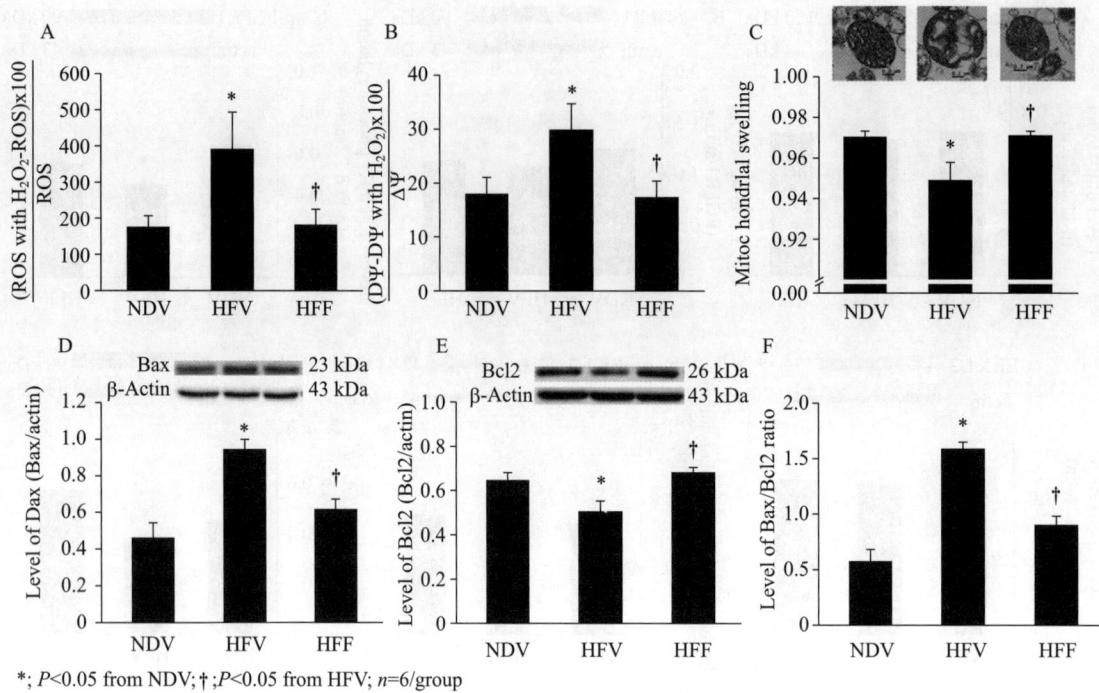

*; *P*<0.05 from NDV; † ;*P*<0.05 from HFV; *n*=6/group

Fig. 4. Effects of FGF21 administration on brain mitochondrial function and cell apoptosis in obese-insulin resistant rats (A) Brain mitochondrial ROS production, (B) brain mitochondrial membrane potential change and (C) brain mitochondrial swelling and transmission electron microscopy (original magnification × 25,000), (D) Bax, (E) Bcl2 and (F) Bax/Bcl2 ratio. NDV; vehicle-treated normal diet fed rats, HFV; vehicle-treated high fat diet fed rats, HFF; FGF21-treated high fat diet fed rats. *P* < 0.05 *vs.* NDV, †*P* < 0.05 *vs.* HFV.

3.7 Obesity caused brain cell apoptosis and FGF21 prevented it

Cells apoptosis in the brain was determined by the expression of Bcl-2 and Bax. The results demonstrated that HFV rats had an increase in the expression of a pro-apoptotic marker (Bax), decreased anti-apoptotic marker (Bcl2) and an increase in Bax/Bcl2 ratio when compared with those of NDV rats (for Bax: $F_{(2,17)}$ = 13.022, P < 0.001, η^2 = 0.605; for Bcl2: $F_{(2,12)}$ = 7.610, P = 0.007, η^2 = 0.559; for Bax/Bcl2: $F_{(2,16)}$ = 36.571, P < 0.001, η^2 = 0.821; Fig. 4D, E, F). These findings suggested that increased brain cell apoptosis was observed in obese-insulin resistant rats.

After FGF21 treatment for 28 days, the reduction in Bax protein expression, increased Bcl2 protein expression and a decrease in Bax/Bcl2 ratio were observed in HFF rats when compared with HFV rats (for Bax: $F_{(2,17)}$ = 13.022, p < 0.001, η^2 = 0.605; for Bcl2: $F_{(2,12)}$ = 7.610, P = 0.007, η^2 = 0.559; for Bax/Bcl2: $F_{(2,16)}$ = 36.571, P < 0.001, η^2 = 0.821; Fig. 4D, E, F). These findings indicated that FGF21 reduced brain cell apoptosis in obese-insulin resistant rats.

4. Discussion

The major findings of the present study demonstrated that FGF21 treated obese-insulin resistant male rats 1) improved metabolic parameters, decreased circulating pro-inflammatory cytokine and serum oxidative stress levels; 2) prevented cognitive decline; 3) restored hippocampal synaptic plasticity; 4) enhanced brain FGF21-mediated signaling; and 5) restored brain mitochondrial function, decreased brain oxidative stress levels as well as brain cell apoptosis.

In this present study, we demonstrated that obesity induced by HFD consumption caused the development of peripheral insulin resistance, which was indicated by increased body mass, plasma insulin levels, HOMA index, total area under the curve (TAUCg) and euglycemia (Table 1). These findings on metabolic parameters are consistent with our previous reports for this model (Pintana *et al.*, 2013; Pipatpiboon *et al.*, 2013; Pratchayasakul *et al.*, 2011). Moreover, the present study demonstrated that long-term HFD consumption increased systemic inflammation indicated by increased pro-inflammatory cytokine level (TNF-α) and decreased adipokine level (adiponectin). Previous studies reported that obesity and adipocyte hypertrophy led to an increased level of pro-inflammatory cytokines and impaired the expression and secretion of adiponectin (Ouchi *et al.*, 2011). Hypo-adiponectinemia can cause insulin resistance and diabetes (Kim *et al.*, 2013; Lin *et al.*, 2013). In addition, previous studies reported that low levels of adiponectin found in obesity and the administration of adiponectin in an animal model of obesity improved peripheral insulin sensitivity (Berg *et al.*, 2001; Diez and Iglesias, 2010). All of those findings and our present findings indicated that HFD consumption led to not only obesity, but also systemic inflammation and hypo-adiponectinemia, in which finally resulted the impairment of peripheral insulin sensitivity. We previously found that the obese-insulin resistant condition led to impaired brain functions (Pintana *et al.*, 2013; Pratchayasakul *et al.*, 2015; Sripetchwandee *et al.*, 2014b). Those findings were confirmed in this study, where we found that long-term HFD consumption caused increased brain oxidative stress, brain mitochondrial dysfunction, impaired hippocampal synaptic plasticity, decreased dendritic spine density as well as impaired cognitive function. Moreover, we found that male rats with long-term HFD consumption had increased brain cell apoptosis which was indicated by an increase in Bax levels, decreased Bcl2 levels and an increased Bax/Bcl2 ratio. An increase in apoptotic markers together with increased mitochondrial dysfunction in the brain of obese-insulin resistant male rats could lead to impaired cognition found in this study.

Our results also showed that obese-insulin resistant male rats had increased serum FGF21 levels. Serum FGF21 levels have been shown to increase in several pathological conditions such as obesity, metabolic syndrome and diabetes (Bobbert *et al.*, 2013; Mashili *et al.*, 2011; Novotny *et al.*, 2014; Zhang *et al.*, 2008), and that this increased level of FGF21 in the obese model cannot restore or improve metabolic function. It has been suggested that when a state of high endogenous level of a metabolic regulator does not have any effects on the physiological function, but can lead to an improvement of metabolic function if under a high pharmacological level, this suggests a state of hormone resistance (Yang *et al.*, 2012). In addition, the study by Fisher and colleagues demonstrated that diet-induced obese (DIO) mice fed with a high fat/high sucrose diet showed increased serum FGF21, decreased FGFR1 mRNA expression in both the liver and white adipose tissue (WAT), decreased β-klotho mRNA expression in the WAT but not in the liver (Fisher *et al.*, 2010). These findings suggested that obese-insulin resistance may lead to FGF21 resistance and may alter the FGF21 receptor expression in liver and WAT.

This present study is the first study that has investigated the FGFR1 phosphorylation and β-klotho level in the brain of obese-insulin resistant male rats. Our results showed that, although there was no change in the protein expression of the receptor, the FGFR1 function was impaired in the brain of obese-insulin resistant male rats. All of the findings from our study suggested that obese-insulin resistant male rats had impaired brain FGF21 signaling.

In this study, FGF21 treatment in obese-insulin resistant male rats improved peripheral insulin sensitivity and decreased systemic inflammation which is possibly due to decreased body mass gain and decreased visceral fat. FGF21 reduced body mass gain in obese-insulin resistant male rats without the reduction of food intake. The possible explanations of this observation may be that 1) FGF21 level could induce an increase in the sympathetic activity as shown in a previous study (Douris *et al.*, 2015; Owen *et al.*, 2014) and 2) FGF 21 could up regulate thermogenesis gene (UCP-1) in adipocytes as demonstrated in a previous study (Douris *et al.*, 2015; Owen *et al.*, 2014). These two possible explanations could increase energy expenditure, which caused body weight loss (Douris *et al.*, 2015; Owen *et al.*, 2014). Moreover, the effect of FGF21 on the improvement of peripheral insulin resistance could be due to the following mechanisms 1) increased rate of glucose uptake in adipocytes, increased insulin synthesis and reduced hepatic gluco-neogenesis (Kharitonenkov *et al.*, 2008; Kong *et al.*, 2013; Kralisch *et al.*, 2013; Liu *et al.*, 2012; Xu *et al.*, 2009b) and 2) reduced levels of pro-inflammatory cytokines such as TNF-α, MCP-1 and PAI-1, and 3) increased adiponectin biosynthesis in adipocytes, as shown in Table 2 and other previous studies (Kim *et al.*, 2013; Lin *et al.*, 2013).

Moreover, FGF21 treatment also improved brain FGF21 signaling, as indicated by an increased p-Erk1/2 level and subsequently to increased PGC-1α expression in obese-insulin resistant male rats (Fig. 3). FGF21 has been shown to improve mitochondrial function in human dopaminergic neurons, by increasing mitochondrial anti-oxidant levels and enhancing mitochondrial respiratory capacity, mediated by sirtuin-1 (SIRT1) and PGC-1α which leads to improved mitochondrial biogenesis and cell viability (Houten and Auwerx, 2004; Johanna Mäkelä *et al.*, 2014; Lin *et al.*, 2005; Wu *et al.*, 1999). Moreover, increasing the activity of PGC-1α has been shown to protect oxidative stress-induced cell death and prevent neurodegeneration in Parkinson's disease (Pacelli *et al.*, 2011; St-Pierre *et al.*, 2006). It is known that oxidative stress caused increased neuronal apoptosis and impaired hippocampal synaptic plasticity as indicated by a decrease in the LTP amplitude and the reduction in dendritic spine density (Avila-Costa *et al.*, 1999; Rivas-Arancibia *et al.*, 2010). Additionally, a recent study found that FGF21 treatment improved behavioral performance in the MWM test and in the step-down test by reducing brain cell damage in the hippocampus and suppressing brain oxidative stress in D-galatactose-induced aging model (Yu *et al.*, 2015). The present study showed for the first time that FGF21 treatment in obese-insulin resistant male rats could restore brain mitochondrial function by reducing ROS production, brain oxidative stress levels and these events led to reduced brain cell apoptosis, restored hippocampal synaptic plasticity, restored dendritic spine density as well as prevented cognitive decline.

In conclusion, the present study demonstrated that the effects of FGF21 on the prevention of cognitive decline in obese-insulin resistant condition is associated with its ability to improve peripheral insulin sensitivity, reduce systemic inflammation, restore brain mitochondrial function, decrease brain oxidative stress, decreased brain cell apoptosis and restore hippocampal synaptic plasticity. These beneficial effects of FGF21 in the brain were mediated by the FGF21 signaling pathway.

Limitation of the study

Although our results showed that FGF21 treatment for 4 weeks effectively improved cognitive function, it is not known whether a 4-week treatment of FGF21 is the optimal duration to see its beneficial effects. The sample size was also small in the present study. Future studies with larger sample size are needed to investigate the time course effects of FGF21 on the cognition in obese-insulin resistant rats.

References

[1] Adams AC, Kharitonenkov A. FGF21: The Center of a Transcriptional Nexus in Metabolic Regulation[J]. Current Diabetes Reviews, 2012, 8(4): 285-293.

[2] Arakawa H. Age dependent effects of space limitation and social tension on open-field behavior in male rats[J]. Physiology & Behavior, 2005, 84(3): 429-436.

[3] Avila-Costa MR, Colin-Barenque L, Fortoul TI, *et al.* Memory deterioration in an oxidative stress model and its correlation with cytological changes on rat hippocampus CA1[J]. Neuroscience Letters, 1999, 270(2): 107-109.

[4] Beilharz JE, Maniam J, Morris MJ. Diet-Induced Cognitive Deficits: The Role of Fat and Sugar, Potential Mechanisms and Nutritional Interventions[J]. Nutrients, 2015, 7(8): 6719-6738.

[5] Berg AH, Combs TP, Du XL, *et al.* The adipocyte-secreted protein Acrp30 enhances hepatic insulin action[J]. Nature Medicine, 2001, 7(8): 947-953.

[6] Bobbert T, Schwarz F, Fischer-Rosinsky A, *et al.* Fibroblast Growth Factor 21 Predicts the Metabolic Syndrome and Type 2 Diabetes in Caucasians[J]. Diabetes Care, 2013, 36(1): 145-149.

[7] Chattipakorn SC, McMahon LL. Pharmacological characterization of glycine-gated chloride currents recorded in rat hippocampal slices[J]. Journal of Neurophysiology, 2002, 87(3): 1515-1525.

[8] Coskun T, Bina HA, Schneider MA, *et al.* Fibroblast Growth Factor 21 Corrects Obesity in Mice[J]. Endocrinology, 2008, 149(12): 6018-6027.

[9] Cournot M, Marquie JC, Ansiau D, *et al.* Relation between body mass index and cognitive function in healthy middle-aged men and women[J]. Neurology, 2006, 67(7): 1208-1214.

[10] den Heijer T, Vermeer SE, van Dijk EJ, *et al.* Type 2 diabetes and atrophy of medial temporal lobe structures on brain MRI[J]. Diabetologia, 2003, 46(12): 1604-1610.

[11] Diez JJ, Iglesias P. The Role of the Novel Adipocyte-Derived Protein Adiponectin in Human Disease: An Update[J]. Mini-Reviews in Medicinal Chemistry, 2010, 10(9): 856-869.

[12] Douris N, Stevanovic DM, Fisher FM, *et al.* Central Fibroblast Growth Factor 21 Browns White Fat *via* Sympathetic Action in Male Mice[J]. Endocrinology, 2015, 156(7): 2470-2481.

[13] Elias MF, Elias PK, Sullivan LM, *et al.* Lower cognitive function in the presence of obesity and hypertension: the Framingham heart study[J]. International Journal of Obesity, 2003, 27(2): 260-268.

[14] Fisher FM, Chui PC, Antonellis PJ, *et al.* Obesity Is a Fibroblast Growth Factor 21 (FGF21)-Resistant State[J]. Diabetes, 2010, 59(11): 2781-2789.

[15] Friedewald WT, Fredrickson DS, Levy RI. Estimation of the concentration oflow-density lipoprotein cholesterol in plasma, without use of the preparative ultracentrifuge [J]. Clinical Chemistry, 1972, 18(6): 499-502.

[16] Fung TT, Rimm EB, Spiegelman D, *et al.* Association between dietary patterns and plasma biomarkers of obesity and cardiovascular disease risk[J]. American Journal of Clinical Nutrition, 2001, 73(1): 61-67.

[17] Gaich G, Chien JY, Fu H, *et al.* The Effects of LY2405319, an FGF21 Analog, in Obese Human Subjects with Type 2 Diabetes[J]. Cell Metabolism, 2013, 18(3): 333-340.

[18] Granholm A-C, Bimonte-Nelson HA, Moore AB, *et al.* Effects of a saturated fat and high cholesterol diet on memory and hippocampal morphology in the middle-aged rat[J]. Journal of Alzheimers Disease, 2008, 14(2): 133-145.

[19] Gulbahar O, Aricioglu A, Akmansu M, *et al.* Effects of Radiation on Protein Oxidation and Lipid Peroxidation in the Brain Tissue[J]. Transplantation Proceedings, 2009, 41(10): 4394-4396.

[20] Gunstad J, Lhotsky A, Wendell CR, *et al.* Longitudinal Examination of Obesity and Cognitive Function: Results from the Baltimore Longitudinal Study of Aging[J]. Neuroepidemiology, 2010, 34(4): 222-229.

[21] Houten SM, Auwerx J. PGC-1 alpha: Turbocharging mitochondria[J]. Cell, 2004, 119(1): 5-7.

[22] Hsuchou H, Pan W, Kastin AJ. The fasting polypeptide FGF21 can enter brain from blood[J]. Peptides, 2007, 28(12): 2382-2386.

[23] Mäkelä J, Tselykh TV, Maiorana F, *et al.* Fibroblast growth factor-21 enhances mitochondrial functions and increases the activity of PGC-1α in human dopaminergic neurons *via* Sirtuin-1[J]. Springerplus, 2014, 3(1): 1-12.

[24] Kharitonenkov A, Dunbar JD, Bina HA, *et al.* FGF-21/FGF-21

receptor interaction and activation is determined by beta Klotho[J]. Journal of Cellular Physiology, 2008, 215(1): 1-7.

[25] Kharitonenkov A, Shanafelt AB. FGF21: A novel prospect for the treatment of metabolic diseases[J]. Current Opinion in Investigational Drugs, 2009, 10(4): 359-364.

[26] Kharitonenkov A, Wroblewski VJ, Koester A, et al. The metabolic state of diabetic monkeys is regulated by fibroblast growth factor-21[J]. Endocrinology, 2007, 148(2): 774-781.

[27] Kim HW, Lee JE, Cha JJ, et al. Fibroblast Growth Factor 21 Improves Insulin Resistance and Ameliorates Renal Injury in db/db Mice[J]. Endocrinology, 2013, 154(9): 3366-3376.

[28] Kong L-J, Feng W, Wright M, et al. FGF21 suppresses hepatic glucose production through the activation of atypical protein kinase C iota/lambda[J]. European Journal of Pharmacology, 2013, 702(1-3): 302-308.

[29] Kralisch S, Toenjes A, Krause K, et al. Fibroblast growth factor-21 serum concentrations are associated with metabolic and hepatic markers in humans[J]. Journal of Endocrinology, 2013, 216(2): 135-143.

[30] Lin JD, Handschin C, Spiegelman BM. Metabolic control through the PGC-1 family of transcription coactivators[J]. Cell Metabolism, 2005, 1(6): 361-370.

[31] Lin Z, Tian H, Lam KSL, et al. Adiponectin Mediates the Metabolic Effects of FGF21 on Glucose Homeostasis and Insulin Sensitivity in Mice[J]. Cell Metabolism, 2013, 17(5): 779-789.

[32] Liu MY, Wang WF, Hou YT, et al. Fibroblast growth factor (FGF)-21 regulates glucose uptake through GLUT1 translocation[J]. African Journal of Microbiology Research, 2012, 6(10): 2504-2511.

[33] Markesbery WR, Kryscio RJ, Lovell MA, et al. Lipid peroxidation is an early event in the brain in amnestic mild cognitive impairment[J]. Annals of Neurology, 2005, 58(5): 730-735.

[34] Mashili FL, Austin RL, Deshmukh AS, et al. Direct effects of FGF21 on glucose uptake in human skeletal muscle: implications for type 2 diabetes and obesity[J]. Diabetes-Metabolism Research and Reviews, 2011, 27(3): 286-297.

[35] Matthews DR, Hosker JP, Rudenski AS, et al. Homeostasismodelassessment: insulinresistance andbeta-cellfunction from fastingplasma glucose and insulin concentrations in man [J]. Diabetologia, 1985, 28(7): 412-419.

[36] Munshi M, Grande L, Hayes M, et al. Cognitive dysfunction is associated with poor diabetes control in older adults[J]. Diabetes Care, 2006, 29(8): 1794-1799.

[37] Nishimura T, Nakatake Y, Konishi M, et al. Identification of a novel FGF, FGF-21, preferentially expressed in the liver[J]. Biochimica Et Biophysica Acta-Gene Structure and Expression, 2000, 1492(1): 203-206.

[38] Northam EA, Anderson PJ, Jacobs R, et al. Neuropsychological profiles of children with type 1 diabetes 6 years after disease onset[J]. Diabetes Care, 2001, 24(9): 1541-1546.

[39] Novotny D, Vaverkova H, Karasek D, et al. Evaluation of Total Adiponectin, Adipocyte Fatty Acid Binding Protein and Fibroblast Growth Factor 21 Levels in Individuals With Metabolic Syndrome[J]. Physiological Research, 2014, 63(2): 219-228.

[40] Ogawa Y, Kurosu H, Yamamoto M, et al. beta Klotho is required for metabolic activity of fibroblast growth factor 21[J]. Proceedings of the National Academy of Sciences of the United States of America, 2007, 104(18): 7432-7437.

[41] Ouchi N, Parker JL, Lugus JJ, et al. Adipokines in inflammation and metabolic disease[J]. Nature Reviews Immunology, 2011, 11(2): 85-97.

[42] Owen BM, Ding X, Morgan DA, et al. FGF21 Acts Centrally to Induce Sympathetic Nerve Activity, Energy Expenditure, and Weight Loss[J]. Cell Metabolism, 2014, 20(4): 670-677.

[43] Pacelli C, De Rasmo D, Signorile A, et al. Mitochondrial defect and PGC-1 alpha dysfunction in parkin-associated familial Parkinson's disease[J]. Biochimica Et Biophysica Acta-Molecular Basis

of Disease, 2011, 1812(8): 1041-1053.

[44] Pintana H, Apaijai N, Chattipakorn N, et al. DPP-4 inhibitors improve cognition and brain mitochondrial function of insulinresistant rats[J]. Journal of Endocrinology, 2013, 218(1): 1-11.

[45] Pintana H, Apaijai N, Pratchayasakul W, et al. Effects of metformin on learning and memory behaviors and brain mitochondrial functions in high fat diet induced insulin resistant rats[J]. Life Sciences, 2012, 91(11-12): 409-414.

[46] Pipatpiboon N, Pintana H, Pratchayasakul W, et al. DPP4-inhibitor improves neuronal insulin receptor function, brain mitochondrial function and cognitive function in rats with insulin resistance induced by high-fat diet consumption[J]. European Journal of Neuroscience, 2013, 37(5): 839-849.

[47] Pipatpiboon N, Pratchayasakul W, Chattipakorn N, et al. PPAR gamma Agonist Improves Neuronal Insulin Receptor Function in Hippocampus and Brain Mitochondria Function in Rats with Insulin Resistance Induced by Long Term High-Fat Diets[J]. Endocrinology, 2012, 153(1): 329-338.

[48] Pratchayasakul W, Kerdphoo S, Petsophonsakul P, et al. Effects of high-fat diet on insulin receptor function in rat hippocampus and the level of neuronal corticosterone[J]. Life Sciences, 2011, 88(13-14): 619-627.

[49] Pratchayasakul W, Sa-nguanmoo P, Sivasinprasasn S, et al. Obesity accelerates cognitive decline by aggravating mitochondrial dysfunction, insulin resistance and synaptic dysfunction under estrogen-deprived conditions[J]. Hormones and Behavior, 2015, 72: 68-77.

[50] Raji CA, Ho AJ, Parikshak NN, et al. Brain Structure and Obesity[J]. Human Brain Mapping, 2010, 31(3): 353-364.

[51] Reaven GM, Thompson LW, Nahum D, et al. Relationship between hyperglycemia and cognitive function in older NIDDM patients [J]. Diabetes Care, 1990, 13(1): 16-21.

[52] Riccardi G, Giacco R, Rivellese AA. Dietary fat, insulin sensitivity and the metabolic syndrome[J]. Clinical Nutrition, 2004, 23(4): 447-456.

[53] Rivas-Arancibia S, Guevara-Guzman R, Lopez-Vidal Y, et al. Oxidative Stress Caused by Ozone Exposure Induces Loss of Brain Repair in the Hippocampus of Adult Rats[J]. Toxicological Sciences, 2010, 113(1): 187-197.

[54] Sabia S, Kivimaki M, Shipley MJ, et al. Body mass index over the adult life course and cognition in late midlife: the Whitehall II Cohort Study[J]. American Journal of Clinical Nutrition, 2009, 89(2): 601-607.

[55] Sripetchwandee J, Pipatpiboon N, Chattipakorn N, et al. Combined Therapy of Iron Chelator and Antioxidant Completely Restores Brain Dysfunction Induced by Iron Toxicity[J]. Plos One, 2014, 9(1).

[56] Sripetchwandee J, Wongjaikam S, Krintratun W, et al. A combination of an iron chelator with an antioxidant effectively diminishesthe dendritic loss, tau-hyperphosphorylation, amyloids-beta accumulation andbrainmitochondrial dynamic disruption inrats with chronic iron-overload [J]. Neuroscience, 2016, 332: 191-202.

[57] Sripetehwandee J, Pipatpiboon N, Pratchayasakul W, et al. DPP-4 Inhibitor and PPAR gamma Agonist Restore the Loss of CA1 Dendritic Spines in Obese Insulin-resistant Rats[J]. Archives of Medical Research, 2014, 45(7): 547-552.

[58] St-Pierre J, Drori S, Uldry M, et al. Suppression of reactive oxygen species and neurodegeneration by the PGC-1 transcriptional coactivators[J]. Cell, 2006, 127(2): 397-408.

[59] Stranahan AM, Norman ED, Lee K, et al. Diet-Induced Insulin Resistance Impairs Hippocampal Synaptic Plasticity and Cognition in Middle-Aged Rats[J]. Hippocampus, 2008, 18(11): 1085-1088.

[60] Tan BK, Hallschmid M, Adya R, et al. Fibroblast Growth Factor 21 (FGF21) in Human Cerebrospinal Fluid Relationship With Plasma FGF21 and Body Adiposity[J]. Diabetes, 2011, 60(11): 2758-2762.

[61] Thirumangalakudi L, Prakasam A, Zhang R, et al. High cholester-

ol-induced neuroinflammation and amyloid precursor protein processing correlate with loss of working memory in mice[J]. Journal of Neurochemistry, 2008, 106(1): 475-485.

[62] Wang H, Xiao Y, Fu L, et al. High-level expression and purification of soluble recombinant FGF21 protein by SUMO fusion in Escherichia coli[J]. Bmc Biotechnology, 2010, 10.

[63] Winocur G, Greenwood CE, Piroli GG, et al. Memory impairment in obese Zucker rats: An investigation of cognitive function in an animal model of insulin resistance and obesity[J]. Behavioral Neuroscience, 2005, 119(5): 1389-1395.

[64] Wu ZD, Puigserver P, Andersson U, et al. Mechanisms controlling mitochondrial biogenesis and respiration through the thermogenic coactivator PGC-1[J]. Cell, 1999, 98(1): 115-124.

[65] Xu J, Lloyd DJ, Hale C, et al. Fibroblast Growth Factor 21 Reverses Hepatic Steatosis, Increases Energy Expenditure, and Improves Insulin Sensitivity in Diet-Induced Obese Mice[J]. Diabetes, 2009, 58(1): 250-259.

[66] Xu J, Stanislaus S, Chinookoswong N, et al. Acute glucose-lowering and insulin-sensitizing action of FGF21 in insulin-resistant mouse models-association with liver and adipose tissue effects[J]. American Journal of Physiology-Endocrinology and Metabolism, 2009, 297(5): E1105-E1114.

[67] Yagi K. Simple assay for the level of total lipid peroxides in serum or plasma[J]. Methods in molecular biology (Clifton, N.J.), 1998, 108: 101-106.

[68] Yang M, Zhang L, Wang C, et al. Liraglutide Increases FGF-21 Activity and Insulin Sensitivity in High Fat Diet and Adiponectin Knockdown Induced Insulin Resistance[J]. Plos One, 2012, 7(11).

[69] Yu Y, Bai F, Wang W, et al. Fibroblast growth factor 21 protects mouse brain against D-galactose induced aging via suppression of oxidative stress response and advanced glycation end products formation[J]. Pharmacology Biochemistry and Behavior, 2015, 133: 122-131.

[70] Zhang C, Shao M, Yang H, et al. Attenuation of Hyperlipidemia- and Diabetes-Induced Early-Stage Apoptosis and Late-Stage Renal Dysfunction via Administration of Fibroblast Growth Factor-21 Is Associated with Suppression of Renal Inflammation[J]. Plos One, 2013, 8(12).

[71] Zhang X, Yeung DCY, Karpisek M, et al. Serum FGF21 levels are increased in obesity and are independently associated with the metabolic syndrome in humans[J]. Diabetes, 2008, 57(5): 1246-1253.

Cerebrospinal fluid FGF23 levels correlate with a measure of impulsivity

Hui Li, Yanlong Liu, Xiaokun Li

1. Introduction

Stress is a natural human response to pressure in the face of challenges. Stress can be a cause and a symptom of mood problems such as anxiety and depression (Hammen, 2005). Anxiety and depression are associated with desperation (Garlow *et al*., 2008). People with anxiety and depression tend to be impulsive (Corruble *et al*., 2003; Tillfors *et al*., 2013).

Fibroblast growth factors (FGFs) are well-known regulators of cell growth, differentiation and morphogenesis in the early stages of neural development (Zhang *et al*., 2012). The FGF system is involved in hippocampal neurogenesis, where it helps mediate the effect of anti-depressants (Turner *et al*., 2006). One study suggests a role for FGF system dysregulation in major depression. Expression of several FGF family transcripts were altered in subjects with major depression (Evans *et al*., 2004).

Fibroblast growth factor (FGF) 23, a member of the FGF19 subfamily, modulates mineral ion homeostasis and bone mineralization. FGF23 is a bone-derived protein mainly produced by osteocytes and osteoblasts, and is expressed at low levels in specific parts of the brain (Guo and Yuan, 2015). The major target of FGF23 is the kidney, where it downregulates luminal expression of sodium-phosphate cotransporters in the proximal tubule to stimulate phosphaturia. It also inhibits 25-hydroxyvitamin D-1a-hydroxylase and stimulates 24-hydroxylase to suppress the production of 1,25-dihydroxyvitamin D (1,25-(OH)2D) (Blau and Collins, 2015; Ding and Ma, 2015; Erben and Andrukhova, 2015; Fakhri *et al*., 2014). A recent study demonstrated that lithium treatment gives rise to a significant increase of serum FGF23 concentration in depressive patients (Fakhri *et al*., 2014). It remains unknown whether this upregulation represents a side effect related to dehydration, or rather if it is a crucial factor in the mood-stabilizing properties of lithium. At least, they suggest the neuroprotective effect of lithium might be partly mediated by an increase of FGF23. In spite of the expression of FGF23 in the brain, the function of this secreted protein is still unknown in neuropsychological regulation. In addition, no direct evidence shows a relationship between FGF23 and mood regulation. In this study, we measured FGF23 levels in human cerebrospinal fluid (CSF), and explored the correlations with a cluster of emotions.

2. Materials and methods

2.1 Subjects

A total of 96 male Chinese volunteers (30.29 ± 9.63 years) participated in this study with an average education length of 12.75 ± 2.61 years. All subjects were recruited from a population of patients who were scheduled to undergo surgery for anterior cruciate ligament injuries, and who were not currently on medication. They were all male Chinese without a history of drug use/abuse (including alcohol and nicotine), according to self-report and as confirmed by next of kin. We excluded subjects with a family history of psychosis and neurological diseases, determined according to criteria based on the Mini-International Neuropsychiatric Interview (Chinese version). Individuals with metabolic, systemic or central nervous system (CNS) diseases were also excluded from the study. The study protocol was approved by the Institutional Review Board of Inner Mongolian Medical University. For each subject, written informed consent was obtained either directly from the participants or from their responsible guardians.

2.2 Assessments

Each participant completed a detailed self-reported questionnaire including sociodemographic characteristics, medical history, and psychological condition. The pain levels of all subjects were assessed by the visual analogue scale before surgery. Each participant was then evaluated on the Barratt Impulsiveness Scale, version 11 (BIS-11), the 13-item Beck Depression Inventory (BDI), and the Self-Rating Anxiety Scale (SAS). The Barratt Impulsiveness Scale (BIS-11) is composed of 30 items describing common impulsive or non-impulsive behaviors and preferences. It is the most widely cited instrument for the assessment of impulsiveness, with excellent validity, reliability, and predictive value. The Chinese Version of BIS-11 includes three factors: (1) attentional impulsiveness (attention and cognitive instability), (2) motor impulsiveness (motor impulsiveness and perseverance), and (3) non-planned impulsiveness (self-control and cognitive complexity) (Yao *et al.*, 2007). All scales were assessed in a blinded manner with regard to subject identity. All of the scales were completed by self-report one day prior to CSF extraction. BDI scores were lower than 12, from 0 to 11, and SAS scores ranged from 28 to 50, except for one score of 56. Higher scores of BIS, BDI, and SAS scales reflect greater impulsivity, depression and anxiety, respectively.

2.3 Cerebrospinal fluid sample collection and FGF23 measurement

Cerebrospinal fluid samples were drawn by lumbar puncture with the spinal needle inserted into the L3/L4 or L4/L5 interspace in the morning before surgery by a licensed anesthetist. All CSF samples were collected after discarding the first drop CSF in order to avoid con-tamination. Time interval between assessments and lumber puncture was less 24 h. Time interval between hospitalization and lumbar puncture was five days at most. Each CSF sample was separated into 0.5 ml Eppendorf tubes and immediately frozen at $-80\,^{\circ}\text{C}$ until analysis. Full-length FGF23 levels (Yamamoto *et al.*, 2016) in CSF samples with blinded subject identity were quantified using a commercial enzyme-linked immunosorbent assay kit (Cloud-Clone, Houston, TX, USA) according to the manufacturer's instructions.

2.4 Statistical analysis

The results are expressed as mean ± standard deviation. Partial correlation analysis was performed using parametric methods for continuous variables with age and education years as covariates. All tests were two-tailed, and the P value less than 0.0073 after Bonferroni correction was considered statistically significant. All analysis was performed using SPSS 19.0 (Statistical Package for Social Studies, Version 19.0, SPSS Inc., Illinois, Chicago). Effect size was calculated using the online platform (http://www.campbellcollaboration.org/ escalc/html/EffectSizeCalculator-R-main.php)

3. Results

3.1 Subject characteristics

CSF FGF23 levels showed considerable inter-individual variations, ranging from 12.8 to 99.3 pg/ml (Table 1). Age and education years of all individuals ranged from 17 to 57 years and from 5 to 18 years, and the mean values were 30.29 ± 9.63 and 12.75 ± 2.61, respectively. The mean value of pain levels was 1.47 ± 0.78. The mean values of BIS scores were 25.53 ± 5.33 for non-planning (from 12 to 40), 27.40 ± 7.76 for action (from 10 to 40), 24.95 ± 4.69 for cognition (from 10 to 37), and 26.04 ± 4.94 for total (from 12.33 to 37). The mean values of BDI and SAS scores were 1.25 ± 0.24 and 41.66 ± 0.52, respectively.

3.2 Correlation analysis of CSF FGF23 with other variables

To explore the role of CSF FGF23 in impulsiveness and depression status, partial correlation was used to analyze the association between CSF FGF23 and scores of BIS, BDI and SAS with age and education years as covariates. Significant correlations were found between CSF FGF23 levels and BIS non-planning scores ($r = -0.243$, $P = 0.022$ and effect size = -0.248), BIS Cognition scores ($r = -0.283$, $P = 0.006\ 9$ and effect size = -0.291) and BIS Total scores ($r = -0.240$, $P = 0.025$ and effect size = -0.245) (Table 1 and Fig. 1). After Bonferroni correction, only BIS cognition scores remained significance ($P < 0.0073$), and no other scores showed significant correlations ($P > 0.0073$). We observed no significant correlations of CSF FGF23 levels with SAS or BDI (*P* > 0.05).

Table 1. Basic characteristics of all subjects and correlations between CSF FGF23 levels and other variables (*n* = 96)

Variables	All subjects (*n* = 96) Mean ± SD	CSF FGF23		Effect size
		r	*P*	
CSF FGF23 (pg/ml)	35.68 ± 21.21	–	–	–
Age (years)	30.29 ± 9.63	–	–	–
Education years (years)	12.75 ± 2.61	–	–	–
Pain level	1.47 ± 0.78	0.093	0.385	–
BIS nonplanning	25.53 ± 5.33	−0.243	0.022	−0.248
BIS action	27.40 ± 7.76	−0.108	0.318	–
BIS cognition	24.95 ± 4.69	−0.283	0.0069*	−0.291
BIS total	26.04 ± 4.94	−0.240	0.025	−0.245
SAS	41.66 ± 0.52	−0.005	0.965	–
BDI	1.25 ± 0.24	−0.002	0.982	–

The data are expressed as mean ± standard deviation. Partial correlation with age and education years as covariates between CSF FGF23 levels and continuous variables were performed, *P < 0.0073.

4. Discussion

We measured FGF23 in human CSF and observed correlations between CSF FGF23 concentrations and BIS non-

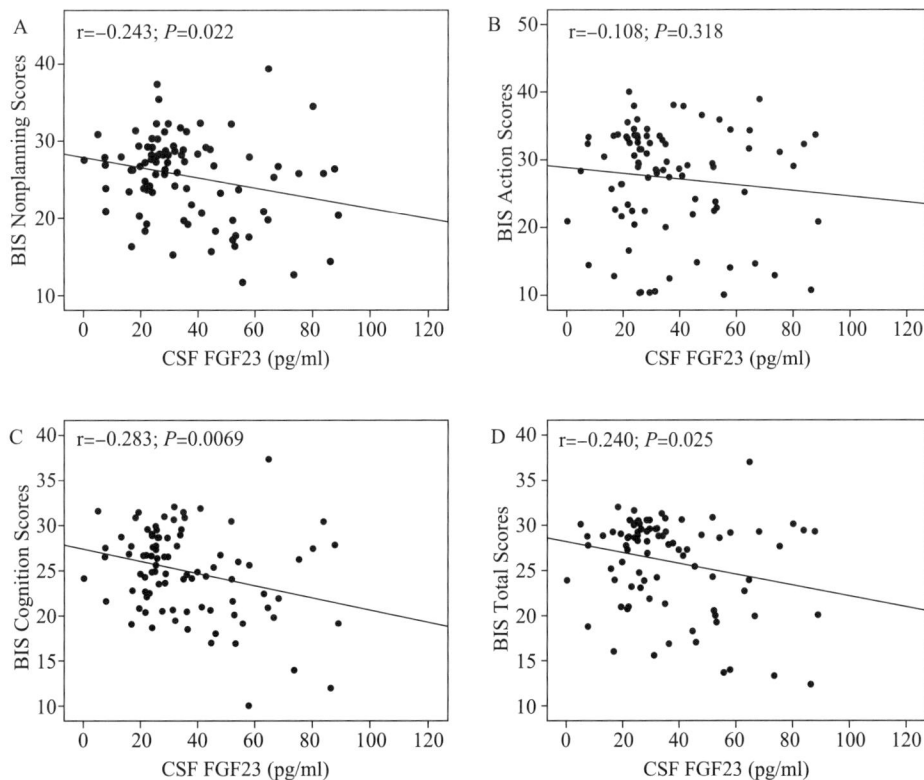

Fig. 1. (A) Correlation between CSF FGF23 levels and BIS Nonplanning scores. (B) Correlation between CSF FGF23 levels and BIS Action scores. (C) Correlation between CSF FGF23 levels and BIS Cognition scores. (D) Correlation between CSF FGF23 levels and BIS Total scores. Partial correlation between CSF FGF23 levels and continuous variables were performed with age and education years as covariates.

planning, BIS cognition and BIS total scores. Correlation analysis showed that CSF FGF23 concentrations negatively correlated with BIS non-planning, BIS cognition and BIS total scores. We show that CSF FGF23 negatively correlated with impulsive behavior in a group of male Chinese subjects.

FGF23 is expressed at low levels in specific parts of the brain (Guo and Yuan, 2015). In the present study, we demonstrated the presence of FGF23 in human CSF. Previous studies have identified FGF21, another endocrine FGF family member, in human CSF (Tan et al., 2011). FGF21 has been shown to have a robust neuroprotective role, and is a key mediator of the effects of mood stabilizers (Leng et al., 2015). Another study showed that lithium treatment results in a significant increase of serum FGF23 concentration in depressive patients (Fakhri et al., 2014). One recent study found no evidence that higher blood FGF23 (FGF23 > 100 RU/ml) was associated with the development of cognitive impairment after accounting for potential confounders (Panwar et al., 2016). This is in agreement with a recent study in individuals with advanced chronic kidney disease, that showed no association of FGF23 with cognitive decline (Jovanovich et al., 2014). However, one animal study showed impaired spatial learning and memory in transgenic mice overexpressing human FGF23. In addition, these mice exhibited impairment of long-term potentiation in hippocampal CA1 region, reduction of hippocampal ATP content, and reduction of choline acetyltransferase-positive neurons in basal forebrain. The authors suggest these are possibly pathogenic factors for the observed cognitive deficits. The central nervous phenotypes of transgenic mice were rescued after correcting hypophosphatemia by the high-phosphate diet intake (Liu et al., 2011). The present study showed that central FGF23 correlated with impulsive behavior in human, which differed from previous study focusing on the relationship between peripheral FGF23 and cognition function.

Recent studies linked metallic ions to regulation of the central nervous system. Magnesium deficiency was found to be related to depression (Rao et al., 2008) or suicide (Banki et al., 1986). Major depression was accompanied by biochemical and immune changes including iron metabolism (Maes et al., 1996). Calcium has been considered to play a role in the etiology of anxiety disorders (Balon and Ramesh, 1996). In fact, blocking calcium channels inhibits aggressive behavior in mice (Kavaliers, 1987). Studies have identified relationships between FGF23 in peripheral blood and various metallic ion deficiencies, including low serum iron associated with elevated FGF23 (Imel et al., 2011), high serum FGF23 levels induced by magnesium deficiency (Matsuzaki et al., 2016), as well as calcium (Andrukhova et al., 2014). Thus, we speculate that the correlation of CSF FGF23 with impulsive behavior might be mediated by metallic ions. In addition, no significant correlation between FGF23 and BDI scores was found, which may be due to the restricted range of BDI scores (<12) located in the relatively healthy range.

Several limitations deserve mention. First, subjects were all male. Analysis of female correlations would be needed to confirm our results. Second, we did not measure serum FGF23 levels. Many pathophysiological factors have been shown to affect serum FGF23, thus FGF23 levels may be regulated by both pathophysiological and neuropsychological factors. In future studies, all these factors should be considered. Taken together, our findings provide evidence of the presence of FGF23 in human CSF, and a correlation of CSF FGF23 levels with impulsive behavior in humans. We propose that CSF FGF23 correlates with a measure of impulsivity. We need further investigations of the potential causative relations between central nervous system FGF23 and mood disorders.

Supplementary materials

Supplementary material associated with this article can be found, in the online version, at doi:10.1016/j.psychres.2018.04.032.

Reference

[1] Andrukhova O, Smorodchenko A, Egerbacher M, et al. FGF23 promotes renal calcium reabsorption through the TRPV5 channel[J]. Embo Journal, 2014, 33(3): 229-246.

[2] Balon R, Ramesh C. Calcium channel blockers for anxiety disorders?[J]. Annals of clinical psychiatry : official journal of the American Academy of Clinical Psychiatrists, 1996, 8(4): 215-220.

[3] Banki CM, Arato M, Kilts CD. Aminergic studies and cerebrospinal fluid cations in suicide[J]. Annals of the New York Academy of Sciences, 1986, 487: 221-230.

[4] Blau JE, Collins MT. The PTH-Vitamin D-FGF23 axis[J]. Reviews in Endocrine & Metabolic Disorders, 2015, 16(2): 165-174.

[5] Corruble E, Benyamina A, Bayle F, et al. Understanding impulsivity

in severe depression? A psychometrical contribution[J]. Progress in Neuro-Psychopharmacology & Biological Psychiatry, 2003, 27(5): 829-833.

[6] Ding H-Y, Ma H-X. Significant roles of anti-aging protein klotho and fibroblast growth factor23 in cardiovascular disease[J]. Journal of Geriatric Cardiology, 2015, 12(4): 439-447.

[7] Erben RG, Andrukhova O. FGF23 regulation of renal tubular solute transport[J]. Current Opinion in Nephrology and Hypertension, 2015, 24(5): 450-456.

[8] Evans SJ, Choudary PV, Neal CR, et al. Dysregulation of the fibroblast growth factor system in major depression[J]. Proceedings of the National Academy of Sciences of the United States of America, 2004, 101(43): 15506-15511.

[9] Fakhri H, Ricken R, Adli M, et al. Impact of Lithium Treatment on FGF-23 Serum Concentrations in Depressive Patients[J]. Journal of Clinical Psychopharmacology, 2014, 34(6): 745-747.

[10] Garlow SJ, Rosenberg J, Moore JD, et al. Depression, desperation, and suicidal ideation in college students: Results from the American Foundation for Suicide Prevention College Screening Project at Emory University[J]. Depression and Anxiety, 2008, 25(6): 482-488.

[11] Guo Y-C, Yuan Q. Fibroblast growth factor 23 and bone mineralisation [J]. International Journal of Oral Science, 2015, 7(1): 8-13.

[12] Hammen C. Stress and depression[A]. In: *Annual Review of Clinical Psychology*, Vol. 1, 2005: 293-319.

[13] Imel EA, Peacock M, Gray AK, et al. Iron Modifies Plasma FGF23 Differently in Autosomal Dominant Hypophosphatemic Rickets and Healthy Humans[J]. Journal of Clinical Endocrinology & Metabolism, 2011, 96(11): 3541-3549.

[14] Jovanovich AJ, Chonchol M, Brady CB, et al. 25-vitamin D, 1,25-vitamin D, parathyroid hormone, fibroblast growth factor-23 and cognitive function in men with advanced CKD: a veteran population[J]. Clinical Nephrology, 2014, 82(5): S1-S4.

[15] Kavaliers M. Aggression and defeat-induced opioid analgesia displayed by miceare modified by calcium channel antagonists and agonists [J]. Neuroscience Letters, 1987, 74(1): 107-111.

[16] Leng Y, Wang Z, Tsai LK, et al. FGF-21, a novel metabolic regulator, has a robust neuroprotective role and is markedly elevated in neurons by mood stabilizers[J]. Molecular Psychiatry, 2015, 20(2):

215-223.

[17] Liu P, Chen L, Bai X, et al. Impairment of spatial learning and memory in transgenic mice overexpressing human fibroblast growth factor-23[J]. Brain Research, 2011, 1412: 9-17.

[18] Maes M, VandeVyvere J, Vandoolaeghe E, et al. Alterations in iron metabolism and the erythron in major depression: Further evidence for a chronic inflammatory process[J]. Journal of Affective Disorders, 1996, 40(1-2): 23-33.

[19] Matsuzaki H, Katsumata S, Maeda Y, et al. Changes in circulating levels of fibroblast growth factor 23 induced by short-term dietary magnesium deficiency in rats[J]. Magnesium Research, 2016, 29(2): 48-54.

[20] Panwar B, Judd SE, Howard VJ, et al. Vitamin D, Fibroblast Growth Factor 23 and Incident Cognitive Impairment: Findings from the REGARDS Study[J]. Plos One, 2016, 11(11).

[21] Rao TSS, Asha MR, Ramesh BN, et al. Understanding nutrition, depression and mental illnesses[J]. Indian journal of psychiatry, 2008, 50(2): 77-82.

[22] Tan BK, Hallschmid M, Adya R, et al. Fibroblast Growth Factor 21 (FGF21) in Human Cerebrospinal Fluid Relationship With Plasma FGF21 and Body Adiposity[J]. Diabetes, 2011, 60(11): 2758-2762.

[23] Tillfors M, Van Zalk N, Kerr M. Investigating a socially anxious-impulsive subgroup of adolescents: A prospective community study[J]. Scandinavian Journal of Psychology, 2013, 54(3): 267-273.

[24] Turner CA, Akil H, Watson SJ, et al. The fibroblast growth factor system and mood disorders[J]. Biological Psychiatry, 2006, 59(12): 1128-1135.

[25] Yamamoto H, Ramos-Molina B, Lick AN, et al. Posttranslational processing of FGF23 in osteocytes during the osteoblast to osteocyte transition[J]. Bone, 2016, 84: 120-130.

[26] Yao S, Yang H, Zhu X, et al. An examination of the psychometric properties of the chinese version of the Barratt Impulsiveness Scale, 11th version in a sample of chinese adolescents[J]. Perceptual and Motor Skills, 2007, 104(3): 1169-1182.

[27] Zhang X, Bao L, Yang L, et al. Roles of intracellular fibroblast growth factors in neural development and functions[J]. Science China-Life Sciences, 2012, 55(12): 1038-1044.

bFGF protects against oxygen glucose deprivation/reoxygenation-induced endothelial monolayer permeability *via* S1PR1-dependent mechanisms

Li Lin, Xiaokun Li, Zhanyang Yu

1. Introduction

Blood-brain barrier (BBB) is a highly selective permeability barrier that separates blood circulation from the brain tissue. BBB is mainly composed of endothelial cells that are connected by tight junction proteins including ZO-1, occludin, and claudin-5 and also adherent junction proteins such as VE-cadherin [1, 2]. Other components of BBB include pericytes and astrocytes. BBB plays a critical role in maintaining brain function by protecting brain tissue from neurotoxins and pathogens in the circulation, in the meantime allowing the passage of small molecules such as water, gas, glucose and amino acids that are crucial for neuronal function [3]. Compelling experimental and clinical evidence has demonstrated that BBB disruption is a critical pathophysiological feature of neurological disorders including stroke and brain trauma [4-6]. BBB dysfunction can persist for a few days through the acute and subacute phase of stroke [4], marked by increased permeability and decreased gene expression of junction proteins [7], and significantly contributes to the severe clinical consequences of stroke such as hemorrhagic transformation (HT), referring to the hemorrhage development within ischemic brain tissue, and motor and cognitive function deficits [3, 8, 9]. It is therefore of tremendous importance to elucidate the mechanisms of BBB disruption after stroke, which will benefit the development of therapeutics targeting BBB protection.

Basic fibroblast growth factor (bFGF), also known as FGF2, is a single-chain polypeptide composed of 146 amino acids and a member of the fibroblast growth factor (FGF) superfamily. Numerous studies have demonstrated that bFGF is a multifunctional growth factor involved in the regulation of neuron survival, neurite growth [10], and angiogenesis [11]. The biological activities of bFGF are mediated through its high-affinity binding to its cell surface receptor, FGF receptor 1 (FGFR1) [12]. In addition, the function of bFGF is also modulated by its binding to heparin and cell surface heparan sulfate proteoglycan [13]. Preclinical studies have shown that administration of exogenous bFGF within hours of stroke onset reduces infarct size and promotes the recovery of sensory motor functions [14] potentially by promoting axon spouting and new synapse formation [15]. In the context of BBB, we recently have demonstrated that exogenous recombinant bFGF administration protects against BBB disruption caused by traumatic brain injury (TBI) in mice [16], and the mechanisms may involve regulation of junction protein expressions, and partially through PI3K-Akt-Rac1 pathway, as blocking this pathway partially blocked the BBB protection effect of bFGF, suggesting that multiple signaling pathways may be involved in this protection effect. Sphingosine-1-phosphate (S1P) signaling pathway plays important roles in vascular system, as experimental evidence has demonstrated that S1P receptor (S1PR1) protects the integrity of BBB against various injuries [17, 18]. In this study, we aimed to further investigate the additional mechanisms, including bFGF receptor and S1PR1, of BBB protection by exogenous bFGF in neurological disorders by testing the permeability of an *in vitro*-cultured primary human brain microvascular endothelial cell (HBMEC) monolayer exposed to oxygen-glucose deprivation and reoxygenation (OGD/R).

2. Material and methods

2.1　Reagents and antibodies

Primary HBMEC was obtained from Cell Systems Corporation (ACBRI376, Kirkland, WA). Recombinant human bFGF was purchased from Sigma (Sigma-Aldrich, St. Louis, MO). Anti-FGFR1 (mouse), anti-pFGFR1 (rabbit), anti-claudin-5 (rabbit), anti-VE-cadherin (rabbit), and anti-S1PR1 (rabbit) antibodies were purchased from Abcam (Cambridge, MA); anti-occludin (rabbit) and anti-ZO-1(mouse) antibodies were purchased from Invitrogen (Carlsbad, CA). S1PR1 inhibitor VPC23019 was purchased from Cayman Chemical (Ann Arbor, MI). S1PR1 activator FTY720 was purchased from Sigma (St. Louis, MO).

2.2　Endothelial monolayer permeability assay

Primary HBMEC was cultured in complete growth media EBM-2 (Lonza, Walkersville, MD). The cells were seeded on the inner surface of collagen-coated Transwell inserts (6.5-mm diameter, 0.4-µm pore size polycarbonate filter; Corning, Corning, NY), which were placed in wells of a 24-well plate with complete EBM-2 media. When the monolayer of cells was confluent, confirmed by ensuring that it is impermeable to media, the cells were serum starved for 8 h with EBM media without growth supplement before OGD/R treatment. Normal control group is the monolayer culture without OGD/R treatment. For OGD/R treatment, EBM-2 media were replaced with DMEM without glucose, and the cells were then put in a specialized, humidified chamber (Heidolph, incubator 1 000, Brinkmann Instruments, Westbury, NY) at 37℃, which contained an anaerobic gas mixture (90% N_2, 5% H_2, and 5% CO_2). After 4-h incubation, the cultures were removed from the anaerobic chamber, and the OGD medium was replaced with EBM-2 complete medium without bFGF. The cells were then allowed to recover in a regular incubator for 20 h (reoxygenation) before permeability measurement. For the bFGF-treated group, recombinant bFGF was added to the medium (final concentration 2.5 µM) during OGD/R. After 20-h reoxygenation, media in both upper and lower chambers were removed and replaced with fresh media without supplement. Permeability was measured by adding 0.1 mg/ml of fluorescein isothiocyanate (FITC)-labeled dextran (MW, 70 000; Sigma, St. Louis, MO) to the upper chamber, with lower compartment containing fresh serum-free media. After incubation for 20 min, 100 µl of sample from the lower compartment was measured for fluorescence at excitation 490 nm and emission 520 nm. All independent experiments were performed in duplicate or triplicate.

2.3　Trans-endothelial electrical resistance

Trans-endothelial electrical resistance (TEER) of cultured HBMEC monolayer was measured using an EndOhm-6 chamber and an EVOM resistance meter (World Precision Instruments, Sarasota, FL) following the manufacturer's instructions. Briefly, the 6 mm Transwell containing cultured endothelial cell monolayer was transferred into the EndOhm-6 chamber containing 0.1 M KCl. The culture media within the Transwell were also replaced with 0.1 M KCl. EndOhm cap was then inserted on the top of the chamber and Transwell and then connected with the chamber using a connector cable, and resistance was then measured using the EVOM resistance meter. A blank Transwell containing 0.1 M KCl but without any cells was used as blank control.

2.4　Cell viability assay

The viability of cultured endothelial cells was assessed by WST assay. Briefly, HBMEC cells were cultured in a 24-well plate in complete EBM-2 medium. After treatment, WST-1 reagent (50 µl) was added to each well (containing 450-µl medium) and the cells were incubated for 2 h at 37℃. The absorbency at 450 nm was measured against a background blank control using a microplate reader (SpectraMax M5, Molecular Devices) according to the manufacturer's protocol.

2.5　Western blot

Western blot was performed following our previously published protocol [22]. Briefly, total protein was isolated from cultured endothelial cells using lysis buffer (Cell Signaling, Danvers, MA). Membrane protein was isolated using the Mem-PER™ Plus Membrane Protein Extraction Kit (Thermo Fisher Scientific, Waltham, MA) following the manufacturer's instructions. The proteins were separated on 4%–20% Tris-glycine gel, followed by blotting to nitrocellulose membrane. The membrane was then incubated with primary anti-FGFR1 (1:200, Santa Cruz), anti-pFGFR1 (1:200, Santa Cruz), anti-claudin-5 (1:1 000, Invitrogen), anti-occludin (1:1 000, Santa Cruz), anti-ZO-1 (1:1 000, Abcam), anti-VE-cadherin (1:1 000, Abcam), and anti-S1PR1 (1:1 000, Abcam) antibodies. After being washed with TBST (250 mM Tris, 27 mM KCl, and 1.37 M NaCl, pH 7.4, 0.1% Tween 20), the membrane was incubated with corresponding horseradish peroxidase-conjugated secondary antibodies and washed with TBST, and immunolabeling was detected by enhanced chemiluminescence (ECL; GE Healthcare) according to the manufacturer's instruction. Optical density of protein bands was quantified with ImageJ.

2.6 Immunocytochemistry

Cultured neurons were washed with cold PBS (pH 7.4) and fixed with 4% paraformaldehyde for 30 min. The cells were then washed with PBS containing 0.1% Tween and further incubated with 5% FBS for 1 h. Next, the cells were incubated with primary antibodies against VE-cadherin (rabbit monoclonal; 1:200; Abcam) and S1PR1 (rabbit polyclonal; 1:200; Abcam) at 4℃ overnight. After PBS washing, the cells were incubated with goat anti rabbit IgG conjugated with FITC (1:150; Jackson ImmunoResearch), respectively, for 1 h at room temperature. Vectashield mounting medium containing DAPI (for nucleic staining) (Vector Laboratory, Burlingame, CA) was used to coverslip the immunocytochemic slides. Immunostaining was analyzed using a fluorescence microscope (Olympus BX51).

2.7 Real-time PCR

Quantitative real-time PCR (RT-PCR) was used to measure S1PR1 messenger RNA (mRNA) levels in cultured HBMEC following the standard protocols. Briefly, total RNA was extracted using miRNeasy kit (Qiagen) following the manufacturer's instructions and quantified spectrophotometrically at 260 nm using a NanoDrop 2000C spectrophotomer (Thermo Scientific); the purity of RNAs was assessed by the ratio of the absorbance at 260 and 280 nm (A260/280) >1.80. One hundred nanograms of total RNAs was reverse transcribed into complementary DNA (cDNA) using random primers and M-MLV reverse transcriptase (Invitrogen) according to the manufacturer's instructions. S1PR1 mRNA levels were tested using specific S1PR1 primer and TaqMan Gene Expression Assays in triplicates (ABI 7500HT, Applied Biosystems). Each reaction was performed with 50 ng of cDNA. B2M was used as an internal control housing keeping gene. Changes in gene expression (fold change) were determined using the $2^{-\Delta\Delta Ct}$ method with normalization to B2M.

2.8 Small interfering RNA-mediated gene silencing

S1PR1 small interfering RNA (siRNA) and control siRNA were obtained from Santa Cruz Biotechnology. siRNA transfection was conducted following the manufacturer's instruction. Briefly, HBMEC was cultured on six-well plates or Transwell for 2 days. siRNA duplex and siRNA Transfection Reagent (Santa Cruz) were separately diluted with Transfection Medium (Santa Cruz) and then mixed together and incubated at room temperature for 40 min. The cells were washed once with siRNA Transfection Medium and then incubated with mixed siRNA and siRNA Transfection Reagent for 5 h at 37℃. The cells on six-well plates were collected for Western blot to detect S1PR1 protein level, and cells in Transwell underwent OGD/R treatment and tested for permeability.

2.9 Statistical analysis

Results were expressed as mean ± SEM. The number of samples was six per group for endothelial monolayer permeability assays and four for western blot experiments. Multiple comparisons were evaluated by one-way ANOVA followed by Tukey-Kramer's tests between all groups. $P < 0.05$ was considered statistically significant.

3. Results

3.1 Recombinant basic fibroblast growth factor reduces oxygen-glucose deprivation and reoxygenation-induced endothelial monolayer permeability through upregulating FGF receptor 1 activity

To examine the effect of recombinant bFGF treatment on OGD/R-induced endothelial monolayer permeability, cultured HBMEC monolayer in Transwells was subjected to 4-h OGD followed by 24-h reoxygenation. Recombinant bFGF (2.5 μM) was used to treat the cells during OGD/R, and then, the permeability of FITC-dextran (70 kDa) was measured.

Our results show that OGD/R significantly increased HBMEC monolayer permeability (2.8 ± 0.25-fold of normal control), while treatment with recombinant bFGF significantly reduced the permeability compared to OGD/R (1.6 ± 0.24-fold of normal control), indicating the protective effect of bFGF on OGD/R-induced endothelial monolayer permeability (Fig. 1A).

To further validate the effect of recombinant bFGF on endothelial monolayer integrity, we tested the TEER using the EndOhm chamber and EVOM resistance meter. We show that OGD/R significantly deceased the TEER of cultured HBMEC monolayer compared to normal control (0.39 ± 0.07-fold of normal control), whereas bFGF treatment significantly rescued the TEER compared to GOD/R condition (0.83 ± 0.09-fold of normal control) (Fig. 1B), further proving the protective effect of bFGF on endothelial monolayer integrity.

Since bFGF normally functions through its receptor FGFR1, we tested the effect of bFGF treatment on FGFR1 activation by measuring the phosphorylation of FGFR1. Cultured HBMEC was subjected to 4-h OGD followed by 4-h reoxygenation, and then, the protein levels of FGFR1 and phosphorylated FGFR1 (p-FGFR1) were examined by Western blot. The results show that total FGFR1 protein level was not changed by OGD/R or OGD/R plus bFGF, whereas the level of p-FGFR1 was significantly decreased by OGD/R, and this decrease was significantly rescued by bFGF treatment (Fig. 1C, D), suggesting that bFGF may function through promoting FGFR1 activation in endothelial monolayer after OGD/R injury.

To test whether FGFR1 activation is involved in the protective effect of bFGF for endothelial monolayer integrity,

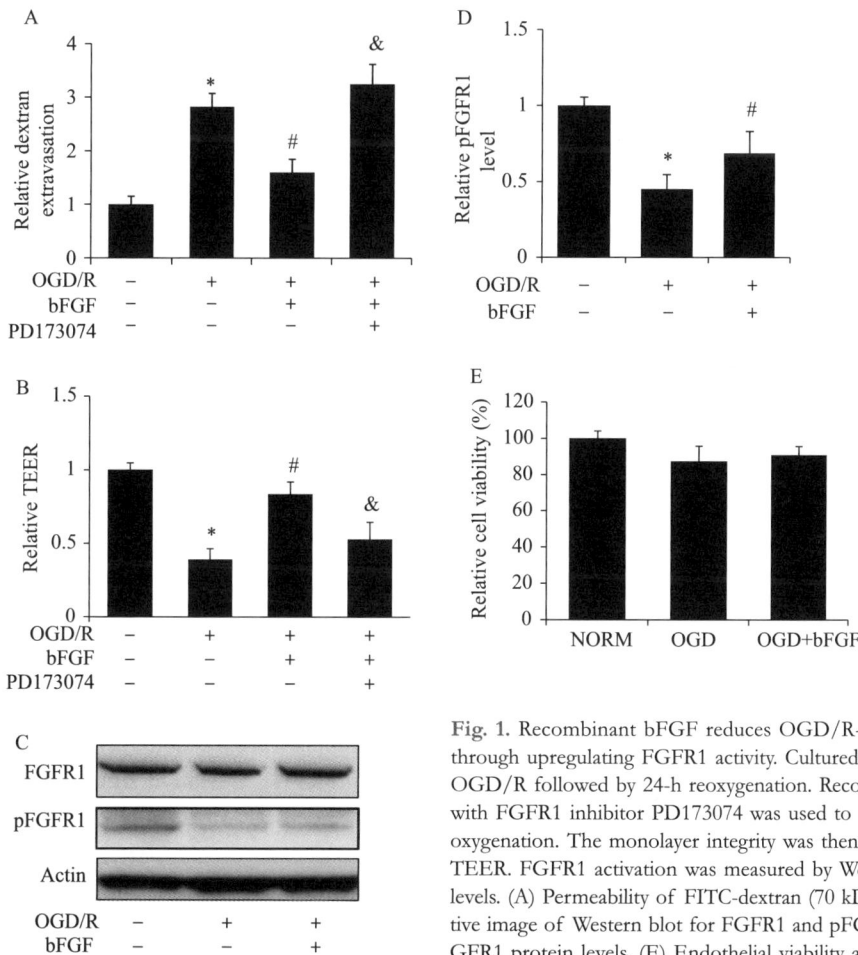

Fig. 1. Recombinant bFGF reduces OGD/R-induced endothelial monolayer permeability through upregulating FGFR1 activity. Cultured HBMEC in Transwells was subjected to 4-h OGD/R followed by 24-h reoxygenation. Recombinant bFGF (2.5 μM) or bFGF combined with FGFR1 inhibitor PD173074 was used to treat endothelial monolayer during OGD/reoxygenation. The monolayer integrity was then measured by FITC-dextran permeability and TEER. FGFR1 activation was measured by Western blot for FGFR1 and pFGFR1 protein levels. (A) Permeability of FITC-dextran (70 kDa). (B) TEER measurement. (C) Representative image of Western blot for FGFR1 and pFGFR1. (D) Quantification of FGFR1 and pF-GFR1 protein levels. (E) Endothelial viability after OGD/R and bFGF treatment measured by WTS assay ($n = 6$, *$P < 0.05$ vs. normal control, #$P < 0.05$ vs. OGD/R group, &$P < 0.05$ vs. OGD/R + bFGF group).

we treated the cultured HBMEC monolayer with bFGF combined with a specific FGFR1 inhibitor, PD173074 (50 nM), and then measured and compared the permeability and TEER with bFGF treatment alone. Our results show that PD173074 blocked the protective effect of bFGF on endothelial monolayer integrity, as the permeability of bFGF and PD173074 cotreated group is significantly higher than bFGF-treated group (Fig. 1A). Furthermore, the TEER of bFGF and PD173074 co-treated group is significantly decreased compared to bFGF-alone-treated group (Fig. 1B). These results suggest that the protective effect of bFGF on endothelial monolayer integrity is mediated by FGFR1 activation.

To test whether the protective effect of bFGF on endothelial monolayer integrity is simply due to protection against OGD/ R-induced cytotoxicity, we further assessed the effect of bFGF treatment on the viability of cultured HBMEC. HBMEC was subjected to 4-h OGD followed by 20-h reoxygenation. Recombinant bFGF (2.5 μM) was used to treat endothelial cells during OGD/R. Cell viability was assessed using WST assay normalized by cell number counting. Our results show that OGD/R did not significantly change the viability of endothelial cells, and bFGF did not significantly change the cell viability either (Fig. 1E), suggesting that the protective effect of bFGF against OGD/R-induced endothelial monolayer permeability is not through increasing cell viability.

3.2 Recombinant basic fibroblast growth factor rescues oxygen-glucose deprivation and reoxygenation-induced downregulation of endothelial junction proteins

Since endothelial tight junction and adherent junction proteins are important regulators of endothelial paracellular permeability, we next examined the effect of bFGF treatment on endothelial junction protein expression after OGD/ R. After 4-h OGD followed by 20-h reoxygenation, total protein levels of tight junction proteins claudin-5, occludin, and ZO-1 and adherent junction protein VE-cadherin were examined by Western blot. Our results show that OGD/R significantly reduced the protein levels of occludin, ZO-1, and VE-cadherin. Recombinant bFGF treatment significantly rescued the expression of these proteins (Fig. 2A–D). Claudin-5 protein level was not significantly changed by either OGD/R or bFGF.

Since adjacent endothelial cells are mainly connected by membrane-localized junction proteins, we further tested the membrane localization of these junction proteins in cultured HBMEC after 4-h OGD and 20-h reoxygenation. Membrane protein was isolated from HBMEC and then subjected to Western blot. NaK-ATPase was used as a membrane internal marker. Our results show that OGD/R significantly reduced the protein levels of occludin, ZO-1, and VE-cadherin in the membrane, while bFGF21 treatment significantly rescued these protein levels (Fig. 2E–H). Claudin-5 protein level in the membrane was not significantly changed by either OGD/R or bFGF. These results suggest that bFGF may protect against OGD/R-induced BBB disruption through rescuing the junction protein expression and localization on cell membrane.

We further performed immunocytochemistry to test the membrane localization of VE-cadherin in HBMEC after 4-h OGD and 20-h reoxygenation. Our results show that VE-cadherin is predominantly localized on endothelial membrane. OGD/R significantly decreased the membrane localization of VE-cadherin, while bFGF treatment significantly rescued the membrane localization of VE-cadherin. Furthermore, the FGFR1 inhibitor PD173074 (50 nM) significantly blocked the effect of bFGF on recovering membrane localization of VE-cadherin (Fig. 2I), indicating that this effect is mediated by FGFR1 activation.

3.3 Recombinant basic fibroblast growth factor rescues oxygen-glucose deprivation and reoxygenation-induced downregulation of sphingosine-1-phosphate receptor 1 protein expression via FGF receptor 1 activation

S1PR1 has been reported to regulate the expression of endothelial junction proteins [19]. We then tested whether bFGF treatment can change the S1PR1 protein expression. HBMEC was subjected to 4-h OGD followed by 4-h reoxygenation, and bFGF was added during OGD and reoxygenation. Total S1PR1 protein levels were measured by Western blot. Our results show that OGD/R significantly reduced S1PR1 protein levels, while bFGF treatment significantly rescued S1PR1 protein expression (Fig. 3A, B). Furthermore, the specific FGFR1 inhibitor PD173074 (50 nM) significantly blocked the upregulation effect of bFGF on S1PR1 protein expression (Fig. 3A, B).

Moreover, we performed immunocytochemistry to examine S1PR1 protein expression in HBMEC after OGD/R and bFGF treatment. We show that OGD/R significantly reduced S1PR1 protein expression in HBMEC compared to normal condition, while bFGF treatment significantly rescued S1PR1 protein expression. Additionally, PD173074 significantly blocked the effect of bFGF in rescuing S1PR1 protein expression (Fig. 3C). These results suggest that bFGF

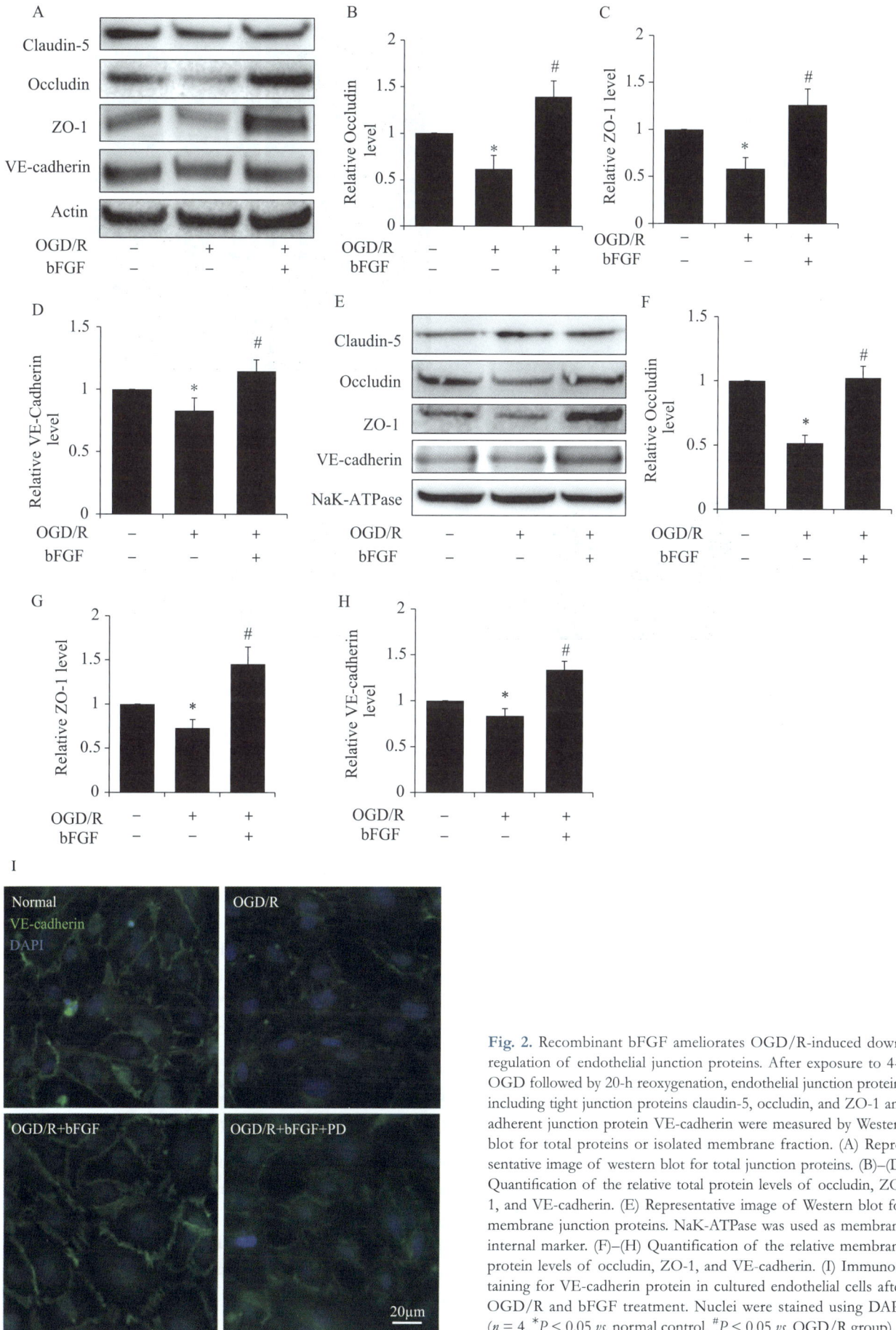

Fig. 2. Recombinant bFGF ameliorates OGD/R-induced down-regulation of endothelial junction proteins. After exposure to 4-h OGD followed by 20-h reoxygenation, endothelial junction proteins including tight junction proteins claudin-5, occludin, and ZO-1 and adherent junction protein VE-cadherin were measured by Western blot for total proteins or isolated membrane fraction. (A) Representative image of western blot for total junction proteins. (B)–(D) Quantification of the relative total protein levels of occludin, ZO-1, and VE-cadherin. (E) Representative image of Western blot for membrane junction proteins. NaK-ATPase was used as membrane internal marker. (F)–(H) Quantification of the relative membrane protein levels of occludin, ZO-1, and VE-cadherin. (I) Immunostaining for VE-cadherin protein in cultured endothelial cells after OGD/R and bFGF treatment. Nuclei were stained using DAPI ($n = 4$, $^{*}P < 0.05$ vs. normal control, $^{#}P < 0.05$ vs. OGD/R group).

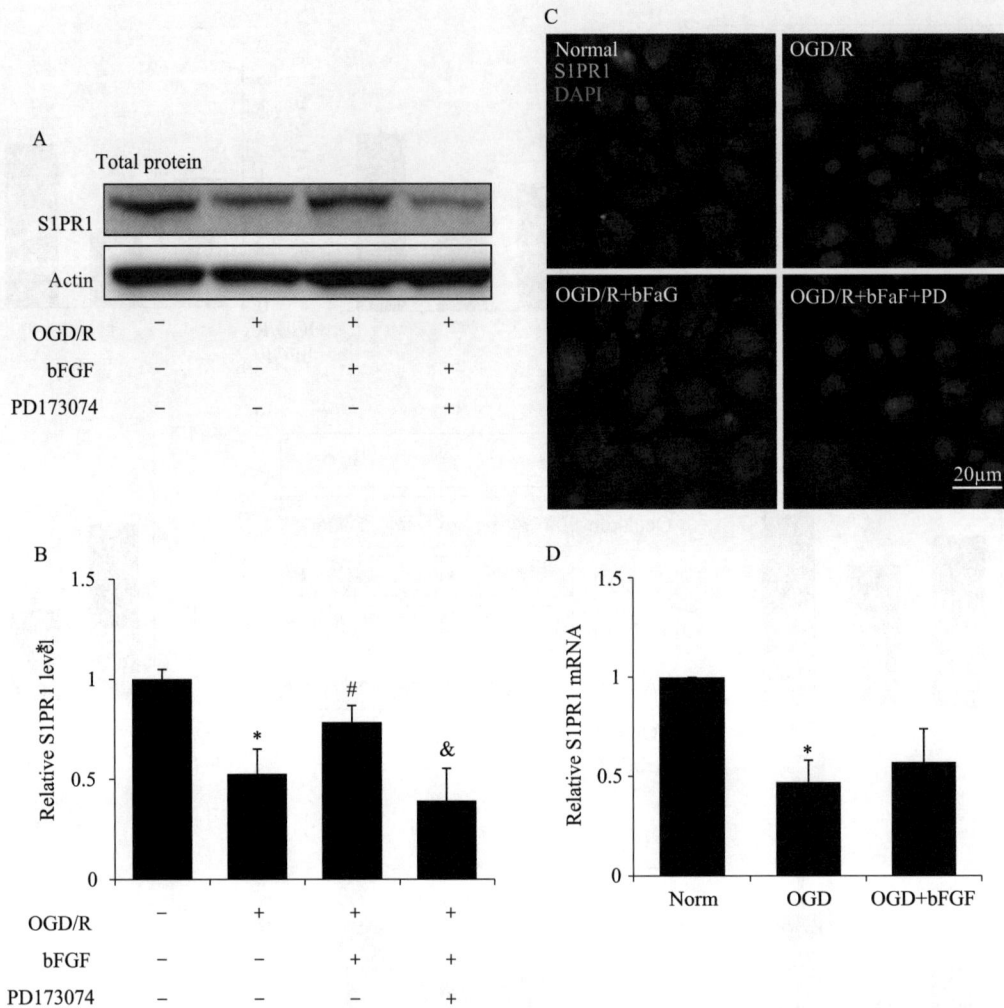

Fig. 3. Recombinant bFGF rescues OGD/R-induced S1PR1 downregulation *via* FGFR1 activation. HBMEC was subjected to 4-h OGD followed by 4-h reoxygenation; bFGF or bFGF combined with PD173074 was treated during OGD/R. The intracellular protein levels of S1PR1 were measured by Western blot, immunocytochemistry, and RT-PCR. (A) Representative image of Western blot for S1PR1. (B) Quantification of S1PR1 protein levels. (C) Immnocytochemistry for measurement of S1PR1 protein. Nuclei were stained using DAPI. (D) RT-PCR to measure the gene transcription of S1PR1. ($n = 4$, [*]$P < 0.05$ *vs.* normal control, [#]$P < 0.05$ *vs.* OGD/R group, [&]$P < 0.05$ *vs.* OGD/R + bFGF group).

can rescue OGD/R-induced S1PR1 downregulation, *via* FGFR1 activation.

We further examined the mRNA expression of S1PR1 gene by RT-PCR in cultured HBMEC after 4-h OGD followed by 4-h reoxygenation, with or without bFGF treatment. Our results show that OGD/R significantly decreased S1PR1 mRNA levels, but bFGF treatment only slightly increased (no significance) S1PR1 mRNA compared to the OGD/R group (Fig. 3D). These data suggest that bFGF may rescue S1PR1 protein expression mainly through increasing protein translation, but not gene transcription.

3.4 *The protective effect of recombinant basic fibroblast growth factor against oxygen-glucose deprivation and reoxygenation-induced endothelial monolayer permeability is dependent on Sphingosine-1-phosphate receptor 1 activation*

We next examined whether S1PR1 is required for the protective effect of bFGF on endothelial monolayer integrity. We first used a specific inhibitor of S1PR1, VPC23019 (final concentration 40 nM) [20], to treat the HBMEC monolayer in combination with bFGF, and then measured the FITC-dextran permeability and TEER. Our results show that bFGF significantly decreased OGD/R-induced HBMEC monolayer permeability, while VPC23019 significantly reversed this effect when cotreated with bFGF (Fig. 4A). Moreover, bFGF significantly rescued OGD/R-induced decrease in TEER, whereas VPC23019 also significantly blocked this effect (Fig. 4B). VPC23019 alone did not significantly change the permeability and TEER of the endothelial monolayer.

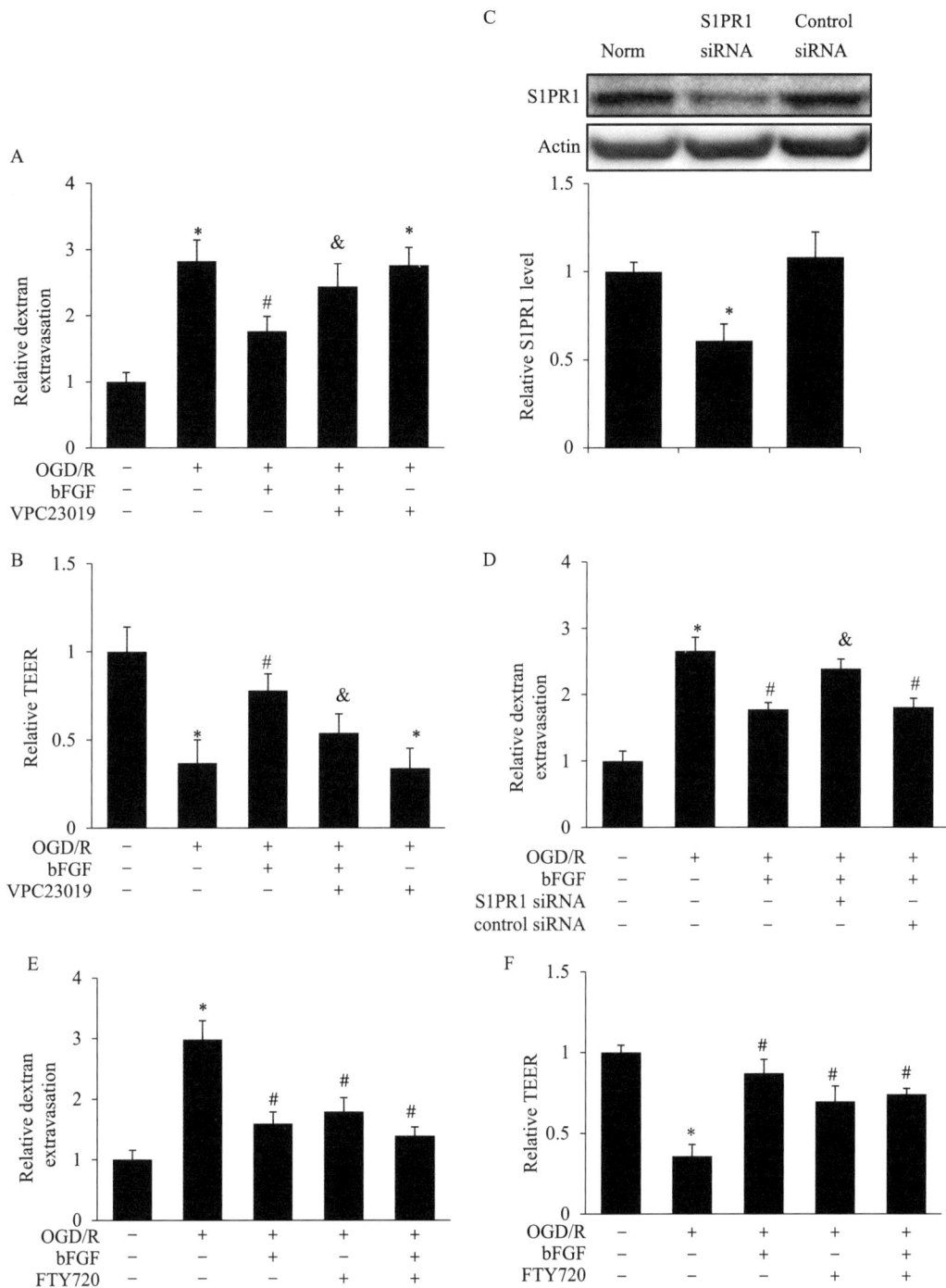

Fig. 4. The protective effect of recombinant bFGF on endothelial monolayer permeability is through S1PR1-dependent mechanisms. To examine whether S1PR1 is required for the protective effect of bFGF on endothelial monolayer integrity, we used a specific inhibitor of S1PR1, VPC23019, and also S1PR1 siRNA to treat the cultured endothelial monolayer in combination with bFGF and then measured the endothelial monolayer permeability and TEER. We also used an S1PR1 agonist, FTY720, to treat endothelial monolayer and compared its effect with bFGF. (A) Permeability of FITC-dextran in cultured HBMEC monolayers after OGD/R treated with bFGF or bFGF combined with VPC23019. (B) TEER measurement of HBMEC monolayers after OGD/R treated with bFGF or bFGF combined with VPC23019. (C) Representative Western blot image and quantification diagram showing the effect of S1PR1 siRNA in silencing S1PR1 protein expression. (D) Permeability of FITC-dextran in cultured HBMEC monolayers after OGD/R treated with bFGF or bFGF combined with S1PR1 siRNA or control siRNA. (E) Permeability of FITC-dextran in cultured HBMEC monolayers after OGD/R treated with bFGF or FTY720 or bFGF + FTY720. (F) TEER measurement of HBMEC monolayer after OGD/R treated with bFGF or FTY720 or bFGF + FTY720 ($n = 6$, $^*P < 0.05$ vs. normal control, $^\#P < 0.05$ vs. OGD/R group, $^\&P < 0.05$ vs. OGD/R + bFGF group).

There are limitations for chemical inhibitors of S1PR1 in that they might have off-target effect; we therefore further validated the involvement of S1PR1 in bFGF protection effect on endothelial monolayer integrity using siRNA-mediated gene silencing. Western blot showed that S1PR1 siRNA significantly decreased S1PR1 protein level compared to normal cells or control siRNA-transfected cells (Fig. 4C). In HBMEC monolayer permeability assay in Transwells, S1PR1 siRNA transfection significantly reversed the protection effect of bFGF on FITC-dextran extravasation, compared to control siRNA (Fig. 4D).

To further validate the roles of S1PR1 in the protective effect of bFGF on endothelial monolayer integrity, we used a widely used S1PR1 agonist FTY720 [21] (final concentration 50 nM) to treat cultured HBMEC monolayer alone or in combination with bFGF. Our results show that FTY720 alone significantly reduced OGD/R-induced HBMEC monolayer permeability, to a degree comparable to bFGF treatment, while cotreatment with bFGF and FTY720 did not further reduce the permeability (Fig. 4E). Moreover, FTY720 alone also significantly rescued OGD/R-induced decrease of TEER, to a degree comparable to bFGF treatment, and bFGF and FTY720 cotreatment did not further increase the TEER (Fig. 4F). Overall, these data suggest that the protective effect of recombinant bFGF against OGD/R-induced endothelial monolayer permeability is at least partially through S1PR1 activation.

4. Discussion

In this study, using cultured HBMEC, we demonstrated that exogenous recombinant bFGF protects against OGD/R-induced disruption of endothelial monolayer integrity. We found that (1) bFGF significantly reduced OGD/R-induced HBMEC monolayer permeability to FITC-dextran and reversed OGD/R-induced decrease of TEER, via FGFR1 activation, (2) bFGF significantly rescued OGD/R-induced downregulations of tight junction proteins occludin and ZO-1 and adherent junction protein VE-cadherin, (3) bFGF significantly recued OGD/R-induced downregulation of S1PR1 protein expression measured, and (4) the protective effect of bFGF on OGD/R-induced endothelial monolayer permeability is dependent on upregulation of S1PR1 demonstrated by both S1PR1 inhibitor and activator.

BBB damage significantly contributes to the pathophysiological progression of neurodegeneration diseases including stroke and brain trauma, thus is an important target for therapeutics development against these diseases. Our recent study has demonstrated that recombinant bFGF protects against BBB disruption caused by TBI in mice [16], potentially through regulation of junction protein expressions and partially through PI3K-Akt-Rac1 pathway. As a continuous study, here we aimed to explore the additional mechanisms of bFGF in BBB protection. We clearly validated the BBB protection effect of bFGF using OGD/R-induced endothelial monolayer permeability and revealed that this protective effect is mediated through FGFR1 activation and S1PR1 upregulation by recombinant bFGF. These findings suggest that bFGF may have BBB protection effect in a wide range of neurological disorders including stroke and brain trauma, and this protection effect may be mediated through multiple mechanisms.

bFGF plays its physiological functions through membrane-bound FGFRs, a family of tyrosine kinase receptors including FGFR1, FGFR2, FGFR3, and FGFR4. FGFR1–3 are predominantly localized in the central nervous system, whereas FGFR4 is mainly expressed in the lung and kidney [22–24]. Although bFGF can also signal through FGFR2 and FGFR3, existing studies up to date suggest that FGFR1 might be the primary mediator for bFGF signaling [25, 26]. However, there is little direct evidence proving the indispensable role of FGFR1 in bFGF signaling in the central nervous system. For example, bFGF has been demonstrated to be essential for cell proliferation and neurogenesis during cortex development, and bFGF gene regulation is synchronized with that of FGFR1, suggesting their functional correlation [27]. A very recent study showed that bFGF protects the integrity of blood-spinal cord barrier (BSCB) after contusive brain injury in the rats, and the interaction of FGFR1 with Cavolin-1 may play important roles in this process [28]. In this current study, we found that bFGF can rescue the activity of FGFR1 ameliorated by OGD/R treatment. Moreover, the specific inhibitor of FGFR1, PD173804, blocked the protective effect of bFGF in OGD/R-induced endothelial monolayer permeability. These results demonstrate the role of FGFR1 as a mediator of bFGF signaling.

Sphingosine-1-phosphate (S1P) signaling pathway, which is mediated by S1P receptors (S1PR), plays important regulatory roles in vascular system including angiogenesis, vascular stability, and permeability [17, 18]. Experimental evidence has demonstrated that S1PR1 protects the integrity of BBB against various injuries. For example, S1PR1 activation is required for the protective effect of activated protein C (APC) on endothelial barrier integrity upon systemic inflammation [29]. A recent study shows that S1PR1 is involved in the protective effect of artesunate, a traditional anti-malaria drug, on BBB integrity in subarachnoid hemorrhage in rats [20]. A more direct evidence arose from the finding that selective S1PR1 agonist protects against intracerebral hemorrhage by enhancing BBB integrity, as well as reducing brain infiltration of lymphocytes, neutrophil, and microglia [19]. Here, we found that recombinant bFGF rescues OGD/R-induced downregulation of S1PR1 protein expression, and the involvement of S1PR1 in the BBB protection effect of bFGF was further confirmed using multiple approaches including S1PR1 inhibitor, siRNA silencing, and agonist. These data strongly support the role of S1PR1 in the protection of BBB integrity. It is worth noting that this S1PR1-dependent mechanism may be just part of the mechanisms underlying the BBB protective effect of bFGF, as S1PR1 inhibitor and gene silencing did not completely abolish the BBB protection effect of bFGF in our study. Other mechanisms may also be involved in bFGF-mediated BBB protection, such as the PI3K-Akt-Rac1 pathway as we demonstrated in our recent report on TBI-induced BBB disruption [16]. These signaling molecules could serve as potential targets in developing therapeutics against BBB disruption in neurological disorders.

There are a few caveats in this study. First, we did not test the roles of other bFGF receptors, i.e., FGFR2 and FGFR3, in the BBB protection effect of bFGF. These factors may also play important roles in the pathophysiological function of bFGF, which warrants further investigation in the future. Second, this is only an *in vitro* study to prove the protective effect of bFGF on OGD/R-induced BBB damage and possible mechanisms. This effect has to be further validated in *in vivo* animal stroke models, which will be investigated in our future study.

In summary, in this study, we clearly demonstrated that exogenous recombinant bFGF treatment protected against OGD/R-induced HBMEC monolayer permeability through rescuing the expression of endothelial junction proteins, and this effect is dependent on FGFR1 activation and S1PR1 up-regulation. These findings, combined with our recent report of bFGF protection for BBB in TBI [16], provide solid evidence for the protective effect of bFGF in neurological disorders including stroke and brain trauma, which may facilitate the development of bFGF as a therapeutic agent for these neurological disorders.

References

[1] Stamatovic SM, Johnson AM, Keep RF, et al. Junctional proteins of the blood-brain barrier: New insights into function and dysfunction[J]. Tissue Barriers, 2016, 4(1).

[2] Weiss N, Miller F, Cazaubon S, et al. The blood-brain barrier in brain homeostasis and neurological diseases[J]. Biochimica Et Biophysica Acta-Biomembranes, 2009, 1788(4): 842-857.

[3] Zhao Z, Nelson AR, Betsholtz C, et al. Establishment and Dysfunction of the Blood-Brain Barrier[J]. Cell, 2015, 163(5): 1064-1078.

[4] Kassner A, Merali Z. Assessment of Blood-Brain Barrier Disruption in Stroke[J]. Stroke, 2015, 46(11): 3310-3315.

[5] Prakash R, Carmichael ST. Blood-brain barrier breakdown and neovascularization processes after stroke and traumatic brain injury[J]. Current Opinion in Neurology, 2015, 28(6): 556-564.

[6] Alluri H, Wiggins-Dohlvik K, Davis ML, et al. Blood-brain barrier dysfunction following traumatic brain injury[J]. Metabolic Brain Disease, 2015, 30(5): 1093-1104.

[7] Fernandez-Lopez D, Faustino J, Daneman R, et al. Blood-Brain Barrier Permeability Is Increased After Acute Adult Stroke But Not Neonatal Stroke in the Rat[J]. Journal of Neuroscience, 2012, 32(28): 9588-9600.

[8] Khatri R, McKinney AM, Swenson B, et al. Blood-brain barrier, reperfusion injury, and hemorrhagic transformation in acute ischemic stroke[J]. Neurology, 2012, 79(13): S52-S57.

[9] Jin R, Yang G, Li G. Molecular insights and therapeutic targets for blood-brain barrier disruption in ischemic stroke: Critical role of matrix metalloproteinases and tissue-type plasminogen activator[J]. Neurobiology of Disease, 2010, 38(3): 376-385.

[10] Abe K, Saitoh H. Effects of basic fibroblast growth factor on central nervous system functions[J]. Pharmacological Research, 2001, 43(4): 307-312.

[11] Rosen L. Antiangiogenic strategies and agents in clinical trials[J]. The oncologist, 2000, 5 Suppl 1: 20-27.

[12] Nugent MA, Iozzo RV. Fibroblast growth factor-2[J]. International Journal of Biochemistry & Cell Biology, 2000, 32(2): 115-120.

[13] Faham S, Hileman RE, Fromm JR, et al. Heparin structure and interactions with basic fibroblast growth factor[J]. Science, 1996, 271(5252): 1116-1120.

[14] Kawamata T, Alexis NE, Dietrich WD, et al. Intracisternal basic fibroblast growth factor (bFGF) enhances behavioral recovery following focal cerebral infarction in the rat[J]. Journal of Cerebral Blood Flow and Metabolism, 1996, 16(4): 542-547.

[15] Kawamata T, Dietrich WD, Schallert T, et al. Intracisternal basic fibroblast growth factor enhances functional recovery and upregulates the expression of a molecular marker of neuronal sprouting following focal cerebral infarction[J]. Proceedings of the National Academy of Sciences of the United States of America, 1997, 94(15): 8179-8184.

[16] Wang Z, Pan X, He Y, et al. Piezoelectric Nanowires in Energy Harvesting Applications[J]. Advances in Materials Science and Engineering, 2015.

[17] Ephstein Y, Singleton PA, Chen W, et al. Critical Role of S1PR1 and Integrin beta 4 in HGF/c-Met-mediated Increases in Vascular Integrity[J]. Journal of Biological Chemistry, 2013, 288(4): 2191-2200.

[18] Gaengel K, Niaudet C, Hagikura K, et al. The Sphingosine-1-Phosphate Receptor S1PR1 Restricts Sprouting Angiogenesis by Regulating the Interplay between VE-Cadherin and VEGFR2[J]. Developmental Cell, 2012, 23(3): 587-599.

[19] Sun N, Shen Y, Han W, et al. Selective Sphingosine-1-Phosphate Receptor 1 Modulation Attenuates Experimental Intracerebral

Hemorrhage[J]. Stroke, 2016, 47(7): 1899-1906.

[20] Zuo S, Ge H, Li Q, *et al.* Artesunate Protected Blood-Brain Barrier *via* Sphingosine 1 Phosphate Receptor 1/Phosphatidylinositol 3 Kinase Pathway After Subarachnoid Hemorrhage in Rats[J]. Molecular Neurobiology, 2017, 54(2): 1213-1228.

[21] Nacer A, Movila A, Baer K, *et al.* Neuroimmunological Blood Brain Barrier Opening in Experimental Cerebral Malaria[J]. Plos Pathogens, 2012, 8(10).

[22] Ford-Perriss M, Abud H, Murphy M. Fibroblast growth factors in the developing central nervous system[J]. Clinical and Experimental Pharmacology and Physiology, 2001, 28(7): 493-503.

[23] Matakidou A, el Galta R, Rudd MF, *et al.* Further observations on the relationship between the FGFR4 Gly388Arg polymorphism and lung cancer prognosis[J]. British Journal of Cancer, 2007, 96(12): 1904-1907.

[24] Singh S, Grabner A, Yanucil C, *et al.* Fibroblast growth factor 23 directly targets hepatocytes to promote inflammation in chronic kidney disease[J]. Kidney International, 2016, 90(5): 985-996.

[25] Schlessinger J, Plotnikov AN, Ibrahimi OA, *et al.* Crystal structure of a ternary FGF-FGFR-heparin complex reveals a dual role for heparin in FGFR binding and dimerization[J]. Molecular Cell, 2000, 6(3): 743-750.

[26] Xuan YH, Bin Huang B, Tian HS, *et al.* High-Glucose Inhibits Human Fibroblast Cell Migration in Wound Healing *via* Repression of bFGF-Regulating JNK Phosphorylation[J]. Plos One, 2014, 9(9).

[27] Raballo R, Rhee J, Lyn-Cook R, *et al.* Basic fibroblast growth factor (Fgf2) is necessary for cell proliferation and neurogenesis in the developing cerebral cortex[J]. Journal of Neuroscience, 2000, 20(13): 5012-5023.

[28] Ye LB, Yu XC, Xia QH, *et al.* Regulation of Caveolin-1 and Junction Proteins by bFGF Contributes to the Integrity of Blood-Spinal Cord Barrier and Functional Recovery[J]. Neurotherapeutics, 2016, 13(4): 844-858.

[29] Feistritzer C, Riewald M. Endothelial barrier protection by activated protein C through PAR1-dependent sphingosine 1-phosphate receptor-1 crossactivation[J]. Blood, 2005, 105(8): 3178-3184.

图书在版编目（CIP）数据

成纤维细胞生长因子 = Fibroblast Growth Factors，
2nd edition：英文 / 李校堃著 . --2 版 . -- 北京：
高等教育出版社，2019.10
  ISBN 978-7-04-052869-5

  Ⅰ . ①成… Ⅱ . ①李… Ⅲ . ①人体细胞学 – 细胞因子
– 研究 – 英文 Ⅳ . ① R329.2

  中国版本图书馆 CIP 数据核字（2019）第 224881 号

| 策划编辑 | 吴雪梅 | 责任编辑 | 张 磊 | 高新景 | 封面设计 | 王凌波 | 责任印制 | 田 甜 |

出版发行	高等教育出版社		网 址	http://www.hep.edu.cn
社 址	北京市西城区德外大街4号			http://www.hep.com.cn
邮政编码	100120		网上订购	http://www.hepmall.com.cn
印 刷	北京信彩瑞禾印刷厂			http://www.hepmall.com
开 本	889mm×1194mm 1/16			http://www.hepmall.cn
印 张	65		版 次	2013 年 4 月第 1 版
字 数	1900 千字			2019 年 10 月第 2 版
购书热线	010-58581118		印 次	2019 年 10 月第 1 次印刷
咨询电话	400-810-0598		定 价	420.00元